Churchill Livingstone

TEXTBOOKS

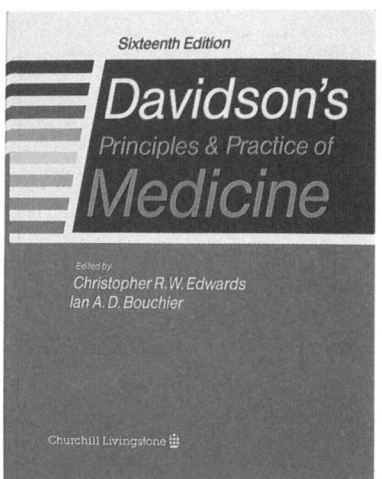

Sixteenth Edition

Davidson's
Principles & Practice of
Medicine

Edited by
Christopher R. W. Edwards
Ian A. D. Bouchier

Churchill Livingstone

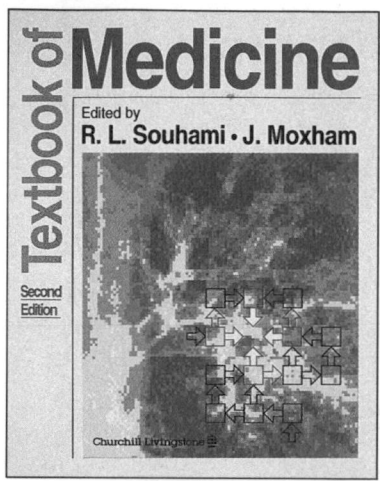

Textbook of Medicine

Edited by
R. L. Souhami · J. Moxham

Second Edition

Churchill Livingstone

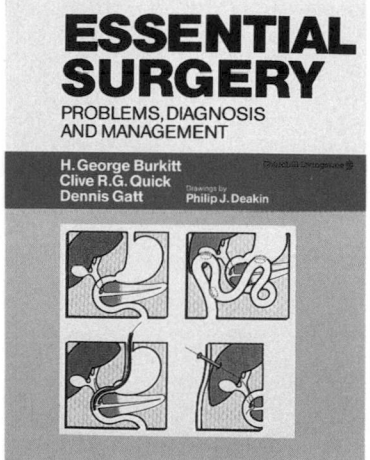

ESSENTIAL SURGERY
PROBLEMS, DIAGNOSIS AND MANAGEMENT

H. George Burkitt
Clive R.G. Quick
Dennis Gatt

Drawings by
Philip J. Deakin

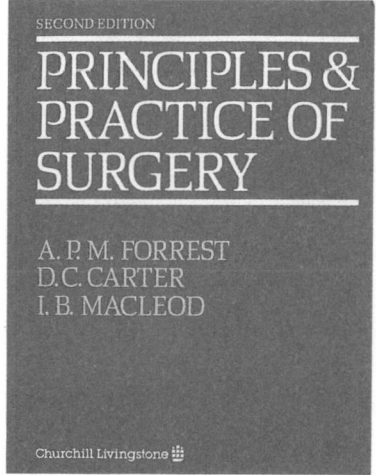

SECOND EDITION

PRINCIPLES & PRACTICE OF SURGERY

A. P. M. FORREST
D. C. CARTER
I. B. MACLEOD

Churchill Livingstone

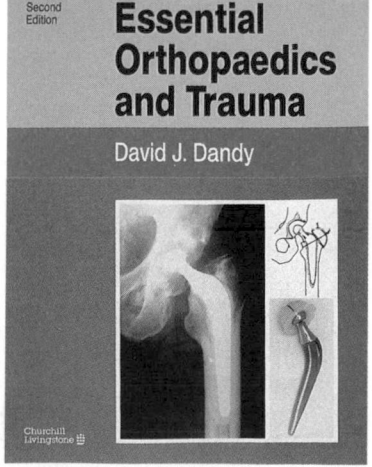

Second Edition

Essential Orthopaedics and Trauma

David J. Dandy

Churchill Livingstone

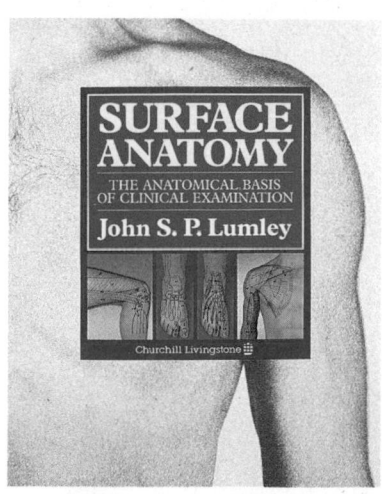

SURFACE ANATOMY
THE ANATOMICAL BASIS OF CLINICAL EXAMINATION
John S. P. Lumley

Churchill Livingstone

Textbook of Medicine

Textbook of Medicine

Medicine

SECOND EDITION

Edited by

R.L. Souhami MD FRCP FRCR

Kathleen Ferrier Professor of Clinical Oncology, University College
London Medical School; Consultant Physician, University College
Hospitals, London, UK

J. Moxham MD FRCP

Professor of Thoracic Medicine, King's College School of Medicine
and Dentistry; Consultant Physician, King's College Hospital,
London, UK

Illustrations by *Chapman Bounford & Associates*

Churchill Livingstone

EDINBURGH LONDON MADRID MELBOURNE
NEW YORK AND TOKYO 1994

CHURCHILL LIVINGSTONE
Medical Division of Longman Group UK Limited

Distributed in the United States of America by Churchill
Livingstone Inc., 650 Avenue of the Americas, New York, N.Y.
10011, and by associated companies, branches and representatives
throughout the world.

First edition 1990
Second edition 1994

ISBN 0-443-04664-6

British Library Cataloguing in Publication Data
A catalogue record for this book is available from the British Library.

Library of Congress Cataloging in Publication Data
Textbook of medicine / edited by R.L. Souhami,
J. Moxham. -- 2nd ed.
      p.   cm.
   Includes index.
   ISBN 0-443-04664-6
   1. Internal medicine.   I. Souhami, Robert L.   II. Moxham, J.
(John)
   [DNLM: 1. Disease.   2. Medicine.   WB 100 T3535 1994]
RC46.T353   1994
616--dc20
DNLM/DLC
for Library of Congress   93-21174
                                                CIP

For Churchill Livingstone:

Publisher: *Laurence Hunter*
Project Editor: *Barbara Simmons*
Editor: *Lesley J Knott*
Indexer: *June Morrison*
Production Controller: *Nancy Arnott*
Design: *Design Resources Unit*
Sales Promotion Executive: *Marion Pollock*

Printed in Hong Kong
C&C/01

The
publisher's
policy is to use
**paper manufactured
from sustainable forests**

Preface

The aim of this textbook is to provide a comprehensive account of clinical medicine incorporating the language and ideas of modern medical science. The rate of growth in the understanding of mechanisms of disease is greater than at any previous period and there has been a corresponding change in the content and form of the pre-clinical teaching of medical science. Many students now undertake basic science degree courses before starting their clinical training. We believe that the new understanding of cellular and physiological processes illuminates medical practice and makes it more exciting and less arbitrary.

The emphasis of the book is clinical, giving a full description of the presentation, investigation and treatment of disease. We have attempted to interpret these clinical aspects by reference to the underlying mechanisms whenever possible. The text is primarily intended for undergraduate students of medicine, but we hope and anticipate that it will be of value to postgraduates and health care professionals in many fields.

In the industrialised world, doctors are now faced with the illnesses of an ageing population. These may not be cured but can be alleviated or, sometimes, prevented. We have included sections on epidemiology and on the particular problems of disease in the elderly. Worldwide, infection continues to pose a formidable challenge and air travel means that doctors all over the world must have a working knowledge of the common tropical diseases. The comprehensive chapter 'Infectious, tropical and parasitic diseases' is designed for doctors in training and practising in this country and overseas. The chapter on nutrition deals with the problems of the elderly and the poor in the industrialised world as well as malnutrition in economically depressed countries. Other general chapters cover genetics, principles of cancer treatment and immunology, all of which are of relevance to every aspect of medical practice. Drugs are the mainstay of medical treatment and for this reason we have included chapters on the principles of drug use as well as the management of drug overdose and addiction.

The range and depth of specialised medical knowledge necessary for a major undergraduate textbook has led us to select our authors from medical schools throughout the United Kingdom. They have been chosen for their acknowledged reputation in clinical and scientific medicine.

In this second edition we have expanded the team of authors and have extensively revised the text to incorporate the important advances which have occurred since the publication of the first edition. By careful editing we have been able to reduce the text in length. We hope that the result is as comprehensive and clear as the first edition. Many of the illustrations have been revised and extended to include the most up-to-date epidemiological data. The text of the new edition is compatible with the associated volume of Multiple Choice Questions.

Undergraduates will find all they need in this book. It is not, however, a syllabus – it contains more knowledge than is required for the final examinations in the UK. All of us would be pleased to receive suggestions which will help the book change and develop for future editions.

London   RLS
1994   JM

Acknowledgements

We wish to express our gratitude to the team at Churchill Livingstone for their enthusiasm and dedication. Trevor Bounford and his team were, as usual, helpful and imaginative in the interpretation of our illustrations. We would also like to thank many colleagues in the UK and abroad who gave us invaluable advice on additions and improvements for this new edition.

Textbook of Medicine MCQs

R.L. Souhami, J. Moxham, S.V. Baudouin,
A.R. Freedman, G.C. Toms, R.A. Watts

Churchill Livingstone 1992

This companion volume of 300 multiple choice questions is based on the contents of this book and is a perfect revision tool to assist learning and preparation for examinations — for undergraduates preparing for their qualifying examinations as well as for junior doctors preparing for the MRCP. The chapters correspond with those in the textbook and full explanatory answers are given.

ISBN   0 443 04663 8

Contributors

David C Anderson MD FRCP MRCPath
Professor of Medicine, The Chinese University of
Hong Kong, Prince of Wales Hospital, Hong Kong

Brian T Cooper BSc MD FRCP
Consultant Gastroenterologist, Dudley Road Hospital,
Birmingham; Senior Clinical Lecturer in Medicine,
University of Birmingham, Birmingham, UK

John F Costello MD FRCP
Consultant Physician, King's College Hospital; Director,
Department of Thoracic Medicine, King's College School
of Medicine and Dentistry, London, UK

John Cunningham MD FRCP
Consultant Nephrologist and Honorary Senior Lecturer,
Royal London Hospital and Medical College, London,
UK

Adrian L W F Eddleston DM FRCP
Professor of Liver Immunology and Dean, Faculty of
Medicine; Consultant Physician, King's College School
of Medicine and Dentistry, London, UK

Jeremy Gibbs MD MRCP
Consultant Neurologist, Royal Free Hospital; Honorary
Senior Lecturer, Royal Free School of Medicine, London,
UK

John Goldstone MD FRCA
Senior Lecturer in Anaesthesia, University College
London Medical School; Honorary Consultant in
Anaesthetics, University College Hospitals, London, UK

Robin A C Graham-Brown BSc FRCP
Consultant Dermatologist, Leicester Royal Infirmary;
Honorary Senior Lecturer in Dermatology, University of
Leicester, Leicester, UK

Brian Hazleman MA FRCP
Consultant Rheumatologist and Director, Rheumatology
Research Unit, Addenbrooke's Hospital; Associate
Lecturer, Department of Medicine, University of
Cambridge; Fellow, Corpus Christi College, Cambridge,
UK

Jeremy Holmes MA MRCP FRCPsych
Consultant Psychiatrist/Psychotherapist, North Devon
District Hopital, Barnstaple, North Devon, UK

Cameron T C Kennedy MA FRCP
Consultant Dermatologist and Clinical Teacher, Bristol
Royal Infirmary, Bristol Children's Hospital and
Southmead Hospital, Bristol, UK

David C Linch FRCP
Professor of Clinical Haematology, University College
London Medical School, London

Richard G Long MD FRCP
Consultant Physician and Gastroenterologist, City
Hospital; Clinical Teacher, University of Nottingham,
Nottingham, UK

Thomas J McManus FRCOG
Consultant in Genitourinary Medicine, King's College
Hospital, London, UK

John P Monson MD FRCP
Consultant Physician and Senior Lecturer in Metabolism
and Endocrinology, Royal London Hospital and Medical
College, London, UK

John Moxham MD FRCP
Professor of Thoracic Medicine, King's College School of
Medicine and Dentistry; Consultant Physician, King's
College Hospital, London, UK

Peter W Overstall FRCP
Consultant in Geriatric Medicine, General Hospital,
Hereford, UK

John H L Playfair DSc PhD
Professor of Immunology, University College London
Medical School, London, UK

Philip A Routledge MD FRCP
Professor of Clinical Pharmacology, University of Wales
College of Medicine; Honorary Consultant Physician,
South Glamorgan Health Authority; Director, Welsh
National Poisons Unit and Consultant Toxicologist,
Welsh Office, Cardiff, UK

John W Scadding MD FRCP
Consultant Neurologist, The National Hospital for
Neurology and Neurosurgery and Whittington Hospital,
London, UK

Robert L Souhami MD FRCP FRCR
Kathleen Ferrier Professor of Clinical Oncology,
University College London Medical School;
Consultant Physician, University College Hospitals,
London, UK

Lip-Bun Tan MRCP DPhil
Senior Lecturer, Leeds University Medical School;
Consultant Cardiologist, Killingbeck and St James's
University Hospitals, Leeds, UK

Andrew Tomkins FRCP
Professor of International Child Health; Head of the
Division of Public Health; Director of the Centre for
International Child Health, Institute of Child Health,
London, UK

Nicholas J Wald DSc FFPHM FRCP FRCOG
Professor and Director, Department of Environmental
and Preventative Medicine, Medical College,
St Bartholomew's Hospital, London, UK

J Malcolm Walker MD FRCP
Consultant Cardiologist, University College Hospitals,
London, UK

Mark H Wansbrough-Jones FRCP
Consultant Physician and Senior Lecturer in
Communicable Diseases, St George's Hospital, London,
UK

Gareth Williams MA MD FRCP
Reader in Medicine, University of Liverpool; Honorary
Consultant Physician, Royal Liverpool University
Hospital, Liverpool, UK

Robin M Winter BSc FRCP
Reader in Clinical Genetics, Institute of Child Health,
University of London, London, UK

Stephen G Wright FRCP
Senior Lecturer, Department of Clinical Sciences,
London School of Hygiene and Tropical Medicine;
Honorary Consultant Physician, Hospital for Tropical
Diseases, London, UK

Contents

1

The Epidemiological Approach

Nicholas J Wald

INTRODUCTION

Epidemiology is the study of the incidence, distribution and determinants of diseases in human populations with a view to identifying their causes and bringing about their prevention.

Epidemiology and clinical medicine are linked, but there is an important distinction between the two. Clinical medicine is concerned with people who already have a disease; it seeks to understand how the disease progresses, what its effects are and how it can be treated. Epidemiology seeks to understand the antecedents of a disease and identify its causes, so making possible its prevention. As such, epidemiology is concerned with populations, which necessarily include not only individuals who have the disease in question but also those who do not, thereby permitting the calculation of the rate of occurrence of the disease and hence the study of factors that influence that rate. Clues to what those factors are may be obtained by seeing:

● whether the disease is more common in one place than in another

● whether its frequency has changed over time or

● whether this differs in people with and without certain characteristics.

Epidemiology has also extended its field of interest into areas directly relevant to clinical medicine, such as clinical trials and the quantitative interpretation of diagnostic or screening tests (p. 10).

Like a detective, the epidemiologist must usually deduce the factors responsible for causing a disease from naturally occurring circumstances over which he/she has no control. The epidemiologist asks, for example, 'Why is coronary heart disease so much more common in the United States than it is in Japan? Does the risk change when Japanese people migrate to the US? Is cholesterol (the principal substance in the atheromatous lesions in the coronary arteries) present in different concentrations in the blood of the Japanese and Americans? And, within each country, is there an association between serum cholesterol concentration and the risk of coronary heart disease? Is there any evidence that serum cholesterol is not associated with the risk of heart disease?' The work of the epidemiologist thus mostly involves observation and interpretation.

CAUSE OF A DISEASE

A cause of a disease is a factor that is *associated* with the disease, such that if the intensity or frequency of the factor in a population is changed, the frequency of the disease also changes.

It is important to note that not all associations are causal. For example, alcohol consumption is associated with lung cancer because cigarette smokers tend to drink more alcohol than non-smokers and smoking is itself associated with lung cancer. The alcohol–lung cancer association is said to be indirect whereas the smoking–lung cancer association is direct and causal. This is supported by noting that the risk of lung cancer varies according to cigarette consumption in persons with a similar alcohol intake but does *not* vary according to alcohol intake in persons with a similar cigarette consumption.

There can be more than one cause of a disease so that, for example, exposure to arsenic, asbestos or nickel can each independently cause lung cancer.

Not everyone exposed to a specific cause of a disease will automatically develop that disease. For example, not everyone exposed to the tubercle bacillus will develop pulmonary tuberculosis (it is not a *sufficient* cause) and nonsmokers can also develop lung cancer (smoking is not a *necessary* cause). Whether a particular individual develops a disease after such exposures will depend on the interplay of several factors, including, for example, exposure to other agents, the influence of factors as yet unidentified, constitutional differences and also the play of chance.

Establishing causality

The most direct way to determine causality is by experiment – adding or withholding the factor and observing whether the frequency of the disease changes. However, such an experiment often cannot be done in humans when investigating a toxic substance; removal of the factor may not be possible, the necessary scale of intervention may be too large or the duration of observation too long, or this too may be considered unethical. In such circumstances, causality needs to be inferred from observational studies. This can be done in two stages:

1. determine that an association between an exposure and a disease is a real one, i.e. unlikely to have arisen by chance
2. assess whether the association is one of cause and effect.

A *real association* (i.e. one not due to chance) is most likely to be detected if:

- the magnitude of the association is large
- the study includes a large number of subjects
- variations in other factors affecting the rate of the disease can be minimised.

A real association between a factor and a disease must either be causal or due to bias. Bias can arise in two ways:

- *Observer bias.* An apparent association between a disease and a study factor may be due to systematic measurement error so that, for example, subjects with the disease are recorded as having more, or less, of the study factor than unaffected subjects even when no such difference exists. This may occur, for example, because an observer who believes that the factor does cause the disease is more likely to diagnose the disease in an individual he knows to have been exposed to the factor. Such observer bias can be avoided by ensuring that the observer who diagnoses the disease is *blind* as to the presence or absence of the factor.
- *Presence of a confounding factor,* i.e. a factor that is associated with both the disease and the study factor. Thus, in the above example involving lung cancer and alcohol consumption, the confounding factor was cigarette smoking.

The magnitude of an association provides an indication of whether the association is causal; big differences are less likely to have been produced by bias than small differences. Establishing causality is facilitated by knowledge of the sequence of events involved; it is always a

---

Summary 1 Criteria and evidence for inferring causality between exposure to a factor and a disease

Essential criteria
- A real association between the factor and the disease, i.e. an association that is unlikely to be due to chance.
- Exposure to the factor precedes the occurrence of the disease.
- The association cannot be reasonably explained by bias, either through systematic measurement error or through the effect of one or more confounding factors.
- The causal explanation is biologically plausible.

Additional evidence
- Demonstration of a dose–response relationship between the factor and the disease in studies of individuals.
- The demonstration of reversibility; elimination or reduction in the intensity of exposure to the factor is associated with a reduction in the risk of disease.
- The distribution and frequency of the disease in different places and in different groups and over time follows the distribution and intensity of exposure to the factor.
- Support from animal or in vitro laboratory experimental evidence.

---

necessary condition of a causal association for the causal factor to precede the effect. This is often clear (e.g. with the association between smoking and lung cancer) but, at other times, it is uncertain. Thus, for example, two equally plausible explanations could apply to the association found between low serum retinol and cancer: either the low serum retinol precedes the cancer and therefore may cause it, or the presence of cancer exerts metabolic effects that lower serum retinol. Only appropriate epidemiological enquiry (a prospective study, p. 5) can determine which explanation is correct.

A causal explanation for an association is supported by the following:

- a dose–response relationship between exposure and the disease
- demonstrating that reduction in exposure produces a reduction in the incidence of the disease
- observing that the variation in the distribution of disease in different places, at different times and in different groups of people, is related to corresponding variations in the distribution of the causal factor.

The above definition of the cause of a disease stresses the central importance of *why* disease occurs rather than how it progresses after it has occurred. In epidemiology, the notion of cause is thus concerned with origins of disease rather than mechanisms. The clinician might regard the cause of diabetes as being a relative lack of insulin; the epidemiologist would wish to know what environmental and genetic factors led to this lack. Both views are correct; to treat diabetes it need only be regarded as a lack of insulin, but to prevent it, it is necessary to understand the factors which led to this lack.

EPIDEMIOLOGICAL ENQUIRY

Epidemiological enquiry initially involves finding clues that will help identify the causes of disease. Such clues can arise from many sources, e.g. clinical observation, inferences drawn from knowledge of the biology involved, or from a more formal description of the epidemiology of the disease concerned. From such observations and inferences, a hypothesis may emerge that a particular disease is caused by a particular exposure. Following such *descriptive* epidemiological studies, two types of investigation can be undertaken – *analytical* epidemiological studies and, in special circumstances, *intervention* (or experimental) studies.

DESCRIPTIVE STUDIES

Descriptive studies involve answering three questions.

- How does the risk of developing a disease vary over *time?*
- How does it vary from *place to place?*
- How does it vary with respect to certain characteristics of the *individuals,* such as age, sex or occupational group?

Incidence and prevalence

Answering these questions requires quantitative measures of the risk of developing a disease. This is done by estimating the incidence or prevalence of the disease in question, both of which involve counting the number of individuals in a defined population with that disease (the numerator) and dividing by the total population (the denominator) so that disease rates can be determined.

The *incidence* of a disease is the number of new cases occurring in a specified period of time and in a defined population. The *prevalence* of a disease is the number of cases of a disorder present at a given point in time in a defined population.

The prevalence of a disease changes according to the product of its incidence and duration. The duration of a disease will be shortened if it either kills the patient or remits completely. Thus, a condition with a high incidence and low prevalence could be either a common disease which has a high fatality rate (e.g. lung cancer) or a common disease with a high remission rate (e.g. measles). A disease with a low incidence and a high prevalence will be a chronic disease with a low fatality rate and a low remission rate (e.g. rheumatoid arthritis).

Age standardisation

The prevalence and incidence of a disease are usually strongly dependent on age, e.g. the incidences of lung cancer and coronary heart disease are relatively high in the elderly and low in the young. When comparing incidence or prevalence across different communities, it can therefore be misleading to compare the overall rates directly, since one population may have a larger number of elderly people. One approach to this problem is to compare rates in specific age groups, although such a comparison across a whole range of specific age groups is usually unwieldy since it does not yield a single summary figure. However, such a summary figure can be obtained by *age standardisation,* in which the age-specific rates of the study population are applied to a standard population (direct standardisation). Alternatively, the age-specific rates for a standard population can be applied to the numbers of individuals in the study population in each age group to derive an *expected* number of deaths for the study population, which is compared with the *observed* number (indirect standardisation). This ratio multiplied by 100 is known as the *standardised mortality ratio,* and it provides a single and widely used index that enables one to compare disease or mortality rates in different populations.

Life expectancy

Another important summary measure for comparing death rates within and between countries over time is *life expectancy.* It is calculated by considering a hypothetical group of, say, 1000 individuals at a given age and applying to the group the age-specific death rates of the population for each year of age until the whole group are estimated to have died. Expectation of life is calculated as the total number of person-years of life lived by the group divided by the number in the group, i.e. the average number of years an individual is expected to live. The calculation assumes that the current death rates will remain unchanged for the lifetime of the group (which, of course, they will not), but expectation of life is a useful single index of *current* death rates.

Use of descriptive studies

Descriptive epidemiological studies are useful not only because they sometimes suggest clues as to the causes of disease, but also because they enable assessment of the burden (in both economic and health terms) of different diseases in different communities. The study of immigrants is especially helpful. For example, the Japanese have a high incidence of stomach cancer but this declines substantially in Japanese migrants moving to the US, the incidence rates approximating to those of the indigenous Americans within one or two generations. The age-specific incidence rates of colon cancer among the Japanese immigrants increase towards those experienced

1 The Epidemiological Approach

Summary 2 Types of epidemiological enquiry

Descriptive studies
Studies of the variation in the incidence of a disease according to time, place and person.

Analytical studies
Studies specially designed to investigate directly the risk of disease in relation to a given exposure.

Intervention studies
Experiments on humans designed to test the efficacy and safety of medical procedures or medications.

by native Americans. There is evidently an important cause of stomach cancer in Japan that is relatively absent in the US. Similarly, an important cause of colon cancer appears to be present in the US but relatively absent in Japan.

Once a hypothesis has been produced that a particular disease is caused by a particular exposure, the epidemiology of the exposure can be described in much the same way as the epidemiology of the disease to see whether the two are correlated with respect to time and place, and whether they tend to occur together in certain groups of people within the same community. Descriptive studies can thus serve as tests of a hypothesis as well as a means of generating aetiological clues.

ANALYTICAL STUDIES

Once descriptive epidemiological studies have pointed to a possible association between an exposure and a disease, the hypothesis can be explored further through analytical studies specially designed to investigate directly the risk of a disease in relation to a given exposure. It is simplest to consider first the measures of risk used and then the usual study designs employed.

Measures of risk used in analytical studies

Incidence rates (or mortality rates) in two groups of people, say, among smokers and non-smokers, can be compared in two ways.

- The *relative risk* of a disease in relation to a particular exposure is the incidence of a disease among exposed persons divided by the incidence among unexposed persons.
- The *absolute excess risk* of a disease in relation to a particular exposure is the incidence of the disease among exposed persons minus the incidence among non-exposed persons.

The relative risk is useful in judging the strength of an association between exposure and disease, and hence whether the association might be causal. If it is causal, the absolute excess risk is a direct measure of how much disease the exposure causes in a particular population. It thus estimates the preventive effect of removing the exposure from the population and is therefore of public health importance. The absolute excess risk depends on the underlying risk of the disease concerned in the unexposed members of a particular population and cannot automatically be generalised to other populations.

Table 1.1 shows the relative and absolute excess risks of mortality from lung cancer, chronic bronchitis and cardiovascular disease in heavy cigarette smokers and non-smokers. Smoking is strongly associated with lung cancer and chronic bronchitis, as evidenced by their high relative risks (25.1 and 38.0 respectively) but it is much less strongly associated with ischaemic heart disease (relative risk 1.9). However, because lung cancer and chronic bronchitis are rare in non-smokers, while ischaemic heart disease is common, smoking causes fewer excess deaths from chronic bronchitis and lung cancer (241 and 111 deaths per 100 000 per year respectively) than from ischaemic heart disease (379 deaths per 100 000 per year). If the incidence of a common disease is increased only two or three times, the final number of deaths can be greater than if a rare disease is increased by as much as, say, 30 times. Another, related measure of risk is the *attributable proportion*. This is the proportion of cases of a disease that can be attributed to an exposure.

A simple hypothetical (but realistic) example illustrates each measure of risk. In a population of 100 000 men aged 45–54 years, 30% (30 000) are smokers; and the risk of dying from coronary heart disease (CHD) is 3 per 1000 per year among smokers and 1 per 1000 per year among non-smokers. The number of deaths from CHD per year is thus 90 ($3/1000 \times 30\ 000$) among smokers;

Table 1.1 Relative and absolute excess risks of deaths from selected causes associated with heavy cigarette smoking (25 or more cigarettes per day) by British male physicians*

Cause of death	Annual death rate per 100 000		Relative risk	Absolute excess risk death rate (per 100 000 per year)
	Non-smokers	Heavy cigarette smokers		
Lung cancer	10	251	25.1	241
Chronic bronchitis and emphysema	3	114	38.0	111
Ischaemic heart disease	413	792	1.9	379
All causes	1317	2843	2.16	1526

* From Doll R and Peto R 1976 Mortality in relation to smoking: 20 years' observations on male British doctors. Brit Med J 1976; ii: 1525–36.

Summary 3 Quantitative measures of risk

- *Incidence* The number of new cases of a disorder occurring in a defined population in a specified period of time (e.g. 5/1000 persons/year).
- *Prevalence* The number of cases of a disorder present in a defined population at a given time (e.g. 5/1000 persons).
- *Relative risk* The incidence among exposed individuals divided by the incidence among unexposed individuals.
- *Absolute excess risk* The incidence among exposed individuals minus the incidence among unexposed individuals.
- *Attributable proportion* The proportion of cases of a disease that can be attributed to a given exposure.

and 70 ($1/1000 \times 70\,000$) among non-smokers, giving a total of 160 CHD deaths overall.

The relative risk of death from CHD in smokers compared to non-smokers is 3/1000 divided by 1/1000 = 3.

The absolute excess risk in smokers is 3/1000 minus 1/1000 = 2/1000, i.e. smoking causes 2 deaths from CHD per 1000 people each year.

If no-one smoked, there would be 100 deaths (100 000 $\times$ 1/1000) each year instead of 160, so that 60 out of the 160 observed deaths are attributable to smoking. The proportion of deaths attributable to smoking in this population is therefore 60/160 or 38%. To estimate the attributable proportion one need not know the absolute death rates in smokers and non-smokers, simply the relative risk, r, and the prevalence of the exposure, p, so that:

$$\text{Attributable proportion} = \frac{p(r-1)}{p(r-1)+1}$$

which, in our example $= \dfrac{0.3\,(3-1)}{0.3\,(3-1)+1} = \dfrac{0.6}{1.6} = 38\%$

Clearly, the attributable proportion will vary from one population to another depending on the prevalence and extent of exposure.

Study designs used in analytical studies

Analytical epidemiological studies are either prospective or retrospective.

Prospective studies

In a *prospective study* (also called a longitudinal or cohort study) we take a group of individuals and categorise them according to whether or not they are, or have been, exposed to a certain factor. We then follow the groups for a period of time, often many years, and record the number who do and do not develop the disease of interest.

A simple 2×2 table of the number of individuals involved can be constructed to show the exposed and unexposed individuals who do and do not develop disease (Table 1.2).

The rates of disease in exposed subjects ($a/a + b$) and in unexposed subjects ($c/c + d$) are then determined. The first divided by the second is the *relative risk* (r). Thus,

$$r = \frac{\dfrac{a}{a+b}}{\dfrac{c}{c+d}}$$

Exposed individuals are then r times more likely than unexposed individuals to develop disease. A value of r that is statistically significantly greater than, or less than, 1 is evidence of an association.

The second rate subtracted from the first is the *absolute excess risk* (e per 100). Thus,

$$e = \frac{a}{a+b} - \frac{c}{c+d}$$

Exposed individuals then have a risk of e per 1000 in excess of that experienced by unexposed individuals.

The figures in the hypothetical (but realistic) study of smoking and lung cancer discussed on page 4 may be used to illustrate the design of a prospective study.

Both the 30 000 smokers and 70 000 non-smokers in the initial population of 100 000 are followed up for, say, 10 years. During this time, there are 42 new cases of lung cancer among the smokers. The rate of disease in exposed subjects is thus

$$\frac{42}{30\,000} = \frac{14}{10\,000}$$

There are 7 new cases among the non-smokers. The rate of disease in non-exposed subjects is thus

$$\frac{7}{70\,000} = \frac{1}{10\,000}$$

Relative risk (r) =

$$\frac{\dfrac{14}{10\,000}}{\dfrac{1}{10\,000}} = 14$$

Table 1.2 Simple 2×2 table used in epidemiological studies to show the exposed and unexposed individuals who do and do not develop disease

	Disease	No disease	
Exposed	a	b	a + b
Not exposed	c	d	c + d
	a + c	b + d	

1 The Epidemiological Approach

Summary 4 Study designs: prospective (cohort) studies

A group of individuals who are categorised according to whether they have or have not been exposed to a certain factor are followed up over a period of time and the incidence of the disease or diseases of interest recorded according to the assigned exposure.

Advantages
- Exposure known to precede development of the disease.
- Direct estimate of incidence, in both exposed and non-exposed groups.
- Permits the study of many diseases so that unsuspected associations can be identified.

Disadvantages
- Long duration (decades).
- Large size (thousands of individuals).
- High financial cost.

Absolute excess risk =

$$\frac{14}{10\,000} - \frac{1}{10\,000} = \frac{13}{10\,000} \text{ per ten years}$$

$$= 1.3/10\,000 \text{ per year}$$

The main advantages of prospective (or longitudinal) studies are: the knowledge that the exposure preceded the occurrence of the disease; the ability to obtain a direct estimate of the incidence of the disease in the exposed and the unexposed groups (allowing both the relative risk and absolute excess risk to be estimated directly); and the ability to detect unsuspected associations.

The main disadvantages of longitudinal studies when studying chronic disorders such as cardiovascular disease and cancer are: their long duration (many years); their large size (thousands of individuals); and therefore their financial cost. For a rare disease, few cases may develop even in a large study of this type.

Retrospective studies

In a *retrospective study* (also called a case-control study) we take a sample of individuals who have the disease (cases) and another sample who do not (controls). The prevalence of exposure in those with the disease and in those without it is determined retrospectively, usually by the administration of a questionnaire.

In a retrospective study, we cannot estimate the relative risk directly because the proportions of diseased and non-diseased subjects sampled from the population are different and unknown. However, if the disease being studied is rare, a simple approximation solves the problem. Referring to the 2 × 2 table on page 5, for a prospective study,

the relative risk (r) = $\dfrac{\dfrac{a}{a+b}}{\dfrac{c}{c+d}}$

Now, since the disease is rare, a and c are much smaller than b and d, so that:

$a + b \simeq b$, and $\qquad \dfrac{a}{a+b} \simeq \dfrac{a}{b}$

$c + d \simeq d$, and $\qquad \dfrac{c}{c+d} \simeq \dfrac{c}{d}$

Therefore,

the relative risk (r) $\simeq$ $\qquad \dfrac{\dfrac{a}{b}}{\dfrac{c}{d}} = \dfrac{ad}{bc}$

For a retrospective study, let s_1 and s_2 be the fraction of the individuals with and without the disease sampled from the underlying population to yield, respectively, the number of cases and controls in the study. Then:

the relative risk (r) $= \dfrac{\dfrac{as_1}{bs_2}}{\dfrac{cs_1}{ds_2}} = \dfrac{as_1}{bs_2} \times \dfrac{ds_2}{cs_1} = \dfrac{ad}{bc}$

i.e. the cross products of the 2 × 2 table. The unknown sampling fractions s_1 and s_2 conveniently cancel out. An example is shown in Table 1.3.

The main advantages of retrospective studies are that they are: quick; require relatively small numbers; and are hence reasonably economical. They are sometimes the only feasible way to conduct an analytical epidemiological study of a rare disease.

Their main disadvantages are: the difficulty, in certain studies, of determining whether the exposure preceded the inception of the disease; avoiding recall bias, e.g. sick people may be more likely to recall a past exposure than healthy controls; avoiding selection bias, so that recruitment of cases and controls is not influenced by whether or not they have been exposed; and the inability to obtain a direct estimate of excess risk.

INTERVENTION STUDIES

Methodological issues

Intervention studies resemble prospective studies in that subjects are followed up to determine their outcome. They differ in that some action or intervention is performed rather than only observing what takes place naturally. Intervention studies are experiments on humans in which something is done to an experimental

Summary 5 Study designs: retrospective (case/control) studies

A sample of individuals who already have the disease of interest (cases) and a sample of similar individuals who do not have the disease (controls) are compared to see if their exposure to the factor under study is or has been different.

Advantages
● Quick.
● Relatively small numbers are adequate.
● Economical.

Disadvantages
● Sometimes there is uncertainty as to whether the exposure preceded the inception of the disease.
● Recall bias.
● Selection bias.
● No direct estimate of excess risk.

Table 1.3 Example of a retrospective study: lung cancer and cigarette smoking*

Smoking habits	Cases (lung cancer)	Control (no cancer)	
Cigarette smokers	647	622	1269
Non-smokers	2	27	29
Total	649	649	1298

Relative risk $(r) = \dfrac{647 \times 27}{622 \times 2} = 14.0$

* From Doll R, Hill A B 1952 The study of the aetiology of carcinoma of the lung. Brit Med J 1952; ii: 1271–86

group and the observed outcome compared with a control group which is not subjected to the intervention. If a difference in outcome between the two groups is demonstrated that is considered unlikely to be due to bias and unlikely to have arisen by chance, cause and effect can be inferred.

In general, three types of control groups can be used:

● *Historical controls:* patients with the same disorder seen in the past before the use of the new intervention
● *Geographical controls:* patients with the same disorder seen at another hospital or clinic where the new intervention is not provided
● *Randomised controls:* concurrent patients chosen at random to be controls while other patients from the same population are chosen at random to receive the new intervention. It is the allocation to receive or not receive the new intervention, e.g. a new treatment, that is conducted at random, not the group of patients for the study. The latter are, rather, often a special subset, e.g. those with a particular complication, those in a particular age group, or those thought likely to comply with the treatment.

Historical and geographical controls

The use of historical and geographical controls is usually unsatisfactory because like is probably not being compared with like. The introduction of a new type of treatment may itself alter the selection of patients referred for the treatment. For example, patients with early disease may start coming from other centres to receive the new treatment. Past patients may have been referred to hospitals at a different stage of the disease and this alone will influence their survival or remission rate. They are also likely to have received different treatments apart from the new one under study and this would have influenced their outcomes. Similar biases affect the use of geographical controls.

Randomised controls

In randomised studies, on the other hand, allocation to treatment is decided at random, and so the study and control groups will, on average, be alike. Randomisation thus removes *allocation bias*. *Observer bias* (where the assessment of response to treatment is influenced by knowledge of treatment group) can be avoided by a single (or observer) blind design. Bias due to patients knowing that they are in a particular treatment (because of the psychological or *placebo* effect or because it would influence habits that may themselves affect prognosis) can be avoided by a double-blind design in which neither observers nor patients know the treatment allocation. Provided sufficient numbers of patients are entered into the trial to avoid chance differences between the treatment and control groups, any observed differences must be due to the new treatment.

To avoid bias some researchers match treated and untreated patients retrospectively on factors known to influence prognosis, rather than allocate patients on a random basis. This is usually inadequate, however, because it can only allow for factors that are known to be related to prognosis. In practice, there are important selective factors relating to both being offered and complying with treatment, and to prognosis, which are usually not known. Matching cannot overcome this problem (one cannot match for unknown factors) but randomisation can.

The statistical analysis of randomised trials should be done by comparing outcome in all the subjects originally allocated to each of the treatment groups, including non-compliers (referred to as an *intention-to-treat* analysis), rather than by comparing outcome only in patients from each group who actually completed treatment (*treatment-received* analysis). It is only with the intention-to-treat analysis that bias can be avoided. Bias could easily be introduced by an actual treatment analysis, e.g. because the more symptomatic patients with a poorer prognosis may be less likely to adhere to the one treatment than the other, particularly if it has side-effects that exacerbate the symptoms from the disease itself, such as nausea. Poor compliance on an intention-to-treat analysis will obviously reduce the ability of the trial to detect a treatment effect if one does exist (as the trial will have little statistical power and may yield inconclusive results), but it will not be biased as may be the case with the treatment-received analysis.

An intention-to-treat analysis also addresses the pragmatic question 'Did the new treatment work in practice, i.e. do patients take the treatment *and* is it effective?' rather than the more limited question 'Does the new treatment work *if* it is taken?' A pharmalogically effective treatment that is rejected because it is so disagreeable is of little value, though knowledge that it may be effective is important because it will keep the door open to further evaluation, both to make it more acceptable and then to reassess, in an unbiased trial, whether it is indeed effective.

A randomised trial can be used to investigate the value of more than one treatment by randomising patients into a control group and several experimental groups. This approach will involve the recruitment of more patients into the trial. A way of avoiding this increased cost is to use a *factorial design*. If two new drugs were being evaluated this would involve randomising the population into quarters; one to receive neither drug, two to receive one drug only and one to receive both. The main advantage is that since each treatment is given to half the available patients, rather than to a third, the statistical power is maintained and in effect two drugs can be assessed using the same number of patients needed to assess one drug. If each drug exerted opposite effects or they interfered with each other in such a way as to reduce the effect of any one alone, this would be a weak design but it is only by using such a design that these and other *treatment interactions* can be studied. Large numbers of patients are usually needed to do this reliably.

An example of a factorial design is the ISIS-2 study (ISIS, 1988). Here, 17 187 patients entering 417 hospitals up to 24 hours after the onset of suspected acute myocardial infarction were randomised, with placebo control, between: (i) a 1-hour i.v. infusion of 1.5 MU of streptokinase; (ii) one month of 160 mg/day enteric coated aspirin; (iii) both treatments; or (iv) neither. Table 1.4 shows the incidence of 5-week vascular mortality (IHD and stroke) following these regimens.

Ethical issues

In an intervention study, there is ethical concern that patients must not be harmed, either by adverse effects of a new treatment or by withholding a treatment which might have been of benefit. Investigators are naturally enthusiastic about the possible benefits of a new 'treatment' with which they have been associated and are often understandably unwilling to carry out a controlled experiment to test its effects. However, it is important to be objective and recognise uncertainty, since many suppos-

Table 1.4 Incidence of 5-week vascular mortality in 17 187 treated cases of suspected myocardial infarction

		Streptokinase		
		Yes	No	
Aspirin	Yes	343 / 4292	461 / 4295	804 / 8587
	No	448 / 4300	568 / 4300	1016 / 8600
Total		791 / 8592	1029 / 8595	1820 / 17 187

The results can be summarised in the following way:

			Odds reduction* with 95% confidence intervals

1. Effect of streptokinase (S)

$$S \text{ vs. no } S = \frac{791}{8592} \text{ (9.2\%) vs. } \frac{1029}{8595} \quad (12\%) \quad 25\% \quad 18\text{–}32\%$$

2. Effect of aspirin (A)

$$A \text{ vs. no } A = \frac{804}{8587} \text{ (9.4\%) vs. } \frac{1016}{8600} \quad (11.8\%) \quad 23\% \quad 15\text{–}30\%$$

3. Effect of both combined (S+A)

$$S+A \text{ vs. no } S+A = \frac{343}{4292} \text{ (8\%) vs. } \frac{568}{4300} \text{ (13.2\%)} \quad 42\% \quad 34\text{–}50\%$$

* Odds compare mutually exclusive groups, e.g. in S category 791/8592–791 instead of 791/8592.

Conclusion: Streptokinase alone or aspirin alone significantly reduces vascular mortality and both together are better than each alone, the effect being nearly additive.

Summary 6 Study designs: intervention studies

A substance is administered to, or a procedure conducted on, an experimental group and the observed outcome compared with a control group that is not subjected to the intervention.

Three types of control groups can be employed:

Historical controls – affected patients seen before the new intervention.

Geographical controls – affected patients seen at another unit which does not have the new intervention.

Randomised controls – intervention is randomly assigned to concurrent patients in the same population.

Advantages of a randomised trial
- Avoids selection bias that may arise through patients with a better (or worse) prognosis being allocated the new intervention.
- Any subject or observer bias can be removed by making the trial double-blind.

edly beneficial treatments have been introduced that have been found subsequently to be of little or no value and sometimes even to be harmful. A formal clinical trial is a practical and ethical way of assessing therapies, and new medical procedures are best evaluated early, before they become universally and uncritically accepted. Diversity of practice is, in itself, evidence of uncertainty and allows a pragmatic justification for conducting a randomised trial to resolve the uncertainty.

PREVENTION

Epidemiology, with its emphasis on identifying the antecedents of disease, offers the opportunity for disease prevention.

Primary prevention is the prevention of the future occurrence of a disorder in unaffected individuals by removing a cause, e.g. preventing lung cancer by avoiding smoking.

Secondary prevention is the prevention of overt (clinical) cases of a disorder through screening and early detection followed by appropriate intervention, e.g. breast cancer screening by mammography.

The treatment of clinical disease, while not normally regarded as prevention, is sometimes referred to as *tertiary prevention,* as effective treatment of overt disease can often prevent disability and pain resulting from the disease.

PRIMARY PREVENTION
General measures

The prevention of disease through general social and economic changes that improve nutrition, increase living standards, lead to smaller families and reduce overcrowding, is extremely important, even if the precise social and economic factors causally involved are difficult to identify. The expectation of life in most countries tends to be positively associated with economic performance as judged, for example, by the gross national product (GNP) per person (Fig. 1.1) although above a certain GNP (about $6000 per person in 1987) the relationship is weak and other factors must operate. Past improvements in life expectancy in developed countries have been largely accomplished by general measures such as those that led to the primary prevention of common infectious diseases; mortality from infectious diseases had thus greatly decreased before the availability of specific methods of prevention or treatment such as vaccination or antibiotics. Some infectious diseases, however, have increased in recent years, particularly venereal diseases such as nongonococcal urethritis and recently the acquired immune deficiency syndrome (AIDS).

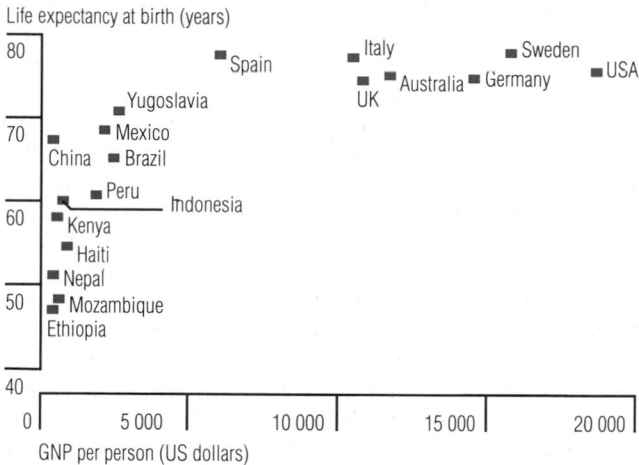

Fig. 1.1 Expectation of life versus gross national product 1987. (Source: World Development Report, 1989, OUP for World Bank)

Specific measures

With the notable exception of AIDS, the major challenge today in the industrialised countries of the world is the prevention of illness due to non-infectious diseases by modification of *specific* cultural and personal patterns of behaviour such as the change in specific dietary components (e.g. lower fat intake), increases in the level of physical activity, reduction in the use of alcohol and the avoidance of tobacco. It has been estimated that the adoption throughout western countries of a diet reducing serum cholesterol levels by 10% would reduce coronary heart disease (CHD) mortality by at least 20%. Since CHD is the leading cause of death in such countries, this would result in a considerable reduction in mortality, approximately equivalent in numbers to the complete eradication of all cases of lung cancer in men and of breast cancer in women. Also important, particularly among young adults, is the problem of death and injury from accidents, especially road accidents.

In general, society can exert an influence on health in various ways, for example by legislation on driving and alcohol consumption, and on the prevention of pollution of air, soil and water; by encouraging the alteration of the composition and quality of the food we eat; by influencing choice through financial incentives (increasing the tax on cigarettes); and by applying engineering principles to build safety into the design of motor vehicles, equipment, buildings and highways.

SECONDARY PREVENTION

Secondary prevention is achieved through screening. *Screening* is the identification, among apparently healthy individuals, of those who are sufficiently at risk from a specific disorder to justify a subsequent diagnostic test or procedure or, in certain circumstances, direct preventive action.

The early detection of disease is only worthwhile for disorders which lend themselves to effective intervention and hence prevention. The identification of either trivial or untreatable conditions may cause anxiety with no useful result, and would therefore not be suitable diseases for screening

Screening may take the form of a simple inquiry, such as determining the age of a pregnant woman when screening for Down's Syndrome (since only older women will be offered the diagnostic test, amniocentesis); or, it may take the form of a special test such as maternal serum alpha-fetoprotein estimation when screening for neural tube defects.

Parameters of a screening test

The performance of screening tests as well as diagnostic tests is characterised by three measures which should be known before the test is used in practice:

- *The detection rate* (or *sensitivity*) of a test is the proportion of affected individuals with positive test results (Table 1.5).
- *The false-positive rate* of a test is the proportion of unaffected individuals with positive test results. This is sometimes given as the *specificity,* which is the false-positive rate expressed as a percentage subtracted from 100; so that, for example, a false-positive rate of 3% is the same as a specificity of 97%.
- *The odds of being affected given a positive result* is the ratio of the number of affected to unaffected individuals among those with positive test results.

The odds of being affected given a positive result depend on the prevalence of the disorder, as well as on the detection rate and the false-positive rate. Figure 1.2 shows a hypothetical flow diagram used to estimate the conse-

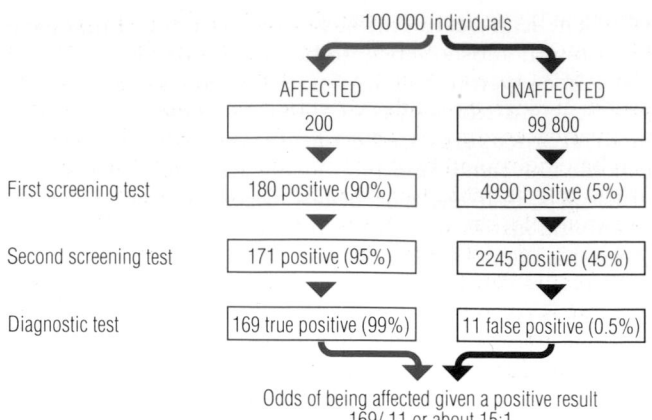

Fig. 1.2 **Hypothetical flow diagram used to estimate the consequences of a screening programme.** (From: Cuckle and Wald in Wald N J (ed) 1984 Antenatal and neonatal screening. Oxford University Press, Oxford.)

quences of two screening tests offered in sequence followed by a diagnostic test. In each case, the detection rate and false-positive rate of each test is applied to the number of affected and unaffected subjects (considered separately) to yield the number of true positives and false positives at each stage of the screening and diagnostic process. The ratio of one to the other gives the odds of being affected given a positive result; in our example, this is 169:11 (about 15 to 1) after the diagnostic test. (This ratio is also known as the *predictive value positive* when expressed as a proportion, i.e. 15/16 or 94%.)

The prevalence of the disorder being screened for has an important influence on the results of screening. The more common the disorder, the more likely it is that a positive test result will be associated with that disorder (the higher the odds of being affected given a positive result). Thus, with a common disorder, a screening test with a relatively poor detection rate and false-positive rate might be acceptable, but the same test might be unacceptable where the disorder is rarer. The detection rate and false-positive rate characterise the ability of an investigation to identify or exclude a particular disorder. They are not affected by the prevalence of the disorder. The probability that a positive test result will be associated with the disorder in question is dependent on the prevalence of the disorder in the setting in which screening is carried out, i.e. the odds of being affected given a positive result is a function of the prevalence of the condition as well as the detection rate and false-positive rate.

Table 1.5 provides a complete description of the detection and false-positive rates for a test which yields *qualitative* (or categorical) results such as cervical smear examinations when screening for cancer of the cervix, or karyotype determinations when making a diagnosis of a chromosome abnormality. It does not provide a complete description for quantitative tests or enquiries that yield

Table 1.5 **Definition of detection rate and false-positive rate of a qualitative test**

Test result	Affected	Unaffected	Total
Positive	a	b	a + b
Negative	c	d	c + d
Total	a + c	b + d	
Detection rate (sensitivity)	= $\dfrac{a}{a+b}$		
False-positive rate (1 – specificity)	= $\dfrac{b}{b+d}$		

results as a continuous variable, such as the measurement of blood pressure when screening for stroke or serum alpha-fetoprotein measurement when screening for spina bifida. In such cases, the detection rate and false-positive rate vary according to the cut-off level chosen. These rates can be determined by reference to frequency distributions of the test variable for affected and unaffected subjects. For example, the use of, say, cut-off level A in Figure 1.3 will have a detection rate given by the area under the curve for affected subjects above cut-off level A; the false-positive rate is given by the area under the curve for unaffected subjects above the same cut-off level. In this example the higher the cut-off level (say, B or C) the lower the detection rate and the lower the false-positive rate.

Requirements for a worthwhile screening programme

Before screening can provide an effective means of disease prevention certain criteria need to be fulfilled. A knowledge of the disorder being screened for, including its prevalence and natural history, is needed to ensure that the disease is sufficiently common and serious to represent an important medical problem. An effective remedy must be available. The performance of the screening test should be known in terms of its detection rate for the disorder concerned and in terms of its false-positive rate. The screening test must be simple, cheap, acceptable and safe, and facilities must be available or could be made available to provide the screening service and the consequent remedy. The whole process from initial screening to application of the remedy must be

---

Summary 7 Secondary prevention of disease: screening

Secondary prevention is prevention through screening and early detection and/or early intervention.

Screening is the identification, among apparently healthy individuals, of those who are sufficiently at risk from a specific disorder to justify a subsequent diagnostic test or procedure, or in certain circumstances, direct intervention.

Terms used in screening:
- *Detection rate (sensitivity)* is the proportion of affected individuals with a positive result.
- *False-positive rate* is the proportion of unaffected individuals with a positive result.
  (False-positive rate is 100 minus specificity expressed as a percentage, e.g. a false-positive rate of 3% is the same as a *specificity* of 97%.)
- *Odds of being affected given a possible result* is the ratio of affected to unaffected individuals among those with a positive result. (Expressed as a proportion, this is also called the *predictive value positive*, e.g. a 4:1 odds is the same as a predictive value of 4/5 or 80%.)

---

ethical and regarded as desirable and offering value for money (Tables 1.6 and 1.7).

PATTERNS OF MORTALITY AND MORBIDITY

A useful description of the pattern of mortality and morbidity in a country can often be obtained by national organisations concerned with the collection of vital statistics. The Office of Population Censuses and Surveys (OPCS) in the UK and similar offices in other countries play a crucial role in providing the intelligence needed for effective public health and the appropriate allocation of resources for medical care.

Obtaining reliable information on the extent of disease in the low income countries referred to loosely as 'the developing world' is frequently difficult.

ENGLAND AND WALES

The pattern of mortality and morbidity in England and Wales is fairly typical of that of an economically rich western nation.

Up to about age 35 there are more males than females; at older ages the number of females exceed males. Over the age of 85 about three-quarters of the population are women.

Birth and induced abortion rates

The *birth rate* is the number of live-births and stillbirths occurring in a given year divided by the estimated total

---

Table 1.6 Requirements for a worthwhile screening programme*

Factor	Requirement
Disorder	Well defined
Prevalence	Known
Natural history	Medically important disorder for which there is an effective remedy available
Financial	Cost effective
Facilities	Available or easily installed
Ethical	Procedures following a positive result are generally agreed and acceptable both to the screening authorities and to the patients
Test	Simple and safe
Test performance	Detection rate and false-positive rates known, i.e. distributions of test values in affected and unaffected individuals known, extent of overlap sufficiently small and a suitable cut-off level defined

* Modified from: Cuckle and Wald in Wald N J (ed) 1984 Antenatal and neonatal screening. Oxford University Press, Oxford.

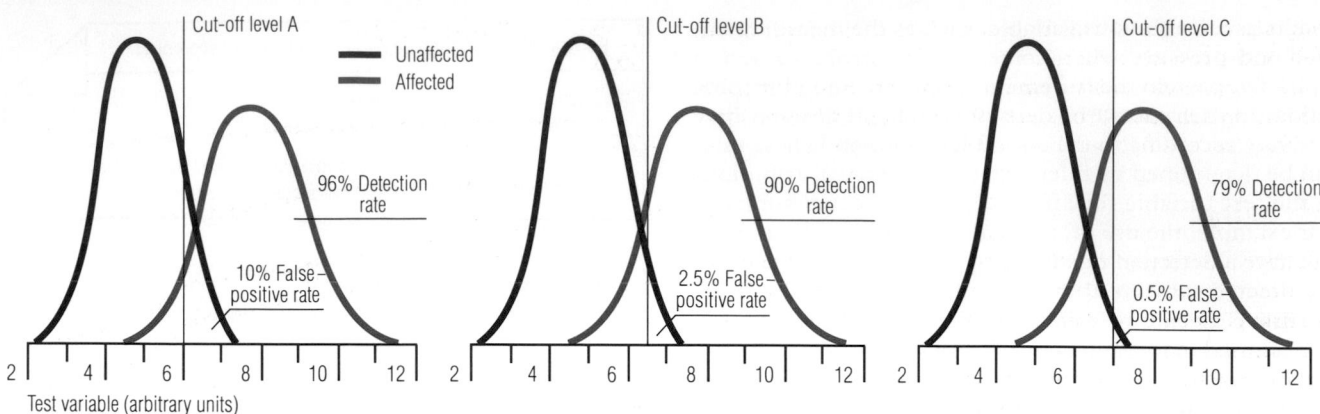

Fig. 1.3 Hypothetical example of the detection rate and false-positive rate of a screening test at three different cut-off levels. (Modified from: Cuckle and Wald in Wald N J (ed) 1984 Antenatal and neonatal screening, Oxford University Press, Oxford.)

Table 1.7 Examples of worthwhile screening procedures

Disorder	Initial screening test or enquiry	Subsequent test	Approximate proportion of disease preventable
Antenatal screening			
Down's syndrome	Maternal age and maternal serum alpha-fetoprotein, unconjugated oestriol and human chorionic gonadotrophin	Amniocentesis and fetal karyotype	60%
Open neural tube defects	Maternal serum alpha-fetoprotein	Amniotic fluid alpha-fetoprotein and acetylcholinesterase, and ultrasound	90%
β-thalassaemia	Red cell mean corpuscular volume	Haemoglobin electrophoresis, DNA analysis	95%
Screening in infancy			
Congenital hypothyroidism (cretinism)	Neonatal serum thyroid stimulating hormone and/or thyroxine	Repeat screening tests	95%
Phenylketonuria	Neonatal serum phenylalanine	Repeat screening test and serum tyrosene	95%
Adult screening			
Mortality from cancer of the cervix	Cervical smear (over 25 years)	Colposcopy	80%
Mortality from cancer of the breast	Age (over 40–50 years)	Mammogram	40%
Mortality from cerebrovascular disease	Age (over 40–50 years)	Diastolic blood pressure above 100 mmHg	50%
Diabetic retinopathy	Identify diabetics	Retinal examination	60%

population at the middle of the year. For England and Wales in 1988 it was 13.8 per 1000. This rate corresponds to an average of 1.8 babies born to each woman during her reproductive years (the *period fertility rate*). The induced abortion rate at present is about one-fifth of the birth rate. In some countries (e.g. Czechoslovakia) the induced abortion rate is low (<10%), whereas in others (e.g. Cuba) it is approximately 50%.

Perinatal and infant mortality

The *stillbirth rate* is the number of stillbirths divided by the total number of births. The term stillbirth, in England and Wales, applies to any infant born after the 28th week of pregnancy and showing no signs of life after birth. The rate in 1986 was 5.3 per 1000 total births.

The *perinatal mortality rate* is the number of stillbirths plus deaths in the first week of life divided by total births.

The rate in England and Wales in 1986 was 9.5 per 1000 total births (i.e. about 1%).

The *infant mortality rate* is the number of deaths in liveborn infants under one year of age divided by total live births. This was 9.4 per 1000 live births in 1986.

Mortality

The introduction of death registration was a landmark in the development of epidemiology. The UK was one of the first countries to collect mortality statistics routinely, and annual figures have been produced since 1838. Figure 1.4 shows that the standardised mortality ratio (SMR) fell steeply from the middle of the 19th century and that infant mortality has declined rapidly from the beginning of the current century. Figure 1.5 shows the reduction in selected age-specific death rates from 1841 to 1985. There has been a decline in all age groups with the greatest percentage reductions in the relatively young. For example, there has been a 90% reduction in mortality in persons aged 25–34, compared to a reduction of 38% in those aged 75–84 years. The most important reason for the decline in mortality in the young is the decline in mortality from infectious diseases. Figure 1.6 shows the decline in the standardised mortality ratio for tuberculosis from about 1500 in the mid-1850s to 60 in recent years. Most of this reduction occurred well before the introduction of specific medical interventions such as the use of antibiotics, immunisation or the use of special investigative techniques such as radiography. It has, instead, been largely due to the improvement in living standards, particularly in housing conditions and nutrition.

With the reduction in age-specific death rates, the expectation of life has increased. From birth, it is now

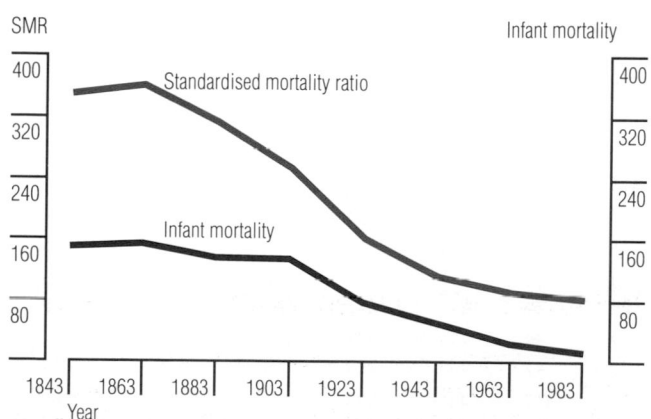

Fig. 1.4 Standardised mortality ratios (SMR) and infant mortality in England and Wales, 1841–1985. Standardised mortality ratios are for all causes, 1950–52 = 100. Infant mortality = deaths under one year of age per 1000 live births. (Source: OPCS, series DH1 No. 19, 1989.)

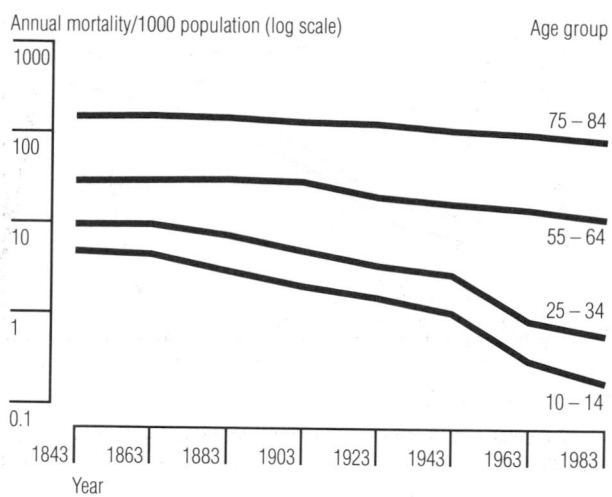

Fig. 1.5 Age–specific mortality in England and Wales, 1841–1985. (Source: OPCS, series DH1 No. 19, 1989.)

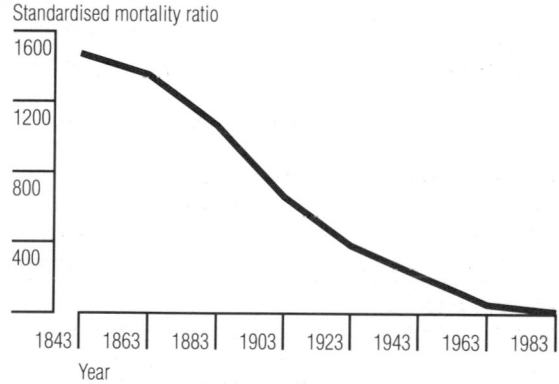

Fig. 1.6 Mortality from tuberculosis in England and Wales, 1850–1985. (1950–52 = 100. Source: OPCS, series DH1 No. 19, 1989.)

about 78 years in women and 72 in men, compared to 42 and 40 years respectively in the middle of the 19th century (Fig. 1.7).

The major causes of death vary considerably according to age. In the first four weeks of life the main causes are those associated with prematurity, congenital malformations and complications of birth. The main causes of death during the remaining part of the first year of life are infectious diseases, congenital malformations, sudden infant death syndrome and accidents. Table 1.8 shows the age-specific death rates in 1987 in England and Wales for selected causes of death.

Accidents are the major cause of death in both children (1–14 years) and young adults (15–34 years), with road traffic accidents accounting for about half of these. In adults aged 35–54 (both sexes combined), ischaemic heart disease is the major cause of death, followed by cancer and cerebrovascular disease. The death rate in

1 The Epidemiological Approach

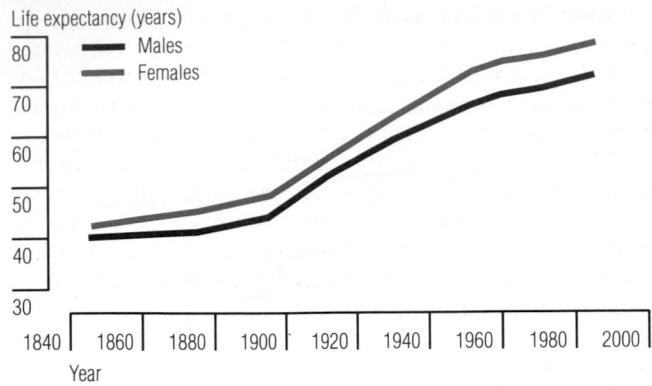

Fig. 1.7 Expectation of life from birth in England and Wales, 1840–1980.
(Source: OPCS, series DH2 No. 15, 1990.)

men has declined somewhat since about 1920, but that in women has declined more. Both ischaemic heart disease and lung cancer have increased rapidly during this century; both are more common in men than in women. Mortality from these two diseases is the main reason for the fact that, among the 55–74-year-old age group, the death rate from all causes in men is about twice that in women (see Table 1.8). The rise in lung cancer mortality during this century (see Ch. 8, Fig. 8.6) is particularly striking, not only on account of its magnitude but also because it is almost all caused by smoking. Although

mortality from lung cancer declined in the 1980s in the UK due to a reduction in smoking and the use of cigarettes with a lower tar yield, during this time the disease overtook stomach cancer as the most common fatal cancer in the world – a completely avoidable world epidemic. In Poland, for example, death rates from lung cancer among 50-year-old men has increased four-fold from 1960 to 1980. About half the world's tobacco production is consumed by economically undeveloped countries. By the year 2000 it is estimated that there will be two million cases of lung cancer per year in the world, nearly two-thirds arising in economically undeveloped countries. Neither the scale of the risk nor of the epidemic is adequately appreciated by the public. The manufacture, sale and promotion of cigarettes represents the greatest threat to public health in our age.

Taking men and women of all ages together, about a quarter of deaths are caused by ischaemic heart disease, a quarter by cancer, an eighth by strokes, and a further eighth by obstructive lung disease and pneumonia, leaving one-quarter attributable to other causes (Fig. 1.8). The distribution of cancer deaths according to the organ affected is shown in Chapter 8, Figure 8.5.

AIDS figures demonstrate the relatively small mortality from this disease in the UK up to 1992. The future of the epidemic in the UK remains uncertain but as yet it has not produced the major toll it has in Africa (in Uganda and Zaire over 15% of adults are infected

Table 1.8 Death rates per million population from selected causes by age and sex in England and Wales, 1987

Cause	Sex	>1	1–4	5–14	15–24	25–34	35–44	45–54	55–64	65–74	75–84	>85
All causes	M	5238	440	225	781	884	1671	5007	15 973	41 225	96 301	191 548
	F	4009	32	161	296	476	1125	3227	9135	22 753	60 065	158 560
Lung cancer	M	0	0	0	1	5	64	415	210	4887	7538	6951
	F	0	0	0	0	4	45	190	831	1504	1660	1406
Breast cancer	F	0	0	0	1	41	206	634	1037	1351	1921	3156
Colorectal cancer	M	0	0	0	0	9	39	181	580	1378	2695	4109
	F	0	0	0	0	5	37	154	434	894	1788	3384
Other cancer	M	35	40	42	69	120	290	920	2801	6585	13 348	20 668
	F	40	48	37	42	115	303	817	1998	3796	6543	9619
Ischaemic heart disease	M	3	1	0	2	44	398	1938	6192	14 501	28 227	45 781
	F	0	0	0	1	11	60	358	1922	6320	16 369	34 256
Cerebrovascular disease	M	19	2	3	10	20	76	247	909	3470	11 777	25 354
	F	30	3	2	9	25	74	212	673	2674	10 572	30 202
Other circulatory diseases	M	61	8	6	24	29	76	226	827	5789	7751	20 641
	F	44	17	4	12	18	41	143	468	1560	5782	21 132
Accidents, injury, violence, etc.	M	170	121	90	526	462	410	434	485	591	1196	2656
	F	128	19	50	129	135	150	194	239	405	916	2431
Chronic obstructive airways disease	M	180	12	6	15	15	23	111	729	1383	7687	14 677
	F	121	11	4	11	12	18	86	405	1025	1875	3702

Source: OPCS Mortality Statistics, Causes 1987, Series DH2 No. 14. HMSO, London 1989.

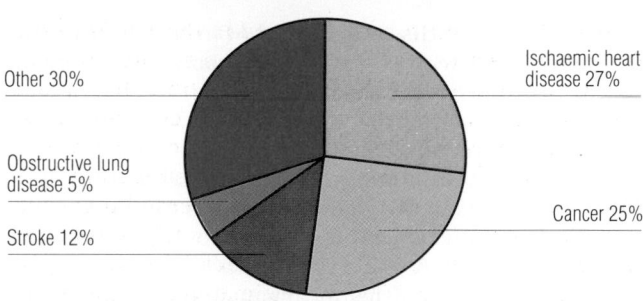

Fig. 1.8 Causes of death in England and Wales, 1987. (Source: OPCS, series DH2 No. 14, 1989.)

with the HIV virus and 5–10% will die of AIDS in the next ten years – mostly heterosexuals) and in cities such as New York and San Francisco.

In all societies, there are inequalities in health. Figure 1.9 shows the SMR in England and Wales classified according to social class. This system of categorising the population according to occupation was devised by the Registrar General in 1875, and has been continued ever since. According to this system, there are five social classes, with class III divided into two subclasses. These are:

I. professional
II. semi-professional
III. skilled – subdivided into non-manual (IIIN) and manual (IIIM)
IV. semi-skilled
V. unskilled.

The differences in mortality among social classes illustrates the extent to which mortality in western countries is due to differences in lifestyle and environmental factors. As Figure 1.9 shows, the mortality of social class V is about two and a half times greater than that in social class I. For accidents in children under 14 years of age, the difference is eight-fold. Nearly all diseases are more

common in social classes IV and V than in I and II, e.g. there are large differences in mortality from ischaemic heart disease and lung cancer, reflecting differences in smoking habit and diet between the social classes. Some diseases, however, are more common in social classes I and II, e.g. breast cancer, multiple sclerosis, malignant melanoma and Hodgkin's disease. This observation suggests some interesting aetiological hypotheses such as the possible link between melanoma and sudden episodes of sunbathing among fair-skinned persons able to afford holidays in the sun.

Morbidity

There are four main sources of information on the extent of illness in the population:

- hospital statistics on the number of episodes of hospital illness and bed occupancy rates (Fig. 1.10)
- registration of all newly diagnosed cases of cancer
- general practitioner consultation rates
- self-reported illness in population surveys.

Mental disorders account for nearly half of inpatient hospital days mainly because these admissions tend to be long-term. Figure 1.11 shows the general practitioner consultation rates according to major disease groups. Consultation rates are, for nearly all conditions, higher for women than for men.

THE DEVELOPING WORLD

The pattern of disease in the developing world is quite different from that of the economically rich western

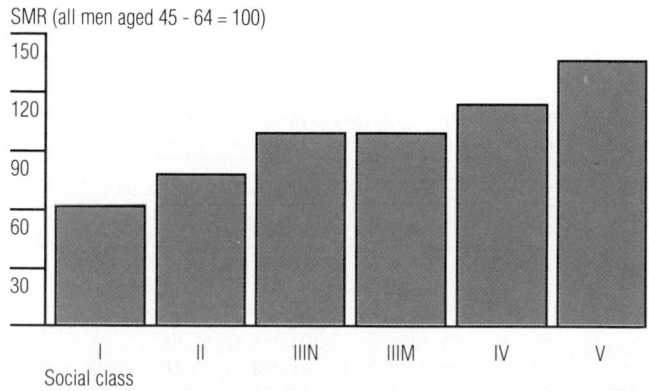

Fig. 1.9 Death rates by social class in England and Wales, 1971. (Source: Goldblatt P Population Trends 56. HMSO, 1989.)

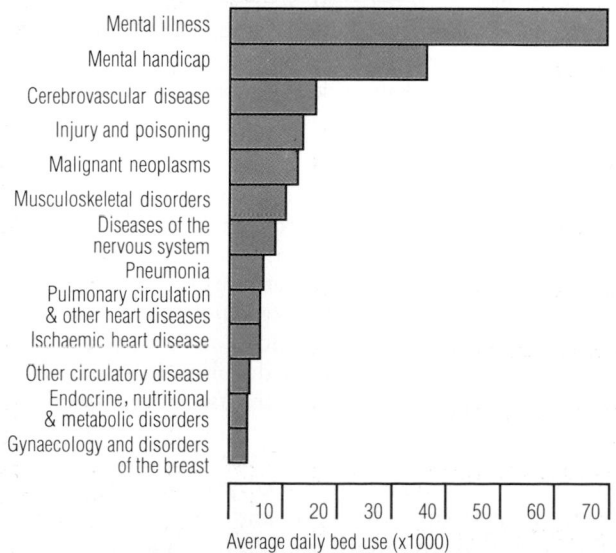

Fig. 1.10 Average daily hospital bed use according to disease in England, 1985. (Source: DHSS/OPCS.)

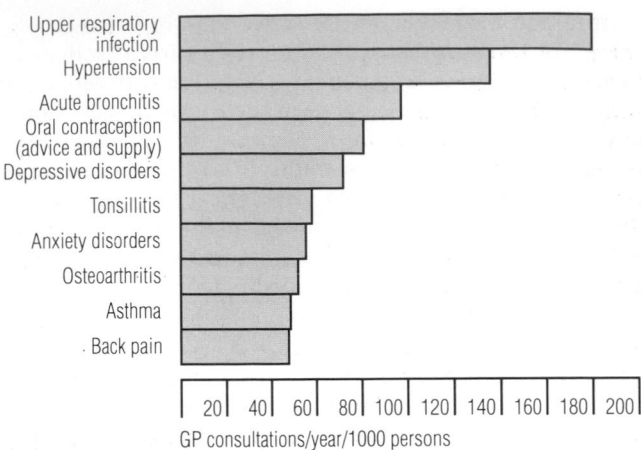

Fig. 1.11 General practitioner consultation rates in England and Wales, 1981–2. (Source: OPCS.)

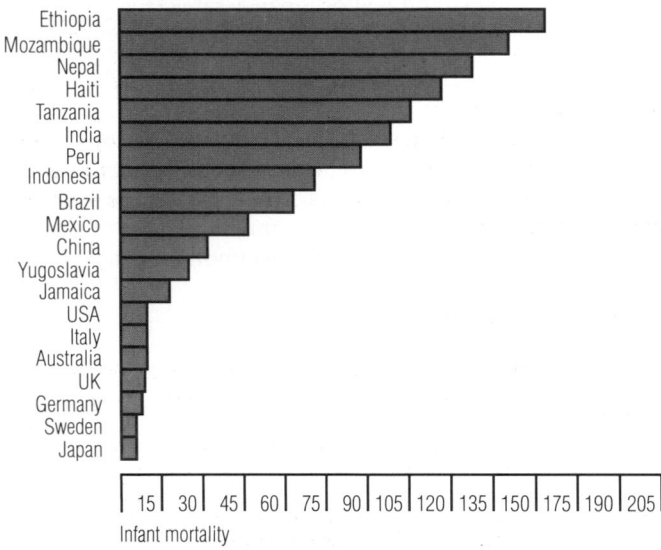

Fig. 1.12 Infant mortality (deaths under one year of age per 1000 live births) for selected countries, 1987. (Source: World Bank, 1989.)

In addition, some diseases typical of industrial societies are being exported to the poorer countries. A prime example is lung cancer through the introduction of cigarette smoking, so that this formerly relatively rare cancer is now the commonest cancer in the world.

A useful way to compare the relative importance of different diseases in different countries is to calculate, for each disease, the years of life lost due to deaths from that particular disease. A disease that kills a person at age 60 results in that person losing fewer years of life than a person who dies at, say, 20. Table 1.9 compares the years of life lost from accidents, circulatory disease and cancer, which are important causes of mortality in the industrialised world, with the years of life lost through these causes in the developing world. Two representative countries, namely Ghana and Canada, have been used for comparison. It may be seen that, while these three causes of death account for only 8% of years of life lost in Ghana, they account for 79% in Canada.

In Ghana, the major causes of years of life lost are quite different (Table 1.10). Malaria is judged to be among the most serious health problems in many parts of tropical Africa and has been estimated to cause over one million deaths a year. Sickle cell disease affects about 1 in 400 Africans and about 1 in 10 people of African descent carry the gene. Measles, while not a typical tropical disease, is an important cause of mortality in the developing world.

Diarrhoeal disease is another important cause of morbidity and mortality in the developing world. In 1975, an estimated 500 million episodes of diarrhoea in children in Asia, Africa and Latin America caused 5–18 million deaths. The problem is largely due to the vicious cycle arising from contaminated water and food and malnutrition. Poorly nourished children are more liable to get diarrhoea, contaminate the water supplies and thereby infect others. In the developing world, it is from this vicious cycle that the greatest disease burden arises, rather than from diseases more generally regarded as 'tropical' such as schistosomiasis, leishmaniasis, leprosy and onchocerciasis.

About a billion people in the developing world are infested by worms. Surveys in Sri Lanka, Bangladesh and

nations. Apart from malaria and certain disorders specific to particular regions, it is similar to that found in the UK in the early part of the 19th century. Infectious disease accounts for the major burden of mortality in developing countries; infant mortality rates are some ten times greater than those now seen in rich countries (Fig. 1.12); and the expectation of life in developing countries is nearly half that seen today in industrialised countries (Fig. 1.1).

The main cause of disease in the economically poor countries of the world – home to three-quarters of the world's inhabitants – is poverty and, unfortunately, most of the poor countries in the world are remaining poor. It is estimated that 80% of deaths in the developing world could be avoided by clean water and improved sanitation.

Table 1.9 Years of life lost by men between ages of 1 and 70 due to accident, circulatory disease and cancer in Ghana and Canada in 1967

Cause of death	Years of life lost (% total)	
	Ghana	Canada
Accidents	3	39
Circulatory diseases	4	24
Cancer	1	16
Total	8	79

(Adapted from Table 3.1 in The Health of Nations, 1985, Open University Press.)

Table 1.10 Major causes of years of life lost in Ghana

Disease	Years of life lost (% total)
● Perinatal disorders	24
Pregnancy complications	(1.6)
Congenital malformations	(1.9)
Prematurity	(9.1)
Birth injury	(6.0)
Neonatal tetanus	(3.7)
Neonatal respiratory disorders	(1.6)
● Malaria	15
● Malnutrition and gastroenteritis	10
● Sickle-cell disease	6
● Measles	6
● Pneumonia	6
Total	67

(Adapted from Table 3.2 in The Health of Nations, 1985, Open University Press.)

Venezuela indicate that over 90% of 6-year-old children are affected. The commonest worm infestations are hookworm and roundworm (ascariasis).

The burden of disease from respiratory illness is largely due to the same infections that arise (or arose before satisfactory control measures were introduced) in industrial countries – mainly pneumonia, whooping cough, influenza, measles, TB and diphtheria. Overall, the important difference between the developing world and the industrialised countries lies not so much in the types of diseases that occur as in the frequency and impact that they have.

Within developing countries, there are important geographical differences in the distribution of disease. These tend to reflect the local ecological conditions. For example, malaria is transmitted by certain kinds of mosquito; and transmission of schistosomiasis (bilharzia) depends on passage of the parasite from urine or faeces through certain kinds of water snail, in which the parasites develop and then emerge in a form that can reinfect people. The prevalence of these two parasitic diseases therefore depends upon a combination of circumstances favourable to the existence of the mosquito and water snail respectively. Many parasitic diseases are restricted to certain locations, e.g. Chagas' disease is confined to South America, and sleeping sickness, transmitted by the tsetse fly, is restricted to Africa.

Disease problems in the developing world cannot be solved by building hospitals with their costly infrastructure of staff and equipment. The greatest need is for simple measures, such as ensuring the supply and quality of food, the provision of clean water, effective sewerage systems and the control of fertility. The World Bank has estimated that the cost of providing clean water to all those in need would be about $260 billion which, although a vast sum, is only about one half of one year's global expenditure on military arms.

The importance of education in improving the health of the world cannot be overestimated. Much of the difficulty in the introduction of measures designed to improve health is due to cultural or religious obstacles which may take the form of traditional practices that are deeply ingrained. In a poor country, people obtain long-term security in large families so that birth control, while of benefit to the community, may not be of help to the individual. Social and cultural changes must progress together with economic development in a way that is sensitive and responsive to all the relevant issues. Few would doubt that the rich industrialised countries of the world have an obligation to provide a lead but, to be effective, they will need to recognise the cultural and political obstacles to the prevention of disease as well as the economic ones.

FURTHER READING

Ahlbom A, Norell S 1984 Introduction to modern epidemiology. Epidemiology Resources Ltd, Chestnut Hill, Maine. *A short, handy textbook.*

Doll R, Peto R 1984 The causes of cancer. Oxford University Press, Oxford. *A good example of how epidemiology can identify causes of diseases.*

ISIS. Randomized trial of intravenous streptokinase, oral aspirin, both or neither among 17 187 cases of suspected acute myocardial infarction; ISIS-2 Lancet 1988; ii: 349–359.

MacMahon B, Pugh T F 1970 Epidemiology: principles and methods. Little, Brown and Company, Boston. *A good basic textbook of epidemiology.*

Mausner J S, Bahn A K 1974 Epidemiology: an introductory text. W B Saunders, Philadelphia. *A monograph presenting the concepts of modern epidemiology in a quantitative manner.*

McKeown T 1984 The role of medicine. Blackwell, Oxford. *A short book dealing with concepts of health and disease, and the role of medicine in influencing our health.*

The U205 Course Team 1985 The health of nations. The Open University Press, Milton Keynes. *OUP coursebook examining contemporary and historical patterns of health and disease in the UK and the rest of the world.*

2
Clinical Pharmacology

Philip A Routledge

PHARMACODYNAMICS AND PHARMACOKINETICS

Pharmacodynamics is the study of the action of drugs on the body, while *pharmacokinetics* describes the action of the body on the drug (i.e. the process by which it absorbs, distributes and eliminates the drug).

Pharmacokinetics has benefited from advances in chemistry which allow the accurate and sensitive determination of even tiny quantities of drugs in biological fluids. Pharmacodynamics, on the other hand, is still in its infancy, as it has proved difficult to measure accurately the effects of drugs on the body. However, because drugs are prescribed not for their pharmacokinetic behaviour but for their pharmacodynamic activity, much effort is now being directed towards improving measurement of drug action.

PHARMACODYNAMICS

There are three major ways by which a drug can produce pharmacological effects:

- by combination with specific receptors
- by alteration of physiological enzyme processes
- by direct physical or chemical action.

Interaction with specific receptors

An increasing number of drugs are being discovered that act through receptors on the cell surface or within the cell. When this combination of a drug with a receptor provokes a biological response, the drug is known as an *agonist*. According to the receptor occupancy theory, the intensity of the pharmacological effect (E) is directly proportional to the number of receptors combined with the drug molecule; thus, the relation between intensity of effect and drug concentration (D) is given by a rearrangement of the law of mass action:

$$E = \frac{E_{max} \cdot D}{K_D + D} \qquad\qquad 2.1$$

where E_{max} is the maximum response and K_D is the dissociation constant of the reaction between drug and receptor site. When the intensity of pharmacological action is plotted as a proportion of maximum response against drug concentration, the relationship in Equation 2.1 results in a rectangular hyperbola (Fig. 2.1A). Logarithmic transformation of drug concentration results in a sigmoid curve, with a log-linear relationship in its central portion (Fig. 2.1B). Most drugs exert their action on the log-linear portion of their dose response curve; maximum drug effect is rarely achievable because of the risk of other adverse effects of the drug. The dissociation constant, K_D, is a measure of the reversibility of the drug–receptor interaction and is low when the interaction is slowly reversible. It is also the concentration at which half the maximum response of the agonist is seen and is thus a measure of drug 'potency'. The E_{max}, on the other hand, is a measure of drug 'efficacy'. The lower the K_D the greater the potency. It is thus possible to have a drug which is more potent than another but less efficacious. Thiazide diuretics, for example, are more potent than frusemide since they usually produce their effects at lower molar drug concentrations, but they are less efficacious diuretics since their maximum diuretic effect is lower.

Antagonists are drugs which will combine with the receptor site to prevent another agent from producing its maximal effect. If the antagonist produces some activity, it is termed a partial agonist. If it has no efficacy of its own, but merely prevents the activity of an agonist at the receptor site, it is termed a full antagonist. When this antagonism is competitive, the dose–response relationship of the agonist is shifted to the right in a parallel fashion. Non-competitive antagonists reduce the number of receptors available for binding of agonists by irreversibly binding to receptors. Maximum efficacy is there-

Figure 2.1 Relationship between drug effect and drug concentration A on linear scale and **B** on logarithmic scale.

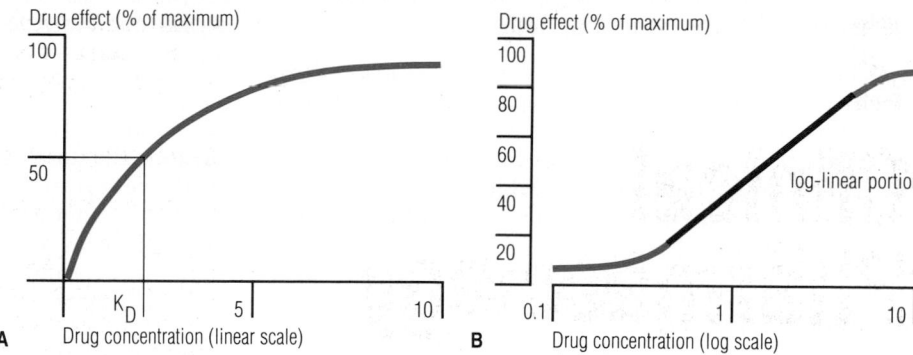

fore reduced and the dose–response relationship, although shifted to the right, is shifted in a non-parallel fashion. Some examples of receptors, their agonists and antagonists are shown in Table 2.1.

Alteration of physiological enzyme processes

The vast majority of drugs acting in this way inhibit (rather than stimulate) enzyme processes either competitively or non-competitively. Thus, neostigmine competitively inhibits the enzyme cholinesterase, which allows the build-up of concentrations of acetylcholine which, in turn, enhances neuromuscular transmission in myasthenia gravis. The dose–response relationship of such drugs often resembles those of drugs acting at receptor sites.

Most monoamine oxidase inhibitors (e.g. phenelzine) inhibit this enzyme irreversibly and only when new enzyme has been synthesised does the effect of these drugs wear off. Similarly, it is probable that the action of some cytotoxic agents is due to intermediate products to which they are metabolised, and which inhibit enzymes responsible for synthesis of DNA and RNA.

Table 2.1 Some receptor types and their agonists and antagonists

Receptor type	Natural agonist	Some effects of agonist	Other agonists	Antagonists
Adrenergic				
α_1	Noradrenaline	Contraction of vascular smooth muscle	Phenylephrine	Prazosin
α_2	Noradrenaline	Inhibition of noradrenaline release at presynaptic receptors in CNS	Clonidine	Yohimbine
β_1	Adrenaline	Increased cardiac inotropism and chronotropism	Dobutamine	Atenolol
β_2	Adrenaline	Relaxation of bronchial, vascular and uterine smooth muscle	Salbutamol	Propranolol (also β_1)
Cholinergic				
Muscarinic	Acetylcholine	Decreased heart rate	Carbachol	Atropine
Nicotinic	Acetylcholine	Neuromuscular transmission	Nicotine	Tubocurarine
Dopaminergic				
D_2	Dopamine	Neurotransmission (CNS)	Bromocriptine	Chlorpromazine
Histaminergic				
H_1	Histamine	Contraction of bronchial smooth muscle	–	Chlorpheniramine
H_2	Histamine	Stimulation of gastric acid secretion	–	Cimetidine Ranitidine
Serotonergic				
(5 HT_2)	5-hydroxytryptamine	Neuronal excitation (CNS)	–	Ketanserin
Opioid	β-endorphins, enkephalins	Modulation of pain perception	Morphine	Naloxone

Direct physical or chemical actions

Bulk purgatives and osmotic diuretics are examples of this mechanism of action. Chelating agents combine chemically with heavy metals to produce less active chelates which are eventually excreted. Local and general anaesthetics, which are highly lipid soluble, appear to change the properties of neuronal membranes and discourage depolarisation by a physical action.

PHARMACOKINETICS

Before a drug can exert a biological effect, it must be absorbed or directly introduced into the body; be distributed through body tissues to its site of action; and, finally, be eliminated from the body either by metabolism and subsequent excretion of the metabolites, or by direct excretion of unchanged drug. These biological processes are often termed *drug disposition*, and *pharmacokinetics* is the mathematical description of these biological events.

When a drug is introduced directly into the circulation (i.e. by intravenous administration), its concentration in plasma declines in an exponential fashion as shown in Figure 2.2. This process is known as *first order elimination*. A fixed proportion of the drug present in the plasma is eliminated per unit time, but the total amount of drug removed per unit time falls. The time necessary for the drug concentration to fall to half of its original value is constant and is known as the half-life of elimination of the drug. Transformation of drug concentration to its natural logarithm results in a linear decline with time, and the slope of the line is the elimination rate constant (K). This is related to the half-life ($t_{1/2}$) of the drug as follows:

$$K = \frac{0.693}{t_{1/2}} \qquad 2.2$$

where 0.693 is the natural logarithm of 2. When common logarithms ($\log_{10}$) are used (Fig. 2.2), the slope of the line is:

$$-\frac{K}{2.303}$$

Apparent volume of distribution

The apparent volume of distribution (V_d) is a measure of the proportion of drug present in the plasma relative to the rest of the body at any particular time. It is calculated by dividing the dose of the drug administered intravenously, by the concentration at zero time (C_0) (Fig. 2.2). Thus a drug given in a dose of 1 g (1000 mg) which produced a concentration of 100 mg/l in plasma immediately after rapid intravenous injection would have an apparent volume of distribution of 10 litres (1000/100). Although this measure has no direct anatomical significance, it does reflect tissue uptake of the drug. Thus, tricyclic antidepressants, which are avidly taken up by tissues, have a very high apparent distribution volume (over 1000 litres in a normal adult); while drugs which remain principally in the intravascular space, such as heparin, have a distribution volume of around 7 litres in the normal adult.

Drug clearance

Clearance (Cl) is the best measure of the efficiency of elimination of a drug. It is defined as the volume of plasma cleared of the drug per unit time, and can be calculated from the equation:

$$Cl = V_d \cdot K \qquad 2.3$$

Thus the clearance of the drug described in Fig. 2.2 is 10 litres multiplied by 0.347 l/hour (3.47 l/hour);

$$\text{or from the equation: } Cl = \frac{D}{AUC} \qquad 2.4$$

where D is the dose and AUC is the area under the plasma concentration curve from time 0 to infinity. Equations 2.3 and 2.4 show that, unlike the elimination rate constant K (and thus also the half-life of elimination), clearance is not dependent on the volume of distribution of the drug. The total plasma clearance of drug is the sum of the clearances by metabolism and excretion. Some drugs (e.g. phenytoin, ethanol and salicylate) undergo concentration-dependent metabolism sometimes known as capacity-limited or *saturation kinetics*. For these

Figure 2.2 Time course of decline of plasma drug concentrations A on a linear and **B** on a logarithmic scale after intravenous injection of 1 g of drug (V_d = 1000/100 = 10 l, K = 0.347–1 hour, $t_{1/2}$ elim = 2 hours, plasma clearance = 3.47 l/hour).

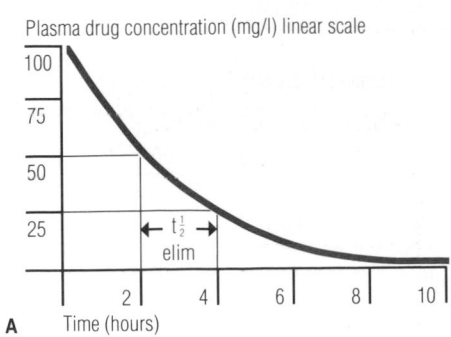

Plasma drug concentration (mg/l) linear scale

A   Time (hours)

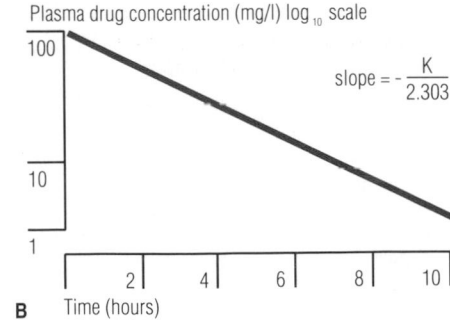

Plasma drug concentration (mg/l) $\log_{10}$ scale

$$\text{slope} = -\frac{K}{2.303}$$

B   Time (hours)

drugs, clearance falls with rising drug concentration. The fall in drug concentration is not log-linear with time, and a true half-life of elimination cannot be calculated.

Absorption and bioavailability

When drugs are given by the oral route they are often absorbed in a first order fashion, so that the plasma concentration rises exponentially to a peak when absorption rate equals distribution or elimination rate and then declines (Fig. 2.3). However, it must be remembered that at the time of peak concentration, absorption is still not complete and continues for some time after this. *Bioavailability* is defined as the proportion of the drug reaching the systemic circulation when administered by any route other than the intravenous route. (By the intravenous route, bioavailability is of course 100%.) The bioavailability of a drug can be calculated by dividing the area under the plasma concentration curve produced after administration by a given route, by the area under the curve produced using the intravenous route. Bioavailability after oral administration may be less than 100% either because the drug is not completely absorbed from the gastrointestinal tract, or because it is metabolised in the gut (e.g. isoprenaline), the liver (e.g. propranolol) or the lung (e.g. noradrenaline) before it can reach the systemic circulation. The reduced bioavailability in these situations is due to presystemic (or *first-pass*) elimination and such drugs are termed high clearance compounds.

Steady state pharmacokinetics

Most drugs are not given as a single dose but are administered on a regular basis. This may result in accumulation of drug depending on the frequency of administration and the half-life of the compound. Eventually, a *steady state* situation will be achieved when the rate of drug administration is equal to the rate of drug elimination. Fifty per cent of the steady state concentration will be achieved in one half-life, 75% in two half-lives and so on, so that it takes approximately five half-lives to reach steady state (Fig. 2.3). Thus, for warfarin ($t_{1/2}$ = 36 hours), steady state will take over a week to achieve; and a similar period will be required for the plasma concentration to decline to undetectable levels after the drug has been discontinued. The steady state concentration (C_{ss}) is defined as the average plasma concentration of drug during the dosage interval; and is calculated using the equation:

$$C_{ss} = \frac{D \cdot F}{Cl \cdot Tau} \qquad 2.5$$

where D is the dosage, Cl the clearance (l/min), Tau is the time interval between doses and F the bioavailability of the drug after the particular route of administration. It is evident from this equation that, if the total dose of drug given per day remains the same, C_{ss} will remain constant, although if larger doses are given at less frequent intervals, the difference between C_{max} and C_{min} (the peak and trough plasma concentrations) will increase. These fluctuations may be important if the adverse effects of the drug are related to peak concentrations, or if there is a threshold concentration below which drug effect is not obtained. For this reason, heparin (which has a short half-life and whose concentration would therefore fluctuate markedly after intermittent intravenous administration), is normally given by continuous intravenous infusion. The longer the half-life of the drug, the longer the interval that can elapse between doses for any given difference between peak and trough concentrations. It is also clear from Equation 2.5 that this steady state concentration (C_{ss}) will be directly proportional to the dose administered under first order conditions. For drugs with saturation kinetics (e.g. phenytoin) where the clearance falls with increasing dosage, the relationship between steady state concentration and dose will be curvilinear, so that increases in dose will produce disproportionate increases in circulating drug concentrations and risk of toxicity.

Figure 2.3 Time course of plasma drug concentrations after repeated oral administration of the same oral dose at 12 hourly intervals. The drug has a $t_{1/2}$ elim of 12 hours and is described by a two-compartment open model. C_{ss} = steady state concentration.

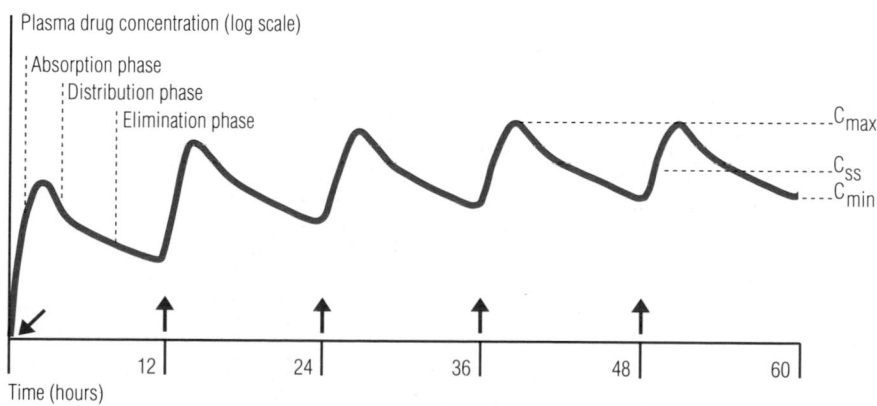

2 Clinical Pharmacology

Summary 1 Clinical pharmacokinetics

● A drug, once introduced into the body, takes five half-lives to reach steady state concentration.

● For drugs undergoing first order elimination, the concentration at steady state is directly proportional to the dose and inversely proportional to the clearance.

● For drugs with saturation kinetics, increased doses cause reduced clearance and therefore disproportionate increases in steady state drug concentration.

● Clearance is independent of the volume of distribution, whereas the $t_{1/2}$ elimination is not.

Multicompartment models

When the natural logarithm ($\log_e$) of drug concentrations is measured against time, a relationship with two or more linear portions may be obtained. The simplest example is the two-compartment open model shown in Figure 2.3. Each portion has its own rate constant with the early component normally due to distribution of the drug throughout the tissues. This means, firstly, that the circulating plasma concentration may fall rapidly after administration of a drug so that a loading dose may be necessary to achieve and maintain an effective circulating drug concentration. Secondly, blood samples taken during the distribution phase will tend to overestimate the steady state concentration of drug. Thirdly, estimates of clearance made using data which do not contain sufficient sampling points soon after drug administration may underestimate the area under the curve (AUC) by missing the distribution phase, and therefore tend to overestimate drug clearance.

Absorption

Drugs are usually given by the alimentary route, and must therefore pass through the bowel wall in order to enter the bloodstream. This occurs by four different mechanisms:

● *Passive diffusion*, which involves diffusion down a concentration gradient from the gut into the bloodstream. For this to occur, the drug must dissolve in the gastrointestinal fluids, traverse the cell membrane and enter the bloodstream. The rate at which it does so depends on both the concentration gradient and the lipid solubility of the drug. This is the most important mechanism of absorption for most drugs.

● *Active transport*, a less important mechanism by which some drugs, because of their resemblance to naturally occurring substances, use existing transport systems. Thus, levodopa is absorbed by the active process responsible for absorption of the amino acid tyrosine.

● *Filtration through pores*, a route generally limited to molecules of molecular weight less than 100 (e.g. urea). Most drugs are too large to traverse the pores between cells.

● *Endocytosis*, by which drugs or particles are engulfed by cells in the bowel wall. This is of relatively little importance to drug absorption.

Factors affecting absorption

Absorption is affected by the chemical nature and formulation of the drug, as well as the physiological characteristics of the absorption site. Thus, some drugs cannot be administered orally because they are broken down by gastrointestinal enzymes (e.g. the polypeptide, insulin) or are unstable at extremes of pH (e.g. benzyl penicillin at gastric pH). Most drugs are either weak acids or weak bases and thus exist in two forms in solution – as ions or as undissociated molecules. The equilibrium between these forms is determined by the pK of the drug (the pH at which 50% of the drug is ionised) and the pH of the medium in which the drug is dissolved. At the low pH encountered in the stomach, a weakly acidic drug exists mainly in its undissociated form; it is thus more lipid soluble, and will tend to be more easily absorbed. Basic drugs, on the other hand, are largely ionised at low pH and exist predominantly in the undissociated form only in the alkaline media of the small bowel. Despite these considerations, both acidic and basic drugs tend to be absorbed predominantly in the small intestine, because they are there for longer and because the inner surface of the intestine provides a much greater absorptive area than the stomach. A few basic drugs have a pK much greater than the highest pH reached in the intestine, and therefore remain ionised throughout the gastrointestinal tract and are poorly absorbed.

Formulation factors are important in determining the rate and extent of drug absorption. Most drugs consist not only of an active agent but also of diluents, granulating and binding agents, lubricants and disintegrating agents, any of which may have a marked effect on absorption. Particle size of the active constituent may also be important, and sustained or delayed release preparations will also delay absorption rate.

Gastrointestinal motility affects the rate of absorption. Delays in gastric emptying will result in delayed drug absorption although the extent of absorption is normally unchanged. *Food* has a variable effect. Some drugs (e.g. propranolol) have greater bioavailability in the presence of food because of reduced pre-systemic elimination, whereas others (e.g. rifampicin) are more poorly absorbed. Such factors may be important in determining the times of administration of drugs.

The *route of administration* is also important. Alternatives to the oral route are:

- *Intramuscular injection,* either to speed the onset of effects or to enhance biovailability when the oral route is suboptimal. Use of the intramuscular route can, however, cause local pain and some drugs (e.g. phenytoin and diazepam) are poorly and variably absorbed when administered in this way, because of poor solubility at tissue pH. Absorption rate varies with the muscle group used (it is usually faster from the deltoid than from the vastus or gluteus muscles) and may be slow in situations of poor tissue perfusion.
- *Rectal administration* can sometimes be used but, because the haemorrhoidal veins drain partly into the portal tract, presystemic elimination is not completely avoided. The suppository may also be variably retained or have poor and erratic absorption.
- *Buccal administration* can completely avoid presystemic elimination and is used for drugs (e.g. glyceryl trinitrate) which are rapidly metabolised after the oral route. Unfortunately, not all such drugs can rapidly penetrate the buccal mucosa and enter the systemic circulation.
- *Transdermal administration* is an alternative to the buccal route for drugs such as glyceryl trinitrate or the antihistamine, hyoscine. The latter is used for motion sickness, but, when given by the oral route, may be ineffective due to delayed gastric emptying associated with nausea. The rate of absorption varies with the skin site used and the extent of absorption is limited, so that only very potent drugs (effective dose <10 mg) can be usefully administered by this route. Absorption is normally rapid but membranes are being developed to control the rate.
- *Intrapulmonary route.* Some drugs, and all anaesthetic gases, are administered by the intrapulmonary route. Non-gaseous compounds are difficult to introduce into the lungs. Only 10% of a drug administered by pressurised aerosol actually enters the lungs; the remainder is deposited in the buccal cavity and subsequently swallowed.

Distribution

If drug distribution did not occur, only those drugs with an action within the vascular compartment would provoke biological effects. Like absorption, distribution is dependent on the physicochemical characteristics of the drug as well as upon biological factors.

The major physiochemical properties determining drug distribution are lipid solubility and (if the drug is a weak electrolyte) the degree of dissociation (ionisation) in

tissues. Highly lipid soluble drugs are generally distributed throughout all fluid compartments and, because they can cross lipid membranes readily, can reach most organs including the brain. Poorly lipid soluble drugs are normally able to enter the interstitial fluid, but if they are weak electrolytes, only the undissociated form can penetrate the cells and then only to a limited extent, depending on the lipid–water partition coefficient.

Biological factors determining the distribution of drugs in the body include the degree of both plasma protein binding and of uptake by tissue, either by binding or by active transport mechanisms. The blood contains approximately 180 g of protein, half of which is albumin. Albumin is thus the most abundant single protein in the plasma and, because of its structure, is able to reversibly bind many drugs by Van der Waals forces, hydrogen bonds or hydrophobic bonds. However, its binding capacity is relatively limited and it has been estimated that only 200 mg of drug of average molecular weight (300) would be bound to albumin in plasma if there were only one binding site available on each albumin molecule. For some drugs, there may be more than one binding site and the binding capacity will relatively greater. Major sites of binding are the so-called site 1 (warfarin site), which also binds the endogenous compound bilirubin; and site 2 (diazepam site), the site at which the endogenous amino acid tryptophan also binds. Drugs may bind to either or both of these sites and can competitively displace each other.

The relationship between the serum albumin concentration and the proportion of two drugs in the free (unbound) form is shown in Figure 2.4. It can be seen that the differences in protein binding are likely to be relatively small over the range of serum albumin concentrations seen in health. In situations of hypoalbuminaemia, however, even small further decreases in serum albumin concentration may cause marked increases in the proportion of drug free in the plasma.

It has recently become apparent that another plasma protein, α_1-acid glycoprotein (AAG) also binds drugs,

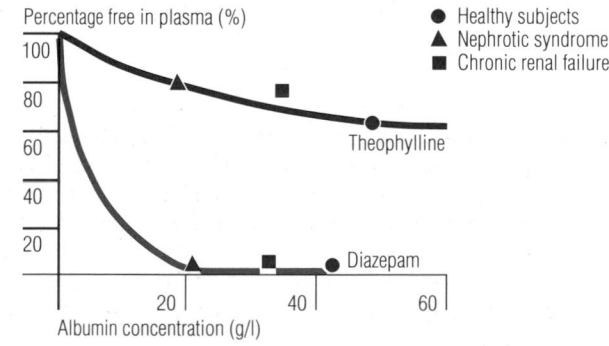

Figure 2.4 Relationship between the percentage of diazepam and theophylline free in plasma and plasma albumin concentration in different disorders. See text for details.

particularly those of a basic nature. Although its plasma concentration is much lower (c.2%) than that of albumin, its affinity for drugs is high and some drugs (e.g. lignocaine, erythromycin and disopyramide) may bind appreciably more to this protein than to albumin. Because of its low concentration, however, its binding capacity is relatively limited and, for several drugs, protein binding falls with increasing drug concentration.

The tissues also contain proteins which combine with drugs (60% of the total exchangeable body albumin is outside the vascular compartment), while body fat can serve as an important reservoir for lipid-soluble agents such as thiopentone. Finally, active transport mechanisms – such as the uptake of adrenergic neurone-blocking drugs by the adrenergic neurone – may also contribute to high tissue concentrations of a drug. Extensive tissue binding tends to result in the drug having a large apparent volume of distribution (V_d), since most of the drug is outside the intravascular space.

Metabolism

The liver is the main organ of metabolism of drugs although some may also occur in the gastrointestinal tract, lung, blood or kidney. Metabolism is particularly important for lipid-soluble drugs which more readily enter cells and are also prevented by their lipid solubility from being excreted unchanged by the kidney. The routes of metabolism are relatively non-specific and are shared by a variety of drugs. In most instances, more water-soluble metabolites (which are more easily excreted by the kidney) are produced. It has been suggested that, without metabolism, a lipid-soluble drug would have a half-life of around 30 days and, if it were also reversibly bound to tissues, its half-life might be as great as 100 years!

Summary 2 Drug disposition

Absorption Most drugs are administered by the alimentary route. Absorption from the gut occurs via passive diffusion (main mechanism), active transport, filtration through pores, or endocytosis.

Distribution Depends on the drug's ability to penetrate cells and bind to plasma proteins and on tissue uptake (cell protein binding or active transport). In the plasma, acidic drugs bind to albumin. Basic drugs may also bind to α_1-acid glycoprotein.

Metabolism The liver is the main site of the metabolism of drugs. Phase I metabolic reactions involve oxidation, reduction, hydrolysis and dealkylation of the drug. Phase II reactions involve conjugation reactions (e.g. with glucuronic acid) to form generally more water-soluble compounds.

Excretion Almost all drugs must be metabolised to more water-soluble compounds before excretion in the urine.

There are two groups of metabolic reactions: phase I and phase II reactions.

Phase I reactions involve the enzyme mono-oxygenase situated in the smooth endoplasmic reticulum of cells with metabolic function, especially the liver. These are called cytochrome P_{450} enzymes and are responsible for oxidation, reduction, hydrolysis and dealkylation of drugs with the relevant molecular structure. A given drug may be metabolised by one or more of these routes to produce more water-soluble (and thus biologically active) metabolites.

Phase II reactions are conjugation reactions of more water-soluble molecules to the drug or metabolite. Conjugation with glucuronide (glucuronidation) is the commonest pathway, but conjugation can also occur with sulphate, amino acids such as glutathione, or acetylCoA (acetylation). Most of these conjugated metabolites (except for some acetylated compounds) are biologically inactive. Although most metabolic processes are controlled by environmental factors, acetylation is under genetic control: 45% of the UK population are slow acetylators and the remainder either intermediate or fast acetylators. Approximately 10% of the British population have a reduced ability to hydroxylate several drugs (e.g. debrisoquine, nortriptyline and phenformin), which may lead to an increased risk of adverse reactions to drugs metabolised by this route.

Excretion

The vast majority of drugs must first be metabolised to more water-soluble compounds before they can be excreted in the urine. Those drugs (e.g. cimetidine, digoxin, aminoglycosides, lithium, cephalosporins, penicillins, atenolol and chlorpropamide) which are largely excreted unchanged, tend to be relatively water-soluble drugs which are not appreciably bound to plasma proteins and can therefore enter the glomerular filtrate. Lipid soluble drugs may also enter the glomerular filtrate, provided they are not extensively plasma protein bound, but they then readily pass back through the proximal tubular cells into the bloodstream by passive diffusion down a concentration gradient. Only when they have been metabolised to more water-soluble compounds will they have difficulty in passing back through the renal tubular cells and therefore be excreted in the urine. Weak electrolytes can also be actively secreted in the proximal renal tubules – weak bases sharing one mechanism and weak acids another – and there is some evidence for an active transport system promoting the excretion of digoxin in the distal renal tubule.

Drugs may also be excreted in the bile, normally as conjugates and particularly if they have a high molecular weight. The drug may, however, be reabsorbed from the intestine, either directly or after deconjugation by intestinal microflora, to create an enterohepatic cycle. This may reduce the clearance of the drug and thus prolong its effect.

CAUSES OF PHARMACODYNAMIC VARIABILITY

Altered sensitivity to a particular drug concentration at its effector site (pharmacodynamic variability) may occur in several situations. The very young and elderly appear to have an increased sensitivity to several drugs, particularly those affecting the central nervous system. An increased sensitivity to drugs acting on the central nervous system is also seen in patients with chronic renal and liver disease. The elderly appear also to have less adaptable homeostatic mechanisms and are therefore more prone to drug-induced postural hypotension or hypothermia. Hyperthyroid patients are more sensitive to the effects of digoxin and oral anticoagulants.

Information in this field is limited because of difficulties in accurately measuring drug effects, but great care should be exercised in prescription of drugs to the very young, the very old, and patients with chronic renal or liver disease.

CAUSES OF PHARMACOKINETIC VARIABILITY

Absorption

Drug absorption is normally so efficient that it is rare to see differences in the extent of absorption of most modern drugs, even in the presence of extensive bowel resection. Reduction in absorption may, however, occur in severe malabsorption syndromes or in severe diarrhoea, and differences in bowel motility may affect the rate (although not the extent) of absorption. Gastric emptying is slow and erratic in the very young and in adults who are shocked or in pain. In such circumstances (e.g. myocardial infarction) threshold concentrations for drug effect may not be achieved rapidly, or at all, and the drug may have to be given by an alternative, non-alimentary route.

Distribution

Drug distribution may be altered by changes in regional blood flow in disease: the volume of distribution of lignocaine, for example, appears to be lower in patients with cardiac failure. Protein binding also determines drug distribution. Albumin concentrations are low in the neonate, begin to decline over the age of 40, and are reduced during pregnancy. Severe hypoalbuminaemia also occurs in nephrotic syndrome (Fig. 2.4) and chronic liver disease. In patients with chronic renal failure, the proportion of drug in the free form is greater than would be expected from the reduction in serum albumin alone, indicating either structural changes in albumin or the presence of endogenous inhibitors of binding.

AAG is reduced in neonates and in pregnancy, but tends to be normal in healthy elderly individuals. It is markedly increased in patients with rheumatoid arthritis and other inflammatory diseases, including chronic renal disease, after myocardial infarction, and in cancer. As with albumin, it may be reduced in patients with nephrotic syndrome or chronic liver disease. Concomitant changes in plasma protein binding also occur – the effects depending on the relative strength of binding of the drug to these proteins and on the disease state in question (Fig. 2.5) – which may alter the amount bound to free drug. Thus, the total plasma concentration of drug (free + bound), which is generally used as an index of drug concentration, may not always reflect the free (presumably active) concentration. Therapeutic ranges for total drug may therefore need to be altered in diseases where plasma protein binding is affected.

Metabolism

Drug metabolism may be diminished at the extremes of age. Neonates have a reduced capacity for phase I and most phase II reactions: impaired glucuronidation of chloramphenicol, for example, may lead to grey baby syndrome in the neonate. In the elderly, impairment of drug metabolism is only slight and tends to be overshadowed by changes in pharmacodynamic response. Dietary and environmental factors, such as smoking, may affect the rate of drug metabolism; and chronic liver disease may be associated with an impairment of metabolism, particularly of phase I pathways. In liver disease, the serum albumin concentration correlates roughly with the

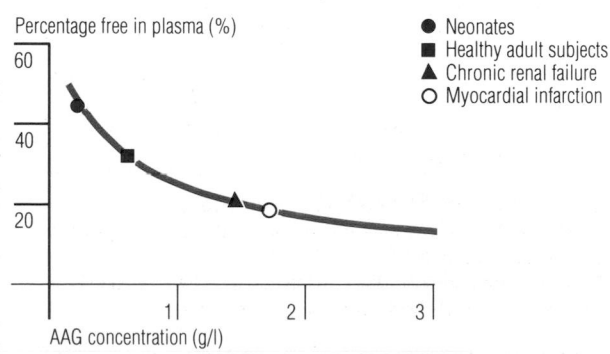

Figure 2.5 **Relationship between the percentage of lignocaine free in plasma and plasma AAG concentration in several disease states and in neonates.**

degree of impairment of drug metabolism (i.e. the lower the albumin the more severe the impairment). The effect of impairment of metabolism in liver disease will be greater for those drugs with extensive presystemic metabolism. The bioavailability of propranolol is much greater in patients with chronic liver disease not because of better absorption (absorption is virtually complete in health) but because it cannot be efficiently metabolised on its first passage through the liver.

The metabolism of high clearance drugs given intravenously is dependent on delivery of the drug to the liver. Thus, because liver blood flow falls in heart failure and shock, the clearance of lignocaine, propranolol and several other high clearance drugs is impaired. Hepatic cirrhosis has a similar effect, due in part to a reduction in the liver's intrinsic metabolic capacity, but also because of intra- and extrahepatic shunting of blood past the liver cells and a consequent reduction in effective liver blood flow.

Excretion

Neonates have a reduced glomerular filtration rate (GFR) relative to their body surface area, and their active tubular secretory mechanisms are also not fully developed. These processes mature relatively rapidly and are fully functional after 6–12 months, but GFR begins to fall again over the age of 40 (the renal tubular secretory mechanisms appear to be less affected by age). Thus, the dose of digoxin or gentamicin (drugs excreted predominantly by glomerular filtration) may need to be reduced in the elderly or very young. Renal disease is associated predominantly with a fall in GFR, with active renal tubular secretion mechanisms less affected. Measurement of serum creatinine or creatinine clearance is therefore useful in calculating the optimum dose of drugs excreted predominantly by glomerular filtration, but it is of less value for drugs such as penicillins, which are actively secreted at the proximal renal tubule.

Summary 3 Causes of pharmacokinetic variability	
Absorption:	Extent of absorption rarely affected Bowel motility may affect rate
Distribution:	Alteration of regional blood flow in disease Altered protein binding, e.g. hypoalbuminaemia in nephrotic syndrome
Metabolism:	Diminished in neonates and the elderly Dietary and environmental factors, e.g. smoking Liver disease
Excretion:	Immature renal function in neonates Impaired in renal disease

ADVERSE REACTIONS

It has been estimated that approximately 5% of all hospital admissions are due to adverse reactions to a drug; 1 in 10 patients admitted for other reasons will develop an adverse reaction to a drug while in hospital; and perhaps 1 in 1000 deaths in hospital are due to an adverse reaction to a drug. Adverse reactions are equally common in general practice. The drug groups most commonly associated with adverse reactions are antihypertensive drugs, anticoagulants, antirheumatic drugs (particularly the non-steroidal anti-inflammatory drugs), cytotoxic drugs, corticosteroids and digoxin.

Although adverse reactions can affect all systems of the body, they are most often described in the skin and central nervous system (where detection tends to be easier). The very young (i.e. under 1 year of age) and the elderly are particularly at risk; and women appear to be at greater risk than men, although the reason for this is unknown. Patients with a history of allergy, or who have had a drug reaction in the past, are more likely to develop further reactions, even to a drug in some other therapeutic group. The presence of disease, particularly heart failure, or liver or renal disease predisposes to a risk of adverse reactions, as may genetic factors, such as enzyme deficiencies.

Types of adverse drug reaction

Adverse reactions have been classified into two major types.

Type A

The most common type is the *dose-dependent adverse reaction (type A)* which is an 'Augmentation' or 'Accentuation' of a known pharmacological effect of the drug – not necessarily always the wanted effect. Thus, beta sympathomimetic agents can cause increased tremor, a recognised pharmacological effect of the drug, but one which may limit its use in bronchodilator therapy. Type A reactions account for about 75% of all adverse reactions and, because they are often insidious in onset, may go unrecognised for some time. They may thus produce considerable morbidity but the mortality from type A reactions is generally low. They may occur because of altered pharmacokinetic or pharmacodynamic factors and are therefore commonest in those diseases (e.g. renal and liver disease) where these are affected.

Type B

Type B reactions are not dependent on the dose given, but are unpredictable or 'Bizarre' reactions to a drug, which may be present only in tiny concentrations. Because of their lack of predictability and their often acute onset, they have a higher mortality than type A reactions; but the morbidity is relatively low if the patient survives the initial event. Like type A reactions, type B reactions can be related to pharmacokinetic or pharmacodynamic factors. There are many ingredients in medications other than the active compound and reactions may occur to the preservative, filler, dye, binder or solubilising agent in the tablet or injection. Type B reactions may occur because individual subjects metabolise the drug through a novel pathway which produces a toxic metabolite. In other cases, the presence of hereditary enzyme deficiencies may predispose the patient to the toxic effects of drugs or their metabolites. Thus, haemolysis caused by dapsone and other oxidising agents is commoner in patients with glucose-6-phosphate dehydrogenase (G6PD) deficiency. Similarly, many agents can precipitate an attack of acute intermittent porphyria (p. 781) in those carrying a gene for this disorder.

Type B reactions are also often related to allergic mechanisms, and may involve any or all forms of antibody-mediated or cell-mediated tissue damage. Thus, anaphylaxis may occur due to immediate (type I) hypersensitivity associated with cell-bound IgE, after administration of drugs such as penicillin. Cell surface (type II hypersensitivity) damage may occur as a result of the combination of methyldopa with red cell membranes and subsequent haemolysis. Toxic immune complexes may be formed in patients receiving gold or penicillamine, with subsequent renal or skin toxicity by a type III hypersensitivity mechanism. Cell-mediated (type IV) tissue damage is thought to be the mechanism of the relatively common (but usually mild) rash associated with ampicillin therapy, or the more serious erythroderma sometimes associated with drugs such as gold.

Diagnosis and management of adverse reactions

Diagnosis

It is rarely possible to make a diagnosis of drug-induced adverse reaction with complete certainty. Erythema multiforme, for example, may be caused by either an infective agent or the antibiotic with which the patient was being treated. It is therefore necessary to weigh up all circumstantial evidence carefully before making the diagnosis. This includes taking a *full drug history*, remembering that patients may not consider over-the-counter remedies, or even the oral contraceptive pill, as medicines or drugs. The brand names of the agents may also be important, since different pharmaceutical formulations may contain different dyes, binders, fillers, preservatives or lubricants, and reactions may occur for only some formulations.

Physical examination provides only limited information. Some physical signs may be directly attributable to drug therapy, e.g. blue discolouration of the skin associated with amiodarone therapy is rarely caused by disease. Similarly, an eruption occurring at a fixed site on the skin may suggest a drug-induced fixed drug eruption. But in most cases, the organs affected have a limited number of responses to noxious stimuli. *Biochemical tests* are also of limited value, but measurement of plasma drug concentration may help to confirm the suspicion of a dose-dependent (type A) adverse reaction. In some cases, measurement of metabolic phenotype may also be of help. It is extremely rare, for example, for patients who are fast acetylators to develop drug-induced lupus erythematosus after hydralazine therapy.

Probably the most helpful indication of the drug responsible for the adverse reaction is the *time course* relative to drug treatment, particularly the rate of resolution of symptoms on stopping a specific drug. Subsequent re-exposure associated with a recurrence of the symptoms or signs gives the strongest evidence of causation; but it is rarely ethically justifiable to rechallenge the patient, unless the patient's need for the drug outweighs the potential risk of the adverse reaction.

Management

The only choice with most type B reactions is to stop the suspected drug completely. With type A reactions, it is sometimes possible to reduce the dose to prevent the unwanted effects whilst still obtaining therapeutic benefit. If an adverse reaction does occur, the patient's medical notes and prescription chart should be clearly marked with an eye-catching label to indicate the nature and date of the reaction. Any serious adverse reaction should also be reported to the Committee on Safety of Medicines using a 'yellow card' (p. 34). In addition, even minor adverse reactions to drugs which have been recently introduced (marked with an inverted black triangle in the British National Formulary) should be reported.

Prevention of adverse reactions

It must be remembered that although drugs provide enormous benefit to patients, all are potentially toxic and should be used selectively, particularly in patients at greatest risk of adverse reactions, i.e. the very young, very old and those with severe disease. The risk of developing an adverse reaction appears to increase disproportionately with increasing number of drugs prescribed concomitantly. Prescriptions should therefore be reviewed and drug therapy rationalised at frequent intervals. When a drug is prescribed, the prescription should be written legibly, in block letters, and preferably using the approved name. Failure to do so may lead to errors in prescribing. In some cases, the risk of adverse reactions to certain drugs is such that they should be avoided if at all possible. There are particular dangers during pregnancy or breast-feeding, when certain drugs may cause an adverse reaction in the fetus or breast-fed child (Table 2.2).

DRUG INTERACTIONS

Drug interactions have been recognised for over 100 years and are described under the classical headings of antagonism, synergism or potentiation. Many of these interactions are beneficial and have been used to therapeutic advantage; but unwanted or adverse interactions also account for 10–20% of all adverse reactions to drugs. Those of clinical importance (the actual number of interactions may be much larger than this) usually

Table 2.2 Drugs to avoid during pregnancy or breast-feeding

	Pregnancy	Breast-feeding
Antibiotics	Tetracyclines Sulphonamides Aminoglycosides Trimethoprim	Tetracyclines Sulphonamides Isoniazid Chloramphenicol
Antithyroids	All, including radioiodine	All, including radioiodine
Analgesics	Opiates NSAIDs	Opiates
Anticoagulants	Warfarin	Phenindione
Antineoplastics	Most	Most
Antidiabetics	Hypoglycaemics	Use with caution
Androgens	All, also oestrogens and high dose progestogens	All, also high dose oestrogens and progestogens
Miscellaneous	Vitamin D and its analogues Live vaccines	Lithium Anthraquinone Laxatives and phenolphthalein

occur in drugs with a relatively low margin between safety and toxicity (i.e. a narrow 'therapeutic ratio'). Thus, they are most often described with oral anticoagulants, anticonvulsants, antidepressants or antihypertensive drugs (Table 2.3). As with adverse reactions in general, the risk of developing an adverse interaction increases disproportionately with the number of drugs prescribed concomitantly; the mechanisms of interaction are also similar, in that both pharmacodynamic and pharmacokinetic interactions may occur. Interactions may also take place, however, before the drugs even enter the body, and these have been termed 'pharmaceutical' interactions.

Pharmaceutical interactions

Interactions may occur prior to the drug entering the body when drugs are mixed together for infusion, or when a drug interacts with the infusion material itself. Guides to intravenous mixture are available, and should be consulted before compounds are given by intravenous infusion or mixed together. In general terms, it is advisable to avoid adding drugs to infusion fluids unless absolutely necessary and certainly to avoid adding more than one drug if at all possible. Infusion fluids particularly likely to be associated with pharmaceutical incompatibilities include blood and blood products, amino acids and lipid solutions, mannitol and sodium bicarbonate.

Pharmacodynamic interactions

Pharmacodynamic interaction occurs where one drug alters the response to another by interacting either at the receptor site or at a different site to enhance or diminish the primary drug effect (Table 2.1).

Partial agonists initiate a minor response but, by occupying a significant fraction of the receptors, they antagonise the action of more potent agonists. Nalorphine, for example, is a partial antagonist but may add to the respiratory depression produced by opiates; whereas naloxone, while having no efficacy itself, antagonises the pharmacological effects of most opiates. Many pharmacodynamic interactions occur when the physician forgets that a drug known to be acting at one receptor may also act at another. Thus, antihistamines, phenothiazines and tricyclic antidepressants may have muscarinic anticholinergic activity in addition to their desired pharmacological effects; and administration of two or more of these agents – particularly in the elderly – may lead to pronounced anticholinergic symptoms and signs.

Pharmacodynamic interaction may also occur when two drugs act at different sites, e.g. the interaction of digoxin and diuretics. Here, hypokalaemia caused by

Table 2.3 Some drug interactions of clinical importance

Drug (A)	May interact with (B)	Effect of interaction	Mechanism
Warfarin	Cholestyramine Colestipol	Reduced anticoagulant effect of A	Impaired absorption and increased elimination of A. Long-term R may cause impaired vit K absorption and enhance anticoagulant effect
	Barbiturates Carbamazepine Primidone Rifampicin	Reduced anticoagulant effect of A	Induction of metabolism of A
	Cimetidine Sulphonamides Erythromycin Metronidazole Mefenamic acid Azapropazone Phenylbutazone Amiodarone Fluconazole Ketoconazole Sulphinpyrazone Chloramphenicol Ciprofloxacin	Increased anticoagulant effect of A	Inhibition of metabolism of A
	Salicylates Clofibrate Bezafibrate Gemfibrozil D Thyroxine L Thyroxine Stanozolol Danazol	Increased anticoagulant effect of A	Pharmacodynamic potentiation of anticoagulant effect
	Oral contraceptives Vitamin K	Reduced anticoagulant effect of A	Pharmacodynamic antagonism of anticoagulant effect

diuretic-induced reduction of potassium reabsorption in the kidney may potentiate the effects of digoxin on the heart.

Pharmacokinetic interactions

Absorption

Drugs may interact with each other to prevent either the rate or the extent of absorption of another compound. Drugs which increase gastric emptying (e.g. metoclopramide) will increase the rate of absorption of many drugs, so that the peak concentration of that drug will tend to be higher. The opposite effect is achieved by agents, such as the anticholinergic compound propatheline, which diminish gastric emptying. These changes are likely to be more important after single dose administration in a situation where threshold concentration for drug effect exists, e.g. for analgesics. Under these circumstances (particularly if the rate of elimination of the drug is high), a delay in absorption may result in an inability to reach therapeutic drug concentrations.

The extent of absorption of the drug may be impaired by the presence of another through the formation of chelates, ion pairs or complexes. Ion exchange resins such as cholestyramine and colestipol combine with warfarin, thyroxine and digitalis glycosides to impair absorption. Similarly, the calcium, magnesium or aluminium ions in antacids or milk may interact with tetracycline. In most cases, these interactions can be prevented by ensuring a time interval of at least 2 hours between administration of the two compounds. In the case of warfarin and digitoxin, however, cholestyramine or colestipol may also affect enterohepatic recirculation and reduce concentrations of these drugs, even if they are administered after absorption has been completed.

Table 2.3 Some drug interactions of clinical importance (cont.)

Drug (A)	May interact with (B)	Effect of interaction	Mechanism
Phenytoin	Amiodarone Isoniazid Cimetidine Chloramphenicol Fluconazole Sulphonamides	Increased effect or toxicity of A	Inhibition of metabolism of A
	Carbamazepine	Reduced effect of A	Induction of metabolism of A
Carbamazepine	Cimetidine Fluoxetine Isoniazid Verapamil Erythromycin	Increased effect or toxicity of A	Inhibition of metabolism of A
Oral contraceptives	Barbiturates Phenytoin Carbamazepine Primidone Rifampicin	Reduced effect of A	Induction of metabolism of A
	Antibiotics (broad-spectrum)		? Interruption of enterohepatic recycling of A
Theophylline	Cimetidine Ciprofloxacin Erythromycin	Increased effect of A	Inhibition of metabolism of A
Digoxin	Amiodarone Quinidine Verapamil	Increased effect of A	? Reduced renal excretion
	Potassium-losing diuretics	Increased effect of A	Pharmacodynamic potentiation by hypokalaemia induced by B
Beta-blockers	Cimetidine	Increased effect of A	Inhibition of metabolism of A
	Verapamil	Increased effect of A	Pharmacodynamic potentiation
	NSAIDs	Reduced hypotensive effect of A	Unclear, ? sodium retention
Angiotensin converting enzyme (ACE) inhibitors	NSAIDs	Reduced hypotensive effect of A	Unclear, ? sodium retention
	Potassium-sparing diuretics	Hyperkalaemia	Additive effects of A and B
Diuretics	NSAIDs	Reduced diuretic effect of A	Unclear
Lithium carbonate	Thiazide diuretics	Increased effect of A	Increased renal tubular absorption of A
Azathioprine Mercaptopurine	Allopurinol	Increased effect of A	Inhibition of metabolism of A
Methotrexate	Aspirin NSAIDs	Increased effect of A	Inhibition of renal tubular secretion of A
Cyclosporin	Erythromycin Ketoconazole	Increased effect of A	? Inhibition of metabolism of A
	Barbiturates Phenytoin Rifampicin	Reduced effect of A	Induction of metabolism of A

Distribution

Drugs may compete for both plasma protein binding sites and active transport processes in the body. The importance of plasma protein binding displacement interactions has been much exaggerated. For most drugs, only the drug free in plasma is available for metabolism. Thus, an increase in the percentage of free drug will result in a concomitant increase in total clearance and the rapid return of the free (biologically active) drug concentration to its original value. (The net result is a lower total drug concentration, but a larger percentage of this is in the free form.) The temporary increase in free drug concentration is only likely to be important if the drug is normally highly protein bound (e.g. >90%) and has a low apparent volume of distribution. If the displacing agent is given by a rapid intravenous injection, the temporary increase in free drug concentration of the displaced agent may also be important, but clinically significant examples of this interaction are difficult to find. At present, whenever significant clinical interactions have been shown to be associated with protein binding displacement, other mechanisms (e.g. competition for metabolism) have been shown to be the major causes of the interaction. It is therefore possible that plasma protein binding displacement merely reflects the physicochemical similarities of the two compounds, which leads to their competing for transport or metabolic processes.

Inhibition of active transport of one drug by another can result in significant interactions. The adrenergic neurone blocking drugs guanethidine, bethanidine and debrisoquine are all substrates for the amine pump, which normally takes up noradrenaline into the adrenergic nerve endings. Drugs which inhibit this process (e.g. tricyclic antidepressants and chlorpromazine) may antagonise the antihypertensive effect of these drugs. Blocking of the amine pump may also potentiate the pressor effect of directly acting sympathomimetics such as noradrenaline or phenylephrine.

Metabolism

Metabolism of drugs by the hepatic mono-oxygenase system can be stimulated by compounds in cigarette smoke and a variety of other drugs (Table 2.4). Enzyme induction is related to an increase in the amount of cytochromes present, and may therefore take 7–14 days to develop fully, and a similar lag period to wear off after

Table 2.4 Some drugs causing induction of drug metabolism

• Barbiturates and primidone	• Dichloralphenazone
• Carbamazepine	• Phenytoin
• Cigarette smoking	• Rifampicin

Table 2.5 Some drugs causing inhibition of drug metabolism

• Allopurinol	• Isoniazid
• Amiodarone	• Ketoconazole/fluconazole
• Cimetidine	• Metronidazole
• Ciprofloxacin and some other quinolones	• Monoamine oxidase inhibitors
• Erythromycin	• Sulphonamides

the inducing agent is discontinued. This time lag tends to disguise any causal relationship between the drug interaction and administration of the inducing agent. Furthermore, if the dose of the active drug has been increased to maintain adequate effects, marked increases in drug concentration and toxic effects may be seen when induction wears off.

Other agents can impair the metabolism of concomitantly administered drugs, either by competing for metabolism or in a non-competitive manner (Table 2.5). Cimetidine is an interesting example in that although not itself metabolised (it is largely excreted unchanged in the urine), it inhibits the metabolism of drugs by the liver. Since the effect of enzyme inhibitors is generally direct, the lag time for this effect to occur is shorter than with enzyme inducers, and the effects disappear more quickly after discontinuation. Allopurinol has little effect on drugs metabolised by the mono-oxygenase pathway but, by inhibiting xanthine oxidase, can impair the metabolism of azathioprine and 6-mercaptopurine and potentiate their toxicity.

Excretion

It is unlikely that drug-induced changes in GFR will markedly alter the excretion of other drugs by the kidney. However, drugs which alter urinary pH may have a marked effect on the renal clearance of weak bases or acids, because of the effects on passive reabsorption in the proximal tubule. The administration of bicarbonate, for example, may enhance the removal of weak acids (such as phenobarbitone and aspirin) by increasing the proportion of drug in the ionised form in the urine, thus preventing passive reabsorption. Similarly, acidification of the urine (using ammonium chloride) reduces tubular reabsorption of weak bases such as amphetamine – an effect which has been used in overdose to enhance renal excretion.

Acidic drugs may compete with each other for the active renal tubular secretory pathway – salicylates and thiazides may potentiate the toxicity of methotrexate in this way. No clinically important interactions involving basic drugs at this site have been reported. Quinidine and verapamil may compete with digoxin for an active tubular secretory mechanism in the distal convoluted tubule. This may result in digoxin toxicity, although quinidine also displaces digoxin from binding sites in tissues and this could also contribute to the interaction.

THERAPEUTIC DRUG MONITORING

Therapeutic drug monitoring refers to the measurement of drug concentrations in plasma to aid in optimising drug efficacy and reducing the risk of toxicity.

The ideal way to monitor drug therapy is, of course, to measure wanted and unwanted effects directly; where good measures of these exist (e.g. in anticoagulant therapy) measurement of plasma drug concentrations has a very limited role. There are, however, situations in which drug efficacy or toxicity are more difficult to measure, and both here, and where the drug is being given prophylactically to prevent serious events (e.g. antiepileptic and antiarrhythmic drugs), therapeutic drug monitoring may have a role to play (Table 2.6). Measurement of plasma (or urine) drug concentration is also of value in detecting overdose (either deliberate or accidental) and in monitoring compliance with therapy in patients who may not be responding normally to the drug.

For therapeutic drug monitoring to be of value in optimising therapeutic benefit, the drug should work by a reversible mechanism without development of tolerance to the therapeutic effect. The possibility of accumulation of active metabolites which are not detected by the drug assay must also be considered. Procainamide, for example, is metabolised to N-acetylprocainamide which also has antiarrhythmic activity, and should also therefore be measured.

Sample collection

Unlike many endogenous compounds, such as creatinine, which are produced at a continuous rate, drugs are normally administered at fixed intervals and the plasma concentration will therefore vary markedly with time after administration. Early after administration, the plasma concentration may be affected by the rate of gastric emptying. However, if there is extensive distribution of the drug, early samples may be higher than the average, or steady state, drug concentration during the dosage interval, and may not accurately reflect the concentration at the site of action of the drug. It is therefore preferable to wait at least 8 hours after administration of an oral dose of digoxin, or 12 hours after lithium, before sampling. If peak levels are important, samples should be taken 2–3 hours after a conventional tablet or later if a sustained-release formulation has been administered; or 30–60 minutes after intramuscular injection. In most cases, however, a trough concentration taken just before the next dose will correlate most closely with the steady state drug concentration.

Since it takes approximately five half-lives before steady state is achieved, sampling before this time will tend to underestimate the subsequent steady state concentration and is only indicated if toxicity due to accumulation of the drug is possible. Details of sampling time, change in dose, and last administration of the dose should always be given on the assay request form to enable the plasma concentration to be interpreted correctly.

Total drug concentrations are normally measured and these generally mirror the free plasma concentration. This may not be true in diseases where changes in plasma protein binding of drugs are likely, such as hepatic and renal disease. For some drugs (e.g. phenytoin and theophylline), the saliva drug concentration may be a closer reflection of the free plasma drug concentration; and in young children, saliva collection (stimulated by a drop of citric acid solution on the tongue) may avoid venepuncture.

SPECIFIC DRUGS

Anticonvulsants

Phenytoin metabolism shows saturation rather than first order kinetics, so that clearance falls with increasing dose

Table 2.6 Drug concentrations associated with optimal efficacy in most patients

	Usual half-life (hours)	Usual therapeutic plasma concentrations	Toxic concentration	Principal route of elimination
Digoxin	30–40	1–2 µg/l	>2 µg/l	Renal excretion
Gentamicin	2	Trough <2 mg/l Peak 4–8 mg/l	Trough >2 mg/l Peak >12 mg/l	Renal excretion
Lithium	7–20	0.6–1.4 mmol/l	>1.5 nmol/l	Renal excretion
Phenytoin	20–60	Plasma 10–20 mg/l Saliva 1–2 mg/l	>20 mg/l >2 mg/l	Hepatic metabolism
Theophylline	4–16	Plasma 10–20 mg/l Saliva 6–12 mg/l	>20 mg/l >12 mg/l	Hepatic metabolism

and the risk of toxicity increases. Half-life also increases with increasing dose and so it will take longer for steady state to be achieved. Most patients tend to be given too small a dose of phenytoin, but therapeutic drug monitoring has reduced the tendency to prescribe a second antiepileptic drug in many patients who initially received sub-therapeutic doses. Therapeutic monitoring of other anticonvulsants is of limited value except in the identification of poor compliance.

Antiarrhythmics

Because of their serious toxicity and the narrow margin between therapeutic and toxic doses, monitoring of several antiarrhythmic drugs may help to reduce adverse effects and improve response. The half-life of most antiarrhythmics is short but that of amiodarone is around 30–45 days. A loading dose is therefore necessary to achieve early therapeutic concentrations of this drug, and prolonged monitoring will help to detect accumulation of amiodarone and its major (and possibly toxic) metabolite, desethylamiodarone.

Digoxin

The plasma digoxin concentration is one of the determinants of toxicity of the drug, particularly the non-cardiovascular toxicity, causing lassitude, depression and anorexia. Monitoring is particularly important in patients with reduced renal function (e.g. in the elderly) and will also help to identify poor compliance.

Theophylline

Patients vary greatly in metabolic clearance of this potentially toxic bronchodilator, and adjustment of dose is facilitated by measurement of plasma theophylline concentrations.

Antibiotics

The aminoglycosides are the most frequently monitored antibiotics. The risk of ototoxicity can be reduced by preventing excessive plasma drug concentrations, but the nephrotoxic effects of the drug are less closely related to the plasma concentration, so that renal function must also be carefully monitored during therapy.

Lithium

Lithium is used in the treatment of hypomania, and because toxicity may occur insidiously (p. 45), therapeutic monitoring is essential.

DRUG REGULATION AND DEVELOPMENT

The importance of drug regulation has grown with the rapid increase in the number of therapeutic agents developed over the last 50 years. Increased efficacy of new compounds is often associated with a risk of serious adverse effects.

The United Kingdom Medicines Act (1968)

In the late 1950s, thalidomide was introduced as a new hypnotic drug and was widely used in Europe in all types of patient, including pregnant women. In 1961 an epidemic of appalling proportions occurred in which hundreds of the babies were born with limb abnormalities (phocomelia). The connection with thalidomide administration was soon realised and the drug was hastily withdrawn. The nature of this adverse reaction and the public pressure which it provoked resulted in the formation, in the UK, of the Committee on Safety of Drugs (the Dunlop Committee) in 1965, and the consequent development of strict legislation concerning all aspects of drug manufacture, testing and selling. This legislation is contained in the United Kingdom Medicines Act (1968). Most countries have comparable systems of vetting and approval.

Licensing authority

The United Kingdom Medicines Act is administered by the Medicines Control Agency (MCA). Together with the Health Ministers, the Medicines Division acts as the *Licensing Authority*. If a pharmaceutical company wishes to market a new product, it requires a *Product Licence*, and this is given only if the Licensing Authority is satisfied of its safety, quality and efficacy. It is illegal for a medicinal product to be sold without a product licence.

A number of advisory committees exist to ensure the Licensing Authority performs its duties properly. The Medicines Commission, established immediately the Medicines Act came into force, was charged by Section 4 of the Act to set up five committees, usually referred to as *Section 4 Committees*. The Committee on Safety of Medicines (CSM), which replaced the Dunlop Committee, is now the best known of these. It reviews all applications for Clinical Trials Certificates (p. 34) and Product Licences for new products (i.e. a new drug or new formulation). Its most publicised activity, however, is in reviewing adverse drug reactions, and it has in recent years often been criticised over decisions to withdraw the Product Licence of a number of drugs.

When the Medicines Act was introduced, a *Product Licence of Right* was given to every product already on the market, as it would have been impossible to review all

36 000 of them simultaneously. The Committee on Review of Medicines (CRM) had the less than exciting task of reviewing all these products, a task completed in 1990. As a result of its activities, many products have been taken off the market, while those which remain have been given a full Product Licence.

The main task of the British Pharmacopoeia Commission is to maintain the *British Pharmacopoeia*, or list of approved drugs. Only drugs listed here can be sold as generic products and have the abbreviation BP in parentheses after their name.

Four sub-committees were also established to provide expert advice to the Section 4 Committees. One of these, the Safety, Efficacy and Adverse Reactions Sub-committee (SEAR) is concerned with the collection and evaluation of information on adverse reactions through the Yellow Card system (see below).

Developing new drugs

Virtually all new drugs are developed within the pharmaceutical industry because of the enormous financial investment (about £50 million for a new product in 1985), and considerable amount of work involved. Because a patent taken out on a new compound lasts for only 17 years, the 10–12 years (or longer) required for most drugs to reach the stage of a Product Licence erodes the patent life alarmingly. The industry therefore has to look very carefully at the likely returns on its investment over the short period that it alone can market the drug under patent. Developing drugs for less common diseases becomes commercially unattractive under these circumstances.

Apart from the basic chemistry and pharmacology required to develop a new drug, a large amount of toxicological data from animal testing is also required from the pharmaceutical company to satisfy the CSM that the drug is unlikely to cause serious adverse

---

Summary 5 Drug development

Synthesis/isolation of new substance

Animal studies
Pharmacological/toxicological studies

Clinical trials

Phase 1	Pharmacological tests in healthy volunteers (20–50)
Phase 2	Tested in patients (50–300). Collection of data on efficacy and safety
Phase 3	Formal, larger-scale trials (250–1000 or more). Efficacy, safety and comparison with other drugs in same therapeutic class
Phase 4	Postmarketing studies on a much larger population of patients (2000–10 000 or more)

---

reactions in man. If it is so satisfied, the Committee will grant a Clinical Trials Exemption (CTX) or Clinical Trials Certificate (CTC), both of which allow the drug to be tested in patients. In the UK, a CTX or CTC is not required for studies in healthy volunteers, however, and thus it is normal for initial tolerance and pharmacokinetic data to be available before an application is made to the CSM.

Clinical trials are usually divided into four phases. In phase 1, healthy volunteer studies are performed. If the results are satisfactory, a small number of patients are given the drug to discover whether the pharmacological effect shown in animals also occurs in man (phase 2). In the third phase, formal and larger-scale clinical trials are performed, in order to confirm the drug's therapeutic benefit, evaluate its adverse effects and compare it with existing drugs in the same therapeutic class. At this point, assuming that the results are satisfactory, an application will be made for a Product Licence so that marketing and promotion of the drug can begin. Postmarketing studies (phase 4) examine its effect on a much larger population of patients.

Monitoring adverse reactions

Following the thalidomide tragedy, the Government set up a voluntary system for reporting suspected adverse reactions (better called *adverse events*, as a cause–effect reactionship has yet to be established at this stage). This is known as the Yellow Card system (because of the colour of the cards used for the reports). Initially, the system was monitored by the Dunlop Committee, but is now the responsibility of the CSM and SEAR sub-committee. If a doctor or dentist sees an unusual or serious reaction to an old drug, or any suspected reaction to a new one (new drugs are marked with an inverted triangle in the British National Formulary (BNF)), he or she is encouraged to fill in a card and send it to the Medicines Division or one of the Regional Monitoring Centres to be assessed by medical assessors. A substantial data bank is thereby accumulated and analysed monthly for associations between adverse events and individual drugs, e.g. venous thrombosis and the contraceptive pill. The main shortcomings of the Yellow Card system are that less than a quarter of registered doctors and dentists use it (the 20 000 reports received in 1991 represent only a small proportion of adverse events occurring), and the lack of case control. The system has therefore seldom identified a new association, but has nevertheless been invaluable in confirming a suspected reaction.

Several other systems of monitoring have been suggested or are under trial and pharmaceutical companies are, in addition, being encouraged (and may in the future be required), to set up a system of postmarketing surveillance. These systems monitor every patient receiving the new drug together with a matched control, and therefore have a much greater power to detect a novel adverse reaction. Nevertheless, large numbers of patients will need to be given a drug before rare adverse reactions can be detected by any system.

Controlling prescribing

While free enterprise leads to a dynamic and healthy pharmaceutical industry, it also leads to the promotion of excessive numbers of similar drugs, as one company vies with another for its share of the lucrative markets. Cephalosporin antibiotics, benzodiazepines and β-adrenoceptor blocking drugs are three such examples. In order to rationalise prescribing, most hospitals and many general practitioners have compiled their own restricted lists. In 1985, however, the Government decided that this voluntary limitation was not happening fast enough and, in order to curb escalating drug costs, introduced the NHS Limited List. At present, this covers mild to moderate pain-killers, indigestion remedies, laxatives, cough and cold remedies, vitamins, tonics and benzodiazepine drugs. An Advisory Committee keeps the list under review and may recommend its extension to other therapeutic classes.

FURTHER READING

Davies D M (ed) 1991 Textbook of adverse drug reactions, 4th edn. Oxford University Press, Oxford. *Reference source for adverse reactions*

Gibaldi M 1991 Biopharmaceutics and clinical pharmacokinetics, 4th edn. Lea and Febiger, Philadelphia. *A clear, relatively non-mathematical introduction to pharmacokinetics*

Hansten P D, Horn J R 1990 Drug interactions and updates, 7th edn. Lea and Febiger, Philadelphia. *A comprehensive reference source for drug interactions*

Speight T M (ed) 1987 Avery's drug treatment, 3rd edn. Churchill Livingstone, Edinburgh. *A large text covering most aspects of clinical pharmacology and drug treatment*

Turner P, Richens A, Routledge P A 1986 Clinical pharmacology, 5th edn. Churchill Livingstone, Edinburgh. *A concise introductory guide to clinical pharmacology*

3

Drug Overdose and Poisoning

Philip A Routledge

DRUG OVERDOSE

Approximately 4000 people die each year of poisoning in England and Wales, a quarter of them of carbon monoxide poisoning. Approximately two-thirds of the remaining deaths occur outside hospital. Nevertheless, more than 100 000 patients are admitted to hospital in England and Wales each year due to poisoning, accounting for 10% of all acute admissions. The unadjusted admission rates in the USA range from 80 per 100 000 in patients aged 65–74 years to 400 per 100 000 in patients aged between 15 and 24 years. Toxic compounds may be ingested or inhaled either accidentally or deliberately or may be administered accidentally or deliberately. This forms the basis for a classification of poisoning incidents separating them into broad epidemiological categories.

The major causes of deaths from poisoning are shown in Figure 3.1.

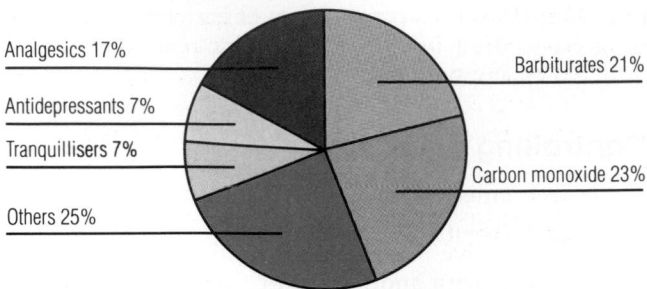

Fig. 3.1 **Agents involved in fatal poisoning episodes.**

Accidental poisoning

Accidental poisoning can occur at any age, but is much more likely to occur in children under 5 years of age (Fig. 3.2). Peak incidence is around 2 years, when children have become independently mobile. Boys appear to be more at risk. This contrasts with other categories of poisoning, in which women are involved more than men. Fortunately, the mortality from accidental poisoning is relatively small. While death from carbon monoxide poisoning predominates, there are approximately 20 accidental deaths per year from other agents, particularly tricyclic antidepressants, aspirin and barbiturates. The incidence of accidental poisoning in childhood is partly determined by availability.

Deliberate self-poisoning

Deliberate self-poisoning is commoner in adults who, unlike children, ingest medicinal agents more readily than they do household chemicals and other non-medicinal

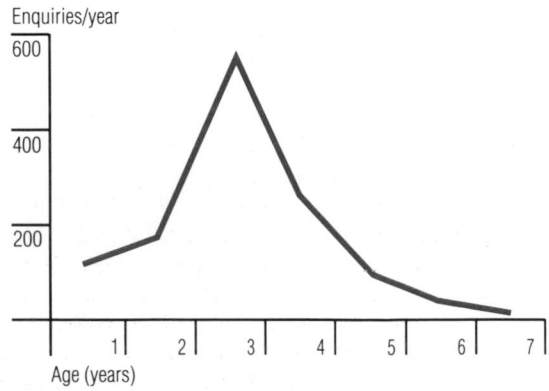

Fig. 3.2 **The relationship between age and the incidence of accidental poisoning in children.** Figures are based on enquiries concerning accidental poisoning made to the Welsh National Poisons Unit in 1984.

compounds. Women are more often involved than men, and the vast majority of instances are not intended to be ultimately fatal. Generally they represent a response to an apparently insoluble personal predicament (Ch. 10), but some have definite suicidal intent. Patients who successfully commit suicide tend to be older and may have been recently divorced or bereaved, may be living alone, suffering from a physical illness, unemployed or abusers of alcohol.

Non-accidental poisoning

Non-accidental poisoning usually involves children and is a form of child abuse. The parents of such children may have suffered child abuse or deprivation themselves, and often have marital or financial problems or difficulties in managing the child at the time of the non-accidental poisoning episode.

Homicidal poisoning

Although often featured in novels and plays, homicidal poisoning is uncommon. When it does happen, it is often caused by a close relative or friend and generally involves the use of poisons producing chronic, rather than acute, symptoms.

DIAGNOSIS OF POISONING

Laboratory tests cannot identify every agent to which an individual might be exposed. A full history and clinical examination is therefore an integral part of the diagnosis.

Since the patient may be unwilling or unable to give a history on presentation, it is important to talk to relatives or friends, to the general practitioner, or to the ambulancemen who brought the patient into hospital. Particular difficulties are encountered with the patient who is found alone and unconscious and in which poisoning is just one of the differential diagnoses.

The first priority in the unconscious patient is maintenance of the airway, ventilation and cardiovascular function. When this has been ensured, the question arises as to whether the patient is poisoned. Other causes of unconsciousness are discussed in Chapter 22. In deep coma due to drug overdose, the pupillary reflexes are often preserved, whilst the oculovestibular responses (e.g. 'doll's eye response') are absent. Focal neurological signs are rare in overdose and, unless they can be accounted for by previous pathology, these should alert the clinician to the possibility of another cause. Papilloedema due to drug overdose is rare, unless the overdose has been associated with cerebral hypoxia and oedema.

If the patient shows no improvement in consciousness level by 12 hours after admission, some other pathology should be suspected.

Clinical examination

It is sometimes possible to identify the poison by the clinical signs on examination, although it may be more difficult if the patient has taken several agents. The most helpful clinical signs which implicate particular toxins are shown in Tables 3.1A and B (p. 38).

Eyes

Pupillary dilatation occurs in poisoning with anticholinergic drugs such as the tricyclic antidepressants, anti-Parkinsonian agents, antihistamines and phenothiazines. It also occurs with agents that stimulate the sympathetic nervous system such as amphetamines, LSD and theophyllines. Unequal pupils are occasionally seen in poisoning. Strabismus is not uncommon, particularly in carbamazepine poisoning. Papilloedema, however, is rare, except as a result of methanol, carbon monoxide or glutethimide poisoning. Nystagmus may be caused by agents affecting the central nervous system (CNS), particularly phenytoin.

Mouth

Acneiform lesions around the buccal cavity may suggest solvent abuse, and the characteristic odour of solvent or alcohol may be present on the breath. Examination of the

Table 3.1A Physical signs suggestive of overdose or poisoning: head and neck

Sign	Possible cause
Dilated pupils	Tricyclic antidepressants Anticholinergics Sympathomimetics
Strabismus	Carbamazepine
Nystagmus	Phenytoin Carbamazepine
Papilloedema	Methanol Carbon monoxide Glutethimide
Perforated nasal septum	Cocaine abuse
Acneiform rash	Solvent abuse
Erythema/burns	Corrosives
Mouth dryness	Anticholinergics
Hypersalivation	Parasympathomimetics

3 Drug Overdose and Poisoning

Table 3.1B Physical signs suggestive of overdose or poisoning: trunk and limbs

Sign	Possible cause
Bronchospasm	Irritant gases NSAIDs
Pulmonary oedema	Irritant gases Opiates Aspirin
Tachycardia	Anticholinergics Sympathomimetics
Bradycardia	Beta-blockers Verapamil Digoxin
Hypotension	Many agents
Hypertension	Clonidine MAOIs
Needle tracks	Drugs of addiction
Absent bowel sounds	Anticholinergics
Bladder distension	Anticholinergics
Hypothermia	Phenothiazines
Hyperthermia	Salicylates Anticholinergics Sympathomimetics MAOIs
Hyperreflexia	Anticholinergics Sympathomimetics Opiates
Blisters	Barbiturates Carbon monoxide Occasionally other hypnotics
Extensor plantar response	Anticholinergics

oral cavity may reveal ulceration due to corrosion by acids or alkalis. The mouth may be abnormally dry because of anticholinergic compounds, and increased salivation may be seen in subjects who have taken agents which stimulate the parasympathetic nervous system, e.g. carbamate insecticides and anticholinesterases.

Cardiorespiratory

Chest wheeze may be caused by inhalation of irritant compounds; pulmonary oedema can also be caused by these agents or by ingestion of drugs such as opiates or aspirin. There may be tachycardia with poisoning due to anticholinergic compounds, salicylates or drugs stimulating the sympathetic nervous system. Bradycardia, on the other hand, may be caused by verapamil, beta-blockers

or drugs stimulating the parasympathetic nervous system. Cardiac arrhythmias may be associated with hypoxia, but are particularly troublesome in patients who have taken tricyclic antidepressants, drugs stimulating the sympathetic nervous system, phenothiazines or quinine. Hypotension can be caused by many agents, but hypertension is rarer and usually associated with monoamine oxidase inhibitors or clonidine, which, in overdose, may act like alpha-adrenoceptor agonists.

Abdomen

Absent bowel sounds or bladder enlargement suggest the possibility of anticholinergic poisoning. Rectal examination should be performed and may reveal melaena due to poisoning by iron, non-steroidal anti-inflammatory agents or other agents which damage the gut mucosa. The rectal temperature should be recorded using a low reading thermometer. This may reveal hypothermia (e.g. with phenothiazine poisoning) or hyperthermia (in poisoning by salicylates, anticholinergic compounds or drugs stimulating the sympathetic nervous system).

Skin

The hands, arms and legs may show needle tracks indicating drug abuse. Blisters over the bony prominences, commoner on the lower limbs, are most often seen in patients who have taken a barbiturate overdose. They are by no means diagnostic, even of a drug-induced coma, and may occur after hypoxia.

Neuromuscular

Examination of the limbs normally reveals hypotonia and hyporeflexia in poisoning, but anticholinergic drugs, some opiates and drugs stimulating the sympathetic nervous system may cause hypertonia, hyperreflexia and, occasionally, myoclonus. Anticholinergic compounds may also produce an extensor plantar response which is usually bilateral.

Convulsions may be caused directly by a variety of compounds including the anticholinergic agents and drugs stimulating the sympathetic nervous system, opiates, mefenamic acid and isoniazid, or may be secondary to hypoxia or hypoglycaemia associated with overdose. Dystonic reactions are much less commonly seen, and are generally related to poisoning with drugs with antidopaminergic activity such as metoclopromide, the phenothiazines and butyrophenones.

Laboratory investigations

Routine laboratory investigations are sometimes helpful in identification of the drug ingested.

Urine

The urine should be examined both macroscopically and microscopically. A specimen should also be stored for possible future analysis even if this is not indicated initially. Red discolouration of the urine may be caused by rifampicin or phenindione, and haematuria by drugs affecting haemostasis or clotting, or by drugs causing haemolysis, such as chlorates. Drugs which contain methylene blue (e.g. some commercial analgesics) may colour the urine blue or green; a greyish discolouration of the urine may indicate poisoning due to phenols or cresols. Microscopic haematuria or albuminuria may be the first sign of renal damage; crystalluria can occur with primidone and some of the sulphonamides.

Blood

Brown discolouration of venous blood may indicate methaemoglobinaemia, which can be caused by oxidising agents such as dapsone. Pink discolouration of the plasma indicates haemolysis, which may be drug induced.

The urea and electrolytes are rarely of diagnostic value. Hypokalaemia can be caused by theophylline and drugs stimulating the sympathetic nervous system, or may indicate potassium loss due to diuretic or purgative overdose. Hyperkalaemia is sometimes seen in severe digoxin overdose. Reduction in the serum bicarbonate may indicate metabolic acidosis and should be investigated by arterial blood gas analysis. The alcohols and glycols, as well as aspirin, may cause metabolic acidosis. Profound hypoglycaemia may indicate overdose with oral hypoglycaemic agents, or be secondary to overdose with alcohols, salicylates or paracetamol. Clinical judgement must be used in deciding which test will give useful diagnostic or prognostic information. It is useful to store blood for future reference.

Specific tests

An increasing number of compounds can now be detected specifically in either urine (which tends to be more useful since it concentrates the drug or its metabolites) or in blood. Toxicological analyses are not a substitute for clinical judgement and the physician should consider whether the result will alter his management.

PRINCIPLES OF MANAGEMENT OF POISONING

General supportive measures to prevent complications are usually more important than specific therapies to treat the particular poison, since the latter are not always available.

Supportive management

Maintenance of respiratory function

Maintenance of an adequate airway and respiration is the first priority in an unconscious patient, since many early deaths from poisoning are due to airway obstruction. Dentures should be removed, the tongue pulled forward and the mouth and pharynx cleared of saliva and vomitus. If the patient has no cough reflex, a cuffed endotracheal tube is necessary to protect the lungs; in other cases, a short oropharyngeal tube should be inserted. The patient is then moved into a semi-prone position and, if there is any suspicion of inadequate ventilation, oxygen should be administered. Assisted ventilation may be necessary.

In less urgent circumstances, arterial blood gas analysis is the best guide to assessing adequacy of ventilation. Drugs which stimulate respiration (e.g. doxapram) should be used cautiously in poisoned patients, since they may provoke convulsions or cardiac arrhythmias. The *'shock lung syndrome'* (adult respiratory distress syndrome, ARDS; see p. 511) may appear at about 24 hours. The patient begins to hyperventilate but remains hypoxic, and develops a respiratory and metabolic acidosis. A chest radiograph may show changes similar to pulmonary oedema and, in severe cases, the lung fields may be completely obscured. Assisted ventilation using positive end expiratory pressure (PEEP) may help to support the patient through this severe complication. The treatment of aspiration pneumonia is discussed on page 468.

Maintenance of circulatory function

Maintenance of circulatory function is essential. Hypotension and reduced peripheral perfusion may be caused by several mechanisms including:

- depression of the vasomotor centre
- a direct cardio-depressant action
- increased venous capacitance, leading to reduced venous return to the heart and a consequent fall in cardiac output
- increased capillary permeability resulting in a reduced circulating blood volume.

In hypotensive patients a central venous pressure line should be inserted. If the venous pressure is low, the blood volume should be increased using a plasma expander, such as haemacell. If the hypotension does not respond, intravenous (i.v.) dopamine or dobutamine may restore the blood pressure; low-dose dopamine may prevent subsequent acute renal failure (see Ch. 14).

Cardiac arrhythmias, which may be a direct effect of the drug or a result of hypoxia and acidosis, may also contribute to hypotension by reducing cardiac output. It is important to correct the predisposing causes if

3 Drug Overdose and Poisoning

Table 3.2 Assessment of level of consciousness (Edinburgh Method)

Grade	Degree of consciousness
Grade 0	Fully conscious
Grade 1	Drowsy but able to obey commands
Grade 2	Responds only to pain
Grade 3	Responds only to maximal painful stimuli
Grade 4	Completely unresponsive to any stimuli

possible (e.g. by charcoal haemoperfusion) before considering specific antiarrhythmic therapy, since many antiarrhythmics may further reduce cardiac output. The choice of an antiarrhythmic agent is generally based on the arrhythmia rather than the specific toxin.

Prevention of complications

Good nursing care of the unconscious patient is essential. Skin and muscle compression injuries associated with prolonged immobility and hypoxia are a particular problem. The bladder can sometimes be emptied by firm suprapubic pressure but, if it is markedly distended, catheterisation may be necessary, particularly when measurement of urine production is required. The level of consciousness should be monitored (see Table 3.2); if it fails to improve after 12 hours, this may indicate neurological complications of the overdose or an alternative diagnosis of the coma. Cerebral oedema is the most life-threatening complication of overdose, and may be caused by hypoxia, hypoglycaemia, hypercapnia or hypotension. It is particularly likely to occur after cardiorespiratory arrest and may respond to dexamethasone or mannitol. Convulsions may also be secondary to hypoxia or cerebral oedema, but otherwise are generally shortlived and do not always require specific therapy. If necessary, intravenous diazepam may be used, but if the patient is vomiting, temporary intubation and mechanical ventilation may be necessary to prevent aspiration pneumonia.

Summary 1 Prevention of further drug absorption

- Gastric lavage may prevent further absorption of drug, if performed sufficiently early
- Emesis induced by syrup of ipecacuanha is the preferred method of emptying the stomach in conscious children
- Emptying the stomach by either lavage or emesis should not be performed if the airway cannot be protected
- Activated charcoal prevents further absorption of many drugs, if administered sufficiently early

---

Gastrointestinal bleeding or paralytic ileus may be seen in patients with drug overdose. Insertion of a nasogastric tube and regular emptying of the stomach help to reveal bleeding early and prevent the aspiration pneumonia or acute gastric dilatation sometimes seen with paralytic ileus.

Measures to prevent further drug absorption

Gastric emptying

Futher absorption of the drug from the gut can be reduced by emptying the stomach, either by inducing emesis or by gastric lavage. These procedures are only indicated if the amount of poison taken is likely to cause serious symptoms, and are of little value if the material ingested has already left the stomach. They should thus be attempted when less than 4 hours has elapsed since ingestion of the toxin, although they may still be worthwhile if the time of ingestion is unknown or if the overdose itself is associated with delayed gastric emptying (e.g. with salicylates, mefenamic acid, opiates and drugs with anticholinergic activity, such as tricyclic antidepressants), or a slow-release preparation.

Emesis and lavage are contraindicated in patients who have taken corrosive agents, unless the danger of systemic toxicity associated with a corrosive agent is greater than the risk of local damage. Lavage and emesis are also usually contraindicated after oral ingestion of petroleum distillates, because of the risk of aspiration pneumonia. Emesis should not be performed in patients whose consciousness is impaired, because of the delay in action of ipecacuanha and the risk of aspiration pneumonia in a subsequently unconscious individual.

Gastric lavage

Gastric lavage is the preferred method of emptying of the stomach in adults. In the unconscious patient, a cuffed endotracheal tube must always be inserted first. Lavage should be carried out in the left lateral position in a bed or trolley raised at the foot. A large-bore Jaques stomach tube (external diameter c. 14 mm) is introduced into the stomach and the gastric contents removed. Aliquots of water warmed to body temperature are then introduced and removed until the returned fluid is clear of particles.

Emesis

Emesis is generally the preferred method in children. Syrup of ipecacuanha is the most reliable agent and produces vomiting in 70% of individuals within 20 minutes. A repeated dose after this time will be effective in most of those patients who did not vomit initially. Salt and water should not be used to produce emesis, since death may occur from hypernatraemia. This is particularly likely in small children.

Oral adsorbents

Activated charcoal is being used increasingly as it may reduce the absorption of many drugs (Table 3.3). It is most effective with high-toxicity agents at low dose, since 10 times as much charcoal as drug is required to provide adequate absorption onto the charcoal. The charcoal must be given soon after the overdose to achieve maximum efficacy. It is of little value in adsorbing organic solvents, lithium, cyanide, corrosive agents and iron. A dose of 50–100 g (proportionally smaller in children) can be administered orally or, in an adult, by nasogastric tube. It is of particular value in accidental poisoning in children, since these cases normally present early enough for the adsorbent to be effective.

In iron poisoning, desferrioxamine is the preferred method to prevent further absorption of iron present in the stomach.

Antidotes

There are only direct antidotes to about 5% of poisons, so supportive therapy remains the mainstay of treatment for the vast majority of patients, including those where an antidote exists.

Antidotes work in several different ways:

- They may speed the metabolism of a toxin, e.g. thiosulphate speeds the metabolism of cyanide by pro-

viding sulphur to form non-toxic thiocyanate, which is then excreted in the urine.

- If a compound is only toxic when metabolised, antidotes may reduce the rate of metabolism. Ethanol is used in poisoning by methanol and ethylene glycol to reduce the rate of production of toxic aldehydes and acids.
- For receptor-mediated toxins, an antagonist which competes for a receptor may be useful, e.g. the use of beta-agonists in the treatment of beta-adrenoceptor blocking drug overdose.
- If the toxin competes with a natural substrate, an antidote may increase the natural substrate's concentration, competitively displacing the poison from the receptor site. Inhibitors of acetyl cholinesterase reverse some of the features of anticholinergic poisoning in this way.
- Antidotes may combine with the poison to form an inactive compound. Thus, specific antidigoxin antibody (Fab) fragments combine with digoxin to produce an inert complex, which can be excreted more rapidly via the kidney.

The availability of a specific antidote does not necessarily justify its routine use. Many are toxic in their own right and should only be used if the severity of the poisoning merits their administration. In general, they are most useful early on in the course of poisoning.

Enhancement of drug elimination

Methods to enhance drug elimination (Table 3.4) are of limited value in the treatment of overdose and are generally only effective when the volume of distribution of the drug is relatively small. This is because drug removal can only occur from the 'central' (intravascular) compartment, which must therefore contain a reasonable proportion of the total body burden of the compound.

Forced diuresis

Forced diuresis can be used to enhance the elimination of those drugs excreted predominantly in an unchanged form by the kidney. It acts by increasing the glomerular filtration rate and by reducing the tubular reabsorption of unchanged drug. This is dependent on renal tubular flow, and on the degree of ionisation of the drug in the tubular fluid. For weak acids, alkalinisation of the tubular fluid by administration of bicarbonate will result in a greater proportion of the drug existing in the ionised, poorly lipid soluble form. It is then unable to diffuse back across the lipid membrane of the tubular cell and be reabsorbed. Conversely, acidification of the urine by administration of ammonium chloride, arginine or lysine hydrochloride will increase the ionisation of some basic

Table 3.3 Drugs for which charcoal may prevent absorption

Hypnotics and tranquillisers	Cardiovascular drugs
Phenobarbitone	Digoxin
	Disopyramide
Antidepressants	Mexiletene
Amitriptyline	Pindolol
	Quinidine
Analgesics	Sotalol
Aspirin	
Dextropropoxyphene	**Respiratory drugs**
Indomethacin	Aminophylline
Mefenamic acid	
Paracetamol	**Antidiabetic drugs**
Phenylbutazone	Chlorpropamide
	Tolbutamide
Anticonvulsants	
Carbamazepine	**Diuretics**
Phenytoin	Frusemide
Valproate	
	Others
Antibiotics	Cimetidine
Tetracycline	Paraquat
Trimethoprim	Thallium

3 Drug Overdose and Poisoning

Table 3.4 Techniques used to enhance drug elimination

Forced diuresis	Haemoperfusion
Alkaline	Barbiturates
Barbitone	Carbamazepine
Phenobarbitone	Glutethimide
Phenoxyacetate herbicides	Meprobamate
Salicylates	Methaqualone
	Phenytoin
Acid	Salicylates
Amphetamine	Theophylline
Fenfluramine	
Phencyclidine	**Enteral adsorbents**
	Charcoal
Dialysis	Amitriptyline
Barbitone	Carbamazepine
Ethanol	Dapsone
Ethylene glycol	Dextropropoxyphene
Isopropanol	Digitoxin
Lithium	Nadolol
Methanol	Nortriptyline
Phenobarbitone	Phenobarbitone
Salicylates	Quinine
	Sotalol
	Theophylline
	Cholestyramine
	Digitoxin
	Phenprocoumon
	Warfarin

drugs, thereby reducing reabsorption from the tubular fluid.

Alkaline diuresis has been used in the treatment of phenobarbitone, barbitone and salicylate poisoning. Forced acid diuresis has been used to enhance removal of phencyclidine (the active ingredient of 'angel dust'), amphetamine and the closely related appetite suppressant fenfluramine.

Forced diuresis should only be used in patients with good cardiac and renal function since fluid overload can lead to water intoxication, pulmonary oedema or severe electrolyte and acid–base disturbances. A careful assessment of fluid status is therefore necessary, and unconscious patients will require catheterisation. Intravenous frusemide is used to maintain the fluid output around 500 ml/hour. In forced alkaline diuresis, sufficient sodium bicarbonate (1.2% solution) is given to maintain the urine pH between 7.0 and 8.0; in forced acid diuresis, the pH is maintained between 5 and 6.5 with oral ammonium chloride. Urine pH should be monitored at least half-hourly and electrolytes every 2–4 hours.

Dialysis

Peritoneal or haemodialysis is useful to remove drugs with low plasma protein binding, poor lipid solubility and relatively low volume of distribution. It is generally reserved for those cases where other methods of removal are contraindicated. Salicylates, phenobarbitone and barbitone, methanol, isopropanol, ethylene glycol and lithium are effectively removed by this process. Haemodialysis is normally the most effective of the two approaches.

Haemoperfusion

Haemoperfusion involves the passage of arterial blood through an extracorporeal column of activated charcoal or ion-exchange resin. This effectively removes a number of drugs where the lipid solubility or plasma protein binding reduces the efficacy of removal by dialysis techniques, but a low volume of distribution is still required. Haemoperfusion is therefore useful in severe poisoning with barbiturates (including the short-acting barbiturates not removed effectively by haemodialysis) and non-barbiturate hypnotics such as glutethimide, ethchlorvynol, meprobamate, methaqualone and chloral derivatives (e.g. chloral hydrate). These agents are now used less frequently as hypnotics. Haemoperfusion using resin columns is particularly effective in removing theophylline and, to a lesser extent, salicylates. Complications of the procedure include thrombocytopenia, bleeding and possible infection, so haemoperfusion should only be used in patients with severe poisoning who fail to improve despite supportive management and who have developed, or are at high risk of developing, complications of the overdose.

Enteral removal

Enteral removal is the most recent approach to the enhancement of drug elimination. It relies on the ability of some non-absorbed agents either to remove drugs which have been excreted in the bile but would have been reabsorbed in the gut, or to remove drugs directly from the splanchnic circulation. Charcoal is the most widely used enteral adsorbent, and markedly enhances the rate of removal of phenobarbitone, digitoxin, theophylline and dapsone. It is given as an initial loading dose of 50 g followed by repeated doses of 20 g every 4–12 hours, together with a laxative to prevent constipation. Oral cholestyramine (an anion-binding resin) increases the rate of removal of digitoxin, warfarin and some other coumarin anticoagulants. This non-invasive procedure usually has no major adverse effects.

Support services

It is impossible for a clinician to be familiar with all the details of management of all toxins. As in other countries, in the UK and Eire, Poisons Information Services have therefore been established in several major cities.

On recovery from an overdose, the patient should undergo thorough psychiatric and, if necessary, social assessment (Ch. 10, p. 182). There appears to be a poor correlation between the severity of the overdose and any underlying psychiatric illness. The general practitioner also plays an important role in supporting the patient once he or she has left hospital. Finally, voluntary services often provide useful emotional and practical support to the patient at risk, and details of these local organisations should be made available.

MANAGEMENT OF SPECIFIC DRUG OVERDOSE

The drugs most commonly involved in acute poisoning are hypnotics and tranquillisers, antidepressants and analgesics.

Hypnotics and tranquillisers

Barbiturates

The incidence of barbiturate poisoning has declined markedly over the past 10 years. However, this group of compounds is associated with high mortality and still accounts for the largest number of deaths of any drug group.

Diagnosis

In overdose, the barbiturates produce an impaired level of consciousness and, in severe cases, hypotension and respiratory depression. Approximately 5% of patients have bullous lesions on the extremities, particularly over the extensor surfaces, but these are not specific to barbiturate overdose.

Summary 2 Management of barbiturate poisoning

- Barbiturate poisoning is now relatively rare but has a significant mortality
- Gastric lavage should be performed if within 4 hours of ingestion
- Supportive care is the most important aspect of treatment
- Charcoal haemoperfusion is effective in enhancing elimination of phenobarbitone, barbitone and other barbiturates and should be considered in severe poisoning
- Activated charcoal may prevent absorption of phenobarbitone and repeated doses may enhance elimination of drug already absorbed

---

Barbiturates can be detected in the urine. Although their plasma concentrations can also be measured, these correlate poorly with the severity of the overdose, partly because of other confounding drugs such as alcohol, and partly because of tolerance, particularly in those taking the drug chronically. Plasma concentrations are therefore of limited value in the management of a particular case, although very high concentrations in the presence of grade 4 coma and other complications of overdose may indicate the need to enhance the removal of the drug.

Management

Gastric lavage should be performed if tablets have been taken less than 4 hours previously, or if the time of ingestion in an unconscious patient is unknown. General supportive management is all that is required in most cases, with particular attention to respiration and cardiovascular function. However, even with these measures, the mortality in grade 4 coma is about 5% and procedures to enhance drug elimination may be considered in such subjects, particularly if complications of overdose are already present. Forced alkaline diuresis has been used to enhance the removal of phenobarbitone and barbitone because these drugs are mainly excreted unchanged in the urine. This procedure is relatively inefficient, however, and has been largely replaced by charcoal haemoperfusion which removes most barbiturates, even those (e.g. many of the short- and intermediate-acting compounds) that are relatively highly protein bound and eliminated by hepatic metabolism. Repeated doses of activated charcoal given by mouth through a nasogastric tube can reduce the half-life of phenobarbitone from over 100 hours to less than 20 hours. This procedure is relatively non-invasive and may replace the use of haemoperfusion for phenobarbitone poisoning. Activated charcoal has not yet been shown to enhance the elimination of any of the other barbiturates.

Benzodiazepines

Benzodiazepines are involved in almost half of the drug overdoses in the UK. There are only a small number of fatal cases each year in which a benzodiazepine is the only drug identified, but they potentiate the effects of other CNS-depressant drugs and can thus contribute to fatal outcome.

Diagnosis

The major effects are on the CNS and include drowsiness, ataxia, dysarthria and nystagmus. Coma then supervenes, although it is rarely greater than grade 2 unless other agents have been ingested. Recovery is normally

3 Drug Overdose and Poisoning

> **Summary 3 Management of benzodiazepine poisoning**
>
> - Benzodiazepine poisoning is common but death is rare, unless other potentiating agents (e.g. alcohol) have also been taken
>
> - Flurazepam, flunitrazepam and triazolam may cause deeper coma than the other agents
>
> - Management is generally supportive
>
> - Flumazenil, a specific benzodiazepine antagonist, may help in the diagnosis of mixed overdose

within 24 hours, although flurazepam and flunitrazepam may cause deeper and more prolonged coma, and clonazepam has been associated with cyclical coma. Lorazepam causes only modest CNS depression but can be associated with restlessness and hallucinations, particularly in children. Respiratory depression occurs rarely in benzodiazepine overdose, although it may occur in patients with pre-existing respiratory disease, particularly with flunitrazepam. Cardiovascular effects are also generally mild although slight hypotension may occur. Flunitrazepam may cause more profound hypotension and a sinus bradycardia. Bullous skin lesions have been reported, but are much rarer than after barbiturate overdose.

Management

Management is supportive; methods to enhance elimination of the parent compound or its active metabolites are of no value. Most patients will recover with no sequelae. Antagonists of benzodiazepines (e.g. flumazenil) may be helpful in the diagnosis of mixed overdose, or in avoiding the need for ventilatory support in severe poisoning. However, they may precipitate benzodiazepine withdrawal in dependent individuals.

Non-barbiturate, non-benzodiazepine hypnotics

These were once widely used but have now been largely replaced by benzodiazepines. Isolated overdoses of these agents still occur, however. Specific effects may be seen in addition to CNS depression.

Methaqualone can cause hypertonia, myoclonus, hyperreflexia, extensor plantar responses and occasionally papilloedema. Pulmonary oedema, coma and convulsions have also been reported. Supportive measures are normally sufficient, but charcoal haemoperfusion is indicated in severely poisoned patients.

Glutethimide may cause fluctuating coma, convulsions and acute respiratory failure. Pulmonary oedema and cerebral oedema may also occur and papilloedema may be a sign of severe overdose. Charcoal haemoperfusion is

indicated in severe overdose, together with management of specific complications.

Chloral hydrate and its relatives (e.g. dichloralphenazone) may cause gastrointestinal irritation, haematemesis and subsequent oesophageal stricture. Cardiac arrhythmias are a particular problem with this group of agents but generally respond well to beta-blockers. Haemodialysis may remove the active metabolite, trichlorethanol, but charcoal haemoperfusion is probably more effective and may be helpful in very seriously poisoned patients.

Chlormethiazole is often used in alcoholic patients, although its value is not proven and it may be dangerous when taken in overdose together with alcohol. Increased salivation is a particular problem which may increase the risk of aspiration pneumonia, and regular oropharyngeal aspiration may be necessary.

Meprobamate is still used in the treatment of anxiety, and particularly with muscle spasm. Signs of overdose are muscular incoordination and weakness and CNS depression. In severe cases, pulmonary oedema may be seen. Haemodialysis may be useful in severe overdose, but haemoperfusion appears to be more effective.

Antidepressants

Antidepressants, particularly those in the tricyclic group, are commonly taken in overdose and are particularly dangerous. They are the commonest cause of death in children aged under 10 years and, in contrast to the situation with barbiturates, adult mortality is also rising.

Tricyclic antidepressants

The tricyclic antidepressants act by blocking the uptake of noradrenaline by neurones both peripherally and in the CNS. They also have an anticholinergic effect and, in overdose, may have direct actions on the heart.

Diagnosis

The first signs are usually due to the anticholinergic effects. Dryness of the mouth and initial stimulation of the CNS is followed by depressant effects. In severe overdose, muscle hypertonia, hyperreflexia and extensor plantar responses are followed by hypotonia and hyporeflexia; convulsions may also occur. Other anticholinergic features are warm dry skin, pupillary dilatation, urinary retention and, in severe cases, paralytic ileus. Depression of respiration may be associated with hypoxia and respiratory and metabolic acidosis. Hypothermia may also occur, and respiratory complications such as aspiration and ARDS (p. 511) can further compromise tissue perfusion.

The most life-threatening complication is cardiotoxicity. Tricyclic antidepressants resemble quinidine in their action on the heart, producing a decrease in myocardial contractility, prolongation of the PR interval and widening of the QRS complex. In severe cases, the T wave may disappear and the ECG may resemble ventricular tachycardia. Severe ventricular arrhythmias occur in some patients (Fig. 3.3), particularly in the early stages, and the ECG should therefore be monitored preferably even before emptying the stomach.

Management

The stomach should be emptied if more than 250 mg of drug has been taken by an adult, and correspondingly less in a child. This may be effective for up to 12 hours after overdose, because of delayed gastric emptying induced by the anticholinergic effects of the drug. Activated charcoal should then be given to prevent further absorption of drug. Repeated administration of charcoal may have only a modest effect on the half-life of amitriptyline, but be slightly more effective in removing its active metabolite, nortriptyline. Other methods of removal such as dialysis are of little value because of the large volume of distribution with only a small proportion in the blood.

Convulsions may be related to anoxia and will sometimes respond to adequate oxygenation, although they may require treatment with anticonvulsants such as diazepam. Physostigmine has been used to reverse the CNS effects, but it may precipitate convulsions, ventricular tachyarrhythmias and increased salivary and bronchial secretions. It is therefore rarely used.

Arrhythmias and hypotension may respond to correction of acidosis, hypoxia, hypothermia and hypovolaemia. Antiarrhythmic agents should be used cautiously since they may worsen already impaired myocardial contractility, but positive inotropes (e.g. dobutamine) may be necessary to correct the hypotension.

Monoamine oxidase inhibitors

The monoamine oxidase inhibitors (MAOIs) are much less frequently taken in overdose than tricyclic antidepressants. They produce features of increased sympathetic activity, with hyperexcitability and hyperreflexia followed by coma and convulsions. A sinus tachycardia is often present, but the patient may be either hypertensive or

hypotensive. Hyperthermia, or more rarely hypothermia, has been reported. The agitation may require treatment with a sedative agent such as diazepam, while hypotension may respond to replacement of the circulating blood volume. Sympathomimetic agents (e.g. dopamine and dobutamine) should be avoided if possible, since they may lead to a severe hypertensive crisis. Severe hypertension should be treated with an alpha-blocker such as phentolamine.

Lithium carbonate

Lithium carbonate is widely used in the prophylaxis of manic-depressive psychosis. It has a low therapeutic ratio, and signs of toxicity are most often due to excessive therapeutic doses.

Diagnosis

Nausea, vomiting and diarrhoea are often the first signs of overdose, followed by dysarthria, ataxia, drowsiness, confusion, coma and convulsions. Renal impairment and nephrogenic diabetes insipidus may occur, and liver damage has also been reported. Cardiotoxicity may be first indicated by ECG findings of non-specific ST segment depression, T wave inversion, atrioventricular block, and prolongation of the QRS and QT intervals.

Management

Rehydration is important, but hypernatraemia (which may indicate nephrogenic diabetes insipidus) may require i.v. dextrose until the serum sodium and osmolality become normal. Hypokalaemia should be treated. Toxicity correlates relatively well with the plasma lithium

---

Summary 4 Overdose of tricyclic antidepressants

- Tricyclic antidepressant poisoning is common and life-threatening

- Anticholinergic signs predominate in the early stages but coma may supervene

- Direct cardiotoxicity may result in ventricular tachycardia or ventricular fibrillation. The ECG should be monitored until recovery

- Gastric lavage may be effective up to 12 hours after overdose and activated charcoal may prevent further drug absorption

---

Fig. 3.3 Rhythm ECG in tricyclic overdose.

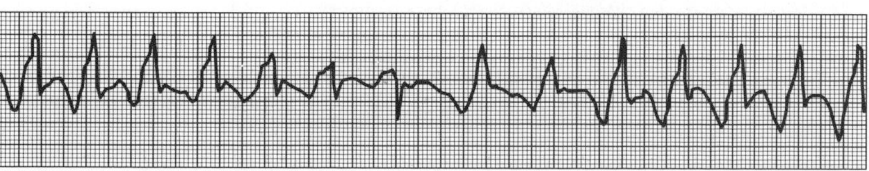

level. Concentrations greater than 5 mmol/l may indicate the need for active elimination of the lithium. Forced diuresis is of little value and carries the risk of fluid overload, particularly if renal failure occurs. Peritoneal dialysis is more effective, but haemodialysis is better. Because of the relatively large volume of distribution, plasma lithium concentrations may increase by up to two-fold shortly after the end of the dialysis. Repeated dialyses may therefore be necessary to maintain the serum lithium level below 1.5 mmol/l. Levels above this may be associated with toxicity.

Other antidepressants

Mianserin is a tetracyclic compound with only weak peripheral anticholinergic activity. It appears to be less likely to cause cardiotoxicity, convulsions or respiratory depression than the tricyclic compounds. Maprotiline is similar to mianserin in its effects, but is more toxic in overdose. In both cases, treatment is supportive.

Analgesics

The dangers of analgesics are not widely appreciated. They are the second commonest group of drugs involved in overdosage in adults and, in children, salicylates are the second commonest cause of drug-related death.

Salicylates

Salicylate overdose is responsible for approximately 200 deaths each year in the UK. In addition to being acids, salicylates also increase circulating lactic and pyruvic acid concentrations by interfering with normal carbohydrate metabolism. Stimulation of fat metabolism causes increased production of β-hydroxybutyric and aceto-acetic acids, and increased protein metabolism results in increased circulating amino acids. Impairment of reab-sorption of these amino acids, by competition with the salicylate for active tubular reabsorption, produces amino-aciduria and increased fluid loss due to the effect of this solute load. Fluid loss is worsened by the vomiting associated with salicylate overdose, and by the uncoupling of oxidative phosphorylation which causes hyperpyrexia and increased sweating. Stimulation of the respiratory centre by salicylates causes a respiratory alkalosis which partly offsets the metabolic acidosis but causes further bicarbonate depletion, electrolyte loss and dehydration.

Diagnosis

The clinical features of salicylate overdose are agitation, tinnitus and deafness, increased sweating and hyperventilation; nausea and vomiting and epigastric pain may also be present. Respiratory alkalosis may occur initially but is quickly followed, particularly in children, by a metabolic acidosis associated with increased production of lactate, pyruvate and ketones. There may be hypokalaemia and hypo- or, more rarely, hyperglycaemia. Impaired clotting factor and platelet function are sometimes seen, but bleeding is rare. Coma may occur before death.

Management

Treatment involves emptying of the stomach, either by gastric aspiration in the adult or induction of emesis in a child. Activated charcoal can be administered after emptying the stomach but may have limited value, partly because an optimum ratio of charcoal to the mass of drug ingested cannot be attained, and partly because the tablets may form a large mass in the stomach which is difficult to remove or adsorb. Emesis or gastric lavage may be of value up to 12 hours and possibly 24 hours after ingestion, because salicylates may cause pylorospasm and delayed gastric emptying.

Correction of any acid–base abnormalities and rehydration should be sufficient in mild or moderate cases of salicylate poisoning. Patients whose blood salicylate level is greater than 700 mg/l should be considered for forced alkaline diuresis. Potassium supplements may be necessary to achieve adequate urinary alkalinisation but, if this cannot be attained without increasing the blood pH to greater than 7.5, haemodialysis or haemoperfusion may prove necessary. The latter procedures are generally the treatment of choice for severely poisoned patients or in those in whom forced alkaline diuresis is contraindicated. Pulmonary oedema may occur due to fluid overload or as a direct effect of the drug on capillary permeability. In the former case, the pulmonary artery pressure will be raised but not in the latter. Ventilation with positive end expiratory pressure may be helpful.

Summary 5 Salicylate poisoning

- Salicylate poisoning is serious because of the derangement of acid–base and electrolyte balance (metabolic acidosis, respiratory alkalosis and dehydration)

- Coma is rare except as a terminal event, and agitation and restlessness, tinnitus, deafness and hyperventilation are characteristic

- Emptying the stomach is indicated up to 24 hours after overdose in adults, and activated charcoal may prevent further absorption

- Correction of acid–base abnormalities and dehydration is usually sufficient in mild to moderate poisoning; forced alkaline diuresis, haemoperfusion or haemodialysis may be necessary in severe poisoning

---

Other non-steroidal anti-inflammatory drugs

Salicylates form one group of non-steroidal anti-inflammatory drugs (NSAIDs) but there are five other groups which can be classified according to chemical structure. These are:

- *The arylalkanoic acids*, which include phenyl propionic acid derivatives like ibuprofen, the naphthyl propionic acid derivatives such as naproxen, and the phenyl acetic acid derivatives such as fenclofenac
- *The anthranilic acids*, which include the fenamates (mefenamic acid and flufenamic acid)
- *The pyrazalone group of compounds*, e.g. azapropazone and phenylbutazone
- *The cyclic acetic acids*, which include indomethacin, sulindac and tolmetin
- *The oxicams*, at present represented by piroxicam.

Diagnosis

The arylalkanoic acids, like all NSAIDs, cause headache, nausea and epigastric discomfort, but coma is rare. Gastrointestinal bleeding may occur and, rarely, bronchospasm. Poisoning with anthranilic acids (e.g. mefenamic acid) is more serious and severe haemorrhagic enterocolitis may occur. CNS effects are also commoner and may include convulsions. Overdose with pyrazolones can produce gastrointestinal and CNS toxicity and hepatic and renal damage. The cyclic acetic acids also produce coma, while piroxicam has been associated with coma and convulsions.

Management

The stomach should be emptied if appropriate. Early administration of charcoal will reduce the absorption of some of the anthranilic and cyclic acetic acids, and may also be of benefit in poisoning with other groups of NSAIDs. Although there is no definite evidence that histamine-2-receptor antagonists (e.g. ranitidine) protect against gastrointestinal haemorrhage, they are often administered prophylactically. Convulsions are generally short-lived but can be treated with diazepam. Blood pressure should be measured regularly and hypotension corrected to prevent subsequent acute renal failure.

Paracetamol

Paracetamol is a remarkably safe drug in therapeutic doses but in overdose may cause fatal hepatic necrosis and is responsible for approximately 200 deaths per year. Toxicity of paracetamol in overdose is related to the metabolism of the drug. In therapeutic doses, approximately 90% of the drug is conjugated with glucuronide or sulphate, with only 10% oxidised by the mixed function oxidase system. The latter pathway produces a highly reactive intermediate compound which is normally conjugated with glutathione and subsequently excreted. In overdose, however, the glucuronidation and sulphation pathways cannot metabolise such a high proportion of the drug so that more is oxidised. The availability of glutathione is not sufficient to detoxify all the intermediate product produced, which instead binds to macromolecules in the liver cell, causing necrosis. Patients on enzyme-inducing drugs (e.g. phenobarbitone, carbamazepine and rifampicin) may develop liver damage at lower plasma concentrations of paracetamol and require antidote treatment at half the usual plasma concentration.

Diagnosis

The clinical features are initially mild and consist of nausea, vomiting and epigastric pain. Liver damage normally manifests itself clinically at 3 days, although the one-stage prothrombin time (INR) is often prolonged in such patients as early as 24 hours after the overdose, before the liver enzymes have started to rise. Liver damage may occur with as little as 12 g of paracetamol and, although individuals vary in their sensitivity to the drug, those with liver disease or on enzyme-inducing drugs may be more susceptible. In severe overdose, metabolic acidosis, hypoglycaemia, hypotension and cardiac arrhythmias have been described. Acute renal failure has also been reported, which is usually associated with severe liver damage but may occur in its absence. Renal function and electrolytes should therefore be measured daily. Finally, there have been very rare reports of pancreatitis associated with severe paracetamol poisoning. A raised serum amylase concentration may, however, be related to inability to clear amylase because of liver damage and does not necessarily indicate pancreatic damage.

Management

Initial treatment is the induction of emesis or gastric lavage within 6 hours of tablet ingestion. Plasma paracetamol concentration should also be checked and, if it is greater than a given concentration (shown in Fig. 3.4), an antidote should be administered. Antidotal therapy should also be used without waiting for the plasma paracetamol concentration if the overdose has been taken at least 8 hours previously, since the efficacy of the antidotes declines markedly with time.

Acetylcysteine is a glutathione precursor which is usually given intravenously because given orally it causes severe vomiting. Acetylcysteine appears to have some efficacy up to 24 hours after a large overdose. Oral methionine is also recommended, but is probably ineffective 12 hours or more after an overdose. Patients may be

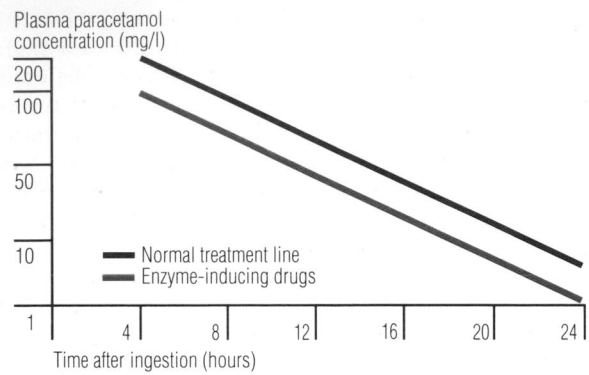

Fig. 3.4 Plasma paracetamol concentrations above which antidotal treatment for poisoning is required.

vomiting as a result of paracetamol ingestion, so it will be difficult to retain in the stomach. Anaphylactoid reactions have been reported after the use of acetylcysteine, in which case the infusion may have to be discontinued and methionine used instead. The anaphylactoid reaction (urticaria and bronchospasm) is more serious in patients who have been inadvertently given an overdose of acetylcysteine, so the dose of this antidote should be checked carefully.

Blood sugar should be measured and any abnormality treated. The INR should be measured daily. An INR of 3 or more at 48 hours or >4 at 72 hours indicates the likelihood of liver failure in which case the patient should be commenced on a low protein diet and oral lactulose to help to remove nitrogenous compounds from the gut. Vitamin K may reduce the INR but this is often ineffective and fresh frozen plasma may be necessary to prevent haemorrhagic complications. Even if acute hepatic failure does occur, the mortality is less than 50% with good supportive management (p. 630).

Opiates

Opiates are used not only as narcotic analgesics but also as constituents of some cough suppressants, antidiarrhoeal products (e.g. diphenoxylate) and veterinary tran-

---

quillisers. The opiate most often involved in poisoning is dextropopoxyphene. Opiates are being increasingly misused in society for their effects on mood, administered intravenously as well as orally.

Diagnosis

Respiratory depression is the commonest cause of death in opiate overdose. The pupils are often pin-point. Depression of the CNS eventually leads to coma and convulsions. The muscles may be hypotonic, but muscular twitching and hyperreflexia have been described. Hypotension is common but hypertension has been described after pentazocine overdose. Non-cardiogenic pulmonary oedema may occur, particularly in methadone overdose.

Management

If the opiate has been taken orally, gastric emptying may be of value for up to 12 hours because of opiate-induced delay in gastric emptying. Naloxone is effective in reversing the symptoms of opiate overdose with all compounds except buprenorphine, which is a partial agonist and not completely antagonised. Repeated doses may be necessary because of the short half-life of naloxone, and, in severe overdose with long-acting agents, such as dihydrocodeine and methadone, naloxone by continuous infusion may be required. In buprenorphine poisoning, naloxone may have only limited benefit and, if doxapram fails to stimulate respiration sufficiently, assisted ventilation may be necessary. Naloxone may precipitate acute opiate withdrawal, with abdominal pain, diarrhoea and pilo-erection, but the dangers of opiate overdose are greater.

Anticonvulsants

The incidence of psychiatric abnormalities is higher in epileptics than in the non-epileptic population. The availability of anticonvulsants to some epileptic patients results in their being taken relatively frequently in overdose. Barbiturates and primidone (which is converted into phenobarbitone and phenylethylmalonamide) are the most toxic anticonvulsants (p. 43).

Phenytoin

Phenytoin is one of the most widely prescribed anticonvulsants. Acute overdosage leads to ataxia, dysarthria, horizontal nystagmus, drowsiness and, in severe cases, coma. Respiratory depression is a rare but potentially serious complication, which is generally only seen after massive overdose. The stomach should be emptied within 4 hours of ingestion and activated charcoal will help to

---

Summary 6 Management of opiate poisoning
● Opiate poisoning is a common, serious medical emergency
● Naloxone reverses the effects of all opiates (except buprenorphine) if given in sufficient dose, since it is a competitive antagonist
● The short half-life of naloxone necessitates repeated doses or even constant infusion in treatment of opiates with long half-lives of elimination (e.g. dihydrocodeine and methadone)
● The association between intravenous opiate abuse and infection (hepatitis B and HIV) should be recognised, and appropriate safeguards taken

prevent further absorption. Because phenytoin is highly protein bound, only charcoal haemoperfusion will effectively remove the drug from the circulation. This should, however, be reserved for patients with severe overdose. Rarely, cases of permanent cerebellar damage with persistent ataxia after phenytoin overdose have been described.

Carbamazepine

Carbamazepine is widely used for the treatment of generalised and partial seizures. The drug is structurally similar to tricyclic antidepressants, and overdose can be associated with anticholinergic effects including dry mouth, hyperreflexia and generalised convulsions. Nystagmus, diplopia, ataxia, hypotension and respiratory depression have been noted, and cardiac conduction disturbances may also occur. The stomach should be emptied if appropriate, and activated charcoal administered. Repeated doses of charcoal speed the elimination of drug in normal volunteers and may be effective in severe overdose. Effective removal of drug by haemoperfusion has also been reported.

Sodium valproate

Sodium valproate poisoning is associated with coma and respiratory depression. The drug is rapidly absorbed, and supportive measures form the mainstay of treatment.

Cardiovascular drugs

Antihypertensives

The major adverse effect is hypotension. With clonidine, hypotension is often associated with bradycardia but severe hypertension caused by the drug's partial alpha-agonist activity is sometimes a major problem. Bradycardia often responds to atropine, and alpha-adrenergic blocking drugs have been used to treat the hypertension. Beta-receptor blocking agents also cause bradycardia and hypotension and, like clonidine, can cause drowsiness, coma and convulsions in overdose. In severe hypotension, glucagon can be used to increase cardiac output by a mechanism separate from beta-receptor stimulation. Beta-agonists, such as isoprenaline or prenalterol, are also effective, although large amounts may have to be given intravenously to competitively antagonise the beta-blockade. Beta-2 agonists (e.g. salbutamol) may be necessary if bronchospasm is present, and the blood sugar should be monitored to detect and treat hypoglycaemia.

Calcium antagonists such as verapamil may also cause severe hypotension and bradycardia and, in the case of verapamil, conduction abnormalities may also be seen. If atropine is ineffective in treating the bradycardia, calcium gluconate (10–20 ml of a 10% solution) may be required.

Digitalis glycosides

Poisoning with the digitalis glycosides is rare, but potentially very serious. Nausea, vomiting and diarrhoea are early features, but the major life-threatening complications are hypotension and cardiac conduction disturbances with brady- and tachyarrhythmias. Hyperkalaemia is often present and mirrors roughly the severity of the overdose. This should be treated with glucose and insulin, or a sodium resonium ion exchange resin, or by haemodialysis if necessary. Digoxin is predominantly excreted by the renal route, and a good urine output should be maintained. Digitoxin is excreted by metabolism with marked enterohepatic recirculation of the drug. Repeated doses of activated charcoal or cholestyramine will speed elimination of the drug. Continuous monitoring of cardiac rhythm is essential; bradyarrhythmias may require temporary cardiac pacing. Ventricular tachyarrhythmias often respond to lignocaine, but phenytoin has been used in resistant cases. Digoxin-specific Fab antibody fragments may be necessary in the treatment of severe digoxin poisoning. In the UK, the National Poisons Information Services can be consulted for information on their availability and applicability to specific cases (see Appendix).

Respiratory drugs

Theophylline

Theophylline is the respiratory drug most often taken in overdose; it causes CNS stimulation, hallucinations and convulsions. A sinus tachycardia may be followed by supraventricular and ventricular arrhythmias with hypokalaemia (often profound), metabolic acidosis and pancreatitis.

The stomach should be emptied to prevent further absorption, and charcoal left in the stomach. The metabolic abnormalities should be treated appropriately, while convulsions may respond to diazepam administered intravenously. Supraventricular and ventricular arrhythmias may respond to the use of beta-1 adrenergic blockers (e.g. metoprolol), but the metabolic abnormalities may only respond to agents which also possess beta-2 agonist activity (e.g. propranolol). Beta-blockers should not be used in asthmatic patients, because of the risk of precipitating bronchospasm. In such patients, verapamil has been used successfully to treat arrhythmias. Haemoperfusion is one of the most efficient ways of enhancing the removal of theophylline from the circulation. It should be considered in severely poisoned patients, particularly those with major arrhythmias, hypotension or convulsions. Repeated enteral administration of charcoal has recently been shown to reduce markedly the half-life of elimination of theophylline and should be considered if haemoperfusion facilities are not readily available.

Ephedrine, salbutamol and terbutaline

Ephedrine, salbutamol and terbutaline are generally safer than theophylline in overdose, but can cause all the same features in severe cases. Treatment is broadly similar to that of theophylline overdose; again, beta-blockers must be avoided in asthmatic subjects.

Drugs with anticholinergic activity

In addition to tricyclic antidepressants, many drugs have anticholinergic activity, including some used to suppress gastrointestinal motility (e.g. propantheline), some antiparkinsonian drugs (e.g. amantidine and orphenadrine) and some antihistamines (e.g. chlorpheniramine and promethazine). The effects of these drugs are similar to those caused by overdosage with tricyclic antidepressants, but they are less likely to cause arrhythmias.

Physostigmine may antagonise the central effects for a short period but may itself produce convulsions and hypersalivation; although physostigmine has been used to treat ventricular arrhythmias, it may also itself induce ventricular tachycardia. Treatment of overdose is otherwise supportive.

Antidiabetic drugs

Poisoning with antidiabetic drugs and insulin produce all the features of hypoglycaemia. The management is described in Chapter 19, page 747. Severe hypoglycaemia has been treated with diazoxide, which inhibits insulin release and raises circulating plasma catecholamines. At the dose used (1.25 mg/kg over 1 hour every 6 hours), it rarely produces hypotension. Once hypoglycaemia has been corrected, the stomach should be emptied if appropriate; activated charcoal will help to prevent further absorption of chlorpropamide and tolbutamide.

Metabolic acidosis may occur after sulphonylurea poisoning, but is more common after poisoning with metformin. Oral antidiabetic drugs may also cause haematemesis and melaena, so patients should be examined carefully for signs of gastrointestinal bleeding. Pulmonary oedema has also been recorded. Methods to enhance drug elimination have not yet been shown to be effective.

Antibiotics

The penicillins and cephalosporins are generally safe in overdose.

Sulphonamides may cause bone marrow depression and renal damage (and haemolysis in glucose-6-phosphate dehydrogenase deficient patients). Maintenance of a high urine output and alkalinisation of the urine may prevent sulphonamide-induced renal damage, by preventing crystallisation of the drug in the renal tubule. Calcium folinate may help to reverse bone marrow depression induced by sulphonamide or trimethoprim.

Isoniazid can cause CNS symptoms with coma and convulsions. Pyridoxine can be used to treat or prevent both convulsions and the metabolic abnormalities; it should be given in a dose of 1 g for every gram of isoniazid ingested.

Rifampicin overdose may be associated with orange discolouration of the skin (although this colour can be removed by washing). Treatment is usually supportive. Although most patients recover completely, occasional deaths have been reported, presumably from cardiac arrhythmias.

Antimalarials

Quinine

Although rarely used for malaria prophylaxis, quinine is the antimalarial agent most often taken in overdose and also the one most likely to cause serious toxicity. In the UK, it has been most often prescribed for 'night cramps'. Children may take tablets belonging to a family member. Early symptoms of overdose are similar to those of aspirin, with nausea, vomiting, bowel disturbances, tinnitus and deafness. Initial respiratory stimulation may be followed by respiratory depression and respiratory arrest. Quinine can cause brady- and tachyarrhythmias, with death from ventricular fibrillation. Its effect on vision is dramatic. Visual acuity is initially impaired, and this may progress to constriction of visual fields or even complete blindness. Retinal examination reveals retinal oedema, optic atrophy and constricted retinal arteries. Most patients recover vision, although some are left with permanent visual field defects.

The management of quinine poisoning is supportive. Stellate ganglion block has been used to treat the visual impairment, but quinine toxicity is likely to be direct on the retina and this procedure is of limited efficacy. As quinine has a large volume of distribution and is predominantly metabolised by the liver, methods to enhance elimination are of limited value, but repeated oral charcoal may be beneficial.

Chloroquine

Chloroquine is widely used as prophylaxis against malaria and can be purchased without prescription. Its toxicity is similar to that of quinine but as little as 5 g may be fatal. Ventricular arrythmias occur early as well as coma and convulsions. Very large doses of diazepam (which may necessitate ventilation) may reduce mortality. Chloroquine is also predominantly metabolised by the liver and has a high volume of distribution; thus, none of the techniques for enhancing removal appear to be effective.

Anticoagulants

The major risk of oral anticoagulant poisoning is haemorrhage; this occurs several days after the overdose because of the delayed effect of these agents. Vitamin K should be administered intravenously and may be necessary for up to a week. Repeated administration of cholestyramine will enhance the removal of warfarin and phenprocoumon and also reduce the length of time for which vitamin K is required.

POISONING WITH GASES AND VOLATILE LIQUIDS

Carbon monoxide

Carbon monoxide is still the most common cause of fatal poisoning in the UK, despite the substitution of natural gas for coal gas in general use. Deaths occur either accidentally (often by inhalation of fumes during fires) or deliberately, from inhalation of car exhaust fumes in a confined space. Methylene chloride, which is widely used in paint removers, is metabolised by the body to carbon monoxide and causes symptoms identical to those of direct carbon monoxide exposure.

Diagnosis

The early symptoms of chronic or acute exposure are headache, mental agitation, nausea and vomiting. The characteristic cherry-pink colour of the skin is rarely present during life, but the patient is not cyanosed, despite considerable hypoxia because of the production of carboxyhaemoglobin. Cerebral oedema and myocardial ischaemia or infarction may also occur.

Management

Oxygen should be given in as high a concentration as possible. Hyperbaric oxygen is even more effective in severe cases, but is not always immediately available, and transfer to this facility should not interrupt the treatment of severely poisoned patients. Oxygen should be administered until the carboxyhaemoglobin concentration in blood falls below 15%; this may take up to 2 days.

Most patients who die of carbon monoxide poisoning do so before they reach hospital; those who do arrive in hospital usually survive. Unfortunately, permanent neuro-psychiatric sequelae may be seen, including intellectual and personality deterioration, Parkinsonism and, in rare cases, akinetic mutism. These severely affected patients often show areas of low density in the area of the globus pallidus on CT brain scans.

Irritant vapours and gases

Carbon disulphide, hydrogen sulphide, sulphur dioxide, hydrochloric acid and ammonia are all highly irritant to the eyes and respiratory tract. Cough and chest pain may be followed by dyspnoea, bronchospasm, haemoptysis and pulmonary oedema.

Management

Treatment is supportive, with bronchodilators for bronchospasm, oxygen for hypoxia and, in severe cases, assisted ventilation (with PEEP if pulmonary oedema is present). Steroids, diuretics and antibiotics have been used but, since the complications are direct effects of the gas, they are unlikely to be of benefit. The metabolic acidosis may improve with adequate oxygenation but if this fails, sodium bicarbonate may have to be administered. Ophthalmological advice should be sought to diagnose and treat corneal abrasions.

Cyanide

Cyanide may be inhaled in the form of hydrogen cyanide. Symptoms appear within a few minutes, firstly with headache, agitation, confusion leading to coma, cardiovascular collapse and respiratory arrest. Cyanide may also be taken orally, in which case symptoms may occur much later, particularly if food in the stomach delays gastric emptying.

Management

Oxygen in high concentrations should be administered and assisted ventilation performed if necessary. Dicobalt edetate is the treatment of choice, but this may cause hypotension and chest pain on i.v. administration, and should therefore only be used if the diagnosis is certain. It acts by forming inert complexes with cyanide, thus preventing the cyanide-induced inhibition of cellular oxidising enzymes. Thiosulphate acts as a sulphur donor to allow conversion of cyanide to thiocyanate via the enzyme rhodanase. Amyl- and sodium nitrites convert haemoglobin to methaemoglobin, which chelates the cyanide ion. Amyl nitrite can be given by inhalation, but it is much less effective than intravenous sodium nitrite.

The latter is often given with intravenous sodium thiosulphate as together they have synergistic action. They are generally used if there is no response to dicobalt edetate, or if the latter is not immediately available.

Hydrocarbons

Poisoning with hydrocarbons is nearly always accidental, generally from industrial or domestic exposure, but also increasingly from solvent abuse.

Aliphatic hydrocarbons

The aliphatic hydrocarbons appear to be less toxic than the aromatic group. The shorter-chain aliphatic hydrocarbons are volatile so that poisoning is usually from inhalation. High concentrations may cause asphyxia and the butane in lighter fluid has been used to produce euphoria by solvent abusers. Coma may occur, with death from respiratory depression or ventricular fibrillation. Renal and liver damage may develop if the patient survives. Pulmonary and cerebral oedema have also been reported. Inhaled hydrocarbons may also produce myopathies, neuropathies and permanent neuropsychiatric damage, although some of these effects may be related to additives to the hydrocarbon. Ingestion of liquid aliphatic hydrocarbons can produce effects similar to the above, either due to a systemic effect or, more likely, to aspiration of the low surface tension solvents. Pyrexia, cough and hyperpnoea may be followed by basal crackles in the chest, consolidation and collapse involving predominantly the middle and lower zones of the lung.

Treatment of solvent inhalation or ingestion is generally supportive. Gastric lavage or emesis should not be performed after ingestion because of the risk of chemical pneumonitis. There is no evidence that steroids and antibiotics are effective in the pulmonary complications but, in severe cases, ventilatory support may enable the patient to recover.

Chlorinated aliphatic hydrocarbons

Chlorinated aliphatic hydrocarbons are widely used as solvents in industry. In addition to the effects described with other hydrocarbons, the chlorinated aliphatics are also more likely to produce hepatic and renal damage (particularly carbon tetrachloride and chloroform), haemolytic anaemia and aplastic anaemia. Methylene chloride is metabolised by the body to carbon monoxide and its systemic toxicity is that of this metabolite, although it is itself locally corrosive. It has been suggested that acetylcysteine may inhibit the metabolism of chlorinated hydrocarbons to reactive intermediate metabolites and thereby reduce hepatotoxicity if given early.

Aromatic hydrocarbons

Aromatic hydrocarbons are less often involved in poisoning. Benzene is the most toxic of these agents and, in acute overdose, produces effects similar to those of the aliphatic hydrocarbons. Chronic exposure may lead to aplastic anaemia and leukaemias. Toluene and xylene are similar in structure and effects to, but less toxic than, benzene; any marrow toxicity is probably related to benzene contamination. Benzene contamination is probably also responsible for the haematological problems sometimes seen with chronic petrol inhalation.

OVERDOSE WITH ALCOHOLS

Ethanol (ethyl alcohol) (see also Ch. 22, p. 979)

Ethanol, present in alcoholic drinks, is the alcohol most often taken in overdose. It is also found as a solvent in some cosmetic and antiseptic preparations. Its major toxicity is related to its central nervous depressant effects. The loss of the gag reflex may result in aspiration of stomach contents. Alcohols inhibit gluconeogenesis and may cause profound hypoglycaemia, particularly in children. Blood ethanol concentrations give a rough guide to the severity of overdose, but may be misleading because of tolerance in chronic alcohol users. Severe intoxication with stupor and marked incoordination is generally associated with blood concentrations above 3000 mg/l. The rate of metabolism is shown in Figure 3.5.

Management

The stomach should be emptied if large quantities have been taken within 4 hours of presentation, but the airway must be protected. Metabolism is saturated even at low

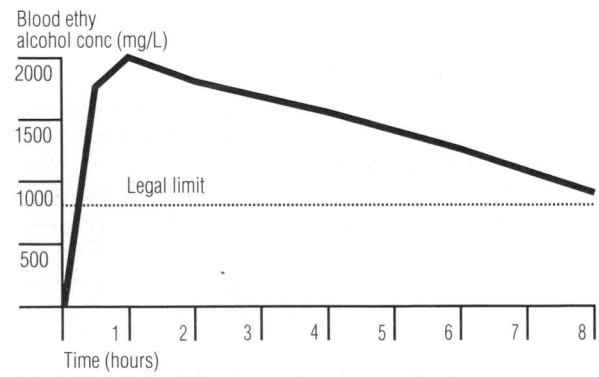

Fig. 3.5 Blood alcohol concentrations after oral administration of ethyl alcohol (2 ml/kg). The concentrations decline in a zero-order fashion at an average rate of 190 mg/l each hour.

doses. Although haemodialysis will remove alcohol efficiently, it is only indicated in severe and complicated cases of poisoning. Fructose accelerates the metabolism of alcohol, but it can potentiate the metabolic acidosis already caused by the alcohol and may therefore be dangerous in overdose. Intravenous dextrose may be necessary to treat hypoglycaemia. The problems of alcoholism are discussed on page 199.

Methanol

Methanol is much more toxic than ethanol and is used widely as a solvent. Methylated spirit is 5% methyl alcohol and 95% ethanol. The mode of toxicity is not clear, but accumulation of formaldehyde and formic acid is partly responsible. As little as 10 ml of methanol may cause serious illness. The initial features are those of mild inebriation, but 8 or more hours later the patient may develop abdominal pain and vomiting, dilated and unreactive pupils, a metabolic acidosis and, sometimes, signs of cerebral oedema. The optic disc is at first hyperaemic and then becomes oedematous; vision is progressively lost.

Management

The stomach should be emptied within 4 hours of methanol ingestion, and intravenous sodium bicarbonate used to correct any metabolic acidosis. Diazepam is indicated if convulsions are a problem. Ethanol competitively inhibits the metabolism of methanol to formaldehyde and formic acid, and is used in less serious poisoning. Haemodialysis may be necessary if the blood methanol concentration exceeds 500 mg/1 or if there is clinical deterioration despite other measures. Haemodialysis also removes ethanol, so that ethanol administration during this procedure has to be increased. Visual impairment often remains permanent, although prompt treatment reduces its severity.

Isopropanol (isopropyl alcohol)

Isopropanol is found in rubbing agents, sterilising fluids and disinfectants, window cleaning fluids and some aftershave lotions. Features of poisoning resemble those of ethyl alcohol poisoning but, because some of it is metabolised to acetone, ketonuria and a characteristic smell of acetone on the breath may be observed.

Management

The stomach should be emptied within 4 hours of ingestion, but treatment is otherwise symptomatic. Haemodialysis will remove isopropyl alcohol but is normally only indicated in severe poisoning.

Ethylene glycol

Antifreeze solutions contain ethylene glycol, a solvent which is sweet-tasting and therefore not unpleasant to drink. Death may occur after ingesting as little as 100 ml of ethylene glycol which, like alcohols, is metabolised by alcohol dehydrogenase. CNS toxicity is similar to alcohol overdose, but ophthalmoplegias, papilloedema and subsequent optic atrophy may also occur and the patient may become comatose and develop convulsions. After 12 hours, respiratory and cardiovascular complications are seen, together with a metabolic acidosis, hypocalcaemia and hyperkalaemia. If the patient survives this phase, he or she may develop acute renal failure after approximately 24 hours.

Ethylene glycol is not itself toxic but is metabolised by alcohol dehydrogenase to aldehydes, glycolates, oxalates and lactate, which are responsible for the toxic features.

Management

The stomach should be emptied within 4 hours and arterial blood gases and serum calcium measured. The metabolic acidosis may respond to intravenous bicarbonate, and calcium gluconate may be necessary to treat hypocalcaemia. Ethylene glycol metabolism can be inhibited by administration of alcohol in doses sufficient to attain blood ethanol concentrations between 1000 and 2000 mg/l. In severe cases (ethylene glycol concentration >500 mg/l, clinical condition deteriorating despite other measures), haemodialysis is necessary to remove ethylene glycol metabolites. Ethanol administration may also be necessary for up to 4 days after the overdose to reduce their production. Dialysis may be required for renal failure.

POISONING WITH CORROSIVE AGENTS

Fortunately, poisoning with corrosive agents is rare, and most incidents are accidental rather than deliberate. The majority of agents produce local tissue damage by protein denaturation, but some (e.g. paraquat) also have serious systemic toxicity. The patterns of damage with acids and alkalis are different and are therefore discussed separately.

Acids

Acids produce severe pain on ingestion. They may cause asphyxia from epiglottal oedema and, although oesophageal damage has been described, they are more likely to cause gastric perforation, particularly in the region of the antrum. Late stricture formation is also a possibility.

Lavage or emesis should not be performed unless the agents also have serious systemic toxicity. Any metabolic acidosis should be treated with intravenous bicarbonate, but weak alkalis should not be given by mouth. Endoscopy is of limited value in the acute phase, and may cause perforation; in later stages, however, it may be helpful in identifying stricture formation. Corticosteroids have been used to prevent stricture formation, but their value is unclear.

Phenol (carbolic acid) can cause systemic toxicity as well as local corrosion. Haemolysis, renal failure, coma and convulsions, myocardial damage and metabolic acidosis may occur, and early gastric lavage is indicated, provided the airway can be protected. Cresols (methylphenols) have similar effects and treatment is therefore as for phenol poisoning.

Formic acid is used in kettle de-scalers and de-staining solutions. It too can produce a metabolic acidosis, intravascular haemolysis and renal failure, as well as local corrosion. Gastric lavage is therefore indicated early after ingestion. As with phenols, aspiration into the lung may cause haemorrhagic tracheobronchitis and the airway must therefore be protected during lavage.

Alkalis

Corrosion by alkalis (e.g. drain and oven cleaners) is generally more severe than by acids and is more likely to cause serious oesophageal, as well as gastric, damage. Treatment is identical to acid ingestion; lavage should not be performed. The risks of perforation should always be considered if endoscopy is performed but it may be useful in identifying alkalis in tablet form which may adhere to the oesophagus (e.g. Clinitest tablets and some denture cleaners).

Bleaches

Most bleaches contain sodium hypochlorite (up to 10%) which may produce corrosion in large or concentrated doses, and laryngeal oedema due to chlorine liberation. The stomach should be emptied and sodium thiosulphate solution (2%) left to prevent further chlorine-liberation. The sodium load resulting from ingestion of large amounts of bleach can cause hypernatraemia and hyperchloraemic acidosis.

Summary 7 Acid poisoning

- Acid ingestion may cause local corrosion, asphyxia due to oedema of the glottis and perforation of the stomach (less commonly the oesophagus)
- Metabolic acidosis and renal failure may also occur
- Lavage should not be performed unless the agent has severe systemic toxicity
- Late stricture formation may occur but the value of corticosteroids in preventing this complication is not proven

---

Disinfectants

Although phenols and cresols have been largely replaced by dichlorometaxylenol in disinfectants, corrosive effects may occur after large or concentrated doses. Metabolic acidosis, coma, myocardial and renal damage and laryngeal oedema may also occur after severe overdose, and the stomach should therefore be emptied and the metabolic abnormalities corrected. Some disinfectants also contain isopropanol (discussed on p. 53).

POISONING WITH INSECTICIDES, HERBICIDES, FUNGICIDES AND RODENTICIDES

Insecticides

The organochlorine group of insecticides (e.g. DDT) have now largely been replaced by safer compounds because of the persistence of the former in the environment. The safer compounds now in use include the organophosphorus and carbamate insecticides.

Organophosphates

The organophosphates act as inhibitors of cholinesterase in man, causing symptoms of excessive cholinergic activity with vomiting, abdominal pain, sweating and hypersalivation. These are followed by muscle fasciculation, diarrhoea, convulsions and coma. Plasma cholinesterase activity, measured in several centres throughout the UK, is useful in the diagnosis of both organophosphate and carbamate insecticide poisoning. Severe toxicity is associated with a reduction in plasma cholinesterase activity to around 10% of normal. Treatment consists of atropine to antagonise the cholinergic (muscarinic) effects. Large doses (up to 30 mg in 24 hours) may be necessary until there are signs of atropinisation (dry skin, tachycardia, dilated pupils and dry mouth). Within the first 24 hours, use of an oxime (e.g. pralidoxime) will help to reactivate cholinesterase. Diazepam may reduce mortality. A clear airway must be maintained and assisted ventilation may be necessary.

Carbamate insecticides

Carbamate insecticides produce identical symptoms and atropine is again the treatment of choice. However, because these compounds have a reversible effect on cholinesterase, their duration of action is much shorter and pralidoxime is contraindicated in poisoning with these agents.

Herbicides

The five major groups of herbicides are: chlorates, triazines, bipyridilium herbicides, dinitro compounds and phenoxyacetic acids.

Chlorates

The chlorates are powerful oxidising agents which can produce haemolysis, methaemoglobinaemia, haemorrhagic gastroenteritis and, in severe cases, renal failure. Treatment consists of emptying the stomach (if appropriate) and methylene blue to reverse methaemoglobinaemia.

Triazines

Triazine herbicides (e.g. simazine) appear to be relatively non-toxic and serious human poisoning has not been reported.

Bipyridilium herbicides (paraquat)

The bipyridilium herbicides, particularly paraquat, are extremely toxic. Not only can they cause local corrosion, but systemic absorption leads to renal and liver damage and later progressive pulmonary fibrosis. Diquat causes similar toxicity although pulmonary fibrosis seems to be slightly less likely to occur. Treatment consists of gastric lavage with care because of the corrosive effects of the toxin. Fuller's earth or bentonite is left in the stomach as an adsorbent for paraquat and magnesium sulphate or mannitol is used to purge the gut and remove any remaining material. Finally, haemodialysis and haemoperfusion have been tried in an attempt to remove the body burden of drug, but there is no evidence that either has any effect on the mortality, particularly when the more concentrated solutions (e.g. Gramoxone) are ingested.

Dinitro compounds

Dinitro compounds (e.g. dinitroorthocresol) are generally used in the form of washes for fruit trees. They cause yellow staining of the skin but can be absorbed subcutaneously and produce toxicity by uncoupling oxidatative phosphorylation. This results in pyrexia, hyperpnoea and tachycardia with subsequent sweating, thirst, dehydration and collapse. Treatment consists of preventing severe pyrexia and replacement of electrolytes and fluid. Pentachlorophenol acts similarly to the dinitro compounds, but does not produce yellow discolouration of the skin.

Phenoxyacetic acids

Phenoxyacetic acids are probably the most widely used herbicides. They are relatively non-toxic unless large doses have been ingested; signs of cholinergic hyperactivity are then evident resulting in coma and occasionally ventricular arrhythmias. The stomach should be emptied if appropriate, contaminated clothing removed and the skin washed with soap and water. With 2-4-D and mecoprop, forced alkaline diuresis may enhance their rate of removal and should be considered in severely poisoned patients.

Fungicides

Organic and inorganic mercurials, organotin derivatives and dithiocarbamates are all used as fungicides in industry and horticultural practice. Organotin compounds are poorly absorbed from the gastrointestinal tract and therefore have low toxicity; dithiocarbamates are also relatively non-toxic.

Organic mercurials

Inhalation or ingestion of organic mercurials can produce severe corrosion and irritation of the respiratory tract. CNS toxicity consists of tremor, memory and psychiatric disturbances, and visual impairment which may lead to blindness. The chelating agent, dimercaprol, may reduce the systemic toxicity.

Inorganic mercurials

Inorganic mercurial fungicides (e.g. mercuric chloride) are also predominantly corrosive. Inorganic mercury salts are sometimes present in disc or button batteries which may break. Severe local corrosion or systemic mercury toxicity can occur. Treatment includes gastric lavage, adequate analgesia and treatment of any complications. Mercurous chloride and mercuric oxide (the most commonly used agents) are poorly absorbed and, although corrosive, systemic toxicity is unlikely. If albuminuria occurs, however, significant absorption may have taken place and plasma mercury concentration should be measured. Treatment is as for organic mercurials.

Metallic mercury

Ingestion of metallic mercury is of no major consequence. However, intramuscular injection of metallic mercury may cause systemic toxicity, and intravenous injection has resulted in pulmonary embolus.

Rodenticides

Many rodenticides contain warfarin or related coumarin anticoagulants and, unless taken in huge amounts, generally cause few symptoms. If the INR does rise, vitamin K should be administered as for warfarin overdose. Alpha-chloralose is a hypnotic agent related to the chloral hypnotics and can cause drowsiness and coma if taken in large amounts by children. Treatment is as for chloral hydrate overdose. Chloroacetic acid derivatives are only used as rodenticides for commercial purposes but are highly toxic. They can be absorbed subcutaneously and orally and produce muscle twitching, tremor, cardiac arrhythmias, convulsions and coma. Cyanides are sometimes used as rabbit killers.

Arsenic is sometimes used as a rodenticide and also as a timber treatment. Symptoms of overdose are similar to those of tetanus. Sensory stimuli should be minimised by nursing in a darkened room; convulsions should be treated with diazepam. In severe cases, neuromuscular blockers may be needed to paralyse the patient while ventilation is supported mechanically.

POISONOUS PLANTS AND FUNGI

Although the number of plants that have been suggested to be poisonous is extremely high, many of these contain only small amounts of toxins and generally do not cause severe poisoning. They can be classified into those:

- producing cholinergic (nicotinic) stimulation
- producing cholinergic (muscarinic) stimulation
- with anticholinergic activity
- with gastrointestinal activity
- with effects on the heart
- with convulsant activity
- with hallucinogenic effects
- with dermatological effects
- with toxicity on other organs.

Plants with cholinergic (nicotinic) activity

Alkaloids similar to nicotine are found in the hemlock (coniine) and laburnum (cytisine). Nausea and vomiting may be followed in severe poisoning by confusion, hallucinations, convulsions and finally coma and respiratory arrest. Treatment for severe poisoning is as for nicotine. The stomach should be emptied and activated charcoal administered. Monitoring of fluid and electrolytes and adequate replacement therapy, together with measures to assist the respiration and cardiovascular functions, are generally only necessary in severe poisoning (rarely caused by laburnum).

Plants with cholinergic (muscarinic) activity

Plants with cholinergic activity include the clitocybe and inocybe fungi. Ingestion produces increased perspiration, abdominal pain and visual disturbances. Treatment is with atropine.

Plants with anticholinergic activity

Plants with anticholinergic activity include the deadly nightshade (*Atropa belladonna*), the thorn apple and henbane. In addition to atropine these plants may contain hyoscine and hyoscyamine. The symptoms are similar to those caused by drugs with anticholinergic activity (e.g. tricyclic antidepressants). Neostigmine is sometimes used to counteract the peripheral anticholinergic effects, but treatment with physostigmine is rarely necessary or indicated.

Plants with gastrointestinal toxicity

Oxalates present in some plants can cause local gastrointestinal irritation and painful ulceration of the mouth if chewed by children. These include the household plants, dumbcane (dieffenbachia) and some of the monstera and philodendron species. Other plants contain irritant resins and saponins (e.g. arum, yew, bryony, and daphne mezereum), which can cause severe vomiting and diarrhoea. Delayed gastrointestinal symptoms can be caused by the beans of the Abrus species (e.g. Ricinus and Robinia) as these contain compounds which can impair RNA synthesis. Solanum species also produce delayed gastrointestinal symptoms; these include potatoes which have been allowed to sprout, and woody and black nightshades. Treatment is supportive, with replacement of fluids and electrolyte loss.

Plants causing cardiovascular disturbances

Digitalis glycosides are found not only in the foxglove but also in lily of the valley (Convallaria). Treatment is as for digitalis poisoning. The aconitine present in the monkshood and delphinium may cause bradycardias and muscular weakness.

Plants with convulsant activity

Cicuta virosa (cowbane) and *Oenanthe crocata* (hemlock water dropwort) contain potent alcohols with effects similar to picrotoxin in antagonising the CNS inhibitory effects of γ-amino butyric acid. In severe cases, nausea, vomiting and hypersalivation are followed by convulsions and respiratory failure. Convulsions can be controlled with either short-acting barbiturates or diazepam; respiration may require support until the effects of the toxin wear off.

Strychnine is an alkaloid present in the seeds of the tree *Strychnos nux-vomica*, native to India. It is used predominantly as a rodenticide and produces severe muscular spasms which may respond to short-acting barbiturates or to diazepam. Sensory stimulation should be minimised, since it may provoke convulsions; assisted ventilation may also be necessary. Once convulsions have been controlled, the stomach should be emptied and charcoal left inside. Acute renal failure and hepatic necrosis may occur after strychnine poisoning.

Plants with hallucinogenic effects

In addition to those anticholinergic agents with hallucinogenic effects, there are several other hallucinogens in plants and fungi. These include the psilocin and psilocybin in psilocybes (magic) mushrooms, the tetrahydrocannabinols in cannabis, and the ibotinic acid and muscimol found in *Amanita muscaria*. Tranquillisers may be necessary if the patient is a risk to himself or to others, and adequate supervision must be given until the hallucinations subside.

Plants which cause dermatological toxicity

Plants contain substances which can either cause direct chemical irritation (e.g. histamine and oxalic acid) or delayed hypersensitivity reactions (e.g. *Primula obconica*, the hogweeds, which can produce photoallergic dermatitis, and several other species). Treatment is symptomatic.

Plants with toxicity on other organs

The lectins present in the seeds of *Ricinus communis* not only cause delayed gastrointestinal tract symptoms but may also lead to liver and lung damage. Ricin is the most potent toxin known to man. Management is purely supportive.

Severe liver damage can also be caused by the phallotoxins and amatoxins found in *Amanita phalloides* and some of the other Amanita species. Vomiting, abdominal pain and diarrhoea often occur 6–12 hours after ingestion, while albuminuria, haematuria, renal failure and liver failure may occur around 2–3 days later. Treatment consists of emptying the stomach and replacement of fluid loss. Specific antidotes are of unproven value, but thioctic acid and high doses of penicillin may be of value in preventing the liver and renal damage.

POISONOUS ANIMALS

Adder evenomation

The adder, *Vipera berus*, is the only indigenous poisonous snake in Western Europe. Only 50% of those bitten develop signs of evenomation, which may occur either immediately, with shock, vomiting and explosive diar-

rhoea, or several hours later. The initial collapse may be due to activation of the kinin system; the later shock is more often due to hypovolaemia, caused by increased capillary permeability and fluid loss into the swollen limb, and direct cardiotoxicity of the venom.

Management

Treatment includes reassurance since shock may be exacerbated by the fear of impending toxicity. The limb should be kept still, but a ligature should not be used unless there is likely to be a delay of more than half-an-hour between the patient having been bitten and transfer to hospital. If a ligature is used, it should only be tight enough to prevent venous return but not to obstruct arterial inflow. The patient should be admitted and observed for at least a day after the bite. Pulse and blood pressure should be recorded, together with urinary output and fluid losses from diarrhoea and vomiting. Local swelling should also be noted and the white cell count, urea and electrolytes should be measured each day.

The use of Zagreb antivenom should be considered if hypotension persists, ECG signs occur, the white count rises markedly to above 20 000/mm^3 or, in an adult, severe swelling has extended up the limb within 2 hours after the bite. Anaphylactic reactions to the antivenom occur in 1% of patients and so antivenom should only be used when the above indications are present. A history of asthma or allergy is a relative contraindication to its use. Antivenom is given by slow intravenous infusion and is stopped at the first signs of allergic reaction. Adrenaline solution must be drawn up prior to administration of the antivenom and given intramuscularly if a reaction occurs (intravenously in the case of a severe reaction).

Deaths from adder bite are extremely rare, but local tissue necrosis may be severe, particularly in adults.

Fish evenomation

In the UK, the only venomous fish regularly found are the Weever fish (*Trachinus vipera*), which is found around the coast in the summer months, and the Lion fish (an aquarium species). Both contain heat labile venom in their spiny dorsal fins, which causes severe local pain. Hypotension, and myocardial and respiratory depression may develop.

Management

Treatment is to remove any barbs and clean the wound, immersing the limb in water as hot as can be tolerated without discomfort to destroy the toxin. The wound should be examined at a later stage for signs of secondary infection.

3 Drug Overdose and Poisoning

Venomous invertebrates

The Portuguese man of war (Physalia) is the only poisonous jellyfish found around the coasts of the UK. Its sting contains substances capable of releasing histamine and other kinins. Local pain is common, but more serious symptoms include abdominal pain, dyspnoea, hypotension, muscular paralysis and convulsions.

Management

The wound should be bathed in vinegar solution (4–6% acetic acid), and any tentacles still adherent to the wound removed with adhesive tape.

Arthropod evenomation

Wasp and bee stings contain amines, kinins, peptides and enzymes which cause local pain, erythema and swelling. Systemic effects are rare unless the stings are numerous or the subject is hypersensitive, in which case even a single sting may kill. Initial symptoms are generalised urticaria, flushing, dizziness, bronchospasm, collapse and coma. Serum sickness may occur after a week or more.

Management

The sting should be removed, taking care not to squeeze it and inject more venom. Severe pain may respond to local anaesthetic or aspirin. Anaphylaxis should be treated immediately with adrenaline (0.5–1 ml of a 0.1% solution). Severe respiratory tract obstruction may be caused by stings in the mouth, even in those patients who are not hypersensitive. In allergic individuals, specific venoms have been used in increasing doses to produce desensitisation.

Poisonous seafoods

Seafood may contain bacteria (e.g. vibrio, salmonella) or viruses (e.g. hepatitis A); toxicity may also occur as a result of contamination by dinoflagellates or decomposition by bacteria.

Antemortem infestation by dinoflagellates of certain subtropical fish (such as groupers and snappers) may occur, but contamination usually involves shellfish, such as mussels, oysters, scallops and clams. The dinoflagellates contain neurotoxins (e.g. saxitoxin) which can cause nausea, vomiting and diarrhoea, followed by circumoral paraesthesiae, ataxia, muscular weakness and, in severe cases, respiratory paralysis. Treatment is symptomatic, with respiratory and cardiovascular support.

Postmortem contamination of some oily fish such as mackerel, skipjack and tuna, sardines and pilchards by Proteus bacteria may result in production of histamine and other unidentified toxins which produce urticaria, flushing, abdominal pain, nausea, vomiting and diarrhoea and, in some cases, bronchospasm. The effects occur around 4 hours after ingestion, last only a few hours and are seldom severe. Treatment is symptomatic. Prevention involves keeping the raw fish frozen or on ice to prevent decomposition by bacteria.

POISONING BY METALS

Iron

Although mortality from iron poisoning has fallen in recent years, it remains one of the most dangerous metals in overdose. Children are particularly sensitive to its effects. Abdominal pain, nausea and vomiting are often followed by gastrointestinal bleeding, encephalopathy, metabolic acidosis, pulmonary oedema, acute renal failure and liver failure. A serum iron level greater than 5 mg/l (90 μmol/l) in a child, or greater than 8 mg/l (145 μmol/l) in an adult, within 4 hours of the overdose, is associated with an increased likelihood of severe poisoning.

Management

The stomach should be emptied if more than 15 tablets have been ingested within the previous 4 hours. Desferrioxamine (2 g/l of warm water) should be used as lavage fluid, and a further 5 g per 50 ml water left in the stomach after lavage. Radiography of the abdomen will reveal whether or not the tablets have been removed. If the patient has clinical evidence of severe iron poisoning, desferrioxamine should also be administered both intramuscularly (2 g/10 ml water) and by slow intravenous infusion (15 mg/kg per hour to a maximum of 80 mg/kg in 24 hours, to prevent hypotension induced by the desferrioxamine). With prompt treatment, the mortality should be less than 5% in severe cases.

Summary 8 Iron poisoning

- Children are particularly sensitive to the toxicity of iron

- Abdominal pain, nausea and vomiting may be followed by gastrointestinal haemorrhage, encephalopathy and renal and hepatic failure

- Severe poisoning is normally associated with plasma concentrations (4 hours after ingestion) greater than 5 mg/l in children and 8 mg/l in adults

- Gastric lavage with desferrioxamine and intra-muscular and intravenous desferrioxamine should be given in severe iron poisoning

---

Heavy metal poisoning

Heavy metals can cause acute or chronic symptoms, depending on the dose and duration of exposure. Acute ingestion of most heavy metals will cause gastroenteritis. Generalised convulsions may also be seen, particularly with lead poisoning, and renal failure and cardiac arrhythmias have also been recorded. Inhalation of heavy metal fumes may cause chemical pneumonitis and, in severe cases, pulmonary oedema and a syndrome known as 'metal fume fever' may occur several hours after the inhalation of some metallic oxides.

Chronic effects of heavy metal exposure are similar but milder. Chronic gastrointestinal symptoms and CNS effects occur, particularly after exposure to lead, manganese and mercury. Lead, thallium, bismuth and arsenic can also produce peripheral neuropathy, and renal damage may be caused by gold, lead, cadmium and mercury. Inhalation of heavy metal fumes can cause pulmonary fibrosis, particularly with beryllium, cadmium, tungsten, titanium and cobalt. An emphysematous picture has been seen with cadmium, and an asthma-like syndrome may occur as a result of sensitivity to chromium, vanadium and platinum. Nickel, chromium, cobalt, platinum and beryllium may also cause skin sensitisation and subsequent dermatitis.

Diagnosis is helped by taking a full occupational history. Clinical examination may reveal specific signs of poisoning, such as the blue line on the gums in chronic mercury poisoning or the raindrop pigmentation of the skin in arsenic poisoning. Toxicological examination of the urine, blood, or hair and nail clippings may also help, but this often has to be performed in specialised centres.

Management

Treatment consists of preventing further exposure to the heavy metal, treatment of the complications of poisoning, and chelation therapy to enhance the elimination of the metal already absorbed. It must be remembered, however, that most chelating agents are toxic and should only be used when their benefits are likely to outweigh the risks of their use. Sodium calcium edetate is the treatment of choice for lead poisoning. It must be given by slow intravenous infusion. Dimercaprol is effective in severe mercury and arsenic poisoning. Penicillamine is the treatment of choice for copper poisoning and has the advantage that it may be given by mouth. Finally, Prussian Blue has been used successfully in the treatment of thallium poisoning.

FURTHER READING

Ellenhorn M J, Barceloux D G 1988 Medical Toxicology: Diagnosis and treatment of human poisoning. Elsevier, New York. *A comprehensive reference text.*

Olson K R ed 1990 Poisoning and drug overdose. Appleton and Lange, Norwalk, USA. *A pocket-sized but relatively detailed guide to management of poisoning.*

APPENDIX

Information, analytical and clinical services in the United Kingdom and Eire.

National Poisons Information Service

Belfast	0232 240503
Cardiff [*+]	0222 709901
Dublin [+]	010 3531 379964
	010 3531 379966
Edinburgh	031 229 2477
	031 228 2441
	(SPIB Viewdata)
London [+]	071 635 9191
	071 407 7600

Other Centres

Birmingham [*+]	021 554 3801
Leeds	0532 430715
Newcastle [*]	091 232 5131

[*] Poisons Treatment Unit
[+] 24-hour Toxicological Analysis

4

Physical and Environmental Causes of Disease

John Moxham, Robert L Souhami
and J Malcolm Walker

DISORDERS DUE TO HEAT AND COLD

Heat produced by metabolism is lost mainly through the skin and, to a lesser extent, through the gut, urine and breath. Inadequate heat loss leads to sweating and vasodilatation. Cold produces cutaneous vasoconstriction and shivering which results in increased muscle metabolism. In moving from a cold to a hot climate, acclimatisation occurs over a period of 1–2 weeks; this process is not well understood. There is increased sweating and the salt content of sweat diminishes. Aldosterone secretion increases, at least at first, causing a low urinary sodium with loss of potassium.

HEAT EXCESS

Three syndromes due to excess heat occur: heat cramps, heat exhaustion and heatstroke.

Heat cramps

Spasms of painful muscular contraction may occur with sudden rises in temperature during strenuous activities such as long-distance running, or during work in very hot environments. Muscles of the legs and arms are usually affected, typically after the exertion or heavy work is over. There is usually hyponatraemia, and severe cramps may be accompanied by a rise in creatine phosphokinase and evidence of rhabdomyolysis. Part of the pathogenesis appears to be due to replacement of fluid and salt loss by water with too low a salt content; the condition is preventable by drinking fluids containing 0.25% saline.

Heat exhaustion

Heat exhaustion or heat collapse is the commonest syndrome and is especially likely to occur in individuals exposed to a hot environment for a few days, before they are acclimatised. The very young and the elderly (especially those on diuretics) are particularly at risk. The syndrome is due in part to salt and water loss, and in part to a failure of circulatory adaptation to heat.

When water loss predominates, there is intense thirst and weakness, agitation and confusion. Haemoconcentration occurs with a rise in haematocrit and blood urea. With salt depletion, there are muscle cramps, headaches, vomiting and myalgia. Usually, salt and water depletion occur together, and the patient has a normal temperature, and appears pale and clammy.

The disorder is treated by rest and oral fluids containing salt; it is seldom necessary to administer intravenous fluids.

Heatstroke

Heatstroke is a serious and sudden disease which may be fatal unless treated urgently. It is due to a failure of thermoregulation, resulting in a rapid rise in body temperature. The patient is usually elderly, often with underlying disease such as cardiac failure, diabetes, obesity or alcoholism. Atropine-like drugs, beta-blockers, phenothiazines and diuretics predispose to the syndrome. Heatstroke can also occur in fit men working in hot environments, and there are some clinical differences in these cases.

Typically the patient develops headache, dizziness and faintness, and abdominal pain and delirium may occur. Sweating stops and the body temperature rises rapidly (and may reach 43°C). Hypotension, renal failure and rhabdomyolysis may occur; the latter is especially common in heatstroke following severe exertion. Sweating may continue in this form of heatstroke.

On examination, the skin is hot and usually dry, and the patient exhibits tachypnoea and flaccidity. Coma and shock are grave signs. The blood shows leucocytosis and respiratory alkalosis (but may be acidotic in the exertional form), the urea is raised and hypokalaemia and hyperphosphataemia occur. Myocardial necrosis may give ST

Summary 1 Clinical features of heatstroke

Symptoms
- Headache
- Dizziness/faintness
- Abdominal pain

Signs
- Increased body temperature
- Hot, dry skin (sweating may be absent)
- Tachypnoea
- Flaccidity
- Hypotension
- Delirium → shock/coma

Results/complications
- Hepatic and renal failure
- Leucocytosis, alkalosis/acidosis, hypokalaemia
- Rhabdomyolysis
- Myocardial necrosis
- Disseminated intravascular coagulation

changes and even an infarction pattern on the ECG. Liver function tests are abnormal, and acute renal failure may occur. Disseminated intravascular coagulation is present in mild degree in the elderly, but may be severe in exertional heatstroke.

Management

Treatment is of the utmost urgency. The patient must be cooled as quickly as possible. The most effective way is immersion in very cold water, the skin being rubbed to increase the efficiency of cooling. An alternative is to blow cold air over dampened skin. Core temperature must be monitored using a rectal thermometer. Hypotension can be treated with small quantities of saline, with care to avoid circulatory overload. Hypoglycaemia, if present, can be treated with glucose, and severe acidosis by sodium bicarbonate. More serious complications, such as acute renal failure and disseminated intravascular coagulation, are treated in the usual way (Chs 20 and 24).

HYPOTHERMIA

Hypothermia is a common problem mainly affecting the elderly population, in whom the response to cold may be defective (p. 149). Hypothermia contributes to the excess mortality of the elderly during winter months. It occurs when the deep body temperature falls below 35°C. As the mouth temperature may fluctuate depending on the ambient air temperature, it is best to use a rectal thermometer when monitoring hypothermic patients. A low-reading thermometer is necessary.

Aetiology

Hypothermia may be due simply to an age-related impaired thermoregulatory response to a cold environment (Ch. 9, p. 149). In the majority of patients, however, there is an associated underying pathological cause, including any cause of autonomic dysfunction (p. 150). Hypothyroidism and hypopituitarism are both associated with hypothermia, and the risk is also higher in immobile or demented patients, or in the presence of an acute illness such as bronchopneumonia. There is a clear association between phenothiazines and impairment of temperature regulation, and hypothermia may also be precipitated by sedative drugs, such as hypnotics and alcohol.

Clinical features

Hypothermic patients typically live alone in poor housing with impaired mobility. A typical case would be that of an old person who gets out of bed in the middle of the night to go to the lavatory, falls, and then lies all night on the cold floor in thin night-clothes until discovered the next morning by a neighbour.

The skin has a greyish look due to a combination of vasoconstriction and cyanosis; the face may appear puffy, resembling myxoedema. The diagnosis is often first suspected during examination when it is found that the patient's skin feels cold in normally warm areas, such as the axilla or the abdomen. The patient is often confused, since drowsiness and loss of consciousness occur when the temperature falls below 32°C. Shivering is absent below this temperature; instead, there is increased skeletal muscle tone with neck stiffness and abdominal rigidity. The heart rate is slowed and the ECG may show a prolonged PR interval and J waves (Fig. 4.1). Respirations are slow and shallow, and there may be hypoxia and hypercapnia. Acute pancreatitis is often found at necropsy, but this is only rarely diagnosed in life.

Impaired renal and respiratory function may lead to a raised blood urea or bicarbonate. Blood sugar levels may be raised, but do not indicate diabetes mellitus, and will fall as the temperature returns to normal. Serum aspartate aminotransferase and creatine kinase may be raised due to muscle damage.

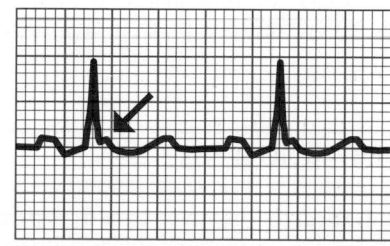

Fig. 4.1 Electrocardiogram showing J wave (arrowed) in a hypothermic patient.

4 Physical and Environmental Causes of Disease

Summary 2 Clinical features of hypothermia

- Confusion/impaired consciousness
- Cold, greyish skin
- Shivering absent
- Increased skeletal muscle tone
- Slow heart rate, prolonged PR interval and J waves
- Slow, shallow respiration, hypoxia and hypercapnia
- Raised blood urea or sugar levels
- Raised serum aspartate aminotransferase and creatine kinase

Management

The lower the deep body temperature, the higher the mortality (about 50% overall). The high mortality is because many hypothermic patients have a serious underlying illness. Patients with mild hypothermia (core temperature 32–35°C) should be wrapped in a space blanket and nursed in a side ward where the ambient temperature is 25–30°C. The patient's temperature should be allowed to rise *gradually*, at a rate of about 0.5°C per hour, as fast surface rewarming carries the risk of hypotension. For this reason, the patient's pulse and blood pressure must be monitored. If the blood pressure drops, the space blanket should be removed or the room temperature lowered so that the patient is temporarily cooled. A broad-spectrum antibiotic is usually given parenterally because bronchopneumonia is nearly always present, even if not clinically apparent. The ECG should be monitored, since both bradyarrhythmias and ventricular fibrillation may occur. The patient is at serious risk of developing a pressure sore and must be nursed on a suitable mattress and turned regularly.

When the deep body temperature is below 32°C, a more aggressive approach to resuscitation is sometimes advocated, although there is little evidence that this reduces mortality. These measures include positive pressure ventilation to correct hypoxia, measurement of central venous pressure, and active rewarming using a radiant heat cradle over the torso or warmed intravenous fluids.

Thyroid hormones should not normally be given to hypothermic patients. If there is good clinical or laboratory evidence of hypothyroidism, then tri-iodothyronine (5 μg) may be given by slow intravenous injection every 12 hours.

RADIATION SICKNESS

Ionising irradiation is of two broad types: photons (gamma and X-rays) and particulate (alpha and beta particles). Radiation dose is defined in a variety of ways.

The energy deposited *in a tissue* is measured in gray (Gy; 1 Gy = 1 J/kg). Since different types of radiation have different tissue effects, a unit called the sievert (Sv) is sometimes used to weight the radiation dose. Particulate radiations are absorbed according to their mass and energy, but do not penetrate deeply into tissues (see also Ch. 8, p. 135).

Exposure

Exposure to ionising irradiation comes about in three ways:

- *Background irradiation.* We are exposed to approximately 2–3 mSv per year from solar and geological irradiation in the form of photons. Of this, 80% is in the form of radon.
- *Medical exposure.* The therapeutic uses of ionising irradiation are described in Chapter 8. Accidental exposure of patients or staff has been rare since the advent of stringent precautions following the radiation-induced damage to skin and eyes in the early days of therapeutic and diagnostic radiation.
- *Military and industrial irradiation.* The atomic bombs dropped on Hiroshima and Nagasaki led to numerous cases of acute leukaemia and other cancers. Fallout from nuclear tests has increased annual background radiation by 1%. Industrial exposures also occur, the most dramatic example of which has been the ingestion of radium by radium dial painters from 1916 to 1926, resulting in a great increase in risk of bone sarcoma and cancer of the air sinuses of the skull. The recent accident in the Chernobyl nuclear power station resulted in many deaths due to acute radiation exposure, and an increase in background radiation over a wide geographical area.

Tissue damage

The tissue-damaging effect of ionising irradiation is probably related mainly to damage to DNA, leading to strand breakage and impaired reproductive integrity of the cell. Following whole-body exposure, there are certain tissues which are damaged acutely by relatively low doses:

- *Bone marrow.* This can regenerate after exposure to 10 Gy, but above this dose permanent aplasia may occur. The white count and platelet count begin to fall within 10 days of exposure.
- *Intestine.* Doses of 10 Gy or over cause severe loss of crypt cells leading to loss of villi and extensive ulceration.
- *Skin.* Erythema occurs at doses below 10 Gy. At 20 Gy, the skin starts to desquamate and ulcerate.
- *Lung.* Above 10 Gy in a single fraction, pneumonitis occurs and is increasingly severe with increase in dose.

Long-term changes include glomerular loss and interstitial nephritis, infertility, pulmonary fibrosis, neuronal loss and gliosis, intestinal stricture and hepatic fibrosis. The development of cancers occurs after a latent interval of several years.

Clinical features

After acute whole-body exposure, the clinical features depend on the received dose.

Following an initial period of nausea and vomiting (sometimes with parotid swelling), the patient may be relatively well for 7–10 days and then develop a syndrome of haematological failure. There is depression of the white count and platelets, with infection, bruising and bleeding. At the same time, skin reactions occur with desquamation, alopecia and ulceration. If the dose is above 15 Gy, the gastrointestinal syndrome may predominate and be the first sign of toxicity. In a patient with severe leucopenia, severe diarrhoea and fluid loss is followed by septicaemia from gut bacteria. This is almost always fatal. Higher doses of radiation (25–60Gy) cause cardiovascular collapse and shock.

Management

Management is supportive. Anti-emetics are given in the acute phase, and fluid losses from diarrhoea are replaced. Blood, platelets and antibiotics are used during the phase of myelosuppression and infection. Allogeneic bone-marrow transplantation may help the minority of patients for whom there is a donor, and in whom the haematological toxicity is the major life-threatening complication.

Accidental exposure to radionuclides is treated according to the isotope. Potassium iodide is given for ^{131}I ingestion, and soluble phosphate for ^{32}P overdose. Overdose with bone-localising isotopes (caesium, radium, strontium) is treated with EDTA and large doses of oral calcium.

Prognosis

With adequate treatment, most patients will survive exposures up to 10 Gy. Above this dose, bone-marrow failure and the intestinal syndrome are usually fatal.

DISORDERS DUE TO EXTREMES OF BAROMETRIC PRESSURE

ALTITUDE SICKNESS

The effects of reduced barometric pressure result from the low partial pressure of oxygen and reduced oxygen-carrying capacity of the blood. Figure 4.2 shows this relationship. Because of the sigmoid shape of the oxygen-dissociation curve, oxygen saturation is reasonably well maintained until an altitude of 5000 metres. A precipitous fall in saturation then occurs with increasing height. Commercial aircraft are maintained at a pressure equivalent to 2500 metres, so that no additional oxygen is needed unless a patient has severe cardiac or respiratory disease. If there is a loss of pressurisation, extra oxygen is made available through masks.

There are four recognised syndromes of altitude sickness:

- acute altitude sickness
- acute pulmonary oedema
- acute cerebral oedema
- chronic altitude sickness.

Acute altitude (mountain) sickness

This syndrome occurs in unacclimatised individuals who ascend rapidly to heights in excess of 2500 metres. People who are unfit, elderly or patients who have respiratory or cardiac disease are especially prone. The symptoms are headache, dyspnoea, malaise, nausea, vomiting and abdominal pain; these slowly subside over a week if not relieved by oxygen or by descent. Acetazolamide can alle-

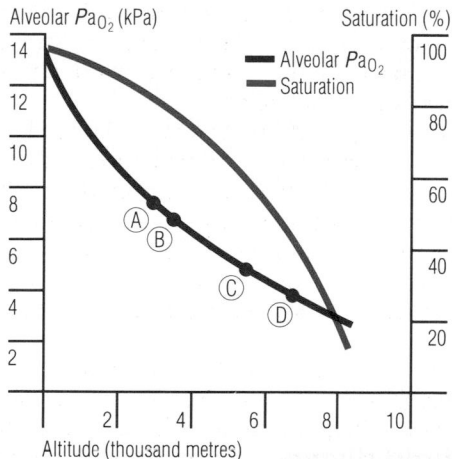

Fig. 4.2 Effect of altitude on alveolar Pa_{O_2} and oxygen saturation. Because of the steep slope of the oxygen dissociation curve, increasing altitude above 5000 metres causes a precipitous fall in saturation. In an unacclimatised person, acute changes occur at: (A) 3000 metres (10 000 feet) – slightly impaired memory and judgement, increased heart rate, abdominal cramps and nausea; (B) 3500 metres (12 000 feet) – headache, nausea, diminished visual acuity, and possible pulmonary oedema; (C) 5500 metres (18 000 feet) impaired consciousness after several hours in many people; and (D) 6750 metres (22 000 feet) – loss of consciousness.

viate the symptoms of acute altitude sickness by acting as a respiratory stimulant, lowering the P_{CO_2} and raising the P_{O_2}. It is advisable to start acetazolamide (250 mg b.d.) before ascent, and climbers should be warned of the side effects, particularly paraesthesiae.

Acute pulmonary oedema

Rapid ascent to heights greater than 3000 metres may provoke the sudden onset of acute pulmonary oedema. Hypoxia is the cause, but the pathogenesis is unclear. The symptoms usually begin 5–36 hours after ascent; acute dyspnoea, haemoptysis and widespread crackles in the lungs occur. Pathologically, there is acute oedema and a 'hyaline' membrane in bronchioles. Treatment is with evacuation to lower altitude and, failing that, oxygen and diuretics.

Acute cerebral oedema

Acute hypoxia increases cerebral blood flow, intracranial pressure, and can cause cerebral oedema. This is associated with headache and brain dysfunction, which can progress to coma and death.

Chronic altitude (mountain) sickness

Individuals who have lived for many years at altitudes above 4000 metres may develop polycythaemia and a chronic insensitivity of the respiratory centre to hypoxia. Such individuals hypoventilate and develop a raised P_{CO_2}. There is central cyanosis, with cough, headache and giddiness. The CNS symptoms are similar to those of polycythaemia rubra vera and are due to decreased cerebral blood flow (a consequence of the raised haematocrit) and hypoxia. Not all people living at high altitude develop this syndrome, which appears in part to be an excessive response to decreased inspired P_{O_2}. The syndrome can only be treated by descent to a lower altitude.

INCREASE IN BAROMETRIC PRESSURE

An increase in barometric pressure is encountered in diving or in mining.

Breathhold diving

During a breathhold dive the body directly encounters the increased pressure (1 atm for every 33 feet descent). The breathhold causes a rise in P_{CO_2} and a fall in P_{O_2}. The main respiratory stimulus is the raised P_{CO_2}, so that hyperventilation *before* diving leads to a lack of stimulus to breathe (due to CO_2 depletion). This may cause fatal loss of consciousness from hypoxia (which does not cause an irresistible urge to breathe and thus terminate the dive).

As the diver surfaces, decompression lowers P_{O_2} and again may cause loss of consciousness.

Decompression sickness

Deep diving and tunnel (caisson) work places a diver under an increased barometric pressure. When breathing air, the nitrogen dissolved in blood (P_{N_2}) increases and, on rapid decompression, forms bubbles which come out of solution in small blood vessels. Ischaemia results, causing pain in joints, spinal cord injury, chest pain, cyanosis, confusion, visual defects, paralysis and fits. Minor confusion occurs with lesser degrees of decompression injury. Treatment is by recompression followed by very gradual decompression over days.

Air embolism

Occasionally, a scuba diver breathing air may hold his/her breath while ascending rapidly, without breathing out. The gas expands in the lung and may disrupt it, causing air embolism with cerebral vascular occlusion leading to paralysis, fits and visual disturbance. Rapid recompression is necessary. Air embolism is a cause of death in these divers. Pneumothorax and air in soft tissues can also occur.

There is some evidence to suggest that some instances of systemic embolisation during diving occur in individuals who shunt blood from the right atrium to the left via a patent foramen ovale.

DROWNING AND NEAR-DROWNING

Drowning is a relatively common cause of accidental death, particularly in children. In adolescents and adults, alcohol and drugs are frequently a contributory factor. There are considerable differences in the osmotic pressure of salt water (5% NaCl), fresh water (0%, NaCl) and plasma (0.9% NaCl). It has been suggested that, when large amounts of salt water are aspirated into the lung, water may be sucked into the alveoli from pulmonary capillary plasma, causing death from pulmonary oedema. When fresh water is aspirated, however, large volumes may pass into the pulmonary circulation causing haemolysis and consequent potassium release, which may lead to cardiac arrest. In fact, in both cases, death usually results from acute reflex laryngospasm, causing asphyxia, most of the water entering the lungs only during the last few moments of life.

Resuscitation from near-drowning

A patient who is nearly drowned needs urgent resuscitation. The basic techniques are the same as for any 'sudden death', but the physiology of drowning raises special issues. In both fresh- and sea-water drowning, gastric aspiration must be performed once a cuffed endotracheal tube is in place. Large volumes of water tend to be swallowed during drowning. Similarly, ventilation with positive end expiratory pressure is required, once in hospital, to attempt to reinflate atelectatic and water-logged lungs.

Sea-water drowning is often associated with cardiac arrest produced by the rapid absorption of Ca^{2+} and Mg^+ into the blood. Treatment by basic life support is frequently effective in sea-water drowning, if begun within five minutes. Fresh-water drowning may produce massive intravascular haemolysis. It is associated with ventricular fibrillation and hyperkalaemia, which can be difficult to treat. Survival after fresh-water drowning during warm weather is unusual, but survival (with normal cerebral function) has been recorded in children, even after 30 minutes' immersion, particularly in low-temperature water.

Sudden death due to a combination of vagal slowing of the heart and intense peripheral vasoconstriction may occur in previously fit individuals who dive into cold water.

ELECTRIC SHOCK

Injury following electric shock depends on the voltage and current. Sudden death is less likely below 1000 volts. Alternating current appears to be much more dangerous than direct, since it produces muscle spasm and is more likely to stop the heart. The direction of flow is also important, as flow from hand to hand or hand to foot traverses the heart. At high voltage, the body heats up as the current flows. This heating is much more severe in a small cross-sectional area (fingers) than in a large one (trunk), and burns and charring are thus mostly found in the hands. Burns occur at the skin, and arcing of the current may ignite clothing, causing further burns.

Clinical features

With high voltage, cardiac arrest occurs. Cardiac resuscitation is essential, as is a careful assessment for burns which may manifest themselves later. Arrhythmias may recur for up to two days after resuscitation.

Intestinal perforation, and liver and gallbladder injury may occur. There may be cerebral and spinal cord damage, and peripheral nerves may be permanently damaged. Spinal cord injury may have a delayed onset, with paraplegia or a tabes-dorsalis-like syndrome. Acute muscle necrosis may result in renal failure.

Treatment

After resuscitation, the cardiac rhythm must be monitored for two days after the last rhythm disturbance. Renal failure due to rhabdomyolysis must be treated. A surgical assessment must be made of burns and charring, and peripheral circulation. Debridement, fasciotomy and even amputation may be necessary.

An extreme example of high-voltage injury is a lightning strike. Cardio-pulmonary resuscitation is essential as described above. Rhabdomyolysis and burns are treated in the same way as in other electric-shock injury. With effective resuscitation, over half the victims will survive.

SMOKE INHALATION

Smoke inhalation causes anoxia, frequently exacerbated by carbon monoxide poisoning and, if plastics are burned, hydrogen cyanide poisoning. Lung and airway injury is mainly chemical rather than thermal. Initial effects are mainly on the airways, including laryngeal oedema and bronchoconstriction; severe pulmonary oedema can develop. Factors predicative of severe injury include fire in an enclosed space, black sputum, burns around the mouth, reduced consciousness, altered voice, symptoms and signs of respiratory distress. In fires involving plastics, carboxyhaemoglobin levels generally reflect hydrogen cyanide levels. Treatment is supportive, including humidified oxygen, bronchodilators and mechanical ventilation in severe cases. Steroids are useful when airways obstruction is severe and persistent. Severe hydrogen cyanide poisoning requires treatment with sodium nitrite and thiosulphate. In patients surviving smoke inhalation injury the long-term prognosis for pulmonary function is good.

Passive smoking

Breathing other people's smoke is a much less serious cause of morbidity and premature death than active smoking, but it does represent one of the most serious causes of indoor air pollution that can affect health. Respiratory symptoms such as wheezing, coughing and the development of respiratory infections are increased in the children of smoking parents. The effect is particularly noticeable in children aged under one year. Various international expert committees have concluded that exposure to environmental tobacco smoke increases the incidence of lung cancer in non-smokers, the observed risk being some 30% higher than expected and contributing approximately 300 cases of lung cancer annually in the UK. There is also evidence that environmental tobacco smoke can exacerbate asthma in adults.

CHEMICAL WARFARE

Chemical weapons were first used on a large scale during the 1914–18 war, and although a wide range of chemicals were subsequently developed they were not used extensively until the Iran–Iraq war. Their use, but not their possession, is banned by an international treaty.

The agents most readily available are nerve gases and mustard gas (see below). Other chemical agents include lewisite, hydrogen cyanide, riot control agents such as CS gas, phosgene and chlorine. Biological weapons such as anthrax and Botulinus toxin are also potential weapons.

When the use of these weapons is threatened, protection of those involved in, or close to, the conflict with respirators and protective clothing is important. Obviously, civilian populations are very vulnerable. Rescue of casualties by medical teams may expose these personnel to risk, so they should also take preventative measures.

For all casualties of poisoning by chemical and similar weapons, decontamination is essential, particularly before they are transferred to areas where unprotected staff may be working.

Mustard gas (sulphur mustard) is on alkylating agent (like nitrogen mustard). It is a 'vesicant', causing skin blistering, sloughing of respiratory epithelium, ocular damage and, in a small number of cases, subsequent bone marrow depression. There is no antidote, and the treatment is supportive, including careful management of the skin damage, which often takes many months to treat.

Overall mortality of mustard gas exposure is only about 2%.

Nerve agents are organophosphorus compounds, closely related to insecticides. They inhibit the action of acetylcholinesterase leading to parasympathetic over-activity and ultimately neuromuscular blockade. Clinical manifestations are meiosis, bronchoconstriction, hypersecretion and hypersalivation, rapidly progressing to general paralysis (including the respiratory muscles), convulsions and death. These events may occur in minutes so rapid treatment is essential; this includes the use of atropine and oximes (which reactivate acetylcholinesterase). If there is a risk of nerve gases being used, pretreatment with pyridostigmine, which binds reversibly to acetylcholinesterase and thus 'protects' it from the effects of the nerve gas, is useful. Many armies now equip personnel with individual antidote packs for use in the field.

FURTHER READING

Callaham M L (ed) 1987 Current therapy in emergency medicine. BC Decker,Philadelphia. *A comprehensive textbook of emergency medicine.*

Howard J, Tyrer F H 1987 Textbook of occupational medicine. Churchill Livingstone, Edinburgh. *A comprehensive and very readable text book describing environmental and work hazards.*

Raffle P A B, Lee W R, McCallum R I, Murray R 1987 Hunter's diseases of occupations. Hodder and Stoughton, London. *A traditional and comprehensive text covering the entire field of occupational medicine.*

Skinner D, Driscoll P, Earlam R (ed) 1991 ABC of major trauma. BMV Books, London. *A concise, practical account of important topics in major trauma.*

5

The Genetic Basis of Disease

Robin M Winter

In the Western World, chronic diseases with a substantial genetic component occur in 5–10% of the adult population. Furthermore, more than one in 50 babies have a recognisable congenital anomaly at birth, many of which will have a genetic cause. Genetic disorders and malformations account for around 30% of paediatric hospital admissions and up to 50% of deaths under the age of 15 years. The relative frequency of the different types of genetic disorders in the United Kingdom is shown in Figure 5.1.

In certain populations, specific genetic disorders are of such high incidence as to represent significant public health problems, e.g. the thalassaemias in Mediterranean and Oriental populations, and sickle cell anaemia and other haemoglobinopathies in Afro-Caribbean populations. The incidence of affected homozygotes with these disorders can be as high as one in 50 births in some areas.

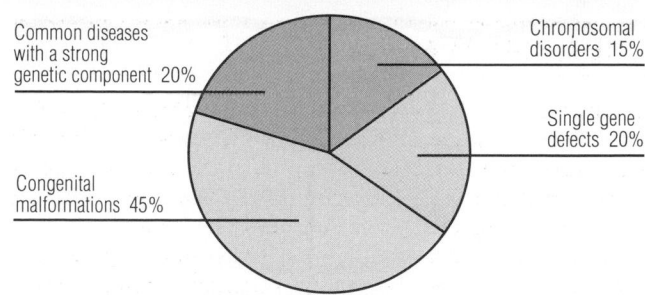

Fig. 5.1 The relative frequencies of different types of genetic disorder in the United Kingdom.

DNA, GENES AND CHROMOSOMES

The basic unit of inheritance is the gene. A gene is a length of *deoxyribonucleic* acid (DNA) which codes for a specific protein.

The DNA molecule is a double helix, i.e. it is formed from two interwoven strands. Each strand consists of a chain of nucleotides, and each nucleotide is made up of a deoxyribose sugar and a nitrogenous base. There are four possible nitrogenous bases: adenine (A), thymine (T), guanine (G) and cytosine (C). The deoxyribose sugars link to form the backbone of each strand, and the bases on each strand face each other and pair by hydrogen bonding. The base pairing is specific: adenine always pairs with thymine and guanine with cytosine. The specific base pairing allows DNA molecules to be copied precisely when cells divide.

A sequence of bases coding for a gene is usually divided into coding regions (exons) and non-coding regions (introns). DNA is *transcribed* by synthesising a single strand *ribonucleic* acid (RNA) molecule, using one of the DNA strands as a template. The resultant *messenger* RNA (m-RNA) molecule is processed, to splice out the noncoding regions and to modify each end, and then migrates into the cytoplasm where it directs the synthesis of a specific protein by a process known as *translation*. This process involves the interaction of the m-RNA with both *ribosomes* in the cytoplasm and a series of molecules known as *transfer* RNA (t-RNA) (Fig. 5.2). t-RNA is a specialised molecule, to which can be attached a specific amino acid. Each t-RNA carries a three-base coding region, which pairs specifically with a corresponding sequence of three bases on the m-RNA. The sequence of three bases is known as a *codon* and is specific for each amino acid. The sequence of codons makes up the *genetic code*. There are also three codons which determine the end of a protein; these are known as *stop codons*.

A gene may occupy a sequence of one to tens of kilobases (one kilobase = 1000 base pairs), depending on the length of the resultant protein and the number of introns

5 The Genetic Basis of Disease

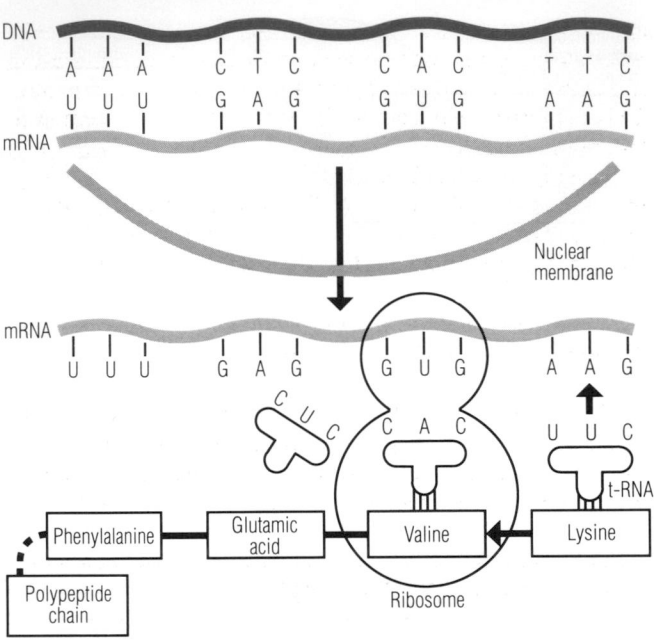

Fig. 5.2 DNA transcription and translation (after Emery A E H. An Introduction to Recombinant DNA, John Wiley, London, 1984). See text for details.

in the gene. A *chromosome* consists of a continuous molecule of DNA coding for many thousands of genes. In a chromosome, DNA is intricately coiled and combined with proteins, including *histones*, which results in a compact structure that can be seen with a light microscope. Often, special stains are used, which create a pattern of light and dark bands. These band patterns are specific for each chromosome, and reflect their macrostructure. Figure 5.3 demonstrates the relative size of a gene, in relation to a chromosome band and the chromosome itself.

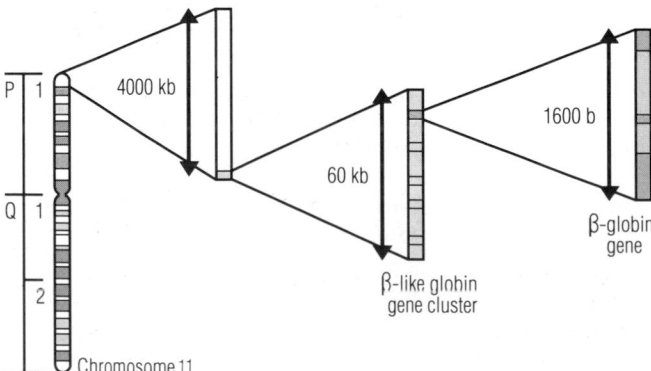

Fig. 5.3 The size of a gene relative to a chromosome and chromosome band, illustrated by the β-globin gene. This is situated on chromosome 11 in band 11p15.5, which may contain around 4000 kb. The gene itself is around 1600 base pairs long and is part of a cluster of similar genes, the ß-like globin gene cluster.

WAYS OF LOOKING AT GENES

There are three basic steps in the analysis of the sequences of DNA that make up genes (Fig. 5.4):

1. *Use of restriction enzymes.* Restriction enzymes, which originate from bacteria, cut double stranded DNA at specific base sequences. The distance between such restriction enzyme recognition sites may range from one to tens of kilobases, so that the genome is cut into fragments of differing sizes.
2. *Electrophoresis and Southern blotting.* Fragments generated using restriction enzymes can be separated by electrophoresis on an agarose gel. The fragments are then denatured (i.e. double stranded DNA separates into single stranded DNA) and a mirror image of the pattern of fragments is made onto nitrocellulose paper by a process known as Southern blotting.
3. *Use of DNA probes.* At this stage, single stranded fragments of DNA have been separated according to size, and fixed onto the nitrocellulose filter paper. A gene probe must now be used to identify the individual gene sequences present in specific bands. A gene probe is a radioactively labelled single stranded length of DNA whose sequence is specific for a particular gene, or length of chromosome. It is sometimes made using m-RNA coding for a specific protein, by a

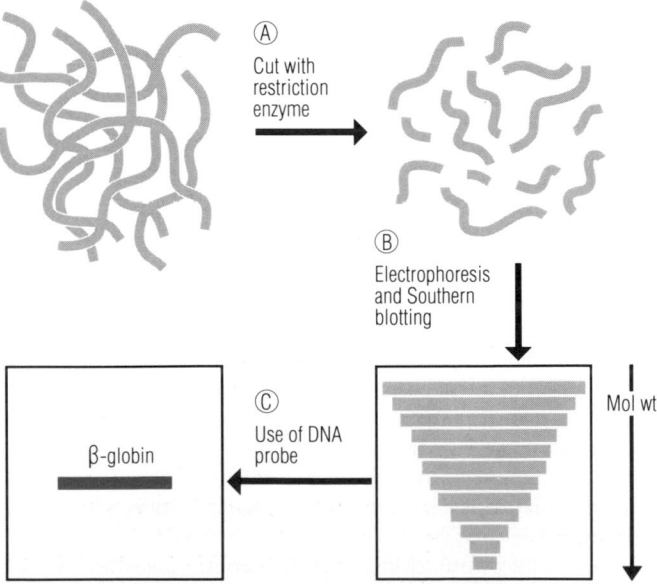

Fig. 5.4 DNA analysis. (A) DNA is cut at specific points by restriction enzymes into different sized fragments. (B) These fragments are separated by electrophoresis on an agarose gel and blotted onto nitrocellulose paper (Southern blotting). Specific genes cannot be visualised at this stage. (C) A radioactive DNA probe is used to locate a specific gene. The position of the gene on the gel depends on the size of the DNA fragment in which it is contained.

process known as reverse transcription. The single stranded probe recognises complementary sequences of DNA on the Southern blot, and anneals to them. Autoradiography can be used to locate the position of the gene probe, which will mark the position of all similar sequences on the Southern blot. If a gene-specific probe has been used, only a few bands will be seen on the autoradiograph, according to how many restriction enzyme recognition sites there are within the gene itself. Different restriction enzymes will generate different patterns, using the same probe. The position of the various restriction enzyme cutting sites within the gene can be inferred, and a *restriction map* produced.

Restriction fragment length polymorphism

The restriction enzyme cutting sites in and around genes are variable, as a common, harmless base change may create or destroy a cutting site. Thus, in some individuals, different patterns may be seen on Southern blotting using the same restriction enzyme and the same gene probe. This is because the gene in question will be contained in fragments of different lengths according to the presence or absence of specific cutting sites. Such *restriction fragment length polymorphisms* (RFLPs) are extremely important because they act as genetic markers, allowing abnormal genes to be tracked through families (Fig. 5.5).

TYPES OF SINGLE GENE MUTATION

At the molecular level, there are many mechanisms that can give rise to a malfunctioning gene (Table 5.1). The haemoglobinopathies best illustrate the full range of molecular defects which can occur.

CHROMOSOME STUDIES

Chromosomes are usually visualised during mitosis, at metaphase (p. 71). At this stage, they consist of two

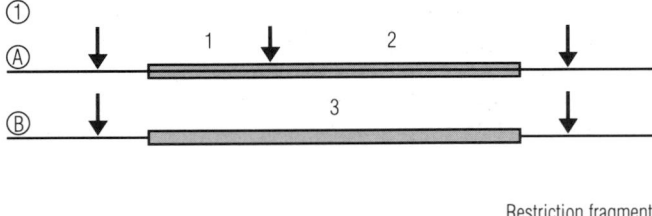

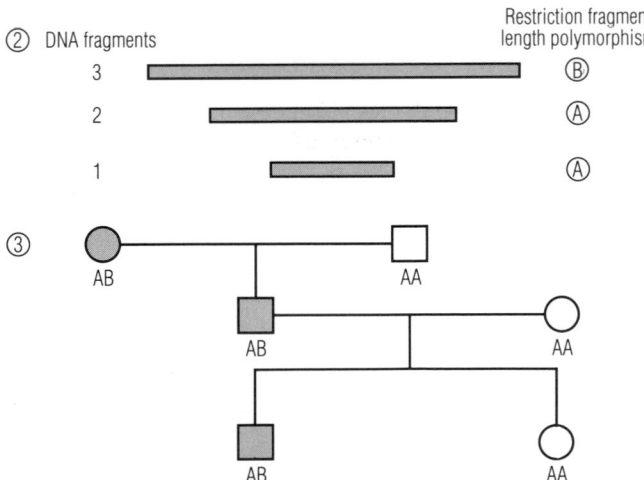

Fig. 5.5 Restriction fragment length polymorphism. (1) Shows the two alleles (A and B) of a gene at a specific locus. The alleles are represented by the coloured blocks on each of the two chromosomes. The arrows indicate restriction enzyme recognition sites. In allele A, there is an extra site in the middle of the gene so that when a DNA sample from this individual is cut with the restriction enzyme and a Southern blot made, three bands will be seen (2). The largest band represents allele B and the two smaller bands allele A. (3) Shows a pedigree where alleles A and B are being passed from generation to generation. Allele B causes an autosomal dominant disorder (e.g. neurofibromatosis) in this family so that the RFLP can be used to track the abnormal gene.

Table 5.1 Molecular mechanisms of single gene mutation, illustrated by the haemoglobinopathies

Abnormality of DNA	Effect	Example
Deletion of gene	Diminished or absent protein, depending on the number of genes involved	Most forms of α-thalassaemia
Point mutation (i.e single base change)	Substitution of a single amino acid in the protein	Sickle cell anaemia, Hb E, C and many other examples
	Creation of a stop codon leading to a short protein chain	Hb McKees Rocks, some forms of β-thalassaemia
	Removal of a stop codon, leading to an elongated protein chain	Hb Constant Spring (α-chain)
	Alteration of splicing signal	Some forms of α- and β-thalassaemia
Insertion or deletion of a number of nucleotides that are not a multiple of three	Frame-shift mutation	Hb Cranston, Tak and Wayne Some forms of β-thalassaemia
Fusion of genes	Absence of normal product and presence of a new protein resulting from the fused genes	Lepore haemoglobins involving β- and δ-globin chains (β-thalassaemias)

identical *chromatids*, joined together at the *centromere*. The position of the centromere is specific for each chromosome. In some chromosomes (1–3) the centromere is close to the centre of the chromosome (metacentric); in others (13–15, 21–22) it is near one end (acrocentric); while in the remaining chromosomes, the centromere is somewhere in between these two extremes (sub-metacentric). By convention, all chromosomes are divided by the centromere into a short arm (p) and a long arm (q).

Chromosome banding

Like other cell structures, chromosomes must be stained in order to visualise them with the light microscope. Using various methods, a pattern of bands can be produced, which is specific for each chromosome. A number of staining techniques are commonly used:

- *G (Giemsa) banding* is the most widely used technique. Light and dark bands are produced.
- *Q (quinacrine) banding* requires a fluorescent microscope. The band patterns are similar to G-banding. Certain chromosome structures, e.g. the long arm of the Y, are particularly well stained.
- *R (reverse) banding* produces a negative image of G-banding.
- *T (telomere) banding* preferentially stains the telomeres (ends of the chromosomes).
- *C (centromere) banding* stains centromeric regions.

Band nomenclature

The banding pattern is specific for each chromosome, and a convention exists for labelling each band. The long and short arms are divided into regions by particularly prominent bands (landmark bands) (Fig. 5.6). Within each region, individual bands are numbered from the centromere distally and landmark bands are included in the distal region they demarcate. Thus, in Figure 5.6, band 1q32 means band 2 in region 3 of the long arm (q) of chromosome 1.

Types of chromosome abnormality

Chromosome abnormalities can be divided into those involving the number of chromosomes, and those involving breakage or rearrangement.

Abnormalities in chromosome number

The normal diploid number of chromosomes in humans is 46. Individuals with chromosome counts that are not multiples of the normal haploid number (23) are said to be aneuploid. A fetus can receive higher multiples of the haploid number of chromosomes to give 69 (×3)

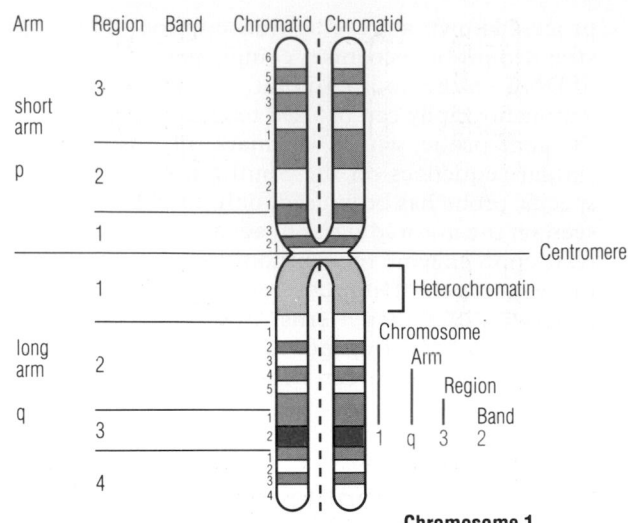

Fig. 5.6 Chromosome nomenclature, using chromosome 1 as an example.

or 92 (×4) chromosomes. Such triploid or tetraploid fetuses usually miscarry early.

If individuals carry one extra chromosome, they are said to be trisomic for the chromosome concerned. Very occasionally, an individual can have two extra chromosomes (double trisomy). Monosomy describes the situation where one chromosome is missing. In liveborn children, it is virtually only seen for the sex chromosomes, giving monosomy X (Turner's syndrome, p. 75).

Translocation, deletion and insertion

Breakage of chromosomes can result in loss of material (*deletion*), exchange of material between two non-identical chromosomes (*reciprocal translocation*), inversion of a segment of chromosome (*pericentric inversions* involve the centromere, *paracentric inversions* do not), and joining of the two ends of the same chromosome (to give a *ring chromosome*). Horizontal splitting of the centromere can result in a chromosome with identical long and short arms, an *isochromosome*. A translocation between the long arms of two acrocentric chromosomes, joined at the centromere, is known as a *Robertsonian translocation*. These possibilities are illustrated in Figure 5.7.

Karyotype nomenclature

The convention in karyotype nomenclature is to give the number of chromosomes first, followed by the types of sex chromosomes, followed by the types of any additional, missing or abnormal chromosomes. Thus, for example:

- 46,XX – normal female
- 45,X – Turner's syndrome

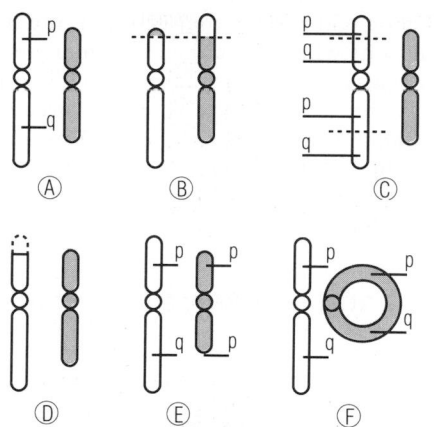

Fig. 5.7 Types of chromosome aberration. (A) Two normal non-homologous chromosomes. (B) A reciprocal translocation between the two chromosomes. Note that material has been exchanged between the short arms. (C) A pericentric inversion of the large chromosome. Breaks have occurred in the long and short arms and the middle segment of the chromosome has become inverted. (D) A deletion. The top part of the large chromosome has been lost. (E) An isochromosome. The small chromosome consists of two identical short arms due to mis-division after replication. (F) A ring chromosome. Both ends of the small chromosome have joined to form a ring.

- 47,XY + 21 – male with trisomy 21
- 69,XXY – triploidy, XXY sex chromosome complement
- 45,X/46,XX – mosaic Turner's syndrome.

For inversions or translocations, the numbers of the chromosomes involved are given in brackets (with the chromosome with the lowest number first). This is followed by the bands or regions involved in further brackets. Symbols are used to indicate the type of rearrangement involved. Thus, 46,XX,t(9;21)(q11;p11) karyotype means that chromosome 9 has broken at band q11 and chromosome 21 has broken at band p11. The small letter t (for translocation) indicates that material has been exchanged between the two chromosomes.

CELL DIVISION

Mitosis

Division of somatic cells is known as *mitosis*. This is divided into four stages (Fig. 5.8). Between cell divisions, in *interphase*, the chromosomes are extremely elongated and cannot be seen with the light microscope.

1. *Prophase*. As a preparation for cell division, the chromosomes replicate, to give the classical structure with two chromatids, and they begin to condense.
2. *Metaphase*. The chromosomes line up at the centre of the cell.

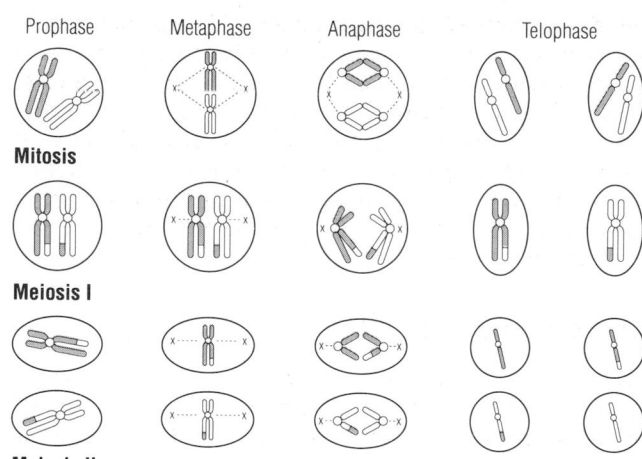

Fig. 5.8 Mitosis and meiosis: see text for details.

3. *Anaphase*. Each chromosome separates longitudinally at the centromere, and the two chromatids pass to opposite poles of the cell.
4. *Telophase*. Two new daughter cells are created by the formation of a nuclear envelope around each new set of chromosomes.

Meiosis

During the production of gametes, the normal diploid complement of 46 chromosomes must be reduced to the haploid number of 23 in the gametes by the process known as *meiosis*. During meiosis, there is the independent assortment of maternally and paternally derived genes in the different gametes of an individual. This is brought about by two separate means:

- Different gametes receive different combinations of maternally and paternally derived chromosomes.
- There is an exchange of genetic material between the two members of an homologous pair of chromosomes, known as *crossing over*. This process results in the creation of a chromosome containing part of the maternal and part of the paternal member of an homologous pair, known as a *recombinant* chromosome. Without crossing over, alleles on the same chromosome would always be inherited en bloc.

Crossing over takes place during the first step of meiosis (meiosis I) which is divided into prophase, metaphase, anaphase and telophase, as in mitosis. However, meiosis I differs in that homologous members of a pair of chromosomes line up and exchange genetic material during prophase, while at anaphase each member chromosome passes to an opposite pole without division at the centromere. Meiosis I is known as *reduction division*, because it results in the formation of two daughter cells containing 23 chromosomes, each of which has two chromatids that may not be identical because of crossing over.

The second step, meiosis II, is similar to mitosis except that each 'parent' cell now has only 23 chromosomes (each with two chromatids), and each 'daughter' cell contains 23 chromatids at telophase. Fusion of parental gametes at fertilisation restores the diploid number of chromosomes.

LOCI, ALLELES AND SEGREGATION

The genes determining a particular trait are situated at identical points or *loci* on each member of a homologous pair of chromosomes. The two genes on each chromosome at a particular locus may not be identical, and are known as *alleles*. If two alleles at a locus are identical, the individual is said to be *homozygous* at that locus; if the alleles are not identical, the individual is said to be *heterozygous*. The chance of a child inheriting one particular allele from a heterozygous parent is 1 in 2 (50%). For autosomal loci, if both parents are heterozygous, the chance of a child being homozygous for one particular allele is 1 in 4 (25%) (Fig. 5.9A).

If a locus is on the X chromosomes, males can only carry one allele (because they only have one X chromosome). They are said to be *hemizygous* for a particular allele. All daughters of a male hemizygous for an abnormal gene will receive that gene; on the other hand, none of the sons will receive the abnormal gene (because a male must pass on a Y chromosome to his sons, and not an X). Each time a heterozygous female has a child, there is a 50% chance it will be a boy, and if it is a boy, a 50% chance that he will be affected. Likewise there is a 50% chance of a girl and a 50% chance she will be heterozygous (Fig. 5.9B).

Dominant and recessive inheritance

Disorders where it is only necessary to carry one abnormal allele in order for an individual to be affected are said to be dominant. In autosomal dominant disorders, the abnormal gene is carried on a non-sex chromosome; in X-linked disorders, the gene is carried on the X chromosome.

In recessive inheritance, an individual is only affected if he or she does not carry a normal allele at all. For autosomal recessive inheritance, affected individuals will be homozygous for the abnormal allele and both of the parents will be heterozygote carriers. In X-linked recessive disorders, males hemizygous for the abnormal allele will be affected, whereas heterozygous females will be unaffected.

Typical pedigree patterns are shown in Figures 5.10 and 5.11.

New mutation, penetrance and gene expression

Abnormal alleles have to arise somewhere in a pedigree by the process of *new mutation*. Sometimes this can be inferred in a case where an affected individual for an autosomal dominant disorder has normal parents. However, many autosomal dominant disorders also display *incomplete penetrance* or *reduced expression*. This means the gene carriers sometimes show no signs, or only a few minor signs, of the condition. The two phenomena are therefore important in the context of genetic counselling.

If a person has an autosomal dominant disorder, but there is no family history, both parents must be examined very carefully in order to determine whether either of them carries the abnormal gene. If they do not carry the gene, the chance of them having a further affected child will be small (as this would require two, unconnected, new mutations). On the other hand, if one parent shows very minor signs of the condition, recurrence risk would be 50% for a further affected child.

Gene maps and linkage

The presence of loci close to one another on chromosomes leads to the phenomenon of linkage. The closer together

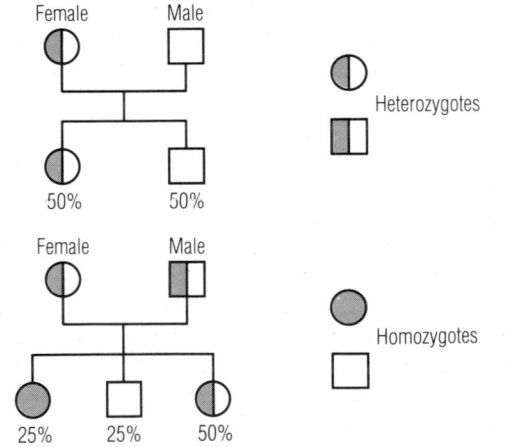

Fig. 5.9A Inheritance of alleles at autosomal loci.

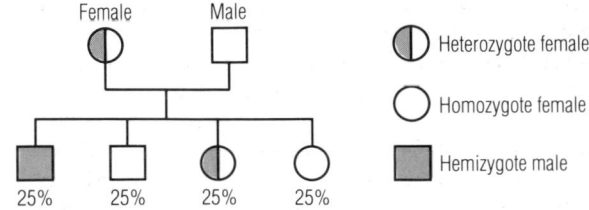

Fig. 5.9B Inheritance of alleles at X-linked loci.

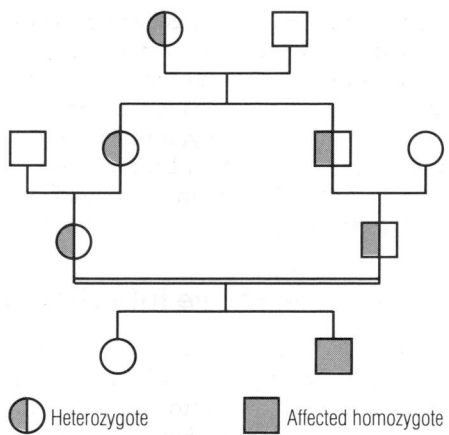

Fig. 5.10A **Autosomal recessive inheritance with first cousin parents**. The boy at the bottom of the pedigree is homozygous for an abnormal gene inherited from the great-grandmother through both parents. The double line indicates consanguineous marriage.

Legend: ◐ Heterozygote ▪ Affected homozygote

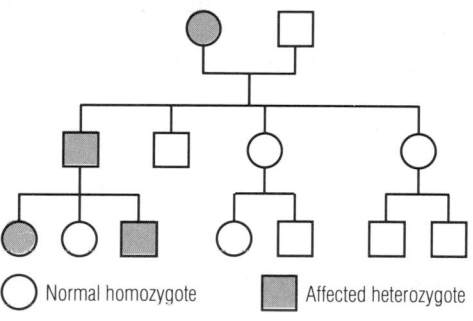

Fig. 5.10B **Autosomal dominant inheritance**. Note that the disease is passed on from parent to child and that both males and females are affected. There is also transmission of the disease from father to son.

Legend: ○ Normal homozygote ▪ Affected heterozygote

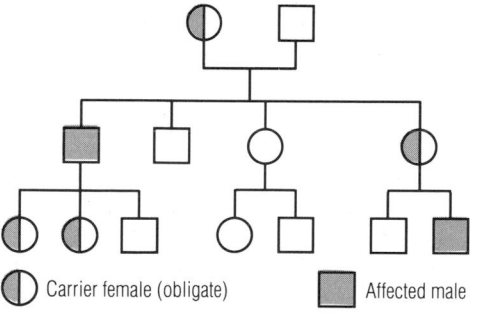

Fig. 5.11 **X-linked recessive inheritance**. Note that half of the sons of a carrier female are affected and half of the daughters are carriers. All the daughters of an affected male are carriers and all the sons are normal, because a male passes on his one X chromosome to his daughters and his Y chromosome to his sons.

Legend: ◐ Carrier female (obligate) ▪ Affected male

loci are on a chromosome, the lower the probability that a crossover will take place between them during meiosis I, and the higher the probability that two alleles inherited from the parent will be passed on *together* to an offspring. Linkage between loci can be studied in suitable families by looking at the joint inheritance of specific traits, and an estimate can be made of the distance separating the loci.

These family studies are informative for linkage but do not give information about the chromosomes on which the loci are situated. This problem is known as *gene assignment* and can be tackled by a number of different methods such as somatic cell hybrids. Using these methods, a human gene map is being constructed giving information about the assignment of various loci and their distance from other loci on the same chromosome.

CHROMOSOMAL DISORDERS

Frequency of chromosomal disorders

About 7 per 1000 babies are born with detectable chromosomal anomalies. Of these, 3 per 1000 will have sex chromosome anomalies, 1.5 per 1000 autosomal trisomies (mainly Down's syndrome) and the remaining 2.5 per 1000 will have chromosomal rearrangements. Most of the latter are balanced, i.e. no genetic material is lost or gained.

Of the autosomal trisomies, only trisomy 21 (Down's syndrome) cases are likely to survive into adulthood. The sex chromosome anomalies will frequently present with infertility or amenorrhoea. Unbalanced chromosomal rearrangements usually cause severe physical and mental handicap. However, balanced rearrangements have no effect on the carrier, although they predispose to recurrent miscarriage and children with unbalanced chromosome complements. An unbalanced karyotype means that there is duplication or deletion of some genetic material.

Down's syndrome

Between one in 700–1000 live births have Down's syndrome. The characteristic physical features are well described in paediatric texts and are present at birth, allowing immediate clinical diagnosis in most cases (Fig. 5.12). The head is foreshortened (brachycephaly) and there are usually three fontanelles. The eyes have an upward slant and crescents of skin are present covering the inner canthi (epicanthic folds). Brushfield spots are commonly seen on the iris. These are small white spots, situated around the outer third of the iris. The nasal bridge is flat and the tongue protuberant and deeply furrowed. A single transverse palmar crease is present on the hand, together with a short, incurved fifth finger (clinodactyly). A wide gap is present between the first and second toes, often with a longitudinal plantar crease. Hypotonia and delayed development are universal. Congenital heart defects (particularly A-V canal defects) and duodenal atresia can occur. It is essential that the chromosomal type of a Down's syndrome child is obtained. There are three possibilities (Table 5.2):

5 The Genetic Basis of Disease

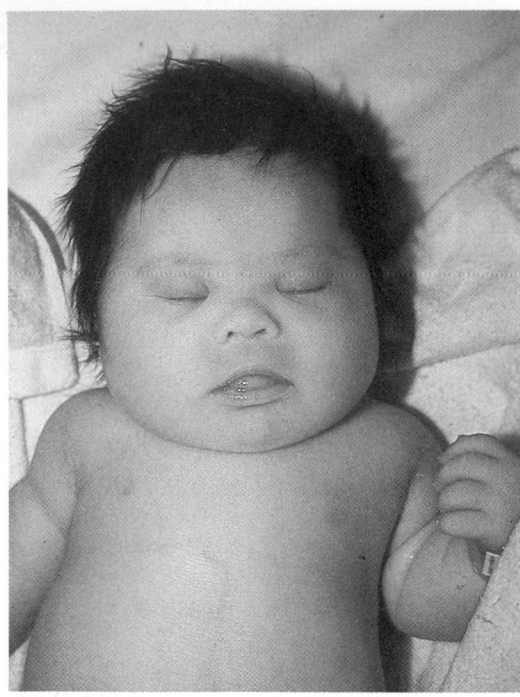

Fig. 5.12 Down's syndrome.

- In about 95% of cases, there is an extra, free-lying chromosome 21. This form of Down's syndrome is associated with increased maternal age. The risk at a maternal age of 37 years is one in 250, at 40 years one in 100, and at 45 years one in 40.
- In 2–3% of Down's syndrome cases, there is a chromosome translocation, usually involving Robertsonian translocation. The parents of such individuals must be checked to see whether they carry a balanced translocation.

Table 5.2 Chromosomal types of Down's syndrome

Types of Down's syndrome	Chromosome complement	Comment
Standard trisomy 21	47,XX,+21 or 47,XY,+21	Approximately 95% of Down's syndrome children
Translocation Down's syndrome	e.g. 46,XY,−14,+t(14;21) 46,XX,−21,+t(21q;21q)	In about 2–3% of cases, an extra chromosome 21 is attached to another chromosome. It is essential to examine the chromosomes of the parents, as one may carry a balanced translocation
Mosaic Down's syndrome	e.g. 46,XX / 47, XX,+21	Can be demonstrated in about 2–3% of cases

- The remaining Down's cases are mosaic. In these cases, the degree of mental retardation can vary according to the proportion of abnormal cells.

The recurrence risks for Down's syndrome are set out in Table 5.3.

Trisomy 18 (Edwards' syndrome)

This autosomal trisomy occurs in approximately one in 5000 live births. There is usually low birth weight, hypotonia, a prominent occiput, a small chin, a short sternum and characteristic hand and foot abnormalities. The index and little fingers of the hand overlap the middle two and the nails are small; in the feet the hallux is dorsiflexed and the lateral profile of the foot is convex with a prominent heel (a so-called 'rocker-bottom foot', caused by a vertical talus). Analysis of the dermatoglyphic patterns of the digits reveals an increased number of arch patterns. Internal malformations are common, especially congenital heart defects (ventricular septal defects, patent ductus arteriosus) and renal abnormalities (horseshoe kidney, hydronephrosis). Aplasia of the radius, facial clefts and exomphalos each occur in about 20% of cases. Prognosis is very poor with 50% of cases dying before two months, 90% before one year and 99% before 10 years; long-term survivors are very severely retarded. Most cases are caused by an extra chromosome 18 (rather than a chromosome translocation) and there is an association with increased maternal age. The risk of recurrence after a trisomic case is about one in 100 for a baby with a chro-

Table 5.3 Recurrence risks for Down's syndrome

Type of Down's syndrome	Risk to sibs of affected patient	Risk to other relatives (excluding offspring of an affected patient)
Standard trisomy 21		
Mother <40 years old	1%	Probably similar to maternal age risk
Mother >40 years old	Maternal age risk	
Translocation Down's (Parents have normal chromosomes)	Maternal age risk	Maternal age risk
Translocation Down's (One parent carries the translocated chromosome)		
Mother carries 14:21 translocation	10%	Depends on chromosomes of relative
Father carries 14:21 translocation	2%	Depends on chromosomes of relative
Either parent 21:21 translocation	100%	Depends on chromosomes of relative
Mosaic Down's	1%	Maternal age risk

mosomal trisomy (not necessarily trisomy 18); however, these risks might have to be modified for older mothers (see section on Down's syndrome).

Trisomy 13 (Patau's syndrome)

This occurs in about one in 8000 live births. There are significant craniofacial abnormalities with punched-out scalp lesions (aplasia cutis), microphthalmia, and low-set, malformed ears. Many cases have severe bilateral cleft lip and palate and some cases have hypotelorism or cyclopia (a single central eye with a proboscis-like nose), indicating underlying holoprosencephaly of the brain (failure of midline separation of the cerebral hemispheres). In the hands and feet an extra, hypoplastic digit on the ulnar or fibular side is common (postaxial polydactyly). Brain, heart and kidney malformations are very common. Survival past the first year of life is very unusual and retardation is severe. Most cases arise by standard trisomy but some are the result of a Robertsonian translocation involving chromosome 13. The risk of recurrence after a trisomic case is about one in 100 for a baby with a chromosomal trisomy (not necessarily trisomy 13); however, these risks might have to be modified for older mothers (see section on Down's syndrome).

Sex chromosome abnormalities

Klinefelter's syndrome

Klinefelter's syndrome (47,XXY) occurs in about one in 1000 males. Adult individuals tend to have eunuchoid proportions with female fat distribution and gynaecomastia. The testes are small. Pituitary gonadotrophins are raised and androgen production is low. Affected individuals are sterile, as they produce no sperm. Androgen therapy may help to improve libido and encourage the development of male secondary sexual characteristics. Intelligence is usually normal, although mild to moderate retardation may be seen.

XYY males

About one in 1500 males are XYY. Such individuals are physically normal although they tend to be tall. Although an increased tendency to psychopathic behaviour has been reported, prospective studies have shown that the majority of affected individuals lead normal lives.

Turner's syndrome

The incidence of Turner's syndrome (45,X) is one in 5000 births. Affected individuals are short, tend to have a web of skin on the lateral borders of the neck (Fig. 5.13), and may have other physical abnormalities such as a

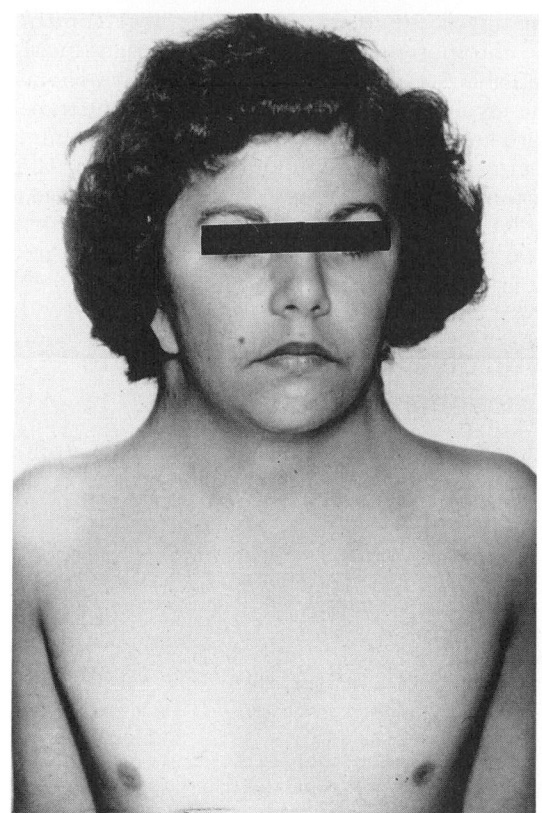

Fig. 5.13 Turner's syndrome (45,XO) showing characteristic facies, webbing of the neck, absent breast development and widely spaced nipples.

broad chest with widely spaced nipples and an increased carrying angle at the elbows. Coarctation of the aorta can occur. The vagina and internal genitalia are normally formed, but the ovaries consist of simple streaks of fibrous tissue without ovarian follicles, so that primary amenorrhoea is the rule. Treatment consists of oestrogen replacement around puberty to promote the development of secondary sexual characteristics.

47,XXX females

Females with a chromosome constitution 47,XXX have no physical abnormalities. However, primary and secondary amenorrhoea may occur, and IQ is 20–30 points below average, so that mental retardation is more common than in the general population. Nevertheless, the majority of affected females (about 70–80%) have normal intelligence.

Chromosome aberrations and cancer

Cytogenetic analysis of any malignant cell will frequently reveal a non-specific chromosome abnormality. However, there are certain malignancies where a characteristic abnormality is found; in others, the development of a specific chromosome change can be of prognostic significance (Table 5.4). In the case of Burkitt's lymphoma and chronic myeloid leukaemia, the chromosome translocations are known to bring together the loci for immunoglobulin genes and specific oncogenes (see p. 126). In other cases, the precise nature of the genetic change is not known. Occasionally, an individual with a specific chromosome abnormality will be predisposed to develop particular types of cancer (Table 5.4).

Genetic disorders predisposing to chromosome breakage

A group of single gene disorders exists, which result in an increased tendency to chromosome breakage, due to

Table 5.4 Chromosome aberrations in different types of malignancies

Chromosome aberration present in tumour cells only	Malignancy	Comment
t(9;22)	Chronic granulocytic leukaemia	These are characteristic changes.
t(8;2)	Burkitt's lymphoma	c-myc and c-abl
t(8;14)	Burkitt's lymphoma	oncogenes are on
t(8;22)	Burkitt's lymphoma	chromosomes 8 and 9. Immunoglobulin genes are on chromosomes 2, 14 and 22.
t(8;21)	Acute myeloblastic leukaemia	Loci involved uncertain
Trisomy 12	Chronic lymphocytic leukaemia	Good prognosis
inv (16)	Acute non-lymphocytic leukaemia	Good prognosis
Complex rearrangements	Acute non-lymphocytic leukaemia	Poor prognosis

Constitutional chromosome abnormality predisposing to specific cancers		
del(13q)	Retinoblastoma	Deletion may be submicroscopic and only revealed by DNA studies.
del(11p)	Wilms' tumour	Deletion may be submicroscopic and only revealed by DNA studies.
Trisomy 21 (Down's syndrome)	Acute lymphocytic leukaemia	

Table 5.5 Genetic disorders predisposing to chromosome breakage

Disorder	Clinical features
Fanconi's anaemia	Short stature, radial defects, patches of skin hyperpigmentation, pancytopenia, malignancies
Ataxia telangiectasia	Telangiectasia of conjunctiva, face and ears, ataxia, malignancies
Bloom syndrome	Short stature, facial telangiectasia, immunodeficiency, leukaemia
Xeroderma pigmentosum	Skin freckles and carcinomata, sensitivity to uv light, sometimes mental retardation

abnormalities of DNA repair after damage by agents such as ultraviolet light and radiation. These disorders, most of which are autosomal recessive, also predispose to malignancies (Table 5.5).

SINGLE GENE DISORDERS

Sir Archibald Garrod first put forward the concept of an 'inborn error of metabolism' in 1908 after studying alkaptonuria, a familial disorder in which patients excrete large amounts of homogentisic acid. This led to the concept that an enzyme controlling a metabolic step can be missing or reduced, leading to failure of production of essential metabolites further down the metabolic chain (e.g. in albinism) or accumulation of toxic substrates of the enzyme (e.g. in alkaptonuria and phenylketonuria) (Fig. 5.14).

Today, McKusick's catalogue of genetic disorders lists over 4000 defects involving every organ system. Only a few important groups of disorders are described here.

Aminoacidopathies

Defects in the metabolism of amino acids include a form of congenital hypothyroidism, albinism, disorders of the urea cycle and organic acid metabolism, as well as the disorders described below.

Phenylketonuria

Phenylketonuria is an autosomal recessive disorder affecting about one in 10 000 infants at birth. It is usually caused by a defect of the enzyme phenylalanine hydroxylase, which converts phenylalanine to tyrosine. The most common clinical presentation, now rarely seen, is vomiting in early infancy, with eczema, depigmentation of skin and hair, hypertonia, seizures, and mental retardation developing during the first years of life. Fortunately,

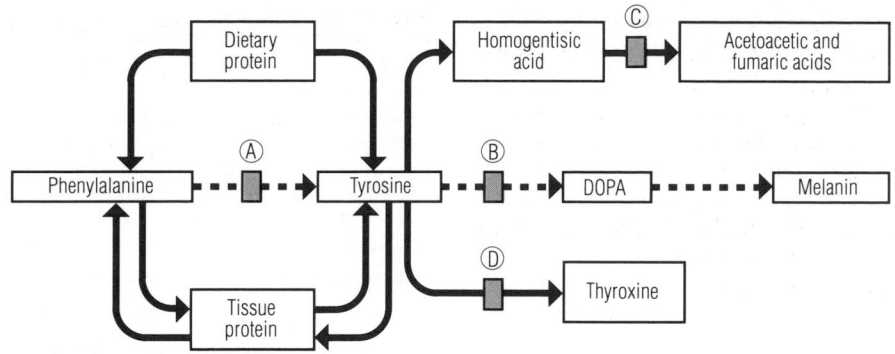

Fig. 5.14 Partial metabolic pathway of phenylalanine, tyrosine and related compounds showing position of 'metabolic blocks' caused by enzyme deficiencies. (A) Deficiency of phenylalanine hydroxylase results in an inability to metabolise phenylalanine, leading to phenylketonuria. (B) Tyrosinase deficiency leads to an inability to produce melanin, thus causing albinism. (C) Deficiency of homogentisic acid oxidase leads to the accumulation of homogentisic acid, and hence to alkaptonuria. (D) Deficiency of any one of several enzymes at this point means that thyroxine cannot be synthesised. The result is familial hypothyroidism.

screening at birth is now widely available, in which a drop of blood, obtained within the first few days of life, is placed on a filter paper and a bacterial inhibition assay used to measure phenylalanine levels (the *Guthrie test*). Affected infants can be treated by giving an artificial diet low in phenylalanine until at least eight years of age. If dietary control is strict, prognosis for mental development is good.

Females with phenylketonuria run a very high risk of having abnormal children, unless a strict diet is re-introduced throughout pregnancy. Their children do not have phenylketonuria themselves, but the abnormal metabolites cross the placenta during pregnancy and affect the developing fetus. Microcephaly, cardiac defects and mental retardation are common.

Phenylketonuria is a heterogenous disorder; the most common form results from a mutation at the phenylalanine hydroxylase locus itself. However, a rarer form due to a defect in dihydropteridine reductase has been described. This enzyme is essential for the recycling of the cofactor, tetrahydrobiopterine.

Homocystinuria

Homocystinuria is an autosomal recessive disorder and affects one in 200 000 infants. It is due to a defect of cystathionine β-synthase and leads to the accumulation of homocysteine, methionine and other metabolites. Clinical manifestations include lens dislocation, mental retardation, osteoporosis and thrombosis of arteries and veins. Affected individuals tend to be long and thin, making Marfan's syndrome part of the differential diagnosis. Treatment involves a low methionine diet, and pyridoxine treatment in that proportion of patients who are vitamin B_6 responsive.

Cystinosis

Cystinosis, an autosomal recessive disorder, should be distinguished from cystinuria (Table 5.6). There are abnormally high intracellular levels of free cystine, which lead to crystal deposition in the kidneys, conjunctiva, bones and leucocytes. Presentation is in childhood with

Table 5.6 Transport disorders

Disorder	Site	Metabolites affected	Clinical features	Inheritance
Intestinal disaccharidase deficiency	Small intestine	Maltose, sucrose, lactose	Abdominal pain and distension, diarrhoea	Autosomal recessive
Hypophosphataemic rickets	Renal tubules	Phosphates	Rickets (vitamin D-resistant)	X-linked dominant
Hartnup disease	Renal tubules	Amino acids (mono-amino-monocarboxylic group)	Red, scaly facial rash, ataxia	Autosomal recessive
Cystinuria	Renal tubules, small intestine	Cystine, ornithine, arginine, lysine	Renal stones	Autosomal recessive
Nephrogenic diabetes insipidus	Renal tubules	Insensitivity to ADH	Polyuria, polydipsia	X-linked dominant

photophobia and crystalline deposits in the conjunctiva, and the effects of renal tubular malabsorption (Fanconi's syndrome). Renal failure can occur before the age of 10 years.

Alkaptonuria

Alkaptonuria is a rare autosomal recessive disorder due to a defect in the enzyme homogentisic acid oxidase (Fig. 5.14). Homogentisic acid, a byproduct of the metabolism of tyrosine and phenylalanine, cannot be metabolised, and so accumulates in the body tissues and is excreted in increased quantities in the urine. Classically, the urine turns dark on standing, and the sweat may be black, but these findings are not invariable. The homogentisic acid and resultant polymers also stain cartilage and other connective tissue; ochronosis is the name given to the generalised blue/grey pigmentation that results and is best seen in the cartilage of the ear and the sclerae. It can also be seen in the tendons of the hands, through the overlying skin, in older patients.

The main clinical problem is arthritis, which affects the hips, knees, shoulders and spine. Onset is unusual before middle age. Radiological changes include narrowing and calcification of the intervertebral discs, together with some fusion of the vertebral bodies. Rarer complications include an increased incidence of ischaemic heart disease, calcification of the cardiac valves, and occasionally arterial aneurysms. Treatment is symptomatic.

Transport disorders

The transport of metabolites across cell membranes often involves specific binding sites and transport proteins. Mutations can disrupt these mechanisms and result in a group of disorders characterised by the failure of essential metabolites to enter the appropriate body compartments. Some important disorders are outlined in Table 5.6.

Storage disorders

Macromolecules in the body are often in a perpetual state of accumulation and breakdown. Thus, if an enzyme needed to break down a macromolecule is deficient, increased accumulation occurs, leading to a variety of symptoms according to the type of molecule and the site involved. Storage material usually accumulates in the lysosomes. Several examples are given in Table 5.7.

Connective tissue disorders

The main protein of connective tissue is collagen. There are at least four different types of collagen, each with its own functions (Table 5.8). Defects of collagen synthesis can cause a wide variety of disorders (Table 5.9). Some of these have been characterised at the molecular level, and various collagen probes are available for precise diagnosis. The specific collagen chain abnormality can sometimes be

Table 5.7 Storage disorders

Type	Example	Symptoms
Glycogen storage disorders	8 types including: Von Gierke's disease (glucose-6-phosphate deficiency) Pompe's disease (acid maltase deficiency)	Hepatomegaly, hypo-glycaemia, muscle weakness, cardiac failure (Symptoms vary according to type)
Sphingolipidoses	Niemann-Pick disease Gaucher's disease Krabbe's disease Metachromatic leukodystrophy	Hepatosplenomegaly (in some), progressive neurological deterioration
Gangliosidoses	Tay-Sachs disease	Progressive blindness and neurological deterioration
Mucopoly-saccharidoses	At least 8 types including: Hurler's syndrome Hunter's syndrome Moroteaux-Lamy syndrome Morquio syndrome	Hepatosplenomegaly, abnormal bones (dysostosis multiplex), corneal clouding, mental deterioration

Table 5.8 Types of collagen and their functions

Type	Function
I	Major collagen in skin, tendon, bones, heart valves and scar tissue
II	Major collagen in cartilage
III	Found mainly in blood vessels and intestine; also in skin
IV	Found mainly in basement membranes

Table 5.9 Connective tissue disorders

Disorder	Clinical features
Ehlers-Danlos syndrome (At least 8 distinct forms)	Hyperextensible skin, loose joints, 'cigarette paper' scars, easy bruising, rupture of blood vessels, internal viscera, etc.
Osteogenesis imperfecta (At least 4 distinct forms)	Multiple fractures of bones, blue sclerae, hyperextensible skin, easy bruising
Cutis laxa (Several different forms)	Loose skin, premature aged appearance, hernias, diverticulae and emphysema
Marfan's syndrome	Tall stature, span greater than height, loose joints, dislocated lens of eyes, aortic and mitral incompetence, dissection and aneurysms of the aorta

deduced from the clinical features (Table 5.9). Thus, some forms of osteogenesis imperfecta are caused by abnormalities of type I collagen; while type III collagen deficiency can result in a form of Ehlers-Danlos syndrome, with thin, atrophic skin and a tendency to spontaneous rupture of blood vessels and other internal organs. Defects of the connective tissue protein elastin are thought to cause the different forms of cutis laxa. Both collagen and elastin are abnormal in pseudoxanthoma elasticum (Ch. 12, Table 12.27). Marfan's syndrome has been shown to be caused by a defect in fibrillin protein.

MULTIFACTORIAL DISORDERS

Many common malformations, some diseases and many normal traits are said to have a *multifactorial* origin, in that both genetic and environmental factors contribute to their aetiology. Furthermore, the genetic component is thought to be due to several genes acting together, so-called *polygenic* inheritance. A good example is the inheritance of height. The genetic component is determined by several genes, and final height correlates between parents and children. Nevertheless, environmental factors (such as nutrition) can play an important role. The contribution of the many factors involved results in a Gaussian (normal) distribution of height in the general population.

Common malformations

There are many clues which suggest that a common malformation has a multifactorial origin:

- After one affected family member, the risk to other first degree relatives is usually in the range 1–5%, depending on the condition.
- The presence of additional affected family members increases the risk to subsequent offspring.
- Where a condition can have varying degrees of severity (e.g. cleft lip, with or without cleft palate), risks are higher for relatives of an individual with a more severe malformation.
- If there is a sex difference in incidence, risks are greater for relatives of an affected individual of the less commonly affected sex.
- The risk declines rapidly as one passes from first to second degree relatives.

It is thought that everyone inherits a *liability* to a partiular malformation. The degree of liability can vary in different individuals and families, according to the number of adverse genes and environmental factors present. If the liability exceeds a given threshold, the malformation is manifested. Individuals from families where there is more than one affected member will, on average, have a higher liability, as will relatives of more severely affected individ-

Table 5.10 Recurrence risk (%) in some common multifactorial malformations

Condition	Normal parent		Affected parent
	Risk of second affected child	Risk of third affected child	Risk of affected child
Cleft palate alone	2	8	7
Cleft lip ± cleft palate	4	10	4
Neural tube defect	4	10	4
Club foot	3	10	3
Dislocation of hip	6	10	12
Congenital heart disease (varies with type)	1–4	5–10	1–10
Hirschsprung's disease (long segment):			
Male index case	8	–	–
Female index case	14	–	–
Pyloric stenosis:			
Male index case	3	–	4
Female index case	7	–	13

uals. Similarly, where a condition is less common in a particular sex, affected persons of that sex must carry a greater liability, as will their relatives.

Some common multifactorial malformations with their recurrence risks are given in Table 5.10.

Common diseases, genetic markers and disease association

Many common diseases, e.g. the common allergies and some forms of epilepsy, have been proposed as candidates for multifactorial inheritance. As more research is carried out into these conditions, heterogeneity is recognised and subtypes are defined. Subdivision is aided by the identification of genetic markers, which may indicate that a major contribution to the disorder is being made by a gene on a specific chromosome. These genetic markers are particular blood groups, tissue types or RFLPs at specific gene loci which are found to occur more commonly in individuals with the disorder (Table 5.11).

A good example of the complex interaction between environmental factors and genetic loci is provided by the various possible causes of atheroma. A proportion of patients with early onset atherosclerosis show abnormalities of lipoproteins or lipoprotein receptors which are determined by various gene loci. In some patients, a single gene defect (e.g. of the cell membrane low-density lipoprotein receptors) can strongly predispose to atheroma. In the majority of cases, however, factors such

5 The Genetic Basis of Disease

Table 5.11 Some common disorders of multifactorial origin, with possible genetic markers

Disorder	Marker
Insulin-dependent diabetes mellitus	HLA haplotypes, e.g. B8, B15, DW3, DW4
Coeliac disease	HLA-A1-B8-DW3
Ankylosing spondylitis Reiter's disease Anterior uveitis	HLA-B27
Peptic ulceration	Blood group O
Atherosclerosis	Apolipoprotein A-1 Low density lipoprotein receptors Apolipoprotein E

as diet, smoking and high blood pressure may play the predominant role, with minor abnormalities of the lipoproteins merely providing an extra predisposition.

Linkage disequilibrium and pleiotropy

There are two possible explanations for the association of a genetic marker and a specific disease: linkage disequilibrium and pleiotropy.

Linkage disequilibrium. If a genetic marker (e.g. an RFLP) is extremely closely linked to a disease locus, specific marker alleles may not be separated from the disease allele by recombination over the generations and

an *association* will be observed in random individuals. This is known as linkage disequilibrium. It should be noted that linkage disequilibrium is a special case, observed only with very close linkage. In most cases of linkage, recombination over many generations will mean that a particular marker allele will not necessarily be associated with the disease in individuals picked at random.

Pleiotropy. The allele at the marker locus itself may predispose an individual to develop the disease, due to some function of the gene. Some of the disorders associated with specific HLA types may be examples of a pleiotropic effect. For example, a specific HLA type may predispose to infection with specific viruses, leading to some forms of insulin-dependent diabetes mellitus.

MANAGEMENT OF GENETIC DISORDERS

Screening

The treatment of many genetic disorders is often most successful if the disorder is diagnosed in an early, presymptomatic stage. In addition, the prevention of genetic disease by genetic counselling and prenatal diagnosis requires the identification of asymptomatic gene carriers. For these reasons, genetic screening programmes have been developed. Depending on the nature and frequency of the condition, screening can involve the entire population, subgroups of the population (for example, particular ethnic groups), or specific families in which a genetic disorder is known to be segregating (Table 5.12).

Table 5.12 Screening for genetic disorders

Disease	Group screened	Method	Purpose
Phenylketonuria	Total population of neonates	Guthrie test	Early dietary treatment of affected homozygotes
Hypothyroidism	Total population of neonates	TSH levels from dried blood spot	Early thyroxine therapy
Cystic fibrosis	Individuals of reproductive age	Direct DNA analysis of gene mutations	Prenatal diagnosis where both parents are carriers
Sickle cell anaemia and other haemoglobinopathies	Offspring of heterozygote mothers (total population of neonates in some regions)	Haemoglobin electrophoresis	Prophylaxis and early treatment of complications. Prevention by counselling and prenatal diagnosis
Tay-Sachs disease	Individuals of Ashkenazi Jewish extraction	Carrier detection by serum enzyme analysis	Prenatal diagnosis where both parents are heterozygous
Adult-onset polycystic renal disease	Relatives of affected individuals	Renal ultrasound, blood pressure, gene tracking in families using DNA probes	Early treatment of hypertension and renal failure
Multiple endocrine adenomatosis	Relatives of affected individuals	Calcitonin, urinary VMA, gene tracking in families using DNA probes	Early treatment of endocrine tumours
Familial polyposis coli	Relatives of affected individuals	Sigmoidoscopy, gene tracking in families using DNA probes, ophthalmoscopy for associated retinal lesions	Identification of gene carriers, early treatment of malignancy

Treatment of genetic disorders

It is still technically difficult to replace missing or defective genes; although it may be possible to isolate and replicate a gene in the laboratory, it is much more difficult to ensure that a replacement gene reaches the correct tissue, and is properly regulated. There are, however, a number of treatment strategies for genetic disorders which aim to ameliorate the phenotypic effects. Many common malformations of multifactorial or chromosomal origin can be corrected surgically; while a variety of treatments have been devised for single gene disorders (Table 5.13).

Table 5.13 Therapy for single gene disorders*

Treatment	Disorder
Replacement therapy	
Replacement of deficient protein	Haemophilias
	Diabetes
Replacement of deficient vitamin or co-enzyme:	
Vitamin B$_{12}$	Methylmalonicacidaemia (some types)
Vitamin D	Vitamin D-resistant rickets
Biotin	Biotinidase deficiency
Replacement of deficient metabolite:	
Cortisone	Adrenogenital syndrome
Thyroxine	Congenital hypothyroidism
Organ or cell replacement	
Kidney	Polycystic renal disease
Bone marrow	Immunodeficiencies
	Osteoporosis
Blood transfusion	Thalassaemias
Amelioration therapy	
Restriction of substrates in diet:	
Phenylanaline	Phenylketonuria
Methionine	Homocystinuria
Galactose	Galactosaemia
Drug therapy to remove harmful metabolites:	
Penicillamine	Wilson's disease
Cholestyramine	Hypercholesterolaemia
Iron chelating agents	Thalassaemias
Avoidance of harmful drugs or dietary factors	G6PD deficiency
	Porphyria
Preventive therapy	
Removal of potentially malignant tissues	Polyposis coli
Removal of site of destruction of diseased cells (e.g. spleen)	Spherocytosis

*After Emery (1984)

Genetic counselling

Most doctors will be faced at some stage with questions about the risk of a genetic disorder in patients or their families. Straightforward situations, such as Down's syndrome or neural tube defect, can be dealt with by the non-specialist; but complex problems, involving the diagnosis of rare disorders or the use of carrier detection tests and linkage studies, require a specialist opinion.

Whatever the problem, there are a number of essential steps in genetic counselling:

1. *Detailed family history.* At least a three generation pedigree should be taken and details of racial background and consanguinity (i.e. whether parents have common ancestors) obtained.
2. *Accurate diagnosis in affected family members.* An accurate diagnosis in affected family members must be made. This should include both a pathological diagnosis (established where possible from original notes and investigations) and an assessment of any genetic subgroup of the disorder.
3. *Ancillary tests.* Chromosome analysis, DNA marker studies or other carrier detection tests may need to be carried out, according to the nature of the problem.
4. *Risk assessment.* For single gene disorders, risk assessment is sometimes straightforward, providing a correct diagnosis is available. For instance, the recurrence of risk for a couple who have had one child with phenylketonuria is one in four, because phenylketonuria is autosomal recessive. Difficulties arise where a disorder has different inheritance types (e.g. retinitis pigmentosa) and with X-linked disorders, where carrier detection tests may need to be applied, new mutations have to be considered and risks must be modified to allow for normal sons in the pedigree. In addition, disorders with a late age of onset (such as Huntington's chorea) or of variable expression (such as tuberose sclerosis) can present problems that may require a specialist opinion. Where linked DNA probes are used, risk assessment can become complex. If a condition is caused by a chromosomal abnormality or is multifactorial, empirical risks derived from follow-up studies must be used.
5. *Prenatal diagnosis.* The availability of prenatal diagnostic tests (Table 5.14) has to be assessed and any possible risks to the mother or fetus weighed against the risk of fetal abnormality.
6. *Communicating risks.* Having marshalled all the facts, sufficient time must be set aside to discuss the risks in detail with the patient. A non-directive approach should be taken, whereby objective risks are given and discussed in detail, in the light of the severity of the condition and the availability and reliability of

5 The Genetic Basis of Disease

Table 5.14 Techniques of prenatal diagnosis

Procedure	Timing	Types of disorder detected
Villus biopsy	Transcervical 9–11 weeks Transabdominal 12–16 weeks	Cytogenetic abnormalities Enzyme defects Single gene defects (DNA probes)
Maternal α-fetoprotein	16-19 weeks	α-fetoprotein Raised: neural tube defects Lowered: Down's syndrome Edwards' syndrome (N.B. These are screening tests; diagnosis must be confirmed by further investigation)
Amniocentesis	16–20 weeks	Cytogenetic abnormalities Enzyme defects Neural tube defects Single gene defects (DNA probes)
Ultrasound	From 16 weeks	Anatomical defects Neural tube/hydrocephalus Body wall defects Limb reduction defects Hydrops Major urinary anomaly Bone dysplasias Cardiac defects Craniofacial anomalies
Fetoscopy/ cordocentesis	16–20 weeks	Fetal blood sample Clotting disorders Haemoglobinopathies Cytogenetic abnormalities Fetal skin biopsy Epidermolysis bullosa Ichthyosis Albinism Fetal liver biopsy Urea cycle enzyme defects Fetal visualisation Craniofacial defects Digital defects Genital defects

prenatal diagnosis. These factors may be crucial in the final decision of the parents.

It is best to give the risks as a proportion (i.e. one in two, one in 100, etc.) and to emphasise that a one in 20 risk of a child being affected means that 19 times out of 20 the child will not be affected. In order to put the risks into perspective, it is also worth pointing out that over one in 50 children is born with significant abnormalities at birth. In comparison to these background risks, a genetic risk of one in 20 is generally regarded as low, and those of greater than one in 10 as relatively high. However, the perception of an 'unacceptable' risk will depend on a large number of factors. The severity of the condition and the availability of treatment will obviously affect the willingness of a couple to have further children. For example, a one in 20 risk of a child with isolated cleft lip and palate will often be seen as acceptable, whereas the same risk for a child with severe, untreatable mental retardation may seem too high.

7. *Sympathy and understanding.* If a couple have given birth to an abnormal child, the genetic counselling clinic is often the place where considerable feelings of guilt are expressed. Alternatively, there may be an understandable tendency to blame poor medical care or environmental factors for the abnormalities. Time should be set aside to discuss all these feelings in a sympathetic and understanding manner, as they are part of the normal reaction to the birth of an abnormal child. Guilt and blame are usually the result of lack of information. Once a couple have been fully informed of the nature and causes of a child's problems, they can be helped to accept the fact that many genetic abnormalities are unavoidable.

Successful genetic counselling requires a combination of communication skills, detailed genetic knowledge, and a sound clinical background in both adult and paediatric medicine, if couples are to be helped to make the most appropriate decisions about childbearing. It is this combination that makes the practice of clinical genetics so rewarding.

FURTHER READING

Emery A E H, Rimoin D L 1990. Principles and practice of medical genetics, 2nd edn. Churchill Livingstone, Edinburgh. *A comprehensive, multi-author text covering most of clinical genetics.*

Gelehrter T D, Collins F S 1990. Principles of Medical Genetics. Williams and Wilkins, Baltimore. *An excellent introduction to basic human genetics and molecular biology.*

Harper P S 1988 Practical genetic counselling, 3rd edn. John Wright & Sons, Bristol. *A comprehensive introduction to the problems of clinical genetics.*

McKusick V A 1991 Mendelian inheritance in man, 10th edn. The Johns Hopkins Press, London. *A catalogue of all known single gene disorders in man.*

6

The Immunological Basis of Disease

John H L Playfair

The immune system exists in order to recognise and eliminate infectious micro-organisms. Its normal working is unobtrusive and can be detected only by cellular or serological changes. However, there are five circumstances in which it comes to the attention of the doctor:

- *Inadequate immunity.* Immunity may be inadequate either because a particular micro-organism is difficult or impossible to eliminate, which leads to persistent infection, or because, in a particular patient, some part of the immune system is deficient, either intrinsically or as a result of medical treatment. In this case, normally mild infections may become severe or fatal, and normally non-pathogenic organisms may cause unusual symptoms (opportunistic infection). Immune function may be improved by vaccination, immunostimulants or replacement therapy, depending on the circumstances.
- *Hypersensitivity.* In the process of responding to a foreign organism, immune mechanisms may produce side-effects which damage normal host tissue. Reactions of this type are collectively known as hypersensitivity and can affect virtually any organ, the skin, joints and kidneys being especially vulnerable.

- *Autoimmunity.* The normal ability of the immune system to discriminate foreign or 'non-self' material from 'self' may break down, leading to autoimmunity. Again, almost any organ can be affected, but autoimmunity is particularly common within the endocrine system.
- *Immunosuppression.* It is sometimes desirable for foreign material *not* to be eliminated, e.g. in a blood transfusion or kidney graft. Immunology therefore makes an important contribution to the practice of transplantation, in minimising and/or *suppressing* the rejection response. Immunosuppression may also be required for severe autoimmunity or hypersensitivity.
- *Immunological techniques.* The sensitive and precise discriminatory power of antibodies to recognise molecules is used, for example, in the measurement of hormone levels by *immunoassay*, and in blood and tissue *typing*. Another special use of antibodies is the targeting of drugs on particular cells.

THE IMMUNE SYSTEM

This section summarises the essential information, but it must be remembered that research into immunology proceeds at an ever-increasing rate and many aspects are still controversial.

One important distinction is between natural and adaptive immune mechanisms.

Natural immunity is based on ever-present and relatively unchanging elements such as *phagocytic cells*, together with *complement* and other tissue and serum factors.

Adaptive immunity is based on the special properties of *lymphocytes*, which include a high degree of specificity of individual cells for individual foreign molecules or *antigens*, rapid proliferation to expand a small specific population and the retention of specific *memory*. The term *immune response* is used to describe the events of adaptive immunity.

Another convenient distinction is between *cellular* and *humoral* immunity. The principal units of function in the immune system are a variety of cells and the molecules they secrete into the blood or extracellular fluids. The principal units of recognition are *receptors* carried by these cells; some of these recognise foreign material, and thus represent the actual interface between *self* and *non-self*, while some recognise other cells and allow them to *interact*. Most cell–cell interactions are ultimately carried out by soluble factors called *cytokines*, usually acting only at close range.

The principal components of the natural and adaptive immune systems are shown in Figure 6.1, which also emphasises the number of important interactions between the two.

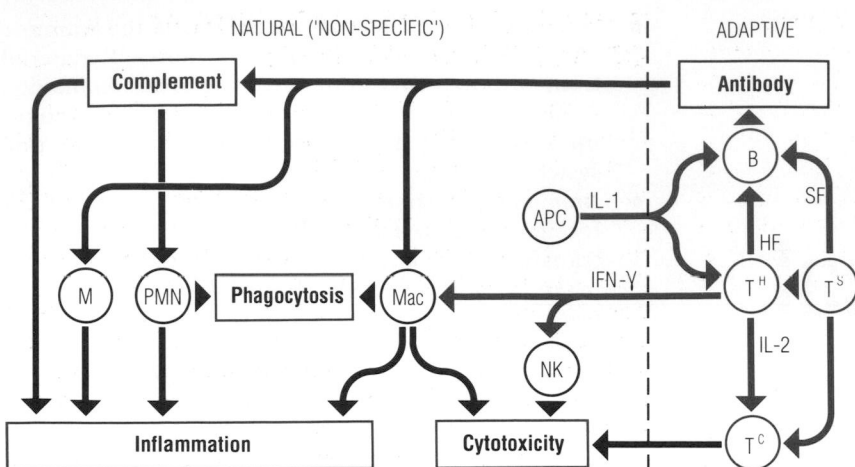

NATURAL ('NON-SPECIFIC') | ADAPTIVE

Fig. 6.1 Natural and adaptive immunity: the principal cells and molecules of the immune system and their interactions. PMN = polymorphonuclear leucocyte, M = mast cell, Mac = macrophage, APC = antigen-presenting cell, NK = natural killer cell. T cells: T^H = helper, T^C = cytotoxic, T^S = suppressor. IFN-γ = gamma interferon, IL-1 = interleukin 1, IL-2 = interleukin 2, HF = helper factor(s), SF = suppressor factor(s). Cells and molecules with high antigen specificity are printed in red. Red arrows indicate secretion of molecules.

NATURAL IMMUNITY

Natural immune mechanisms are responsible for a great deal of resistance to infection, and deficiencies in them can be extremely serious.

The intact skin and mucous membranes constitute a barrier to the entry of many micro-organisms, which have to rely on injuries, insect bites, etc. in order to gain access to the body. However, some micro-organisms can penetrate these barriers by means of specific attachment and penetration mechanisms.

Numerous antimicrobial substances (e.g. unsaturated fatty acids) are secreted onto the skin or into other secretions (e.g. lysozyme). Of particular importance in viral infections are the *interferons*, a family of molecules made by a variety of cells, which lead to the blocking of viral replication.

Once in the tissues, many micro-organisms are rapidly *phagocytosed* by polymorphonuclear leucocytes (PMN) or macrophages. Some bacteria (e.g. pneumococci) can resist phagocytosis by virtue of their capsules, while others (e.g. staphylococci) release toxins that destroy phagocytes. Certain bacteria, fungi and protozoa can survive within phagocytic cells, giving rise to chronic infection and, often, chronic inflammation, but most organisms are killed by a combination of acid pH, oxygen metabolites (e.g. hydrogen peroxide) and various cytotoxic proteins. Although it is over a century since the discovery of phagocytosis, the exact nature of the recognition between the phagocyte and its target is still not properly understood.

Complement system

A second line of defence is the *complement* system (Fig. 6.2). This is a series of 20 serum proteins activated in succession to give three important effects:

- the release of small peptides that stimulate inflammation and attract phagocytes
- the deposition of a component (C3b) on microbial membranes which promotes their phagocytosis by virtue of attachment sites for C3b on phagocytic cells
- the activation of lytic components which puncture cell membranes.

This activation 'cascade' can be triggered by numerous microbial surfaces, notably the endotoxins of

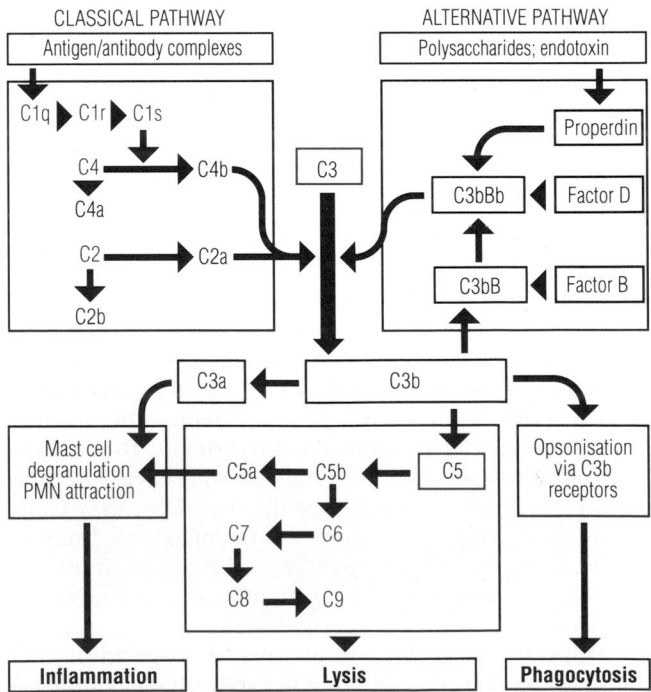

Fig. 6.2 Complement activation pathways. Components normally present in serum are shown outlined in red. Note the central role of C3→C3b conversion in both classical and alternative pathways.

Gram-negative bacteria, and, together with phagocytic cells, constitutes a rapid, integrated defence system against many bacteria, viruses, fungi, etc. However, as will be seen (p. 90), both phagocytosis and other complement functions can be greatly enhanced by the presence of *antibody*. Also, many of the inflammatory effects of complement operate via *mast cells* which, scattered throughout the tissues, respond rapidly to injury of all kinds. Here, again, antibody can augment mast cell activation, sometimes to dangerous levels, as in allergies (p. 94).

Macrophage and PMN secretions

Not all killing is intracellular. With large targets, e.g. worms, and perhaps tumour cells, the secretion of toxic molecules by macrophages or PMN may contribute to killing. Macrophages are particularly active in this respect, and more than 80 secreted products have been identified, of which the most important are lysozyme, some complement components, oxygen and nitrogen metabolites, interferon and a variety of cytotoxic proteins. In the case of viruses and tumours, *natural killer (NK) cells* are also thought to play a part.

ADAPTIVE IMMUNITY

The adaptive immune system represents a great advance over natural immune mechanisms in terms of both precision and flexibility. It is based on the *lymphocyte*, a type of cell found essentially only in vertebrates (whereas natural immunity is also found in invertebrates and, indeed, in the earliest life forms). By virtue of its *specificity* for individual chemical shapes or antigens and its extensive proliferative capacity, this cell confers the property of *memory* of particular infections. This, in turn, forms the basis for immunity to reinfection and the efficacy of vaccines. In both cases, a small *primary response* is followed, on subsequent contact with the same microorganisms, by a greatly augmented and biologically more effective *secondary response*.

Lymphocytes are of two main kinds and give rise to two corresponding types of immune response:

- B (bone-marrow derived) lymphocytes give rise to the *antibody-mediated (B)* immune response.
- T (thymus-derived) lymphocytes give rise to the *cell-mediated (T)* immune response.

However, some T lymphocytes are also involved in antibody formation and in the complex regulation of all immune mechanisms, including many 'natural' ones. The T lymphocyte can thus be regarded as the central cell of the whole adaptive system.

THE GENETIC AND MOLECULAR BASIS OF ADAPTIVE IMMUNITY

The specificity of lymphocytes for individual antigens is mediated by specific surface *receptors*, which are complementary to and 'recognise' small portions of the antigenic molecule. B cells use, as their receptors, antibody molecules essentially identical to those they secrete when stimulated. T cell receptors are smaller, but more complex, since they recognise not only portions of antigen but also normal molecules found on the surface of cells with which they interact. These molecules, known as *class I* and *class II major histocompatibility antigens*, are of great importance in normal immune responses and also, unfortunately, in transplant rejection.

Three sets of highly polymorphic genes code for these recognition molecules (Fig. 6.3). They are spread over several chromosomes, but the amino acid sequences of the proteins they code for show a degree of homology that suggests they have all evolved from a single precursor gene. These proteins are:

- the antibody, or immunoglobulin (Ig) molecule
- the T cell receptor
- the major histocompatibility antigens (HLA in man).

Antibody genes

The antibody genes are found on three separate chromosomes; two code for light (L) chains (kappa and lambda type) and one for heavy (H) chains. Each gene consists of four main regions:

- V (variable)
- D (diversity)
- J (joining)
- C (constant)

separated by untranslated introns. The V region contains several hundred copies, each slightly different, of a gene coding for the variable region of the antibody molecule; parts of the latter (the 'hypervariable regions') are responsible for antigen recognition, and thus specificity. The C region is much larger for heavy chains than for light chains because it includes, in tandem, the genes for all the immunoglobulin classes and subclasses (IgM, IgG, etc.; see p. 86).

In B lymphocytes, but not in other cells, rearrangement of DNA occurs so that particular V and D genes are brought next to a particular J gene. The RNA transcribed from this is further spliced, so that the VDJ and one of the C regions are brought together to code for a complete polypeptide chain. Finally, two identical H chains and two identical L chains (either both kappa or both lambda) are disulphide-bonded and glycosylated, to form the antibody molecule, which is now ready either for secretion

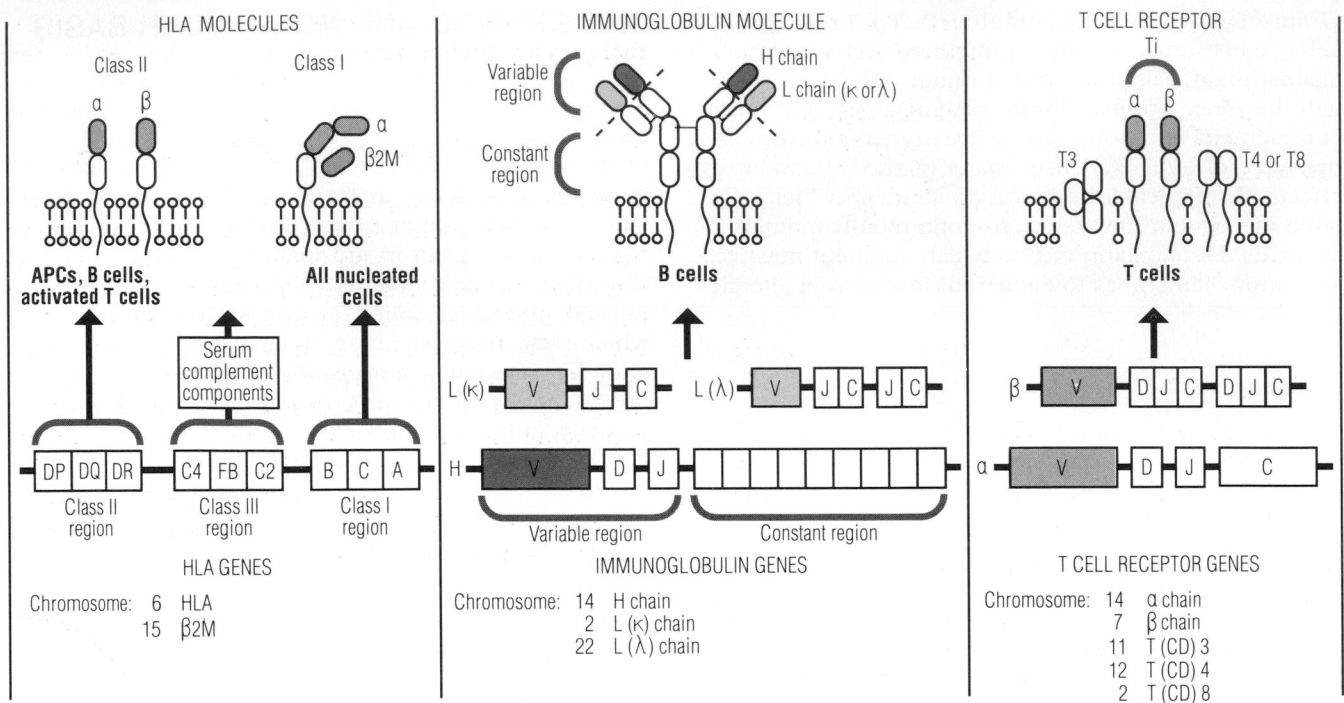

Fig. 6.3 Genes and molecules involved in immune recognition. The genes are shown in the centre, the molecules they code for at the top, inserted in the plasma membrane of the respective cells. Domains showing high variability and involved in antigen recognition are shown in red. Note that T and CD are alternative nomenclatures for T cell surface molecules, but the CD terminology also applies to molecules on other types of cell. APC = antigen-presenting cell; H = heavy; L = light.

into the blood, or insertion into the B lymphocyte membrane as a specific receptor.

Individual B lymphocytes and their progeny retain transcription of the same V gene, but can switch from one C gene to another, usually in the direction IgM→IgG. The enormous diversity of V genes ensures that an antibody molecule can be produced to fit virtually any shape of antigenic determinant. It is now agreed that the combinatorial possibilities of one heavy and two kinds of light chain plus, within each chain, a number of different V, D and J genes, to which is added the occasional mutation, are sufficient to code for about 10^8 different antibody specificities.

Genetic differences between antibody molecules are known as *isotypic* if they reside in the constant region (the various classes and subclasses are thus isotypes), and as *idiotypic* if they reside in the hypervariable regions; the idiotype of an antibody is the portion which is unique to that variable region, and may include either the antigen combining site or the adjacent regions. There are also allelic differences known as *allotypes*, which enable the antibody molecules of one individual to be distinguished from those of another, just as with blood groups on red cells.

The antibody molecule

The antibody or *immunoglobulin* (Ig) molecule is ideally suited to its function of promoting the removal of foreign antigens. Its basic structure is seen in antibodies of the IgG class (Fig. 6.4).

The N-terminal half is composed of H and L chains and is responsible for binding to antigen (Fab portions); the C-terminal half (Fc portion), which consists of heavy chains alone, determines the *class* of antibody and is responsible for the biological functions of the molecule.

- *IgG*. In the case of IgG, these functions include activation of complement, attachment to phagocytic cells, passage into the tissues and transport across the placenta. The four IgG subclasses vary somewhat in these functions, while the other classes of Ig show more substantial differences.
- *IgM* is a large molecule confined to the bloodstream, but is very efficient at activating complement and agglutinating foreign material by virtue of its 10 combining sites.
- *IgA* is secreted into, and can survive in, such locations as the eyes, nose, gut and urine.
- *IgE* attaches to mast cells causing them to release the contents of their granules, which leads to increased local vascular permeability and acute inflammation.
- *IgD* is found mainly on B lymphocyte membranes, where it may have a role in triggering their responses.

The properties of the various Ig classes and subclasses are summarised in Table 6.1.

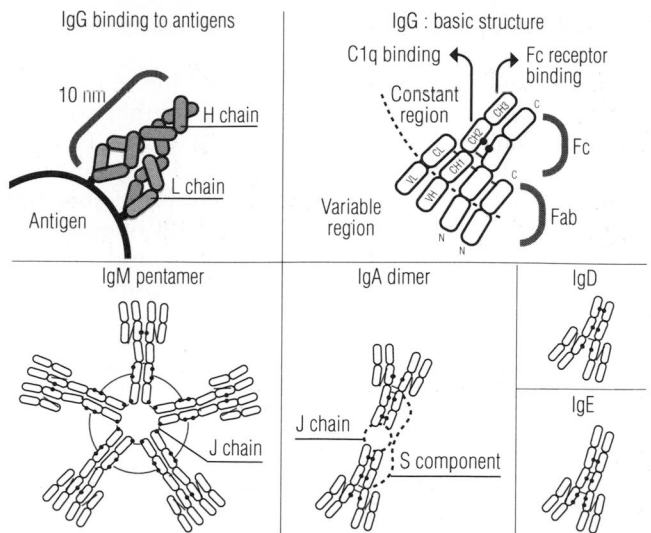

Fig. 6.4 Antibody structure and function: the five classes of immuno-globulins showing their main structural and functional differences. The basic domains of about 110 amino acids are shown as ellipsoids. Except in the top left figure, interchain disulphide bonds are in red (intrachain disulphide bonds are not shown). J chain = joining chain, which stabilises the pentameric and dimeric structure of IgM and IgA respectively; S component = secretory component, which allows IgA to be secreted and to avoid digestion by proteolytic enzymes. L chains are shown in red, and H chains in grey. Solid black circles represent carbohydrate side-chains. Clq = the first component of complement.

The T cell receptor

The T cell receptor is a two-chain (α and β or γ and δ) molecule, rather like a shortened immunoglobulin. In this case, DNA rearrangement occurs only in T lymphocytes. However, the T cell receptor has a more complicated combining site than antibody, and recognises combinations of small foreign peptides and molecules of the major histocompatibility complex (MHC; see below and Fig. 6.5). Associated with the T cell receptor are smaller molecules, named CD3, CD4 and CD8, which also play a

part in cell–cell interaction. Their main practical value is that the corresponding monoclonal antibodies can be used to identify different kinds of T lymphocytes (p. 89).

The major histocompatibility complex

The important set of genes comprising the major histo-compatibility complex (MHC) is so named because, in all higher animals, it dominates transplant rejection responses (p. 97). However, its normal function is to control cell–cell interactions in adaptive immunity (see below). The human MHC is known as HLA and its genes lie on the short arm of chromosome 6. They are grouped in two sets, referred to as class I and class II, each set containing three genetic loci, each of which has a large number of alleles coding for HLA antigens (Fig. 6.3). The genes for certain complement components also lie within the MHC, but their products are quite unrelated to class I and class II molecules.

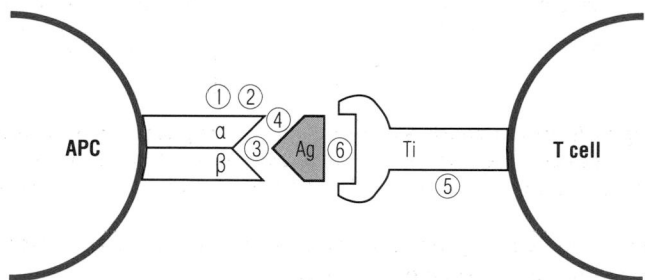

Fig. 6.5 HLA and disease: a simplified scheme to show the probable interactions between antigen HLA molecules and the T cell receptor. The numbers indicate points at which abnormalities may lead to unduly high or low responses to a foreign antigen and so predispose to disease. (1) General high or low responsiveness associated with particular HLA combinations. (2) Linkage disequilibrium between HLA and other disease-associated genes. (3) Failure of an antigen to associate with a particular HLA molecule. (4) Suppressor-inducing epitopes on an antigen. (5) Lack of a specific T cell receptor for an antigen. (6) Resemblance between an antigen and particular HLA molecule.

Table 6.1 Classes and subclasses of immunoglobulin and their major features

Class	Subclass	Mol. wt (sedimentation coefficient)	Normal serum level (g/l)	Functions	
				Complement	Opsonisation
IgM		900 000 (19S)	0.5–2	+	
IgG	G1	150 000 (7S)	9 ⎫	+	+
	G2	150 000 (7S)	3 ⎪	+	
	G3	170 000 (7S)	1 ⎬ 7–19	+	+
	G4	150 000 (7S)	0.5 ⎭		+
IgA	A1	160 000 (7S) or a dimer of	3 ⎫ 0.8–5	Protects mucous surfaces	
	A2	320 000 (11S)	0.5 ⎭		
IgE		190 000 (7S)	50 mg/l	Mast cell activation	
IgD		180 000 (7S)	30 mg/l	B cell surface receptor	

Class II HLA molecules are two-chain (α and β) structures somewhat resembling the T cell receptor. Class I molecules consist of a larger α chain and a small β chain known as β-2-microglobulin, whose gene lies on a different chromosome and shows no variability. In order for a T lymphocyte to respond to a foreign antigen, its receptor must interact with both the antigen and an HLA molecule.

Class I antigens (i.e. alleles at the A, B and C loci) are expressed on all nucleated cells (two from each locus on diploid cells), and are mainly concerned with the recognition of viral antigens by cytotoxic T cells (p. 90). Class II antigens (alleles at the DP, DQ, and DR loci) are expressed on a more limited range of cells, namely those with which T lymphocytes are required to interact – principally antigen-presenting cells, B lymphocytes and certain other T lymphocytes – and are concerned with the initiation and control of the immune response (p. 89).

Apart from their importance in matching transplants, certain HLA antigens are associated with particular diseases (Table 6.2). Sometimes, as with antigen B27 and ankylosing spondylitis, this association is so strong as to be of value in diagnosis; more often, however, it is only relative. The combination of B8 and DR3 is associated with a variety of autoimmune diseases, and possible reasons for this are discussed on page 96. Figure 6.5 illustrates the probable interactions involved.

LYMPHOCYTES

Like all other haemopoietic cells, lymphocytes originate from stem cells in the bone marrow; unlike other cells, however, they have the ability to leave and re-enter the circulation repeatedly. This facilitates the contact between a foreign antigen and the tiny minority of lymphocytes specific for it, which would otherwise be a very rare event. Differentiation and maturation of lymphocytes, and most of their functions, are carried out in specialised *lymphoid organs*.

Lymphoid organs

Primary

The B lymphocytes complete their maturation in the *bone marrow*, but T lymphocytes require passage through the *thymus* where, under the influence of peptide hormones probably secreted by epithelial cells, they acquire full immunocompetence. At the same time, they appear to 'learn' to recognise the individual's own HLA specificities and to avoid self-reactivity.

Secondary

The secondary lymphoid organs contain mature lymphocytes and are strategically placed where foreign antigens are likely to be encountered: *lymph nodes* for antigens in the tissues; the *spleen* for those in the blood; *Peyer's patches* for the small intestine; *tonsils* and *adenoids* for the nose, mouth and pharynx. The structure of secondary lymphoid tissue is best seen in the lymph node, where the cortex contains mainly B lymphocytes, and the paracortex T lymphocytes, while antibody-secreting plasma cells are found in the medulla. Other lymphoid organs show a similar demarcation, which is also seen in the aggregates of lymphocytes that can develop wherever there is a focus of infection. The lymphoid tissues of the gut and lungs behave, to a certain extent, autonomously, in that particular B cells (largely IgA-secreting) and T cells recirculate selectively through them. They are sometimes referred to as the *mucosal immune system* (Fig. 6.6).

Table 6.2 Major HLA-associated diseases

Disease type	Associated HLA antigen	
	DR	B
Joints		
Ankylosing spondylitis		27(87)
Reiter's		27(37)
Juvenile RA		27
Rheumatoid arthritis	4(6)	
Gut		
Ulcerative colitis		5
Atrophic gastritis		7
Haemochromatosis		14
Coeliac disease	3(11)	8
Chronic active hepatitis	3(14)	8
Endocrine and autoimmune		
Addison's	3(6)	8*
IDDM	3(5), 4(7)	8(10)
Sjögren's	3(10)	8
Graves'	3(4)	8
Hashimoto's	5(3.2)	
Myasthenia gravis		8(4)
Cancer		
Thyroid	3(3), 1(6)	
CNS		
Multiple sclerosis	2(5)	7
Skin		
Alopecia		12
Behçet's		5
Psoriasis	HLA C–W6(13)	

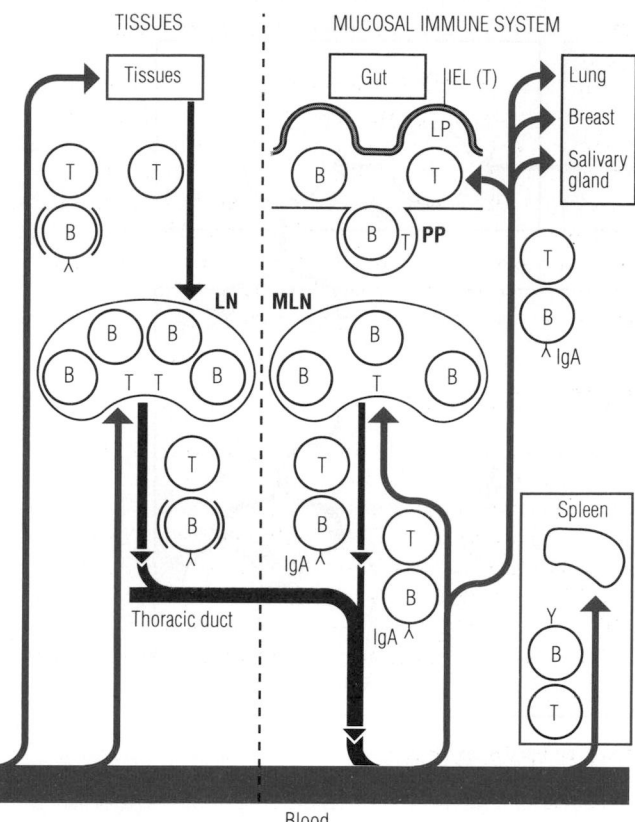

Fig. 6.6 Lymphocyte recirculation. In this stylised diagram, blood vessels (arterial side only shown) are in red, lymphatics in black. LN = lymph node; MLN = mesenteric lymph node; PP = Peyer's patch; IEL = intra-epithelial lymphocytes; LP = lamina propria.

Table 6.3 Some useful lymphocyte markers and their functional significance*

Cell type	Standard name*	Distribution and functional significance
T lymphocyte	TcR	Receptor for antigens
	CD3	All T cells
	CD2	Receptor for sheep RBC
	CD4	Helper cells, HIV receptor
	CD8	Cytotoxic/suppressor cells
	CD5	Thymocytes
	CD25 (Tac)	Receptor for IL-2 (activated cells)
B lymphocyte	Ig	Receptor for antigens
	CD25 (Tac)	Receptor for IL-2
	IL4 receptor	
	IL5 receptor	Involved in 'help'
	IL6 receptor	
	CD21	Receptor for C3 and EB
	C3d receptor	virus
	CD5	? Autoimmune B cells

*CD numbers refer to 'clusters of differentiation', a standard nomenclature.

Lymphocyte subpopulations and markers

B lymphocytes are identified by the possession of surface Ig, usually detected by immunofluorescent staining with anti-Ig sera. T lymphocytes lack surface Ig, but conveniently form 'rosettes' when centrifuged lightly with sheep red blood cells. However, using these two techniques, about 10% of blood lymphocytes still cannot be classified; these are referred to as *null*.

The use of monoclonal antibodies against the CD3, CD4 and CD8 molecules (p. 90), combined with immunofluorescence, makes it possible to identify subpopulations of T cells with important functional differences. In general, CD4 is found on *helper* T lymphocytes, CD8 on *cytotoxic* and *suppressor* lymphocytes, and CD3 on all types (Fig. 6.7). Further subdivisions can be made using other antibodies (Table 6.3).

THE IMMUNE RESPONSE

The term 'immune response' covers all responses of lymphocytes to antigen, whether involving T or B cells or both. All immune responses have certain features in common.

- *Presentation*, i.e. the requirement for antigens to be *presented* by specialised cells.
- *Selection* of lymphocytes whose receptors are specific for determinants on the antigen.
- *Clone formation*: proliferation of these lymphocytes to form a *clone* of cells with identical specificity. This process was predicted by Burnet in his clonal selection theory of 1959, but received full confirmation only recently, with the development of methods of growing clones of T and B cells in culture.
- *Differentiation*. Interactions between lymphocytes leading to their differentiation into effector cells.
- The generation of *memory*.
- *Regulation*, i.e. control of the magnitude and duration of the response by various regulatory mechanisms.

On the basis of the type of effector cell generated, immune responses can be classified into three types:

- antibody responses
- cytotoxic T cell responses
- responses involving activation of macrophages and other non-specific cells.

Types 2 and 3 are often somewhat confusingly lumped together as *cell-mediated immunity*.

Antigen presentation and T cell triggering

Antigen-presenting cells (APC) include the dendritic cells of spleen and lymph nodes, the Langerhans cells of the

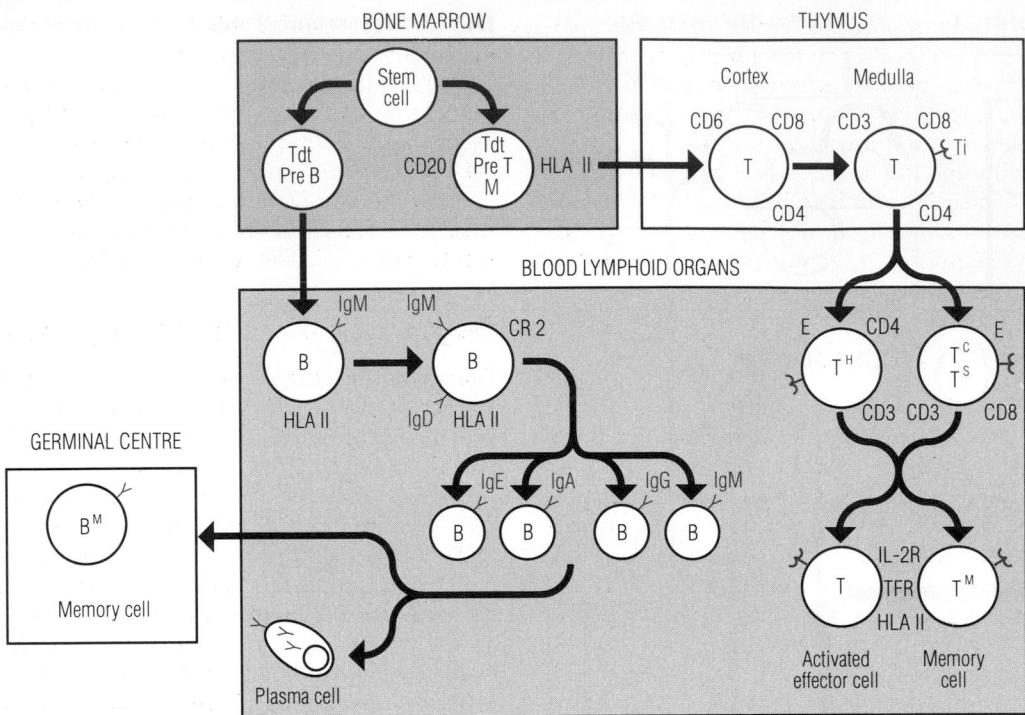

Fig. 6.7 T and B lymphocyte differentiation markers. Diagram shows the principal stages in the T and B cell lineages, with some of the surface and cytoplasmic molecules that help to differentiate them. Tdt = terminal deoxynucleotidyl transferase (possibly involved in receptor gene rearrangement); E = receptor for sheep erythrocytes (= CD2); Ti = T cell receptor for antigen; T^H = T helper cell; T^C, T^S = cytotoxic or suppressor T cell; T^M, B^M = T or B memory cell; IL-2R = receptor for interleukin 2 (= CD25); TFR = transferrin receptor; M = cytoplasmic IgM heavy chain; CR2 = complement receptor (= CD21); CD20 = a useful B cell marker, possibly involved in triggering. Antigen-specific receptor molecules are shown in red.

skin and related cells in other organs, and B cells. Macrophages can also often present antigen, especially when some degree of preliminary antigen breakdown is needed, as with large or particulate antigens. Presentation is by digestion of proteins to small peptides, which are then orientated with MHC molecules on the cell surface.

When APC make contact with specific lymphocytes, they secrete a protein known as interleukin-1 (IL-1) and perhaps other factors, which cause lymphocytes to proliferate. In the case of CD4 (helper) cells, recognition of class II MHC molecules, as well as antigen, is required, so that only cells expressing these can act as APC. In the case of cytotoxic (CD8) cells (p. 91), antigen, usually of intracellular origin (e.g. from viruses), is recognised in association with class I MHC molecules. In both cases, other soluble mediators are required for proliferation and expansion of the specific clone of T cells, notably interleukin 2 (IL-2), which is made by T helper cells and for which activated T cells of all types express surface receptors. The half-life of IL-2 is very short (due in part to serum inhibitors), so that its action is highly localised and predominantly restricted to antigen-specific cells.

The antibody response

Both B and T cells are required for the antibody response. The exceptions are some large polymeric antigens (e.g. bacterial capsular polysaccharides), which stimulate B cells directly and are known as *T-independent*. With all other antigens, B cells are triggered to proliferate by interaction between their surface Ig and the antigen, plus factors secreted by the APC; however, they require additional signals from T helper cells in order to differentiate into plasma cells and secrete antibody. These signals consist of non-antigen-specific cytokines, principally the *interleukins* 1–6. The T helper cells also need antigen to be presented, in this case in association with MHC class II molecules.

During T-dependent responses, some B lymphocytes are retained in *germinal centres* instead of differentiating 'terminally' into plasma cells; these are called *memory B cells*. These, together with memory T cells, form the basis for the vigorous *secondary response* that follows subsequent exposures to the same antigen. Typical features of secondary as compared with primary responses are: more rapid onset, higher level of antibody, higher average affinity, and relatively more IgG.

Antibody is predominantly effective against micro-organisms free in the blood or tissue spaces; in practice, this means viruses in their extracellular stage and many bacteria. Pneumococcal pneumonia is a good example of a disease in which a rapid antibody response can make the difference between life and death. The predominant role of antibody in such cases is to improve phagocytosis by virtue of the attachment of the Fab portion to the microbe and the Fc portion to Fc receptors on phagocytic cells; this process is known as *opsonisation*.

The cytotoxic T cell response

The cytotoxic T cell response is mainly useful against viruses in their intracellular stage, though it unfortunately also contributes to transplant rejection. The final effector cell is a T cell, usually of CD8 phenotype, which recognises viral antigens on the surface of infected cells in association with class I MHC molecules. Rather like a B cell, it usually requires help from T helper cells for clonal proliferation, in this case mainly in the form of IL-2. The mechanism by which cytotoxic T cells act is not exactly known, but it involves contact with the virus-infected cell which is subsequently destroyed by lysis.

T cell–macrophage interactions

The third group of responses is somewhat more heterogeneous and includes all those in which a specifically activated T cell modifies the function of another, non-specific, cell via the secretion of soluble molecules collectively known as *cytokines* (Table 6.4). Many of the cytokines act on macrophages, to improve their ability to terminate, or at least control, infection by intracellular bacteria such as mycobacteria and several important fungi and protozoa. However, there are also cytokines that affect eosinophils, NK cells, other lymphocytes (e.g. IL-2), haemopoietic precursors in the bone marrow, osteoclasts and even mucus secretion. In all these types of response, memory resides entirely in the specific T cells.

Regulation of immune responses

Both T and B cells require specific antigens for triggering, so that *elimination of antigen* constitutes the most effective way of terminating a response. However, there are other ways in which a prolonged response can be damped down, presumably as an attempt to limit hypersensitivity and autoimmunity (pp. 93–96). These include the stimulation of suppressor T cells and the production of anti-idiotypic antibodies. Suppressor T cells resemble cytotoxic T cells in their usual phenotype (CD8), and appear to use similar receptors, but their triggering requirements are not clear. Antibody itself can also regulate antibody production, and this may be idiotype-specific or antigen-specific. In general, IgG antibodies are more inhibitory than IgM.

TOLERANCE

Immune responses are not normally triggered by the body's own antigens; this is known as *self-tolerance* and is thought to be due to a combination of several mechanisms including:

- the elimination of self-reactive lymphocytes in the primary lymphoid organs (thymus and bone marrow)
- suppressor T cells, specific for self-antigens
- antigen–receptor interactions that lead to unresponsiveness instead of responsiveness.

None of these mechanisms is fully understood, and they clearly are not foolproof because *autoantibodies* (antibodies against self) are quite often found (p. 96).

The same mechanisms are apparently also responsible for the unresponsiveness to foreign antigens found in special circumstances and also known as *tolerance*. This can occur with:

- very *large* amounts of antigen
- an *immature* or compromised immune system
- antigens that for any reason are not properly *presented*
- antigens absorbed through the *gut* (of particular interest in relation to food allergies).

The induction of tolerance against foreign MHC antigens is one of the aims of research into transplant rejection (pp. 96–98).

Table 6.4 The major cytokines and their functions

Cytokine*	Principal cellular source	Principal effects
IL-1	APC	T cell proliferation; fever etc. (as TNF)
IL-2	T	T, B proliferation
IL-3	T	T, B, mast cell growth
IL-4	T	T, B proliferation
IL-5	T	Eosinophil growth; B differentiation
IL-6	T	B differentiation; acute-phase proteins
IL-7	T	B, T proliferation
IL-8	T	PMN activation
IL-10	T,B,Mac	Inhibits other cytokines
IFN-α	Mac	Anti-viral
IFN-β	Fibroblast	Anti-viral
IFN-γ	T	Anti-viral; MHC; activates macrophages
GCSF	Mac	Granulocyte growth and maturation
MCSF	Mac	Monocyte growth and maturation
GMCSF	T	As GCSF and MCSF
TNF (TNF-α)	Mac	Anti-tumour; vascular damage; anti-viral; PMN
LT (TNF-β)	T	activation; bone absorption; etc.

IL = interleukin; IFN = interferon; TNF = tumour necrosis factor; LT = lymphotoxin; CSF = colony-stimulating factor; APC = antigen-presenting cell; Mac = macrophage; MHC = major histocompatibility complex

6 The Immunological Basis of Disease

IMMUNODEFICIENCY

Deficiencies of immunity can be classified as *primary* (i.e. cause unknown) or *secondary* to some known cause such as infection, cancer, malnutrition, drugs or X-radiation. Alternatively, they can be described in terms of the component which is faulty, the most important being defects of phagocytic cells, complement, B cells and antibody, and T cells, or combinations of these (Table 6.5).

Table 6.5 Some immunodeficiency syndromes

System affected	Syndrome	Clinical effects
Primary		
Antibody	Hypogamma–globulinaemia	Bacterial infections
	Transient (neonatal)	Bacterial infections
	Congenital X-linked (Bruton's disease)	Bacterial infections
	Selective IgA	Gut infection; allergies
	Selective IgM	Septicaemia
T cells	Thymic aplasia (Di George)	Viral infections
	PNP deficiency	Viral infections
	Ataxia telangiectasia	Viral infections
	Wiskott-Aldrich syndrome	Viral infections
T and B cells	Common variable	Childhood infection
	Severe combined ADA deficiency	Childhood infection
Myeloid cells	Chronic granulomatous disease	Abscesses; granulomas
	Chediak-Higashi syndrome	Pneumonia
	MPO, G6PD, deficiency*	Pneumonia
Complement	C1,2,4 deficiency	Immune complex disease
	C3 deficiency	Infection
	C5,6,7,8,9 deficiency	Neisserial infection
Other	Opsonisation defect	Infection
Secondary		
Antibody	Splenectomy	Pyogenic infections
	Myeloma, CLL*	
	Cyclophosphamide	
	Malnutrition	
	Nephrotic syndrome	
T cells	AIDS	Pneumocystis; TB; Kaposi's sarcoma
	Hodgkin's disease	Fungal infections; TB CMV
	Azathioprine (Imuran)	Infections rare
	Cyclosporin A	
	Measles, CMV, IM*	
	Malnutrition: zinc	
Myeloid cells	Steroids	
	Gentamycin	
	Malnutrition: iron, zinc	

MPO= myeloperoxidase; G6PD = glucose 6 phosphate dehydrogenase; CLL = chronic lymphatic leukaemia; CMV = cytomegalovirus; IM = infectious mononucleosis.

Phagocytic cell deficiencies

PMN are especially prone to genetic deficiencies usually involving particular enzymes, e.g. *chronic granulomatous disease* (CGD) in which oxygen metabolites are not generated. There are also deficiencies of myeloperoxidase, G6PD, pyruvate kinase and other enzymes. There is also a defect of phagosome-lysosome fusion known as Chediak-Higashi syndrome. In general, PMN defects are associated with recurrent bacterial (especially staphylococcal) and fungal infections.

Complement deficiencies

Almost any of the complement components may be absent or reduced, the most serious (but extremely rare) being C3 and the commonest, C2. Defects of the (lytic) components of C5–8 are associated mainly with Neisserial (meningococcal and gonococcal) infection, suggesting that lysis is not a major killing mechanism for most other organisms, and that phagocytosis is more important overall. Deficiencies of the 'classical' components (C1, C2 or C4) are associated with an increased risk of immune complex disease, because this pathway plays a role in reducing the size of complexes. An interesting defect is that of a C1 inhibitor associated with hereditary angio-oedema. There is also a poorly characterised deficiency of a serum opsonising activity apparently distinct from complement.

Antibody deficiencies

The newborn baby relies on IgG transferred across the placenta, and is protected from common infections for about 6 months. Any delay thereafter in endogenous Ig synthesis may lead to recurrent pyogenic infection. Occasionally, the synthesis of IgA is selectively reduced or absent, often in association with allergies or autoimmune disease. Sometimes, all Ig classes are affected (*common variable immunodeficiency*). More rarely, B lymphocytes are absent altogether, leading to agammaglobulinaemia. When inherited on the X chromosome, this is known as Bruton's disease. Pneumonia is the commonest presenting condition, but repeated infections can occur almost anywhere. Treatment is by immunoglobulin replacement and, where appropriate, antibiotics (see p. 216). Immunoglobulin is prepared from pooled donor plasma and given i.v. or i.m. It is screened for hepatitis B and HIV; reactions are rare.

T cell deficiencies

AIDS, in which the virus infects T helper cells using the CD4 molecule as receptor, represents the extreme end of the spectrum of T cell deficiency (see p. 216). However, a mild lowering of T cells is probably quite common, particularly during other virus infections, such as measles. Very rarely, absence of the thymus leads to a total lack of T cells; if associated with absence of the parathyroids, this is known as the Di George syndrome. Severe T cell deficiency leads to fatal infections with micro-organisms of all kinds, including normally non-pathogenic *opportunists*, such as cytomegalovirus, pseudomonas, pneumocystis and candida, and also, in some cases, to the development of tumours. Treatment is unsatisfactory, but bone marrow and/or thymus grafting have had some success.

Combined deficiencies

In *severe combined immunodeficiency* syndromes (SCID) both B cells and T cells are affected in various proportions. Sometimes, the defect appears to be in an enzyme of the purine salvage pathway, such as adenosine deaminase (ADA) or purine nucleoside phosphorylase (PNP); in these cases, replacement of the missing enzyme is a practical possibility. There are a number of very rare syndromes in which immunodeficiency is found alongside abnormalities of the CNS (e.g. ataxia telangiectasia), of platelets (Wiskott-Aldrich syndrome) or of the entire haemopoietic system (reticular dysgenesis).

IMMUNOPATHOLOGY

Dangerous and even fatal conditions can be due to the activity of the immune system, whose function is normally to protect life and health. In evolutionary terms, however, these conditions are evidently less of a threat to survival than is infectious disease. Immunopathology is the price paid for the possession of a vigorous immune system.

Immunopathological reactions are usually classified in terms of the *mechanism* responsible for the damage. This is the basis of the Gell and Coombs classification shown in Table 6.6 and used throughout this book. An alternative approach would be a classification based on the *antigen* concerned. This has the virtue of clearly distinguishing responses to foreign antigens from those to self antigens, the former being essentially 'normal' responses and the latter inherently abnormal. Responses to foreign antigens are loosely referred to as *hypersensitivity*, and to self antigens as *autoimmunity*; however, there is a substantial overlap.

HYPERSENSITIVITY

The word hypersensitivity was coined over 100 years ago, to describe differences in immune status detectable by skin testing. A patient immune to (that is, recovered from) a disease, who is subsequently injected intradermally with an appropriate antigen, might show an *immediate* reaction (a wheal and flare within minutes), a slower *acute* reaction (swelling and redness within hours), or a *delayed* reaction (swelling and redness 2 days or more after the injection). Immediate and acute reactions indicate that the patient possesses antibody to the antigen in question, while the delayed reaction indicates the presence of specific memory T cells. Skin testing is still widely used in diagnosis, but, confusingly, a positive result may be either good or bad for the patient depending on circumstances; a knowledge of the underlying mechanism is thus essential.

Table 6.6 Immunopathological mechanisms (the Gell and Coombs classification)

Type	Mediators	Result	Examples	Basis of diagnosis
Hypersensitivity				
I	IgE, mast cells	Allergy Anaphylaxis	Hay fever Bee sting	Immediate skin reaction Specific IgE (RAST)
II	Ig bound to cell-surface antigens	Phagocytosis Cytotoxicity Lysis	Transfusion reactions Rh disease Autoimmune diseases	Antiglobulin tests (see p. 1072)
III	Ag-ab complexes, PMN, complement	Vascular damage	SLE Post-streptococcal glomerulonephritis	Complexes in serum (see p. 817)
IV	T cells, macrophages	Granuloma Oedema	TB Contact sensitivity	Delayed skin reaction
Other mechanisms (Designated IIa or V)	Ig bound to hormone receptors	Stimulation or blocking of hormone effect	Graves' disease Myxoedema	In vitro assays
	Cytokines	Vascular damage	Gram-negative shock	Plasma cytokine levels

6 The Immunological Basis of Disease

Anaphylaxis and allergy

The commonest forms of hypersensitivity are hay fever and other allergies, up to 15% of the population being affected to some degree. The crucial steps in the allergic response are:

1. the formation of *IgE antibody* specific to the inducing antigen or 'allergen'
2. binding of this antibody to *mast cells* and basophils
3. attachment of further molecules of the allergen to the cell-bound IgE
4. degranulation of the mast cells and release of a number of *mediators* with a variety of inflammatory effects.

The symptoms of allergy depend partly on the type of mediators released, but mainly on the site at which it occurs.

The serum IgE level, which normally constitutes only a few millionths of total Ig, is regulated by T cells and by genetic factors, including HLA. The level is usually raised in allergic subjects, but why individual patients often make high levels of IgE to only a single allergen is not clear.

Mast cells are found in most organs and there is a special subpopulation in the mucosa of the gut and the lung. Together with basophils, these cells have very high affinity receptors for the Fc region of IgE. If two molecules of IgE bound to a mast cell or basophil are cross-linked by a molecule of antigen, membrane changes occur, leading to Ca^{2+} influx, a fall in intracellular cAMP and release of mediators. The same result can also be produced by stimulation of adrenergic receptors by noradrenalin or cholinergic receptors by acetylcholine; β receptor stimulation has the opposite effect.

The main effect of the released mediators is to increase vascular permeability and to cause bronchial constriction. *Histamine* has both of these effects, while the *leukotrienes* and *prostaglandins* tend to bring about one or other of them. There are also some important chemotactic molecules which attract other cells, such as PMN, eosinophils and platelets, to the site of inflammation. Eosinophils may play a regulatory role by releasing molecules that counteract many of the mast cell products.

Allergic responses may be localised to the site of entry of the allergen, e.g. the nose and eyes in hay fever, the bronchi in asthma and the skin in eczema. When allergens enter the circulation, as with insect venoms or injected drugs, the reaction may be widespread and lead to vascular collapse, vomiting and even death; this is known as *systemic anaphylaxis* and calls for immediate treatment with adrenalin. For localised allergies, treatment consists of removing the cause if possible, or the use of drugs that inhibit mast cell degranulation. Numerous desensitisation regimes are in use and these undoubtedly work sometimes, but the effect is variable.

While asthma is frequently allergic, there are numerous other contributory factors. Some chemicals, e.g. anaesthetics, can cause mast cells to degranulate in the absence of IgE antibodies; the resulting reactions are called *anaphylactoid*, the key difference being that, unlike true anaphylactic reactions, they can occur without previous exposure to the inciting agent.

Acute inflammation is beneficial in increasing the local availability of blood components such as antibody, complement and PMN, and it is possible that IgE antibody has evolved to enhance and accelerate this in an antigen-specific fashion. A particularly important case may be intestinal worm infections, where contact between potentially cytotoxic cells and their target would normally be extremely limited.

Antibody-mediated cytotoxic hypersensitivity

Antibody-mediated cytotoxic hypersensitivity refers to reactions in which antibody attached to a cell surface leads to damage by complement and/or PMN or other Fc-receptor-bearing cytotoxic cells. This is one of the predominant mechanisms by which antibody destroys infectious micro-organisms and, in the majority of cases, is purely beneficial. Because of the specificity of antibody, the damage is normally focused on the foreign organism, but ill-effects to the host can result in two particular situations:

- when the foreign cell is one whose destruction is not desirable, such as a blood transfusion or an organ graft
- when the antibody is directed not against foreign but against *self*-antigens. It follows that most type II 'hypersensitivity' reactions are, in fact, aspects of either transplant rejection (p. 96) or autoimmunity (p. 94). They are dealt with more fully in these sections.

Immune complexes and disease

Damage to tissues or blood vessels by the deposition of antigen–antibody complexes is a very important cause of disease, but there is nothing inherently abnormal in the formation of such complexes. Millions of antigen–antibody complexes are removed from the blood and tissues every day in normal health, chiefly by phagocytic cells but also by the solubilising effect of complement. When such clearance is inadequate, complexes become deposited elsewhere and cause disease.

Pathogenesis

The commonest reasons for inadequate clearance and thus deposition of complexes are *persistent* antibody responses, e.g. chronic infections, inhalation of antigens in special occupations or passive immunotherapy with foreign serum. A special case is when the antibody is directed against *self*-antigens, which obviously can never be totally eliminated. Such autoimmune reactions are considered on page 96.

The mechanism of damage is essentially the same for all immune complex-mediated diseases. The activation of complement releases the inflammatory peptides, C3a and C5a, generating local vascular permeability, attraction of platelets, basophils and PMN, microthrombus formation and PMN degranulation; the lysosomal enzymes released by the PMN do most of the damage. Complexes tend to deposit in sites of turbulent blood flow or filtration, such as the renal glomerulus, but it is probable that the nature of the antigen is also important; thus, anti-DNA complexes (e.g. in systemic lupus erythematosus) are especially prone to deposit in the glomerulus, and anti-Ig complexes (e.g. in rheumatoid arthritis) in the joints. However, very widespread complex deposition, as used to be seen in *serum sickness*, can affect both sites.

Investigation

Most laboratories use a combination of tests that depend on the size of the complex (such as precipitation with polyethylene glycol) and the ability of the antibody in the complex to bind complement (C1q binding assays). However, except in bacterial endocarditis, the level of complexes in the serum *per se* is not usually of much diagnostic value. On the other hand, when tissue biopsies are available, the demonstration of Ig and/or complement in a particular site can be most informative. A striking example of this is the difference between the linear deposition of anti-glomerular basement membrane complexes of Goodpasture's syndrome (an autoimmune disease) and the more granular appearance of immune-complex glomerulonephritis, which may be due to a variety of infections, such as hepatitis B virus, streptococci and malaria, to drugs or to an autoantigen such as DNA.

Delayed-type and cell-mediated hypersensitivity

Delayed-type hypersensitivity

A delayed-type hypersensitivity (DTH) skin test indicates the presence of T cell-mediated immunity to the antigen in question, the best known example being the Mantoux (tuberculin) test for previous exposure to tuberculosis. Changes in the skin include: contact between the antigen and circulating specific helper T lymphocytes; release of cytokines by the latter; and the consequent accumulation and activation of non-specific cells, particularly monocytes, in the vicinity. Most of these steps can also be

reproduced in tissue culture, and it is assumed that they represent the 'cell-mediated' changes that would take place at the site of the actual reinfection, e.g. in the lung for tuberculosis. DTH tests are useful for diagnosis of a number of infections, particularly those involving chronic intracellular organisms. They can also be of prognostic value, e.g. in leprosy, where strong DTH correlates with effective immunity to the bacterium, but also with tissue-damaging and truly immunopathological reactions.

Other forms of delayed reaction

The relationship between cell-mediated immunity, DTH and resistance to infection is, however, more complicated. In the first place, very similar changes can be found in *contact sensitivity*, an eczematous skin reaction to, for example, dyes, metals and plants, which has no beneficial value. In addition, there are other forms of delayed reaction where the cellular changes are somewhat different. These range from the slightly earlier (24-hour) Jones-Mote response, in which vascular changes and basophil accumulation are more prominent, to the much slower-developing granulomatous and necrotic lesions originally noted by Koch. It is assumed that different T cells and cytokines are responsible for these different patterns of response.

Granuloma formation

Granuloma formation is the most serious manifestation of cell-mediated hypersensitivity. A granuloma is a solid mass of macrophages, some of which may fuse to form *giant cells*, while others become specialised for protein synthesis (the *epithelioid cells*). Eosinophils are often prominent, as are lymphocytes. The latter include T cells, whose lymphokines initiate and maintain the lesion, though there is evidence that T cells can also suppress granuloma formation.

The clash of interests faced by the cell-mediated immune system is illustrated by the deposition of eggs in the liver during the worm disease schistosomiasis. In the absence of a cellular reaction (e.g. in T cell-deficient mice) enzymes secreted by the eggs (in a vain attempt to escape into the intestine) lead to damage and destruction of liver tissue. A granulomatous reaction around each egg, with ultimate fibrosis and calcification, protects liver function but can result in cirrhosis with portal hypertension, oesophageal varices and fatal haematemesis.

Anti-receptor antibodies

Although not part of Gell and Coombs' original classification, antibodies against cell-surface receptors for hormones can cause important pathological effects in one of two ways:

- by blocking the binding of the natural hormone and thus preventing cell stimulation
- by actually mimicking the action of the hormone and leading to overstimulation of the cell.

Such antibodies are autoantibodies, and both types are found in thyroid disease (p. 684).

Lymphocytes can also be inhibited or stimulated in a similar way by antibodies against their own surface receptors. An example is the ability of anti-idiotype antibodies to trigger a B lymphocyte, by combining with its antigen-binding site in the same manner as antigen. Such idiotype–anti-idiotype interactions form the basis for artificial manipulations of the immune response with exciting prospects for the future.

AUTOIMMUNITY

The immune system can react against the host's own antigens. Details of particular autoimmune diseases will be found in the relevant chapters, this section being concerned with the general principles underlying self-tolerance and its breakdown in autoimmunity.

Self-tolerance and experimental autoimmunity

It is clearly impossible to prevent the *genes* for a self-antigen and an antibody which recognises it occurring in the same individual. For example, the blood group AB child of an A father and B mother inherits the genes for both anti-B and anti-A but must not make either of these antibodies. The mechanisms preventing this appear to be a combination of clonal elimination of lymphocytes, suppressor T cells, receptor-blocking and anti-idiotypic interactions (p. 91). Antigens present in high concentrations, such as the blood groups or serum albumin, may lead to clonal elimination, whereas in normal individuals, B lymphocytes are demonstrably present against thyroglobulin, of which there are only trace amounts in the serum. With T lymphocytes, the situation is more complicated, since part of their normal triggering involves recognition of self MHC molecules (p. 90). However, recent work with cultured monoclonal T cells suggests that fully self-reactive T cells also exist in normal individuals. This implies an important role for *regulatory* mechanisms in maintaining self-tolerance, and suggests that when autoimmunity does develop, it is these that may have failed.

Classification of autoimmune diseases

The traditional classification of human autoimmune diseases is based on the site affected, ranging from highly localised damage to single organs, frequently endocrine glands (*organ-specific*), to multi-site disease with lesions disseminated throughout the blood vessels, kidney, skin and joints (*non-organ-specific*). Generally speaking, the pathological mechanisms in organ-specific disease are of the cytotoxic or anti-receptor type, while non-organ-specific disease is due to immune complex deposition (p. 94). Table 6.7 lists some common autoimmune diseases in these two categories. Interestingly, the organ-specific as well as the non-organ-specific diseases tend to be grouped in individuals or families; an example of the latter is the association of anti-DNA and anti-Ig (rheumatoid factor) antibodies in connective tissue diseases, such as rheumatoid arthritis, SLE and Sjögren's syndrome, and of the former, the association of antibodies to stomach, thyroid and other endocrine organs.

It must be emphasised that the finding of an autoantibody in a patient does not mean that it is the cause of the presenting disease; it may be purely secondary, such as the anti-cardiolipin (Wasserman) antibodies in syphilis. Nor does the absence of detectable autoantibodies rule out an autoimmune cause; it may be a purely T cell-mediated disease. The strongest evidence for a direct link between autoantibodies and disease comes when the symptoms can be transferred by antibody, as can occur in the newborn babies of mothers with thyrotoxicosis or myasthenia gravis.

The influence of HLA

Autoimmune diseases make up the largest group of conditions associated with particular HLA phenotypes (p. 87 and Table 6.2). The B8-DR3 combination is particularly interesting, in view of the range of quite different organ-specific diseases to which it is linked; it has been suggested that people with this combination are immunologically 'high responders' to a variety of antigens. In the case of ankylosing spondylitis, actual cross-reaction between the B27 molecule and an antigen on certain enterobacteria, such as *Klebsiella* and *Yersinia*, may be an element in the disease.

A second aspect of HLA is the finding of class II molecules on the cells of affected organs where they are not normally expressed, the most striking example being the thyroid in Graves' and Hashimoto's disease. It remains to be established whether this anomalous expression is a primary phenomenon leading to presentation of self-antigens to T cells, or whether it is secondary to T cell infiltration and release of mediators such as interferon.

TRANSPLANTATION

The understanding of transplant rejection began in 1900, when Landsteiner discovered the ABO blood groups. Donor and patient had to be matched so that no antigens were present in the donor that were absent in the recip-

Table 6.7 Major autoimmune diseases

Category	Area affected	Disease	Auto-antibodies found	Page reference
Organ-specific	Thyroid	Hashimoto's	Thyroglobulin	690
		Graves'	TSH receptor	689
	Stomach	Atrophic gastritis	Parietal cells	573
		Pernicious anaemia	Intrinsic factor	1054
	Adrenal	Addison's	Adrenal cell	699
	Pancreas	Juvenile diabetes	Islet cells	745
	Liver	Chronic active hepatitis	Smooth muscle; LSP	638
	Gut	Ulcerative colitis	Colon antigen (?)	596
	Skin	Pemphigus	Desmosomes	1145
	Blood	AIHA	Red cells	1066
		ITP	Platelets	1107
	Nerve-muscle	Myasthenia gravis	Acetylcholine receptor	950
	Salivary gland, eye, joints	Sjögren's syndrome	Salivary cells and ducts	999
	Kidney, lung	Goodpasture's syndrome	Basement membrane	823
	Liver, salivary gland	Primary biliary cirrhosis	Mitochondrial	641
Non-organ-specific	Joints	Rheumatoid arthritis	IgG (→Immune complexes)	993
	Lung	Polymyositis		
	Blood		DNA (→Immune complexes)	1029
	Skin	Scleroderma		1028
	Kidney	SLE	Red cells, platelets	1023

LSP = liver-specific protein; AIHA = autoimmune haemolytic anaemia; ITP = idiopathic thrombocytopenic purpura; SLE = systemic lupus erythematosus.

ient: apparent exceptions turned out to be due to other 'minor' antigenic systems. Tissue transplants obey similar rules, with the MHC playing the dominant role, and a still unknown number of minor histocompatibility antigens making their contribution to rejection.

Here, however, the parallel with blood transfusion ends because:

- a blood transfusion is rejected purely by *antibody*, while with most organ and tissue grafts, *cell-mediated* immunity also plays a crucial part
- the degree of complexity and polymorphism at the MHC are such that matching of donor and recipient are seldom perfect; thus, the resulting rejection response usually has to be *suppressed* by drugs or other means.

HLA typing and matching

Class I antigens (A, B and C) are typed using monospecific antisera and complement in a micro-cytotoxic assay. Of the class II antigens, those at the DQ and DR locus can be typed in the same way, but DP antigens seem to be recognised only by T lymphocytes and are typed by *mixed lymphocyte reactions* (MLR). For convenience, B lymphocytes from a blood sample are normally used, since those cells carry all the class I and class II antigens of the individual. All MHC alleles are expressed *co-dominantly*, so that it should be possible to detect two antigens at each locus, unless the patient happens to be homozygous for one of them. Because of the large number of alleles at each locus, the number of possible permutations is enormous (at least 10^{13}), but some alleles are very rare so that, in practice, the chance of a perfect match between unrelated people is around 1 in 10^5. This chance is higher in relatives, rising to 1 in 4 in siblings and, of course, 1 in 1 in identical twins. Retrospective studies on large groups of kidney-grafted patients suggest that class II matching is the most important.

Mechanisms of rejection

The mechanisms of transplant rejection (Fig. 6.8) depend to some extent on the tissue concerned. Transplants introduced via the circulation, such as blood and bone marrow, are highly vulnerable to the lytic and phagocytic actions of antibody. Skin grafts are destroyed by purely cell-mediated reactions, probably a combination of cytotoxic T cells and activated macrophages. Well-vascularised organs, such as the kidney and heart, are susceptible to damage by both mechanisms: antibody against MHC class I or ABO blood group antigens on the

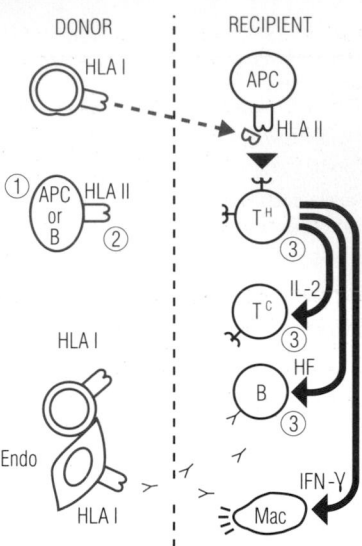

Fig. 6.8 Transplant rejection and immunosuppression. Donor cells and moleculues are shown in red. On the right are the principal mechanisms by which the recipient recognises and responds to donor antigens. APC = antigen-presenting cell; Endo = vascular endothelium; Mac = macrophage; T^H and T^C = helper and cytotoxic T cells; IL-2 = interleukin 2; HF = helper factors; IFN-γ = gamma interferon. Immunosuppression: (1) Removal of HLA class II bearing cells (organ culture; anti-HLA class II antibodies). (2) Blocking of recognition (anti-HLA class II antibodies). (3) Elimination of specific lymphocytes (antigen suicide; anti-idiotype antibodies). In addition to these specific mechanisms, there are also non-specific means of suppressing rejection: irradiation; anti-lymphocyte antibodies; cytotoxic drugs, e.g. azathioprine; anti-T cell agents, such as cyclosporin A; and anti-inflammatory drugs, e.g. steroids.

vascular endothelium leads to platelet and PMN accumulation and vascular obstruction; while T cells infiltrate and damage the organ much as they do a skin graft. Liver grafts are unusual, in that HLA matching seems to make no difference.

Bone marrow transplants pose an additional problem because they contain competent T lymphocytes which can react against the HLA antigens of the recipient – the *graft versus host* (GVH) reaction. GVH disease is frequently fatal, but progress has been made in developing methods for removing T cells from the transplanted marrow, e.g. using monoclonal anti-T cell antibodies.

IMMUNOSUPPRESSION

The mainstay of management of transplant patients is immunosuppression. Many drugs can suppress one or other aspect of the immune response (Table 6.8). Cyclosporin A is rapidly becoming the drug of choice for transplantation, and perhaps also for severe autoimmune diseases; it acts by selectively suppressing activated T lymphocytes, mainly by blocking cytokine production. Other drugs still widely used are antiproliferative agents

Table 6.8 Commonly used immunosuppressive drugs and their effects

Drug	Mode of action (principal target)	Major side-effects
Steroids (e.g. prednisone)	Anti-inflammatory (macrophage)	Infections Diabetes Osteoporosis Cushing's syndrome
Azathioprine (Imuran)	Anti-mitotic (T cell)	Infections Marrow aplasia Hepatotoxicity Hair loss
Cyclophosphamide	Anti-mitotic (B-cell)	Infections Sterility (male)
Cyclosporin A	Inhibits T cell cytokine formation, especially IL-2	Nephrotoxicity Lymphomas
FK 506	As cyclosporin A	Few reported so far

such as *azathioprine* (Imuran) which kill dividing cells, including lymphocytes, and corticosteroids, such as *prednisone*, which act mainly by depressing macrophage function. All these drugs have the unwelcome side-effect of rendering the patient susceptible to infection. In addition, the antiproliferative drugs can cause agranulocytosis and thrombocytopenia (by inhibiting cell division in the bone marrow), unless carefully monitored.

Plasma exchange can be life-saving, where the aim is to remove pre-existing antibody, e.g. Rhesus antibodies (p. 1077), or autoantibodies in myasthenia gravis or Goodpasture's syndrome.

IMMUNOLOGICAL TECHNIQUES

Antibodies are highly discriminatory and highly sensitive in their reactions with antigens. This makes them valuable reagents for typing cells or micro-organisms, and for detecting very small amounts of materials such as hormones. Antigen–antibody interactions can be visualised by the use of a fluorescent dye, a radioisotope or a specific enzyme attached to the antigen or the antibody. In the case of tissue sections, *immunofluorescence* is commonly used to identify the sites to which a particular antiserum binds, e.g. in autoimmune diseases. For hormone estimation, *radioimmunoassay* can be used. Here, the unknown sample is allowed to compete with the binding of a standard antibody/labelled antigen mixture. Enzyme-linked (ELISA) assays, in which an enzyme (such as peroxidase) which induces a colour change in its substrate is used in place of the radioisotope, are increasingly popular because of their cheapness and safety.

At present, considerable hopes are attached to the use of monoclonal antibodies as reagents for 'finding' particular antigens in vivo and directing other compounds to the site. Examples would be the localisation of tumours by isotope-labelled antibody, or the anti-tumour effect of antibodies coupled to cytotoxic drugs, such as ricin molecules. The same idea can be applied in reverse, by using a toxic preparation of antigen to seek out and destroy lymphocytes whose receptors recognise the antigen.

FURTHER READING

Bibel D J 1988 Milestones in immunology. Springer-Verlag. *A fascinating history of immunology since the first vaccine (1798) with excerpts from classic papers.*

Chapel H, Heaney M 1989 Essentials of clinical immunology, 2nd edn. Blackwell Scientific Publications, Oxford. *The best short textbook of clinical immunology, predominantly systems-based.*

Lachman P J, Peters D K, Rosen F S, Walport M J, 1992 Clinical aspects of immunology, 5th edn. Blackwell Scientific Publications, Oxford. *The bible of British clinical immunology, now with an Anglo-American editorial panel. A massive and authoritative reference book.*

Playfair J H L 1992 Immunology at a glance, 5th edn. Blackwell Scientific Publications, Oxford. *A simple illustrated introduction to the subject.*

Roitt I M 1991. Essential immunology, 7th edn. Blackwell Scientific Publications, Oxford. *An up-to-date and stimulating textbook, including many experimental details.*

Stites D P, Terr A I 1991. Basic and clinical immunology, 7th edn. Appleton and Lange, Connecticut. *An excellent multi-author volume, one of the few to combine basic and clinical aspects.*

7

Nutrition in Clinical Medicine

Andrew M Tomkins

FOOD AND ITS USE

Nutrition is the process by which food is eaten and utilised by the body. This chapter is concerned with the ways in which nutrient supplies — especially energy — are utilised, and how dietary factors and deficiencies may produce specific clinical syndromes or contribute to the development of disease.

Energy

Without energy, maintenance of metabolic processes, physical activity and growth could not occur. The majority of dietary energy is needed for pumping ions across cell membranes, e.g. in red blood cells, cardiac muscle or intestinal epithelium. Energy expenditure can be measured as the basal metabolic rate (BMR) in the early morning in a resting subject having last eaten the previous evening. More recent methods measure energy expenditure in free-living adults using stable isotopes.

The energy requirement of an individual subject depends primarily on body size and composition, but age, physical activity, environmental temperature and physiological state (whether pregnant, lactating or suffering from systemic infection) are also important. Energy expenditure may be considerably increased in situations of metabolic stress such as pyrexia and burns. Energy is expressed as kilocalories (kcal) or kilojoules (kJ) (1 kcal = 4.18 kJ). Energy requirements are highest — on a body weight basis or by comparison with 'lean body mass' — in infants and young children. Energy expenditure starts to drop in the twenties and declines steadily thereafter into old age. Because the factors affecting energy requirement vary considerably between individuals, it is impossible to give an exact ideal nutrient intake, but there are clearly differences in daily energy expenditure between adults with different lifestyles (Table 7.1). Table 7.2 shows how this expenditure is partitioned between different activities, and Table 7.3 shows the energy required for various physical activities. As the total time in each 24 hours spent in such activities is often rather short, significant increases in energy expenditure are hard to sustain. Weight reduction by increasing physical activity is hard to achieve. However, there are

Table 7.1 Average daily energy expenditure in various lifestyles

Occupation (age in years)	Expenditure in kcal (MJ)			
	Men		Women	
Retired elderly (65+)	2300	(9.5)	1900	(7.8)
Housewife (25–45)	–		2200	(9.0)
Office worker (20–50)	2500	(10.4)	2100	(8.6)
Laboratory technician (20–50)	2800	(11.7)	2200	(9.0)
Factory worker (20–45) (Heavy industry)	3200	(13.2)	2400	(9.9)
Labourer (20–45) (Heavy physical work)	3600	(14.8)	–	

Table 7.2 Breakdown of average daily energy expenditure in clerks and miners

	Clerks		Miners	
	kcal	MJ	kcal	MJ
Sleep	500	2	500	2
Work	900	4	1750	7
Non-work activity	1400	6	1400	6
Total	2800	12	3650	15

Table 7.3 Average energy expenditure in various degrees of physical activity

Degree of activity	Expenditure (kcal/min)
Minimal (e.g. sitting, slow walking)	1
Moderate (e.g. walking, gardening)	5
Intermediate (e.g. swimming, brisk walking)	7
Heavy (e.g. digging, squash, running)	10

indications that energy expenditure remains elevated for 12–24 hours after vigorous exercise, and even resting energy expenditure may be increased by fitness.

Energy is required for growth, and measurements of weight gain or height gain are useful indicators of dietary insufficiency. During the first few weeks of catch-up growth from severe protein-energy malnutrition (PEM), the energy cost of weight gain is about 5 kcal/g. There-after, it becomes more energy expensive to lay down tissue, as fat rather than protein is stored.

Almost all components of the diet — fat, carbohydrate, protein and alcohol — provide energy. In the UK, fat and carbohydrate each provide between 40% and 50% of dietary energy whereas in developing countries the propor-tion from fat may be less than 15% and from carbohy-drates more than 75%. The proportion of energy from protein is around 10% in an average UK diet. If protein is given without sufficient energy — e.g. in parenteral feeding regimes using amino acid solutions alone, or in athletes in training on very high protein diets — a large proportion is used up in oxidation. This also occurs in certain synthetic micro-diets providing 400 kcal/day or less, where protein is supplied in otherwise adequate quantities, but without adequate calories. At least some of the resulting weight loss is due to loss of body protein as it is oxidised.

Protein

Tissue growth, repair and atrophy depend on protein. The relative efficiency of proteins from different sources in promoting tissue growth depends on the presence or otherwise in the protein of the nine essential amino acids (which cannot be synthesised by the body). If one or more are in low concentration, food is less efficient at building protein (i.e. more has to be eaten). Dietary proteins are usually scored for their efficiency in compar-ison with whole egg or milk protein. However, it is impor-tant to remember that foodstuffs with a low score such as maize (which scores 47% because of low levels of trypto-phan) or beans (which score 47% because of low levels of sulphur-containing amino acids) may complement each other in terms of amino acid level. A maize/beans mix — which is eaten by millions of people all over the world —

has a score of 57%, i.e. this diet is not really 'protein limiting' provided there is enough of it.

Adequate protein intake can be achieved either by eating more of the cereals or by increasing the intake of foods with a higher protein score. The protein content of some common foods is shown in Table 7.4. Most of the world's population (i.e. those in developing countries) practises the cereals strategy. Their diet is, of necessity, very bulky because of the high viscosity and low energy density of most cereal porridges (Fig 7.1). Some cereals, such as cassava, have a very low protein content, but most populations take a mixed vegetarian diet well balanced with respect to protein and energy. The major problem is that millions of people do not get enough of it.

There is considerable debate as to how much protein we require. A useful strategy in all nutritional states is to consider the nitrogen balance — the difference between the dietary intake and obligatory losses of nitrogen (e.g. in the urine, faeces, sweat and sputum). Positive balance is achieved when intake exceeds losses, such as occurs in normal infant and child growth or during recovery from malnutrition in adulthood. Negative balance occurs when losses exceed intake, as in systemic infection or diarrhoea, or when dietary intake is reduced. The greatest require-ments for protein (relative to body weight) occur in young infants. Those less than three months of age require about 2.5 g protein/kg body weight/day, and the older

Table 7.4 The protein content of some common foods

Protein source	Proportion of energy from protein (%)
Poor	
Cassava	3.3
Cooked bananas (plantains)	4.0
Sweet potatoes (*Ipomoea batatas*)	4.4
Taros	6.8
Adequate	
Irish potatoes	7.6
Rice (home-pounded)	8.0
Maize (wholemeal)	10.4
Millet (*Setaria italica*)	11.6
Sorghum (*Sorghum vulgare*)	11.6
Wheat flour (medium extraction)	13.2
Millet (*Pennisetum glaucum*)	13.6
Good	
Groundnuts (peanuts)	18.8
Cows' milk (3.5% fat)	21.6
Beans and peas	25.6
Beef (lean)	38.4
Cows' milk (skimmed)	40.0
Soya bean	45.2
Fish (fatty)	45.6
Fish (dried)	61.6

7 Nutrition in Clinical Medicine

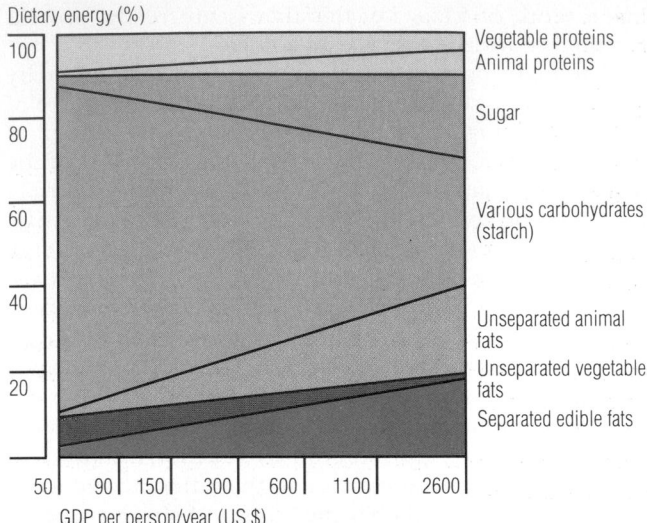

Fig. 7.1 Breakdown of total dietary energy related to income (GDP of countries).

infant (9–12 months age) requires 1.5 g protein/kg body weight/day. Children need less than infants but more than adults. Rates of protein synthesis vary with age, being highest in the newborn and declining with time (Table 7.5).

Carbohydrates

There are three major groups of carbohydrates in the diet: sugars, starches and cellulose and related materials.

- *Sugar.* The monosaccharides glucose, fructose and galactose are readily absorbed at the jejunal surface. The disaccharides, sucrose, maltose and lactose, are usually well absorbed as the monosaccharide component parts, provided that there has been effective hydrolysis by the disaccharidases. Sucrose intolerance and lactose intolerance may occur during diarrhoeal disease as a result of secondary disaccharidase deficiency. All sugars are absorbed as monosaccharides.
- *Starches.* These are a group of polysaccharides containing large numbers of glucose units linked together

Table 7.5 Variation in rate of protein synthesis with age

Age group	Body weight (kg)	Total body protein synthesis (g/kg body weight/day)
Newborn (premature)	2.0	15.0
Infant	9.0	7.0
Young adult	70.0	3.0
Elderly	55.0	2.0

to form straight branched chains. They are hydrolysed as a result of cooking, and are then further hydrolysed within the intestine. The commonest are the dextrins amylose and amylopectin.
- *Cellulose and related materials.* Most plant substances contain a range of celluloses that may or may not be digested in the intestine. Some celluloses are degraded by intestinal bacteria in the colon. Fibre has an important physiological function in influencing the absorption of sugars and fat, and contributes to intestinal bulk. Fibre content of different foods is shown in Table 15.28.

Several varieties of non-sugar sweetener exist. Sorbitol is sometimes used in diabetic foods because it is absorbed slowly. However, its energy value is the same as that of any other carbohydrate. Saccharin has no chemical or nutritional relationship to sugars and provides no energy; it is about 500 times as sweet as sucrose. Aspartame is also used as a sweetener; EEC regulations control the amount that is permitted in foods.

Fat

Fats provide the chief store of energy in the sub-cutaneous tissue, are important in the development of all cell membranes and some tissues, and are essential components of some hormones. The most common storage fats are the *triglycerides*. These are esters of glycerol and three fatty acids, which exist in a variety of forms according to the length of the carbon chain and the degree of saturation. This affects their solubility in water (shorter chain triglycerides are more soluble), fluidity and melting point. Vegetable oils have a greater proportion of polyunsaturated fats and are more fluid than the more saturated fats from animal sources, which are often hard (Fig. 7.2). *Phospholipids* — esters of glycerol with two fatty acids — are important for stability of cell membranes and deficiency may affect satisfactory psychomotor development. *Cholesterol* is the most important sterol. It is the precursor of the bile acids (which are essential for mixed micelle formation in the intestinal absorption of fat) as well as of adrenal and sex hormones and vitamin D. Cholesterol is also linked to the development of atheroma.

Lipoproteins are the chemical complexes, formed by the triglycerides, phospholipids and cholesterol with proteins, that circulate in the blood. These lipoproteins can be separated by electrophoresis or according to density on ultra-centrifugation (p. 776).

The body is efficient at synthesising triglycerides, sterols and phospholipids. Many populations whose diet provides only 15% of total energy as fat are able to lay down good stores of subcutaneous fat. Requirements for essential fatty acids are rather low and deficiency is there-

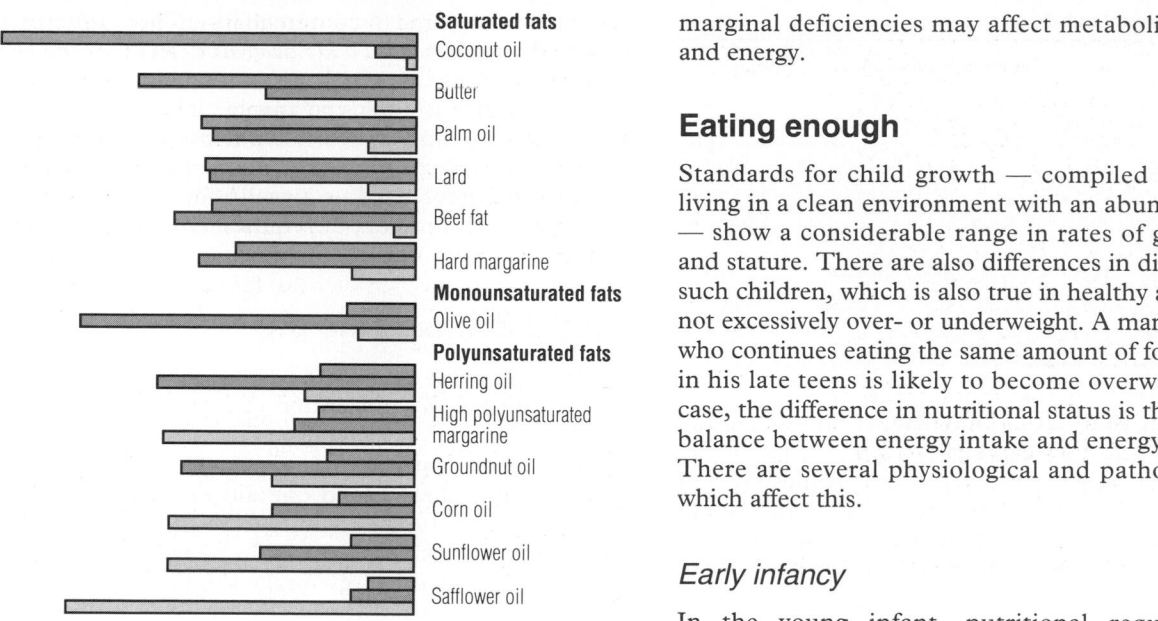

Saturated fats
Coconut oil
Butter
Palm oil
Lard
Beef fat
Hard margarine
Monounsaturated fats
Olive oil
Polyunsaturated fats
Herring oil
High polyunsaturated margarine
Groundnut oil
Corn oil
Sunflower oil
Safflower oil

☐ Saturated fatty acids
▨ Monounsaturated fatty acids
☐ Polyunsaturated fatty acids

Fig. 7.2 Fatty acid composition of some common fats and oils.

fore uncommon. However, low fat diets are often less palatable, which sometimes limits dietary intake and may lead to malnutrition. Low fat diets may also limit the absorption of carotene (the precursor of vitamin A found in green leafy vegetables). Fats provide twice as much energy per unit weight as protein or carbohydrate, and are thus useful sources of energy in diets designed to increase the rate of weight gain, e.g. in malnourished children. Conversely, a reduction in the fat content of the diet is a relatively efficient way to lose weight.

Micronutrients

Deficiencies of individual vitamins result in specific biochemical and clinical responses, but vitamins are also involved in metabolism in more general ways. Folate, for example, is necessary for cell division and the transfer of methyl groups in protein synthesis; thus, a deficiency may impair tissue repair or growth, even if dietary energy and protein are adequate. Thiamine is important in carbohydrate metabolism, and lactic acidosis may occur in deficiency states. A number of trace elements, such as zinc, are important in protein metabolism; deficiency of zinc is associated with an increased energy requirement for deposition of lean tissue. Children receiving nutrient supplements for PEM grow more slowly relative to the number of calories given, if they are not also supplemented with zinc. Severe individual micronutrient deficiencies may have recognizable clinical features, but even

marginal deficiencies may affect metabolism of protein and energy.

Eating enough

Standards for child growth — compiled from subjects living in a clean environment with an abundance of food — show a considerable range in rates of gain in weight and stature. There are also differences in dietary intake in such children, which is also true in healthy adults who are not excessively over- or underweight. A man in his thirties who continues eating the same amount of food that he ate in his late teens is likely to become overweight. In each case, the difference in nutritional status is the result of the balance between energy intake and energy expenditure. There are several physiological and pathological states which affect this.

Early infancy

In the young infant, nutritional requirements for protein are particularly high in relation to body weight (Table 7.5). Breast milk certainly provides enough protein for at least the first four months, and also has immunological advantages over cows' milk. Cows' milk formulae, while nutritionally adequate, are frequently dangerous when prepared under unhygienic conditions, as in many poor families in developing countries.

Later infancy and early childhood

Nutritional requirements are also high in infants over four months of age, when children often begin to receive solid foods in addition to breast milk. In developing countries, the growth rate frequently falters at this state — either because the energy given is not enough (the energy density of weaning foods in traditional societies is often low); or because there is so much gut infection that the food is not so well absorbed. Specific nutrient deficiencies (e.g. zinc, protein, folate) may also play a role.

Later childhood and adolescence

Nutritional requirements for protein and energy are usually met in older children, but there tend to be micronutrient deficiencies (e.g. of iron, folate and zinc), which may lead to anaemia, impaired intellectual performance and short stature.

Pregnancy

The nutritional stress of pregnancy is created by the need to produce both an infant and a placenta, plus some maternal fat stores. The generally accepted idea of a

Table 7.6 Average weight gain during pregnancy

	Increase in weight (g)			
	Up to 10 weeks	20 weeks	30 weeks	40 weeks
Fetus, placenta and liquor	55	720	2530	4750
Uterus and breast	170	765	1170	1300
Blood	100	600	1300	1250
Fat	325	1915	3500	4000
Total gain	650	4000	8500	12 000

9–12 kg weight gain during pregnancy requires (on the assumption of 5 kcal/g weight gain) an increased dietary intake of 150 kcal/day during the first trimester, and about 300 kcal/day thereafter, including extra protein (Table 7.6). Several studies show that the baby is rather small at birth if this is not achieved. In UK women there is evidence of decreased birth weight in those with low energy and protein intakes, a situation found especially among Asian immigrants. There are also increased demands on maternal stores, especially of iron, zinc and folate. However, despite such considerable increases in requirement, there are populations of women in developing countries with rather poor diets and very unfavourable lifestyles who produce babies of reasonable weight. Similarly, there are many women in the UK who date their obesity from their pregnancy. The reason for these findings is the markedly increased efficiency of metabolism during pregnancy so that dietary energy is stored more easily.

Lactation

The need to produce breast milk (up to 800 kcal/day) for many months has obvious nutritional implications. Some of this can be provided from maternal stores laid down in pregnancy, but an additional 500 kcal intake and extra protein is often recommended. Again, many women are able to produce adequate volumes of breast milk despite poor dietary intakes. However, when maternal nutritional status is severely decreased, there is a corresponding decrease in the volume and nutritional content of the milk. It is thus essential to improve the diet and lifestyle of women in developing countries if breast-feeding is to be promoted. A high proportion of women in the UK on the other hand eat more than they need during lactation and pregnancy.

Recommended daily allowances

In view of the considerable variation in nutrient metabolism between both population groups and individuals, accurate nutritional recommendations are difficult to make. The *recommended daily allowance* (RDA) is the level of nutrient intake at which nobody would be deficient; there are various tables available. The RDA is thus set to prevent undernutrition but may, if adhered to slavishly, contribute to overnutrition. The term *safe level* is also sometimes used — usually for nutrients where accurate measurements of requirements have not been performed.

Food patterns in the UK

There is currently an increased awareness of the importance of diet in the prevention of coronary thrombosis, hypertension and colon cancer. The National Advisory Committee on Nutrition Education (NACNE) proposed that a healthy diet should contain no more than 35% of energy from fat, that dietary fibre should increase to 25 g daily, that salt intake should be reduced by about 30% and that total energy intake should maintain body weight within normal levels (Fig. 7.3). The Coronary Prevention Group seeks to publicise the NACNE recommendations, which are summarised in Table 7.7.

ASSESSMENT OF NUTRITIONAL STATUS

The body is made up of lean body mass (the bony framework, muscle and dense connective tissue), adipose tissue

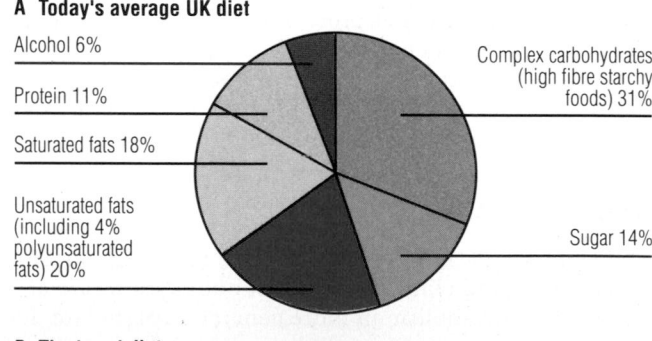

A Today's average UK diet

Alcohol 6%
Protein 11%
Saturated fats 18%
Unsaturated fats (including 4% polyunsaturated fats) 20%
Complex carbohydrates (high fibre starchy foods) 31%
Sugar 14%

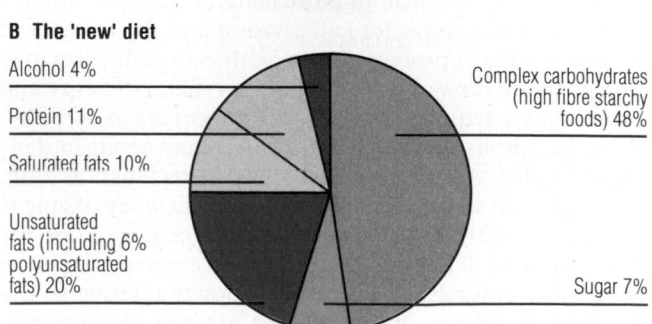

B The 'new' diet

Alcohol 4%
Protein 11%
Saturated fats 10%
Unsaturated fats (including 6% polyunsaturated fats) 20%
Complex carbohydrates (high fibre starchy foods) 48%
Sugar 7%

Fig. 7.3 Composition of an average UK diet, compared with that recommended by NACNE.

Table 7.7 Summary of proposals for dietary change to lower disease prevalence*

Nutrient	Current intake	Proposals
Energy	Increasing prevalence of obesity in UK indicates excessive intake.	Energy intake such as to keep body weigh within healthy limits (BMI 20–26)
Fat	Above 40% of energy taken in the form of fat.	Reduce, such that intake is <35% of energy intake.
Saturated fats	About 18% of energy taken in form of saturated fat.	Reduce, such that <15% of energy intake comes from saturated fats.
Polyunsaturated fats	About 4% of energy taken in form of polyunsaturates.	Increase to >5% of energy from polyunsaturates.
Fibre	About 15 g daily	Increase to above 25 g
Sugar	Very variable	Reduce by 10%
Salt	Very variable	Reduce by 10%
Alcohol	Very variable	Not more than 4 alcohol units per day

*National Advisory Committee on Nutrition Education, 1983; DHSS Diet and Cardiovascular Disease, 1984. BMI = Body Mass Index = weight/height^2.

Table 7.8 Assessment of nutritional status: body size, protein and fat

Method	Comments
Body size	
Weight and height	
Weight as % of standard weight/age in children	A child who is chronically underweight (compared to international standards) may still achieve good rates of weight gain.
Weight as % ideal body weight in adults	Weight varies by 0.5–1.0 kg/day in healthy adult subjects.
Weight/height^2 (BMI) in teenagers and adults	BMI is difficult to interpret in the elderly – use length of humerus as index of height.
Degree and rate of weight loss	More than 10% loss usually indicates PEM.
Protein	
Mid-arm circumference (MAC)	
Use the absolute value in children aged 1–5 years because there is little change with age. In adults there is considerable variation but <22 cm usually indicates loss of muscle mass	See Table 7.9.
Urinary creatinine/height	
Use 24 hour urine collection which indicates how much muscle mass is present	Creatinine excretion is affected by pyrexia. Incomplete 24 hour collections invalidate the method.
Plasma concentrations of hepatic export proteins (e.g. albumin, prealbumin, retinol binding globulin, thyroid binding globulin, transferrin)	All are affected by dietary intake in 2 weeks prior to test. 'Leak' of proteins (e.g. albumin in intestinal disease) may occur. Acute and chronic infections may decrease synthesis of the export proteins. Plasma albumin of <35 g/l or plasma transferrin of <1.5 g/l usually indicates PEM.
Tests of cellular immunity	
In vitro lymphocyte studies or skin tests	Considerable amount of laboratory work. No more sensitive than anthropometry.
Fat	
Skin fold thickness	
Measured at mid-triceps, subscapular and supra-iliac sites and expressed as absolute values or percentage of standard	Considerable sources of error in repeat measurements by different observers. Triceps skin fold thickness is the least variable.

and water. In weight terms, the composition of the constituents is 16% protein, 10–25% fat in men (15–30% in women), 5% minerals, 1% carbohydrate and the rest water (about 60%). This total body water is either in the cells (intracellular water, 35%) or in the vascular system and tissues (extracellular water, 25%). Measurement of nutritional status seeks to determine how these body compartments compare with one another and whether nutrient deficiencies or excesses are affecting the function of tissues.

Anthropometry

Measurements of weight in childhood can be compared with the weight of a child of the same age in tables of reference standards (thus, for example, a child's weight for its age may be 70% of the standard; see Table 7.8). The standards recommended by the World Health Organisation are those of the National Centre for Health Statistics (NCHS) which are based on the measurements of a large number of North American children. Similar NCHS standards exist for height, and an index of thinness can be expressed by calculating a child's weight as a proportion of that expected for a child of that height.

Among adults the range of body proportion is considerable. This can be expressed in a number of ways:

- As a weight as a percentage of ideal body weight from tables constructed from life assurance tables, or
- As the body mass index (BMI = weight/height^2).

- The mid-arm circumference (MAC) relates closely to weight/height measurements. Plastic strips to measure MAC using coloured bands have been used with great success in screening for children with severe PEM in developing countries (Table 7.9).
- A reasonable measurement of body fat can be made from measurement of skin fold thickness using

Table 7.9 Mid-arm circumference (MAC) in children aged 12–60 months

MAC (cm)	Level of nutrition
More than 13.5	Normal
12.5–13.5	Mild/moderate protein-energy malnutrition
Less than 12.5	Severe protein-energy malnutrition

Table 7.10 Classification of severe protein-energy malnutrition

Weight for age*	With oedema	Without oedema
60–80%	Kwashiorkor	Undernutrition
Less than 60%	Marasmic kwashiorkor	Marasmus

*Weight as % of standard (NCHS) weight of child of that age

Harpenden calipers, which apply a constant spring-loaded pressure to the fold. There is, however, considerable variation both between observers and within the same observer.

- Functional tests of muscle, such as dynamometry and measurement of the response to electrical stimulation, are said to measure muscle mass, but results are only abnormal when the level of nutrition is very poor.
- Urinary creatinine, on the other hand, is a very reliable index of muscle mass and is a useful marker for completeness of 24 hour urine collections.

Biochemical

A series of proteins produced by the liver may be used in the assessment of protein status, namely albumin, pre-albumin, transferrin, retinol binding globulin and thyroid binding globulin. These indicators are of limited value on their own because they are affected by short term energy intake as well as by protein stores. However, low levels (of albumin in particular) suggest decreased synthesis due to poor dietary intake, increased metabolism as in systemic infection, or a leak of protein as occurs, for example, in intestinal disease. Table 7.8 shows the tests available to assess individual nutrients.

PRIMARY NUTRITIONAL DISORDERS

PROTEIN-ENERGY MALNUTRITION

The term *protein-energy malnutrition* (PEM) is used to describe a variety of clinical syndromes which result from a diet inadequate in both energy and protein. It is often accompanied by micronutrient deficiencies, electrolyte imbalance and metabolic disorders. When it occurs in the UK, it is usually precipitated by a severe illness (e.g. gastrointestinal disease, surgery); in developing countries, it is the result of a poor diet often exacerbated by the added stress of infection (especially diarrhoea and measles). Indeed, the presence of infection is so common in children with PEM that the term *malnutrition/infection syndrome* is often used to describe the condition. Classification of the severe clinical syndromes of PEM (Table 7.10) depends on the child's weight calculated as a percentage of the median international standard for a child of the same age. Milder grades of PEM also exist

according to weight/age. Undernourished children may be further classified according to whether, or to what degree, they are short for their age *(stunting)*; alternatively they may be underweight and thin, i.e. a low weight/height *(wasting*, see Table 7.11 and Fig 7.4). The inference is that children who are stunted are likely to have been deprived of an adequate diet for many months (sufficient to cause linear growth retardation). The child who is wasted has lost body tissues, often, though not always, because of a recent infection or poor diet, for example due to harvest failure.

PEM in children

PEM is the end result of several processes. Thus, a child may become marasmic because of total lack of food in a

Table 7.11 Classification of stunting and wasting

Degree	Stunting (height/age)	Wasting (weight/height)
Normal	Over 95	Over 90
Mild	87.5–95	80–90
Moderate	80–87.5	70–80
Severe	Less than 80	Less than 70

*Weight (or height) as percentage of standard (NCHS) weight of child of that age

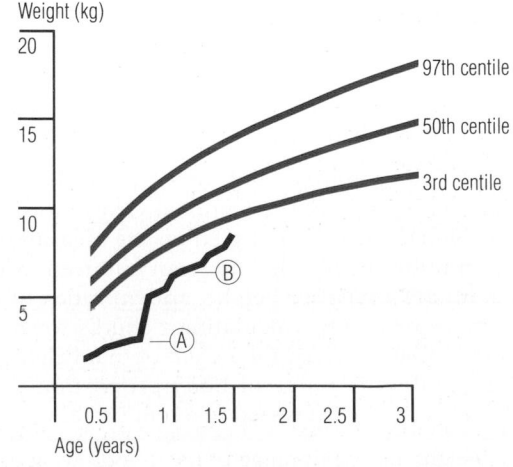

Fig. 7.4 Growth chart of a severely malnourished child. A. Start of nutrition rehabilitation. **B.** After discharge from nutrition rehabilitation centre.

famine, or because he has severe giardiasis, intestinal parasites or tuberculosis. A child may develop kwashiorkor at the time he is weaned off the breast and has to rely instead on inadequate quantities of solid food. There is only limited evidence that dietary differences explain why some children develop kwashiorkor and others become marasmic; kwashiorkor is often precipitated by measles and intestinal infection.

Marasmus

In marasmus, there is loss of both lean tissue and subcutaneous fat with characteristic wrinkling of the skin. This is sometimes difficult to differentiate from dehydration. The child is usually very cachectic, and has long eyelashes and lanugo hair on the forearms despite loss of hair on the head. However, the child is generally alert. The plasma albumin is usually maintained but plasma sodium and potassium levels are low.

Kwashiorkor

The main feature of kwashiorkor is oedema, which conceals the loss of lean tissue. The oedema usually starts in the legs but may extend to the trunk and head. There is often an associated scaly cracking of the skin and some children have discoloured or orange hair. The liver is sometimes enlarged, as it becomes infiltrated with fat which cannot be removed because of inadequate production of lipoproteins (see Ch.19, p. 777). Plasma albumin is low, as are plasma sodium and potassium. The low plasma potassium indicates a reduction in total body potassium, due to the loss of muscle mass. The low plasma sodium, however, is misleading, as it is due to an excess of body water. The total body sodium is in fact elevated.

Several factors contribute to the development of oedema. A decrease in plasma albumin decreases colloid osmotic pressure; while an increase in the generation of free radicals by infection (from systemic or intestinal pathogens, or toxins such as aflatoxin) can damage the capillaries sufficiently to cause them to leak fluid into the tissues. The deleterious effects are greatest in children with impaired scavenging mechanisms for free radicals, due to a deficiency of zinc, copper and vitamin A.

Associated deficiencies

Zinc deficiency is common in severe PEM, and may account for the skin lesions and impaired cellular immunity. Vitamin A deficiency is frequently precipitated by PEM, probably because of lack of synthesis of retinol binding globulin by the liver, and anaemia often occurs as a consequence of folate and/or iron deficiency and systemic infection (especially malaria). Cellular immunity is frequently depressed, permitting infections such as tuberculosis to become rampant. Antibody production is also impaired, but to a lesser extent, so that even severely malnourished children generally produce satisfactory levels of antibodies following immunisation. However, the general reduction in immunity is a key factor in the development of bacterial overgrowth syndromes in the intestine, pneumonia and septicaemia. The decreased heat production in PEM is often severe enough to cause hypothermia and prevents a pyrexial response to infection.

Specific organ changes

There is atrophy of the lining of the alimentary tract causing hypochlorhydria and flattening of intestinal villi. Nearly all children are heavily colonised by intestinal parasites and bacteria. Renal function is often impaired, leading to difficulties in excreting sodium and water. Experimental studies show marked effects of PEM on brain size and psychomotor development, but longitudinal studies of severely malnourished children show that the social environment is more important than nutrient deficiency in determining subsequent intellectual achievement.

Management

Several principles should be followed:

- Resuscitation for dehydration (in most cases using oral rehydration therapy).
- Antibiotics (such as procaine penicillin or chloramphenicol) should be given for systemic infections, together with treatment for malaria.
- Nutritional therapy depends on the introduction of special feeds providing maintenance requirements (100 kcal/kg body weight and 3 g protein/kg body weight). This should be accompanied by mineral mixes (especially potassium and zinc). In children with kwashiorkor, maintenance requirements are given until the oedema is cleared, then energy intakes are increased. In marasmic children, the intake can be increased earlier, until — ideally — about 200 kcal/kg body weight/day are given (Table 7.12). Table 7.13 shows some mixes which can be given during different stages of nutritional rehabilitation.

PEM in adults

PEM in adults is surprisingly common in medical and surgical practice. Inadequate intake is the most important factor, whether due to psychological factors (such as anorexia nervosa), pain (oral or intestinal cancer), nausea/vomiting (liver metastases, chemotherapy, gastrointestinal

7 Nutrition in Clinical Medicine

Table 7.12 Predicted rate of weight gain* in malnourished child weighing 7 kg

Total intake (kcal/day)	Excess (kcal/day)	Weight gain (g/day)	Days to gain 3000 g
700	0	0	–
760	60	10	300
820	120	20	150
940	240	40	75
1180	480	80	38
1660	960	160	19

*Assuming maintenance requirements of 100 kcal/kg/body weight/day

Table 7.13 Suitable high energy/protein mixes for children with severe protein-energy malnutrition

Type of milk (g)	Sugar (g)	Oil (g)	Water (ml)
Dried skimmed milk (86)	67	86	811
Evaporated milk (443)	67	52	488
Lactogen (183)	14	43	813
Complan (100)	67	71	812
Cows' milk (885)	67	56	42

disease) or fever (which often causes anorexia). Nutrient intakes are often reduced drastically in those who can only take fluids. Nutrient requirements may be considerably increased by sepsis. Energy expenditure increases by at least 10% for every 1°C rise in body temperature, and muscle protein is mobilised to provide amino acid precursors for the inflammatory response. Infection also increases the production of acute phase proteins such as C-reactive protein, but levels of plasma albumin may decrease due to decreased synthesis by the liver and increased catabolism of circulatory albumin. Any cause of malabsorption may cause a serious decrease in absorption of protein and energy. Disease of the lower small intestine and colon may cause serious leakage of endogenous protein and protein loss from blood. A checklist for nutritional assessment is given in Table 7.14. An approximate

Table 7.14 Assessment of causes of protein-energy malnutrition in adults

Food intake	Energy and protein intakes can be assessed by dietitian using memory recall or direct weighing. Reasons for decrease can be assessed by clinical history.
Nutrient requirements	Assessment of inflammatory response by measurement of body temperature and C-reactive protein.
Malabsorption	Use degree of steatorrhoea to assess energy losses approximately if unable to measure faecal energy losses directly.
Nutrient losses	Estimates of faecal protein losses can be made approximately from measurement of stool blood/mucus losses.

nitrogen balance can be obtained by measurement of urinary urea (the form in which 80% of urinary nitrogen is excreted).

VITAMIN DEFICIENCIES

A checklist for the methods of assessment of vitamin deficiencies is given in Table 7.15. The important food

Table 7.15 Assessment of nutritional status: vitamins*

Vitamin	Method	Comment
A	Clinical	Night-blindness is a good indicator. Corneal lesions are very late stage findings.
	Plasma carotene	
	Plasma retinol	Sensitive indicator of liver stores but reduced in infection.
Thiamine	Clinical	Neuropathy and optic atrophy are late stage findings.
	Erythrocyte transketolase	Sensitive but rapidly altered by amount of dietary thiamine.
Riboflavin	Clinical	Mouth lesions are non-specific.
	Erythrocyte glutathione reductase	Difficult to know physiological significance of low enzyme levels.
Niacin	Clinical	Glossitis, stomatitis, dermatitis.
	Urinary n-methyl-nicotinamide/creatine excretion	Sensitive. Difficult assay.
Folate	Serum folate	Marked changes after dietary intake.
	Erythrocyte folate	Sensitive assay of body stores.
B₁₂	Plasma vitamin level	Sensitive assay of body stores.
C	Clinical	Specific but occur at late stage only.
	Plasma or leucocyte ascorbate	Sensitive. Rapid response to diet.
D	Clinical	Rickets, osteomalacia.
	Plasma alkaline phosphatase	Non-specific. Sensitivity may be improved by isoenzyme analysis.
	Plasma 25-hydroxycholecalciferol	Very specific.
	Bone marrow histology	Specific.
E	Plasma or erythrocyte tocopherol	Sensitive and specific.
K	Prothrombin time	Non-specific, as it is influenced by hepatocellular dysfunction.

*Pyridoxine is omitted as this is not a routine assay.

sources of the various vitamins are shown in Table 7.16, and their roles in the body in Table 7.17.

Vitamin A deficiency

Dietary sources of carotenoids are green leafy vegetables and certain fruits, which provide beta carotene. Vitamin A deficiency leads to night blindness and xerophthalmia (damage to the conjunctiva): it also affects the immune system — increasing the severity of respiratory infections and diarrhoea — and the formation of epithelium in the sweat glands, lung and gut. It may also contribute to the high rates of child mortality in certain populations, particularly among poor communities where dietary intakes of carotene are low, and where the availability of the nutrient may be further reduced by intestinal parasites and diarrhoea. Vitamin A deficiency sometimes complicates inflammatory bowel disease, coeliac disease and cirrhosis. Measles is an important factor in xerophthalmia because of its effect (a) directly on the conjunctiva, where it increases the local requirement for vitamin A needed to repair the damaged conjunctiva; and (b) by its effect on

Table 7.16 Vitamins and their important food sources

Vitamin	Food sources
A	Carotenoids (esp. β-carotene), in carrots, dark green leafy vegetables, pumpkin, mango. Preformed vitamin A, in fish oils, liver, eggs, margarine.
Thiamine (B$_1$)	Fortified wheat flour (much of the thiamine in flour is removed by milling, but is then replaced in most flours), fortified breakfast cereals, milk, eggs, yeast extract, fruit.
Riboflavin (B$_2$)	Milk, cheese, eggs, fortified breakfast cereals, liver, kidney, whole grain cereals.
Niacin	Liver, kidney, milk, cheese, eggs, beef, chicken, pork, yeast extract, instant coffee, peas, beans.
Pyridoxine (B$_6$)	Liver, meat, fish, whole grain cereals, milk, peanuts.
Folate	Liver, kidney, green leafy vegetables, peas, beans, oranges, bananas.
Cobalamine (B$_{12}$)	Liver, kidney, fish, beef, pork, lamb, eggs, cheese.
Ascorbic acid (C)	Oranges, lemons, potatoes, green vegetables, fortified fruit drinks.
D	Fortified milk (e.g. evaporated), fatty fish, fortified margarine, eggs, liver.
E	Vegetable oils, wholegrain cereals, eggs, margarine.
K	Vegetables, peas, beans, liver.

Table 7.17 Role of vitamins in the body

Vitamin	Function
A	Maintenance of mucosal surfaces; production of mucus; immune system and retinal function.
Thiamine (B$_1$)	Metabolism of carbohydrate to provide energy; maintenance of cardiac muscle and peripheral nerves.
Riboflavin (B$_2$)	Control of intracellular oxidation; maintenance of skin, especially around the mouth.
Nicotinic acid	Utilisation of energy from food; maintenance of skin, especially in light-exposed areas.
Pyridoxine (B$_6$)	Metabolism of amino acids, especially tryptophan to nicotinic acid.
Folate	Cell multiplication, in the blood and mucosa.
Cobalamine (B$_{12}$)	Cell multiplication, esp. blood cells; control of fatty acid synthesis in myelin sheaths of nerves.
Ascorbic acid (C)	Maintenance of connective tissue; stimulates iron absorption.
D	Maintenance of calcium and phosphate levels in the blood; control of absorption of dietary calcium and movement of calcium between blood and bone.
E	Contributes to anti-oxidant capacity of body; important in maintenance of erythrocyte membranes in neonates.
K	Control of blood clotting.

synthesis of retinol binding protein which carries vitamin A from the liver stores to the eye.

Night blindness alone is easily reversible, but xerosis (the dry appearance of the conjunctiva) and Bitot's spots (heaped up desquamated cells causing flecks on the conjunctiva) are signs that, unless treatment is started soon, the lesion may progress to irreversible corneal ulceration.

In those areas where dietary vitamin A intake cannot be increased by horticulture and nutrition education programmes, the administration of vitamin A capsules (100 000 IU every four months) will largely prevent xerophthalmia. Vitamin A capsules should not, however, be given to pregnant women because of their teratogenic effect. Breast feeding tends to prevent vitamin A deficiency. In established xerophthalmia, retinol palmitate (100 000 IU) is given intramuscularly.

Thiamine deficiency

Thiamine is an essential factor in many glycolytic pathways and is especially important for proper function of the peripheral nervous system and the heart. Deficiency can cause a peripheral neuropathy, especially in the legs, with ataxia and optic atrophy. Most cases in the UK occur in malnourished alcoholics. Such patients may develop two additional syndromes. In *Wernicke's encephalopathy* nuclear or supranuclear ophthalmoplegia occurs with nystagmus, pupillary abnormalities, aphasia and mental confusion. In *Korsakoff's psychosis* a confused state characterised by memory loss and confabulation develops. Cardiac beri-beri (a high-output cardiac failure) sometimes occurs, particularly in populations who change to eating rice which is highly milled as this process removes the thiamine.

Diagnosis is usually made on clinical history and examination, but elevated levels of erythrocyte transketolase activity and blood pyruvate occur. Thiamine (100 mg) may be given intravenously or orally, followed by repeated doses of 20 mg three times daily. Cardiac beri-beri improves rapidly, but nutritional neuropathies tend to recover only partially, especially if present for a long time.

Niacin (nicotinic acid and nicotinamide) deficiency

Nicotinic acid occurs in many plant and animal foods and can also be synthesised from tryptophan. Nicotinic acid deficiency tends to occur in those who eat a monotonous maize diet (which is low in tryptophan), such as is often supplied to refugees. The resulting deficiency syndrome is *pellagra*.

Pellagra often starts with either a sore mouth, mild diarrhoea or confusion. The full clinical syndrome of 'dermatitis, diarrhoea and dementia' is not striking, except in well-established cases. The skin lesions are initially erythematous, but dry, cracked appearances then occur, especially in areas exposed to the sun, producing 'Casal's necklace' around the neck. There may be villus atrophy in the small intestine and malabsorption. If untreated, later stage deficiency may cause severe encephalopathy and spasticity. Pellagra is rare in the UK, but may occur in malabsorption syndromes such as coeliac disease, in patients treated with isoniazid, in Hartnup disease, in the carcinoid syndrome, in patients with very low protein diets, or in conditions giving rise to considerable loss of protein such as the nephrotic syndrome. Deficiency responds rapidly to daily doses of nicotinic acid (500 mg).

Riboflavin deficiency

Riboflavin deficiency occurs whenever a diet is continually deficient in legumes, pulses and animal products. It may thus accompany PEM or alcoholism and is especially liable to occur during pregnancy. The main lesions are mucosal dryness and cracking around the mouth, ears and eyelids, with the genital region also affected. Red blood cells are affected, causing a normochromic anaemia. Diagnosis is usually on clinical grounds but can be confirmed by reduced glutathione reductase activity in red blood cells. Lesions respond rapidly to riboflavin (6 mg daily).

Pyridoxine deficiency

Pyridoxine deficiency occurs in malabsorption syndromes, alcoholism and secondary to drug toxicity (especially isoniazid), but rarely as a primary deficiency disorder. Clinically, there is mental confusion, glossitis, dry skin lesions and peripheral neuropathy. There are also a number of rare metabolic disorders in which pyridoxine deficiency is associated with infantile convulsions and sideroblastic anaemia. Pyridoxine deficiency is popularly believed to be a cause of premenstrual syndrome but there is no scientific evidence for this. Treatment of deficiency in adults is by 5–20 mg doses daily. Excess leads to neurotoxicity.

Folate deficiency

Folate deficiency occurs in those whose diet lacks fresh vegetables or meat, or in which the vitamin is destroyed by overcooking. It may also occur secondary to upper small bowel malabsorption; in situations of increased requirements (i.e. pregnancy or haemolytic conditions); or in patients taking anti-folate drugs (e.g. methotrexate, trimethoprim). Clinical features, diagnosis and treatment are described in Chapter 24, page 1052.

Vitamin B$_{12}$ deficiency

Vitamin B$_{12}$ deficiency is described in Chapter 24, page 1054.

Vitamin C deficiency

Scurvy was well known among those on long-distance sea voyages for centuries. In the 18th century, Lind carried out a controlled trial treating scurvy with citrus fruits and using mouthwashes of dilute vinegar or sea water as a control. Complete recovery occurred in the treated group but none in the controls.

Today, deficiencies occur in the elderly — especially those on a 'tea and toast' diet — and in food faddists. It may also occur in young children during the first years of life when requirements are high. The clinical features of tiredness, hyperkeratosis of the hair follicles, petechial haemorrhages and bleeding gums are only present in severe deficiency; bleeding gums in malnourished children are more usually due to poor oral hygiene than to vitamin deficiency. The classical features of infantile scurvy — irritability, pain on moving the legs, and tenderness and enlargement of costochondral epiphyses together with megaloblastic anaemia — are now rarely seen.

Diagnosis is by measurement of leucocyte ascorbate content, but as leucocytes are rapidly renewed, normal levels are usually acquired within a few days of eating a hospital diet. Ascorbic acid 100 mg three times per day is rapidly effective in clinical deficiency. There is no consistent scientific evidence that large doses of vitamin C are effective in the prevention or treatment of the common cold.

Vitamin D deficiency

Vitamin D deficiency occurs in those who fail to produce enough in their skin (from the precursor 7-dehydrocholesterol in response to UV light), or who have inadequate dietary intake. In the UK, the high risk group are immigrant Asians who tend not to expose themselves to the limited sunlight available. Although they do eat fatty fish (a good source of vitamin D), their consumption of vitamin D fortified foods, e.g. margarine, is low, and the high phytate content (in chapatti flour) of the diet decreases its bioavailability. The result of vitamin D deficiency is rickets (in children) or osteomalacia (in adults), described in Chapter 18, page 727.

Vitamin E deficiency

Vitamin E deficiency occurs in low-birth-weight infants, malabsorption syndromes (especially cystic fibrosis) and abetalipoproteinaemia. Deficiency permits free radical damage to a number of membranes such as red blood cells (causing haemolytic anaemia) and nerve cells (causing ataxia and peripheral neuropathy). These conditions are exacerbated if extra nutrients, such as linoleic acid and iron, are given without vitamin E. There is no consistent scientific evidence of any effect of vitamin E on athletic success, sexual potency or atheroma. The only indication for therapy is if the level of plasma tocopherol is shown to be low in an appropriate clinical setting. Deficiency can be treated by 200 mg daily doses in adults.

Vitamin K deficiency

This may occur in neonates because placental transfer is limited and breast milk is often deficient; it also occurs in obstructive jaundice and certain malabsorption syndromes (see pp. 633 and 576). The result is hypothrombinaemia and bleeding, which is rapidly reversed by injections of vitamin K (phytomenadione).

Summary 1	Vitamin deficiency syndromes
Vitamin	*Deficiency syndrome*
A	Night blindness; xerophthalmia
Thiamine	Wernicke's encephalopathy; Korsakoff's psychosis
Niacin	Pellagra
Riboflavin	Mucosal lesions
Pyridoxine	Glossitis; neuropathy
Folate	Megaloblastosis; villus atrophy
B_{12}	Megaloblastosis; neuropathy
C	Scurvy
D	Rickets; osteomalacia
K	Hypoprothrombinaemia

Trace elements

The precise role of trace elements in health is uncertain but zinc deficiency appears important. Zinc, and probably also copper, are important in protecting cell membranes against free radical damage. Deficiency is seen most clearly in the congenital disorder *acrodermatitis enteropathica*, which is characterised in children by a scaly skin rash, secondary bacterial and fungal infection, diarrhea and severe growth faltering. All are rapidly reversed by zinc therapy. Deficiencies are also seen in children with severe PEM and were formerly seen in patients receiving parenteral nutrition without sufficient trace element mixes.

Iodine deficiency

Most iodine deficiency is due to low levels in the soil and water. There are many regions in the world, e.g. Nepal, Peru and Bangladesh, where iodine intakes are so low (<50–75 mg/day) that thyroid function is impaired. There is a high prevalence of cretinism in neonates in these regions, which may present as deaf mutism, mental retardation and ataxia with the characteristic morphological features of thickened facial appearance, stunted stature and enlarged tongue. The brain damage is irreversible if not treated early. It is now also realised that the poor intellectual performance and deafness (without any unusual morphological features) found in many children in iodine deficient areas is due to marginal iodine deficiency. This may be partially reversible. In some areas, an already limited iodine availability is made worse by the consumption of goitrogens, e.g. certain brassicas, cassava or soya beans. The extent of the problem can be assessed by measuring the prevalence of goitre (enlargement of the thyroid gland) which is particularly common among adolescents and pregnant women. Measurements of urinary iodide and iodine/thiocyanate levels can determine if the problem is primary dietary iodine deficiency (low iodine) or a result of a dietary goitrogen (high thiocyanate).

Richer people in goitrous areas generally obtain enough iodine by eating food (e.g. fish) brought in from other areas, but the main strategy is to iodise salt. Where this is impractical, injections of iodised oil (lipiodol) may be given, especially to women of childbearing age. A single dose (5 ml) will usually last for up to five years. Oral doses (400 mg) of iodine preparations may provide enough to last for two years.

VITAMIN EXCESS

In addition to the variety of illnesses now attributed to vitamin deficiency, there are also several toxicological syndromes associated with vitamin excess (Table 7.18).

Vitamin A

Toxicity occasionally occurs acutely in children given large doses (e.g. 200 000 IU) of vitamin A intramuscularly. It takes the form of irritability, and even convulsions, as a result of increased intracranial pressure. Recovery occurs within a few days.

Levels of vitamin A in liver consumed in the UK appear to have risen in recent years. It is quite possible to consume, in a single meal containing liver, much more than the maximum permitted of 10 000 IU per day for a woman during pregnancy. Large doses of vitamin A are associated with increased prevalence of cranio-facial abnormalities of the infant. For this reason it is recommended that pregnant women do not eat liver at the present time. It is especially important therefore to ensure that the diet of pregnant women contains adequate amounts of iron as liver is a major source in many people's diets.

Table 7.18 Main consequences of vitamin toxicity

Vitamin	Symptoms of toxicity
A	Headache, convulsions, muscular stiffness, hepatomegaly, teratogenic effects
Thiamine (B$_1$)	Not described
Riboflavin (B$_2$)	Not described
Nicotinic acid	Vasodilatation
Pyridoxine (B$_6$)	Peripheral neuropathy
Folate	Not described
Cobalamine (B$_{12}$)	Not described
Ascorbic acid (C)	Increased urinary oxalate
D	Hypercalcaemia, renal failure
E	Nausea
K	Hyperbilirubinaemia

Pyridoxine

Pyridoxine toxicity has been occurring more frequently in recent years due to its use — successful or otherwise — in the alleviation of severe premenstrual syndromes (depression and fluid retention). A peripheral neuropathy is likely if the daily dose exceeds 500 mg. Some cases have neurological abnormalities, e.g. peripheral neuropathy, which persist even after stopping the drug.

Vitamin C

Toxicity occurs among those who take large doses of vitamin C in the unfounded belief that it will prevent the common cold or cancer. Doses above 2 g/day may cause abdominal discomfort and osmotic diarrhoea. There is increased urinary oxalate excretion — which may predispose to oxalate stones — and some evidence of damage to the intestinal epithelium.

Vitamin D

Vitamin D toxicity occurred in the UK after World War II in some children given too much fortified milk. (The quantities added are now more strictly controlled.) Mild forms of vitamin D toxicity are characterised by weakness, weight loss and growth failure. Severe forms cause nephrocalcinosis, radiological changes in the epiphyses and mental retardation.

OBESITY

Everybody who is obese must necessarily be eating more than he or she needs, but it is not clear in every case why this is so.

Causes

There are certain obvious causes of obesity. Many people eat excessively in response to stress or lack of satisfaction in their lives. A sympathetic request for a two-week diary of everything the patient eats may be very revealing, but most obese people underestimate their intake and so a brief history in the outpatient clinic will usually fail to give an accurate assessment. A careful history taken by a dietitian is often invaluable.

Obesity may be the result of an obvious decrease in energy expenditure due to a change in lifestyle (e.g. to a more sedentary job) or an injury or arthritis which limits mobility. However, in most obese individuals it seems that intake and expenditure problems occur together.

The metabolism of food energy has been studied in detail over the last 20 years, and the evidence to date would suggest that some individuals are more prone to weight gain than others with a similar energy intake.

● Certain thin people eat more than fat people.
● When volunteers are given extra calories some put on weight faster than others.
● Prolonged, severe dieting may lead to an adaptive decrease in energy expenditure.
● Obese people appear to have a decreased thermogenic response to stimulation by norepinephrine; this persists even when they have lost weight.

Studies with genetic strains of experimental animals provide strong evidence for a metabolic basis for obesity. Although convincing evidence for a metabolic basis for obesity in man has not yet been obtained, the improved energy efficiency during pregnancy and lactation, and the weight gain that some experience while on the contraceptive pill, do point to some form of hormonal control of energy metabolism.

Whatever the nature of the metabolic processes which cause obesity, there is little doubt that a variety of metabolic consequences occur, including an increased risk of diabetes mellitus and atheroma (Table 7.19).

Assessment

Before any advice is given it is important to assess how fat the patient is. The body mass index (BMI = weight/height^2) is an objective index of size by which the level of

Table 7.19 Metabolic changes in obesity

Glucose tolerance	Decreased
Plasma insulin	Increased
Sensitivity to insulin	Decreased
Response to starvation:	
production of ketone bodies	Decreased
plasma free fatty acids	Increased
Plasma triglycerides	Increased
Plasma cholesterol	Increased
Plasma uric acid	Increased
Sensitivity to growth hormone	Decreased
Urinary 17-hydroxycorticoids	Increased

Table 7.20 Classification of Body Mass Index

Grade	W/H^2	Proportion of population (%)	Description
0	19–25	60	Normal range of weight
I	26–29	34	Overweight
II	30–39	6	Obesity
III	40 or more	6	Severe or morbid obesity

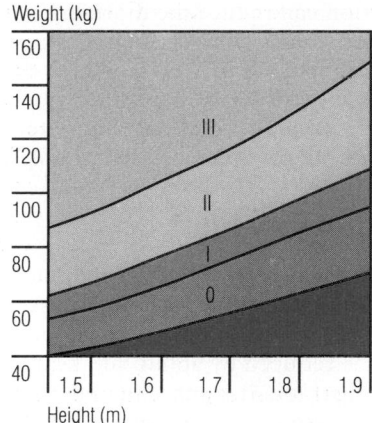

Fig. 7.5 Grades of obesity as measured using the body mass index (BMI = weight/height^2). Grade 0 is the desirable range, and grade III morbid obesity.

risk of morbidity and mortality can be estimated from graphs derived from insurance company data (Table 7.20 and Fig. 7.5). 'Acceptable weights' are in the range BMI 20–25; obesity is anything above BMI 30. This index may also be used in children and adolescents but, as there are some age effects, it is best to compare their measurements with the NCHS data.

Why diet?

There are many thousands of people in the UK who seem to themselves and/or to other people to be excessively fat. A number of studies in school-children, army recruits or housewives show that, as a nation, we are indeed much heavier than in previous decades. At the same time, a considerable proportion of the population is on diets of various types, many of them low energy 'crash' diets. Before the doctor recommends or condemns such approaches to weight reduction, it is important to consider the social and medical implications of obesity.

There are three main reasons why people wish to lose weight:

● Self-esteem. Mass media images of 'thin is beautiful' foster the idea held by many that they would be more attractive if they were thinner.
● A concern that life should be lived to the full, unaffected by the diseases associated with obesity, such as coronary thrombosis, arthritis and gallstones.
● A crisis response to a medical condition which requires weight reduction for its improvement (e.g. an operation which has been postponed until weight is lost).

Most people succeed at weight reduction without help from others. Many are helped by a variety of group approaches. The failures consult dietitians and/or doctors. Patients should be encouraged by the information that weight reduction can reduce the mortality rate. They may also be warned of the increased prevalence of diseases associated with obesity. These include diabetes, gallbladder and liver disease, degenerative joint disease, impaired respiratory function, hypertension, gout, ischaemic heart disease and increased prevalence of stroke.

How to reduce weight

- Of the three factors — food intake, metabolism and exercise — affecting weight gain or loss, *food intake* is quantitatively the most important. Food energy intake needs to be reduced by about 500 kcal/day for recognisable weight loss (i.e. more than 0.5 kg per week) to occur. Most people — patients and doctors included — want rapid results, and more severe dietary restriction, e.g. an intake of less than 600 kcal/day may be used. This undoubtedly leads to weight loss, but a high proportion of the initial loss is water. In addition, there is likely to be loss of body nitrogen from breakdown of skeletal muscle. There has been a vogue in recent years for 'nitrogen sparing modified fasts' in which high protein/low calorie formula feeds are given. These may help the patient to remain in positive nitrogen balance, and are a successful means of weight reduction in the short term; the long-term benefit is very uncertain, partly because of an adaptive decrease in energy expenditure. People find that they regain weight rapidly once they return to their customary diet. Undoubtedly the best approach to weight loss is to reduce customary intake by 500–1000 kcal/day and to set realistic long-term goals. Advice from a dietitian is frequently useful in setting diets and identifying previously unrecognised sources of high energy foods, especially fats and alcohol.
- *Exercise* should be encouraged, primarily to increase energy expenditure, but also because it increases fitness and well-being, and may be a useful diversion from thinking about the unpleasantness of dieting. It is also possible that the thermogenic effect of a meal is increased after exercise. People taking regular exercise generally have less illness and longer lives.
- Many obese people have emotional problems, but formal psychiatric treatment is not particularly effective in most cases. *A positive, caring and supportive approach* by the dietitian or doctor is often invaluable in assisting the obese patient regain his confidence, a key factor in success; continuity of visits and regular supervision are essential. It is striking how many patients' emotional crises seem to lessen as they lose weight.
- *Appetite suppressants* are of very limited value. Fenfluramine and diethylpropion have been tried, but individual responses vary greatly and, as they are drugs to which it is possible to become habituated, they should not be prescribed.

- *Thyroxine* is initially effective, but the rate of weight loss always slows as endogenous thyroid hormone ceases to be produced and thyroxine should not, therefore, be prescribed.
- *Jaw-wiring,* when liquids only are taken, has been used with some success, but many find the weight lost is rapidly regained once the wires are removed, and damage to teeth and gums is common.
- Some particularly unfortunate individuals have severe obesity (BMI > 40). Such patients have often tried — and failed — every diet possible, usually because they cannot sustain the effort. In the past, a jejunoileal bypass operation was performed, but this has now been abandoned because of severe side-effects (diarrhoea, liver disease, arthritis and osteomalacia). The main *surgical approach* is now the vertical banded gastroplasty, in which the stomach is stapled to reduce its size, thus inducing satiety at an early stage of the meal. This appears to be both effective and relatively safe; however, it does not cure hunger completely and selection of patients for this procedure requires very careful consideration.

FOOD SENSITIVITY

The clinical importance of food allergy is difficult to assess as little is known of the scientific basis for hypersensitivity to food, there have been few controlled clinical trials of exclusion diets, and the mechanisms by which they work are not understood. A variety of foods have been implicated in food intolerance (Table 7.21).

A number of food allergies are associated with immunological reactions — usually an IgE response. A radio allergosorbent test (RAST) may detect antibodies in plasma against a specific food protein, but there is little correlation between the clinical features and the results of a variety of RAST tests. Skin tests of purified antigens

Table 7.21 Foods associated with food intolerance*

Food	% of cases
Milk	25
Egg	22
Nuts/peanuts	12
Fish/shellfish	12
Wheat/flour	6
Chocolate	5
Artificial colours	3
Pork/bacon	3
Chicken	3
Tomato	3
Soft fruit	3
Cheese (but not milk)	3

*From: Truswell AS 1986 ABC of nutrition.

may detect an urticarial response within a few minutes of intradermal inoculation, but positive skin tests do not correlate well with sensitivity reactions in other organs, such as lungs and the gastrointestinal tract. In short, there is as yet no defined mechanism in most cases of food sensitivity and very few laboratory tests are of any use. Management therefore depends on careful history-taking and a critical approach to elimination diets.

Clinical symptoms

The major clinical symptoms associated with food sensitivity are shown in Table 7.22.

Eczema

Exacerbations of eczema are frequently associated with reactions against eggs and milk. Infantile eczema is sometimes improved by withdrawing eggs and cows' milk products; families with a strong history of eczema are advised to breast-feed as long as possible and delay the introduction of eggs and cows' milk. Dietary manipulation in older children and adults is also worth trying but is often disappointing, and must be supervised.

Gastrointestinal symptoms

The best defined gastrointestinal hypersensitivity syndrome is coeliac disease (p. 576). Onset is sometimes precipitated by a gut infection, especially in children. Transient gluten intolerance following mucosal damage from giardiasis or rotavirus infections may occur.

A more frequent problem is cows' milk protein intolerance. Here, mucosal damage permits access to mucosal lymphocytes which become sensitised to the dietary protein. Subsequent exposure then produces a severe response in which lymphokines are released, damaging enterocytes. Villus atrophy occurs and malabsorption develops. There is also some evidence of exacerbation of symptoms of ulcerative colitis by cows' milk; it is sometimes suggested — though reliable evidence is lacking —

that infantile colic is caused by dietary factors transmitted across breast milk or contained in cows' milk.

Many patients with severe intestinal infections complain of a relapse of diarrhoea in the convalescent period after eating certain foods (e.g. chocolate, alcohol, coffee, certain fruits). Their symptoms differ from irritable bowel syndrome (IBS) in which abdominal pain dominates. There are no specific patterns of food intolerance in IBS.

Migraine

Migraines sometimes appear to be precipitated by foods such as chocolate, cheese, red wine, nitrates, cows' milk and wheat. Some of these contain amines or stimulate histamine release which may produce an effect on cranial arteries.

Respiratory tract responses

Respiratory tract responses — including excessive production of tears, nasal secretions, sneezing and asthma — may all be related to environmental factors, e.g. chemical sprays, cosmetics and food or plant pollens, but eggs, cows' milk and chocolate may also precipitate symptoms. Recent studies suggest that a variety of food preservatives, including tartrazine and sulphur dioxide, may also be responsible.

Urticaria

Acute or chronic urticaria may occur in response to eggs, fish (particularly shellfish) and cows' milk, as well as certain fruit, wine and cheese.

Management of food sensitivity

If the patient suffers a reaction each time exposure to the allergen occurs, the latter should be easily identifiable. However, in the case of the general system symptoms described above, identification of the allergen is more difficult. There are two approaches:

- exclude a suspected allergen for at least four weeks and then re-introduce it (this is mostly satisfactory where the condition is mild); or
- work out an elimination diet (one based on lamb, rice and pears is sometimes effective) as advised by a dietitian. Then re-introduce a potential allergen every two weeks and observe the response.

MALNUTRITION IN DISEASE STATES

Weight loss and deficiency of individual nutrients are common in a variety of illnesses and frequently occur

Table 7.22 Symptoms in 100 patients with food intolerance*

Symptom	Number of patients affected
Asthma	58
Gastrointestinal	41
Eczema	37
Urticaria	35
Rhinorrhoea	31
Angio-oedema	8

*From: Truswell AS 1986 ABC of nutrition.

Table 7.23 Factors causing weight loss in surgical patients

Reduced appetite

Anxiety, pain
Infection and sepsis
Drugs, e.g. anaesthetics, chemotherapy
Radiotherapy, metabolic disturbances

Reduced intake of nutrients

Difficulty in feeding
Inability to sit up or use arms
Damage to CNS and impaired consciousness
Damage to upper alimentary tract
Inadequate provision by medical/nursing staff

Increased need for nutrients

Raised energy expenditure
Metabolic response to injury
Increased protein synthesis

Replacement for extraneous losses

Haemorrhage
Serous exudates, especially after burns
Fistulae and sinuses

after major surgery (Table 7.23). There are a multiplicity of factors leading to nutritional deficiency in disease.

Dietary intake

Decreased appetite is the commonest cause of weight loss. In patients who have lost weight it is often helpful to ask a dietitian to take a careful history of the recent food intake. Modern microcomputer software programmes can process data on energy, protein, fat, fibre, iron intake, etc. very quickly, and certain patterns may emerge. For example, patients with malabsorption often avoid fat; adolescents with early forms of anorexia nervosa may become very fussy over food; and painful abdominal conditions (e.g. pancreatitis) may cause the patient to avoid solid foods altogether. In addition to identifying the specific food items avoided, the strictness with which a patient keeps to a diet should also be assessed. In all cases, patients' relatives should be interviewed to corroborate the dietary history. Dietary diaries kept by patients, relatives or nursing staff can be very valuable.

Maldigestion

Following partial gastrectomy, food may not be completely digested in the small bowel. Short-term maldigestion may complicate intestinal infection (such as with rotavirus or giardiasis) as a result of impaired hydrolysis of lactose due to temporary lactase deficiency. The presence of undigested lactose in the intestinal lumen causes severe osmotic diarrhoea, and a consequent loss of some nutrients.

Malabsorption

This term is often used to describe steatorrhoea (excessive fat in the faeces), but carbohydrate and vitamin malabsorption are also important. The mechanisms of malabsorption are described in Chapter 15. With some nutrients, such as iron, folate and vitamin B_{12}, malabsorption may present as a clinical deficiency syndrome with excessive losses of dietary protein and energy in the faeces. However, metabolic balance studies show that weight loss in some malabsorption patients is due more to a decrease in dietary intake than to malabsorbed nutrients.

Increased nutrient requirements

Energy requirements are often increased in pyrexial conditions — usually about 10% increase for every 1°C in body temperature. The rate of protein synthesis (e.g. of acute phase reactant proteins or antibodies) is also increased in systemic infections. As nutrient intakes are often decreased rather than increased during infection, these processes lead to energy deficiency. There may be mobilisation of muscle protein for oxidation as a fuel and thus increased urinary losses of nitrogen. At the present time, various chemical messengers — such as interleukins and prostaglandins — are thought to control all of these processes, but it has not yet proved possible to reverse them successfully by pharmacological means.

Losses of endogenous nutrient

Losses of albumin, electrolytes and blood may occur in intestinal diseases, particularly those such as Crohn's disease or ulcerative colitis where the mucosa is 'leaky'. Systemic infection may also lead to loss of zinc and other minerals in the urine.

NUTRITION SUPPORT

Many patients leave hospital weighing considerably less than when they came in. This can be regarded as a form of PEM if the body weight is less than 80% of the ideal weight for a person of that height or the BMI is less than 20. The majority of cases of PEM are the result of poor appetite due to illness and the experience that eating tends to make the pain and diarrhoea worse. Individual reasons for PEM should always be investigated.

Severe degrees of PEM delay wound healing and recovery of muscle tone after an operation, and may increase susceptibility to infection. Adults with a BMI below 16 have three times the postoperative mortality of better nourished patients. The striking changes in body composition from partial starvation in illness are shown in Figure 7.6. It is better to avoid PEM than treat it and it is essential to make a nutritional assessment of every patient. If any of the criteria for PEM are present, some form of nutrition support, such as dietetic supplements, enteral feeding or parenteral feeding, can be used to prevent further deterioration (Table 7.24). In deciding which technique of nutrition support to use, it is often advisable to use a nutrition team comprising a physician or surgeon with special experience in clinical nutrition, a nutrition nurse/technician and a dietitian, together with strong support from the pharmacy and pathology laboratory.

Enteral feeding

Many patients find hospital food unappetising even when they feel relatively well. In such cases, it may be possible to increase energy and protein intake by snacks provided by the diet kitchen between main meals; food and drink may be fortified by a range of supplements available from the dietician (Table 7.25). A 24 hour calorie count performed by the dietitian is a good way of monitoring intake. If solid food is not well accepted, it is often

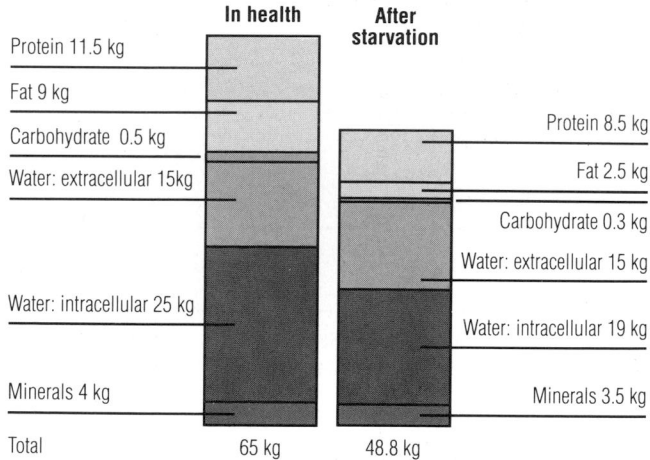

Fig. 7.6 Body composition of a man in health and after partial starvation.

Table 7.24 Examples of conditions in which nutrition support is necessary

Illness associated with nausea and abdominal pain	Intestinal disease
Gastrointestinal disease	Malabsorption
Malignancy	Inflammatory bowel disease
Chemotherapy	Fistulae
Inability to eat	**Increased requirements**
Coma	Burns
Weakness	Sepsis
	Trauma

Table 7.25 Examples of commercially available nutritional supplements

Commercial name	Nutrient source	Nutrient content
Maxipro	Whey protein	Protein 88 g/100 g Energy 390 kcal/100 g
Maxijul/Caloreen	Maltodextrin powder	Carbohydrate 96 g/100 g Energy 375 kcal/100 g
Prosparol	Peanut oil	Energy 450 kcal/100 g

Table 7.26 Examples of commercially available enteral feeds

Name	Osmolality (mosmol/kg)	Non-protein energy/nitrogen (kcal/gN)
Ensure	380	149
Ensure Plus	460	140
Clinifeed	255	142
Special feeds		
Osmolite	Lactose and gluten free	
Enrich	Lactose and gluten free plus fibre	

possible to give liquid feeds for sipping. A considerable range of commercially prepared feeds are available, presented as 200 ml cartons (Table 7.26). These should be served chilled and their volumes recorded accurately.

If the intake is still not satisfactory, a fine-bore silastic tube may be passed per-nasally. Enteral feeding solutions are passed down the tube at controlled rates from a reservoir situated above the patient's head. Small battery operated pumps can control the exact flow rate but they are not essential. The commercially available enteral feeds are made up from a variety of protein sources including casein, soya and mixtures of amino acids, with glucose polymers and triglycerides added to increase the energy content. Most feeds provide about 1 kcal/ml and have an osmolality of 280–420 mosmol/kg. Low lactose and cows' milk-free feeds are available. Flavour and consistency vary considerably and a tasting session is generally advisable before prescribing large quantities. The feeds should be started in small volumes, and no more than 1000 ml given in the first 24 hours, otherwise diarrhoea may develop. The volume is then increased to the desired amount (probably a maximum of 2500 ml/day). The feed should be stopped for one hour before meals and continued throughout the night.

Enteral feeding can be performed at home; the reservoir bottles and lines should be changed every 24 hours to avoid the risk of contamination of feeds but the silastic tubes can remain in situ for several weeks. Even so, complications of enteral feeding occasionally occur and should be anticipated. Oesophagitis caused by the tubes is rare with modern silastic tubing, but the tube may be misplaced and an X-ray should be performed before feeding is commenced. A few patients suffer abdominal distension and pain, and the volume infused should then be decreased. Diarrhoea is best controlled by codeine phosphate (30–60 mg t.d.s.) or imodium (2–4 mg t.d.s.).

Parenteral feeding

If enteral feeds cannot be given (e.g. due to severe ileus) then parenteral feeding is an option, but the dangers of infection and metabolic problems with this method are considerable. There are various commercial preparations; these should be mixed in a 3 l bag system in sterile laminar airflow conditions in the pharmacy.

The regime used varies with the patient's clinical condition (Table 7.27). In general, regimes 1–4 are administered through a central venous catheter. Where central venous access is impossible, regime 5 may be used, administered through a butterfly needle on the back of the hand or forearm. The site of this needle should be changed every 24–48 hours to avoid thrombophlebitis.

A number of metabolic complications may occur in patients receiving parenteral nutrition (Table 7.28).

- Hyperglycaemia is common in patients with severe surgical stress (e.g. burns and trauma) and sepsis, but plasma glucose levels can be controlled with carefully monitored insulin. Rebound hypoglycaemia may occur if intravenous feeding is abruptly halted.
- Metabolic acidosis is rare if fructose and excessive quantities of amino acids are avoided.
- Parenteral feeding, especially with lipid solutions, has been blamed for hepatic abnormalities. However, most patients receiving parenteral feeding have many other potential causes for hepatic damage and there is rarely any indication for parenteral nutrition to be stopped on account of mild biochemical changes.
- Fat is metabolised more favourably than glucose by septic patients.
- Patients with respiratory failure should not receive large glucose loads because of their impaired ability to excrete the extra CO_2 produced.
- Mineral and electrolyte abnormalities occur variously according to the underlying disease processes. Fortunately, deficiencies can be made up relatively easily during preparation of the 3 l bag which contains the feeding solutions.

Monitoring nutrition support

The measurements available for monitoring nutrition support are shown in Table 7.29.

Regular measurements of weight are necessary but are difficult to perform in the very sick without special bed balances. Changes in body weight may indicate alterations in fluid balance rather than an increase in lean body mass.

Table 7.28 Metabolic complications in patients receiving parenteral nutrition

- Hyperglycaemia
- Rebound hypoglycaemia
- Electrolyte and mineral imbalance
- Metabolic acidosis
- Disturbed liver function
- Raised plasma CO_2

Table 7.27 Standard parenteral nutrition regimes*

Composition	Regimen 1 (central line)	Regimen 2 (central line)	Regimen 3 (central line)	Regimen 4 (central line)	Regimen 5 (peripheral)
Nitrogen (g)	9.4	9.4	13.5	14.1	9.4
Carbohydrate (g)	200	200	250	350	240
Fat (g)	50	100	100	100	100
Non-protein energy (kcal)	1350	1800	2000	2400	1900
Sodium (mmol)	80	80	122.5	122.5	80
Potassium (mmol)	60	60	80	80	60
Calcium (mmol)	5	5	5	5	5
Magnesium (mmol)	5	7	8	8	7
Zinc (μmol)	100	100	100	100	100
Phosphate (mmol)	27.5	27.5	37.5	37.5	35
Chloride (mmol)	85	85	107.5	107.5	108
Trace elements (Additrace) (ml)	10	10	10	10	10
Vitilipid N Adult (ml)	10	10	10	10	10
Solivito N (vial)	1	1	1	1	1
Volume of feed (ml)	2560	2560	2540	2540	3050

*Regimen 1 is indicated for a patient of weight 35–54 kg; regimen 2, 46–59 kg; and regimens 3–5, 60–75 kg.

Table 7.29 Measurements for monitoring nutrition support

- Anthropometric: weight, mid-arm muscle circumference (MAC)
- Plasma proteins: albumin, transferrin, retinol binding globulin
- Minerals and electrolytes: uric acid, phosphate, sodium, potassium, zinc
- Nitrogen balance: corrected 24 hour urinary urea excretion
- Glucose

Plasma proteins are useful indicators of progress in nutrition support, but are subject to considerable change by underlying disease processes. *Glucose* should be measured regularly.

Plasma phosphate levels may decrease rapidly and even precipitate cardiac arrhythmia if nutrition support is given rapidly in large quantities to a severely malnourished subject who has previously received very little dietary intake. Most modern amino acid solutions, however, have sufficient phosphate to avoid this.

A low plasma *sodium* is often present in severely malnourished subjects. Total body sodium, however, is often high and extra sodium should only be given with great caution.

An approximate assessment of urinary *nitrogen* loss can be obtained by measurement of the 24 hour urinary urea excretion, corrected according to the formula

$$\text{Nitrogen (g/24 h)} = \text{urinary urea (mmol/l)} \times \text{urine volume (1)} \times 0.028 \times 6/5.$$

This formula allows for the conversion of mmol of urea to grams of nitrogen and corrects for the fact that urea accounts for approximately five-sixths of total urinary nitrogen loss.

The previously high prevalence of infection has been reduced by the 3 l bag system, but high standards of nursing and medical care of the lines are essential if sepsis is to be prevented. Different types of intravenous catheters are available — the best are those tunnelled subcutaneously (e.g. Hickman). Blood samples should never be taken from this line as the clot at the tip is a major source of infection. Specialist texts should be referred to before any central venous feeding is attempted, to reduce the complications of catheter insertion, which include pneumothorax, central vein thrombosis, nerve injury, haematoma and arrhythmias. Similarly, only staff trained in the care of central venous feeding lines should be allowed to touch them, and aseptic changing of sets and meticulous care of the catheter entry site should be emphasised. Efforts to reduce infection rates are particularly important among immunocompromised patients.

Parenteral feeds are made up from mixtures of L-form amino acids to which glucose (20%) or lipid emulsions (10% or 20%) are added as energy sources. An ideal calorie to nitrogen ratio is around 150:1. Electrolytes, minerals and vitamins are then added to this basic solution. If large quantities of glucose are given, the patient may become hyperglycaemic; this is best managed by subcutaneous insulin administered by a pump. Considering the relative costs, risks and nutritional benefit from total parenteral nutrition (TPN) it seems best to confine its use to those who need it for at least two weeks; anything less is not really justified.

NUTRITION AS A COFACTOR IN DISEASE

There are several diseases in which dietary factors are implicated. Dietary fat in coronary heart disease and dietary salt in hypertension are two good examples. However, the importance of such single factors in human disease is not clear-cut, because most studies have not allowed for the degree of variance in other cofactors (e.g. cigarette smoking in coronary heart disease and genetic factors in hypertension).

Hypertension

International comparisons show a direct relationship between sodium intake and blood pressure. There is a threshold effect of additional salt in volunteers, with those on very high doses showing an increased blood pressure. However, there are also important cofactors including family history, stress, obesity and potassium intake which may obscure the relationship in an individual. In the UK, the average daily salt intake in adults is around 20 g. This is more than twice the amount associated with lower rates of hypertension experimentally.

Atheroma

International comparisons of mortality rates from coronary heart disease (CHD) show that rates are highest in populations with the highest fat intakes. This is true even when the effects of obesity, hypertension, cigarette smoking, diabetes, stress and family history are allowed for. The major risk factors for the development of atheroma are high levels of plasma cholesterol and low density lipoproteins (VLDL). Consumption of fat in the saturated form is particularly likely to increase both VLDL and cholesterol. Diets in which fats are consumed mainly in the unsaturated form lead to lowering of these levels. In practice, saturated fats are present in butter, lard, sausages, meat pies, pastries and chocolates, while unsaturated fats predominate in margarines prepared from maize, sunflower or soya. Not all margarines are unsaturated — those which contain coconut oil (used in many hospital canteens in the UK), for example, are highly saturated. It

Summary 2 Nutrition as a cofactor in disease

Disease	Associated dietary factors
Hypertension	High sodium intake
Atheroma	High consumption of saturated fats; obesity, insufficient fibre (all lead to high cholesterol and VLDL)
Diabetes (Type II)	High fat, low fibre
Oesophageal cancer	Preservatives, e.g. nitrosamines; dietary deficiencies, e.g. zinc, carotenoids, retinol. Also alcohol, mycotoxins
Stomach cancer	Nitrosamines (derived from nitrates in diet); fat
Cancer of large intestine	High protein and fat; low fibre
Gallstones	High cholesterol due to obesity, high sugar, low fibre
Cirrhosis	Alcohol
Liver cancer	Aflatoxins (in badly stored cereals)
Pancreatitis	PEM
Dental caries	Sugar in prolonged contact with teeth
Urinary calculi (oxalate)	High phosphate

should be remembered that plasma cholesterol indicates the production of cholesterol by the liver; cholesterol-containing foods (such as eggs) do not necessarily increase the synthesis of cholesterol in the liver. In the UK, only a relatively minor proportion of the population have a high plasma cholesterol and VLDL; why only some people respond to a high fat diet in this way is unknown.

Two main dietary strategies have been proposed to reduce CHD mortality in the UK.

● Encourage everybody to eat less fat. This is the approach recommended by the National Advisory Committee for Nutrition Education (NACNE). At the present time, the population eats over 45% of its daily energy in the form of fat; they should be encouraged to eat less fat (say 35% of energy) and eat more starch and carbohydrates.

● Screen high risk groups (e.g. men between 35 and 55 years of age) for plasma cholesterol and VLDL, and select out those with high levels for individual dietary counselling. The second approach is perhaps the more logical, but has not been widely adopted because of administrative and financial constraints.

The best advice is to eat fat in as unsaturated form as possible. Certain polyunsaturated fats, such as eicosapentaenoic acid, present in cod-liver oil, mackerel and pilchards, tend to inhibit thrombosis and should be particularly encouraged. Increasing dietary fibre intake may also reduce plasma cholesterol. Obesity is often associated with high levels of plasma cholesterol and triglyc-

erides; successful weight reduction by moderately or severely obese subjects is followed by a decreased risk of mortality from CHD.

Diabetes

Non-insulin dependent diabetes (Type II) is closely linked with diet. In nearly every society, those who are overweight and whose diet is high in fat and low in dietary fibre have a significantly increased risk of diabetes. The current epidemics in middle income countries, as they eat more polished rice and white bread, are striking. The benefits conferred by dietary fibre are probably due to its effects on gastric emptying and the rate of carbohydrate hydrolysis.

Gastrointestinal disease

There are striking differences in the prevalence of cancer of the oesophagus, stomach and large intestine between populations on different diets. A variety of carcinogens such as nitrosamines (which are widely available in preserved food such as pickled foods, continental sausage and certain types of fish), together with dietary deficiencies (e.g. of zinc, carotenoids and retinol) appear to be associated with cancer of the oesophagus. Other toxins include alcohol (especially from spirits), silica derived from grinding cereals (as in parts of China) and mycotoxins (e.g. in Transkei, South Africa).

Cancer of the stomach may also be associated with high levels of dietary nitrosamines. There is evidence that high levels of dietary nitrates (both in food and in water) may be converted into nitrites by the gastric microflora. The nitrites then react with amino acids to form nitrosamines which are carcinogenic in experimental studies. When gastric acidity is low — as in the elderly and those with pernicious anaemia — there is greater opportunity for bacterial metabolism of nitrates to nitrites and this may account for the higher incidence of gastric cancer in these subjects. Other dietary factors, such as fat, have been implicated in explaining the changes in stomach cancer rates observed among Japanese migrating to the USA.

High rates of cancer of the large intestine have been associated with diets high in fat and protein and low in dietary fibre. A series of carcinogens are produced as a result of bacterial metabolism of endogenous bile salts and dietary fat. It may be that prolonged contact between carcinogen and mucosa in subjects with a low fibre diet accounts for the high rate of large bowel cancer in some communities.

Gallstones

The deposition of cholesterol to form gallstones depends on the relative concentrations of total bile salts, lecithin and cholesterol. The fine balance between these is a fected by obesity, high dietary sugar intake and low dietary fibre intake but the precise mechanisms of the imbalance or of the formation of gallstones are not clear.

Liver disease

The most important association between dietary factors and liver disease is that between alcohol and cirrhosis. However, mycotoxins may also affect the liver: aflatoxins — which are widely prevalent in cereals kept under poor storage conditions — may be a factor in causing primary liver cell cancer and may also contribute to the development of the fatty liver in kwashiorkor. Temporary PEM in children does not account for the high prevalence of cirrhosis in developing countries; hepatitis B infection seems to be the major cause.

Pancreatic disease

Chronic pancreatitis is found frequently among populations where PEM is rife. Periods of undernutrition may cause stasis of exocrine juices within the pancreas, leading to acinar cell destruction and loss of digestive function. Pancreatic calcification often follows. However, alcohol excess seems more important than PEM as a cause of chronic calcific pancreatitis.

Dental caries

There has been a marked decrease in dental caries among children in certain social groups in the UK over the last 20 years. This has been associated with: an increase in the use of fluoride (in toothpaste, in drinking water or as tablets); reduced consumption of sticky sweets; and possibly also an increased prevalence of cleaning the teeth. Dental caries occur when *Streptococcus viridans* adheres to teeth and metabolises sugar into lactic acid. All sugars can act as substrate; thus 'natural' sugars such as fructose are just as cariogenic as sucrose. The most important factor is the length of time that sugar-containing foods remain in contact with teeth; adhesive foods are thus particularly damaging.

Urinary calculi

Calcium or oxalate stones are sometimes precipitated in the urinary tract as a result of increased dietary intake. Oxalate stones are those most frequently associated with dietary factors, occurring most commonly in populations with high phosphate intakes. In Thailand, for example, oxalate calculi occur most commonly in the rural populations, where the high phosphate intakes associated with a predominantly vegetarian diet contrast with the lower phosphate intakes of the better off, urban families. Oxalate stones may also be precipitated by dehydration in extremely hot climates.

NUTRITIONAL FACTORS IN HEALTH PROMOTION

There is increasing public awareness of the importance of attention to lifestyle in avoiding the development of disease. In the UK, many of the diseases — coronary artery disease, hypertension, lung cancer, cancer of the large intestine, gallstones, diabetes, irritable colon syndrome and varicose veins — that now cause premature death or years of discomfort were far less prevalent a hundred or so years ago, and are rare today in developing countries. The reasons for the differences in disease patterns between communities are complex but some factors, such as cigarette smoking, obesity and lack of exercise, are clearly implicated. This should be emphasised by both GPs and community health programmes in routine medical examinations and screening of high risk groups.

There is now a reasonable consensus that the risk of developing certain diseases is reduced if the diet contains:

- sufficiently few calories to avoid obesity (BMI > 30)
- less than 35% of energy in the form of fat
- more than 25 g of fibre daily
- about 30% less salt than in the average UK diet
- 50% less sugar than in the average UK diet
- daily alcohol consumption less than four units of alcohol for men and three for women.

To achieve this overall change in diet it is necessary to increase the consumption of wholegrain cereals, pasta and vegetables such as potatoes. The introduction of numerous diet and health magazines over the last 10 years means that appropriate menus and dietary information are readily available. Some of this information is conflicting and many community dietitians produce booklets designed to clarify the situation.

In recent years, there have been many claims of an association between many commercial food additives and cancer, food allergy, skin conditions and behaviour disorders. These include preservatives (such as nitrates, chromates, sulphur dioxide), emulsifiers (such as lecithin), antioxidants, colourants (such as tartrazine) and flavourings. While the quantitative degree to which any of these contributes to disease in man is unknown, it is probably minimal compared with the risks associated with current dietary levels of fat, fibre, salt and sugar.

7 Nutritional factors in health promotion

There are, in additional, specific disorders associated with nutrient deficiencies. Thus, neural tube defects are associated with folate deficiency; coronary heart disease is associated with dietary selenium deficiency in some communities; and iron deficiency is associated with poor intellectual performance at school. Unfortunately, it is difficult to obtain rigorous proof for some of these associations and even more difficult to evaluate critically the value of dietary additions. This leaves much scope for those favouring approaches such as micronutrient therapy in microdoses, megadoses of vitamins, etc. The proliferation of 'health consultants' and 'nutrition counsellors' in the UK and elsewhere reflects public anxieties about food and health fuelled by intensive information in the media. The wise clinician will respect this anxiety, ensure that he or she is as well informed as possible on new developments and — at all times — maintain the same critical approach to the claims of the health stores as to the claims made for new pharmaceuticals.

FURTHER READING

Dickerson J W T, Lee H A 1988 Nutrition in the clinical management of disease, 2nd edn. Edward Arnold, London. *A comprehensive textbook of a range of disease states in which nutrition is involved.*

Eastwood M A, Passmore R 1986 Human nutrition and dietetics, 8th edn. Churchill Livingstone, Edinburgh. *Still the classic textbook of human nutrition.*

Garrow J S 1988 Obesity and related disorders. Churchill Livingstone, Edinburgh. *A personal account of in-depth studies of obese subjects by a single author. Stimulating and instructive.*

Silk D B A 1983 Nutritional support in hospital practice. Blackwell Scientific Publications, Oxford. *A scientific review of the principles of nutrition support, with a strong emphasis on practical management.*

Tomkins AM, Watson F Malnutrition and infection ACC/SCN State of the Art Series Nutrition Policy Discussion Paper No 5 pp 1–135.

Truswell A S 1992 ABC of nutrition, 2nd edn. British Medical Association, London. *A well-illustrated series of articles first published as weekly reviews in the British Medical Journal.*

8

Cancer Medicine

Robert L Souhami

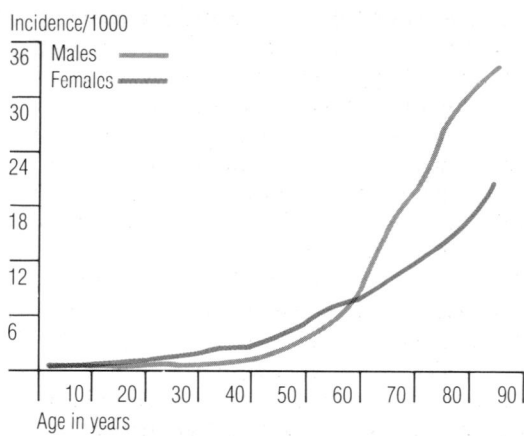

Fig. 8.1 **Age-specific incidence of cancer (England 1990).**

discussion with patients. Cancer medicine therefore demands a combination of a high degree of technical competence and a sympathetic insight into the feelings of the patients. It is this double challenge which makes it a most rewarding part of medical practice.

Each year in the UK there are approximately 220 000 new cases of cancer. Almost one-third of the population will develop cancer during their lifetime and 70% of these will die of the disease – 150 000 deaths a year. As a cause of mortality, cancer is second only to cardiovascular disease. It is most common in the elderly: the age-specific incidence rates for men and women are shown in Figure 8.1. The frequency of cancer and the increasing complexity of management mean that every clinician must have a firm grasp of the principles of diagnosis, investigation and management. In recent years, the approach has been changing rapidly as a consequence of fundamental advances in cancer biology, increasing accuracy in diagnosis and staging, and major developments in the use of radiotherapy and chemotherapy. At the same time, clinicians have developed a better awareness of the problems faced by patients who are incurable, and professional attitudes have changed in direction of more open

INCIDENCE AND EPIDEMIOLOGY

Incidence means the proportion of a defined population developing a disease in a stated period of time; *prevalence* is the proportion which has the condition at a single point in time. *Crude* incidence or prevalence rates refer to a whole population and *specific* rates to selected groups, for example those defined by age or sex.

The age-specific incidence rates of some cancers are shown in Figures 8.2 to 8.4. It can be seen that adenocarcinomas in women have quite different age-specific incidence rates. Cancer of the breast increases rapidly in incidence before the menopause, and at a slightly slower rate thereafter (Fig. 8.2). Uterine and ovarian cancer also show an increasing incidence premenopausally but the rate does not rise in later life. Gut cancers (Fig. 8.3), on the other hand, show no relation to the menopause but rise rapidly in incidence in old age in both sexes. The biphasic age-specific incidence of Hodgkin's disease (Fig. 8.4) contrasts markedly with the findings in adenocarcinoma. Lung cancer is at present more common in men. Cancer is the second main cause of death in childhood, with acute lymphoblastic leukaemia accounting for nearly half the deaths.

The commonest sites of cancer in the West are lung, skin, large bowel, prostate, stomach and rectum in men; and breast, large bowel, skin and lung in women. The mortality rates are, however, different from incidence rates (Fig. 8.5), with skin cancer having a low mortality rate and lung cancer a very bad prognosis. However, the

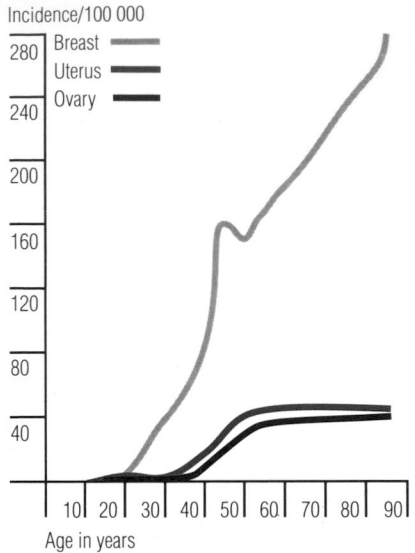

Fig. 8.2 Age-specific incidence of carcinomas of the breast, ovary and uterus. Note change in rate of increase at the time of the menopause.

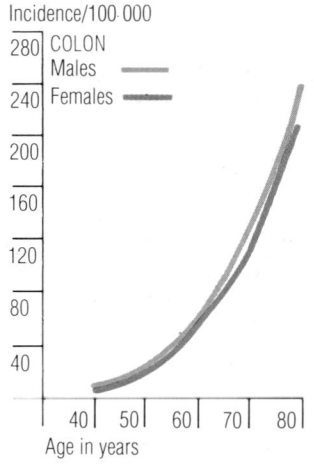

Fig. 8.3 Age-specific incidence of adenocarcinoma of the colon.

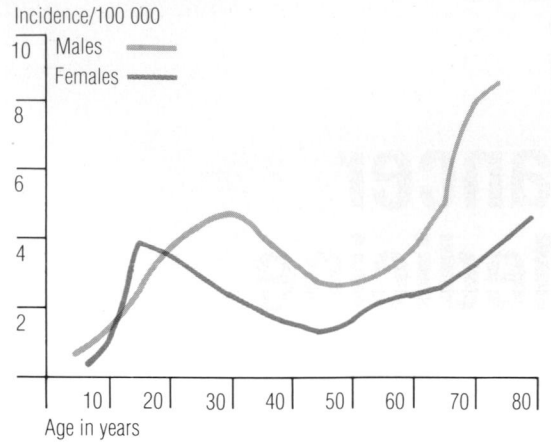

Fig. 8.4 Age-specific incidence of Hodgkin's disease.

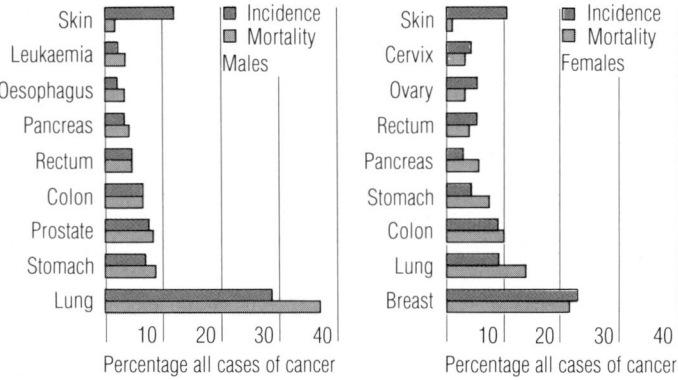

Fig. 8.5 Incidence and mortality of common cancers in men and women in England and Wales. Note that while skin cancer is common, its mortality is low. Cancer of the lung is common and accounts for a large number of total cancer deaths.

relative incidence of cancers is changing with time. For example, the incidence of lung cancer has been rising rapidly since the mid-1960s, especially in women; while that of stomach cancer has been falling for both men and women (Fig. 8.6). The rise in incidence of lung cancer is undoubtedly due to smoking, but the reason for the decline in stomach cancer is not clear.

Cancer incidence varies in different countries (Table 8.1) and this variation may provide insights into aetiology. Carcinoma of the oesophagus has a high incidence in an area extending from the Caspian Sea to Central Asia and the Far East; it is also more common in the Transkei. In these areas, it has an incidence 200 times that found in the UK. In Japan, gastric carcinoma is 30 times more common than it is in the UK, but pancreatic cancer is much rarer. The reasons for these variations are as yet unknown, but dietary and nutritional factors are suspected to play a part. The migration of populations has helped to determine how much of the geographical variation is genetic and how much is environmental. When Japanese people settle in the USA, the incidence of cancers in their offspring resembles that of the adopted country – the high incidence of gastric cancer falls, and the lower incidence of cancers of the breast, colon, ovary, and prostate rises. These findings suggest that environ-

Table 8.1 Geographical incidence of cancer

Cancer	High incidence	Low incidence	Ratio (high:low)
Oesophagus	Transkei, Kazakhstan	Holland	200:1
Liver	Mozambique	UK	100:1
Nasopharynx	Far East (China)	Europe	100:1
Stomach	Japan	UK	30:1

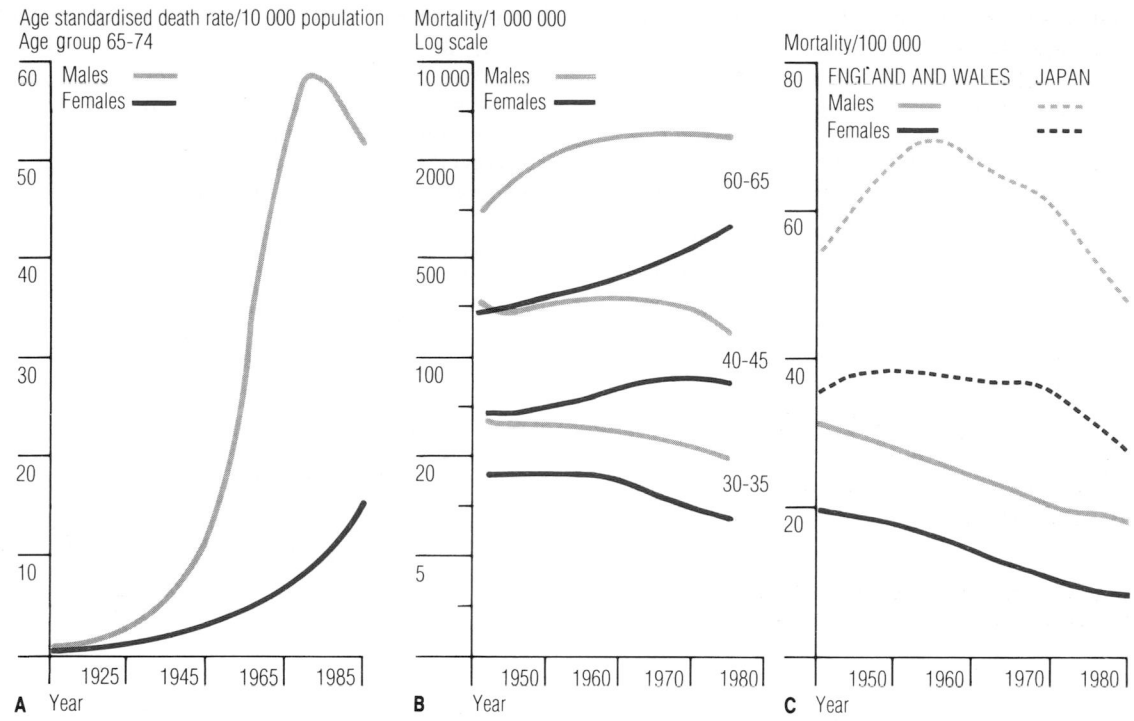

Fig. 8.6 Cancer of the lung and stomach. A. Cancer of the lung – age-standardised death rate/10 000 in age group 65–74, 1905–85 in the UK. **B.** Cancer of the lung – mortality 1940–80 for different age groups. **C.** Cancer of the stomach – change in mortality in England and Wales and in Japan, 1940–1980.

mental, rather than genetic, causes account for most of the observed differences between countries.

AETIOLOGY

Evidence suggesting aetiological factors in cancer has come from epidemiological and laboratory investigation. It is probable that, for many types of neoplasm, an interaction of genetic and environmental factors is responsible for the development of a cancer.

Table 8.2 Chemical carcinogens

Class	Example	Source
Polycyclic hydrocarbons	Dibenzanthracene	Smoke, cigarettes
Aromatic amines	Beta naphthylamine	Aniline dyes
Azo dyes	Dimethylaminobenzene	Butter yellow
Nitrosamines	Dimethylnitrosamine	? Food
Toxins	Aflatoxin	*Aspergillus flavus*
Alkylating agents	Melphalan	Drug treatment of cancer
Chromates		Industrial exposure
Asbestos		Insulation and heating installations

Chemical carcinogens

The frequency of scrotal carcinoma in chimney sweeps was noted by Sir Percivall Pott in 1775, and the high incidence of bladder cancer in dye workers in 1895. The mechanisms of action of chemical carcinogens have been intensively studied. There are several classes of experimental carcinogens (Table 8.2) which are possible causes in humans:

- *Polycyclic hydrocarbons* are formed from combustion of organic compounds. They are present in cigarette smoke, soot, car exhaust fumes and some foods. Dibenzanthracene was one of the first to be shown to be carcinogenic. The carcinogenic effect is thought to result from a reaction with bases in cellular DNA.
- *Aromatic amines and azo dyes*, such as beta naphthylamine and benzidine, are metabolised to an active form. In the case of beta naphthylamine, this is then glucuronated in the liver and excreted in the urine where glucuronidases liberate the carcinogen in the bladder.
- *Nitrosamines* are formed when nitrites in food are converted to nitrates which react with amines in food. The substances can cause stomach cancer experimentally.
- *Alkylating agents*, such as those used in cancer management, bind to DNA. Use of these drugs in

cancer has been associated with the development of secondary malignancies.

- *Organic toxins* include the best studied example, aflatoxin, produced by the mould *Aspergillus flavus* growing on grain. This substance has been suggested as an aetiological agent in liver cancer in Africa, but the hepatitis B virus is perhaps a more important agent.

When carcinogens act on a cell, they may cause a permanent change which predisposes to cancer – a process known as *initiation*. Other agents can then produce transient changes which lead, with continued exposure, to cancer; this is known as *tumour promotion*. This two-stage process has been shown in some experimental cancers, where mutagens act as initiators and hormones or dietary constituents act as promoters.

Irradiation

The carcinogenic effect of ionising irradiation was indicated by the skin cancers that developed on the hands of early radiologists, and by the increased frequency of acute and chronic leukaemia, breast and thyroid cancer in Hiroshima during the 30 years after the atom bomb was dropped. The mechanism of carcinogenesis is probably related to the chromosomal damage caused by X-rays. It seems likely that 'background' ionising irradiation does not contribute greatly to common cancers in humans.

Ultraviolet light probably plays a role in the development of skin cancers. This is seen most clearly in the autosomal recessive disorder, xeroderma pigmentosum, where a defective DNA repair mechanism is associated with the early development of skin cancers on skin exposed to sunlight. Malignant melanoma and other skin cancers are uncommon in black people but are particularly frequent in fair-skinned Celts. In Australia, skin cancers are common among the non-indigenous population and increase in incidence in the north nearer the Equator.

Viruses

Ribonucleic acid (RNA) viruses can cause a variety of cancers in animals. These viruses contain a gene which codes for the enzyme reverse transcriptase, which is produced in the infected cell and results in the cellular synthesis of DNA complementary to the viral RNA and thus to the production of more viruses. For this reason they are called *retroviruses*. Tumours caused by these viruses include avian erythroblastosis, rat sarcoma, feline leukaemia and murine leukaemia. The insertion of the viral genome into DNA leads to malignant transformation, but the steps involved are not yet clear. A growth-factor receptor is encoded by the erythroblastosis-B virus (v-erb B); a phosphokinase by Rous sarcoma virus (sis).

The relationship between these gene products and cancer remains to be elucidated and promises to be one of the most fruitful areas of cancer research. Until recently, RNA viruses had not been shown to cause cancer in humans. There is now strong evidence that an RNA virus is involved in the development of some forms of T cell leukaemia and lymphoma (human T cell leukaemia virus, HTLV types 1 and 2). The human immunodeficiency virus (HIV) is the cause of the Acquired Immune Deficiency Syndrome (AIDS) in which there is a greatly increased frequency of skin sarcoma and B cell lymphoma. These tumours are probably not caused by the virus but are a consequence of oncogenesis in patients with greatly reduced immunity.

Research into RNA viruses led to the discovery that the viral oncogenes had homologues in normal cellular DNA. These cellular *proto-oncogenes* appear to code for products very similar to those produced by the equivalent virus. These findings have led to the search for increased expression of cellular oncogenes in human cancers, for the gene products, and for the link between carcinogenesis and oncogene activation.

There is strong circumstantial evidence implicating DNA viruses in the pathogenesis of some malignant neoplasms. For example, Epstein-Barr virus (EBV) was first isolated from cells from a case of Burkitt's lymphoma. The virus causes proliferation of normal human B lymphocytes; EBV-coded proteins are found in Burkitt's lymphoma cell lines; and African children with the lymphoma have high titres of antibody to viral antigens. Despite this evidence it is not clear if the virus is a cause of the lymphoma or whether other oncogenic stimuli produce the cancer in infected cells. Infection with two other DNA viruses has been linked to cancer: Herpes simplex II (HSV II) with cervical carcinoma and cytomegalovirus (CMV) with Kaposi's sarcoma. In both these cases the evidence is inconclusive.

Although uncommon in the West, hepatoma is a common cancer in Africa. Infection with hepatitis B virus (HBV) is associated with its development both in Africa and in Europe. Hepatoma is particularly likely to occur in chronic active hepatitis associated with HBV, and in alcoholic cirrhosis where there is evidence of previous HBV infection. Cancer of the uterine cervix is increasing in frequency in young women. There is strong evidence that human papilloma virus is associated with this disease, possibly as a result of sexually transmitted infection.

Genetic factors

Numerous *inherited*, rare, genetic abnormalities predispose to the development of malignancy (Table 8.3). These syndromes include examples of autosomal dominant and recessive inheritance, and X-linked disorders. Inherited chromosomal abnormalities may also predis-

Table 8.3 Inherited genetic abnormalities and malignancy

Inherited disorder	Cancer
Skin disorders	
Neurofibromatosis (AD)	Sarcoma, phaeochromocytoma, medullary carcinoma of thyroid
Tylosis palmaris (AD) (keratosis of palms and soles)	Oesophageal cancer
Peutz-Jehger's syndrome (AD)	Intestinal and ovarian cancer
Immune deficiency	
X-linked agammaglobulinaemia (XLR)	Lymphoma
Wiscott-Aldrich syndrome (XLR)	Lymphoma
Ataxia telangiectasia (AR)	Lymphoma and stomach cancer
X-linked lymphoproliferative syndrome (XLR)	Lymphoma
Gut disorders	
Polyposis coli (AD)	Colonic carcinoma
Gardner's syndrome (AD)	Colonic carcinoma Duodenal carcinoma
Neurological disorders	
Tuberose sclerosis (AD)	Glioma
Retinal/cerebellar angiomatosis (von Hippel-Lindau syndrome) (AD)	Hypernephroma, ependymoma, phaeochromocytoma
Other syndromes	
Bloom's syndrome (AR) (short stature, telangiectasia)	Leukaemia Many other cancers
Hemihypertrophy	Wilm's tumour, hepatoblastoma
Fanconi's anaemia (AR) (skeletal abnormality, patchy pigmentation, mental retardation)	Acute leukaemia
Multiple enchondromata (S) (Ollier's syndrome)	Chondrosarcoma
Chromosomal abnormalities	
Down's syndrome (trisomy 21)	Acute leukaemia
Klinefelter's syndrome (47,XXY)	Breast cancer
Aniridia-Wilm's syndrome (11p⁻)	Wilm's tumour
Mosaicism (45XO/46XY)	Gonadoblastoma
13q⁻ (multiple malformations)	Retinoblastoma
Li-Fraumeni syndrome (17p⁻)	Sarcoma in children Breast cancer in mother

AD	Autosomal dominant	XLR	X-linked recessive
AR	Autosomal recessive	S	Sporadic

pose to cancer (Table 8.3). The most common is Down's syndrome (trisomy-21), where there is an increased incidence of acute leukaemia. In some cases the relationship between the genetic abnormality and the induction of cancer has become clearer. In hereditary retinoblastoma the retinoblastoma gene (Rb) acts as a growth suppressor gene. Inherited loss of this gene is followed by mutation in the other allele, which sets the scene for malignant transformation. Germ-line mutation followed by loss of heterozygosity of the p53 gene occurs in the Li-Fraumeni syndrome, in which the families of children with sarcoma show an excess of other cancers. There may be an important inherited genetic component to many other common cancers, but the candidate genes are not yet identified.

Acquired genetic abnormalities are frequently found in cancer cells with mutation transposition and deletion of genetic material. These abnormalities are sometimes consistent, such as the translocation from chromosome 22 in chronic granulocytic leukaemia, and the reciprocal translocation involving chromosome 8 in Burkitt's lymphoma. In many tumours (lung cancer, leukaemia, hepatoma) there is mutation of the p53 gene, which codes for a growth regulatory transcription factor. In colon cancer, a cascade of genetic events appears to accompany the transformation of polyps to invasive cancer.

TUMOUR GROWTH AND DEVELOPMENT

Some tumours exhibit properties which imply that they have arisen as a result of clonal expansion caused by an oncogenic event in a single cell. Lymphomas, for example, usually show restriction to one type of surface immunoglobulin light chain; and studies in individuals who are heterozygotes for the enzyme glucose-6-phosphate dehydrogenase have shown that tumours contain only one form of the enzyme. Whether all cancers are monoclonal in origin is not known, and development of some carcinomas in a polyclonal field of premalignant change remains a possibility. Even if many tumours are monoclonal, heterogeneity of structure and function arises during the course of tumour growth. Cells from a tumour are diverse with respect to resistance to damage by irradiation or cytotoxic drugs, surface antigen expression, growth rate, and expression of biochemical markers such as embryonic proteins or peptide hormones. The mechanism of acquisition of this diversity is ill understood, but heterogeneity within tumours presents a formidable problem for treatment.

In normal tissues, self-renewing stem cells replenish a proliferating population of cells which follow a pathway of differentiation resulting in a mature tissue (Fig. 8.7). Cell death is balanced by formation of precursors, and the tissue is static in size or else grows and diminishes in response to such external controls as hormonal environment. This model of tissue growth can be applied to tumours but it is not certain whether, in cancer, renewal comes from a small stem-cell population. In cancers, the

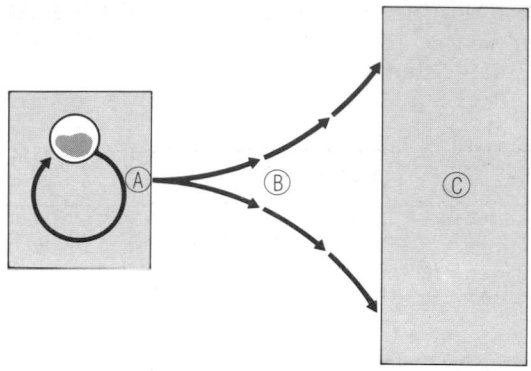

Fig. 8.7 Diagrammatic representation of cellular proliferation in a tumour. A. Pluripotent self-renewing stem cell. **B.** Proliferative compartment in which cell number increases but gradually loses reproductive potential. **C.** Mature tissue.

restraint on growth is disrupted so that sustained expansion of the tumour occurs.

For clinically detectable cancers, the kinetics of growth appear to be exponential and the rate of tumour volume doubling varies widely. In Burkitt's lymphoma, the doubling time of visible tumour may be as short as one to two days, in contrast to 100–400 days for some squamous carcinomas and adenocarcinomas. It seems unlikely that growth is exponential from the beginning of the cancer, since this would imply very long sub-clinical growth periods for some tumours (Fig. 8.8). Cancers are clinically apparent after about 32 doublings, and lethal after 36–38. It is possible that tumours grow more rapidly when they are very small and slow progressively as they enlarge (Gompertzian growth). If true, this may have implications for therapy, since the more rapidly dividing small tumour might be more susceptible to chemotherapy.

During growth, the tumour becomes vascularised and lymphatic drainage is established. Cells more than 150 μm from a capillary are relatively hypoxic, and such cells are resistant to radiotherapy. They are also exposed to a lower

concentration of cytotoxic agents. The vascularisation may be insufficient to sustain viability and areas of necrosis and haemorrhage are frequently found in large cancers. The process of vascularisation allows tumour cells to penetrate blood and lymphatic channels, and thence to metastasise to regional lymph nodes and distant sites.

Metastasis

Metastasis is a remarkable process and one which is still very poorly understood. The risk of metastases increases as tumours become larger. The cells must survive tissue invasion, circulation, passage across the capillary wall, and establishment in tissues. The process of tissue penetration appears to be by secretion of enzymes known as metalloproteinases (such as collagenase). The precise location of a metastasis is probably due in part to chance. Nevertheless, clinical patterns of blood-borne metastasis are apparent: gut cancers spread through the portal venous system to the liver; ovarian cancers seed into the peritoneal space; breast cancer has a predilection for bones of the axial skeleton; sarcomas characteristically spread to the lungs.

PATHOLOGY

The major categories of malignant tumours are:

- *carcinomas* which arise from ectoderm or endodermal cells;
- *sarcomas* which arise from mesodermal cells making up bone and connective tissue;
- *leukaemias and lymphomas* which arise in cells of the bone marrow and immune system.

The distinction between benign and malignant neoplasms is based histologically on the cellular pleomorphism, frequent mitoses and tissue invasion which are characteristic of malignancy. The clinical manifestations of malignancy are tissue infiltration and lymphatic and blood-borne metastasis.

The degree of differentiation of a tumour is often an important guide to prognosis and therefore to therapy. Poorly differentiated carcinomas have a worse prognosis than well-differentiated tumours. This is due in part to an association with a more rapid growth rate and more early and widespread metastases. About 5% of cancers present as metastases where the primary site of the tumour is unknown. The histology is usually a poorly differentiated carcinoma often with features suggestive of adenocarcinoma, but the pathologist may find the tumour difficult to classify.

The development of monoclonal antibodies has led to a greater precision in diagnosis by using immunocyto-

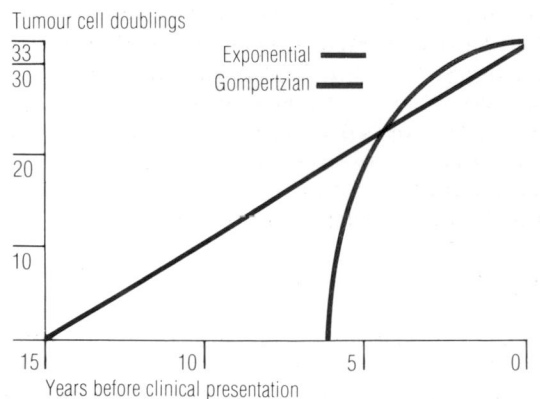

Fig. 8.8 Diagrammatic representation of exponential and Gompertzian growth.

chemical methods. Many anaplastic tumours can now be diagnosed as epithelial tumours, melanomas or lymphomas by using antibodies against epithelial antigens, or antigens associated with melanoma, leucocytes or T and B lymphocytes. The correct identification of lymphoma will lead to important changes in management of a patient (Fig. 8.9). Many antibodies will not bind to antigens on formalin-fixed and paraffin embedded sections, and require fresh tissue. Other specialised investigations can be carried out on fresh tumour tissue – measurement of hormone receptor content (e.g. oestrogen and progesterone receptors) for example, which may be of importance in prognosis and in deciding treatment. Using immunocytochemical techniques, the presence of such substances as alphafetoprotein can be detected in the tumour. The increasing complexity and versatility of histopathological diagnosis means that it is now essential for there to be close collaboration between clinician and pathologist before specimens are obtained.

Ultrasound and computed tomography (CT) scanning now allow accurate needle biopsy and aspiration cytology of hitherto inaccessible intra-abdominal and intrathoracic tumours. Cytological diagnosis does have some limitations: in the diagnosis of lymphoma, for example, it may be difficult to distinguish tumour cells from normal reactive lymphocytes. For this reason, histological diagnosis is preferred, especially in situations in which there is clinical doubt about the diagnosis.

CLINICAL FEATURES

Cancers cause symptoms due to the local spread of the primary tumour, and as a result of metastasis and of metabolic and remote effects of the malignancy.

Symptoms due to local disease

The primary tumour is clinically silent either until it becomes a visible painless lump which the patient notices (this is a common presentation of breast cancer and Hodgkin's disease and other lymphomas) or until it impinges on surrounding tissues. Thus, carcinoma of the lung will cause increasing bronchial narrowing, with breathlessness, cough and collapse of the distal lung; colonic carcinoma may present with disturbed bowel habit and obstruction; brain tumours may cause raised intracranial pressure or focal neurological signs; cancer of the head of the pancreas will cause obstruction of the bile duct leading to jaundice. As the primary tumour gets larger, it may ulcerate and bleed. Haemoptysis is a common symptom of bronchial carcinoma, and chronic blood loss leading to iron deficiency anaemia frequently occurs with carcinoma of the colon. The tumour may infiltrate nerves and bone leading to pain, or pain may arise from stretching of the capsule of an organ – for example, pain over the liver with advanced hepatoma. Nerve entrapment frequently occurs with pelvic tumours such as carcinoma of the cervix. Similarly, carcinoma of the bronchus occurring in the superior sulcus (Pancoast tumour) may be accompanied by intense pain in the arm, due to involvement of the brachial plexus.

Metastatic disease in bone causes pain which is often intense and distressing. Bone pain may occur in the absence of a pathological fracture or vertebral collapse, but it becomes worse when this occurs. In the liver, metastases cause pain by stretching the capsule. Cerebral metastases give rise to raised intracranial pressure, fits, focal signs and symptoms, and mental confusion. Pulmonary spread may cause breathlessness due to large intrapulmonary tumour masses, diffuse lymphatic permeation (lymphangitis carcinomatosa) and massive pleural effusion.

Systemic symptoms

Primary and metastatic cancer may cause a variety of metabolic and other disturbances which are important causes of symptoms. In general, these are produced in one of three ways:

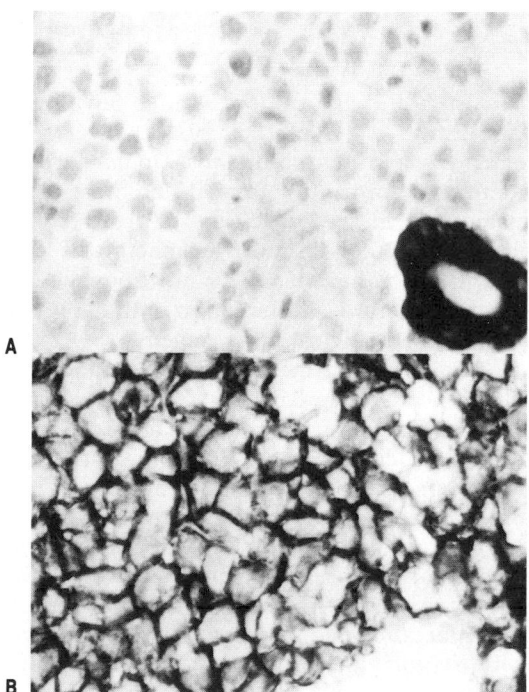

Fig. 8.9 Section of nasopharyngeal tumour. A. Staining with anti-cytokeratin; the epithelium of normal respiratory gland stains strongly but tumour cells are negative. **B.** Staining with antibody to the leucocyte common antigen reveals that the tumour cells are expressing the leucocyte antigen and that the tumour is a lymphoma.

- as a result of the tumour mass, both primary and metastatic;
- as a result of secretion of hormones by the tumour (Table 8.4);
- by ill-understood mechanisms which give rise to specific cutaneous, neurological and other syndromes remote from the tumour and not due to metastasis – *paraneoplastic syndromes* (Table 8.5).

The commonest metabolic disturbance associated with advanced cancer is cachexia. This is a state of profound weight loss, muscle wasting and weakness. Many factors contribute to the state, of which anorexia is perhaps the major cause. Loss of appetite occurs early with tumours of the upper gastrointestinal tract, even before metastases have occurred. For most tumours, loss of appetite is an accompaniment of advanced disease, particularly hepatic metastases. Anorexia may be made worse by treatment with radiation and cytotoxic drugs, by psychological factors such as depression, and by unrelieved pain. The tumour may promote weight loss by direct metabolic effects. For example, there may be excess lactate production by the tumour which is recycled into glucose (a process wasteful of energy), and an increased glucose consumption at a time when carbohydrate intake has declined. Some tumours may cause malabsorption (carcinoma of pancreas) or intestinal obstruction (colon cancer) which contributes to weight loss. Unlike patients who are starving, many cancer patients have a normal or high metabolic rate but the reason for this is not clear.

Fever may accompany cancer – not always due to infection, although this must always be excluded. Fever is particularly likely to occur with lymphomas, renal carci-

Table 8.4 Hormonal syndromes in non-endocrine cancers

Hormonal syndrome	Tumour	Mechanism
Hypercalcaemia	Squamous carcinomas	? Tumour-derived growth factors
	Carcinoma of kidney	? Other calcium mobilising factors
Hyponatraemia	Small cell lung cancer Lymphoma Pancreatic carcinoma	Ectopic ADH produced by tumour
Cushing's syndrome	Small cell lung cancer Bronchial and thymic carcinoids	Ectopic ACTH produced by tumour
Gynaecomastia	Teratoma Hepatoma Large cell bronchial cancer	? Excess oestrogen activity
Hyperpigmentation	Small cell lung cancer	? Ectopic MSH produced by tumour

Table 8.5 Paraneoplastic syndromes

Syndrome	Associated tumours
Neurological	
Neuropathy (usually sensory)	Small cell lung cancer Cancers of breast and ovary
Cerebellar degeneration	Small cell lung cancer
Eaton-Lambert syndrome	Small cell lung cancer
Musculoskeletal	
Clubbing Hypertrophic pulmonary osteoarthropathy	Carcinoma of the lung (particularly squamous cell)
Dermatomyositis	Lung cancer Oesophageal cancer Other cancers
Polyarthritis	Adenocarcinomas of breast, gut and ovary
Haematological	
Multiple venous thrombosis	Pancreatic cancer Other adenocarcinomas
Erythrocytosis	Renal carcinoma Hepatoma Cerebellar haemangioblastoma Uterine cancer
Disseminated intravascular coagulation	Mucinous adenocarcinomas

noma, sarcomas and any tumours which have metastasised to the liver.

Anaemia may be due to blood loss, malabsorption or dietary deficiency of iron or folate. The most common mechanism is a failure of release of iron (stored in macrophages) into the plasma – the anaemia of 'chronic disease' (p. 1070). This anaemia is unresponsive to iron therapy. Chemotherapy and radiation both depress bone marrow function and contribute to anaemia.

The hormonal syndromes which accompany cancer (Table 8.4) are important because they are a cause of symptoms which are frequently treatable. In many patients, hypercalcaemia is due to bone destruction by metastases, but some cancers produce hypercalcaemia by a hormonal mechanism. In these cases, the calcium level falls if the tumour is removed. The tumour elaborates a peptide (parathormone-related peptide) and other factors (such as growth factors) which can mobilise bone calcium. Hypercalcaemia associated with cancer can be very severe, requiring urgent management (see Ch. 18, p. 733). Hyponatraemia, due to production of antidiuretic hormone (ADH) by the tumour, is a frequent accompaniment of small cell lung cancer. Malaise, fatigue leading to fits, and coma may result. The condition can be reversed by demeclocycline and water restriction (Ch. 21). Adrenocorticotrophic hormone (ACTH)-like peptides may also be produced by small cell lung cancer. In this disease, the high levels of ectopic ACTH produce profound metabolic disturbances, with proximal muscle weakness, hyperglycaemia and hypokalaemic alkalosis. These symptoms can be reversed by management of the tumour.

The paraneoplastic syndromes (Table 8.5) can cause diagnostic difficulty in two ways. Firstly, the syndromes have to be distinguished from other diseases causing a similar clinical picture. For example, the peripheral neuropathy accompanying cancer may be clinically indistinguishable from other causes. Secondly, the underlying carcinoma may not always be clinically apparent. Tumours such as carcinoma of the ovary or pancreas may be associated with multiple migratory venous thromboses at a time when the primary disease is not detectable.

The diversity of symptoms caused by primary and metastatic cancer, together with the hormonal, metabolic and paraneoplastic syndromes which accompany many malignant tumours, mean that a diagnosis of cancer must be considered in any unexplained illness, particularly in a middle-aged or elderly patient.

STAGING AND INVESTIGATION

Once a diagnosis of cancer has been established, further investigation is usually needed to establish the degree of spread of the primary tumour and to determine if metastasis has occurred. It has been known for many years that the prognosis of a patient depends, among other things, on the size of the tumour and the presence of metastases. Our ability to locate the tumour and distant metastases accurately has improved immeasurably in recent years with the introduction of radionuclide and ultrasound scanning, CT scanning and magnetic resonance (MR) imaging. These techniques have shown that, in many patients, the cancer is metastatic at the time of presentation. This realisation has led to a greater emphasis on systemic treatments such as hormone therapy and chemotherapy and, in some cases (e.g. breast cancer), a tendency towards less radical surgical procedures for the primary tumour. The determination of the degree of spread at presentation is generally known as *staging*. The international acceptance of staging systems has meant that, in treatment trials, comparable groups of patients can be treated allowing a comparison between different methods.

TNM classification

A generally accepted system, which is applicable to some (but not all) cancers, is the TNM (*Tumour, Nodes, Metastases*) classification. The *T* component defines certain characteristics of the primary tumour such as its size, site or depth of invasion; the defining criteria will be different with each type of cancer. *N* refers to the presence or absence of involved nodes; the degree of node involvement may be designated as N0 (no involved nodes) and N1, N2, N3, as more nodes are involved. If no metastases are present, the designation is M0, and M1 if they are detected. Clearly, the TNM stage assigned to a tumour will depend on the thoroughness of the clinical and radiological investigation, and this will change as new techniques are invented and perfected.

The TNM stages can be grouped into categories which have prognostic significance. These categories or 'stage groups' have been of great value in the design of treatment trials. The TNM stages and related stage groupings for carcinoma of the kidney are shown in Table 8.6 and the prognosis related to the stage grouping in Figure 8.10.

The TNM system is not applicable to some tumours and is of limited value in others; it is clearly inappropriate, for example, in acute leukaemias, and prognostic factors in these diseases are based on other criteria (see Ch. 24). Nevertheless, staging classification is possible and useful in diseases such as chronic lymphatic leukaemia and myeloma. The criteria have nothing to do with a TNM system, but are related to tumour mass. In lung cancer, the TNM system is useful and widely used in squamous carcinoma, but is of considerably less value

Table 8.6 Renal carcinoma TNM staging and stage grouping

Stage	Definition		
	T stage		
T1	Small tumour surrounded by normal kidney		
T2	Large tumour with kidney deformity		
T3	Perinephric infiltration or renal vein extension		
T4	Invasion of local structures (e.g. abdominal wall)		
	N stage		
N0	No nodes involved		
N1	Ipsilateral nodes involved		
N2	Contralateral nodes involved		
N3	Fixed nodes		
	M stage		
M0	No distant metastases		
M1	Distant metastases		
	Stage grouping		
Stage I	T1	N0	M0
Stage II	T2	N0	M0
Stage III	T3	N0–2	M0
Stage IV	T4	N0–3	M1

(The stage grouping refers to the worst prognostic feature of the case: e.g. a T1 N1 tumour would be Stage III)

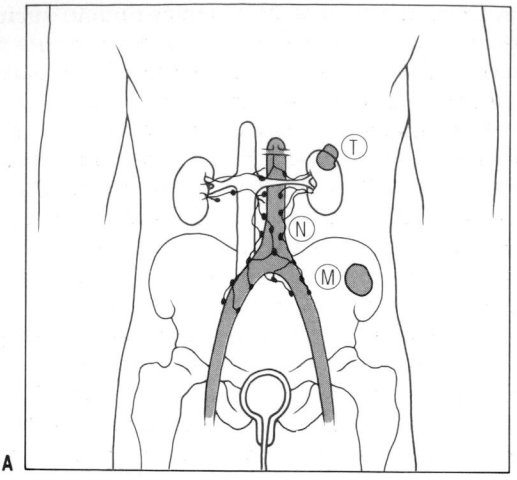

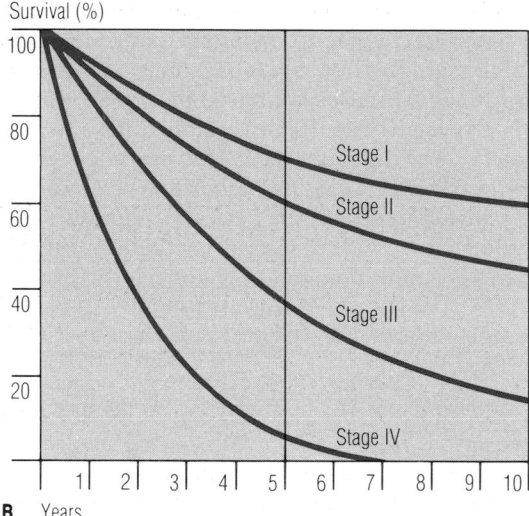

Fig. 8.10 A. Carcinoma of the left kidney. T = degree of local spread; N = involvement of adjacent lymph nodes; M = metastasis to bone or other sites. **B. Prognosis according to stage grouping.**

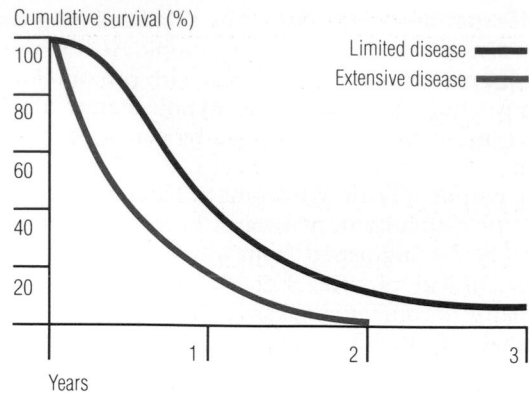

Fig. 8.11 Prognosis of small cell carcinoma of the lung related to the disease extent at presentation. Limited disease = disease confined to one hemithorax. Extensive disease = more widespread local extent or metastasis.

in small cell carcinoma. In this disease, a rough categorisation is made into *limited* disease (confined to one hemithorax) and *extensive* disease (spread beyond one hemithorax including metastases). There is a clear difference in prognosis in these two categories (Fig. 8.11).

Staging investigation

As techniques are developed, the *sensitivity* (ability to detect an abnormality if it is present) and *specificity* (ability to distinguish a metastasis from other pathologies) of the investigations changes. At present, radionuclide bone scanning is the most sensitive method of detection of bone metastases. CT scanners are better than, or at least equal to, ultrasound scanning in detection of hepatic

metastases, but ultrasound is much cheaper and can be repeated regularly to assess response. CT scanning is the best method of detecting pulmonary and brain metastases. MR is superior to CT scanning in detecting deep-seated brain tumours, especially in the brainstem and spinal cord, and in delineating the extent of soft-tissue involvement in tumours such as sarcomas.

CT scanning has proved of value in detecting lymph node enlargement in the thorax and the abdomen. Unfortunately, nodes can be replaced by secondary tumour and yet not be enlarged. Lymphography – in which contrast material is injected into lymphatics in the dorsum of the feet – can show filling defects in normal size nodes, as well as node enlargement. For those tumours which spread transperitoneally, such as carcinoma of the ovary, laparoscopy (peritoneoscopy) is the most sensitive method of detecting spread of tumour if a laparotomy is not carried out. Although invasive, this procedure can also be used to obtain liver biopsy material under direct vision.

Tumour markers

Tumours may secrete substances into the blood which can be used both diagnostically (to detect the presence of disease) and in therapy, to monitor the effects of treatment. A variety of biochemical disturbances may be induced in the body by a tumour, such as the rise in alkaline phosphatase caused by liver or bone metastases, but these are crude and insensitive guides to the effect of treatment. The markers in common clinical use (Table 8.7) are oncofetal antigens, placental products, isoenzymes, ectopic hormones and some cellular antigens usually derived from the cell membrane.

Ideally, the tumour marker should always be produced by the cancer in question. In choriocarcinoma, human chorionic gonadotrophin (HCG) is produced in over 95% of cases; and 75% of germ cell tumours secrete either

Table 8.7 Tumour markers present in blood

Marker	Tumour
Oncofetal antigens	
Alphafetoprotein	Germ cell tumours of ovary and testis Hepatoma
Carcinoembryonic antigen	Gastrointestinal cancer
Pancreatic oncofetal antigen	Pancreatic carcinoma
Placental products	
Human chorionic gonadotrophin	Choriocarcinoma Teratoma
Placental lactogen	Choriocarcinoma
Placental alkaline phosphatase	Seminoma Ovarian cancer
Isoenzymes	
Alkaline phosphatase	Osteosarcoma
Lactic dehydrogenase	Neuroblastoma, many cancers
Acid phosphatase	Prostatic carcinoma
Neurone specific enolase	Small cell carcinoma of lung
Ectopic hormones (see Table 8.4)	
Other cellular antigens (defined by antisera) Antigens of ovarian carcinoma, e.g. Ca125	
Antigens of cervical carcinoma	

alphafetoprotein (AFP), HCG or both. Carcino-embryonic antigen (CEA) is found in the serum in 65% of cases of colorectal cancer. With some markers, e.g. HCG, AFP and placental alkaline phosphatase (PLAP), the serum level of the marker is a reasonably accurate and sensitive reflection of the tumour mass in an individual patient, and can therefore be used as a guide to therapy. In other cases, e.g. alkaline phosphatase in osteosarcoma, the relationship to tumour response is inconsistent.

The serum marker may be a valuable guide to tumour recurrence and, in most cases of germ cell tumours (such as teratoma of the testis), is a more sensitive indicator of tumour recurrence than any other technique. There is, of course, little value in knowing when relapse is occurring if there is no effective treatment. However, in the case of early-stage germ cell tumours, the markers have allowed a policy of observation following initial surgery, since highly effective chemotherapy is available for relapse. An example of the use of tumour markers is shown in Figure 8.12.

The tumour marker may be produced in other diseases; for example, serum AFP is raised in early pregnancy, and CEA may be present in inflammatory bowel disease. Other markers, such as ADH, are too difficult to measure for routine use. AFP is produced in the fetal liver, in the malignant yolk-sac cells in teratoma, and in hepatoma. It has a plasma half-life of 5–7 days. HCG is produced by the placenta and by choriocarcinoma, and by the trophoblastic elements in teratoma. The plasma half-life is 30 hours. CEA is a group of glycoprotein antigens produced by epithelial tumours and by normal colonic mucosa.

PRINCIPLES OF CANCER MANAGEMENT

Surgery and radiotherapy are the principal methods of treating the primary tumour. For many early-stage cancers – e.g. in cancer of the breast, squamous cancer of the lung, and cancers of the ovary, kidney, testis and gastrointestinal tract – surgery alone has a good chance of cure. Unfortunately, many patients cannot be cured surgically, either because the tumour is so advanced locally as to make resection impossible, or because investigation has revealed metastases.

Advances in radiotherapy technique and the recent developments in combination cytotoxic chemotherapy have meant that, for many patients, a combined approach

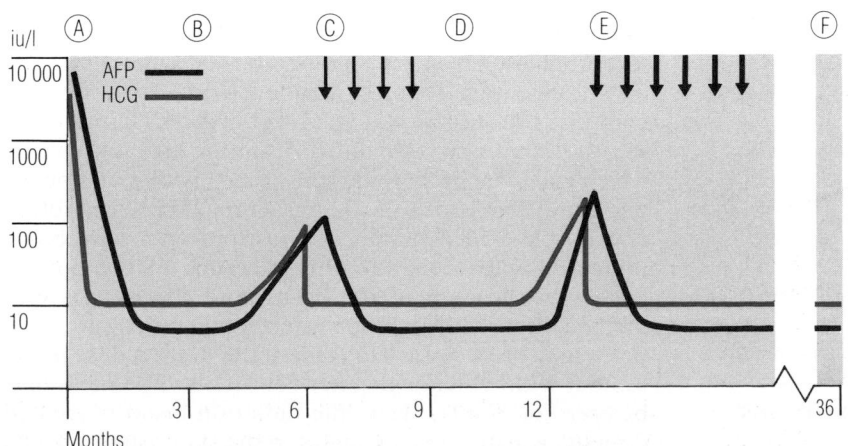

Fig. 8.12 Tumour markers in management of testicular cancer. A. Both HCG and AFP markers are elevated before orchidectomy but fall following operation (HCG more rapidly because of its short half-life). **B.** No evidence of recurrence, followed by a rise in marker levels. **C.** Combination chemotherapy for recurrence is followed by a fall in levels to normal (**D**). **E.** A further rise in marker levels is treated more intensively and the patient is disease-free at three years (**F**).

to management is needed to achieve the best results. This in turn involves close collaboration between surgeon, radiotherapist and medical oncologist. Before treatment begins, it is essential to decide if there is a possibility of cure or whether the intention should be palliative. Many factors will influence this decision, including the degree of spread of the tumour locally, the presence of distant metastases, and the patient's age and state of health. It may be very difficult to decide on the best policy if the chances of cure are relatively small and the toxicity of treatment considerable. In a young patient, the aim of cure would probably overcome doubts about toxicity, but this would not be so in the elderly.

If the clinical evidence makes it quite clear that there is no hope of cure, then it becomes unnecessary and wasteful to undertake elaborate staging investigations since these are unlikely to alter management. Investigation, as previously outlined, will be necessary in all other patients to determine the degree of spread of the disease before deciding on the treatment plan. The principles of surgical management of cancer are beyond the scope of this chapter, but it is important for all physicians to have an understanding of the basis of management using radiotherapy, chemotherapy and hormone therapy.

RADIOTHERAPY

Most radiotherapy treatment involves the use of electromagnetic waves with very high energy and short wavelength – gamma rays and X-rays. Some modern radiotherapy machines use ^{60}Co as a source which decays to a more stable form with a half-life of 5.3 years. The process of decay (with loss of a neutron) is accompanied by emission of gamma rays with a high energy (1.2 MeV). X-rays were first produced by Roentgen, who heated an electrode in a sealed vacuum tube. The electrode produced electrons which bombarded a target, resulting in emission of electromagnetic waves which were desig-

nated 'X-rays' and whose nature was the same as gamma rays. By increasing the voltage, X-rays of shorter wavelength and higher energy are produced which have greater tissue penetrating power than those produced from low voltage machines (Fig. 8.13). Modern machines accelerate the electrons almost to the speed of light, which results in a high-energy beam. These machines (linear accelerators) have become standard equipment in most departments. They provide a sharper beam than that obtained from ^{60}Co sources and greater depth doses. When the target is moved out of the path of the electrons, the high-energy electron beam can be used for the treatment of superficial tumours.

The tissue penetrating power of high-energy X-rays and gamma rays means that normal tissues will be irradiated as well as the tumour. With lower voltage X-rays, the penetrating power is less and more energy is deposited in superficial tissues, especially bone. With electrons, the radiation decays rapidly in tissue, the depth of penetration depending on the energy of the beam (Fig. 8.13).

The important site of radiation damage is nuclear DNA. The damage appears to be induced indirectly. The radiation first produces highly reactive radicals which in turn damage the DNA, impairing the reproductive integrity of the cell. The damaging effects of radiation are less marked in cells which are hypoxic. Some areas of tumour may not be well vascularised and these cells are relatively radio-resistant. The mechanisms of resistance are not well understood. The amount of cell death following exposure to irradiation is also proportional to the dose administered. At low doses the damage is sublethal. Nevertheless, radiation administered as a few large fractions may not be as effective as multiple fraction regimens using smaller daily doses. This technique may be more effective because it allows the tumour to shrink and become less hypoxic, may be easier to tolerate, and allows normal tissues to recover at a faster rate than the tumour. In treating tumours, multiple fractions are usually employed and the total dose administered depends on what is known of the radiosensitivity of the neoplasm (Table 8.8). The total dose received by the tumour is measured in Gray (Gy:1 J/kg) or rad (100 rad = 1 Gy).

The planning of the radiation field is often a highly complex procedure that has been greatly facilitated in recent years by the use of CT scanning and simulators, which allow the fields to be constructed with precision. In planning the fields, the radiotherapist must therefore consider the localisation of the tumour, its probable inherent radiosensitivity, the tolerance of the normal tissues in the path of the beam, and the necessity to include draining lymph nodes in the treatment. Multiple fields may be necessary to achieve the desired dose in the tumour without damaging normal tissues. The fields may be *open* (or *direct*). Here, the radiation beam is applied directly, usually at right angles to the skin. Alternatively,

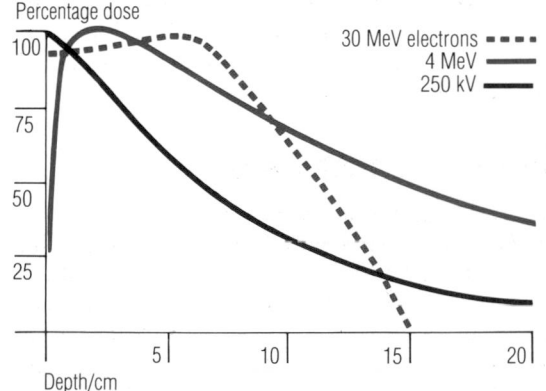

Fig. 8.13 Diagrammatic representation of tissue penetration of different types and energies of radiation.

Table 8.8 Relative radiosensitivity of tumours

Highly radiosensitive	Relatively resistant
Lymphomas	Squamous cell lung cancer
Ewing's sarcoma	Hypernephroma
Seminoma	Bladder carcinoma
Wilm's tumour	Rectal carcinoma
Myeloma	Soft tissue sarcoma (adults)
	Cervical carcinoma
Moderately radiosensitive	
	Very resistant
Breast cancer	
Small cell lung cancer	Melanoma
Ovarian cancer	Osteosarcoma
Medulloblastoma	Pancreatic carcinoma
Basal cell carcinoma	
Teratoma	

Table 8.9 Complications of radiotherapy

Tissue	Complication	
	Immediate	Delayed
Skin	Erythema, desquamation	Fibrosis Telangiectasia Squamous carcinoma
Oral cavity	Mucosal ulceration	Loss of saliva
Gut	Nausea, diarrhoea	Fibrosis and stricture
Bone	Bone necrosis	Loss of bone growth in children
Kidney	Acute nephritis	Chronic nephritis Hypertension
CNS	Radiation myelitis and encephalitis	Demyelination Possible alteration of personality and intellect
Eye	Conjunctivitis	Dry eye Cataract formation
Gonads	Sterility	Sterility
Bone marrow	Leucopenia	Suppression of haemopoiesis in area irradiated

if several fields are used, the field may be *wedged*. These wedges, inserted into the beam, alter the dose distribution so that the tumour dose is homogeneous and problems of irradiation of normal tissue are minimised where fields overlap. An example of a multiple field is shown in Figure 8.14. The treatment area is immobilised and for some tumours, such as head and neck cancers, moulds and shells are used to ensure accurate and reproducible positioning. The radiation source is mounted in a gantry which moves isocentrically about the patient.

Radiotherapy may also be given by placing a sealed source containing a radioactive isotope inside a body cavity or in tissues. This is known as *brachytherapy*. Examples of such isotopes are ^{137}Cs, which is widely used as an intracavity source of radiation in treating carcinoma of the cervix; and iridium wires, which may be placed in breast tissue to provide interstitial irradiation when radical radiotherapy is used following conservative surgery for breast cancer. Unsealed sources of radioac-

tivity may be taken by mouth, e.g. ^{131}I in the treatment of thyroid cancer, or given intravenously, e.g. ^{32}P in the treatment of polycythaemia rubra vera.

The complications of radiotherapy depend on the radiation sensitivity of normal tissues in the path of the beam, and may be immediate or delayed. A summary of some of these is given in Table 8.9.

SYSTEMIC TREATMENTS

In the last 40 years, there has been a dramatic increase in interest in the use of drugs to kill cancer cells. So many cancers are either disseminated at diagnosis or too advanced locally to resect, that a systemic approach to treatment offers the only chance of remission or cure. The two treatments in general use are *cytotoxic chemotherapy* and *hormone therapy*.

Cytotoxic chemotherapy

The earliest compounds to be introduced were nitrogen mustards, which were shown to be cytotoxic to lymphoid tissue and then to have activity against lymphomas in humans. In 1948, Farber demonstrated remissions of leukaemia using the antifolate aminopterin, and this led to the development of a wide variety of antipurines and antipyrimidines. Anti-tumour antibiotics were first developed in 1940 (actinomycin A) with a significant step forward in 1963 with the isolation of anthracyclines.

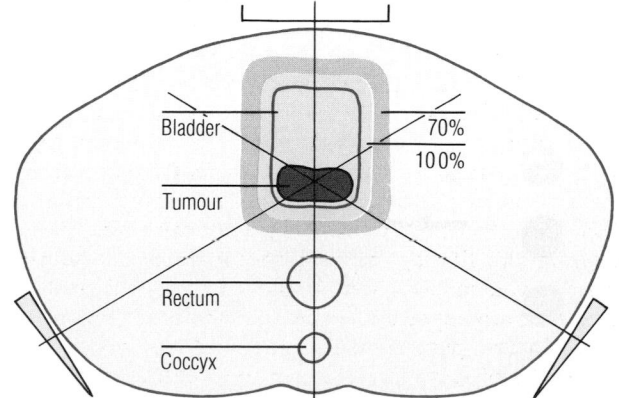

Fig. 8.14 Radiation planning for carcinoma of bladder, showing relationship of the three beams to the tumour and the dose levels (% of maximum) achieved within the tumour and surrounding normal tissue.

More recent developments include platinum complexes and epipodophyllotoxins. There are now about 35 cytotoxic drugs of proven value in routine use, and the increasing complexity of medical treatment of cancer has led to the development of medical oncology as an important specialty in cancer management.

Mechanisms of action

Cytotoxic drugs produce their effect mainly by damaging the capacity of the cell to divide, and also by interfering with synthesis of essential proteins. For many of these agents, the most important toxicity concerns DNA, with impairment of DNA synthesis, reaction with the DNA helix or damage to DNA repair mechanisms. This and other sites of damage are shown in Figure 8.15.

During cell division there is a phase (G_1) which precedes the phase of DNA synthesis (S). Following the S phase there is a postsynthetic phase (G_2) which is followed by mitosis (M). The daughter cells then either enter into the cycle of division or remain in a non-reproductive stage (G_0). Because of their action on DNA, most

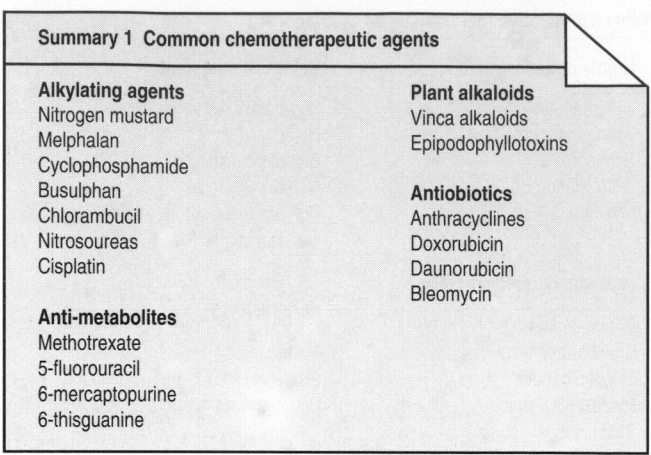

Summary 1 Common chemotherapeutic agents

Alkylating agents
Nitrogen mustard
Melphalan
Cyclophosphamide
Busulphan
Chlorambucil
Nitrosoureas
Cisplatin

Anti-metabolites
Methotrexate
5-fluorouracil
6-mercaptopurine
6-thisguanine

Plant alkaloids
Vinca alkaloids
Epipodophyllotoxins

Antiobiotics
Anthracyclines
Doxorubicin
Daunorubicin
Bleomycin

cytotoxic drugs exert their maximum effect on replicating rather than resting cells. If, after damage to DNA (e.g. by alkylation), the cell does not divide, there will be time for DNA repair mechanisms to excise the attached alkyl groups and to repair strand breaks. Rapidly proliferating cells are thus more susceptible to cytotoxic damage, but

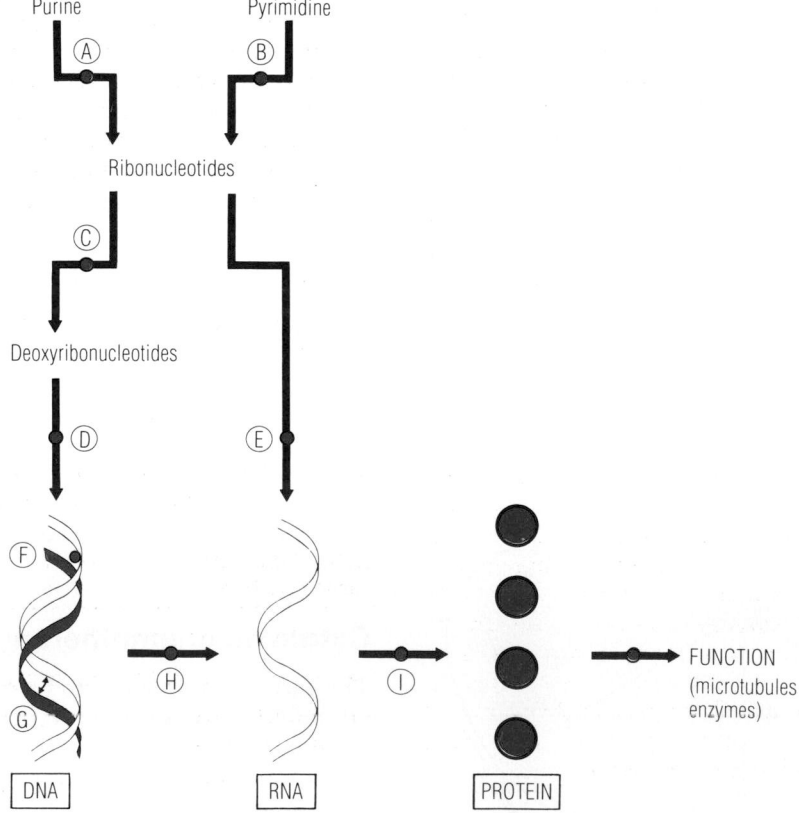

Fig. 8.15 Sites of action of some cytotoxic drugs. A, B. Blocks to purine (6MP) and pyrimidine metabolism (azaribine). **C.** Block of ribonucleotide reductase (hydroxyurea). **D.** Inhibition of DNA polymerase (cytosine arabinoside). **E.** Alteration of synthesis and function of RNA (5FU, azacytidine). **F.** Intercalation with DNA and inhibition of topoisomerase II (anthracyclines, epipodophyllotoxins). **G.** Cross-linking of DNA (bifunctional alkylating agents). **H.** Impaired synthesis of RNA (actinomycin, anthracyclines). **I.** Impaired protein synthesis (asparaginase). **J.** Impaired function of proteins (vinca alkaloid blocking of microtubule formation).

this is not the only determinant of susceptibility since, as with radiation, different tissues and tumours show inherent differences in susceptibility, the biochemical basis of which is poorly understood.

Alkylating agents are very reactive compounds which exert their effect by the linkage of the alkyl group to DNA bases, particularly guanine. If the drug is bifunctional (having two alkyl groups), inter- and intra-strand crosslinks will form. Nitrogen mustard, phenylalanine nitrogen mustard (melphalan), cyclophosphamide, busulphan and chlorambucil are commonly used alkylating agents. Cyclophosphamide itself is inactive but is metabolised by the liver to 4-hydroxycyclophosphamide, which is transported to the tissue and there releases the active alkylating compounds. Nitrosoureas and cisplatin probably act mainly as alkylating agents.

Methotrexate inhibits dihydrofolate reductase, thus preventing the formation of tetrahydrofolate which is necessary for thymidine synthesis. Other antimetabolites include: 5-fluorouracil (5FU), which also blocks thymidine formation; 6-mercaptopurine (6MP), which interferes with purine nucleotide biosynthesis; and 6-thioguanine, which has a similar mechanism of action to 6MP.

Several plant alkaloids have anticancer activity. The vinca alkaloids interfere with the formation of the mitotic spindle by blocking the assembly of tubulin. The epipodophyllotoxins, which have been introduced more recently, damage DNA through topoisomerase II, which results in the drug/enzyme complex cleaving the DNA strand.

Anthracycline antibiotics intercalate between DNA bases, as does actinomycin, which has the additional action of interfering with RNA synthesis. Bleomycin causes DNA strand breaks.

Testing a new drug

When a new drug has shown activity in the laboratory, it is tested in patients with cancer. At first, it is given in gradually increasing doses to patients with advanced drug-resistant cancer. These trials are called *Phase I* studies and the aim is to monitor toxicity and to study metabolism and distribution of the drug as well as to note any activity. In *Phase II* studies, patients with a wide range of tumours are then treated in order to determine the spectrum of activity of the drug. Later, *Phase III* studies are performed in which the drug is tested, usually in previously untreated patients, either alone or in combination with other drugs and often as part of a randomised comparison.

Combination chemotherapy

In recent years, it has become standard practice to use cytotoxic drugs in combination. The aim is to produce a variety of different biochemical lesions in the tumour, if possible without increasing toxicity. It quickly became apparent that quadruple therapy in, for example, advanced Hodgkin's disease, produced a far higher *complete response rate* (disappearance of all symptoms and signs of the tumour) than single-agent therapy. Furthermore, many of these complete responses were sustained, about 40% of patients being disease free between five and 10 years later. This had not been observed with single-agent therapy. Similar results were reported with non-Hodgkin's lymphoma and, later, with testicular teratoma, Ewing's sarcoma and other childhood tumours. In the common tumours of adults (such as cancer of the breast and small cell lung cancer), an increased response rate is also obtained with drugs in combination, but most of these responses are partial (greater than 50% reduction in size) and not sustained for long.

Most of the regimens used today have been derived empirically by oncologists with knowledge and experience. There are, however, some general principles governing selection of the drugs (Table 8.10). Using these general principles, combination chemotherapy has been introduced into the treatment of many cancers, and forms the mainstay of management in an important minority of uncommon tumours. Unfortunately, most of the common adult cancers are only moderately sensitive to these drugs, and some are very resistant (Table 8.11). Cancer is a disease of the elderly and many patients are not fit enough to risk the toxicity of chemotherapy, especially if the intention is to palliate rather than cure.

Complications of chemotherapy

There are both immediate and long-term complications of chemotherapy.

Immediate

The most troublesome immediate side-effects of chemotherapy are nausea and vomiting, mucosal ulceration,

Table 8.10 General principles governing the selection of drugs used in combination therapy

- The drugs are known to be effective when used as single agents.
- Where possible, drugs with differing modes of action are combined.
- The major toxicity of each drug should be as different as possible from that of other agents.
- Pulsed intermittent treatment is used to allow recovery of the gut and bone marrow.
- If possible each drug should be used in its optimum dose and schedule, although in practice some reduction in dose is nearly always necessary.
- There should be no known synergistic toxicity.

Table 8.11 Relative chemosensitivity of tumours

Highly sensitive tumours (which may be cured by chemotherapy)

Teratoma of testis
Hodgkin's disease
High grade non-Hodgkin's lymphoma
Wilm's tumour
Embryonal rhabdomyosarcoma
Choriocarcinoma
Acute lymphoblastic leukaemia in children
Ewing's sarcoma

Moderately sensitive tumours (in which chemotherapy may sometimes contribute to cure and often palliates)

Small cell carcinoma of lung
Breast carcinoma
Low grade non-Hodgkin's lymphoma
Acute myeloid leukaemia
Ovarian cancer
Myeloma

Relatively insensitive tumours (in which chemotherapy may sometimes produce palliation)

Gastric carcinoma
Bladder carcinoma
Squamous carcinoma of head and neck
Soft tissue sarcoma
Cervical carcinoma

Resistant tumours

Melanoma
Squamous carcinoma of lung
Large bowel cancer

bone marrow depression and alopecia. Nausea and vomiting are probably initiated by a centre in the medulla. Intravenous alkylating agents tend to produce nausea at 12–18 hours, and cisplatin and doxorubicin typically produce nausea about six hours after administration. Nausea is often accompanied by vomiting and the symptoms usually last 12–24 hours. These symptoms can be very troublesome but are tolerated by the majority of patients. Skilled, meticulous and flexible use of antiemetics is essential. Piperazine phenothiazines (e.g. prochlorperazine) are of some help when given in full dose, but aliphatic phenothiazines (e.g. chlorpromazine) have less antiemetic effect. Metoclopramide is of some value, and its effect may be increased by giving it in high dosage. Benzodiazepines enable the patient to sleep during the period of maximum nausea. $5HT_3$ receptor antagonists have been a big advance in controlling nausea and vomiting.

Mucosal ulceration in the mouth and gut is a complication of chemotherapy which is particularly likely to occur following methotrexate and anthracyclines. It is dose related, but some individuals are especially susceptible and the dose may then need to be lower than usual. Alopecia is

very common with many drugs, especially doxorubicin and cyclophosphamide, and is due to damage to the proliferating cells of the hair follicle. Although the hair regrows when treatment is finally stopped, many patients find this a distressing side effect. With anthracycline, the hair loss can be minimised by scalp cooling during drug administration. The patient must be warned of the likelihood of hair loss, and a wig ordered if desired.

Bone marrow depression results in acute leucopenia and thrombocytopenia and the slower onset of anaemia (because of the greater lifespan of red cells). The nadir of the leucocyte count often comes at 7–9 days after intravenous chemotherapy and it is at this time that the patient is most susceptible to serious infection. Increasingly, oncologists are adjusting the dosage in each cycle of very myelosuppressive regimens according to nadir counts, even though this involves an extra blood count between visits. Patients must be forewarned of their susceptibility to infection and bleeding, so that they can report symptoms promptly.

Long-term

The long-term sequels of cancer chemotherapy are now becoming better defined as more children and adults are surviving previously incurable cancers. One in 1000 adults now has been cured of cancer in childhood or adolescence. While complications may be an inevitable risk of regimens that are potentially curative, they are a reminder of the risks attached to increasing the intensity of treatment.

Cytotoxic drugs impair fertility in adults. In men, complete and irreversible loss of fertility occurs with many regimens, particularly those which include an alkylating agent or procarbazine. Prepubertal boys do not become infertile, but Leydig cell function may be impaired and testosterone levels may fall. It is important to inform men of this risk and to arrange sperm storage before chemotherapy begins. Curiously, in Hodgkin's disease, where there is greatest experience of this problem, patients are often subfertile even before chemotherapy begins. For women, the problem is more complex. Amenorrhoea is common during chemotherapy, especially if an alkylating agent is used. Menstruation will usually return when treat-

Summary 2 Complications of chemotherapy

Immediate	Long-term
Nausea and vomiting	Impairment of fertility
Mucosal ulceration	Secondary cancers
Bone marrow depression	Pulmonary fibrosis
Alopecia	Cardiomyopathy
	Nerve damage
	Loss of hearing
	Renal impairment

ment is finished, although subfertility is common. Chemotherapy may, however, induce the onset of menopause and this is more likely to occur in older women who are nearer the natural menopause. In both sexes, patients who are receiving chemotherapy should be advised of possible short-term teratogenic effects and to use a contraceptive during treatment.

Second cancers are increasingly recognised as a long-term consequence of chemotherapy, particularly in ovarian cancer or Hodgkin's disease. In both cases, the risk is especially of acute myelomonocytic leukaemia. Second cancers are also more common in patients receiving immunosuppressive therapy with cytotoxic drugs, and in these patients there is an increased incidence of brain lymphoma, cervical carcinoma and skin cancer.

Pulmonary fibrosis is a complication of treatment with busulphan (e.g. for chronic myeloid leukaemia), and acute pneumonitis leading to fibrosis is a dose-related complication of bleomycin. Other cytotoxic agents rarely produce lung damage, although pulmonary fibrosis is a long-term complication of cyclophosphamide and nitrosoureas treatment.

Anthracyclines such as doxorubicin cause a cardiomyopathy, the risk being dose related. Above a total dose of 400 mg/m^2 about 50% of patients will have measurable impairment of cardiac function, but only 5% will develop cardiac symptoms. Established cardiomyopathy leads to cardiac failure which is irreversible on stopping the drug.

Vinca alkaloids cause damage to peripheral and autonomic nerves. The earliest symptoms are of tingling paraesthesiae. There is loss of tendon reflexes and, later, sensory loss and motor weakness. Autonomic neuropathy produces ileus and postural hypotension. Vincristine and vindesine are particularly likely to produce neuropathy, and vinblastine less so. The neuropathy is usually reversible, is total-dose related and more common and severe in the elderly. Cisplatin may cause irreversible loss of hearing, particularly of high frequencies, and peripheral neuropathy. Renal impairment is also common and irreversible.

These toxic effects are a reminder that the treatment of cancer with cytotoxic drugs is a matter requiring skill and judgement if the benefits are not to be outweighed by the disadvantages. Nevertheless, the improvement in prognosis in some cancers as a result of cytotoxic drug treatment fully justifies the acute and long-term risks involved.

Hormone therapy

The growth of many normal tissues is under hormonal regulation, and the cancers which arise in them often retain sensitivity to changes in the hormone environment. Hormone therapy is an essential part of management of cancers of the prostate, breast and endometrium. In these cases, the steroid hormone binds to a hormone binding molecule (*receptor*) in the cytoplasm and the receptor/hormone complex is transported to the nucleus where it modifies the activity of DNA. There is an increase in RNA polymerase activity, resulting in increasing production of cytoplasmic proteins followed by cell division (Fig. 8.16). In some cases, the hormone provokes the increased synthesis of receptors for other hormones; oestrogen, for example, increases the synthesis of progesterone receptor in breast epithelium.

It has been found that the likelihood of response to hormone therapy is strongly associated with the presence of cytoplasmic receptors. In breast cancer, the presence of oestrogen receptors is associated with a 60% likelihood of response to hormone manipulation, with only a 5% chance of response if the cancer contains very low levels of receptor. The likelihood of response is even more strongly associated with progesterone receptor status.

The following general approaches are taken in hormone-sensitive tumours.

Blocking the action of circulating hormones

In breast cancer, the use of tamoxifen has been a major advance. It appears to exert most of its effect by binding to the oestrogen receptor, thereby preventing the activity

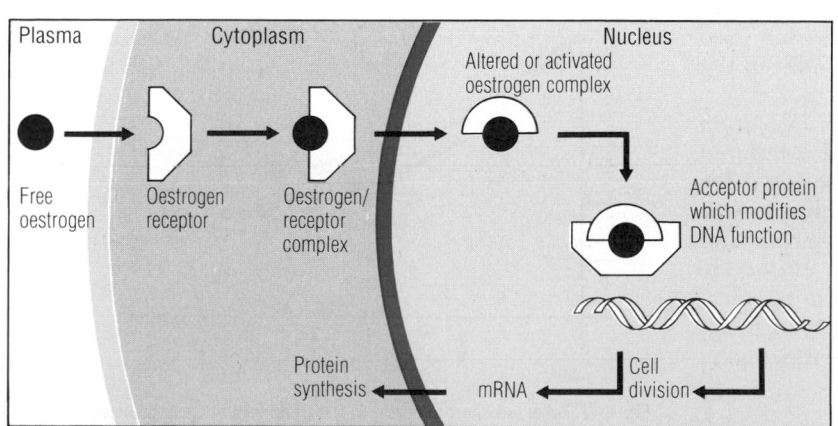

Fig. 8.16 Diagrammatic representation of mechanism of oestrogen action on cell growth. Tamoxifen acts by binding to the oestrogen receptor and blocking its action.

of circulating oestradiol. Paradoxically, the drug is effective in postmenopausal women whose tumours are receptor-positive, but in whom circulating levels of oestrogen are likely to be low. A direct growth regulatory effect of the drug may be responsible.

Reduction in concentration of circulating hormones

Until recently, this was the mainstay of hormone therapy and was usually accomplished surgically. In breast cancer, oophorectomy was performed, or a radiation menopause induced in premenopausal women. In those who showed an initial response, but then relapsed, further responses could be obtained by adrenalectomy, which prevented sex hormone synthesis in the adrenal, and by hypophysectomy which produced a similar effect.

The advent of aminoglutethimide has led to a decline in frequency of these operations. This drug blocks the formation of pregnenolone in the adrenal, which diminishes the production of cortisol and androstanedione. Androstanedione is converted in peripheral tissues (and in the breast itself) to oestradiol by enzymes known as aromatases, and aminoglutethimide is a powerful aromatase inhibitor thus preventing oestradiol formation. In prostate cancer luteinising-hormone releasing hormone (LHRH) agonists cause a spurt of LH release followed by a profound fall, which reduces plasma testosterone levels to those seen after castration. Prostatic cancer is usually very sensitive to a fall in testosterone levels. LHRH agonists are a medical alternative to orchidectomy.

Addition of hormones

The hormonal environment can be altered by administration of hormones which are judged to provide an unfavourable environment for the tumour. Stilboestrol has, for many years, been used to produce regression in carcinoma of the prostate; while androgens, glucocorticoids and progestogens may all slow the growth of the tumour in breast cancer. Progesterone derivatives will also produce regressions in about 20% of carcinomas of the endometrium.

In breast cancer, endocrine therapy has the great advantage of low toxicity and low cost when compared with chemotherapy. Tumour responses are often more complete and more durable than those achieved with cytotoxic drugs. On the other hand, the proportion of responding patients is lower (30% with endocrine therapy, 60% with chemotherapy). For these reasons, many physicians prefer to start treatment with hormone manipulation, moving to chemotherapy when the disease becomes unresponsive and progresses.

Adjuvant chemotherapy and hormone therapy

There are many situations in which a cancer has been removed surgically or treated with radiotherapy, but the risk of local or systemic recurrence is high. Examples include: breast cancer, where there is involvement of axillary nodes; gastric and other cancers, where the regional nodes are involved; or Ewing's sarcoma of bone, where the tumour is highly sensitive to radiotherapy but the risk of metastasis is very great. In these situations, advances have been made by the use of cytotoxic drugs or hormones in an attempt to delay or prevent recurrence. Even if these treatments are not very effective against advanced cancer (of the stomach or breast), they may be more so when the residual tumour mass is small, when the penetration of the drugs may be better and the degree of cell kill may lead to cure rather than temporary tumour regression.

In recent years, many large-scale trials have been undertaken to assess the value of adjuvant cytotoxic or endocrine therapy. For the results to be accepted with confidence, there must be both sufficient numbers of patients in the study, and prospective randomisation of the allocation of the treatment policy. (The difficulties involved in these trials are discussed below.)

In patients with stage II breast cancer, both adjuvant endocrine therapy (using tamoxifen) and cytotoxic therapy (using drug combinations such as cyclophosphamide, methotrexate and 5-fluorouracil) have been shown to give a survival advantage of about 7% at five years and 10% at 10 years (Fig. 8.17).

Adjuvant drug therapy after surgery or irradiation has become an essential part of management in most childhood tumours (rhabdomyosarcoma, Wilm's tumour, osteosarcoma, Ewing's sarcoma), and in a number of adult tumours, such as some stages of breast cancer and ovarian cancer. There are many other tumours (gliomas, gastric carcinoma, colorectal carcinoma, operable lung cancer) in which adjuvant chemotherapy has not yet been

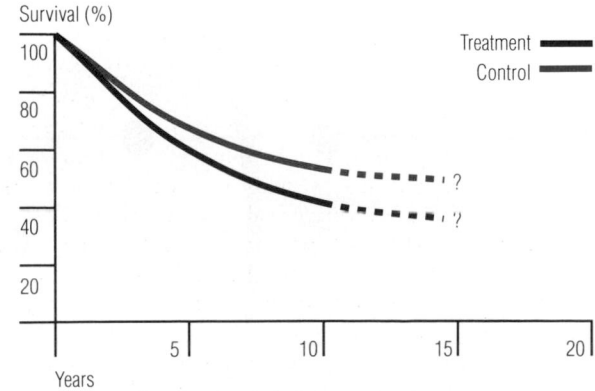

Fig. 8.17 Adjuvant chemotherapy in the treatment of breast cancer.

adequately evaluated. Since the survival benefit is likely to be small, it will only be demonstrated in very large-scale trials, which are still to be undertaken. Even a 5% improvement in survival in colorectal cancer would be worthwhile since the disease affects 1 million people a year in Eastern and Western Europe.

SUPPORTIVE CARE IN CANCER MANAGEMENT

Patients with cancer need supportive care for both the psychological impact of the disease and the physical effects of the tumour and its management. Even if there is no prospect of cure, the quality of life of the patient can be greatly improved by the attitude of the medical staff and by meticulous attention to the management of pain, anaemia, infection, nausea and anorexia.

Psychological support

The last 20 years have seen an increasing readiness, on the part of doctors, to discuss the diagnosis of cancer with their patients and to explain the principles of management. Indeed, the complexities of modern cancer management make it difficult to withhold the facts of the diagnosis, even if it were desirable to do so. Nevertheless, the manner in which the diagnosis is explained and the words used is of great importance, and must be carefully judged in each case. Cancer is the only word which conveys the nature of the complaint accurately, other words used are often misinterpreted by patients as implying a less, or even more, serious condition. The problem is that in the mind of many patients, cancer is an invariably fatal disease. Explanation of the diagnosis must, therefore, be accompanied by an unhurried and easily comprehended account of management and the possibilities of cure. It is nearly always wrong to offer no hope of either cure or a period of normal life. Usually, the physician will need to talk to the patient on several occasions, since the patient's understanding of the problems may be incomplete at the beginning. Time taken in unhurried, private conversation is always well spent and greatly appreciated. One of the advantages of having specialised oncology units in hospitals is that all members of the medical team – nurses, doctors, social workers and counsellors – become familiar with the problems that are associated with malignant disease and skilful in dealing with them. It is important that all members of this team know what has been said to the patient in the way of explanation, in order to avoid conflicting advice.

A relapse of the disease or the appearance of a new symptom will often cause a slump in morale and confidence which will require more explanation and reassur-ance. The emotional demands of this aspect of cancer medicine are considerable and are one reason why some doctors are reluctant to spend time in discussion with their patients.

Pain relief

This is a very important aspect of management, particularly in patients with widespread disease who are terminally ill. No single analgesic will suit all patients all of the time. A patient will need to change from one to another depending on the severity of pain. A brief classification of some of the most useful analgesics is given in Table 8.12. When using opiates, the dosage should be adjusted to the patient's requirements. A wide range of dosage is encountered. Long-acting morphine and heroin are especially useful and should be given regularly rather than 'as required'. The constipating effects of opiates can be partly relieved by regular laxatives.

If pain is at a particular site, it may be possible to give relief by local measures, such as radiotherapy to a bone metastasis, a nerve block or a coeliac plexus block. The advice of colleagues specialising in these forms of pain relief is often helpful, and the procedures may allow a reduction in dosage of opiate.

Nutritional support

Patients lose weight because of the local effects of the tumour (especially if this is in the alimentary tract),

Table 8.12 Useful analgesics

Drugs	Duration of action (hours)
Mild analgesics	
Aspirin	4–6
Paracetamol	2–4
Indole derivatives (e.g. indomethacin)	6–8
Proprionic acid derivatives (e.g. ibuprofen)	4–6
Moderate analgesics	
Codeine (and dihydrocodeine)	4–6
Pentazocine	3–4
Dipipanone	6
Oxycodone	8
Strong analgesics	
Morphine sulphate	4–6 (up to 12 with sustained release forms)
Diamorphine	4–6
Dextromoramide	4–6
Pethidine	3
Methadone	12–30

metastases and as a result of treatment. Successful treatment of the primary tumour (e.g. by surgery) will be accompanied by a return of appetite and weight gain. During radical treatment with surgery, radiotherapy and intensive chemotherapy, weight loss is common.

Calorie supplements can be given to patients undergoing cancer treatment both in the form of oral supplements and intravenously. However, the value of nutritional support is difficult to demonstrate. It is usual practice to consider total parenteral (intravenous) nutrition in patients undergoing exceptionally intensive treatment, such as high-dose chemotherapy or total-body irradiation with bone marrow transplantation, or during the intensive phases of chemotherapy for acute leukaemia, where there is prolonged hypoplasia. At these times, mucosal ulceration, nausea and diarrhoea make it difficult to feed the patient by mouth, and nasogastric tubes may produce monilial infection or exacerbate acid reflux and oesophagitis. Parenteral nutrition is also used for patients undergoing extensive surgery, particularly gut resection. The aim is to maintain the patient's weight and nutritional status so that recovery is more rapid, allowing further treatment with chemotherapy or irradiation to begin as soon as possible. There is no evidence that additional enteral or parenteral feeding is of value in the management of advanced cancer where cure is impossible. It is, however, important to encourage the patient to eat by giving food which appeals (often in the form of smaller more frequent meals), by controlling nausea with drugs such as metoclopramide, and by the careful use of corticosteroids which improve well-being and stimulate the patient's appetite.

Tumour lysis syndrome

In some very sensitive untreated cancers, chemotherapy may produce massive tumour breakdown when treatment is first given. This process may be accompanied by severe metabolic disturbances which constitute the *tumour lysis syndrome*. The syndrome is usually associated with the early phases of treatment of lymphoma and leukaemia in children and, less frequently, in other chemosensitive childhood tumours. In adults, the syndrome is infrequent but may occur with treatment of lymphoma, especially if there is impairment of renal function (such as ureteric obstruction by lymph nodes) which diminishes renal excretion of the tumour products.

Tissue destruction releases large amounts of urate, phosphate and potassium. The urate may be deposited in the renal tubule causing reversible renal failure which, in turn, diminishes further urate excretion. Severe hyperuricaemia and renal failure may necessitate dialysis. This complication can largely be avoided by using the xanthine oxidase inhibitor allopurinol (100–200 mg eight-hourly) before and during the early phase of treatment, and by

establishing and maintaining a diuresis during the first 24–48 hours. Hyperkalaemia may be severe, particularly if renal failure occurs, and may need treatment with glucose and insulin (see Ch. 19). Hyperphosphataemia can be partly prevented by hydration and diuresis before and during the initial treatment.

NEW APPROACHES TO MANAGEMENT

Progress in cancer treatment is slow, and results usually improve after many small refinements in therapy rather than by sudden steps forward. Since the late 1970s, only modest progress has been made and the search for new drugs and new approaches continues.

High-dose therapy and bone marrow transplantation

Allogeneic (from one individual to another) bone marrow transplantation was introduced for the treatment of acute myeloblastic leukaemia in the early 1970s. Allogeneic marrow was infused after an attempt had been made to eradicate the leukaemia by total-body irradiation and high-dose cyclophosphamide. The results (Ch. 24) showed that the leukaemia might be eradicated. This finding led to the consideration of total-body irradiation in the management of other disorders, such as lymphomas and myeloma. More recently, attempts have been made to eradicate leukaemia, lymphoma and some solid tumours with very high-dose chemotherapy (rather than total-body irradiation) using *autologous* (taken from, and re-infused into, the same individual) bone marrow, harvested just before treatment, as a means of preventing life-threatening myelosuppression. These approaches are based on the assumption that increasing doses of chemotherapy will eradicate residual disease when multiple conventional doses will fail. Uncontrolled trials show promising survival rates, but, as yet autologous bone marrow transplantation remains an unproven method of management in any tumour.

Half-body irradiation

Stimulated by the effects produced by a single fraction of whole-body irradiation in the eradication of leukaemia, radiotherapists have begun to explore the use of a single fraction of irradiation given first to one half of the body and then the other, allowing time for bone marrow recovery between treatments. Significant responses can be seen in radiosensitive tumours such as lymphoma or myeloma, and palliation of pain from widespread bone metastases can be achieved in diseases such as carcinoma of the prostate. There is much more to be discovered about the use of radiation as a 'systemic' treatment of cancer.

Monoclonal antibodies to cell surface antigens

There is little evidence that human tumours express unique antigens, but many tumours appear to express oncofetal or differentiation antigens not usually found in the normal tissue from which the cancer is derived. An example is the common acute lymphoblastic leukaemia antigen (CALLA) found on the surface of both acute lymphoblastic leukaemia cells and normal lymphatic progenitor cells. The development of monoclonal antibodies of defined specificity has resulted in the production of monoclonal reagents, which bind preferentially to antigens on the surface of some tumour cells (and to those normal cells which express the antigen). Cytotoxic drugs, cell poisons such as ricin or abrin, and radioactive isotopes can be attached to such antibodies in the hope of selectively destroying the tumour. There are considerable difficulties with this approach – heterogeneity of antigen expression within the tumour; variable uptake and distribution of antibody in normal and malignant tissue; and the production of antibodies by the patient against the foreign (usually mouse) protein. Nevertheless, there are interesting future possibilities for therapy and tumour localisation using this approach.

TRIALS OF TREATMENT

Many cancers have a long and unpredictable natural history: cancer of the breast, for example, is associated with an excess mortality for over 25 years after diagnosis. If survival is the endpoint of treatment then assessment of therapy in this disease will mean prolonged periods of observation. In small cell lung cancer or acute myeloblastic leukaemia, on the other hand, a majority of patients are dead within two years, and relapse in those that survive is less frequent beyond that point. Treatment trials will therefore give answers quickly. In assessment of therapy of a cancer (such as breast cancer), there may be more than one endpoint to be considered: does the treatment give effective local control; does the treatment influence the onset of metastasis; is the proportion of survivors at five and 10 years or longer increased?

Comparison of a treatment with historical controls is very unreliable, since diagnostic and staging criteria are changing constantly and selection of cases is thereby altered. Randomised, prospective, studies are now regarded as the only reliable way of making a comparison between two treatments. Such studies must include sufficient numbers of patients to allow the questions to be answered with confidence statistically. The studies require careful documentation and prolonged observation of the patient groups. The treatments being compared must be justifiable ethically and the design of the study capable of giving a clear answer to the central question.

These considerations mean that treatment trials in cancer are complex and usually demand collaboration between many different centres; even, in the case of rare tumours, between different countries. To detect a 5% difference in survival with confidence, may require many hundreds or even thousands of patients in a study. Nevertheless, a 5% difference in long-term survival in breast cancer, if achieved by a non-toxic hormonal means, would mean 1000 lives saved a year in the UK alone – greater than the number of patients cured of Hodgkin's disease. However, a 5% difference achieved by means of toxic chemotherapy might be regarded with less enthusiasm. At present, because progress in cancer management is slow and achieved only by small improvements, large-scale clinical trials are the only reliable way of validating new treatments.

CARE OF THE DYING

Many patients with cancer die from their disease, and it is the responsibility of the oncologist to be sure that aggressive management of the tumour is not thoughtlessly continued beyond the point at which cure is possible. This does not mean that treatment is discontinued but that the aim of management becomes palliative rather than curative. Palliative treatment can often, in skilled hands, give the patient a period of happy life free from distressing symptoms. Palliation may require radiotherapy, e.g. for painful bone metastases or bronchial obstruction; chemotherapy at low dose to suppress constitutional symptoms in lymphoma; aspiration of ascites or pleural effusion; or surgical pinning of a bone weakened by metastasis. There is more to palliative management than pain relief. Nevertheless, relief of pain, control of nausea and treatment of depression become increasingly important as the disease progresses.

The most important component of management at this stage is the psychological support of the patient and his or her family. Support comes from the nature of the relationship that the patient has established with the medical team throughout the illness. Extra help may be needed from domiciliary nursing teams, which are increasingly providing expert and readily available advice on symptom control to patients in their own homes. Many patients prefer to remain at home in the last few weeks of life, and the family doctor and specialist nurses can often make this possible. Alternatively, the patient's wishes or family circumstances may make admission to a hospital or hospice necessary. The nursing practices and the approach to symptom control that have been developed in hospices are now being incorporated into hospital practice. In some hospitals, nurse specialists have been appointed to advise on these aspects of management.

The gradual awareness of death produces many different reactions. The patient may become angry and direct this at the medical or nursing staff. Feelings of apathy, hopelessness and fatigue are common, and depression may be severe enough to need treatment with antidepressants. The support of relatives and friends is essential.

Meticulous attention to detail and a willingness to take time to talk to the patient are just as important at this stage in management as during the early stages when the intention may have been curative. Even though management has finally failed, this does not mean it was not worthwhile, nor is it a reflection on the abilities of the medical or nursing staff. The fact of treatment failure leads some doctors to avoid seeing their patients at this stage. This is bad practice and increases the patient's feeling of isolation and helplessness.

Many non-medical agencies are able to help the patient and his or her family. Patients with religious beliefs may gain great comfort from their clergyman and other members of their local religious community. Counselling and support groups have been set up in many towns to provide help during the illness and to the bereaved relatives afterwards.

ALTERNATIVE THERAPY

A multitude of unorthodox approaches to management of cancer have been offered to patients over the years. These usually have echoes of current medical practice. Serotherapy was used after antitoxins were introduced for infectious disease; tooth extraction was practised, based on the interwar notions that dental sepsis was responsible for chronic inflammation. Nowadays, psychological ideas are translated into visualisation therapy, and concern over pollution and diet are transmuted into strict vegetarian or fat-free diets. The uncritical assumption that answers will be found in nature has led to a wide range of herbal remedies some of which (e.g. laetrile) are somewhat dangerous. As with many chronic diseases, the practitioners of homeopathy and faith healing offer their remedies.

Most of these approaches share certain recognisable characteristics. These include a tendency to borrow the jargon of medicine without its science; a belief that all tumours can be treated by the same or similar remedies; a tacit or explicit assumption that there exists a medical conspiracy to conceal the truth about the remedy in question; and a complete failure to adopt any of the proven methods of validation of the results of treatment.

What these approaches offer distressed and anxious patients is a feeling that they can themselves do something to combat their disease, a glimmer of hope that they might be cured, and relief from the side-effects of conventional treatment if this is abandoned. These benefits are often a reflection of inadequacy in the relationship of the patient and doctor, rather than a clearly held view by the patient and family. The damaging aspects of these approaches are that they may induce the patient to abandon a worthwhile treatment, weaken the relationship between doctor and patient, and impose unpleasant constraints on the patient's life, such as rigid dietary control. These disadvantages should be discussed with the patient and, if patients are thinking of abandoning a potentially curative treatment, every attempt should be made to persuade them not to do so. Nevertheless, the doctor's role in management is to offer help, advice and expertise; the patient has the right to choose what to do. In many cases, no great harm will be done and an experienced doctor will make it clear that the patient is welcome to continue under his or her care in the future.

FURTHER READING

Cancer Surveys 1986 Hormones and cancer. Vol 5, No 3. Oxford University Press, Oxford. *One of a series of reviews of cancer topics.*

DeVita V T, Hellman S, Rosenberg S 1989 Cancer: principles and practice of oncology, 3rd edn. Lippincott, Philadelphia. *A comprehensive cancer textbook.*

Easson E C, Pointon R C S 1985 The radiotherapy of malignant disease. Springer-Verlag, Berlin. *A textbook of radiation treatment.*

Peckham M, Pinedo H, Veronesi V 1994 Oxford Textbook of Oncology. Blackwell, Oxford. *A comprehensive textbook of oncology*

Saunders C M 1985 The management of terminal malignant disease 2nd edn. Edward Arnold, London. *An excellent account.*

Souhami R L, Tobias J S 1994 Cancer and its management 2nd edn. Blackwell, Oxford. *A medium-sized text covering most aspects of cancer treatment.*

9

Ageing and Disease

Peter W Overstall

Most ill health in developed countries now occurs in elderly persons. Not only are the elderly more prone to illness, but the proportion of elderly people has increased considerably this century. The response of an individual to growing old depends more upon the previous pattern of life than upon anything in the ageing process itself, so that one of the features of old age is increased differences between individuals.

Life expectancy

Life expectancy is the average observed years of life from birth or from any stated age. Since 1900, life expectancy

at birth in the UK has increased from 49 to 73 years for men and from 52 to 78 years for women (Fig. 9.1, see also Ch. 1, p. 13). This is mainly the result of reductions in infant mortality from the major infectious diseases. Tuberculosis, acute rheumatic fever, smallpox, diphtheria, tetanus and poliomyelitis now account for less than 2% of the ill health they caused in 1900. These changes are largely due to improvements in nutrition and to public health measures which have reduced water- and food-borne diseases. The influence of immunisation and treatment on mortality is comparatively much smaller.

Changes in the elderly population

The age structure of a population is affected by infant mortality and by fertility rates, late-age mortality and migration. Demographic ageing, i.e. a shift towards a larger proportion of elderly people in the population, began in Europe in the early 20th century, as a result of falling fertility. This change has already occurred in the UK so that during the 1990s the projected increase in the population aged 60 years or more will be only 0.08% per year. After 2001, the cohort of the post-1945 'baby boom' reach retirement and there will then be a further rise (see Table 9.1). The proportion of elderly in the

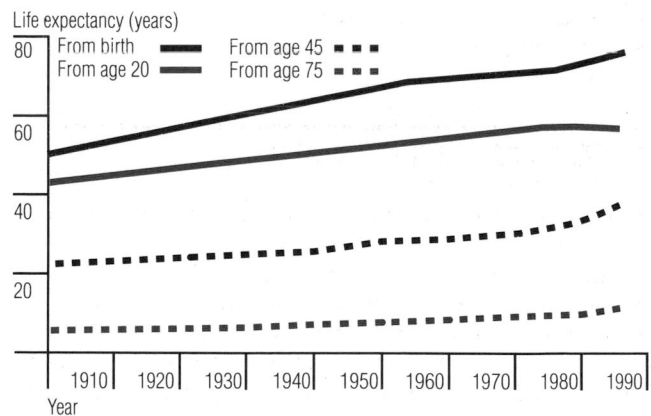

Fig. 9.1 Changes in life expectancy this century. Most of the increase in life expectancy at birth results from reductions in infant mortality rather than an extension of the natural lifespan.

Table 9.1 Projected growth in the elderly population in developed countries, 1990–2025

Country	%
UK	25
Italy	40
France	60
USA	100
Japan	136
Canada	200

9 Ageing and Disease

Table 9.2 Projected increase in the elderly (over 60) population in major world regions

| | Proportion of total population % | | | No. (m) |
	1950	2000	2025	2000
Africa	5.0	5.0	6.6	42.8
S. America	5.4	7.3	10.8	41.0
N. America	12.1	15.0	22.3	44.3
E. Asia	7.5	11.5	19.6	168.8
S. Asia	7.6	6.4	10.9	133.4
Europe	12.9	19.9	24.7	101.6
USSR	9.0	17.5	20.1	54.4
Oceania	11.3	12.5	17.8	3.7

population will not increase thereafter unless there are further substantial falls in both fertility and late-age mortality.

Fertility rates are declining worldwide and we can anticipate the most rapid changes in age structure of the population to be in the developing world. At present only half the world's elderly population live in developing areas but by the end of the century this will have increased to 61%. Between 1980 and 2000, the world's elderly population will increase by 66%, ranging from 100% in central America to 2.7% in northern Europe. By 2025, 14% of the world's population will be aged over 60 with 71% of these 1135 million people living in developing countries and fewer than 12% in Europe (Table 9.2).

One factor contributing to the current increase in the number of very old people is the decline in late-life mortality. Between 1961 and 1986 in England and Wales, mortality after the age of 65 years declined by around 20% for men and 25% for women.

THEORIES OF AGEING

Ageing is a complex process resulting from intrinsic and extrinsic damage to the organism at a rate dependent on each particular individual's genetic background and environment. The resulting disability is not fixed or inevitable. For example, high tone deafness and high blood pressure are common in elderly Britons, but are absent among elderly persons in the Easter Islands. Osteoporosis is common in western Europe and the USA but rare in China. Thus descriptions of physical decline are too variable to be useful for defining ageing. A better approach, which allows populations to be compared and so highlights differences in environmental or intrinsic ageing factors, is to define ageing as a process which brings about an ever-increasing age-specific mortality (i.e. the older the individual becomes the more likely he/she is to die). In the UK, mortality is at its lowest around puberty and ageing can be said to begin at this point, rising progressively throughout adult life.

There is general agreement that ageing is, at least in part, genetically determined. Each animal species has a specific lifespan: the maximum recorded longevity of Marion's tortoise, for example, is over 152 years, for man approximately 115 years and for golden hamsters two or three years. In species of *Drosophila*, the F1 hybrid has a greater longevity than either parental strain. Female sex also generally confers increased longevity in a number of different species. Individuals whose parents live to the age of 75 years or more live longer than those whose parents died before the age of 60. The mean difference in longevity in dizygotic twins is twice that of monozygotes.

Current theory sees the ageing process as non-adaptive, with ageing evolving as a late by-product of processes which benefit the individual during its earlier, more fecund lifespan. With limited energy resources, an organism has to strike the right balance between investing in bodily maintenance and repair, and producing and rearing its young.

SOCIOLOGICAL ASPECTS

Retirement age is an administrative measure without relation to the capacity of individuals. Most people, at retirement, can expect good health for several years, and for developed countries the World Health Organisation has introduced a new demographic indicator of 'life expectancy without incapacity'. At age 65 this is estimated to be between eight and 11 years for men and between nine and 12 years for women. Nonetheless, medical costs are four times greater in the first decade of retirement than during working life and by the second decade of retirement they are nine times as great.

Attitudes to the elderly

In Europe the falling birth rate, increased longevity and trend to early retirement has reduced the worker–

Summary 1 Epidemiology of ageing

- In the UK, the increase in life expectancy at birth seen in the early part of this century was largely due to a decrease in infant mortality.

- The rising percentage of elderly in the population is due to falling fertility and lower mortality rates, particularly in the very old.

- During the 1990s there will be a pause in the growth of the elderly population in the UK. This is expected to rise again in 2001.

- In some developing countries, the increase in the elderly population over the next 10 years may be as much as 100%.

pensioner ratio. Between 1961 and 1981 the number of people aged over 65 increased by a third in the UK without causing economic strain or intergenerational strife.

Discrimination against elderly people springs from three main impulses: a fear of death and dying, a social belief that falsely associates success with productivity, and misconceptions about the inevitability of senility. There is, in fact, little or no sign of a significant decline in happiness or life satisfaction with age. Over 80% of elderly people maintain independent households, three-quarters of those over 85 can wash all over unaided, 95% can go to the WC alone and only 5% of people over 75 have significant dementia. It is true that institutionalisation rates for the very old have increased considerably in the last 30 years due to a decline in the amount of family support available to the elderly. Women aged between 45 and 60 have carried the brunt of community care, and since the start of the century when there were 83 women in this age group for every 100 people over 65, there are now only 45. Nonetheless families do still care for their elderly relatives and indeed provide far more support than is available from health or social services.

Retirement

Retirement is now a well established part of life in developed countries and is starting to appear in developing countries among government employees and urban workers. Most people no longer see it as a traumatic event marked by major losses to the individual but instead prepare for it as a normal and expected part of the life cycle and welcome it as a time of opportunity and increased leisure. The rate of early retirement is, therefore, rising. Over the past 20 years the proportion of men aged 55 to 64 in full employment has fallen in the UK from 87% to 57%, in Germany from 81% to 51% and in France from 74% to 47%. Of course, not all of these early retirements are voluntary and there has been a noticeable trend for businesses in economic difficulties to make their older rather than their younger workers redundant.

The period of active retirement, in which many take up part-time or voluntary work, ends when the person becomes disabled by declining physical or mental ill health. The difference between these two stages of old age depends on functional capacity, not on chronological age.

Some people do find that retirement produces troublesome stresses. The most frequent problem is adjustment to a lower level of income. Some suffer from a loss of self-esteem, others fear onset of ill health or are distressed by their idleness. Most of these problems fade as the new pattern of activity is taken up and serious depression is not a particular feature of retirement.

Claims of large numbers of super-centenarians living in certain geographical regions – such as Vilcabamba in Ecuador, Hunza in Pakistan and Abkhasia in Georgia

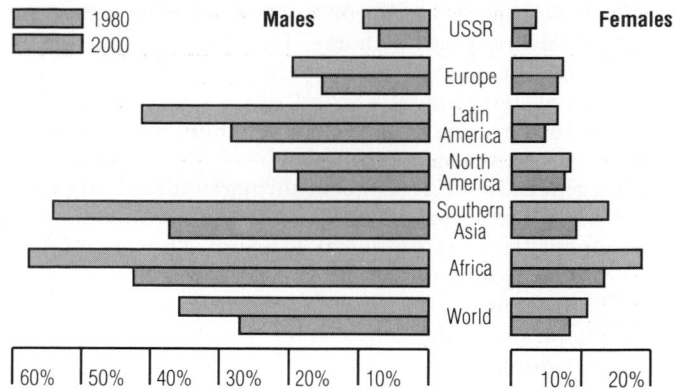

Fig. 9.2 Percentage of the population aged 65 years and over that is economically active worldwide. The developed countries have still to find a satisfactory role for their unemployed elderly.

have been shown to be exaggerated. However, it is true that the inhabitants of each of the above areas are relatively long-lived, and in each case the esteem and merit enjoyed by a person increases with age. There is no retirement age and old persons continue to play an active role in the economic and social life of their communities (Fig. 9.2).

SPECIAL FEATURES OF DISEASE IN OLD AGE

Measurement of physiological functions in healthy young adults gives fairly uniform results, with a narrow range between the upper and lower limits of normal. From about 30 years of age, a functional decline in performance can be detected in most organs and body systems (Fig. 9.3). However, the organs and systems age differ-

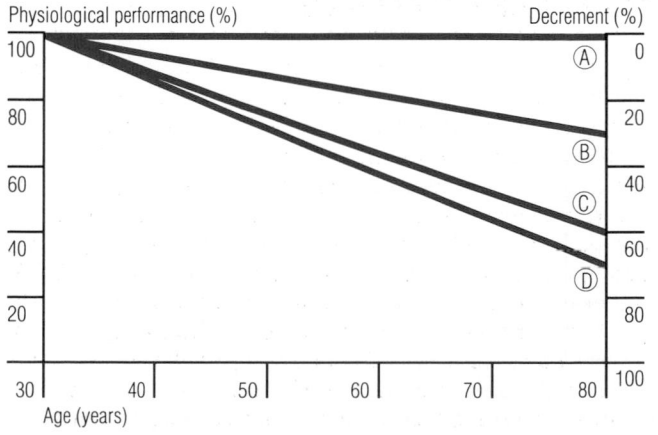

Fig. 9.3 Age decrements in physiological functions in males. A. Fasting blood glucose; **B.** Resting cardiac index; **C.** Maximum breathing capacity; **D.** Maximum work rate.

entially so that the variation both within, and between, individuals increases with age. The chronological age of an old person may therefore bear little relation to their functional age (Fig. 9.4), and the response of an old person to the stress of illness will be more unpredictable than that of a young adult.

Degenerative changes occur throughout the body with increasing age, but these may become sufficiently marked to constitute a pathological process. The distinction between this and normal physiological ageing is often difficult to make. These changes have an important bearing on the management of the patient, as will be seen in the examples that follow.

The ageing eye

The force required to focus the eye increases considerably at about 40 years of age and, by 45 or 50, accommodation will be so poor that for most persons small print can be read only at arm's length (*presbyopia*). This is a result of both a reduction in elasticity of the lens capsule, and also a thickening of the lens which prevents it adapting its shape to focus on near objects. Whether the change is regarded as pathological or physiological is unimportant, since the defect can be readily corrected with spectacles.

The ageing ear

Impaired hearing increases with age and can contribute to poor health, social isolation, depression and (probably) paranoid psychosis. About 30% of the elderly regard themselves as having a hearing impairment but audiometric testing reveals a much higher prevalence (60%) in those aged over 70. *Presbyacusis* is age-related loss of high frequency hearing, but this cannot be reliably distinguished from the effect of ototoxic drugs, diuretics or

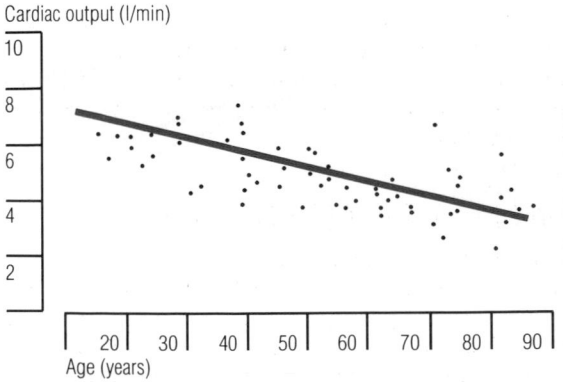

Fig. 9.4 The relation between resting cardiac output and age in men without circulatory disorders. Note that several men over the age of 70 have values similar to men in their 30s.

vascular disorders. Some of the hearing loss usually regarded as an inevitable part of old age may be due to our noisy environment or hypertension.

Osteoporosis

Bone loss from the skeleton begins around 35 years of age and can, when sufficiently advanced, be detected on X-ray by a loss of density of the bone and thinning of the cortex of the long bones. For the majority of elderly persons, this age-related osteoporosis is asymptomatic, but a minority suffer 'accelerated' osteoporosis and will develop fractures. The causes of this pathological osteoporosis are not well understood but it appears to be related to a number of factors, particularly the skeletal status at maturity, the rapid bone loss occurring after the menopause, hyperadrenocorticism and immobility. Oestrogen supplements provide partial protection against postmenopausal bone loss. However, because only 25% of women will have suffered one of the common osteoporotic fractures (distal forearm, vertebral compression or femoral neck) by the age of 80, it is difficult to decide whether or not to treat all women with oestrogens, given the inability to predict at the menopause who will develop accelerated osteoporosis later.

Dementia and normal ageing

Cross-sectional studies consistently demonstrate a decline in cognitive function with increasing age. Differences in educational levels between populations can confound age-associated changes. A decline of cognitive ability is not confined to old age and tests which measure the ability to solve novel problems rapidly (fluid intelligence) show a fall in performance by the late third and early fourth decades. Age-related changes in cognitive function appear to be related to a general decline in the speed at which information is processed. Thus, highly practised skills, such as vocabulary test scores, alter very little with age but timed novel problem solving, reaction time tests and ability to learn new material decline with increasing age. Ill health undoubtedly affects cognitive performance, particularly anything interfering with cerebral oxygenation such as cardiovascular disease and chronic obstructive pulmonary disease.

The major cause of intellectual loss in old age is senile dementia of the Alzheimer's type (SDAT). Characteristic pathological findings – neurofibrillary tangles, senile plaques and lipofuscin pigment in the brain – also occur, albeit to a much less extent, in very old persons, but it is probable that SDAT is a distinct entity rather than a mere exaggeration of normal ageing. The early stages of dementia in a patient with SDAT are often difficult to distinguish from the simple forgetfulness of old age.

Impairment of biochemical homeostasis

Most normal old persons can, under resting conditions, maintain their internal environment at levels similar to those in the young. When stressed, however, it is apparent that homeostatic mechanisms in the elderly are impaired. Blood glucose control and osmoregulation are two good examples of this.

The control of blood glucose

The average fasting blood glucose level increases only slightly with advancing age. When a glucose load is imposed, however, the rise in maximum blood glucose levels is clearly greater, and the return to resting levels slower, in old persons (Fig. 9.5). The upward drift of blood glucose with age produces diagnostic difficulties. If criteria used to diagnose diabetes in young populations were applied to the elderly, there would be a considerable increase in the number of those diagnosed as diabetic from the glucose tolerance test. Thus, elderly patients with an impaired glucose tolerance test (i.e. a 2 hour post-glucose load of 7–11 mmol/l) should probably not be regarded as diabetic if they are asymptomatic, but they do carry a higher risk of developing frank diabetes.

Osmoregulation

On average, young adults maintain their blood osmolality in the range 280–295 mmol/kg. Although resting plasma osmolality is unchanged in the elderly, the osmoregulatory response to 24 hour water deprivation is impaired, even in good health. Old subjects develop higher plasma osmolality and sodium concentrations in response to dehydration, and their maximum urine osmolality is lower, but the sensation of thirst is less. Care is needed in

Summary 2 Normal vs pathological decrements in physiological performance in old age	
Normal age-related functional decline	*Pathological process*
Impaired sight (presbyopia)	Pathological in extreme cases
Impaired hearing (presbyacusis)	Effects of ototoxic drugs, diuretics or vascular disorders
Bone loss	'Accelerated' osteoporosis
Decline in intellectual function	Reduced cerebral oxygenation (e.g. in cardiac failure); SDAT
Impaired glucose tolerance	Diabetes
Impaired balance (increased sway), shorter steps, slower gait	Parkinson's, Alzheimer's or cerebro-vascular disease; dementia; vestibular lesions; cervical spondylosis; visual problems
Altered sleep pattern	Insomnia due to nocturia (due to detrusor instability); pain, depression etc.

correction of hypernatraemia with hypotonic fluids in the elderly, because of the risk of cerebral oedema.

AUTONOMIC DYSFUNCTION

This results from a number of factors: a reduction in nerve density and neurotransmitter concentrations in the autonomic nerves; reduced responsiveness of effector organs such as blood vessels and stretch receptors in arterial walls; and a decline in cellular beta adrenergic sensitivity.

Dysfunction may follow central lesions such as cerebrovascular disease, Parkinson's disease, Shy-Drager syndrome, Wernicke's encephalopathy (due to thiamine deficiency associated with alcoholism) and SDAT. Peripheral autonomic neuropathy may occur in diabetes mellitus, chronic alcoholism and malignancy. Autonomic dysfunction may also be caused by drugs such as phenothiazine, tricyclic antidepressants and haloperidol. The important clinical consequences are postural hypotension, bowel and bladder disturbances, impotence and impaired thermoregulation.

Ageing and thermoregulation

Under normal circumstances the body core temperature is about 37°C with, under normal conditions, a skin temperature of 33°C, giving a core/skin temperature gradient of 4°C. Thermoregulatory responses are impaired in old age due to disordered autonomic function. This usually passes unnoticed; but in times of environmental stress, the old person is less able to maintain a constant deep body temperature. Surveys of old persons living at home in

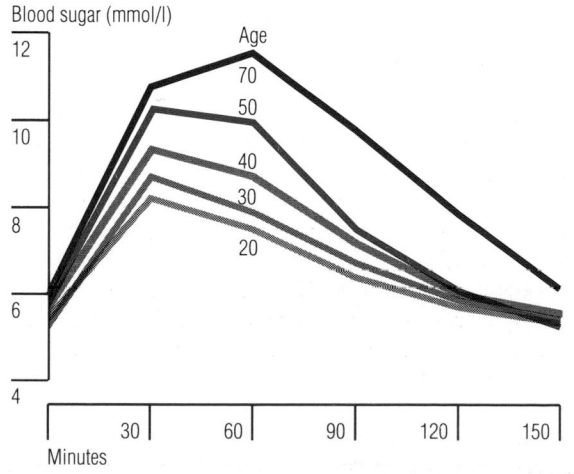

Fig. 9.5 Mean blood sugar levels after a 50 g oral glucose load in a cross-sectional population study. Known diabetics have been excluded.

winter show that only 0.5% had frank hypothermia (deep body temperature less than 35°C) but 10% had a deep body temperature below 35.5°C. The latter individuals had impaired thermoregulation – as shown by a core/skin temperature gradient only half that of normal individuals.

The elderly may also suffer impairment of thermal perception. Young persons can detect temperature differences as small as 0.8°C, but old persons only perceive differences of 2–5°C. Furthermore, the elderly shiver less efficiently in response to cooling, with little more than half the metabolic heat production seen in young subjects. Old people are thus not only less able to maintain their deep body temperature when subjected to cold stress, but may also be less aware of cold conditions and therefore fail to take the appropriate steps. This may explain why some old people can tolerate cold living conditions without discomfort. Indeed, a survey in the winter of 1972 showed that 75% of old persons had a living room temperature at or below 18.3°C. Poverty is, of course, another reason for these low levels of heating.

About 80% of the variation in mortality rates throughout the year is associated with changes in temperature (Fig. 9.6). For every degree change in the average winter temperature, the number of annual winter deaths rises or falls by about 8000. Thus, in the mild winter of 1983/4, about 30 000 more elderly people died than during the summer months (a 14% increase). In the cold winter of 1984/5, this figure rose to 46 000 (an increase of 20%). However, the majority of these 'excess' deaths are directly due not to hypothermia, but to coronary and cerebral thrombosis resulting from haemoconcentration and hypertension after cold exposure. The diagnosis and treatment of hypothermia are discussed in Chapter 4, page 61.

The elderly are also less able to cope with excessive heat, and the mortality rate during heat waves rises with

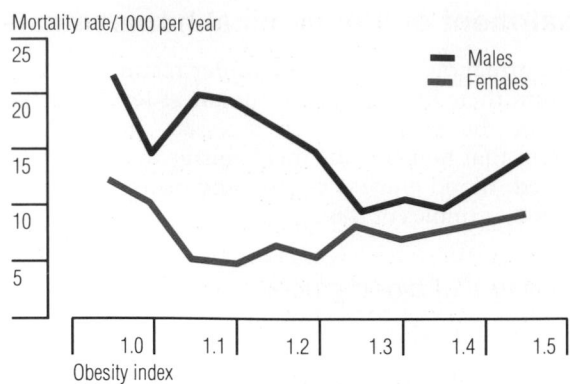

Fig. 9.7 Relation of obesity to mortality found in the Framingham study. The obesity index is the ratio of the subject's weight to a reference weight obtained from height and frame charts compiled by large insurance studies. Note that the lowest mortality occurs at an obesity index rather above 1.0.

increasing age. Heat illness is only rarely recognised as a contributory factor, however, and the cause of death is usually recorded as cerebrovascular or ischaemic heart disease.

NUTRITION AND AGEING

At retirement age in developed countries the average person is more likely to be obese than undernourished, but subsequently body weight and nutrient intake falls and for the very elderly the main concern is with undernutrition. Moderate overweight is not associated with a high mortality in old age (Fig. 9.7) but low body weight is associated with a higher mortality in both fit old people and those admitted to hospital.

Nutritional surveys have shown a marked decrease in energy requirements and intakes of nutrients with

Table 9.3 Risk factors for malnutrition

- Unexpected weight change of more than 3 kg
- Physical disability
- Lack of sunlight
- Gastrectomy
- Mental confusion
- Chewing or swallowing difficulties
- Fewer than eight main meals, hot or cold, in a week
- Absence of fruit or vegetables in diet
- Food wastage
- Alcoholism
- Receiving supplementary benefit
- Depression or loneliness

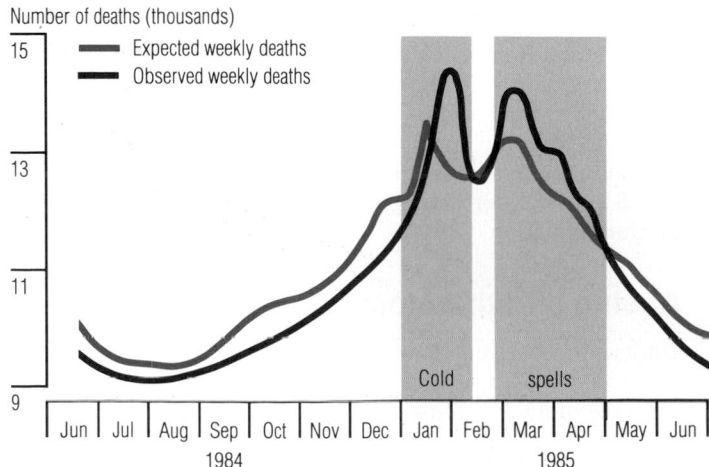

Fig. 9.6 Observed and expected deaths in the UK during the cold winter of 1984/5. Note the rise in death rate during the winter months and the excess deaths during the two exceptionally cold periods in early 1985.

increasing age. However, this is mainly due to physical illness and reduced physical activity, which reduce appetite and energy expenditure. With increasing age there is a gradual decline in metabolism at rest but this is relatively unimportant. For healthy, active persons over 60 years of age, the energy and nutrient requirements are similar to those of a 30-year-old. Longitudinal studies have shown that nutrient intakes are maintained in old people who remain in good health. Housebound elderly women consume 15% less carbohydrate and 46% less vitamin C than active age-matched controls.

Nutritional deficiencies

A survey of old people living at home found that 3% were suffering from malnutrition, including protein-calorie malnutrition, iron deficiency and specific vitamin deficiencies. In most cases, this was the result of some underlying medical problem and was only rarely due primarily to economic or social factors (see Table 9.3). Social factors are, however, likely to be important in cases of subclinical malnutrition. For example, 31% of those living alone had leucocyte ascorbic acid levels below 7.0 $\mu g/10^8$ wbc compared with 8% of those living with a spouse. Scurvy remains rare even amongst the most isolated patients.

Megaloblastic anaemia due to a folate-poor diet is rare in old people in the UK. However, low serum folate levels are found in about 8% of elderly hospital patients and are often found in patients with physical disability and dementia.

Osteomalacia may contribute significantly to the skeletal rarefaction seen in old age (although this is more commonly due to osteoporosis). There are many causes of osteomalacia, but two of the most important are reduced vitamin D intake and low exposure to sunlight – two factors often present together in the elderly. Housebound old people with poor exposure to sunlight are four times more likely to have a dietary intake of vitamin D less than the recommended level (30 i.u./day) than ambulatory women of the same age.

BALANCE AND FALLS

Normal balance is maintained by keeping the body's centre of gravity within its supporting base. In a normal standing position, the centre of gravity – which lies on average a few centimetres in front of the transverse axis of the ankles – tends to pull the body forwards. This is corrected by active contraction of the calf muscles, so that even during quiet standing the body sways slightly in the anterior-posterior plane.

Threats to balance are detected by vision, by proprioception (particularly from the ankle) and by vestibular sensors. Coordinated muscular activity is then initiated to move neck, trunk and limbs so that balance is restored. Disease in any part of this system will impair balance, but single lesions are rarely completely disabling because of good overall reserve. Effective balance control depends on both unimpaired sensory input and a stable support base. When the eyes are closed there is generally a slight increase in postural sway, and it appears that peripheral vision in particular is necessary for normal balance.

Changes in balance in old age

With increasing age the first change in balance detected in normal persons is increased sway. Sway is measured in the antero-posterior plane with the person standing still, and is a way of quantifying the Romberg test (see Fig. 9.8). There is also a change in gait with age (Fig. 9.9). Normal, active older people have a shorter step length as compared to the young; the step length is also more variable and they walk more slowly.

FALLS

Elderly persons who have had falls have significantly impaired sway and gait when compared with age-matched controls. Fallers are usually found to have significant impairment of one or more sensory input as well as disease affecting central coordination, such as cerebrovascular or Parkinson's disease. Demented elderly persons are more likely to fall than non-demented and, though mobility appears unimpaired, demented patients also sway more, have a shorter and more variable step length, and slower walking speeds.

Wearing an artificial limb following an above-knee amputation only affects postural sway when the subject's eyes are closed, indicating that the instability of the base and loss of proprioception is compensated for by increased

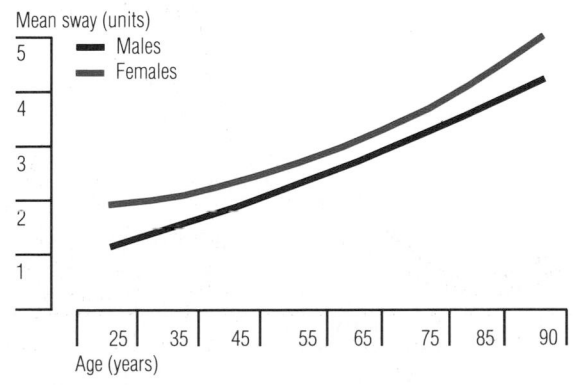

Fig. 9.8 Postural sway (measured as movement in the anterior/posterior plane with the subject standing) increases with age. At all ages, women sway significantly more than men. 1 unit = $3\frac{1}{3}^{\circ}$ of angular movement.

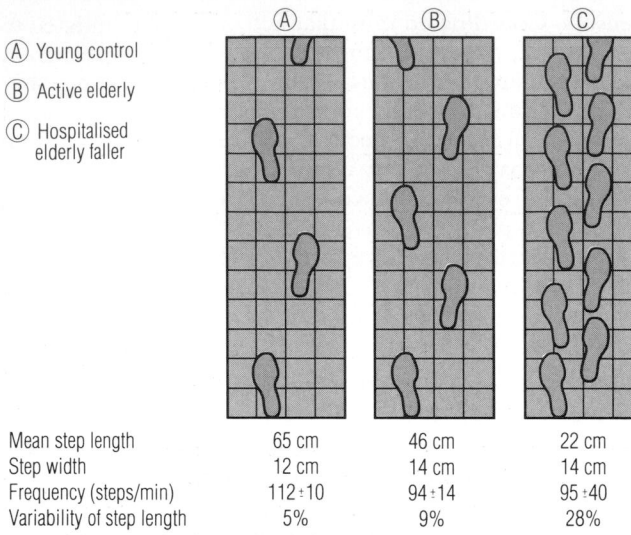

Ⓐ Young control
Ⓑ Active elderly
Ⓒ Hospitalised elderly faller

	Ⓐ	Ⓑ	Ⓒ
Mean step length	65 cm	46 cm	22 cm
Step width	12 cm	14 cm	14 cm
Frequency (steps/min)	112 ÷ 10	94 ÷ 14	95 ÷ 40
Variability of step length	5%	9%	28%

Fig. 9.9 Changes in gait with age. A step where the heel of the leading foot comes to just beyond the midpoint of the trailing foot is about 30 cm. The hospitalised faller walks with a slow, short paced gait: the step length is very variable. This indicates considerable instability and poor confidence.

Table 9.4 Causes of spontaneous falling

Patient usually impaired in more than one of the systems concerned with balance control:

- Vision, e.g. poor illumination
- Impaired proprioception, e.g. cervical spondylosis, osteoarthritis of ankles, knees or hips
- Vestibular lesions, e.g. Ménière's disease
- Impaired central coordination, e.g. cerebrovascular disease
- Unstable support base, e.g. turning quickly, walking downstairs or arising from a chair

If balance already impaired, falls are precipitated by:

- Acute illness, e.g. chest infection, worsening of heart failure
- Drugs, e.g. tranquillisers
- Occult ill health, e.g. anaemia, hyponatraemia

dependence on vision. Similarly, patients with chronic bilateral impairment of vestibular function walk normally when their eyes are open. They can still walk satisfactorily when blindfolded unless they are also on uneven ground. An important contribution to postural control is provided by the activity of mechanoreceptors in the apophyseal joints of the cervical spine. These exert a reflex influence on the activity of neck and limb muscles, and damage to this mechanism – typically from cervical spondylosis – can cause a feeling of unsteadiness during movements, often worse on turning the head. In man, the vestibular system plays little part in static posture or in the righting reactions. It is, however, important if the supporting base is uneven (e.g. when walking on a cobbled street) or if the body is unstable.

Balance is usually only seriously impaired if more than one of these sensory systems is affected. Patients with spontaneous falls (see below) nearly always have multiple defects and their identification allows a rational treatment programme to be planned.

Examination of the patient

The history will often allow differentiation between a straightforward trip or accident and a spontaneous fall (Table 9.4). Patients with trips or accidents are generally younger and more active, and their balance and gait no worse than non-fallers of the same age.

Patients who suffer spontaneous falls often have difficulty in describing why they fell, and may try to rationalize the fall by saying 'I must have tripped'. Comments such as 'All of a sudden I fell' or 'I felt peculiar and down I went'

are common. Some may say that they felt dizzy (particularly if prompted by the doctor). However, only very rarely does the patient experience true vertigo (a sensation of the patient's surroundings or the inside of his head spinning around). They do not so much feel dizzy as unsteady when standing or walking, and are frightened that they are going to fall over (see Ch. 22, p. 884). Some of these patients suffer drop attacks. These are falls which occur without warning; the patient suddenly crumples to the ground and there are no neurological sequelae. Like other spontaneous falls, their aetiology is multifactorial. Regardless of their precise nature, patients with spontaneous falls tend to have certain characteristics in common. They are usually older and more frail, their gait and balance noticeably impaired, and their general health poor. They are also more likely to be taking drugs such as sedatives and diuretics, and to have incontinence of urine or mental impairment. Their mortality is about five times that of non-fallers.

Points to note in the history are:

- Whether the patient felt unsteady and fell after turning their head (which suggests cervical spondylosis or vestibular disease).
- If the fall occurred soon after standing up (raising the possibility of postural hypotension).
- Loss of consciousness (can the patient remember hitting the floor?). This suggests an arrhythmia causing syncope or epilepsy. If there are focal symptoms or signs (dysphasia, motor or sensory loss), transient ischaemic attacks should be considered.
- The patient's drugs will need to be checked. Sedatives or hypnotics frequently slow the patient down and may precipitate a fall. Hypotensive drugs may cause postural hypotension, with the patient complaining of feeling faint when getting out of bed or standing up from a chair.
- Mental state should be assessed if there is a suspicion of dementia or depression.
- A history of tinnitus, deafness or vertigo should be sought. If present, this may indicate a vestibular lesion,

either peripheral (e.g. Ménière's disease) or central (vascular disease in the brain stem or cerebellum).

In the general examination:

- The lying and standing blood pressure should be measured (a drop in systolic pressure of more than 20 mmHg indicates postural hypotension).
- The range of neck movements should be assessed.
- The patient should be observed standing and walking.
- Normal old persons should not have a positive Romberg test (i.e. closing the eyes when standing should not markedly impair balance).
- Patients with spontaneous falls will often be unsteady even with eyes open, and their righting reflex may be so poor that they fall following a very light tap with the examiner's finger on their sternum.
- Such patients walk with short steps (sometimes these are very short, a gait known as a *marche à petits pas*).
- In severe cases, there will be manifest anxiety and fear of falling, with the patient reluctant to move without clutching onto furniture or onlookers for support.

In addition to routine investigations:

- A 24-hour ambulatory ECG should be obtained for patients suspected of having Stokes-Adams attacks (although without a reliable witness at the time of the fall, this is a difficult diagnosis to make). Palpitations before the fall or loss of consciousness are important pointers, but a useful clue is that, despite repeated falls, the patient's gait, balance and confidence are normal.
- An EEG for patients suspected of having epilepsy (see Ch. 22, p. 859).
- Early morning falls in patients taking a long-acting hypoglycaemic drug (e.g. chlorpropamide) raises the possibility of hypoglycaemia.
- Patients suspected of having a vestibular lesion can have this accurately localized only by specialist examinations, which include electronystagmography and caloric tests.
- The patient's vision, both with and without spectacles, should be noted.

Management

Many patients with spontaneous falls have multiple defects and their balance is precarious. Sometimes a minor illness such as a chest infection or a newly prescribed sedative drug can simply prove too much for a frail patient. Identification of precipitating factors enables the patient to be appropriately advised. Cervical spondylosis should be treated with neck exercises, not a cervical collar which often makes the patient feel more unsteady. Faulty spectacles should be replaced and everything possible done to improve the patient's vision, including better illu-

---

Summary 3 Typical features in patients with spontaneous falls

- Older, frailer and in poorer health than patients with trips or accidents
- Significantly impaired gait and balance (normal in some Stokes-Adams patients)
- Difficulty in accounting for how they fell
- Positive Romberg's test; often very unsteady even with eyes open
- Short steps, *marche à petits pas*
- Generally have multiple defects both in the sensory systems concerned with balance control (vision, proprioceptors and the vestibular system) and in central coordination centres

---

mination in the home. Peripheral vestibular lesions may be improved with cinnarizine (15 mg tds) or betahistine (8 mg tds), but these drugs may have troublesome sedative effects. Central vestibular lesions are rarely helped by drugs and the latter therefore should be avoided if this diagnosis is definitely made. Phenothiazines should not be prescribed for vague complaints of dizziness, because of the risk of drug-induced Parkinsonism.

The patient's chair should be at the right height (the seat level with the top of the knee) so that getting out of it is not difficult. A walking frame may initially help both mobility and confidence, but should be removed once the patient's walking is better. Balance exercises and measures to improve confidence and well-being are often very helpful. If the falls have been such as to warrant hospital admission, then follow-up for a few weeks in a day hospital is helpful. In case of another fall, the patient should be taught how to get up off the floor, and advised of the various alarm systems that can be installed in the home. An occupational therapist should also visit the home and correct obvious hazards, such as unguarded fires or a broken light bulb over the stairs.

URINARY INCONTINENCE

Although more common in the elderly, the causes and management are similiar to those in the young (see Ch. 20). The major difference is that elderly patients are more likely to suffer in silence or even to deny the problem. Age has little effect on prognosis and the majority of patients can expect to become dry following treatment.

Detrusor instability

The majority of patients are incontinent because of idiopathic detrusor instability. The symptoms are often aggravated by emotional stress. The cortical centre for this willed control over the hindbrain–sacral reflex lies in the frontal premotor area. In old age these tracts are vulnerable to normal ageing processes, to cerebrovascular disease and Alzheimer's disease. An early sign of detrusor instability in old age is nocturia, which may progress to symptoms of urgency, urge incontinence, daytime frequency and, in women, stress incontinence. Genuine stress incontinence due to laxity of the pelvic floor support is uncommon and most women who leak when they cough or sneeze do so because the rise in intra-abdominal pressure triggers an unstable detrusor contraction. A cystometrogram is needed to distinguish between the two causes and patients with genuine stress incontinence can expect good results from pelvic floor exercises and surgery.

Whether the detrusor instability is idiopathic or due to cortical damage (e.g. from a stroke), the response to bladder retraining is good provided that the patient can comprehend the instructions and is well motivated. About 80% of patients will be dry after six weeks' treatment. Bladder retraining (see Table 9.5) depends on asking the patient only to urinate after a certain fixed time, the underlying assumption being that asking the patient to 'hold' in this way strengthens cortical inhibition over the sacral reflex.

Retention with overflow

Even elderly men should be considered for a prostatic transurethral resection and, if too frail for surgery, may be suitable for insertion of a stent into the prostatic urethra under local anaesthetic. Acontractile bladders sometimes respond to distigmine bromide 5 mg on an empty stomach. Failing this, intermittent self-catheterisation or a permanent indwelling catheter will be needed.

Postoperative urinary retention

This may happen to any elderly man following surgery. It is commonly assumed to be due to prostatic outflow obstruction, but is much more likely to result from a combination of postoperative pain, preoperative opiates, anticholinergic anaesthetic agents, a bladder overdistended with intravenous fluids and lying immobilised in bed. If the patient doesn't respond to indoramin 20 mg

Table 9.5 Principles of bladder retraining

1. Explanation of condition
2. Establish baseline micturition pattern using chart
3. Select appropriate time for patient to wait between urination, e.g. 1–2 hours
4. Provide patient with a suitable pad to wear in case of incontinence
5. Gradually extend interval as patient improves
6. Concomitant relaxation therapy for stressed or anxious patients

Table 9.6 Causes of faecal incontinence

- Secondary to colo-rectal disease, e.g. infective diarrhoea, carcinoma of the rectum
- Idiopathic weakness of the anal sphincter and pelvic floor muscles
- Faecal impaction
- Neurological causes, e.g. dementia, impaired consciousness and rectal instability

b.d. then the bladder should be emptied with intermittent catheterisation until normal detrusor activity returns.

Catheters

A permanent indwelling catheter is the last resort for urinary incontinence, but is not necessarily a bad solution. Some patients clean, dry and comfortable for the first time in years are very relieved. The gauge should be 14f or 16f and the retaining balloon should contain no more than 5 ml of water to reduce the risk of provoking unstable contractions, which will cause urine to leak out around the catheter.

FAECAL INCONTINENCE

Faecal incontinence is distressing for the elderly patient and carer and is a major reason for care breaking down in the home. The prevalence in the community is less than 1% rising to 10% in residential homes and 25–30% in nursing homes or on long-stay wards. The causes are given in Table 9.6.

Faecal impaction

This is the commonest cause of faecal soiling. Rectal sensation is impaired, probably aggravated by chronic rectal distension and the patients often leak before experiencing a call to stool. Problems result not only from a large hard stool in the rectum, but also from a mass of soft stool, which is not readily recognised. Repeated enemas are necessary until the rectum and lower colon are completely clear and the rectal tone has returned to normal. Thereafter, the patient is kept regular with appropriate diet, high fluid intake and judicious use of laxatives. Patients who are unable to defaecate regularly may need a daily suppository or twice weekly enema, the aim being to prevent chronic rectal distension.

SLEEP AND INSOMNIA

Insomnia is a common complaint in the elderly and there is great pressure on doctors to prescribe hypnotics.

The elderly receive more hypnotics than any other age group.

It is often assumed that hypnotics are both harmless and effective, but for the elderly neither assumption is true. Elderly patients taking hypnotics regularly rate the quality of their sleep as worse than those not on hypnotics; and more than one in ten persons aged 70 or over taking nitrazepam (10 mg) at night have troublesome daytime sedation. Any patient complaining of insomnia – but particularly an elderly one – needs careful assessment and not just a prescription for an hypnotic.

Normal sleep

A person falling asleep 'descends' rapidly through progressively deeper stages of sleep. Slow wave sleep–which occupies about 20% of the night in the young–is reduced to only 5% by 70 years of age, and stage four is almost completely absent.

The elderly wake more frequently and take longer to fall asleep so that, even for the normal old person, sleep becomes increasingly fragmented. Thus, the doctor needs to decide whether an elderly patient's complaint of insomnia is an unrealistic expectation of what constitutes a good night's sleep. Less physical activity and daytime catnaps will further reduce the ability to sleep well at night.

Causes of insomnia

Insomnia may be age related as discussed above. Nocturia is another common reason for an old person waking up, a condition which may be caused by prostatism, renal failure or diabetes but is most likely due to detrusor instability (especially if associated with some urgency). Pain is also an important cause of insomnia, and the akinetic Parkinsonian patient who cannot turn over in bed will find their sleep is disturbed. Anxiety and depression commonly cause sleep disturbances, and are best managed by psychiatric treatment directed at the primary condition.

Insomnia may be drug induced. The most familiar example is alcohol, which, if taken in the evening, will quickly induce sleep but results in rebound insomnia with

awakening later the same night because of its rapid metabolism. A similar effect can be seen after hypnotics are withdrawn, when the patient complains of anxiety, tension and insomnia. If these withdrawal effects are not understood by the doctor and patient then a hypnotic may be needlessly represcribed.

Choosing a hypnotic

Hypnotics should only be used when insomnia is impairing the patient's daytime performance. There should be a clear indication, such as a recent bereavement or impending major surgery, and the prescription should be limited to seven or ten days wherever possible.

The drug should have a rapid onset of action, particularly if the patient's main complaint is difficulty in falling asleep. There should be no daytime sedation, although this may occur due to accumulation of long-acting hypnotics and their active metabolites, or because of an age-related alteration in sensitivity to the drug.

Benzodiazepines

Diazepam has a half-life in hours approximately equivalent to the person's age, but the constant clearance rate means that the average steady state plasma level of diazepam is unaffected by ageing. However, the half-life of its major active metabolite, desmethyldiazepam, is prolonged due to reduced plasma clearance. The dose necessary to produce sedation is therefore inversely correlated with age, due partly to an increased sensitivity to the drug in old age and also to accumulation of the active metabolite. Diazepam (2 mg or 5 mg) may be a suitable hypnotic for anxious old people where a daytime anxiolitic effect is required. Daytime drowsiness, confusion and falls, however, may be a problem.

Nitrazepam also produces more sedation in the elderly, probably as a result of increased receptor sensitivity (since the pharmacokinetics remain unaltered). The unwanted daytime sedation is largely dose dependent (Fig. 9.10); 2.5 mg is the maximum dose that should be given to an old person.

Temazepam has a half-life of only 5–10 hours in young persons but may be as long as 30 hours in the elderly. Accumulation therefore occurs and, after a week of continuous dosing at 20 mg each night, subjects show a significant slowing of reaction times. The effect is likely to be dose related; 10 mg at night rarely causes serious problems.

Lormetazepam has a good pharmacokinetic profile for use in the elderly. Although the elimination half-life is prolonged to about 14 hours in elderly subjects, accumulation does not occur and there is no impairment of daytime performance with a nightly dose of either 0.5 mg or 1.0 mg.

Summary 4 Causes of insomnia
• Age-related changes in sleep pattern
• Nocturia (probably due to detrusor instability)
• Pain
• Anxiety and depression
• Drug induced, e.g. alcohol, withdrawal from hypnotics
• Specific problems, e.g. sleep apnoea, myoclonus

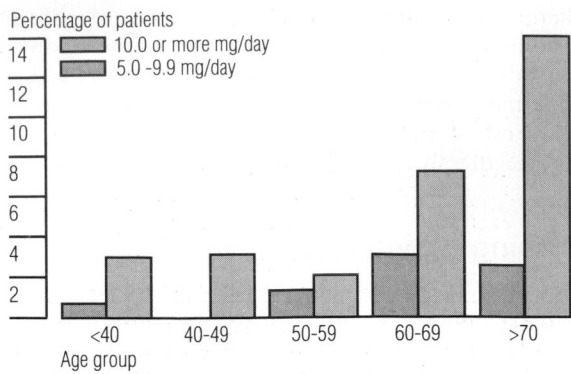

Fig. 9.10 Relationship of daily dose (5.0–9.9 mg/day and 10.0 or more mg/day) to the frequency of unwanted CNS depression attributed to nitrazepam, with the population stratified according to age.

Other hypnotics

Chloral hydrate is a syrup with an unpleasant taste. The usual dose in the elderly is 1 g and it is largely free from side-effects although it potentiates the effect of warfarin. It is particularly useful for treating confused patients, many of whom are made worse by benzodiazepines.

Chlormethiazole is valuable in the elderly. Its pharmaco-kinetics are unaltered by age and its short plasma half-life of 3–4 hours prevents accumulation. It is metabolised by the liver, and should be used with caution in patients with cirrhosis of the liver or in alcoholics. One capsule (192 mg of chlormethiazole base) may be sufficient but two capsules is still safe.

Restless and confused patients are often best sedated by a *phenothiazine* such as thioridazine (25–75 mg nocte) or haloperidol (0.5–3 mg nocte). Both drugs carry a long-term risk of extrapyramidal side-effects.

SEXUAL FUNCTION

In Western society, sexuality amongst adolescents and young adults is studied and discussed openly. No such liberal attitude exists towards sex in old age and, unfortunately, the stereotype of the sexless old persists. Although sexual activity does decline with advancing age, much of this is due to ill health or the death of the marriage partner. Old age itself causes very little impairment of sexual enjoyment. Overall, it would appear that continued sexual activity in old age depends on the frequency and enjoyment it afforded in middle age, the availability of a suitable partner and (particularly in men) continuing good health.

The main physical changes in women result from a lack of oestrogen, which may cause vaginitis with reduced lubrication and painful intercourse. Length of orgasm may be reduced but many postmenopausal women report increased desire and arousability. Male fertility is usually maintained into extreme old age although the volume of prostatic secretions reduces, it takes longer to achieve an erection, orgasm is briefer and the following refractory period is longer.

Many doctors are reluctant to discuss sexual practice with their elderly patients and thereby lose the opportunity for helpful counselling. Vaginitis due to oestrogen deficiency responds to dienoestrol cream. Complaints of impotence in the male should prompt a thorough physical examination, including a blood sugar estimation. Many drugs interfere with sexual function and the elderly should be warned about this when they are prescribed. Propranolol and thiazide diuretics may produce impotence. All of the phenothiazines may cause impotence, while thioridazine may also cause lack of ejaculation; haloperidol is free of these problems.

Sexuality – or the lack of it – in old age should not be seen in isolation. The need for affection, tenderness and caressing may be more important than intercourse, and counselling as to what is normal and appropriate may dispel fears of inadequacy or embarrassment.

ALTERED REACTIONS TO DISEASE

In the elderly, acute illness may present in ways which are different from the young and non-specific presentations are of great importance.

Confusional states

A toxic confusional state is the ageing brain's response to a number of insults: the stress of a physical illness, a variety of powerful drugs, and alterations in the old person's familiar environment. It tends to occur more commonly in persons whose mental state is already impaired, for example by Alzheimer's disease, or who have communication difficulties because of defective hearing and vision.

Typically, the onset is abrupt over hours or days. This and the clouding of consciousness are the main points of differentiation from dementia (see Table 9.7). Typically, the acutely confused patient is drowsy; it is difficult to get their attention and there are fluctuations in the level of consciousness. The patient's agitation and confusion are usually worse at night. About 15% of elderly admissions to acute medical wards are delirious. One third die within a month, and of the survivors, 80% will have recovered mentally within a month.

Investigations

Proper assessment and diagnosis are essential, which require a careful history from a reliable witness. Physical

Table 9.7 Differential diagnosis of confusion and dementia

	Differential diagnosis	
	Acute confusional state	Dementia
Onset	Abrupt	Gradual, months or years
Clouding of consciousness	Yes	No (but there may be drowsiness due to sedation)
Course	Fluctuates, lucid intervals during day. Worse at night	Stable over course of day
Disorientation and cognitive impairment	Yes (may be intermittent)	Yes
Alertness	Increased or impaired	Usually normal
Hallucinations	Yes (common)	Yes (uncommon)
Duration	Hours or days	Steadily progressive

N.B. None of the clinical features of the acute confusional state is reliable and a confident diagnosis depends on the history.

illness, co-existing dementia, recent emotional stress, alcohol abuse, change of drugs, or head injury are important precipitating factors. In hospital, surgery is an important cause of confusional states. Physical examination should concentrate on identifying possible causes. The commonest are congestive cardic failure, Gram-negative septicaemia and pneumonia.

Management

After treatment of any underlying cause, management of the confused patient relies mainly on the correct environment and sedation should be kept to a minimum. The patient is best looked after in a side-ward so as to avoid disturbing other patients. A relative or nurse should stay with the patient at all times to reassure, comfort and explain to the patient what is happening. The light should be kept on in the room at night. Sedation may be needed if the patient is very restless, e.g. thioridazine up to 100 mg t.d.s. or haloperidol 1–3 mg t.d.s. by mouth. Droperidol 2.5–5.0 mg by i.m. injection is fast-acting and effective.

Falls

Old persons who suddenly start to fall frequently, often have an underlying physical illness as well as an age-related balance impairment (see pp. 151–3).

Urinary incontinence

A patient may become incontinent due to a confusional state, in which bladder function cannot be controlled normally, or because of immobility as a result of physical illness (see pp. 153–4).

Absence of pain

For reasons not clearly understood, pain due to illness or trauma which would be expected in a younger individual, is often minimal or absent in the elderly. Thus, myocardial infarction is commonly pain free, and the patient presents instead with dyspnoea or non-specific illness. Similarly, abdominal pathology such as gastric ulcers or mesenteric thrombosis may be silent; however, acute appendicitis often has a fulminating course in older patients, with the rapid development of gangrene and peritonitis. Even a fracture of the neck of femur may cause the patient only slight discomfort, evidenced by a disinclination to walk.

Multiple pathological processes

The explanation of all symptoms, signs and abnormal investigations by one diagnosis is seldom possible in older patients. The usual pattern is one of multiple disorders. Thus, a momentary cardiac arrhythmia which may produce only a slight feeling of dizziness or palpitations in a young person may cause loss of consciousness or even a stroke with hemiplegia in an old patient. Similarly, a chest infection may precipitate heart failure because the cardiac reserve is already impaired by ischaemic heart disease. Common conditions such as obesity, osteoarthritis, diverticular disease, hypertension, diabetes, dementia and presbyacusis may all be present in a single individual, and the aim then is to decide which are causing important functional disability.

Unreported illness

The early identification of disease or disordered function allows treatment to be initiated or social support organised before things have gone too far. Studies in general practice show that an elderly person has, on average, at least three disabilities; and for every one known to the general practitioner there is another which is not. Typically, cardiac, chest and neurological disabilities are known to the GP, but incontinence, difficulty in walking, painful feet, dementia and depression often go unreported.

CLINICAL APPROACH

When assessing an elderly patient it is generally more useful to think in terms of functional ability than to lay emphasis on the underlying pathology. For example, the distinction between rheumatoid and osteoarthritis in a patient with arthritis of the knees may be largely academic; the fact that the patient has poor mobility is much more important. Emphasis is placed on physiotherapy, walking exercises and possibly surgery to improve mobility and independence.

History

A full history remains the primary investigation. In a confused patient, it is necessary to get additional information from a relative, community nurse, or someone who knows the patient well.

The tempo with which the symptoms have developed is particularly important. Forgetfulness gradually increasing over two or three years suggests senile dementia of the Alzheimer's type (SDAT) whereas a sudden onset of confusion over a day or two indicates a toxic confusional state, and requires a search for underlying physical problems such as an infection or myocardial infarct. A sudden onset of headaches or recent change in bowel habit is never normal in old age, whereas gradually failing hearing and vision may be.

The history must include: a full list of the patient's medication, including details of dose and frequency; details of the patient's functional ability (to do shopping, cooking, cleaning and attend to personal toilet); and social circumstances. The main carer at home should be identified, as well as additional support which might be provided by family, neighbours and social services.

Assessment

The chances of successfully discharging an elderly, frail person, if their homelessness, anxiety and inadequate personality are ignored, are remote. Seeing the patient as a whole is thus not only good for the patient, it is essential if limited health service resources are to be used effectively. An overall view of the patient includes assessment of medical, functional, social and psychological status, and usually brings together the professional views from several disciplines.

The doctor attends to the physical and mental diagnosis and appropriate treatments. The nurse notes to what extent the patient can wash and feed him/herself or use the lavatory, and also particular problems such as incontinence, pressure sores or nocturnal confusion. The physiotherapist is concerned with whether the patient can get in and out of bed, rise from a chair, balance and walk; and as the patient improves, the occupational therapist assesses how well the patient can dress, bathe, cook and care for him/herself. As soon as possible after admission, the social worker inquires into the patient's social background to find out what circumstances are like at home – whether the old person is already receiving support from relatives or neighbours, and whether this support will be

---

Summary 5   Assessment of an elderly patient

- Main stress is on functional disability, rather than underlying pathology.

- Overall view essential:
  Medical status – manner of onset of symptoms is important. Full drug history required.
  Functional ability – washing, cooking, shopping, etc.
  Psychological status – depression, anxiety, confusion, etc.
  Social circumstances – support available at home from family and friends.

- Involves a multidisciplinary team of doctors, nurses, occupational and physiotherapists and social workers.

---

continued or needs to be increased once the patient returns home.

The aim is to ensure that patients are speedily and effectively treated and returned to their own home in a planned and thoughtful manner, so that the gains resulting from treatment are likely to be maintained. A similar process of assessment can be initiated by GPs using community staff, for patients living at home.

Physical examination

An extensive and detailed examination of every system can exhaust a frail patient. However, the examination can, with practice, be thorough, informative and quick if the doctor concentrates on identifying disabilities and assessing loss of function.

General appearance

The examination should begin with an observation of the patient's general appearance and clothes, noting any signs of self neglect. Facial pallor is frequently present and so is a poor indicator of anaemia. Pupil size is often small with reduced response, and upward gaze is often limited. Angular stomatitis – if not due to ill-fitting dentures – suggests multivitamin deficiency or iron deficiency anaemia, but a black hairy tongue or sublingual varicosities are of no significance.

Skin changes

Loose, dry, scaly skin is a common finding, as are senile purpura due to increased capillary fragility on the dorsum of the hands and extensor surface of the arms. Sun-exposed skin should be searched for basal cell carcinomas or actinic keratoses which are potentially malignant. The incidence of both conditions increases with years of exposure to the sun, and are common in the elderly.

Intertrigo – sore, inflamed patches of skin under the breasts or in the abdominal folds of obese patients – is often the result of poor personal hygiene. A keratinised transverse crease across the abdomen is the consequence of long-standing kyphosis, following osteoporotic spinal wedging. The breasts should be examined for lumps.

Feet

The ankles and feet should be inspected for signs of oedema and the need for chiropody.

Cardiovascular

Abnormalities of cardiac rhythm are frequently present: occasional ectopic beats occur in about one-sixth of elderly persons, but any other arrhythmia should be regarded as abnormal and investigated by electrocardiography. Systolic and diastolic blood pressure increases with age although there is little change over the age of 65; values up to 160/90 can be regarded as normal. Above this level, the risk of cardiovascular disease increases, but the value of treatment needs to be set against the risk of unwanted drug effects (see p. 163). Systolic murmurs – usually of the ejection type and present at the left sternal edge and aortic area are found in up to 60% of the elderly. They are commonly associated with significant disease such as cardiac failure, ischaemic heart disease, arrhythmias and hypertension and should not therefore be regarded as always benign.

Bowels and bladder

A rectal examination is essential: carcinoma of the rectum or prostate is common in the elderly, and there may be loading of the rectum with faeces – a common cause of faecal incontinence. The presence of urinary incontinence should be noted and – particularly in bedridden patients – the pressure areas inspected for sores.

Eyesight and hearing

The patient should be asked whether their vision is satisfactory and, if not, should be tested with eye charts. Hearing is probably adequate if the patient can hear a normal conversational voice. Examination of the eardrums for wax should be a routine, particularly where a hearing aid is worn, since the earpiece may compress wax into a hard, impenetrable lump.

Neurological changes

Ankle jerks tend to be absent in about 10% of elderly patients. Superficial abdominal reflexes are also often absent, but the presence of extensor–plantar responses is best regarded as pathological.

Vibration sense in the lower limbs is reduced, and may be absent at the ankles, in up to a half of patients over 75.

However, joint position sense is usually normal. Appreciation of pain, temperature and light touch is very variable, but one or other of these sensations is impaired in about a quarter of the elderly. Both the glabellar tap, and primitive reflexes such as the pout reflex (tap the upper lip and the lips pout), grasp reflex and palmomental reflex (the palm is scratched and the chin wrinkles on the same side), can often be elicited in the elderly, particularly in those who have dementia. Hearing loss of old age (presbyacusis) is a sensory neural loss of high frequencies and affects perhaps 60% of persons over 70.

Gait and balance

Changes in posture and gait with old age follow an essentially extrapyramidal pattern. The stance of an old person is one of general flexion with increased muscle tone, poverty of movement and bradykinesis. These changes are also seen in Parkinson's disease but, in normal old age, are of a much milder degree. Postural control is impaired, as shown by the increased number of falls occurring in the elderly (see pp. 151–3).

INVESTIGATION IN THE ELDERLY

Potentially remediable conditions cannot be ignored simply because the patient is elderly, but it is not good medicine to order invasive, uncomfortable and possibly expensive tests when the potential benefit to the patient is minimal.

Overall state of health

Does the patient have the physical and mental capacity to benefit from a proposed treatment? If surgery is an option, would the patient be fit for operation? If the patient is debilitated and being looked after by family at home, then the views of these relatives must be included when assessing the benefits and risks of investigation and treatment. For example, an active old person who is having repeated falls associated with transient loss of consciousness should have 24-hour ambulatory ECG monitoring to detect whether the falls are related to a cardiac arrhythmia. If they are, then a pacemaker can be safely inserted – even in the very elderly – with the potential for a considerable improvement in the quality of life.

Will the investigation influence management?

Before ordering an investigation it is necessary to consider whether the result is likely to usefully influence management. For example, a severely demented patient with an abdominal mass and positive faecal occult bloods could have the presumptive diagnosis of carcinoma of the colon confirmed by a barium enema. However, if surgery is not being considered (because of the patient's poor general condition and inability to cope with a colostomy), there is little point in the barium enema. On the other hand, if the same patient is found to be unable to walk following a fall, the patient's hips should certainly be X-rayed. Repair of a fractured neck of femur will not only relieve the patient's pain, it is also much easier to nurse an ambulant patient than one who is bedridden.

Will the diagnosis affect prognosis?

It is important to consider whether the investigation will establish a diagnosis which significantly affects prognosis. A very frail patient with severe dyspepsia can be treated easily with an H_2 antagonist. But if symptoms persist it may be important for the patient and relatives to know if the diagnosis is peptic ulceration or carcinoma of the stomach.

Routine screening

Most patients seen in clinic or admitted to hospital will have a full blood count, ESR (or viscosity), urea and electrolytes, glucose and free T4. Urine should be analysed for protein, glucose and blood. All of these tests can usefully detect treatable disease where the clinical diagnosis is unsuspected or doubtful. This is particularly true of thyroid disease, which is found on screening in about 4% of elderly in-patients in whom classical symptoms and signs of hypo- or hyperthyroidism may be absent. Thyroid function tests can be considerably distorted by systemic illness or drugs: the best screening test is the free T4 with the TSH as a confirmatory test.

A routine chest X-ray is usually taken since about 5% of patients over 65 admitted to hospital are found to have an unexpected lesion on chest X-ray. It is particularly valuable in patients presenting with falls, immobility, incontinence or deteriorating mental function; nearly a quarter of these have cardiopulmonary disease without classical features.

An electrocardiogram is not routine, but is required for patients with cardiopulmonary disease, strokes (quite commonly associated with a myocardial infarct) and falls (which might be caused by a cardiac arrhythmia).

Investigation of dementia

The main concern in the investigation of dementia is not to miss a cause for which there is specific treatment. Although rare among elderly patients referred to a geriatrician or general physician, such reversible dementias are relatively common amongst referrals to specialist neuro-

logical centres. Conditions which may respond to treatment include:

- depression and other psychiatric disorders
- normal pressure (communicating) hydrocephalus
- resectable tumours
- subdural haematoma
- toxic drug effects
- thyroid disease
- pernicious anaemia
- syphilis.

In addition to the routine blood tests, the patient should have the serum B_{12} level checked and a VDRL test to exclude syphilis. Although it cannot positively diagnose dementia or Alzheimer's disease, a CT scan is a valuable – though expensive – screening test as it can identify multiple infarctions, space-occupying lesions and hydrocephalus. However, only 2% of all demented patients could expect an improvement in their mental state from treatment following a CT scan. Thus, they are only indicated in patients with mild to moderate dementia of less than one year, who are fit enough for surgery if a remediable lesion is found.

Investigation of gastrointestinal lesions

In the investigation of upper gastrointestinal lesions, both barium meal and endoscopy give accurate results. However, endoscopy has the advantage of providing a tissue diagnosis where a tumour is suspected, and tends to be better tolerated by a frail elderly patient. It is thus probably the investigation of choice when readily available but needs to be preceded by a barium swallow (to check if a blind sac is present) when investigating dysphagia.

For lower bowel disorders, the first steps are usually rectal examination, sigmoidoscopy, stool culture, examination of the stool for occult blood and – finally – barium enema and possibly colonoscopy. Treatment of non-metastatic colonic malignancies gives a good prognosis; vigorous investigation of fit and active elderly patients is therefore justified. In the frailer patient, however, more caution is necessary before ordering a barium enema. Both the preparation (laxatives and sodium citrate enema) and the barium enema itself are uncomfortable and difficult procedures for elderly patients to undergo. Ultrasound scans have the advantages of being noninvasive, quick and relatively cheap, and are particularly useful for investigating jaundice, abdominal masses, pancreatic tumours and possible liver metastases. Investigation of faecal incontinence is described on page 154.

Investigation of bacteriuria

A routine mid-stream urine (MSU) test in elderly patients admitted to hospital will show significant bacteriuria (bacterial count of more than 100 000 organisms per ml) in 20–30% of women. In particular, elderly incontinent patients frequently have bacteriuria. This is not the cause of the incontinence but the result of detrusor instability, which often leads to residual urine thus encouraging bacterial growth. Over half will be asymptomatic and antibiotics seem to have only a temporary effect on clearing the urine – eventually another, more resistant organism usually appears. Routine MSUs in asymptomatic patients are not recommended and it is advisable to have a clear management policy when a positive MSU is found (Fig. 9.11). Half the patients with bacteriuria have a renal infection rather than cystitis so there is a possibility of renal damage. However, little is known about the natural history of these infections and their recurrence rate with or without antibiotics.

ASSESSMENT OF FITNESS FOR OPERATION

Advanced age is no longer a contraindication to surgery yet the risks are undoubtedly higher. The mortality rate for surgical patients over the age of 65 is about 5%. This doubles to 8–10% in those aged over 75 and rises to 15–20% in those over 85. Such high risks are only justified if surgery offers a reasonable prospect for improving the quality of the patient's life, or of preventing loss of function. Surgery for relief of severe pain or complete bowel obstruction would probably be indicated even in the most severely disabled patient. However, a patient would need to be relatively fit and active before removal of a non-obstructive malignant bowel tumour, repair of

Table 9.8 Selecting patients for surgery or intensive care

Chronological age alone is a poor indicator of outcome:
- Good results in the elderly reflect good selection criteria
- Consider the patient's previous health, level of physical independence, exercise tolerance and mental state
- Patients' and families' views must be considered; they may be much less enthusiastic than the doctor about major surgery

Increased mortality is associated with:
- The presence of unsuspected heart disease
- Reduced pulmonary and cardiac reserve (making a postoperative chest infection or myocardial infarct more likely)
- Greater susceptibility to anaesthetic drugs
- Greater risk of developing pressure sores postoperatively

an aortic aneurysm or a coronary artery bypass would be considered.

The increased surgical mortality in the elderly is due to several factors, which are shown in Table 9.8.

The mortality risk must be weighed against the likely final outcome of surgery. Total hip replacement has transformed the lives of many old people and is now a routine operation. However, if chronic lung disease or an old stroke has reduced the patient's exercise tolerance to a few yards, the operation is unlikely to be worthwhile. Before surgery, heart failure and diabetes should be controlled, dehydration and electrolyte disturbance corrected, and severe anaemia remedied by blood transfusion.

A routine preoperative ECG is worthwhile. Its major use is in detecting a recent myocardial infarct which would mean postponement of surgery for six months (if this is practicable). Many patients will have a minor ECG abnormality which provides a useful baseline measurement for comparing postoperative changes. Preoperative ECG abnormalities do not reliably predict postoperative cardiovascular complications, which can be expected in about one-fifth of elderly patients and consist mainly of heart failure with some cases of myocardial infarction. Cardiovascular disease is the major cause of increased mortality following general surgery in the elderly.

Impaired mental function and poor motivation are also barriers to postoperative rehabilitation. If concentration and short-term memory are poor, the patient may be unable to grasp the physiotherapist's instructions; episodes of mental confusion and agitation may also occur.

PRESCRIBING FOR THE ELDERLY

A general rule when prescribing drugs for the elderly is 'not too many and not too much'. Thus, while the elderly make up only 18% of the total population, they receive almost one-third of all prescriptions issued.

About 75% of persons over the age of 65 and living at home are taking some kind of medication, with 15%

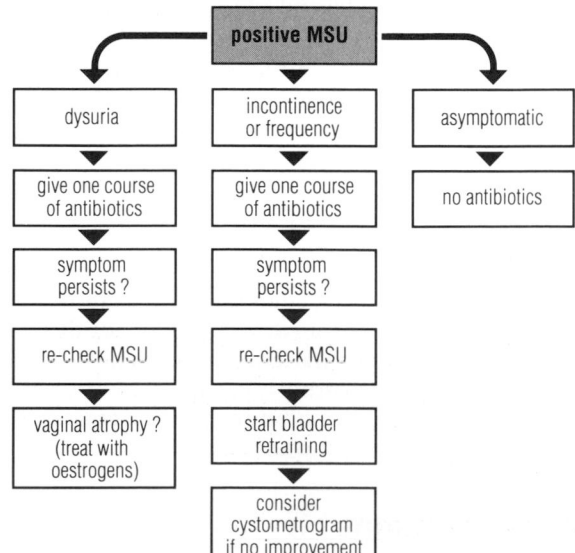

Fig. 9.11 Suggested approach to bacteriuria in elderly women.

receiving four drugs or more. However, multiple prescriptions increase the risk of drug interactions and adverse effects, and compliance is likely to be poor. Only in exceptional circumstances can the prescription of more than four drugs to an older person be justified.

Adverse reactions are two or three times more common in the elderly than in those under the age of 60. This is due primarily to slower rates of inactivation and excretion but also, with some drugs, to increased sensitivity of the target organ. Thus, many drugs need to be given in lower dosage.

Altered pharmacokinetics

Drug absorption

Changes in gastrointestinal function with increasing age include: a rise in gastric pH, decreased gastric emptying time, decreased splanchnic blood flow, and loss of small bowel mucosal surface area. Although these changes are theoretically rate-limiting for drug absorption, none appears to be important for passively absorbed drugs.

Distribution

There are a number of theoretically important changes that affect drug distribution in the elderly.

- A decrease in lean body mass and total body water reduces the distribution of water soluble drugs.
- Increase in body fat results in an increased volume of distribution of lipid-soluble drugs such as lignocaine, chlordiazepoxide and diazepam.
- The small decrease in plasma albumin that occurs in the elderly will reduce drug binding and may thus result in an increased distribution of the drug. Since it is the unbound fraction that is clinically active, there may be an increased pharmacological effect. This may be important in sick or malnourished patients who have a greater reduction in plasma albumin concentration.
- Conversely, if the drug binds predominantly to α-1 acid glycoprotein (e.g. lignocaine and disopyramide) then protein binding is likely to be normal, or even slightly increased, in the elderly.

Metabolism

There is a reduced rate of hepatic metabolism with increasing age. This reduces presystemic metabolism and causes a marked increase in the bioavailability of drugs metabolised by the liver, such as propranolol, labetalol, lignocaine, chlormethiazole and verapamil. In the case of propranolol, the age differences in plasma concentrations are large, with the mean concentration in the elderly about twice that found in the young. However, because of reduced sensitivity, the dosage need not be lowered. Age-related effects on drug metabolism are variable, so that even some extensively metabolised drugs, e.g. warfarin or diazepam, may show no change in clearance.

Excretion

Advancing age is accompanied by a reduction in both glomerular filtration rate and tubular function. At 60 years of age, renal function is about half that at age 30, and will be further impaired by dehydration, congestive cardiac failure and urinary retention, as well as by diseases such as diabetic nephropathy. Normal elderly persons may have significant reductions in glomerular filtration rate and tubular function yet have a normal blood urea and serum creatinine.

For those drugs excreted by glomerular filtration, the rate of excretion correlates with glomerular filtration rate. Some of these drugs, e.g. digoxin, gentamicin, lithium, cimetidine and chlorpropamide, have a low therapeutic index and their dosage therefore needs to be carefully chosen in the elderly. In general, a lower dose will be needed than in young patients. The drug plasma concentration should be measured.

Altered pharmacodynamics

The most clinically important result of altered pharmacodynamics occurs with drugs acting on the central nervous system. Sedatives and tranquillisers are more likely to produce drowsiness and hangover effects in the elderly. Although nitrazepam and diazepam have similar plasma concentrations in young and old, psychological testing shows that the elderly make more mistakes and have longer reaction times for 36 hours after a single dose. They also show increased sensitivity to anaesthetic agents such as halothane.

A reduced sensitivity to adrenergic agonists is seen in the elderly heart. Sensitivity to propranolol also decreases so that – despite the higher plasma propranolol concentrations seen in elderly subjects – the degree of beta blockade is reduced.

The dose of warfarin needed to produce anticoagulation in the elderly is reduced, but this is not due to an age-related rise in plasma warfarin concentration. Warfarin acts by inhibiting the synthesis of vitamin K-dependent clotting factors, and this inhibitory effect is greater in the elderly, resulting in an increased sensitivity.

Adverse reactions

Whenever a reduction in drug elimination or increase in receptor sensitivity occurs, there is the likelihood of an excessive drug effect and hence an adverse reaction. The risk of these adverse reactions increases with age (Fig. 9.12A). About 3% of all admissions to geriatric units in the UK are solely due to unwanted drug effects; in a further 8% of cases, an adverse reaction is a contributory cause. Two-thirds of all reactions are caused by two groups of drugs.

- Cardiovascular drugs – diuretics, digoxin and hypotensive drugs.
- Drugs acting on the central nervous system – anti-Parkinsonian drugs, antidepressants, hypnotics and tranquillisers.

Although more than 70% of patients taking the cardiovascular drugs make a full recovery from the adverse reaction, only 46% recover from the ill effects of anti-Parkinsonian drugs.

The risk of an adverse reaction increases with the number of drugs taken (Fig. 9.12B). Elderly persons are more likely to have multiple diseases than the young, and the likelihood of polypharmacy is therefore high. Not only is the patient apt to be muddled by a large number of drugs and inadvertently take the wrong dose; but drug interactions lead directly to an increased adverse reaction rate. This is particularly likely to occur when drugs with a low therapeutic index, e.g. anticoagulants, antidepressants, anticonvulsants and antihypertensives, are used in combination.

There are a number of important causes of adverse drug reaction in the elderly other than altered pharmacokinetics and pharmacodynamics. Inadequate clinical assessment is perhaps the most common. Dependent leg oedema, for example, is more often due to immobility rather than to congestive cardiac failure, and a diuretic is thus not an appropriate treatment. Similarly, old persons who complain of dizziness are often expressing a sensation of unsteadiness and fear of falling rather than true vertigo. Prochlorperazine – an effective vestibular sedative – is frequently prescribed in this situation but is quite useless and also carries a serious risk of Parkinsonian side effects.

Loneliness and social problems often present as minor aches and pains, unhappiness or insomnia. Although both difficult and time-consuming, it is far better to deal with the underlying problems than simply issue a number of drug prescriptions.

Compliance

There is no evidence that the elderly are less compliant than the young, but they do make more medication errors. These errors occur in up to three-quarters of old persons taking drugs, but only about a quarter are potentially serious, usually because of underdosage. Medication errors are more commonly made in patients over the age of 75 who are living alone and are confused. Poor visual acuity often prevents an old person from reading the instructions correctly, and impaired manual dexterity may make it difficult or even impossible to unscrew the cap on the bottle (particularly if it is one of the child-resistant types). Compliance can be improved, and errors in medication reduced, by careful counselling and an explanation of when and how to take the drug. Written instructions or a calendar pack can be helpful.

REHABILITATION

The aim of the rehabilitation team is to help restore maximum capability within the limits of the elderly patient's needs and disability.

Principles of rehabilitation

When setting a realistic rehabilitation goal, it is important to consider the patient's needs. For a very elderly and frail amputee, wheel-chair independence may be perfectly satisfactory, but this would not be acceptable for a fit 65-year-old amputee who is a keen golfer.

The principles of rehabilitation in the elderly are essentially the same as for young patients, but some special features of old age should be noted. Multiple pathology is likely to be present, so that the speed with which a stroke patient can be mobilised is often hampered by shortness of breath due to chronic lung or heart disease. The mental barriers to recovery may also be greater, whether due to dementia or to the increased feelings of passivity and dependence sometimes shown by older persons. There may be difficult social problems due to lack of family support or poor housing.

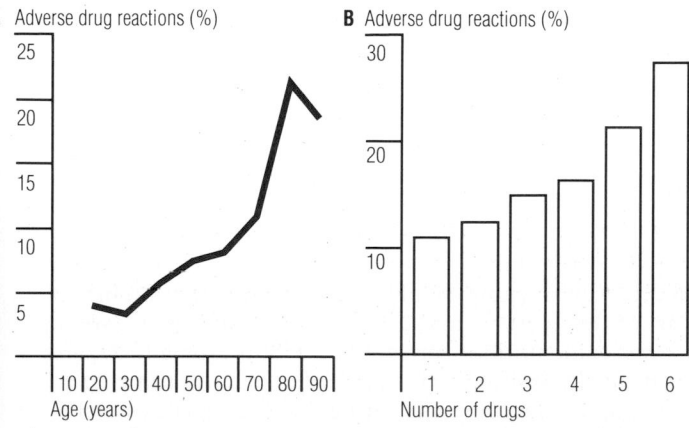

Fig. 9.12 Adverse drug reactions. A. The increase in adverse drug reactions with age. **B.** Prevalence of adverse reactions related to number of prescribed drugs. The risk in a patient taking only one drug is about 11% but is 27% if six drugs are taken.

Rehabilitation is concerned with helping the patient to learn to do things for him/herself: better for a stroke patient to spend half an hour trying to feed himself – even if most of the food ends up on the floor – than to have a well-meaning relative or nurse spoon it in with speed and efficiency. Patients enjoy exercising their painfully regained skills and it is essential to regain independence before leaving hospital and returning home.

The multidisciplinary team

The most effective approach to rehabilitation is through a multidisciplinary team, with each member contributing their special skills and working together with the patient and family towards an agreed goal. The team meets regularly to discuss the patient's progress and review future plans. With a good team, the patient is undergoing rehabilitation all the time and not just during the half an hour a day spent with the physiotherapist or occupational therapist. Although elderly patients can be successfully rehabilitated on a busy general medical ward, there are definite advantages in grouping them together in one ward. The nurses develop greater expertise, the pace of treatment can be better geared to the patient's needs, and it is easier to create an atmosphere of 24-hour-a-day rehabilitation. Correctly positioning a stroke patient is something all nurses and doctors should be aware of (Fig. 9.13).

Before discharge, the occupational therapist will take the patient on a home visit to see how well the patient copes in familiar surroundings. This also allows assessment of the need for a specific aid – e.g. a grab handle on the wall next to the lavatory – and the opportunity to have it fitted before the patient arrives home. The social worker has a valuable role to play over and above organising a home help or arranging a place in a residential home.

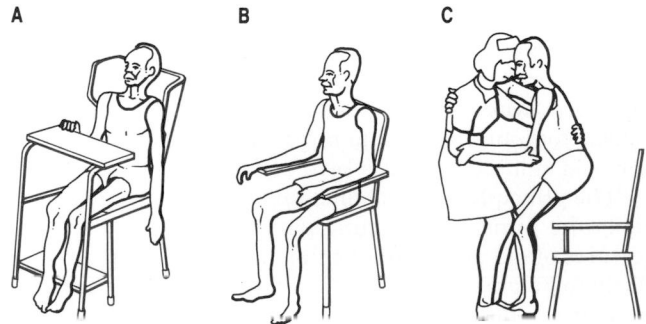

Fig. 9.13 Positioning the stroke patient. A. Incorrect. **B.** Correct. The forearm on the affected side should be supported and should point straight forwards with wrist and fingers extended and thumb abducted. The arm must not be allowed to hang from the shoulder in internal rotation. Choosing a suitable chair – with unrestricted view and with arm rests – is important. **C.** Transferring the stroke patient to a chair. Note the support given to the affected arm.

COMMUNITY CARE AND LONG-STAY CARE

In Western industrialised countries, there have been considerable changes in the way that these services are organised. In the UK these have followed the NHS and Community Care Act of 1990. The aim is to coordinate domiciliary, day care and respite services so that the old person can live in their own home for as long as possible and when that becomes no longer feasible they are cared for in private residential or nursing homes.

In the UK the practical details have still to be worked out. The aim is that an old person, living at home in need of support, has a case worker who identifies the patient's needs and plans a package of care. This may involve a home help, care assistant, district nurse, bathing attendant and meals on wheels. Respite care, to give the carers a break, may be arranged either at a local authority home or in the local geriatric department. Day care is available at local authority centres, where the needs are mainly social, or at the geriatric day hospital if the needs are medical. Geriatric day hospitals may be used either to investigate or to treat patients living at home and attendance sometimes avoids the need to admit a patient to hospital or, through close follow-up, may enable an early discharge from hospital.

If, despite full support, the patient is no longer coping at home, a decision will be made, following an assessment by a geriatrician, whether to admit the patient to a private residential or nursing home (which is paid for, like the package of care at home, by the local social services department). Long-stay hospital beds have now completely disappeared from some health districts in the UK although other districts retain a small number to improve the choice open to patients and to provide a refuge for those patients who are too physically or mentally disabled to be managed in a nursing home.

There is enthusiasm for these changes (a more efficient, coordinated and patient-orientated service) as well as uncertainty (particularly over the ability of social services to properly fund adequate numbers of residential or nursing home places). There are two points which should not be forgotten. First, the bulk of community care in the UK as in other countries is carried out by six million unpaid carers made up of relatives, friends and neighbours. Advising and helping these carers is an important part of the doctor's role. Secondly, the quality of care in long-stay institutions, private or NHS, is crucially dependent on the visiting doctor's vigilance and enthusiasm. This applies not only to ensuring that high quality nursing standards are maintained but that the environment for the patients is made homely, pleasant and comfortable as possible. The emphasis should be on educating patients to do as much for themselves as possible and physiotherapy and occupational therapy may be entirely appropriate for certain patients.

FURTHER READING

Almeida J, Fottrell E 1991 Management of the dementias. Reviews in Clinical Gerontology 1:267–281. *An excellent wide-ranging review*

Andrews K 1991 Rehabilitation of the older adult 2nd edn. Edward Arnold, London. *A good mix of practical advice and learned discussion*

Brocklehurst J C, Allen S C 1987 Geriatric medicine for students. Churchill Livingstone, Edinburgh. *A short introduction; good value for money*

Fairweather D S 1991 Ageing as a biological phenomenon. *Reviews in Clinical Gerontology 1: 3–16. A very readable short review*

Mandelstam D 1988 Understanding incontinence. Routledge, Chapman and Hall, Andover, Hants. *The best small book on the subject*

Seymour D J, Vaz F G 1987 Aspects of surgery in the elderly. British Journal of Hospital Medicine 37: 102–113. *Review article*

10
Psychological Medicine

Jeremy Holmes

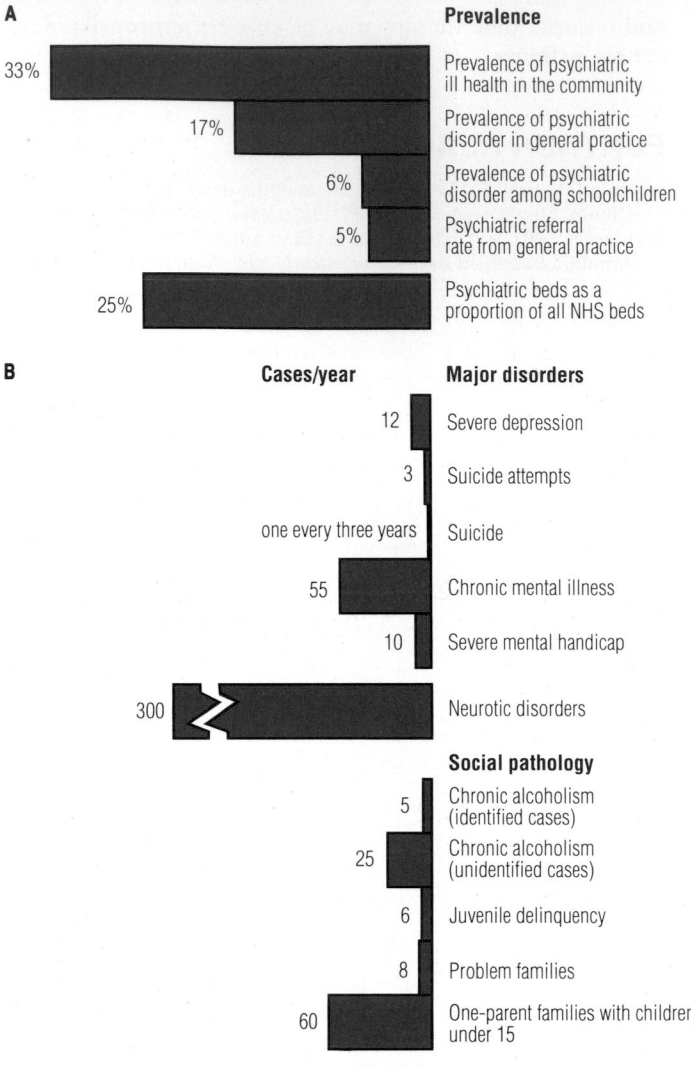

A Prevalence

33% — Prevalence of psychiatric ill health in the community

17% — Prevalence of psychiatric disorder in general practice

6% — Prevalence of psychiatric disorder among schoolchildren

5% — Psychiatric referral rate from general practice

25% — Psychiatric beds as a proportion of all NHS beds

B Cases/year — Major disorders

12 — Severe depression

3 — Suicide attempts

one every three years — Suicide

55 — Chronic mental illness

10 — Severe mental handicap

300 — Neurotic disorders

Social pathology

5 — Chronic alcoholism (identified cases)

25 — Chronic alcoholism (unidentified cases)

6 — Juvenile delinquency

8 — Problem families

60 — One-parent families with children under 15

Fig. 10.1 Epidemiology of psychiatric disorders. A. Prevalence of, and provision for, psychiatric ill health in the community. **B.** Cases per annum of various psychiatric disorders in a general practice population of 2500.

Psychiatric disease constitutes a large proportion of disability and illness within society (Fig. 10.1). Although in their origins psychiatry and medicine were not divided, from about 1850 onwards they went separate ways. Medicine became dominated by a powerful but sometimes narrow scientific approach, while psychiatry became increasingly isolated, both institutionally in the mental hospitals, and intellectually set apart from the rest of medical science through its low status and the esoteric nature of its subject matter. Part of the challenge of present-day psychiatry is to bring this division to an end. The large mental hospitals are closing and acute psychiatric illness is now treated in general hospital units and the community alongside the other medical disciplines. Patients and their illnesses are no longer seen by physicians purely as scientific puzzles to be solved; and psychological aspects of physical illness are, through *liaison psychiatry*, now recognised to be of great importance. Medical science is, in turn, making an increasingly important impact on psychiatric knowledge and practice. The basic disciplines underlying psychiatry are psychology, psychoanalysis and sociology; but biochemistry and the new genetics are making important contributions to the subject.

The central meeting ground for medicine and psychiatry is the *doctor-patient relationship*. All patients, whatever their illness, have feelings and fears which the doctor needs to understand and know how to handle. The *meaning* to the patient of a particular symptom – chest pain, for example, whether due to angina or anxiety in a 40-year-old man whose father died suddenly of a heart attack in middle age – needs to be *understood,* in order to appreciate its impact on the patient, as well as *diagnosed* and investigated. Psychiatry is concerned with meaning as well as explanation, and with methods of communication with the patient, as well as the technology of treatment.

Despite this intimate association with everyday medicine, many doctors find psychiatry difficult and confusing. This is partly because the subject is inherently complex and multifaceted, but also because psychiatry involves the doctor's own feelings and attitudes in a way that can often be avoided in other branches of medicine. In approaching psychiatry, doctors have to learn to deal not just with the patient, but also with themselves.

CLASSIFICATION AND OVERVIEW

A simple classification of psychiatric illness is summarised in Table 10.1. Psychiatry of old age is also considered in Chapter 9.

MINDS AND BRAINS

An eminent neurologist once stated that 'psychiatry is neurology without physical signs'. This would be true if psychiatry were simply concerned with the *brain* and its disorders, and the problem of psychiatric diagnosis and classification would, in this case, be no different from that of any other system of the body. A significant part of psychiatry is indeed concerned with diseases of the brain

Table 10.1 Classification of psychiatric illness

Organic syndromes	**Others**
Delirium	Addictions
Dementia	Alcohol
Intoxication and withdrawal syndromes	Drugs
	Eating disorders
Functional psychoses	Sexual dysfunction and deviation
Schizophrenia	
Manic-depressive psychosis	**Personality disorders**
Paranoid states	(Axis II in DSM)
	A. Paranoid
Neuroses	Schizoid
Anxiety	B. Antisocial
Phobias	(psychopathic)
Depression	Histrionic
Obsessive-compulsive neurosis	Borderline
Somatoform disorders	C. Avoidant
Conversion	Dependent
Somatisation	Obsessive-compulsive
Hypochondriasis	

– the organic psychoses such as confusional states for example, or the affective symptoms caused by adrenal disorders. The 19th century discovery that the psychosis known as general paralysis of the insane (GPI) was caused by syphilis, stimulated Emil Kraepelin to search for other physical causes of insanity, with the expectation that all mental illness would soon be found to be caused by diseases of the brain. The attempt has failed, not simply because brain research is difficult, but because psychiatry is concerned with *minds* as well as brains.

Mind has three main properties:

● the ability to experience emotions
● intentionality (i.e. having desires and goals)
● self-awareness.

Although psychiatric diagnosis approaches the mind as if it were an organ, this is often merely an analogy. When we speak of psychiatric illness we may be speaking about a brain disease, e.g. GPI, Alzheimer's disease or (possibly) some forms of schizophrenia, in the same way we speak of pneumonia as a disease of the lungs. On the other hand, while conditions such as personality disorders or agoraphobia are in some ways like illnesses, they also differ in many important respects because they affect the mind.

This important distinction between mind and brain may help to explain the discomfort which some feel when confronted with the essentially rather simple issue of psychiatric diagnosis. The categories of mental illness are few and not difficult to memorise. The main problem is philosophical rather than one of classification.

A number of other difficulties may also be encountered on first approaching psychiatry. Firstly, psychiatric diagnoses tend to be at a rather general level. They are *symptomatic/syndromic* rather than *pathological/specific*. The diagnosis of anxiety neurosis or schizophrenia bears more resemblance to that of heart failure than that of mitral stenosis.

Secondly, with the exception of the organic psychoses, the underlying pathology of psychiatric disorders is usually complex and *multifactorial*. This follows from the nature of mental phenomena. Just as there is usually no simple reason why an individual chooses medicine as a career, so there is rarely a single 'cause' of depression. There may be many explanations for a particular symptom or problem.

A third difficulty encountered in psychiatric diagnosis is that of deciding what is normal or abnormal, sometimes more a political or ethical question than a technical one. The doctor's own standards and feelings are involved in assessing a psychiatric patient. This also leads to two errors commonly made by psychiatric novices: either the student identifies the patient with himself, and so decides there is nothing much wrong; or identifies himself with the patient and worries that he must be psychiatrically ill!

(Please note that throughout this chapter 'he' is used to mean 'he or she'.)

Two systems of classification are widely used in psychiatry: *ICD* (international classification of diseases), which is favoured in Europe, and *DSM* (diagnostic and statistical manual), which has been developed in the USA by the American Psychiatric Association. The latter is interesting in that it is a multi-axial classification: Axis I diagnoses classify the psychiatric disorder; Axis II classify any personality disorder that may or may not accompany the psychiatric illness; while Axis III allows for the diagnosis of any concomitant physical disorder.

PSYCHOSIS AND NEUROSIS

The distinction between psychosis and neurosis is fundamental to psychiatric classification, although neither is easily defined on its own. The difference turns on four main issues:

- relationship to reality
- severity
- relationship to normality
- insight.

Relationship to reality

The essence of psychosis is that the patient loses contact with everyday reality. This may happen as a result of either hallucinations or delusions, or both.

Delusions and hallucinations are not a feature of neurosis. The neurotic's feelings and beliefs about himself may be distorted, but perception and understanding of the external world remains intact.

Hallucinations

An hallucination is a false perception. The patient undergoes a sensory experience in the absence of an external stimulus, for example hearing a voice when there is nobody there. For this to be diagnostic of psychosis it should be clear-cut; hearing an 'inner voice' which the person recognises as really part of himself is not an hallucination. An *illusion* should be distinguished from an hallucination in that it is an elaboration of a real percept, e.g. 'seeing faces in the fire', and is of less, if any, pathological significance. Any of the five senses may be involved in the patient's altered perception of reality.

Hearing. Auditory hallucinations are probably the commonest type of hallucination, found especially in paranoid states, in schizophrenia and occasionally in psychotic depression.

Sight. Contrary to popular belief, schizophrenic patients rarely 'see things'; visual hallucinations occur most commonly in drug and alcohol withdrawal states, temporal lobe epilepsy, and hysterical psychosis.

Smell and taste. Olfactory hallucinations are usually a sign of organic disease, e.g. temporal lobe seizures.

Touch. Tactile hallucinations are rare, but can occur in schizophrenia and drug withdrawal.

Hallucinations are not always a sign of pathology. After bereavement, visual or auditory hallucinations of the lost loved one are common.

Delusions

A delusion is a fixed and firmly held false belief. The patient's perceptions are unaltered, but his interpretation of them is, and is at variance with common experience. The patient sees people chatting at a bus-stop and is convinced they are talking about him, saying he is homosexual or a spy. These beliefs may be well concealed and not evident in superficial conversation.

We normally assume that our thoughts are private, that individuals are autonomous, that the non-human world is indifferent to our existence, that we are not in any special danger, and that we are not of any particular importance or interest to strangers. The deluded patient (e.g. in schizophrenia) has experiences which conflict with these everyday beliefs. The patient may feel that his thoughts can be interfered with from outside, or that his movements can be controlled by others; he may believe there is some special significance in the number plate of a passing car, that he is in great danger from hostile forces, or that television programmes or public events are caused by, or directed at, himself.

Severity

In general, psychotic disorders are more severe, more disabling and produce greater overall disturbance of mental functioning than neuroses. There are exceptions to this. An obsessional neurosis, for example in which the individual may spend many hours a day engaged in complicated washing or dressing rituals, can be incapacitating.

Relationship to normality

In psychosis there is a clear departure from normality. In contrast, minor neurotic symptoms, e.g. depression, anxiety, obsessional symptoms and hysteria, are common in normal people. The neurotic population is best seen as an extreme end of a normal distribution curve in which quantitative, but not qualitative change has taken place.

Insight

It is commonly stated that the difference between neurosis and psychosis is that the psychotic 'lacks insight'. The psychotic patient attributes his symptoms to reality

Summary 1 The distinction between psychosis and neurosis

Feature	Psychosis	Neurosis
Relationship to reality	Loss of contact with reality. Delusions and/or hallucinations	Perception of external reality intact. Problem is with the self
Severity	More severe, more global disturbance	Areas of normal function remain
Relationship to normality	Clear distinction between normal and psychotic experience	Represents extremes of normal difficulties
Insight	Usually lacking	Present

rather than illness, and cannot be persuaded out of these delusions or hallucinations; the neurotic, on the other hand, can usually see that his view of the world might be mistaken. However, while it is undoubtedly true that the psychotic lacks insight, there are several reasons for giving less prominence to insight than is customary. Firstly, if the psychotic is identified on the basis of a loss of touch with reality, then he will, by definition, lack insight. If the patient knew that his delusions or hallucinations were false, he would not be deluded or hallucinating. Secondly, the patient often tacitly accepts that he is ill by coming for help despite the apparent illogicality of complaining to a doctor about a delusion. Thirdly, the word 'insight' has two distinct meanings in psychiatry: one, given above, refers to the patient's relationship to reality and his illness; another more literal meaning refers to the ability to look into oneself and one's emotions and motives without denial or self-deception. While insight in this second sense may be desirable, it bears no relationship to the presence or absence of illness. It is possible to be perfectly healthy yet lack self-knowledge, or to be profoundly insightful yet mentally ill.

THE PSYCHOSES

Psychoses may be divided by their features and causes into two main groups: *organic* and *functional* (or, more accurately, 'of unknown origin'). In organic psychosis there is established biochemical, infective or structural brain disease. In functional psychosis no such disease process can be demonstrated. Organic psychoses can be divided into acute organic psychoses (also known as acute confusional states, delirium, or 'acute brain syndrome')

Summary 2 Classification of psychosis

Organic	Functional
Acute (delirum)	Manic-depressive psychosis
Chronic (dementia)	Schizophrenia

and chronic organic psychoses (also known as dementia and 'chronic brain syndrome') (see also Ch 22).

Functional psychosis vs. acute organic psychosis

It is essential to be able to distinguish functional psychoses from acute confusional states since the former require psychiatric, the latter medical, treatment. The key difference is the state of consciousness. In functional psychosis consciousness is clear, and patients fully orientated: it is possible to complete a complicated crossword puzzle while suffering from paranoid schizophrenia. In organic psychosis, however, there is almost always some disturbance of consciousness; this is usually variable ('fluctuating level of consciousness') and is often worse at night. Some causes of acute organic psychosis are given in Table 10.2.

Functional psychosis

One hundred years ago, Kraepelin divided the functional psychoses into two main groups: manic-depressive psychosis, and schizophrenia (or, as he called it, 'dementia praecox'). Manic-depressive psychosis is primarily a disorder of *mood*. The patient becomes psychotically depressed or elated ('unipolar manic-depression') or experiences episodes of both ('bipolar manic-depression'). There are usually periods of normality between episodes of illness. Schizophrenia is primarily a disorder of *thinking* and it produces, on the whole, a more severe and more general disturbance of mental functioning. The prognosis is less good than for manic-depression.

THE NEUROSES

Unlike psychosis, in neurosis the patient experiences no alteration of external reality. Instead, the patient is troubled by, and tries to avoid, some unacceptable aspect of himself or of his internal reality.

Table 10.2 Some causes of acute organic psychosis

Cause	Examples
Systemic infection	Malaria, HIV, pneumonia (especially in the elderly)
Metabolic disturbance	Electrolyte imbalance, renal failure, liver failure
Vitamin deficiency	Thiamine deficiency (Wernicke-Korsakoff syndrome in alcoholics, and beri-beri)
Endocrine	Hypoglycaemia, hypothyroidism, steroid administration
Drug intoxication	Anticonvulsants, hypnotics, anti-depressants, LSD, amphetamines
Intracerebral	CVA, subarachnoid haemorrhage, tumour, cerebral abscess
Withdrawal syndrome	DTs, benzodiazepine withdrawal

There are four main patterns of neurosis:

- anxiety neurosis and phobia
- depressive neurosis
- hysteria
- obsessive-compulsive neurosis.

Anxiety neurosis and phobia

Anxiety is an almost universal feature of all psychiatric illness. It is the psychic equivalent of pain. Anxiety is normally a response to external threat or unpredictability in the environment. In *anxiety neurosis*, the patient is not alerted and mobilised into action by anxiety, but is paralysed or overwhelmed by it. Where anxiety is experienced only in specific situations, the patient is said to suffer from a *phobia*. In phobic disorders the patient attempts to master anxiety by avoidance (e.g. an agoraphobic patient avoids public places).

Depressive neurosis

If anxiety is the psychic equivalent of pain, depression is the equivalent of disability (although anxiety can also of course be disabling, and depression intensely painful). In depression, the patient has lost not a limb or a function but a relationship. It is usually a person who is lost, but the 'lost object' can also be a job or a house, or the patient's own self-esteem. Depression can be seen as an attempt to avoid painful reality by withdrawal.

Hysteria

The basic themes of hysteria are *denial, dissociation, displacement* and *dependency*. The patient denies a painful conflict and thus avoids anxiety or depression, but at a price: she (most hysterical patients are female) dissociates herself from her feelings and displaces the latter into her body instead. Psychic pain is thereby converted into physical symptomatology, and the patient becomes dependent on doctors and others.

Obsessive-compulsive neurosis

Here the patient deals with anxiety – often aroused by fear of his own feelings of aggression, sexuality or wish for power or independence – by an attempt at control. A ritual action or a repetitive thought is performed over and over again in the magical hope that this will keep the patient safe from imagined danger. The patient knows it is absurd (thus has insight and is not psychotic), tries to resist, but still has, say, to wash in a particular way every morning to feel safe to start the day.

Summary 3 Classification of personality

Dimensional approaches
e.g. extrovert/introvert

DSM Categorisation

A. Paranoid	B. Antisocial	C. Avoidant
Schizoid	(psychopathic)	Dependent
	Borderline	Obsessive-compulsive
	Histrionic	

PERSONALITY DISORDER

Individuals are recognisable not just by their appearance but by their personality which, despite ageing and change, remains relatively constant through time.

Personalities can be classified dimensionally or categorically. A dimensional approach is exemplified by Hans Eysenk who, following his intellectual opponent Jung, devised a method for assessing personalities along the dimensions of *extrovert* (outgoing, gregarious, stimulus-seeking) and *introvert* (inner-directed, shy, stimulus-avoiding).

The problem of differentiating between normal and abnormal personality is even more difficult than for neurosis. There are undoubtedly individuals whose personalities are very unusual, at least in the statistical sense, but they are not necessarily abnormal. An alternative approach to the classification of personality uses psychiatric categories to describe different types of individual. The *schizoid personality*, for example, is withdrawn and aloof, preoccupied with material objects or intellectual pursuits rather than people, lacking in close emotional contact, and is defensive and easily hurt. These features may only be a personality trait, and may even be advantageous: many creative people have schizoid tendencies. However, when taken to extremes they become a personality disorder. Here, the individual is so handicapped by his personality that he seeks, or is brought for, help, e.g. the schizoid personality who suffers from severe social isolation.

Unlike psychosis and neurosis, a personality disorder is not an illness. Its features date back to childhood or adolescence and so there is no premorbid period of normality. However, personality disorder often co-exists with, and may predispose to, psychiatric illness. Personality disorders are grouped in DSM into three main types. Group A have some of the features of schizophrenia and paranoia, but without any overt signs of psychosis. They may, however, predispose to a psychotic illness, and eventually develop into one. Thus the paranoid personality may, in later life, develop *paraphrenia*. Group B are patients with social difficulties that often bring them into conflict with authority. For *histrionic* personality disorder, see page 192, and for *antisocial* personality disorder, page 203. Group C are neurotic personalities typified by anxiety, avoidance of threat or challenge, and dependent relationships. An example is that of *obsessional personality disorder*. Here the individual is meticulous, controlled, orderly and rigid, and may find the sloppiness of others unbearable. Such characteristics may be advantageous in certain circumstances, e.g. the armed forces or the operating theatre, but may also bring the individual into conflict with others when flexibility is needed, e.g. under stress and in intimate relationships.

THE CAUSES OF PSYCHIATRIC ILLNESS

The complexity of the interactions underlying psychiatric illness can be confusing. A causal model of the type 'one pathogen–one disease' rarely applies in psychiatry.

There are three types of causal factor in psychiatric illness: genetic/biochemical; developmental; and social. All play at least some role in most psychiatric disturbance, and part of the art of psychiatry lies in assigning the appropriate weight to each factor and identifying which may be the most important.

Genetic/biochemical ('organic')

Occasionally a single genetic defect can determine a psychiatric illness, e.g. the psychiatric manifestations of Huntington's chorea. However, although genetic inheritance may, as in schizophrenia, be a necessary cause of illness, it is rarely sufficient. Biochemical, viral, immunological and nutritional factors may well be important in a number of psychiatric illnesses; few have so far been convincingly demonstrated as a unique cause.

Developmental ('intrapsychic')

Each individual is a product of, and in a sense contains and continues, his past. Psychological development, especially that shaped by early childhood experience and family relationships, plays a crucial part in determining personality and ways of reacting to stress in later life.

Social ('interpersonal')

Many psychiatric illnesses are triggered by recent social events, such as bereavement, divorce or unemployment. The patient's social and family situation can play a major role in both initiating his illness and helping or hindering his capacity to recover. The quality of family relationships is itself influenced by the personality, which is in turn a product of both genetic and developmental factors.

THE PSYCHIATRIC EXAMINATION

The psychiatric examination, although similar to the medical examination insofar as it is a systematic gathering and ordering of fact and observations, is unique in a number of important ways. First, it consists of a detailed account of a person's biography and current circumstances. Second, in gathering the history the interviewer uses a much more open style than is usual in the closed-question, 'checklist', approach of conventional history-taking. The 'facts' of psychiatry are often feelings and these are often most effectively elicited by open questions such as 'how do you feel about...?' or 'what was the worst moment...?'. Third, the interviewer's own reactions and thoughts, rather than being put aside, should be recognised as relevant data to be noted and recorded. The interviewer should maintain a non-judgemental, balanced, compassionate but neutral position. The interviewer should also be gentle but firm and should not avoid eliciting material (e.g. sexual or traumatic) that may be painful for the patient simply because of his own scruples or anxiety.

The *psychiatric history,* which may have to be supplemented by interviewing close friends or relations, should include the following.

- *Reason for referral.* Did the patient ask for help, were they encouraged to seek it, and if so by whom, or were they brought unwittingly or unwillingly to the doctor?
- *History of present complaint.* A detailed account, as far as possible in the patient's own words, of what he/she experiences as 'wrong', unusual or bizarre, or would like to change in his/her life.
- *Previous psychiatric and medical history.*
- *Drug and alcohol history.*
- *Family history.* A detailed description of the patient's 'family of origin' and 'family of procreation' (if they have one) can conveniently be recorded in the form of a family tree or 'genogram'.
- *Personal history.* Detailed biography, starting at birth, recording all significant memories and events, including early separations, family atmosphere, school experiences and achievements, work history, psychosexual and marital history.
- *Personality.* A person's likes and dislikes, interests, attitudes and aptitudes should be recorded to establish a premorbid state against which to evaluate the present condition.

MENTAL STATE EXAMINATION

This is a systematic compilation of the abnormal phenomena observed and elicited by the interviewer or complained about by the patient.

- *General appearance and behaviour.* How is the patient dressed? How does the patient relate to the interviewer – relaxed and friendly, or suspicious and taciturn? Does the patient sit immobile in the chair or is he/she fidgety and restless?

- *Speech.* Is the speech normal in form and content, slowed down or accelerated? Does it follow a logical progression, jumping from idea to idea ('flight of ideas'), or is there evidence of a disorder of the logical progression of thoughts?
- *Mood.* Is the mood normal, depressed or elated? Is the person troubled by feelings of guilt and unworthiness and suicidal thoughts, or is the patient grandiose and overexcited? Is the patient anxious or agitated?
- *Abnormal beliefs (delusions).* Does the patient feel he/she is being spied on, talked about or got at? Are his/her thoughts or actions being interfered with?
- *Abnormal experiences (hallucinations).* Has the patient had any bizarre or unusual sensations? Is the patient hearing noises or voices when no-one is around?
- *Cognitive assessment* (for mini-mental state examination, see p. 862). What is the general level of intelligence? Is there evidence of impairment of consciousness, immediate memory or recall? Is the patient fully oriented in time, place and person?
- *Insight.* What is the patient's self-appraisal and theory about what is happening to him/her?
- *Response of the interviewer.* How does the patient make the interviewer feel? Sympathy? Anger? Irritation? Boredom?

The examination should be concluded by a *formulation* containing the salient points of the history and mental state, with a differential diagnosis and some ideas about possible aetiological and precipitating factors.

ANXIETY

Anxiety, like pain, is an unpleasant necessity. A person unable to feel anxious would be severely incapacitated. Arousal, which may be experienced subjectively as anxiety, leads to an adaptive response to threat: fight or flight.

AROUSAL AND ANXIETY

There are three main components of the arousal response:

- psychophysiological
- psychological
- interpersonal.

The psychophysiological component

This is mediated by the autonomic nervous system and is accompanied by increased adrenalin, noradrenalin and corticosteroid secretion. These result in: tachycardia, piloerection, sweating and pupillary dilatation; and subjective manifestations of autonomic activity including paraesthesiae, giddiness, 'butterflies in the stomach',

---

Summary 4 Manifestations of anxiety	
Physical	*Psychological*
Tachycardia	Irritability
Tightness/pain in chest	Inability to memorise
Difficulty in breathing	Inability to concentrate
Headache	Fear of impending death
Paraesthesia	Fear of madness
Muscular pains	(depersonalisation)
Muscular weakness	
Dizziness	
Difficulty in swallowing	
Abdominal discomfort	
Diarrhoea	
Frequency	

breathing difficulties, a sensation of painful pressure in the chest, and muscular tension, especially around the head and neck. These symptoms may be mistakenly attributed by both patients and doctors to organic illness.

The psychological component

There is a continuum of arousal responses to threat, running from alertness and readiness, through mild fear, to severe anxiety and incapacitating panic. Effective action depends on an optimal state of arousal; little can be achieved when an individual is either barely aroused or in a state of panic. Examination nerves, if not too great, improve results.

During a panic attack, the patient experiences a sense of threat, or even of impending death. Chronic anxiety states may produce irritability, lack of concentration and a subjective sense of failing memory. Anxious patients fail to habituate to stimuli and so remain chronically over-aroused; this can result in extreme sensitivity to sudden noises or movements. In extreme anxiety, a state of detachment may supervene in which anxiety suddenly disappears, to be replaced by a feeling of being outside of oneself *(depersonalisation)* and cut off from one's surroundings, which appear unreal and distant *(derealisation)*. These experiences may be misinterpreted by the patient as signs of 'going mad'.

The interpersonal component

A frightened individual clings to those he loves and on whom he depends. This is part of 'attachment behaviour' and, like anxiety, is adaptive: species survival depends on secure bonding. The dependency and excessive demands on others that so often accompany anxiety states (and can be trying to both relatives and doctors) can be understood as part of the attachment response to threat.

ANXIETY SYNDROMES

Anxiety may be a primary diagnosis, or secondary to a psychiatric or physical illness. It is a non-specific symptom which occurs in a wide range of psychiatric syndromes, including benzodiazepine withdrawal, depression, alcoholism and schizophrenia. It can also be an important manifestation of organic illness, particularly thyrotoxicosis, paroxysmal tachycardia, carcinoid syndrome, hypoglycaemic attacks, phaeochromocytoma, and temporal lobe seizures.

CLASSIFICATION

Primary anxiety syndromes may be classified as shown in Table 10.3.

Generalised anxiety

Individuals who experience anxiety symptoms, either chronically or intermittently, without a clear stimulus or an obvious focus of fear suffer so-called 'free-floating' anxiety.

Situational anxiety

In situational anxiety there is an identifiable precipitant to which the anxiety is related. Phobias are closely related to anxiety syndromes because in a phobia the patient avoids the feared situation and is thus restricted by the underlying anxiety. Situational anxiety syndromes include:

- *Specific phobias*, e.g. snake or spider phobia or fear of heights. These have a good prognosis, are found in otherwise healthy individuals and respond well to behavioural treatment (p. 174).
- *Agoraphobia* is named after the Greek *agora*, or meeting place. In agoraphobia the patient is frightened to leave home unaccompanied, avoids public places like supermarkets and department stores and cannot travel on public transport, especially underground railways and aeroplanes. (Claustrophobia is usually part of agoraphobia.) The patient is usually female and may be very dependent on her mother, daughter or husband. The prognosis is less good than with specific phobias, but behaviour therapy can be helpful. Agoraphobic symptoms may develop as part of a depressive illness (p. 177).
- *Social phobia*, fear of meeting people in social situations, e.g. parties, canteens. This affects mainly young people and is an extreme form of normal 'shyness'. Patients can be helped by social skills training in groups with fellow-sufferers in which they 'role-play' the feared situations.
- *Hypochondriasis*, a morbid fear of illness, leading to a frequent need for reassurance by family, friends and doctors.

Panic attacks (hyperventilation syndrome)

These may be part of a specific syndrome, e.g. agoraphobia, or may occur on their own. They frequently present to physicians as medical emergencies and are usually self-limiting. The patient presents in a state of terror, over-breathing, complaining of chest pain and often feeling he is dying. The diagnosis can be established by provoking these symptoms by voluntary overbreathing, which are then relieved by rebreathing from a paper bag. Tetany may be a feature. Organic causes (e.g. hyperthyroidism) must be eliminated and a positive psychiatric history should be established (i.e. a history of recent stress/conflict or background of chronic difficulty).

Aetiology

There is no single cause of anxiety syndrome. Individuals vary in their tendency to become over-aroused: *genetic factors* may play a part in this. Anxiety may also arise from *faulty learning*. A child who senses his mother's tension in social situations may become socially phobic himself. Repeated avoidance of a feared stimulus then exaggerates the threat associated with it, since there is no opportunity for mastery through repeated exposure.

Attachment theory explains how early childhood relationships may predispose to anxiety in later life. A developing child must, in order to survive, bond to an attachment figure (usually the mother). If the mother is consistently present, reliable in her handling and 'good

Table 10.3 Classification of anxiety syndromes

Primary anxiety	Secondary anxiety
Generalised	Psychiatric illness, e.g. depression
Situational	Organic illness, e.g. thyrotoxicosis
Agoraphobia	Alcohol-related withdrawal symptoms
Social phobia	Benzodiazepine-related withdrawal
Hypochondriasis	symptoms
Specific (e.g. spiders)	
Panic attacks	
(hyperventilation syndrome)	

enough' in her emotional responsiveness, then a bond of secure attachment will develop. This enables the child to engage in exploratory behaviour, to deal with new situations without becoming over-anxious, and so gradually to separate, safe in the knowledge that the mother is available if necessary. The child builds up an internal image of a good parent which provides a sense of security. If, on the other hand, the early relationship with the parent is disrupted – by separation or by inconsistent handling, for example – the child may develop a bond of anxious attachment. Rather than being able to explore and become autonomous, the child clings to the mother, at first physically and later emotionally, showing signs of distress when separation is threatened. This childhood experience then acts as a template for separations in later life. Faced with threat, the anxious individual clings to attachment figures – spouse, parent, child or doctor.

The following factors should be considered in cases of anxiety:

- *The nature of the current external threat.* This may be obvious, such as major illness in the patient or a close relative. The 'threat' may, on the other hand, appear as trivial or 'normal' as an adolescent leaving home, or a family holiday. For an anxiously attached individual these can be major hurdles.
- *The relationship to attachment figures, past and present.* A pattern of anxious attachment in childhood, now repeated in relationship to spouse or children, is often found.
- *'Internal threat'.* Anxious patients often experience an inner conflict between their need for dependency and their feelings about those on whom they depend. The patient is threatened not so much by external circumstances as by himself. A patient who feels angry, for example with an unfaithful spouse, but is unable to express this because of fear of separation and loss, may develop anxiety symptoms. He fears to bite the hand that feeds. The patient is frightened by his own inner impulses: sexual or aggressive feelings, or the wish for independence and autonomy. Anger in particular often co-exists with anxiety; the angry patient is often a frightened one and vice versa.

MANAGEMENT

Michael Balint, a psychoanalyst who pioneered the use of psychotherapeutic methods in medicine, wrote 'the doctor is a drug: the question is in what dose, and with what frequency it should be prescribed'. The two drugs most commonly prescribed for anxiety are tranquillisers and 'doctor'. Both can be effective in the short term, but can in the long term produce the complication of dependence, and may even exacerbate the symptoms of anxiety.

Exploratory psychotherapy

Normal individuals who become anxious are usually relieved of their fears by *reassurance,* and the ability to reassure is thus an important part of a doctor's skill. Reassurance in neurotic individuals is often ineffective, however, because it deals only with the surface fear and not with the underlying conflict. A man who develops repeated attacks of pain, in which he is convinced that he is about to die of a heart attack, can be reassured that his ECG is normal and that he is a fit man, and be discharged. Yet a few days later, he may develop another attack and present again to the doctor. *The underlying fear,* and root cause of his anxiety, of which he may be unaware or unconscious, may be that his mother, on whom he is very dependent and who has recently had an illness, will die and that he will be left alone. Only when this fear is exposed and when he has learned to accept the dependent part of himself, will his panic attacks cease.

This kind of exploration is helpful in the evaluation of most cases of anxiety. In some cases, it may need to be followed by longer-term psychotherapy. If the patient can learn to resolve his inner conflicts through his relationship with a doctor or therapist, and so move from a position of anxious attachment to one of secure attachment, he will be relieved of the symptoms.

Cognitive–behavioural psychotherapy

In exploratory psychotherapy the doctor aims to be understanding, but is non-directive. In behavioural psychotherapy, on the other hand, the doctor aims to change the patient's behaviour directly. A phobic patient *associates* the feared stimulus (e.g. a spider or department store) with unpleasant feelings. The therapy aims to *desensitise* the patient by gradual exposure to the feared stimulus, often in the reassuring presence of the therapist. An important feature of behavioural treatment for anxiety is *relaxation training.* Here the patient learns to control anxiety through muscular relaxation and deep breathing, sometimes with the aid of tape-recorded instructions. Physiological measures of arousal – galvanic skin response and pulse rate – may provide objective evidence of anxiety

Summary 6 Management of anxiety syndromes	
Exploratory psychotherapy	Exploration and resolution of underlying conflict. Non-directive.
Cognitive–behavioural psychotherapy	Aims to change patients' behaviour directly, through desensitisation, and/or challenge their underlying assumptions.
Psychotropic drugs	Antidepressants Minor tranquillisers Beta-blockers

reduction. When self-administered, this is known as *autogenic training*.

In cognitive therapy the patient's underlying assumptions and view of the world are challenged: for example, someone with fear of flying is asked to consider rationally the probabilities of an aircraft crashing and to compare them with accident rates for road and rail travel. Their tendencies to *catastrophise* (i.e. fear the worst) and *dichotomise* (divide the world into black and white, good and bad) are pointed out, and alternative strategies suggested.

Psychotropic drugs

When anxiety is a manifestation of depressive illness, the treatment of depression with antidepressants (many of which are sedative) also relieves the anxiety. Short-term (up to 10 days) prescription of minor tranquillisers such as benzodiazepines is occasionally justified for the relief of stress-related anxiety. Longer-term prescription of tranquillisers should be avoided. Beta-receptor blocking drugs relieve the peripheral symptoms of anxiety and may also occasionally be useful. Side-effects of benzodiazepines are common (see Table 10.4) (see also p. 43).

DEFENCE MECHANISMS

Life is beset with threat. A variety of social and psychological defence mechanisms exist which keep anxiety within manageable limits. Many of these can be observed on hospital wards, where both patients and staff face the daily threat of illness and death and yet usually manage to remain cheerful and efficient.

Denial

'Everything's wonderful'.

One way of dealing with fear or pain is simply to pretend it does not exist. Men are particularly prone to this in everyday life, but false cheerfulness (sometimes known as *manic denial*) may conceal unvoiced fears or sadness.

Table 10.4 Side-effects of benzodiazepines

Tolerance
Drowsiness
Incoordination, ataxia
Emotional blunting
Anger and irritability
Diminished sexual response (women)
Withdrawal syndrome: insomnia
anxiety
depression (may be profound)
irritability
muscular pains and twitching
perceptual distortion
fits

Dissociation or conversion

'I'm not worried about anything doctor, it's just that I keep getting this pain...'.

Akin to denial is dissociation, in which a fear is displaced or converted into a bodily symptom. Patients who have inexplicable and elusive pains, in addition to established physical disease, may well be harbouring unspoken fears and conflicts.

Splitting

'You're wonderful doctor, not like those terrible doctors at the other hospital'.

As Trojans should fear Greeks bearing gifts, so doctors should beware the patient who heaps excessive praise (as opposed to expressing genuine gratitude). The patient may be dealing with anxiety by splitting his world into good and bad, and clinging to the good in the vain hope of absolute security. As with the Trojans, the tables may suddenly turn and *we* may be seen as bad, and *they* good. Patients can sometimes split ward staff in this way; physicians and nurses must learn to take both praise and condemnation with a pinch of salt.

Projection

'It's the psychiatrists who are mad, not me'.

Closely linked to splitting is projection, in which unwanted feelings are attributed instead to a convenient other.

Idealisation

'The doctors here are the best in the world'.

The defence of idealisation is closely linked to splitting and projection. It is probably best seen as an example of positive *transference*, in which past childhood feelings towards one's parents are, under the threat of illness, transferred on to present medical attendants.

Regression

'Nurse...nurse...'.

The sick, like children, are tucked up in bed, fed, pampered and waited on. This sometimes helps the physiology of recovery, but can also lead to helpless behaviour on the part of the patient, who may deal with the fear

---

Summary 7 Defence mechanisms against anxiety

- Denial
- Dissociation or conversion
- Splitting
- Projection
- Idealisation
- Regression
- Obsessional defence
- Intellectualisation

associated with illness by becoming more and more child-like, regressed and demanding.

Obsessional defences

'I always have my bowels open at such-and-such o'clock doctor'.

The *'malade-à-petit-papier'*, the patient who presents with a written list of symptoms, is a familiar figure in medical folklore. The obsessional defence is an attempt to deal with fear by *control*. This may produce feelings of irritation and discomfort in the doctor that mirror the way the patient feels. This is an example of how the doctor's subjective response to the patient (technically known as *counter-transference*) can be a useful guide to what the patient is feeling.

Intellectualisation

'Just a few more tests should clinch the diagnosis'.

This defence applies more to doctors than their patients. Incurable illness and death are inescapable reminders of the limitations of medicine. The feelings of inadequacy and sadness that this creates may be defended against by preoccupation with diagnostic precision and excessive investigation and treatment.

LOSS, GRIEF AND BEREAVEMENT

Man is not an island, and human beings are inevitably vulnerable to loss. The mourning response – a patterned sequence of psychophysiological reactions to the loss of a loved one – is as deeply embedded in our psyche as are the phases of inflammation in our pathophysiology. Common to both are the experience of pain, immobility and gradual recovery.

MOURNING

The mourning response is divided for convenience into a number of stages, which can be summarised as *denial*, *despair* and *detachment*, but emotional reality does not conform to any such neat sequence. Grief is characterised by surges and cycles of often confused feelings rather than an orderly progression of recognisable developments.

Denial

The initial reaction, especially to sudden bereavement, may be denial: 'Oh no...'. This attempt to resist the reality of death may persist long after the bereaved have consciously and rationally accepted their loss; they find themselves talking to their lost loved one, or may 'hear' or

'see' them in one of the hallucinatory experiences that occur after bereavement.

Numbness

Another early response to bereavement is a complete absence of feeling. The bereaved person may appear to be coping very well because of this emotional shutdown, which, like the analgesia of a soldier injured in battle, enables him to get through the initial phase of loss. When this is prolonged, however, it produces chronic impoverishment of emotional life.

Searching

Part of the 'work' of grief involves a mental combing-through of events leading up to the loss of the loved one. This phase is often accompanied by intense anxiety and restlessness. Searching, a form of separation anxiety, may lead to apparently aimless wandering or visits to familiar spots associated with the lost one. The bereaved person appears to be struggling to negate the reality of the loss, or to rewrite history with a different, happy ending. Acceptance of loss only occurs when this impossible task has been attempted countless times.

Guilt

Pangs of guilt or self-blame are a very common feature of bereavement. Survivors blame themselves, often quite irrationally, for the loss of their beloved. 'If only', they say, 'I had phoned the doctor earlier/not gone on holiday/been kinder...'. This response can be seen as an example of *omnipotence*, a relic of childish thinking which attempts to deny human vulnerability to fate and fortune.

Anger

Anger and guilt go together in bereavement. Outbursts of anger towards medical staff or close relatives often occur after a death, and should be met by acknowledgement of the underlying pain rather than retaliation.

Detachment

As mourning proceeds, so the grieving individual begins to separate himself from the loss and develop new interests and attachments. Pangs of grief recur, particularly at times of stress and on special dates like birthdays, Christmas, and anniversaries of loss.

Acceptance

When mourning is 'successful' and circumstances favourable, the bereaved individual may come to accept that death and loss are part of life and may even be enriched by the experience. This mature state is rare. More usually, scars remain, and many bereaved people continue to struggle with feelings of meaninglessness and diminished vitality for many years.

Physiological changes

Psychological reactions to loss are accompanied by physiological changes, including disturbance of corticosteroid metabolism and depression of T lymphocyte response. Death from 'a broken heart' is a reality: mortality rates, mainly from coronary artery disease, are higher in widowers and widows than their non-bereaved counterparts.

DELAYED OR PATHOLOGICAL MOURNING

Return to near-normality after a major loss generally takes from nine to 18 months. However, chronic states of depression, numbness, anger, anxiety and hopelessness can continue for much longer following a bereavement. The patient becomes stuck in one of the phases of mourning and is unable to progress towards detachment and acceptance.

The likelihood of pathological grief depends on four main factors:

- *Type of death.* A sudden, untimely (for example, of a child) or horrifying death is especially hard to accept.
- *Nature of the relationship.* An *ambivalent* relationship (one in which love and hate co-exist) is more likely to lead to pathological mourning than a straightforward one. Feelings of guilt (associated perhaps with past phantasy-wishes that the person would die) are more intense in such cases. 'Symbiotic' relationships, such as those involving unmarried daughters living with their mothers, are also often difficult to recover from when they are severed.
- *Personality of the survivor.* Dependent, insecure or depression-prone individuals are more vulnerable to prolonged grief, as are those with difficulty in expressing feelings. The latter may in part account for the greater vulnerability of men to lasting problems after bereavement.

Summary 8 Mourning responses

- Denial
- Numbness
- Searching
- Guilt
- Anger
- Detachment
- Acceptance

- *Social circumstances of the survivor.* The lack of close family, friends, religious beliefs or employment all make recovery from loss more difficult.

MANAGEMENT

About one-third of bereaved persons may be in need of professional support or intervention. Support groups, such as those for widows or for parents whose children have died, can be very helpful. Brief psychotherapy may be necessary in order to recapture and work through buried feelings associated with the loss. Sometimes this is systematised as *guided mourning*, in which the sufferer is encouraged to think about his lost one, talk about the details of his or her death, look at photographs of him or her, visit the grave, and so face and accept loss with diminished denial.

DEPRESSION

The complaint of 'depression' can refer to a number of different feelings and reactions – anger, boredom, frustration, anxiety, hopelessness and helplessness – as well as the specific psychophysiological state which psychiatry recognises as 'depressive illness'.

DEPRESSIVE ILLNESS

Clinical features

Clinical depression can be distinguished from both 'ordinary' depression or sadness (transient depressive moods) and depressive personality by three main features:

- Depressive illness is a *sustained* depression of mood lasting for weeks or months.
- The *severity* of the depression is great enough to interfere with normal functioning.
- The depression has a definite onset with a distinct *change* from normal to depressive thinking.

Summary 9 Features of depressive illness (as opposed to unhappiness)

- Sustained lowering of mood
- Severe
- Definite onset
- Depressed mood
- Low self-esteem
- Physiological changes: disturbance of sleep, appetite, weight, libido
- Sometimes atypical features brought to the surface by depressive illness: pain, obsessional thoughts, violence

---

Depressive illness involves an alteration of many different aspects of mind, body and behaviour. It is nearly twice as common in women as in men. The features of depression may be summarised under four main headings:

- *Depressed mood.* The patient feels weepy and miserable, 'low-in-spirits', anxious, lacking in concentration and irritable, and takes no pleasure in anything. The patient feels he has no future and that it is pointless or impossible to make plans. Suicide attempts are common and thoughts of suicide almost invariably present, although the patient may try to resist these by saying 'I would not have the courage'.
- *Low self-esteem.* The patient feels worthless, inadequate, unwanted and useless. He feels intense guilt and plagues himself with thoughts of past failures and mistakes. He can only see himself in a negative light and emphasises his weaknesses and faults.
- *Physiological changes.* The most important of these is sleep disturbance. Anorexia, weight loss, loss of libido, constipation, retardation (slowing of thought and movement) or occasional agitation are all important features, especially in severe or psychotic depression.
- *'Atypical' features.* Sometimes a depressed patient may present atypically, with physical symptoms such as unexplained pain, obsessional thoughts, agoraphobia, criminal behaviour (such as shoplifting) or episodes of anger and violence. These may have been brought to the surface by a depressive illness. In a so-called 'smiling' or 'masked' depression, the patient conceals severe depressive feelings behind a cheerful facade.

Although the presentation of depressive illness can vary greatly, there are two common clinical pictures (Table 10.5).

Neurotic depression

Here the patient, despite depressive feelings, remains in contact with reality: 'I know it is stupid, but I feel *as though* I have let everybody down'. The patient might be a woman in her thirties with several small children, living in poor housing and with a husband who drinks and is having an affair which she has just discovered. She is tearful, has lost weight and cannot fall asleep at night. She feels she is not coping with her job or housework, and no longer enjoys company or television.

Psychotic depression

Depressive psychosis is a part of manic-depressive psychosis, an *affective psychosis*. The depth of the depression is here much greater than in neurotic depression.

Table 10.5 Clinical features of neurotic and psychotic depression

Clinical features	Psychotic	Neurotic
Severity of depression	More severe	Less severe
Delusion/hallucinations	Yes	No
Sleep disturbance	Early morning wakening	Difficulty in getting off to sleep
'Vegetative features', e.g. weight loss, constipation	Yes, prominent	Yes/No
Diurnal mood variation	Worse on wakening and a.m.	No, or worse p.m.
'Reactive', i.e. precipitated by loss	Yes	Yes
Genetic factors, e.g. family history of manic-depressive psychosis	Yes	No
Dexamethasone suppression tests	Sometimes	No
Response to tricyclic antidepressants	Yes	Yes
Response to ECT	Yes	No

The ratio of women to men affected is more equal. The patient becomes immobilised both in thought and action. He wakes very early in the morning and may have diurnal mood variation, feeling at his worst in the morning and improving slightly towards the evening. Depressive delusions develop, the patient becoming convinced that he has, for example, brought ruin on his family, that he is evil or ugly or radioactive. Depressive hallucinations may occur: the patient may hear a voice telling him that he is evil, or he may feel that his insides are rotting and complain that he smells. Endocrine disturbance may occur in psychotic depression, with disruption of the pituitary–adrenal axis. The normal diurnal variation of cortisol output is abolished, providing the basis of the *dexamethasone suppression test.* Dexamethasone is administered but fails to reduce urinary steroid levels in many, but not all, cases of severe/psychotic depression.

DIFFERENTIAL DIAGNOSIS OF DEPRESSION

The differential diagnosis of depression includes:

- *organic illness,* especially hypothyroidism
- *drug administration,* especially steroids and some antihypertensive drugs
- *alcohol-induced depression,* where depression is secondary to alcoholism (or drug addiction), and withdrawal of the intoxicant results in lifting of depressive symptoms

Summary 10 Factors contributing to depression

- Loss
- Genetic
- Biochemical, e.g. reduced catecholamine levels at postsynaptic nerve endings
- Social, e.g. lack of close relationships, unemployment, lack of good childhood experiences to build self-esteem, learned helplessness.

- *anxiety states,* as anxiety is a common feature of depression. When they co-exist, treatment of the depression usually, but not always, removes the anxiety
- *depressive psychoses,* which must be distinguished from other psychoses, especially schizophrenia.

THE CAUSES OF DEPRESSION

Depression is often divided into:

- *Reactive depression,* whose symptoms correspond with neurotic depression and which is said to be a response to external events
- *Endogenous depression,* where the symptoms are psychotic in character and where there is no clear environmental precipitant.

The distinction is misleading. Psychotic depression is usually also 'reactive', in the sense that it is triggered by a painful event in the patient's life; and neurotic depression can be 'endogenous', in the sense that genetic and personality factors influence the likelihood of an individual developing depression in response to misfortune.

Loss

Loss plays a central role in the origins of depression, and is the link connecting *grief* with depression. The grieving person is in pain not only because of the loss of an external relationship, but because he has lost a part of him/herself. His internal world as well as his external world has been impoverished. The similarity between the clinical features of grief and those of depression are striking. In grief, an external loss dominates the picture; in depression, it is an internal feeling of loss. In 70% of depressions, there has been a preceding external loss or stress: a bereavement (delayed grief is best seen as a special case of depression), loss of job, break-up of a relationship, child leaving home or a theft, for example. It is when this then leads to a feeling of internal loss – of optimism, vitality and (especially) of self-esteem – that a depression occurs.

Whether or not a particular individual reacts to loss by developing depression depends on a number of inter-related factors: genetic, social, developmental and psychological.

Genetic/biochemical make-up

Twin studies have shown that genetic factors play an important part in manic-depressive psychosis. Changes in neurotransmitter biochemistry in depression are important: current views emphasise reduction of catecholamine levels at postsynaptic nerve endings. Anti-depressant drugs may work through the prevention of breakdown (monoamine oxidase inhibitors), or reduction in re-uptake (tricylic drugs), of cerebral amines at central nerve endings.

Current social situation

The presence of a close confiding relationship, usually with a spouse, protects individuals from developing depression after the experience of loss. Employment is another protective factor; the unemployed are thus doubly vulnerable to depression, the loss of a job being a precipitant and lack of a job being a vulnerability factor. Women with three or more children under 15 and long-term social and financial difficulties are more vulnerable to depression following loss.

Early childhood experience

Women who have lost their mothers before the age of 11 – whether through death, separation (for example, due to illness) or divorce – are especially vulnerable to depression in later life. A reservoir of good experiences in childhood is needed for an individual to develop a lasting sense of self-esteem. This provides a child with a good and secure internal world which can withstand the inevitable separations and losses of later life, and enables an individual to respond to such situations with appropriate sadness rather than by developing depression.

Psychological factors

Recent studies of depression have focused on the vicious circle of depressive thinking and its accompanying negative assumptions about the self and the world. The depressed individual has developed *learned helplessness,* feeling that nothing he can do will make any difference to the situation. Actions and experiences are avoided which *might* make the individual feel better, and he continues to view himself in a negative light. His depression thus becomes a self-fulfilling prophecy.

Management
Mild depression

This is best dealt with by psychotherapy, which may take one of three forms.

Exploratory psychotherapy. Here, the patient is encouraged to express depressive feelings, to vent anger and despair and – through the relationship with the therapist (who may be a GP, social worker, psychotherapist or physician) – to experience the containment that was lacking in childhood and so to recognise and recapture some of the good experiences which the depression has blotted out.

Cognitive behaviour therapy. This counteracts learned helplessness and negative depressive thinking by challenging the erroneous assumptions on which they are based, and by considering positive features of the self. The patient is encouraged to set himself small, easily accomplished tasks and to feel pleased if he succeeds.

Family and marital therapy. Here, the aim is to improve the marital relationship which can then provide a bulwark against depression in response to loss.

Moderate depression

A combination of antidepressant drugs and psychotherapy can be more effective than either alone in treating moderate depression. Both depressed mood and biological symptoms improve with drugs; low self-esteem and social difficulties improve with psychotherapy. Tricyclic anti-depressants such as *amitriptyline* (75–200 mg/day) should always be tried when sleeplessness and guilt are prominent features. They take 10–14 days to produce full effect. Side-effects include parasympathomimetic symptoms of dry mouth and urinary retention, constipation, blurred vision and 'muzziness'; and cardiac arrythmias can occur. *Dothiapin* and *lofepramine* have fewer side-effects. *Imipramine* and *clomipramine* are less sedative. Tricyclics should be avoided in patients with prostatism or a history of heart disease. *Mianserin*, a tetracyclic, has fewer side-effects but can produce haematological reactions and is possibly also less effective in its antidepressant action. If mianserin is used, a blood count should be carried out every four weeks. Newer antidepressants which selectively inhibit serotonin (5 HT) re-uptake are *fluoxetine* and *fluvoxamine*, with fewer antimuscarinic side-effects and low cardiotoxicity and are therefore preferable when the suicide risk is strong. The latter may cause nausea and vomiting. Monoamine oxidase inhibitors (MAOIs) such as tranylcypromine are still occasionally useful as second-line drugs, especially when phobic symptoms are present; but dietary restrictions (e.g. no cheese or yeast-extract) are needed because of harmful (hypertensive) interactions with tyramine-containing substances.

Severe depression

Depressed patients who are severely ill, psychotic or actively suicidal require hospital admission. Tricyclics, which may have to be given in large doses (up to 250 mg

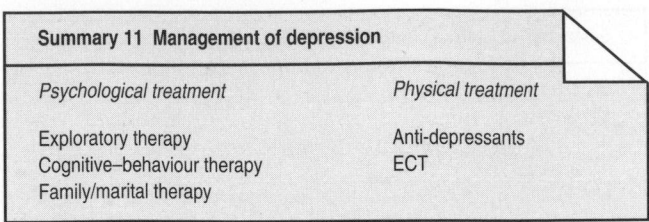

Summary 11 Management of depression

Psychological treatment	Physical treatment
Exploratory therapy	Anti-depressants
Cognitive–behaviour therapy	ECT
Family/marital therapy	

of amitriptyline or equivalent daily), are the first line of treatment.

ECT

Despite debate about its mode of action and efficacy, controlled trials of electroconvulsive therapy (ECT) have shown it to be an effective and rapid treatment for depressive delusions and hallucinations (see Fig. 10.2); it is also free from side-effects, apart from the dangers of the anaesthetic and some short-term memory impairment. ECT is a first-line treatment in depressive stupor or where the patient is refusing food and drink. In the UK it can only be given without the patient's consent after Section 3 of the 1983 Mental Health Act has been applied and a second, independent, psychiatric opinion obtained.

ECT produces rapid improvement in severe depression and is especially effective in elderly patients in whom tricyclics may produce confusion and cardiac arrhythmias. The basis of ECT is the delivery of a convulsion or fit, and its effectiveness depends on an adequate fit of around 25 seconds. A 'course' of ECT, given twice or thrice weekly, should deliver a total of around 250 seconds of fit if relapse is to be avoided. ECT can be given to both hemispheres (bilateral) or to the non-dominant one (unilateral) depending on the position of the electrodes. Unilateral ECT produces less memory impairment but may also be less effective.

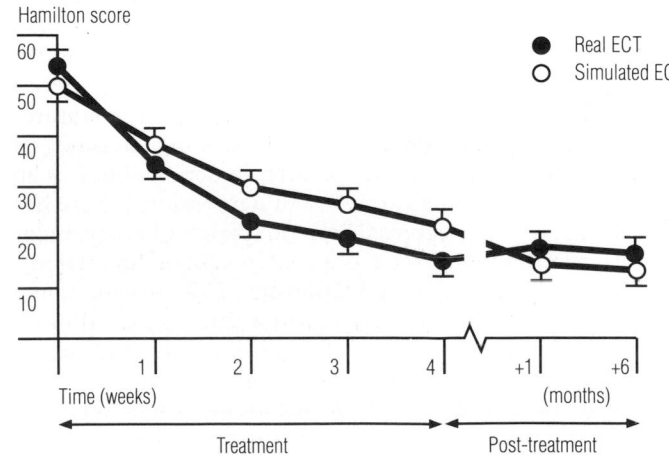

Fig. 10.2 Effect of ECT on severity of depression.

Chronic or recurrent depression

Most depressive illness has a tendency to remit, but relapse is common. Prolonged treatment with tricyclics may have a prophylactic effect, as may psychotherapy. Relapse of depressive psychosis may in some cases be prevented by prophylactic lithium carbonate. Chronic depressive states are rare but disabling, and prolonged attendance at a supportive day hospital may be required.

SUICIDE AND PARASUICIDE

Suicide has a long history and is an integral part of human psychology. There are few individuals lucky and happy enough never to have had even a fleeting thought of suicide at some point in their lives. There has been a recent increase in suicide in young men (Fig. 10.3).

'Parasuicide', a syndrome of *deliberate self-harm*, appears to be a relatively recent phenomenon, and has reached epidemic proportions over the past 25 years. It is the commonest cause of hospital admission for women under 65, and the second commonest for men. Many cases of deliberate self-harm go unreported; probably only about one-third reach hospital.

Clinical profiles

The clinical profiles of suicide and parasuicide are, on the whole, distinct (Table 10.6). A person who commits suicide could be a middle-aged man with a previous history of depression and alcoholism, recently divorced or made redundant, living alone and with few close friends or relations. He deliberately tells the neighbours and milkman that he is going away for the weekend and then takes a bottle of aspirin or shoots himself. A parasuicidal

Table 10.6 Clinical profiles of suicide and parasuicide

	Suicide	Parasuicide
Central theme	Despair, depression	Anger, frustration
Epidemiology	Slight decline 1963–83	Fourfold increase 1963–83
Age, sex, class	Commoner over 50; commoner in men than women; no class preference; recent increase in death by suicide in young men	Commoner in women aged 18–35 and in social classes IV and V
Social circumstances	Isolated, e.g. unemployed, retired, divorced, children left home, few friends or religious/social groups	Disturbed but not isolated, e.g. teenager unhappy with parents or boyfriends
Method and build-up	Planned. Usually leaves a note; method often violent, e.g. hanging, shooting, drowning	Impulsive. Commonest method is swallowing pills. Cutting (usually wrists) a more disturbed subgroup
Alcohol	May play a part – 'Dutch courage'	Attempt very commonly associated with alcohol/drugs, i.e. reduced impulse control
Illness	90% of suicide cases are mentally ill, usually with depressive illness. Physical illness also common	Only about 30% are mentally ill. Some have personality disorder. Majority normal or with 'minor affective illness'
Outcome	Not all 'succeed'. Survivors need hospital admission for treatment of mental illness	Not all survive, but most do. About 5% repeat. May benefit from counselling or psychotherapy

person might be a woman in her late teens living with her mother and stepfather, and getting on badly with her boyfriend. After a row with him, in which both have been drinking, she goes home, swallows some of her mother's sleeping tablets, and is then noticed to be drowsy. When challenged about what has happened, she immediately 'confesses' and is rushed to hospital.

The central theme of suicide is *despair* and depression; in parasuicide it is *anger* and frustration. Although there are important differences there are also psychological similarities. Both involve a physical attack on self, on the body. In both cases the patient feels a combination of personal inadequacy and anger towards friends and family. This anger is directed inward but there is often a wish to punish or harm those to whom the patient feels close. This is done indirectly via the suicide or suicide attempt.

A second point of contact is the wish to die. It is often said that parasuicide cases 'do not really mean it'. This is only partially true, and can sometimes be used by staff as justification for adopting a punitive attitude. It is best to assume that both suicide cases and parasuicide cases want *both* to die, *and* not to die. The relative proportion of the two feelings varies greatly but both feel both.

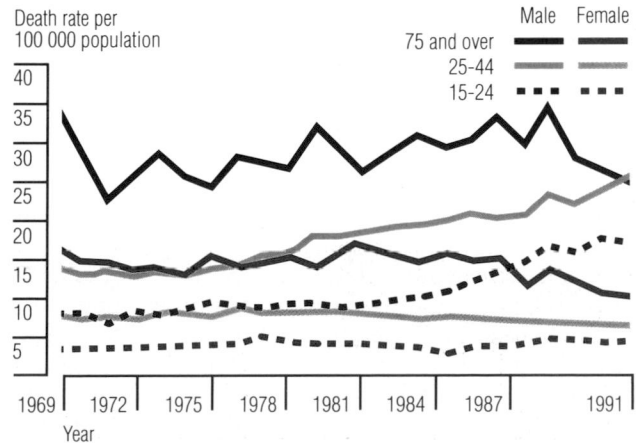

Fig. 10.3 **Death rates for suicide and undetermined injury in England 1969–91.**

A third point of overlap follows from this. Not all suicide cases succeed, and conversely it is possible in parasuicide to die by mistake. Patients who have made major suicide attempts may recover and, with the help of drugs, psychotherapy and time regain the will to live. In the majority of parasuicide cases the attempt resolves the difficult social situation which prompted it and so is not repeated. In a minority, about 5%, the attempts are repeated, and a proportion of these will eventually 'succeed'. Parasuicide repeaters are more likely to have a personality disorder, be addicted to drugs or alcohol, or to have been in trouble with the law.

Management of 'failed suicide'

The causes of suicide are essentially the causes of depressive illness and the management of attempted suicide is that of prevention, and particularly the early detection, of depression. About one-half of successful suicide cases have contacted a helping agency – a counselling organisation, a general practitioner, social worker or priest – in the month before they kill themselves. It is important to ask troubled, unhappy or depressed patients about suicidal feelings. Fleeting suicidal thoughts, 'I would like to sleep' or 'I would like to be dead but would never have the courage to do anything', are less worrying than a definite suicide plan. Talking about suicidal thoughts may in itself be a relief. Suicidal patients with symptoms of depressive illness should be admitted to a psychiatric unit. Patients who are managed as outpatients need to be seen frequently while they are in a suicidal state. Antidepressants can be prescribed but only in small amounts, as hoarding of tablets can be a danger.

Although the prevention of suicide remains the ideal this is in practice difficult to achieve. Counselling organisations such as the Samaritans seem not to have had a major impact on overall suicide rates, but the incidence of suicide in the UK has fallen slightly over the past 30 years as compared with the rest of Europe.

Suicide is a reminder of the limitations of psychiatric and social care. When a patient who is receiving treatment commits suicide, it is especially stressful for the doctors and nurses involved, as it always is for the patient's family. Feelings of guilt and anger are inevitable. Suicide, like any death, is a reminder that doctors are not omnipotent. In dealing with suicide or the threat of it, it should be remembered that, ultimately, a person determined or ill enough can always find a way to end his life.

PARASUICIDE

Causes

The causes of attempted suicide cannot be found solely within the individual. Social factors which need to be considered in understanding the increase in parasuicide rates include:

- *Complex family structures* without clear rules or roles, such as unsupported one-parent families; adolescents who want freedom but lack the emotional or financial resources to leave home; families with stepparents.
- *Drugs* being a socially acceptable means of dealing with *distress:* the commonest tablets taken in parasuicide are mild analgesics and minor tranquillisers.
- *An epidemic factor.* Deliberate self-harm is often behaviour learned from friends, fellow-patients, relatives or television.

Management

The medical management (p. 43) of the parasuicide patient takes initial precedence over the social and psychiatric assessment. Medical staff often feel angry with overdose patients compared with those whose illness is not self-inflicted and, like alcoholics and drug addicts, these patients may become scapegoats. Their irresponsibility affronts the overworked nurses and doctors who are often similar in age and maturity to the patient. In addition, medical staff work in a stressful and hierarchical situation in which they can at times feel angry or frustrated; and these emotions can be displaced into a punitive attitude towards parasuicide patients. This can be avoided if ward procedures give time for discussion of these patients and the feelings they arouse.

History

A careful history must be taken from the overdose patient, who should be kept in hospital until alert and co-operative enough for this to be possible.

The presence of depressive illness and suicidal rather than parasuicidal features must be identified. The risk of repeat has to be assessed (Table 10.7). Social isolation, marked sleep disturbance preceding the attempt, strong feelings of guilt or unworthiness, evidence of pre-planning, inability to look to the future, and previous psychiatric history – especially if there are drug or alcohol problems – all point to serious disturbance and should lead to referral to a psychiatrist.

A detailed account of the attempt itself and of events surrounding it should be taken. It is often unhelpful to ask the patient 'why' he harmed himself. If the patient knew he might not have had to do so. In attempted suicide one often finds an *acting-out* of feelings rather than the capacity to contain or verbalise them. The patient will find it much easier to answer questions about 'what happened, and how'. This provides an 'action replay' of the attempt which will contain the clues to the question of

Table 10.7 Deliberate self-harm: assessment of severity of disturbance. Ideally, all cases should be referred for psychiatric assessment. Psychiatric referral essential if any of the following are present:

Circumstance of the attempt
Evidence of pre-planning (e.g. suicide note, use of car exhaust)
Violent method used (e.g. attempted hanging)

Social circumstances of patient
Alone
Away from home

Personal history of patient
Recent loss (e.g. bereavement, divorce/separation, unemployment)
Physical illness
Previous attempts
Alcohol or drug addiction
History of depressive illness

Family history of patient
Suicide
Depressive illness

Mental state examination
Sleep disturbance, low mood before attempt
Low self-esteem, hopelessness
Psychotic features (e.g. 'I deserve to die')

Future
No relatives or other support
Unresolved crisis
Continued determined suicidal intent

'why'. Most commonly the patient feels *angry* but is unable to express this directly, usually for fear of rejection by a partner, spouse or parent on whom he feels dependent. As in depression, he dare not bite the hand that feeds, so attacks himself instead. It can be useful to ask the patient who he thinks would have been most distressed if he had died. Later, it is often helpful to discuss alternative strategies with the patient, to examine what he could have done in the same situation other than attempt suicide. Follow-up counselling after discharge either as an individual or in a family, by a social worker, psychiatrist or psychotherapist may be offered, although less than half of patients accept such help. However, even without follow-up the prognosis of parasuicide, in the absence of depressive illness or personality disorder, is fairly good.

MANIA AND HYPOMANIA

Clinical features

In depression, mood is abnormally lowered. In *mania*, or its milder form *hypomania*, it is abnormally elevated. In *unipolar manic-depressive psychosis*, the patient may have recurrent depressive, or recurrent manic episodes. If both manic and depressive episodes occur, the patient has *bipolar manic-depressive psychosis*.

There are three main groups of symptoms in mania and hypomania:

- *Psychological symptoms.* The patient feels elated, cheerful and expansive, and his thoughts are speeded up. He may develop *grandiose delusions* of wealth, potency and fame. He is full of optimistic (and unrealistic) plans for the future.
- *Physical symptoms.* The patient is restless, sleeps little, eats voraciously or not at all, often loses weight, has poor concentration and tries to do several things at once.
- *Behavioural symptoms.* The patient often spends large amounts of money, dresses flamboyantly and may behave in an outrageous, disinhibited and promiscuous manner. Outbursts of irritability and aggression are common. Speech is rapid, may be incoherent and flits from subject to subject (known as *flight of ideas*). The patient is often humorous in an irreverent and infectious way.

Hypomania frequently co-exists with depressive symptoms: the patient laughs and cries almost simultaneously. This is known as a *mixed affective state*.

Hypomanic episodes may, like depression, be triggered by a painful rejection or loss. This has led to the concept of *manic defence*, whereby the patient escapes into mania as a way of avoiding unhappy or sad feelings.

Management

A hypomanic patient can cause havoc to both himself and his family. Hospital admission is often indicated but may be hard to achieve voluntarily as the patient denies illness, often indeed claiming to have never felt better, or to have discovered the secret of life. Immediate management is with tranquillisers such as chlorpromazine (100–600 mg daily) or haloperidol (15–60 mg daily). Subsequent relapses may be prevented by prophylactic lithium carbonate (800–1600 mg daily). Lithium also has a mild immediate antimanic effect. Blood levels should be monitored regularly and be in the range 0.8–1.5 mmol/l. Lithium may produce hypothyroidism and renal damage leading to nephrogenic diabetes insipidus, and thyroid and renal function should be monitored. Other side-effects include abdominal pain, fine tremor, subjective memory impairment, thirst and lowered zest for life. Patients should be encouraged to keep up fluid intake in hot weather. *Carbamazepine* (400–1600 mg daily) is a useful second-line antimanic prophylactic if lithium is ineffective or not tolerated.

SCHIZOPHRENIA

Just under 1% of the population develop schizophrenia at some point in their lives, a statistic that appears to hold true for all cultures and countries. Chronic major mental illness in people under 65 is mainly due to schizophrenia. Until the move towards community care began, about half of all hospital beds in the UK were in mental hospitals, and the majority of these (for the under 65s) were occupied by patients with a schizophrenic illness. As the number of hospital beds has fallen, a significant proportion of the vagrants living in large inner-city hostels and prison recidivists are schizophrenic.

Aetiology

It is probable that schizophrenia is not a single entity, but a group of related conditions. Both genetic and environmental factors are important in the aetiology of schizophrenia. It is best seen as a developmental disorder of the brain to which genetic and perinatal factors (birth trauma or maternal viral infection) contribute, but manifesting itself in late adolescence when brain maturation is finally completed.

- Twin and adoption studies have demonstrated the role of heredity in schizophrenia (Fig. 10.4). The concordance rate for identical twins is about 50%, for non-identical twins around 15%.
- The efficacy of antipsychotic drugs like chlorpromazine, with its inevitable Parkinsonian side-effects, suggests a disturbance of mid-brain dopaminergic pathways in schizophrenia.
- A subgroup of patients shows ventricular abnormalities on CT scan. These patients lack a family history of the illness, suggesting that non-genetic organic factors, perhaps associated with perinatal brain injury, may be important in some cases.

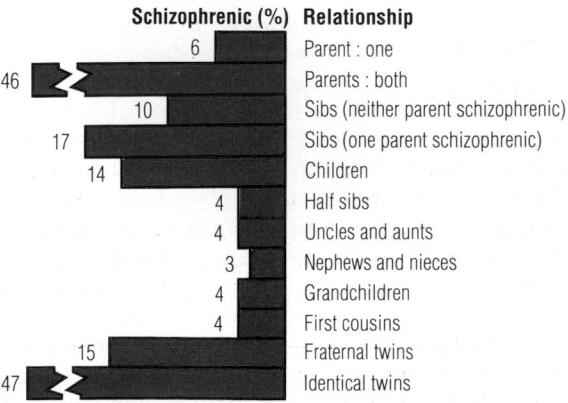

Fig. 10.4 Expectation of schizophrenia in relatives of schizophrenics.

Table 10.8 Relapse rate for schizophrenia

A. At nine months	
	Relapse rate
High EE homes	50%
Low EE homes	12%

B. In high EE homes		
Face-to-face contact	Maintenance therapy	Relapse rate
High	No	92%
High	Yes	53%
Low	No	42%
Low	Yes	15%

- Family and social factors have also been shown to be important although not pathognomonic. In established schizophrenia, relapse rate is high when the patient is living in an over-involved family where there is a negatively charged emotional atmosphere (high 'expressed emotion' or 'EE') (Table 10.8).
- Schizophrenic patients have a high state of psychophysiological arousal, possibly related to family stress. This may reflect limbic system dysfunction and lead to a difficulty in processing sensory stimuli.

Clinical features

Schizophrenia usually starts in young adulthood (the exception being *paraphrenia*, a form of paranoid schizophrenia affecting the elderly). There is a slight preponderance of men. The features of the illness can be divided into two parts: the effects on mental processes, and the effects on social functioning.

Mental disturbance

There is a general disturbance of mental functioning in schizophrenia. The normal progression of logical thought is disrupted ('thought disorder'). The privacy of the self is breached. Certain patterns of disorganisation of thinking are characteristic of schizophrenia, and are known as *Schneider's first-rank symptoms*.

Hallucinations

These are usually auditory. Characteristic of schizophrenia are 'third person' hallucinations, in which more than one person is heard discussing the patient and referring to him as 'he', 'she' or 'it'. Voices commenting on a person's actions like a 'running commentary' are also characteristic, as are voices that echo the patient's thoughts. Tactile or 'kinaesthetic' hallucinations, for

Summary 12 Schneider's first-rank symptoms

- Delusional perception
- Auditory hallucinations
  Audible thoughts (thought echo)
  Voices arguing or discussing ('third person')
  Voices commenting on the patient's actions
- Thought disorder
  Thought withdrawal
  Thought insertion
  Thought broadcasting
- Passivity experiences: delusions of control
  'Made' feelings (includes somatic hallucinations)
  'Made' actions
  Somatic passivity (body invaded from outside)

example electric shock feelings in the limbs, are rare but pathognomonic.

Delusions

In schizophrenia these include the feeling that one's thoughts originate from outside ('thought insertion'), that they are being interfered with, removed ('thought block') or transmitted to outsiders as though on a loudspeaker ('thought broadcasting'). 'Passivity feelings' are the feeling that one's thoughts or actions are 'made' from outside.

Delusional perception

In delusional perception, a neutral stimulus (e.g. a car number plate or a traffic light) suddenly acquires special and often frightening significance for the patient.

Social deterioration

The second main feature of schizophrenia is social deterioration. This is known as a *negative feature* of the illness, as opposed to the *positive features* of thought disorder, delusions and hallucinations. The patient may withdraw from social contact, give up his job, shun his friends and family, and spend many hours in isolation.

Differential diagnosis

An important subtype of schizophrenia is *paranoid schizophrenia* characterised by paranoid delusions. Here the onset is later (around 30–40 years of age), social deterioration is much less marked, and the personality is relatively well preserved. *Schizoaffective disorder* has features of both schizophrenia and an affective illness, e.g. first-rank symptoms plus considerable depression. Its diagnosis is intermediate between that of the two 'parent' disorders.

Not all madness is schizophrenia. The differential diagnosis includes:

- organic psychosis, such as acute confusional states and drug- and alcohol-related psychosis
- manic or depressive psychosis (in which auditory hallucinations occur but are more often 'second person', in which voices speak directly to the patient)
- hysteria
- stress-induced or 'psychogenic' psychosis
- severe personality disorder.

Prognosis

The course of schizophrenia is very variable. About 30% of patients have only one episode. A good prognosis is more likely if the psychosis has an acute onset, a clear precipitant, florid symptoms, marked mood change in addition to disturbance of thinking, and good previous social adjustment and personality. At the other end of the scale, about 15% remain severely disabled and will still be in hospital after a year ('new long-stay' patients). In these patients the negative features of schizophrenia (withdrawal and inertia) may predominate. In the middle group, representing the majority of patients, the illness has a fluctuating course but relapse and some residual disability are likely to occur.

Management

Acute schizophrenic symptoms respond well to phenothiazines. There is some evidence that prompt treatment is associated with a good prognosis. The patient will normally be admitted to a psychiatric unit and treated initially with 100–1000 mg daily of chlorpromazine or its equivalent. The longer-term management of schizophrenia is difficult. It involves both prevention of relapse, and management of chronic disability.

Antipsychotic drugs

These can be divided into three main groups:

- A group characterised by profound sedative effects, and moderate antimuscarinic and extrapyramidal effects, e.g. chlorpromazine (50–1000 mg daily).
- Moderate sedative effects, marked antimuscarinic effects, but fewer extrapyramidal effects, e.g. thioridazine (25–250 mg daily), often used as a sedative in the elderly.
- Fewer sedative and antimuscarinic effects but more pronounced extrapyramidal effects, e.g. trifluoperazine (2–30 mg daily); haloperidol (2–80 mg daily); flupenthixol (2–100 mg daily).

A wide range of side-effects and idiosyncratic reactions may be produced with the antipsychotic drugs (see Table 10.9). Perhaps the most serious of these is the rare but potentially fatal *neuroleptic malignant syndrome*, characterised by hyperthermia, confusion, muscular rigidity and autonomic disequilibrium (tachycardia, labile BP, sweating). All antipsychotics should be discontinued and bromocriptine and dantroline are often given.

Prevention of relapse

Long-term maintenance on phenothiazines (often given in the form of a weekly or fortnightly injection because of problems of compliance) has been shown to prevent relapse. Phenothiazines can, however, have unpleasant and serious side-effects, especially a feeling of tiredness and extrapyramidal syndromes of stiffness and involuntary movements (Table 10.9). Anti-Parkinsonian drugs such as orphenadrine (100 mg t.d.s.) or kemadrin (5 mg t.d.s.) should be given to counteract these. Reducing family tension has also been shown to prevent relapse. This can be achieved by family counselling sessions and by physical separation of the patient from an over-involved family through provison of hostel accommodation and/or attendance at a day centre.

Table 10.9 Side-effects and toxic effects of antipsychotic drugs (e.g. chlorpromazine, flupenthixol)

Type of effect	Examples
Autonomic (antimuscarinic)	Blurred vision
	Dry mouth
	Constipation
	Precipitation of glaucoma
	Postural hypotension
	Inhibition of ejaculation
	Urinary hesitancy
Extrapyramidal	Akinesia (Parkinson-like)
	Acute dystonia
	Tardive dyskinesia (involuntary repetitive movements)
	Akathisia (motor-restlessness)
Endocrine effects	Weight gain
	Galactorrhoea and amenorrhoea
	Gynaecomastia
Hypersensitivity reactions	Agranulocytosis
	Cholestatic jaundice
	Skin rashes
Neuroleptic malignant syndrome	
Provocation of epileptic fits	
Hypothermia (especially in the elderly)	
Skin photosensitivity	

Summary 13 Management of schizophrenia

- First attack: admit to hospital or day hospital for assessment, confirm diagnosis, establish contact and initiate treatment.

- Treat symptoms with neuroleptics.

  Chlorpromazine 100 mg. t.d.s. by mouth
  Trifluoperazine 5 mg. t.d.s. by mouth } example of moderate doses

  Flupenthixol ('Depixol') 40 mg. 2 weekly
  Fluphenazine ('Modecate') 25 mg. 2 weekly }

  Treat side effects as necessary with anti-parkinsonian agents, e.g. Kemadrin 5 mg. t.d.s.

- Assign 'community keyworker' as part of community care programme who will offer supportive psychotherapy and co-ordinate care package.

- Assess family situation: offer psycho-educational programme to lower 'EE' if indicated.

- Rehabilation: attend day hospital, day centre, sheltered workshop, live-in-hostel, sheltered housing.

- Where resistant to medication consider newer neuroleptics: Clozapine and Remoxipride.

Management of chronic disability

Chronic mentally ill patients are severely handicapped. Their prospects of employment are poor; they may have little or no family support; and their capacity to care for and occupy themselves may be very limited. They are sometimes also shunned or made scapegoats by society which tends to fear and despise madness. For at least 150 years these problems were dealt with by removing patients from society and locking them away in mental hospitals, thereby reinforcing the helplessness and isolation produced by the illness. Because of this, and also because mental hospitals are expensive to run and often sited on valuable land, government policy in England has now shifted away from the mental hospitals and towards *community care*. Patients are supposed to be cared for within the local community, in a network of hostels, sheltered houses, day hospitals and day centres, and Community Mental Health Centres. These are run by a locally based team of professionals, the *'multidisciplinary team'*, including community psychiatric nurses, social workers and general practitioners as well as psychiatrists. However, although this pattern of care is desirable for many patients, and already a reality for some, it is not necessarily suitable for all patients, who will continue to need highly staffed or secure facilities, and as far as the UK is concerned, it is still not yet clear whether adequate funds and facilities will be made available to replace those previously provided in the mental hospitals.

PARANOID STATES

Paranoia means literally 'to be beside oneself', or 'out of one's mind'. In psychiatry, it refers to a psychosis whose central theme is a feeling of persecution and fear of being attacked. Paranoid states are common in general medical and hospital settings. A postoperative patient may suddenly rip out an intravenous cannula and attack one of the nurses. A patient may refuse all drugs, convinced that the staff are torturers dressed up as doctors and nurses.

The conditions resulting in paranoid states are as follows:

- *Organic psychosis.* This is by far the commonest cause in the hospital setting. Paranoid delusions are frequently found in patients with acute confusional states. Any of the causes of organic psychosis (p. 169) may be responsible, with steroid-induced psychosis, alcohol withdrawal syndrome and amphetamine psychosis particularly common. Alcoholism may also produce a chronic paranoid state in which auditory hallucinations predominate (p. 201).
- *Manic-depressive psychosis.* Feelings of being disliked and shunned are common in depression, and may assume psychotic proportions if the patient feels he/she is so wicked that he/she is deservedly in danger of attack. Paranoid ideas can occur in mania, but elation and over-activity are usually more prominent features.
- *Paranoid schizophrenia* (see p. 185).
- *Paranoid psychosis.* Sometimes the patient develops paranoid delusions and hallucinations without the full range of features of schizophrenia. There is often a sexual content to the psychosis. The patient may, for example, become convinced that his spouse is having an affair (morbid jealousy or *Othello syndrome*). The feeling that workmates or strangers are accusing the patient of homosexuality is often a prominent feature of paranoid psychosis.
- *Paranoid personality.* The paranoid personality has a tendency to mistrust and blame others and thus frequently becomes involved in complaints and battles with authority. The patient is often sensitive, isolated, insecure and quick to take offence and misinterpret the behaviour of others as hostile. When his fragile self-esteem is threatened by illness or rejection, he may develop a paranoid psychosis.
- *Paranoia in the elderly.* Elderly patients may develop a paranoid psychosis *(paraphrenia)* with schizophrenic features. Deafness, social isolation and previous paranoid personality are important predisposing factors.

Common to all the different forms of paranoia are isolation, insecurity, mistrust and misperception. In some cases the defence of *projection* seems to be operating. A cancer patient may refuse to leave hospital, attributing the 'hostility' felt from the cancer within to the outside world as well. Paranoid states can be treated symptomatically with phenothiazines, but the underlying cause itself should be treated whenever possible.

SOMATOFORM DISORDERS

Somatoform disorders are conditions in which (a) physical symptoms are present for which no organic or physiological basis can be found, and (b) where there are demonstrable underlying psychological factors or conflicts, i.e. *the physical symptoms may be manifestations of underlying psychological distress or disease.*

Terminology and definitions

There are several terms commonly used to describe physical disorder in which psychological mechanisms may be important.

The outmoded, but still widely used, term *psychosomatic* illness refers to conditions in which there is definite *structural* physical illness (e.g. bowel inflammation in ulcerative colitis) but whose precipitant or maintaining factors are considered to be in part psychological.

The term *functional* is sometimes used to describe symptoms produced by changes in organ *function* in the absence of structural change. Functional illness may or may not be psychological in origin. Functional bowel disease (irritable bowel syndrome, see p. 601), for example, may result from faulty diet or disturbance of the autonomic system (potentially stress-related) or both.

The term *psychogenic* usually implies that the symptoms are entirely psychological in origin. Many of the ill-defined conditions seen in general practice and medical outpatients could be labelled as psychogenic, although this term may obscure the fact that physical factors (e.g. muscular tension) are also important.

Summary 14 Conditions resulting in paranoid states
• Organic psychosis
• Manic-depressive psychosis
• Paranoid schizophrenia
• Paranoid psychosis
• Paranoid personality
• Paranoia in the elderly

The concept of *hysteria* (p. 190) has a long history and has become differentiated from the more non-specific psychogenic symptoms. Hysteria is divided into two types:

- *Conversion disorders.* These are psychogenic illnesses – often simulating neurological disorders – based on unconscious mechanisms, in which mental conflict is avoided both by converting anxiety into physical symptoms (hence *conversion* hysteria) and by *dissociation* (i.e. a split between the mental self and the physical self).
- *Somatisation disorders.* These are polysymptomatic disorders in which the patient experiences multiple unexplained symptoms without physical disease and in the context of a disturbed personality.

In psychosomatic illness psychological factors may well aggravate, prolong or cause relapses in an illness whose basis is physical (just as a poor ward atmosphere has been shown to delay postoperative wound healing). Psychogenic symptoms are often based on circular patterns in which, for example, emotional conflict produces muscular tension, which results in pain which leads to greater emotional stress, or anxiety (e.g. fear that the pain may be due to cancer) which results in more muscular tension and so on.

MIND–BODY MODELS

There are two extreme but widely held views on the nature of psychosomatic illness. The first, corresponding to the philosophical position of *materialism,* holds that all phenomena are physical in origin and denies the existence of the mind. For the materialist, there are no psychogenic conditions, only illnesses whose physical cause has yet to be determined. The second, *idealist,* view holds that psychosomatic illness is mental in origin.

There are problems in both these models. The materialist might point to the numbers of patients labelled as hysterical who have subsequently died of carcinoma or multiple sclerosis; but the existence of mind cannot altogether be denied. The idealist, on the other hand, tends to confuse the symbolic *meaning* of an illness with its *cause,* claiming, for example, that a man who developed oesophageal cancer did so because he could not *swallow* his wife's infidelity. A classic error of this type was the pre-1956 theory of Down's syndrome. This held that Down's syndrome was caused by physical or mental trauma in pregnancy, since mothers of Down's syndrome babies regularly reported such traumatic incidents. Only when the chromosomal abnormality responsible was found, was it realised that the trauma theory was a retrospective rationalisation rather than a causal explanation.

In reality, the relationship between mind and body is far more complicated than either the pure materialist or idealist models allow. The interesting questions concern the *interactions* between the mental and the physical, just

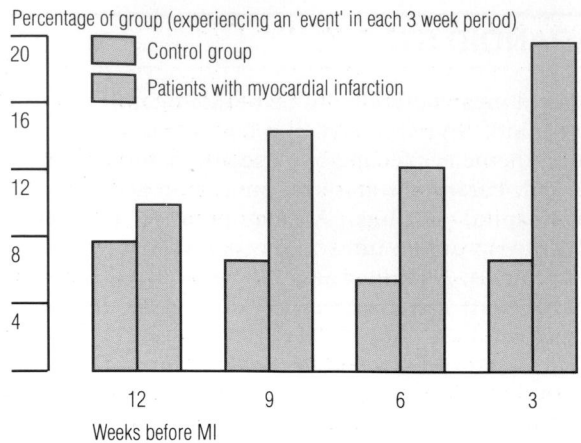

Fig. 10.5 **Experience of potentially stressful life events by myocardial infarction patients in the 12 weeks before MI occurred.**

as the interesting problems in genetics involve interactions between heredity and environment.

Experimental evidence

There is evidence that painful events in a person's life can precipitate physical illness. The link between stress and myocardial infarction, for example, is well documented (Fig. 10.5). Bowel disease, such as ulcerative colitis or even appendicitis, may also be triggered by a preceding painful or stressful life event.

Personality plays an important part in determining the impact of such events. Individuals with 'type A personality' (competitive, driving) are, other factors being equal, more likely to develop coronary artery disease than those with more placid temperaments. Similarly the prognosis of breast cancer may depend in part on personality; women who are emotionally inhibited appear to have, on average, a less good prognosis than those more able to express anger and sadness. The *intervening variables* that link the psychological to the physical are largely unknown. Autonomic and corticosteroid responses to stress play their part, as do changes in the immune system (especially T-lymphocytes), but the precise pathways and links remain to be elucidated. Current evidence does not support the view that psychosomatic diseases are *primarily* psychological in origin; nor that any *specific* relationship exists between personality type and a particular disease or target organ.

PSYCHOLOGICAL APPROACHES TO SOMATOFORM DISORDERS

The contribution of psychiatry to the understanding of psychosomatic and psychogenic illness can be considered under two headings: the development of the body image; and repression and the unconscious.

Development of the body image

In adult life mind and body are separate realms. The body is experienced as an object among other objects in the world; but is also, for its 'owner', the source of knowledge and sensation, and the means by which contact and communication with others is possible. The mind, though experienced as a separate domain, is indissolubly connected to the body. As Freud pointed out, it only takes a toothache to feel that 'the molar hole contains my soul'.

The adult state in which the self comfortably inhabits both mind and body, experiencing each as separate and yet connected, is a complex product of health, maturity and culture. The infant is born in a state of psychosomatic unity: pain for a young child is both mental and physical. In adult life physical illness may produce *regression* to a child-like state. Childhood experiences may play a crucial part in determining later relationships between mind and body. In early childhood, the parents' love and care for the child and his body sow the seed of healthy self-love in later life. A girl who was 'meant' to be a boy may have to struggle with the effects of her parents' disappointment for years to come. Later, the adolescent has to learn to accept his or her body and sexuality. Self-acceptance is an essential precondition of loving others. When this process is disturbed, some individuals may, when anxious, ask their doctor for an examination, complaining that there is something wrong with their body or even asking for it to be changed by plastic surgery. The patient is looking for the acceptance and care he feels he missed from his parents. If external relationships fail, the patient may turn for interest and gratification to his own body and this too can lead to development of, and preoccupation with, psychogenic physical symptoms.

Repression and the unconscious

Repression is the active removal from consciousness of painful or disturbing thoughts, feelings or memories. The mind's eye is blinded to problems and conflicts. The difficulties and the feelings they evoke remain, however, even though the patient is *unconscious* of them. They may then manifest themselves in physical symptoms, by the process of displacement.

'MINOR' PSYCHIATRIC ILLNESS

Minor psychiatric illnesses are hard to classify and often go undetected, hiding behind and contributing to physical symptoms (Tables 10.10 and 10.11). In these illnesses a somatic 'facade' conceals difficulty in adjustment to social stress ('adjustment disorders'), symptoms of anxiety and/or depression, or personality difficulties. Once these are explored, and the patient reassured, the physical symptoms may be relieved.

In considering patients with somatisation disorders, a number of psychosocial factors should be explored:

- *Stress factors,* especially recent losses such as bereavement, unemployment, children leaving home, financial difficulties, divorce and termination of pregnancy.
- *Social support,* relationship with partner (including sexual relationship), parents, children and friends, housing conditions.
- *Personality,* how the person has reacted to stress in the past, previous stressful or painful experiences, especially in childhood, and whether the patient is able to respond with appropriate anger or sadness.
- *Alcoholism, drug abuse and eating disorders,* which frequently present indirectly via physical symptoms.

Table 10.10 Characteristics typical of doctors who frequently detect psychological problems

- Show empathy
- Sensitive to emotional cues
- Use appropriate psychiatric questions and probes
- Tend to ask for clarification of the patient's complaints
- Make early eye-contact with the patient
- Do not bury themselves in notes
- Good at dealing with interruptions and garrulous patients

Table 10.11 Psychiatric illness in general practice: how much goes undetected?

Category	All patients	Probability of detection by GP
Physical illness without psychiatric disorder	67%	n/a
Physical illness and unrelated psychiatric disorder	8%	19%
Physical illness with secondary disorder	1%	74%
Somatisation	**19%**	**47%**
Physical with symptoms exacerbated or caused by psychiatric disorder	13.5%	33%
Somatised psychiatric illness (no diagnosable physical illness)	5.5%	85%
Psychiatric disorders presenting with psychological symptoms	5%	95%

HYSTERIA

The three essential features of hysteria are: physical symptoms, absence of organic pathology, and psychological conflict.

CLASSIFICATION AND CLINICAL FEATURES

There are three main patterns of hysteria: monosymptomatic, polysymptomatic and epidemic.

Monosymptomatic hysteria (conversion disorder)

Typically there is gross loss of neurological function. This may involve:

- the limbs, e.g. paralysis, anaesthesia or dystonia
- the higher functions, e.g. hysterical fits, hysterical blindness, *fugue states* (in which the patient has complete memory loss), or even *hysterical psychosis* (where the patient develops a short-lived and dramatic psychosis in response to external stress).

The pattern of dysfunction follows the patient's 'idea' of how the body works rather than anatomy. Similarly, in hysterical psychosis the patient behaves in the way he/she thinks a madman ought to behave, rather than demonstrating the specific symptoms of schizophrenia. A neurologist can usually determine the integrity of the nervous system either by subtle physical examination (extensor activity in apparently paralysed limbs) or by investigation (intact visual-evoked potentials in hysterical blindness). The patient may also exhibit the *belle indifférence* described by Janet, i.e. an apparent lack of anxiety in the face of crippling disorder. Psychophysiological measures of arousal show that hysterical patients are in fact often highly aroused despite the absence of manifest anxiety.

Polysymptomatic hysteria (Briquet's syndrome, somatisation disorder)

Polysymptomatic hysterics (usually women in their thirties) develop a wide variety of physical complaints with no organic basis over a number of years. These often involve pain centering around the abdomen, back and pelvis. Such patients have often been extensively investigated by physicians and frequently admitted to hospital. Their medical notes are thick but inconclusive. Unlike patients with monosymptomatic hysteria, their prognosis is poor and is related to general personality difficulties rather than a specific conflict.

Epidemic hysteria

This rare and self-limiting condition occurs in schools and other situations where young people are in close proximity. Fainting, nausea and paraesthesia brought on by overbreathing are common presentations. The condition is sometimes, wrongly, assumed to have an infective cause.

Diagnosis

Hysteria is not an easy diagnosis to make. A proportion of patients diagnosed as hysterical turn out to have genuine organic disease: multiple sclerosis or occult cancer, for example. Others may develop another psychiatric condition such as a depressive illness or even schizophrenia. However, it is important to recognise and diagnose hysteria when it does occur, so as to spare the patient unnecessary investigation. Hysteria and organic illness can also, and often do, co-exist; establishing one diagnosis should not prevent searching for another.

Meaning and aetiology

The manifestations of hysteria are often dramatic, and therein lies a clue to its nature. Most people, especially as children, have the capacity to act a role. This involves an internal *splitting*, or *dissociation*, between the actor and his part. The actor is not really Hamlet, yet becomes Hamlet as he acts the role. The hysteric is not paralysed and yet, psychologically, can become so.

According to Freud, the symptoms in hysteria have a *meaning* which can be understood in terms of the patient's life. Psychological theories of hysteria also highlight several other important aspects of the illness:

- *Defence.* Hysteria is a defence against the anxiety created by conflict. A young man from an academically minded family was facing exams which he feared he would fail; he became paralysed.
- *Unconscious behaviour.* Although a conflict is often obvious to others, the patient is *unconscious* of it.
- *Personal gain.* There are two kinds of gain for patients in being ill. The *primary gain* is the fact that they are unaware of their conflict and thus do not experience anxiety. The *secondary gain* is the care and attention they get from family, friends and relatives. This is only possible if the family to some extent go along with, or allow the patient to *manipulate* them. Here they may be meeting their own needs, e.g. the husband who only feels potent when he has a sick wife to look after. 'Manipulation' is a normal process in childhood, and hysteria always has childlike aspects. The child who does not want to go to school develops a tummy-ache; his mother lets him stay at home with her. A

similar process is at work in hysteria. The child is not consciously making himself ill or *malingering* (as, for example, the soldier is, who deliberately shoots himself in the foot to avoid going to battle). There really is a pain, even if it clears up quickly once the danger of having to go to school has passed.

- *Identification.* A common finding in the histories of hysterical patients is that there has been a close relative who has suffered illness, often serious. The young man who became paralysed because he feared his exams had had a younger brother who had died with cerebral palsy and on whom his parents had lavished all their care and attention. The patient often has such a model of illness and its accompanying behaviour which influences him. Sociologists speak of 'illness behaviour' to describe the socially sanctioned behaviour which accompanies illness and which is not strictly related to the pathophysiology of the disease. Sick people are allowed to retire temporarily from work and spend time in bed; they receive flowers, cards and gifts from relatives and are treated with special consideration; they are allowed to be childish and demanding. Their medical attendants also adopt a particular role, usually one of reassurance, benevolence and quasiomniscience. One of the rules of illness behaviour seems to be that the patient should recover, or at least attempt to recover. When this does not happen there may be a sudden switch: the previously privileged patient may be seen as manipulative, attention-seeking and deviant, and be shunned or covertly punished by irate relatives and medical attendants. In hysteria this often results in a worsening of the symptoms.

Management

It is tempting to try to argue a hysterical patient out of his illness. Occasionally this can be helpful, but more often it entrenches the patient more deeply in his symptoms and an escalating battle between doctor and patient may then ensue. There is, moreover, a sense in which the patient is right. There is something wrong, namely a psychological conflict, albeit one of which the patient is unconscious.

A more helpful approach is therefore to adopt a *psychosomatic attitude*. This involves explaining to the patient that stress can cause illness, that he may have a psychological conflict, and that there may be a connection between this and the physical problem, both of which are real. The patient who has committed himself to a physical illness should be offered appropriate physical treatments (e.g. physiotherapy, massage) and should not be deprived of it out of spite. When recovery does take place the temptation to say 'I told you so' should be resisted. Instead, the patient needs a face-saving formula; the paralysed person must be allowed to put his crutch down gradually, inadvertently even, not have it knocked from under him.

The psychological principles of treatment are:

- *Exploration of conflict.* With allowance for face-saving, this is perhaps the most helpful strategy. If the conflict is removed (e.g. the time for exams past) the symptoms will usually remit.
- *Behavioural approaches.* These are often useful. They (a) aim to avoid reinforcement of the symptoms, e.g. by suggesting to ward staff or relatives that they respond positively to any signs of movement in the paralysed patient, but as far as possible ignore (non-punitively) helpless behaviour; (b) are directed towards helping the patient overcome his cognitive responses (e.g. of panic and catastrophe) towards the imagined illness.
- *Drugs.* Where hysteria is secondary to a depressive illness antidepressants should be prescribed. In general, however, drug treatment should be avoided in hysteria as the patient is often very suggestible and tends to develop dramatic reactions and side-effects. Hysterical amnesia can sometimes be approached by *abreaction,* in which painful experiences are 'relived' with the help of an intravenous injection of a sedative drug such as diazepam.
- *Psychotherapy.* Some patients will benefit from long-term psychotherapy.

HISTRIONIC PERSONALITY AND RELATED CONDITIONS

There are a number of conditions which are related to hysteria, but take the form of a life-long personality disorder rather than an illness. These conditions share with hysteria the capacity for *dissociation* and the use of illness for *manipulation* of those around them.

HISTRIONIC PERSONALITY

A patient with histrionic personality (usually female) finds it difficult to form close attachments and when she does they are highly dependent. Her emotions are often superficial and rarely satisfying. She may be very alluring and attractive to men, but finds it difficult to enjoy sex herself. She carries with her an atmosphere of drama: her life is often a series of emotional or practical crises. Her feelings are dramatised and exaggerated; her headaches are always 'migraines', her diarrhoea 'dysentery' and her pains invariably 'excruciating'. She uses her crises to coerce those around her (including doctors and nurses) and sometimes has a husband whom she abuses and yet clings to, and who appears to submit willingly to all her demands. As a child she may have felt emotionally neglected and insignificant, helpless and dependent. The anger and manipulation which manifest themselves in adult life can be seen as a continuation of this, an attempt, through the coercive power of illness, to keep attached to her those whom she feels may otherwise ignore or abandon her. Patients with histrionic personality sometimes develop the physical symptoms of hysteria.

MULTIPLE PERSONALITY

The adult personality is made up from a number of elements:

- Some come from *identifications* based on parents ('he has his father's temper and his mother's charm').
- Some represent different aspects of the *self*: the caring self, the aggressive self, the childish part of the self and so on.
- Some can be defined in terms of *relationships:* in a marriage a partner may be expected to be a spouse, lover, parent, colleague and friend.

Eric Berne has summarised these different aspects of the self as 'parent', 'adult' and 'child', all of whom co-exist within one person. In the mature personality, there is a blending together of the different aspects into a coherent whole so that a person is all of a piece, although minor

discontinuities and splits in the personality are common. The fascinating but rare clinical condition of multiple personality, in which several quite separate personalities appear to inhabit the same individual (fictionalised in such works as *Dr Jekyll and Mr Hyde* and *The Three Faces of Eve),* is an extreme example of this everyday splitting. In multiple personality, the different personalities have lives of their own which are entirely *dissociated* from one another; the good self is totally unaware of the bad self and would be horrified by its activities. This enables, say, a prudish aspect of the self to live alongside the sexual side without being aware of it, thereby avoiding anxiety or guilt. Patients with multiple personality can occasionally be helped towards integration with psychotherapy.

FACTITIOUS ILLNESS

Patients with unexplained symptoms are sometimes found – often after lengthy investigation – to have caused their own illness. A patient with unexplained and extensively investigated 'haemoptysis' was found to be venepuncturing herself, swallowing blood and then spitting into a sputum pot; a person with unexplained intestinal bleeding may be inserting foreign bodies into the rectum; hypoglycaemic attack can be produced by insulin injections in non-diabetics; and dermatitis artefacta (p. 1165) is yet another example of such factitious illness. Occasionally, such behaviour is due to psychosis but more often it is a manifestation of a personality disorder. These patients are often very 'nice'; they may be nurses or members of the other caring professions. They are often on good, even intimate, terms with medical staff. They may induce incomprehension, abhorrence and anger once they are discovered. Factitious illness is best seen as an extreme example of histrionic personality disorder. The patient has split off an angry, destructive, defiant part of herself which acts semi-autonomously and of which the 'good' self may be partially unaware. The principles of management of hysteria may be applied in these cases. A full history will reveal underlying conflicts, and the patient can then be told, in as gentle and unconfrontational a way as possible, that these conflicts may be responsible for her symptoms and that she may thus be playing a part in causing her own illness. Although the patient may become angry, the results of such an approach are rarely disastrous. The patient will often be relieved and even begin to accept psychological help.

FICTITIOUS ILLNESS: MUNCHAUSEN SYNDROME

Baron von Munchausen was an 18th century fictional character who travelled extensively and told fantastic stories. His name is now used to describe a group of patients with characteristic features:

Summary 17 Conditions related to histrionic personality	
Multiple personality	Aspects of the self entirely dissociated from one another, with lives of their own
Factitious illness	Self-inflicted illness
Fictitious illness (Munchausen syndrome)	Patient travels from hospital to hospital with ficitious illnesses. Pseudologia phantastica.

- The patients often experience recurrent unexplained symptoms, especially abdominal or chest pain, which are often thought to be due to renal colic, myocardial infarction or intestinal obstruction. The patient may be given opiates and have had several inconclusive laparotomies which reveal themselves as multiple abdominal scars.
- These patients travel from hospital to hospital, usually discharging themselves after a brief admission, and using a variety of assumed names.
- They give dramatic accounts of their lives, for example stories of heroic wartime feats or tragic losses, none of which can be corroborated and none of which quite adds up. These stories are sometimes labelled *pseudologia phantastica*.

Munchausen patients may be seen as the male counterparts of factitious illness patients. They are hard if not impossible to manage or help but awareness of the diagnosis will avoid unnecessary or dangerous investigations. Most doctors have had at least one experience of being hoodwinked in this way and this may be a necessary learning experience. The doctor must be friendly but firm in refusing to treat these patients as though they are ill. The patient usually disappears, but may occasionally accept social help.

EATING DISORDERS

Eating is not just about physiology. Food has great psychological and sociological significance. Morality starts with the child's discovery of what is good and bad to eat and a mother's self-evaluation may continue to depend on how well she feels she feeds her family. Birth, the reaching of adulthood, marriage and death are all marked by a meal. In addition, there are two factors, specific to many highly industrialised Western societies, of especial relevance to eating disorders: the role of the food industry with its large marketing system; and the emphasis on a slim body image as a mark of vitality and attractiveness.

Eating disorders are increasingly common, especially among women (Fig. 10.6). Although the overall incidence of anorexia nervosa is only 1 per 100 000 population, 1% of 16–18-year-olds are affected; 2% of women attending a family planning clinic suffer from bulimia nervosa; and the prevalence among dance students is 20%.

ANOREXIA NERVOSA

Aetiology and pathogenesis

No single cause of anorexia nervosa has been found. A number of factors appear to be involved:

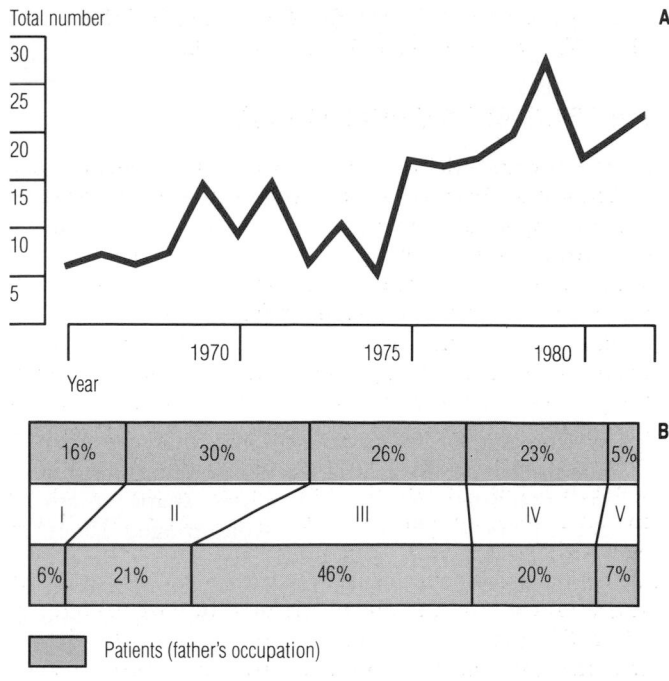

Fig. 10.6 Epidemiology of anorexia nervosa. A. New cases of anorexia nervosa appearing on the Aberdeen Psychiatric Register, 1965–82 (both sexes and all ages). **B.** Social class distribution of anorexic patients (father's occupation) compared with that for general population.

- *Social pressures* towards both eating and thinness, though contradictory, are important.
- *The fear of losing control* – both of eating and of sexuality – and a feeling of inadequacy and of not being a separate person are characteristic of the anorexic's inner world. Anorexia is an attempt by the individual to remain in complete control by regulating her food intake and her weight, and thereby putting her sexuality into reverse.
- *Family function* in anorexia is often abnormal. The families (where food is frequently a central theme) tend to be 'enmeshed', i.e. mutually overdependent. This causes little difficulty in early childhood, but with the advent of adolescence the family may be threatened by the possibility of autonomy and separation.
- *Endocrine abnormalities* occur in anorexia nervosa. Hypothalamic function is disturbed with reduced luteinising hormone (LH) and gonadotrophic hormone output, but this is more probably a consequence rather than a cause of weight loss. Low levels of plasma thyroxine and plasma TSH are also common. There may be alkalosis if there is surreptitious vomiting.

Clinical features

Four features are characteristic of anorexia nervosa.

- The most important is *phobic avoidance of normal weight*. The patient is terrified by the idea of her normal weight.
- With this goes a distortion of body image, known as *overperception*. By asking women to choose a silhouette that they feel represents their shape, it can be shown that it is normal for women aged 15–30 to perceive themselves as up to 50% fatter than they really are. Patients with anorexia nervosa see themselves as at least 100% bigger than they are: an emaciated girl of 35 kg may be disgusted by what she perceives as her gross obesity.
- The consequence of phobic avoidance and overperception is *relentless dieting*, especially the renunciation of carbohydrates.
- *Amenorrhoea* is an essential diagnostic feature. In males (10% of all anorexics) there is *disturbance of sexual function*, usually with loss of libido.

Anorexia nervosa usually starts in early or mid-adolescence. There is frequently an initial period of mild overweight, which may appal the girl, who then begins to pursue thinness. Her thoughts are dominated by food and how to avoid it. She absents herself from family meals although she may pride herself on providing food for others, whilst secretly despising and envying those who eat normally, or as she sees it, gluttonously. As long as she is thin she will be happy. To be thin is to be good; fat, bad. She may augment her efforts at dieting by taking laxatives, amphetamines or diuretics, and by self-induced vomiting. Battles about food may develop with her parents. *Denial* of weight loss (p. 175) is an important feature: she may conceal her emaciation within voluminous and floppy clothes. She is physically active or over-active as part of her secret plan for weight loss. Sometimes, deliberately *excessive exercise* may be a major factor in the weight loss. She complains of a feeling of 'fullness' in her stomach which prevents her from eating. She will be emotionally and socially, but not intellectually, less mature than her peer-group.

Physical examination will reveal thinness, scanty secondary sex characteristics, possibly peripheral cyanosis, a soft downy covering of the face and body *(lanugo hair)*, hypotension and bradycardia.

Differential diagnosis

The clinical picture may be one of two types:

- In *typical* anorexia the only obvious psychological abnormality is the difficulty in eating. Here, the main differential diagnoses are organic causes of weight loss in a young woman, for example, malabsorption syndrome, thyrotoxicosis or occult neoplasm.
- An *atypical* picture also occurs. Here the woman is often older (in her twenties) and her anorexic symptoms co-exist with other psychiatric features, such as depressive symptoms of misery and withdrawal; obsessional symptoms centering, for example, around cleanliness; and personality difficulties.

Management

A patient weighing less than 35 kg should be admitted to hospital. A behavioural regimen in which the patient agrees on a target weight and is rewarded with privileges (watching television, being allowed visitors) in return for weight gain is usually effective in the short run. Occasionally, a small dose of a phenothiazine (e.g. chlorpromazine 50 mg b.d.) is helpful. However, the patient will often lose weight again once she is discharged unless psychotherapy is also started. Psychotherapy is the treatment of choice for outpatients. Mild anorexia can respond to simple counselling. In more severe cases, family therapy is the best treatment for those under 17; while for older patients (especially if they have left home) individual psychotherapy is the preferred treatment. In each case, the aims of therapy are:

- to help both patient and family to move away from the area of food as a focus for all conflicts and difficulties
- to help the patient accept herself as she is, both her body and her feelings.

Prognosis

Twenty-five per cent of anorexic patients spontaneously recover; 25% make a full recovery with medical intervention; about 25% continue to experience some difficulties with eating but can lead a normal life; 25% remain quite severely handicapped. About 5–10% of anorexics die of the condition. Poor prognosis is associated with later onset, 'atypical features' (see above), marked body image disturbance and self-induced vomiting. Recovery is accompanied by reversal of the hormonal abnormalities and the onset of normal menstruation.

BULIMIA NERVOSA

Bulimia nervosa is a syndrome of 'binge eating' (bulimia: to stuff oneself with food) and self-induced vomiting in the presence of normal weight. There is an overlap here with anorexia nervosa, where binge–vomit cycles can also occur, but in anorexia the patient is always abnormally thin and also amenorrhoeic. The usual age of presentation in bulimia also tends to be older, with patients (usually women) in the 20–30 age range, rather than the teens.

The bulimic is frightened of becoming fat, but can accept her normal weight. She is terrified by her greed and tries to avoid its consequences by making herself sick. She normally feels deeply ashamed about this. She lives in a state of *dietary chaos* in which she is determined to fast, succeeds for a while, then succumbs to hunger and starts eating. She binges, then feels guilty, makes herself sick and then starves; and so the cycle starts again.

The physical consequences of bingeing and vomiting include erosion of dental enamel from exposure to gastric acid, Mallory-Weiss oesophageal tears, and even oesophageal rupture. Repeated vomiting causes hypokalaemia which may in turn produce tetany, paraesthesiae, ileus, cardiac arrhythmias, and epileptic fits.

Bulimic symptoms are common: 20% of women attending a family planning clinic admitted to bingeing, while 2% had the full syndrome. Like anorexia, bulimia may exist either on its own, or as part of a general disturbance of personality and be associated with alcoholism, deliberate self-harm or shoplifting, all of which make the prognosis less good.

Treatment of bulimia nervosa is usually successful and involves helping the woman to re-establish a regular eating pattern, and to feel less guilty. The bulimic often feels a great relief when dietary control is re-established, unlike the anorexic, who feels threatened at the idea of giving up her own control. In addition to a behavioural approach, exploration of the conflicts underlying the bulimia (such as marital difficulties or feelings of anger which the patient is unable to express) is also necessary. A proportion of bulimics have experienced sexual abuse in childhood and this too needs psychotherapeutic exploration.

OBESITY

Obesity in itself is not a psychiatric problem, but morbid obesity can be experienced as a severe handicap, compa-

---

Summary 20 Treatment of bulimia nervosa

- Keep a diary of everything eaten and all episodes of vomiting
- Re-establish dietary control; eat three meals per day *even if bingeing*
- Identify triggers to bingeing (anger, loneliness)
- Challenge erroneous assumptions, e.g. 'if I eat a chocolate bar I will become grossly obese and no-one will love me'

---

rable to amputation or disfigurement. Respiratory, endocrine and cardiovascular complications are common and serious, and gross obesity should, like anorexia nervosa, be considered a life-threatening condition. Obese people feel ostracised, and experience self-disgust. They long to be 'normal' and may become depressed by unsuccessful efforts at dieting. There are often marital and family difficulties which are both a cause and a consequence of their obesity. Prognosis for weight loss, either by dieting or surgery (e.g. intestinal by-pass) is not good. Psychotherapy can be a precursor to weight reduction if it helps the patient to accept him/herself as he/she is. The patient may then find it easier to diet, being less inclined to resort to the comfort of food whenever an emotional upset occurs.

DRUG DEPENDENCE

Addiction to illicit drugs, especially opiates, is a source of widespread medical and social concern. There are three main reasons for this. Firstly, there has been an epidemic increase in opiate abuse over the past 50 years. In 1936, there were about 500 known addicts in the UK (of whom one-quarter were doctors); by the mid-1970s this figure had risen to 6000; and in 1988, following the introduction to the UK of cheap heroin, the number of known addicts was estimated to be at least 50 000 (Fig. 10.7), of whom 9000 were registered with the Home Office.

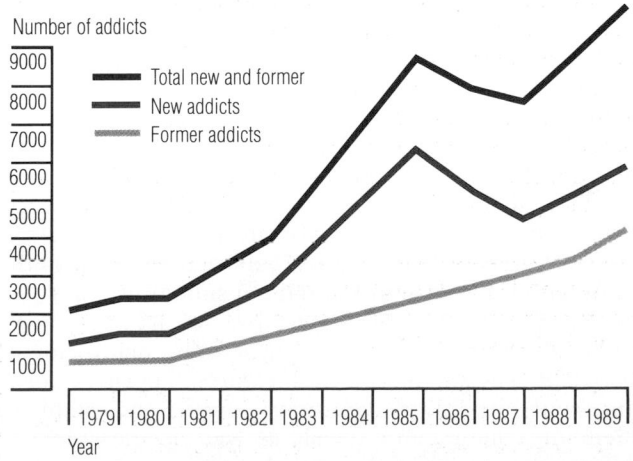

Fig. 10.7 New and former addicts notified to the Home Office.

Secondly, the impact of opiate addiction has profound medical and social consequences. Within five years, 10% of addicts will have died from drug-related causes, including AIDS, hepatitis B and overdose. Thirdly, 'drug addiction' is a microcosm of a much wider social problem.

Nature and causes of drug dependence

In the past, definitions of drug abuse have concentrated on a contrast between the harmful and the beneficial effects of drugs, thus dividing drugs into 'good' drugs (prescribed by doctors) and 'bad' ones (self-administered by addicts). This distinction does not take account of the fact that almost all drugs, even when medically prescribed, have harmful effects and can be misused; analgesics and tranquillisers are the best examples of this. Conversely, opiates can be of great benefit in the treatment of severe pain.

Current definitions of drug dependence are based on the interaction between the individual and the drug leading to a compulsion to take it:

- in order to experience its psychic effects and/or
- to avoid the unpleasant effects of its withdrawal (abstinence syndrome).

There is no single cause of drug addiction. The prevalence of addiction is determined by:

- the *availability* of the drug. The greater the availability, the greater prevalence of addiction. In Hong Kong, where heroin is widely available, 8–10% of the adult male population is addicted
- the *accessibility* of the drug. This explains the relative commonness of drug addiction among doctors and nurses, and in inner-city and coastal areas
- the *susceptibility* of individuals to addiction or misuse.

Management of drug addiction is equally multifaceted and involves a combination of physical, psychological and social rehabilitation.

OPIATE ADDICTION

Causes

The most important cause of opiate addiction is its availability. Susceptible individuals expose themselves to the drug, either because they inhabit a subculture in which drug taking is prevalent, or because they are psychologically vulnerable due to family difficulties, depression or boredom. The pharmacological features of opiates – tolerance and withdrawal syndrome – ensure the establishment of a habit, and social, as well as physiological factors, then maintain the addiction and make rehabilitation difficult.

Biochemical factors

The discovery in 1977 of the encephalin neurotransmitters was a major advance in the understanding of opiate addiction. Endorphins are naturally occurring, opiate-like substances which mediate pain and other sensations in the mid-brain. It is possible that individuals susceptible to addiction may genetically be deficient in endorphins and so 'opiate hungry'. Both opiates and endorphins reduce the amount and effects of other cerebral neurotransmitters such as acetylcholine. This has led to the 'supersensitivity' theory of withdrawal syndrome, which postulates that addicted individuals have reduced amounts of transmitter reaching postsynaptic receptors. Stopping the drug then results in a sudden increase in transmitter and stimulation of the already supersensitive receptor.

Psychological factors

Drugs can be administered ('dropped') by injection ('fixing') either subcutaneously ('skin-pop') or intravenously ('mainline'); or by smoking ('chasing the dragon'). All these methods are powerful reinforcers in the Pavlovian sense:

- *primary* reinforcement from both the pleasure ('buzz') and removal of withdrawal symptoms
- *secondary* reinforcement from the associated rituals of administration, e.g. filling the needle
- *social* reinforcement from fellow-addicts.

Psychiatric factors

Opiate addiction is more likely to be a cause than a consequence of psychiatric illness. 'Loners' may well be suffering from anxiety and depressive symptoms which they are trying vainly to treat with opiate drugs. Hospitalised addicts (as opposed to the generality of addicts) tend to be suffering from personality disorder and to have difficulty in forming close relationships. Addicts are caught in a vicious circle in which their primary relationship comes to be with the drug, which is felt to be more accessible, reliable and instantly gratifying than a person. There is some evidence that family discord and alcoholism is commoner in the childhood histories of addicts than in controls. The anxiety associated with the early stages of opiate withdrawal may mirror early childhood experiences of separation from desired, but inaccessible, parents.

Social factors

There is no particular social class preponderance for opiate addiction.

Presentation

Addiction to opium and its derivatives, morphine and heroin (diacetyl morphine), can be considered as a model of drug addiction in general. The physical signs which should arouse suspicion of opiate abuse are listed in Table 10.12. Addicts present to doctors in one of four ways:

- With infective complications of self-administered injections, e.g. septic abscess at injection site or septicaemia, infectious hepatitis or manifestations of HIV.
- With confusion or unconsciousness due to overdose of the drug, deliberate or accidental.
- Wanting, or apparently wanting, help with their habit.
- With a withdrawal syndrome. This consists of a craving for the drug together with physiological features which include rhinorrhoea, lacrimation, yawning, perspiration, irritability, gooseflesh, nausea, diarrhoea, cramps, muscle pains, tachycardia, flushing and involuntary movements. It is not life-threatening and the symptoms begin to recede at about 72 hours after last taking the drug.

Opiate users are heterogeneous; only a minority correspond to the social stereotype of the addict. Lifestyles can be divided into four types:

'Stables'. Addicts in whom the habit exists with a fairly conventional life, e.g. regular employment, family and marriage.

'Junkies'. Here, the addict inhabits a drug subculture in which all activities – social, financial, sexual – are subsidiary to the need to obtain drugs.

'Loners'. The addict is socially isolated and inhabits a solitary world of addiction.

'Two-worlders'. These contain elements of stables and junkies, often leading a 'normal' life at work but returning to a 'junkie' world when not working.

Management

Legal requirements

In the UK, any doctor attending a patient who is known, or suspected, to be addicted to opiates is required to inform the Home Office Drug Branch. Only specially licensed doctors are permitted to prescribe morphine and diamorphine (heroin) for the maintenance of addiction. Other opiates, such as methadone, may be prescribed by any doctor for the management of withdrawal syndrome, but this should be done only with great constraint and in an emergency.

General management

Drug abusers may not be open about their habit, which should be suspected in unexplained cases of psychosis, sepsis, serum hepatitis or HIV infection. Scapegoating should be avoided, and drug users should be treated with the same concern and courtesy as any other patient. At the same time, caution should be exercised: addicts may steal prescription pads and syringes, and exaggerate their drug needs in order to obtain drugs which are then sold. In an initial interview, a urine screen should be carried out to confirm that the patient is a user, and blood should also be tested for hepatitis B and HIV (the latter normally with the patient's consent). Whenever possible, the patient should then be referred for specialist help. Occasionally (e.g. in a casualty department at a weekend) withdrawal symptoms have to be treated and a dose of methadone given equivalent to the average daily intake which the doctor calculates is being used. The usual dose is between 20 and 70 mg of methadone. Typical detoxification schedules are given in Table 10.13. Where heroin intake is low, diphenoxylate and chlormethiazole can be used. Prescriptions should be on a daily basis for not more than two days. A clear management policy should be instituted and explained to the patient.

Table 10.12 History and examination of suspected opiate abuser

History
Previous contact with a prescribing doctor or clinic
History of recent use (doses, frequency, legal, illegal)
Assessment of demands or requests
Assessment of withdrawal symptoms
Current legal problems

Examination
Injection sites: needle marks, tracks, bruises, thrombosed veins, abscesses, skin ulcers
Arterial spasm or gangrene (caused by, e.g. dipipanone, cyclizine)
Jaundice from hepatitis A or B
Emaciation

Investigation
Urine for drug assays
Liver function tests
Hepatitis A or B serology
HIV test (with consent)

Table 10.13 A typical detoxification schedule for opiate addiction

10 day detoxification (volume kept at 25 ml)		28 day detoxification (volume kept at 25 ml)	
Methadone	25 mg/day – 2 days	Methadone	30 mg/day – 4 days
	15 mg/day – 2 days		25 mg/day – 3 days
	8 mg/day – 2 days		20 mg/day – 4 days
	4 mg/day – 2 days		13 mg/day – 3 days
	2 mg/day – 2 days		10 mg/day – 4 days
			6 mg/day – 3 days
			3 mg/day – 7 days

Treatment of medical complications of addiction

The main medical complications of addiction are septi-caemia (p. 220), hepatitis (p. 641), endocarditis (p. 413) and HIV infection (p. 243).

Rehabilitation

In the UK, all regions have drug clinics to which the addict should be referred. Here, the patient may be offered an oral methadone maintenance programme (see Table 10.14) in the hope, not always realised, of reducing use of illicit drugs. An attempt is made to form a rapport with the user. After establishing a baseline habit, some addicts will be gradually withdrawn from the drug over a 10-week period either as an outpatient or, more rapidly, as an inpatient. Others will be stabilised on a mainte-nance methadone programme as a way of facilitating a period of stability in the addict's life (reduces the need for crime; forms a relationship with the drug clinic team). Withdrawal is an essential, but by no means sufficient, aspect of treatment. Addicts exposed to enforced absti-nence, e.g. in prison, almost always relapse when released. Psychotherapeutic and social help are also needed if the addict is to remain drug-free.

ADDICTION TO NON-OPIATES

Dependence on non-opiate drugs has become a major health problem in recent years. The changing pattern of dependence is shown in Figure 10.8.

Barbiturates

Barbiturate addicts now comprise a small number of older patients (mostly women) who are relics of the barbi-turate era, and a number of young multiple drug users for whom barbiturates are one of a number of drugs in their repertoire.

The effects of barbiturates are similar to those of alcohol, viz. intoxication, ataxia and depression of con-

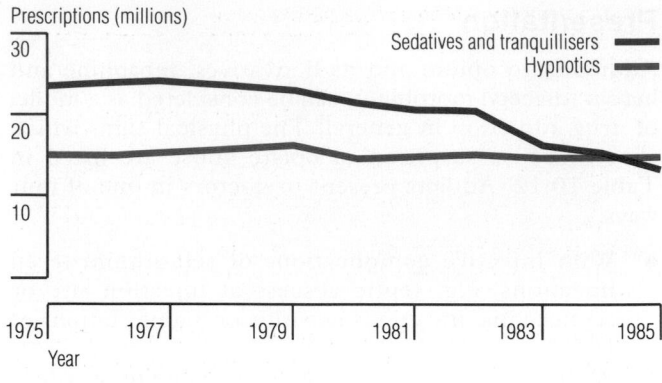

A

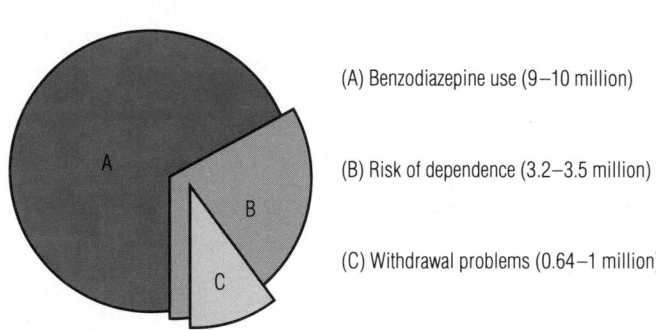

(A) Benzodiazepine use (9–10 million)

(B) Risk of dependence (3.2–3.5 million)

(C) Withdrawal problems (0.64–1 million)

B

Fig. 10.8 Changing patterns of consumption of non-opiate drugs in the UK. A. Prescriptions for sedatives/tranquillisers and hypnotics, 1974–1985. **B.** Current benzodiazepine use and dependence in the UK. In one year, (A) 9–10 million people use benzodiazepines. (B) Of these, 3.2–3.5 million use them for more than four months and are at risk of dependence. (C) Of these, 0.64–1 million are likely to suffer withdrawal problems.

sciousness. Respiratory depression due to overdose is a frequent cause of death. A *withdrawal syndrome* occurs in which convulsions are common. This should be controlled by pentobarbitone (short-acting) 4–6 hourly. Withdrawal should be carried out slowly over several weeks.

Benzodiazepines

Benzodiazepines have now replaced barbiturates both in popularity and as a cause for widespread addiction. Although the three million annual prescriptions cause less mortality than barbiturates (as they do not produce respi-ratory depression), they are an important source of morbidity (see p. 175). There is an increased incidence of road traffic accidents in benzodiazepine-takers. A with-drawal syndrome occurs in patients who have taken more than 20 mg daily over six weeks (see Table 10.15).

The symptoms of minor affective disorder (often self-limited), for which benzodiazepines are initially prescribed, may also then become part of a withdrawal syndrome which can be mistaken for the original illness and lead to further prescriptions. Like barbiturates,

Table 10.14 Characteristics of methadone linctus which justify its use as a treatment

- Non-injectable
- Not attractive to users looking for buzz
- Low street retail value
- Controlled drug – able to be prescribed on daily collection
- Long half-life for established users, hence reliable urine testing and stabilises drug-taking experience
- If it does 'leak' from the drug service to the streets is likely to only be used by established users for whom it is a safer preparation. Some of these will use purchased methadone for detoxification
- As a 'linctus', consumption can be supervised if necessary

Table 10.15 Symptoms of benzodiazepine withdrawal

● Insomnia	● Sweating
● Anxiety	● Tiredness
● Depression	● Perceptual abnormalities
● Outbursts of anger	Visual disturbance
● Muscular pains	Depersonalisation
● Tremor	Vertigo
● Headache	● Fits
● Nausea, weight loss, anorexia	● Psychosis

benzodiazepines are best withdrawn in a slowly reducing dosage over several weeks. Antidepressants or even ECT (q.v.) may be needed to treat the depression associated with withdrawal.

Stimulants

Amphetamines do not appear to cause physiological dependence, but produce a psychosis which is clinically very similar to paranoid schizophrenia. Tactile hallucinations ('formication') are a feature of cocaine intoxication. Withdrawal from amphetamines often leads to a severe state of depression.

Hallucinogens

Hallucinogenic drugs like LSD (lysergic acid diethylamide) and 'magic mushrooms' produce a toxic psychosis characterised by vivid hallucinations and delusions. Prolonged psychosis may be precipitated by taking LSD in susceptible individuals. 'Flash-backs' may occur for several months after an LSD 'trip'.

Cannabis

Cannabis, like alcohol, appears to have few harmful effects if taken in moderation. Ten per cent of all young people have tried cannabis at some time, and 25% of students use it at least once a week. In some cultures and subcultures (e.g. Rastafarians), regular cannabis use, especially among males, is the rule. The active principle is THC (tetrahydrocannabinol) which is sometimes used as an antiemetic in terminal care. As with LSD, excessive use (or occasional use in susceptible subjects) produces a psychosis, and a withdrawal syndrome may occur. It has been suggested that regular use of cannabis may produce a state of apathy or *amotivational syndrome.*

Solvent abuse

Inhalation of solvents such as toluene and acetone (used as vehicles for glue and other agents) produces a temporary state of euphoria. Glue-sniffing is common in certain youth subcultures. It is dangerous: an appreciable mortality has been recorded from direct cerebral damage as well as asphyxia due to the use of polythene bags to concentrate the vapour. Morbidity includes hepatitis, renal damage, cardiac arrhythmias, polyneuropathy and aplastic anaemia.

Drug screening

Urine can be analysed for benzodiazepines, cannabis, amphetamines and opiates (but not LSD) and this is a useful test in cases of psychosis where drug abuse may be a possible cause.

ALCOHOLISM

Alcohol is a major cause of medical and psychiatric morbidity in the UK (Table 10.16) and world-wide. In the UK, a 200% increase in alcohol consumption since 1950 (Fig. 10.9) has been accompanied by a 25-fold increase in

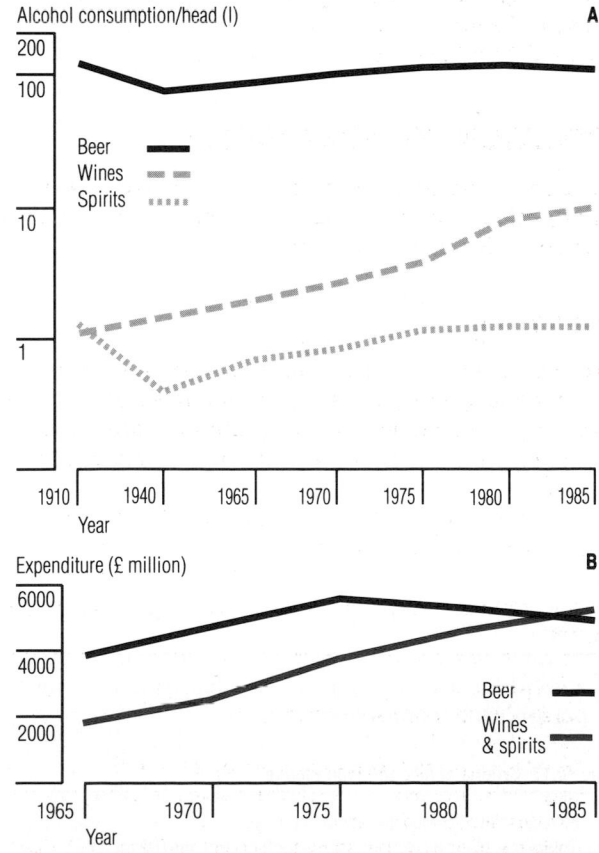

Fig. 10.9 Trends in alcohol consumption and expenditure in the United Kingdom. A. Alcohol consumption 1916–1986. **B.** Consumer expenditure on alcohol, 1950–1985.

Table 10.16 Alcohol consumption and alcoholism in the United Kingdom (population 55 million)

Alcohol consumption	Estimated numbers
Regular drinkers	36 M
Heavy drinkers	2 M
Problem drinkers	700 000
Addicted drinkers	200 000

admissions for alcoholism to psychiatric hospitals between 1960 and 1980. About 20% of admissions to medical wards are due to alcohol or alcohol-related diseases. Forty per cent of male attenders at hospital casualty departments have drink-related problems (p. 637).

Definitions

Some criteria for alcohol dependence are given in Table 10.17. Two important patterns of alcoholism require definition, problem drinking and alcohol dependence.

Problem drinking

The WHO defines alcoholism as drinking that causes emotional, social or physical damage to the individual. Problem drinkers may suffer from all three, e.g. anxiety or depression related to alcohol; divorce, unemployment or financial difficulties; and gastritis or physical trauma associated with drinking.

Alcohol dependence

The essential feature of alcohol dependence is the development of a *withdrawal syndrome* when the drug is removed. The dependent alcoholic will drink, usually early in the day, in order to stave off withdrawal symptoms such as nausea, tremor, sweating or agitation. Other features of alcohol dependence include:

- *Narrowing of the drinking repertoire.* The ordinary drinker's consumption varies from day to day. The dependent alcoholic has a daily drinking routine which must be followed.
- *Predominance of drinking over other activities.* For the alcoholic, drink, even if it is clearly damaging the person's life, comes first.

Table 10.17 Criteria of alcohol dependence

- More than 80 g of alcohol consumed daily
- Tolerance: blood alcohol levels greater than 150 mg/100 ml
- Withdrawal symptoms
- Continued drinking in spite of psychological, social, and physical problems
- Abnormal blood tests, e.g. macrocytic anaemia and raised γ-GT

- *Tolerance.* The capacity of the dependent individual to drink large quantities of alcohol is an expression of physiological tolerance.

Presentation: the hidden alcoholic

Alcoholics have to be very ill or very brave to complain of their condition directly. Only about 10% of alcoholics in the community are in contact with psychiatric services, while about half are known to other agencies such as general practitioners, social services or parish priests. The remainder are unknown and untreated. Doctors need a high 'index of suspicion' if they are to diagnose these hidden alcoholics correctly. The following factors should alert the examining doctor:

- unexplained gastrointestinal complaints
- complaints of anxiety and depression or panic attacks without obvious external precipitants
- social difficulties, e.g. marital disruption, absenteeism
- unexplained accidents
- smelling of alcohol at unexpected times
- single males over 40, socially isolated females
- certain occupations, e.g. publicans, journalists, doctors
- unexplained macrocytosis, or elevated liver enzyme values.

Where alcoholism is suspected, a detailed alcohol history should be taken. Vague questions, such as 'How much do you drink?', are unlikely to be informative, while positive answers to two or more of the CAGE questions (Table 10.18) suggest a drinking problem. A detailed account of a typical 'drinking day' is required. Alcohol intake is measured in units. One unit equals half-a-pint of beer, quarter-of-a-pint of strong lager, one 'short' or one glass of wine. Regular intake of six units or more per day puts men at risk of alcohol dependence. Women need half as much (i.e. three units per day) for half as long (e.g. as little as two years) for dependency to occur. The patient should be asked when he last had a day without a drink; about the longest period without a drink in the preceding five years; about withdrawal symptoms; and about blackouts. A 'drink diary' in which the patient records his drinking behaviour for a week can be a useful aid to history-taking. Raised serum γ-glutamyl transpeptidase (γ-GT) and increased mean corpuscular volume

Table 10.18 The CAGE questions*

- Have you ever felt you ought to cut down on your drinking?
- Have people annoyed you by criticising your drinking?
- Have you ever felt bad or guilty about your drinking?
- Have you ever had a drink first thing in the morning to steady your nerves or get rid of a hangover (eye-opener)?

*Positive answers to two or more of these suggests a drinking problem

(MCV) are useful supportive evidence of abnormal drinking and are also helpful in monitoring progress. A blood alcohol concentration may confirm suspicions of recent excessive intake.

Aetiology

Mutually interacting genetic, psychological and cultural factors underlie alcoholism. Adoption studies show that adopted children of alcoholics are four times as likely to develop alcoholism as adopted children of non-alcoholics. The biochemical mediator of an inherited tendency to alcoholism is unknown: however, active alcohol dehydrogenase leading to higher (and unpleasant) acetaldehyde levels has been postulated as protective against alcoholism.

Psychological factors operate in two ways in alcoholism.

- *Imitation learning.* An individual's tendency to drink follows that of his subculture, parents and peer group (Table 10.19).
- *Alleviation of unpleasant feelings.* Alcohol reduces unpleasant feelings such as social anxiety and guilt. Each time an individual drinks the experience of reduction of unpleasant mood ('drowning your sorrows') is reinforced. Family disruption is a common experience in the history of alcoholics.

The true aetiology should be distinguished from the reasons for drinking offered by the patient, as the alcoholic's explanation of why he drinks is often a rationalisation. The alcohol addict drinks because of his physiological state of addiction.

Physical complications

The physical complications of alcoholism (see Chs 12, 16, 22) include liver disease (Ch. 16), neurological syndromes (Ch. 22) (including peripheral neuropathy, cerebellar

Table 10.19 Factors associated with risk of alcoholism

Factor	Examples of occupations affected
Availability of alcohol	Workers in the drink trade, caterers, business executives
Social pressure to drink	Coal miners, seamen, medical students, journalists
Freedom from supervision	Company directors, lawyers, GPs
Separation from normal social or sexual relationships	Commercial travellers, seamen, oil-rig workers, service personnel
Strains, stresses, and hazards	Coal miners, doctors, military personnel, actors, saxophonists
High or low income	Doctors, the unemployed
Collusion by colleagues	Doctors, workers in the drink trade

Summary 21 Some presentations of undeclared alcohol abuse (should raise 'index of suspicion')

Psychological	Physical
Memory lapses	Gastrointestinal symptoms
Depression	Dyspepsia
Anxiety	Pain
Outbursts of unprovoked anger	Nausea
Suicide attempts	Haematemesis
Morbid jealousy	Neurological symptoms
Paranoia	Tremor
Acute confusional state (DTs)	Paraesthesia
Unpredictability	Muscular weakness
	Unexplained fits

Social
Marital difficulties
Problems at work
Accidents at home or on the roads
Delinquency, crime
Violence

degeneration, myopathy and convulsions), cardiomyopathy, pulmonary tuberculosis, anaemia, hypoglycaemia and pancreatitis. Children of alcoholic mothers may be born with a syndrome of low birth-weight and developmental retardation known as the *fetal alcohol syndrome*.

Psychiatric complications

There are three levels of severity at which psychiatric complications of alcoholism occur. In the initial stages, the patient may present with minor psychiatric symptoms of panic attacks, anxiety, depressions or sexual difficulties. The alcoholic addict will develop delirium tremens and sometimes alcoholic hallucinosis. Prolonged and severe alcohol addiction leads to alcohol-related dementia including Korsakoff psychosis (Ch. 22.)

Delirium tremens (DTs) is discussed on page 979.

Alcoholic hallucinosis. Alcoholics may experience auditory hallucinations, usually derogatory or persecutory, in the presence of clear consciousness (consciousness is always clouded in DTs). These usually stop when drinking ceases but occasionally persist, suggesting coexisting schizophrenia.

Morbid jealousy. Alcohol is a frequent cause of a syndrome of morbid jealousy, in which an individual (usually male) becomes convinced that his spouse is unfaithful.

Wernicke-Korsakoff syndrome (q.v.) and alcoholic brain damage are discussed in Chapter 22.

Management

The outcome of treatment for alcoholism (Table 10.20) depends less on the nature of the treatment than on the

Table 10.20 Outcome of treatment for alcoholism

Outcome	1 year (%)	2 year (%)
Improved	35	25
Still drinking	53	43
Dead	3	1
Lost to follow-up	19	21

social situation and personality of the patient. Addicts with stable family and employment and a good personality do best. The impulsive or psychopathic drinker lacking home, family or job has a very poor prognosis for sobriety.

The aim of treatment should almost always be abstinence. Any doctor who attempts to help alcoholics must be prepared for disappointment as relapses ('slips') are common. A combination of limit-setting and acceptance is needed in all of the following treatment approaches.

Psychotherapy

A supportive relationship, either with a spouse, peer (e.g. through Alcoholics Anonymous) or a professional helper is probably essential. Formal psychotherapy or social help should be conditional on sobriety, on the principle that whatever an alcoholic's problems (and they will be many) drink makes them worse. Wherever possible, the spouse and family should be included in any psychotherapy programme.

Inpatient treatment

Brief admission for 'drying-out', or longer admission to a therapeutic community with group therapy can help maintenance of sobriety. Patients who need admission are by definition more disturbed, and the long-term prognosis is therefore often poor.

Drug treatment

Disulfiram (Antabuse) reacts with alcohol to produce acetaldehyde, producing unpleasant feelings of flushing and nausea. Some patients find it helpful to have this internal 'chemical fence' to discourage drinking.

Alcoholics Anonymous

Alcoholics Anonymous (AA), started in the 1930s by an alcoholic doctor ('Bob'), is a worldwide self-help organisation for alcoholics run by ex-alcoholics. It offers a structured personal and group psychotherapy programme aimed at sobriety. An important feature of AA is that it provides a social life that is not based on pubs or drinking. A parallel organisation, Al-Anon, offers support to the families of alcoholics.

'Shop-front'/'dry house' programmes

The 'skid-row' alcoholic has usually lost everything – job, home, family, possessions, friends – through drinking, and special facilities are needed for this group of patients (about 10% of alcoholics). These include non-threatening 'drop-in' day centres, after-care hostels and long-term medical and social support.

Prevention

There is a direct relationship between per capita consumption and the price and availability of alcohol. As the real cost of alcohol has fallen steadily in the UK over the past decade, so per capita alcohol consumption and hence alcoholism rates have risen accordingly (Fig. 10.9). Governments, through pricing policies and licensing laws, can have a direct effect on alcoholism rates. Well-funded education programmes are also needed to alert the public to the dangers of alcohol.

MENTAL HANDICAP

Mental handicap can be defined as the arrested or incomplete development of the cognitive (i.e. intellectual) part of the mind. Such a broad definition covers a wide range of individuals:

- *Severely mentally handicapped*, who lack speech, are unable to learn, cannot dress or feed themselves, may be incontinent, and may have stereotyped movements such as rocking or thumb-sucking. The majority are looked after in institutions.
- *Moderately mentally handicapped*, who have a considerable handicap (e.g. very restricted speech) but are able to live in sheltered accommodation in the community.
- *Mildly mentally handicapped*, who have the capacity to learn and to live normal, if somewhat restricted, lives. Their primary problems are social and educational rather than medical. Most can live independently in the community.

Mental illness and mental handicap

It is only recently that mental illness and mental handicap have been properly distinguished. It is now understood that the majority of mentally handicapped people are not psychiatrically ill, and that they should be cared for by the social, rather than medical, services. Nevertheless, the mentally handicapped are particularly vulnerable to mental illness due both to their physical handicap and to emotional and social immaturity. They can develop the full range of mental illness including schizophrenia, manic depression, anxiety states and hysteria. Distress is likely to be expressed behaviourally, for example through withdrawal, temper tantrums, compulsive masturbation or law-breaking (e.g. shoplifting or self-exposure) rather than verbally.

Causes of mental handicap

Moderate and *severe* mental handicap usually has a distinct cause. This may be:

- *A single gene disorder,* e.g. untreated phenylketonuria, tuberous sclerosis, mucopolysaccharidoses, untreated galactosaemia and Tay-Sachs disease.
- *Chromosomal,* e.g. Down's syndrome, fragile-X mental retardation, deletion and duplication syndromes.
- *Traumatic,* e.g. birth injury or anoxia. Here, the mental handicap is usually associated with spasticity.
- *Infective,* e.g. maternal toxoplasmosis, cytomegalovirus and rubella; bacterial and viral meningitis. All may cause severe mental handicap.
- *Other causes* include rhesus incompatibility, lead poisoning, and maternal drugs such as anticonvulsants or alcohol.

Mild mental handicap usually lacks a specific inherited or environmental cause. It is thought to be a result of polygenic inheritance, often coupled with an impoverished environment.

Management

The principles of management of adult mental handicap are shown in Table 10.21.

Prevention

Primary prevention is exemplified by rubella inoculation and the provision of lead-free paint. Secondary preven-

Table 10.21 Principles of management of adult mental handicap

- Accurate diagnosis
- Treatment of co-existing mental and physical illness
- Provision of training facilities, day centres, sheltered workshops and social clubs
- Residential provision, e.g. hostels for those whose relatives cannot cope or are not available
- Provision of emotional support for carers who, for example, worry about what will happen when they are no longer able to care for their mentally handicapped dependant

tion is made possible by genetic counselling and by prenatal diagnosis and screening (see Ch. 5, p. 81).

PSYCHIATRY AND THE LAW

Mental illness may be associated with crime in one of three ways:

- *Psychosis.* The most famous example of a crime being the result of a psychosis is the 19th century McNaughten case in which a man who had tried to shoot the American President was acquitted 'by reason of insanity'.
- *Neurotic disorder.* Depression, for example, may make a criminal act such as shoplifting more likely ('diminished responsibility').
- *Psychopathic personality.*

Psychopathic personality disorder

People with a psychopathic personality disorder may be described as those with persistent social difficulties (often, but not always, involving law-breaking) in the absence of a psychosis or neurosis. Their crimes, if they do occur, may be as trivial as repeatedly breaking shop windows; or they may be serious, such as murder. In the 19th century these individuals were classified as 'morally insane'; they were not deluded or hallucinated, but they appeared not to know right from wrong or to be aware of the consequences of their actions. The term *sociopathic* is now sometimes used in order to avoid the derogatory connotations of 'psychopath'.

The concept of psychopathy implies:

- a persistent abnormality extending backwards to a childhood which was often disrupted and poor ('depraved because deprived')
- a major problem of social adjustment
- the absence of another psychiatric disorder.

A psychopathic individual has trouble not just in relationship to himself, or to immediate family (although this usually does happen), but also to institutions like the law, school, the armed services, employment and marriage. He is both dependent on institutions, and unable to coexist peaceably with them. There is usually associated alcohol and/or drug abuse.

The dividing line between normal and abnormal is harder to draw in psychopathy than any other psychiatric category and it is not a diagnosis that should be applied lightly. It is also important not to make such patients scapegoats. Sociopaths sometimes benefit from psychotherapy (providing firm limits are set), and from help with the social consequences of their psychopathy, such as homelessness and unemployment.

10 Psychological Medicine

MENTAL HEALTH LEGISLATION

Psychotic patients lack insight and may, occasionally, be dangerous either to themselves or to others. In the UK, until the 1930s, nearly all psychiatric inpatients were legally detained in hospital. Today, less than 10% of patients are detained on a 'Section'. While compulsory admission is sometimes necessary for the protection of the patient and the public, this power is open to misuse or even abuse. The United Kingdom Mental Health Act of 1983 aimed to provide safeguards against such abuse, and the Sections of the Act of particular relevance to general physicians are described below. In all cases, it is a duty of the hospital administration to inform the patient of his Section and a statutory right of the patient to appeal against compulsory detention.

Admission for assessment (Section 2)

The patient may be detained for up to 28 days if (a) he is suffering from mental disorder which warrants assessment; or (b) he is a danger to himself or others. The *application* for such assessment must be made by a social worker or the patient's nearest relative. There has also to be a *medical recommendation* from two medical practitioners. One of these must be a doctor officially approved as having special psychiatric experience; the other should if possible have known the patient previously (and is thus usually the patient's GP). In an emergency, the patient may be detained for up to 72 hours (Section 4) on the basis of only one medical recommendation which need not necessarily be by a psychiatrist.

Admission for treatment (Section 3)

The patient may be detained for up to six months. The conditions of the application and recommendation are therefore more stringent, and the rights of appeal greater than under Section 2. The patient must have a defined mental disorder, be thought likely to improve, and be unable to be cared for within the community.

Emergency detention of patients already in hospital (Section 5)

An informal patient may be held in hospital for up to 72 hours on the recommendation of the doctor in charge of his treatment without a Section 2 or 3 being instituted. Under Section 5(4), a psychiatric nurse can detain an informal patient already being treated for mental illness for up to six hours. Under Section 5(2), a patient in a general hospital who is being treated by a non-psychiatrist can be detained, under the report of the doctor in charge of the case, for up to 72 hours. A psychiatrist should see the patient as soon as possible to decide whether further detention is needed. Section 5(2) cannot be renewed.

Powers of the Courts (Sections 36, 37, 38)

Under these sections, mentally ill offenders can be compulsorily admitted to psychiatric units for assessment and treatment, rather than going to prison.

Place of safety order (Section 136)

Police officers have the power to remove to a place of safety any person whom they find in a public place who appears to be suffering from mental disorder, and who is in immediate need of care and control for his own sake, or that of others. Once removed, the patient must be medically examined and assessed. The place of safety is often a police station but may also be a hospital casualty department.

Consent to treatment (Sections 57, 58)

An important feature of the Act is a tightening of the procedure surrounding consent to treatment. Compulsorily detained patients can still be treated without their consent (e.g., given ECT or phenothiazine drugs), but a second opinion must first be obtained from a doctor appointed by the Mental Health Commission. Patients may not undergo *psychosurgery* (a brain operation occasionally undertaken in cases of depression or phobic anxiety) if they do not consent to it. Even if they do, a doctor and two non-medical appointees of the Mental Health Commission must scrutinise the case to ensure that consent has been validly given.

MEDICINE AND THE EMOTIONS

There are two basic types of mental activity. One is pictorial, non-rational and emotional, and concerns the biological fundamentals of birth, attachment, sex, separation and death as well as art and creativity; the second is rational, verbal and logical and concerns the achievement of specific goals and solving of particular problems. Freud called these the primary and secondary processes. Non-rational thinking is primary because it precedes rational thinking developmentally: infants and young children think in feelings and pictures. The secondary processes are only gradually acquired. In healthy adult life both co-exist. Much of waking life is dominated by secondary processes, but in dreams, daydreams and instinctual activity the primary processes take over. In mental illness the balance of primary and secondary processes may be disturbed: the psychotic, for example, is dominated by primary processes, while the patient with obsessional neurosis is trying to apply the false logic of secondary processes to his emotions.

Modern medicine is based on scientific rationality. This means that, at times, doctors may find it difficult to comprehend the emotional reactions of the patient to illness, death or sexuality. For the doctor, the patient who needs a routine hernia operation presents a technical problem to be solved; meanwhile, the patient may, at some level, be wondering whether he will survive the operation and, if so, whether his sex life will continue. Medical training is predominantly a training in rationality, in learning to set feelings aside. In order to understand the 'irrational' anxieties that trouble patients the doctor has to remain in touch with and respect the primary processes. The following sections on sex, and on death and dying, highlight some of these issues.

SEX AND MEDICINE

Sex matters for three main reasons: identity, attachment and continuity. Sexual abuse in childhood threatens all three and is an important underlying cause of psychiatric disturbance.

Identity

Gender is fundamental. When a baby is born the mother asks 'Is it alright?' then 'Is it a girl or a boy?'. Gender is essential to a sense of identity, and this can be threatened by illness at any of the stages of development. Hypospadism, hirsutism, hernia, delayed puberty, amenorrhoea, infertility, hysterectomy, prostatectomy, diabetes-related impotence – these are just a few of the many medical conditions which may threaten the sense of identity that is rooted in gender and sexual functioning.

Attachment

Human attachment occurs through the body. Even when communication is at a distance, hands are needed to write a letter, a voice to speak on the telephone. Sexual bonding is a powerful and rewarding form of attachment. The adolescent worries whether his or her body is 'good', 'big' or attractive enough to find a partner.

Where sexuality is threatened by illness and disability, the patient fears that the basis of his or her attachment may be undermined: 'who will want me if... I have a colostomy... a mastectomy... am impotent...?'

Psychogenic symptoms such as lower abdominal discomfort, pruritus or back pain may both arise from, and lead to, sexual difficulties. Such symptoms may draw attention to an underlying sexual anxiety, and at the same time provide the patient with the care and attention which

he fears may be lost through sexual failure. Occasionally, guilt about masturbation may be based on the misconception that it is 'wrong' or harmful and this too may lead to psychogenic symptoms.

Continuity

Psychologically, sex and reproduction may serve as an insurance against the fear of extinction. The idea of personal death is more acceptable if there is family continuity, or if an individual feels he has contributed something: that children, memories, ideas or objects will live on in the next generation. Threat to this sense of continuity can lead to feelings of anxiety or depression.

Taking a sexual history

Sex is, at least in theory, no longer a taboo subject, but in practice both doctor and patient are likely to feel anxious about some aspects of their sexuality. It is important that the doctor feels reasonably comfortable when asking about a patient's sexual life. All human beings have a sexual life – in the sense of thoughts, fantasies and feelings about sex regardless of whether or not they are celibate. The doctor needs to be sensitive to the common anxieties about sex and to be aware of those that may apply to a particular patient's age and situation (Table 10.22).

SEXUAL AND MARITAL DIFFICULTIES

Divorce and family disruption are becoming increasingly common. More than one in three marriages in the UK now ends in divorce, while in the USA the figure is one in two. The effects on developing children are unknown but are likely to be considerable. Partly in response to this there is now great interest in marital and family therapy.

The commonly encountered sexual difficulties are impotence, premature ejaculation and delayed ejaculation for men; and vaginismus and lack of sexual enjoyment (including anorgasmia) for women. Both sexes may suffer diminished libido. Transient difficulties are common; it is only when they are persistent and cause distress that they

Table 10.22 Common anxieties about sex

Adolescence	Middle-aged
Masturbation	Extramarital affairs
Homosexuality	Sex and illness
Genital inadequacy	
	Any age
Young adults	Incest
Impotence	Fetishism
Anorgasmia	Non-consummation
Infertility	of marriage
Lack of libido	

> **Summary 22 The Masters and Johnson approach**
>
> - Treatment in couples
> - Physical examination/history-taking (to reassure they are 'normal')
> - Instruction in sexual arousal
> - Instruction initially not to make love (to dispel anxiety)
> - Graded exercises based on sensate focus
> - Psychotherapy if necessary

constitute a problem. Sexual problems may be primary, i.e. present from the onset of sexual life, or secondary, i.e. develop after a period of satisfactory sexual functioning.

The Masters and Johnson approach

Current thinking about sexual dysfunction has been greatly influenced by the work of Masters and Johnson, who studied the physiology of sexual response and introduced a new classification and treatment for sexual difficulties.

General principles of the Masters and Johnson approach include the following:

- Treatment is in couples. Sexual difficulties are often complementary (e.g. premature ejaculation and anorgasmia) even though one member may present as the person with the problem. The non-presenting partner is given the role of co-therapist.
- Physical examination and careful history-taking of both partners are required both to rule out organic causes of sexual dysfunction and to reassure the patients that they are 'normal'.
- There is more to sex than penetration. Sexual arousal depends – especially in women – on a series of steps, and a man may need to learn that foreplay cannot usually be omitted if full sexual arousal in his partner is to occur.
- Anxiety is seen as a central element in sexual dysfunction. Anxiety is antagonistic to sexual arousal and a vicious circle can arise in which the patients fear they will fail (for example, to maintain erection, not to ejaculate prematurely, or to have an orgasm), which makes them 'try' harder, which makes them less able to relax and respond to sexual stimuli and thus more rather than less likely to fail.
- The aim of treatment is to break this circle. Paradoxically, the couple are initially instructed not to make love, in order to prevent performance anxiety. They are given a series of graded exercises based on sensate focus or stroking, in which they learn to give and receive pleasure. Initially this is non-genital, but later moves on to 'genital sensate focus', i.e. mutual masturbation. It is ironic that whereas masturbation was viewed (wrongly) by 19th century psychiatry as a major cause of insanity, it is now considered impor-

tant that both sexes are able to masturbate without guilt.
- Psychological factors in sexual dysfunction may also need treatment, through either individual or marital therapy. Unexpressed anger is a common cause of sexual disharmony: a couple who cannot row may also not be able to make love. Fear of loss of control, ignorance or guilt may also affect sexual pleasure.

The results of the Masters and Johnson approach are generally good, with 60–70% improvement rates reported in well-motivated couples.

DEATH AND DYING

Death is an integral part of medicine, but doctors and other medical staff often feel confused by the psychological and ethical questions it poses. Should a terminally ill patient be kept alive as long as possible, or allowed to die in peace? Should every patient with a fatal illness be told of his/her diagnosis, and if so how should the patient be told? Can a dying patient be helped to come to terms with death and how can this happen? What are the psychological reactions in the relatives of dying patients, and what support do they need?

These questions are problematic not only because of a lack of training and technique, but also because death is an intrinsically difficult subject which all but the exceptionally compassionate find it hard to face. Patients and doctors alike deny the reality of death in order to carry on with life.

Reactions in the patient

The response of the patient to the knowledge that he/she has a terminal illness can be compared to a bereavement reaction. The patient enters a state of grief for the loss of his/her own life. The initial reaction to discovering that one has a terminal illness is usually one of numbness and shock, a struggle between denial and acceptance. The patient attempts to fight off what is happening, and cannot believe it is true, that it is happening to him. This is often followed by a period of severe anxiety, in which the patient becomes dependent on visitors, family and medical staff, and finds it very hard to be alone. A period

> **Summary 23 Emotional reactions in terminally ill patients**
>
> - Numbness and shock
> - Struggle between denial and acceptance
> - Severe anxiety
> - Sadness and weeping
> - Anger
> - Eventual calmness

of sadness and weeping is inevitable. Anger is also a normal feature of this phase and the patient may become difficult, complaining, ungrateful and demanding. With time, however, the patient gradually becomes calmer, and during this phase the opportunity to talk may be very helpful. This series of reactions may be compressed into a few hours or spread over months, and, as with bereavement, does not follow a neat, orderly course.

Talking to dying patients

Breaking bad news and talking to dying patients is an art which can be learned through watching others, and through discussion of the feelings and difficulties it arouses. The patient can often be helped if staff and family recognise the subsequent reactions for what they are and then let the patient talk about his anger, panic and sadness. When this has happened the patient may feel better.

The issue of 'to tell or not' is a false alternative. Some patients want to know their diagnosis in great detail; others would rather not know. It is unnecessary and inappropriate to confront all patients with the stark reality of their illness. On the other hand, far more patients than are officially 'told' want to know their diagnosis or know it already. The patient needs space and time in which to discuss his feelings and ask questions. Gentle probing may be needed to help the patient make use of this opportunity.

Reactions in the family

Like the patient, families also go through an anticipatory grief reaction when a loved one is dying. The death of a child or adolescent is especially painful and unsupportable. Spouses of dying patients are particularly vulnerable. They may, for example, feel angry with their husband or wife for being ill, and feel very guilty about having such unvoiced thoughts. The stress of death may lead to tense and angry outbursts, either within the family or outside it at medical staff. Doctors and nurses should be prepared for this. Family counselling can help with these grief reactions and help to make death and bereavement, when they come, more bearable.

FURTHER READING

Clare A 1980 Psychiatry in dissent, 2nd edn. Tavistock, London. *A stimulating discussion of contemporary issues in pychiatry.*

Edwards G 1987 Treatment of drinking problems: a guide for the helping professions. Blackwell, Oxford. *A helpful, common-sense approach.*

Edwards G 1987 Drug scenes. Royal College of Psychiatrists, London. *A good guide to the problems and management of opiate addiction.*

Gelder M (ed) 1989 Oxford textbook of psychiatry, 2nd edn. OUP, Oxford. *Good, standard, medium-size textbook.*

Holmes J (ed) 1991 A textbook of psychotherapy in psychiatric practice. Churchill Livingstone, Edinburgh. *Covers the main psychiatric disorders from a psychodynamic point of view, with many case examples.*

Holmes J, Lindley R 1989 The values of psychotherapy. OUP, Oxford. *A discussion of the uses and abuses of psychotherapy.*

Malan D 1979 Individual psychotherapy and the science of psychodynamics. Butterworth, London. *Very readable account of brief psychotherapy.*

Wolff H, Bateman A, Sturgeon D (eds) 1989 The UCH handbook of psychiatry, 3rd edn. Duckworth, London. *Comprehensive up-to-date textbook with a psychodynamic slant.*

11

Infectious, Tropical and Parasitic Diseases

Mark H Wansbrough-Jones,
Stephen G Wright and Thomas J McManus

The relationship between humans and micro-organisms is usually one of balanced conflicts. In the first months of life encounters with micro-organisms are both a threat and a stimulus to the development of complex immune responses. In many parts of the world micro-organisms appear to have the upper hand, particularly over children. Worldwide, infectious gastroenteritis is the most common cause of death in children below the age of 1 year. The causative organisms are similar in underdeveloped and Western countries, but there is more frequent exposure from water supplies, methods of food preparation and poor standards of hygiene, including disposal of sewage. The outcome is worse, due to severity of dehydration.

Table 11.1 shows how the frequency of some infections varies in different areas of the world. The figures illustrate differences attributable to climate (malaria), standards of hygiene (typhoid) and immunisation (poliomyelitis, measles and diphtheria). The mortality associated with these diseases is also higher in underdeveloped countries because of a poor nutritional state at the onset of illness and limited access to medical facilities.

The pattern of infections is constantly changing. Infectious diseases become less important as a cause of death as the standard of living improves. England in 1860 was much the same as parts of Africa and Southeast Asia today with respect to some infectious diseases (Table 11.2). Improvements in standard of living and immunisation account for the change in many of these diseases but sometimes the pathogen itself changes in virulence. Scarlet fever (scarlatina) is no longer the feared disease it was 50 years ago due to erythrogenic toxin-producing streptococci becoming less virulent. Changes in micro-organisms may produce little change in the clinical disease but are of no less significance. The type of meningococcus most commonly incriminated in bacterial meningitis in the UK has been group B for many years, but recently there has been a resurgence of group C infections. Meningococcal vaccine will protect against group A or C infection but group B meningococci are poor immunogens. Similar antigenic variation occurs repeatedly in influenza virus.

Most of the changes in the pattern of infections are gradual. New infections are extremely rare but can have an enormous impact; an example is human immunodeficiency virus (HIV), the cause of the acquired immunodeficiency syndrome (AIDS). All of the infections encountered in temperate and developed areas of the world will be found in tropical regions. Certain infections

Table 11.1 Cases of infection reported to WHO from different geographical regions and countries

Region or country	Malaria (1989)	Poliomyelitis (1988)	Measles (1989)	Typhoid (1980/1)	Diphtheria (1989)
Americas (all)	1 114 000	341	142 242	42 160	1014
USA*	1277	9	18 193	390	2
Europe	2000	213	330 478	7810	886
E. Mediterranean	531 000	2170	62 810	75 203	5953
Africa	7000	1187	117 820	28 418	204
S.E. Asia	2 810 000	22 567	194 592	329 980	1321
W. Pacific	709 000	3135	115 485	145	359
England and Wales†	1474	2	26 180	177	2

(Data supplied by Communicable Diseases Surveillance Centre, Colindale.) All figures are to nearest 100. *All figures for USA are for 1984. †All figures for England and Wales are 1985.

Table 11.2 Deaths from infection in England in 1860 (all age groups)

Cause	Number
Measles	9557
Scarlatina (scarlet fever)	9681
Smallpox	2749
Diphtheria	5212
Typhus	13 012
Whooping cough	8553
Cholera	327
Tuberculosis	58 564

are exclusive to the tropics because of climate, and the presence of animal reservoirs and insect vectors.

THE RELATIONSHIP BETWEEN MAN AND MICRO-ORGANISMS

Micro-organisms which can cause disease in man are widely distributed in nature and man is colonised by vast numbers of organisms. Whether a particular organism causes disease is determined by its natural distribution, its pathogenicity and the state of the host defence systems.

With common pathogens it is likely that immunity will develop at an early age. The age at which this occurs can influence the outcome of infection. At extremes of age the immune system is either immature or in decline and the patient is highly vulnerable. Paradoxically, during childhood many viral infections are silent or mild but the same infection in an adult may be severe and complicated. This may reflect a difference in the vigour with which inflammatory responses are generated.

PATHOGENICITY

Microbial pathogenicity, that is, the potential of a micro-organism to cause disease, is determined by its ability to enter the host and colonise, to penetrate tissues, to evade host defences and to damage tissues. The *virulence* of an organism is its degree of pathogenicity. An organism is described as highly virulent if a small number of microbes can cause severe disease.

Skin is an effective barrier to most organisms and they usually enter either through a breach or via more delicate mucosal surfaces such as those of the oropharynx and respiratory tract. Attachment to the cell membrane is essential for viruses, and bacterial colonisation is also often facilitated by a specific attachment mechanism. Examples are *Vibrio cholerae* or *Escherichia coli* in the intestine and *E. coli* in the urinary tract. In each case a determinant on the bacterial surface interacts with a specific receptor on epithelial cells.

Some pathogenic organisms cause disease at the site of colonisation by producing toxins (*V. cholerae*) but most traverse the epithelium and their further success depends on their ability to avoid host defences. If this is the first encounter between man and organism innate immunity is man's only defence. In the case of bacteria this centres on phagocytosis and some bacteria are equipped with capsules which confer resistance to phagocytosis. Interferons play a major part in first-line resistance to viruses but viruses differ both in their ability to stimulate interferon production and in their susceptibility to its effects.

The mechanisms of disease provoked by bacteria are very complex but a distinction can be made between effects caused by exotoxins (tetanus or diphtheria toxins, for example) and those resulting from release of bacterial components such as endotoxins.

SUSCEPTIBILITY TO INFECTION

Effects of even virulent microbes are curtailed by an immune response. Infections therefore typically result from a small number of identifiable situations:

- first encounter with a virulent organism, in sufficient numbers, entering by an appropriate route
- breach of normal anatomical barriers, e.g. by surgery, injury and in-dwelling lines
- impairment of innate immune responses
- impairment of adaptive immune responses.

11 Infectious, Tropical and Parasitic Diseases

When anatomical barriers are breached by surgery, tissues which are usually sterile are exposed to normal microbial flora at the adjacent site. Similarly accidental injury often results in exposure to environmental organisms such as *Clostridium tetani* present in the soil.

Impairment of immune responses leads to susceptibility to infection by organisms of low pathogenicity as well as to virulent organisms. Infection by organisms of low pathogenicity is called *opportunistic*. Patients with impaired immunity may therefore present with frequent infections, infection caused by opportunist micro-organisms, unusually severe disease caused by infection, or repeated infection by the same organism.

PRINCIPLES OF DIAGNOSIS AND MANAGEMENT

The principles guiding the clinician in the diagnosis and treatment of an infective illness can be considered by asking some simple questions:

- Is the disease caused by infection and, if so, where is the site of infection?
- What is the micro-organism responsible?
- Which drugs can eliminate the organism and will treatment benefit the patient?

This approach will often lead to a simple plan for management of the patient. It may also be necessary to establish the source in the community. In some cases the doctor has a legal obligation to notify the disease (see 'Control of infection', p. 218).

Is the disease caused by infection and, if so, where is the site of infection?

A careful history and examination will provide important indicators that the patient is suffering from infection.

History

Three aspects of the history are likely to be helpful:

- pattern of the illness
- history of contact with patients with a similar illness or types of behaviour that confer risk of infection
- history of travel to places where particular infections are known to be common.

Illnesses caused by infection tend to have a form which is reproduced in most individuals and which is characterised by the following features:

- *incubation period:* time from contact with micro-organisms to onset of symptoms (Fig. 11.1)
- *prodromal illness:* minor symptoms preceding the definitive illness
- *overt disease*
- *resolution (convalescence).*

This pattern is often influenced by the immune state of the patient and may be altered by drug therapy.

Some symptoms, such as sore throat and fever, are more commonly associated with infection than with other disease processes. The pattern of fever may be helpful, but patients may say that they have had a fever when they have not measured their temperature. They may mean an aching sensation in the limbs, sweatiness, or true rigors. Of these, a rigor is a good indicator. It is a sensation of coldness accompanied by shivering (associated with a rise in temperature) followed by a hot sensation and marked sweating.

While there is no symptom which is specifically associated with infection there are many symptom complexes which are highly suggestive of an infective aetiology. For example, while headache has many causes, the combination of headaches with fever, photophobia and vomiting strongly suggests infection of the meninges (meningitis).

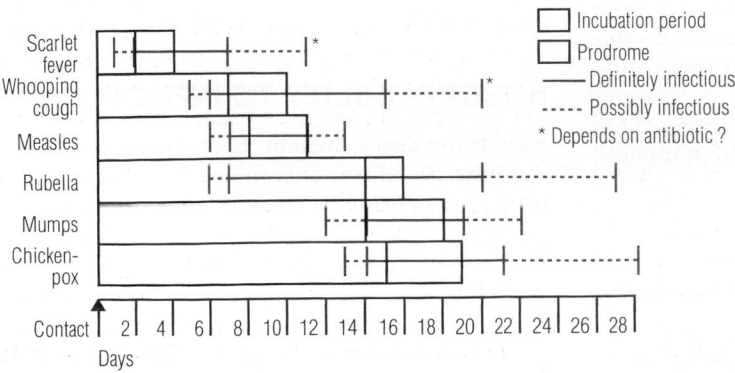

Fig. 11.1 Incubation periods and periods of communicability of common infectious diseases.

Examination

The findings on examination may be helpful in three ways:

- Some infections are associated with signs which are specific or which suggest only a short list of differential diagnoses. Examples are the rash of chickenpox or measles, neck stiffness caused by acute meningitis or the characteristic cough of whooping cough.
- More commonly a combination of signs is highly suggestive of an infection. For example, exudative tonsillitis, generalised lymphadenopathy and splenomegaly together suggest infectious mononucleosis; fever, relative bradycardia, splenomegaly and rose spots suggest typhoid.
- Physical signs may indicate the site of infection. Consolidation in the lungs suggests pneumonia; loin tenderness is associated with pyelonephritis; inflammation, swelling and fluctuance beneath the skin suggest an abscess.

What is the micro-organism responsible?

A careful history and examination may point to a diagnosis of infection and can be specific for a particular infection. More frequently, infection is strongly suspected but the site and the organism responsible are unknown. Imaging techniques are often helpful in finding the site of infection, e.g. ultrasound or CT scanning can demonstrate an abscess in soft tissues. A gallium scan or indium[111] (^{111}In) leucocyte scanning frequently demonstrates a soft tissue abscess. In the latter technique the patient's leucocytes are labelled with ^{111}In and reinjected (Fig. 11.2). Labelled leucocytes enter sites of acute inflammation such as an abscess, surgical wounds and the bowel wall of patients with inflammatory bowel disease.

Before appropriate treatment can be started the right samples must be collected and sent to the laboratory. The laboratory can give most help if the correct samples are taken and are accompanied by a brief summary of the patient's illness. The drug history is particularly important since antibiotic in the sample may inhibit growth of bacteria in vitro. There are simple rules for the collection of samples:

- Avoid contamination of the sample with irrelevant organisms by careful cleaning, e.g. clean skin with iodine before taking blood for culture and wear gloves during venepuncture.
- When infected fluid is to be cultured (e.g. pus) send a fluid sample in a sterile bottle rather than a swab if the volume of fluid permits. The yield will be higher and a Gram stain can be performed.
- Think of culture before allowing a tissue specimen to be immersed in fixative such as formalin.

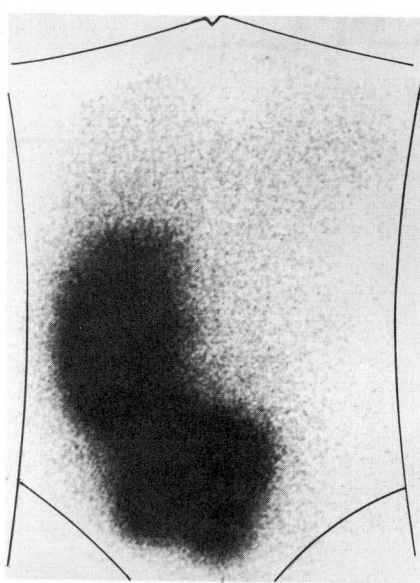

Fig. 11.2 ^{111}In white cell scan in a paracolic abscess. At 24 hours after the intravenous injection the activity is localised, indicating the accumulation represents an enclosed abscess rather than inflamed bowel. (Reproduced by kind permission of Dr Seth Saverymuttu.)

- Ensure that specimens for culture are transported to the laboratory without delay. Micro-organisms must be nurtured and all too often they die waiting for transport or are outgrown by contaminant organisms.

Specimens for viral or fungal culture often require special techniques of collection and the laboratory should be consulted before obtaining the specimen.

Which drugs can eliminate the organism from the infected site and will treatment benefit the patient?

Some guidelines for the choice of antimicrobial drugs are given on page 212. Whether treatment is to be started immediately or after the results of laboratory tests are available depends on the severity of the disease and the likely consequences of delay. There is virtue in waiting until the precise diagnosis is known if the clinical situation permits, and this applies particularly when antibiotics have been given before admission to hospital. Acute meningitis and septicaemia are obvious exceptions because the patient may die before a final result is available but even then it is vital that the correct specimens are obtained before treatment is started. Valuable preliminary information can be obtained by Gram staining and microscopy of specimens such as sputum or pus. Direct testing for microbial antigens may increase in importance for disease caused by a limited range of organisms such as acute meningitis.

Treatment is not always beneficial to the patient, even when an antimicrobial drug with appropriate activity can be delivered to the site of infection in adequate concentration. Faecal excretion of salmonellae may be prolonged by treatment with some antibiotics.

ANTIMICROBIAL AGENTS

The choice of antimicrobial drugs is central to the management of infection. General measures should not be neglected; these include use of analgesics, attention to nutrition and hydration, and cleaning, debridement or drainage of infected areas.

The term 'antimicrobial agent' can be applied to any substance which is active against micro-organisms. Strictly, an antibiotic is a substance produced by a micro-organism which inhibits the growth of another. In this chapter 'antibiotic' will be used (inaccurately) to refer to antibacterial drugs, whether synthetic or naturally produced.

Choice of appropriate drugs

Selection of a suitable antimicrobial agent is fairly straightforward when the micro-organism responsible is known (Table 11.3), but often this is not the case and a sensible guess has to be made as to the organisms responsible. In the case of a urinary tract infection in a previously healthy young woman, for example, faecal organisms such as *E. coli* would be the most likely pathogens and this would guide initial therapy.

The information required to make an appropriate choice can be summarised:

- probable organism/s
- probable antimicrobial sensitivities of the organisms
- ability of the chosen drugs to reach the site of infection
- history of allergy to drugs
- interaction of these drugs with any other drugs the patient is taking
- side-effects of the chosen drug
- cost of the drug.

An example of the process of decision is shown in Fig. 11.3. This logical sequence assumes a considerable

Table 11.3 Common sensitivities of some bacteria to antibiotics

Bacteria	1st choice	2nd choice
Streptococci (except anaerobic)	Penicillin	Erythromycin
Staphylococci	Flucloxacillin	Erythromycin
Neisseria meningitidis	Penicillin	Chloramphenicol
Neisseria gonorrhoeae	Penicillin	Tetracycline
Gram-positive bacilli	Penicillin	
Escherichia coli (urinary tract)	Trimethoprim	Nitrofurantoin
Pseudomonas aeruginosa	Gentamicin and azlocillin (usually requires a combination)	Gentamicin and ceftazidime
H. influenzae (respiratory infection)	Pivampicillin	
Gram-negative (septicaemia)	Cefotaxime	Ampicillin and gentamicin Ciprofloxacin Piperacillin

knowledge of antibiotics, including the known sensitivity of particular organisms to them. The latter are not constant, so treatment is often started on the basis of an intelligent guess and modified later according to laboratory results.

Bacterial sensitivity is tested using discs impregnated with antibiotic and measuring the size of the ring of inhibition on culture plates. Other factors are also important in the choice of antibiotic, such as absorption and penetration to the site of infection. Whenever possible the antibiotic chosen should have a spectrum of antibacterial activity limited to a few organisms, since the broader the spectrum, the greater the chance of side-effects due to disturbance of the normal microbial flora. The choice between a bactericidal and a bacteriostatic drug is not usually critical but it may be important when the organisms are fairly inaccessible, as in infective endocarditis, or when host defences are impaired (Table 11.6).

Combinations of antibiotics are used for one of three purposes:

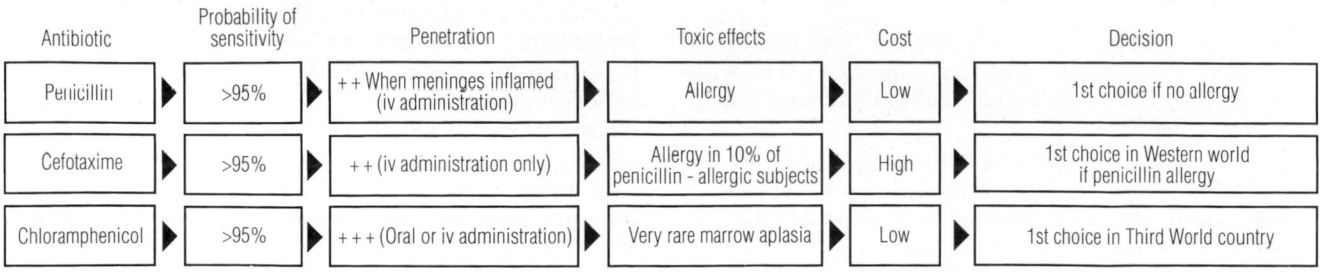

Fig. 11.3 Choice of antibiotic in a patient with acute pneumococcal meningitis.

- to obtain a spectrum of antibacterial activity which could not be achieved with a single agent (e.g. treatment of septicaemia when the causative organism is not known)
- to take advantage of synergism between drugs (e.g. during the initial treatment of infective endocarditis)
- to prevent the emergence of resistant organisms (e.g. treatment of tuberculosis).

Route of administration

The ideal drug would give adequate serum levels after oral administration, whatever the state of the patient. However, an ill patient often cannot swallow tablets and absorption from the gut may be unreliable. The choice between intravenous (i.v.) and intramuscular (i.m.) administration is determined by the form in which the drug is available and its pharmacokinetics; the discomfort of intramuscular administration; and practical issues such as accessibility of veins and other drugs being administered.

Topical antibiotic treatment is sometimes useful in the eye (Ch. 25), on the skin (p. 252) or in the respiratory tract (e.g. in cystic fibrosis, see p. 477) but development of resistance is a problem.

Mechanism of action of antibiotics

Antibiotics act in one of the following ways:

- inhibition of bacterial cell wall synthesis (penicillins and cephalosporins)
- inhibition of particular aspects of bacterial cell function: *protein synthesis* (aminoglycosides, chloramphenicol, tetracyclines, macrolides, clindamycin); *DNA replication* (rifampicin, 4-quinolones); *microbial enzymes* (sulphonamides, trimethoprim, isoniazid).

Resistance to antibiotics

There are two major ways in which resistance occurs:

- Production of an enzyme which inactivates the antibiotic. The best-known example is β-lactamase which alters the β-lactam ring of penicillins and cephalosporins (Fig. 11.4). Aminoglycosides and chloramphenicol are other drugs broken down by bacterial enzymes.
- The bacterium itself may alter such that the antibiotic is rendered ineffective. This occurs either by a change in the permeability of the bacterial cell wall or by an alteration at the target site of the antibiotic.

Resistance tends to emerge by natural selection in a population of bacteria exposed to antibiotic. This may be acquired by mutation but more often it is the result of

incorporation of new genetic material into the bacterial nucleus or transfer of genetic material from other organisms in the form of extrachromosomal DNA as plasmids (episomes).

ANTIBIOTICS IN COMMON USE

β-lactams

These are the most commonly used antibiotics and have in common the β-lactam ring (Fig. 11.4). There are two major groups, the penicillins and cephalosporins.

Penicillins

Benzyl penicillin or *penicillin G* is a highly potent bactericidal natural penicillin which was the forerunner of all the other penicillins. Long-acting forms, procaine and benzathine penicillins, allow longer intervals between doses. Its disadvantages are that it can only be given parenterally, it has little activity against Gram-negative organisms, and many staphylococci are resistant to it. Semi-synthetic and synthetic penicillins have been developed to circumvent these problems. Doses are now usually expressed in mg ($600 \text{ mg} = 10^6 \text{ units} = 1 \text{ megaunit}$).

Phenoxymethyl penicillin is a natural penicillin which is acid-resistant and can therefore be taken by mouth for treatment of minor infections with streptococci which are

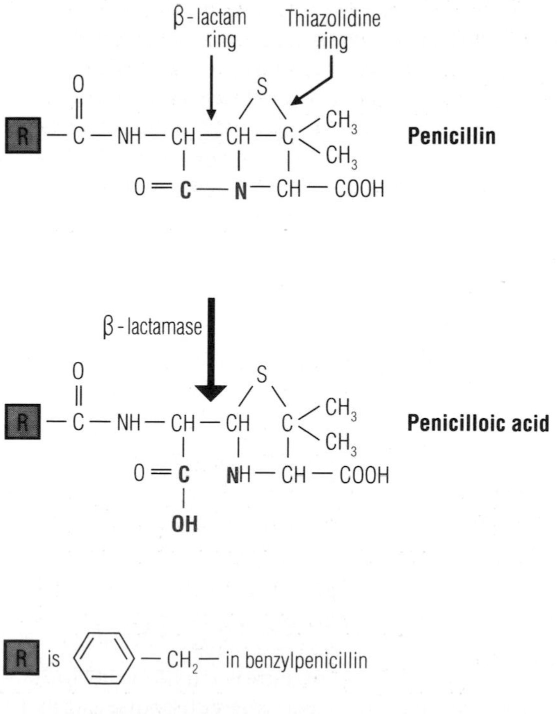

Fig. 11.4 Structure of β-lactam ring.

highly sensitive. Absorption is variable so it should not be used for more serious infections.

Broad-spectrum penicillins, such as ampicillin, amoxycillin and pivampicillin, have useful activity against Gram-negative organisms excluding *Pseudomonas* species. They are well absorbed from the intestine.

β-lactamase-resistant penicillin, such as flucloxacillin and methicillin, are used mainly to treat penicillinase-producing staphylococci.

Antipseudomonal penicillins: carbenicillin, ticarcillin and the ureidopenicillins (azlocillin, mezlocillin and piperacillin) are all distinguished by their activity against *Pseudomonas* species but the ureidopenicillins have a broader spectrum of activity against Gram-negative organisms.

Cephalosporins

Cephalosporins have a similar structure and mode of action to penicillins but modifications to their structure have produced a range of drugs with a broader spectrum of activity. Examples are cephradine, which has a broad spectrum of activity, including some against staphylococci, and can be taken orally; cefotaxime, a parenteral drug with a very broad spectrum excluding *Pseudomonas;* and ceftazidime, similar to cefotaxime but including *Pseudomonas* activity. These drugs are expensive and should only be used when there is no alternative.

Other β-lactams

Imipenem is a carbapenem which differs from other β-lactams in its remarkable spectrum of antibacterial activity and resistance to hydrolysis by most β-lactamases and other enzymes. At present Imipenem is a reserve drug only prescribed when conventional drugs have failed.

Aztreonam is a monolactam with a spectrum of activity limited to some aerobic Gram-negative bacteria.

Erythromycin

Erythromycin is an extremely useful drug with a macrolide structure. It can often be used as an alternative to penicillin when the patient is allergic. In addition it is active against *Haemophilus influenzae, Mycoplasma, Legionella, Bordetella pertussis* and *Campylobacter.*

Chloramphenicol

Chloramphenicol is a cheap drug, well absorbed and distributed, with useful activity against Gram-positive and negative cocci, *H. influenzae* and *Salmonella typhi.* Its major drawback is the very rare but usually fatal induction of marrow aplasia. It is also difficult to use safely in babies.

Tetracyclines

Tetracyclines were widely used to treat exacerbations of chronic bronchitis until resistance became common. Now their main use is for treatment of chlamydial infection but they are also active against *Mycoplasma, Brucella,* rickettsiae and *Coxiella.* They should not be used in pregnant females and children under 9 years old.

Aminoglycosides

Aminoglycosides such as gentamicin, amikacin and tobramycin are used in serious Gram-negative infections. They are ototoxic and blood levels have to be monitored carefully, especially when there is renal impairment, since they are excreted purely by the kidneys. Peak blood levels are measured 15 minutes after intravenous or 1 hour after intramuscular administration, and trough levels immediately before the next dose.

Sulphonamides

Sulphonamides were the first synthetic antimicrobial drugs but their use is now limited by the development of resistance and by the frequency of troublesome side-effects. Sulphamethoxazole is still widely used in combination with trimethoprim since they were thought to be synergistic, but it now seems that trimethoprim alone is just as effective in the treatment of Gram-negative urinary infection. Trimethoprim can cause thrombocytopenia and megaloblastic anaemia.

Clindamycin

Clindamycin is a lincosamide with activity against Gram-positive organisms, including resistant staphylococci, but also against anaerobic organisms. It achieves good penetration into bone and can be used to treat osteomyelitis.

Metronidazole

Metronidazole is an excellent drug for the treatment of anaerobic infection. It is cheap when administered orally or rectally and the more expensive intravenous preparation is rarely indicated. It is also the first choice in treatment of *Giardia lamblia,* amoebic disease and *Trichomonas vaginalis.*

Sodium fusidate

Sodium fusidate is highly bactericidal against staphylococci, including penicillin-resistant ones, but resistance develops during treatment unless another drug is given concurrently. It is expensive and is therefore reserved for treatment of serious infections such as septicaemia and osteomyelitis.

Vancomycin

Vancomycin is another expensive drug reserved for serious, penicillin-resistant staphylococcal infection.

4-Quinolones

Nalidixic acid has been used exclusively in the treatment of urinary infection by Gram-negative organisms, since adequate levels are only found in the urine. Resistance to this group of drugs is rare since they are not susceptible to plasmid-mediated resistance. A new generation of 4-quinolones includes ciprofloxacin, which is well absorbed from the intestine and widely distributed. It is the only drug active against *Pseudomonas* and may become important for this reason.

Rifampicin

Rifampicin, a synthetic derivative of rifamycin, is central to the treatment of tuberculosis (p. 473) but it is also very active against staphylococci, streptococci and *E. coli.*

ANTIFUNGAL DRUGS

Most fungal infections of the skin are treated with topical preparations but cuticular infection requires prolonged systemic therapy. Visceral infections also require systemic therapy.

Amphotericin B and nystatin

Amphotericin B and nystatin are polyene antibiotics produced by *Streptomyces* species. They exert a fungistatic effect by binding to sterols in the fungal cell membrane, causing leakage of cell components. Amphotericin B acts synergistically with the unrelated compound flucytosine, probably by increasing permeability to flucytosine.

Neither amphotericin B nor nystatin is absorbed from the intestine but amphotericin B can be administered intravenously, after which there is wide tissue distribution but little penetration to brain and meninges. The plasma half-life is 24 hours and it is excreted very slowly in the urine, 40% of the infused dose appearing in the urine during the following week.

Amphotericin B has a broad spectrum of activity and it is used against the agents of candidiasis, aspergillosis, histoplasmosis, blastomycosis, coccidiomycosis, cryptococcosis and some organisms causing mucormycosis. Minor symptoms following infusion are common and a wide variety of symptoms may be unpleasant enough to require suppression with analgesics, anti-emetics, etc. More serious side-effects occur when there is impairment of renal function which is exacerbated by the resultant rise in plasma drug levels. Renal and haematopoietic toxicity are the main problems. Therapy has to be interrupted to allow a fall in plasma level.

A test dose of 1 mg is given to assess side-effects, followed by 0.8 mg/kg body weight per day infused i.v. over 6 hours, withdrawing treatment intermittently as required to maintain plasma level at 1–1.5 mg/litre.

Nystatin is not absorbed from the intestine, but it is useful as a topical or mucosal preparation, particularly for treatment of *Candida* infections. It is available as a suspension or pastilles for oral infection; cream and pessaries for vaginal infection; and cream or ointment for skin infections.

Flucytosine

Flucytosine is a synthetic fluorinated pyrimidine which enters fungal cells and inhibits metabolism by interfering with DNA and RNA synthesis. It is usually given in combination with amphotericin B for treatment of systemic fungal infections and it adds a fungicidal effect to the fungistasis caused by amphotericin. Resistance develops rapidly when it is administered alone.

Flucytosine is well absorbed from the intestine and widely distributed, giving a cerebrospinal fluid (CSF) concentration 75% of plasma level. Intravenous infusion is difficult and confined to patients unable to take oral medication. Excretion is in the urine, so dosage must be reduced in the presence of renal failure. Side-effects are gastrointestinal disturbance, neutropenia and thrombocytopenia.

Imidazoles

Ketoconazole, miconazole and clotrimazole are imidazole drugs. Most are available only topically and have activity against dermatophytes and *Candida*. Imidazoles have no place in treatment of systemic fungal infections. The mode of action is not fully understood but imidazoles interfere with synthesis of sterols and other fungal membrane lipids, resulting in defective cell wall synthesis. In vitro they enhance killing of *Candida* by leucocytes.

Ketoconazole is an oral preparation which is useful for treatment of severe mucosal infections, such as oesophageal candidiasis which is not responsive to topical treatment. The major toxicity is drug-induced hepatitis, which can progress to irreversible hepatic failure.

Triazoles

Triazoles are a new group of antifungal agents including fluconazole and itraconazole. Early results suggest that they will be useful in treating some systemic mycoses; for example, fluconazole has been used successfully in *Candida* oesophagitis and cryptococcal meningitis. Side-effects appear to be rare.

Griseofulvin

Griseofulvin, produced by *Penicillium griseofulvum*, is absorbed from the gastrointestinal tract and deposited in keratin, where it inhibits growth of dermatophytes. It is relatively non-toxic and can be used in extensive dermatophyte infections which are unresponsive to topical treatment. It is particularly useful for nail and scalp infections (p. 1127).

ANTIVIRAL TREATMENT

In recent years considerable progress has been made in synthesising agents which specifically inhibit an essential step in virus replication (Table 11.4), without causing host toxicity. This has been achieved:

- by using an agent which is activated by the virus, thus localising its action within infected cells
- by using an agent which inhibits virus metabolism specifically. Usually this is achieved when the agent inhibits a viral enzyme.

Acyclovir, the most widely used agent presently available, produces its specific effects using both of these mechanisms. It is inactive until phosphorylated to a triphosphate by viral thymidine kinase in infected cells. In this form it produces its main antiviral action by inhibiting viral DNA polymerase, essential for synthesis of viral DNA. Acyclovir triphosphate is a more powerful inhibitor of viral than of host DNA polymerases. Acyclovir seems to be a safe drug but is expensive. Its use is restricted to situations in which it is clearly beneficial (Table 11.5).

During acute viral infections much of the inflammation is caused by the host response in the later part of the illness and antiviral treatment must be started early to be effective. Antiviral treatment does not affect virus integrated into the host genome and treatment of the primary herpes simplex infection does not influence subsequent viral reactivation. Ganciclovir, an antiviral drug licensed for treatment of

Table 11.4 Current antiviral treatment

Treatment	Example	Uses	Route
Contact inactivation	Dry ice	Warts	T
Inhibition of virus metabolism			
Uncoating	Amantadine	Influenza A	O
Replication	Acyclovir	HSV, VZV	O,P,T
	Zidovudine	HIV	O
	Ganciclovir	CMV	P
	Vidarabine	HSV, VZV	P,T
	Idoxuridine	HSV, VZV	T
Assembly	Interferons	VZV, HBV	P

HSV = herpes simplex virus: VZV = varicella zoster virus; HIV = human immunodeficiency virus; CMV = cytomegalovirus; HBV = hepatitis B virus; T = topical; O = oral; P = parenteral

Table 11.5 Treatment of herpes virus infections with acyclovir

Virus	Infection	Route
Herpes simplex virus	Encephalitis	IV
	Neonatal infection	IV
	Primary genital infection	O
	Keratoconjunctivitis	T
	Prophylaxis: bone marrow transplantation	O
Varicella zoster	Shingles in immunocompromised patient	IV
	Chickenpox in immunocompromised children	IV
	Chickenpox in neonates	

IV = intravenous; O = oral; T = topical

cytomegalovirus (CMV) infection, is activated by phosphorylation in a similar way to acyclovir, but depends on human cellular enzymes for this process. Since phosphorylation occurs in infected and normal cells, toxicity is greater than that of acyclovir and it causes bone marrow suppression. Zidovudine is an inhibitor of HIV replication which is achieved by inhibition of reverse transcriptase activity.

INFECTION IN THE IMMUNO-COMPROMISED PATIENT

An immunocompromised patient is defined as a patient in whom any part of the innate or adaptive immune response is defective. Defects of the immune system are physiological (neonates and the aged), and primary or secondary. Primary immune deficiency diseases are rare and an account is given in Chapter 6. Secondary immune deficiency is more common and of increasing importance (Table 6.5, p. 92). Causes of secondary immune deficiency are:

- *malignant disease and its treatment*
- *drug-induced chronic immune suppression*, e.g. in organ transplantation or chronic inflammatory diseases such as systemic lupus erythematosus (SLE)
- *infection;* the most severe infection is HIV (p. 243) but many other viruses cause a milder deficiency of cell-mediated immunity (CMI)
- *splenectomy*
- *chronic diseases*, e.g. chronic renal failure, malnutrition, protein deficiency, diabetes mellitus.

These conditions cause varying combinations of neutropenia and impairment of humoral and cellular immunity. Deficiencies of antibody or neutrophils are associated with infection by encapsulated bacteria, yeasts and fungi. Deficient CMI causes infection by a wider range of pathogens including Gram-positive and negative bacteria, viruses, yeasts, fungi, protozoans and helminths (Table 11.6). In all these situations immunisation with live viral vaccines is dangerous since the attenuated organism may behave as a pathogen.

Table 11.6 Some micro-organisms causing infection in immuno-compromised patients

Type	Micro-organism	Remarks	Deficiency
Bacteria	Gram-positive, e.g. Pneumococcus	Encapsulated	Ab/Neut/S
	Gram-negative, e.g. H. influenzae	Encapsulated	CMI
	Mycobacteria, e.g. avium intracellulare	Both typical and atypical	CMI
Viruses	Herpes, e.g. Herpes simplex virus Varicella zoster virus Cytomegalovirus	Reactivation	CMI
	Echo	Encephalitis	Ab
	Live vaccines, e.g. Measles	Virulent	Ab/CMI
Yeasts	Candida	Septicaemia/ pneumonia	Ab/Neut
		Mucosal	CMI
Fungi	Aspergillus	Systemic	CMI
	Cryptococcus	Meningitis	CMI
Protozoa	Pneumocystis	Pneumonia	CMI/Ab
	Toxoplasma	Cerebral	CMI
	Cryptosporidium	Gut	CMI
	Giardia lamblia	Gut	CMI/Ab
	Malaria	Systemic	Ab/S
Helminths	Strongyloides	Systemic	CMI

Ab = antibody; Neut = neutrophil; CMI = cell-mediated immunity; S = post-splenectomy

The pattern of infection in immunocompromised patients is unusual in several respects. Bacterial infections in splenectomised patients are of sudden onset and rapidly progressive, fulminant pneumococcal septicaemia being the most common. Cellular immune deficiency causes viral infection to be more severe, prolonged and widely disseminated than is usual.

Fever in the neutropenic patient

During periods of neutropenia, the onset of fever should be taken to indicate serious infection unless there is an obvious alternative explanation. 'Blind' treatment with antibiotics is started immediately after collection of specimens including blood cultures. Blood cultures are negative in over half of such fever episodes but the choice of antibiotics is guided by positive results in which Gram-negative bacteria, including *Pseudomonas* species, predominate and a combination of a broad-spectrum penicillin with activity against *Pseudomonas* (e.g. piperacillin) and gentamicin is often used (p. 214).

New pulmonary infiltrates on chest radiograph

New pulmonary infiltrates may be due to infection with a wide range of possible pathogens (Table 11.7). Sputum induction, bronchoscopy and lavage, and transbronchial

Table 11.7 Organisms causing pneumonia in immunocompromised patients

Bacteria
Gram-positive, e.g. *Strep. pneumoniae*
Gram-negative, e.g. *H. influenzae, Klebsiella pneumoniae*

Viruses
Cytomegalovirus, herpes simplex, varicella zoster
Measles (giant cell pneumonia)

Protozoa
Pneumocystis carinii

Fungi/yeasts
Candida
Aspergillus

biopsy may provide diagnostic information. Invasive procedures have a risk in neutropenic and thrombocytopenic patients.

Reactivation of herpes viruses

Patients with impaired CMI may suffer severe herpes virus infection. Shingles (varicella zoster) in patients with Hodgkin's disease tends to involve more than one dermatome and there may be dissemination of virus causing widespread chickenpox lesions on the skin and occasionally in viscera. Within affected dermatomes lesions are dense and heal slowly. Reactivation of herpes simplex virus (HSV) may cause extensive perioral ulceration and occasionally visceral dissemination. CMV reactivation causes pneumonia in renal transplant recipients.

NOSOCOMIAL INFECTION

Hospital patients may be particularly susceptible to infection and hospital bacteria are often resistant to common antibiotics. Susceptibility is increased in postoperative patients, patients with burns, patients on ventilators, in malnourished patients and in disease states which compromise immunity specifically. Hospital acquired infections are known as 'nosocomial' and are a particular problem on intensive treatment units. The bacteria associated with particular situations can sometimes be predicted, e.g. staphylococci and streptococci are common causes of surgical wound infections and *Pseudomonas* frequently infects burns. In ventilated patients difficulties arise in deciding whether bacteria such as *Pseudomonas* are merely colonising the respiratory mucosa or whether they are pathogenic. Antibiotic treatment of colonising organisms is undesirable since the local flora then change to more resistant organisms.

With increasing use of antibiotics in recent years there has been a resurgence of outbreaks of nosocomial infection with methicillin (and flucloxacillin)-resistant *Staphylococcus aureus* (MRSA). MRSA colonise the skin and nose of normal or diseased subjects but they are

11 Infectious, Tropical and Parasitic Diseases

particularly persistent in patients with any form of skin lesion. In most cases MRSA do not cause disease but occasionally vulnerable patients can develop septicaemia or local suppuration which necessitates the use of vancomycin. Since MRSA spreads rapidly from patient to patient it is important to isolate infected patients and to screen staff for carriage. Colonised subjects are treated with topical antiseptic preparations and, in the case of staff, removed from work until repeated swabs are clear.

The use of antibiotics must be controlled both in hospitals and in the community. Most hospitals have antibiotic control policies which recommend the antibiotic to be used in a particular situation and restrict administration of some drugs to special situations.

CONTROL OF INFECTION

Containment of outbreaks of infection is required when susceptible subjects may develop a serious illness if they become infected. It is not always desirable to contain infection. Chickenpox, a mild disease in normal children, is usually severe in adults and so outbreaks among schoolchildren should not be controlled. In a hospital where non-immune patients are liable to develop severe manifestations, however, it is important to prevent cross-infection to non-immune individuals (about 10% of the adult population).

Isolation of patients in single rooms greatly facilitates control of infection. Other measures are determined by the mode of transmission and the degree of infectivity of the organism. Transmission is by:

- respiratory secretions (e.g. measles, pulmonary tuberculosis)
- excretions and secretions (e.g. gastroenteritis, hepatitis A, typhoid)
- skin contact and fomites (e.g. MRSA).

Respiratory transmission can be prevented by having the patient and/or the attendants wear appropriate masks. Organisms transmitted in respiratory secretions usually infect others through the upper or lower respiratory tract, and gowning and hand washing are of minor importance.

When *excretions and secretions* are infectious the most important containment measure is hand washing. When close contact is necessary with a highly infectious patient, such as a patient excreting *Shigella* in the faeces, gowns and gloves are worn. Special arrangements are needed for disposal of excreta, contaminated dressings and contaminated clothing and bedding.

When micro-organisms are found in significant number on the skin, in fomites and in dust around the patient, as when MRSA colonise patients in hospital, additional precautions must be taken, including the use of overshoes together with gowns and gloves.

Table 11.8 Notifiable diseases (UK, October 1988)

Under the Public Health (Control of Disease) Act 1984	Under the Public Health (Infectious Disease) Regulations 1988
Cholera	Acute encephalitis
Plague	Acute poliomyelitis
Relapsing fever	Anthrax
Smallpox	Diphtheria
Typhus	Dysentery (amoebic or bacillary)
	Leprosy
	Leptospirosis
	Malaria
	Measles
	Meningitis
	Meningococcal septicaemia (without meningitis)
	Mumps
	Ophthalmia neonatorum
	Paratyphoid fever
	Rabies
	Scarlet fever
	Tetanus
	Tuberculosis
	Typhoid fever
	Viral haemorrhagic fever
	Viral hepatitis
	Whooping cough
	Yellow fever

AIDS is not a statutorily notifiable disease but doctors are urged to participate in a voluntary confidential reporting scheme

In many countries some infections are notifiable (Table 11.8); that is, the medical attendant is obliged by law to report the case to the authority which controls the area in which the patient lives so that steps can be taken to trace contacts. Notification also allows surveillance of the incidence of these infections. Most patients have ceased to be an infectious risk by the time they are discharged from hospital but intestinal pathogens often remain in the stools for several weeks. Carriers of such pathogens are advised to avoid handling food for others, to wash hands regularly and to avoid towel sharing. Following notification, stool samples will be checked by the local authority until they are pathogen-free.

IMMUNISATION

Active immunisation

Active immunisation is the administration of antigen to induce a protective immune response in the host. Antigens used include crude preparations of killed organisms, extracellular products of organisms and live, attenuated organisms. The immunisation schedule in the UK in 1990 is shown in Table 11.9. Mumps vaccine was introduced as part of the routine childhood immunisation schedule in 1988. The policy of immunising only females

Table 11.9 UK immunisation schedule (1990)

Age	Immunisation	Type of vaccine	Route
2 months	Diphtheria	Toxoid	IM or SC
	Tetanus	Toxoid	IM or SC
	Pertussis	Killed	IM or SC
	Polio	Live attenuated	O
	H. influenza type b	Capsular antigens	IM or SC
3 and 4 months	As above	As above	As above
12–18 months	Measles, mumps, rubella (MMR)*	Live attenuated	IM
5 years	Diphtheria	As above	As above
	Tetanus		
	Polio		
10–14 years	BCG	Live attenuated	ID
10–14 years (girls only)	Rubella†	Live attenuated	IM
School-leaving	Tetanus	As above	As above
	Polio		
Adults	Rubella	For seronegative women	"
	Polio	For non-immunised	"
	Tetanus		
	Hepatitis B	High-risk groups	IM
	Influenza		

*MMR introduced into UK in October 1988
†Retained in UK until MMR established
IM = intramuscular; SC = subcutaneous; O= oral; ID = intradermal

against rubella has also been changed since there is still a notable incidence of congenital rubella. BCG (bacille Calmette-Guérin) immunisation for protection against tuberculosis is more important among children of racial groups with a high incidence of the disease, such as Asian immigrants to the UK. In North America the incidence of tuberculosis is not high enough to justify its routine use. In contrast BCG vaccination of neonates is a common practice in the tropics.

Contra-indications to immunisation

- Live vaccines should not be given to anyone with untreated malignant disease or with any form of immunodeficiency, including those receiving immunosuppressive therapy, or to pregnant women.
- Live vaccines should not be given within 3 weeks of another injected live vaccine.
- Coincidental severe febrile illness may limit the response to immunisation. Immunisation should therefore be postponed *but not forgotten.*
- Significant documented allergy to any component of the vaccine may be a contra-indication to its use.

- Rubella vaccine should not be given in pregnancy and pregnancy should be avoided for 1 month after immunisation against rubella.

Passive immunisation

Passive immunisation is the administration of antibody preparations to prevent or ameliorate infection. Pooled human immunoglobulin is the crudest form which is used commonly to protect travellers against hepatitis A virus infection. More defined preparations of hyperimmune globulin contain high levels of antibodies to particular organisms, usually viruses, which are not present in sufficient concentration in pooled human immunoglobulin to provide protection. Examples are hepatitis B immune globulin given following needle-stick injuries; varicella zoster immune globulin used in neonates born to mothers who have recently developed chickenpox (p. 228), and tetanus immune globulin used for patients at risk of developing tetanus. Most current antibody preparations are derived from human serum. Passively administered antibody has a short half-life, giving protection for only a few weeks. Treatment has to be given soon after exposure to be effective.

PREVENTIVE MEASURES FOR OVERSEAS TRAVEL OR RESIDENCE
Protection of skin

The skin must be protected against biting insects. This is not only important for the prevention of malaria, but also for protection against viral, rickettsial, protozoal and filarial diseases transmitted by insect vectors.

Exposure to ticks occurs mainly in rural bush areas and so appropriate clothing and footwear is needed to prevent ticks getting on to the skin. Evening and night hours are times for maximum frequency of biting by many insects and at these times the skin should be covered as much as possible and insect repellants applied to exposed areas or as impregnated wrist and ankle bands. Mosquito nets should be used in malarious areas if doors and windows are not screened. It is also useful to spray bedrooms with insecticide last thing at night.

Schistosomiasis is acquired by contact between skin and slow-flowing or still water containing cercariae. Swimming and paddling in fresh water are best avoided in endemic areas.

Protection against malaria

Preventing the bite of the mosquito is very important (see above). The traveller should be told that there is *no* vaccine against malaria and that none of the vaccines received prior to travel is of any benefit in this regard.

Chemoprophylaxis against malaria is the other mainstay of protection (details in Table 11.34, p. 295).

Immunisation for travellers or overseas residents

A range of vaccines is available and the commonly used ones are listed in Table 11.10. *Poliomyelitis* is still common in many areas of the world and so adequate vaccination should be assured in all travellers. *Yellow fever* vaccination is essential for those visiting tropical Africa, the Caribbean and South America. Oral poliomyelitis and yellow fever vaccines should be given either together or separated by an interval of 3 weeks. *Hepatitis B* vaccination is only recommended for those who are likely to be at particular risk, i.e. health care and hospital laboratory workers. Pre-exposure *rabies* vaccination is needed by those who may have any contact with animals. Increasingly tourists undertaking overland travels are having pre-exposure vaccination. The intradermal route allows more economical use of the vaccine.

Tetanus vaccination is needed for any who may be at particular risk of trauma, e.g. military personnel, construction workers, etc. *Typhoid* vaccination is a sensible precaution for many areas but those vaccinated should be told that having the vaccine does not mean they are 100% protected and can be careless about sources of water and food. Cholera vaccination is not effective.

Protection of the gut

Gastrointestinal infection is the most common affliction faced by the traveller. Boiled water used to make tea and coffee or left to cool in a covered, clean container is safe to drink. Bottled drinks are safe. Water from the tap or water used to make ice cubes may not be safe. Tincture of iodine (2%) can be used to sterilise water, adding 0.5 ml per litre and allowing it to stand for 30 minutes. Iodine is more potent than chlorine-based sterilising tablets.

SYNDROMES OF INFECTION

SEPTICAEMIA

Septicaemia is uncontrolled bacterial infection in the blood. In contrast to septicaemia, transient *bacteraemia* is fairly common in normal subjects. Septicaemia is a much more serious condition which is likely to lead to death if untreated.

Aetiology

A wide range of bacteria can cause septicaemia but they can be divided into those which do so as *part of a primary infection* by a single organism acquired in the community, and those which cause septicaemia as a *complication of another process,* such as abdominal sepsis following surgery, when there is often a mixed infection. Community acquired infections are usually recognised as part of a specific illness, as when *Strep. pneumoniae* septicaemia complicates pneumonia, meningococcaemia with meningitis, or *E. coli* septicaemia with pyelonephritis. The other kind of septicaemia is usually seen in hospitals, often in a debilitated patient, and the likely bacteria can often be predicted from the clinical situation.

Pathogenesis

Whole bacteria and substances released by bacterial lysis trigger a complex series of events. A major component is endotoxin, the lipopolysaccharide component of Gram-negative bacterial cell walls, of which lipid A is thought to be responsible for most of the toxic effects. Lipid A can activate complement and Hageman factor and can cause the release of cytokines including tumour necrosis factor. Important pathological consequences ensuing from activation of the potent inflammatory pathways are hypotension, increased vascular permeability and consumptive coagulopathy.

Less attention has been paid to the effects of Gram-positive organisms, but activation of inflammatory processes can certainly be triggered by cell membrane components of these organisms. An example is alternate pathway complement activation (Fig. 6.2, p. 84) by teichoic acid found in *Staph. aureus* membranes.

Table 11.10 Immunisation for travellers to and residents in the tropics and subtropics

Vaccine	Route	Duration of protection	Comments
Poliomyelitis			
Live attenuated	O	Lifelong	Not in pregnancy or immune-suppressed
Killed	SC	Several years	
Yellow fever	SC	10 years	Not in infants or pregnancy
Hepatitis A	IM	Unknown	Endemic areas
Hepatitis B	IM	Not yet known	For health care workers
Rabies	IM or ID	Not known	For workers with animals
Tetanus	SC	10 years	
Typhoid	SC	3 years	
Meningococcal	SC	3 years	Types A and C only

O = oral; SC = subcutaneous; IM = intramuscular; ID = intradermal

Clinical features and diagnosis

The manifestations depend on the age of the patient, the illness being more featureless and more lethal at extremes of age. Signs are usually non-specific but there are signs in the skin suggestive of the diagnosis, such as purpuric lesions associated with meningococcaemia and pustular lesions in staphylococcal septicaemia. Usually there is a rapid deterioration in the patient's condition, including a change in mental state. Fever is often present, with tachycardia and bounding pulse, but as the condition progresses the patient becomes hypothermic with a rapid thready pulse and peripheral vasoconstriction. The latter situation is often considered to be typical of Gram-negative septicaemia, but it also occurs with Gram-positive septicaemia. For this reason the general term 'septicaemic shock' is usually used. Prolonged hypotension leads to acute renal failure and disseminated intravascular coagulation causes bleeding. Adult respiratory distress syndrome (p. 511) frequently complicates hospital-acquired septicaemia.

The diagnosis is based on clinical assessment but blood cultures, urine cultures, wound swab and any aspirate from an infected site should be obtained at the time the patient is seen, so that antibiotic treatment can be started without undue delay. The antibiotic regimen can be changed if necessary when culture results are available and the response to treatment has been assessed. Blood cultures should be taken whether the patient is febrile or not.

Management

Treatment is urgent because of the high mortality. Antibiotics and circulatory support are the mainstays of management. The use of plasma expanders and selective vasoactive drugs is discussed on page 539.

Antibiotics

The initial choice of antibiotics is based on a logical guess at the bacteria responsible (p. 212). As few antibiotics as possible are given to achieve the necessary cover. At present a common choice is a combination of a broad-spectrum penicillin such as ampicillin, with an aminoglycoside such as gentamicin. One problem is that many patients are in incipient renal failure, which enhances the toxicity of gentamicin. Newer drugs, like cefotaxime and piperacillin, are active against Gram-positive and Gram-negative bacteria, and lack the toxicity of gentamicin, but they are more expensive. If anaerobic septicaemia is suspected metronidazole is often used, and for hospital-acquired staphylococcal infection a β-lactamase-resistant penicillin, such as flucloxacillin, is added. *Pseudomonas* infections are treated with a combination of drugs, e.g. azlocillin and gentamicin.

PYREXIA OF UNKNOWN ORIGIN

When a patient has an elevated body temperature for a period of longer than 3 weeks without a cause being found the diagnostic problem is called pyrexia (or fever) of unknown origin (PUO).

A febrile patient may lose the normal diurnal variation in body temperature or may sometimes have an exaggerated diurnal pattern, with a rise during the night causing drenching night sweats (common in tuberculosis and lymphoma) followed by a rapid fall. Many patterns of fever are described but they are rarely helpful in diagnosis.

Causes of PUO

The most common causes of PUO vary according to the age of the patient, and published incidences vary with the type of institution at which the problem is studied. Infection is usually the most common cause in children, whereas infection and neoplastic disease are equally important in adults. Connective tissue disease can present with fever at any age. Still's disease and SLE are commoner causes in children and young adults, and polymyalgia and giant cell arteritis more frequent in the elderly.

Infection

Most bacterial infections cause an illness which is clinically manifest within 3 weeks, but there are some exceptions. Bacterial endocarditis can cause low-grade illness, particularly in the elderly. Most cases can be diagnosed by blood culture but occasionally blood cultures are repeatedly negative. Infection in the biliary tract may be associated with only minor clinical signs and little abnormality of liver function tests.

Intracellular bacteria, such as *Brucella* and some *Salmonella* species, can cause recurrent septicaemia, but this can usually be diagnosed by blood culture. Deep-seated abscess is a possible cause of PUO and modern imaging techniques are helpful in locating the collection (p. 211).

Tuberculosis is still a major cause of PUO in developing countries and in some temperate countries such as the UK, especially in Asian patients. Often the granulomatous lesions of tuberculosis are too small to cause pulmonary radiological abnormalities and the site of infection is often outside the lungs. In recent years, tuberculosis has become a common feature of HIV infection.

Viral infections rarely cause PUO (within the definition), with the important exception of HIV. The history should therefore enquire into sexual practices, intravenous drug abuse and transfusions.

Fungal infections rarely cause PUO without a predisposing cause but they may do so as a complication of immunosuppressive disease or therapy. An exception is histoplasmosis.

Neoplasia

Lymphomas frequently produce a prolonged period of fever before any other manifestation emerges. Leukaemias can also cause PUO but this is sometimes caused by a complicating infection. Many occult solid tumours can present as PUO, among them hypernephroma, pancreatic carcinoma, intestinal tumours, bronchial carcinoma, ovarian tumours and sarcomas. Fever is particularly likely when there are hepatic metastases. Atrial myxoma is a rare benign tumour (p. 421) which occasionally produces an illness similar to bacterial endocarditis.

Connective tissue (autoimmune) disease

Most diseases in the category of connective tissue disease can present with PUO before the characteristic disease pattern emerges. SLE, rheumatoid arthritis and Still's disease (including the adult form), polyarteritis nodosa, temporal arteritis and polymyalgia rheumatica should be considered according to the clinical setting.

Miscellaneous

Granulomatous conditions. Granulomatous conditions include sarcoidosis, granulomatous hepatitis and Wegener's granulomatosis. Sarcoidosis often lacks overt signs in the early phase of the disease and should be considered, particularly in ethnic groups with a high prevalence, such as West Indians.

Factitious. One of the most odd forms of human behaviour is the habitual feigning, or deliberate inducement of, illness. Factitious fever is caused in two ways:

- In the first the fever disappears when the temperature is measured by someone other than the patient, with the patient under continuous observation. The patient is either saying that fever exists when it does not, or is manipulating the thermometer.

- In the other, more serious, form the patient induces true fever by self-injury or self-infection. The methods used are diverse, but faeces are the usual source of organisms and infection is induced by rubbing or injecting organisms into the skin or blood. Suspicion is aroused when mixed and varying organisms which could be faecal are found in an unexpected site, or when infection persists despite treatment which would normally be effective.

Patients are often nurses or young women associated with medical work and there are sometimes personal problems which suggest that this behaviour is a plea for attention or help. When suspicion grows that fever is factitious it

---

Summary 1 Causes of pyrexia of unknown origin in UK

Frequency is given in parentheses

- Infection (30%)
- Neoplasia (25%)
- Connective tissue (autoimmune) disease (20%)
- Miscellaneous (12%)
- Undiagnosed (13%)

---

is wise to avoid directly confronting the patient with the possibility. Usually it will be denied and sometimes confrontation can precipitate a psychiatric crisis, even resulting in suicide. It is preferable to attempt to solve the associated problems if they can be identified and to create a situation in which it is difficult for the patient to continue to provoke sepsis, e.g. by removing intravenous catheters or covering inflamed sites. The patient should be made to realise that the manoeuvres are understood, if possible without a direct accusation. The best efforts to resolve factitious fever often fail and patients either return intermittently or present themselves to another medical team.

Inflammatory bowel disease. Inflammatory bowel disease is usually associated with incriminating symptoms such as weight loss and diarrhoea, but these may be slow to emerge.

Drug reaction. Once thought of, drug reaction is a straightforward cause of PUO. The possibility that the fever is caused by a drug is tested by withdrawal.

Multiple pulmonary emboli. When frequent small embolic events occur, pyrexia may be the sole manifestion before the pulmonary circulation is greatly compromised.

Other causes. Other occasional causes of PUO are alcoholic hepatitis, familial Mediterranean fever, Whipple's disease and occult haematoma. There are some young women whose normal evening temperature runs above the normal range by up to 0.5°C. This usually comes to light after an infection with slow recovery. Once it is established that there is no underlying pathology the patient can be reassured. Tropical causes are discussed on page 223.

Diagnosis

A careful history and examination of the patient is essential and it is important to return to the patient repeatedly to go over parts of the history and to look for emergent physical signs. Simple screening tests which may need to be repeated at intervals include full blood count and ESR, routine biochemistry of blood and urine, cultures of blood, urine and other relevant samples, and chest radiograph.

Additional investigations are guided by the clinical findings. There are two approaches. One is to perform tests which are more or less specific for particular diseases, e.g. the Kveim test for sarcoid, autoantibodies in autoimmunity or antibodies to particular pathogens. The other is to investigate a particular site which seems to be generating symptoms or signs. The latter is more often helpful and it is in this area that advances in imaging techniques have changed the methods for diagnosing PUO. *Ultrasound* is particularly useful for abdominal examination, both in detection of solid tissue abnormalities, such as tumours of the kidney or pancreas, lymph node enlargement or infiltration of the liver, and in locating collections of pus (subphrenic, perinephric, intrahepatic, etc.). *CT scanning* supplements, and is in some situations superior to, ultrasound. A further use of these techniques is to guide the needle during *tissue biopsy*. The use of ^{111}In labelled leucocytes is described on page 211. Even if no localised lesion has been found by imaging techniques, certain biopsy procedures are sometimes rewarding. If the liver enzyme tests are abnormal, percutaneous *liver biopsy* should be considered, since diffuse granulomatous or infiltrative diseases such as sarcoidosis or lymphoma may be detected. *Marrow aspiration and biopsy* may reveal cryptic tuberculosis, or lymphomatous or carcinomatous infiltration. The marrow and liver biopsy should be cultured for *Mycobacterium tuberculosis*.

Patience and persistence are essential in managing PUO. Neoplasia is the major cause of death among PUO patients, so exclusion of treatable neoplastic disease is a priority. In most studies about one-fifth of cases remain unsolved despite the best efforts.

The approach to the patient with fever in the tropics

Febrile illness is common in the tropics, or after travel to the tropics. The causes encompass infectious and non-infectious sources. Infections include those peculiar to tropical regions and those common worldwide (such as urinary tract infection).

Clinical features

A detailed history is essential. This should include accurate recording of the dates of travel, duration of stay, countries visited, with information on the places involved (cities, rural areas, beach resorts, etc.) and the reasons for travel. Information about sexual contact during travel is also important. It should also include details of vaccination prior to travel and malaria prophylaxis, with some assessment of the regularity of taking prophylaxis.

The chronology of events should be recorded, particularly noting the interval between the end of the patient's travels and the onset of illness where this has occurred after return home. This gives an idea of the incubation period of the disease (Table 11.11). Physical examination should pay attention to the presence of skin lesions, oral lesions, jaundice, adenopathy, hepatosplenomegaly and involvement of the nervous system. After initial assessment it is vital to reassess the patient at frequent intervals, looking for the appearance of diagnostic symptoms and signs.

Investigations

The investigations done will depend on the clinical diagnosis or the differential diagnosis, but *blood films* should be examined for malaria parasites in any febrile patient who has been to a malarious area. *Blood films* may also be examined for trypanosomes. A *full blood count* is useful for

Table 11.11 Incubation periods for some tropical diseases

Type of organism	Short (less than 2 weeks)	Intermediate (2–6 weeks)	Long (more than 6 weeks)
Viruses	Arbovirus infections Marburg virus disease	Poliomyelitis Hepatitis A virus Arenavirus infection Ebola virus infection Lassa fever virus infection Haemorrhagic fever with renal syndrome	Hepatitis B Non-A, non-B hepatitis Rabies
Rickettsia		Q fever	
Bacteria	Typhoid	Typhoid Brucellosis Leptospirosis Relapsing fever Lymphogranuloma venereum	
Protozoa	*Trypanosoma cruzi* infection	Malaria Toxoplasmosis *Trypanosoma rhodesiense* infection	Visceral leishmaniasis *Trypanosoma gambiense* infection
Helminths		Schistosomiasis (Katayama syndrome)	

looking for leucocytosis (suggesting bacterial infections), leucopenia (typhoid, viral infections), pancytopenia (visceral leishmaniasis) or eosinophilia (helminthiasis: schistosomiasis, fascioliasis, visceral larva migrans, clonorchiasis, Bancroftian filariasis). A *Mantoux test* should be done early on. *Blood cultures* should be taken and, if brucellosis is a possibility, kept under observation for up to 6 weeks, as the organism grows slowly. *Serological tests* that may be useful include those for syphilis, leptospirosis, rickettsial diseases, brucellosis, amoebiasis, leishmaniasis, trypanosomiasis, toxoplasmosis, filariasis and schistosomiasis. They should be used selectively in relation to the clinical presentation. A serum sample should be taken on admission and saved, and a second sample taken 10 days later. This pair of sera can then be used to look for a change (usually a rise) in titre. A *chest radiograph* should be obtained. The scanning procedures mentioned under PUO are used as clinically indicated, as are the more invasive tests such as liver and marrow biopsy (see PUO above). Bone marrow should be stained for Leishmania.

Management

Ideally treatment will follow from the specific microbiological diagnosis of the cause of fever. Occasionally it may be necessary to treat the patient for a disease suspected clinically but not proven by laboratory tests. This may be treatment for malaria, or typhoid or rickettsial infection, or tuberculosis in fevers of longer duration.

GASTROENTERITIS

Gastroenteritis is defined as an acute disease with diarrhoea and/or vomiting and a variable degree of systemic illness. 'Food poisoning' is a term used to describe a self-limiting form of gastroenteritis, which is caused by eating contaminated food.

Aetiology

A large variety of micro-organisms can cause gastroenteritis (Table 11.12) but the causative organism cannot be identified in over half of all cases. *Salmonellae* and *Campylobacter* species are among the most frequent causes. In children the spectrum of organisms is slightly different and rotavirus is the most frequently recognised agent.

Epidemiology

Gastroenteritis is a common infection in all parts of the world, occurring sporadically or in epidemics. Epidemics occur when a common source of food or drink is contaminated with micro-organisms and when infection spreads from person to person by the faecal–oral route. For example, *Salmonella enteritidis* species frequently colonise

Table 11.12 Common causes of gastroenteritis

Cause	Clinical presentation
Tissue-damaging bacteria	
Salmonella enteritidis	Diarrhoea, vomiting
Campylobacter jejuni	Diarrhoea predominantly
Shigella species	Dysentery
E. coli	Diarrhoea predominantly
Toxin-producing bacteria	
E. coli (enterotoxigenic)	Secretory diarrhoea
Vibrio cholerae	Secretory diarrhoea
Clostridium difficile	Pseudomembranous colitis
Staphylococcus	Vomiting (short incubation)
Bacillus cereus	Vomiting (short incubation)
Tissue-damaging viruses	
Rotavirus	Infantile diarrhoea
Norwalk virus	Winter vomiting
Adenovirus	Diarrhoea, vomiting
Enterovirus	Diarrhoea, vomiting
Protozoa	
Cryptosporidium	Diarrhoea
Entamoeba histolytica	Dysentery
Giardia lamblia	Chronic diarrhoea (steatorrhoea)

the gut of chickens bred in battery conditions and may infect the oviduct and eggs of hens in batteries. During evisceration in the factory the meat is contaminated and the salmonellae survive freezing and thawing. If such chickens are not thoroughly cooked, salmonellae are ingested and colonise the intestine.

Some forms of gastroenteritis show striking seasonal variations in frequency but these are usually significant only in temperate areas. Rotavirus is the most common cause of infantile diarrhoea worldwide. In Britain and the USA its peak incidence is in 2 or 3 months during the winter, but in tropical climates there is little seasonal variation. Outbreaks of food poisoning caused by *Salmonella*, *Campylobacter* or toxin-producing *Staph. aureus* are more common in summer.

Pathogenesis

Organisms must evade the host defences and colonise the intestine before they can cause disease. Gastric acid is an important defence and patients with a partial gastrectomy are susceptible to intestinal infection. The bacteria adhere to intestinal epithelium. Some bacteria have on their surface determinants which bind to epithelial receptors. Examples are *V. cholerae* and some strains of *E. coli*.

The known mechanisms by which micro-organisms cause diarrhoea can be divided into two groups: toxin secretion and mucosal damage. These are not mutually exclusive and the precise mechanism is unknown for many organisms.

Toxin secretion

Cholera is a good example of small intestinal, toxin-mediated, secretory diarrhoea (see p. 296). Enterotoxigenic strains of *E. coli* secrete a heat-labile enterotoxin which acts in a similar way. In staphylococcal food poisoning enterotoxin-secreting staphylococci multiply in food, and the toxin causes vomiting and diarrhoea within hours of ingestion. Staphylococci are not detected in the stools of patients with this type of food poisoning. *Bacillus cereus*, which contaminates reheated rice, causes vomiting by a similar mechanism.

Mucosal damage

Shigellae invade the colonic mucosa and cause local inflammation, so the faeces contain blood and inflammatory cells. Impairment of water absorption from the colon is the cause of fluid stools. Salmonellae, *Campylobacter* and rotavirus are also invasive and cause tissue damage but the precise mechanisms are not understood. Damage to the brush border of the enterocytes causes temporary disaccharidase deficiency which may prolong the diarrhoea after small intestine infection, even after the pathogen has been eliminated.

Clinical features

Most episodes of gastroenteritis are mild and self-limiting. The incubation period is usually short, ranging from a few hours with staphylococcal food poisoning up to 5 days with *Campylobacter* infection. Vomiting, diarrhoea and cramping abdominal pains are typical features. Large-volume stools suggest a small bowel diarrhoea. The stools are fluid without blood or pus in toxin-mediated disease (e.g. cholera), but when invasion and mucosal damage occur in *Salmonella*, *Shigella* and *Campylobacter* infections blood and mucus may be seen in the stool. The appearance of the stools is an unreliable guide to the type of organism.

The major consequence of gastroenteritis is dehydration with electrolyte imbalance. Babies are more vulnerable and can rapidly become severely dehydrated. It is essential that the clinician can make a reasonably accurate assessment of the degree of dehydration and Table 11.13 gives some guidelines.

Fever and signs of systemic illness suggest invasive pathogens. Some invasive organisms can cause septicaemia (e.g. *Salmonella typhimurium*), and some shigellae produce neurotoxins which enter the circulation in the absence of septicaemia and, reaching the central nervous system (CNS), cause headache and meningism.

The illness is usually over within 7 days but symptoms are liable to persist for longer with shigellae and *Campylobacter*. Persisting diarrhoea suggests *Giardia*

Table 11.13 Assessment of degree of dehydration

	Degree of dehydration		
	Mild	Moderate	Severe
Body weight loss	4–5%	6–9%	>10%
Thirst	Present	Present	Present
Conscious level	Normal	Irritable, lethargic (infants and young children)	Drowsy/coma
Skin turgor	Normal	Reduced	Inelastic
Mucosae	Moist/dry	Dry	Very dry
Fontanelle	Normal	Sunken	Sunken
Pulse rate	Normal	Increased	Increased (may be impalpable)
Blood pressure	Normal	Normal or reduced Postural hypotension (older children/ adults)	Reduced (unrecordable)
Urine output	Normal	Reduced	May be anuric

infection, especially if steatorrhoea is present. Persistent diarrhoea and bleeding suggest amoebic dysentery.

Diagnosis

The diagnosis is usually clear but problems arise when there is vomiting in the absence of diarrhoea; when abdominal pains are accompanied by localised tenderness, suggesting pelvic inflammatory disease or appendicitis; and when blood in the stools is taken to indicate inflammatory bowel disease. A positive diagnosis is established by identification of the organism in stools by microscopy, antigen assay (for rotavirus) or culture.

Management

Rehydration can usually be achieved by administration of oral fluids containing glucose and electrolytes. Oral rehydration therapy is discussed in more detail on page 269. In the home, a simple method of preparation is to add 1 heaped teaspoon of sugar and a pinch of salt to a beaker (250 ml) of water. Fruit squash drinks can exacerbate diarrhoea because of excess sugar (secondary disaccharidase deficiency is common), but a very dilute solution is occasionally helpful when a child finds the salty rehydration fluid unpalatable. In children milk is completely withdrawn in the first 24 hours and is re-introduced as rapidly as possible. Breast-feeding should be maintained, especially in tropical countries.

Intravenous fluid replacement is rarely required but persistent vomiting or severe dehydration with circulatory collapse is an indication for its use.

Antibiotics are normally not required but there are some situations in which their use is justified:

- septicaemic *Salmonella* infection
- severe shigellosis
- severe *Campylobacter* infection
- infection with *Yersinia, V. cholerae, Entamoeba histolytica* or *Giardia lamblia*.

Problems associated with use of antibiotics are exacerbation of diarrhoea, prolonged carriage of some organisms (e.g. salmonellae) and development of resistance to multiple antibiotics (e.g. shigellae).

ACUTE UPPER RESPIRATORY INFECTION

Common cold and pharyngitis

The common cold has an incidence of 1–4 episodes per person per year. Large gaps remain in our knowledge of pathogenesis although it is clear that many viruses can cause the same clinical entity. There is considerable overlap between organisms causing colds and those causing pharyngitis (Table 11.14). Pharyngitis is more important, since it is often part of a more systemic illness. The majority of episodes of pharyngitis are caused by viruses. Antibiotic treatment should be reserved for culture-proven cases of streptococcal pharyngitis. In the developed world, group A streptococcal pharyngitis is now rarely complicated by rheumatic fever or glomerulonephritis. Penicillin, as a single i.m. dose or orally for a minimum of 10 days, is the treatment of choice for strep-

Table 11.14 Causes of upper respiratory infection

Disease	Causative organism
Common cold and pharyngitis	Rhinovirus Coronavirus Influenza virus Para-influenza virus Respiratory syncytial virus Adenovirus Unknown
Pharyngitis/tonsillitis	As above, plus: Epstein-Barr virus β-haemolytic streptococcus group A *Mycoplasma pneumoniae* Mixed anaerobes and spirochaetes* *Corynebacterium diphtheriae** *Neisseria gonorrhoea**
Stomatitis	*Candida albicans* Herpes simplex virus Coxsackie A and other enteroviruses Mixed anaerobic bacteria

* Less common.

tococcal pharyngitis, with erythromycin for penicillin-allergic subjects. Ampicillin and related drugs should be avoided, since they often cause a rash in patients with infectious mononucleosis.

Upper respiratory infections are frequently complicated by otitis media in children and, less often, by sinusitis in adults or children. These are usually caused by secondary bacterial infection and it is therefore important to recognise them and treat with antibiotics.

Common bacterial causes of otitis media include *Strep. pneumoniae, H. influenzae* (mainly untypable), group A β-haemolytic streptococci and *Branhamella catarrhalis*.

The bacteria which cause acute sinusitis are similar to those incriminated in otitis media but anaerobes, Gram-negatives and *Staph. aureus* should also be considered. Upper respiratory anaerobic bacteria are usually penicillin-sensitive in contrast to those found in the large bowel.

Acute stomatitis

In contrast to pharyngitis, the microbial cause of acute stomatitis can often be diagnosed from the appearance of lesions in and around the mouth. *Candida* is a common pathogen, particularly in debilitated patients, patients receiving broad-spectrum antibiotics and patients with HIV infection. White plaques occur on an erythematous background. The distribution is wide, including the buccal mucosa. Ulcers are usually superficial and not easily confused with primary herpes simplex infection. The latter is often associated with perioral clusters of vesicles. Severely painful ulceration of the mouth and lips in a young immunocompetent patient is usually due either to Stevens-Johnson syndrome or to primary herpes simplex infection. Coxsackie virus infection may cause small, scattered vesicles and ulcers but they are more sparse than those of herpes simplex and less painful. Other, non-infective causes of ulcers must also be considered, such as aphthous ulcers and, rarely, Behçet's disease (p. 1010).

Infections in the subcutaneous tissue spaces of the face and neck often originate from periodontal infection. Ludwig's angina is an anaerobic bacterial infection of the submandibular and sublingual spaces, which causes firm swelling of the tissues below the chin. These may press inwards and compromise the airway. There is accompanying fever and tachycardia and the patient requires urgent antibiotic treatment, usually penicillin and metronidazole.

SEXUALLY TRANSMITTED DISEASES

Sexually transmitted diseases (STDs) are infections commonly transferred through sexual contact. Our appreciation of the range of agents capable of being transmitted sexually has increased.

Epidemiology

The prevalence and incidence of sexually transmitted infections varies in different parts of the world. This is due to a variation both in the diseases found and in the methods of reporting such infections. The type of sexual behaviour and the sexual orientation of the person involved also influence the transmission of the infectious agents.

For England and Wales there has been an increase in some STDs in recent years (Fig. 11.5). In the UK there was a fall in incidence of syphilis and gonorrhoea after the introduction of penicillin, but the number of reported infections rose again during the 1960s. Figure 11.6 shows the most commonly found STDs treated at genito-urinary medicine clinics. This is an underestimate of the problem. Morbidity associated with STD is more common in women and the agents responsible are more difficult to identify.

Reported STDs are observed mostly in the 20–24-year-old age group, followed by 25–29 and 15–19-year-olds. In the Western world male homosexuals are more likely to contract hepatitis B, syphilis and HIV infection than their heterosexual counterparts. However, the incidence of newly acquired syphilis and gonorrhoea in homosexual men is falling as trends in sexual behaviour change.

The basis of any STD service is the control of sexually transmitted infections. There are basic requirements:

- The patient needs ready access to a specialist centre for accurate diagnosis and treatment of any infection. Attendance needs to be voluntary. Treating the index case only partly helps in controlling an infection, therefore sexual partners need to be identified and treated.
- The patient's co-operation in all these matters is optimum if he/she is assured of absolute confidentiality. The STD service is the most confidential in the present health service and details are generally only released with the patient's consent.
- Education about STDs, both for an individual and as part of a general health education, is important in helping to control the spread of infection.
- The clinics keep a record of the number of patients seen with each infection and these figures form part of a detailed national epidemiological report.

CHRONIC FATIGUE SYNDROME (POST-VIRAL SYNDROME, 'MYALGIC ENCEPHALOMYELITIS')

This syndrome is seen most often in young adults. There is a prolonged period of lethargy, often with muscle pains and fatigability, usually after an episode reminiscent of a viral illness but sometimes in the absence of an evident acute illness. The problem causes great distress to patient and relatives because an explanation is lacking and there is prolonged inability to work or play at expected levels, often coupled with an unreasonable need for sleep. Doctors are frustrated by their inability to establish a positive diagnosis or to give any specific treatment and the patient often turns to alternative medicine.

Aetiology

The syndrome is heterogeneous and no single explanation will fit all patients. The term 'myalgic encephalomyelitis' is misleading since there is no evidence of encephalitis and myalgia may not be present. A number of infections have been associated with this syndrome and they are not all viral. Infectious mononucleosis is the best known and studied but CMV infection and toxoplasmosis have been suspected, and it is likely that many other organisms can act as triggers in susceptible individuals. Enteroviruses, particularly of the Coxsackie group, have also been suspected but evidence is inconclusive. Often the only

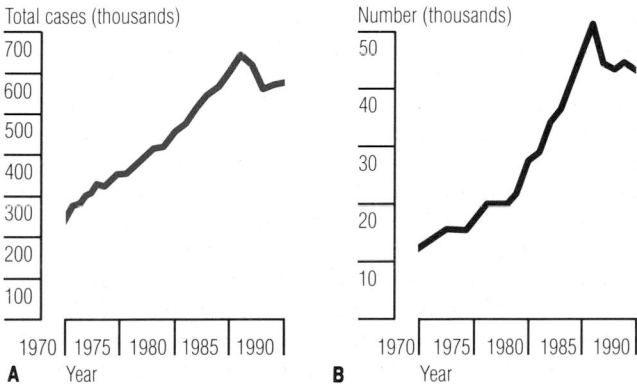

Fig. 11.5 Sexually transmitted diseases. A. Total numbers of cases of sexually transmitted diseases in England and Wales, 1970–1990. **B.** Incidence of non-specific genital infection in women, 1970–1990 (Communicable Diseases Surveillance Centre, Colindale).

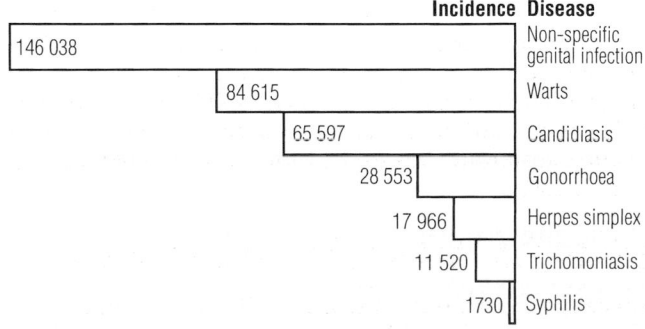

Fig. 11.6 Incidence of sexually transmitted diseases in the UK, 1990 (Communicable Diseases Surveillance Centre, Colindale).

evidence for infection at the onset is a history of febrile illness, perhaps with pharyngitis or lymphadenopathy, and a full blood count may have revealed some atypical mononuclear cells.

The relationship of postviral syndrome to depression is complex. There is no doubt that some patients develop the symptoms and signs of depression and benefit from antidepressant treatment. More commonly the patient becomes depressed as a result of the illness but lacks many of the features of primary depression. In this situation antidepressant therapy is unlikely to be beneficial.

Clinical features

The central symptoms are profound lethargy and easy fatigability. Often these are accompanied by muscular pains, headaches and symptoms suggestive of fever, such as sweating. This is usually mild, and when the temperature is recorded it is normal or only minimally elevated in the evenings. Exertion exacerbates tiredness and the patient often goes to bed early and wakes late still feeling tired.

Management

Patients benefit greatly from having their illness taken seriously and if a precipitating infection can be positively identified this also helps. Sometimes the greatest problem is anxiety about the outcome or about whether there is an underlying disease which has not been diagnosed, so reassurance is important. When patients have restricted their activity it is worth trying to rehabilitate them by a programme of daily exercise, starting with something light like walking or swimming and gradually increasing it in a documented way. The patient is assured that exercise is not harmful and advised to sleep as required.

Most patients recover spontaneously within weeks rather than months, but a few continue to suffer for over a year.

VIRUS INFECTIONS

Viruses are usually classified according to their nucleic acid content and morphology. The classification of viruses used in this section is shown in Table 11.15. Arboviruses (*ar*thropod-*bor*ne) are viruses transmitted by the bite of an insect vector. Most arboviruses are togaviruses, but bunyaviruses and orbiviruses (RNA viruses in the reovirus family) are also included.

ENVELOPED DOUBLE-STRANDED DNA VIRUSES

HERPES VIRUSES

Six herpes viruses cause disease in man:

● varicella zoster virus (VZV)
● *two* herpes simplex viruses (HSV 1 and 2)
● Epstein-Barr virus (EBV)
● cytomegalovirus (CMV)
● human herpes virus 6.

Morphologically, herpes viruses are very similar and indistinguishable by electron microscopy. They are similar in some aspects of their behaviour, notably their ability to establish latent infection with the potential for reactivation. During latency in dorsal root ganglia VZV shows no demonstrable evidence of viral replication for many years. With HSV there is evidence of a low level of replication and reactivation is more frequent. EBV infects B lymphocytes, and EBV and CMV replicate at a low level continuously. CMV can often be detected in the

Table 11.15a Classification of viruses: DNA

Morphology	Virus

Enveloped double-stranded	Herpes viruses
	  Varicella zoster (VZV)
	  Herpes simplex (HSV I, II)
	  Epstein-Barr (EBV)
	  Cytomegalovirus (CMV)
	  Human herpes virus 6 (HHV6)
	Pox viruses
	  Vaccinia
	  Variola (smallpox)
	  Orf

Enveloped single-stranded	Parvovirus

Non-enveloped double-stranded	Adenoviruses
	Papovaviruses
	  Papilloma
	  Polyoma

urine of asymptomatic carriers, and herpes simplex in saliva. The mechanisms by which virus replication is suppressed are incompletely understood but CMI probably has an important role, since all the herpes viruses are liable to reactivate in patients with depression of CMI.

Varicella zoster virus infection

Chickenpox (varicella)

This illness is easy to recognise, common and highly infectious. It is a febrile illness with a vesicular rash (Plate 1, p. 247).

Table 11.15b Classification of viruses: RNA

Morphology	Virus
Enveloped single-stranded	Orthomyxoviruses
	Influenza
	Paramyxoviruses
	Para-influenza
	Respiratory syncytial
	Mumps
	Measles
	Togaviruses
	Rubella
	Alpha
	Flavi
	Bunyaviruses
	Rift Valley fever
	Arenaviruses
	Lassa
	Marburg-Ebola
	Retroviruses
	Human immunodeficiency (HIV) 1, 2
	HTLV1, 2
	Rhabdoviruses
	Rabies
Non-enveloped double-stranded	Reoviruses
	Rota
Non-enveloped single-stranded	Picornaviruses
	Rhino
	Entero
	Coxsackie A, B
	Echo
	Polio

During the primary infection there is a viraemic phase when VZV becomes widely disseminated in white cells. In normal subjects it only produces significant lesions in the skin and mucous membranes, but infection of cutaneous sensory nerves leads to infection of dorsal root ganglia and here the virus enters a latent state. Reactivation later causes herpes zoster (shingles). During primary infection VZV is present in nasopharyngeal secretions and is transmitted readily by coughing and sneezing. It is also in vesicle fluid in chickenpox and shingles and this can be a source of transmission.

The incubation period of chickenpox is 15–18 days and the patient is infectious from a few days before the rash erupts until new lesions cease to appear.

The severity of chickenpox is determined by the age and immunological state of the patient. It is most severe in neonates if they have no maternal antibody to VZV, and in patients immunocompromised by disease such as leukaemia or by immunosuppressive therapy. It is usually a mild disease in children but it becomes increasingly severe after puberty.

Clinical features

In children chickenpox starts with the appearance of the rash, which is often sparse and not accompanied by constitutional symptoms. The most troublesome feature of the illness is itching. In adults there is a notable prodromal illness lasting 2–3 days, during which headache, backache, shivering and fever occur, sometimes with sore throat and cough. The more severe the prodromal illness, the more profuse is the rash which follows.

The rash starts on the trunk and spreads to the face and limbs (Plate 1, p. 247). Lesions appear in crops which progress rapidly through the sequence macule, papule, vesicle, pustule, scab. Often the first visible lesions are vesicles containing clear fluid with little surrounding erythema, but the pustular stage is reached within 24 hours. Vesicles on the palate, tonsils and pharynx rapidly burst, leaving superficial ulcers. Crops of skin lesions erupt over 2 or 3 days, but it takes several more days for them all to heal. Constitutional symptoms, if present, lessen with the onset of the rash and disappear within 2 days.

Complications

Secondary infection of the skin lesions, including the scalp, occurs because of scratching, but it usually responds to cleaning and bathing and rarely requires antibiotics. Chickenpox pneumonia occurs in one-fifth of adults and more frequently in immunocompromised patients. It varies in severity from transient dyspnoea to a fulminant pneumonia.

Postinfectious encephalitis is extremely rare and has a variable course, but it is often severe or fatal. Its onset is within a week of the rash and cerebellar involvement is characteristic.

Bleeding into the skin, nose or intestine, also rare, is due either to steroid-responsive thrombocytopenia or to consumptive coagulopathy, when the prognosis is much worse.

Neonatal chickenpox

Most women are immune by the time they reach childbearing age but if a mother develops chickenpox within a few days of having a baby the child is born without the protection of maternal IgG antibodies transferred across the placenta, and it is immediately exposed to the virus. If the child becomes infected during the first 5 days of life disease is severe, with multi-organ involvement.

Disease can be prevented or modified by administration of varicella immune globulin. Acyclovir is given.

Congenital chickenpox

Rarely, VZV can cross the placenta during the first 20 weeks of pregnancy, causing fetal damage or death.

Diagnosis and management

A clinical diagnosis of chickenpox suffices in most cases. Electron microscopy is the quickest way to establish that a herpes virus is present in vesicle fluid but does not establish its type. The virus can be identified by tissue culture inoculation, and antibodies are detected by a complement fixation test.

Treatment with acyclovir (p. 216) is required only in severe cases with complications such as chickenpox pneumonia, in patients with inadequate CMI (such as children with malignant disease), and in neonates (Table 11.5, p. 216). The virus is sensitive to intravenous acyclovir.

Shingles (zoster)

When VZV reactivates within a dorsal root ganglion it migrates down the nerve into the skin and causes a crop of lesions identical to those of chickenpox but confined to the dermatome (Plate 2, p. 247). Pain within the dermatome may precede the eruption by a few days and is often severe. One or two adjacent dermatomes on the trunk are most commonly affected but involvement of the ophthalmic division of the fifth cranial nerve is important because the eye can be damaged by the virus or by secondary bacterial infection.

In the elderly it is common for a mild viraemia to occur, causing a few scattered lesions to appear outside the involved dermatome. More serious dissemination with visceral involvement is seen in immunocompromised patients. Patients with Hodgkin's disease are particularly susceptible to shingles, especially during chemotherapy.

The skin heals over 2–3 weeks and there is often some residual pain for a few weeks. Rarely, intractable pain continues for years (post-herpetic neuralgia). This is more common following ophthalmic zoster and after severe infections in immunocompromised patients.

Management

Most patients do not require admission to hospital and treatment of pain is the main concern. Continuous treatment with simple analgesics such as paracetamol is often effective and should be tried before drugs which have more side-effects.

Topical treatment of the skin with antiviral drugs is of limited benefit, but an increase in the rate of healing has been demonstrated when high-dose oral acyclovir is used. This benefit must be weighed against the cost of treatment. When the ophthalmic division of the trigeminal nerve is involved, prophylactic topical treatment with an antibiotic such as chloramphenicol and an antiviral drug such as acyclovir is advisable.

Systemic antiviral treatment, e.g. with intravenous acyclovir, should be given to immunocompromised patients. It reduces pain, shortens the healing time and limits dissemination of the virus.

Herpes simplex virus infection

HSV 1 and 2 cause patterns of disease which differ clinically and epidemiologically but share some characteristics. Both establish permanent, latent infection within sensory nerve ganglia following primary infection, with reactivation causing episodes of disease in the area supplied by the nerve. These viruses are indistinguishable morphologically but can be separated by differences in antigen expression.

Infection with HSV 1 is more common. Antibodies are detectable in 80–100% of adults in lower socio-economic groups, and 30–50% in higher socio-economic groups.

Both viruses are readily transmitted, mainly in vesicle fluid. HSV 1 is usually acquired during childhood but HSV 2 infection is mainly transmitted sexually and is most common in sexually promiscuous adults.

Clinical expression of infection with these viruses is strongly influenced by age, nutrition and the immunological state of the patient. An immunologically immature neonate is overwhelmed by disseminated HSV infection acquired during parturition. Infection in older children is often asymptomatic or causes localised disease which is most severe in the presence of malnutrition.

Primary infection with HSV 1

Acute herpetic gingivostomatitis in children 2–4 years old presents with fever, sore throat and submental and anterior cervical lymphadenopathy. Clusters of vesicles appear around the lips and in the mouth from gums to pharynx (Plate 3, p. 247). Inside the mouth, lesions rapidly ulcerate, causing pain and dysphagia with consequent drooling of saliva. The child is miserable and may become dehydrated if not encouraged to drink through a straw. The lesions heal over 1–2 weeks.

Primary infection can occur anywhere on the skin and, on the finger, a *herpetic whitlow* can closely mimic a bacterial paronychia. Widespread involvement of the skin can occur in individuals with atopic dermatitis (eczema herpeticum, p. 1138), and, particularly in infants, this can be associated with systemic symptoms. In the eye *keratoconjunctivitis* can cause scarring of the cornea and loss of vision.

Summary 2 Varicella zoster and herpes simplex infection		
	Primary	**Reactivation**
VZV	Chickenpox	Shingles
HSV 1	Acute or asymptomatic gingivostomatis Keratoconjunctivitis Encephalitis	Cold sores Keratoconjunctivitis
HSV 2	Genital	Genital

Herpetic encephalitis in adults presents a characteristic clinical picture due to necrotic lesions in the temporal lobe. This rare manifestation of primary HSV infection is described on page 968.

Primary infection with HSV 2

Although HSV 1 and 2 can cause identical disease, HSV 2 is largely associated with genital infection. Primary genital infection is most common in young, sexually active adults and the risk of infection is proportional to the number of sexual partners. After an incubation period of 2–7 days, clusters of vesicles with surrounding erythema appear at the site of virus entry, on the glans or penile shaft in men or on the vulva and vaginal mucosa in women. Homosexual men may develop rectal and perianal lesions. The lesions are usually painful and there may be systemic illness with headache, myalgia, fever and local lymphadenopathy.

Occasionally paraesthesiae develop in areas supplied by infected nerves and there may be urinary retention or constipation. Skin and mucosal lesions resolve over 2–3 weeks. Virus may be shed from the lesions for up to 12 days.

Infection of neonates can occur during parturition when the mother has genital herpes, particularly if her infection is primary rather than recurrent. The infant develops scattered clusters of vesicles which recur in the same sites subsequently. Alternatively there may be rapid deterioration as the virus disseminates to all the viscera, causing encephalitis, pneumonia and hepatitis with a high mortality. Usually this severe illness starts in the few days after birth but occasionally onset is delayed several weeks.

Reactivation of HSV 1 and 2

The mechanisms involved in maintaining latency are not fully understood. Reactivation may occur after exposure to ultraviolet light, an episode of infection or trauma to the sensory nerve. Many episodes have no identifiable precipitant. Reactivation is more common in immuno-compromised patients, particularly leukaemics undergoing treatment.

The characteristic lesion of reactivated HSV 1 is a *cold sore*. Patients often experience minor discomfort in the form of tingling or itching up to 24 hours before a lesion appears. Lesions can occur anywhere on the skin or mucous membranes but are commonly adjacent to the lips. A macule rapidly progresses to a papule and then to a cluster of vesicles which involute, ulcerate and scab. The whole process takes 1–2 weeks.

Reactivation of genital HSV causes lesions similar to but milder than those of the primary episode, with more localised lesions occasionally accompanied by shooting pains in the buttocks or legs.

Reactivation in immune deficient patients causes more severe local disease which may become disseminated, causing pneumonia or hepatitis. Patients with AIDS may develop oesophagitis or proctitis.

Asymptomatic secretion of virus can occur in the mouth (HSV 1) or in the vagina (HSV 2) but this is rarely a source of transmission.

Management of herpes simplex

HSVs are highly sensitive to acyclovir and other DNA polymerase inhibiting drugs. Only serious primary infections with HSV 1, such as encephalitis in adults, severe eczema herpeticum or disseminated neonatal infection, warrant treatment with systemic antiviral drugs. Appropriate forms of treatment are shown in Table 11.5. Initial attacks of genital herpes are treated with 5 days of acyclovir, with an antibiotic if secondary infection has occurred. For recurrences attention to local hygiene is all that is required and 5% acyclovir ointment may be helpful for local lesions.

Epstein-Barr virus infection

Epstein-Barr virus (EBV) is a herpes virus which is transmitted by close oral contact. Infection is frequently acquired asymptomatically during early childhood in underdeveloped countries and in crowded living conditions, but infection is delayed in more prosperous environments. Infection in adolescents and adults usually causes infectious mononucleosis (glandular fever).

Other diseases related to EBV infection are nasopharyngeal carcinoma, Burkitt's lymphoma, the very rare syndrome of X-linked recessive progressive combined variable immunodeficiency, and lymphoid interstitial pneumonitis in children with AIDS.

Infectious mononucleosis

Infectious mononucleosis is an acute febrile illness caused by EBV, characterised by severe sore throat and generalised lymphadenopathy.

Pathology and pathogenesis

EBV enters through the pharyngeal epithelium and replicates in B lymphocytes, causing them to proliferate. Fifteen per cent or more of blood mononuclear cells appear 'atypical' during acute infection; these cells are T lymphocytes reacting to the presence of infected B lymphocytes. EBV does not establish a true latent state but maintains a low level of replication throughout life. During infectious mononucleosis, the spleen and lymph nodes are intensely infiltrated with mononuclear cells and the spleen is unusually friable. Haemorrhage may occur into the subcapsular area and rarely this leads to intraperitoneal haemorrhage.

Clinical features

Infectious mononucleosis is most common in adolescents and young adults, but children as young as 5 years old may be affected. The illness is more severe in older patients.

The incubation period is uncertain but is probably 1–2 weeks. There is gradual onset of malaise, general aching and fever. The throat becomes painful and engorged with enlarging lymphoid tissue so that speech is nasal and swallowing is inhibited by pain. The tonsils are large and coated with thick, white exudate (Plate 4, p. 247). Petechiae may be seen on the soft palate. There is generalised lymphadenopathy in most patients and splenomegaly is common. Uncommon features (occurring in less than 15% of patients) are rash, jaundice and tender hepatomegaly. Thrombocytopenia or autoimmune haemolytic anaemia occur rarely. The acute stage of the illness lasts 2–3 weeks and most patients are entirely well within a month. A small proportion of patients, particularly when older, make a slower recovery, continuing to feel lethargic for a variable period (see chronic fatigue syndrome, p. 227).

Differential diagnosis

Other viral causes of sore throat and lymphadenopathy, such as adenovirus, influenza virus and rhinovirus, must be considered (Table 11.14). Streptococcal infections can cause an identical appearance in the throat but the lymphadenopathy is mainly in the anterior cervical region. Streptococci are found on throat swabs in 10% of patients with infectious mononucleosis and their role is unclear.

Many virus infections are associated with atypical lymphocytes on the blood film but these can be distinguished from 'glandular fever cells' by an experienced observer. The latter are also seen in acute CMV infection and occasionally in toxoplasmosis. Both of these conditions can cause lymphadenopathy but they rarely produce sore throat.

Laboratory features

Atypical mononuclear cells are usually present in the blood film at some stage of the disease. Tests for heterophil antibodies, i.e. antibodies to heterologous erythrocytes are the Paul Bunnell and Monospot tests. Heterophil antibodies are present in 90% of patients by the third week of illness but in only 30% during the first week. Specific IgM antibody measurements are not reliable. Liver function tests are often abnormal.

Management

No specific treatment is available. Simple analgesic therapy is used to relieve discomfort in the throat and frequently the patient can only take fluids in the early stages. Occasionally the degree of congestion is such as to threaten the airways and a short course of prednisolone starting at 30 mg daily, tailing off over 2 weeks, can produce a rapid reduction in size of the tonsils.

If penicillin therapy is indicated for treatment of concurrent streptococcal infection, ampicillin and amoxycillin should be avoided, since they cause a severe maculopapular rash.

X-linked recessive progressive combined variable immunodeficiency (Duncan's disease)

This rare inherited disease is now recognised as an abnormal response to EBV infection. Patients either die of overwhelming EBV infection in the acute stage or develop a progressive immunodeficiency following infection. Lymphoma may complicate the late stages.

Cytomegalovirus infection

CMV is a herpes virus which rarely causes significant disease in immunologically competent subjects. Infection is usually asymptomatic but it may be associated with a mild febrile illness during which atypical mononuclear cells appear in the blood; these cells are similar to those seen in infectious mononucleosis.

Primary infection in the neonate causes serious disease, and primary infection of pregnant women can cause congenital defects in the fetus. As with other herpes viruses, infection is lifelong. CMV replicates at a low level throughout life, but when immunity is suppressed the rate of replication increases. Patients with kidney or heart transplants are particularly at risk and CMV sometimes causes severe disease in patients with AIDS (p. 243).

Transmission

The virus is present in blood during primary infection and can cross the placenta. It can also be transmitted in blood used for transfusion.

Infected organs transplanted from seropositive donors can cause primary infection in the recipient, but most CMV disease in renal transplant patients is caused by reactivation.

The virus is shed from the cervix during active infection and is also present in semen and urine.

Acute infection in normal adults

There may be a mild febrile illness which is recognised as viral infection when atypical mononuclear cells are seen in a blood film. Sore throat, generalised lymphadenopathy and splenomegaly occur in less than one-third of patients. Abnormal liver function tests show that there is usually a mild hepatitis but jaundice is rare. The average age for symptomatic infection is 30 years, about 10 years older than for infectious mononucleosis.

Complications are rare in immunocompetent patients and, when they occur, they are mild. Pneumonitis, myocarditis, meningo-encephalitis, Guillain-Barré syndrome, thrombocytopenia and haemolytic anaemia have all been described.

Infection in immunosuppressed patients

Both primary infection and reactivation can cause disease in immunosuppressed patients, but in renal transplant recipients the more severe disease is seen during primary infection. Asymptomatic reactivation is common and is shown by culture of virus from urine. Fever, sometimes with atypical mononucleosis, is the most common presentation of disease, followed by interstitial pneumonitis.

Interstitial pneumonitis presents with insidious onset of fever, non-productive cough and dyspnoea. Chest radiograph shows bilateral diffuse interstitial changes indistinguishable from those of many other opportunistic infections. Diagnosis is usually made by transbronchial biopsy. *Hepatitis* is usually mild but occasionally causes hepatic failure.

CMV may be a harmless passenger in the gastrointestinal tract of patients. Its association with *enteritis* is strongly suggested by the coincidence of seroconversion and haemorrhagic lesions anywhere from the stomach to the rectum, causing a severe diarrhoeal disease and blood loss. A response to treatment with antiviral drugs supports the existence of this clinical entity.

Severe *choroidoretinitis* causes progressive loss of sight starting in one eye and then affecting the other. Large white exudates containing haemorrhagic areas occur.

Diagnosis

Virus can be cultured from urine, throat washings or buffy coat during active replication and IgM antibodies are detectable in serum by an immunofluorescence test. In histological sections 'owl's eye cells' are strongly suggestive of CMV infection.

Management

Drugs such as phosphonoformate (foscarnet) or ganciclovir are available for treatment of CMV pneumonia, retinitis and enteritis, but disease may recur if immunity remains depressed. Hyperimmune globulin containing high titre antibody to CMV has been used to treat neonates with CMV pneumonia with possible success.

Human herpes virus 6 infection

Human herpes virus 6 (HHV6) has recently been identified in patients with AIDS and has subsequently been found to be widely distributed. It is the cause of roseola, a common febrile illness of young children characterised by the appearance of a rash when the fever and illness are resolving. The temperature is high but the child is relatively well. There is often cervical and postauricular lymphadenopathy. When the temperature starts to fall, or within 2 days, a maculopapular erythematous eruption appears on the trunk; this lasts for a few days. Blood count reveals neutropenia initially, which may be followed by mild leukocytosis. The illness resolves without complications.

POX VIRUSES

Variola and vaccinia

Variola virus is the cause of smallpox, an infection of low infectivity transmitted between humans by close contact. Immunisation introduced globally using the refined vaccine containing vaccinia virus led to the eradication of smallpox in 1979. Only accidental laboratory infections have occurred since then. Vaccination against smallpox is no longer justified.

Orf virus infection

Orf virus causes a single nodular lesion at the site of an abrasion which has been in contact with an infected lamb.

Molluscum contagiosum

Molluscum contagiosum is an infection of the skin caused by a pox virus. The incubation period is variable and may be up to 6 months. A typical lesion is a smooth, firm papule, with the vertex of the papule umbilicated and containing a waxy substance.

Lesions commonly appear on the genitalia, suprapubic area and inner thighs but can appear anywhere on the skin surface. They appear to be more common in people who are HIV positive, in whom the face, including the eyelids, may be involved.

Spontaneous regression may occur. Therapies include curettage and liquid nitrogen cryotherapy or application of phenol, podophyllin or iodine after disruption of the lesions.

ENVELOPED SINGLE-STRANDED DNA VIRUSES

PARVOVIRUS

The association between infection with human parvovirus and disease has only been recognised in the last decade. The virus was first noticed in sera from normal subjects during screening by electron microscopy (1975), but in 1983 it was reported to be the cause of erythema infectiosum ('slapped cheek disease' or 'fifth disease'). A more serious consequence is that the virus can cause aplastic crises in patients with sickle cell disease.

Clinical features

Parvovirus infection is probably transmitted from human to human by nasopharyngeal secretions and causes a range of illness ranging from asymptomatic to a febrile systemic illness with a rash. After a mild prodromal illness consisting of fever, headache, upper respiratory symptoms and myalgia lasting 2–4 days, a rash appears on the arms and chest, spreading peripherally, even to the palms and soles. The classic 'slapped cheek' appearance of erythema infectiosum is seen in less than half of infected patients. Elsewhere the rash is maculopapular and fluctuates in intensity. It often develops a lacy reticular pattern on the limbs and leaves a short-lived pale brown pigmentation as it fades over a week. The rash is frequently pruritic. Other features during the rash are generally mild but include fever, malaise, headache and sometimes arthralgia, lymphadenopathy and splenomegaly.

Complications

Complications are rare. Adult women may develop symmetrical peripheral polyarthritis, which can be the sole manifestation of infection. Although it usually resolves within 3 months it may continue for several years.

Aplastic crises are not a feature of infection in patients who are otherwise normal haematologically, but when the red cell life is reduced, as in sickle cell disease or hereditary spherocytosis, arrest of erythropoiesis for 5–10 days causes a significant fall in haemoglobin level.

Diagnosis and management

IgM serum antibodies detected by enzyme linked immunosorbent assay (ELISA) or radioimmunoassay (RIA) are diagnostic of recent infection and persist for about 2 months. A change in titre of IgG antibodies also indicates recent infection. Virus isolation is not feasible and detection of viral protein is reserved for research purposes.

There is no specific treatment at present.

NON-ENVELOPED DOUBLE-STRANDED DNA VIRUSES

ADENOVIRUSES

Adenoviruses are a common cause of upper respiratory infection in children, and cause a variety of other illnesses depending on the serotype of virus and the age of the patient. Over 40 serotypes have been isolated from man and many of these are known to have pathogenic potential. Virus can frequently be isolated from the posterior pharyngeal lymphoid tissue of asymptomatic subjects, suggesting that it can remain latent for long periods.

Upper respiratory infection. Common cold and pharyngitis occur in all age groups and serotypes 1–6 are the usual cause.

Lower respiratory infection. Tracheobronchitis and pneumonia are rare in children but young adults may be affected. This is one of the differential diagnoses of atypical pneumonia. Types 4 and 7 are the most common causes.

Pharyngo-conjunctival fever. An acute infection spreads among young children in close contact, often caused by adenovirus type 3.

Epidemic keratoconjunctivitis. Epidemic keratoconjunctivitis is a more severe form of eye infection which affects adults and often follows minor trauma to the eye. Type 8 is the usual pathogen.

Haemorrhagic cystitis. Caused by types 11 and 21, haemorrhagic cystitis is a childhood infection.

Adenoviruses are also uncommonly associated with diarrhoeal disease, intussusception and meningitis or encephalitis.

There is as yet no effective antiviral treatment for adenoviruses.

PAPOVAVIRUSES

The important members of the papovavirus group are *papilloma* or wart viruses and *polyoma* viruses, one of which, the JC virus, causes progressive multifocal leucoencephalopathy, a rare neurological disease (p. 970).

Palmar and plantar warts are benign infections, common in childhood, which often spontaneously regress with increasing age. They are caused by viruses which are distinct from the anogenital warts viruses; the latter are sexually transmitted (p. 1131) and are regarded as important in view of increasing evidence associating them with cervical cancer.

Genital warts

In men warts can appear on any part of the genitalia but especially the frenum, coronal sulcus and the inner surface of the foreskin. They are called condylomata accuminata. They may involve the male urethra and appear as bright red lumps at the meatus.

In women the vulva, vagina, cervix and perineal area can be involved. Cervical condylomata may be flat and identifiable only by colposcopy. They may be associated with dyskaryosis and koilocytosis and with cervical cancer.

Management

Local application of cytotoxic agents such as podophyllin and 5-fluorouracil, or destructive agents or methods such as trichloracetic acid, cautery, diathermy or cryosurgery, are still the main therapeutic approaches. Ablation of cervical warts by laser therapy is effective.

ENVELOPED SINGLE-STRANDED RNA VIRUSES

ORTHOMYXOVIRUSES

Influenza virus infection

Influenza types A and B are the main viruses in this family but there is also a type C virus. Influenza is an ancient disease characterised by regular winter epidemics with occasional much larger outbreaks (pandemics) when there is a major shift in antigenic type against which there is little immunity in the population. Although the disease is normally mild and self-limiting, the elderly and those with chronic chest disease are susceptible to complications resulting in a considerable mortality.

Epidemiology

Epidemics of influenza start with cases in children and spread to the adult population. As the epidemic progresses, vulnerable adults start to present in hospitals and the size of the epidemic becomes apparent when absenteeism causes problems at work and in schools. Epidemics usually peak within three weeks and last about six weeks. They occur in winter, December to April in the Northern hemisphere and May to September in the Southern hemisphere. In tropical countries, virus isolates can be obtained year round but epidemics tend to occur after changes in weather whereas in temperate climates it is rare to find the virus in the community between epidemics.

Surprisingly, several variants of the virus are found to be circulating during an epidemic but they are sufficiently similar to previously recognised viruses for some cross immunity to exist. Variants which appear late in the course of an epidemic are sometimes the ones responsible for an outbreak during the following winter.

Pandemics have occurred infrequently over the last century in 1889, 1918, 1957, 1968 and 1977. They result from the emergence of new viruses in which there are major changes in the surface proteins, mainly neuraminidase and haemagglutinin, against which the populations of the world have no immunity. The mechanism for these changes is likely to be genetic reassortment and some evidence suggests that this occurs in animal reservoirs, such as birds and lower mammals. Two neuraminidases and three haemagglutinins have been detected at various times in the last century and these are recognised in the name given to a sub-type of virus. For example the virus responsible for the 1918 epidemic was H1N1 and another severe epidemic in 1957 was caused by H2N2. The severity of an outbreak is determined by the extent of change in antigenicity of the virus so that if the neuraminidase and the haemagglutinin both undergo a major change, the severity of disease and the size of the epidemic are greater than if only one determinant changes.

After a major antigenic *shift* causing a pandemic, smaller variations in antigenicity known as antigenic *drift* occur over a variable period (nine to thirty years in the past century) and the population gradually builds up immunity to the possible variants of the new virus sub-type. The scene for the next major antigenic shift may be set by the level of herd immunity to the sub-type variants but other factors probably make a contribution also.

Clinical features

Influenza is transmitted by droplets of respiratory secretions and the incubation period is one to three days. Influenza A and B cause a similar illness but influenza C only gives rise to sore throat.

The onset of influenza is rapid with symptoms of fever including chills, sweats and sometimes rigors accompanied by malaise, anorexia, headache and marked myalgia. The severity of general symptoms varies greatly between individuals from mild to prostrating. They are worst in the first three days and usually disappear within a week. Cough and sore throat are variable features which tend to increase as other symptoms subside and resolve over two to three weeks.

On examination the patient is initially febrile, flushed and tachycardic with minor nasal discharge. The pharynx may be inflamed and cervical lymph nodes palpable and tender.

Complications

The elderly are more vulnerable to all complications. The most common is exacerbation of chronic bronchitis and this is responsible for most adult admissions to hospital in influenza epidemics. Asthma is also exacerbated. Bacterial pneumonia, often caused by *S. pneumoniae*, *S. aureus* or

11 Infectious, Tropical and Parasitic Diseases

H. influenzae, can occur in chronic bronchitics or patients with no previous history of chest disease but it is more common in smokers.

Viral pneumonia caused by influenza virus itself is a severe complication which usually occurs in patients with underlying disease of the chest or cardiovascular system although in some epidemics it has affected previously healthy adults suggesting that virus virulence is a factor. This type of pneumonia is bilateral, with opacities on the chest radiograph which do not correspond to clinical signs, low diffusing capacity and a progressive course.

Other rarer complications include myositis, myocarditis, pericarditis, Guillain-Barré syndrome and encephalitis.

Other clinical syndromes

Diagnosis

Influenza virus can be cultured from respiratory secretions but the diagnosis is more often made by serum antibody measurement using paired samples in a complement fixation test. When an epidemic is in progress a clinical diagnosis suffices.

Management and prevention

The only available antiviral drug, amantidine, is active against influenza A virus but not influenza B. It has been shown to reduce the severity of symptoms but it is rarely used since the effect is small and there is a considerable incidence of minor side-effects such as insomnia and loss of concentration. Treatment is therefore symptomatic using analgesics such as paracetamol. (Aspirin should be avoided in children because of the danger of precipitating Reye's syndrome.)

Amantidine has been shown to be effective in prophylaxis also but vaccination is much more widely used. Inactivated viral vaccine containing the currently prevalent strains of influenza A and B is recommended for persons at special risk, especially the elderly and those suffering from chronic pulmonary, heart or renal disease, diabetes, and those with some forms of immunosuppression. The vaccine is usually given in the autumn and confers about 70% protection for a year.

PARAMYXOVIRUSES

Para-influenza virus infection

There are four types of para-influenza virus and the organisms are a common cause of mild upper respiratory infection in children under 2 years of age (Ch. 13). Types 1–3 occasionally cause more severe lower respiratory tract disease, such as croup and bronchiolitis. Although there is little antigenic variation in para-influenza viruses, immunity is poor and reinfection causing mild disease is common.

Respiratory syncytial virus infection

Respiratory syncytial virus (RSV) is the most important cause of lower respiratory tract infection in young children. Outbreaks occur annually, usually in late winter or spring, and about half of primary infections result in pneumonia, bronchiolitis or tracheobronchitis. Upper respiratory involvement is also common and otitis media is a frequent complication. Children over the age of 3 usually suffer milder disease and adults are occasionally infected. RSV is highly infectious and is commonly transmitted to other patients in hospital. Respiratory isolation procedures should be applied (but rarely are). Successful therapy for RSV has been described using ribavirin administered as an aerosol, but in practice this is difficult to apply.

Mumps

Mumps is a systemic paramyxovirus infection which commonly causes inflammation of salivary glands. It is transmitted by droplets from the mouth. Infection in childhood is common but infectivity is low and many people reach adulthood without becoming affected.

Clinical features

The incubation period is about 18 days (Fig. 11.1, p. 209). Mumps is a mild disease in childhood and about one-third of children infected have no symptoms. In its mildest form there is fever with discomfort and swelling in the parotid glands, which lasts a week or less. In more severe forms there is considerable malaise, the glands are painful and there may be trismus. Other salivary glands are often inflamed and glands are sometimes involved sequentially. Swollen parotid glands can be distinguished from lymphadenopathy because the angle of the mandible is obliterated by the former. The mouth is dry and there may be redness around the orifices of the parotid ducts, but there is no purulent discharge.

About 20% of adult males develop *orchitis* in the course of mumps but *oophoritis* is rare. Usually orchitis starts a few days after the onset of parotitis, but it may be earlier and may occur in the absence of parotitis. The swollen inflamed testicle is exquisitely tender and remains so for 3–4 days before gradually recovering. Orchitis is accompanied by fever and malaise and the latter often persists for some weeks.

Orchitis is bilateral in 15–30% of cases but even in these patients sterility is extremely rare. Although some shrinkage of involved testicles may be detected shortly after the illness, this does not imply complete loss of function and it is important to reassure patients on this point.

Mumps virus is highly neurotropic and involvement of the CNS is the most common complication of this infection. There are two distinct entities, *meningitis* and *encephalitis*.

Lymphocytic meningitis occurs in about 5% of patients with mumps parotitis, but this figure underestimates its prevalence since it also occurs in the absence of parotitis. There is some seasonal variation in the clinical manifestations, meningitis with parotitis being more common in spring whereas meningitis alone is seen more in summer. The time of onset of meningitis varies but it usually becomes apparent a few days after parotitis. The CSF shows a lymphocytic pleocytosis and virus can be isolated from it. The course is invariably benign.

Encephalitis is rare. It either occurs during parotitis as a result of direct viral invasion of the brain, or its onset is 7–10 days after that of parotitis, when it represents a postinfectious encephalitis. Most patients recover completely but there is a mortality of 1–2%.

Pancreatitis is rarely severe but may account for some of the abdominal symptoms in mumps. Some degree of abdominal pain is not infrequent and may be accompanied by vomiting. In severe cases there is marked abdominal tenderness and the serum amylase level is elevated.

Diagnosis

A clinical diagnosis usually presents little difficulty, but if necessary the virus can be isolated from saliva and throat washings or from CSF in cases of meningitis. Complement-fixing antibody detection can be used to make a retrospective diagnosis.

Management

There is no specific treatment, but oral hygiene is important both for comfort and to prevent secondary infection. Orchitis requires testicular support and adequate analgesia. There is little evidence that corticosteroid treatment is beneficial in orchitis.

Prevention

Vaccination with a live attenuated vaccine was adopted as part of the routine programme in the UK from 1988. It is given in combination with measles and rubella in the second year of life.

Measles

Measles is an easily recognised, highly infectious disease of childhood caused by measles virus, an RNA virus of the paramyxovirus group.

Epidemiology

Infection is spread by droplets coughed on to mucosal surfaces of the conjunctiva and nasopharynx, and since cough is a feature of the illness from the onset it is not surprising that infection spreads rapidly between non-immune subjects. One of the interesting features of the disease in older epidemics was the high mortality rate. It is not clear whether measles virus has changed to a more benign form or whether environmental factors are responsible, but the latter is more likely since the disease is still severe in Africa. The size of the pool of non-immune humans determines whether there is an epidemic of measles. In the past, epidemics have occurred in Britain every 2 years or so, but immunisation has made this pattern less apparent.

Pathogenesis

Measles virus can infect many different cell types and during the incubation period, which is 8–11 days from infection to the onset of prodromal symptoms (Fig. 11.1, p. 210), the virus multiplies, becoming widely disseminated. It reaches most tissues, including skin, mucous membranes, lungs, gut, brain and lymphoreticular tissue.

The lesions of measles, containing mononuclear and giant cells, are caused by a combination of viral cytopathic effect and non-specific and specific inflammatory reactions. The role of immune mechanisms is demonstrated by the modified or absent skin rash in immunodeficient subjects, who may nevertheless die from a giant cell pneumonia. Antibody is detectable in serum 24–48 hours after the onset of rash and virus is rapidly cleared during this period.

Clinical features

In Britain measles is most common at the age of 3–5 years but the age is lower in underdeveloped countries. In the period 2–4 days before eruption of the rash the features are similar to many upper respiratory infections. The patient feels unwell and has a fever, red eyes, swollen eyelids, congested streaming nose, diffuse redness in the mouth and a hacking cough. Koplik's spots, 1–2 mm white spots like a grain of salt on a red background, may be seen on the buccal mucosa. Their number varies from a few to hundreds and they often persist after the rash appears.

The worst of the illness is during the first few days after eruption of the rash, when there is a spiking fever and the child is irritable and miserable. Spots appear first behind the ears and on the forehead, and then spread to the rest of the face, on to the trunk and out to the limbs over 24–72 hours. This pattern of spread is characteristic but the rash of rubella (German measles) spreads in the

---

> **Summary 3 Clinical features of measles**
>
> - Incubation period 8–11 days
> - Initial symptoms of upper respiratory infection
> - Koplik's spots on buccal mucosa
> - Rash spreads from face to trunk to limbs
> - Complications (pneumonia, otitis media, encephalitis) more common in malnourished children

same direction. Measles spots are red macules and maculopapules initially a few millimetres in diameter, which enlarge and coalesce to form irregular blotches, the most striking of which are on the cheeks. As the rash fades and the patient starts to feel better there is transient brown staining of the skin and sometimes fine desquamation.

At the height of the eruptive stage the mucous membranes and eardrums are red, and there is generalised lymphadenopathy, a barking cough and widespread crackles in the chest.

Complications

Major complications are rare in Britain today. All complications are more common in malnourished children, and severe skin desquamation with secondary bacterial infection, diarrhoea, appendicitis, laryngitis, stomatitis and major weight loss all occur frequently in Africa. Measles sometimes precipitates the onset of kwashiorkor. Secondary bacterial infection usually manifests itself 3–4 days after the rash and prolongs the illness. The timing is an important clue, as renewed fever heralds a third phase of illness. Bronchopneumonia and otitis media are examples. Giant cell pneumonia is rare and usually affects immunocompromised children, such as leukaemics.

Febrile convulsions may occur as the temperature rises in the incubation period or at the beginning of the eruptive phase. Encephalitis is rare and varies in severity. It occurs in the convalescent phase and in fatal cases virus is not recovered from the brain, so encephalitis may be caused by an immune reaction to viral antigen in neural tissue. Subacute sclerosing panencephalitis (SSPE) is a progressive fatal form of encephalitis affecting older children who had measles many years before. High titres of measles antibodies and recovery of a measles-like virus from the brain suggest that it is related to measles.

Diagnosis

Clinical diagnosis of measles is usually straightforward. The rash of rubella has a similar distribution, but lesions are smaller and they tend to remain discrete. Rubella is a milder illness with a characteristic distribution of lymphadenopathy (occipital and posterior cervical). Laboratory confirmation of measles is rarely necessary, but measles virus can be cultured from nasopharyngeal specimens during the prodrome and for about 2 days into the eruptive phase. A blood count normally shows leucopenia, and neutrophilia suggests secondary bacterial infection. Antibody titres are measured by a complement fixation test.

Management

Most children with measles are looked after at home but if hospital admission is required for social reasons, or because of complications, the patient should be nursed in isolation. Antiviral treatment is not available at present and management is directed at providing comfort and maintaining hydration. Prophylactic antibiotics have no place but appropriate antibiotics must be given for secondary bacterial infection. Important organisms in respiratory infection and otitis media are *Strep. pneumoniae*, *H. influenzae* and, less commonly, *Staph. aureus*. Therefore the usual first choice of antibiotic is a broad-spectrum penicillin (e.g. amoxycillin) or erythromycin.

Management of encephalitis is described on page 969. Passive immunisation with 500 mg normal human immunoglobin intramuscularly (250 mg for children less than 1 year old) attenuates or prevents clinical manifestations if it is given within 6 days of contact. This is useful in children under 18 months and in those whom immunosuppression makes susceptible to severe forms of measles. Protection lasts for about 3 weeks.

Active immunisation

Live attenuated measles virus vaccine is given in the second year of life in Britain. In parts of the world where the disease is common in younger children immunisation is recommended at an earlier age. A single subcutaneous or intramuscular dose gives prolonged protection.

Contra-indications are immune deficiency disease (primary or secondary), immunosuppressive therapy, and severe egg allergy. Atopy and febrile convulsions do not preclude use of the vaccine. The uptake rate for measles immunisation has increased since the introduction of MMR vaccine and measles could become a rare disease, as it has in the United States.

TOGAVIRUSES

The togavirus group comprises the rubella virus, alphaviruses and flaviviruses. *Rubella* is the commonest togavirus infection in the Western world. *Alphaviruses* are the cause of Eastern, Western and Venezuelan equine encephalitis. *Flaviviruses* cause dengue and yellow fever.

Rubella

Postnatal rubella (German measles) is a mild illness occasionally complicated by arthritis or encephalitis. By contrast, infection in utero can have devastating effects on the fetus.

Pathogenesis

Rubella virus infects nasopharyngeal secretions, where it is found during subclinical as well as overt infection. During the viraemic phase it is disseminated widely and, as for measles, the clinical illness corresponds in time with the development of immunity. The incubation period for rubella is 14–16 days.

Clinical features

Like measles, rubella is associated with fever, lymphadenopathy, rash and conjunctival suffusion, but it is a mild, short-lived illness which may be asymptomatic. The lymphadenopathy of rubella is characteristically suboccipital, postauricular and posterior cervical. It may persist long after the rash has faded. Although, as in measles, the rash starts on the face and behind the ears, spreading downwards and outwards over the trunk and limbs, the spots are paler red, circular macules which remain discrete and do not coalesce into brighter irregular blotches. The rash varies from hour to hour, fading and reappearing for up to 4 days. It is common to find petechiae on the soft palate (Forscheimer spots) but these are not diagnostic.

Complications

Arthritis is the only common complication of rubella. It usually affects young women, who develop polyarthritis of small joints, especially those of the fingers and wrists, although larger joints may be affected. It is easily confused with acute rheumatoid arthritis, especially in the absence of rash. It usually subsides within a few days but can last up to 3 months. Encephalitis and thrombocytopenic purpura are very rare complications.

Congenital rubella

Both the risk and the severity of damage to the fetus are closely related to the time of infection. Following infection during the first month of pregnancy, over half of fetuses are affected, whereas by the fourth month only 5% have defects, although this is still twice the frequency in control groups. Minor damage can result from later infection.

During the viraemic phase of the maternal illness rubella virus invades the placenta, causing villous placen-

titis, and then disseminates through the fetal circulation. The degree of damage is variable, even in twins infected at the same time.

The common major abnormalities resulting from infection in the first trimester are cataracts, patent ductus arteriosus with or without pulmonary stenosis, and deafness. Rubella virus can be isolated from the baby's pharynx for several months, a much longer period than in acquired rubella. The virus is present in all other secretions and these babies can readily infect nurses handling them.

Diagnosis

Serology is the mainstay of diagnosis in both congenital and acquired rubella. In the haemagglutination inhibition (HAI) test, the virus agglutinates chick red cells. Serum antibodies inhibit this agglutination. A rise in total antibody titre or the presence of specific IgM antibodies indicates recent infection.

In acquired infection antibody is detectable by HAI 14–16 days after infection and reaches a peak 6–12 days later. The fetus starts to produce IgM antibody at about the twentieth week of life, and since only IgG antibody can cross the placenta, the presence of IgM antibodies to rubella virus in the fetus or infant implies active infection. Rubella virus can be cultured from clinical specimens but this is rarely used for diagnosis.

Immunisation

Live attenuated virus vaccine is given routinely as part of the measles/mumps/rubella (MMR) vaccination to boys and girls aged 15 months. This was introduced in 1988 and replaces the policy of immunising girls aged between 11 and 13 years. Vaccine virus can cross the placenta so it should not be given during pregnancy, and pregnancy should be avoided for 2 months after immunisation.

Exposure to rubella during pregnancy

Definite exposure to rubella of a non-immune, pregnant woman during the first trimester is an indication for termination of pregnancy. If the woman does not know whether she is immune to rubella, the following course of action is recommended:

- if possible, establish by serology the diagnosis of rubella in the patient with whom the pregnant woman was in contact. Find out whether contact was close enough to allow transmission of virus.
- Test the pregnant patient for rubella antibodies:
  If positive by HAI within 14 days of exposure to rubella, the patient was immune previously and she can be reassured.

If negative by HAI then test a further sample 2–3 weeks from contact. If the second serum is positive or if IgM antibodies are detected, discuss risks and offer termination. Some women prefer to continue with the pregnancy despite the risk to the fetus. In this case intramuscular rubella immunoglobulin should be given as soon as possible after exposure.

ARBOVIRUSES

Arboviral infections are a group of virus infections of man that are transmitted by the bite of an arthropod vector. There are two main diseases: dengue and yellow fever.

Dengue

Dengue is an acute febrile illness with severe bone pain, rash and lymphadenopathy. The vectors are *Aedes* mosquitoes. The dengue virus is a 50 nm RNA-containing flavivirus. Four serotypes are recognised, and these can be differentiated in a range of standard serological tests. The serotypes are closely related antigenically but cross-protection between serotypes is lacking. The dengue shock syndrome and haemorrhagic fever occur in patients experiencing reinfection with a different serotype.

Distribution and incidence

Dengue occurs throughout tropical and subtropical areas of the world closely related to the distribution of the *Aedes* mosquito vector.

Transmission and epidemiology

The most common vector is *Aedes aegypti* but other species have more limited roles in transmission. Eight to eleven days after ingesting dengue virus in a human blood meal the mosquito is infective to a receptive host by biting; it remains infective for the rest of its life.

Both sexes and all age groups are susceptible to dengue provided they have not been infected before with that serotype. Dengue haemorrhagic fever is predominantly a disease of children.

Pathology and pathogenesis

After inoculation, virus replicates in local lymph node cells. Viraemia follows and reticulo-endothelial cells in skin and other tissues become infected. Local inflammatory changes occur around small vessels in the skin. The pathogenesis of dengue haemorrhagic fever is poorly understood. It is characterised by hypovolaemia, due to increased vascular permeability, and coagulation defects.

Clinical features

The incubation period is about 7 days prior to the onset of high fever, headache, eye pains, backache and chills. Limb pain is often severe in dengue and this gives rise to its common name, 'breakbone fever'. A blanching, erythematous, macular rash may appear on the third or fourth day of the illness. Lymphadenopathy may be present. Leucopenia is usual in the peripheral blood.

In dengue haemorrhagic fever the patient is more ill, and the peripheral blood shows thrombocytopenia and increased haematocrit. There may be spontaneous bleeding into the skin and at other sites. The loss of circulating blood volume causes shock with low blood pressure, rapid pulse, restlessness and abdominal pain (the dengue shock syndrome), which can have a mortality of 50% untreated. This occurs most often in children but occasional cases are reported in adults.

Diagnosis

Virus can be isolated from blood using *Aedes* or mammalian cell lines. A rising antibody titre in paired sera obtained 10–14 days apart is diagnostic, although the serological response may not be so clear-cut in areas where populations are exposed to other flaviviruses.

Management

Patients with uncomplicated dengue require simple supportive measures, such as attention to nutrition and hydration and relief of pain. Paracetamol should be used in preference to aspirin. Dengue haemorrhagic fever and dengue shock syndrome require early intensive therapy with intravenous fluids, which greatly reduces mortality.

Control

Vaccines are not yet available. Vector control comprises removal of breeding sites, which are often collections of water in tins, tyres, tubs and water storage vessels around homes, and larviciding.

Yellow fever

Yellow fever is an acute arboviral infection caused by the yellow fever virus, a flavivirus. The illness is characterised by high fever, jaundice and encephalopathy in its severe form. The disease occurs in focal outbreaks in Africa, the Caribbean and Central and South America.

Distribution and incidence

Sub-Saharan tropical Africa (especially West Africa), the Caribbean islands (most recently Trinidad) and South

America (Brazil, Peru, Bolivia, Ecuador, Venezuela and Colombia) are the areas affected by yellow fever. Relatively small numbers of cases occur every year in these areas, although cases in isolated areas may go unreported.

Transmission and epidemiology

Transmission is shown in Figure 11.7. In South America, and Central and East Africa, a jungle cycle involves monkey–mosquito–monkey and maintains the virus in the mosquito reservoir. *Haemagogus* mosquitoes are the vector. The epidemiology in savannah and forest-savannah areas involves other *Aedes* species with man and monkeys. The insect vector passes infection to the next generation of mosquitoes by transovarial transmission.

Non-immune persons of all races, all ages and both sexes are susceptible to infection. Prior exposure to other flaviviruses produces some degree of cross-protection. Men are at particular risk of infection because of occupations which take them into forests.

Pathology and pathogenesis

The liver is the main organ involved and shows mid-zonal necrosis of hepatocytes. Councilman bodies result from the degeneration of hepatocytes. The kidneys show acute tubular necrosis which may relate to shock and hypovolaemia. There may be haemorrhage into mucous membranes and the skin, associated with the bleeding tendency that is common in yellow fever. The underlying pathogenic mechanisms are poorly understood.

Clinical features

There is a range of severity of disease from mild to severe, life-threatening illness. The latter constitutes a minority of all those infected. The incubation period is about 6 days before the onset of headache and fever. More severe illness is associated with marked limb pains. Proteinuria is usual. High fever, headache, severe limb and back pain, chills

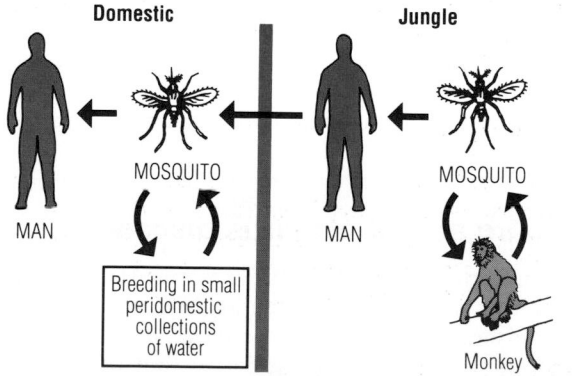

Fig. 11.7 Cycle of transmission of yellow fever virus. Infected humans bring the virus from the jungle. Mosquitoes can breed peridomestically in small collections of water such as puddles and water pots.

associated with fetor, haemorrhages in the gums, and nosebleeds are early features in severe cases. There may then be a short period of remission of symptoms for up to 24 hours before the recurrence of fever with vomiting and jaundice. Bleeding into the gut, skin and other sites is usual in severe cases. Occasional cases are seen with organ damage limited to heart or kidneys, causing cardiac or renal failure. Bleeding and renal failure are the main causes of the high mortality (up to 50%) in severe cases. Resolution in severe cases can take from 3 days to 6 weeks.

Diagnosis

The clinical features in severe cases suggest the diagnosis but in milder cases without evidence of organ dysfunction the diagnosis may not be made. Virus can be isolated most often from blood taken in the first 4 days of clinical illness. Rising antibody titres in paired sera may also give the diagnosis, but serological tests may not be easy to interpret in people exposed to related viruses.

Differential diagnosis

In mild cases the range of febrile illnesses to be considered is extensive and includes malaria, typhoid, the prodromal phase of viral hepatitis, leptospirosis and rickettsial diseases. The presence of jaundice with fever prompts consideration of leptospirosis, malaria, East African trypanosomiasis, typhoid, biliary tract sepsis and Marburg virus diseases. Ebola virus disease and Lassa fever are other causes of haemorrhagic fever, although marked jaundice is not usual.

Laboratory features

Anaemia, leucopenia and thrombocytopenia are usual features in more severe cases. Conjugated bilirubin levels and transaminases are high in jaundiced cases. Coagulation abnormalities comprise prolonged prothrombin time, reduced fibrinogen levels and detectable fibrin degradation products. Renal failure with proteinuria, oliguria and raised creatinine and urea may occur.

Management

More severe cases are likely to come to medical attention. Paracetamol may be helpful symptomatically and in relief of fever. Severe cases require intensive care but this is rarely available in the endemic areas.

Prevention and control

All travellers to endemic areas, apart from pregnant females, infants under 1 year and immunosuppressed patients, should receive the attenuated 17D yellow fever vaccine. Patients with yellow fever should be nursed under mosquito nets to prevent mosquitoes becoming infected.

Other arboviral infections

There are a considerable number of arboviruses which affect man. In these infections the main clinical manifestations are fever, chills, joint pain and a maculopapular rash. Mild forms of the diseases are frequent. Vaccines are not available.

VIRAL HAEMORRHAGIC FEVERS

The viruses causing viral haemorrhagic fevers, a group of clinically similar infections, mainly comprise togaviridae and arenaviridae (Table 11.16). The diseases have a wide geographic distribution. They are characterised, in the clinically severe cases, by a bleeding tendency evident by purpura and ecchymoses in the skin, bleeding from the gums and rapidly falling haemoglobin level, often associated with bleeding into the lungs, gut and other internal organs. The onset is abrupt with rigors, headache, myalgia and an erythematous flush of face and thorax. Progressive renal failure may occur with a rapidly declining haemoglobin, often due to bleeding into the lungs. It should be noted that not all patients infected with these viruses develop severe disease; many have a febrile illness which resolves spontaneously. Treatment in severe cases is mainly supportive, comprising restoration of blood volume, transfusion, platelet support, and dialysis where there is renal failure.

Lassa fever

Lassa fever is an acute febrile illness first described from the region of Lassa in north-eastern Nigeria in 1969. It is an arenavirus (RNA) infection characterised by high sustained fever, ulcerative pharyngitis and swelling of the neck and face in typical cases.

Transmission and epidemiology

The multimammate rat, *Mastomys natalensis*, is the peridomestic reservoir and persistently excretes virus in its urine. Man is infected by ingesting food contaminated with urine containing virus.

Person-to-person spread can occur through contact with vomit, urine, faeces, blood and serum. The virus may enter the body through cuts, abrasions or mucous membranes. Studies in endemic areas indicate that mild infections commonly occur, with a low mortality. The disease may be milder in children than adults. Virus replication occurs in many organs with cell death and necrosis.

Clinical features

The incubation period can be up to 17 days. Gradual onset of fever with anorexia, lethargy and headache is usual, followed by prostration and ulcerative pharyngitis. Cervical lymphadenopathy and swelling of the neck and face may appear. Bradycardia is often present. Vomiting, diarrhoea, cough and chest pain are common features. A maculopapular rash on face, trunk and upper limbs is seen in the second week of the illness. Bleeding from gums and other mucosal sites occurs during the third week of the illness but convalescence may be protracted. Nerve deafness is a common sequel. Fatal cases usually show declining renal function and oliguria, declining conscious level and secondary bacterial infection. Laboratory investigations show leucopenia, low albumin, raised blood urea and elevated transaminases. Platelet counts are normal but function is impaired.

Diagnosis

In the endemic areas this will be based on the clinical features plus the exclusion of important treatable causes of fever. The specific laboratory diagnosis is made by finding the virus in blood, urine or throat washings, using electron microscopy or culture, or by detecting antibodies or antigen in serum.

Management

Hydration and nutrition should be maintained. Oral toilet and analgesics such as paracetamol may be helpful. Volume replacement is necessary in shocked patients. Ribavirin given intravenously or orally reduces mortality.

Diagnosed cases of Lassa fever in Europe and North America are managed in secure isolation facilities to give maximum protection to the attendant nursing and medical team, although standard barrier nursing precautions are adequate.

Marburg and Ebola virus disease

Marburg and Ebola virus diseases are African diseases caused by morphologically identical arenaviruses; they are distinguished from each other serologically. The course of Marburg virus disease is similar to that of Lassa, with sudden onset of fever, headache and general systemic upset, progressing to prostration with watery diarrhoea and dehydration. The diarrhoea may last for a week and

Table 11.16 Causes of viral haemorrhagic fever

Type of virus	Disease	Frequency and distribution
Togaviridae	Dengue haemorrhagic fever Yellow fever	Relatively common
Arenaviridae	Lassa fever Argentine haemorrhagic fever	Epidemics/endemic
Marburg-Ebola group	Marburg virus disease Ebola virus disease	Rare, focal epidemics

be associated with cramping abdominal pain. Haemorrhagic manifestations may be seen at the end of the first week of the illness with bleeding from mucosal surfaces. A maculopapular rash also occurs. Recovery occurs after 2–3 weeks in those surviving.

Management in supportive and symptomatic, with fresh blood transfusions for significant haemorrhage.

RETROVIRUSES

Acquired immunodeficiency syndrome (AIDS) and human immunodeficiency virus (HIV) infections

AIDS was first described in the USA in 1981. Homosexual men were reported as having opportunistic infections, such as *Pneumocystis carinii* pneumonia, and Kaposi's sarcoma. The spread of the condition resembled that of hepatitis B. The causal agent, called human immunodeficiency virus (HIV; previously HTLV III) was isolated in 1983.

Epidemiology

The epidemic is now traced in two ways: the number of people showing antibodies to HIV, and those with clinically defined AIDS (Fig. 11.8). Many people have opted not to be tested for HIV antibodies and the overall prevalence of HIV infection will not be known until anonymous surveys have been conducted.

In Europe and the USA most AIDS cases are found in metropolitan areas. Homosexual men and injecting drug users are at highest risk. Haemophiliacs contracted HIV infection when clotting factor concentrates made from cryoprecipitates pooled from a large number of donors contained HIV.

HIV and AIDS are now increasingly reported in heterosexual men and women and in babies. In the

Table 11.17 Causes of genital ulceration

- Genital herpes
- Trauma
- Syphilis
- Chancroid
- Lymphogranuloma venereum

Western world sexual intercourse with an injecting drug user, or a past user, is still the major risk factor for heterosexuals contracting HIV. In Africa, however, the epidemic is spread heterosexually. The high prevalence of other sexually transmitted diseases, particularly those causing genital ulceration (Table 11.17) may be a factor in the spread of HIV. In some areas of Africa up to 10% of women of childbearing age are infected.

HIV is not transmitted by saliva, although the virus has been cultured from saliva and tears as well as from blood and semen. Breast milk may rarely transmit infection. HIV is *not* transmitted by normal household contact and only very rarely by needle-stick injury.

Human immunodeficiency virus

HIV has a lipid envelope and is about 100 nm in diameter. It has a dense cylindrical nucleoid containing core protein, genomic RNA, and the reverse transcriptase enzyme which classifies HIV as a retrovirus. HIV is closely related to a group of viruses called the lentiviruses; this includes the visna virus, which is capable of causing chronic neurodegradation in sheep. There are also similarities with lymphotropic retroviruses HTLV I and II. There are many minor variations between HIVs but only two major variants, HIV 1 and 2, have been identified. HIV 2 was first found in West Africa and exists both as a single infection and as a co-infection with HIV 1. It is much less common than HIV 1 and it may be less pathogenic.

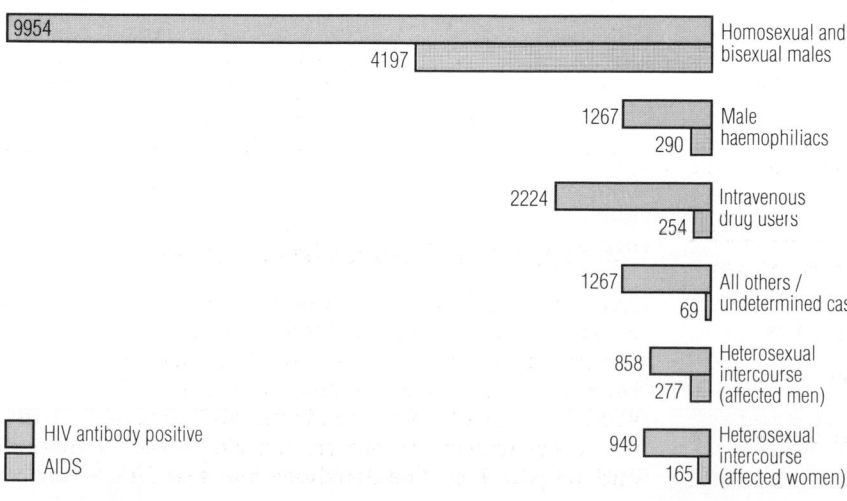

Fig. 11.8 Totals of HIV antibody positive persons and AIDS cases reported in the UK to December 1991 (Communicable Diseases Surveillance Centre, Colindale).

The main action of HIV is to cause depletion of the CD4+ helper or inducer lymphocytes. The CD4 molecule appears to be the HIV receptor. After HIV enters the cell, the genomic RNA is transcribed into DNA by the reverse transcriptase. The DNA is then integrated into the host genome. HIV replication remains at this stage till the infected cell is activated. After activation, transcription occurs, followed by protein synthesis, and the CD4+ cell dies. The virus spreads to infect other cells. As well as CD4+ lymphocytes, other cells of the immune system can be infected by HIV. The monocytes and macrophages are vulnerable. The monocytes may carry HIV to the CNS. B cell abnormalities are also seen as an effect of HIV infection. There is polyclonal activation, with high immunoglobulin levels but a poor antibody response to newly acquired antigens, leading to susceptibility to bacterial infections which are common in HIV-infected individuals.

Clinical features

HIV infection is asymptomatic and produces no abnormal physical signs in over half of affected subjects. The remainder are often described as having persistent generalised lymphadenopathy (PGL), symptomatic HIV disease (formerly called AIDS-related complex — ARC) or AIDS. Their relationship is shown diagrammatically in Figure 11.9. The time from infection to development of AIDS is from a few months to a mean of 8–10 years.

AIDS is defined as a reliably diagnosed disease that is indicative of cellular immunodeficiency, such as an opportunistic infection or Kaposi's sarcoma in a patient (aged less than 60) who has serum antibodies to HIV and no other cause of deficient CMI. This definition does not embrace the neurological manifestations or recognise the bad prognosis of symptomatic HIV infection. The following classification groups are more useful in this respect; group IV contains patients with symptomatic HIV infection.

Group I: acute seroconversion illness

Some people infected with HIV develop a febrile illness about 6 weeks after infection. With the fever they have

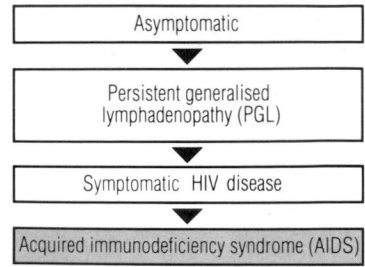

Fig. 11.9 Usual evolution of HIV infection to AIDS. Individual stages may be bypassed in some patients; for example, an asymptomatic carrier may present with AIDS without going through the intermediate stage.

oral ulcers (Plate 5, p. 247), rash, lymphadenopathy and arthralgia. After 2 weeks the majority become asymptomatic (group II) but a few have persistent generalised lymphadenopathy (group III).

Group II: asymptomatic infection

The majority of people, for at least the first 2 years after infection, are completely well. They are seropositive and can transmit infection.

Group III: persistent generalised lymphadenopathy

PGL is diagnosed when lymph nodes in extrainguinal sites remain enlarged for more than 3 months. Commonly the posterior cervical, anterior cervical, submandibular, posterior occipital and axillary nodes are involved. The nodes may swell up and cause pain intermittently. Biopsy of the nodes usually shows reactive hyperplasia. A large single node or rapidly enlarging nodes are an indication for biopsy to exclude opportunistic infection or tumour. About one-third of patients with PGL develop AIDS within 5 years.

Group IV A: constitutional disease or symptomatic HIV disease

Symptomatic HIV disease is a collection of symptoms and signs including chronic fatigue, unexplained weight loss, night sweats and recurrent fever, a variety of cutaneous manifestations including recurrent HSV infections, oral candida, chronic tinea infection, seborrhoeic dermatitis, molluscum contagiosum (p. 1131), intermittent diarrhoea, and myalgia.

Many of these infections are treatable but there is an inevitable progression to AIDS.

Group IV B: HIV-related neurological disease

Psychoneurological defects are associated with HIV infection for which HIV itself may be responsible. Peripheral neuropathy and subacute encephalitis (AIDS encephalopathy or dementia complex) occur. Clinically, subacute encephalitis is characterised by poor memory, inability to concentrate, apathy and psychomotor retardation. There may also be focal motor abnormalities and behavioural changes. For the majority of patients, before the use of zidovudine, dementia rapidly followed subacute encephalitis.

Group IV C: opportunistic infection

Table 11.18 shows part of the spectrum of opportunistic infections in patients with AIDS. The incidence of these infections varies considerably in different parts of the world. *Pneumocystis carinii* pneumonia (PCP) was the most common presentation of AIDS in the UK and

Table 11.18 Opportunistic infection in AIDS

Syndrome	Organism
Pneumonia	*Pneumocystis carinii*
	Mycobacterium tuberculosis
	Cytomegalovirus*
Stomatitis	*Candida*
	Herpes simplex
Oesophagitis	*Candida*
	Herpes simplex
	Cytomegalovirus
Enterocolitis	Cytomegalovirus
	Cryptosporidium
	Isospora belli
Proctitis	Herpes simplex
Retinitis	Cytomegalovirus
CNS disease	
Meningitis	*Cryptococcus neoformans*
Encephalitis	Cytomegalovirus
	JC virus and SV40
Mass lesion	Toxoplasma
Septicaemia	*Salmonella typhimurium*
	Mycobacterium avium intracellulare

*This is a questionable cause of pneumonia.

other Western countries until prophylaxis became routine. There is a history of slowly increasing dyspnoea and fever, sometimes accompanied by dry cough. The patient is often hypoxaemic and chest X-ray changes lag behind the clinical signs. In a developed pneumonia the radiological changes are classically a bilateral ground glass appearance.

Diagnosis is made by identifying trophozoites in bronchial lavage fluid or in sputum induced by inhalation of nebulised hypertonic saline. The organisms can be seen with a silver stain or by immunofluorescent staining using a monoclonal antibody.

Therapy consists of high-dose co-trimoxazole (20 mg trimethoprim per kg body weight per day) for 3 weeks. There is a high incidence of skin rashes during treatment and alternative treatment with trimethoprim plus dapsone is sometimes used. Addition of corticosteroids has been advocated for moderate to severe cases (p. 289).

Many other organisms can cause pneumonia in AIDS but tuberculosis caused by *M. tuberculosis* is a common initial presentation in poor countries. Whereas PCP and Kaposi's sarcoma are common in the Western world, tuberculosis and weight loss are the main features in Africa. Candida albicans infection is a common feature in both continents (Plate 6, p. 247).

Intestinal infection is common, particularly in African patients, in whom weight loss is so striking that AIDS is sometimes referred to as 'slim disease'. HIV infects gut epithelial cells and it may be this or an as yet unidentified secondary infection which causes malabsorption and weight loss. Profuse watery diarrhoea occurs with several unusual protozoal infections such as *Cryptosporidium* or *Isospora belli*.

CNS opportunistic infection presents major problems because of inaccessibility to diagnosis. *Toxoplasma* is the most common cause of a mass lesion within the brain and when CT scanning is available, the main differential diagnosis is from a cerebral lymphoma. This distinction may require a stereotactically directed brain biopsy. Meningeal infection is most often caused by the yeast *Cryptococcus neoformans*.

Retinitis is the most frequent manifestation of CMV infection in AIDS (Plate 7, p. 247); this can be bilateral, resulting in loss of sight.

Blood and bone marrow are affected by septicaemia, which is caused by conventional bacteria, particularly in children, but *Candida* or atypical mycobacteria may be responsible. *M. avium intracellulare* also infects bone marrow and causes a pancytopenia. This is usually a late complication.

Group IV D: secondary cancers

Kaposi's sarcoma (KS), the most common secondary cancer, shows initially as a purple nodule or plaque on the skin or mucous membranes (Plate 8, p. 247).

In the early stages, patients with KS alone are relatively well. Later there may be rapid spread over the skin and then to lymph nodes, gut and lung associated with constitutional symptoms. In the UK and the USA, KS is almost confined to gay men. Diagnosis is by biopsy and histological examination. The lesion consists of a mixture of spindle cells and vascular spaces which are infiltrated by plasma cells.

Therapy is unsatisfactory at present. Skin cream can be used to camouflage unsightly lesions and local radiotherapy will shrink large nodules. In the later stages, treatment with cytotoxic agents or drugs acting on the immune system like alpha interferon may be of value.

There is an increased incidence of high-grade lymphomas of either a Burkitt's or immunoblastic B cell type. CNS spread is frequent. Treatment is outlined in Chapter 24 but is complicated by the profound immune suppression.

Group IV E: other conditions

This heterogenous subgroup contains other symptomatic conditions which have not been classified elsewhere. *Lymphoid interstitial pneumonitis* is a descriptive term for a common pneumonia of unknown aetiology in children with AIDS. It has a variable course, sometimes responding to corticosteroid therapy. Oral leucoplekia is a common feature of AIDS (Plate 9, p. 247).

11 Infectious, Tropical and Parasitic Diseases

Thrombocytopenia may occur during an asymptomatic or a symptomatic phase of infection. When it is early it often remits without having any apparent influence on the subsequent prognosis.

Other patients are included in this group when they have infections, tumours or other conditions which do not fit into one of the other subgroups. An example would be an HIV positive drug addict with frequent bacterial (i.e. not opportunistic) chest infection.

Diagnosis

The diagnosis of AIDS rests on the demonstration of infections or tumours associated with immunodeficiency.

The presence of HIV is usually determined by demonstration of antibody to the HIV envelope or core proteins. HIV antigen can be measured in serum.

Identification of a patient as having HIV-related disease usually requires the demonstration of HIV antibody or antigen. Clinical examination and follow-up for symptoms or signs of symptomatic HIV disease or AIDS is necessary.

The level of CD4+ cells in the blood correlates with the risk of infection and is a guide to the institution of co-trimoxazole prophylaxis of PCP.

Paediatric HIV infection

About 15% of babies born to HIV positive mothers are infected; the baby is usually infected in utero but can also be infected from contact with the mother's blood at birth. HIV antibody passively acquired from the mother can be demonstrated in the baby's blood for several months after birth. The presence of HIV antigen confirms active infection but its absence does not exclude infection. If the antigen is present the baby is likely to show signs of HIV infection within the first year of life. Signs of HIV infection in a baby include failure to thrive, loss of weight, psychomotor retardation, interstitial pneumonitis, skin rashes and many of the infections seen in adult AIDS.

Management

There is no curative therapy for AIDS or HIV infection. Patients are advised to have all associated infections, such as candida, treated promptly. Zidovudine, an antiviral drug effective against HIV, is a thymidine analogue inhibiting reverse transcriptase, which terminates the viral DNA-chain elongation. It increases life expectancy and reduces the incidence of opportunistic infections, particularly PCP in patients with AIDS or symptomatic HIV disease. The main side-effects of zidovudine are megaloblastic anaemia unrelated to vitamin B_{12} or folate deficiency and neutropenia. Regular full blood counts are necessary.

Counselling

Severe distress is experienced by patients with HIV infection. Trained counsellors have an important role at all stages of the disease. Counselling prior to antibody testing is important so that people are aware of what they are being tested for and to discuss the health education aspects of HIV disease. Counsellors can also help people who are HIV positive or have AIDS to cope with the many problems caused by having a fatal infection.

HTLV infection

See page 1096.

RHABDOVIRUSES

Rabies

Rabies is an acute encephalomyelitic illness, caused by an RNA-containing rhabdovirus. It is characterised by paroxysms of muscle spasm, particularly of muscle groups associated with inspiration and swallowing, in response to attempts to drink water as well as at the sight, sound or mention of water. It is almost invariably fatal.

Aetiology

The rabies virus is an RNA rhabdovirus which, with five related viruses, comprise the *Lyssavirus* genus. It is pathogenic for all mammals. The virus can be grown in cell culture.

Distribution and incidence

Antarctica and Australasia are the only continents free of rabies. It is endemic in the rest of the world, with the exception of the UK, the Scandinavian countries, Japan and Taiwan. The incidence of human rabies is difficult to estimate. Occasional cases occur in Europe and North

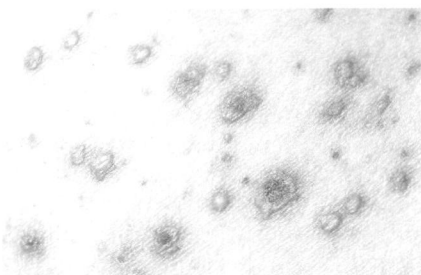

1. Vesicles and pustules in a patient with chickenpox.

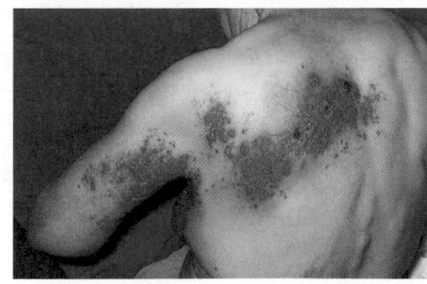

2. Dermatomal distribution of varicella zoster lesions.

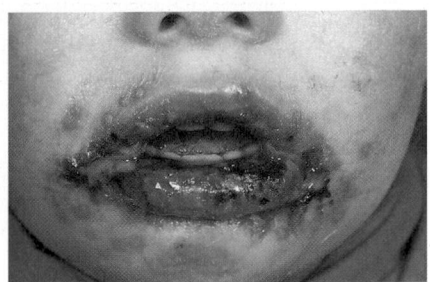

3. Gingivo-stomatitis caused by primary herpes simplex I.

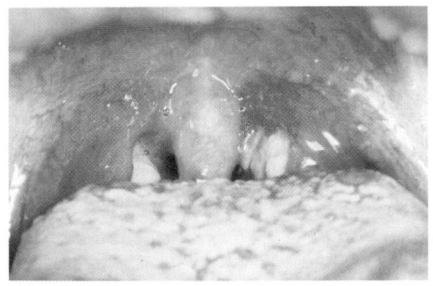

4. Acute tonsillo-pharyngitis caused by primary Epstein-Barr virus infection.

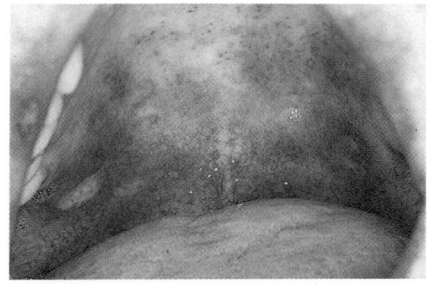

5. Acute oral ulceration during HIV seroconversion.

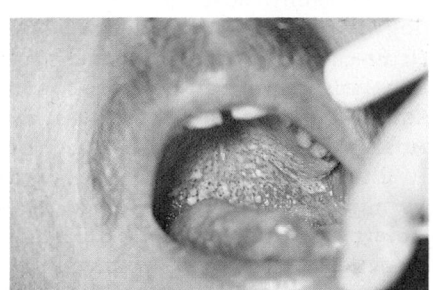

6. Candida albicans in a patient with AIDS.

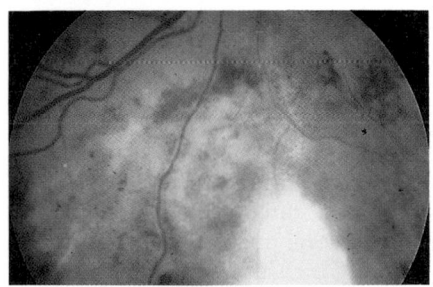

7. Cytomegalovirus retinitis in a patient with AIDS.

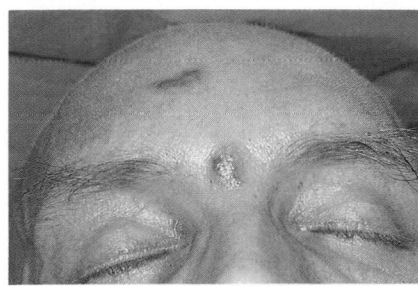

8. Kaposi's sarcoma in a patient with AIDS.

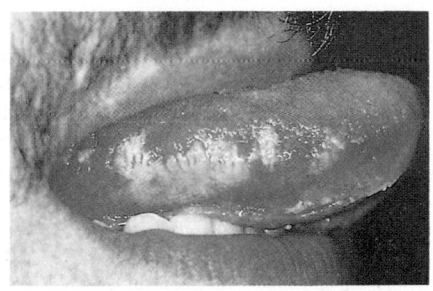

9. Leucoplakia in a patient with AIDS.

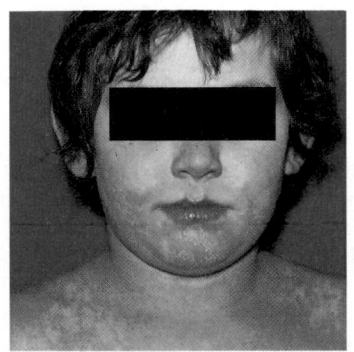

10. Scarlet fever rash.

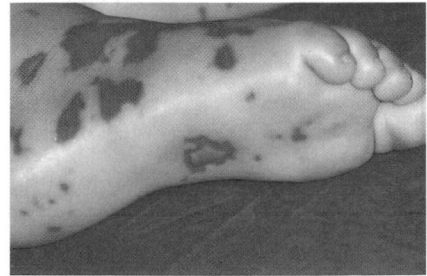

11. Necrotic haemorrhagic lesions in meningococcal septicaemia.

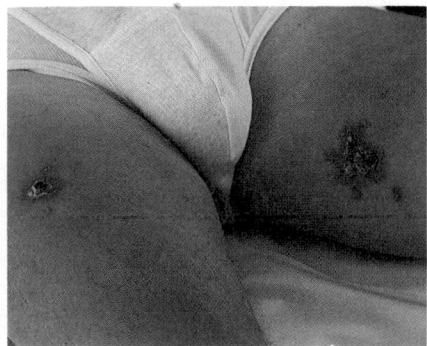

12. Cutaneous Leishmaniasis.

America. It is a considerable health problem in Asia, Africa and Central and South America.

Transmission and epidemiology

Rabies virus is inoculated in saliva by the bite of a rabid animal; this is most often a dog, less often a cat (Fig. 11.10). Licking of abraded or cut skin can transmit infection. Virus can penetrate the mucous membranes of mouth and eye. Endemic canine rabies is the major determinant of risk for human infection.

All mammals can become infected but transmission to man is mainly caused by biting animals, most often stray dogs in the tropics. Wolves, jackals, mongooses, bats (fruit-eating, insectivorous and vampire), monkeys and ungulates (sheep, cattle and deer) can all become infected and to a greater or lesser extent transmit the infection. Apart from bats, all infected species die from the disease. In Europe the red fox is the reservoir of infection. Vampire bats infect cattle in the countries of South America, causing considerable economic losses through cattle rabies. These bats painlessly incise veins around the lower legs of cattle and lap the blood. Human rabies has been acquired from vampire bats.

Pathology

Virus first penetrates skeletal muscle cells. It then enters nerves through the fibres supplying muscle spindles and travels centripetally to infect nerve cells. Virus replication occurs and cell rupture releases new virions to infect other neurones. The neuropathological changes are not gross. Collections of inflammatory cells around small vessels, dead neurones and phagocytosis of degenerating neurones are seen, especially in the medulla and midbrain. Viraemia is not thought to contribute to dissemination of virus. There is centrifugal spread of virus via autonomic nerve fibres to cornea, skin and salivary glands.

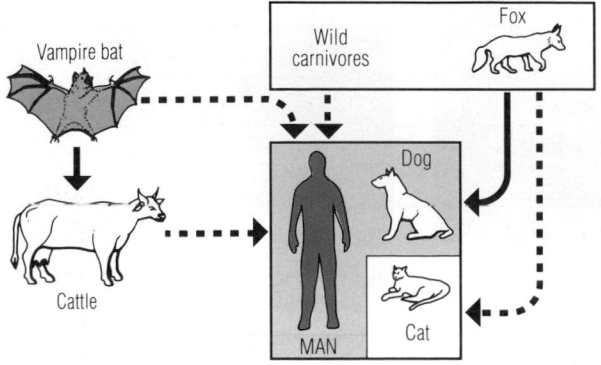

Fig. 11.10 Cycle of transmission of rabies. The commonest routes of spread are shown in solid lines. Man is usually infected by dog bites.

Clinical features

The incubation period is 20–60 days on average, with a range of up to 1 year.

Initial symptoms are headache, fever, anorexia, insomnia and paraesthesia or altered sensation at the site of biting or some peripheral site. After 2–3 days the patient may become markedly agitated, hyperexcitable, anxious, confused and lucid in turn. The earliest hint of fear of water may be evident at this stage; this rapidly progresses to typical hydrophobia, with involuntary contraction of main and accessory inspiratory muscles in a sustained spasm, brought on by attempts to drink water or the sight, sound or mention of water. Variations in mood persist. Saliva may continuously be spat out as it cannot be swallowed. The spasms may be provoked by fanning air across the face. Cranial nerve palsies, paralysis and bizarre patterns of breathing follow. Ascending paralysis without hydrophobia occurs in a few patients and this may pose problems in diagnosis. Death occurs within 7–14 days, due to respiratory failure or cardiac arrhythmias.

Differential diagnosis

Tetanus, other causes of ascending paralysis and encephalitis, and rabies hysteria form the main differential diagnosis.

Laboratory features

Virus particles may be grown from saliva, nasal washings, CSF or urine. Viral antigen can be identified in skin biopsies, or less easily, in corneal impression smears using direct fluorescent antibody techniques. Rising titres of antibody to rabies virus in blood or CSF also confirm the diagnosis.

Prevention, control and management

Correct management at the time of biting prevents rabies. First aid treatment consists of thorough washing of the wound with soap and water for 5 minutes, followed by washing with clean water. This is followed by application of 40–70% alcohol, povidone iodine or 0.01% aqueous iodine. Extensive areas of necrotic tissue should be excised. An occlusive dressing should not be applied and the wound should not be sutured, as this may inoculate virus into skeletal muscle. Delayed suture may be appropriate. Tetanus prophylaxis should be started. Antibiotics are given as needed.

The need for rabies vaccination must be considered. Following licks on abraded skin or minor scratching or nibbling of skin without bleeding, vaccination should be started but discontinued if the cat or dog involved remains healthy through 10 days' observation or if the animal is killed and its brain is free of rabies virus on reliable testing. Vaccination is continued if the animal becomes rabid or if the animal is not available for observation or examination. Following single or multiple bites or scratches that penetrate the skin or contact between animal saliva and mucosal surfaces, anti-rabies immunoglobulin and rabies vaccine should be given immediately. If the animal is a dog or cat and it remains healthy through 10 days' observation, vaccination can be stopped. If the animal is killed and virus is not found on reliable testing, vaccination can be stopped. In all other circumstances vaccination should be continued.

Reactions to horse and mule antirabies serum are common and so a test dose should be given first. The vaccine is killed virus grown in human diploid cells.

The problem of controlling reservoirs of infection remains. The capturing and killing of stray dogs in endemic areas has reduced an important source of human rabies. Vaccination of household dogs and cats is a helpful measure but does not exclude the possibility of the animal contracting rabies. The spread of rabies in Europe has been uncontrolled so far.

NON-ENVELOPED SINGLE-STRANDED RNA VIRUSES

PICORNAVIRUSES

Rhinovirus infection

Rhinoviruses are the most common cause of colds (p. 463). There are over 90 serotypes and reinfection with the same serotype can occur. Infection is usually confined to the nasal mucosa, but complications such as sinusitis and otitis media can occur as a result of mucosal swelling and obstruction to drainage of secretions. Rhinoviruses can also cause exacerbations of chronic bronchitis but the mechanism for this is not clear.

Enterovirus infection

Coxsackie A, Coxsackie B and *Echoviruses*, of which there are 24, 6 and 34 types respectively, cause a wide variety of clinical infections, but overall most are asymptomatic. A febrile illness with upper respiratory symptoms is another common manifestation of infection with many different serotypes. More specific disease associations are shown in Table 11.19. *Polioviruses* types 1, 2 and 3 cause poliomyelitis, which is described on page 969.

Acute meningitis

Enteroviruses are a common cause of lymphocytic meningitis (more than 70% of cases), which is a benign disease. Enteroviral meningitis is common in young children and rare over the age of 40. The clinical features are described on page 968.

Other neurological disease

Encephalitis is a rare manifestation of enteroviral infection which may occur with or without meningitis. Flaccid motor paralysis is only seen with any frequency in poliomyelitis.

Fever and exanthem

A variety of skin rashes occur. Maculopapular eruptions associated with fever are more common with Echo than Coxsackie viruses. Petechial or purpuric eruptions are uncommon.

The most distinctive exanthem is the vesicular eruption of hand, foot and mouth disease caused by Coxsackie

Table 11.19 Enterovirus types and their disease associations

Disease	Virus types most commonly associated		
	Coxsackie A types	Coxsackie B types	Echo types
Acute meningitis	Most	All	Most
Encephalitis	One-fifth	Most	One-third
Herpangina (pharyngitis)	2–6, 8, 10, 22	None	None
Hand, foot and mouth disease	5, 7, 9, 10, 16	None	None
Pleurodynia (Bornholm disease)	None	1–5	None
Pericarditis/myocarditis	None	1–5	None
Chronic meningo-encephalitis in hypogammaglobulinaemics	None	None	One-third

virus A16 (and occasionally others). Lesions are found in the mouth consistently and on the palms, soles and extensor surfaces of the hands and feet. Vesicles are sometimes surrounded by a ring of erythema and lesions may be slightly tender. The child feels unwell for 1 or 2 days and has a fever but recovers completely. Virus can be isolated from vesicles, throat washings or stools.

Respiratory tract infection

Most enteroviruses can cause non-specific upper respiratory infection but group A Coxsackie viruses are the common cause of herpangina, an acute painful vesicular eruption on the fauces and soft palate, associated with fever, malaise and myalgia and lasting up to 10 days.

Pleurodynia

Pleurodynia (sometimes known as Bornholm disease) is an acute febrile illness characterised by 'pleuritic' chest pain; it is usually caused by group B Coxsackie viruses. The pain is due to infection of muscle and there is no pleural inflammation. About half of patients have pain in an area of the thorax but upper abdominal pain occurs in others, especially children, and this may mimic an abdominal emergency. Tenderness over involved muscles is the characteristic sign.

The illness is usually over in 5 days but it may last up to 3 weeks and it sometimes recurs.

Myopericarditis

Enteroviruses, mainly group B Coxsackie, are an important cause of acute myocarditis and pericarditis in young adults. Usually the two conditions occur simultaneously but one predominates in the clinical presentation. The clinical features are described on page 409.

Epidemic haemorrhagic conjunctivitis

This epidemic form of acute conjunctivitis, which is associated with pain, subconjunctival bleeding and oedema of the eyelids, lasts about 1 week and is usually caused by enterovirus 70. The virus is highly infectious and is spread by contact and fomites rather than by droplet.

NON-ENVELOPED DOUBLE-STRANDED RNA VIRUSES

REOVIRUSES

Rotavirus diarrhoea

Rotavirus diarrhoea is an acute dehydrating diarrhoeal disease caused by a 70 nm RNA-containing virus. This organism is the commonest cause of diarrhoea in children up to 2 years old in the tropics. It is spread by the faecal–oral route and possibly by droplet transmission. The infection occurs in both endemic and epidemic forms worldwide.

Clinical features

After an incubation period of up to 5 days (most often 2 days) anorexia, vomiting, diarrhoea and fever begin suddenly. There may also be a blocked nose and sore throat. The stools are watery and non-dysenteric. The illness is self-limiting, terminating in about 5 days in most cases. Moderate dehydration is the usual consequence of the illness but a number of fatalities from severe dehydration have occurred. The organism may be found in faeces by immune electron microscopy and viral antigen detection using an enzyme-linked immunosorbent assay.

Management

Management comprises assessment of the degree of dehydration (Table 11.13, p. 225) and replacement of that volume of fluid in the first 4–6 hours after presentation. Continuing fluid losses must also be replaced until diarrhoea ceases.

Oral rehydration solution (ORS) can be used for rehydration. The standard WHO/UNICEF formulation comprises glucose 20 g (or sucrose 40 g), sodium chloride 3.5 g, sodium bicarbonate 2.5 g (or sodium citrate 2.9 g) and potassium chloride 1.5 g made up to a volume of 1 litre with clean water. Additional water, not ORS, must be allowed for insensible losses and obligatory urinary losses. When there is shock, intravenous rehydration is necessary. As soon as the child wishes to start eating again, they should be allowed to do so.

CHLAMYDIAL, MYCOPLASMA AND RICKETTSIAL INFECTIONS

CHLAMYDIA

Chlamydia are bacteria which contain both DNA and RNA (unlike viruses) but are unable to replicate extracellularly (Table 11.20). They are Gram-negative and have a lipopolysaccharide endotoxin.

Chlamydia psittaci, a common pathogen of birds and animals, can infect man, causing psittacosis (ornithosis). *Chl. trachomatis* is transmitted between humans by sexual contact or from a mother's infected genital tract to her newborn infant, causing conjunctivitis or occasionally pneumonia. Different serotypes of *Chl. trachomatis* cause lymphogranuloma venereum (LGV) and trachoma.

Psittacosis

Although ornithosis is a commonly used name for infection with this organism, this is a misnomer because a wide range of animals other than birds are infected by *Ch. psittaci*.

Epidemiology

Psittacosis is worldwide and occurs sporadically, but it is most frequent in people closely associated with birds. Infected birds are usually ill but continue to shed organisms in excreta and feathers for months after recovery. Humans are infected by inhalation.

Clinical features

After an incubation period of about 2 weeks there is fever, malaise, headaches, myalgia and sometimes arthralgia. Dry cough and variable dyspnoea occur with confusion and clouding of consciousness if severe hypoxia develops. There are few abnormal signs in the chest, although there may be fine crackles in the lower zones. The chest radiograph shows unilateral or bilateral patchy infiltrates, especially in the lower zones, but occasionally there is the appearance of lobar consolidation. Gastrointestinal symptoms occur uncommonly. Rarely the disease is complicated by aortic or mitral valve endocarditis. Abortion in pregnant women may occur.

Diagnosis and management

Diagnosis is suspected from the history and evidence for atypical pneumonia, and confirmed by testing for serum antibodies by immunofluorescent or complement fixation tests. Tetracyclines given for at least 10 days are the most effective treatment.

Non-specific genital infection (NSGI)

Urethritis, cervicitis and proctitis are most commonly caused by organisms that are not identifiable by routine staining of the exudate. Among the relevant organisms are *Chlamydia*, mycoplasmas and *Ureaplasma*. Chlamydial infection appears to account for more than 50% of NSGI in the UK.

Chl. trachomatis is an obligatory intracellular parasite whose replication results in the death of the infected cell. During its life cycle the infectious particle changes to an actively dividing form, which later reorganises into the infectious form which is released on cell lysis.

Clinical features

Men usually have a urethral discharge and dysuria about 10 days after exposure to infection. In women the infection is usually silent. If uncomplicated rectal infection occurs there may be anal discharge, perianal dampness, irritation and tenesmus.

Complications are more common in women than in men. In women they include bartholinitis, salpingitis and perihepatitis; in men epididymoorchitis, prostatitis and sexually acquired reactive arthropathy (Reiter's syndrome, p. 1008).

Table 11.20 Chlamydial infections

Type	Transmission	Disease	Clinical features
Chlamydia psittaci	Zoonosis	Psittacosis	Pneumonia
Chlamydia trachomatis			
Types A, B, C	Fingers, flies, fomites	Trachoma	Keratoconjunctivitis
Types D–K	Sexual	Non-gonoccal urethritis, salpingitis	Urethritis, pelvic inflammatory disease, Reiter's syndrome, perihepatitis (rare)
	Mother-to-infant		Conjunctivitis, pneumonia (rare)
Types L$_1$, L$_2$, L$_3$	Sexual	Lymphogranuloma venereum	Suppurative inguinal lymphadenitis

11 Infectious, Tropical and Parasitic Diseases

Diagnosis

In men a Gram-stained urethral smear shows excess of polymorphonuclear leucocytes but no gonococci. In men and women chlamydial infection is diagnosed by identifying antigen at the site of infection or serum antibody.

Management

Most NSGI responds to tetracycline therapy. The usual therapy is oxytetracycline (250 mg four times daily) or doxycycline (100 mg daily) for at least 10 days. Erythromycin (500 mg twice daily) may be used as an alternative and is the first choice in pregnancy and tetracycline allergy.

Relapse or recurrent infection is common in both sexes. There may be symptoms of a postinfective urethritis with no signs of infection. Sexual partners of both sexes should always be examined and treated.

Congenital Chlamydia trachomatis infection

Chl. trachomatis infection is now frequently seen as a cause of ophthalmia neonatorum. The infected baby develops a conjunctivitis about 10 days after birth. Investigation should include culture of pus or monoclonal antibody test for *Chl. trachomatis*. The organism may be a cause of pneumonia in the neonate.

Treatment is with erythromycin syrup. The baby's parents should always be examined for *Chlamydia* and other genital infections.

Trachoma

Trachoma is a chronic infection of the conjunctiva of the globe and eyelids caused by *Chl. trachomatis* serotypes A, B, Ba and C. It is widespread throughout the tropics and subtropics, and is primarily a disease related to poor personal and public hygiene. It is one of the commonest causes of blindness in the world, with 500 million affected, 2 million blind and 100 million with severe visual impairment.

Transmission and epidemiology

The organisms present in ocular secretions infect other people by direct contagion on contaminated fingers or clothes. Absence of water for washing means that infected secretions are wiped on to hands and clothes. Flies may also carry the organisms from one person to another. Infection occurs early in life and subsequently there are episodes of reinfection and secondary bacterial infection.

Pathology and pathogenesis

Acute inflammation is present in the conjunctiva. This progresses to a chronic state, with lymphoid aggregates around infected conjunctival cells. It is likely that damage due to trachoma is exacerbated by repeated bacterial infections. The tarsal plates fold inwards due to fibrosis (entropion) and the cornea is continually damaged by the inverted eyelashes, resulting in corneal opacity from scarring.

Clinical features

The earlier features are hypertrophic follicles on the upper tarsal conjunctiva and at the corneo-scleral junction superiorly. With time and repeated reinfection, this inflammatory response leads to fibrosis. The scarring disorganises the arrangement of Meibomian glands, and their orifices are pulled away from the lid margin. The eyelid is inverted and sites of eyelash trauma on the cornea are seen. New vessels grow into the cornea (pannus formation) and corneal scarring follows.

Diagnosis

Diagnosis is made on the appearances described above. Giemsa staining of scrapings from the affected conjunctiva shows intracytoplasmic inclusion bodies. Antigen can be detected by enzyme-linked immunoassay.

Management and prevention

Tetracycline (2.0 g per day in divided doses) is given for 3 weeks to all patients apart from pregnant women and children under 8 years. Erythromycin is an effective alternative (250 mg or 4 mg/kg four times daily for 3 weeks). Topical 1% tetracycline eye ointment, applied two to four times daily for 3 weeks and repeated at 1-month intervals up to six times, is effective.

Continued trauma to the cornea must be prevented. Removal of offending eyelashes helps. Surgical reconstruction of the eyelid may be needed.

Education concerning the importance of washing with soap and water is an important measure in preventing transmission. This depends on the availability of an adequate water supply sufficient for all domestic needs. The use of antibiotics in infected persons reduces the inflammation in their eyes and prevents progression of the disease, while eradicating sources of infection for others.

Lymphogranuloma venereum

Lymphogranuloma venereum (LGV) is caused by L_1, L_2, or L_3 serotypes of *Chl. trachomatis*. It is most prevalent in parts of Africa, Asia and South America.

Clinical features

The most common primary lesion of LGV is a shallow ulcer appearing on the genitals of men or women 3–10 days after exposure to infection. In men there may be an associated lymphangitis of the dorsal penis. More commonly in men there may be an inflammation and swelling of the inguinal lymph nodes 10 days to 6 months after infection. The inguinal bubo is unilateral in about 60% of cases and may enlarge, causing pain, and rupture. About 20% also have involvement of femoral lymph nodes. This creates a groove over the inguinal ligament, the characteristic 'groove sign'.

LGV may also cause a rectal infection. After initial inflammation of the rectal mucosa a chronic inflammatory process may follow; this invades the bowel wall, with non-caseous granulomas and crypt abscesses forming. A partial or complete stricture of the rectum may develop.

Diagnosis and management

Diagnosis is based on a positive complement-fixation or micro-immunofluorescent (micro-IF) test. Doxycycline (100 mg daily for 2–4 weeks) is the therapy of choice.

MYCOPLASMAS

Mycoplasmas are the smallest organisms able to grow in cell-free media, wherein they differ from viruses. They differ from bacteria in lacking a cell wall. *Mycoplasma pneumoniae* is an important cause of atypical pneumonia and a number of other clinical syndromes described in Chapter 13. *M. hominis* and *Ureaplasma urealyticum* can cause non-gonococcal urethritis, prostatitis, pelvic inflammatory disease and postpartum fever. They are sensitive to tetracycline, the treatment of choice (p. 251).

RICKETTSIA

Rickettsial infections comprise a group of acute infectious diseases caused by small bacteria. They include the typhus group of infections, the spotted fever group of infections, scrub typhus, Q fever (*Coxiella burnetii*) and trench fever (*Rochalimaea quintana*). These organisms produce diseases with a range of severity from mild to severe and life-threatening.

Apart from *Rochalimaea* all are obligate intracellular parasites and can only be grown in cells in vitro. *Rochalimaea quintana* grows in cell-free cultures. They are Gram-negative organisms and, like Gram-negative

bacteria, produce endotoxin which may contribute to the pathogenesis.

Q fever

Q fever is an acute illness caused by *Coxiella burnetii*; it is transmitted between animals by ticks and to humans from domestic animals by close contact, particularly with aborted placentas or with infected carcasses in abattoirs or, more often, by inhalation of the endospores.

The main clinical features of acute infection are high fever with severe headache and myalgia, after an incubation period of about 20 days. Hepatosplenomegaly is common, with biochemical evidence of hepatitis. Pneumonia is less common but may be severe and bilateral. Q fever may present as PUO (p. 223).

The natural history of the disease is to resolve spontaneously within 2 weeks in most patients, but a slower recovery with progression to chronic disease may occur. The main feature of chronic Q fever is endocarditis, which is usually fatal if left untreated (p. 413).

Diagnosis

Diagnosis is usually made by serology, since laboratory handling of the organisms is dangerous. Tetracycline is the treatment of choice but it is not known whether it prevents progression. Endocarditis is very difficult to eradicate and surgery is often required.

Typhus

Distribution and incidence

Typhus group

Louse-borne typhus (*Rickettsia prowazekii*) occurs in louse-infested populations. These are usually relatively poor people living at high altitude, who wear as much clothing as they can to keep warm, and do not change or wash their clothing. Mountainous areas of South America, the Himalayas and highland regions of Ethiopia are endemic areas. Louse-borne typhus is less common than it used to be. Murine typhus (*R. mooseri*) is widely distributed where rat and man live close together.

Spotted fever group

Rocky Mountain spotted fever (*R. rickettsii*) occurs most often in the hills and mountains of the eastern seaboard of the USA. South American countries are also affected.

African tick typhus affects the countries of North Africa, and eastern, central and southern Africa. The incidence is unknown. African tick typhus is the commonest imported rickettsial infection in the UK. Rickettsial pox infections occur in Asia, Asian regions of the CIS (former USSR) and Korea.

Scrub typhus

Scrub typhus (*R. tsutsugamushi*) occurs throughout Asia and is probably one of the commonest causes of fever there. Studies in Malaysia showed that it accounted for 23% of patients with febrile illnesses presenting at rural hospitals.

Trench fever

Trench fever is not common now. It is thought to have a focal distribution in Africa and Central America.

Transmission and epidemiology

Typhus group

Louse-borne typhus is transmitted by *Pediculus humanus*. The louse defecates after taking a blood meal, and *R. prowazekii* in the faeces of an infected louse is scratched into the bite site or abrasions in the skin. Man is the reservoir for *R. prowazekii* and infection passes from one person to another.

Epidemic disease occurs when infection is introduced into a large group of people not previously exposed. Refugee camps present an ideal situation for such epidemics.

Spotted fever group

These are transmitted by the bite of infected ticks which are also the reservoir of infection. Occupational and leisure exposure, such as walking, camping, farming, lumber work and hunting, take man into tick-infested areas in North America. Tourism, tending animals and gathering wood take people into similar areas in Africa.

Scrub typhus

Scrub typhus is a zoonosis transmitted by chiggers – larvae of leptotrombiculid mites. Occupational exposure in rural areas (farming, animal tending, rubber plantation work, etc.) is the usual means of infection.

Trench fever

Trench fever is transmitted by rubbing infective louse faeces into the bite or a skin abrasion. Man is the reservoir and conditions which favour human lousiness will favour the occurrence of trench fever. In World War I, it occurred among men during trench warfare.

Pathology and pathogenesis

These organisms replicate within vascular endothelial cells of small vessels in many tissues. The vasculitic responses and blood vessel damage underlie the pathogenesis. *R. rickettsii* infection is more invasive than the other organisms, and causes more severe illness due to full-thickness vessel wall damage.

The effect of blood vessel damage is a rash that may become purpuric and haemorrhagic, even ecchymotic in louse-borne typhus and *R. rickettsii* infection. Leakage of protein-rich fluid from the vascular compartment into the interstitium causes hypovolaemia, hypotension and reduced tissue perfusion. Thrombotic lesions occur in a variety of organs, including the brain. Renal and liver damage from vasculitis occur in severe cases.

Clinical features

Typhus group

The incubation period is usually about 12 days with a range of 10–14 days. Headache and mild fever are usual initial symptoms, followed after 48 hours by a sharp rise in temperature to 40°C, which is sustained. Conjunctival suffusion is seen. Meningism and photophobia also occur. The rash occurs at about the sixth day and begins as red macular lesions on the axillary folds and trunk, spreading on to the limbs, with palms, soles and face affected in the most severe cases. The rash may evolve through purpuric stages to form ecchymoses. Initial bradycardia progresses to tachycardia in hypotensive patients. Haemorrhagic manifestations and hypotension lead to renal involvement, with rising blood urea and falling urine output. Mild cases get better in the second week of the disease but untreated severe cases may go into the third week before recovery begins. Death from shock, cerebral involvement or renal failure occurs in the second or third week.

Brill-Zinsser disease is a mild form of louse-borne typhus due to recrudescence of latent infection. Recovery is the rule.

Spotted fever group

The incubation period is about 7 days for Rocky Mountain spotted fever (RMSF) and African tick typhus, and rather longer – around 13 days – in rickettsial pox. Fever and headache with generalised limb pains are usual early in the course. The clinical features are similar to typhus. There is early deterioration in those with severe RMSF. Death may occur between 3 and 6 days of onset.

African tick typhus is generally mild and self-limiting. Fever, systemic upset and headache are the usual presenting features. Rash may occur, causing macular lesions which have a widespread distribution on trunk and limbs. Palms and soles may be affected. A black, ulcerated eschar is usually found marking the site of the tick bite.

Scrub typhus

The incubation period is about 10 days (range 6–18). Fever, headache, chills and general body pains are usual symptoms. Conjunctival suffusion, macular skin rash, pneumonitis and hepatosplenomegaly may occur.

Trench fever

The incubation period may be as long as 22 days or as short as 4 days. Fever, headache and chills are usual symptoms, appearing and usually settling over about 5 days. Relapses may occur.

Diagnosis

The clinical features usually lead to suspicion of a rickettsial infection. This can be confirmed by serological tests using group-specific rickettsial antigens. The main differential diagnosis in RMSF is meningococcal septicaemia, which also requires urgent treatment.

Laboratory features

Severely affected patients with all forms of rickettsial disease will show generalised derangement of coagulation and evidence of liver and renal dysfunction. Platelet counts are low, in association with prolongation of the prothrombin time, reduced fibrinogen levels and elevated levels of fibrin degradation products. Anaemia is usual.

Plasma albumin levels fall. Declining urine output indicates renal failure.

Management

Tetracycline (500 mg 6-hourly for 7 days) is very effective (30 mg/kg/day) for typhus and scrub typhus. Pregnant women and children under 8 years should receive chloramphenicol (50 mg/kg/day in divided doses for 7 days; 25 mg/kg/day in divided doses for infants under 1 month). Doxycycline, 100 mg (single dose) for adults or 50 mg for children, is the ideal treatment for louse-borne typhus. Tetracycline or chloramphenicol are effective for spotted fever. In vitro sensitivities suggest a good response to tetracyclines in trench fever but there is little clinical experience.

Supportive measures

Prompt administration of antibiotics is essential. Management comprises restoring blood volume with infusions of plasma and fluids, and restoring coagulation mechanisms by fresh blood transfusions or fresh frozen plasma.

Prevention and control

Delousing is the main way to control louse-borne typhus. Thorough and regular washing of clothes in hot water with detergent kills lice and their eggs. DDT 10% or malathion 1% can be applied to clothed people with good effect. Appropriate clothing should be worn to prevent ticks getting to the skin. In tick-infested areas the skin should be carefully inspected at the end of the day. Any that are found should be removed by gentle pulling to keep the tick intact.

BACTERIAL INFECTIONS

A classification of bacteria is given in Table 11.21.

GRAM-POSITIVE COCCI

STREPTOCOCCI

β-haemolytic streptococci are classified by the Lancefield grouping system which detects polysaccharide antigens on their surface by a panel of antisera. Table 11.22 shows these and other streptococci which are α-haemolytic or non-haemolytic. Not all group D streptococci are β-haemolytic. Cutaneous streptococcal infections are described in Chapter 25.

Scarlet fever

Scarlet fever is a febrile illness with a characteristic rash caused by infection with an erythrogenic toxin-producing strain of *Strep. pyogenes*. Infection is usually in the throat, but the skin or genital tract may be the primary site.

It is now a much milder disease than it was 50 years ago. The severity of disease is probably determined by variations in the micro-organism but host factors also play a part. The same bacterium may be a harmless passenger in one subject, or produce a sore throat or scarlet fever in another. Host antibodies are largely responsible for these differences. Antibodies to the erythrogenic toxin prevent the rash of scarlet fever but not tonsillitis.

Table 11.21 Classification of bacteria

Gram-positive cocci	Gram-positive bacilli
Streptococci	Bacilli
Strep. pneumoniae	*B. anthracis*
Strep. pyogenes	*B. cereus*
Strep. viridans group	*Corynebacterium diphtheriae*
Anaerobic	*Listeria monocytogenes*
Staphylococci	Clostridia (anaerobic)
Staph. aureus	*Cl. tetani*
Staph. epidermidis	*Cl. botulinum*
	Cl. perfringens
	Cl. difficile
	Cl. septicum

Gram-negative cocci	Gram-negative bacilli
Neisseria	Enterobacteria
N. meningitidis	*Escherichia coli*
(meningococcus)	*Klebsiella*
N. gonorrhoeae	*Proteus*
(gonococcus)	*Salmonella*
	Shigella
	Parvobacteria
	Haemophilus
	Bordetella
	Brucella
	Yersinia
	Pseudomonas
	P. aeruginosa
	P. pseudomallei
	Francisella tularensis
	Bartonella bacilliformis
	Cat-scratch bacillus
	Vibrios
	V. cholerae
	Campylobacter jejuni
	Anaerobic bacteria
	Bacteroides
	Fusobacteria

Mycobacteria

Spirochaetes
Treponema
T. pallidum
T. pertenue
T. carateum
Borrelia
Leptospira icterohaemorrhagiae

Table 11.22 Streptococci

Group and name	Characteristics	Disease/syndromes
Group A *S. pyogenes*	β-haemolytic Secrete enzymes, e.g. hyaluronidase, and toxins, e.g. erythrogenic	Pharyngitis Scarlet fever Otitis media Sinusitis Erysipelas/impetigo Lymphangitis Puerperal sepsis
Group B *S. agalactiae*	β-haemolytic Common vaginal commensal	Neonatal infection (puerperal sepsis)
Group D Enterococci, e.g. *S. faecalis*	β- or non-haemolytic Anaerobic Normal bowel flora Antibiotic resistance	Urinary tract infection Septicaemia Endocarditis
S. pneumoniae (pneumococcus)	α-haemolytic Common throat commensal More than 80 serotypes	Pneumonia Acute meningitis Otitis media/ mastoiditis
S. viridans group, e.g. *S. milleri, mitior, mutans, salivarius, sanguis*	α- or non-haemolytic Dental commensals	Endocarditis Cerebral abscess and empyema (*S. milleri*)

The rash (Plate 10, p. 247) appears within 2 days on the face. It is a diffuse erythema often with perioral pallor (not specific for this condition). On the trunk it is a punctate erythema which is less brightly coloured. Superficial peeling of the skin starts on about the fourth day. The illness resolves within a week, although the patient may continue to feel unwell for several more days.

Complications

Complications are now rare. Septic complications include otitis media. Late complications are rheumatic fever (p. 419) or acute glomerulonephritis (p. 818), which may develop 2–3 weeks after the infection.

Diagnosis and management

Strep. pyogenes can be cultured readily from a throat swab, and the presence of neutrophilia helps to distinguish from infectious mononucleosis, which can cause an identical appearance. Retrospective diagnosis can be made by measuring antistreptolysin O antibodies. Treatment with oral penicillin is commonly used, but may not eliminate streptococci unless given in high dose for 10 days. Eradicating the organism is less important since complications have become so uncommon.

Clinical features

Infection is spread by droplets. After an incubation period of 2–4 days there is abrupt onset of sore throat, pain on swallowing and fever. There is tender cervical lymphadenopathy. The tonsils are enlarged, congested and often covered with exudate. The tongue is coated and initially red papillae are visible, but later the fur is lost, leaving the classical 'strawberry tongue' appearance.

Erythromycin is an alternative agent for penicillin-allergic patients.

STAPHYLOCOCCI

Staph. aureus and *Staph. epidermidis* are the clinically important staphylococci. Both are common skin commensals but *Staph. aureus* is more virulent and is commonly associated with disease.

Staphylococcus aureus *infection*

There are two distinct mechanisms by which *Staph. aureus* can cause disease. Most often it is by *direct invasion of tissues* (Table 11.23), when some of the enzymes produced by *Staph. aureus* may be important in pathogenesis, e.g. catalase, coagulase, hyaluronidase. Less often, the major disease manifestations are the result of *toxin secretion* (Table 11.24).

Staph. aureus often produces β-lactamase, particularly in hospital-acquired infections, so treatment is usually started with a β-lactamase-resistant antibiotic such as flucloxacillin. Methicillin-resistant *Staph. aureus* (MRSA) has reappeared recently in European hospitals. The cutaneous syndromes of staphylococcal infection are described on page 1124. The management of septicaemia is discussed on page 221. Lung abscess is described on page 474.

Staphylococcus epidermidis *infection*

Staph. epidermidis is a skin commensal. It is now clear that it causes serious infections in patients who are immunocompromised and in patients with intravenous cannulae, prosthetic heart valves, pacemaker wires, CSF shunts and other foreign materials in place for long periods. *Staph. epidermidis* produces β-lactamase and is usually resistant to a wide range of antibiotics including methicillin. Resistance to methicillin is mediated by alteration to penicillin-binding proteins. The mainstay of treatment is vancomycin.

Table 11.23 Invasive disease due to *Staph. aureus*

Site of infection	Disease
Skin	Impetigo Boils and carbuncles Surgical wound infections
Blood	Septicaemia
Lungs	Pneumonia with abscesses
Liver, bone and other	Abscess
Heart	Acute endocarditis

GRAM-NEGATIVE COCCI

NEISSERIA

Neisseria meningitidis (meningococcus) infection

There are three types of meningococcus – groups A, B and C – which are the most common cause of acute bacterial meningitis (p. 961). They also cause septicaemia with or without meningitis (Plate 11, p. 247). Disease occurs sporadically or in epidemics and the epidemiology is poorly understood.

Neisseria gonorrhoea (gonococcus) infection

Gonorrhoea is an important STD causing urethritis, endocervicitis or proctitis. The annual incidence of cases reported by clinics in the UK declined after the introduction of penicillin treatment but soon rose again (Fig. 11.11). The different reported incidence for females is largely artefactual, since 70% or more of female cases are asymptomatic. The incubation period is between 2 and 7 days.

Table 11.24 *Staph. aureus* toxin-mediated diseases

Disease	Manifestations	Organism	Pathological effect	Site of infection
Staphylococcal scalded skin syndrome	Skin erythema; may progress to bullae, exudate, crusting, positive Nikolsky sign	*S. aureus* phage group II, often phage type 71 (produce epidermolytic exotoxins)	Split skin at stratum granulosum	Skin
Toxic shock syndrome	Diarrhoea and vomiting Hypovolaemia Erythema of mucosae and skin leading to peripheral desquamation Fever and myalgia	*S. aureus* phage group I, often phage types 29 and 52 (Produce enterotoxin F, identical to exotoxin C)	Uncertain	Vagina, skin or other (occurs mainly in young women using tampons)
Food poisoning	Vomiting and diarrhoea	*S. aureus* phage group III (produce enteroxins A, B, C, D, E)	Uncertain	Food (toxin ingested)

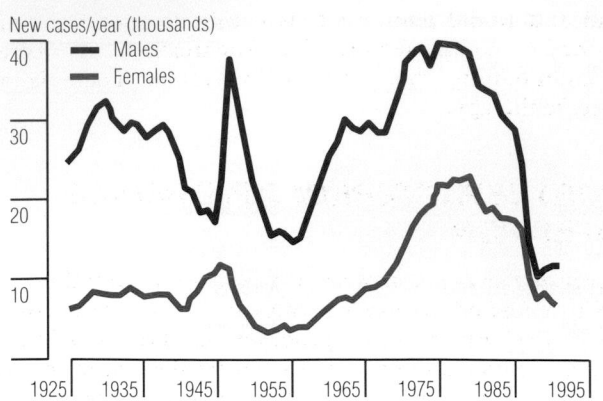

Fig. 11.11 Annual incidence of gonorrhoea in England and Wales, 1925–1990 (Communicable Diseases Surveillance Centre, Colindale).

Clinical features

In men there is urethritis, with creamy discharge, dysuria and frequency. Homosexual men also develop proctitis, with pruritus, tenesmus and rectal discharge often containing blood.

In women the infection is usually asymptomatic (discovered by contact tracing) or causes vaginal discharge, dysuria, frequency and lower abdominal pain. Pharyngeal infection follows oral sex but is usually asymptomatic.

Complications

Ascending infection causes pelvic inflammatory disease, with salpingitis, peritonitis or abscess formation in 10–20% of infected women. Septicaemia may occur, with a rash on the extremities. Gonococcus is an important cause of acute septic arthritis (p. 1012). Perihepatitis (Fitz-Hugh Curtis syndrome) is rare. Disseminated gonococcal infection is commoner in women than in men. Signs include fever, pustular rash and arthritis.

Infection in pregnancy may cause abortion or premature labour and is associated with high perinatal mortality. The baby is infected in utero, at birth or postnatally, and at worst develops disseminated infection. Ophthalmia neonatorum is a sign of infection.

Diagnosis

Microscopy of Gram-stained smears shows pus cells and both intra- and extracellular Gram-negative diplococci. Specimens should be taken from the endocervix in women; a high vaginal swab is inadequate. Culture is essential since β-lactamase-producing gonococci are becoming more common. Serology is not helpful in diagnosis.

Management

Treatment is with amoxycillin (3 g) plus probenecid (1 g orally), or procaine penicillin (2.4 g i.m.) with probenecid (2 g orally). These combinations allow single dose treatment, probenecid delaying excretion of the penicillin. If the patient is allergic to penicillin, kanamycin (2 g i.m.) or co-trimoxazole (4 tablets twice daily for 2 days) is an alternative. Neither of these preparations has any antitreponemal activity.

β-lactamase-producing strains of gonococcus comprise about 2% of isolates in the UK at present. If a resistant strain is cultured, appropriate drugs are spectinomycin (2 g i.m.) or cefuroxime (1.5 g i.m.). Follow-up is essential, since 50% of patients have concurrent non-specific urethritis. This is suspected if symptoms persist a week after treatment of gonococcal infection. Contacts should be traced, examined and treated.

GRAM-POSITIVE BACILLI

BACILLI

Bacillus anthracis: anthrax

Few cases of anthrax are seen in Western countries but about 100 000 cases occur in the world each year. The Gram-positive rods of *B. anthracis* give rise to spores in conditions unfavourable for replication, and spores survive for many years. The spores can contaminate the hides, hooves and bones of herded animals, and contact with these can cause cutaneous anthrax both in the endemic areas and in industrialised countries to which these animal materials are taken for processing. Bacilli are found in the tissues of animals dying of systemic infections. Transmission to man is by skin contact with infected material such as hides or meat, by inhalation of spores or by ingestion of infected meat, causing skin, respiratory and gastrointestinal disease respectively. Disease onset is within 5 days in all forms and usually about 2 days.

Cutaneous anthrax

Cutaneous anthrax is the most common form of the disease and the most benign. A red macule or papule develops at the contact site, e.g. the neck of a meat carrier in a slaughterhouse. A pruritic vesicle develops, satellite lesions appear, and the whole evolves into an ulcer, then a black eschar. There is usually some surrounding oedema, but occasionally there is a severe local reaction with gross oedema, and general toxaemia ensues.

Inhalation anthrax

At first there are mild general symptoms and non-productive cough. Improvement over a few days is followed by abrupt decline. Rapidly the patient becomes very ill, with cough, fever, tachypnoea, cyanosis, tachycardia, vomiting and chills. Diffuse crackles are heard over the affected lung fields. The spleen may enlarge. There is massive enlargement and oedema of the neck and chest wall. Untreated, the patient often dies within 24 hours.

Gastrointestinal anthrax

Following ingestion, lesions can occur anywhere in the gastrointestinal tract, including the throat. There is severe gastroenteritis with haemorrhage, and mortality is high.

Haematogenous dissemination of organisms can sometimes cause meningitis with bloody CSF.

Diagnosis

Many cases may go undiagnosed in the tropics and subtropics. The cutaneous form is probably most often diagnosed on the clinical appearances. Occupational exposure may be suspected from the nature of the patient's job. The severity of a pneumonic illness may prompt consideration of pulmonary anthrax.

The organisms are readily found in Gram-stained smears from skin lesions and grow well in blood culture samples.

Management

The cutaneous form may resolve without treatment. Benzyl penicillin is very effective and is given for 7–10 days. For mild cutaneous disease 2 g/day is given; 4–6 g/day are required for more severe infection. When the patient is allergic to penicillin, tetracycline or chloramphenicol can be used. The latter is given to children and pregnant women. Pulmonary or intestinal cases will require supportive care, with maintenance of oxygenation and infusions to maintain blood volume and hydration.

Prevention is by elimination of the infection from animals. Immunisation is available when there is danger of occupational exposure.

Bacillus cereus infection

B. cereus is one of the causes of food poisoning (see Gastroenteritis, p. 224). Two illnesses are associated with different incubation periods. Short incubation (1–6 hours), vomiting and abdominal pain caused by heat-stable enterotoxin are often related to ingestion of reheated rice. Longer incubation (8–16 hours), diarrhoea

and abdominal pain are caused by a heat-stable toxin formed in the infected intestine. The treatment is directed at maintaining the patient's hydration. There is no specific therapy.

CORYNEBACTERIUM DIPHTHERIAE INFECTION

Corynebacterium diphtheriae is the cause of diphtheria, a toxin-mediated disease which is rare in countries with an effective immunisation programme. Transmission is mainly person-to-person by nasopharyngeal droplets, but skin infection is also important in tropical countries.

Pathogenesis

C. diphtheriae infects the throat and causes minor local disease, but its major effects result from production of a protein toxin of MW 62 000. The toxin is elaborated only by *C. diphtheriae* strains infected by a bacteriophage. Its main effects are on the myocardium and nervous tissue.

Clinical features

After an incubation period of 2–6 days there is slow onset of malaise and fever, sometimes with mild sore throat. At an early stage the predominant findings are profound weakness, restlessness and irritability, with fever, pallor and a rapid thready pulse. The pharynx shows the characteristic membrane which is adherent; attempts to scrape it off result in bleeding. In laryngeal diphtheria, the membrane involves the larynx and trachea, causing respiratory obstruction which may require tracheostomy. The primary infection may also involve the nose, larynx or bronchi. ECG abnormalities suggesting myocarditis appear in the first week (flattening or inversion of T waves most commonly) and acute circulatory collapse may occur. Neurological complications start later, with paralysis of the palate, followed by the ocular muscles, then the pharynx, larynx and respiratory muscles, and lastly the limbs.

Management and outcome

Administration of antitoxin is essential. Intensive nursing is necessary and the patient must be isolated, with respiratory precautions to avoid spread of infection. Penicillin or erythromycin will eradicate the organism from the primary infection site. Contacts must be traced, treated if infected, and immunised. If the patient survives the acute illness, recovery from complications such as paralysis is complete.

LISTERIA MONOCYTOGENES INFECTION

Listeria monocytogenes is a Gram-positive bacillus which is commonly dismissed as a diphtheroid contaminant on examination of CSF specimens. Microbiologists are now aware of its significance as a cause of serious disease, particularly in immunocompromised patients, pregnant women and neonates. The bacillus is a common contaminant of soft cheeses, especially if these are unpasteurised. It causes septicaemia, often associated with meningo-encephalitis. Ampicillin or penicillin is the drug of first choice, with erythromycin in reserve for penicillin-allergic patients.

CLOSTRIDIA

Clostridia are a group of obligate anaerobic bacteria; they cause illness largely through toxins which act locally or enter the circulation. Clostridia are frequent wound contaminants without necessarily causing disease; when disease occurs, however, it is severe.

Tetanus

Tetanus is a potentially fatal disease dominated by muscle spasm caused by an exotoxin, tetanospasmin, produced by *Clostridium tetani*.

Epidemiology and pathogenesis

Cl. tetani is found in the faeces of man and animals, and its spores abound in soil. It is anaerobic and proliferates in ischaemic or necrotic tissue, usually in a poorly tended wound. In rural areas farm workers or gardeners are infected, but in cities the disease has been observed in drug addicts. Since immunisation against tetanus toxin is standard in Western countries, tetanus is rare. In poorer countries immunisation is variable.

Tetanospasmin is a neurotoxin which acts in several different ways. It inhibits the release of acetylcholine from nerve endings in muscle but, more importantly, it interferes with synaptic reflexes in the spinal cord, causing disinhibition which results in muscle spasms.

Clinical features

The incubation period can be up to 3 weeks, depending on inoculation dose and site. A short incubation and rapid onset of first spasm indicate a severe infection. Symptoms are most severe at either extreme of age.

The first (and sometimes sole) sign of tetanus is often muscle spasm local to the wound; in most, the CNS is involved and trismus (lockjaw) heralds the onset of generalised tetanus. The patient notices difficulty in opening the mouth and swallowing, followed by stiffness in the neck and back. Examination reveals the initial site of infection and 'risus sardonicus', the facial expression caused by trismus and contraction of facial muscles. Muscles of the back and abdomen become stiff, and painful spasms, provoked by sudden movement or noise, occur in the back muscles, causing opisthotonos. Autonomic involvement causes sweating and cardiovascular instability. Death is from exhaustion, aspiration or secondary infection.

Management

Further toxin production is prevented by local debridement of wounds and parenteral treatment with benzyl-penicillin (tetracycline in penicillin-allergic patients). Human immune globulin containing antibodies to tetanus toxin in high titre is given to neutralise free toxin. If surgery is indicated, it should be delayed for an hour after administration of antibody.

The patient is nursed in a quiet room to avoid stimuli likely to provoke spasms. Neuromuscular block is indicated when spasms become generalised, and then the patient is ventilated. Since prolonged ventilation is usual, tracheostomy is performed early. In countries where intensive care is not available, anticonvulsant drugs such as diazepam are used as an alternative to paralysis. Nutrition is maintained enterally or parenterally.

An attack of tetanus does not render the patient immune and a full course of immunisation should be given after recovery.

Prevention

Immunisation with tetanus toxoid is the only way to prevent the disease altogether. A full course of toxoid confers immunity for at least 5 years. Neonatal tetanus can be prevented by immunising the mother during pregnancy.

Patients with wounds at risk from *Cl. tetani* infection are managed according to their state of immunity. All patients require local wound toilet. Fully immunised patients receive a booster dose of toxoid. Unimmunised patients with a wound considered susceptible to *Cl. tetani* receive human tetanus immune globulin and, simultaneously, active immunisation with adsorbed tetanus toxoid is started. Injection of long-acting penicillin, followed by a course of oral penicillin, is also indicated in these cases.

Botulism

Botulism is a virulent form of food poisoning caused by enterotoxins of *Cl. botulinum*. The toxins cause disease when produced in contaminated food, usually tins of meat. These highly potent poisons interrupt cholinergic neurotransmission. The initial illness is an afebrile gastroenteritis developing within 12–36 hours of ingestion in one-third of patients, but the remainder have only malaise and dizziness (with postural hypotension), progressing to extreme dryness caused by autonomic paralysis. Other neurological symptoms appear during the next 3 days: diplopia followed by bulbar signs, then symmetrical weakness of the limbs – usually in that order. Bulbar and respiratory muscle weakness may lead to inhalation pneumonia. Treatment is supportive and recovery is very slow, taking several weeks. Polyvalent horse antitoxin is available but it is poorly tolerated by many patients and of uncertain value.

Other clostridial syndromes

Gas gangrene

Cl. perfringens (welchii) is one of a number of gas-producing clostridia which contaminate wounds containing necrotic, anoxic material. *Cl. perfringens* produces 12 toxins, alphatoxin being the one associated with gas gangrene. It proliferates rapidly, producing myonecrosis. Gas infiltrates neighbouring tissues, causing crepitus. Toxins entering the circulation cause profound toxaemia with a high mortality.

Skin and soft tissue infections

Local infections, often involving muscle, occur in amputated stumps, diabetic ulcers of the foot, decubitus ulcers, perirectal abscesses and in abscesses at injection sites of drug addicts. Such infections frequently contain multiple organisms, including clostridia.

Gut infections

Pseudomembranous colitis is caused by toxin-producing strains of *Cl. difficile* which colonise the large intestine after antibiotic therapy. Although the early association was with clindamycin therapy, most antibiotics have caused this disease. Watery diarrhoea (without blood) and abdominal pain are associated with severe systemic toxicity. Treatment is with oral metronidazole or vancomycin.

Suppurative intra-abdominal infection caused by clostridia is particularly associated with carcinoma of the colon or pancreas. Neutropenic patients may develop severe *enterocolitis* caused by *Cl. septicum*.

GRAM-NEGATIVE BACILLI

ENTEROBACTERIA

The enterobacteria group comprises *Escherichia coli (E. coli)*, *Klebsiella*, *Proteus*, *Salmonella* and *Shigella*.

E. coli causes a wide variety of diseases, usually as a result of autoinfection. Urinary tract infection is the most common, but systemic infection is a major problem in hospitals. Septicaemia arises from the bowel when there is a bowel disease or surgery has been carried out, or from the urinary tract as a complication of infection or surgery there. In neonates, *E. coli* is a common cause of septicaemia and meningitis. Several strains of *E. coli* cause gastroenteritis by a number of mechanisms; they are referred to as enteropathogenic, enteroinvasive, enterohaemorrhagic, enteroadherent and enterotoxigenic. The latter produces toxins, one of which acts in a similar way to cholera toxin.

Klebsiella causes urinary tract infection, septicaemia and pneumonia. *Kl. pneumoniae* causes an acute, severe, cavitating pneumonia most frequently seen in alcoholics (p. 467).

Proteus is mainly associated with urinary tract infection.

Salmonella is found in several hundred strains. Salmonellae other than *S. typhi* and *S. paratyphi* are amongst the most common causes of gastroenteritis related to food poisoning (see Gastroenteritis, p. 224). They cause disease by direct invasion of the intestinal mucosa, and some strains, e.g. *S. typhimurium*, cause septicaemia, but usually disease remains localised. Typhoid (enteric fever) is caused by *S. typhi*, and is described below.

Four strains of *Shigella* are the cause of bacillary dysentery, a form of acute diarrhoeal disease characterised by severe, bloody, purulent diarrhoea and abdominal pain.

Shigella dysentery

Shigella sonnei and *S. flexneri* are the common organisms in the UK, the incidence of *S. flexneri* infection having increased in recent years; the other species are *S. dysenteriae* and *S. boydii*. Shigella infections occur worldwide, and epidemics are common where conditions are crowded and hygiene poor. Faecal–oral transmission results from lack of hand washing, and the organism is highly infectious, ingestion of less than 200 organisms causing disease in healthy adults.

The infection localises in the colon, where the epithelium is invaded and becomes inflamed. There is an acute inflammatory exudate which produces diarrhoea containing large numbers of leucocytes. Enterotoxin production contributes to the intestinal damage and the organisms may also produce a neurotoxin.

Clinical features

After an incubation period of 2–3 days there is rapid onset of vomiting, abdominal colic and diarrhoea, which is usually bloody and purulent. Severity ranges from mild to fulminant. The most severe illness is caused by *S. dysenteriae*. Although the main illness is usually over within 1–2 weeks, diarrhoea and abdominal discomfort may persist for several weeks. Fever is common in the first few days and dehydration can occur rapidly, especially in children.

Postinfective aseptic arthritis and Reiter's syndrome (conjunctivitis, urethritis and arthritis) are complications which vary in frequency in different epidemics but are more common in HLA-B27 positive individuals.

The diagnosis is made when organisms are cultured from faeces.

Management

Patients are managed as for any severe form of gastroenteritis, rehydration being the key factor. Antibiotics are usually given to severely ill patients, although plasmid-mediated resistance is common and transfers rapidly. Ampicillin, ciprofloxacin or co-trimoxazole is usually effective.

Typhoid

Typhoid (enteric fever) is a serious, prolonged, systemic infection with the Gram-negative bacillus *S. typhi*.

Epidemiology

Typhoid is endemic in many poor countries, and although uncommon in Britain (about 200 cases reported per year), it is an important cause of fever in returning travellers. Humans are the reservoir of infection and spread of infection is by contamination of water or food by human faeces. Epidemics usually occur when a common water supply is contaminated. Small outbreaks sometimes result when a chronic excreter of the organism works as a food handler.

Pathogenesis

Ingested organisms invade the small intestinal mucosa. In the absence of specific immunity, organisms phagocytosed by macrophages survive and proliferate. After an incubation period varying from 1 to 3 weeks (usually 10–14 days), determined by the infecting dose, septicaemia develops and foci of infection may be established in any organ.

The gall bladder is an important site, since it is the source of chronic excretion when this occurs. Focal inflammation of Peyer's patches may be so vigorous as to cause intestinal perforation or haemorrhage.

Clinical features

In Britain typhoid usually presents as a pyrexia of insidious onset in a patient returning from abroad, often travelling from the Indian subcontinent.

The classic stepwise rise in temperature is rarely seen but the untreated illness has a remorseless progression. Headache and dry cough are common in the first week, and the patient is often vague and withdrawn. Constipation is usual. In the second week the spleen is often palpable and the elusive rash consisting of rose spots is seen in less than half of patients. The rash is sparse, less than a dozen spots in all, and consists of 1–2 mm pale red macules, which are hard to discern on a pigmented skin. By the third week diarrhoea may develop and the patient, now extremely ill, may lapse into coma.

The overall mortality in untreated typhoid is about 10%, but with appropriate antibiotic therapy it is less than 5%. Spontaneous remission is often followed by relapse within 2 weeks.

Typhoid in children

Typhoid is even more featureless in children than in adults and presents as an abrupt severe septicaemic illness. The mental state is striking, the child initially being irritable but later frankly delirious. Febrile convulsions may be the presenting feature and some degree of meningism is not uncommon. Diarrhoea is perhaps more frequent than in adults with typhoid, although intestinal infection with other organisms complicates the issue.

Complications

The most serious complications in the acute phase are intestinal haemorrhage or perforation. In severe cases there may be myocarditis or bone marrow suppression. Later complications are relapse, even after correct antibiotic treatment, in 15% of cases, and local sepsis in any organ as a result of septicaemia. Osteomyelitis is slow to cause symptoms.

Chronic carriage

Faecal excretion of *S. typhi* often continues several weeks after resolution of the illness and, rarely, patients excrete the organism for years. The organism is not detected in faeces during antibiotic treatment but reappears after therapy is stopped. The source of organisms in long-term carriers is probably the gall bladder, and gallstones readily become infected. Chronic excretion has obvious epidemiological consequences.

> **Summary 5 Antibiotics for typhoid in adults**
>
> Minimum 2 weeks
>
> *Chloramphenicol* 500 mg 4-hourly initially, then 500 mg 6-hourly
>
> *Co-trimoxazole* 2 tablets (trimethoprim 80 mg, sulphamethoxazole 400 mg each) 12-hourly
>
> *Amoxycillin* 500 mg 6-hourly
>
> *Ciprofloxacin* 500 mg 12-hourly

Diagnosis

The diagnosis is usually made by blood culture. The organism is not present in stools initially but can be isolated in the second to third week. It may also be cultured from urine in 30% of patients. Serology is rarely helpful in diagnosis. The blood count is helpful since neutropenia is common.

Management

Patients must be barrier nursed, preferably in an isolation unit. Person-to-person transmission is not common. Attention must be paid to management of fluid balance. Chloramphenicol, co-trimoxazole, trimethoprim alone, amoxycillin and ciprofloxacin have all been used successfully. Although duration and severity of symptoms, as well as mortality, are reduced by treatment, the response to treatment is not immediate. Treatment is continued for a week after resolution of fever and in any case for at least 2 weeks. Relapse can be treated with the original antibiotic, provided the organism was sensitive. Prolonged carriage is difficult to treat but success has been reported with high-dose amoxycillin and ciprofloxacin. Cholecystectomy may be necessary.

Perforation of the intestine is dangerous and carries a high mortality. Good results have been achieved by laparotomy and perfusion of the peritoneum and intestinal lumen with chloramphenicol.

Prevention

A monovalent vaccine to protect against *S. typhi* is more effective and has fewer side-effects than the old TAB vaccine, which included *S. paratyphi A* and *B* antigens. An oral vaccine which uses the mutant strain of *S. typhi*, Ty 21a, is now available and has given good protection in endemic areas.

Salmonella paratyphi infection

S. paratyphi B is the most common paratyphoid infection in Britain. Other strains are called *S. paratyphi A* and *C*.

Paratyphoid has a shorter incubation period than typhoid and is a milder disease with fewer complications. Diarrhoea tends to occur early, in contrast to typhoid. Treatment is with co-trimoxazole.

PARVOBACTERIA

Haemophilus infection

Haemophilus organisms are normal colonisers of the upper respiratory tract. *H. influenzae* is a major human pathogen; other *Haemophilus* species rarely cause disease, although *H. para-influenzae* can cause illness similar to *H. influenzae*.

A small proportion of *H. influenzae* isolated from humans are encapsulated and six antigenic types are recognised. The most important is type b, which can cause septicaemia and several clinical syndromes in children under 5 years old (Table 11.25). Older children acquire immunity to the capsular antigens. Untypable (non-encapsulated) *H. influenzae* are potential pathogens in the lower respiratory tract.

Strains of *H. influenzae* have become increasingly resistant to antibiotics in recent years: 5–15% of strains are resistant to amoxycillin. This is particularly relevant to children with life-threatening diseases such as acute meningitis, in which a delay in treatment with the right antibiotic could be fatal. Resistance is mediated by β-lactamases.

Vaccine containing the polysaccharide capsular antigens has now been introduced in the UK for children below the age of 4 years old.

Whooping cough (pertussis)

Whooping cough is a prolonged lower respiratory tract infection caused by the Gram-negative coccobacillus *Bordetella pertussis*. It is highly infectious and is transmitted by droplet.

Table 11.25 Diseases caused by *H. influenzae*

Type	Disease	Age
Type b	Acute meningitis Epiglottis Septic arthritis Orbital cellulitis Pneumonia	Up to 5 years
Non-encapsulated	Exacerbations of chronic bronchitis Otitis media and sinusitis Conjunctivitis	Any age
Other encapsulated types	Rarely pathogenic	

11 Infectious, Tropical and Parasitic Diseases

Epidemiology

Spread of infection is entirely human-to-human and the disease is endemic, cases occurring continuously. Epidemics in susceptible children occur every 4 years in the UK (Fig. 11.12). Since reports of a possible association between pertussis immunisation and encephalopathy in 1973, the rate of immunisation has fallen off and epidemics have been larger.

The disease may affect any age group, but it is most common in children under 5 years and most severe in those below 1 year.

Pathogenesis

The infection is concentrated in the bronchial walls, producing damage to the epithelium and accumulation of viscid mucus. Toxins produced by *B. pertussis* probably have a role in the tissue damage. Collapse of segments of lung distal to obstructed bronchioles is common.

Clinical features

After an incubation period of 7–10 days there is sometimes a prodromal illness resembling a cold and lasting 2–3 days (catarrhal stage). This is followed by onset of the characteristic cough, with long spasms of coughing interrupted by rapid inspiration, which sometimes produces a whooping sound. This is often followed by vomiting.

During a spasm of coughing the child becomes pink and then blue, and small babies may become apnoeic after a spasm. Between spasms the child looks and feels deceptively well.

Whooping cough lasts about 2 months on average and in the later stages the cough is mainly at night. It is distressing to watch small children rendered helpless by the spasmodic cough, and anxiety and disruption of sleep cause a major disturbance to family life.

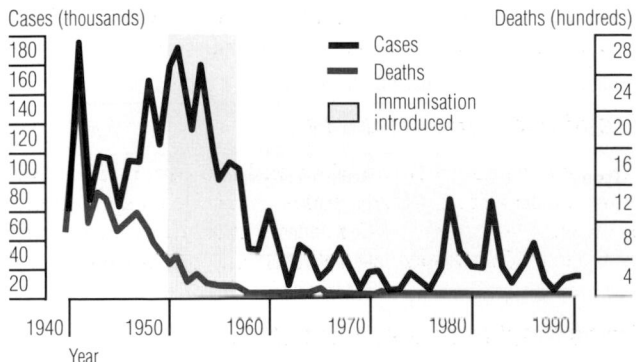

Fig. 11.12 Incidence of whooping cough in England and Wales, 1940–1990. Note the effect of immunisation on incidence. The death rate was falling before immunisation was introduced (Communicable Diseases Surveillance Centre, Colindale).

Complications

Secondary bacterial infection causing pneumonia or mucus plugging with segmental collapse are the most common serious complications. Cerebral hypoxia during prolonged coughing spasms may cause convulsions. Minor complications are subconjunctival haemorrhages, periorbital bruising and frenal ulcer, all of which result from prolonged spasms of coughing.

Diagnosis

Clinical diagnosis rests on recognition of the pattern of cough and is fairly simple when whooping is heard. However, in the early stages in babies and in adults, the whoop may be absent.

Laboratory support comes from the lymphocytosis and culture of *B. pertussis* from a pernasal swab; the latter is taken by passing a special swab through the nostril to the nasopharynx.

Management

Attentive nursing is the most important aspect of treatment and parents need help and reassurance to learn to manage coughing spasms. Babies frequently feed poorly and lose weight, necessitating feeding through a nasogastric tube.

The organism is sensitive to erythromycin and early treatment may be beneficial, although the effect is seldom pronounced. Antibiotic treatment of secondary bacterial pneumonia is along conventional lines.

Prevention

Pertussis vaccine is a crude preparation of killed organisms, but it is 80% effective in preventing whooping cough and often ameliorates the disease if not wholly preventing it. There is a small risk of convulsions after immunisation (1 in 6000 doses) and a minute incidence (1 in 100 000 doses) of encephalitis with lasting consequences. Since there is severe morbidity and a small mortality in whooping cough epidemics the vaccine is strongly recommended. Prophylactic erythromycin treatment of close contacts has proved ineffective.

Brucellosis

Brucellosis (undulant fever) is a septicaemic infection caused by *Brucella abortus*, *Br. melitensis* or *Br. suis*. *Br. abortus* is acquired from cattle, *Br. melitensis* from sheep or goats (Malta fever), and *Br. suis* from swine. Most northern European infection is by *Br. abortus* acquired during occupational exposure of vets, farm workers and slaughterhouse employees, by ingestion of raw milk or by accidental infection in the laboratory. Most herds in the UK are brucella-free and pasteurisation is an additional insurance against infection of milk. As a result of control measures the disease is now very rare in the UK but it remains a major problem in parts of Europe, the Middle East, Central and South America and perhaps elsewhere.

Brucellae are Gram-negative coccobacilli, which proliferate intracellularly. The incubation period of the disease is about 3 weeks.

Clinical features

Some patients are infected asymptomatically but the common presentation is an acute illness with swinging fever and profuse sweats. Back pain is common. There are no specific physical signs but 40% of patients have hepatosplenomegaly, 20% have splenomegaly only, and 20% have arthritis in one large joint. Less common manifestations are epididymo-orchitis, spondylitis, an erythematous papular eruption on the extremities, and neurological involvement with meningitis, encephalitis or radiculitis.

If no treatment is given, fever may persist for weeks or months, although it gradually declines, only to relapse again in many cases. A prolonged debilitating illness can be associated with depression. Depressed patients with moderate brucella antibody titres rarely have chronic brucellosis in the absence of a preceding history suggestive of acute brucellosis.

Diagnosis

There is neutropenia and lymphocytosis in the acute phase, and brucellae can be cultured from blood in 50–60% of cases and also from bone marrow. Complement fixing and agglutinating antibodies can be detected in rising titre following acute infection.

Management

Inadequate treatment is associated with a high rate of relapse within 3 months, and some relapses occur despite the best known therapy. Tetracycline combined with rifampicin or streptomycin gives the lowest relapse rates. Co-trimoxazole has also been used but should not be given alone.

Preventive measures are concentrated on elimination of brucellae from domestic animals and avoiding contact with infected materials.

Yersinial infection

Yersinial infections are zoonoses. The important human pathogens are Y. enterocolitica and Y. pseudotuberculosis, which are enteric pathogens, and Y. pestis, the cause of plague.

Y. pseudotuberculosis and Y. enterocolitica

Infection with Y. pseudotuberculosis and Y. enterocolitica (see also p. 600) is less common in the UK than in some other European countries, notably Scandinavia and Belgium. The organism is a common commensal in the pharynx and tonsillar tissue of pigs, which are included in ground pig meat. Other foods, including milk and seafoods, have been incriminated in human outbreaks.

Y. enterocolitica causes febrile enterocolitis in young children (less than 5 years old), but in adolescents an illness which is difficult to distinguish from acute appendicitis is caused by mesenteric adenitis. The latter is also the most common manifestation of Y. pseudotuberculosis infection. The presence of exudative pharyngitis may give a clue in Y. enterocolitica infection. Many laparotomies have been carried out for these self-limited infections, which may be partially responsive to gentamicin therapy (often given as blind treatment or prophylaxis for surgery).

Reactive polyarthritis and erythema nodosum are well-recognised complications which are more common with Y. enterocolitica.

Plague

An acute severe infection caused by Y. pestis manifests by either lymphadenitis with suppuration (bubonic plague) or necrotising pneumonitis (pneumonic plague). It is a zoonosis.

Aetiology

The organism is a Gram-negative aerobic bacillus in the parvobacteria family. It grows well at 28°C. At 37°C it produces an antigen which inhibits phagocytosis. It has a lipopolysaccharide capsular endotoxin.

Distribution and incidence

Asia, Africa, the Middle East and the Americas (South America and the southern states of the USA) are endemic areas with comparatively small numbers of reported cases each year. The disease is probably under-reported.

Transmission and epidemiology

The infection is transmitted to man by the bite of the rat flea (Fig. 11.13). The natural hosts are rodents and the vector is the rat flea, Xenopsylla cheopis, which takes blood meals from its rodent hosts. Infected rats die and the fleas

11 Infectious, Tropical and Parasitic Diseases

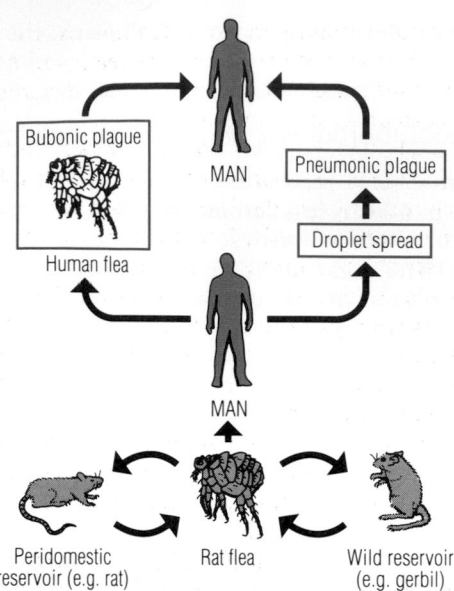

Fig. 11.13 Cycle of transmission of plague.

leave the dead rats for other hosts. The organisms produce a coagulant which prevents the flea taking a full blood meal. The flea bites the host repeatedly, encouraging transmission. The coagulant is inactive above 28°C and transmission diminishes.

Pathology

Necrosis and haemorrhage are the main features, together with marked inflammatory changes. An eschar at the bite site is occasionally found. Buboes are grossly enlarged, inflamed lymph nodes draining the site of the flea bite. The normal lymph node architecture is destroyed and necrotic, with large numbers of bacilli. The pathological changes in pneumonic plague are very similar, with haemorrhagic necrosis of lung tissue.

Clinical features

The incubation period is 2–8 days before the onset of systemic upset, fever, chills and headache. Within 24 hours of this, the patient finds a bubo which is exquisitely tender. Any group of lymph glands can be involved. Tachycardia and high fever are usual, with hypotension and shock in severely affected patients. Purpura may occur.

Pneumonic plague results from haematogenous spread of organisms to the lungs. Cough, chest pain and haemoptysis in a severely ill patient are usual features. Patchy shadowing is seen on the chest X-ray. Aerosol spread of plague can occur from patients with pneumonic plague. Septicaemic plague has a high mortality.

There is a neutrophil leucocytosis. Some degree of disseminated intravascular coagulation is common, although spontaneous bleeding is uncommon.

Diagnosis

The organism may be found in material aspirated from the necrotic centre of buboes and in blood films. Smears made on slides can be stained with Giemsa stain, which shows the Gram-negative coccobacilli. The organism grows readily on standard media.

Management

The high mortality in untreated plague (over 50%) has been altered by antibiotics. Streptomycin (15 mg/kg twice daily i.m.) for 10 days is the treatment of choice. Defervescence occurs by the third or fourth day. Tetracycline and chloramphenicol are alternative choices. Supportive treatment is needed in those with low blood pressure and shock, with volume replacement using saline or plasma. Buboes should be aspirated.

Prevention and control

A vaccine is available for those working with plague in the laboratory or in the field. Proven cases are not infectious unless there is pneumonic involvement, when isolation of cases, with respiratory precautions to avoid aerosol spread, is necessary. Antibiotics rapidly reduce infectivity. Vector control with insecticides and rat control will minimise transmission in towns and cities.

PSEUDOMONAS

Pseudomonas aeruginosa infection

Pseudomonas aeruginosa is an opportunist organism which rarely causes disease in immunocompetent subjects. It causes serious infection in patients with deficient immunity and in patients who have had surgery. Septicaemia, osteomyelitis, infection of burns and pneumonia are examples. Skin changes due to *P. aeruginosa* are described in Chapter 25. Patients in intensive care units may become colonised superficially and treatment with antibiotics is often counterproductive, since resistance develops rapidly.

Melioidosis

P. pseudomallei is a Gram-negative, aerobic bacillus that is found contaminating surface water. The south-east Asian countries and northern Australia are endemic areas. Infection occurs by ingestion or inhalation of contaminated water, or by contact of infected water with abraded skin. If health is good, then there may be subclinical infection shown by seroconversion without systemic upset. Debilitating illness and immunosuppression enhance susceptibility and the development of clinical infection, which can be acute or chronic, may follow.

After some days' incubation there is fever, myalgia, vomiting, confusion or delirium. Diarrhoea may also occur, as may shock with features of endotoxic shock. Pustular skin lesions may occur. The lungs may be involved, with consolidation, cavitation and pus formation. Chronic and relapsing sepsis may occur, with abscess formation affecting lymph glands, lungs, skin, liver, genito-urinary tract and bones.

The organism is a dangerous pathogen which may be grown from pus, lymph gland biopsies, liver biopsy material and bone marrow aspirate. Serological responses using indirect haemagglutination (IHA) or complement-fixing antibody techniques are available.

Treatment is with ceftazidime (30 mg/kg i.v. 8-hourly) and co-trimoxazole (5 mg trimethoprim/kg; 25 mg sulphamethoxazole/kg) 12-hourly, given for 4 weeks.

TULARAEMIA

Francisella tularensis is a Gram-negative bacillus that infects a wide range of wild animals; man is occasionally infected in rural areas of the northern hemisphere (North America, Sweden, Norway, northern Europe, Russia and Japan). Infection occurs by the bite of an infected insect, by mucosal or skin contact with an infected animal, by inhalation, and by eating inadequately cooked meat.

The effects in man may be localised cutaneous pustular disease with regional adenopathy, a pneumonic illness, or a systemic illness sometimes with diarrhoea. Inapparent (subclinical) infections occur.

The North American rabbit strain produces severe disease, with a mortality of up to 10% without treatment. Mortality is negligible (except for the American rabbit strain) even without treatment.

The diagnosis is made by finding the organisms in material from infected tissues. Direct immunofluorescence may be used. Serological tests may also be used to detect antibodies to the organism by ELISA and agglutination techniques. Great caution is needed in handling specimens to avoid the risk of laboratory infection.

Streptomycin (10 mg/kg twice daily for 14 days) is very effective. Tetracycline and chloramphenicol are effective. Patients need to be isolated until they have been on treatment for 48 hours to minimise the risk of cross-infection.

BARTONELLOSIS

Bartonella bacilliformis is a Gram-negative aerobic bacillus transmitted by the bite of the female sandfly, *Lutzomyia verrucarum*. The disease is limited to the valleys of the western Andes, mainly in Peru, Colombia and Ecuador, between 2500 and 8000 feet above sea level. Man is the reservoir of infection. There are two manifestations of the disease: *haematological* and *cutaneous*.

After a 21-day incubation period there is sudden onset of systemic upset. The onset of fever is often followed by acute severe intravascular haemolysis which may last up to 4 weeks before resolution. Several weeks to several months later the eruptive phase of the disease appears, with nodular lesions of various sizes over the body in the miliary form, or fewer nodular, deep lesions particularly concentrated on the extensor aspects of the limbs. Mucous membranes of the mouth and gut, and serous cavities can be affected.

The organisms can be grown in blood cultures taken in the first week of the illness and can be readily found in Giemsa-stained thick and thin blood films, or in material obtained from skin lesions.

Treatment with antibiotics kills the organisms and produces rapid defervescence and clearance of organisms from the blood. Penicillin, streptomycin and chloramphenicol are effective; the latter is recommended in view of the reported association between systemic salmonellosis and bartonellosis.

CAT-SCRATCH DISEASE

Cat-scratch disease (CSD) is a benign lymphadenopathy in a site determined by an area scratched by a cat, most often in the neck or axilla.

Aetiology and pathogenesis

Histology of affected lymph nodes reveals scanty small pleomorphic rod-shaped bacilli which stain erratically with Gram stain. The other histological features are micro-abscesses and sometimes necrotic granulomas.

The infection is transmitted by scratching or licking by a cat which does not itself appear ill. The cat is probably infectious for only about 3 weeks. It is not clear how cats transmit the infection.

Clinical features

Most cases occur in children or young adults. There is gross enlargement of a single group of lymph nodes, which are usually tender. Lymphadenopathy develops about 2 weeks after the scratch and usually lasts for 2–4 months, but it may persist for up to a year. A papule may occur at the site of the scratch; it appears about a week after the scratch and persists for 1–3 weeks. Although most patients remain well, one-third have a low-grade fever for a few days and may experience malaise, headache and sore throat. Rare manifestations are conjunctivitis and preauricular lymphadenopathy (oculoglandular syndrome), encephalopathy, thrombocytopenic purpura, osteomyelitis and pneumonia.

Diagnosis

The diagnosis is usually based on the histology of excised lymph node with negative cultures for bacteria and mycobacteria. The Warthin-Starry silver impregnation stain may reveal the CSD bacilli but they are present in small numbers.

There may be a mild neutrophil leucocytosis but other tests are unhelpful. Antibody tests are being developed.

Management

Since the disease resolves spontaneously the only treatment usually required is analgesia if the lymph nodes are painful, and reassurance. Antibiotics do not help.

VIBRIOS

Cholera

Cholera is due to infection with the Gram-negative bacillus *Vibrio cholerae*, which causes acute secretory diarrhoea with death due to dehydration.

Aetiology

V. cholerae is a curved Gram-negative motile bacillus. Two biotypes are recognised, the *classical biotype* and the *El Tor biotype*. The organism is present in vast numbers in the faeces of infected patients. The El Tor biotype tends to cause more asymptomatic and mild infections, which resolve spontaneously and leave the patient excreting vibrios to infect others. The organism is sensitive to desiccation but survives in saline waters.

Distribution and incidence

Distribution and incidence are shown in Figure 11.14. Cholera has been imported into European countries but no outbreaks have resulted, apart from that in Naples in 1974.

Transmission and epidemiology

Organisms are ingested in contaminated food and water. In India, Bangladesh and Pakistan, where cholera is endemic, it is predominantly a paediatric disease. All ages are affected in epidemic cholera. Individual susceptibility is governed by the infecting dose and by the gastric acid barrier.

Pathogenesis

V. cholerae secretes an exotoxin which binds to the GMI ganglioside, a glycolipid on the surface membrane of jejunal enterocytes (Fig. 11.15). The effects of cholera toxin are mediated by several mechanisms, one of which may be accumulation of cyclic AMP in the cell. Local neurohumoral stimuli may also contribute to the diarrhoea.

The outcome is that the upper small intestine becomes a site of net secretion with accumulation of isotonic fluid containing Na^+, Cl^-, HCO_3^- and water. This fluid passes down the intestine and in the colon K^+ exchanges for Na^+ under the influence of aldosterone. Stooling rates of 500 ml/hour are common and up to 1 litre/hour may be produced. The effect of cholera toxin lasts for the duration of the life of the enterocyte, which is 3–4 days; during this time the cell migrates from the crypt to villous tip, where it is desquamated into the gut lumen.

There are no histological changes in the affected mucosa. Cholera is a secretory diarrhoea with no mucosal inflammation. Secondary changes in a range of

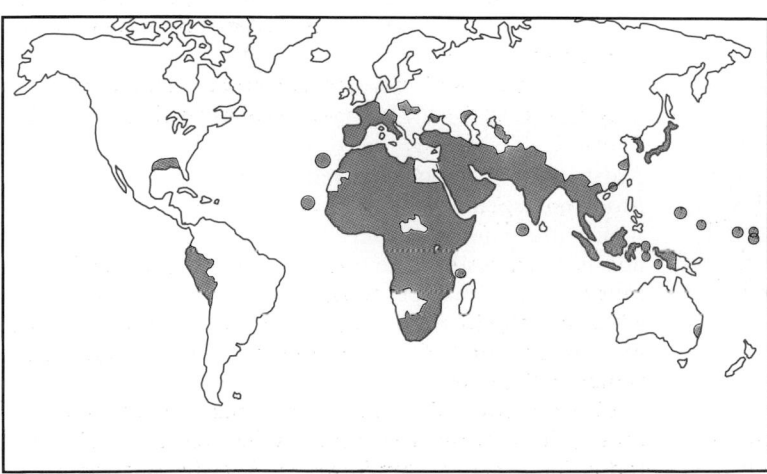

Fig. 11.14 World distribution of cholera 1961–1991 (WHO).

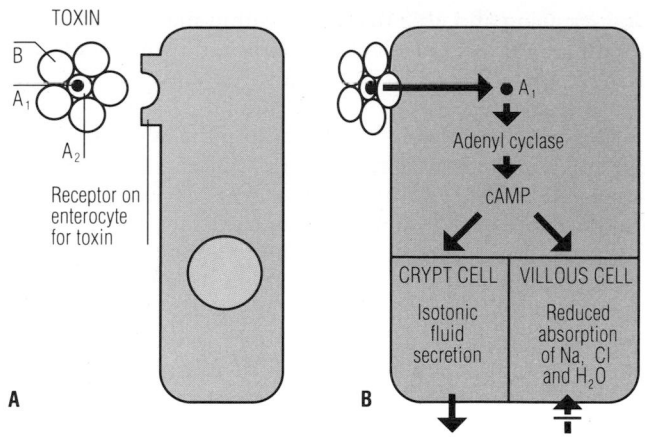

Fig. 11.15 Mechanism of action of cholera toxin on intestinal cells. A. Attachment of cholera toxin to receptor in enterocyte. **B.** Activation of cAMP – note different effects on villous and crypt cells.

tissues, e.g. kidney, occur as a result of hypovolaemia and shock.

Clinical features

The incubation period is about 2 days. Diarrhoea begins suddenly, with vomiting during the first 24 hours of illness. Faecal residues disappear, and opalescent, rice-water stools are passed. There are no pus cells in faecal smears. The abdomen may be distended and bowel sounds are increased. Stool losses are maximal within the first 48 hours of the illness and decline thereafter spontaneously, but death can occur from dehydration within 24 hours in the most severe cases.

The clinical features are due to isotonic volume depletion (Table 11.13, p. 225). Haematocrit and plasma specific gravity rise with haemoconcentration. Hypoglycaemia may occur in young children and may be associated with convulsions. Loss of bicarbonate causes acidosis. There is prerenal uraemia.

There is a considerable range in the severity of diarrhoea in cholera, particularly the E1 Tor biotype.

Diagnosis

Severe diarrhoea causing rapid progression to dehydration suggests that cholera is the cause in severe cases. Milder cases will not be diagnosed unless a stool is cultured, or immediate dark ground microscopy of a fresh faecal smear shows the characteristic mortality of *V. cholera*.

Differential diagnosis

Al the acute infective causes of diarrhoea need to be considered, including ingestion of staphylococcal entero-toxin, invasive bacteria, such as *Salmonella*, *Shigella* and *Campylobacter*, and enterotoxigenic strains of *E. coli*. Rotavirus infection may also be difficult to distinguish from cholera.

Management

Mild to moderate dehydration can be managed with oral rehydration solution (ORS) (p. 250), while those with severe dehydration need intravenous infusions, e.g. Ringer's lactate, to restore blood volume. The aims of rehydration are:

- to replace estimated fluid losses in the first 6 hours after presentation
- to replace continuing intestinal fluid losses with equal volumes until diarrhoea stops.

Frequent small amounts of ORS are better tolerated than less frequent large volumes, especially if the patients is vomiting. Additional fluid, such as water, fruit juice, tea or breast milk but *not* ORS, should be given to allow for insensible losses and obligatory urinary losses. The glucose in ORS is not sufficient to counter hypoglycaemia and so extra sugar should be given orally.

Antidiarrhoeal and antisecretory drugs have no part to play in the management of dehydrating diarrhoeal disease. Tetracycline (250 mg q.d.s. for 4 days) reduces the duration of diarrhoea and reduces the duration of faecal excretion of *V. cholerae*. Pregnant women and children under 8 years can be given furazolidone. Co-trimoxazole is also effective.

Prevention and control

Adequate clean water supplies and safe disposal of faecal wastes would do much to prevent the occurrence of cholera. Concurrent education of the population about the relationship of infective diarrhoea disease to personal and general sanitation practices is essential. The widespread use of ORS early in the course of all diarrhoeal illness reduces mortality.

Vaccination with the present killed vaccine is of no benefit, either for prophylaxis in the traveller or for the control of epidemics.

CAMPYLOBACTER

Campylobacter are morphologically similar to *Vibrios* but are now regarded as a separated genus since they have different biochemical characteristics. There are six species, of which *C. jejuni* and *C. fetus* are important human pathogens.

C. jejuni is a major cause of prolonged, severe entero-colitis, frequently associated with bloody stools and abdominal pain and tenderness suggestive of peritonitis.

Infection may be acquired from food or drinks but there is often a relationship with domestic animals, many of which are normally colonised (e.g. dogs and cattle).

C. fetus rarely infects normal subjects but can cause septicaemia in debilitated patients. Like many gastrointestinal pathogens *Campylobacter* may cause of reactive arthritis.

C. jejuni is sensitive to erythromycin in vitro, and oral treatment tenders stool specimens culture-negative, but its effect on the rate of resolution of disease is disappointing. Nevertheless it is sometimes used in ill patients.

ANAEROBIC BACTERIA

Bacteroides fragilis is the most commonly encountered pathogenic anaerobe but many other anaerobes are found among the normal flora of the gastrointestinal tract and genital tract; these include other *Bacteroides*, *Fusobacteria* and some *anaerobic cocci* such as peptostreptococci and micro-aerophilic streptococci. Anaerobic organisms often cause wound infection, abscesses and septicaemia in patients who had abdominal surgery or intestinal perforation. Antibiotic sensitivity is restricted; metronidazole is very useful, since it is well absorbed orally or rectally and *B. fragilis* is usually sensitive to it. Clindamycin is also useful.

Mixed infections

Infection may involved several different bacteria including anaerobes. Abscesses associated with the bowel, especially the colon, or vagina are examples and, less obviously, cerebral patients. Some tissue infections, especially in debilitated patients, may also contain multiple pathogens. Severe stomatitis, one from of which is known as *Vincent's angina*, commonly occurs in malnourished patients with poor dental hygiene. The pathogens responsible are members of the normal mouth flora, including anaerobes and spirochaetes which are sensitive to penicillin. Metronidazole is an alternative.

Necrotising fasciitis is a rapidly spreading subcutaneous infection; it results in extensive necrosis, which may involve any part of the body but most often involves the periphery, particularly in diabetic patients, and the perineum. Scrotal infection is called *Fournier's gangrene*. The organisms involved are mixed anaerobic bacteria, mainly *Bacteroides* or peptostreptococci. Treatment is by a combination of aggressive surgery and antibiotics aimed mainly at anaerobes.

MYCOBACTERIA

Mycobacteria are classified as a group because they contain mycolic acids. They are bacilli which are mostly slow-growing and able to survive within macrophages. On staining by the Ziehl-Neelsen method they are acid- and alcohol-fast. The most important pathogens within the group are *Mycobacterium tuberculosis* and *M. leprae*.

Tuberculosis is now uncommon in the Western world but still a major problem in less developed countries. The disease is discussed fully on page 471. *M. bovis* is rarely incriminated now but can cause similar disease. Other mycobacteria, sometimes called atypical, such as *M. kansasii*, are less pathogenic than *M. tuberculosis* but can cause disease. *M. avium intracellulare* has become more familiar in recent years because it is one of the infection which afflict patients with AIDS. Mycobacteria other than *M. tuberculosis* are often resistant to standard antituberculous drugs, so their treatment presents difficult problems in immunocompromised patients.

LEPROSY

Leprosy is a chronic infection of skin and cutaneous nerves caused by *M. leprae*. The manifestation in the patient may be localised or generalised, and are determined largely by the host response to the infecting organism.

Aetiology

M. leprae is an acid-fast bacillus. It cannot be cultured in vitro. Ziehl-Neelsen staining of smears of the organism differentiates viable (solid staining) from granular (non-viable) organisms. In man the cooler superficial regions of the body are the preferred sites for bacterial proliferation. The generation time is about 13 days.

Distribution and incidence

Leprosy is mainly a disease of the tropics and subtropics (Fig. 11.16). It is relatively common is Africa and Asia with a prevalence of 2–9 per 1000 in most areas and higher rates in a few countries. Lepromin skin test positivity rates in endemic areas are much higher than rates of clinical cases, suggesting that host factors do much to influence to outcome of the disease. The disease has almost completely disappeared from Europe.

Transmission and epidemiology

There is little evidence to support skin-skin contact as the route of infection. Aerosol spread from the upper respiratory tract of patients with multibacillary (lepromatous) leprosy may be a source of infection.

There is considerable variation in the course of infection from person to person, and the majority of those infected develop no clinical disease.

Among those developing clinical disease there appears to be a racial variation in the type of leprosy occurring: up

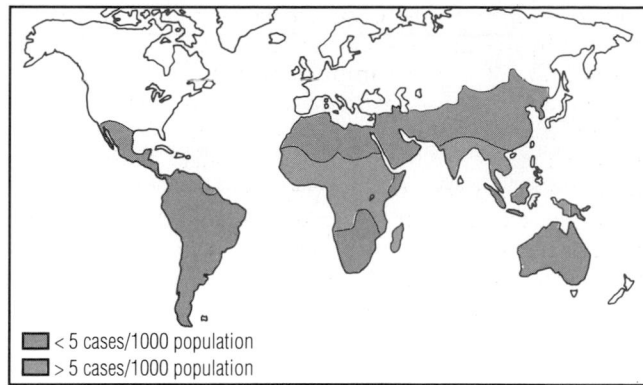

Fig. 11.16 Geographical distribution of leprosy.

to 50% of cases in Asia have lepromatous disease, compared with 10% in Africa. The male-to female ratio is 2:1 in adults and unity in children.

Pathogenesis and pathology

The host's cellular immune response determine the outcome of infection. If macrophages are able to kill the infecting organisms there is either no clinical disease or the lesions of indeterminate leprosy at most (Fig. 11.17). Those in whom the infection progresses further develop one of the forms of disease described in Table 11.26 and classified as one of the following:

- tuberculoid (TT)
- borderline tuberculoid (BT)
- borderline (BB)
- borderline lepromatous (BL)
- lepromatous (LL).

Few bacilli are found in the tuberculoid forms while large numbers are found in patients with lepromatous leprosy. Host cellular responses to mycobacterial antigens determine the form of disease that develops, with delayed type *hypersensitivity* at the tuberculoid end of the spectrum and anergy at the lepromatous end. The borderline forms are immunologically unstable and without treatment will deteriorate to the lepromatous end of the spectrum.

The earliest lesions in leprosy begins in cutaneous nerves. The most severe damage to nerves is seen in TT leprosy. At the lepromatous end of the spectrum the involved nerves are not so large. The auriculo-temporal, ulnar, median, radial cutaneous, lateral popliteal and sural nerves are preferentially involved at sites where the nerve trunks are close to the skin and therefore cooler.

The bacterial load and the morphology of the organisms need to be assessed, initially for classification purposes and subsequently to determine the response to treatment. Slit skin smears are obtained from the edges of lesions. Numbers of bacilli and their viability can be graded. Lepromin is a skin test antigen obtained from *M. leprae*. The antigen is injected intradermally, and the test is read at 3 weeks, when a nodule at the site of injection indicates a positive response supporting a classification at the tuberculoid end of the spectrum.

Two types of acute reaction are recognised in leprosy:

- *Erythema nodosum leprosum* (ENL) is an immune-complex-mediated vasculitis occurring in LL patients and, less often, in BL, either while on treatment or in the untreated patient. The inflammation with oedema and a prominent infiltrate of neutrophils.
- A *reversal reaction* indicates a change in cellular responsiveness to the infecting organism, either increasing or decreasing responsiveness. Skin lesions and affected nerves become more inflamed. The swollen lesion resolves completely in time, becoming smaller in 'upgrading' and bigger with 'down-grading'.

Clinical features

Indeterminate leprosy

Indeterminate leprosy is manifest as a hypopigmented macule on a dark skin, and as a slightly reddened macule on a light skin, with either normal or mildly reduced

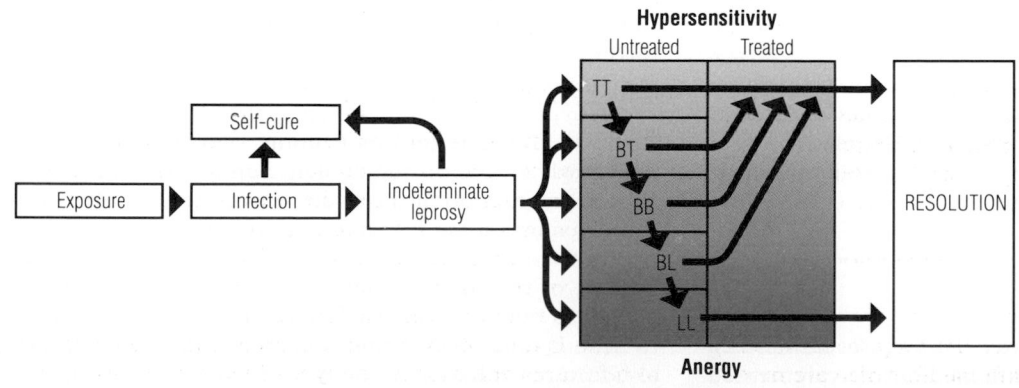

Fig. 11.17 Evolution of leprosy lesions with and without treatment. (TT = tuberculoid; BT = borderline tuberculoid; BB = borderline; BL = borderline leppromatous; LL = lepromatous) (After Ridley D S 1977 Skin Biopsy in Leprosy. Ciba-Geigy, Basle.)

11 Infectious, Tropical and Parasitic Diseases

Table 11.26 Major features in leprosy

Feature	Tuberculoid leprosy (TT)	Borderline leprosy (BB)	Lepromatous leprosy (LL)
Lesions	Few (1–3)	More numerous	Large numbers
Nerve involvement	Local	Present in nerves of predilection	Diffuse, symmetrical late in disease
Numbers of bacilli	Fragmented only	Viable bacilli present in lesions	Vast numbers of viable bacilli
Lepromin test	+++	–	–
Reactions			
Upgrading/ downgrading	–	+++	–
Erythema nodosum leprosum (ENL)	–	–	+++

sensation. There lesions may regress spontaneously or progress to one of the stages described below.

Tuberculoid leprosy

Tuberculoid leprosy (TT) is characterised by a hairless, hypopigmented, anaesthetic lesion with a flat centre and a well-defined, raised edge with minimal inflammation. The skin of the lesion does not sweat. Single lesions are usual but up to three may be found. Common sites are the extensor aspect of the arm, around the elbow and the knee. A thickened cutaneous nerve supplying the affected area may be felt. The examiner should run his/her finger over the nerve trunk in a direction at right angles to that of the nerve trunk. Neural TT leprosy occurs with a single thickened nerve as the only physical sign.

Borderline tuberculoid leprosy

Borderline tuberculoid (BT) lesions are similar to those of TT but more numerous and asymmetrically distributed. The edges of the lesions are inflamed and irregular. The nerves preferentially involved in leprosy are usually thickened and damaged, causing anaesthesia, loss of function and deformity to a variable extend in hands and feet. Penetrating ulcers in the soles of the feet, burns and skin sepsis are often present. There may be osteomyelitis of the bones of the feet due to an infected penetrating ulcer.

Borderline leprosy

Borderline leprosy (BB) produces multiple lesions that vary in form, size and shape. Papules, plaques and lesions with elevated wide outer rims and depressed, well-defined, anaesthetic centres are seen. The lesions may be hypopigmented or hyperpigmented. There is diffuse involvement of the peripheral nerves.

Borderline lepromatous leprosy

Borderline lepromatous leprosy (BL) causes numerous, asymmetrically distributed, inflamed or hyperpigmented lesions which may be papules, nodules or plaques. Sensation over the lesions may be normal. Vague macules that ary in size are present in some patients. Peripheral nerves may only show slight enlargement.

Lepromatous leprosy

Lepromatous leprosy (LL) is associated with numerous symmetrically distributed skin lesions. At the earliest stage, numerous slightly reddened hypopigmented macules and nodules occur. There evolve into papules and plaques without treatment. The eyebrows are lost and the skin of the face and ears becomes diffusely thickened (leonine facies). Involvement of the nasal mucosae may block the nose and cause a bloodstained nasal discharged. Destruction of the nasal cartilage may occur later. Iritis and keratitis are often present. The voice may later because of inflammation and thickening of the laryngeal mucosa. Testicular atrophy and gynaecomastia occur because of testicular damage. Bilateral oedema if the legs is often present. Nerve involvement occurs late in the course of the disease. Renal failure due to glomerulonephritis and amyloid disease are late complications in LL.

Reactional states

The skin lesions and involved nerves become more inflamed and swollen in *reversal reactions*. There reactions may also be accompanied by swelling of face, hands and feet. Involved nerves become very tender, often with further deterioration in function. This type of reaction may persist for 2–3 months before subsiding.

ENL produces acute inflammation of existing skin lesion in BL. The lesions become swollen and painful and slowly evolve through a livid appearance to residual hyperpigmentation of the affected skin. Bullae form over some lesions, these ulcerate and are slow to heal. New papules appear in LL cases, typically on the extensor aspects of the limbs. They may evolve over 2–3 days, through a bullous stage, to indolent ulcers which are slow to heal. Uveitis, lymphadenitis, orchitis and neuritis are also features of ENL.

Diagnosis

Diagnosis is based on the clinical features, characteristic histology, a positive lepromin test (at the tuberculoid end of the spectrum) and acid-fast bacilli in slit skin smears taken from the edge of lesions and other sites, the ear lobes, elbows and knees (BB and LL). In pure neural leprosy the diagnosis can be made from a biopsy of a few fascicles of an effected distal cutaneous nerve with no motor functions, such as the radial cutaneous nerve at the wrists, or sural nerve.

Management

Multidrug therapy is now the rule and the current WHO recommendations are set out in Table 11.27. These drugs are generally well tolerated. Dapsone occasionally causes haemolysis. Clofazimine may stain the skin a rather reddish hue. Ethionamide and prothionamide may cause hepatitis.

Mild upgrading reactions may be controlled with aspirin or non-steroidal anti-inflammatory drugs. More severe reactions that threaten nerve function require oral steroids. ENL may be controlled by steroids but sometimes thalidomide is needed.

The patient needs careful instruction regarding the care of hands and feet, prevention of cracking and infection of the skin of the feet and appropriate footwear. Where the cornea is exposed as a result of facial nerve palsy, early lateral tarsorrhaphy is essential to prevent corneal damage. Tendon transplants may help in managing foot and hand deformities.

Prevention and control

There is still a considerable stigma attached to leprosy; this is based on ignorance. Education of the public regarding the disease and the efficacy of treatment is being attempted. BCG vaccination reduces the incidence of leprosy. Currently there are efforts to define protective antigens which may result in a genetically engineered vaccine.

MYCOBACTERIUM ULCERANS

M. ulcerans causes chronic ulceration, usually on an exposed area of the body, often the lower limbs. The condition has a wide distribution in the tropics and is often called *Buruli ulcer*. The lesion may begin as a subcutaneous nodule which ulcerates through the skin. Lateral, subcutaneous extension produces an ulcer with markedly undermined edges. The organisms (acid-fast bacilli) are numerous and can be grown in Löwenstein-Jensen medium at 30–33°C.

Prior to ulceration, rifampicin is of help. Local heat will encourage healing, as the bacteria are killed by temperatures over 33°C. When the lesion affects a region near to a joint, active and passive movement of the joint must be encouraged to prevent contractures.

SPIROCHAETES

SYPHILIS

Spyhilis is caused by *Treponema pallidum* (TP), one of a small group of treponemes. TP is a bacterium 6–15 μm in length, and is narrow, with regular tight spirals, and mobile in all axes. Transmission is usually by sexual contact although transplacental infection may occur. Exposure to moist mucosal or cutaneous surfaces is required; transmission is commonly during the first 1–4 years of infection.

The incidence of syphilis in England and Wales fell after the introduction of antibiotic therapy but there was a resurgence during the 1970s in males (Fig. 11.18). There cases were mainly in homosexual men with numerous sexual partners. More recently there has been a decline in the incidence of syphilis.

Table 11.27 Treatment of leprosy

Type	Drugs
Paucibacillary Tuberculoid (TT) and borderline tuberculoid (BT)	Rifampicin, 600 mg monthly, supervised + dapsone, 100 mg daily, unsupervised both for 6 months
Multibacillary Borderline (BB), borderline lepromatous (BL), lepromatous (LL)	Rifampicin, 600 mg monthly, supervised + dapsone, 100 mg daily, unsupervised + clofazimine, 300 mg monthly, supervised + clofazimine, 50 mg daily, unsupervised
	Ethionamide or prothionamide may also be added. All drugs are continued for 2 years from time of diagnosis and thereafter until slit skin smears contain no bacilli

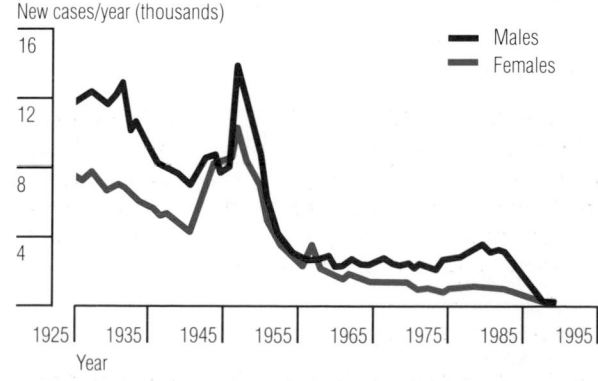

Fig. 11.18 **Incidence of syphilis in England and Wales, 1925–1990.**

Clinical features

There may be signs of active infection, or the disease may be latent. Clinically, syphilis may be divided into four stages: primary, secondary, tertiary and quaternary.

Primary

The primary lesion is a chancre, which starts as a painless pink papule and may develop into an ulcer. The ulcer has a button-like feel on palpation. The base is initially pink and shiny, becoming grey later. Painless inguinal lymphadenopathy is common and may be uniteral. On occasions the chancres may be multiple and painful. A chancre usually appears about 3 weeks after exposure to infection (range 10–90 days), and heals. Men, especially homosexual men, are infected more often than women.

In the male the common genital sites of infection are coronal sulcus, glans penis and prepuce. In the female chancres may be found in the vagina, and on the labia, fourchette and cervix.

In both sexes infections can occur in the pharynx and anus. In the anal area a chancre resembles a fissure and may be painful. Chancres, because they can be small and painful, are often missed.

Secondary

The secondary stage may take 3 months or more to appear after infection (average 6 weeks). At this stage there is a bacteraemia. Systemic upset is common, including low-grade fever, malaise, headache, generalised lymphadenopathy including epitrochlear glands, and rarely hepatosplenomegaly and transient proteinuria. Arthragia, acute meningitis and cranial nerve palsies are rare features.

The skin is most frequently involved; a non-pruritic rash is common. The lesions are usually papules or plaques and early on tend to be symmetrical and widespread. The palms, soles and face are often involved. Scalling is common and the lesions can resemble proriasis. Later lesions tend to be fewer and asymmetrical. Patchy

```
+--------------------------------------------------+
| Summary 6  Sites of involvement in secondary     |
|            syphilis                              |
+--------------------------------------------------+
| The proportion of cases is given in parentheses  |
|                                                  |
| Skin (90%)                                       |
| Lymph glands (50%)                               |
| Mouth and throat (35%)                           |
| CNS                                              |
|     symptomatic (20%)                            |
|     asymptomatic (2%)                            |
| Kidneys (Rare)                                   |
| Gastrointestinal tract and liver (Rare)          |
| Bones and joints (Rare)                          |
+--------------------------------------------------+
```

and partial hair loss can occur, giving a moth-eaten appearance. Other signs include patchy alopecia, erosive lesions of the mucous membranes (mucous patches) common in the mouth, and soft, flat-topped and highly infectious warts found in the perianal area, known as condylomata lata. At this stage all tests for syphilis are positive. The venereal disease research laboratory slide test (VDRL, see below) shows a very high titre.

Latent period

Syphilis, if untreated, will go into a latent phase, when clinical symptoms and signs are absent, approximately 2 years after the initial infection. Before this, there may be periods of infectivity; over 90% occur in the first year. There relapses may be characterised by rashes and lymphadenopathy. During the latent phase, sexual transmission is rare, although feto-maternal transmission may occur. Transplacental passage becomes unlikely in late latent syphilis. The VDRL will be negative or have a very low titre, e.g. 1:8. The *T. pallidum* haemagglutination assay (TPHA) and fluorescent treponemal antibody absorption test (FTA-Abs) – see below – are always positive.

Late (tertiary) syphilis

Tertiary syphilis is now rare, since effective treatment prevents progression.

The characteristic pathological lesion at this stage is a gumma, which is a destructive granuloma sometimes associated with vasculitis. Treponemes are very scanty and not usually seen under the microscope. Gummas can involve any organ. They cause punched-out skin ulcers, and may destroy the nasal septum. Lesions in bones and joints lead to fractures and joint destruction. Liver involvement causes fever and local tenderness. Gummas respond remarkably rapidly to treatment.

Quaternary

Quaternary syphilis is either neurosyphilis (p. 970) or cardiovascular syphilis, which is due to endarteritis obliterans of the vasa vasorum of the aorta. This causes aneurysm, most commonly of the ascending aorta (p. 438)

Congenital syphilis

TP crosses the placenta after the third month of pregnancy, usually when the mother has early disease. If she is not treated, infection of the fetus may cause abortion, stillbirth or the birth of a child with congenital syphilis. The child may have signs of infection at birth, similar to those of secondary syphilis in adults, or may be asymptomatic but develop signs of late congenital syphilis, equivalent to adult tertiary, after the age of 2 years. The predominant signs in early presentation are snuffles and rash which may vesiculate.

Possible late signs are facial abnormalities, including frontal bosses, saddle nose, protruding mandible, Hutchinson's incisors (peg-shaped, splayed), interstitial keratitis, eighth nerve deafness, periostitis and Clutton's joints, juvenile neurosyphilis, and paroxysmal cold haemoglobinuria.

As in adult syphilis diagnosis depends on serology in the later stages.

Diagnosis

Primary syphilis is diagnosis by identifying TP with dark ground microscopy. TP can be identified in serous exudate from the surface of the chancre. A negative result does not exclude the diagnosis, as topical (e.g. antibiotic ointments) or systemic therapy may alter the findings. The FTA-Abs is positive in approximately 70% of cases at this stage.

Later stages require serological testing for confirmation of the diagnosis. Serological examination of the CSF is necessary if neurosyphilis is suspected. Antibodies to treponemal antigens are present, i.e. positive TPHA and FTA-Abs, in 80% of cases of primary syphilis.

Two types of antibody tests are employed (Table 11.28):

● *Non-treponemal tests* (e.g. VDRL; rapid plasma reagin card test or RPR). These detect cardiolipin antibodies in serum. A high titre indicates an active infection. They become negative after therapy or during the latent phase of untreated syphilis. False positive results may be found in acute febrile illness, autoimmune diseases and after immunisations.

Table 11.28 Serological tests for syphilis

Disease/stage	Test		
	VDRL or RPR*	TPHA[†]	FTA-Abs[†]
Primary syphilis	Negative	Positive/negative	Positive
Secondary syphilis	>1:64	Positive	Positive
Latent (over 2 years) syphilis	<1:16	Positive	Positive
Latent (over 2 years) late syphilis	Negtive/<1:2	Positive	Positive
Yaws	Negative/<1:2	Positive	Positive
Treated syphilis	Negative/<1:2	Positive	Positive

* Tests for cardiolipin antibodies: VDRL = Venereal Disease Research Laboratory slide test; RPR = rapid plasma reagin card test.
[†] Tests specific for treponemal antibodies: FTA-Abs = fluorescent treponemal antibody absorption test; TPHA = *T. pallidum* haemagglutination assay

Table 11.29 Treatment of syphilis

Stage	Drug*	Dose and route[†]	Duration (days)
Early (incl. latent for under 1 year)	Procaine penicillin	600–1200 mg/day, IM	14
Late (incl. latent for over 1 year)	Procaine penicillin	600–1200 mg/day, IM	21
Congenital	Procaine penicillin	30 mg/kg per day, IM	10
Penicillin-allergic patients			
Early	Oxytetracycline	500 mg 4 times/day, O	15
Late	Oxytetracycline	500 mg 4 times/day, O,	30

* Probenicid is usually added for treatment of neurosyphilis and cardiovascular syphilis.
[†] 1 megaunit penicillin = 600 mg; IM = intramuscular, O = oral

● Trepnemal tests (e.g. FTA-Abs; TPHA). These detect antibodies against the treponemal antigen. They are positive earlier in the infection, but remain positive after therapy and in latent syphilis.

Yaws, another treponemal disease caused by *T. pertenue* (see below), gives a serological picture similar to that of untreated syphilis. Careful history is necessary to differentiate the cause, and if doubt about the diagnosis persists, treatment for syphilis is given.

Management

Table 11.29 shows acceptable treatment regimens.

Benzathine penicillin does not effectively cross the blood-brain barrier. Patients may, but do not commonly, experience Jarisch-Herxheimer reaction (a transient fever) 1–2 hours after the first does of penicillin. This reaction is more commonly seen in secondary syphilis.

In cardiovascular syphilis the inflammatory response to antibiotic therapy may result in small vessel occlusion in the coronary ostia. The use of prednisolone (24 hours before and up to 48 hours after commencing therapy) may prevent this. Serological examinations are repeated for at least 1 year after treatment. This is of especial value in primary and secondary syphilis. Tracing the partners of patients is an integral part of treatment.

If the erythromycin regimen is used for a pregnant patient, it is always advisable to treat the baby at birth with procaine penicillin (30 mg/kg daily for 10 days). Since erythromycin is not a fully reliable treatment, the mother should be treated with doxycycline after delivery; doxycycline is, of course, contra-indicated during breast-feeding.

YAWS

Yaws is a chronic infection due to *Treponemal pertenue*; it is characterised by a primary site of skin infection, with later dissemination to other cutaneous sites and perosteum. Unlike syphilis, cardiovascular and nervous systems are not affected and congenital infection does not occur.

Distribution, incidence and transmission

Following mass eradication campaigns, yaws became very uncommon, but there has been a resurgence of cases in South America, West and Central Africa, Indonesia and the Pacific region. The organism must be introduced into the skin by contact between an infective lesion and an abrasion in the skin of the recipient.

Clinical features

The primary papilomatous lesion or 'mother yaw' develops at the site of infection. This lesion is highly infectious. Other forms are a localised area of dry papules or a localised maculopapular rash. Regional lymp nodes are often enlarged. Secondary infectious lesions appear within a few weeks, either before or after the primary lesion has healed. Rashed continue to appear over the next 5 years. Condylomata form at moist sites, and are highly infectious. Later periostitis may occur, affecting fingers, tibia (causing sabre tibia) and nose (a destructive lesion called gangosa). Painful, deep fissures in the soles of the feet also occur.

Diagnosis and management

The organisms are readily found in serous material from primary and secondary lesions examined by dark ground microscopy. Serological tests for syphilis are positive.

Penicillin aluminium monostearate is very effective given once only in a single does of 1.5 g (0.75 g for children under 10 years). Tetracycline (2.0 g per day in divided doses for 14 days) can be used in those allergic to penicillin, apart from pregnant women and children under 8 years, who should receive erythromucin for 2 weeks.

ENDEMIC SYPHILIS (BEJEL)

Endemic syphilis is due to non-venereal infection with an organism that is intermediate between *T. pallidum* and *T. pertenue*. It is present in the desert regions of North Africa and the Middle East. Infection probably occurs by person-to-person spread among children and older females who look after children.

The first lesions are mucous patches in the mouth. Later, moist raised lesions of various sizes in axillae, groins, perineum and between the buttocks are seen. Hyperkeratotic lesions, like those of yaws, affect palms and soles. Bone involvement (periostitis) is associated with pain in the knees and shins. Destructive lesions of the nose, similar to gangosa in yaws, may occur. Congenital transmission does not occur, and late disease affecting the cardiovascular and nervous systems is very rare. Treatment with penicillin aluminium monostearate, as in yaws, is effective.

PINTA

Pinta is a treponemal infection caused by *T. carateum*. Geographically it is localised to the drier regions of Central and South America. Transmission occurs by direct contagion from infectious skin lesions, and breaks in the skin may be a route of entry for the organism.

The primary skin lesion is a papule sited on the extremities, around which smaller, similar lesions appear. Spirochaetes may be found in serous material expressed from the erythematous and violaceous lesion. Serological tests for syphilis are positive. Treatment is with a single does of benzathine penicillin (1.5 g intramuscularly, or 0.75 g for children under 10 years).

RELAPSING FEVER

Relapsing fever is an acute infectious illness caused by spirochaetes of the genus *Borrelia*. *Borrelia recurrentis* is the cause of louse-borne relapsing fever, while a range of other species cause the tick-borne variety.

Aetiology and transmission

Borrelia are spiral organisms which can be identified in peripheral blood smears using Giemsa and Leishman stains; they can also be readily identified using dark ground microscopy and cultured on artificial media.

Man is the reservoir of infection of louse-borne relapsing fever. The human body louse, *Pediculus humanus*, is the vector. Sudden mass migrations of people grouped together in adverse conditions encourage the spread of lice and louse-borne diseases, relapsing fever and typhus. Tick-borne relapsing fever is a sporadic zoonosis in man in areas where there is a cycle of transmission between ticks and wild rodents. The disease has a worldwide distribution, except for Australia and the Pacific region.

Pathogenesis and pathology

During the incubation period spirochaetes divide intravenously. Platelets are sequestered, intravascular coagulation occurs, and a bleeding tendency results. After 4–5 days of symptoms there is a crisis associated with massive phagocytosis of *Borrelia* helped by opsonising antibody. Following the crisis there is an afebrile period during which numbers of organisms expressing different surface antigens build up and symptoms recur. This can occur up to five times.

The spleen, liver, heart and brain are the main sites of pathological lesions, which consist of macrophages surrounding and ingesting large numbers of organisms.

Clinical features

After an incubation period that varies from 4 to 18 days the illness begins suddenly with rigors and a fever which rises rapidly to 40°C. Headache, joint pains, anorexia, malaise, nausea and vomiting are usual features, with mental confusion frequently present. Hepatospleno-megaly is common, with jaundice present in some patients. A petechial rash, most prominent on the trunk, is seen. Bleeding from the nose, the respiratory tract or the gut may occur, as may focal neurological signs.

The first febrile period lasts about 5 days before spontaneous defervescence. This follows a severe febrile paroxysm with cold extremities, a rising pulse rate and blood pressure, and tachypnoea. An afebrile period lasting about 7 days recurs before the first relapse.Tick-borne disease is milder than louse-borne disease. In both, death can occur during the initial rigor or during defervescence.

Diagnosis

Organisms can be found in Giemsa-stained peripheral blood smears. Dark ground microscopy can be used to demonstrate the motile spirochaetes in a fresh blood smear.

Management

Antibiotics kill spirochaetes readily. Tetracycline can be used in patients over 8 years old. Erythromycin can be used in pregnant women and young children. Louse-borne relapsing fever requires a single dose of 500 mg of either drug. Tick-borne relapsing fever requires treatment for 10 days.

Supportive care is needed, particularly in patients with louse-borne disease, as they can develop severe reactions after being treated. Central venous pressure monitoring is essential if facilities are available. Hypoxia is corrected by giving oxygen continuously. Vitamin K is given if the prothrombin time is prolonged.

Prevention

Delousing by washing with soap and water, followed by dusting with 10% DDT, is effective. Clothes should be washed with soap in water at 55°C to kill live and nits (lice eggs) which are found in the seams of clothes. Lice cannot survive on a person who has two sets of clothes worm on alternate weeks.

LYME DISEASE

Lyme disease is due to infection with *Borrelia burgdorferi*, transmitted by the tick *Ixodes dammini*. It is described on page 1013.

LEPTOSPIRAL INFECTION

Infections with *Leptospira icterohaemorrhagiae* is discussed on page 653.

ACTINOMYCOSES

Actinomyces species, despite their name, are bacteria which are often confused with fungi because of their fila-mentous appearance and their propensity to produce chronic suppurative infection with sinuses discharging purulent material. Most human disease is caused by *Actinomyces israelii*, an oral commensal, and occurs in the presence of chronic lack of dental hygiene. The characteristic pathological feature is that tissue boundaries are crossed and bone is infected. There is a fibrotic reaction around suppurating areas, which accounts for the indura-tion detected in palpable lesions. Three major forms of disease occur: cervicofacial, thoracic and disseminated actinomycosis.

In *cervicofacial actinomycosis* the characteristic lesion is a painless swelling below the border of the mandible, bluish, fluctuant and slowly enlarging. Sometimes the abscess is painful and is usually apparent long before there is any spontaneous discharge.

Thoracic actinomycosis may result from aspiration of oral debris, or may occur after thoracic surgery; it is easily confused with carcinoma. The chest radiograph shows unilateral consolidation with evidence of chest wall involvement. Nowadays the disease is usually diagnosed before discharging sinuses develop.

Actinomycosis may become *disseminated* haemato-genously. Lesions may occur at almost any site. The

---

Summary 7 Actinomycosis

- Cervicofacial form associated with poor dental hygiene
- Thoracic form may follow surgery
- Adbominal form is usually ileocaecal
- Discharging sinuses occur
- Prolonged penicillin treatment is needed

abdomen is the most common, usually in the ileocaecal region. Because of the chronic course and difficulty in diagnosis, sinus or fistula formation is still seen in abdominal actinomycosis.

Diagnosis and management

Microscopy of tissues reveals the Gram-positive organisms, with surrounding acute or chronic inflammatory reaction and foamy macrophages. The organism can be cultured from tissues and rarely from blood.

Penicillin is the drug of choice and *prolonged* treatment is necessary, with intravenous treatment for 4–6 weeks, followed by oral treatment for at least 6 months. Tetracycline, erythromycin and choramphenicol are alternatives in penicillin-allergic subjects.

MADUROMYCOSES

Maduromycosis is a descriptive term for a group of chronic infections of the subcutaneous tissues and bone of the limbs. Two groups of organisms cause this condition:

- *actinomycetes*, causing 60% of cases, which are bacteria and response to antibiotics
- true fungi such as *Madurella mycetomatis* which are almost totally unresponsive to antifungal drugs.

These two groups of organisms are found in the soil and enter the skin by penetrating injuries.

Pathology and clinical features

The main features are chronic inflammation with microabscesses and granulomatous reactions around collections of the organisms. Sinuses form and organisms are extruded. There may be localised erosion of bone. Infection spread along fascial tissue planes. Progressive destruction of affected tissue occurs.

Investigations and management

The most important investigation is an adequate surgical biopsy of diseased tissue. This specimen is divided to give samples for histology and culture for the two groups of organisms.

Actinomycetoma responds well to prolonged courses of antibiotics. Co-trimoxazole for 9 months, plus streptomycin for the first 2 months, is effective. Fungi respond poorly to antifungal drug, even though there may be in vitro sensitivity. Wide local excision with grafting may be effective in early lesions, but amputation is necessary in more advenced cases.

NOCARDIOSES

Nocardiosis is a systemic infection due to species of *Nocardia* (*N. asteroides* and, less often, *N. brasiliensis* and *N. caviae*). *N. brasiliensis* is the common cause of actinomycetoma in the tropics and subtropics. *Nocardia* are higher bacteria which exist in a filamentous and coccobacillary form, depending on culture conditions.

Aetiology, pathogenesis and epidemiology

Nocardia are aerobic, filamentous, branching Gram-positive bacteria and grow well on standard culture media. The organisms are found in rotting vegetation, and infection is acquired by inhalation in most cases, although inoculation in the skin occurs. Initial pulmonary lesions may lead to dissemination of infection by the bloodstream. Necrosis and suppuration are the typical pathological changes.

Adults are most often affected. Infection mainly occurs in immunosuppressed individuals.

Clinical features

Acute and sometimes fulminant or chronic suppurative pulmonary disease occurs in nocardiosis. Fever, cough with viscid sputum, night sweats and weight loss are usual features. Pleural thickening and empyema may develop, and the affected lung may cavitate. Haematogenous dissemination to cause brain abscess, kidney lesions, bone lesions and subcutaneous sepsis is reported.

Actinomycetoma due to Nocardia presents with longstanding swelling of the extremity, most often foot or ankle, and sinuses discharging on to the skin.

Diagnosis

Diagnosis depends on finding the organism in discharges, exudates, bronchial washing or biopsy sections. *Nocardia* grow well on media used for growing tubercle bacilli and on Sabouraud's medium. Serological tests are of help in diagnosis and can give information about the response to treatment. An adequate deep biopsy will give the best chance of isolating the organism concerned.

Management

A sulphonamide is given in combination with trimethoprim (co-trimoxazole) or with ampicillin or erythromycin. Prolonged treatment (6–12 months) is needed, continuing for 6 weeks after apparent resolution of the condition.

SYSTEMIC MYCOSES

Mycosis are infections caused by organisms classified morphologically as yeasts or filamentous fungi. Yeasts are round or oval and reproduce by budding. Filamentous fungi grow by branching and longitudinal extension of hyphae. This is not a simple distinction, as several organisms can grow in either form, depending on conditions.

CANDIDA INFECTIONS

The range of disease caused by *Candida albicans* is very broad. It is a common commensal of the oral and vaginal mucosae at one extreme. At the other it can cause pneumonia, endocarditis, septicaemia and death.

Candida can become a pathogen on damaged skin, in severely ill patients, in patients who have specific immune deficiency, especially AIDS, and in patients receiving broad-spectrum antibiotics when the local microbial ecology is disturbed. Both cell-mediated and humoral immunity participate in control of *Candida*. Inherited deficiency of T cell function causes severe but localised disease. In combined immune deficiency the infection becomes disseminated. Severely ill patients under intensive care frequently have a mixed immune deficiency and are also receiving antibiotics which predispose to *Candida* infection. Disseminated infections are also seen in intravenous drug abusers. Cutaneous and mucosal surface candidiasis is described in Chapter 25.

Diagnosis of systemic Candida infection

Candida septicaemia is often a terminal event and over half of patients are diagnosed at post-mortem. Clinical signs are usually minimal, but there may be *endophthalmitis* with fluffy yellow/white retinal spots resembling cotton-wool spots, or small *abscesses* may be detected elsewhere, such as in the liver, where ultrasound-guided biopsy or aspiration can clinch the diagnosis. *Pulmonary infiltrates* may occur on chest X-ray, with *Candida* in bronchial washings. Isolation of *Candida* from a single site on one occasion does not necessarily indicate serious infection, even when it comes from a blood culture. The judgement that *Candida* is responsible for disease manifestations remains clinical. In view of the difficulty in diagnosis, treatment is given for disseminated Candida infection if *Candida* is cultured from more than one site in a severely ill patient in whom there is new evidence of infection (e.g. fever) but bacterial infection is judged to be unlikely.

Management

Amphotericin B administered intravenously is the only effective treatment for disseminated candidiasis. Acute toxicity with hypotension and collapse can occur so a test dose is given. The full dose is then given by slow intravenous infusion. If the blood urea level rises, treatment is withheld temporarily. Oral flucytosine is synergistic with amphotericin. Fluconazole is an alternative treatment which is less toxic.

ASPERGILLUS

Aspergillus is a less common fungal pathogen which can cause disseminated disease in terminally ill patients. However, its more common manifestations are a range of respiratory diseases, the mature of which is determined by the immune response of the host (Ch. 13).

CRYPTOCOCCOSIS

Cryptococcosis (torulosis) is a systemic infection with the yeast-like fungus *Cryptococcus neoformans*. The organism is commonly found is soil contaminated by bird droppings, notably those of pigeons. Disease occurs following inhalation of the organism, but it is unusual in immunocompetent people and currently is seen most often in patients with AIDS.

Clinical features

CNS infection causes chronic meningitis with very low-grade symptoms at presentation. Cranial nerve palsies may cause visual abnormalities, loss of acuity or diplopia, or facial weakness and numbness. The course is slow or rapidly progressive, depending in the patient's immune status. Corticosteroid therapy accelerates progression.

Respiratory infection usually occurs in the absence of CNS involvement. It is more chronic and may regress spontaneously.

Skin lesions are found in 10% of patients. The face and scalp are the most common sites of the painless lesions, which are variable nodules, sometimes ulcerating.

Diagnosis

Routine culture is often negative. In the CSF little abnormality is found, apart from a few cell, mainly lymphocytes, mildly reduced glucose compared with the blood, and slightly raised protein. The organisms are shown by India ink preparations but the most sensitive method of diagnosis is by detection of antigen in CSF and sometimes in blood.

11 Infectious, Tropical and Parasitic Diseases

Management

Amphotericin B is the most useful drug. Successful treatment is reported with some of the new triazoles such as fluconazole.

HISTOPLASMOSIS

Histoplasma capsulatum is a common environmental fungus found in the soil in a filamentous form, but it behaves as a yeast when it infects humans. It multiplies rapidly in soil containing the droppings of birds and bats, and humans are usually infected by inhalation of spores in infected dust. Infection has been shown to be common by skin test surveys in the eastern central part of the USA, but there are also scattered areas of infection in both temperate and tropical areas of the world. *H. capsulatum* var. *duboisii* is a variant found in central Africa.

H. capsulatum infects macrophages and the pathogenesis of disease is similar to that tuberculosis. Delayed hypersensitivity skin tests show that the majority of infected individuals are asymptomatic.

Clinical features of H. capsulatum

Acute pulmonary infection in normal hosts causes of febrile illness with headache, often accompanied by cough and chest pain, with malaise, myalgia and weight loss. Erythema nodosum or multiforme may occur. Symptoms usually last less than a week, but occasionally severe infection is seen following a large infecting dose and it may even be fatal. Radiological changes occur in only 25% of acute infection, with scattered pulmonary infiltrates and hilar and mediastinal lymphadenopathy. The histoplasmin skin test is not helpful in diagnosis but a complement fixation antibody test may be useful. Treatment is not usually required, as spontaneous resolution is the rule, but in severe cases amphotericin B is given intravenously for 2 or 3 weeks. Ketoconazole and itraconazole have been used successfully.

Chronic pulmonary histoplasmosis affects normal individuals with structural defects of the lung. Infection of emphysematous lesions causes chronic destructive disease in the lung apices, similar to tuberculosis. Fever may be accompanied by night sweats or one-third of patients have chest pain. Diagnosis requires repeated sputum cultures. Antibody and skin tests are usually unhelpful.

Treatment is problematic, since it is impractical to give long courses of amphotericin B intravenously, but imidazoles have now been shown to be of value. The need for treatment is judged on the basis of clinical severity.

Disseminated histoplasmosis is a rare and often fatal manifestation of infection in immunocompromised hosts. It may be acute, subacute or chronic, depending on the age of the patient (acute is more frequent in infants) and the degree of parasitisation of macrophages (more severe parasitisation causing more acute disease). Fever, hepatosplenomegaly, anaemia, leucopenia, thrombocytopenia and interstitial pneumonia are most common in the acute disseminated form. Intestinal ulceration, Addison's disease, meningitis and endocarditis in the subacute form, and oropharyngeal ulcers occur in the chronic disseminated disease. Diagnosis is by histology and culture of relevant tissues and treatment is as for the other forms of the disease but with a poorer prognosis.

Histoplasma capsulatum var. duboisii

H. capsulatum var. *duboisii* infection occurs in Africa. The route of infection is poorly defined; asymptomatic pulmonary infection, with later spread to the skin and bones or inoculation into the skin, is a possibility. Skin, subcutaneous tissues and underlying bone can be affected causing:

● superficial, cutaneous granulomas (papules or ulcers)
● subcutaneous granulomas and abscesses
● osteomyelitis with discharging sinuses which heal intermittently.

Smears from exudate or discharges show numerous large yeast cells. Histological sections of infected tissue show giant cell granulomas with the large yeast cells. Treatment with ketoconazole or amphotericin B may be needed in lesions which show no signs of regression.

COCCIDIOIDOMYCOSIS

Coccidioidomycosis is a fungal infection caused by *Coccidioides immitis*. Its distribution is confined to arid areas of the western hemisphere, including the southwest USA, Central America and some countries of South America. Dust contaminated with fungal spores is the source of infection. Granulomatous responses occur around fungal spherules, while suppurative lesions with leucocytes characterise the tissue response to endospores.

The host response to the organism determines the outcome of disease. Asymptomatic infection occurs in about three-fifths of patients and is detected by skin testing. A smaller number of those infected present with respiratory symptoms, cough, fever and chest pain, with malaise, muscle pains, night sweats and chills. A macular erythematous rash, erythema nodosum and erythema multiforme also may be seen (pp. 1141 and 1142). Radiograph appearance include pneumonitis, hilar adenopathy and pleural effusion. In most of these patients the disease resolves spontaneously. In some patients pulmonary infiltrates and systemic symptomis persist, sometimes with cavitation. The diagnosis is made by finding the endospore of the organism in material from affected lung. There is a considerable risk of laboratory infection with this organism. Serological tests are an aid to diagnosis.

Dissemination of infection from an initial site of pulmonary disease may occur. Pregnant females show increased incidence of dissemination. All tissues and organs of the body may be affected. Meningitis is one of the most severe manifestations of disseminated infection.

Amphotericin B is used in treatment. The main difficulty lies in deciding which patients will benefits from treatment. Persistent, symptomatic pulmonary infection and disseminated infection require chemotherapy.

PARACOCCIDIOIDOMYCOSIS

Paracoccidioidomycosis, or South American blastomycosis, is unrelated to coccidiodomycosis. It is caused by *Paracoccidioides brasiliensis* and occurs exclusively in the area between Mexico and Argentina. The natural environment of the pathogen is uncertain. Its mode of acquisition is probably through inhalation.

Clinical features, diagnosis and management

Adults usually present with progressive respiratory symptoms, sometimes accompanied by ulcers in the mouth and nose, dysphagia, voice changes, skin lesions and cervical lymphadenopathy.

Diagnosis is usually made by culture or histology, and treatment is with imidazole (particularly itraconazole), sulphonamides or amphotericin B.

BLASTOMYCOSIS

Blastomycosis is a primarily pulmonary disease caused by the dimorphic fungus *Blastomyces dermatitidis*. It is much less common than histoplasmosis, and it occurs mainly in the eastern USA. The organism has been isolated from soil, and infection may be by inhalation of dust.

Clinical features

Primary infection may be asymptomatic, or it may lead to an acute pneumonia which either resolves spontaneously

or progresses to chronic pulmonary disease which may be confused with tuberculosis. Extrapulmonary manifestations are caused by haematogenous spread from the lungs, and the most common is skin disease with verrucous or ulcerative lesions.

Diagnosis is by demonstration of the yeasts in sputum or other specimens, or by culture of the organism. Amphotericin B is the mainstay of therapy but imidazoles have been used successfully.

SPOROTRICHOSIS

Sporothrix schenckii is a dimorphic fungus found in soil, on plants and on plat debris. Infection is uncommon and is seen in the Americas and Africa. Disease usually results from traumatic inoculation into the skin, and the common form is a red painless papule at the site which enlarges and forms a gramulomatous plaque that commonly ulcerates. Further lesions often appear proximally along the course of the lymphatics, and regional lymph nodes can be involved. Disseminated disease is rare and usually only occurs in immunosuppressed patients.

Diagnosis is by culture of the organism from skin lesions. Cutaneous lesions are treated with oral potassium iodide, and extracutaneous disease with amphotericin B.

MUCORMYCOSIS

Mucormycoses are a group of similar diseases caused by members of the order Mucorales. The organisms are common in the environment, often growing on fruit or bread. They cause disease almost exclusively in immunosuppressed patients.

Clinical features

In rhinocerebral disease in an uncontrolled diabetic, the fungus invades the palatal, nasal and paranasal sinus mucous membranes, and destructive lesions spread directly back towards the brain. Black necrotic lesions are visible, and from these a variety of secondary bacterial pathogens are often isolated. Pulmonary, cutaneous and intestinal disease may occur.

Diagnosis is made by examination of scrapings and biopsies and cultures are often negative. Successful treatment depends on management of the underlying cause. Amphotericin B is the only useful drug in treatment, but the response is often poor.

PROTOZOAL INFECTIONS

Table 11.30 Classification of protozoa

Gut protozoa
Giardia lamblia
Crytosporidium
Entamoeba histolytica
Blastocystis hominis
Balantidium coli
Isospora belli
Sarcocystis

Genital tract protozoa
Trichomonas vaginalis

Free-giving protozoa causing human disease
Naegleria fowleri
Acanthamoeba

Non-pathogenic gut protozoa
Entamoeba coli
Entamoeba hartmanni
Endolimax nana
Iodamoeba beutschlii
Chilomastix mesnili

Tissue and blood protozoa
Toxoplasma gondii
Pneumocystic carinii
Plasmodium species
Babesia species
Trypanosoma gambiense, rhodesiense and cruzi
Leishmania species

Protozoa are single-cell organisms, and have adapted to a range of ecological niches in the human host (Table 11.30). They are a major cause of human disease, especially in Third World countries.

PROTOZOAL INFECTION OF THE GUT

GIARDIASIS

Infection with the flagellate protozoan *Giardia lamblia* can cause asymptomatic infection or diarrhoeal disease of variable severity from mild to severe with malabsorption.

Aetiology

The parasite is a flagellate, pear-shaped protozoan (Fig. 11.19), which is found in the lumen of the upper small intestine. Some trophozoites encyst to be passed in the faeces. The cyst is infective and can survive for 2 months at 8°C in water. It is resistant to normal levels of chlorination, and sand filtration is used to clear municipal water supplies of this and other parasites. The parasite can now be grown in culture.

Distribution and incidence

The distribution is worldwide, although it is more common in the tropics. It is endemic in the countries of Eastern Europe. Epidemics have occurred at day care nurseries, on cruise ships and in towns in the USA. Giardiasis is fairly common in children in some inner-city populations in Britain, and can cause diarrhoea in the elderly.

Transmission and epidemiology

Spread is by the faecal–oral route. As few as 10 cysts will cause infection, while 1000 cysts consistently cause infection. Contaminated food and water are vehicles of infection. Person-to-person spread is common in childhood, particularly when children are not toilet-trained. Mothers are often infected by changing nappies of an infected child. Any circumstances in which standards of personal and public hygiene (such as water treatment) are low lead to transmission.

In the tropics children are most often infected, although both indigenous and visiting adults can develop symptomatic disease. Male homosexuals and retarded children are other risk groups. Hypogammaglobulinaemia and reduced gastric acid secretion are host factors that increase susceptibility.

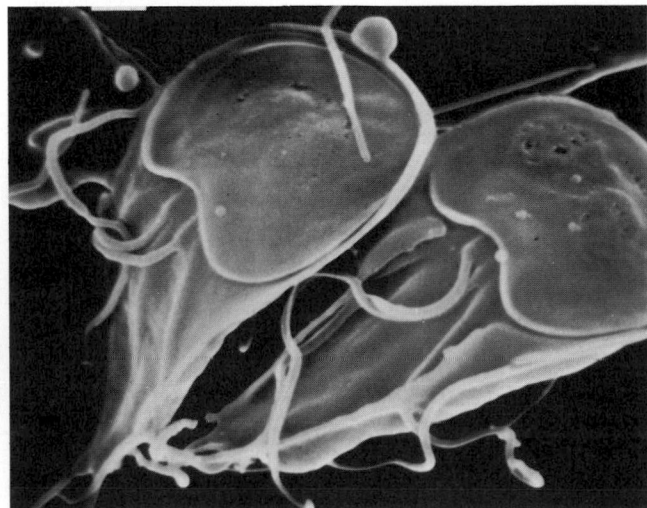

Fig. 11.19 Scanning electron micrograph of *Giardia lambia*. (Reproduced by kind permission of Dr David Warhurst.)

Pathology and pathogenesis

The main abnormalities relate to the function and morphology of the upper small intestine. Markedly symptomatic patients have impaired absorption of fat, d-xylose and vitamin B_{12}, and lactose maldigestion. The jejunal mucosa is abnormal, with a ridged or convoluted mucosa, reduced villous height with increased crypt depth, and an increased infiltrate of plasma cells in the lamina propria. Subtotal villous atrophy may occur with giardiasis but is uncommon. Patients with mild or no symptoms have normal jejunal morphology and function. Lactose maldigestion may be present.

The pathogenesis is not well understood. The parasites itself may damage the enterocyte surface membrane to impair function and fat digestion intraluminally. Jejunal colonisation with bacteria may also contribute to some of the mucosal dysfunction. Antigiardia IgA from the mucosa and in bile may control parasite numbers.

Clinical features

The incubation period is usually about 10–14 days, although it can be much longer. Many patients with giardiasis are asymptomatic or have minimal bowel upset. Acute giardiasis is characterised by the sudden onset of anorexia, nausea abdominal distension, discomfort and diarrhoea with frequent yellow, offensive, frothy stools by day and night. Lethargy is often severe and weight loss is usual. After about 3 weeks there may be the beginnings of spontaneous improvement. This may progress to complete resolution over a month while some remain mildly symptomatic, often because of continuing lactose intolerance.

Some patients remain markedly symptomatic, and fail to regain lost weight or continue to lose weight. The abdomen is distended and bowel sounds are prominent. The stools are yellow and offensive. Testing confirms malabsorption. Children are occasionally brought to medical attention because of failure to thrive. Giardiasis has been reported as a cause of chronic diarrhoea in elderly persons in the UK. It is not a major cause of diarrhoea in AIDS.

Diagnosis

Diagnosis depends on finding the parasites. Stool microscopy shows cysts in most patients, although examination of several samples may be necessary. Trophozoites may be found in diarrhoeal stools. When the parasite is not found and symptoms are marked, investigation of intestinal morphology and function is indicated. Jejunal juice and jejunal mucus obtained at the time of biopsy can be examined for trophozoites. Giardia may be seen in the intervillous space of the sections of the biopsy.

Giardia antigens can be detected in stools by immunological techniques.

Differential diagnosis

Other cause of gastroenteritis are discussed on page 224. Cryptosporidiosis causes self-limited diarrhoea in healthy persons (see below). *Campylobacter* species can cause a small bowel type of diarrhoea but usually cause systemic upset. The differential diagnosis of malabsorption syndrome is discussed in Chapter 15.

Laboratory features

Laboratory investigations show malabsorption of fat, d-xylose and vitamin B_{12} in severely affected patients. D-xylose malabsorption and lactose maldigestion may be present in those with mild symptoms. Occasional patients are seen who have marked malabsorption and folate deficiency. Barium follow-through examinations show non-specific changes, with dilatation of small bowel loops and thickened mucosal folds in patients with malabsorption.

Management

Metronidazole is the drug of first choice, given either as a low dose (200 mg 3 times a day) for 10–14 days, or as a high dose (2 g daily) for 3 days. Tinidazole is more expensive but can be given as a single dose of 2 g (50 mg/kg in children). Both drugs cause nausea in high dose and have a disulfiram-like interaction with alcohol. Asymptomatic giardiasis in pregnancy need not be treated. When there is symptomatic disease in pregnancy associated with weight loss or failure to gain weight, then metronidazole (200 mg 3 times a day for 10 days) may be given. Symptoms due to giardiasis improve rapidly after treatment. Dietary measures are sometimes helpful for continuing gut symptoms. Avoidance of alcohol, spicy foods and lactose is often helpful. Repeat stool microscopy 6–8 weeks after treatment provides a test of cure. Abnormalities in intestinal structure and function disappear over 6–12 weeks after treatment.

Prevention and control

Travellers in areas where the tap water is not safe to drink should avoid salads, uncooked foods, unpeeled fruits and ice cubes in drinks. Sterilising drinking water with 2% tincture of iodine (0.5 ml/l of water and allow to stand for 30 minutes) may be necessary. Treatment of asymptomatic cyst excretes is worthwhile, particularly in a non-endemic area, as it reduces the risk of transmission to others.

CRYPTOSPORIDIOSIS

Cryptosporidiosis is an infection of the gastrointestinal tract with the sporozoan parasite *Cryptosporidium*. It causes enteritis in man and a range of other animals. It is a zoonosis with a worldwide distribution.

Its life cycle is complex, with asexual and sexual cycles. Infection is by the faecal–oral route. Ingested oocysts are disrupted in the intestinal lumen, liberating four sporozoites which enter the apical regions of intestinal cells within a membrane-bounded vacuole. Trophozoites develop from the sporozoites and undergo asexual reproduction. Merozoites liberated by schizogony can undergo further asexual cycles, or become gametocytes which fuse to form oocysts which are passed in the faeces.

Transmission and epidemiology

Early reports recognised this organism as a gut pathogen causing persisting watery diarrhoea in immunosuppressed patients, especially those with AIDS. Later studies showed that cryptosporidiosis was associated with diarrhoea in 4–9% of otherwise healthy children and adults. Children at nursery school may transmit infection person-to-person. Susceptible animals include calves, lambs, goats and birds, although a history of contact with animals is often absent.

Clinical features

An acute watery diarrhoeal illness, often with offensive stools, is the usual history. There may be fever and vomiting. The disease is self-limiting, with a median duration of about 12 days, but prolonged diarrhoea with weight loss occurs in patients with humoral and cellular immunodeficiency states, especially AIDS.

Diagnosis and management

Faecal smears stained by the modified Ziehl-Neelsen technique shoe the pinkish-red-staining oocysts. Other forms of the parasite are seen at the luminal surface of enterocytes in intestinal biopsies.

In most patients the disease is self-limiting and symptoms resolve spontaneously in 10–12 days. There is no effective drug therapy for the chronic infection seen in AIDS patients. Rehydration, nutritional support and symptomatic treatment may be needed.

Hand washing is the most important factor in limiting the spread of infection by the person-to-person route.

AMOEBIASIS

Amoebiasis is infection with *Entamoeba histolytica*. The infection may be:

- non-invasive and confined to the lumen of the colon
- invasive, causing colonic ulceration (amoebic dysentery)
- invasive, causing amoeboma
- invasive, with spread to the liver to cause amoebic liver abscess (ALA).

Aetiology

Entamoeba histolytica has two forms, a motile trophozoite (Fig. 11.20) and an encysted trophozoite. The motile trophozoite is found in the stools of a person with amoebic dysentery and contains ingested red cells. The cyst is the effective form. It is resistant to the chlorine in potable domestic water supplies. Sand filtration is the best method of removing cysts from water.

Distribution and incidence

Amoebiasis has a worldwide distribution. It is common in those areas of the world where standards of sanitation are low. most instances of invasive disease occur either in endemic areas or in travellers who have recently been exposed. Occasional cases are seen in people who returned from endemic areas years before, or who have never left a country such as Britain.

Transmission and epidemiology

Faecal–oral spread by ingestion of amoebic cysts in contaminated food and water or on fingers or other direct

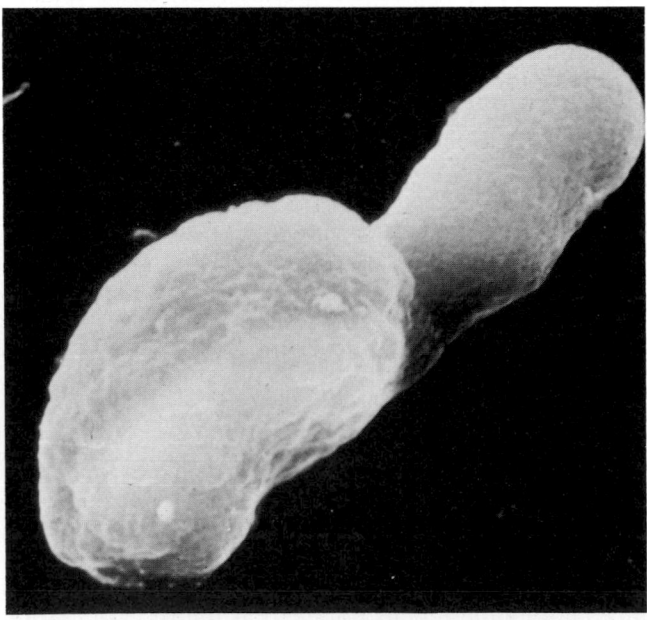

Fig. 11.20 Scanning electron micrograph of *Entamoeba histolytica*.
(Reproduced by kind permission od Dr David Warhurst.)

personal contact is the route of infection. Asymptomatic amoebiasis is not uncommon in male homosexuals in Britain with transmission by person-to-person spread, and this route of infection also occurs in the mentally retarded.

Amoebiasis is more common in adults than children. Men are affected by ALA more often than women but dysenteric disease occurs in both sexes. Invasive amoebiasis can be more severe in pregnancy.

Pathology and pathogeneosis

There are no pathological changes in asymptomatic cyst excreters. Their amoebae live on the colonic mucosa but do not invade. Not all organisms are capable of causing invasive disease, but the reasons for this are not well understood. In amoebic dysentery trophozoites invade the colonic epithelium and lyse host cells causing necrosis. Areas of the mucosa are excavated, leaving multiple flask-shaped ulcers. Amoebae are found in the slough and in the advancing edge of the lesions. The rectum and caecum are commonly affected areas, but the extent can vary from localised proctitis to a pancolitis with a diffusely inflamed ulcerated mucosa.

Amoeboma is an uncommon late complication occurring after amoebic dysentery has resolved. The lesion consists of a mass of granulation tissue containing few amoebac. The caecum is a usual site but any part can be involved and lesions may be multiple.

ALA results from the haematogenous spread of amoebae from the colonic mucosa via the portal vein. Amoebae reach the liver, and liver cells are lysed on contact with amoebae. The affected area enlarges progressively and the necrotic cells liquefy in the abscess cavity, which may be unilocular or multilocular. A single abscess in the right lobe is usual. The pus is typically odourless, pinkish-brown, sterile on culture and with few pus cells.

Clinical features

No symptoms are attributable to the commensal amoeba. In the patient with amoebic dysentery, symptoms vary according to the extent and site of colonic involvement. The usual symptoms are abdominal discomfort and increased frequency of bowel action, with softer stools. Blood may be noticed in the stools, especially when the rectum is involved. Physical signs usually consist of mild colonic tenderness. Sigmoidoscopy may show the typical appearance of scattered ulcers surrounded by mucosal erythema with normal mucosa intervening, but the mucosa may be diffusely inflamed and ulcerated. With increasingly extent of colonic disease, symptoms and signs are more marked.

Dehydration, anaemia and septicaemia may occur in severe disease, and perforation, toxic dilatation and significant haemorrhage may complicate the clinical course. Rarely the superficial part of the mucosa may be sloughed over a variable length of colon and passed per rectum. Late complications of amoebic dysentery are colonic stricture and amoeboma, where a mass of granulation tissue forms in response to the presence of relatively few amoebae. Localised pain and blood in the stools are usual symptoms and one or more masses may be felt in the abdomen or rectally.

Symptoms and signs in ALA

Symptoms and signs in ALA relate to the site and size of the abscess. There may be no history suggest past or present intestinal amoebiasis and many patients do not have amoebic cysts in their stools. Fever, swears, lethargy and anorexia are usual early symptoms and examination may reveal no abnormal physical signs, or only tenderness on springing the right lower ribcage. With larger abscesses pain becomes a more prominent feature related to the site of the abscess. Abscesses sited laterally or superiorly cause chest pain which may be pleuritic, or referred pain in the right shoulder indicating diaphragmatic irritation. Rigors occur with multiple large abscesses. Some patients have no systemic symptoms.

The liver may be enlarged and tender, with a localised tender mass on the surface. With superiorly sited abscesses, there may be dullness to percussion and impaired movement at the right lung base. Left lobe abscesses may present with symptoms and signs related to the epigastrium of left hypochondrium.

Complications

The main complication in ALA is extension outside the liver (Fig. 11.21). Spread to the brain may occur, producing a mecrotising abscess-like lesion. Rarely the skin of the perianal region is ulcerated by local extension of amoebic proctitis, and the skin of the chest or abdominal wall is involved after percutameous rupture of ALA.

Diagnosis

Cyst passers are usually diagnosed when stool microscopy is carried out during screening after overseas travel or residence, investigation of diarrhoea due to some other microbial pathogen, or examination of other groups at risk of infection, e.g. male homosexuals. Serological tests for amoebiasis are negative.

Amoebic dysentery is diagnosed by finding motile trophozoites with ingested red cells in faecal smears or scrapes from ulcerated colonic mucosa. Amoebae can be

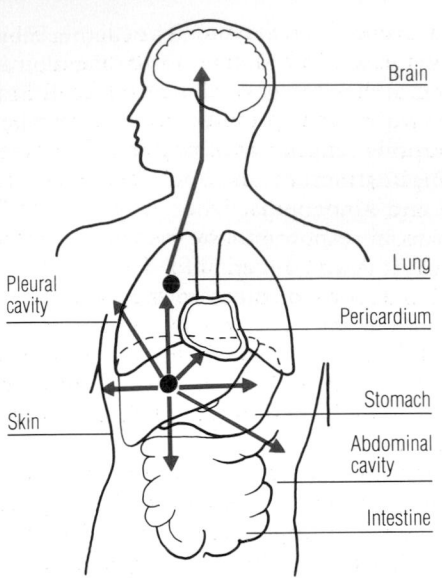

Fig. 11.21 Sites of spread of amoebic liver abscess.

Summary 8 Amoebiasis

- *Cyst passers.* Asymptomatic. Cysts in stools.
- *Amoebic dysentery.* diarrhoea, dehydration, anaemia. Motile trophozoites in faeces and scrapes from ulcers.
- *Amoebic liver abscess.* fever, pain, tendermess. Ultrasound shows abscess. Positive serology.

seen in the edges of ulcers in rectal biopsies. Serological tests for amoebiasis (e.g. indirect fluorescent antibody test, or IFA) are positive in 60% of cases. Diagnosis depends on finding the parasite.

With *amoeboma*, cysts may be found in the stools. Colonoscopy allows the lesion to be visualised and biopsied. Serology for amoebiasis is positive in over 90% of cases and is a reliable test in this situation.

Disgnosis of *ALA* depends on the clinical features suggesting an intrahepatic lesion and strongly positive amoebic serology (found in over 95% of cases). Cases seen early in the course of disease occasionally have a negative IFA but have a definitely positive test 7 days later.

Additional investigations

Intestinal disease

With increasing extend of colonic involvement there is increasing exudation of protein-rich fluid into the gut. Plasma albumin levels fall; normochromic, normocytic anaemia and a raised ESR develop. These investigations are normal in more localised disease. Barium enema studies show non-specific features with ulceration in dysentery. Amoeboma appears as one or more mass lesions causing narrowing of the colon, simulating colon cancer.

Amoebic liver abscess

There is neutrophil leucocytosis, a normochromic, normocytic anaemia and raised ESR. Bilirubin levels are usually normal, while aminotransferase levels are slightly raised; alkaline phosphatase levels are raised and plasma albumin levels are low.

A chest X-ray will show elevation of the diaphragm above an abscess in the right lobe superiorly, and sometimes basal linear atelectasis or consolidation or plueral effusion. Ultrasound scanning and CT scanning give more accurate information about and abscess, and its precise site and size. Ultrasound scanning can be repeated to assess changes and to guide insertion of a needle for percutaneous aspiration.

Differential diagnosis

Intestinal disease

Shigella, Salmonella, Campylobacter and *Yersinia* infections all may cause colitis. Non-specific inflammatory bowel disease. Crohn's colitis and ulcerative colitis must be considered. Amoebic infection should be rigorously excluded in an at-risk patient before treatment for inflammatory bowel disease, as steroids may promote rapid progression of invasive amoebiasis with perforation and death. Carcinoma of the colon, tuberculosis of the ileo-caecal region or colon, and schistosomiasis are possible causes of the colonic mass.

Amoebic liver abscess

Subphrenic and intrahepatic pyogenic abscesses cause similar symptoms and signs. Often the history is more acute and the patient more toxic with chills and rigors, but their presence does not exclude amoebic infection. Hepatocellular carcinoma and bacterial infection of a hydatid cyst may present like ALA.

Management

The drug treatment of amoebiasis is set out in Table 11.31. Symptoms and signs improve rapidly within 48 hours. Surgical treatment of amoebic dysentery is rarely needed, except where large areas of mucosa are sloughed; in this case resection of the affected colon can be like-saving.

When ALAs are very large, pointing or likely to rupture, percutaneous aspiration is needed. This is done using a large-bore needle inserted under local anaesthetic, if possible under ultrasound guidance. Variable amounts

Table 11.31 Drug treatment of amoebiasis

Clinical situation	Drug
Cyst passer	Diloxanide furoate for 10 days 500 mg 3 times a day (8 mg/kg 3 times a day)
Amoebic dysentery Amoeboma Amoebic liver abscess	Metronidazole 800 mg 3 times a day for 5–10 days (40 mg/kg per day in 3 divide doses) or Tinidazole 750 mg twice a day for 5–10 days 2 g (50 mg/kg) single for 3 days followed by Diloxanide furoate 500 mg 3 times a day (8 mg/kg 3 times a day)

of fluid can be removed. Amoebae are sometimes found in the material aspirated from the edge of the abscess. Aspiration has a low morbidity. Rupture of ALA dramatically increase the mortality, which is low in uncomplicated cases.

Preventive and control

The provision of clean water and safe disposal of faecal wastes would do much to prevent transmission. Patients with invasive amoebiasis should always receive diloxanide furoate as well as metronidazole to eradicate any pathogenic amoebae remaining in the gut lumen. Where water supplies are not treated, boiling and filtering drinking water is advised. Tincture of iodine (2%) is effective in killing amoebae used as above. Salads unpeeled fruits and ice cubes are possible sources of infection and should be avoided in endemic areas.

BALANTIDIUM COLI INFECTION

The coliate *Balantidium coli* is the largest of man's protozoan parasites. It can be seen with the naked eye in cultures. It is a parasites of pigs, and humans who have close contact with pigs become infected. It causes no disease in most infected humans. Occasional cases of enteritis affecting small and large intestine due to *B. coli* are reported. Death occurs as a result of bacterial peritonitis after ulceration and perforation of the gut. Metronidazole is effective in symptomatic cases.

ISOSPORA BELLI INFECTION

Isospora belli is a sporozoan parasite of the gastro-intestinal tract in man. It has a worldwide distribution and man is the only reservoir of infection. The life cycle has asexual and sexual phases. Infection occurs by ingestion of oocysts containing sporozoites which are released in the small intestine and invade epithelial cells; there they undergo asexual reproduction, or schizogony. The host cell ruptures, releasing merozoites which invade other epithelial cells and reproduce asexually to form oocysts. These are released into the gut lumen by the normal desquamation of epithelial cells and passed in the faeces. Infection occurs by ingesting oocysts in contaminated food and water.

Most infections cause no symptoms. Some cause a diarrhoeal illness, with weight loss, pale stools, lethargy and low-grade fever. Patients with immunodeficiency syndromes including AIDS exhibit chronic diarrhoea with more marked symptoms.

The diagnosis is made by finding oocysts in stools, jejunal juice and in stained sections of jejunal biopsies.

Co-trimoxazole appears to be effective in treatment, giving 2 tablets twice daily for 10 days. Longer courses of treatment may be needed in patients with immunodeficiency.

SARCOCYSTOSIS

The two parasites of man are *Sarcocystis bovihominis* and *S. suihominis*, which have cattle and pigs as their respective intermediate hosts. They have a worldwide distribution, with high infection rates in cattle and pigs. However, the infection is probably uncommon in man. The parasites have a complex life cycle involving both asexual and sexual reproduction.

Abdominal discomfort, distension, nausea and diarrhoea occur within hours of infection, and sporocysts are found in the stools 14–18 days later. Diagnosis is by finding the small numbers of cysts shed in the faeces.

Treatment with pyrimetamine and sulphadiazine or nitrofuranacion has been successful in patients with chronic symptoms. Freezing meat reduces the infectivity of muscle cysts, and thorough cooking of meat prevents infection.

GENITAL TRACT PROTOZOA

TRICHOMONIASIS

Trichomonas vaginalis (TV) is a pear-shaped, flagellate protozoan. It causes vaginal discharge and urethritis in women and urethritis in men. It is a sexual transmitted infection.

Clinical features

Most women with TV have an offensive vaginal discharge associated with vulvovaginal pruritus, and occasionally dysuria and dyspareunia. Clinically the vulva is erythematous and excoriated; the vaginal discharge may be seen at the introitus. The discharge is grey, yellow or green and may be frothy. Vaginal erythema and punctate haemorrhages of the cervix may be seen.

It is a rare cause of non-specific urethritis in men.

Diagnosis and management

Examination of the discharge on a wet mount is essential. The trichomonads are easily seen.

Metronidazole (200 mg 3 times a day for 7 days, or 400 mg twice daily for 5 days) is effective but recurrences are common. Sexual partners should be treated. Single doses of tinidazole (2.0 g, or 50 mg/kg) are effective only for treating male partners.

FREE-LIVING PROTOZOA CAUSING HUMAN DISEASE

NAEGLERIA FOWLERI INFECTION

Naegleria fowleri is a free-living amoebo-flagellate which causes primary amoebic meningo-encephalitis. It is found in water from hot springs as well as in ponds and pools, and has a worldwide distribution. Amoebae in fresh water are carried into the nasal passages by activities like swimming. They adhere to areas of the nasal mucosae bearing terminal filaments of the olfactory nerves, and then migrate through the cribriform plate along the nerve fibres. The amoebae replicate asexually and spread through the subarachnoid space.

Pathology

The olfactory bulbs show massive invasion with amoebae and necrotic changes. There is a superficial encephalitis of the effected area. In the meninges there is a prominent fibrinous and purulent reaction that is most marked over the inferomedial regions, with particular involvement of the basal subarachnoid cisterns. The amoebae are circular, 6–9 μ in diameter and have a fine cell membrane.

Clinical features

The patients are often children or young adults. Fever, headache, nausea, vomiting and lethargy are usual early features, followed by deterioration of conscious level. Neck stiffness is usual. Papilloedema may be present.

Lumber puncture in these patients shows features suggesting acute pyogenic meningitis. The CSF is turbid, with a very high cell count, predominantly neutrophils. Protein levels are very high and sugar levels are reduced or normal. The amoebae are readily seen on phase

contrast microscopy if a direct smear of CSF is examined. They stain well with iron haemotoxylin and can be grown in special culture media.

Management

Amphotericin B is effective in treatment, possibly in combination with miconazole. The high mortality in this condition is probably related to delay in diagnosis and initial trials of antibiotics as for pyogenic meningitis.

ACANTHAMOEBA INFECTION

Acanthamoebae are free-living amoebae. Infection may occur by ingestion or inhalation of cysts, which are very light and may be distributed on the wind.

A considerable range of clinical features has been reported for this infection. Cerebral abscess, meningitis and involvement of the scalp, orbit and middle ear have occurred. Acanthamoebae have been identified in corneal ulcers. Lung involvement has also been reported. Amoebae may be identified in smears from CSF or from corneal ulcers, or in stained tissue sections. Amphotericin B is used in systemic infections, and 5-fluorocytosine and clotrimazole can be used topically on corneal ulcers.

NON-PATHOGENIC GUT PROTOZOA

There are a number of protozoa which infect man but cause no disease. There are listed in Table 11.30. When they are found in patients with abdominal symptoms, the symptoms should not be ascribed to these parasites and further investigations should be undertaken.

TISSUE AND BLOOD PROTOZOA

TOXOPLASMOSIS

Toxoplasmosis is caused by *Toxoplasma gondii*. It is a zoonosis, the definitive host in the life cycle being cats. Primary human infection is acquired by ingestion of oocysts derived from animal excreta or from undercooked meats such as pork or mutton, the pig or sheep having acted as an intermediate host (Fig. 11.22). Infection is common, 20–40% of adults in Britain having antibodies. The most serious effects are seen after congenital infection or in immunocompromised patients.

Pathology and pathogenesis

Trophozoites released at the site of entry multiply and spread via blood and lymphatics to all tissues. They can

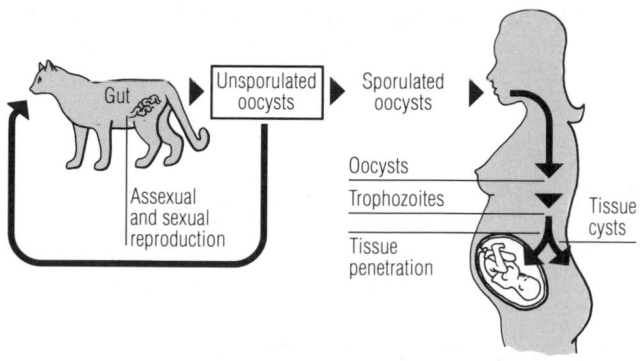

Fig. 11.22 Transmission of toxoplasmosis. Infection can occur in either sex and at any age. Reactivation causes disease in immunosuppressed patients.

invade any cells, and intracellular proliferation leads to cell death. Development if immunity results in restriction of proliferation and the organism is eliminated, or forms tissue cysts. Cysts 10–200 μ in diameter, containing several thousand organisms, may remain in the tissues for life. Depression of CMI results in reactivation.

Clinical features

Congenital infection

Congenital infection usually follows primary asymptomatic infection of the mother during the third trimester of pregnancy. The effect on the fetus may be spontaneous abortion, stillbirth, premature birth or norman birth with subsequent illness. The latter is most frequent and results in disease of the eye, usually bilateral choroidoretinitis, or of the brain, with hydrocephalus, microcephaly, cerebral calcification or convulsions. Fever, lymphadenopathy, hepatosplenomegaly and rash may also occur.

Acquired infection

Asymptomatic infection is common in adults, but there may be a mild chronic febrile illness with lymphadenopathy. Often a group of enlarged lymph nodes in a single area is the only finding, although more diffuse adenopathy may occur with splenomegaly. Sore throat does not occur. Choroidoretinitis is a rare manifestation of acquired infection.

Reactivation in the immunosuppressed patient

Most toxoplasmal disease in patients with deficient immunity is caused by reactivation of latent cysts. The most common manifestation, especially in AIDS, is necrotising lesions in the brain, often presenting as intracerebral mass lesions. Myocarditis and possibly pneumonitis also occur.

Diagnosis

This is by serology. The Sabin-Feldman dye test, indirect haemagglutination or fluorescent antibody test (FAT) are used to measure IgG antibodies, and an FAT is also available for measurement of IgM antibodies. Histology of affected lymph nodes shows reactive changes which are not specific for toxoplasmosis. The organisms are rarely seen in tissue sections. Diagnosis of cerebral lesions is by CT or MR scan.

Management

Treatment of acquired infection in normal adults does not affect outcome and is rarely required. Severe infections are treated with a combination of pyrimethamine and sulphadimidine (e.g. Sulphatriad), which are synergistic in their action against trophozoites. Pyrimethamine is a folic acid antagonist and causes bone marrow suppression, which can be prevented by concurrent administration of folinic acid. There is no treatment for tissue cysts.

PNEUMOCYSTIS CARINII INFECTION

Pneumocystic carinii is a common organism that is found worldwide. Although previously classified as a protozoan, recent evidence suggests that it may be fungal in nature. In infects the lungs and causes no problems in normal human hosts. The organism is found in autopsy material from healthy people in up to 4% of cases and serological studies in Europe have shown up to 75% seropositivity in healthy children. The reservoirs of infection and the mode of transmission are poorly defined, but it seems likely that human-to-human droplet infection occurs.

It causes interstitial pneumonitis in premature and young infants, in children with protein-energy malnutrition, in immunosuppressed patients during treatment for haematological malignancies, and in AIDS patients in the West. It is uncommon in AIDS in Africa.

In normal lung the organisms are found singly or in clusters on the alveolar septal wall, with no surrounding host response. When there is pneumonitis large numbers of parasites are found in the alveoli, with desquamation of alveolar cells and accumulation of proteinaceous material in the alveolar spaces.

Clinical features and diagnosis

The clinical features of *Pn. carinii* pneumonia are progressive dyspnoea, cough, fever and weight los. Chest examination is often normal; chest radiographs may be normal initially but progress fairly rapidly to show extensive interstitial shadowing. The diagnosis should be suspected in any immunosuppressed patients, especially those with

AIDS, and confirmation is obtained from examination of bronchial washings obtained at bronchoscopy or in sputum induced using nebulised hypertonic saline.

Management

The treatment is adequate oxygenation and vestilatory support when necessary, and chemotherapy with either high-dose co-trimoxazole (4 tablets 4 times a day) or pentamidine given by intramuscular injection or slow intravenous infusion in 250 ml of normal saline or 5% dextrose over 1–2 hours. Nebulised pentamidine is effective in treatment and prophylaxis in AIDS patients. There is no difference in outcome with either drug. Fever, rash and leucopenia have been seen in AIDS patients after about 7–10 days on co-trimoxazole, and a change to pentamidine may be necessary, as treatment for at least 21 days in required. Pentamidine side-effects include renal and hepatic failure and prolonged hypoglycaemia. There is a 20% mortality in AIDS patients in their first episode of *Pn. carinii*, irrespective of treatment. Prophylaxia with co-trimoxazole for this infection has been effective in patients with acute leukaemia. Primary prophylaxis in AIDS patients with the combination of an antifolate and a sulphonamide/sulphone may be of value, and nebulised pentamidine has also been used successfully.

MALARIA

Malaria is an acute febrile illness characterised clinically by paroxysms of fever, these are the consequence of asexual reproduction by species of *Plasmodium* within red cell (schizogony). *Plasmodium vivax*, *P. ovale* and *P. malariae* are associated with morbidity but no major mortality, while *P. falciparum* causes both morbidity and considerable mortality. The infection is transmitted by the bite of the female anopheline mosquito.

Distribution and incidence

Malaria occurs widely throughout the tropical areas of the world, in the Americas, Africa, Asia and the Pacific area (Fig. 11.23). *Falciparum* malaria is particularly common in tropical Africa, where it causes about 1 000 000 deaths per year, mainly in children. The resurgence of malaria in the Indian subcontinent was led by a rising incidence of *vivax* malaria in the 1970s, and now *falciparum* infection is more widespread in the region. *Ovale* malaria is predominantly an African disease. *Malariae* malaria is the least common form.

Malaria is imported into temperate regions by tourists, people employed overseas, business travellers and immigrants. The numbers of cases have progressively risen over the past 20 years (Fig. 11.24).

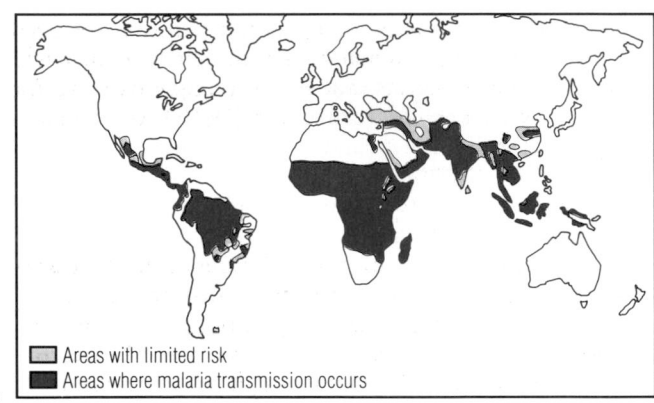

A

☐ Areas with limited risk
■ Areas where malaria transmission occurs

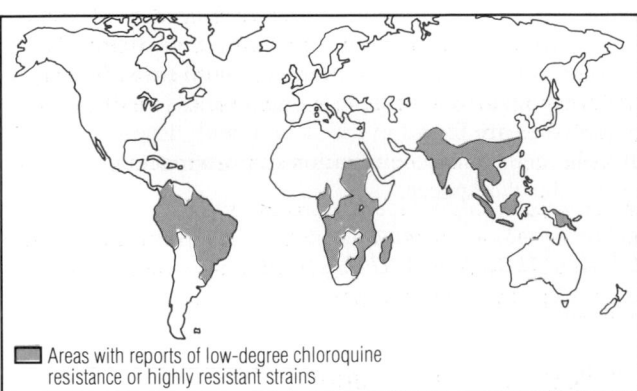

B

▨ Areas with reports of low-degree chloroquine resistance or highly resistant strains

Fig. 11.23 Malaria. World distribution of malaria, 1986. Chloroquine-resistant malaria occurs in all areas.

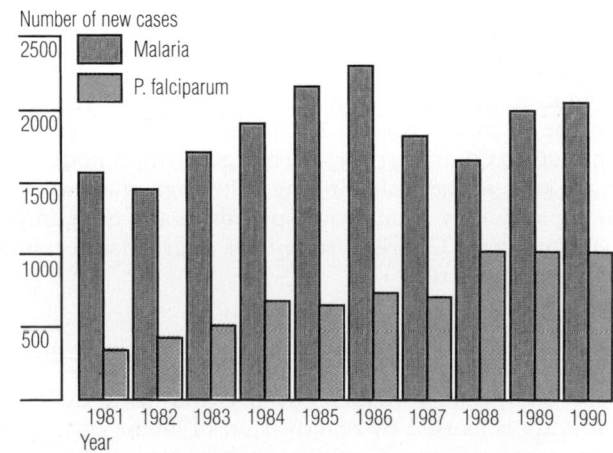

Fig. 11.24 Malaria in the UK 1981–90 showing the progressive rise of *falciparum* **importations** (Communicable Diseases Surveillance Centre, Colindale).

Transmission and epidemiology

Life cycle

The life cycle is shown in Figure 11.25. *Vivax* and *ovale* life cycles are similar, with primary exo-erythrocytic schizogony (EES) in hepatocytes leading to infection of the peripheral blood with merozoites. These enter red blood cells (RBCs) and undergo erythrocytic schizogony (ES) every 48 hours; this is benign tertian and *ovale* tertian malaria. Some of the sporozoites produce latent forms, the hypnozoites, within liver cells, which produce EES and then ES up to 2 or 3 years after infection, i.e. relapsing malaria.

Falciparum malaria has no hypnozoite form, and so the infection is cured when parasites are cleared from the blood by treatment. ES has a periodicity of less than 48 hours ('subtertian'). *Malariae* parasites lack the hypnozoite stage but can cause reappearance of parasitaemia (parasites in peripheral RBCs) up to 20 or more years after infection, i.e. recrudescence. Small numbers of parasites persists in RBCs to cause this. The periodicity of ES is 72 hours (quartan malaria).

Vivax, *ovale* and *malariae* parasites invade 1–2% of RBCs at most. *Falciparum* parasites invade any propor-

tion of RBCs, accounting for the severity of disease and high mortality.

Host

A baby born of an indigenous mother in an endemic *falciparum* area will be protected against infection during the first year of life by maternal antimalaria IgG crossing the placenta in the last trimester of pregnancy. After the first year, the child is fully susceptible. Without chemoprophylaxis the child experiences repeated attacks of malaria, and by the age of 4 or 5 years will have acquired protective immunity; this persists while he or she remains in the endemic area. Parasites are often found in the peripheral blood of an asymptomatic child. The immunity declines if an individual leaves the endemic area. Maternal immunity declines during pregnancy, particularly in primipara, with trasplacental transfer of IgG. Anaemia, fever and intense parasitisation of placenta make miscarriage, premature labour and low birth weight common, especially in areas such as West Africa where there is heavy, seasonal transmission with a high risk of infection. Where transmission is not so intense, effective immunity is not built up and all ages in the exposed population are at risk.

Any individual, of any age, from a malaria-free area may contract severe malaria. Sickle cell trait protects against severe malaria, and the heterozypous state for glucose-6-phosphate dehydrogenase (G6PD) deficiency is also protective.

Vector

Climatic factors have a profound influence on the transmission of malaria through effects on survival and reproduction of the mosquito population, and on the development of the parasite in the vector. Mosquitoes survive up to several months and their lifespan is not affected by malaria parasites. Ambient temperatures in the range 20–30°C, with a relative humidity of 60% or more, are ideal. Sporogony will not occur below 16° or above 33°C. The vector species vary considerably in different localities. *Anopheles gambiae* is one of the most effective vectors.

Additional routes for transmission of malaria are:

- *transplacenta,*, which is uncommon
- *transfusion-associated*, which is uncommon in Europe and North America but common in endemic areas
- *syringe-transmitted*, among intravenous drug abusers.

Pathogenesis and pathology

The pathogenesis of malaria is complex and incompletely understood. The initial step is adhesion of the merozoite

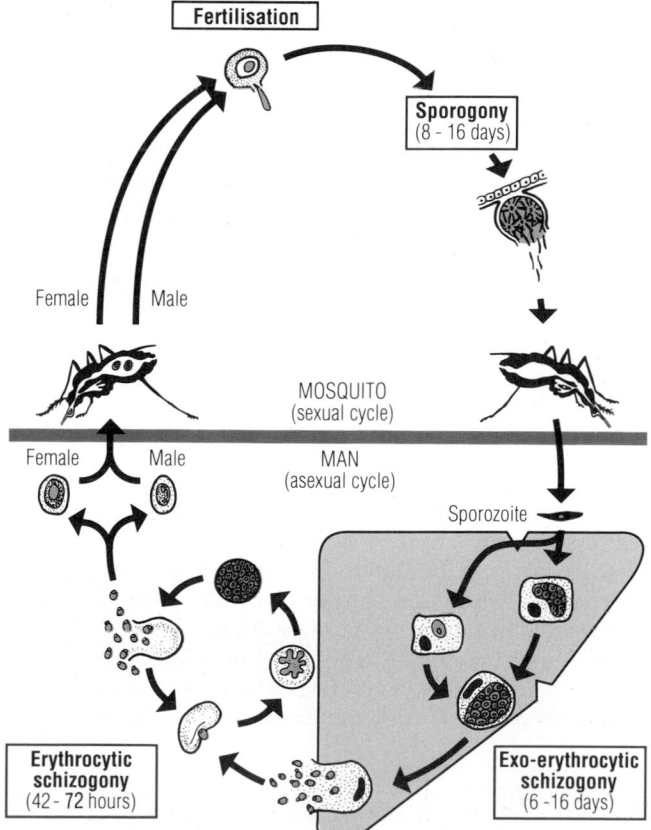

Fig. 11.25 Life cycle of malaria.

Fertilisation

Sporogony
(8 - 16 days)

Female   Male

MOSQUITO
(sexual cycle)

MAN
(asexual cycle)

Female   Male

Sporozoite

Erythrocytic
schizogony
(42 - 72 hours)

Exo-erythrocytic
schizogony
(6 - 16 days)

11 Infectious, Tropical and Parasitic Diseases

to the erythrocyte membrane. Glycophorin A, the major glycoprotein on erythrocyte membranes, is a receptor for binding specific surface proteins of the merozoites. RBCs deficient in glycophorin A are resistant to invasion. The Duffy blood group antigen is a specific receptor for invasion by *P. vivax* merozoites.

Changes in the parasitised RBC result in sequestration of RBCs containing *mature* trophozoites in the postcapillary venules. Mature trophozoites are not seen in peripheral blood films. Maximum numbers of adherent RBCs are found in venules in brain, liver, spleen, kidney and lung. The trophozoite matures into the schizont and at schizogony the RBC membrane bursts, releasing merozoites, malaria antigen, malaria pigment and RBC cytoplasmic constituents. The cycle continues, progressively building up the numbers of parasitised RBCs.

How these changes lead to altered consciousness in cerebral malaria is not clear. CT of the brain in patients with cerebral malaria has not shown oedema. Diffuse irreversible vascular obstruction is also an unlikely cause, in view of normal cerebral flow and complete recovery without neurological deficit in most survivors. CSF lactate levels are increased in cerebral malaria, which may indicate some degree of anaerobic cerebral glycolysis.

Renal damage occurs because of prerenal and renal factors. Acute tubular necrosis is the usual effect of severe malaria on the kidney. This may occur both with and without severe intravascular haemolysis. Vessels in the heart are parasitised but cardiac function is well preserved. Reduced peripheral vascular resistance, dehydration from sweating, vomiting and reduced fluid intake may contribute to hypotension.

In cerebral malaria post morten the brain shows swelling with small haemorrhages throughout the white matter. The spleen is enlarged and has a slate-grey hue over the normal red colour. Centrilobular necrosis is seen in the liver with the accumulation of malaria pigment in Küpffer cells. The pulmonary venules contain large numbers of parasitised RBCs. Pulmonary oedema may occur but the cause is not understood. The placenta is usually heavily parasitised.

The anaemia of malaria has several causes which include rupture of parasitised RBCs in schizogony, sequestration of RBCs in tissue venules, destruction of parasitised RBCs in the reticulo–endothelial system (especially the spleen), haemolysis due to the presence of malaria antigen, antibodies and complement on RBCs, and marrow suppression. Abnormalities of coagulation are usual with low platelet counts due to peripheral consumption and consumption of clotting factors. Disseminated intravascular coagulation does occur in a few patients with severe malaria but is probably not a major factor in pathogenesis.

Clinical features

Vivax and ovale

After an incubation period of about 13 days (*vivax*) or 18 days (*ovale*), prodromal symptoms – headache, fever, shivering without rigors, and general aches – begin. These last for up to 3 days before the first paroxysm of coldness, then extreme heat, then defervescence with a profuse sweat. Forty-eight hours later the full paroxysm occurs, with a feeling of extreme coldness and a rigor beginning in the late afternoon. Headache, nausea and vomiting are usually present. The temperature is high, the pulse rapid and of low volume, and the skin is cold. This phase lasts for 45 minutes to 1 hour. When the rigor ceases, peripheral dilatation occurs; the patient feels very hot and thirsty. The pulse is rapid and of full volume. The skin is hot and dry. This lasts about 1 hour and defervescence follows, with a profuse sweat. The symptoms settle completely and the patient will usually sleep. The following day there may be a little weakness. One day later the malaria paroxysm recurs. Daily paroxysms occur when parasite broods are undergoing schizogony on successive days. Untreated, the paroxysms continue for 6 weeks and die out spontaneously, only to recur 2–3 months later. By the time symptoms have been present for a week the spleen is usually palpable and there may be mild anaemia. Rupture of the enlarged spleen is reported in *vivax* malaria.

Malariae malaria

The incubation period is usually about 28 days. Nonspecific prodromal symptoms last for 2–3 days before the onset of the first paroxysm, which is accompanied by a rigor. The periodicity of symptoms is every 72 hours. The spleen is enlarged when symptoms have been present for 7–10 days.

Falciparum malaria

The incubation period is about 12 days. Headache, anorexia, nausea, vomiting, weakness and fever are prominent symptoms. The periodicity of symptoms is less than 48 hours, but periodicity is an unreliable clinical feature, present in only 30% of cases. The patient feels ill all the time, with exacerbation of symptoms at the time of paroxysms, which are similar to those described above but usually more severe. Convulsions may occur in children . Vomiting and diarrhoea are sometimes prominent features in the history. Herpes simplex vesicles may appear on the lips during the illness.

Complications

Complicated malaria occurs in *falciparum* infections. Altered consciousness in the presence of *falciparum*

Summary 9 Organ involvement in complicated falciparum malaria

Brain	Impaired consciousness: drowsiness, progressing to coma
	Convulsions
Kidney	Oliguria
	Blood urea raised, K$^+$ raised, pH lowered
Liver	Upper abnormal tenderness from enlarged liver
	Marked jaundice
	Bilirubin and aminotransferases elevated
Lungs	Dyspnoea
	Tachypnoea
	Cyanosis
	Scattered bilateral crackles
Intravascular haemolysis	Haemoglobinuria
	Tachycardia
	Blood pressure lowered
	Jaundice
	Oliguria

malaria must be taken as a clinical indication of cerebral malaria. Neck rigidity is not a feature, although mild neck stiffness may be present. Raised intracranial pressure is not a feature, and focal neurological signs are uncommon. Generalised convulsions occur in children and adults. Hypoglycaemia occurs in children, pregnant women with severe malaria and, less often, in adults with severe infection.

Jaundice may be a prominent physical sign in some patients with severe malaria. Haemolysis can cause this, but tender hepatomegaly and abnormalities of liver function suggest liver involvement. Some degree of ureamia is common but this resolves after treatment. Uraemia with oliguria indicates renal involvement. Pulmonary oedema can result from overhydration, but can also occur in the patient whose infection is coming under control. Blackwater fever, due to acute massive intravascular haemolysis, became less common after chloroquine replaced quinine in the prophylaxis and treatment of malaria, suggesting that quinine itself contributed to pathogenesis. It does, however, occur in people who have not taken quinine. The urine is black, the haemoglobin falls rapidly and jaundice appears. Hypotension and tachycardia are usual, and renal failure may follow. Gram-negative septicaemia has been reported in patients with severe malaria and may be responsible for hypotension.

Late complications

Tropical splenomegaly syndrome (TSS) occurs in areas of endemic *falciparum* malaria. There is considerable splenomegaly, a lesser degree of hepatomegaly, anaemia and pancytopenia. Malaria antibody titres are high, with polyclonal elevation of serum IgM.

Quartan nephrotic syndrome is related to *P. malariae* infections, and presents with gross oedema and proteinuria in children aged 4–6 years. The histological features are segmental endothelial proliferation with obliteration of capillary loops by periodic acid-Schiff (PAS) positive material. There is segmental thickening of the basement membrane. Progression of the glomerular lesion leads to diffuse glomerulosclerosis. Immunoglobulins and complement are deposited in the glomerulus, and *P. malariae* antigen is detectable in 25% of biopsies. The prognosis is poor, with progressive deterioration in renal function. Treatment of malaria and chemoprophylaxis do not influence the course of established disease.

Diagnosis

The clinical diagnosis of malaria is based on the history of a febrile illness after exposure in an endemic region. Differential diagnosis is shown in Table 11.32. Cases in non-endemic areas present most often in the first 3 months after leaving the endemic area. *Ovale* and *vivax* infections may present later, and the latencyin *malariae* malaria may be prolonged. The diagnosis is confirmed by the finding of parasites in stained blood films. If *falciparum* malaria is diagnosed, the percentage of RBCs parasitised should be determined and the film should be carefully examined for schizonts which are seen in the blood film from patients with severe malaria. Severe malaria is defined parasitologically as over 5% of RBCs parasitised, although complicated malaria can occur with only 1% parasitised; clinical assessment is therefore very important. The blood film is positive on the first occasion in most cases.

A blood film should be made and examined as soon as the diagnosis of malaria is considered. It is not necessary to wait for fever to occur. An antimalaria drug taken before blood films are obtained may clear the blood of parasites. I necessary further blood films should be made and examined once or twice daily until the febrile illness either is diagnosed or resolves. During a period of observation in hospital, prophylactic antimalarial drugs should be stopped to give the best chance of demonstrating parasites. It may be necessary to start treatment as soon as blood films have been taken.

Table 11.32 Differential diagnosis of malaria

Fever alone	Fever and renal failure
Any cause of pyrexia of unknown origin (see p. 221)	Septic shock
	Leptospirosis
	Viral haemorrhagic fevers
Fever and jaundice	
Yellow fever	**Fever and impaired consciousness**
Typhus	Meningitis
Leptospirosis	Encephalitis
Biliary sepsis	Brain abscess
Septicaemia	

Laboratory features

Laboratory investigations are normal or mildly abnormal in *vivax*, *ovale* and *malariae* malaria, but consistently abnormal to some degree in *falciparum* malaria. Haemoglobin levels may be normal or slightly reduced at presentation but they fall thereafter. Reticulocyte counts may be low before and after treatment, suggesting a period of marrow suppression, followed by recovery and reticulocytosis. White cell counts are normal but leucocytosis occurs in severe malaria. Platelet counts are reduced, often below $100 \times 10^9/L$. The prothrombin time and other measures of blood coagulation may be abnormal, particularly in *falciparum* infections, but gross clotting abnormalities are not usual.

Plasma sodium levels are low in *falciparum* malaria and urea may be raised. Abnormalities in liver function tests are frequent, and there may be a minor elevation in both total and unconjugated bilirubin in mild infections or greater elevation in more severe *falciparum*. Serological tests for malaria have no place diagnosis of individual cases but may be helpful in assessing previous exposure.

Management

Drug treatment

The prime of treatment is to stop further ES cycles (Table 11.33). There is usually a prompt response in *vivax*, *ovale* and *malariae* malaria. The fever in *falciparum* infections may take 2–4 days to settle. Where radical cure of relapsing malaria is required, G6PD levels should be checked and, if normal, primaquine is given. When there is severe G6PD deficiency, primaquine should not be given, because of the risk of severe haemolysis, chemoprophylaxis can be given to prevent relapse, e.g. pyrimethamine (25 mg weekly). Primaquine is not recommended in pregnancy and a chemoprophylactic should be given.

P. falciparum malaria is a serious infection demanding urgent treatment. Chloroquine resistance in *P. falciparum* is now so widespread that quinine is the drug of first choice for treatment. The route of administration must be chosen carefully. A patient who is vomiting will need parenteral treatment. Intravenous treatment is needed when there is severe *falciparum* malaria – judged either on the clinical condition of the patient or on the presence of complication – of high parasitaemia (2% or more of the RBCs parasitised) or schizonts in the peripheral blood. The dosage regimens used are set out in Table 11.33. Impairment of renal or hepatic function will prolong the half-life of the two main schizonticidal drugs, and so the dosage regimen will need to be modified, reducing the amount given and, if necessary, the frequency of administration. As soon as the patient's condition has improved sufficiently, oral treatment should be given. Tinnitus, deafness and headache are common side-effects of quinine and if they are very troublesome, the frequency of administration of the drug can be reduced.

Quinine alone will not cure *falciparum* malaria and another drug is needed. Fansidar, a combination of pyrimethamine with the long-acting sulphonamide, sulphadoxine, has been effective but Fansidar resistance is becoming more common. Mefloquine is being used with very good results.

Chloroquine is generally well tolerated by mouth; nausea and blurring of vision are transitory side-effects. Upper abdominal discomfort may occur after taking the

Table 11.33 Treatment of malaria

Type of malaria	Drug	Dose	Additional treatment
Vivax and ovale	Chloroquine base	600 mg (100 mg/kg) start, then 300 mg (5 mg/kg) 6 hours later, then 300 mg (5 mg/kg) daily for 2 days given daily	Primaquine, 7.5 mg twice a day for 14 days (children 250 μg/kg per day)
Malariae	Chloroquine	As above	Nil
Falciparum Chloroquine-resistant or sensitivity unknown			
Mild	Quinine salt	600 mg max (10 mg/kg) 3 times a day for 7 days orally	Fansidar, 3 tablets as a single dose for adults; reduced doses for children
Severe*	Quinine salt	600 mg max (10 mg/kg) by i.v. infusion in 250–500 ml fluid over 4 hours given 12-hourly until the patient can take oral quinine, giving a total of 7 days' treatment	Fansidar as above (Mefloquine is an alternative to Fansidar)
Known chloroquine-sensitive			
Mild	Chloroquine base	As above	Nil
Severe	Chloroquine base	300 mg (5 mg/kg) given by i.v. infusion in 250–500 ml fluid, repeated 12-hourly. Change to oral chloroquine as soon as the patient's condition permits	

*Quinine resistance is emerging in south east Asia and there a loading dose of 20 mg/kg by i.v. infusion is needed.

drug. Pruritus is common in Africans taking chloroquine. This is not associated with a rash and is not a manifestation of allergy. Chloroquine can be used in pregnancy. The route of administration of the drug is determined by the severity of the illness, judged by the criteria detailed above.

Additional measures

Patients with severe or complicated malaria should be managed in an intensive care unit. Convulsions should be controlled with diazepam. Apart from effective treatment of the malaria and the usual care of the unconscious patient, no additional treatment is needed in cerebral malaria. Hypoglycaemia has been reported in severe cases, both before and during treatment with quinine, particularly in young children and pregnant women. Quinine causes insulin release. Blood sugar should be monitored regularly and 50% glucose given i.v. as needed. Dialysis is needed when there is renal failure. Attention to fluid balance is essential to prevent fluid overload. Pulmonary oedema can occur because of fluid overload, but can also occur without evidence of heart failure. Mechanical ventilation may be needed when pulmonary oedema occurs. Transfusion is indicated when there is acute intravascular haemolysis and when the haemoglobin falls below 7.0 g/dl. Fresh frozen plasma and platelet transfusions are given when there are major clotting defects. Whole blood exchange transfusion appears to be effective in severely ill patients, and is indicated when more than 20% of RBCs are parasitised and when complications are present.

Management of other complications

Quartan nephrotic syndrome has a poor prognosis, with progressive deterioration of renal function to end-stage renal failure. Fluid restriction, diuretics and albumin infusions may be of help in relieving the oedema and fluid retention.

The idiopathic *tropical splenomegaly syndrome* is treated with maintenance antimalarial chemoprophylaxis. With this, the splenomegaly regresses, haematological indices improve, and abnormal serological findings return towards normal. Cessation of chemoprophylaxis may cause relapse.

Prevention and control

Everything possible must be done to prevent mosquito bites (p. 219). With the increasing problems posed by drug-resistant malaria, these measures occupy a central place in prophylaxis and their importance must be stressed to travellers and residents in endemic areas. This applies particularly to infants, children and pregnant women. The drugs currently used are listed in Table 11.34 but up-to-date information should be obtained by those advising travellers to endemic areas.

Eradication is no longer perceived as an achievable goal and control is the current aim. Insecticide resistance among mosquitoes, particularly to the cheapest compound, DDT, and chloroquine resistance among *falciparum* parasites, have contributed to the problems of controlling malaria. The main methods used are:

- reduction of vector breeding sites
- larviciding pools that cannot be drained
- spraying insecticides inside houses and on other sites where mosquitoes rest
- treating cases in man.

BABESIOSIS

Babesia are intracellular protozoa that invade, divide asexually within, and finally rupture host erythrocytes. There are 70 species, affecting a wide range of vertebrates including cattle (*B. divergens*) and rodents (*B. microti*). The parasites are transmitted by the bite of hard-bodied (ixodid) ticks. *Babesia* are widely distributed geographically, with reports of cases in humans from many countries including Scotland and the USA.

The incubation period is up to 4 weeks, less in patients who have had a splenectomy. There is a considerable range in the severity of infection, from mild to severe. Asymptomatic infections also occur. Prodromal features include headache, malaise and gastrointestinal upset prior to the onset of fevers and rigors, with jaundice, haemoglobinuria and renal impairment in *B. divergens* infections. *B. microti* produces a more prolonged but less severe illness. Increasing age is associated with more severe clinical illness.

Table 11.34 Malaria prophylaxis

General measures
Protection against mosquito bites (insect repellants, nets, clothing)

Chemoprophylaxis
Low risk of malaria – chloroquine-sensitive
   Chloroquine or proguanil
High risk of malaria – chloroquine-resistant
   Chloroquine and proguanil
High risk of malaria – multiple drug resistance
   Chloroquine and proguanil or mefloquine (for up to 3 months; exceptionally
   for up to 1 year)

Points to note
- Where the risk of drug-resistance malaria is high, severe malaria may occur despite regular prophylaxis, but this is *not* a reason to omit prophylaxis.
- Prophylaxis should be started 1 week before entering the area, and continued for 4 weeks after leaving.
- Mefloquine is a new drug and there is limited experience of its use for prophylaxis.

The laboratory diagnosis is made by finding organisms similar to malaria parasites in Giemsa-stained peripheral blood films.

There is no treatment of proven value in the management of babesiosis. Survival in the rapidly progressive *B. divergens* infections depends largely on supportive measures such as renal dialysis according to the usual criteria, with transfusion and/or exchange transfusion. Treatment with quinine and clindamycin in standard doses appears to be effective. *B. microti* infection is usually self-limiting and requires only symptomatic treatment.

TRYPANOSOMIASES

African trypanosomiasis (sleeping sickness)

Infection with *Trypanosoma gambiense* causes an initial febrile illness which progresses slowly to a chronic phase dominated by infection of the CNS, causing neuronal death and a variety of organic neurological syndromes. Neurological involvement occurs early in *T. rhodesiense* infections within weeks of inoculation of parasites and, untreated, there is rapid deterioration and death. The two species cannot be distinguished on morphological grounds. Various species of tsetse fly, *Glossina*, are the vectors.

Distribution and incidence

The specific names of these parasites suggest a West African (*T. gambiense*) or East African (*T. rhodesiense*) origin for the infections, but there is a considerable overlap of the distribution of the two species in Central Africa (Fig. 11.26). The total numbers of cases are far fewer than malaria, but *rhodesiense* infections have a considerable economic impact as valuable farming and grazing lands cannot be used because of the high risk of infection.

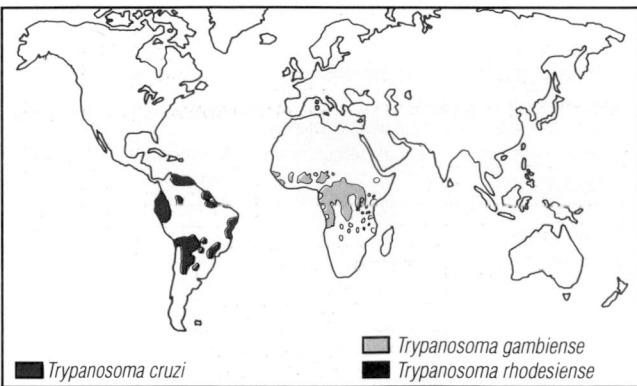

Fig. 11.26 World distribution of trypanosomiases.

Transmission and epidemiology

Tsetse flies become infected by ingesting trypanosomes in a blood meal. Once infected, a fly remains infective for life. About 1% of flies in an area are infected. Man is the reservoir in *gambiense* infections, while a variety of wild mammals, including bush buck and hartebeest, are the reservoir if *rhodesiense* infection and man is an incidental host. Transmission of *gambiense* trypamosomiasis occurs in wooded areas around rivers and streams that are water sources for local populations. Blood transfusion and transplacental transmission are also possible routes of infection.

Pathology and pathogenesis

There is an early marked inflammatory response at the site of inoculation and in the lymphoid tissues of the body, lymph glands, liver and spleen. Trypanosomes may be seen in tissue sections. *Rhodesiense* infections progress rapidly to involve the heart and brain. Myocarditis and pericarditis are common. An obliterative endarteritis with vascular occlusion is found in the CNS, causing the degenerative changes. The neuropathological features include thickening of the meninges, which are infiltrated by lymphocytes and plasma cells. This infiltrate extends into brain substance in a perivascular distribution.

The parasites continuously shed surface antigens which evoke antibody responses in the host, but the antigens change in sequence – a possible mechanism of evading host immune responses. Autoantibodies to brain and heart may cause tissue damage. Disseminated intravascular coagulation can occur in *rhodesiense* infections.

Clinical features

With both species, fever, chills and weakness are usual initial symptoms, beginning about 10 days after the bite. An inflamed lump is present at the bite site and there is regional adenopathy. On white skins it is possible to see transient irregular areas of erythema in both types of disease. Posterior auricular and posterior cervical adenopathy develop after 1–2 months of infection in *gambiense* infections. Unpleasant dysaethesia follows squeezing of the calf muscles. Hepatosplenomegaly is often present in both infections early on. Jaundice occurs in *rhodesiense* infections. Purpuric rashes on the extremities are occasionally seen in severe *rhodesiense* infections.

Neurological involvement appears within weeks of infection in *rhodesiense* infections, but it may be months or years later with *T. gambiense*. Indifference, lassitude, personality changes and altered behaviour are early features. Sleep rhythm is reversed. The basal ganglia, cerebellum and brainstem regions are most affected, producing tremor, incoordination, and problems with speech, balance and walking. Parkinsonian features may be prominent. Epilepsy occurs. In the terminal stage the patient is scarcely rousable, unable to swallow or feed him/herself. Bronchopneumonia is a common cause of death.

Diagnosis

Diagnosis depends on finding trypanosomes. Early in the course of infection with either species, parasites may be found in peripheral blood films. There are usually many more parasites in *rhodesiense* than *gambiense* infections. Repeated examinations must be made to detect the low levels of parasitaemia in *gambiense* infection. *Gambiense* parasites may be seen in bone marrow smears. Smaller number of parasites can be detected in smears of the buffy coat. Material aspirated from a lymph node can be smeared on a slide and stained.

CSF must also be examined. The cell count is determined and the stained deposit examined for trypanosomes. An increased white cell count ($>5/mm^3$) and/or an increased CSF protein ($>250mg/l$) indicates CNS infection in a patient with parasites in the blood or tissues. Serum immunoglobulin concentrations are increased, with IgM levels very high. Increased CSF IgM indicates nervous system involvement. Serological tests do not have diagnostic value for individual patients.

Management

Suramin is used to kill parasites in blood and lymphoid nodes, and cures patients early in the disease. It does not cross the blood-brain barrier and so is ineffective when the CNS is involved. Pentamidine is a second-line alternative to suramin.

The arsenical compound, melarsoprol (Mel B), is used when there is CNS involvement. It will also kill blood forms but its high toxicity prohibits its use as a first-line drug. Eflornithine is a new drug effective against CNS infections with *T. gambiense*.

Examination of blood films, IgM levels, CSF and the patient's condition are helpful in assessing the response to treatment. Improvement in the patient's condition and resolution of the abnormalities indicate a good response. Relapse is indicated by a rise in the CSF protein or cell count and further treatment should be given.

When patients are treated early, complete recovery is the rule. In more advanced cases treatment arrests progression of the disease.

Prevention and control

Appropriate clothing in endemic areas is essential to minimise the area exposed to biting. Tsetses can bite through thin material. Pentamidine has been used as a prophylactic agent against *gambiense* infection in those heavily exposed. Efforts to control vectors by destruction of habitats may be helpful.

American trypanosomiasis (Chagas' disease)

Aetiology

American trypanosomiasis is an infection caused by *T. cruzi*. The parasite exists in several forms during its life cycle. The trypomastigote is found in the blood and has similar appearances to the African trypanosome. Amastigotes are found within host cells. Human blood forms are ingested by the vector, a species of reduvid bug, when it takes a blood meal. The bug defaecates infective faeces on the skin after taking a blood meal, and the metacyclic forms enter the host through the bite or other skin abrasion, or through the conjunctiva if the faeces are carried to the eye on fingers.

Distribution and incidence

American trypanosomiasis is most common in the countries of South America among people living in poorly constructed housing, as the bugs live in roof thatch and cracked mud walls. Many people are infected in South America, with about 6 000 000 cases in Brazil, although not all those infected develop disease (Fig. 11.26).

Transmission and epidemiology

Contact with infected bugs, transplacental infection and blood transfusion are the routes of infection (Fig. 11.27). Infected bugs are the most important source. Infection in bugs is maintained from a reservoir of *T. cruzi* in dogs. Infection of children in the first decade of life is common.

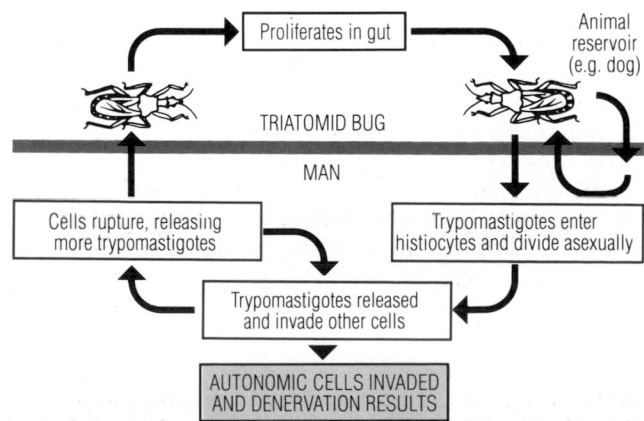

Fig. 11.27 Life cycle of *Trypanosome cruzi*.

Pathology and pathogenesis

Trypasomes invade cells, including mycocardial and gut smooth muscle cells. Rupture of the cell releases trypomastigotes and evokes inflammatory responses in the surrounding tissues. The trypomastigotes circulate, invade other cells and replicate as amastigotes. Phagocytic cells in any tissue, as well as heart muscle, skeletal and smooth muscle, and CNS, are among the tissues involved. Pericarditis and cardiomegaly are often present.

The heart and the gut are the organs severely affected in chronic Chagas's disease. The heart is enlarged, with apical ventricular aneurysm commonly present. Thrombus is often present in the atrial appendage and in the ventricles. There is diffuse myocardial cell necrosis, with fibrosis and involvement of the conducting system. Parasymphathetic plexuses of the gut are destroyed, causing dilatation of the intestine, frequently the oesophagus or colon (the mega-syndrome).

The pathogenesis of the disease is complex. There are several different strains of *T. cruzi*, some of which cause the cardiac and mega-syndromes. Other strains cause lifelong infection but no disease. Autoimmune mechanisms are probably involved in damaging tissues.

Clinical features

Acute infection may be inapparent in young children, but in older children and adults there may be an acute febrile illness. The patient may find a lump in the skin marking the site of the infected bite and initial parasite replication (the chagoma). Unilateral periorbital oedema indicates a conjunctival route of infection. Local adenopathy and hepatosplenomegaly are found. Cardiomegaly, heart failure, arrhythmia and conduction defects indicate myocarditis in the acute illness. This may cause sudden death. Meningo-encephalitis may occur. The local signs at the bite size, hepatosplenomegaly and fever subside in 6 weeks.

Chronic Changas' disease presents with heart and gut disease. Right and left sided cardiac failure are common. There may be signs suggesting pulmonary or systemic embolisation from thrombus in the cardiac chambers. Conduction abnormalities are often present and may cause Stokes-Adams attacks and sudden death. Mega-oesophagus causes dyphagia and aspiration pneumonia in the most severely affected. Megacolon causes constipation and faecal impaction. Volvulus of sigmoid megacolon may occur.

Diagnosis

Acute infections can be diagnosed by finding parasites in the peripheral blood film. Trypanosomes may also be found on microscopy and culture of CSF, even when evidence of CNS involvement is lacking. Serological tests are usually positive in both acute and chronic cases by indirect immunofluorescence, indirect haemagglutination and complement fixation techniques.

Management

Treatment is unsatisfactory. Two drug are available, nifurtimox and benznidazole. Both will clear the blood of parasites in the acute phase but prolonged follow-up suggests that neither gives a radical cure. Control of arrhythmias and heart failure is all that can be done for cardiac disease in the chronic phase. Relief of obstruction at the oesphagogastric junction by dilatation or surgery may help the patient with mega-oesophagus. A dilated segment of small or large intestine can be excised.

prevention and control

Improvement to housing would do much to prevent this disease. Residual spraying with gamma benzene hexachloride is a useful method of vector control.

LEISHMANIASIS

The Leishmania are obligate intracellular protozoan parasites that infect man and other mammals, including dogs, foxes, gerbils and rats. Infection is transmitted by the bite of infected sandflies. The generalised life cycle is shown in Fig. 11.28. These organisms parasites cells of the reticulo-endothelial system and evoke granulomatous

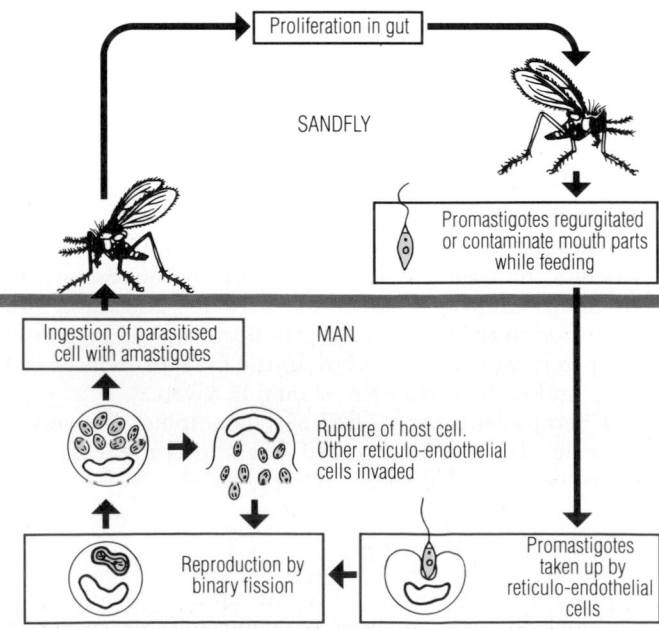

Fig. 11.28 Generalised life cycle of Leishmania.

responses in infected tissue. Genetic factors controlling the host cell-mediated responses determine the outcome of infection, with only a proportion of those infected developing clinically apparent disease.

The geographical distribution is shown in Figure 11.29. Two forms of disease are recognised. *Cutaneous leishmaniasis* denotes infection with species of *Leishmania* that affect primarily reticulo–endothelial cells in the skin, while *visceral leishmaniasis* denotes infection with a species that primarily infects reticulo–endothelial cells of deeper tissues (Table 11.35). The species causing cutaneous disease are geographically distinct between the Old and New World.

Cutaneous leishmaniasis

Cutaneous leishmaniasis is a granulomatous infection of the skin caused by various species of *Leishmania*, which results in one or more chronic ulcerating skin lesions (Plate 12, p. 247). In time, the ulcers usually heal with scarring.

Aetiology

The organisms causing cutaneous leishmaniasis are listed in Table 11.35. Morphologically they are all identical.

Distribution and incidence

The incidence is difficult to estimate, as many self-healing cases never come to medical attention. World Health Organization figures put the incidence ar 100 cases per 10 000 of the population in endemic areas (Fig. 11.29).

Transmission and epidemiology

Female sandflies of the genera *Phlebotomus* (Old World) and *Lutzomyia* (New World) transmit these infections by their bite. Apart from *L. tropica* (transmitted in towns and cities with man as the reservoir), these are zoonotic infec-

Table 11.35 Forms of Leishmania infection

Location	Cutaneous leishmaniasis	Visceral leishmaniasis
Old World	Leishmania tropica	Leishmania donovani
	Leishmania major	
	Leishmania aethiopica	Leishmania infantum
	Leishmania infantum	
New World	Leishmania mexicana	Leishmania donovani
	Leishmania braziliensis	
	Leishmania peruviana	

tions; humans are infected when they move into areas where there is a mammal–sandfly cycle. Urban infections tend to be more common among children.

Pathology and pathogenesis

Promastigotes change to amastigotes after inoculation into the skin, and the amastigotes are very rapidly phagocytosed by macrophages where they replicate (Fig. 11.28). The local granulomatous reactions produce a subcutaneous nodule and then the overlying skin ulcerates. The lesion persists as long as amastigotes proliferate within macrophages. This occurs despite the presence of sensitised T lymphocytes, shown by a positive delayed hypersensitivity reaction to a leishmanin skin test antigen. Healing occurs spontaneously in time in most infections.

Clinical features

Persisting cutaneous ulceration on an exposed part of the body continuing for more than a month is the usual feature. The ulcer is painless and may crust over, only for the crust to separate again. Regional adenopathy is not seen unless there is secondary infection. Around the main ulcer, which has well-defined indurated margins, a number of smaller nodular lesions may be present. These infections will heal spontaneously in 2–8 months, leaving a residual scar.

Recidivans leishmaniasis caused by *L. tropica* infection is characterised by a chronic relapsing course in spite of T cell immunity. In contrast, *diffuse cutaneous leishmaniasis* causes numerous nodular or plaque-like lesions which tend not to ulcerate. These patients represent a kind of 'lepromatous' cutaneous leishmaniasis (p. 271). It is caused by *L. aethiopica* in Africa and *L. mexicana* in Central and South America. Leishmanin tests are negative. The South American species cause lesions similar to those of *L. major*. *L. braziliensis* causes an initial ulcerating skin lesion which heals, but may subsequently produce a recurrence of disease with destruction of tissues at a mucocutaneous junction (*mucocutaneous leishmaniasis*).

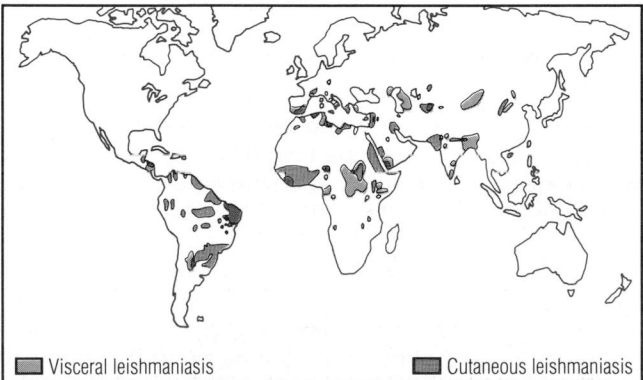

| ▨ Visceral leishmaniasis | ▨ Cutaneous leishmaniasis |

Fig. 11.29 World distribution of leishmaniasis.

Diagnosis

Parasites can usually be found in Giemsa-stained smears of material from slit skin smears, material aspirated from the edge of the lesion or touch impression smears from the surface of a biopsy. Material from the biopsy can also be cultured in Novy-McNeal-Nicolle (NNN) medium. Serological tests for leishmaniasis are positive at low titre in most forms of cutaneous leishmaniasis.

Differential diagnosis

A variety of infective disorders can cause indolent ulceration. Among these are yaws, tertiary syphilis, lupus vulgaris, *Histoplasma duboisii*, diphtheritic ulcers (desert sore) and blastomycosis. Malignant ulcers and tropical ulcer should also be considered. Diffuse cutaneous leishmaniasis can be mistaken clinically for lepromatous leprosy unless the causative organism is demonstrated in skin smears.

Management

The treatment of cutaneous leishmaniasis is unsatisfactory, not least because the commonly used drug, sodium stibogluconate, has to be given by daily intravenous injection for 20–30 days. Intralesional antimonials, emetine and γ-interferon have been used successfully. Self-cure is a feature of infection with *L. tropica* and *L. major*, and so a single lesion caused by these parasites in a site that will not produce disfiguring scarring or be particularly exposed to secondary bacterial infection may be left to heal spontaneously. Patients with multiple lesions, large lesions or lesions in exposed places should receive treatment. Patients in areas where diffuse cutaneous leishmaniasis or mucocutaneous leishmaniasis occurs must be treated.

Sodium stibogluconate (Pentostam) is the first choice of drug for both Old and New World leishmaniasis, and usually results in healing in most types of disease. Diffuse cutaneous leishmaniasis is often resistant and pentamidine is the alternative drug.

Prevention and control

Among Old World cutaneous leishmaniasis, cure is usually associated with immunity to reinfection with the same strain, but vaccination is not yet available. Destruction of burrows of rodent vectors can be successful in removing reservoirs. Removal of sandfly breeding sites around houses and spraying with insecticides will help to control peridomestic transmission. Protection against the bites of sandflies may be helpful, e.g. mosquito nets and insect repellants, although the insects will bite through a shirt.

Visceral leishmaniasis (kala-azar)

Visceral leishmaniasis, an infection due to *L. donovani*, is spread by the bite of an infected female sandfly and causes a prolonged febrile illness with wasting, hepatosplenomegaly and lymphadenopathy.

Distribution, incidence and transmission

The areas affected are shown in Figure 11.29. This condition is endemic in some countries of southern Europe and Mediterranean islands that are regularly visited by tourists. Infections acquired in these areas are seen in the UK. Children are commonly affected in the endemic areas. Subclinical cases probably exceed clinical cases by 5 to 1. Endemic, epidemic and sporadic forms of the disease occur. All ages and both sexes are susceptible to infection.

The dog seems to be an important reservoir throughout the endemic areas. Man is the reservoir in northeastern and eastern India.

The vectors are female sandflies of the genus *Phlebotomus* in the Old World and *Lutzomyia* in the New. These insects, guided by scent plumes, bite at night-time.

Pathology and pathogenesis

Amastigotes (Fig. 11.28) replicate asexually within macrophages and are carried to lymph nodes drainin the site of the bite; they then disseminate to macrophages in other tissues, particularly the liver, spleen, nodes and marrow. There is progressive enlargement of liver and spleen. Wasting of the muscles and low plasma albumin are metabolic responses to the infection. The malnutrition will impair immune responses to the parasite and to other diseases such as tuberculosis or pneumococcal pneumonia, which may complicate the patient's illness. Leishmanin tests (a delayed hypersensitivity skin test) are negative before treatment and become positive after cure.

Clinical features

The incubation period is very variable, from 2 weeks to 2 years or more. Early symptoms are lethargy, sweats, and fever with a typical pattern of two peaks in a day. Within weeks of onset the liver and spleen are palpable and progressively enlarge. Body weight falls. Lymphadenopathy may be found. Emaciation is obvious in more long-standing cases. Darkening of the skin of hands, feet, face and abdomen is common in eastern India ('kala-azar' means 'black sickness'). Lymph glands may be enlarged. Poorly nourished patients should be carefully examined for coexisting tuberculosis or other infection such as pneumonia. Leishmaniasis has been recognised as one of the infections that may complicate the course of AIDS.

Investigation shows anaemia and pancytopenia due to hypersplenism, low plasma albumin and high globulin (e.g. 50 g/l) with polyclonal elevation of IgG. Serological tests for leishmaniasis are positive in most cases.

Diagnosis

The clinical features, together with exposure in an endemic area, suggest visceral leishmaniasis. The parasites are usually found on examination of Giemsa-stained smears of bone marrow aspirate, which should also be put into NNN culture medium. Percutaneous splenic aspiration has a high yield of positive results (95%); it can be done safely in a co-operative patient whose prothrombin time is not more than 5 seconds greater than the control, and whose platelet count is 40×10^2/L or more. Again, material should be cultured and used for making smears.

Management

Sodium stibogluconate (Pentostam) is the drug of first choice, given by daily intravenous injection for about 30 days depending on the response. Fever settles quickly and there is progressive improvement in the clinical and laboratory findings. Relapse occasionally occurs and the options are to give more sodium stibogluconate continuing for longer periods, or to give a second-line drug, e.g. pentamidine or amphotericin B (this is effective and less toxic in a liposomal formulation). One of these is certainly needed if there is no response to a second course of sodium stibogluconate.

Prevention and control

Prevention is difficult. Where man is the reservoir, finding and treating cases and insecticiding homes may help in control. Control of canine reservoirs can be of help. Vaccines are under study but not in clinical use yet.

HELMINTH INFECTIONS

A large number of helminthic parasites affect man. Man is the definitive host in most instances and the sexual phase of the life cycle takes place in the human host. A classification is given in Table 11.36. Less commonly man is an inadvertent intermediate host infected either with larvae that do not develop any further because they are in the wrong host, e.g. *Toxocara canis*, or with larvae that are unlikely ever to be consumed by the definitive host, e.g. hydatid disease.

The life cycles of these parasites differ markedly faecal–oral transmission or percutaneous infection by infective larvae is characteristic of the soil-associated gut nematodes. In contrast the filariases have blood-sucking insect vectors in which there is development to infecting larvae that will infect man when later blood meals are taken. The life cycles of the trematode platyhelminths are more complex, involving more than one intermediate host in many instances.

The climatic conditions favouring transmission are warmth and humidity. These factors promote the survival of the soil-transmitted helminths and the insect vector of the filarial parasites. Local traditions in food preparation and consumption are important in transmission of a number of parasites, such as eating raw meat or lightly cooked or raw fish and crabs. Among sheep- and goat-herding communities where dogs are used, definitive and intermediate hosts of *Echinococcus granulosus* are brought together, and it is common for sheep and goat offal containing hydatid cysts to be fed to dogs. Dog faeces then contaminate the environment around houses.

The effect of helminthic infections on the health of communities is difficult to assess. *Ascaris lumbricoides* is one of the most common helminthic infections. It undoubtedly causes disease, but these events probably do not happen very often among the 290 million people infected worldwide. In contract, *Onchocerca volvulus* in the

Table 11.36 Classification of helminth infections

Nematodes (roundworms)

Human intestinal	Filarial	Animal intestinal
Ascaris	Onchocerca	Trichinella
Ancylostoma	Wuchereria	Toxocara
Necator	Brugia	
Strongyloides	Loa loa	
Enterobius		
Trichuris		

Trematodes (flukes)

Schistosoma
Clonorchis
Opisthorcis
Fasciola
Fasciolopsis
Paragonimus

Cestodes (tapeworms)

Human intestinal	Larval tissue cestodes
Taenia species	Taenia solium (cysticercosis)
Diphyllobothrium	Hydatid (Echinococcus)
Hymenolepis	

savannah belt of West Africa causes significant morbidity through the ocular complication, sclerosing keratitis, which can progress to blindness.

The chemotherapy of helminthic infections has become progressively simpler. The benzimidazoles – thiabendazole, mebendazole and albendazole – are broad-spectrum antihelminthics active against the soil-transmitted helminths. The incidence of side-effects decreases in the order given; albendazole, the newest, has much better absorption from the gut than mebendazole, but lacks the nausea and vomiting associated with thiabendazole. Praziquantel has actions in a range of cestode and tremetode infections, with a low incidence of side-effects. It is the first drug to be effective in cysticercosis.

NEMATODES

HUMAN INTESTINAL NEMATODE INFECTION

Ascariasis

Ascariasis is infection of the gut lumen with the nematode parasite, *Ascaris lumbricoides*.

Aetiology

The adult female worm measures up to 400 mm long by 6 mm wide at its thickest. The male is up to 300 mm long by 2–4 mm. They live for about 1 year. Both are a greyish-white colour. The female lays up to 200 000 eggs per day. The worms do not attach themselves to the gut mucosa but maintain their position by actively moving against the flow of intestinal contents. The eggs survive well in warm moist soil but are killed by heating to 50°C.

Distribution and incidence

Ascariasis is common in the tropics and subtropics, and up to 90% of people may be infected. Poor or absent sanitation and frequent faecal contamination of the environment with vast numbers of ascaris eggs lead to a high frequency of infection, often with large worm loads in children.

Transmission and epidemiology

Eggs are ingested in food or water or from fingers, and the larvae are released in the small intestine. They enter the mucosa and then blood vessels to reach the lungs, where they leave blood vessels and enter air spaces. Here they undergo two further moults and then ascend the bronchial tree to the pharynx. They migrate down the oesophagus and through the stomach to reach the small intestine.

Pathology

No intestinal mucosal lesions are attributable to the adult worms. Pulmonary infiltrates with eosinophils are found during the larval migratory phase of the life cycle.

Clinical features

Symptoms due to the migrating phase of ascariasis are very uncommon. Pulmonary infiltrates on X-ray, eosinophilia and restrictive pulmonary function defects can occur.

There are also few symptoms attributable to established infection. Worms may be vomited, or passed with the stools, or may even emerge from a nostril. Bolus obstruction of the small intestine occurs, particularly in children with very heavy infections. An adult worm in the bile duct causes pain and obstructive jaundice with ascending cholangitis. Pancreatitis may result from ascaris obstruction of the pancreatic duct. Ascarids can also migrate through intestinal suture lines to cause leakage from an anastomosis.

Diagnosis

Diagnosis is made by finding eggs in faecal samples. The complications of ascariasis are usually diagnosed at surgical exploration or endoscopic examination. Eosinophilia is uncommon, apart from at the stage of tissue migration.

Management

Mebendazole (100 mg twice daily for 3 days) or albendazole (400 mg as a single dose) is effective. Both drugs are relatively expensive.

Piperazine hydrate elixir (750 mg of hydrate per 5 ml) is effective. The dose depends on age and weight. Where a mixed infection of ascaris and hookworm is being treated with piperazine and tetrachlorethylene (TCE) for hookworm, it is usual to treat the ascaris first, as TCE may stimulate ascaris migration into biliary or pancreatic ducts.

Prevention and control

The use of latrines would prevent infection. Faecal contamination of the environment and the use of human faeces as fertiliser on crops encourage transmission. Before use as fertiliser, faeces can be treated with sodium nitrate or calcium superphosphate to kill the eggs of gut parasites. Education of the community about the control efforts, and its active co-operation, are essential to the success of control programmes

Hookworm

This is infection of the gut with either *Ancylostoma duodenale* or *Necator americanus*. Both grip the wall of the mucosa with their mouth parts and take a small amount of blood from the host each·day. A relatively small number of people develop disease related to hookworm infection.

Aetiology

The worms are about 9 mm long. The female *Ancylostoma* produces 30 000 eggs per day and *Necator* 9000 eggs per day. Eggs must be passed into warm, moist soil for the ovum to develop into the larval stage. The life cycle is shown in Figure 11.30. Larvae of *Necator* grow in the lungs. *Ancylostoma* larvae can be ingested with food and develop in the gut lumen without tissue migration.

Epidemiology

Both species occur worldwide where temperature and soil conditions are suitable. *Ancylostoma* eggs are capable of resisting desiccation to some extent. Infection rates of 80–90% are common in endemic rural areas. The use of untreated faeces as fertiliser on crops accounts for the high infection of farm workers.

Pathogenesis and pathology

Each worm takes a small amount of blood from the host. Nutrients are removed by the parasite and the residue passes into the gut, where it can be digested and absorbed. Iron deficiency anaemia occurs when iron losses exceed intake and iron stores are depleted. Anaemia may be severe, with haemoglobin levels of less than 5.0 g/dl. Hypoalbuminaemia is usual at this stage but malabsorption does not occur.

Clinical features

No symptoms are attributed to hookworm infection. Hookworm anaemia appears to cause few symptoms until oedema due to hypoproteinaemia develops. Salt retention and water retention exacerbate the oedema and cause some degree of exertional dyspnoea. The findings are those of severe iron deficiency anaemia, with mucocal pallor and koilonychia. Some patients present with high-output congestive cardiac failure.

Diagnosis and investigation

Diagnosis is confirmed by finding eggs in the faeces. Worm burden van be assessed from 24-hour faecal egg outputs.

Hypochromic microcytic anaemia is present. It is important to distinguish between iron deficiency and β-thalassaemia trait. Eosinophil counts may be normal or increased. Plasma albumin levels are low.

Management

Mebendazole (100 mg twice daily for 3 days) or albendazole (200 mg twice daily for 2 days) is effective. Bephenium hydroxynaphthoate granules (5.0 g) are given on an empty stomach. The cheapest treatment is tetrachlorethylene (TCE), giving 0.5 ml/kg to a maximum single dose of 5.0 ml.

Eradication of the worms is not the priority if anaemia is present. Packed cell transfusion after giving diuretics may be needed. Where there is heart failure, diuretics and cautious blood transfusion with packed cells are needed. Exchange transfusion is another way of correcting anaemia without risking adverse effects of fluid overload. Later, iron stores will need replating.

Prevention and control

Safe disposal of faeces prevents transmission. Where night soil must be used to fertilise crops, prior chemical treatment kills ova (see ascariasis above). Wearing shoes or sandals also prevents infection. Where possible, vegetables with a high content of ferrous iron, e.g. soya beans, should be introduced into the diet.

Cutaneous larva migrans

The hookworm parasite of dogs and cats, *Ancylostoma braziliense*, produces eggs which are passed in the animal

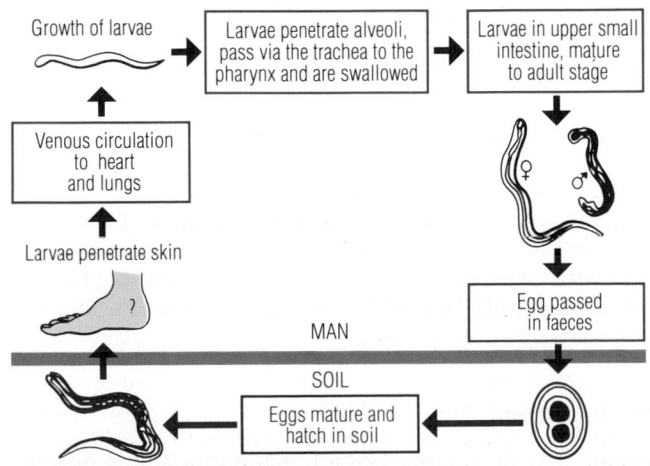

Fig. 11.30 Life cycle of hookworm.

faeces; they hatch in warm, moist soil conditions to release larvae which mature to the infective stage and can penetrate the skin of humans. The larvae cannot follow their usual migration in man and instead meander around in the subcutaneous tissues close to the site of entry until they die. The feet are the most common site for this condition, but any part in contact with contaminated soil or sand can be affected.

The appearances are readily recognised. A red papule marks the tip of the track produced by the migrating worm. The papule is in fact a little way behind the migrating worm. A raised, red, serpiginous track, about 3 mm across, stretches out behind. The affected skin is itchy and may be blistered. Secondary bacterial infection can occur. The lesion can be active for several months.

The diagnosis is made on the appearances. Treatment is with thiabendazole, either orally, or topically as a cream. Albendazole is also effective. Following effective treatment the migration of the worm ceases and the track will slowly disappear. Secondary bacterial infection requires treatment with antibiotics.

Strongyloidiasis

Strongyloidiasis is an infection of the small intestine with the nematode parasite *Strongyloides stercoralis*. Most people are asymptomatic. A small number have cutaneous manifestations and immunosuppressed patients may develop massive systemic invasion with filariform larvae.

Aetiology

Strongyloides stercoralis adult females are small, 2 mm long, and are found in the intestinal lumen, where they insinuate their anterior ends between the villi. The life cycle is described in Figure 11.31.

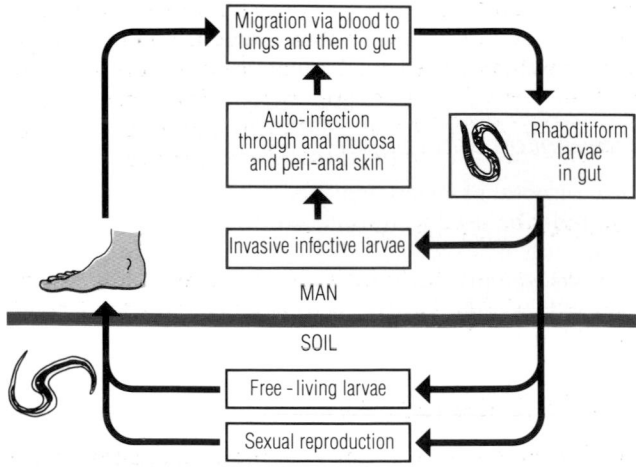

Fig. 11.31 Life cycle of *Strongyloides stercoralis*.

A variation of the life cycle involves rhabditiform larvae developing into filariform larvae during transit down the gut. These larvae penetrate the rectal or anal mucosa or the perianal skin, and then enter the usual migratory tissue phase.

Transmission and epidemiology

Transmission and epidemiology are broadly the same as those of hookworm but tend to be focal depending on soil conditions. The occurrence of autoinfection in strongyloidiasis allows infection to persist for 30 years or more, successive generations of adults maintaining infection.

Pathology

The migrating larvae in lung evoke some degree of eosinophilic pneumonitis. Adult larvae provoke a mild inflammation in the gut. Malabsorption may occur but the mechanism is not understood. Diarrhoea, hypoproteinaemia and oedema of the small bowel wall occur in children. Massive autoinfection with filariform larvae can occur in immunosuppressed patients, with dissemination of larvae to gut, lungs and CNS.

Clinical features

Most patients are asymptomatic and the diagnosis is made by stool microscopy or in the investigation of eosinophilia. Some patients present with a transient, linear or serpiginous urticaria that comes and goes within 40–60 minutes. This is caused by subcutaneous migration of infective filariform larvae. The massive autoinfection syndrome occurs most often in people on steroids or immunosuppressive drugs. Fever, abdominal distension, diarrhoea, vomiting and ileus are common presenting symptoms. There may be signs of meningitis. Dyspnoea, cyanosis and pulmonary infiltrates indicate pulmonary involvement. Septicaemia with organisms from the colonic microflora is common. The prognosis is poor.

Diagnosis

Diagnosis is usually made by finding rhabditiform larvae in stools or juice obtained from the duodenum by intubation. Eosinophilia is usual in normal persons but absent in patients with massive autoinfection. Larvae are readily found in sputum, jejunal aspirate or faeces in patients with massive autoinfection.

Management

Thiabendazole (25 mg/kg to a maximum single dose of 1.5 g) is given twice daily for 3 days. Albendazole (400 mg twice daily for 3 days) is also effective; it causes fewer side-effects and may become the drug of first choice. Treatment is continued for 7 days in massive auto-infection. Intensive care is also needed for these patients.

Prevention

Safe disposal of faeces would prevent *S. stercoralis* infection. Sandals would help to prevent skin/soil contacts. Treatment with cytotoxic or immunosuppressive drugs for leukaemia, lymphoma and other malignancies, reactional states is leprosy or organ transplantation should be preceded by thiabendazole treatment in patients from or in the tropics.

Threadworms

Infection with the intestinal nematode, *Enterobius vermicularis*, causes pruritus ani. Children are most often affected but adults can also become infected. The life cycle is described in Figure 11.32. The full cycle can take 14 days.

Transmission

Autoinfection maintains the parasite in the host. Person-to-person spread is the likely route of infection in children and other family members, or by handling pyjamas, sheets or towels with adherent eggs.

Clinical features

Intense pruritus ani is the usual symptom of this infection. The pruritus often disrupts sleep. When symptoms are present the worms may be seen on the perianal skin. In females vulvo-vaginitis and vaginal discharge may occur.

Diagnosis

Diagnosis is made either by identifying a female obtained from the perianal skin or the faeces, or by finding eggs. The perianal skin should not be washed before the swab is taken. Eosinophilia does not occur.

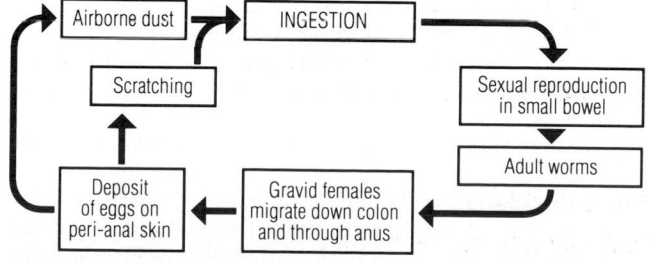

Fig. 11.32 Life cycle of threadworm.

Management

A number of drugs are available and it is usual to treat the whole family. Mebendazole (100 mg as a single dose, followed by a second dose 2 weeks later) is effective. Piperazine citrate (65 mg/kg to a maximum dose of 2.0 g/day for 6 days, repeated after 3 weeks) can be used. Pyrvinium pamoate (5 mg of base/kg as a single dose) is also used.

In addition to chemotherapy it is helpful to prevent finger sucking and nail biting. The importance of head washing after going to the lavatory and before eating should be stressed. Occasionally one child is chronically afflicted by enterobiasis, and this causes both child and family great distress. This may occur in families that are particularly careful about washing. Reassurance is needed that this is not uncommon and that enterobiasis is occasionally difficult to treat.

Trichuriasis

Trichuriasis is infection of the intestinal lumen with the nematode, *Trichuris trichiuria*. Most patients are asymptomatic. Malnourished children suffer heavy infections with this parasite, causing symptomatic disease. Eggs are swallowed and larvae hatch. They mature during their transit down the small intestine, and adults are found in the terminal ileum and colon. The eggs mature in soil and are ingested. The adult worm has a long, thin anterior end and a short, thick posterior end. This appearance is described by the common name of the parasite, the whipworm. The thick posterior end grips the colonic mucosa.

Clinical features

Most people are asymptomatic and eggs are found on faecal microscopy. Malnourished children may become infected with large numbers of these worms, and diarrhoea with blood in the stool may result. By proctoscopy large numbers of worms can be seen adhering to the rectal mucosa. Rectal prolapse is sometimes seen in these malnourished children. It is difficult to know if the worm burden is the cause or the result of malnutrition.

Diagnosis and management

Diagnosis is made by finding eggs in faecal smears or concentrates. Mebendazole (100 mg twice daily for 3 days) is effective.

FILARIAL INFECTION

The filariae are a group of helminthic parasites whose adult and larval forms are found in man, the sole reservoir of infection for all but one species. Transmission occurs by the bite of blood-sucking insects. The larvae, referred to as microfilariae, develop into infective stages by two further moults. The infective microfilariae migrate out from the insect's mouth parts on to the skin when the insect is taking a blood meal, and then enter the skin through the puncture site. Development from the infective larval form to the adult then takes about 6 months.

The adult worms are very long-lived; shedding of microfilariae begins about 6 months after infection and lasts for many years. The severity of disease relates to the burden of adult worms in the host.

Onchocerciasis

Infection with the filarial parasite *Onchocerca volvulus* causes chronic intense pruritus with a papular eruption. This is caused by the death of microfilariae in the skin. Death of microfilariae in the cornea over a prolonged period results in scarring of the cornea and unilateral or bilateral blindness.

Aetiology and transmission

Infective larvae escape on to the skin from the proboscis of an infected *Simulium* blackfly, when it takes a blood meal, and enter the skin through the bite site (Fig. 11.33). The infection is maintained in the vectors when adult blackflies ingest microfilariae in blood meals. These develop into infective larvae over about 9 days. In humans the larvae develop into adults over 6 months. Adult worms survive for up to 15 years and may shed microfilariae for most of that time.

Distribution

Tropical Africa and Central America are the main endemic areas, with foci of disease in Yemen, Colombia,

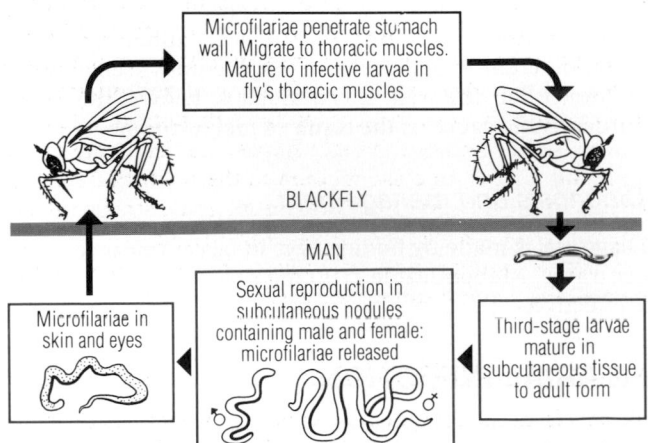

Fig. 11.33 Life cycle of *Onchocerca*.

Microfilariae penetrate stomach wall. Migrate to thoracic muscles. Mature to infective larvae in fly's thoracic muscles

BLACKFLY

MAN

Microfilariae in skin and eyes

Sexual reproduction in subcutaneous nodules containing male and female: microfilariae released

Third-stage larvae mature in subcutaneous tissue to adult form

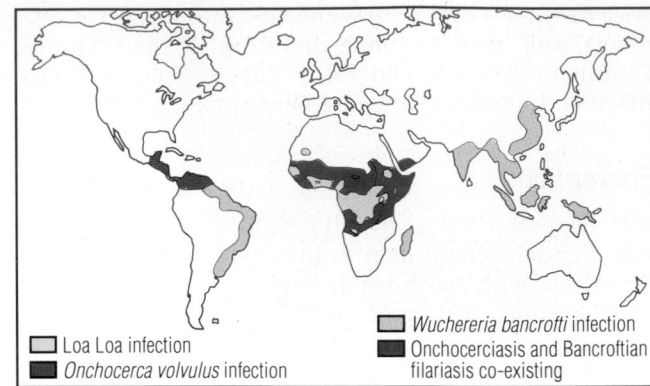

Loa Loa infection
Onchocerca volvulus infection
Wuchereria bancrofti infection
Onchocerciasis and Bancroftian filariasis co-existing

Fig. 11.34 World distribution of filariasis. Onchocerciasis distribution is very focal and not uniform over the areas shown.

Venezuela and the northern Amazonian region of Brazil. In Africa, two distinct areas are affected: the savannah area throughout West Africa where ocular involvement is common, and the tropical rainforest area where ocular involvement is less common (Fig. 11.34).

Epidemiology

The distribution of the disease relates closely to the ecology of the *Simulium* vector, which requires fast-flowing, freshwater streams and rivers for breeding. Most human cases occur in people who live close to those water sources and visit the stream or river to collect water, wash clothes or play.

Pathology and pathogenesis

The changes in the skin and eyes are caused by the death of microfilariae. Following an acute response to the worm there is granuloma formation and fibrosis. Over a number of years the result is destruction of elastic fibres, fibrosis and thickening in the affected skin. Microfilariae die in the cornea, leading to irreversible corneal scarring. Worms also may die in the iris and ciliary body, causing uveitis with secondary glaucoma as a further complication.

Some heavily infected patients have no symptoms, while others have marked symptoms and signs. Antibody and eosinophils are the principal effectors in killing microfilariae.

Clinical features

The earliest symptom is pruritus. The itch may be made worse by a hot bath. Examination shows a papular eruption with excoriation. When the arm or leg is affected, the limb may be obviously swollen in the early phase of the infection. Regional glands are often enlarged and non-tender. The lateral corneo-scleral junction should be examined with a slit-lamp for keratitis, which appears first as small diffuse white spots. Slit-lamp examination may show microfilariae in the anterior chamber. The posterior segment of the eye should be examined for retinal lesions.

The papular rash is less apparent in chronic cases where fibrosis has produced inelastic thickened skin. There may be patchy destruction of the pigment layer in a black skin, giving a 'leopard skin' appearance. Destruction of the elastic fibres of skin in the inguinal region creates pouches containing enlarged inguinal glands, and the same process predisposes to inguinal hernia. Onchocercal nodules may be seen and felt over bone prominences.

Diagnosis

The parasitological diagnosis is confirmed by examining skin shavings from affected areas for microfilariae. Eosinophilia and a positive serological test for filariasis are usually found in the peripheral blood but are not diagnostic for onchocerciasis.

Differential diagnosis

Scabies and lichen planus are common or relatively common itching skin diseases in the tropics and should be considered. Nodules and ocular disease are not found, and the appearance and distribution of lesions in both conditions is different. Loa loa infection (p. 309) causes transient soft tissue swelling that produces short-lived pruritus. The lymphatic filarial infections cause unilateral limb swelling with regional adenopathy but no pruritus or papular rash.

Treatment

Diethylcarbamazine (DEC) has been the mainstay of treatment for many years. The starting dose is 25–50 mg, increasing on alternate days to a maximum of 200 mg 3 times a day, maintained for 21 days. This drug causes gross exacerbation of the symptoms and signs of the disease, even at the lowest doses. When this is severe, doses should be increased more slowly. When ocular disease is exacerbated, topical or systemic steroids may be needed. Nutrition should be improved and infection treated before DEC is given, as reactions on treatment may be fatal in malnourished or infected persons. Without reinfection about 50% of patients relapse by 1 year after treatment. This does not indicate parasite resistance, as DEC kills microfilariae effectively but does not kill adults.

Suramin (Antrypol) is effective against adult worms and microfilariae but is used mainly for its ability to kill adult worms when ocular involvement is present. Anaphylaxis to the drug can occur and the drug is nephro-

toxic. Ivermectin is now the drug of choice because it kills microfilariae with much less exacerbation of symptoms and signs than are caused by DEC. Adult worms are not killed but there is evidence of reduced fecundity after ivermectin. Relapse rates are about 50% over a year after treatment. Excision of onchocercal nodules is recommended, particularly those on the head and shoulders.

Prevention and control

The Onchocerciasis Control Programme in West Africa has been very successful in reducing transmission of the disease by application of insecticides to vector habitats and by treating cases. The success is evidenced by a striking reduction in infection rates among children. The costs involved are considerable. Insecticide resistance may become a serious handicap to further progress.

Lymphatic filariasis

Lymphatic filariasis is a group of filarial infections in which adult worms, found in major abdominal lymphatic vessels, shed microfilariae which are carried to the bloodstream. In contrast to onchocerciasis, it is the adults that cause the pathological changes resulting in lymphoedema. This occurs in a relatively small proportion of those infected. The three species involved are *Wuchereria bancrofti*, *Brugia malayi* and *B. timori*. Geographical distribution of *W. bancrofti* is shown in Figure 11.34.

Aetiology and transmission

W. bancrofti (Fig. 11.35) females measure 80–100 mm long by 0.3 mm. The males are smaller, 40–5- mm long. The adults live in lymphatic channels and the female sheds about 50 000 sheathed microfilariae per day; these are carried to the bloodstream in lymph. They circulate in the blood and are taken up by mosquito vectors of the genera *Culex*, *Anopheles* and *Aedes*. The infective larvae moult twice after they enter a human host when the insect bites. *W. bancrofti* exhibits periodicity of microfilaraemia throughout most of its geographic distribution, releasing microfilariae during the night hours; maximal counts are at about 1 a.m., in close relation to the nocturnal feeding habits of the mosquito vectors. Subperiodic strains release microfilariae throughout the 24-hour period.

Brugia malayi and *B. timori* have similar adult morphology and a similar life cycle.

Distribution and incidence

Bancroftian filariasis has the widest geographical distribution, covering tropical Africa, Asia east of Pakistan as far as eastern China, Indonesia, the Philippines, Papua New

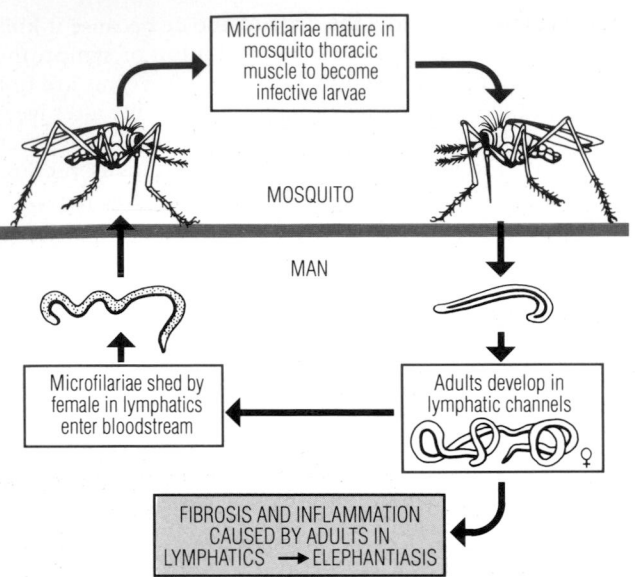

Fig. 11.35 Life cycle of lymphatic filariasis.

Guinea, the Caribbean and the north-eastern regions of South America (all periodic forms). Subperiodic forms are widely distributed in S.E. Asia and the Pacific.

Current estimates indicate that about 905 million people live in endemic areas, of whom about 10% are infected. Of these, 90% have *W. bancrofti*. Two-thirds of all those infected live in China, India and Indonesia.

Pathology and pathogenesis

Obstructive lymphoedema of arm, breast, genitalia or legs is the main outcome of inflammatory changes in main lymphatic channels elicited by the presence of adult worms. Adult worms may be found in lymphatics or lymph nodes. Distal to this obstruction the lymphatics are dilated. Inflammatory changes in the epididymis can be an early manifestation of the host response to *W. bancrofti*. Similar histological features occur in infection with *Brugia* species but these most often affect the legs. In established infections, episodic non-bacterial lymphangitis and lymphadenitis occur, evoked by allergy to filarial antigens. Eosinophils, giant cells, dead adult worms and fibroblasts are seen in the affected lymphatics and glands.

In the chronic phase lymphatic channels are obstructed by fibrosis with distal lymphoedema. There is fibrosis in the lymphoedematous tissue.

Clinical features

Many infected people have no symptoms related to the disease. The earliest feature is often generalised painless swelling of the leg. There is no rash and inguinal glands may be normal. The swelling is worst in the evening and declines while the patient is recumbent overnight. This occurs within months of infection before microfilariae are shed, which indicates a response to adult worms. Without treatment this swelling may progress to the chronic lymphoedema of filariasis. Recurrent lymphangitis is another presentation of filariasis. Lymphatics are red and tender, and inguinal glands are swollen and painful. The lymphangitis may spread distally in a limb, which is the opposite of spread in bacterial lymphangitis. Epididymitis which may or may not relapse is another manifestation of the same process.

The end stage is non-pitting lymphoedema with thickened, lichenified skin. The penis, scrotum or labia may be involved. The breast is sometimes involved. Infection with *Brugia* species tends only to affect the lower limbs. Filarial abscesses can develop along the line of lymphatic channels, more often proximally in the limb. These rupture and discharge, and the ulcerated area heals well.

W. bancrofti infection may cause intermittent chyluria, in which anastomoses between intestinal and renal lymphatic channels are open, these are due to more proximal obstruction in main lymphatics leading to the cisterna chylae and thoracic duct.

Diagnosis

Diagnosis is usually made on the history, physical signs and marked peripheral blood eosinophilia when patients are seen at the early lymphoedema stage. Later, when there is relapsing lymphangitis or epididymitis, microfilariae are found in the blood, maximally at 1 a.m. in the periodic forms, and by day and by night in the subperiodic forms. When there are many microfilariae they are readily found in stained blood smears. Filtration of blood through a filter to retain the microfilariae may demonstrate parasites in lighter infections. The parasitic infection may have died out in patients with end-stage disease, and so parasites cannot be found. Serological tests are not specific for filarial infections and cross-reactions with *Strongyloides* are common, so that a positive test should stimulate a further search for parasites.

Differential diagnosis

Tuberculosis, malignancy and chronic bacterial lymphangitis may all cause lymphoedema in the tropics.

Management

Diethylcarbamazine (DEC) is used, as for onchocerciasis (p. 307). Reactions due to death of worms do occur. Lymphoedema is best controlled by elevation of the affected limbs at night and pressure bandaging. Surgery is not satisfactory and is only a final resort. Prophylactic penicillin (penicillin V, 250 mg twice daily) is helpful in patients who have had repeated attacks of bacterial lymphangitis.

Prevention and control

Traditionally these have depended on vector control and treating cases. Recent work in Indonesia and Kenya has shown that low-dose DEC can be used to control the infections.

Loiasis

Loiasis is a filarial infection characterised clinically by transient soft tissue swellings at sites of adult loa loa worm death. *Chrysops* files are the vectors.

Aetiology

Loa loa adults measure about 60 mm by 0.5 mm (female) and 30 mm by 0.4 mm (male). They migrate freely in subcutaneous tissues. Six months after infection adults have developed, and fertilised females start to shed microfilariae which are found in peripheral blood during the daytime. *Chrysops* flies ingest microfilariae in blood meals. Development to adult worms takes place in subcutaneous tissues, and shedding of microfilariae begins by 90 days after infection. Adults live for up to 15 years.

Epidemiology

The endemic areas (Fig. 11.34) cover the tropical rain forest regions of West and Central Africa, extending as far east as the southern Sudan and Uganda.

The vectors live in the forest canopy and descend to lower levels to feed. The prevalence in some populations is 100%. Animal reservoirs do not play a part in the cycle of transmission.

Clinical features

Transient itchy soft tissue swellings up to 7 cm across, on the limbs or less often the face, are a common presentation; these are called 'Calabar swellings'. Occasionally an adult worm migrates across the globe of the eye beneath the conjunctiva, causing local irritation, a feeling of movement and some alarm. Occasionally a worm dies immediately beneath the skin, producing a linear swelling in the skin.

Problems can arise in patients who have large numbers of microfilariae in the peripheral blood (over 25–50/mm³), beginning a short time after starting treatment with DEC. Encephalitis or encephalomyelitis can occur, probably due to death of microfilariae occluding vessels of the brain and spinal cord. Cerebral oedema and granulomatous reactions around microfilariae are found in fatal cases.

Diagnosis

The diagnosis is confirmed by finding typical sheathed microfilariae in peripheral blood samples taken during the day. When there are few microfilariae, millipore filtration of blood may show parasites (see above). Eosinophilia in the peripheral blood is usual and a positive serological test, e.g. filaria indirect fluorescent antibody test, provides only indirect evidence of infection.

Management

DEC is the most active drug in the treatment of loiasis. It kills microfilariae very well and adults more slowly. While the patient is on DEC, Calabar swellings may appear. Also, worms dying close to the skin may be seen. When microfilariae counts are above 25–50/mm³ DEC cannot be given alone because of the danger of precipitating cerebral complications. Removal of microfilariae from circulation is recommended. Whole blood exchange transfusion or apheresis using a blood separator can be used to remove large numbers of microfilariae. This makes it safe to give DEC is the usual way. Steroids may be given before DEC.

Prevention and control

Measure for control of loiasis have not been successful. Vector control is difficult. Mass chemotherapy is not appropriate because of the need for individual supervision of treatment in people with heavy infections, and because of the co-existence of onchocerciasis in the same endemic areas. Other measures include protection from biting by clothing and the use of insect repellents.

Tropical pulmonary eosinophilia

Tropical pulmonary eosinophilia (TPE) occurs most often in India but can occur wherever there is transmission of Bancroftian filariasis. It is thought to represent pulmonary hypersensitivity to the microfilariae of *W. bancrofti*.

The patients present with a range of nocturnal respiratory symptoms, including unproductive cough, dyspnoea waking the patient from sleep, and wheezing (not common). The severity ranges from mild to severe. The physical signs may be minimal, with pulmonary crackles or minimal wheeze. Radiological changes are prominent, with linear and nodular shadowing that may alter with time. Pulmonary function tests show a predominantly restrictive defect.

Gross eosinophilia is usual, with absolute counts often in the range of $2-10 \times 10^9$/l. Serological tests for filariasis are strongly positive. Studies in TPE patients using species-specific antigens showed the highest titres to *W.*

bancrofti antigens. Blood samples contain no microfilariae. It is thought that these hypersensitive patients sequester the microfilariae in the pulmonary circulation, clearing the blood before it passes to the left heart. Post-mortem studies have shown microfilariae in lung with surrounding inflammatory responses in lung vessels.

Treatment with DEC is effective but there may be initial exacerbation of pulmonary symptoms. If there are particularly bad, oral prednisolone may be given. Symptoms and signs regress, and radiological changes and eosinophil count return to normal.

ANIMAL INTESTINAL NEMATODE INFECTION

Trichinosis

Aetiology

Trichinella spiralis is a nematode parasite with very low host specificity. It will infect over 100 species of animals, particularly carnivores. Infection of man occurs by eating undercooked meat containing encysted larvae (Fig. 11.36). These hatch in the human gut and mature to the adult stage. Fertilised females shed vivaparous larvae for up to 14 weeks until the adults are expelled. The larvae penetrate the gut mucosa to reach the circulation and are disseminated to all the tissues, where they excite inflammatory responses. Larvae encyst and survive in skeletal muscles.

Distribution, incidence and transmission

T. spiralis is widely distributed in nature through the Americas, Asia, Africa and the Arctic. Sporadic cases and epidemics occur. Outbreaks occur in Europe.

All ages and both sexes are susceptible but children seem to have milder attacks, probably related to a lower

infecting dose of larvae in their smaller meals. Exposure to infection is more likely among those nationalities whose cuisine involves eating raw or lightly cooked meats.

Pathology

Granulomata form around worms dying in the tissues. Focal interstitial myocarditis is found in the heart, with a marked infiltrate of eosinophils. A non-suppurative meningitis with granulomata and capillary thromboses is seen in fatal cases. Invasion of the eye muscles may contribute to the periorbital oedema. Skeletal muscles show encysted larvae, myositis with marked eosinophil infiltrate, and patchy degeneration of muscle fibres. Calcification may occur in the capsule of the cyst or in the larvae by 6 months after invasion, but larvae can remain viable in muscle for 10–15 years.

Clinical features

Four main features of the disease are fever, orbital oedema, myalgia and eosinophilia. Bowel upset is variable. Vomiting occurs, and the alteration in bowel habit may be diarrhoea or constipation. In the phase of muscle invasion the affected muscles are tender on movement. Fever, urticaria, splinter haemorrhages in fingers and toes, difficulty with swallowing and difficulty with breathing may all be present. Invasion of the nervous system can cause a meningitis-like picture. Fits, paralysis, disturbed conscious level, difficulty with balance and personality disorders may occur. Heart failure can result from severe cardiac involvement. Symptoms due to reactions to larvae in the tissues start to resolve gradually from about 14 days onwards in milder cases, but can take several months to settle completely.

Diagnosis

Trichinosis is suspected clinically and confirmed by examination of muscle biopsy for encysted larvae. Muscle biopsies can be obtained under local anaesthetic using a Trucut needle and are examined immediately, squashed between microscope slides. Eosinophil counts are very high, over $2 \times 10^9/l$, and muscle enzymes are raised. Trichinella serology is strongly positive. Differential diagnosis includes polyarteritis and other causes of eosinophilia.

Management

Thiabendazole is used in doses of 25 mg/kg, up to a maximum single dose of 1.5 g, twice daily for 5 days. Mebendazole is recommended (200 mg twice daily for a similar time). It eradicates adult worms from the gut lumen but does not affect larvae. Steroids should be given

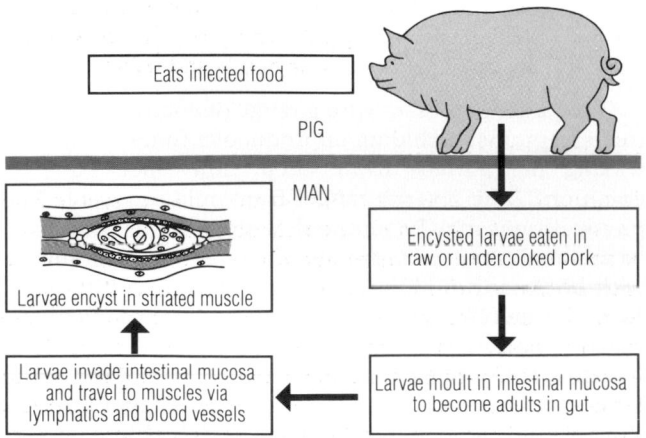

Fig. 11.36 Life cycle of *Trichinella spiralis*.

Eats infected food

PIG

MAN

Encysted larvae eaten in raw or undercooked pork

Larvae encyst in striated muscle

Larvae invade intestinal mucosa and travel to muscles via lymphatics and blood vessels

Larvae moult in intestinal mucosa to become adults in gut

to those who have marked systemic upset and muscle tenderness.

Prevention and control

Thorough cooking or freezing ($-15°C$ for 20 days) of meat will prevent trichinosis. Public health measures include boiling pig swill and inspecting meat.

Toxocariasis

Aetiology

Toxocariasis is caused by infection with larval forms of *Toxocara canis* or *T. cati*, which are primarily parasites of dogs and cats. The adult worms are found in the gut lumen. Eggs are shed in the faeces. Humans are infected by ingesting eggs, and the larvae released burrow into the gut wall to enter vessels and disseminate. Larvae mature outside the host over 14 days and then are infective to the definitive host or to man.

Distribution, incidence and transmission

The distribution is worldwide in dogs and cats, although there is considerable variation in the frequency of animal infection and contamination of the environment. Studies in Britain showed that 17% of soil samples were contaminated with toxocara eggs. Moist soil conditions are more suitable for transmission than hot, dry conditions.

Children are most often infected. Infection is likely to occur when fingers contaminated with soil or sand containing eggs during play are put in the mouth. Dog faeces deposited in public parks, especially around playgrounds, represent a potential source of infection. Dog breeders and people who work in kennels are at risk of infection. Toxocariasis due to *T. cati* is much less common.

Pathology and pathogenesis

Disease in man relates to the number of infecting larvae and the host response. Clinical manifestations are due to dying and dead larvae, which evoke granuloma formation with eosinophils, macrophages and lymphocytes. The eye, brain, liver, spleen and lungs may be involved in toxocariasis, but granuloma formation may occur in any organ of the body.

Clinical features

Ocular toxocariasis and visceral larva migrans (VLM) are two clinical presentations of this disease, which is often a subclinical infection. Unilateral visual impairment is the usual symptom is ocular toxocariasis. Lesions directly on the visual axis will cause severe impairment. A child may develop a squint. The granuloma can form in relation to the lens and ciliary body, or on the retina itself. A cataract may develop secondary to a granuloma affecting the ciliary body. Visceral larva migrans is due to a heavy infection with larvae. Fever, anorexia, chills, night sweats and weight loss are usual features. Examination shows hepatosplenomegaly as the main physical sign. Pneumonitis may be present as well.

There is usually a marked eosinophilia in the peripheral blood in VLM, but eosinophilia is less common with ocular disease. Serological testing is valuable, the ELISA technique using a toxocara secretory antigen being a sensitive and specific test.

Differential diagnosis

Toxoplasmosis usually causes bilateral choroidoretinitis with destruction of the retina. Lymphoma, tuberculosis and sarcoidosis are usually considered in the differential diagnosis of VLM, although the gross eosinophilia is against the former conditions and supports a helminthic infection. The toxocara antibody test is strongly positive.

Management

DEC is the usual treatment, giving initial doses of 50 mg and doubling the dose on alternate days till the maximum dose (10 mg/kg per day in 3 doses for 21 days) is reached. Ocular disease is not specifically affected by DEC because the worm is dead. There may be some spontaneous improvement as inflammation and granuloma size reduce. DEC is given in these cases to kill any worms that are still migrating.

Prevention and control

Regular deworming of dogs, particularly pregnant bitches and puppies, reduces the numbers of eggs contaminating the environment. Dog owners should try to ensure that their dogs defaecate in a place where the faeces will not contaminate open spaces, playgrounds and parks.

Dracunculiasis

Dracunculus medinensis, the Guinea worm, is a tissue nematode widely distributed through Africa and Asia. Man is infected by drinking water containing minute crustaceans of the *Cyclops* genus infected with Guinea worm larvae. The larvae penetrate gut tissues and migrate through host tissues, maturing to the adult stage. The female is fertilised by the male, which dies, and the gravid female migrates out into a limb, producing a painful, fluid-filled blister about 3 cm across. The blister bursts and about 5 cm of the female protrudes. Vast numbers of larvae are released from the worm. Patients often put the affected limb into cold water to relieve the pain; this stimulates discharge of larvae to provide the opportunity for larvae to continue the life cycle by infecting other cyclops. The diagnosis is made on the clinical appearances. Treatment comprises:

- relief of pain
- treatment of secondary bacterial infection with antibiotics
- administration of thiabendazole.

This does not have any direct effect on the worm, but reduces inflammation around the worm, allowing it to be gently wound out of the subcutaneous tissues on a stick.

TREMATODES

Schistosomiasis

Infection with digenetic flukes of the genus *Schistosoma* affects the bladder and urinary tract (*S. haematobium*) or intestine (*S. mansoni, S. japonicum*). These worms cause disease because of the host's response to eggs retained in the tissues. The severity of disease relates to the number of eggs in the tissues, which is proportional to the worm burden.

Aetiology

Eggs are passed in stools or urine; those deposited in still or slow-flowing fresh-water hatch to release the ciliate miracidium, which can survive for up to 48 hours before it dies (Fig. 11.37). During this time it must find an aquatic snail of the appropriate genus, *Biomphalaria* for *S. mansoni, Bulinus* for *S. haematobium*, and *Oncomelania* for *S. japonicum*. Cercariae are released from the snail and these penetrate the skin of a suitable host, almost always man, becoming schistosomules during penetration. These migrate via the blood vessels to the pulmonary vasculature, where some traverse the pulmonary circulation to enter the systemic circulation. Schistosomules of *mansoni* and *japonicum* mature in the hepatic branches of the portal vein, and by 6 weeks after infection they are mature. They migrate out of the liver against the flow of blood in the portal vein to small veins around the colon and small intestine. The colon is mainly involved in mansoni infections, and both colon and small intestine are involved in *japonicum* infections. The life cycle of *S. haematobium* is similar, but maturation takes place in pelvic veins; the worm pairs migrate into small branches of the internal iliac vein around the bladder principally, although other pelvic structures – the prostate and seminal vesicles in men, and the uterus and adnexal structures in women – may be involved. Adult worms

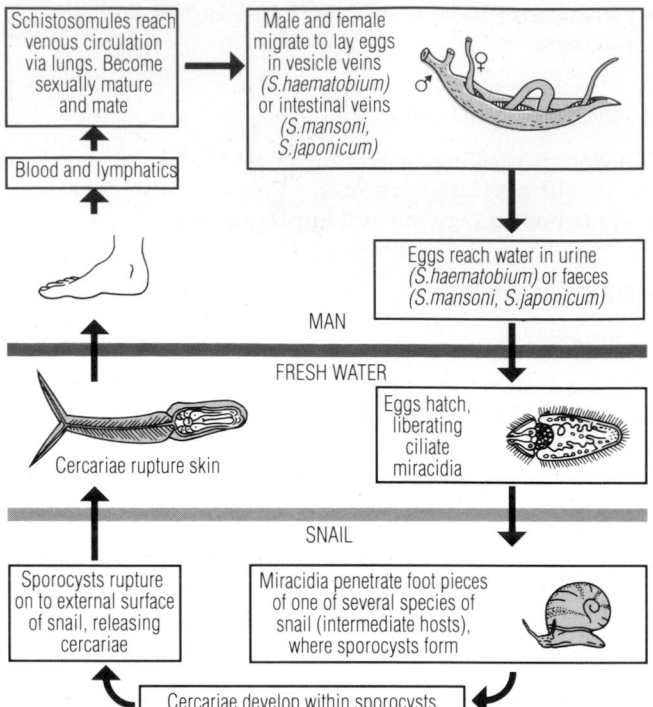

Fig. 11.37 Life cycle of schistosome parasites.

survive for about 7 years on average, but survival of over 30 years has been reported.

Distribution and incidence

The distribution is shown in Figure 11.38. There is considerable overlap in the endemic areas of *haematobium* and *mansoni*, but *japonicum* has a distinct, Asian distribution. The prevalence and incidence of infection vary considerably, with rates up to 70% or more in the endemic areas. Infection rates tend to be highest in children and decline with increasing age.

Transmission and epidemiology

Freshwater contact is the major factor in becoming infected and maintaining transmission. Children are infected early in life by playing in infected water. They are also likely to urinate and defaecate in and around pools and streams, further enhancing the local intensity of transmission. The highest rates and intensities of infection are found in the second and third decades of life.

Pathology and pathogenesis

The pathological changes relate to the presence of eggs in the tissues. Eggs lain in the small branches of veins may:

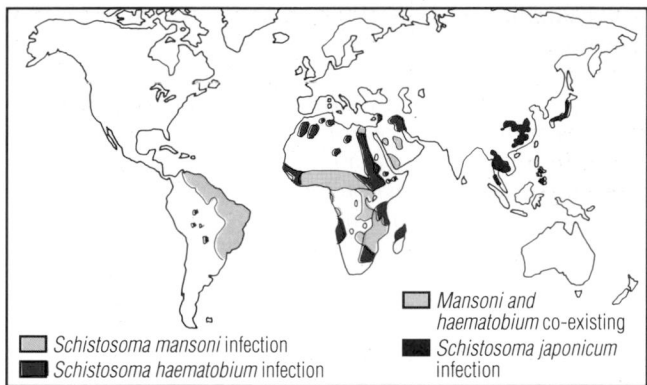

Fig. 11.38 World distribution of schistosomiasis

- pass through the wall of the viscus to reach the exterior in faeces or urine
- be retained in the tissues
- embolise through vessels to lodge in presinusoidal branches of the portal vein in *mansoni* and *japonicum* infections, or in pulmonary arterioles in *haematobium* infections.

The egg excites a granulomatous response with macrophages, lymphocytes, plasma cells and eosinophils. Granuloma formation is important for the transition of the egg through the mucosa to the lumen of the viscus. The chronic inflammation they may cause in the epithelium may be a factor in carcinogenesis in the bladder (*haematobium*) and the colon (*japonicum*).

Eggs retained in the tissues within granulomata gradually break down until all that may remain is remnants of the egg case. The granuloma heals by fibrosis. Early in the course of infection exuberant granuloma formation can cause colonic polyps in *mansoni* and *japonicum* infections, and bladder polyps in *haematobium* infection. These resolve after treatment and may also resolve spontaneously.

Fibrotic polyps and strictures are not often seen in *mansoni* infection, although they are more common in *japonicum* infection. *Haematobium* infection causes fibrosis of the bladder, which is often shrunken with a thick wall. Bladder stones may form and cystitis is common. Unilateral or, less commonly, bilateral ureteric strictures cause obstructive uropathy. Stones may form in the dilated ureters. Distortion of the ureterovesical junction may allow vesico-ureteric reflux of urine with associated recurrent pyelonephritis.

Squamous cell carcinoma of the bladder is common in highly endemic *S. haematobium* areas. It is suggested that schistosomiasis acts with dietary factors to produce malignancy. Reports from China have associated colonic cancer with *S. japonicum* infections. Chronic schistosomal colitis causing epithelial cell dysplasia, a premalignant stage, and later carcinoma is the suggested sequence of events. This has not been found in *S. mansoni* infection.

Mansoni and *japonicum* eggs embolise to the liver. The granulomas add to the volume of the liver and increase its size, and obstruct the flow of blood through the portal circulation in the liver, causing congestive hepatosplenomegaly in those with heavy worm burdens. Over a period of years periportal fibrosis results, causing irreversible portal hypertension. The anatomy and architecture of the hepatic lobules are not altered and there are *no* regenerating nodules, therefore cirrhosis is not caused. In the lungs granulomatous reactions in the vessels cause fibrosis and pulmonary hypertension.

Involvement of the CNS occurs in *S. japonicum*, *S. mansoni* and *S. haematobium*, in descending order of frequency. Granulomas form around eggs that have embolised to the brain or spinal cord.

Clinical features

Cercarial invasion of the skin may cause a local, irritant, papular eruption but this is uncommon. Most patients have no symptoms related to the phase of migration and maturation. Occasionally non-immune people develop the *Katayama syndrome* with the phase of worm migration. There is malaise and lethargy, while fever, profuse sweats, muscle pain, abdominal pain, joint aches, unproductive cough, urticaria, swollen eyelids and hepatosplenomegaly occur in more severely affected patients. These symptoms begin 3–4 weeks after exposure and persist for up to 3 months with reducing severity.

Chest X-rays may show coin lesions due to worms dying in vessels and evoking local inflammatory reactions. Marked eosinophilia is common. Eggs are not found until 3–6 weeks after infection.

S. mansoni and S. japonicum

Many infected patients go through life without any symptoms related to this infection. Rectal examination is normal; sigmoidoscopy is normal or shows scattered mucosal haemorrhages. Occasional patients present with anaemia and oedema because of bleeding and protein loss from schistosomal polyps. The most common physical sign in infected patients in endemic areas is hepatomegaly, which correlates with the intensity or infection in the first two decades but not in older age groups. Similar findings are noted in *S. japonicum* infection. Abdominal pain and subacute intestinal obstruction occasionally occur in the rare patients who develop fibrotic strictures in the colon or, less often, the small intestine. Hepatosplenomegaly with congestive splenomegaly suggests end-stage schistosomal hepatofibrosis. These patients often present with haematemesis and ascites. Porto-systemic encephalopathy is not a usual feature after variceal bleeding in schistosomiasis. Severe pain over a grossly enlarged spleen may indicate splenic infarction.

S. haematobium

Dysuria, frequency and haematuria occur in some patients at the start of egg laying. More commonly, the presenting symptom is terminal haematuria. The last drops of urine passed are blood-stained. Physical examination is usually normal. Most persons have light infections and suffer no long-term adverse effects. Reversible granulomatous polyps and obstructive uropathy occur in the early stages of heavier infection. This appears to be spontaneously reversible and it is certainly reversible after treatment. Those with heavy infections develop fibrotic and obstructive complications which can cause recurrent urinary tract infections, stone formation and finally renal failure. In these patients the infection is associated with an increased risk of bladder cancer. Excretion urography often shows bladder polyps and obstructive uropathy, either unilateral or bilateral, in older children and teenagers.

Chronic infection causes 'sandy' patches on the trigone as a typical cystoscopic finding. Calcification in retained eggs is seen in the bladder wall as a rim of calcium in the pelvis on a plain abdominal X-ray. Tramline calcification in the ureter may also be seen.

Other manifestations

Pulmonary involvement may be subclinical up to the stage when significant pulmonary hypertension develops. Right heart failure develops and this is difficult to treat. Cutaneous involvement is indicated by a collection of subcutaneous papules. The skin of the scrotum and perineum may be affected in haematobium infection.

Symptomatic involvement of CNS is uncommon. Intracranial disease occurs with S. japonicum infections, with a frequency of 2–4% among those infected. It is much less common in mansoni and haematobium infections. Focal signs and Jacksonian epilepsy may occur with involvement of the cerebral hemispheres, while posterior fossa lesions are associated with raised intracranial pressure, cerebellar signs and brainstem compression.

Lesions of the spinal cord may present with features suggesting cord compression. transverse myelitis or spinal artery occlusion. Granulomas may also form around the cauda equina. The occurrence of focal signs in the neuraxis in a patient in or from an area endemic for schistosomiasis should prompt a search for schistosome eggs in stools and urine that would indicate active infection. Eosinophils in the CSF suggest the possibility of schistosomiasis affecting the CNS. The use of antischistosomal drugs also needs to be considered.

Diagnosis

Diagnosis is made by finding schistosome eggs. Eggs of S. mansoni and S. japonicum are found in concentrates of faecal samples. Eggs of S. haematobium are found in the centrifuged deposit of terminal urine samples. Eggs of all three species may be found in rectal snips. Squash preparations can also be made from fragments of bladder mucosa obtained at cystoscopy.

Eosinophilia is a common finding in the peripheral blood but occurs in several helminthic infections. Serological tests can be helpful. An ELISA for antibodies to schistosome egg antigens is useful because it indicates that infection has progressed to the stage of oviposition. The test takes 18 months to revert to negative after treatment and so is not helpful is assessing cure.

Excretion urography, isotopic renography, ultrasound and CT scanning give anatomical and functional detail of the urinary tract in chronic schistosomiasis. Colonoscopy and barium enema can be used to examine the colon in more detail. Ultrasound scanning of the liver demonstrates the presence of periportal fibrosis. Chest radiographs show dilatation of the pulmonary arteries and right ventricular hypertrophy in pulmonary hypertension. Myelography and CT allow localisation of schistosomal lesions of the neuraxis. Eosinophilia in the CSF supports the diagnosis of CNS involvement in schistosomiasis.

Management

Three safe, effective drugs are available for use in schistosomiasis (Table 11.37). Their safety has not been confirmed in pregnancy and so treatment should be delayed until after delivery unless there are urgent indications for prompt treatment. All cases should be treated, even the advanced cases, as further oviposition causes further urinary tract, intestinal, liver or pulmonary damage. Ideally stools and rectal snips should be examined for viable ova 3 months after treatment.

Prevention and control

Control measures are expensive and require a change in the behaviour pattern of the exposed population. Education regarding the reasons for the measures is essential. Dams and irrigation projects for the improvement of the economy of an area may create new habitats for snail hosts of schistosome parasites. Molluscicides can be used, but are expensive and may have detrimental effects on other water creatures. Biological methods of snail control are an attractive concept but are not yet effective.

Clonorchiasis

Aetiology

Clonorchis sinensis is a hermaphroditic trematode parasite of the biliary tract in man. The adult fluke is 10–25 mm

Table 11.37 Drug treatment of schistosomiasis

Drug	Active against	Dose	Side-effects/contra-indications
Oxamniquine*	*Schistosoma mansoni*	West Africa and South America 15 mg/kg x 1 (adult) 20 mg/kg x 1 (child) Elsewhere 20 mg/kg per day x 3	Occasional febrile episode 5 days post-treatment
Metrifonate*	*S. haematobium*	7.5 mg/kg x 3 (2 weeks between doses)	Anticholinesterase actions may prolong neuromuscular blockade after surgery. Avoid elective surgery for 3 days post-treatment and provide ventilatory support after emergency surgery within 48 hours of administration
Praziquantel*	*S. mansoni* *S. haematobium* *S. japonicum*	20 mg/kg b.d. x 3 20 mg/kg x 3 (4 hours between doses)	Dizziness, nausea and occasional vomitting beginning 1 hour after dosing, lasting up to 4 hours

* The safety of these drugs has not been confirmed in pregnancy; treatment should be delayed until after delivery unless there are urgent indications for prompt treatment.

long by 3–5 mm wide. The life cycle is shown in Figure 11.39.

Transmission and incidence

Fish-ponds into which human faeces are poured as fish feed are an important source of infection as eggs, snails and fish are conveniently found together. The disease occurs in Asian countries. Dogs and cats are also important hosts.

Pathology

The worms obstruct small branches of the biliary tree, and bile accumulates in cysts proximal to the obstruction.

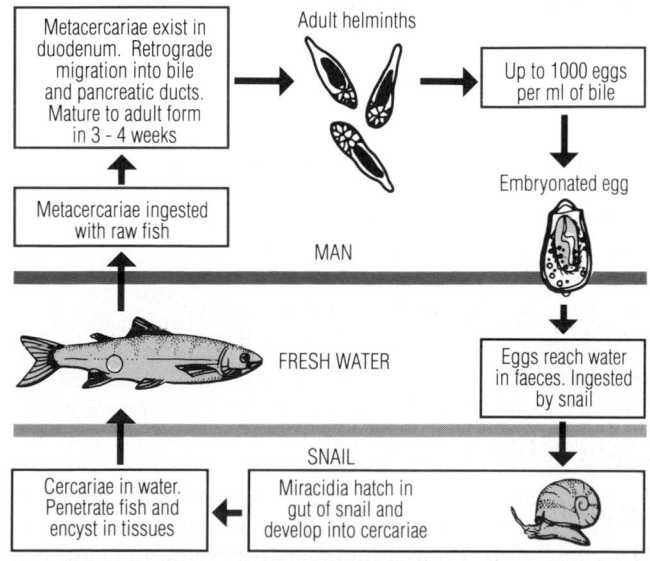

Fig. 11.39 Life cycle of *Clonorchis* and *Opisthorcis*.

Hypertrophy of the bile epithelium with adenomatous proliferation occurs. Later there is cellular infiltrate of the bile duct wall with chronic inflammatory cells. Pigment stones and biliary sludge form. Flukes obstructing the pancreatic ducts can cause pancreatitis. Long-standing heavy infections are associated with malignant change in the adenomatous hyperplasia, leading to cholangiocarcinoma.

Clinical features

Clinical features relate to the worm burden. Mild infections cause no symptoms. Upper abdominal discomfort, diarrhoea and weakness occur with heavier infections; with the heaviest worm burdens upper abdominal pain, diarrhoea, weight loss, obstructive jaundice, hepatomegaly, cholangitis and Gram-negative septicaemia occur.

Diagnosis

The eggs are found in faeces or in duodenal aspirate. Eosinophilia is usual in the peripheral blood. Endoscopic retrograde cholangiopancreatography or percutaneous transhepatic cholangiography shows dilated branches of the biliary tree, and the worms appear as filling defects.

Management

Praziquantel is the treatment of choice, giving 25 mg/kg on three occasions 4 hours apart on one day. When there is obstructive jaundice with cholangitis and septicaemia, relief of biliary obstruction, vigorous treatment of the bacterial infection and circulatory support for the patient are needed.

Prevention and control

Transmission can be interrupted by safe disposal of faecal wastes. Usually this involves a major change in social habits, which is difficult to achieve. Thorough cooking of fish before it is eaten prevents infection, as does freezing fish, −10°C for 5 days, and salting in 10% saline.

Opisthorciasis

Opisthorcis viverrini and *O. felineus* have similar life cycles to that of *C. sinensis*, and in man they parasitise the intra- and extrahepatic branches of the biliary tree (Fig. 11.39). Raw, pickled, smoked and undercooked fish are the sources of infection. The pathological change and consequences are those of chronic irritation and obstruction of the biliary tree with ascending cholangitis in severely affected patients. Cholangiocarcinoma occurs in *O. viverrini* patients.

The diagnosis is made by finding eggs of the parasite in stools or duodenal aspirate. Praziquantel is used for treatment as for clonorchiasis.

Fascioliasis

Fascioliasis is an infection of the biliary tree with the hermaphroditic trematoda, *Fasciola hepatica*. It is primarily an infection of sheep. The life cycle is similar to that of *Clonorchis* (Fig. 11.39).

Aetiology and distribution

The parasite measures 3 cm by 1.5 cm. Eggs are released in the biliary passages and pass to the exterior in the faeces. The miracidium hatches in fresh water and penetrates the tissues of a freshwater snail (*Lymnaea* species). After a cycle lasting 4 months in the snail, cercariae are released. These encyst on the leaves of watercress and other types of aquatic vegetation. Man is infected by eating watercress with encysted metacercariae. Maturation to the adult stage in bile ducts takes about 4 months until egg laying starts. Sheep are the normal hosts of this infection, and human infections are likely wherever sheep are herded in wet pasturelands.

Pathology

There is hepatic parenchymal necrosis in the phase of migration through the liver. The liver tissue regenerates. The worm burden determines the severity of disease. In the bile ducts there is chronic inflammation with regenerative hyperplasia of the epithelium and some degree of duct obstruction.

Clinical features

Pain in the liver area, fever, chills, tender hepatomegaly and marked eosinophilia are usual features during the tissue migration phase. Upper abdominal discomfort and hepatomegaly are present in mild to moderate infections, while heavy infections may cause obstructive jaundice and cholangitis in addition to pain and hepatomegaly.

Diagnosis

Eggs of the parasite are found in stools or duodenal aspirate. Eosinophilia is usual and serological tests for this infection are usually positive.

Management and prevention

Bithionol is effective (40 mg/kg in two divided doses after food on alternate days for 15 dosage days).

Watercress production must be separate from sheep pastures. Wild watercress should not be sold for human consumption.

Fasciolopsiasis

Fasciolopsis buski is the largest trematode parasite, measuring up to 7.5 cm long by 3.0 cm wide. It has a wide geographic distribution through eastern Asia with a reservoir of infection in pigs. The metacercariae are found on bamboo shoots or water chestnuts, and infection occurs when these are eaten uncooked. After about 3 months the adult has matured in the small intestine; egg production begins and lasts for most of the 6-month lifespan of the adult. Upper abdominal discomfort, diarrhoea, preprandial upper abdominal pain relieved by food, and symptoms and signs of intestinal obstruction may occur, more marked symptoms being found with heavier infections. Eggs are found in the faeces. Tetrachlorethylene is effective in treatment. Praziquantel may prove to be effective.

Paragonimiasis

Paragonimus westermani is a hermaphrodite fluke usually found in the lungs but occasionally in other sites, e.g. CNS. It has a wide distribution in South America, West Africa, South-east Asia and the Pacific. Human infection occurs when raw or undercooked freshwater crustacea with metacercariae encysted in their muscles are eaten. The development cycle outside the host involves a freshwater snail: from the snail the cercaria is released and this finds a suitable crustacean host.

In man the metacercaria excysts and penetrates the full thickness of the gut wall to enter the peritoneal cavity. The phase of tissue migration continues with the parasites reaching and crossing the diaphragm to enter the lungs.

Where the worm finally comes to rest in lung tissue it elicits first a cellular response and then fibrosis, so that the worm is enclosed but for a connection to an airway. Dead worms calcify.

Radiological appearances comprise pleural thickening, infiltrates at the site of recent invasion, nodular lesions (encysted adults), fibrosis and finally calcification.

Eggs released by the worms are coughed up or swallowed. Cough productive of sputum, dyspnoea and chest discomfort are usual features. Bacterial infection of the affected area causes fever, systemic upset, purulent sputum and haemoptysis on occasions. Abdominal organs and brain are affected less often.

Diagnosis and management

Eggs are found in the sputum in most cases. Serological tests are available. Praziquantel is effective in doses of 25 mg/kg given three times daily for 3 days.

CESTODES

HUMAN INTESTINAL CESTODE INFECTION

Taenia saginata

Human infection with *T. saginata* is common in Africa, the Middle East, Asia and South America. The infective stage is the cysticercus in beef, and man is infected by eating rare or undercooked beef (Fig. 11.40). The cyst is released in the gut and the scolex everts from the cyst. It adheres to the gut wall and proglottids start to develop. Each segment has testis and ovaries, and is self-fertile. The worm may be 5–10 m long. The distal segments are full of eggs. Lengths of worm are passed in the stools, and when defaecation occurs in pasture, cattle may eat the gravid segments and develop cysticercosis bovis.

The infection causes no symptoms in man, although often a variety of vague abdominal symptoms have been attributed to it. Occasionally a patient will present with pruritus ani and find segments in underwear. The motile segments have wriggled out of the anus.

The diagnosis is confirmed by examining segments. *T. saginata* segments have 15–20 lateral branches to the uterus. The eggs are occasionally found in the stools or on the perianal skin, but are identical in *saginata* and *solium* infections (see below).

Treatment with praziquantel (10 mg/kg as a single dose) is effective in 96% of patients. Niclosamide is also effective. Both praziquantel and niclosamide destroy the scolex and it is not present in the expelled worm remnants. If segments have not been passed by 4 months after treatment the infection is cured.

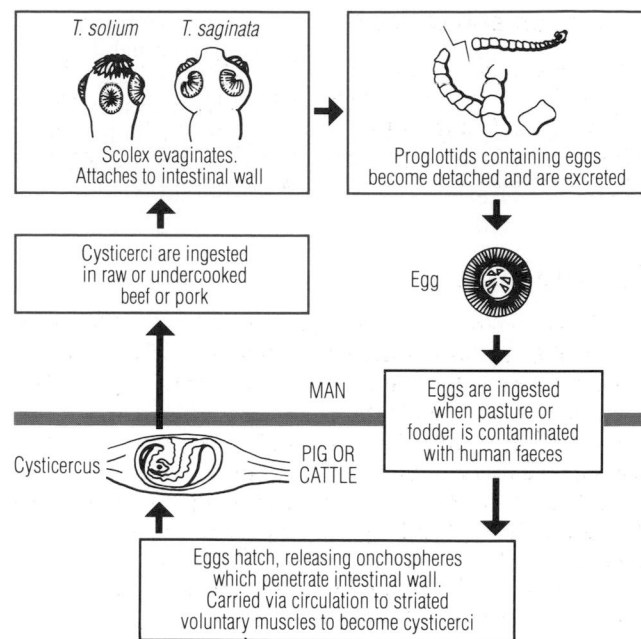

Fig. 11.40 Life cycle of *Taenia* species.

Thorough cooking of meat and freezing meat to –10°C for 10 days kills cysticerci. Meat inspection is also an effective control measure.

Taenia solium

The life cycle is the same as that of *T. saginata*, except that the pig is the intermediate host (Fig. 11.40). Infections with *T. solium* adults cause no symptoms. The segments are distinguished from those of *T. saginata* by the small number of lateral branches of the uterus, 7–13. Treatment is the same as for *T. saginata*, with the addition of an antiemetic prior to dosing and giving a purge 2 hours after dosing. Thorough cooking of pork or freezing to –10°C for 10 days prevents infection. Cysticercosis is discussed below in the section on larval cestodes.

Diphyllobothrium latum

The fish tapeworm has a more complex life cycle than the other intestinal cestodes: coracidia released from eggs infect water fleas (copepods). Further development takes place in fish that eat the copepods and in bigger fish that eat plerocercoid-infected fish. Mammals are infected by eating the plerocercoid-infected fish. Digestion releases the plerocercoid, which adheres to the gut wall and starts to produce proglottids. Proglottids break up, releasing eggs which are passed in the stools. Man is infected by eating uncooked fish.

A variety of abdominal and general symptoms are attributed to this infection, including abdominal discomfort, fatigue, weakness, sensations of hunger and diarrhoea. It is associated with deficiency of vitamin B_{12} and, less commonly, with overt megaloblastic anaemia. When the worm is sited in the upper gastrointestinal tract, it can take up both free and intrinsic factor-bound vitamin B_{12}. Features of vitamin B_{12} deficiency appear when body stores are exhausted.

The diagnosis is made by finding eggs or, less often, typical segments in faecal samples. Purging may provide a sample of segments. Praziquantel gives a high cure rate. Niclosamide is also effective. Thorough cooking of fish and freezing fish to $-10°C$ for 48 hours kills plerocercoids.

Hymenolepiasis

Hymenolepis nana and *H. diminuta* are two species of small tapeworm. *H. nana* is predominantly a parasite of man with person-to-person transmission, while *H. diminuta* is predominantly a rodent parasite with man as an occasional host.

Children are most often infected with *H. nana*. Heavy infection causes abdominal pain, anorexia, diarrhoea, irritability, pruritus ani and urticaria. Eosinophilia is found in heavy infections. Treatment with praziquantel (15 mg/kg as a single dose) is effective.

H. diminuta has a more complex life cycle involving an insect intermediate host which ingests eggs with rodent faeces. Most infections cause no symptoms and are diagnosed when eggs are found in faeces. Treatment with niclosamide is effective.

LARVAL CESTODE INFECTION

Cysticercosis

Infection with the intermediate state of the *T. solium* parasite (see above) can occur in two ways:

- by ingesting eggs of the worm, which hatch in the gut to release the cysticercus
- by regurgitation of gravid segments into the stomach to initiate the process of egg digestion and release of cysticerci.

The cysticerci released by either route of infection then invade host tissues. The first route is more likely.

The development of subcutaneous lumps is a common presentation. Uniocular disturbances of vision occur with cysticerci in the eye. The most serious consequences occur in cerebral cysticercosis, causing epilepsy, raised intracranial pressure and localising signs related to space occupation. Frequently numerous cysts are found in the brain. The diagnosis is based on the geographic history, a positive serological test for cysticercosis on serum, and the finding of cystic lesions on CT of the brain. In endemic areas where CT is not available, the diagnosis would be made on the clinical picture. Antibodies to cysticerci can be detected in CSF, which contains increased amounts of protein, a normal glucose and normal or increased cell count. Skeletal muscles are often involved in cysticercosis. Usually this causes no symptoms and calcified cysticerci are seen on X-rays. There may be muscle pain at the time of invasion. If cysticerci are found at any site in the body a CT brain scan should be done to detect cerebral involvement.

Praziquantel is effective against living cysticerci. The dose is 50 mg/kg per day in three equal doses for 14 days. Dexamethasone is also given is doses of 4 mg three times daily prior to the start of treatment and tailed off after treatment. Follow-up shows that two-thirds of cerebral cysts will disappear, and symptoms and signs will improve. This treatment should be given in centres where neurological expertise is available.

Hydatid disease

Aetiology and distribution

Echinococcus granulosus is a tapeworm of dogs. The life cycle is shown in Figure 11.41. The ingested eggs release the onchosphere, which penetrates the gut mucosa and spreads by vascular or lymphatic channels to other organs, most often the liver, with lung, spleen, brain, eye, bone and other tissues infected less often. Cyprus, Turkey, Middle Eastern countries, the Turkana area of Kenya, and South America are among the endemic areas.

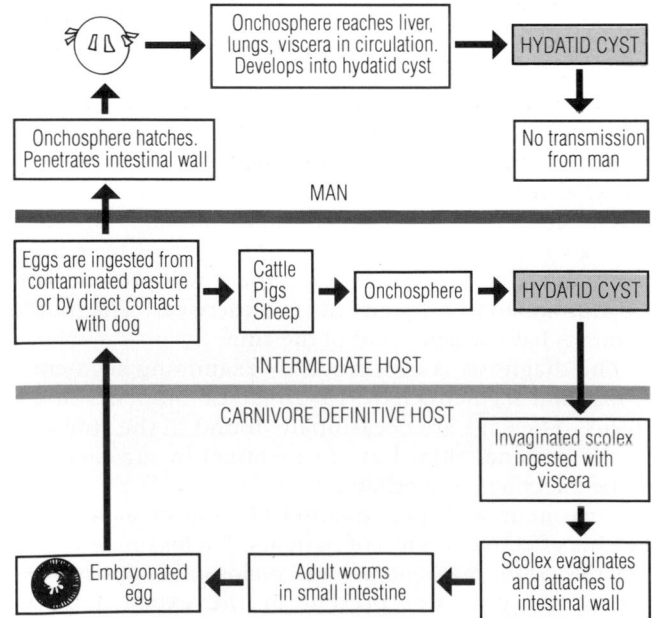

Fig. 11.41 Life cycle of *Echinococcus granulosus*.

Clinical features

The clinical presentation is very variable. Unexplained painless hepatomegaly is fairly common, but an expanding cyst can cause right upper quadrant abdominal discomfort. Rupture of the cyst may produce pleuritic discomfort, abdominal pain and tenderness, and allergic manifestations such as urticaria and anaphylaxis. Rupture of hydatid cysts is infrequent, although the consequences of release of daughter cysts to seed the peritoneal cavity are serious.

Pulmonary hydatids may be symptomless and may be found on chest X-rays. They may rupture spontaneously. Hydatid material, membranes and scolices with hooklets may be coughed up and disseminate endobronchially to seed the lungs bilaterally, causing numerous small cysts in both lung fields. Bone and joint hydatids cause pain, swelling and sinuses discharging hydatid material. The latter may follow surgical exploration. The cyst wall may calcify.

Diagnosis

There may be blood eosinophilia and positive serological tests. Ultrasound and CT scanning allow accurate localisation and measurement of hydatid cysts in internal organs. Bone hydatid produces areas of lucency surrounded by sclerosis. Joints are destroyed.

Management

Management is difficult. Mebendazole in high doses has been successful in occasional cases where cysts are young and newly formed. Albendazole, which is much better absorbed, is currently being evaluated and may prove effective. Surgical treatment is difficult. Solitary pulmonary hydatids can often be excised with the relevant segments or lobe. Excision of hepatic hydatids is more difficult. Surgery for hydatids of the CNS requires great care to avoid rupture.

Complications

Secondary bacterial infection of a hydatid cyst is not uncommon. Amoebic abscess, pyogenic abscess and perihepatic sepsis must be considered in the differential diagnosis when liver cysts are concerned. Gallium scanning may help to indicate bacterial infection and blood cultures should be taken. Amoebic serology is strongly positive in amoebic liver abscess. When infected hydatid cyst is probable, vigorous antibiotic treatment is first needed, followed by safe surgical drainage of the cysts.

Prevention and control

Regular deworming of dogs, killing of stray dogs, and safe disposal or boiling of offal are important control measures. These measures, plus effective communication of the dangers of hydatid disease among populations in Iceland and New Zealand, have controlled the disease.

FURTHER READING

Adler M W (ed.) 1990 ABC of sexually transmitted diseases, 2nd edn. British Medical Association, London. *The only book a medical student needs on STD: summarises the important facts*

Adler M W (ed.) 1991 ABC of AIDS, 2nd edn. British Medical Association, London. *This BMA booklet gives a clear summary, with good pictures, of all aspects of HIV disease*

Lambert II P, Farrar W E 1982 Infectious diseases illustrated. W B Saunders, London. *Illustrations of a wide variety of infections*

Lambert H P, O'Grady F 1990 Antibiotic and chemotherapy, 6th edn. Churchill Livingstone, Edinburgh. *A comprehensive guide to antimicrobials and their use*

Mandell G L, Douglas R G, Bennet J E 1989 Principles and practice of infectious diseases, 3rd end. Churchill Livingstone, New York. *A major reference work*

Strickland G T (ed.) 1991 Hunter's tropical medicine, 7th edn. W B Saunders, London. *A major reference work*

Wilcox R R, Wilcox J R (eds) 1982 Venerological medicine. Grant McIntyre (now Blackwell, Oxford). *A major reference work*

12
Cardiovascular Disease

J Malcolm Walker and Lip-Bun Tan

Ischaemic heart disease is the most important cause of death in the Western World. It causes more than a million deaths per year in the USA and about 160 000 deaths annually in the UK (Fig. 12.1), where it accounts for 40–50% of all deaths and is the main reason for men not reaching their seventh decade.

A recent concerted effort to change life-styles with respect to smoking, diet and exercise, as well as better control of hypertension, appears to have led to a decline in coronary artery disease deaths in the USA and the more affluent Northern European countries, but has yet to make a major impact in the UK.

Rheumatic heart disease has declined rapidly in importance in the West over the last 30–40 years (p. 419). It now accounts for less than half the cases of heart valve disease coming to surgery and, with only a

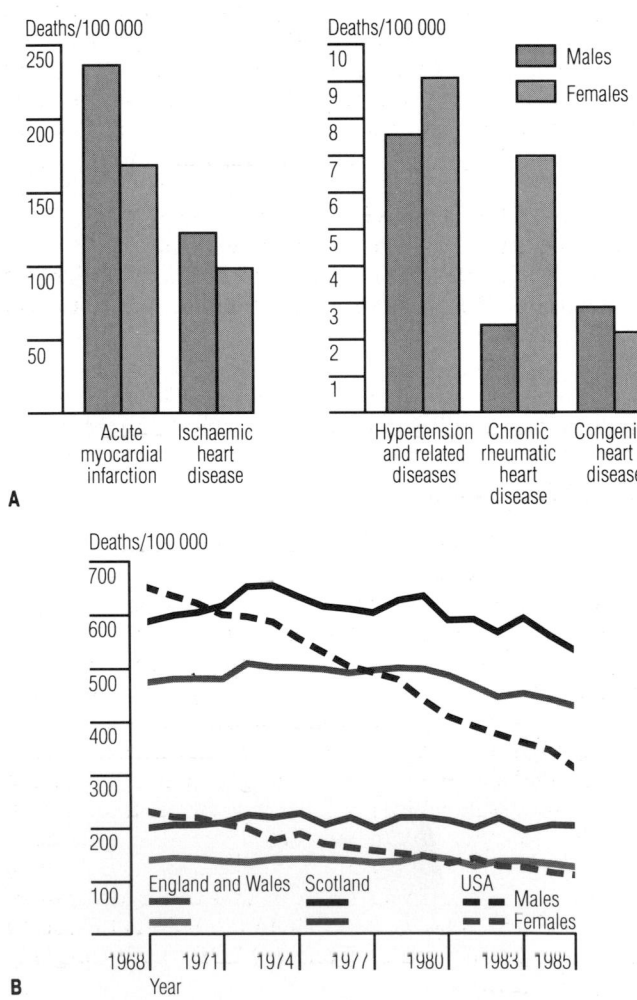

Fig. 12.1 Mortality from cardiovascular disease. A. Causes of death from cardiac disease (England and Wales, 1987). **B.** Deaths due to coronary artery disease in Scotland, England and Wales, and the USA in the years 1968–1985. Note the steep decline in mortality in males and females in the USA. (Source: WHO)

THE SCOPE OF MODERN CARDIOLOGY

More than 40% of patients admitted to medical wards in the UK have some form of heart disease. Coronary artery disease, heart failure and cardiac arrhythmias are among the commonest causes of emergency hospital admission.

small number of new cases presenting, its importance will probably decline further. However, it is still a major cause of morbidity and mortality in the developing world.

Congenital heart disease is one of the principal causes of neonatal death and is likely to remain a significant cause of morbidity and mortality in childhood. However, more cases are now treatable by cardiac surgery in childhood, and major cardiac defects can now be detected during pregnancy, raising the possibility of neonatal, or even antepartum, cardiac surgery.

The development of sophisticated methods of investigation in cardiology now allows great precision in diagnosis, enabling full advantage to be taken of the advances in cardiac surgery and catheter-based treatments. Diagnostic methods have expanded from simple ECG and X-ray to include an ever-widening range of techniques, using ultrasound (both imaging and Doppler), isotope imaging, angiography, intracardiac electrophysiology and 24-hour ECG recording, pressure measurement and magnetic resonance imaging. Therapeutic options have also increased, to include complex cardiac surgery possible at all ages, pacemaker therapy and non-surgical interventions such as angioplasty. The efforts of cardiac surgeons and bioengineers have produced a generation of patients with prosthetic heart valves, implanted pacemakers, modified congenital heart disease and heart transplants. These present a new spectrum of pathology and altered natural history.

NORMAL AND DISORDERED PHYSIOLOGY

CONTRACTION

Cardiac muscle is striated and shares with skeletal muscle the same basic contractile unit, the *sarcomere*. The components of the sarcomere are the myosin thick filaments, and the thin filaments composed of actin, troponin and tropomyosin. A local increase in calcium concentration allows an interaction to occur between the heads of myosin molecules and the thin filaments which produces cross-bridges between the filaments. A conformational change between the globular head of the myosin molecule and its rod-like tail causes a tension in the cross-bridge, making the filaments slide past each other (Fig. 12.2). Relaxation is brought about by a decrease in intracellular calcium and the hydrolysis of adenosine triphosphate (ATP) by myosin ATP-ase to produce adenosine diphosphate (ADP) and inorganic phosphate (Pi).

Energy for contraction

ATP is only stored in small amounts in heart muscle, so its production must occur at a rate equal to its consump-

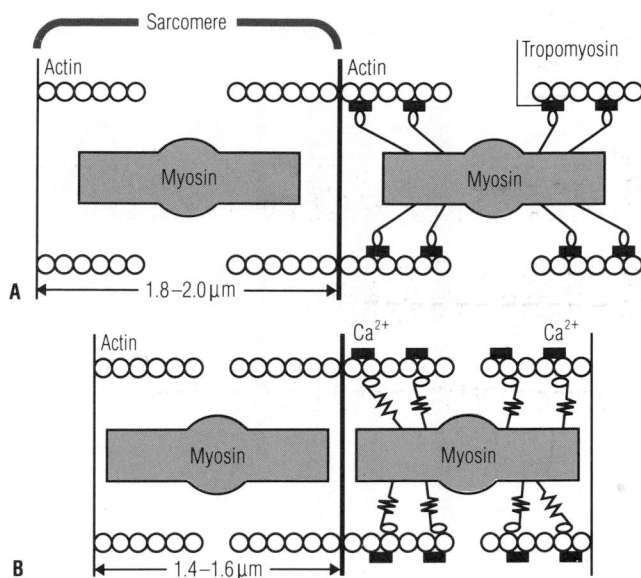

Fig. 12.2 Diagrammatic representation of sarcomere contraction. A. In the relaxed state (diastole) tropomyosin inhibitory subunits prevent the interaction of the myosin heads with actin. **B.** In the presence of calcium, this interaction can take place enabling contraction (systole) to occur.

tion. Free fatty acids (FFA) are the major source of myocardial energy, yielding 2.5 times more ATP per gram weight than glucose. Glucose breakdown can occur in the absence of oxygen, but only two molecules of ATP are produced per molecule of glucose metabolised to pyruvate (instead of the 36 obtained by aerobic metabolism of glucose to carbon dioxide and water). The normal heart consumes lactate, which, by the action of lactate dehydrogenase, yields pyruvate.

The action potential

Rhythmic contraction and relaxation of myocardial cells is achieved by the sequential release of calcium near the myofibrils and its subsequent removal. The sequence of events is outlined in Figure 12.3.

The action potentials from different regions of the heart have different configurations, the most important of which is the spontaneous depolarisation during diastole in the *pacemaker cells* of the sino-atrial and atrio-ventricular nodes (Fig. 12.4, action potentials A and C). This rise in membrane potential in diastole triggers the next depolarisation and sets the heart rate.

Areas distal to the sino-atrial node are inhibited from showing their intrinsically slower pacemaker potential, but will do so if the impulse from the sino-atrial node is absent or delayed. The rate of sino-atrial node depolarisation is greatly influenced by beta adrenoreceptors. Sympathetic stimulation increases this rate and therefore speeds the heart rate, whereas parasympathetic stimulation produces

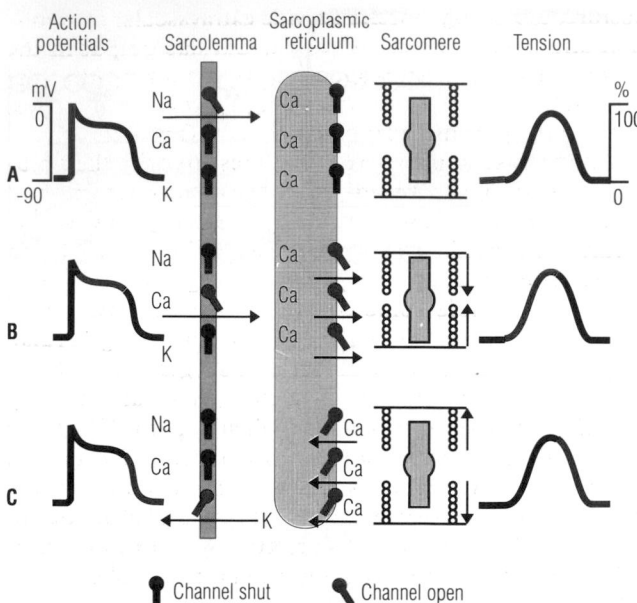

Fig. 12.3 Relationship between action potential, transmembrane ionic movements, sarcomere contraction and muscle tension. A. With the onset of the action potential, sarcolemmal sodium channels open. **B.** This is followed by release of calcium from the sarcoplasmic reticulum into the cytosol and sarcomere shortening. **C.** Relaxation follows resequestration of calcium into the sarcoplasmic reticulum. Repolarisation is accompanied by loss of potassium from

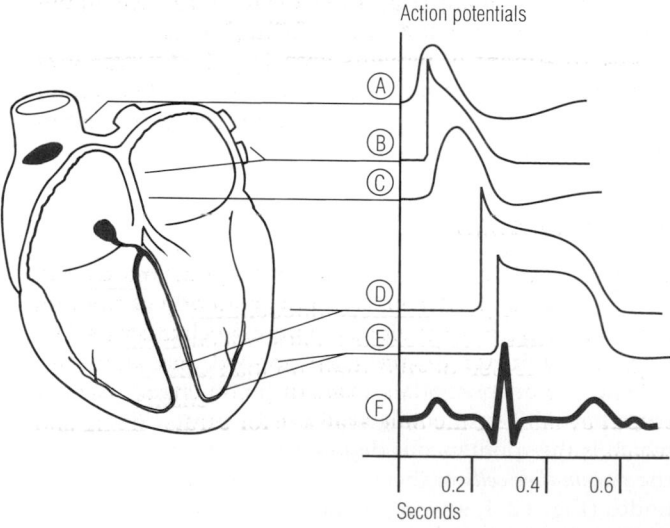

Fig. 12.4 Action potentials from different regions of the heart. (A) Sino-atrial node; (B) atria; (C) atrio-ventricular node; (D) Purkinje network; (E) myocardium; (F) is the electrocardiogram.

opposite effects mediated by acetylcholine. Circulating catecholamines and changes in serum potassium and magnesium are amongst the other factors that affect the basic electrophysiological properties of cardiac cells.

In non-pacemaker cells, the wave of depolarisation from adjacent cells is the stimulus for the inward flow of sodium ions, which starts the cardiac cycle. Periods of absolute and relative refractoriness follow the prolonged plateau phase. Average action potential durations are about 300 milliseconds, but shorten in response to increasing heart rate and adrenaline.

The rate of conduction of impulses through the heart is determined by the action potential shape. Depolarisation is accompanied by a short-lived and very rapid current, producing the fast upstroke of the classical cardiac action potential (Fig. 12.4, B, D, E). The fast inward current is maximal when the foregoing resting membrane potential (Vm) is most negative, the situation found in the Purkinje cells of the ventricle, where conduction velocities are at their highest. Depolarisation of cells occurs in diseased and injured tissue and therefore causes slowing of conduction until, eventually, conduction block occurs. In the specialised tissues of the sino-atrial and atrio-ventricular nodes the upstroke of the action potential is slow and dependent on calcium influx (Fig. 12.4, A and C). These features account for the slow conduction through the sino-atrial node.

HEART PUMP PERFORMANCE

Normal function

Many physiological factors can influence the power of the contraction and pump performance:

- *Inotropy*: dependent on the hormonal and ionic environment
- *Preload*: the myocardial fibre length at which the contraction begins
- *Afterload*: the force against which the muscle contracts
- *Force–interval effects*: dependent on the rate and pattern of stimulation.

Inotropy

The myofibrils produce tension in proportion to the free calcium released into the cytosol, until saturation is reached and tension rises no further. Calcium entry into the cell occurs during the action potential plateau, and variations in contraction strength occur by the release of variable amounts of calcium from intracellular stores, or by a change in sensitivity of the myofilaments to calcium. In a steady state, calcium entry into the cell with each action potential is balanced by a loss to the extracellular space. Accumulation of calcium in intracellular stores is facilitated by increased levels of extracellular calcium or by high intracellular sodium, which may occur when the sodium pump is blocked by digoxin. Under normal conditions, extracellular calcium concentration plays no part in the beat-to-beat control of the heart's performance. This is mainly affected by sympathetic discharge and circulating catecholamines, which produce an increased heart rate (*chronotropic drive*) and also enhance myocardial contraction. The final common pathway of this latter effect is achieved by increased myofibrillar calcium sensitivity. Changes in extracellular concentrations of potassium and pH affect myocardial contraction, but, since those concentrations are generally kept constant by homeostatic mechanisms, they do not control heart activity in normal circumstances, although they may do so in disease.

Preload

Venous return to the heart is dependent on right atrial pressure. During inspiration, intrathoracic pressure falls, causing an accentuation of venous return to the right heart. Standing up tends to diminish this but, in the upright posture, exercising muscles provide extravascular compression and maintain venous return. Cardiac output in the normal heart is very responsive to venous return (the *Frank-Starling curve*), but the failing heart is less sensitive, due to a flatter ventricular function curve (Fig. 12.5).

An increase in intrapericardial pressure with the accumulation of an effusion impedes venous return and cardiac filling, and, with marked elevations, a low stroke volume and cardiovascular collapse follow, a condition called *tamponade* (p. 426). Some drugs affect venous tone, for example some of the therapeutic benefits of nitrates are related to venodilatation, lowering cardiac output and thus reducing myocardial oxygen demand.

Normal ventricular filling occurs principally in early diastole, with atrial systole giving a final 'top-up'. The latter may be particularly important in hypertrophied hearts, which fill poorly in early diastole. Here atrial systole provides a much greater fraction of ventricular filling. In these patients, loss of atrial contraction (due to atrial fibrillation) may lead to marked reduction in stroke volume.

Afterload

During systole, the ventricles eject blood once the diastolic pressure in the arterial circuits is exceeded. *Afterload* is the load during ejection. This can be equated with the peripheral vascular resistance, which, together with vessel wall elasticity, determines the diastolic arterial pressure. Increasing afterloads (Fig. 12.6) decrease cardiac output and this relationship is steeper in failing hearts.

The treatment of patients with impaired ventricular performance now includes the use of drugs that reduce the peripheral vascular resistance and hence reduce afterload (p. 349).

Rate and rhythm

Changes in the rate of stimulation of the heart muscle can alter contractile performance, independently of changes in muscle length (or preload). These mechanisms affect output to a lesser degree than preload and afterload. However, increases in heart rate may also change cardiac output by altering the time available for cardiac filling and coronary flow.

Ventricular dilatation

The cardiac chambers dilate either with abnormal volume loads or as a consequence of impaired myocyte function, as in cardiomyopathy. The larger volume ventricle is an adaptive response, allowing the maintenance of stroke volume despite a reduction in the shortening capability of the myofibrils. However, although the response is initially adaptive, there is a cost. From the Laplace equation, a

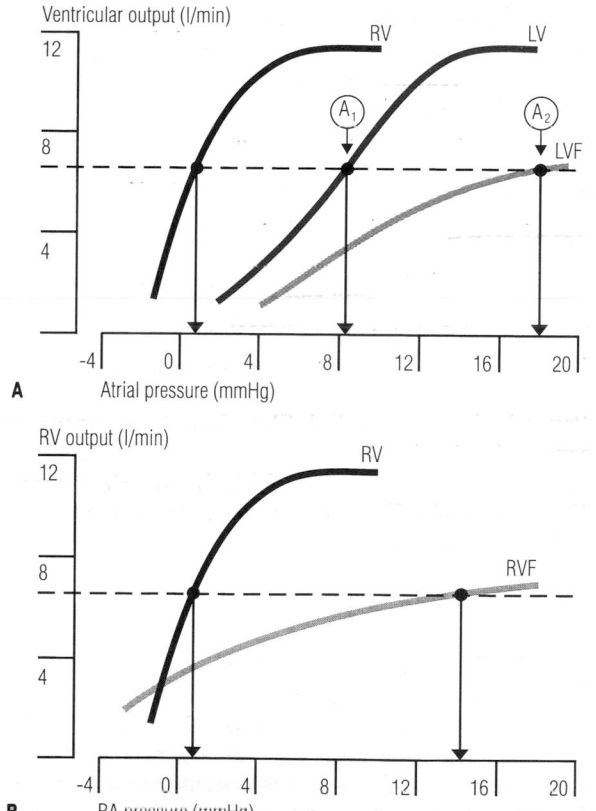

Fig. 12.5 Relationship between ventricular output and filling pressure.
A. The black line shows a normal right ventricular (RV) function curve, where an RV output of 7 l/min (dotted line) is achieved with a filling pressure of 1 mmHg. The left ventricle (LV) must produce the same output (A1), so that the normal LV (red line) requires a filling pressure of 8 mmHg. If the LV is failing (LVF, pink line), a filling pressure of 18 mmHg (A2) is required to maintain this output. **B.** A similar relationship is shown for the normal (black line) and failing (grey line) right ventricle.

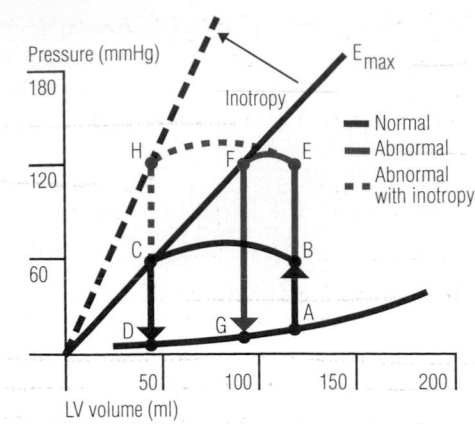

Fig. 12.6 The relationship of LV volume to pressure in a normal cardiac cycle (A-B-C-D). At (A) systole begins. The pressure rises isovolumically until at (B) the aortic valve opens. The ventricle ejects to (C) and then isovolumic relaxation occurs until (D), at which point filling occurs. With acute elevations in aortic diastolic pressure (red line), pressure in the ventricle rises to (E) before the aortic valve opens. Ejection occurs to (F). The pressure–volume relationship at the end of systole is defined by the black line (E_{max}) passing through (C) and (F). The beat A-E-F-G has a low stroke volume (A minus G). For this to be restored to the original volume (A minus D), the line E_{max} must shift to the left (dotted line); i.e. a positive inotropic effect is required, where a given end-systolic pressure is associated with a lower volume and more complete ejection.

dilated ventricle with an increased diameter can only generate the same pressure with an increased wall tension. This increased wall tension can only be produced by an increase in oxygen consumption, which may outrun the supply, leading to further ischaemia and dilatation.

Ventricular hypertrophy

Cardiac myocytes hypertrophy in response to:

- Loss of adjacent myocytes.
- An increase in ventricular wall stress – the resultant increase in wall thickness effectively reduces the stress each sarcomere has to generate. With mild hypertrophy, the capillaries increase in density proportionally to the hypertrophy, but beyond a certain extent the capillary growth lags behind the hypertrophic process, thus rendering the less well-supplied subendocardium liable to ischaemia. The hypertrophic process accompanied by deposition of more collagen fibres, leads to reduced compliance and impairing diastolic function.

SYMPTOMS AND SIGNS OF CARDIAC DISEASE

Heart disease may cause chest pain, shortness of breath, palpitations, syncope and presyncope, oedema and fatigue. These symptoms are not specific to heart disease. A careful history is essential and should reveal that the patient's symptoms are more likely to arise from the heart than from, say, a combination of indigestion and bronchitis. It also provides an opportunity for the patient to indicate the degree of disability and intrusion into normal life. A direct question into the extent to which the patient has had to his or her activities is helpful. Some patients avoid symptoms by grossly restricting their activities; others take their symptoms as a matter of course without realising their significance. It can also be very useful to ask for a history of heart disease in the family or a close acquaintance, since cardiac symptoms may follow dramatic cardiac events in close relatives or contacts (but are not always neurotic in origin). Some diseases, such as hypercholesterolaemia, are familial.

Chest pain

There are several types of chest pain arising from the heart and great vessels. The pain may be from cardiac ischaemia, pericarditis, aortic dissection, massive pulmonary embolism or, in introspective patients, from ectopic beats, when the patient may describe apical, stabbing pain.

Cardiac ischaemic pain

The typical pain of angina pectoris or myocardial ischaemia is a squeezing, gripping pain, usually felt in the praecordium but often felt in the throat (hence *angina* — to choke). It may radiate down the arms, usually the left, up into the jaw and lower teeth, or even through to the back. The pain is reproducible in its location and distribution, except that mild attacks may not gain the full distribution of more severe attacks. For example, an anginal attack may always start in the praecordium and only go through to the back if it becomes more severe.

The discomfort may be very severe and be associated with frightening feelings of impending death, an inability to get enough air and sweating. It can also be a mild discomfort or ache in the chest which may be thought trivial and ignored. Some patients do not experience their angina as a pain, and feel it as a faint constriction in the chest. Many attacks of cardiac ischaemia are unaccompanied by any discomfort (*silent ischaemia*).

Angina usually disappears fairly rapidly if the patient rests, or takes glyceryl trinitrate (GTN). Angina builds up over a few seconds and is usually not greatly influenced by posture, unlike musculoskeletal chest pain (which may also occur with exertion). Although similar in nature and radiation, the pain of myocardial infarction lasts much longer than angina. It is more intense and does not pass off with rest or GTN. In an attack, a patient with cardiac ischaemia usually looks pale and sweaty, unlike someone with an attack of indigestion, who often appears flushed.

Other causes of chest pain

Pericardial pain (p. 426) is very similar to anginal pain but is often influenced by posture, sometimes being relieved by leaning forwards, and aggravated by swallowing. It is more often described as a burning pain, and is less likely to be associated with breathlessness than is cardiac ischaemia.

The pain of *dissection of the ascending* aorta (p. 438) is a severe, tearing pain, often starting suddenly, usually felt retrosternally at first and sometimes radiates through to the back.

Massive pulmonary embolism can also produce a retrosternal constricting discomfort (p. 498).

Oesophageal spasm due to reflux can also produce a severe retrosternal pain which may be confused with that of myocardial ischaemia. The pain of oesophageal rupture can be confused with myocardial infarction.

Jabbing precordial pains are common in highly strung patients. They may have a muscular origin, but, on occasion, coincide with the accentuated postectopic contraction of the heart which is perceived by the patient as a stabbing pain.

Dyspnoea or shortness of breath

This symptom is a feeling of laboured, or unnaturally difficult, breathing. In heart failure, it is due to a decrease in compliance of the lungs owing to the congestion that occurs with a rise in pulmonary venous pressure. The reduced cardiac output limits the oxygen-carrying capacity of the circulation; during mild activity, anaerobic metabolism occurs with the muscles producing lactic acid. The acidosis causes increased ventilation which persists for longer than normal after exertion. Thus, even minor exertion produces disproportionate and prolonged dyspnoea. Finally, in severe left heart failure with pulmonary oedema, the dyspnoea may be caused by arterial oxygen desaturation.

Dyspnoea (or angina) can be categorised using the New York Heart Association scale (Table 12.1). Severe forms of left heart failure are associated with dyspnoea at rest, closely related to posture. This degree of pulmonary venous hypertension is commonly accompanied by a dry, non-productive cough. Dyspnoea at night can be graded on the basis of the number of pillows required to enable the patient to sleep (*orthopnoea*). Patients with left heart failure may be woken from their sleep by severe dyspnoea resulting from pulmonary congestion. This passes off on sitting up, or walking about slowly, and is known as *paroxysmal nocturnal dyspnoea*. This may be the first

Table 12.1 New York Heart Association grading of dyspnoea or angina

Grade	Criteria
1	Symptoms only occur on severe exertion. Almost normal life-style possible
2	Symptoms occur on moderate exertion. Patient has to avoid certain situations, such as carrying shopping up several flights of stairs
3	Symptoms occur on mild exertion. Activity is markedly restricted
4	Symptoms occur frequently, even at rest

symptom of left heart failure, and may be difficult to distinguish from nocturnal asthma, as some patients with left heart failure develop a considerable degree of wheeze with bronchospasm.

Palpitations

The term 'palpitation' is used by patients to describe a wide variety of disorders in which there is an awareness of the heart beat. A careful interpretation of what the patient means is therefore essential. It may be simply an awareness of the normal heart beat, which may be more forceful or faster than usual because of anxiety. It may, however, be indicative of a serious cardiac arrhythmia. It is useful to ask the patient to tap on the table to indicate the rate and rhythm during the attack. Many patients can do this remarkably accurately, especially if they have had a true paroxysmal tachycardia. It is helpful to determine the following:

- Do the attacks stop suddenly or gradually, or with a forceful thump on the chest (ectopic beat)?
- Were there symptoms of cardiac insufficiency (e.g. faintness or dyspnoea, suggesting low cardiac output and blood pressure, and pulmonary venous hypertension respectively)?
- Was there irregular thumping (ectopics or atrial fibrillation)?
- Was there chest pain (the occurrence of angina implies a very fast and potentially dangerous heart rate)?

True syncope indicates an urgent need for investigation, as the arrhythmia is potentially fatal. Polyuria sometimes occurs on cessation of supraventricular tachycardias, but is not usually described by the patient unless a leading question is asked.

Syncope and presyncope (dizziness)

Sudden collapse with loss of consciousness *during* exertion almost always has a cardiac cause. It is due either to an obstruction to outflow from the left or right ventricle, which prevents an adequate increase in cardiac output on

12   Cardiovascular Disease

exertion, or to a cardiac arrhythmia, such as heart block, induced by the exertion. Both may result in a sudden fall in blood pressure and cerebral perfusion.

Syncope *after* exertion is not uncommon and may simply be due to blood pooling in the legs and a poor venous return. However, syncope under other circumstances may be cardiac, and an eye-witness account is invaluable. Cardiogenic syncope usually occurs without warning; the collapsed patient is vasoconstricted and grey and the pulse is either absent or very slow. In a classical 'Stokes-Adams' attack, the unconscious patient blushes dramatically with the return of circulation and subsequent return of consciousness. Syncope may also occur in severe tachycardia.

Some mental confusion after cerebral anoxia is almost invariable. A prolonged period of unconsciousness is, however, unlikely to be cardiogenic, since cardiac asystole or a malignant cardiac arrhythmia sufficiently rapid to cause unconsciousness is unlikely to last long without proving fatal.

Other forms of syncope

'Common' syncope. The common faint, often triggered by pain or an unpleasant sight, gastrointestinal upset, haemorrhage or pyrexial illness, is a vagal phenomenon, and the syncopal episode is followed by profuse cold sweat, a feeling of sickness or actual vomiting, and bradycardia.

Micturition syncope and *cough syncope* are rarely cardiogenic, but are probably triggered by a Valsalva manoeuvre, the first when initiating micturition with a full bladder and the latter after repeated bouts of coughing, which inhibit venous return.

Presyncope or *dizziness* is a common and much less defined symptom, and has a variety of causes as well as heart disease. It may result from a cardiac arrhythmia, but, even then, is much more common in elderly patients with associated cerebrovascular disease.

Oedema

Right heart failure causes pitting oedema of the feet and legs, worse at the end of the day and relieved by rest and elevating the legs. Unlike other causes of oedema, it may be associated with other symptoms of heart failure, such as dyspnoea and fatigue. The oedema may spread to thighs, abdominal wall, sacrum and back. There may be ascites and hepatic congestion, with abdominal distension. The hepatic congestion may be worse on exertion, with pain over the liver (usually epigastric) during exercise and for several minutes after.

The differential diagnosis of cardiac oedema includes fluid retention from other causes, such as nephrotic syndrome and cirrhosis of the liver, oedema of one or both legs from venous insufficiency or lymphatic insufficiency.

Fatigue

Fatigue is a non-specific and often neglected symptom. It is, however, a very real feature of heart disease, a result of the reduced effort tolerance and lactic acidosis produced by anaerobic muscle metabolism and changes in the skeletal muscle. It is a prominent feature of low cardiac output.

EXAMINATION OF THE CARDIOVASCULAR SYSTEM

Position

The patient should lie on a couch or bed with the head and thorax supported at about 45° to the horizontal. There should be a good light and a minimum of competing noise.

General examination

Dyspnoea. The patient may be breathless on lying down (orthopnoea) or on undressing.

'Mitral' facies. The pulmonary hypertensive patient with a long-standing low cardiac output may develop a loss of subcutaneous fat from the face and the appearance of dilated cyanosed blood vessels over the cheek-bones. This characteristic appearance is seen in patients with longstanding mitral valve disease, but is not pathognomonic.

Peripheral cyanosis. A low cardiac output results in poor perfusion of the skin, particularly of the peripheries, such as the hands and nose, which become cyanosed and cold.   *handwritten: shunt / failure*

Central cyanosis. An intracardiac right-to-left shunt of blood causes central cyanosis, with a blue tongue as well as blue peripheries. In this situation, the peripheral circulation may be adequate with warm extremities and there will usually be clubbing of the fingers and toes. In cardiac failure, central cyanosis is not associated with clubbing and the extremities are cold and cyanosed.

Pallor. A low cardiac output causing vasoconstriction can lead to generalised pallor, including the mucous membranes, fingernails and skin.

Oedema. There may be pitting oedema of the legs, scrotum, trunk and sacrum. This is demonstrated by firm finger pressure for 5–10 seconds. There may be abdominal distension from ascites.

Cardiac cachexia. Although acute weight gain is common with development of oedema, in the long term the cardiac patient usually loses fat and muscle bulk with prolonged heart failure and low cardiac output.

Hands

Clubbing may occur in cyanostic congenital heart disease or infective endocarditis.

Splinter haemorrhages are small dark subungual petechiae. They are not specific to infective endocarditis and can be found in other conditions, e.g. polyarteritis nodosa. In infective endocarditis, when recurrent, they are a sign of continuing infection.

Blood pressure

Although usually recorded early in the examination, it may be worth repeating when the patient is more relaxed and hypertension due to anxiety is likely to have settled. Hostility, anxiety and unfamiliarity cause a rise in blood pressure. Measurement should be made with the patient standing and lying.

The interpretation of the Korotkoff sounds and a detailed description of blood pressure measurement are given on page 429.

Arterial pulses

The radial pulse is examined to establish rhythm, volume and character. Each peripheral and central pulse is then examined in turn. Auscultation of carotid and femoral arteries may reveal bruits due to localised narrowing, or transmitted murmurs.

The pulse contour is influenced by the state of vasodilatation of the peripheral vascular bed. However, the carotid pulse supplies a vascular bed with a less variable blood supply, and is therefore more constant in its contour. It is most easily examined with the patient reclining at about 45° with the head fully supported and the chin central. The pulse is most easily felt half-way up the sternomastoid muscle at the level of the major skin crease. If the carotid pulse cannot be examined, any large artery such as the femoral, subclavian or brachial may give similar information, but, being more remote from the heart, they are less reliable as indicators of aortic valve disease.

The carotid pulse is used to time the first heart sound, which immediately precedes the upstroke. It gives an indication of the pulse volume and ejection time, and abnormalities of the waveform indicative of aortic valve disease can also be detected. A thrill may be present, caused by turbulence in the flow.

Rhythm

With a regular pulse the examiner can predict when the next beat is coming, e.g. by counting or tapping the foot. There may be slight variation in rate with respiration, particularly in young patients (*sinus arrhythmia*).

An irregularity of the heart rhythm may occur infrequently, or regularly after a number of normal beats; both are likely to be caused by ectopics. If the heart rate and pulse volume is totally irregular, the patient is likely to be in atrial fibrillation or having a large number of multifocal ectopics. If the pulse is irregular, the heart rate is best counted by auscultation, as observers vary considerably in their ability to feel weak beats. The difference between the heart rate at the apex (by auscultation) and radial pulse rate at the same time is called the apex/radial deficit, but is of limited diagnostic value, as there is always a deficit if the apex rate is fast and irregular.

Pulse volume

The pulse volume at the wrist depends on the stroke volume, which varies with cardiac output and pulse interval. It also depends on the state of vasodilatation of the skin of the hands, with a smaller radial pulse volume when cold than when warm. A thready, low-volume and rapid pulse may be felt in shock due to haemorrhage and a large-volume pulse in thyrotoxicosis or CO_2 retention in pulmonary disease.

Pulse character

The characteristic arterial pulse waveforms are best appreciated in the carotid pulse. *Pulsus alternans* (alternating pulse volume with a regular pulse) is a feature of left ventricular dysfunction. *Pulsus paradoxus* (exaggerated diminution of pulse pressure and volume with respiration) is found when ventricular filling is embarrassed by pericardial constriction, tamponade or a cardiomyopathy. *Pulsus bigeminy* and *trigeminy* are found with regular ventricular ectopics.

Plateau (slow rising, or anacrotic) pulse. The characteristic pulse of aortic stenosis is a small-volume, sustained pulse which rises slowly to its peak displacement, often with a palpable thrill.

Collapsing pulse. This is a sign of aortic regurgitation but may be found in any patient with a low impedance to aortic outflow in diastole (e.g. persistent ductus arteriosus, arterial venous fistula or immediately after exercise). The pulse has a very large volume with an abrupt fall following the upstroke. This is best appreciated by gripping the forearm muscle and raising the arm, when a muscle 'knock' can be felt. There is a large pulse pressure with a low diastolic reading, and the carotid pulse may be visible in the neck (Corrigan's sign).

Bisferiens pulse. There is a double peak to the bisferiens pulse, which is characteristic of aortic regurgitation accompanied by some stenosis of the valve. However, it may also be found in aortic regurgitation without a measurable aortic valve gradient.

12 Cardiovascular Disease

'Jerky' pulse. This occurs with hypertrophic obstructive cardiomyopathy (which may produce a type of bisferiens pulse) and in severe mitral regurgitation.

Jugular venous pulse

The jugular venous pulse (JVP) is visible in most patients. The height of the JVP is dependent on central venous pressure; it is therefore low in states of fluid depletion and haemorrhage, and raised in right heart failure and fluid overload. The waveform of the JVP can be a useful diagnostic aid in heart disease.

The patient should be reclining with the head at about 45°. Jugular pulsation is often better seen with side-lighting, and is often better appreciated from the foot of the bed, when widening of the neck can be seen in time with the JVP.

The JVP falls on inspiration and rises on expiration. Patients with increased airway resistance may be difficult to assess, but should be requested to stop breathing with their mouths open for a few seconds while the height of the JVP is assessed.

If the JVP cannot be seen, the patient can be positioned more horizontally, when the pulse usually becomes visible. Alternatively, abdominal compression can be used to see whether the patient has a low JVP which then becomes visible. *Gentle* pressure anywhere on the abdominal wall, or over the liver, temporarily increases the venous return (hepato-jugular reflux). The normal right ventricle increases its stroke volume within 2 or 3 s, so there is a transient (if any) increase in venous pressure. The failing right ventricle, however, cannot increase its stroke volume, so that abdominal pressure produces a sustained rise in the venous pressure.

Discrimination of arterial from venous pulsation

Venous pulsation has a sinuous quality due to the low pulse-wave velocity and its variation with respiration. Arterial pulsation is always palpable, whereas venous pulsation is only palpable when there is tricuspid regurgitation.

Height of the JVP

The height of the JVP is measured vertically from the sternal angle and is normally less than 3 cm above it. It can be increased slightly in pregnancy.

Jugular venous waveform

The principal components and classical waveforms are shown in Figure 12.7. The *a* wave is generated by atrial systole (there is no valve between the atrium and the jugular vein). It is absent in atrial fibrillation and exagger-

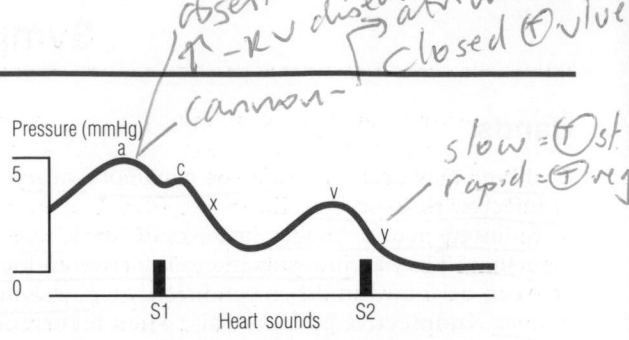

Fig. 12.7 Relationship of venous waveform to heart sounds. The *a* wave of atrial contraction is followed by the *x* descent. The *c* wave is not usually visible. The *v* wave coincides with ventricular systole.

ated in right ventricular disease with a raised right ventricular filling pressure. The *v* wave coincides with ventricular systole, when the tricuspid valve bulges into the right atrium.

Extra-large *a* or cannon *a* waves are seen when the atrium contracts against a closed tricuspid valve as in complete atrioventricular block, ventricular ectopics and nodal rhythm. Regurgitation through the tricuspid valve causes a giant *v* wave (sometimes called an *s* wave) with a very rapid *y* descent. A slow *y* descent is characteristic of tricuspid stenosis.

The precordium

On inspection, there may be thoracic deformity. This is sometimes due to congenital heart disease. The apex beat may be visible.

Palpation is performed to detect cardiac hypertrophy and the presence of palpable heart sounds and thrills. Palpation over the lower end of the sternum, with the heel of the hand and light pressure applied, may reveal a parasternal heave, evidence of right ventricular hypertrophy or occasionally a large left atrium due to severe mitral regurgitation. The position of the apex beat is defined as the furthest laterally and caudally that the pulsation can be felt. The cardiac apex is normally in the fifth space in the midclavicular line, but can be displaced by cardiac hypertrophy or mediastinal shift.

The *character* of the apex beat is often best appreciated with the patient tipped to the left, but the *position* of the apex must be judged with the patient supine. The left ventricle usually makes up the apex, but in severe right ventricular enlargement it may be pushed posteriorly and the apex can be right ventricular. Left ventricular hypertrophy produces an apex beat which displaces the palpating fingers. The impulse may be generated by a pressure-loaded left ventricle (e.g. aortic stenosis or hypertension), in which case the apex impulse feels very muscular and thrusting but is not markedly displaced; alternatively, it may be generated by a volume-loaded left ventricle (e.g. mitral or aortic regurgitation), in which case the left ventricle feels very dynamic and the apex beat may be displaced considerably.

Left ventricular aneurysm may produce a rocking feeling at the apex, from a double or dyskinetic impulse. A grossly dilated damaged heart may have a very diffuse impulse with a presystolic thrust from a prominent *a* wave. In dextrocardia, the impulse will be on the right. Abnormal praecordial pulsation due to other types of heart disease is described in the relevant section below. Aortic aneurysm can produce pulsation retrosternally and 'tracheal tug'.

Auscultation

A quiet environment and well-fitting earpieces on the stethoscope are essential. The diaphragm of the stethoscope is used for mid-range and high frequency sounds – normal valve closures, heart sounds, systolic murmurs and early diastolic murmurs. The bell favours low frequencies and should only be applied gently to the chest wall (or else the skin becomes a diaphragm). It is used for atrial and third heart sounds and the low-pitched, mid-diastolic murmurs of mitral stenosis, tricuspid stenosis and atrial septal defects.

Heart sounds

The timing of the heart sounds is shown in Figure 12.8.

First and second

The first heart sound, S1, signals the onset of systole and is produced by a variety of events, principally closure of the atrio-ventricular valves and tensioning of the left ventricle wall. It is identified by palpating the carotid pulse. The upstroke of the carotid pulse follows closely after S1. The second heart sound, S2, separates systole

and diastole and is due to closure of the aortic and pulmonary valves and the sudden tensioning of their leaflets, like a sail flapping.

The normal sequence is S1 (mitral before tricuspid) and S2 (aortic before pulmonary). Splitting of S1 into its components is not usually very obvious, but splitting of S2 increases with inspiration so that S2 may become two distinct sounds which resynchronise with expiration. This is called normal splitting of S2 (Fig. 12.9). As the pulmonary valve closure sound (P2) is usually much softer than the aortic valve closure sound (A2), this normal splitting is heard most easily over the pulmonary area.

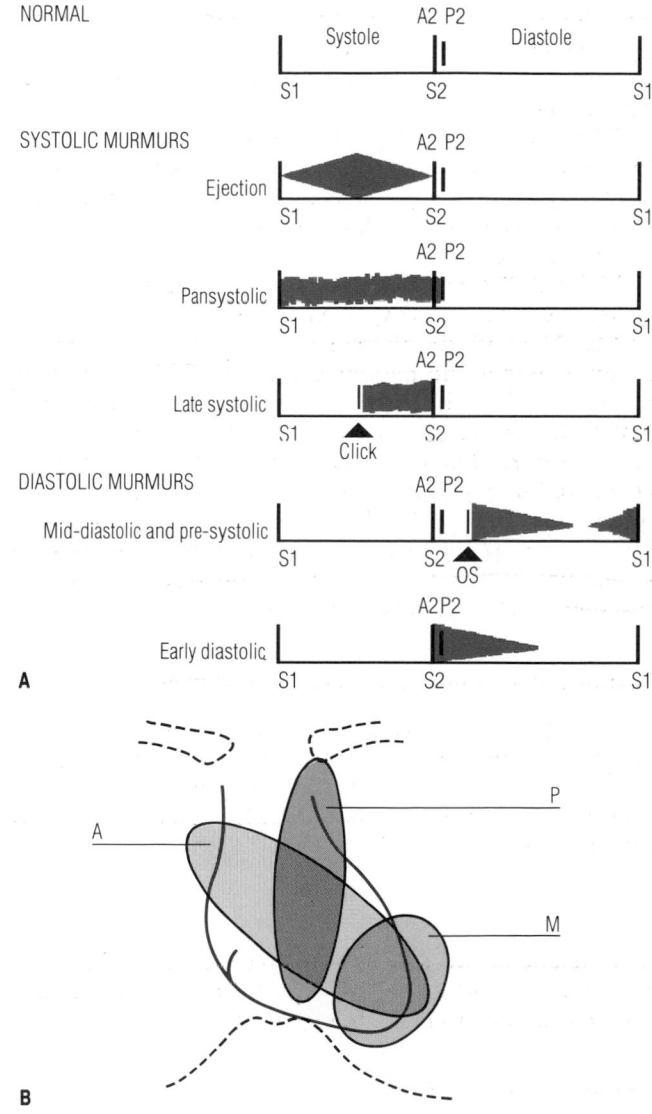

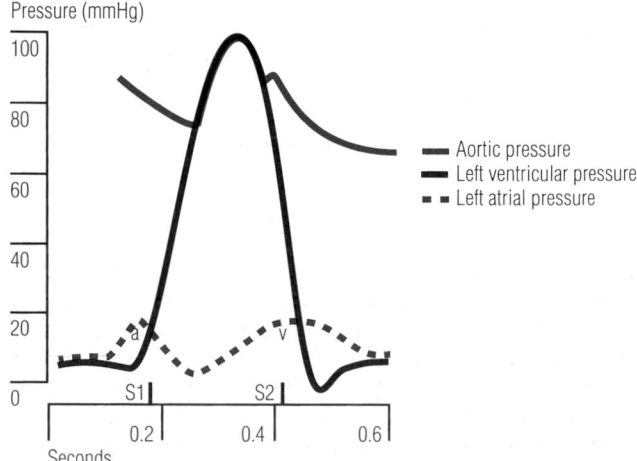

Fig. 12.8 Relationship between pressures in the aorta, left ventricle and left atrium. The timing of the heart sounds (S1 and S2) are shown.

Fig. 12.9 Heart murmurs. A. Diagrammatic representation of murmurs. S1 and S2 = first and second heart sounds; A2 = aortic valve closure sound; P2 = pulmonary valve closure sound; OS = opening snap. **B.** The precordial areas where murmurs are usually heard maximally. A = aortic; P = pulmonary; M = mitral.

12 Cardiovascular Disease

Third and fourth

The third and fourth heart sounds, S3 and S4, are low-pitched and not usually heard. However, they may be audible in fit young patients with bradycardia, such as athletes, and become audible in patients with heart failure or a high ventricular filling pressure. They may arise from either side of the heart, but more usually from the left. S3 coincides with rapid ventricular filling and occurs in early to mid-diastole. Various mechanisms, such as tensioning of the chordae tendinae or ventricular wall, have been proposed. A loud S3 is common in a dilated left ventricle with rapid diastolic filling, such as severe mitral regurgitation. A much higher-pitched S3 is heard in pericardial constriction, as ventricular filling is suddenly truncated in early diastole.

S4, or atrial sound, coincides with atrial systole in patients with a high ventricular filling pressure. It is absent where there is no atrial systole and in mitral stenosis. In sinus rhythm, it immediately precedes S1 and may be heard (and sometimes felt) at the apex of the heart. Typically, it is heard in hypertension and heart failure.

Gallop (triple) rhythm. If either S3 or S4 are very loud, a triple rhythm or gallop results, which almost invariably accompanies heart failure. With an associated tachycardia, S3 and S4 come together in a *summation gallop*. This is particularly common in hypertensive heart disease with left heart failure.

Added sounds

Ejection clicks are heard in young patients with aortic and pulmonary stenosis, where there is 'doming' of a mobile stenotic valve.

Mid-systolic click is heard in mitral valve prolapse, where the redundant chordal length allows mid-systolic prolapse of a mitral valve cusp. This may be single or multiple.

Opening snap. Normally an inaudible event, the opening snap becomes audible and, indeed, as loud as a heart sound in mitral stenosis (and tricuspid stenosis) where the tethered valve cusps cannot separate adequately and the raised atrial pressure forces the valve to open to its full extent with sudden development of tension.

Other added sounds include pericardial rub and pericardial clicks, which may be found in pneumothorax.

Heart murmurs

Murmurs are generated along the path of turbulent flow and radiate in the direction of flow. The same murmur may sound different at different sites on the precordium. A *thrill* is a murmur radiating to the chest wall with sufficient low-frequency components to be palpable. The classical valve 'areas' (mitral, aortic, tricuspid and pulmonary) for auscultation were defined in the 19th century, and reflected the findings in rheumatic and infective cardiac disease (Fig. 12.9B). They are not, however, always the sites where murmurs arising from those particular valves are best heard.

Causes of murmurs

Murmurs may be generated by a high-velocity jet, such as a stenotic or regurgitant jet, passing from a high-pressure to a lower-pressure chamber or vessel. They may occur with increased flow velocity in a normal vessel or with flow into a dilated or distorted vessel, such as the aorta in hypertension or the pulmonary artery in sternal depression. Murmurs therefore do not always indicate valve pathology. They may indicate a high flow, such as in pregnancy, or a minor anatomical distortion not amounting to true pathology, so-called *innocent murmurs*.

Description of murmurs

Murmurs are described in terms of their timing, precordial location, radiation, relative intensity and, if warranted, the influence of respiration and posture (Fig. 12.9). It is possible to grade the *loudness* of murmurs from 1/6 (almost inaudible) to 6/6 (a murmur which can be heard in a quiet room without using a stethoscope). These grades are, however, of limited value, as they are highly subjective and the loudness of a murmur varies considerably depending on circumstances. The *length* of a diastolic murmur can be expressed on a scale of quarters, 1/4 being very short, and 3/4 an almost full-length diastolic murmur.

Systolic murmurs

Ejection murmurs are crescendo-decrescendo (diamond-shaped) and are characteristic of flow across a stenotic aortic or pulmonary valve, or flow into a dilated aorta or pulmonary artery. They may also occur with increased flow across these valves (innocent murmur). Sometimes, in severe stenoses, it is impossible to distinguish an ejection from a pansystolic murmur. The associated signs will often help.

Pansystolic murmurs are generated by jets passing from a high-pressure to a low-pressure chamber throughout systole, including the normally isovolumic phases of contraction and relaxation. The best example is mitral regurgitation, but tricuspid regurgitation and ventricular septal defects produce similar murmurs. The murmur obscures both S1 and S2 and is of almost even intensity throughout systole.

Late systolic murmurs. Mitral valve prolapse and papillary muscle dysfunction give rise to a high-pitched murmur of even intensity starting halfway through systole, often preceded by a mid-systolic click. Posterior papillary muscle dysfunction can give rise to a mitral pansystolic murmur which may be loud in the aortic area.

Diastolic murmurs

Diastolic murmurs are always pathological, but are often much harder to detect than systolic murmurs.

Mitral and tricuspid mid-diastolic murmurs. The mitral (and tricuspid) stenotic jets induce a low-frequency, largely subsonic vibration. These are heard as low-pitched, rumbling murmurs starting after the opening snap, best heard with the bell. They are localised and are often missed by the inexperienced, who are expecting to hear a much higher-pitched sound. The mitral diastolic murmur is accentuated by the patient lying on the left. If short, it can be confused with a third heart sound.

Early diastolic murmurs start immediately after the second heart sound. They are high-pitched noises, which can be very short or persist throughout diastole. Aortic diastolic murmurs are often faint and are best heard with the patient leaning forwards in expiration. A soft aortic diastolic murmur is often missed.

Other types of murmur

Musical or *mewing murmurs* may occur in systole or diastole if a valve cusp adjacent to a jet vibrates at a characteristic frequency. These murmurs can be very loud, but the jet causing them may be small. A mewing murmur is characteristic of a small hole in an aortic valve cusp as a complication of endocarditis.

'Innocent' murmurs

Many mid-systolic and ejection systolic murmurs are unaccompanied by any signs or features of heart disease. These murmurs are common in children and pregnancy. They are maximal in the pulmonary area, but may also be heard along the left sternal edge and at the apex, and often have a low-pitched vibratory quality. They are usually of low intensity. If there is doubt as to their 'innocent' nature, an echocardiograph and, particularly, a Doppler study can rule out a small ventricular septal defect, pulmonary stenosis or unsuspected trivial mitral regurgitation.

Bringing out a murmur

Murmurs can be accentuated by exercise; this increases cardiac output and is best accomplished by asking the patient (if well enough) to lie on the couch and do, say, 20 cycles of toe-touching and then resting back. Murmurs in mitral valve prolapse and hypertrophic cardiomyopathy commonly come and go, and are best assessed both with patient in the usual auscultatory position and when

standing and squatting. If the patient has severe emphysema, heart sounds and murmurs can be so faint as to be inaudible. The location and characteristics of murmurs and other methods of accentuating them are described in more detail below, in the sections dealing with the clinical conditions giving rise to them.

Concluding a cardiovascular examination

The examination is incomplete without examination of the lung bases for signs of cardiac failure, the sacrum and ankles for oedema, assessment of the peripheral pulses, dentition, skin and nails.

- The lungs are examined not only for signs of failure, but also because chronic lung disease can complicate and add to the symptoms and signs generated by heart disease.
- A patient with angina may well have atheromatous peripheral vascular disease, shown by loss of pulses in the legs. Examination of the carotid arteries for signs of atheromatous carotid stenosis may reveal loss of a carotid pulsation, a carotid bruit or loud systolic murmur. Atrial fibrillation may have caused embolic loss of some pulses. If the patient is hypertensive with a systolic murmur, radial and femoral pulses should be felt to detect any delay and weakness of the femoral pulse indicating coarctation. Possible aortic aneurysm should lead to careful assessment of the pulses and the blood pressure in both arms.
- Tricuspid regurgitation is confirmed by finding a pulsatile liver. If the patient has hypertension, the abdomen is examined for renal enlargement or bruits. A patient in right heart failure may well have ascites and considerable liver enlargement.
- Atrial fibrillation or tachycardia may be caused by thyrotoxicosis, so the thyroid is examined for goitre and signs of thyroid overactivity.
- If the patient is hypertensive, the optic fundi are examined for hypertensive retinopathy. They should be examined regularly in patients suspected of having endocarditis.

CARDIAC INVESTIGATION

THE ELECTROCARDIOGRAM

The electrocardiogram (ECG) is now a fundamental part of cardiovascular assessment. It provides information on the heart rhythm and underlying cardiac morphology. A 'normal ECG' (Fig.12.10) at rest can be reassuring but also misleading, as it can be found even with life-threatening coronary disease; in the absence of symptoms, a routine ECG is thus of limited value.

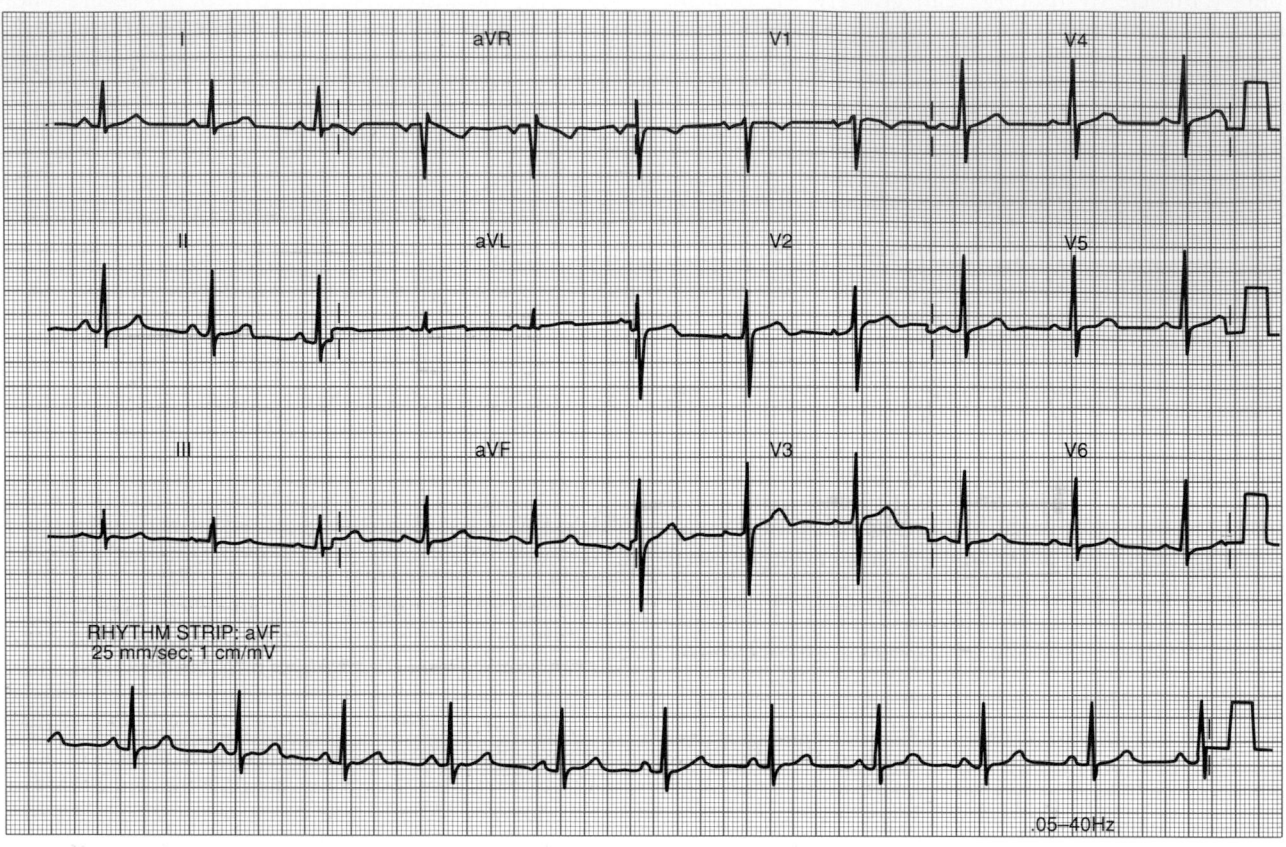

Fig. 12.10 Normal ECG.

Recording an ECG

The patient should be relaxed and warm (not shivering) before the 10 skin electrodes are applied to skin previously mildly abraded with spirit. The six limb leads provide an electrical 'view' around the heart in the frontal plane, while the six ventricular leads view the heart from the complementary horizontal plane (Fig. 12.11). By convention, the lead connections have been made to show a positive deflection as a wave of depolarising electrical activity travels towards the electrode. The final shape of the ECG is determined by the lead being sampled and by the angle (vector) at which it 'views' the activity in the heart; the magnitude of the recorded deflection is affected by the mass of tissue undergoing electrical activation. Understanding the ECG thus requires that the anatomy of the heart, the route taken by electrical activation and the viewpoint of the electrode are known. Differences in anatomy and minor variations in lead positions can account for some of the variability in clinical ECGs; pathological processes account for the rest.

Standard gain settings (1 cm/mV deflection) and paper speed (25 mm/s) complete the ECG recording.

Atrial activity and the P wave

In the normal heart, the dominant pacemaker is to be found in the high right atrium at the sino-atrial node. The depolarising wave front moves through the right atrium first and arrives at the left atrium fractionally later. The wave front moves in a general direction towards +60°. The surface ECG records a P wave which is positive and best seen in leads II, V1 and I. Right atrial hypertrophy produces a tall (>2.5 mm) peaked P wave, sometimes called the *P pulmonale* from its association with the pulmonary hypertension of pulmonary disease. Left atrial hypertrophy (*P mitrale*) produces a broad notched P wave (>0.12 s duration) in lead II or III, with a negative secondary deflection in V1 which exceeds the right atrial positive deflection in that lead (Fig. 12.12). P waves that are inverted in lead II are caused by an abnormal direction of the depolarising wave front, and may be seen when atrial activation is initiated at the atrio-ventricular (AV) node low in the right atrium. Other ectopic atrial rhythms may produce P waves of varying shapes.

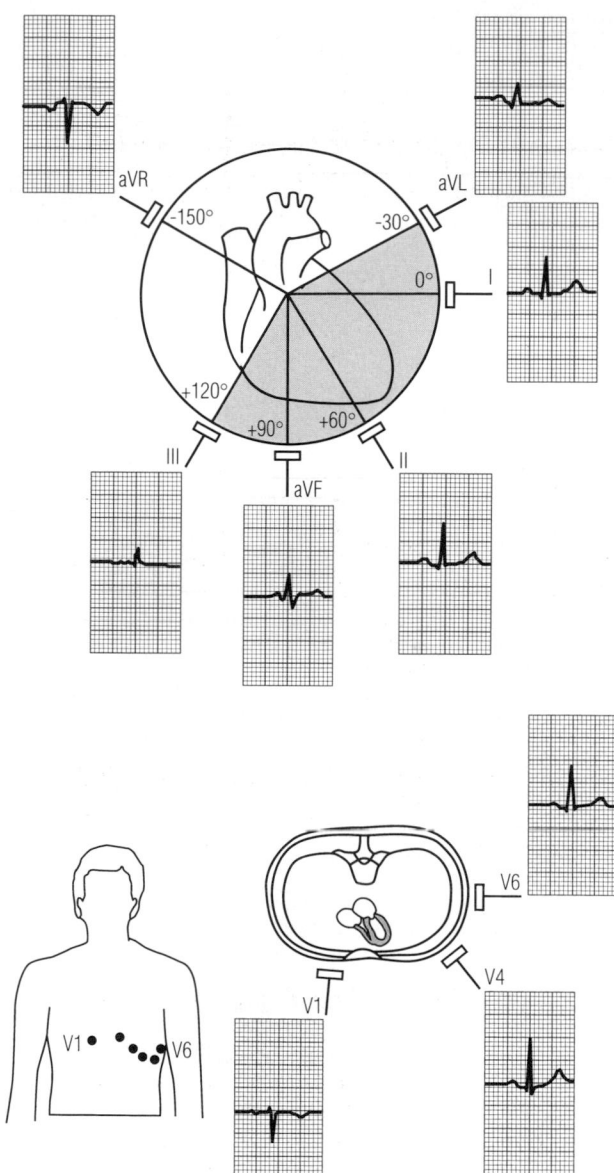

Fig. 12.11 Position of leads and electrodes in the ECG. A. Frontal plane. **B.** Horizontal plane. Four limb leads and six precordial leads are routinely used, the anatomical landmarks for the latter being: V1, right sternal edge, 4th intercostal space; V2, complementary position to left of sternum; V3, between V2 and V4; V4, mid-clavicular line, 5th space; V5, anterior axillary line; V6, mid-axillary line, horizontally in line with V4.

The PR interval

Between atrial and ventricular depolarisation, the ECG signal records a flat isoelectric line for 0.12–0.20 s (Fig. 12.13). This is the delay encountered by the depolarising wave front in the AV node before rapid propagation to the ventricular myocardium. The PR interval

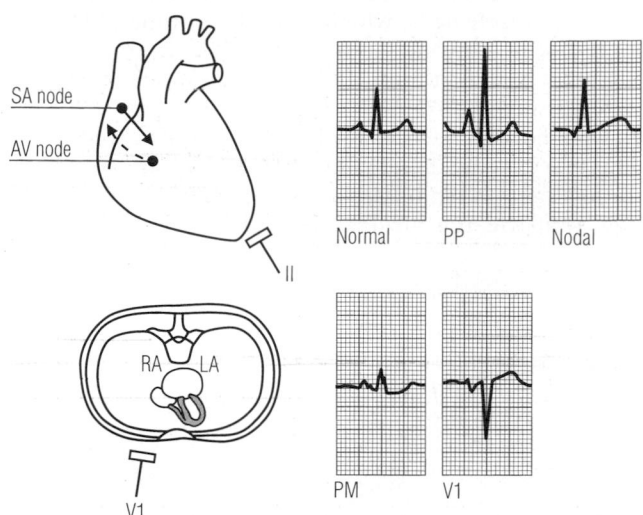

Fig. 12.12 Normal and abnormal P waves. On the left is shown the direction of atrial activation that produces the normal P waves shown in lead II. In P pulmonale (PP) the P wave is abnormally tall and peaked. When activation is retrograde (nodal rhythm shown by dashed line), the P wave is inverted. In left atrial hypertrophy (e.g. in mitral stenosis) a broad bifid P wave is seen in lead II and a prominent negative deflection in lead V1; this is P mitrale (PM).

will diminish at increased heart rates and under the influence of adrenaline. It increases in diseased AV nodes, with certain drugs and, occasionally, in normal people.

The QRS complex and ventricular activation

Normal QRS

The normal QRS parameters are shown in Figure 12.13. Ventricular activation is complete within 0.12 s with virtually simultaneous activation of the left and right ventricles due to the system of specialised rapidly con-

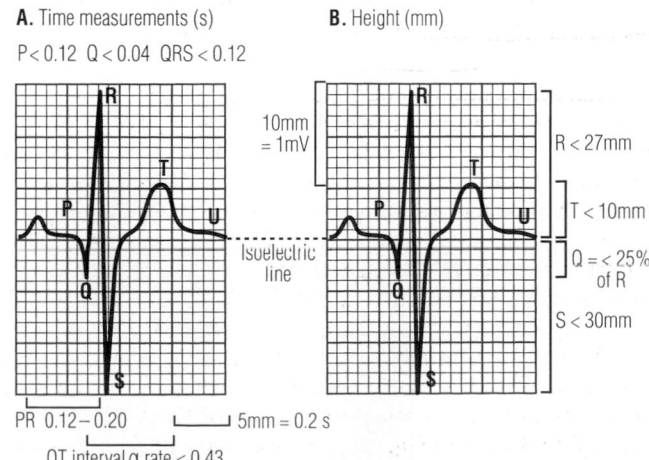

Fig. 12.13 Normal PQRST parameters. A. Duration. **B.** Height.

ducting muscle cells, which form the bundle of His and the Purkinje network. Activation of the interventricular septum begins first from left-to-right and accounts for the small q wave (duration <0.04 s and depth $<25\%$ of R wave height) seen in leads V5, V6 and, usually, V4. This wave is matched by the r wave in V1 and V2. Since the left ventricular muscle mass is greater than that of the right ventricle, it is the left ventricular forces which domi-

nate the chest leads, with rS waves in leads V1 and V2 and qR waves in leads V5 and V6, with an intermediate transition zone to be found between leads V3 and V4.

The mean frontal plane vector (QRS axis)

This is obtained from the six limb leads and describes the direction of the dominant electrical forces. It can be

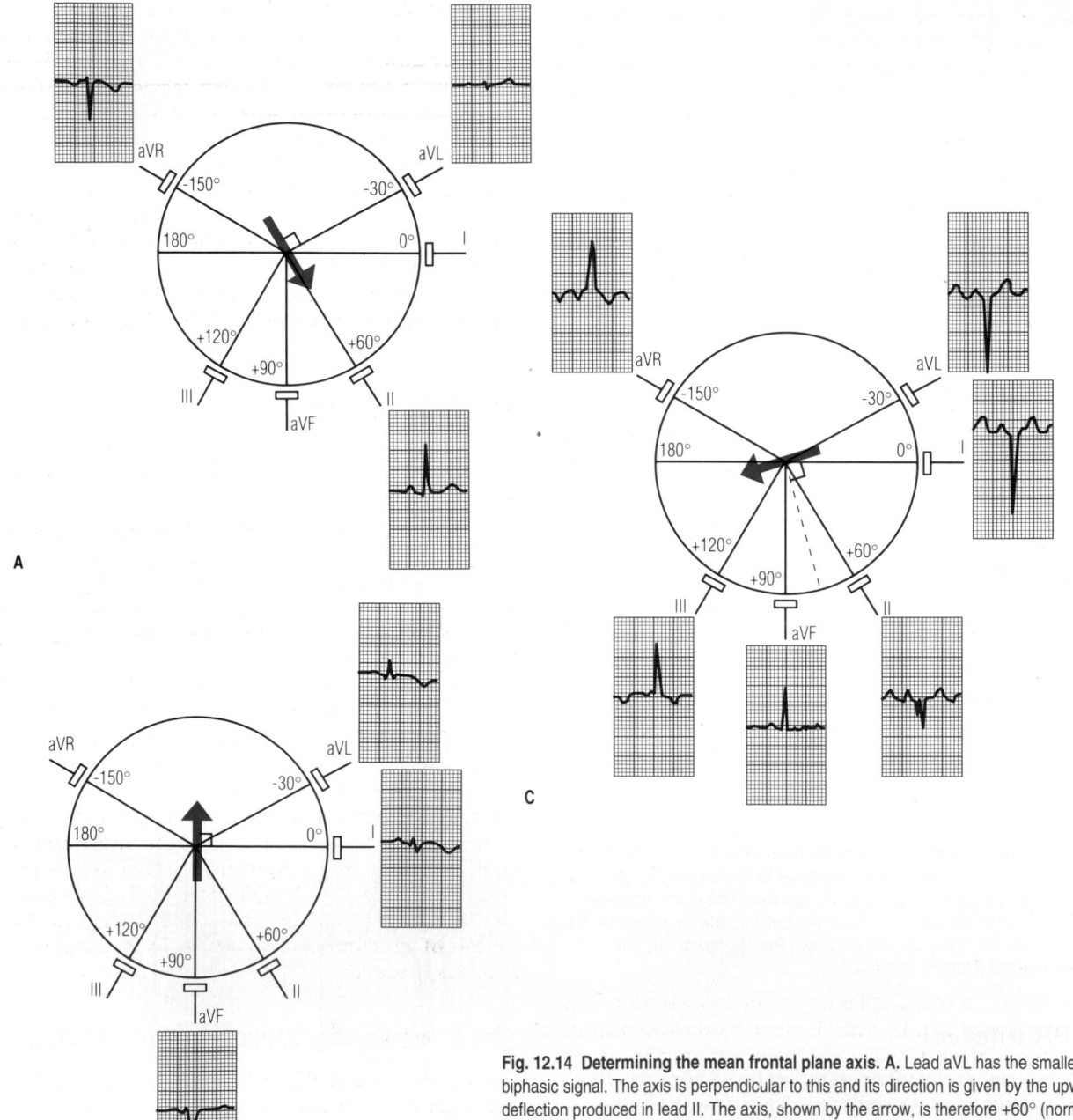

Fig. 12.14 Determining the mean frontal plane axis. A. Lead aVL has the smallest biphasic signal. The axis is perpendicular to this and its direction is given by the upward deflection produced in lead II. The axis, shown by the arrow, is therefore +60° (normal axis). **B.** The axis is –90° (perpendicular to I and away from aVF). This is left axis deviation. **C.** The smallest and most biphasic complex lies between II and aVF and the axis is therefore greater than 120° (severe right axis deviation).

determined for all the major ECG deflections (P wave, QRS complex and T wave) but is mainly used to summarise ventricular depolarisation as the *mean QRS axis*. It is roughly estimated by choosing the lead with the smallest equiphasic deflection, and assuming the vector is at 90° to this lead. On this vectorial line the limb lead which shows a positive deflection indicates the direction of the axis. The units are degrees, with values above the equator (0°) being prefixed negative (Fig. 12.14).

The vector is normally about +60°. Left axis deviation is variously defined, but a shift further than −30° is definitely abnormal; right axis deviation is definite at greater than 120°. The latter can be due to right ventricular hypertrophy or, less commonly, to abnormal patterns of activation caused by interruption of the posterior fascicle of the left bundle branch, in left posterior hemiblock. Left axis deviation is an 'electrical' phenomenon, caused by interruption of the anterior fascicle of the left bundle branch. It is associated with the loss of the normal septal depolarisation and hence the loss of q waves in V5 and V6. This is called left anterior hemiblock; in these conditions, the QRS duration remains less than 0.12 s.

Bundle branch block

Interruption of the right or left bundle branches produces a bundle branch block pattern characterised by broad QRS complexes of greater than 0.12 s duration. With *right bundle branch block*, an rSR or 'M'-shaped pattern is seen in the right facing chest leads V1, V2 ± V3, as right ventricular forces occur late and unopposed by left ventricular contraction; this is also manifested by late deep slurred S waves appearing in V4 to V6. *Left bundle branch block* causes a delay in left ventricular activation, which occurs from right to left, causing a marked axis shift (greater than −60°) and loss of q waves in V5 and V6. Lead V1 shows only a qS wave and the lateral leads (V5 and V6) the characteristic slurred RsR or 'M' pattern.

Left bundle branch block is virtually always pathological, the commonest cause being ischaemic heart disease. Right bundle branch block may be a normal finding, but the change from normal conduction to one or other of these patterns implies heart disease.

Rate-dependent bundle branch block

Occasionally, normal QRS morphology is present at low heart rates, but a bundle branch block pattern appears at faster rates. This is usually right bundle branch block, as its refractory period is generally longer than that of the left bundle branch. Rate-dependent bundle branch block may occur with a supraventricular tachycardia, where the broad QRS complexes may wrongly suggest the diagnosis of ventricular tachycardia.

Ventricular hypertrophy

The tallest R wave should not exceed 27 mm nor the deepest S wave 30 mm, and the sum of the tallest R wave and deepest S wave should not exceed 40 mm (Fig. 12.13). Left ventricular hypertrophy (LVH) is diagnosed when these criteria are exceeded, with a normal total QRS duration of less than 0.12 s. The intrinsic deflection is delayed by more than 0.04 s in the left-facing leads, this measurement being taken from the onset of the QRS deflection to the point at which the R wave swings abruptly downwards. Associated ST segment depression and T inversion occur in the left-facing limb and praecordial leads, particularly with pressure-overloaded ventricles, and is said to represent ventricular 'strain'.

Right ventricular hypertrophy (RVH) is suspected when there is a dominant R wave in V1, associated with a rightward QRS axis shift (> +90°) in a QRS complex of less than 0.12 s duration. There is also ST segment depression and T inversion in the right precordial leads, and often also clockwise rotation of the ventricular leads with the normal transition zone (V3–V4) moving towards V5–V6.

The ST segment

The ST segment begins where the QRS ends, and is normally on the isoelectric line curving upwards into the T wave (the J or *junction point*). There may be 1–2 mm of elevation in the high anterior chest leads (V1 and V2), but greater elevation is seen with myocardial infarction, the so-called current of injury (p. 400, Fig. 12.59) and pericarditis (p. 427, Fig. 12.62). A normal variant, in which there is marked anterior ST elevation, is frequent in young black men.

Depression of the ST segment (p. 394, Fig. 12.55) is the hallmark of cardiac ischaemia. This can vary from subtle loss of the normal slight upward curvature and acute angulation with the T wave origin, to more marked depression, sloping downwards before abruptly changing direction with the T wave onset. The degree of depression of the ST segment is a rough indication of the severity of the myocardial injury. The ST segment is encompassed within the QT interval. This shortens with increasing heart rate, but may be prolonged (> 0.40 s or > 50% of previous R–R interval) by hypocalcaemia or hypomagnesaemia.

The T wave: myocardial repolarisation

There is more variability in T wave amplitude and orientation than in other parts of the ECG, so that criteria for normality have to be more flexible. The T wave may be flat or abnormal in non-cardiac disease and in some normal patients. It is asymmetrical in shape, with a slower upstroke than downstroke and a smooth rounded peak. Symmetrical, peaked T waves may indicate ischaemia, whereas notching may be a feature of pericarditis. T wave height should not exceed 10 mm in the precordial leads; larger heights without LVH suggest acute myocardial infarction or hyperkalaemia. T wave orientation is normally upright in leads with R waves over 5 mm in height, so that, in the normal adult, T waves are upright in I, II and V3 to V6, are always inverted in aVR and may be inverted in aVL, aVF, III, V1 and V2. The evolution of acute infarction (Fig. 12.59, p. 400) involves T inversion in leads affected by the injury, and these changes may persist.

The U wave

The U wave follows the T wave (Fig. 12.13), is of small amplitude and shares the T wave orientation. It is best seen in lead V3 and is enlarged in hypokalaemia. Its genesis is uncertain.

Exercise electrocardiography

The normal 12-lead resting ECG often shows no abnormalities in patients who develop symptoms on exercise. The exercise test, on a treadmill or cycle ergometer, may be performed for the following reasons:

- to reproduce the symptoms of which the patient is complaining, so that he or she can describe them as they happen under standardised exercise conditions
- to assess the patient's 'functional capacity', i.e. the amount of work that can be performed before the patient becomes limited by symptoms, and also how rapidly the patient recovers from exercise
- to ascertain whether the symptoms are accompanied by any objective evidence of myocardial ischaemia, cardiac arrhythmia, hypertension or other events which would make unsupervised exercise hazardous
- to monitor treatment with serial studies
- to assess prognosis in patients with known cardiac disease.

The exercise load is started at an easily managed level, kept stable for 1.5–3 minutes at each load, and then serially increased with the aim of 'exhausting' the subject within 15 minutes (although, in submaximal tests, exhaustion is not usually the end point).

The patient is connected to an ECG monitor and the blood pressure is also recorded. A defibrillator is available.

The *absolute* indications for stopping the test are:

- severe ischaemic symptoms
- fall in systolic blood pressure >10 mmHg
- ST depression >3 mm
- new arrhythmia
- patient requests it.

The *relative* indications for stopping are:

- achieves target heart rate
- systolic blood pressure >220 mmHg
- ill or exhausted patient
- angina.

Interpretation

The exercise test is conclusively positive if the patient develops classical anginal pain and downsloping ST segment depression (≥2 mm) is shown on the ECG (Fig. 12.55, p. 394). Minor degrees of ST segment depression are common, particularly in anxious individuals and especially young women, but are usually upsloping. T wave inversion is not necessarily ischaemic in origin. A commonly used criterion is 1 mm ST depression more than 0.08 s after the previous QRS complex. Severe ischaemia is shown by widespread ST depression in several leads which takes several minutes to return to normal. There may be a sudden drop in blood pressure during exercise; this may be unaccompanied by ECG changes but is diagnostic of severe ischaemia and an absolute indication to stop the test.

CHEST X-RAY

Because of the almost uniform density of its components, the cardiac shadow on a PA chest film is a silhouette of a three-dimensional structure displayed on a two-dimensional film (Fig. 12.15).

Examination of a cardiac X-ray requires a logical approach, and includes the following:

- a check of the technical quality of the film, and the position of the thoracic skeleton (PA film, full inspiration)
- an assessment of heart size (and changes from previous films if available)
- a search for evidence of specific chamber enlargement and abnormalities of cardiac anatomy
- an examination of the lung fields and vessels
- identification of valve or other calcification.

An AP film is only of value in assessing the lung fields or gross changes in heart size. There may be evidence of thoracotomy, rib resection, scoliosis or severe kyphosis which may result in an abnormal appearance of the heart. Lateral films may show a depressed sternum or abnormal sternal segmentation. There may be rib notching, suggesting coarctation.

Heart size and cardiothoracic ratio

Minor variations in heart size can be technical in origin. It is usual to measure the *cardiothoracic ratio* (the maximum

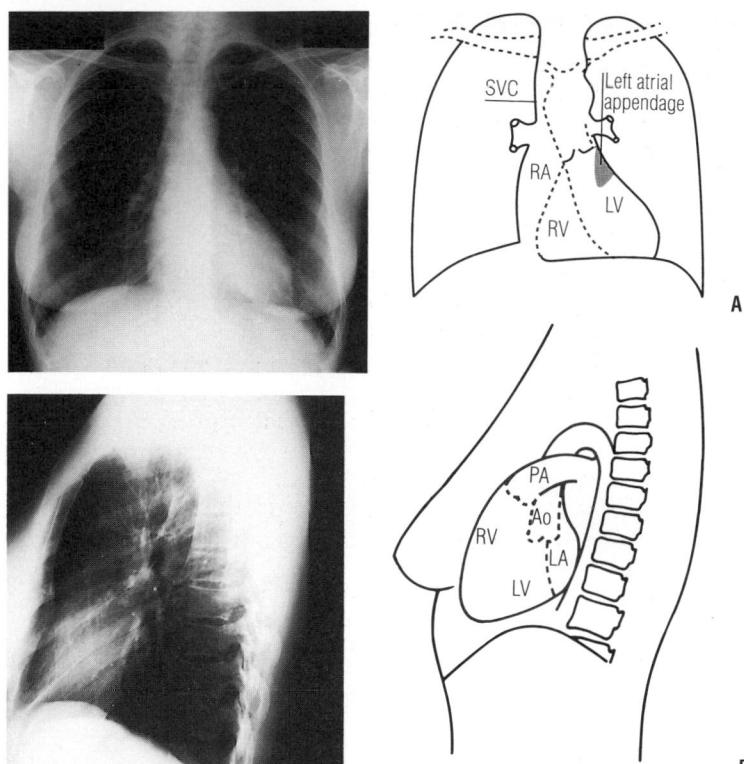

B

Fig. 12.15 Composition of the normal cardiac silhouette on chest X-rays. A. PA view. RV and LV = right and left ventricles; RA = right atrium; SVC = superior vena cava. **B.** Lateral view.

transverse diameter of the heart compared with that of the ribcage) which is 0.5 or less in normals. This commonly accepted criterion is, however, rather rigid and needs to be modified with athletes and people of African descent, many of whose hearts exceed this limit, but are by other criteria physiologically normal. When comparing successive chest X-rays, an increase in transverse diameter of the heart of more than 1.5 cm is regarded as significant.

Anatomy and specific chamber enlargement

The border-forming structures of the cardiac silhouette in the PA and lateral views are shown in Figure 12.15. The approximate positions of the heart valves are also shown.

Left atrium (LA)

LA enlargement may produce widening of the angle of bifurcation (carina) into the main bronchi with lifting of the left main bronchus. The increased density of an enlarged LA may make it visible within the right heart border, or it may protrude beyond it. Enlargement of the LA can cause straightening, and even bulging, of the left heart border.

On lateral chest X-ray, enlargement produces posterior displacement of the upper posterior cardiac border.

Left ventricle (LV)

The LV makes up the cardiac apex and part of the left heart border on PA X-rays, and much of the posterior heart border on lateral views. LV enlargement usually displaces the apex of the heart downwards and laterally on the PA view, while on the lateral view, the LV produces a prominent convexity of the lower half of the posterior border of the heart.

Aorta

In young adults, the upper right cardiac border may not include the ascending aorta, but with ageing the aorta elongates and becomes more tortuous and prominent on chest X-ray. Prominence of the ascending aorta may thus be due to age as well as hypertension, poststenotic dilatation or aortic dilatation from aortic valve disease, aneurysm or dissection. Computed tomography (CT scan), ultrasound or angiography may be needed to define the cause of a prominent aorta. The aortic arch may also be prominent in any of these conditions. Calcification of the ascending aorta occurs in syphilis, but is very common in the arch and descending aorta in normal individuals.

Right atrium (RA)

Enlargement of the RA is seen as prominence of the lower half of the right heart border, and is usually accompanied by superior vena cava (SVC) prominence. The SVC forms the highest part of the right border of the cardiac silhouette and is prominent in right heart failure, SVC obstruction or displacement of the SVC by the aorta.

Right ventricle (RV)

The RV is an 'internal' structure on the PA X-ray unless there is massive RV dilatation with the LV rotated posteriorly. RV dilatation results in a more globular appearance to the heart on PA film, with the cardiac apex being more elevated.

Pulmonary conus and trunk

The pulmonary trunk is more prominent in young subjects than later in life. A dilated pulmonary trunk may indicate a poststenotic dilatation, pulmonary hypertension, increased pulmonary flow or can be idiopathic. It therefore needs to be interpreted along with the appearance of the lung fields.

Lung fields and vessels

Assessment of pulmonary vascularity tends to be subjective and demands a good quality film. Normal pulmonary vascularity will show larger vessels in the lower zones, with symmetry between the two lungs. There is a steady diminution in vessel size peripherally.

Pulmonary venous hypertension

If the pressure in the pulmonary veins rises above about 15 mmHg, the upper lobe vessels dilate and become larger than the lower lobe vessels, which constrict with perivascular cuffing. There is redistribution of flow to the upper lobes. If the venous pressure rises higher than about 20–25 mmHg, the pulmonary lymphatics become engorged, and appearances of interstitial oedema are seen on the chest X-ray. These are the appearance of *Kerley B lines* (horizontal septal lines best seen at the costophrenic angles) and increased haziness of the perihilar regions, sometimes resulting in the classical but uncommon 'bat's wing' appearance of the chest X-ray, often with small effusions (Fig. 12.16). Further rise in pressure above 30 mmHg results in alveolar oedema with dense opacification of the lung from fluid collection.

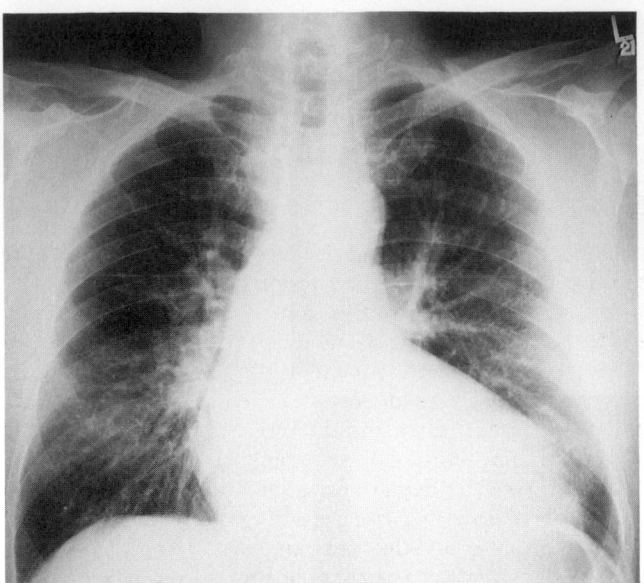

Fig. 12.16 Radiological features of left heart failure. PA chest X-ray showing bilateral shadowing spreading from the hila, typical of acute pulmonary oedema. The heart size is inreased.

Increased lung blood flow

With increased blood flow to the lungs (as in a left to right shunt), the lungs are vascular, with quite large vessels running to the periphery of the lungs. This can be distinguished from left heart failure by the lower lobe vessels remaining larger than the upper lobe vessels.

Pulmonary oligaemia

Pulmonary oligaemia (as in severe pulmonary stenosis) is associated with an avascular appearance of the lung fields but normal size central pulmonary arteries (although the pulmonary trunk may be dilated as a poststenotic dilatation in pulmonary stenosis).

Pulmonary arterial hypertension

The presence of pulmonary arterial hypertension gives rise to large central pulmonary arteries which are rapidly pruned peripherally with relatively avascular-looking lung fields.

Calcification

Calcification is usually best seen on penetrated PA and lateral films, as much of the calcification seen within the heart overlies the spine on PA films. The mitral and aortic valve may both calcify. On lateral films, the latter is usually lying above a line joining the tracheal bifurcation and the costophrenic angle, whilst the mitral is predominantly below the line. Calcification is also sometimes seen in the great vessels, the wall of a rheumatic LA, the pericardium and within the LV in thrombus in an LV aneurysm.

ULTRASOUND TECHNIQUES

Echocardiography

If a beam of ultrasound is directed into the thorax through a suitable 'acoustic window' it travels through the soft tissues and blood at an almost uniform velocity of 1340 m/s. The various tissue interfaces in the line of the ultrasound beam reflect some of the sound back towards the transmitting transducer, and the red blood cells in its path scatter the ultrasound. The reflected ultrasound takes varying times to get back to the transducer, depending on the depth of the interface from which the reflection occurs. As the velocity of the ultrasound is constant, the time of the returning echoes is an indication of their depth, while their strength is an indication of the change in acoustic impedance producing the echo. The beam ultrasound can be pulsed, using the same transducer as transmitter and receiver, to give a map of the tissue interfaces in one or various beam direction(s).

M mode echocardiography

The technique of M mode electrocardiography is illustrated in Figure 12.17. If the beam is maintained in a single direction, an M mode display is produced, where the line of echoes of varying strength at different depths is shown as a vertical line of varying intensity on a cathode ray tube, this line being swept across the tube with time. Signals of differing depth and intensity are therefore displayed against time with centimetre and second calibration markers. Hard copy of the display can be produced simultaneously.

Since both the fronts and backs of tissue interfaces reflect the ultrasound, M mode echocardiography can be used to display the cardiac chambers, the valves and the wall thickness of the LV throughout the cardiac cycle. Their size and thickness can be measured with a resolution of about 2 mm (depending on the ultrasound frequency). An ECG is used for timing the cardiac cycle.

Two-dimensional or sector echocardiography

If the beam of ultrasound is swung through an arc, a two-dimensional (2D) 'sector scan' is produced; this can be recorded as a moving image on videotape, or stored and recorded as hard copy in frozen images (Fig. 12.18). Two-dimensional echocardiography is useful for 'real time' dynamic records, but does not give as high a resolution as M mode.

Echocardiography is particularly useful for demonstrating valve thickening, calcification and vegetations, as well as chamber size and wall thickness and LV function. It is the method of choice for demonstrating pericardial

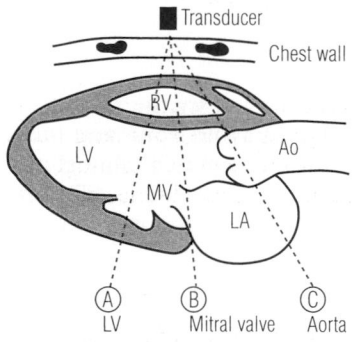

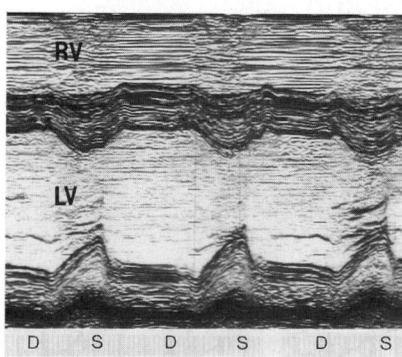

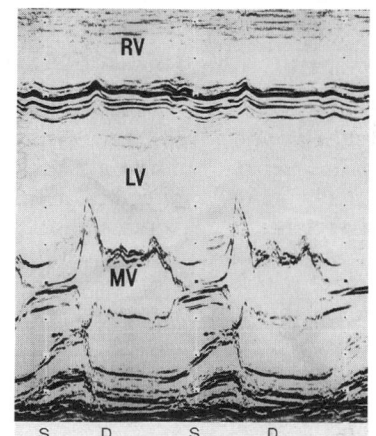

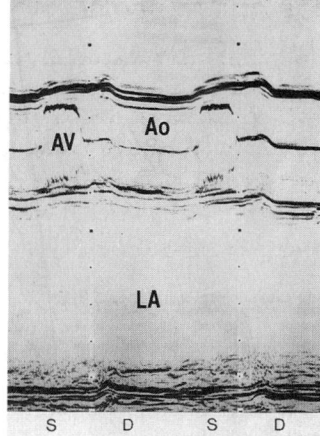

Fig. 12.17 M mode echocardiography. The diagram shows the position of the transducer and directions of the ultrasonic beam. In **A** the beam traverses the left ventricle (LV) below the mitral valve. Systole (S) and diastole (D) are indicated. In **B** the beam is aimed to demonstrate the mitral valve (MV). In **C** the aortic valve (AV) and aorta (Ao) are shown.

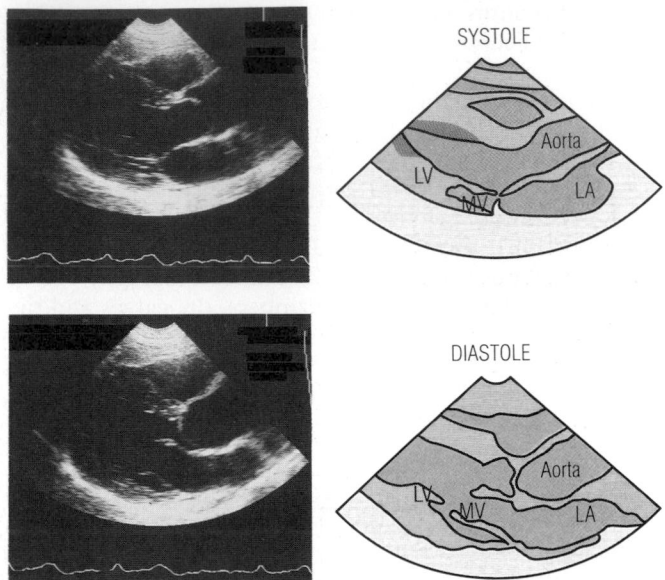

Fig. 12.18 Two-dimensional echocardiography. Parasternal long axis views of the heart in systole and diastole are shown. (The direction of the beam is equivalent to that shown by line B in Figure 12.17A.) The opening and closure of the aortic and mitral valves are clearly shown.

effusion. Under good conditions, 2D echocardiography can demonstrate the presence of thrombus in the heart and can also be used with injected saline contrast to demonstrate intracardiac shunting.

Doppler ultrasound

The technique of Doppler ultrasound makes use of the change in frequency of the backscattered ultrasound energy from the red blood cells. This change of frequency is proportional to the blood velocity; thus, if the beam of ultrasound is aligned with the jet of blood within the heart, accurate measurements of blood velocity can be made and

the gradient across the valve calculated (Fig. 12.19). The relation between the pressure gradient across the valve (P, in mmHg) and the increase in velocity (V, in m/s) is $P = 4V^2$. The predicted pressure gradient from Doppler measurements is the instantaneous pressure gradient, whereas cardiac catheterisation often measures only the peak-to-peak pull-back gradient (Fig. 12.21).

Doppler ultrasound is used predominantly for measuring pressure gradients and can also be used to demonstrate the presence and severity of valvular regurgitation. It is extremely sensitive in detecting minor degrees of regurgitation, which are often unexpected. The combined techniques of echocardiography and Doppler ultrasound save many patients, particularly children, from invasive studies, as in many cases the complete pathology can be demonstrated with ultrasound. These techniques cannot, however, measure chamber pressures, such as the left ventricular end diastolic pressure, or show the coronary arterial anatomy.

Colour Doppler

Colour Doppler is a form of pulsed Doppler in which the blood velocity is colour-coded and superimposed on a 2D sector echo image. The colour code demonstrates whether the mean velocity of the sample is towards or away from the transducer, and the hue can be changed depending on the velocity. Its main use so far is in providing a non-invasive type of colour angiogram which makes the rest of Doppler technology easier to use and appreciate.

Limitation on use

All ultrasound techniques are limited by the size of the acoustic windows, which have to avoid bone and lung. These are large in babies and young children (almost infinite in the fetus) and can be supplemented, if justified, by a transoesophageal approach. The windows become smaller with age and can become particularly limited in

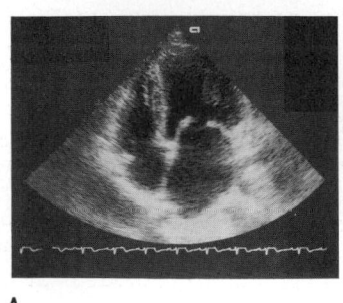

A

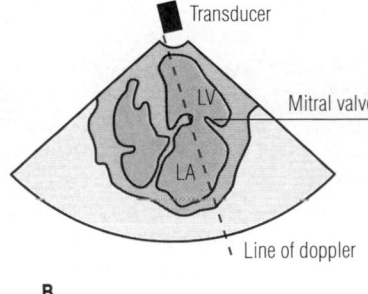

B

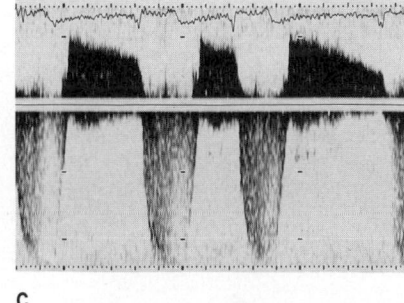

C

Fig. 12.19 Two-dimensional echocardiogram and Doppler ultrasound. A. Apical four-chamber view of the heart. **B.** Diagrammatic representation of A; the transducer position and beam direction of Doppler signal (dotted line) are shown. **C.** The continuous wave Doppler signal that is obtained from position B shows a diastolic jet (upwards towards the transducer). An abnormal systolic jet away from the transducer, due to mitral regurgitation, is also shown. The velocity trace indicates peak velocities of 2 m/s and 5 m/s respectively (corresponding to peak gradients of 16 and 100 mmHg).

people with lung disease, denying the benefits of these techniques to many who would be helped by a non-invasive diagnosis. The usual windows are parasternal, apical, subxiphoid and suprasternal.

NUCLEAR IMAGING

The development of gamma cameras and relatively short-lived nuclear isotopes (most commonly ^{99m}Tc) with suitable emission characteristics has led to a rapid increase in the diagnostic and imaging capability of isotopic techniques.

Nuclear angiography

Nuclear angiography uses intravenously injected radionuclides in the cardiac blood pool. This provides a non-invasive assessment of ventricular wall motion and ejection fraction and demonstrates valvular regurgitation and shunts. In the *first pass technique*, a discrete bolus of labelled blood is followed through the heart, and data collected by an externally placed gamma camera for 30–50 s. A fresh injection is required for each view. Short-lived isotopes such as ^{195}Au enable rest and exercise studies to be performed with relatively low cumulative exposure and background.

In an *equilibrium study* the whole of the circulating blood is labelled and data collection can take much longer, with serial views obtained at leisure. Resolution of the gamma camera image is increased by taking a large number of images over several cardiac cycles and the images from different phases of the cardiac cycle are averaged. This process is accomplished by 'gating' with reference to the ECG as a time marker and dividing the cardiac cycle into a series of time intervals each of, for example, 30–50 ms (Fig. 12.20).

Derived images and measurements

End diastolic and end systolic volumes. Ejection fraction and stroke volume (and thus cardiac output) can be calculated. The ejection fraction is normally above 50%, and should rise with exercise by at least 5%.

Regional wall motion abnormalities are shown by quantitative colour-coding of emission over the heart. This identifies areas showing little change in counts compared with the rest, or showing decreasing counts when the rest of the ventricle is increasing.

Limitations of nuclear angiography

In severe right heart failure, a peripheral venous injection of isotope is dissipated through a large mixing volume before it reaches the heart. Tricuspid regurgitation aggravates the

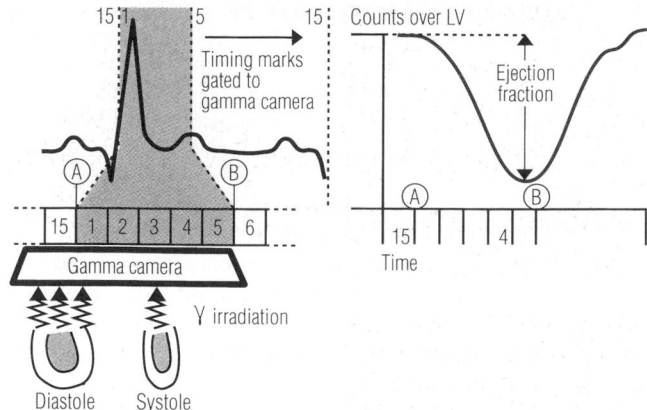

Fig. 12.20 Radionuclide ventriculography: the multiple uptake gated acquisition (MUGA) scan. The blood pool is labelled and counts over the left ventricle are related to defined proportions of the cardiac cycle (1–15 in the diagram). These are summated to give an average radioactivity for end systole (B) and end diastole (A) from which the ejection fraction can be calculated.

problem, leading to greatly degraded imaging. An injection into the pulmonary artery by means of a transvenous catheter overcomes this problem, but changes a non-invasive technique into one requiring cardiac catheterisation.

Time-gating over many cycles is not usually possible in patients with atrial fibrillation or other significant arrhythmias. More than a minor degree of movement of the thorax relative to the gamma camera also tends to limit studies during exertion.

Thallium perfusion scan (myocardial scintigraphy)

The technique of myocardial scintigraphy depends on thallium (^{201}Tl) being taken up by viable myocardium which is normally perfused. These tests are more difficult to perform than nuclear angiography, and ^{201}Tl is not as easily available as ^{99m}Tc. Generally, exercise is incorporated in the protocol. Areas of viable myocardium which are not perfused during exercise appear as cold spots which 'fill in' during the rest scan. Cold spots on the scan that do not perfuse after exercise represent infarcted myocardium.

MAGNETIC RESONANCE IMAGING (MRI)

MRI can now be used for studying flow velocity patterns as well as structure of the heart and great vessels. It produces detailed anatomical and flow images of particular use in complex congenital heart disease, without the need to expose patients to radiation. It is a very valuable tool in diagnosing dissection of the aorta, but although the technique promises much, its high capital cost has limited its availability.

COMPUTED TOMOGRAPHY

X-ray technology using ultrafast CT scanners has developed to the point of allowing rapid scans of the heart, flow and morphological detail can be obtained. However, the newer equipment remains costly and is not widely available.

CARDIAC CATHETERISATION

Cardiac catheterisation is a diagnostic procedure in which a flexible tube is passed, under local anaesthetic, from brachial or femoral superficial veins into the right side of the heart, or from the brachial or femoral arteries to the left side of the heart. In children, the procedure may require a general anaesthetic. In *right heart catheterisation* the catheter tip can be passed to all the right heart chambers. Using an end-hole catheter, an indirect LA pressure can be obtained by wedging the catheter in a small pulmonary artery. *Left heart catheterisation* from a peripheral artery enables cannulation of the aorta, the coronaries and the LV cavity, by passing the catheter retrogradely through the aortic valve.

Uses of cardiac catheterisation

Catheterisation allows pressure measurements to be made and cine angiograms performed by the injection of contrast agents. Selective catheterisation of the *coronary arteries* provides high-quality angiographic views of the coronary tree to demonstrate its anatomy. This has become the major use of cardiac catheterisation, complementing non-invasive techniques which can be used for diagnosis and quantitative assessment in most patients with valvular and congenital heart disease.

In valvular heart disease, the objectives of cardiac catheterisation are as follows:

- *To measure pressures in the chambers of the heart*, and so establish the presence of valve stenosis or ventricular disease (Fig. 12.21).
- *To measure valve pressure gradients*. Although the gradient across a normal valve is trivial and cannot be measured with conventional fluid-filled catheters, pathological pressure gradients are very much larger. An aortic valve pressure gradient is considered surgically significant when it reaches about 50 mmHg if the cardiac output is normal. A mitral valve gradient of less than 5 mmHg is considered insignificant.
- *To enable radio-opaque contrast to be injected selectively* in the different chambers of the heart and thus demonstrate by cine *angiography* the presence of valvular regurgitation, intracardiac shunts and abnormal morphology or contractility of the ventricles.
- *Measurement of oxygen content for demonstration of shunts* (Fig. 12.22). Sampling in the different chambers of the right side of the heart can be used to

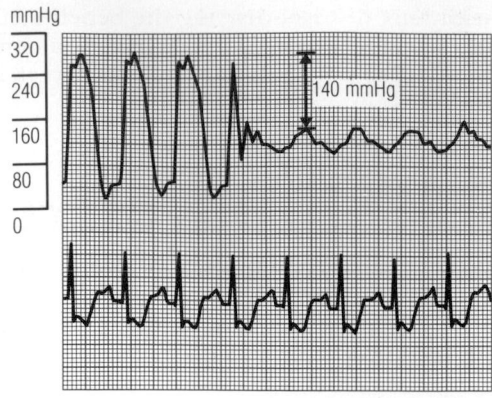

Fig. 12.21 Cardiac catheter pressure tracing in aortic stenosis. As the catheter is withdrawn from the left ventricle into the aorta, there is an abrupt drop in pressure demonstrating a gradient across the aortic valve of 140 mmHg. Lower tracing is the ECG.

demonstrate the presence and size of a left-to-right shunt by the rise in oxygen content (saturation) of the blood. Persistent arterial desaturation, despite the patient breathing 100% oxygen, demonstrates the presence of a right-to-left shunt. Measurement of pulmonary artery and systemic arterial blood oxygen content, together with measurement of oxygen uptake by timed expired air gas collection (or, in many centres, estimated oxygen uptake from normograms of patient's surface area), are used to calculate cardiac output.

Complications of cardiac catheterisation

The complications of cardiac catheterisation are shown in Table 12.2. The risks are small ($<0.1\%$), and are minimised by current techniques. They are increased if

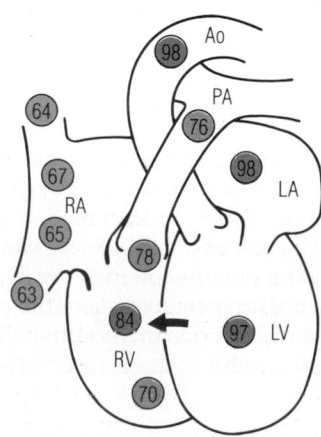

Fig. 12.22 Oxygen saturation in the cardiac chambers and great vessels in ventricular septal defect. A step up in saturation occurs in the right ventricle. Ao = aorta; PA = pulmonary artery; RV = right ventricle; LV = left ventricle; RA = right atrium; LA = left atrium.

Table 12.2 Complications of cardiac catheterisation

- Peripheral arterial damage (dissection, haematoma)
- Cardiac arrhythmia (SVT, VT, VF)
- Cardiac tamponade
- Dissection of a coronary artery
- Heart failure due to hyperosmolar contrast agents
- Thromboembolism, due to clot on catheter, air embolism, dislodged atheroma

the patient has small vessels, is in heart failure, or has very severe coronary artery or valvular disease.

HEART FAILURE

Heart failure can be defined simply as failure of the heart to function as it should to maintain an adequate circulation. Such failure has several physiological consequences, which together are manifested as the clinical syndrome of heart failure. It is not enough to define heart failure as a clinical syndrome consisting of combined features of congestion and hypoperfusion. Firstly, this might lead to the wrong assumption that the definitive treatment of heart failure is solely to correct these secondary defects and to relieve the symptoms. Secondly, pathological states of the vasculature may produce syndromes similar to heart failure, but the heart may not actually be failing. Examples are severe hypertension (when there is excessive vasoconstriction) and the so-called 'high output failure' (such as produced by significant arterio-venous shunting). In these conditions the heart is required to perform supernormal function, and is unable to do so. To refer to these conditions as 'heart failure' is a misnomer, and to treat these as other forms of heart failure, e.g. administering positive inotropic agents to augment cardiac pumping, is inappropriate.

The spectrum of cardiac performances

The main difference between the hearts of an elite athlete, a sedentary healthy subject and a heart failure patient lies not in their cardiac performance at basal resting states (they all have comparable cardiac outputs of 5–7 l/min and cardiac power outputs of 0.8–1.3 W), but in their peak cardiac performance. Elite athletes can attain cardiac outputs of up to 35 l/min and power outputs of up to 11 W, whereas the values for normal subjects are 20 l/min and 6 W, and for patients with moderate heart failure, 10 l/min and 2.5 W. It is the deterioration in peak cardiac performance that heralds the onset of heart failure and this deteriorates progressively. A point will be reached when, even at maximal stimulation, the hearts of some patients in severe heart failure or in

cardiogenic shock are not able to attain the basal resting values observed in normals. These patients have a very grave prognosis.

PATHOPHYSIOLOGY OF HEART FAILURE

The major sequelae of heart failure are organ hypoperfusion, arrhythmia, congestion, vasoconstriction and redistribution of regional blood flow. Arrhythmia in heart failure may be secondary to ischaemia, abnormal mechanical loads and the production of areas conducive to formation of re-entry circuits (see p. 357).

It is important to remember that the primary defect lies in the heart. The secondary defects, such as fluid retention and excessive vasoconstriction, are compensatory, adaptive mechanisms invoked to maintain as normal a circulation as possible. They are mediated by neuroendocrine activation and are sequelae of the primary cardiac dysfunction. Together with the primary defects, they produce the symptoms and signs of heart failure (see below). The tertiary defects are the detrimental effects produced as a result of attempts (or failure) to treat the condition. Categorising the defects in this way is helpful in planning treatment (Table 12.3).

Primary defects

The definitive treatment of heart failure should be directed at diagnosing and correcting the primary defects. Examples might be the removal of cardiodepressant drugs, aspiration of pericardial fluid in tamponade, control of arrhythmias, insertion of pacemakers in complete heart block and severe bradycardia, repair or replacement

Table 12.3 Defects in heart failure and their management

Defect	Clinical response
Primary Pump dysfunction	Establish a cause and remedy if possible
Secondary	
Fluid retention	Diuretics
Vasoconstriction	ACE inhibitors; other vasodilators (eg flosequinan)
Hypoperfusion	Volume replacement (if acute); decrease diuretics
Flow redistribution	Inotropes (if acute); ACEi
Arrhythmia	Correct tertiary defect; anti-arrhythmic drugs
Tertiary (usually due to treatment)	
Electrolyte imbalance	Monitor biochemistry, potassium-sparing diuretics
Arrhythmia	Review drug (pro-arrhythmic effects, e.g. digoxin)
Skeletal muscle deconditioning	Exercise training

of faulty valves, stripping of pericardium in constrictive pericarditis or surgical closure of intracardiac shunts.

By far the most common defect causing heart failure is cardiac myocyte loss, as a consequence of myocardial infarction or cardiomyopathy. Since cardiac myocytes are unable to undergo regeneration, the necrotic myocytes are replaced by connective tissue. The remaining viable myocardium contracts harder and undergoes hypertrophy to compensate for the loss. There is as yet no definitive therapy for this type of defect. Ultimately cardiac transplantation or cardiomyoplasty may be necessary.

The extent to which a primary defect compromises overall cardiac performance can be measured by how much cardiac reserve is reduced. A schematic representation of progressive damage to the heart by sequential myocardial infarctions is shown in Figure 12.23.

Secondary defects

In the event of heart failure or a normal heart facing excessive haemodynamic burden, the heart relies on cardiovascular *compensatory* mechanisms to maintain an adequate circulation. The main mechanisms are:

- fluid and salt retention invoking the Starling effect through an increase in ventricular filling (Fig. 12.24). (The stretching of atrial walls releases atrial natriuretic peptide or factor (ANP or ANF) which counterbalances to an extent fluid and salt retention)
- neuroendocrine responses (sympathetic stimulation followed by activation of the renin-angiotensin-aldosterone system) to increase cardiac pumping rate and force, and increase vasoconstriction to maintain

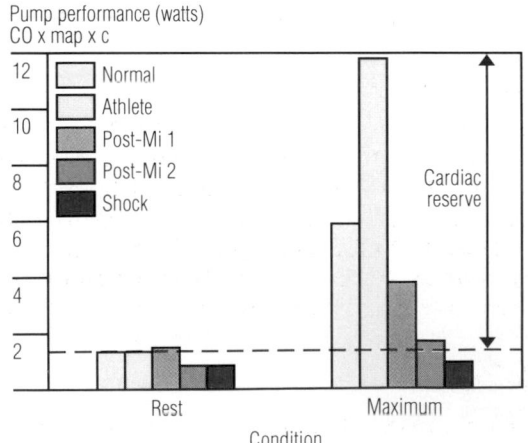

Fig. 12.23 Progressive damage to the heart by sequential myocardial infarctions. With the first infarction there is initial loss of cardiac functional reserve with no compromise of cardiac performance at rest. Further damage results in more loss of reserve, which may be accompanied by depressed cardiac function at rest. Finally, when the cardiac reserve is insufficient even to maintain adequate output at rest (cardiogenic shock), death ensues. CO = cardiac output; map = mean arterial pressure; c = constant.

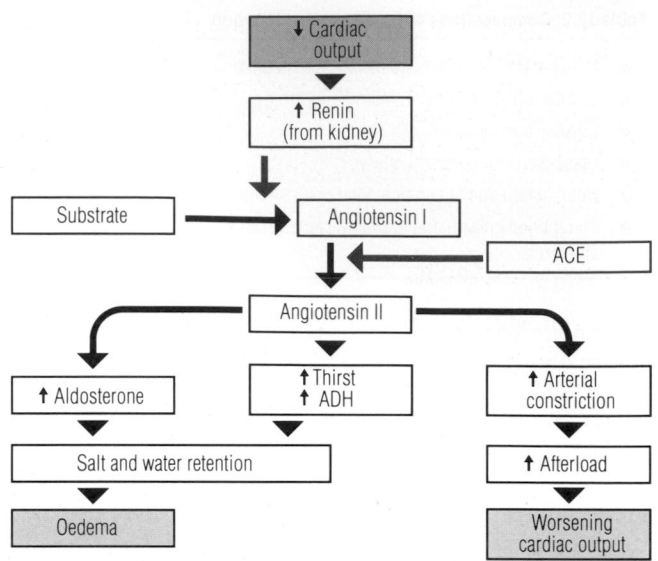

Fig. 12.24 The renin-angiotensin-aldosterone system in cardiac failure. Activation of the renin-angiotensin system by failing cardiac output leads to salt and water retention and worsening cardiac output (ACE = angiotensin-converting enzyme).

normal blood pressure and divert the limited blood flow to the vital organs
- myocardial hypertrophy, which is variable and incompletely understood but may reduce ventricular wall stress and thus augment function
- readjustment of skeletal muscle metabolism such that the same physical work can be performed with a reduced cardiac effort.

Decompensation occurs in heart failure when some of these compensatory mechanisms become excessive. Too much fluid and salt retention results in tissue oedema, which impedes tissue perfusion and reduces vasodilatory capacity. Gut and hepatic congestion impair absorption and metabolism, contributing to cardiac cachexia (and rendering enteral medication less effective). The ensuing hypoalbuminaemia further worsens the oedema. Pulmonary oedema causes orthopnoea and dyspnoea, impairs gaseous exchange and increases the work of ventilatory muscles, which in turn imposes extra demand on cardiac performance. Excessive cardiac dilatation causes functional AV valve regurgitation, further reducing ventricular pumping efficiency.

Excessive vasoconstriction (due to activation of the sympathetic, renin-angiotensin and vasopressin systems) imposes a higher afterload on the heart. Vasoconstriction is exacerbated by diuretic therapy which stimulates the renin-angiotensin system and the release of vasopressin. Excessive vasoconstriction of the renal arterioles leads to reduction in renal blood flow and glomerular filtration rates. The resulting azotaemia and oliguria compounds the management of heart failure. Chronic overstimulation of the sympathetic system depletes myocardial noradrenaline and causes β-receptor downregulation, reducing myocardial chronotropic and inotropic reponses. Excessive myocardial hypertrophy causes cardiac diastolic dysfunction and makes the subendocardial region more prone to ischaemia.

Tertiary defects

Pharmacological treatments that alter physiological homeostatic controls lead to complications, some of which can be detrimental. The commonest is probably electrolyte imbalance. The powerful loop diuretics lead to loss of potassium and magnesium, both of which can increase the likelihood of tachyarrhythmias. Dietary replenishment of potassium supplements does not fully compensate for the losses. A better way of avoiding this complication is to use the so-called potassium-sparing diuretics, which also conserve magnesium. Diuretic therapy in severe heart failure can also lead to significant hyponatraemia which is particularly difficult to treat and associated with a poorer prognosis. Diuretics must be used carefully to avoid this pitfall.

Arrhythmia is an important consequence of electrolyte imbalance. Hypokalaemia, hypomagnesaemia and hyponatraemia all cause arrhythmia, the latter being especially hard to treat. Overdiuresis can also produce hypovolaemia. This leads to further hypoperfusion and postural hypotension.

Vasodilators have preferential effects on different vascular beds. Such selective vasodilation may counter the 'natural' redistribution of blood flow which preserves flow to vital organs in low output states. For example, α-adrenergic blockers such as prazosin counteract the redistribution of blood flow effected by noradrenaline, but prazosin does not improve exercise tolerance or prognosis of heart failure patients. Vasodilators that redistribute blood into the splanchnic or cutaneous vasculature may help in acute severe heart failure, but do not improve exercise capacity or mortality in chronic heart failure. Angiotensin-converting enzyme (ACE) inhibitors are immensely useful but can be counterproductive by worsening renal function in patients dependent on the angiotensin-induced renal efferent arteriole vasoconstriction to maintain glomerular filtration rates. Certain positive inotropic agents (e.g. catecholamines) are toxic, causing arrhythmias and cardiac myocyte necrosis.

CLASSIFICATION

There are three main ways of classifying heart failure:

- *Acute vs. chronic heart failure.* Although this temporal classification may seem clinically obvious, the patho-physiology and therapy of the two conditions have important differences. In acute heart failure, the haemodynamic derangement is severe enough to result in obvious symptoms at rest. In chronic heart failure, however, the circulation at rest is adequate, but there is inadequate cardiac reserve to pursue daily activities.
- *Systolic vs. diastolic (or forward vs. backward) heart failure.* Systolic or forward failure results in low output and low arterial pressure states, whereas diastolic or backward failure results in congestion. Systolic failure is due to inadequate overall myocardial contractile capability, and diastolic failure relates to abnormalities in relaxation. Although heart failure is due most often to systolic dysfunction, some patients have normal systolic function, and the failure is due to abnormal diastolic function. This is due to an inability of the ventricle to relax normally. The cause is either a problem within the heart muscle itself (hypertrophy, restriction) or in the pericardium (effusion or constriction). In ischaemic heart disease, systolic and diastolic dysfunction often coexist, because ischaemia also impairs myocardial relaxation.
- *Left- vs. right-sided heart failure.* This classification arose from a simplistic clinical division into whether there is pulmonary congestion (left heart failure) or systemic congestion (right heart failure). However, the right and left sides of the heart are connected in series, and in juxtaposition, enclosed in the pericardium. This complicates the simple division into right and left heart failure. Marked hypertrophy and dilatation of the left ventricle can impinge on right ventricular filling (the Bernheim effect) and cause systemic congestion without intrinsic right ventricular dysfunction.

Epidemiology

In Western countries, approximately 0.5–2% of the population is affected by heart failure, and the prevalence is greater with increasing age to about 10% in those over 75 years old. The annual incidence of heart failure is about 3 per 1000 for men aged 45–65 years and 8 per 1000 for men aged 65–75 years. Both the prevalence and incidence have more or less doubled since the 1960s.

Aetiology

The main causes of heart failure are ischaemic heart disease, idiopathic cardiomyopathy, hypertension and myocarditis. In the Framingham (Massachussetts, USA) population study (1955–1971), over 75% of those who developed heart failure had antecedent hypertension. More recently the incidence of hypertensive heart failure has decreased markedly, which is probably due to improved antihypertensive treatment.

Prognosis and natural history

Like neural cells, cardiac myocytes do not undergo division; growth is by hypertrophy. In adulthood there is a natural attrition rate of cardiac cells with increasing age. It has been estimated that there is an aggregate loss of about 35% of myocyte cells in the ventricles from young adulthood to old age. This rate is increased by disease.

The prognosis of patients with heart failure is poor and it is worse in those with advanced heart failure. Overall, the 5-year survival rate of patients with all degrees of heart failure is approximately 50%. In patients with severe heart failure, the 1-year mortality rate is greater than 50%. About half of these patients die suddenly and the other half die of progressive heart failure.

CLINICAL FEATURES

The main symptoms and signs of heart failure are those related to congestion and hypoperfusion, either at rest (as in acute heart failure) or during exertion (as in chronic heart failure). In taking a history, the symptoms and signs must be noted, and information about the likely cause of heart failure and the severity of its effect on the patient's life should be sought.

Symptoms and signs

The symptoms of congestion in the lungs are exertional dyspnoea, orthopnoea (dyspnoea and cough on lying down), paroxysmal nocturnal dyspnoea (breathlessness that wakes the patient from sleep), 'cardiac asthma' (wheeziness due to congestion of the bronchial mucosa) and, rarely, haemoptysis (see p. 370). In some patients the dyspnoea at rest may be episodic, raising the possibility of paroxysmal arrhythmia.

The physical signs of pulmonary congestion are fine inspiratory crackles at the lung bases, but throughout the lung fields in severe cases. These are usually associated with tachypnoea. Inspiratory wheeze may be present and should not be assumed to be due to airways disease. Occasionally, dyspnoea is atypical, more like Kussmaul respiration (deeper and slower), and is due to lactic acidosis secondary to marked tissue hypoperfusion. Some of these patients may be labelled 'hyperventilators' until the severity of the underlying left ventricular dysfunction is appreciated. In severe pulmonary oedema due to acute left heart failure the patient is in respiratory distress and producing white frothy sputum through mouth or nostril, pale and cyanosed, and if unrelieved progresses to a moribund or unconscious state.

The clinical features of systemic congestion are raised JVP, peripheral pitting oedema, abdominal distension with discomfort or pain, and dyspnoea due to pleural effusion. In mild failure, the oedema only involves the

---

Summary 1 Symptoms and signs of heart failure

Symptoms	Sign
• Fatigue	• Raised JVP
• Shortness of breath	• Gallop rhythm
on exertion	• Pitting oedema
on lying flat	• Hepatomegaly
• Paroxysmal nocturnal dyspnoea	• Basal crackles
• Haemoptysis	• Positive hepatojugular reflux
• Weight gain	• Cardiomegaly
• Swollen ankles	• Ascites
• Abdominal distension	• Pallor
• Abdominal pain	• Peripheral cyanosis
	• Pulsus alternans

---

ankles and feet, and it may be dependent (occurring after prolonged upright posture). Patients with chronic leg oedema may develop lower leg ulcers with or without cellulitis. With more severe failure, the oedema may involve the thighs, sacrum, abdomen and upper body. Abdominal distension may be due to ascites or hepatic congestion. The latter may induce pain, especially during exercise (*hepatic angina*). Long-term hepatic congestion and gut oedema leads to weight loss and *cardiac cachexia*. Occasionally, there may be sparing of lower limb oedema, and the patient presents with abdominal and/or upper body congestive features. In bed-ridden patients oedema may only be found on the sacrum.

The symptoms of hypoperfusion include fatigue, lethargy, cold peripheries, and dizziness. The dizziness is often due to postural hypotension. The physical signs include tachycardia, hypotension with a small pulse pressure, pallor and feeble peripheral pulses. In more severe failure or cardiogenic shock, the signs are of cool, clammy and cyanotic peripheries, oliguria or anuria and blunted mental function.

Cardiac examination and the history alone may reveal the cause of heart failure (valvular lesions, acute infarction, rhythm or conduction defects, pericardial effusion or constriction). Frequently, a chest X-ray, ECG, and, increasingly, echocardiography are needed to diagnose the primary defect.

ACUTE HEART FAILURE

Diagnosis and management

Pulmonary oedema

Although the commonest cause of pulmonary oedema is acute left ventricular failure following acute myocardial infarction, there are many important non-cardiac causes. These include overtransfusion, shock lung in septicaemia, aspiration of gastric acid, paraquat poisoning and inhalation of certain toxic fumes. The common feature is accumulation of oedema fluid in alveolar spaces leading to dyspnoea. The lungs become stiff, increasing the work of breathing. Gas exchange is impaired and, if unrelieved, progressive hypoxaemia and hypercapnia follow as the patient tires; this can lead to eventual death.

In acute left ventricular failure, initial management consists of manoeuvres to decrease left atrial pressure, increase oxygenation and diminish fear and anxiety which increase the sympathetic drive leading to increased myocardial work demands. A simple regimen is summarised in Table 12.4.

In general, the reduction in preload with diuretics and nitrates is associated with some impairment of tissue perfusion demonstrated by minor elevation in urea and creatinine. This is usually transient. If the reduction in preload by diuretics and nitrates is prolonged tissue perfusion may become greatly compromised and the patient develop multiple organ failure that is more difficult to treat than the original oedema. These situations can be avoided by maintaining adequate systolic pressures, with inotropic support if necessary, avoiding excessive use of diuretics and consideration of vasodilators such as ACE inhibitors early in treatment.

Acute right heart failure

Pulmonary embolism (see p. 496), *cor pulmonale* (see p. 487) and acute inferior or posterior myocardial infarction are the usual causes. The features of acute right heart failure in myocardial infarction include a raised JVP associated with a low blood pressure and usually clear lung fields. The right ventricular function curve has flattened (Fig. 12.5, p. 323) so that a higher right atrial filling pressure is needed to support the same cardiac output. These patients need expansion of the circulating volume with albumin or synthetic plasma expanders to improve output and blood pressure. Injudicious use of diuretics or nitrates to 'treat' the high JVP can lead to serious falls in cardiac output.

Table 12.4 Heart failure: treatment of acute pulmonary oedema

Posture – sit patient up (legs over edge of bed): reduces preload

Oxygen – high concentration, with positive end-expiratory pressure

Ventilate if pco_2 >7 kPa (positive pressure ventilation)

Diamorphine with antiemetic (with care)

Reduce preload i.v. nitrates if SBP ≥100 mmHg or i.v. diuretics (frusemide/bumetanide)

SBP ≤100 mmHg – positive inotropic agents: e.g. dobutamine or i.v. phosphodiesterase inhibitors

Establish diagnosis. Control arrhythmia and heart rate, lower BP if hypertensive, seek surgically treatable conditions

Cardiogenic shock

In cardiogenic shock, tissue perfusion is inadequate to meet basal metabolic demands, as a result of severe cardiac pump dysfunction. Clinically it is recognised by hypotension (systolic BP <80 mmHg; mean BP <60 in normotensives, and <110 in chronically hypertensive subjects), associated with oliguria or anuria, cold sweaty skin, mental confusion and lactic acidosis. It is not necessary for all these features to be present before making the diagnosis of cardiogenic shock.

Causes of cardiogenic shock are massive myocardial infarction (usually loss of ≥40% of total myocardial muscle), mechanical complication of infarction (e.g. VSD and papillary muscle rupture) severe brady- or tachyarrhythmia, rejection in the transplanted heart, myocarditis and infiltration of the previously normal myocardium. It is important to exclude the effects of any myocardial depressant or vasodilatory agents (e.g. diamorphine, beta-blockers, phosphodiesterase inhibitors). In the presence of right ventricular infarction, a fluid challenge to raise the pulmonary wedge pressure to >18 mmHg should be made before making the diagnosis of cardiogenic shock.

The incidence of cardiogenic shock in patients admitted with acute myocardial infarction is 5–20%. The advent of thrombolytic therapy has not altered the incidence significantly. The hospital mortality rate is still 50–70%.

The continuation of function in the heart is also dependent on its own output. When the aortic pressure falls below the critical pressure for coronary perfusion (mean 60 mmHg), left ventricular myocardium becomes ischaemic, further impairing performance.

Medical therapy of cardiogenic shock is described on page 408. The following general principles are the basis of management:

- Optimising heart rate, ideally between 80 and 130 bpm, with pacing if necessary (preferably AV sequential pacing; see p. 355).
- Treating tachyarrhythmia using agents with minimal negative inotropic effects (e.g. therapeutic dose ranges of lignocaine, mexiletine, procainamide, tocainide, digoxin and amiodarone). Direct-current cardioversion is preferred over 'cocktails' of antiarrhythmic drugs provided the patient can be maintained in sinus rhythm afterwards.
- Correcting metabolic acidosis with bicarbonate is rarely necessary. Intermittent positive pressure ventilation may be required (although this may worsen the haemodynamic status).
- In right ventricular infarction and failure, elevating the legs should be tried to increase right atrial filling. If this improves the blood pressure, then fluid can be infused.
- Avoiding pure vasodilators.
- Using positive inotropic agents (see p. 349).

12 Cardiovascular Disease

Summary 2 Clinical features of cardiogenic shock

Hypotension (<60 mmHg mean aortic pressure)

Oliguria/anuria (<60 ml/h)

Cold sweaty skin

Mental confusion

Lactic acidosis

Biventricular heart failure is the rule

Cardiac power output (<1.0 W)

In managing cardiogenic shock it is important to investigate whether the heart, which is obviously depressed at basal resting state, possesses any reserve function, and whether this reserve exceeds that necessary to sustain normal body basal metabolism (e.g. peak cardiac power output > 1 W, Fig. 12.23, p. 344). Cardiac reserve can be measured by stepwise infusion of dobutamine with or without phosphodiesterase inhibitors and noting if the peak cardiac power output attained. If the peak is > 1 W, medical therapy including the use of inotropic agents to maintain adequate pressure and flow can be sufficient. Nevertheless, remediable defects should be dealt with. If the peak is below 1 W (or simple bedside observation of peak attainable systolic BP is <80 mmHg despite maximal dobutamine stimulation), then death is expected unless urgent and definitive treatment of primary defects is obtained (e.g. urgent coronary angioplasty, bypass surgery, other curative operation or cardiac transplantation). If the definitive treatment is delayed, artificial circulatory support in the form of intra-aortic balloon counterpulsation should be instituted (p. 408). If the surgical option is ruled out, frantic therapeutic efforts should be avoided and the patient allowed to die peacefully.

CHRONIC HEART FAILURE

Management

The cause of heart failure must be established and remediable causes sought and treated. These might include the replacement or repair of valves, stripping of the pericardium in constriction and the closure of significant intracardiac shunts.

The overall aim of treatment in chronic (non-surgical) heart failure is to relieve symptoms, to improve quality of life and functional capacity, and lastly to improve prognosis. The general measures should include stopping smoking, reducing alcohol intake, fluid restriction and possibly regular exercise training.

Bed rest is helpful only in acute myocardial infarction, active myocarditis and intractable congestion unresponsive to conventional doses of diuretics. The disadvantages of bed rest (skeletal and myocardial deconditioning, muscular atrophy and weakness, bedsores, deep vein thrombosis, autonomic maladjustment) outweigh the benefits. Patients who are symptomatic at rest should be encouraged to mobilise as soon as possible, since exercise rehabilitation may improve functional capacity even in severe chronic heart failure. A treatment strategy is:

- mild failure – thiazide or loop diuretics (ACE inhibitors, digoxin)
- moderate failure – loop and potassium-sparing diuretics, ACE inhibitors, nitrates, digoxin
- severe failure – as above plus intermittent metolazone therapy with i.v. diuretics and i.v. inotropes
- haemofiltration and ultrafiltration can be used for resistant oedema
- cardiomyoplasty or cardiac transplantation.

Improvement in functional capacity has been shown with diuretics (most effective), vasodilators (ACE inhibitors, nitrates, nitrate–hydralazine combination) and digoxin. Long-term (> 6 months) low-dose beta-blockade may be effective in idiopathic dilated cardiomyopathy, but this form of treatment should be supervised very closely.

Drug therapy to improve prognosis is now possible, and ACE inhibitors and nitrate–hydralazine combinations are the most effective, although the prolongation of survival only averages 6 months. About 20–50% of patients in heart failure die suddenly. However, no antiarrhythmic agent has been shown to be effective in reducing this incidence, although preliminary results using amiodarone appear promising.

DRUG TREATMENT

Diuretics

These agents are still the mainstay and first-line pharmacological treatment of acute and chronic heart failure.

Thiazide diuretics

- used only in the mildest forms of heart failure, and should generally be avoided in elderly patients
- liable to cause significant metabolic upsets (electrolyte imbalance, insulin resistance, lipid disturbances)
- potassium supplements alone may not be sufficient; combination with a potassium-sparing diuretic is recommended.

Loop diuretics (frusemide and bumetanide)

- more powerful than thiazide
- less liable to cause metabolic disturbances

- cause hypokalaemia; regular checks of serum electrolytes are essential
- magnesium loss occurs; better to combine loop diuretic treatment with a potassium-sparing diuretic (e.g. amiloride); significant hyponatraemia may occur and is difficult to treat.

In *acute heart failure* treatment aims to relieve dyspnoea and peripheral congestion, by inducing a gradual fluid loss of no more than 1 litre negative balance each day (body weight reduction of ≤1 kg). Fluid intake should be less than 1.5 litres. The diuretics are given intravenously initially and dosage should be reduced once a stable balance is achieved.

In *chronic heart failure* the aim is to relieve the congestive symptoms without compromising renal function or causing postural hypotension. Patients already on oral diuretics who have slipped back into congestion are best admitted to hospital for a period of treatment with i.v. diuretics. Combination with a thiazide diuretic (especially metolazone) can result in marked diuresis in intractable congestion. However, such therapy may induce severe electrolyte imbalance, especially hyponatraemia. Another way of dealing with intractable congestion is the concurrent use of low-dose dopamine. Congestion unresponsive to this may need more drastic treatment, such as addition of positive inotropic agents, haemofiltration or dialysis.

Vasodilators

Vasodilator drugs are used to decrease both preload and afterload. Excessive preload reduction may result in loss of Starling's effect and compromise ventricular output. Excessive afterload reduction can reduce coronary perfusion and exacerbate myocardial ischaemia.

ACE inhibitors are the vasodilators of first choice in the treatment of chronic moderate and severe heart failure. There are many ACE inhibitors available. The only short-acting agent is captopril (6.25–50 mg t.d.s.). If more prolonged effects are required, then long-acting drugs should be used (e.g. enalapril, lisinopril, ramipril). It is still unclear whether the different properties exhibited by the different ACE inhibitors make any significant difference to the clinical efficacy. There are, however, important adverse effects:

- About 10% of all patients do not tolerate ACE inhibitor therapy due to unacceptable cough.
- Hypotension with the first dose can be avoided by careful introduction, sometimes hospital admission for close BP monitoring is required. Patients should not be dehydrated or hyponatraemic at the introduction of these drugs. A suitable regimen might start with 6.25 mg of captopril, increased over successive days to a maintenance dose of 12.5 or 25 mg t.d.s.

Discharge on a long-acting preparation is then possible.

- The most problematic adverse effect is impairment of renal function. In a significant minority inhibition of angiotensin-induced constriction of the efferent glomerular arteriole and overall renal function is affected. Rising creatinine is a reason to reconsider this therapy.

In those patients unable to use ACE inhibitors, an alternative treatment would be long-acting nitrates. Moreover, since ACE inhibitors do not have direct antianginal effects, nitrates may be preferentially used in ischaemic heart failure. A drug-free period of at least 6 hours in the day is recommended (e.g. sustained release isosorbide mononitrate 30–80 mg o.d.).

The use of other vasodilators, e.g. calcium antagonists, α-adrenoreceptor blockers, hydralazine, minoxidil, have not been shown to be truly beneficial in heart failure, unless hypertension is also a prominent feature. However, there is evidence in favour of a combination of nitrates with hydralazine.

Inotropic agents

Positive inotropic agents are not without potential dangers (e.g. arrhythmogenicity and liability to induce worsening cardiac myocyte necrosis). In viral myocarditis they should be avoided, unless as a bridge to transplantation. With the exception of digoxin (see below), chronic oral inotropic therapy (with β_2 stimulants and phosphodiesterase inhibitors) has been very disappointing. In heart failure following acute myocardial infarction, the indications and rationale for using inotropes are:

- cardiogenic shock (see below)
- precardiogenic shock – because the prognosis of cardiogenic shock is very grave, every effort should be made to avoid the patient progressing into cardiogenic shock, and this includes early use of inotropes. Inotropes are the only agents that can prevent undue loss of coronary perfusion pressure.

Although dopamine is a positive inotropic agent, in low doses it acts as a renal vasodilator, and should be used whenever there is oliguria or anuria after myocardial infarction.

Following myocardial infarction, dobutamine, preferably in combination with low-dose dopamine are the inotropes of choice. In patients with chronic severe heart failure and β-adrenoreceptor downregulation, a combination of phosphodiesterase inhibitors and dobutamine may produce synergistic and thus enhanced inotropic effects.

Digitalis preparations (digoxin, medigoxin, digitoxin, ouabain) are now well established as of value as mild positive inotropic agents in chronic heart failure. Digoxin is still the only oral positive inotropic agent available.

Antiarrhythmic agents

These drugs often have to be used in heart failure patients. Most intravenous antiarrhythmic agents are cardiodepressant to varying degrees. The most negatively inotropic are beta-blockers, verapamil and disopyramide, and are generally avoided in severe heart failure. In therapeutic doses, the following intravenous agents exert little negative inotropism, and may be used in heart failure: lignocaine, mexiletine and procainamide. Orally, amiodarone, digoxin, mexiletine and procainamide are virtually devoid of negative inotropic effects.

CARDIAC TRANSPLANTATION

Since the first human heart transplantation in 1967, the technique has become an accepted form of treatment for patients dying of heart failure, and for whom no other form of treatment offers any help. The current annual rate of cardiac transplantation worldwide is approximately 3000. The number of patients requiring cardiac transplantation each year in the USA alone is estimated to be 35 000–70 000. The shortfall is mainly due to the shortage of donor hearts and is responsible for the plateauing of the rates of transplantation in the USA and the UK. Cardiac transplantation will not become the panacea of heart failure treatment, and strict selection of recipients will necessarily remain.

Indications

The vast majority of patients who undergo cardiac transplantation have either terminal idiopathic dilated or ischaemic cardiomyopathy. Other indications include intractable ventricular tachyarrhythmias, hypertrophic cardiomyopathy, peripartum cardiomyopathy, congenital heart disease and cardiac tumours. The patient must have reached end-stage heart failure and have a very limited life expectancy. The best available method of measuring the prognosis of these patients is by estimating their cardiac reserve (see p. 348).

Contraindications to transplantation of the heart alone include increased pulmonary vascular resistance, blood group incompatibility or any coexisting systemic illness that may significantly limit life expectancy.

Surgery

There are two main surgical procedures:

- *Orthotopic transplantation.* The recipient's heart (except the venous attachment side of the atria) is excised and replaced by the donor's heart. This is the commonest procedure.
- *Heterotopic transplantation.* The recipient's heart is not excised and the donor's heart is anastomosed side to side to the corresponding atria and great vessels of the recipient's heart.

Contrary to popular belief, the surgery itself is simpler than most open-heart surgical procedures. The main operative problem is the preservation of the donor heart during transit.

Management

By far the most difficult part of cardiac transplantation is the postoperative care. The two major complications are graft rejection and infection, which account for most of the early mortality. There is as yet no early and accurate method of detecting rejection non-invasively. Apart from clinical suspicion and loss of R wave in the ECG, the most reliable method of diagnosing rejection is by percutaneous endomyocardial biopsy. Preliminary data suggest that imaging with radiolabelled monoclonal anticardiac myosin antibody may be of help in future.

Immunosuppressive regimens include combinations of cyclosporin, azathioprine, corticosteroids, cyclophosphamide, antithymocyte globulin (ATG), use of monoclonal antibody against the CD3 molecule on mature T cells and occasionally vincristine or methotrexate. The need for immunosuppression means that patients are at increased risks from bacterial infection. Opportunistic fungal infections and reactivation of primary viral infection (notably cytomegalovirus) occur. Late complications include accelerated coronary disease in the donor heart, hypertension, and increased incidence of malignancies (especially lymphoproliferative), and bone diseases (osteoporosis, avascular necrosis).

Prognosis

Current survival rates of cardiac transplantation are as good as renal transplantation, with overall 1- and 5-year survival rates of about 80% and 70% respectively for orthotopic transplantation. The survival rate for heterotopic transplantation is less good, with a 5-year survival of about 50%. Factors that negatively influence prognosis include major HLA mismatch, prolonged cold preservation of donor heart, presence of preformed circulating antibodies and advanced donor age.

Heart–lung transplantation

Patients with end-stage pulmonary vascular hypertension (primary or Eisenmenger's syndrome) and with parenchymal lung disease (mostly cystic fibrosis) have the option of heart and lung transplantation. The two classes of disease each constitute about half of the transplanted cases. The 1- and 3-year survival rates are currently about 65% and 50%. A major difficulty in management is that the diagnosis of rejection is more difficult in the lung than in the heart.

ARRHYTHMIA

Arrhythmia is a general term for any cardiac rhythm or conduction abnormality. Anatomically the arrhythmia may originate supraventricularly (atria or AV junction) or ventricularly. The most compelling clinical feature is whether the arrhythmia causes haemodynamic disturbance, however its implications depend more on the type of arrhythmia, so that ventricular tachycardias have a poorer prognosis compared to supraventricular tachycardias.

INVESTIGATIVE TECHNIQUES

The principal method of analysis of arrhythmia is the 12-lead ECG. The correct interpretation of the ECG may depend on comparison with previously acquired recordings.

24-hour ECG (Holter monitor)

Recorders can monitor two channels of an ECG in ambulant patients over a continuous 24-hour period (Fig. 12.25). Some rhythm disturbances may occur very infrequently and require alternative equipment. One recorder can be applied by the patient during symptoms and records 30 s of ECG in a solid state memory. This can be replayed subsequently through an ECG machine,

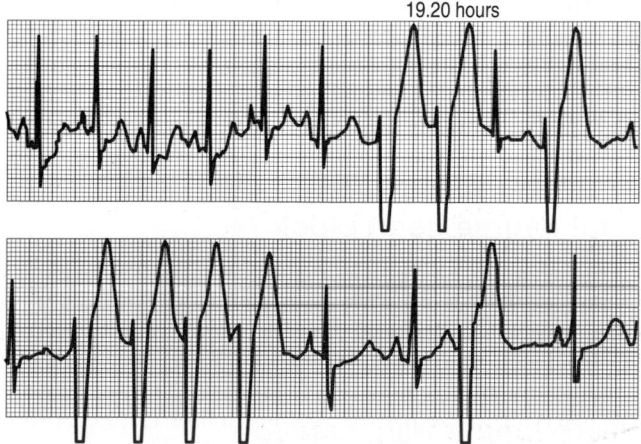

19.20 hours

Fig. 12.25 24-hour continuous ambulatory ECG monitoring. At 19.20 hours, the sinus rhythm is interrupted by ventricular ectopic beats and a short run of ventricular tachycardia.

or transmitted by telephone to a central station, where a doctor can advise on the nature of the event. For those patients who receive no warning of impending rhythm disturbance, there are newer automatic solid state recorders that continually sample the ECG over long periods but only memorise significant events.

Exercise ECG

The exercise test has a role in managing certain patients with arrhythmia. Those with recurrent ventricular tachycardia, or Wolf-Parkinson-White syndrome, may undergo exercise testing to check the efficacy of their drug treatment. However, not all these patients have exercise-induced arrhythmia, and may instead require more sophisticated EP studies.

Intracardiac electrophysiological (EP) testing

The techniques of cardiac catheterisation enable localised intracardiac ECGs to be recorded, using catheters similar to pacing catheters but with electrodes mounted distally. The activity of the atria, AV node, bundle of His and ventricles can be recorded independently. By combining recording with artificial stimulation from intracardiac pacemakers, a detailed analysis of intracardiac conduction can be made. This has proved useful in studying patients with tachycardia, in whom the abnormal rhythm may be induced and its origin (ventricular or supraventricular) confirmed. The site, number and potential danger from accessory AV bypass tracts (e.g. in Wolff-Parkinson-White syndrome) can be mapped and the tracts ablated. The effectiveness of drug regimens and the potential for using antitachycardia pacemakers are also tested using EP studies.

NORMAL SINUS RHYTHM

Each ventricular (QRS) complex is preceded by a P wave with a normal P wave axis (i.e. from the sinus node, P wave axis = 0° to +90°) and normal PR interval (0.11–0.20 s). In some circumstances, sinus rhythm may control the atrial, but not the ventricular, activity; this is most commonly encountered in complete heart block (p. 353 and Fig. 12.29).

Sinus arrhythmia is the quickening of the heart rate which occurs cyclically with each inspiration. It is most marked in individuals (often young) with high vagal tone.

ECTOPIC OR EXTRASYSTOLIC BEATS

These are defined as beats which arise outside the normal heart pacemaker. They may be generated in the atria, the

AV node, bundle of His or the ventricles. They may also arise as 'escape' beats in sinus bradycardia.

Atrial ectopics

Atrial ectopics or atrial premature beats (Fig. 12.26) are usually preceded by a P wave of different shape, different PR interval and, frequently, a different axis to the sinus P wave. The following QRS complex is normal. Atrial ectopics are common even in normal hearts, although, like all extrasystoles, they may be felt as uncomfortable fluttering, palpitation or 'skipped beats' in the chest. Stimulants, such as alcohol or caffeine-containing drinks and cigarettes, may be precipitants.

Junctional ectopics

Junctional ectopics may arise from the AV node or proximal bundle of His, although this differentiation cannot normally be made, hence the less specific term 'junctional' rather than the older 'nodal beat'. Atrial activation occurs retrogradely so that the P wave is positive in aVR and negative in II, III and aVF. The delay between ectopic activation and ventricular activity depends on its site of origin and will vary the timing of the P wave. This can precede, be buried in, or follow the QRS complex, which has a configuration identical to that in sinus rhythm.

Ventricular ectopics

Ventricular ectopic (VE) beats, by definition, are not preceded by a P wave and have a broad QRS configuration (Fig. 12.26). There is no prognostic significance attached to whether the ectopic beat has a left or right bundle branch block pattern. However, when frequent or multiform VEs are found in association with underlying ischaemic heart disease or cardiomyopathy, there is an increased risk of sudden death. Control of VEs with drugs may improve symptoms, but may not improve the prognosis; the severity of the underlying heart disease is probably a more important influence on survival. In addition, the drugs used to suppress VEs may themselves precipitate serious ventricular arrhythmias.

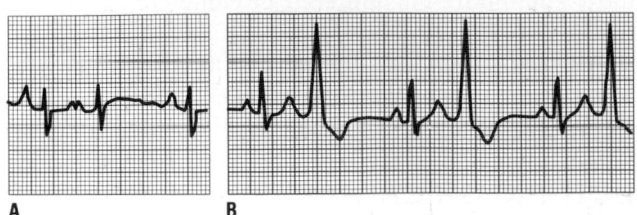

Fig. 12.26 ECGs showing ectopic beats. A. An atrial ectopic beat, demonstrated by the varying shape of the P wave. **B.** Coupled ventricular ectopics (bigeminy).

Clinical features

Ectopic beats, whether from atria or ventricles, are commonly found in normal individuals and generally not perceived by the patient. In some patients the frequency of ectopics is increased and they may produce the feelings of a 'missed beat' or even atypical chest pain (see p. 324).

Explanation of the cause of the symptom and avoidance of certain common precipitants of ectopics, such as alcohol, caffeine and cigarette smoke, may be all that is needed to treat the patient.

BRADYCARDIA AND HEART BLOCK

Bradycardia

Defined as a heart rate less than 60 bpm, bradycardia may be due to vagal tone in athletes or, more commonly, as an unwanted effect of beta-adrenoreceptor blocking drugs. It generally requires no treatment, unless severe and producing symptoms. In an emergency (e.g. severe bradycardia complicating a myocardial infarction), it responds to atropine (600 μg i.v. repeated to a maximum of 2.4 mg in 2 hours). If persistent, a temporary artificial pacemaker should be implanted. Chronic bradycardia may be a manifestation of the sick sinus syndrome (p. 364) and may benefit from permanent pacemaker implantation.

Sinus node block and sinus arrest

Both sinus node block and sinus arrest are associated with a pause in the normal train of sinus rhythm, leading to a delay in the appearance of the P wave. In *sinus node block*, the resultant pause between P waves is approximately double the preceding sinus (P–P) interval. The essential pacemaker rate remains constant but a normal discharge does not occur. In *sinus arrest*, the pause is not a multiple of the sinus interval, implying a transient change in pacemaker automaticity which has led to the loss of the P wave.

First degree heart block

In first degree heart block (Fig. 12.27), the PR interval is prolonged (>0.20 s). This may occur in otherwise normal patients and is caused by delayed propagation within the AV node. A modestly prolonged PR interval may also accompany vagally induced bradycardia. However, long PR intervals in the presence of normal or fast heart rates imply an intrinsic defect in the AV node. This is generally benign. The development of first degree heart block in the context of infective endocarditis usually means aortic root abscess formation. Similarly, widespread conducting

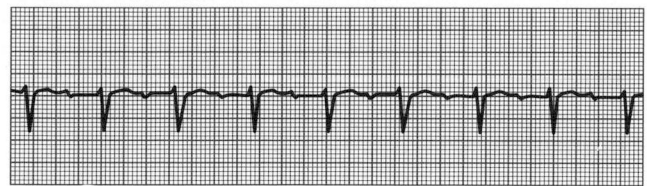

Fig. 12.27 ECG showing first degree heart block. Note prolonged PR interval (0.28 s).

tissue disease is suggested by the combination of first degree block, left axis deviation and bundle branch block. First degree block may also occur following a myocardial infarction (p. 406).

Second degree heart block

Second degree heart block (Fig. 12.28) is defined as intermittent failure to conduct an impulse from the atria to the ventricles, and may be temporary or permanent. It occurs in two major forms.

The Wenckebach phenomenon or Mobitz type I block

The Mobitz type I block (Wenckebach phenomenon) produces successively increasing PR intervals until a P wave is not conducted; the cycle then repeats itself. There are usually 3–5 beats in a cycle. This block occurs *within* the AV node, and is probably relatively benign. It may complicate acute inferior myocardial infarction and generally does not require specific treatment. It may also be seen in patients with generalised conducting tissue disease and as part of the sick sinus syndrome (p. 364).

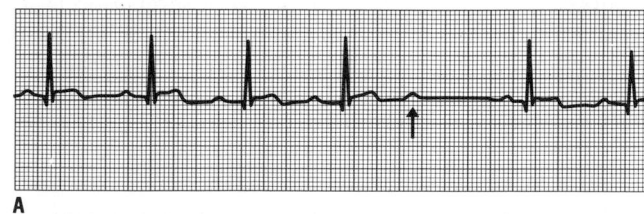

A

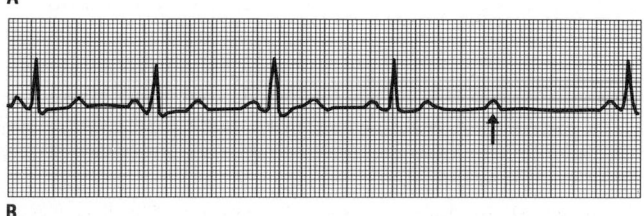

B

Fig. 12.28 ECGs showing second degree heart block. A. Mobitz type I showing progressive lengthening of the PR interval until the P wave is not conducted to the ventricles (arrow). **B.** Mobitz type II. Four sinus beats are followed by cessation of conduction following the P wave (arrowed).

Mobitz type II block

In the Mobitz type II block, an unheralded failure to conduct a P wave occurs. The site of the block is *below* the AV node in the proximal bundle of His. This condition has a tendency to progress unpredictably to complete block, which may cause Stokes-Adams' attacks or even death. This conduction disturbance is much less common than type I block and, because of its implications, usually requires treatment with an artificial pacemaker.

Other special forms of second degree block

During atrial tachycardia (e.g. atrial flutter), there may often be conduction of alternate beats to the ventricles in a ratio of 2 P waves : 1 QRS complex. When a tachycardia is present, this block constitutes the normal physiological function of the AV node, and block can often be increased further (to 3:1 or 4:1 or more) by manoeuvres which stimulate vagal activity such as carotid sinus massage. In the absence of an atrial tachycardia, established 2:1 conduction represents a form of second degree block. High-grade block is present when the ratio of P waves to QRS is 3:1 or greater. In either case, artificial permanent pacemaker implantation is the treatment of choice when the arrhythmia persists.

Complete or third degree heart block

In complete or third degree block (Fig. 12.29), the atrial impulses fail to be conducted to the ventricles. The block may be within the AV node, when the escape ventricular rhythm will be within the lower regions of the node or bundle of His, giving narrow, normal configuration QRS complexes and heart rates of about 40 bpm. Complete heart block may also occur at the level of the bundle of His, so that ventricular or distal bundle pacemakers control the heart rate, producing a much slower pulse (about 30 bpm) and wide, bundle branch block QRS complexes.

Clinical features

Symptoms

First degree heart block is asymptomatic, as are many cases of second degree heart block, but patients may be aware of the dropped beat and the stronger post-pause beat in Mobitz types I and II. In complete heart block, the most dramatic symptoms are related to recurrent asystole or the common ventricular arrhythmias that complicate severe bradycardia. However, complete heart block may present without any symptoms, despite a marked bradycardia; with heart failure secondary to a low cardiac output; and, often, as a confusional state secondary to poor cerebral perfusion and multiple syncopal episodes.

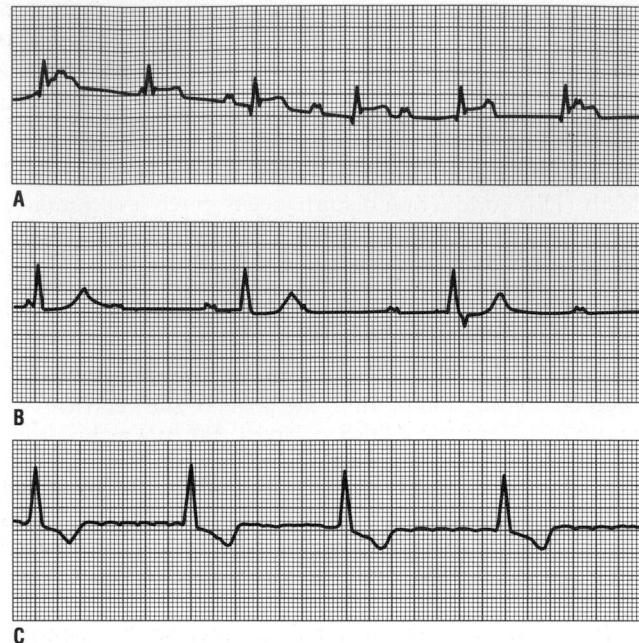

Fig. 12.29 Three rhythm strips demonstrating complete heart block. A.
Atrioventricular dissociation with a relatively rapid ventricular rate and narrow QRS
complex (with acute inferior infarction). **B.** A slow idioventricular rate with broad
QRS complexes. **C.** The unusual combination of complete heart block and atrial
fibrillation (no P waves).

Stokes-Adams' attack

The Stokes-Adams' attack can be caused by transient
asystole or a transient burst of tachycardia. The attacks
are usually unheralded. The patient may first be aware of
lying on the ground or falling. Recovery is usually rapid
and complete. Skin pallor may be followed by flushing. If
the anoxia lasts more than a few seconds, a convulsion
may occur and, on occasion, incontinence. Incomplete
attacks are common, presenting with transient giddiness
(without true vertigo) or near fainting (presyncope).

Attacks are sporadic and random. There may be
months to years between symptoms in some patients with
intermittent block, so that 24-hour ambulatory ECG
recordings may have to be made repeatedly for the diagnosis to be made. Occasionally, treatment with a pacemaker is warranted on the basis of the history alone,
although intracardiac electrophysiological studies may
help in these patients.

Signs

There are few clinical signs in heart block. The first heart
sound is quiet in first degree block, and intermittent
dropped beats will be felt at the pulse in second degree
block. In complete heart block, a slow pulse and intermittent cannon waves will be seen in the JVP, due to occa-

sional simultaneous contraction of the atria and ventricles. The large stroke volume and collapsing pulse with a
systolic murmur may mimic aortic valve disease.

Management

In congenital complete heart block, there is a surprising
degree of tolerance to the slow heart rate, which may
show modest rate responsiveness with exercise. Nevertheless, adults with this condition may risk sudden death,
and permanent pacemaker implantation is warranted.

In acute inferior myocardial infarction, complete heart
block is due to transient ischaemia of the SA and AV
nodes, and may not need a temporary pacemaker unless
symptoms or heart failure occur (p. 406). In extensive
anterior myocardial infarction, complete heart block is
related to extensive muscle damage and carries a poor
prognosis. Temporary pacemaker implantation may not
improve the outlook.

Drug treatment of complete heart block with isoprenaline slow-release capsules is now hardly ever justified,
and permanent pacemakers should be offered to virtually
all patients.

THE PERMANENT ARTIFICIAL PACEMAKER

The basic pacemaker consists of a small battery container
which can be implanted under the skin and connected by
an insulated electrode to the heart. Small electrical
impulses can be transmitted through the electrode to
stimulate the heart to contract. Since 1960 there has been
a great increase in their use, and 1 million people worldwide now live with an implanted pacemaker. The initial
sole indication for pacing was the treatment of chronic
complete heart block, but now a major indication is the
treatment of the sick sinus syndrome (p. 364). More
recently, units able to treat tachycardias and administer
internal DC cardioversion have been developed.
Pacemakers that respond to the patient's activity by
changing the pacing rate are now in common use.

Early pacemakers were fixed rate. Modern pacemakers, however, are almost exclusively demand (or
standby) units, providing a pulse only when the heart rate
falls below certain predetermined limits, and have battery
lives of 8–15 years. They may offer considerable adjustment and analysis via transcutaneous telemetry. The
complexity of cardiac pacemakers has increased for a
number of reasons:

● To increase battery life by reducing unnecessary
  pacing and by reducing output to the lowest safe
  limit.
● To allow fine control of the pacing heart rate, and,
  with dual-chamber devices, to restore the atrial con-

tribution to filling, which may be very important to individuals with impaired ventricular function or valve disease.

- To detect when the patient needs an increase in heart rate (e.g. with exercise).
- To detect tachycardias and abort them by programmed bursts of pacing (antitachycardia).

A letter coding system, used internationally, describes the type of pacemaker used. In some pacemakers, a facility allows the interval between the last natural beat and the paced beat to be longer than the pacing interval. Thus, only when a pause corresponding to a very low heart rate is exceeded will the pacemaker step in and gradually accelerate to its programmed paced rate. This stops the pacemaker inserting beats for trivial slowing of the heart (e.g. during sleep).

Dual-chamber pacemakers

Dual-chamber pacemakers have been developed to achieve a more physiological situation than is possible with ventricular pacing alone. These require implantation of electrodes in the right atrium and right ventricle. They use more complex, and therefore more expensive, generators. In addition, the capacity to 'fine-tune' the multiplicity of programmable functions to each individual patient requires both time and the availability of skilled pacemaker technicians or doctors in pacing clinics. Nevertheless, these units are justified in certain groups of patients:

- Patients with AV block but normal SA activity, in whom a true physiological situation can be achieved, with normal rate increase with activity, and maintained AV sequential contraction. This is usually reserved for young, or very active, elderly patients.
- Patients with poor ventricular function or valve disease where the atrial contribution to filling is of prime importance.
- Patients with the 'pacemaker syndrome'; a small number of patients develop severe symptomatic hypotension with pacing of the right ventricle alone.
- Patients with carotid sinus sensitivity.

Dual-chamber pacemakers should be avoided in patients with unstable SA activity or atrial fibrillation.

Pacemaker implantation and complications

Permanent pacemakers are almost always inserted by a cardiologist using local anaesthesia and full surgical sterile technique. Like temporary pacemakers (p. 406), the pacing electrode is passed down a central vein (usually the cephalic or subclavian) to the right heart. The electrode and generator box are then buried subcutaneously,

above pectoralis major on the high anterior chest wall. Complications of implantation are similar to those of temporary pacemakers. Infection is rare, but when it occurs, it requires major revision of the entire system and accounts for considerable morbidity and a small mortality. Lead displacement and fracture are very rare with modern pacing systems.

Specific pacemaker malfunction is now very rare. With current telemetry, the pacemaker (and lead) function can be assessed transcutaneously, so that premature battery failure can be predicted, problems with lead impedance (electrical resistance), current leak and failure to sense can often be diagnosed, and the unit reprogrammed to compensate for problems until replacement is required. Failure to sense the patient's electrical activity and intermittent failure to capture may sometimes cause problems. Dual-chamber pacemakers, although potentially much closer to normal physiology, carry their own problems, the most serious being the capacity to generate pacemaker-induced arrhythmia. Fortunately, these problems are rare.

Interference with pacemaker function by external sources of high magnetic and electromagnetic fields is less of a problem than might be expected; few problems arise in the normal environment of most patients. However, magnetic resonance imaging is contraindicated, and cautery during surgery has to be performed with care, avoiding placing the ground electrode near the generator and altering the unit to a fixed rate mode.

THE TACHYCARDIAS

Tachycardias are defined as a heart rate above 100 bpm, and are divided according to the origin of the pacemaker impulse. A classification is given in Table 12.5, and a guide to the use of antiarrhythmic agents in Table 12.6. A decision tree to aid in diagnosis is shown in Figure 12.30.

Mechanisms of production of tachycardias

Three basic mechanisms have been established: abnormalities of automaticity; early after-depolarisations and triggered activity; and abnormal impulse conduction and re-entry.

Abnormalities of automaticity

Under normal circumstances, only SA and AV node cells display automaticity. Abnormal automaticity may be displayed by diseased atrial and ventricular muscle. Stretch, alkalosis, temperature increases and hypoxia all increase the rate of repolarisation and reduce the resting membrane potential (Vm), thereby accentuating the tendency to abnormal automaticity. Cardioactive drugs

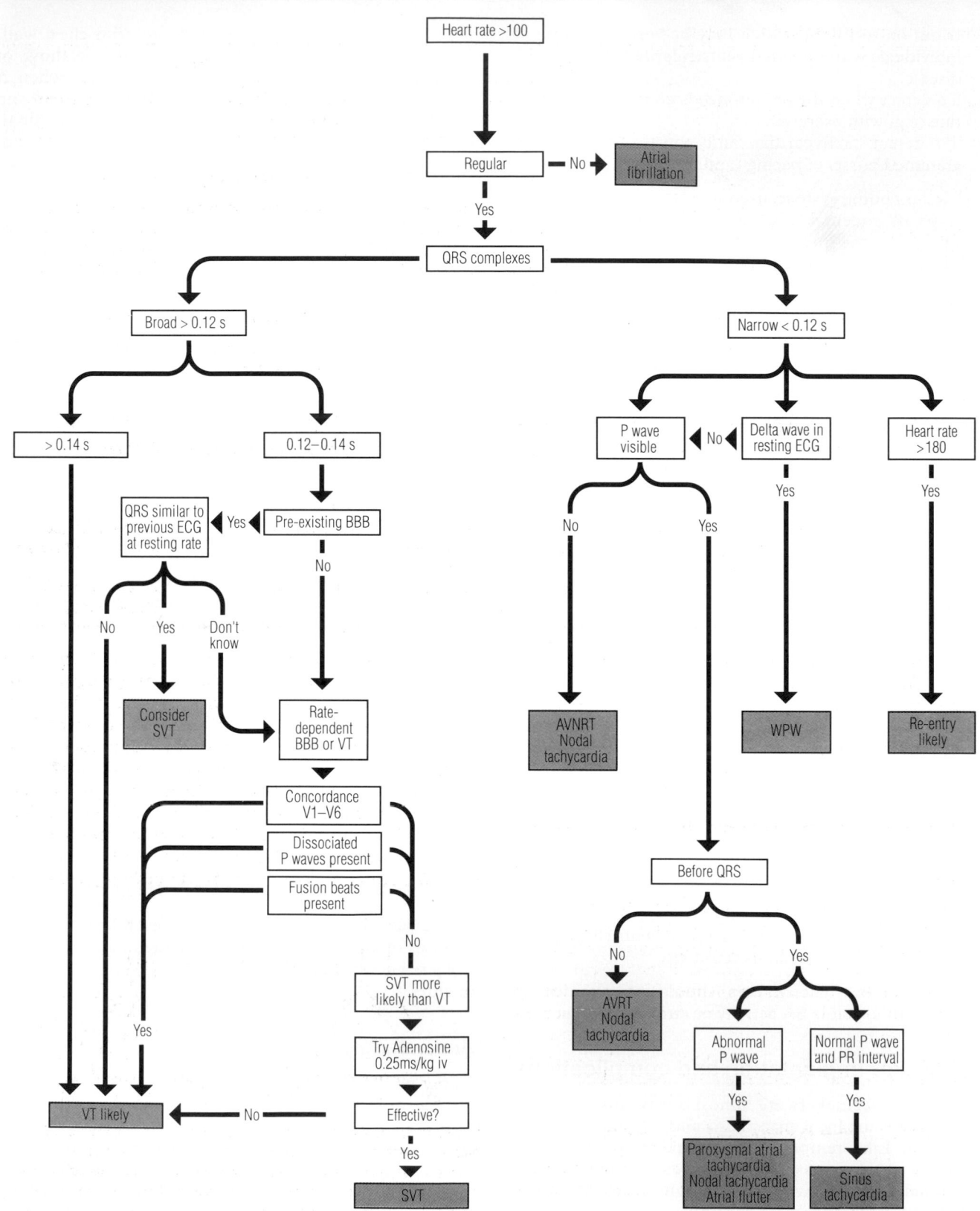

Fig. 12.30 Decision tree for diagnosis of tachycardia.

Table 12.5 Features and classification of tachycardias

Type	Rate (bpm)	ECG		Clinical	
		P-waves	QRS complex	Response to carotid sinus pressure	Symptoms and signs
Supraventricular					
Sinus	>100	Normal	Normal	Transient minor slowing	Palpitation
Atrial Paroxysmal atrial tachycardia	120–250	Abnormal shape	Regular and normal aberrant conduction produces broad QRS of RBBB or, less commonly, LBBB type. Broad QRS also if BBB already present	May terminate tachycardia	Palpitation, dizziness, breathlessness, chest pain may occur. Diuresis on cessation
Atrial fibrillation	>140	Absent	Irregular	Transient slowing	As above
Atrial flutter	150	Flutter waves; saw-tooth pattern in lead V1	Very regular QRS complexes	Conduction may decrease from usual 2:1 to 4:1 or less	As above
Junctional AVNRT	180–240	None seen (buried in QRS)	Normal and regular	None, or abrupt cessation	As above
AVRT	180–240	Inverted P waves after QRS; QP interval ≤ PR	Normal and regular	None, or abrupt cessation	As above
Ventricular					
Ventricular tachycardia	150–250	Dissociated P waves diagnostic, but can be difficult to see	Regular broad QRS >120 ms sometimes ≥ 140 ms. QRS look similar in V-leads 'concordance'	No response	May cause collapse; sometimes well tolerated
Ventricular fibrillation Ventricular flutter	150–300	None seen	Loss of regular discernible QRS features	Inappropriate	Collapse with rapid loss of consciousness

also influence heart rate and rhythm via these mechanisms. Therapeutic doses of some antiarrhythmics achieve their beneficial effects by decreasing the rate of depolarisation (Table 12.8). Toxic doses may cause atrial and ventricular tachyarrhythmia by increasing the diastolic depolarisation slope and lowering Vm.

Early after-depolarisations and triggered activity

Following an action potential, there may be a further spontaneous depolarisation which can occur early during repolarisation or late. Single 'after-depolarisations' can precipitate further spontaneous beats, to produce a rapid cycle of spontaneous activity. Factors which encourage their occurrence include hypoxia, hypercapnia, high circulating catecholamines, non-specific muscle injury and stretch. There is evidence that this activity occurs frequently and is important in producing tachycardia, particularly in the long QT syndrome (p. 365) and with drugs of the Vaughan-Williams classes IA and III.

Abnormal impulse conduction and re-entry

A wave of depolarisation may sometimes circle endlessly around a loop of cardiac tissue. The mechanism of re-entry are shown in Figure 12.31.

The loops of myocardial tissue may be found as a combination of alterations in anatomy (congenital or acquired), and abnormal function of parts of the heart. The best-known is that due to the presence of anomalous pathways connecting the atria with ventricular myocardium. This is the basis of the *pre-excitation syndromes*, so-called due to the tendency of the aberrant pathways to excite areas of adjacent ventricle and produce the *delta* wave on the ECG (Fig. 12.32); the clinical syndrome that results is the Wolff-Parkinson-White (WPW) syndrome (p. 365). Slow conduction in the anomalous pathways is

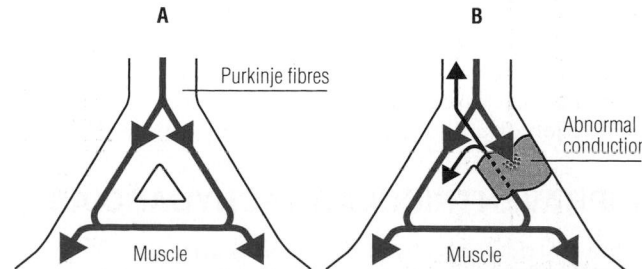

Fig. 12.31 Mechanism of re-entry tachycardias. A. Normal conduction. **B.** An area of abnormal conduction affects one limb of the circuit. This interrupts the antegrade conduction (large red arrow) but is able to conduct retrogradely some moments later (black dashed line). This combination allows re-entry of the impulse (black arrow) and a tachycardia ensues.

Table 12.6 Guide to use of antiarrhythmic drugs

Vaughan-Williams classification	Electrophysiological action		Indications	Toxic effects
	On action potential	On ECG		
Class I: Membrane stabilising drugs				
IA Quinidine			Toxicity now limits use. Effective in VT, and may convert AF or A flutter to sinus rhythm	GI disturbance Pro-arrhythmogenic Interacts with digoxin and numerous other drugs
Procainamide	Increase threshold for activation Slow rate of rise of action potential ? (Inhibit fast sodium channel)	QRS and QT prolongation, especially quinidine	Not used long-term, due to side-effects. Acute i.v. for ventricular and supra-ventricular arrhythmia	Lupus syndrome Other autoimmune disorders
Disopyramide			Ventricular and supra-ventricular arrhythmia Prophylaxis in paroxysmal AF	Negative inotropy Anticholinergic side-effects
IB Lignocaine Mexiletine Phenytoin	Inhibit fast sodium channel Shorten action potential	Usually none	Ventricular arrhythmia during and after myocardial infarction Phenytoin useful for digoxin toxicity arrhythmia	CNS side-effects
IC Flecainide Propanfenone	Inhibit fast sodium channel Inhibit His-Purkinje network with QRS widening	QRS duration prolongation and QT lengthening	Mainly ventricular arrhythmia	Major pro-arrhythmic potential with flecainide
Class II: Beta-adrenoreceptor blockers				
e.g. Propanolol Atenolol	Slow diastolic depolarisation	Bradycardia	SVT Exercise-induced VT Rate control of AF, as adjunct to digoxin	Hypotension, wheeze Negative inotropy Claudication worsens
Class III:				
Amiodarone	Prolong action potential	QT prolongation	Extremely wide-spectrum against SVT, VT and VF For life-threatening arrhythmia	Pneumonitis, pro-arrhythm, interference with thyroid function, photosensivity
Bretylium tosylate	Prolong action potential	QT prolongation	i.v. for resistant VF	Profound hypotension
Sotalol	Additional beta-blocking effects	QT prolongation	SVT and VT	Beta blocker side-effects
Class IV: Calcium antagonists				
e.g. Verapamil Diltiazem	Inhibit slow calcium channel	None	SVT, except acute AF	Hypotension Profound AV nodal block
Unclassified				
Digoxin	Inhibits Na/K ATPase	None	Control of AF, rate	Digoxin toxicity Pro-arrhythmic
Adenosine	AV nodal block	None	SVT. Differentiation of SVT and VT	Transient block; angor animi

the basis for the arrhythmia in WPW, while, in ischaemia, segments of diseased ventricular muscle with slow conduction or unidirectional block is the cause.

SUPRAVENTRICULAR TACHYCARDIAS

Supraventricular tachycardias (SVT) arise in the atria or AV node. They are characteristically associated with *narrow* QRS complexes, but there are important exceptions:

- when there is pre-existing bundle branch block – a situation impossible to diagnose with certainty unless

there are ECGs available in normal sinus rhythm – before or after the arrhythmia
- when there is rate-dependent bundle branch block
- in the pre-excitation syndromes (although the delta waves often do not show during tachycardia, as the anterograde conduction may be normal).

Clinical features

Common symptoms of SVT are an unpleasant awareness of rapid heart beats or palpitations in the chest. Associated cardiac disease may dominate the picture

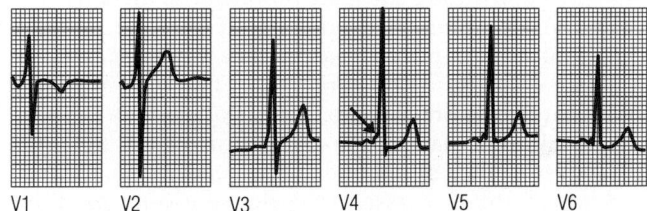

V1   V2   V3   V4   V5   V6

Fig. 12.32 ECG characteristics of the Wolff-Parkinson-White syndrome. Note the short PR interval and pre-excitation of the ventricle producing the slurred upstroke of the R wave (delta wave, arrowed in V4).

causing the arrhythmias to lower cardiac output, producing complaints of breathlessness, dizziness, fatigue or chest pain. The tachycardia may precipitate acute LV failure. Patients who suffer paroxysmal SVT, particularly those with structurally normal hearts, may notice polyuria during, or after, the attack.

Diagnosis

Differentiating between the many forms of SVT may, occasionally, be difficult. The ECG is the basic diagnostic tool, although aspects of the history and, occasionally, physical examination can give clues to the diagnosis. Very fast heart rates may produce ST and T wave changes on the ECG which persist for some hours after cessation of the arrhythmia.

Sinus tachycardia

Sinus tachycardia is a persistent sinus rate over 100 bpm. It is regarded as pathological when inappropriate and chronic, e.g. with diseases such as thyrotoxicosis, or when secondary to heart failure. Under these circumstances, treatment consists of control of the underlying disorder. A number of diseases of sinus node function produce a chronic sinus tachycardia, such as the dysautonomia of diabetes, cardiac infiltration with amyloid and extrapyramidal disease of the Shy-Drager syndrome.

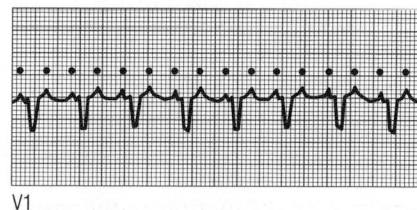

V1

Fig. 12.33 ECG showing atrial tachycardia with 2:1 conduction. Dots indicate position of P waves. (Atrial rate is 300/min.)

Atrial tachycardia

In atrial tachycardia (Fig. 12.33), the ECG shows abnormal P waves at rates from 120 to 250 bpm. The mechanism of the arrhythmia is usually enhanced, or abnormal, automaticity in the SA node or other site in the atria. Causes include ischaemic heart disease, cardiomyopathy, rheumatic heart disease and the sick sinus syndrome. The normal AV node may not conduct at rates much greater than 200 bpm, so that very fast atrial rates may be associated with intermittent failure of contraction. This may lead to an atrial tachycardia with 2:1 conduction or higher degrees of block. Conduction through the AV node may be further impaired by disease or drugs such as digoxin. Indeed, one of the manifestations of digoxin toxicity is atrial tachycardia (at a relatively slow rate) with block.

Management

Withdrawal of digoxin is important if toxicity is suspected. Otherwise, measures to control ventricular rate include intravenous verapamil (slow bolus of 5 mg repeated to a maximum of 10–20 mg in 20 min), when there has been no prior beta-blocker therapy, and intravenous digoxin when glycoside toxicity is not the cause. Patients who have received beta-blocker therapy should be given verapamil with great caution, for fear of precipitating severe bradycardia or high-grade AV block. Intravenous beta blockade may also terminate the tachycardia, as will DC cardioversion or atrial overdrive pacing.

Atrial fibrillation

Atrial fibrillation (AF) is probably the most common arrhythmia, and may be permanent in many patients. It is characterised by a chaotic, rapid and low-amplitude waveform on the ECG (Fig. 12.34). The ventricular response is characteristically completely irregular in rhythm, and usually shows a narrow QRS complex unless there is pre-existing disease or rate-dependent bundle branch block. Despite an atrial activity of 350–600 impulses/min, the AV node conducts only intermittently and randomly. The nodal rate is usually less than 200 impulses/min, or even less in the presence of AV nodal disease or drugs suppressing nodal activity (e.g. digoxin). An exception to the rule of irregular ventricular activity in AF is when it co-exists with complete heart block, when a subnodal pacemaker provides a slow, regular ventricular complex (Fig. 12.29).

The rhythm is believed to be caused by localised re-entry circuits within the atria, and is a frequent consequence of chronic atrial distension from any cause. The

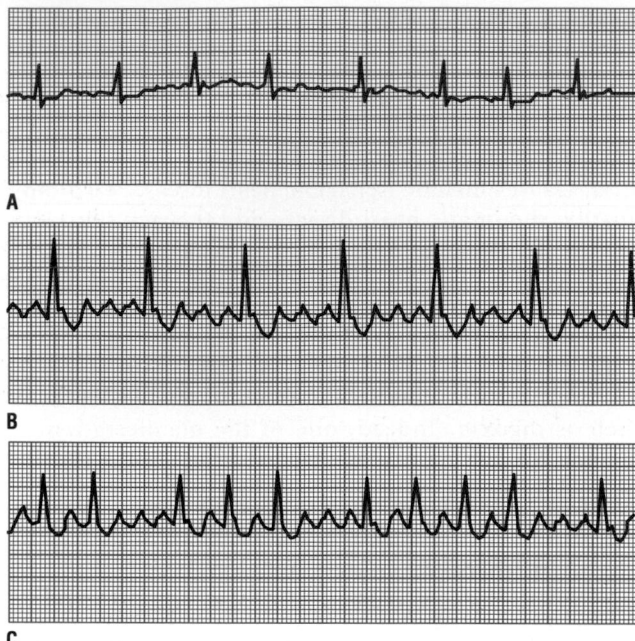

Fig. 12.34 Rhythm strips showing atrial fibrillation and flutter. A. Atrial fibrillation. Note the irregular ventricular rate. **B.** Atrial flutter with typical saw-tooth P waves and a regular ventricular response (4:1). **C.** Atrial flutter with a variable ventricular response.

causes of AF are shown in Table 12.7. The most common underlying condition is probably hypertension. Some patients develop the rhythm for no discernible reason and are said to be suffering *lone atrial fibrillation*; they appear to have a normal prognosis. For other patients, the immediate consequence of the arrhythmia and its long-term prognosis are determined by the underlying condition.

AF may be paroxysmal or permanent. Even when structural heart disease is absent, paroxysms of AF can sometimes be symptomatically disabling and, although drug therapy to control the ventricular rate during an

Table 12.7 Causes of atrial fibrillation

With structural heart disease	Without structural heart disease
● Rheumatic mitral valve disease	● Alcohol
● Hypertension	● Thyrotoxicosis
● Cardiomyopathy 　　Dilated 　　Hypertrophic	● Acute pericarditis
	● Constrictive pericarditis
● Atrial septal defect	● Pulmonary embolism
● Ischaemic heart disease	● Sick sinus syndrome
	● Myocarditis
	● Ischaemic heart disease

attack is reasonably effective, there may be considerable difficulty in providing adequate prophylactic therapy.

The loss of a mechanical atrial systole can be very important in patients with severe heart disease, and, in some, is sufficient to precipitate heart failure. The loss of atrial contraction predisposes to stasis of blood in the atria and atrial appendages. Thrombi form which pose the threat of systemic embolisation. This tendency is accentuated where there is associated rheumatic mitral valve disease, especially mitral stenosis. Stroke due to embolism is nearly five times commoner in patients with AF than in those in sinus rhythm, and this relative risk rises to seventeen-fold if there is associated mitral valve disease.

Clinical features

Clinically, the symptoms are determined by the rate of the arrhythmia and the underlying cardiac state, but they do not differ significantly from those of any SVT. The pulse is of variable rhythm and volume. Very early beats, especially with fast AF, may not produce sufficient stroke volume to produce a pulse at the wrist, producing an apex to radial pulse deficit in 'uncontrolled' AF. The venous pulse shows only a single waveform, corresponding to ventricular systole (the *v* wave).

Management

The aim of treatment is control of the ventricular rate; ideally, this is achieved by re-establishing sinus rhythm. Many patients are, however, likely to remain in AF permanently, and the goal is then to control the ventricular rate both at rest and during exercise. In individuals with paroxysmal AF, prevention of recurrences is attempted.

Acute

Ventricular rate control is achieved by digoxin. When fast AF is causing symptoms or cardiac decompensation, oral digoxin is the drug of choice. Loading is achieved by stat doses of 0.15 mg to a total of 0.75–1.0 mg in 24 hours. Other drugs which may be used acutely include verapamil (5–10 mg i.v., bolus or slow infusion) and amiodarone (up to 5 mg/kg over 20–30 min, diluted and infused through a central venous catheter). Where fast AF has caused severe haemodynamic disturbance, DC cardioversion can be used successfully. There is an increased risk of inducing malignant ventricular arrhythmia when there is digitalis intoxication, but this risk is small in patients without digoxin toxicity who have normal serum potassium.

The commonest maintenance dose is digoxin 0.25 mg by mouth daily. Renal function is the most important determinant of digoxin dosage, which also has to be reduced in the elderly, even if a normal plasma creatinine is present. Verapamil by mouth (80–120 mg) can achieve rapid rate response (within 2 hours), but it has negative inotropic effects.

Chronic

Chronic treatment of AF aims to reduce the resting rate to about 90 bpm, with a modest increase in rate with exertion. Digoxin alone, although effectively controlling the resting heart rate, is insufficient to control the rate response to exercise in a large proportion of patients. A combination of digoxin with verapamil (or digoxin with a beta-blocker) is superior to digoxin alone in these circumstances.

Anticoagulation with warfarin reduces the risk of emboli and is essential when rheumatic valve disease is present, or if the heart, particularly the left atrium, is enlarged. It is probably indicated in patients with a previous history of systemic emboli, and where the cause is thyrotoxicosis. If AF has been present for more than 1 week, anticoagulation for at least 3 weeks should precede attempts to restore sinus rhythm.

Paroxysmal AF can be disabling. Digoxin is less effective at preventing attacks, but disopyramide, quinidine and amiodarone used alone, or in combination with digoxin, have some effectiveness against relapses in paroxysmal AF. The symptoms may be helped by verapamil, which lowers the peak heart rate during a paroxysm of AF. Ablation of the AV node and pacemaker implantation have been used with some success.

Atrial flutter

Atrial flutter is an arrhythmia due to multiple re-entry circuits producing atrial contraction at 300 ± 50 bpm. Conduction block at the AV node (most commonly 2:1) is almost always present, producing a regular pulse of 150 bpm. This pulse rate should always lead to the clinical suspicion of atrial flutter. Vagal slowing of AV conduction produced by carotid sinus massage will temporarily increase the degree of AV block, and the sudden halving or more of the ventricular rate can easily be detected at the bedside. On the ECG monitor, P waves previously concealed within T waves become visible as a saw-tooth pattern, thus establishing the diagnosis (Fig. 12.34). Physical examination may show flutter waves in the neck. The causes of atrial flutter are the same as those of AF (Table 12.7), but flutter is rarely permanent. Drugs are less effective in flutter compared with fibrillation and DC cardioversion is the therapy of choice. Energies of 25–50 J are frequently sufficient to achieve successful cardioversion to sinus rhythm. Intravenous verapamil will successfully convert many patients to sinus rhythm, as will pacing the atria at, or below, the tachycardia rate (underdrive pacing) or rapidly for a few minutes (overdrive pacing).

Chaotic atrial tachycardia and wandering atrial pacemaker

Chaotic atrial tachycardia is characterised by multiple P wave shapes and PR intervals. It is quite common in elderly patients, while in younger patients it is usually associated with severe respiratory disorders. It requires no specific intervention, except for control of any associated illness and withdrawal of digoxin if this has previously been prescribed. Conversely, a sustained rhythm may be slowed by digoxin or verapamil.

The wandering atrial pacemaker is a slower arrhythmia often associated with variations in vagal tone, allowing various subsidiary atrial pacemakers to become established. It requires no special treatment.

JUNCTIONAL TACHYCARDIAS

Atrioventricular nodal re-entry or paroxysmal supraventricular tachycardia

The mechanism involved in AV nodal re-entry tachycardia (AVNRT) is re-entry through a functionally distinct area of the AV node or tissues surrounding it. This is a common arrhythmia, particularly in (young) patients with structurally normal hearts. There is a 1:1 relationship between atrial and ventricular activity. P waves generally cannot be identified; if they can be seen, they will be buried within the QRS or immediately follow it (Fig. 12.35). The onset is abrupt, usually precipitated by an atrial extrasystole, and an equally abrupt cessation is the rule, although the latter may not be appreciated by the patient since a sinus tachycardia may follow the arrhythmia. The usual rates are about 180–240 bpm, with narrow QRS complexes, except if there is pre-existing, or rate-dependent, bundle branch

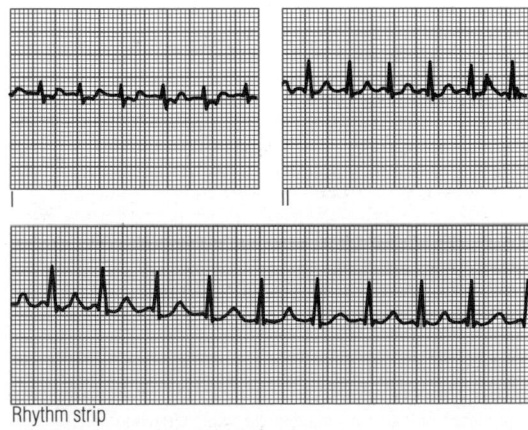

Rhythm strip

Fig. 12.35 AV nodal re-entry tachycardia. Note rapid narrow QRS complex tachycardia (rate 185 bpm).

block. If manoeuvres or drugs induce a lower degree of conduction than 1:1, AVNRT is excluded and a paroxysmal atrial tachycardia or flutter is the more likely diagnosis.

Management

Treatment may not be necessary if the attacks are transient and infrequent. Several vagotonic manoeuvres may be helpful (Table 12.8), all of which can be taught to the patient who suffers paroxysmal attacks. Failing these simple approaches, drug therapy is usually successful. Intravenous adenosine is the drug of choice, although intravenous injections of verapamil beta-blocker, disopyramide and amiodarone may also prove useful. Atrial and ventricular pacing may also be used, the former following a similar procedure to that used to convert atrial flutter. A more elegant approach is to interrupt the re-entry circuit with critically timed ventricular or atrial ectopic impulses using chronically implanted antitachycardia pacemakers.

Long-term prevention can often be achieved with beta-blockers, disopyramide, digoxin or amiodarone. Failing this, antitachycardia pacemakers have been used for disabling symptoms. Finally, disruption by transcatheter ablation of accessory pathways or the AV node can be undertaken. These latter techniques need a prior definitive intracardiac electrophysiological study (p. 351) but with the advent of radio-frequency catheter ablation, may rise to become the treatment of choice in significantly symptomatic patients.

Atrioventricular re-entry tachycardia

The hallmark of atrioventricular re-entry tachycardia (AVRT) – a less common rhythm than AVNRT – is the occurrence of retrograde P waves immediately after the QRS complex.

Non-paroxysmal AV nodal or junctional tachycardia

Non-paroxysmal AV nodal tachycardia is a narrow complex tachycardia associated with inverted P waves in

Table 12.8 Simple procedures to terminate paroxysmal SVT

- Carotid sinus massage. If effective, the rhythm is abruptly stopped; occasionally only moderate slowing occurs
- Cold water splash on face (to mimic the diving reflex). This may be effective, but is often difficult to administer
- Performance of Valsalva's manoeuvre (often effective)
- Swallowing cold drinks

II, III and aVF. Characteristically, it is caused by ischaemia and digoxin toxicity, although junctional rhythms may be precipitated by most forms of heart disease; the mechanism is enhanced automaticity. Since the atria and ventricles are stimulated virtually simultaneously, the P waves may precede the QRS complexes with a short PR interval. Alternatively, they may be buried within the QRS complex or follow after it. The onset of the tachycardia is gradual and the established rates, between 60 and 130 bpm, considerably slower than the paroxysmal forms of tachycardia. Therapy is along the same lines as for AVRT, although lignocaine may also be useful. Withdrawal of digoxin may be all that is required when toxicity is implicated.

BROAD-COMPLEX TACHYCARDIAS

The hallmark of ventricular rhythm is the broad QRS complex. Ventricular fibrillation and flutter do not cause diagnostic difficulties, but ventricular tachycardia (VT) is often wrongly diagnosed as SVT with rate-related aberration, or with pre-existing bundle branch block. There is often a reluctance to diagnose VT, particularly on the part of less experienced physicians, probably because the implications for the patient are so much worse for VT than for SVT. Guidelines for their differentiation are given in Table 12.9. In the context of acute infarction, or when there is severe underlying myocardial disease, the observation of a broad-complex tachycardia should always be assumed to be ventricular in origin until proved otherwise.

Ventricular tachycardia

VT (Fig. 12.36) is defined as the appearance of three or more ventricular ectopic beats in a sequence. When sustained, the rate is between 150 and 250 bpm and regular. Unsustained VT can be seen in people with normal hearts, but organic heart disease is suspected if the rhythm is sustained or produces symptoms. Causes are ischaemic heart disease, cardiomyopathy or myocarditis. VT carries the risk of sudden death, usually due to degeneration of the rhythm to ventricular fibrillation (VF). *VT can → VF & death.*

Even with the guidelines to diagnosis given in Table 12.9, VT can, in some circumstances, be difficult to diagnose, and prolonged examination of the ECG or the use of an oesophageal ECG lead may be necessary. In about one-half of patients, the sinus node continues to fire independently, so that atrial P waves dissociated from ventricular activity can sometimes be observed, if not buried within the QRS complex. In a few patients, retrograde activation of the atria occurs; this may be recognised by finding inverted P waves.

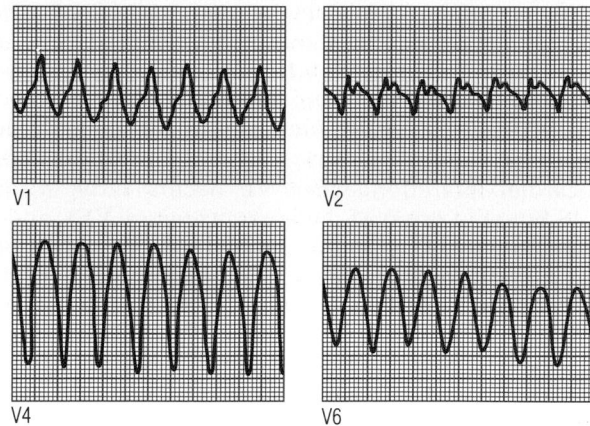

Fig. 12.36 Ventricular tachycardia (Monomorphic). A rapid, broad QRS complex tachycardia illustrating the similarity of appearance in complexes from V1 to V6 (concordance).

In paroxysmal VT (150–250 bpm) the onset is abrupt, usually following a critically timed ectopic beat. A slower form of VT, *accelerated idioventricular rhythm* (rate 60–130 bpm), occurs as an enhanced automatic rhythm during periods of suppressed sino-atrial activity. It is usually seen in acute infarction and its prognosis – unlike that of paroxysmal VT – is generally good.

Management

Acute

[handwritten: DC cardioversion i IV lignocaine.]

In the presence of acute haemodynamic disturbance or acute myocardial infarction, immediate DC cardioversion with a synchronised shock is the treatment of

Table 12.9 Differentiation of VT from SVT with aberration or bundle branch block (BBB)

Feature	Value in differentiation
Broad QRS complex (> 120 ms)	Very broad (> 160 ms) – almost always VT Broader than 140 ms favours VT, but may be due to pre-existing BBB
Bizarre QRS morphology, similar in V1–V6 and not resembling any BBB pattern	Characteristic of VT when present
Independent P wave activity	Diagnostic of VT, when found
QRS between sinus and tachycardia morphology in VT, fusion beat	Diagnostic of VT, when found
Variability of rate from 10 ms to 20 ms; except for fusion/capture beats	Not good
Hypotension, shock and collapse	No value
When V–A conduction occurs with 2:1 block	When ventricular rate is shown to be greater than atrial, the rhythm is VT

Summary 3 Treatment of tachycardia where doubt persists as to SVT or VT

- DC cardioversion if haemodynamics are compromised.
- Oesophageal ECG electrode or ECHO/Doppler may help by detecting dissociated atrial activity – if time allows.
- Do not use verapamil.
- Try i.v. adenosine (0.05–0.25 mg/kg) – it will terminate an SVT but will not affect VT or haemodynamics.
- Try i.v. lignocaine (1 mg/kg bolus) – it may terminate VT.

choice; this is followed by an intravenous lignocaine bolus dose of 100 mg (or 1 mg/kg), followed by an infusion, starting at 4 mg/min for 30 min, reducing to 2 mg/min for 2 hours and continued at 1 mg/min thereafter, for approximately 24 hours. This approach is generally successful, particularly in acute infarction, when there is rarely any indication to continue to chronic oral antiarrhythmic therapy. In resistant or recurrent cases, an alternative therapy is amiodarone. Mexilitene, flecainide or bretylium may be required in certain instances, although the acute use of many different antiarrhythmic drugs should be avoided. The serum potassium must be maintained at, or above, 4.5 mmol, and acidosis and hypoxaemia reversed.

Chronic

Episodic or paroxysmal VT complicating organic heart disease (e.g. hypertrophic cardiomyopathy, chronic ischaemic heart disease and cardiomyopathy), requires prophylactic therapy. In choosing the drug, information on its efficacy in the individual patient should be taken into account. The response to exercise testing and monitoring the effectiveness of therapy with Holter 24-hour ECG recordings is helpful. In those patients in whom VT is inducible by exercise, beta-blocking drugs may be useful; sotalol, with its class III effects (Table 12.6), may be the rational first choice. Patients with poor ventricular function are probably most at risk from VT. The choice of drug for these patients is very limited, due to the negative inotropy of most antiarrhythmic agents. Amiodarone or mexilitene are the most useful in these patients.

A new form of therapy for those patients in whom drug therapy fails is the use of small implantable automatic defibrillators which detect the arrhythmia (VT or VF) and, after an appropriate pause, deliver a DC shock.

Surgery and catheter ablation

Certain patients have an anatomical basis for their ventricular arrhythmia, either a ventricular aneurysm or localised area of ischaemically injured myocardium.

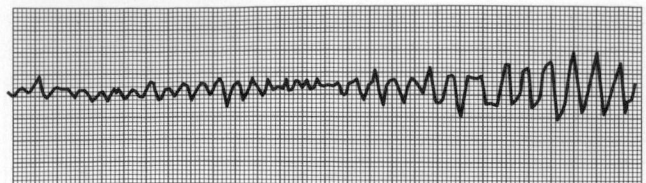

Fig. 12.37 Rhythm strip showing ventricular fibrillation.

Treatment options now include excision of the aneurysm or electrically abnormal tissue by surgery or ablation using catheters capable of delivering radio-frequency ultrasound.

Torsade de pointes ventricular tachycardia

Torsade de pointes VT is an uncommon but important arrhythmia, characterised by a VT, often of modest rate but associated with an undulating QRS height due to a slow but continual variation in the QRS axis (Fig. 12.37). Its importance is due to its precipitation by antiarrhythmic drugs, particularly if electrolyte disturbances coexist.

Management

Acquired forms are treated by withdrawal of the offending agent and correction of electrolyte abnormalities. In less stable situations, infusion of isoprenaline, or increasing the heart rate with a temporary pacemaker, are the appropriate remedies. Congenital syndromes can be caused by abnormalities in sympathetic supply to the heart. These are best treated with beta-blocking agents.

Ventricular fibrillation and ventricular flutter

VF is characterised by rapid, irregular and uncoordinated electrical activity in the ventricles, probably due to re-entry circuits within localised areas of myocardium. The ECG shows more or less coarse, irregular waveforms, without discernible P, QRS or T waves (Fig. 12.38). In ventricular flutter, the entire tracing appears as a rough saw-tooth with a rate of 160–250 bpm, without normal QRS morphology. If either rhythm occurs, effective contraction and cardiac output cease, leading to uncon-

sciousness within seconds. These rhythms do not usually revert spontaneously and are often precipitated by an ectopic beat or runs of VT, particularly when they complicate acute myocardial infarction. VF is probably the arrhythmia responsible for most cases of sudden death in the community (p. 405). In the context of acute myocardial infarction, when VF occurs early, within 24–48 hours of onset of the illness (*primary* VF), and is successfully treated, the prognosis for the patient is not adversely affected. However, VF occurring late in the course of acute infarction (*secondary* VF) often follows extensive muscle damage and carries a grave prognosis.

Management

Witnessed collapse due to VF (usually seen only in coronary care units) requires immediate action; a precordial chest thump (p. 367) may convert up to 15% of cases without the need for electrical defibrillation. In all other circumstances, basic cardiopulmonary resuscitation should begin until the treatment of choice is available, namely defibrillation by application of an external DC shock (p. 367). Correction of acidosis, hypoxaemia and electrolyte imbalance improves the likelihood of conversion to a stable rhythm. Drug treatment and long-term prophylactic therapy are the same as for VT. Primary VF does not generally require subsequent prophylactic therapy.

OTHER ARRHYTHMIC SYNDROMES

Sick sinus syndrome

The sick sinus syndrome (SSS) is a relatively common condition, characterised by episodic arrhythmias combining episodes of profound bradycardia and heart block with episodes of tachycardia (it is sometimes called the tachycardia-bradycardia syndrome). The bradycardias may be paroxysmal or sustained sinus bradycardia, episodes of sinus arrest, or SA block producing long pauses in pulse rate and pauses after atrial ectopics. Immediately following a tachycardia there may be a prolonged pause or very slow sinus rhythm sufficient to cause dizziness or a Stokes-Adams' attack. The tachycardias are mostly supraventricular, with AF, flutter, chaotic atrial rhythm and atrial tachycardia being the most

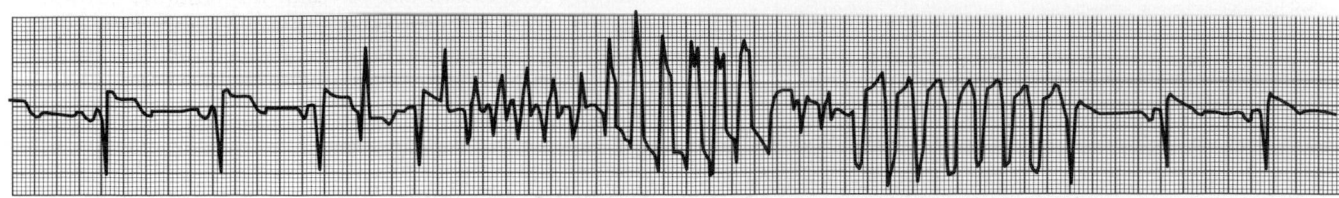

Fig. 12.38 Rhythm strip illustrating torsade de pointes, a broad-complex ventricular tachycardia. Note the fluctuation in size of the complexes.

common, although VT (especially torsades de pointes) is occasionally seen, as is chronic AF with a slow ventricular rate.

The pathology is probably degeneration and fibrosis in the sinus node and conducting tissues. The AV node is often involved in the degenerative process. Ischaemic heart disease and amyloid infiltration of the heart may be the cause in some patients and SSS has also been associated with many other pathologies, from cardiomyopathy to Friedreich's ataxia. Drugs such as digoxin, beta adrenoreceptor blockers or quinidine may mimic SSS.

Apart from discomfort and Stokes-Adams episodes, the condition carries a risk of systemic embolisation and is the cause of episodic heart failure.

Management and prognosis

Treatment is with antiarrhythmic drugs and pacemaker implantation. The prognosis is generally good but mainly dependent on any underlying condition; it is not greatly influenced by pacemaker implantation.

Wolff-Parkinson-White syndrome

The ECG abnormality of short PR interval (<0.12 s) with abnormal QRS widening due to delta-wave (Fig. 12.32) is relatively common. The clinical syndrome, Wolff-Parkinson-White syndrome (WPW), with paroxysmal tachycardias is much less common, although the precise incidence of arrhythmia in individuals with the ECG abnormality is not clearly established. The syndrome generally occurs in an otherwise normal heart, although it may complicate Ebstein's anomaly (p. 387) or mitral valve prolapse (p. 373). The abnormality is due to an accessory pathway between the atrium and ventricle allowing a re-entry or reciprocating tachycardia to develop (p. 357). The tachycardia produces narrow QRS complexes without the delta-wave, because conduction is anterograde through the AV node. Thus, the diagnosis of WPW may not be made until an ECG in sinus rhythm is obtained. There is an increased incidence of AF. In a small proportion of patients who have a short refractory period in the accessory pathway, AF may conduct very rapidly (1:1) to the ventricles; this may degenerate to VF and is the usual cause of sudden death in these patients.

Investigation and management

Electrophysiological studies establish the site, number and refractory period of the accessory pathway or pathways. Treatment may include antiarrhythmic drugs, but sometimes requires ablation of localised accessory bundles; catheter techniques are generally used, although surgical interruption of these tissues may sometimes be required. Digoxin and verapamil should be avoided, since they can increase accessory pathway conduction.

Lown-Ganong-Levine syndrome

Patients with Lown-Ganong-Levine syndrome (LGL) have short bypass tracts that connect the atria to various portions of the proxmal bundle of His or distal AV node. The ECG manifestation is of a short PR interval (<0.12 s) without pre-excitation (no delta-waves). Such patients are subject to paroxysmal tachycardias, but are less commonly threatened by rapidly conducted AF.

Long QT syndrome

Several congenital disorders (Romano-Ward and Jervell-Lange-Nielsen) are described characterised by a long (>0.45 s) QT interval and associated with VT, syncope and sudden death. Children respond to treatment with beta-blocking agents. The QT interval may also be prolonged by amiodarone and quinidine treatment.

Table 12.10 Emergency drug treatment of common arrhythmias

Arrhythmia	First line therapy	Second line therapy
Atrial fibrillation	Digoxin i.v., then oral DC cardioversion if blood pressure low	Verapamil DC cardioversion Beta-blockers
Atrial flutter	DC cardioversion (50–100 J)	Verapamil Vagotonic manoeuvres Atrial pacing
Atrial tachycardia and junctional tachycardia	Vagotonic manoeuvres Adenosine Verapamil	DC cardioversion Digoxin (if not digoxin toxicity)
SVT of AVNRT or AVRT type	Vagotonic manoeuvres Adenosine Verapamil	Beta-blocker Disopyramide Flecainide Amiodarone DC cardioversion
SVT in WPW with narrow QRS	Adenosine	DC cardioversion
SVT in WPW with broad (delta-wave) QRS	Amiodarone Flecainide Adenosine	DC cardioversion
VT and VF	DC cardioversion Lignocaine	Bretylium Amiodarone Flecainide Mexiletine
Bradycardia	Atropine Isoprenaline	–
Complete heart block	Pacemaker Isoprenaline	–

Table 12.11 Doses and methods of administration of drugs commonly used in acute arrhythmia

Drug	First dose	Method	Maintenance	Side-effects
Amiodarone	2–5 mg/kg	i.v. slow bolus	Usually required 600–1200 mg/day i.v. infusion	↓ BP Need central venous access
Atropine	0.6–1.2 mg	i.v. bolus	Not used	Anticholinergic side-effects
Beta-blockers				
Atenolol	5–10 mg	i.v. bolus	50–100 mg oral/day	↓ Heart rate; ↓ BP; bronchospasm
Metoprolol	5–15 mg	i.v. bolus	100–400 mg oral/day	
Propranolol	0.1 mg/kg	i.v. bolus	120–360 mg oral/day	
Bretylium	5–10 mg/kg	i.v. rapid in emergency	Optional 1–2 mg/min (i.v. infusion)	↓↓ BP; nausea
Digoxin	0.5 mg	i.v. slow bolus	Optional 0.75–1.0 mg for first 24 h, then 0.25 mg/day (oral)	Toxicity: lower dose in renal impairment and in elderly
Flecainide	1–2 mg/kg	i.v. bolus over 10 min	Optional 0.15–0.25 mg/kg/h (i.v. infusion)	↓ BP; cardiac failure
Isoprenaline	50 μg	i.v. rapid in emergency	Optional 0.02–0.18 μg/kg/min	↑↑ Heart rate
Lignocaine	100 mg	i.v. bolus	Essential 4 mg/min reducing to 2 mg/min for 24 h (i.v. infusion)	CNS toxicity
Verapamil	5 mg, repeat with 10 mg after 10 min	i.v. slow bolus	Optional 0.005 mg/kg/min for 1 h (i.v.) or 80–120 mg/8-hourly (oral)	↓ BP; ↓ Heart rate; AV block
Adenosine	0.05–0.25 mg/kg (3–18 mg)	i.v. bolus (fast)	Not usual	Transient ↓ BP; chest pain; angor animi

SYNOPSIS OF DRUG TREATMENT OF ARRHYTHMIAS

A decision tree for the diagnosis of tachycardias is shown in Figure 12.30. Summaries of the treatment of, and drug doses used in, arrhythmias are given in Tables 12.6, 12.10 and 12.11.

RESUSCITATION

Within 20 seconds of cardiac inactivity the victim falls unconscious, breathing soon ceases and the pupils dilate. Sudden death affects about 50 000 people a year in the UK. One-half of these are not previously known to have coronary artery disease.

About 60% of deaths due to myocardial infarction occur within an hour of the first symptom (Fig. 12.58), the majority occurring outside hospitals. The commonest rhythm disturbance (over 60% of cases) is VF.

Cardiopulmonary resuscitation (CPR) may involve:

- *basic life support*, requiring training but no special equipment
- *advanced life support*, which requires equipment and specialised skills.

Many cities in the UK and other industrialised countries are involved in training the public in basic life support skills, and provide specialised ambulances with very rapid response times and facilities for advanced life support and DC cardioversion. Examples are Belfast and Brighton in the UK, and Seattle in the USA. With basic life support available to the victims of cardiac arrest, about 20% of victims may reach hospital and 11% live to be discharged. These numbers are halved when basic life support is not available. Survival is worse in older patients, and when arrest occurs at home or in the street. In hospital, when cardiac arrest due to VF occurs within 4 hours of symptoms and is successfully treated, 80% of patients are alive 3 years later.

BASIC LIFE SUPPORT

The basic cardiac arrest procedures are given in Table 12.12. Initial assessment is rapidly followed by establishing a clear open airway. This is done by head tilt with chin lift and jaw thrust. In the absence of airway obstruction, rescue breathing begins with the mouth-to-mouth technique. Recommendations vary, but in the UK, four quick breaths are advocated. In the USA, two slow breaths (1–1.5 s each) have been suggested, in order to

Table 12.12 Basic cardiac arrest procedures

A	**Assessment**
	Patient unconscious or asleep? Call for help if unconscious.
	Is airway clear? Clear it, pull chin up.
B	**Breathing**
	If patient is breathing: turn to recovery position.
	If patient is not breathing, but is choking: Heimlich manoeuvre.
	If patient is not breathing, but is not choking: start mouth-to-mouth resuscitation. Call for assistance
C	**Circulation**
	If no pulse: start external cardiac massage
	call for assistance
	continue ventilation

diminish the likelihood of gastric distension with air, and subsequent vomiting (risking inhalation of vomit into the unprotected airway). Protective masks and airway equipment should be provided for personnel most often exposed (ambulance and paramedical staff), even though the risk of infection (such as from hepatitis B or HIV) is likely to be very small. Bag mask techniques are taught to nursing and medical staff, but are frequently more difficult to use and less effective in inexperienced hands than is mouth-to-mouth ventilation.

Closed cardiac compression follows at a rate of 60–80 compressions/min. Training in the technique is essential. Mid-sternal compression is carried out with the heel of one hand to depress the sternum by 2–4 cm. The patient should be on a rigid, flat surface with the resuscitator kneeling alongside. The arms are kept straight, and compression produced primarily by body weight movement. Closed chest compression achieves a cardiac output by virtue of cyclical changes in intrathoracic pressure, rather than by squeezing the heart.

A single-handed resuscitator should provide 15 chest compressions for every two mouth-to-mouth breaths. If two people are available, the ratio should be 5:1. CPR must be continuous, and pauses to reassess the situation or allow for advanced life support techniques should not be greater than 10 seconds.

The first response to a *witnessed* arrest should be a forceful precordial thump. This may be sufficient to convert VF or VT to a more stable rhythm by localised myocardial depolarisation, or even to initiate a rhythm in cases of acute asystole.

ADVANCED LIFE SUPPORT

Advanced life support (summarised in Fig. 12.39) consists of defibrillation with DC shock, endotracheal intubation, the use of drugs and pacemakers.

DC defibrillation

In VF, the earlier DC shock is given, the more successful the outcome. When defibrillators are immediately available, such as in coronary care units, the first procedure following the precordial thump should be defibrillation at 200 J. This will be sufficient to revert 85% of cases to a more stable rhythm. In 10% of patients, a further 200 J shock is required and is successful. If these approaches are unsuccessful, life support must be begun immediately. Outside coronary care units, basic life support must be begun and interrupted only when the defibrillator is ready to produce the first shock of 200 J. If no monitor is available, major pulses are checked and, if absent after 3 s, 15 chest compressions are given with the appropriate mouth-to-mouth breaths. A second shock follows the same pattern of events and, if VF persists, intravenous lignocaine (100 mg i.v. bolus) is given before the third shock at 400 J. Adrenaline may be given before the fourth shock at the highest energy and, if an acidosis is demonstrated by arterial gases, bicarbonate (1 mmol/kg) is given before the fifth high-energy shock (Fig. 12.39).

The technique of DC shock administration can be taught to nursing and paramedical personnel. Early defibrillation administered out of hospital by ambulance crews has been shown to improve survival from VF. Defibrillation paddles are placed on the chest with firm pressure, one under the right clavicle and one just lateral to the usual cardiac apex. Skin impedance is reduced with conducting gel or pads, and the administrator of the shock ensures that no-one is touching the patient before the shock is delivered. Complications are remarkably few,

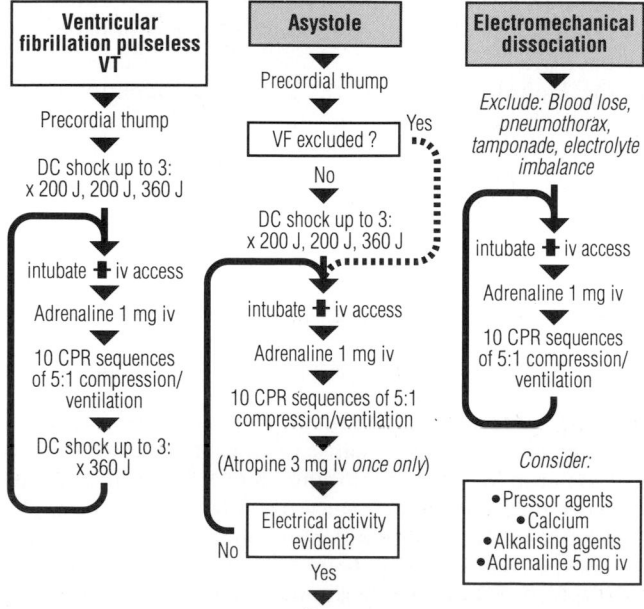

Fig. 12.39 Flow diagram of resuscitation procedures. (Based on recommendations of the UK Resuscitation Council.)

although very high-energy shocks or many repeated shocks carry the risk of some myocardial damage.

Endotracheal intubation

If there is no recovery after a few minutes of basic life support, endotracheal intubation is necessary. This is a skilled technique which can be mastered by medical and paramedical staff alike, but which requires frequent practice. After the cardiac arrest, it may be necessary to continue ventilation, via a mechanical ventilator, of seriously ill patients, those with damaged ribcage from cardiac massage and those who sustain cerebral damage.

Drugs in advanced life support

The number of drugs of proven benefit is small, despite the large number available to treat ventricular arrhythmia.

- *Adrenaline* is the inotropic and chronotropic agent of choice. It is given intravenously in a dose of 1 mg (1 ml of 1/1000) or 2 mg via the endotracheal tube.
- *Lignocaine* is routinely given after VF and during attempts to treat VF. A bolus of 1 mg/kg (or 100 mg) is followed by an infusion (4 mg/min reducing to 2 mg/min over 24 hours). A second half-dose bolus can be given 10–20 min after the first.
- *Sodium bicarbonate.* Bicarbonate infusion is only used in established acidosis, which is a relatively late event. An average dose is 1 mmol/kg of 4.2% sodium bicarbonate solution.
- *Calcium chloride* is useful in specific circumstances, such as resuscitation after cardiopulmonary bypass and in calcium antagonist overdose. The usual dose is 10 ml of 10% calcium chloride.
- *Other drugs.* The treatment of resistant VF or ventricular tachyarrhythmias may require the use of one or other of the alternative drugs available (p. 365). None, however, has a proven role as 'standard' therapy in CPR, and their indications have to be determined individually at the time of the resuscitation attempt.

Special techniques

Cardiac pacing

Cardiac pacing can be used to treat bradycardia, heart block and, sometimes, asystole. Asystole, unless it has been caused by drugs, rarely responds to cardiac pacing.

Intra-aortic balloon counterpulsation

Highly specialised techniques such as intra-aortic balloon counterpulsation have a very limited role in specialised centres, where they can be used to support the circulation until a definitive procedure can be performed.

Intracardiac injection

Intracardiac injection has been used to administer calcium or adrenaline during cardiac arrest with asystole. Central venous cannulation delivers drugs to the heart with much less hazard.

When to stop

Rigid rules cannot be given, but guidelines are possible. Resuscitation is almost never successful in patients who have a cardiac arrest complicating another serious illness, such as pneumonia or malignancy. It is important, therefore, that the staff likely to be first to witness a collapse should have had clear guidance concerning the desirability of resuscitation in individual patients.

In general, the outlook for a useful neurological recovery is poor if the arrest occurred out of hospital and was not witnessed, or if more than 4 min passed without even basic life support being attempted. If no spontaneous respiration or cardiac output is achieved after 30 min of adequate advanced life support, then further attempts at resuscitation are questionable. The state of the pupils, whether widely dilated and reacting or not, is unreliable with respect to outcome. Age should not be used as the sole determinant of policy on resuscitation.

RESUSCITATION FROM CHOKING

Collapse due to acute airway obstruction is often due to a lump of food. In the UK, it is still recommended that active coughing with gravity drainage be encouraged whilst the subject is still conscious. This is supplemented by back blows and, finally, the abdominal thrusts known as the Heimlich manoeuvre. The latter depends upon gripping the subject from behind and, with clenched fist, producing a rapid, powerful upward thrust in the upper abdomen. This produces rapid airflow which may be sufficient to dislodge the offending obstruction.

VALVULAR DISEASE OF THE HEART

AETIOLOGY AND NATURAL HISTORY

In Western countries, rheumatic heart disease was, until recently, the commonest cause of valve disease, and this is still the case in most developing countries. Various forms of degenerative valvular disease are now seen increasingly, some based on congenital abnormalities of the valve, others apparently arising de novo in middle-age or later.

For both rheumatic and congenital heart disease, it is often difficult to predict the progression of what initially may seem a trivial lesion of no consequence, to one that may be life-threatening 30 or more years later.

What dictates progression of the valve lesion? Mechanical forces must be involved; pressure and shear forces on the valve probably make it thicken and even calcify. The tolerance of the myocardium and the advent of myocardial disease add to the difficulty in prognosis.

THE EFFECTS OF STENOSIS AND REGURGITATION

Heart valve disease can occur either due to a narrowing of the valve (*stenosis*), causing obstruction to blood flow through the valve, or when the valve leaks, when the lesion is termed *regurgitant, incompetent* or *insufficient*. A *combined* or *mixed* lesion is common.

Valve stenosis

Mild degrees of stenosis may produce an audible murmur and also a risk of endocarditis, but place an insignificant physiological burden on the heart. For significant symptoms to result, stenosis has to progress until the valve is narrowed to less than 30% of its normal area. Flow through the valve is maintained at close to normal levels by a compensatory increase in pressure in the chamber of the heart upstream of the stenotic valve. This chamber therefore hypertrophies.

The severity of the stenosis is quantified by the pressure drop across the valve. In a normal valve, this pressure drop is not measurable by conventional techniques. However, in severe aortic stenosis, the left ventricular pressure may rise to as much as 200 mmHg more than the aortic pressure, and the valve area may be less than 25% of normal. In mitral stenosis, the left atrial pressure cannot rise above 40 mmHg because the pulmonary capillaries are unable to withstand a higher pressure. Thus, the mitral valve gradient is usually much less than the aortic valve gradient in significant stenosis, and the residual valve area accordingly greater.

It follows that there are three ways of assessing the severity of a valve stenosis:

- *The pressure gradient across the valve.* This indicates the additional work required to push blood through the valve. However, this is flow-dependent (no flow, no gradient); if there is heart failure, with low flow, the valve gradient is smaller.
- *The valve area.* Formerly, this could only be calculated from cardiac catheterisation data, but direct measurement is now possible from ultrasound. There is, however, controversy over the accuracy of the measurements, because of the beam spread and lateral resolution of the ultrasound.
- *The peak blood velocity across the valve.* Measured by Doppler ultrasound, this bears a very simple relationship to the pressure gradient (Fig. 12.13).

Valvular regurgitation

Normal human valves are highly efficient. The aortic valve closes as the flow decelerates, and is fully closed with about 97% efficiency. However, severe mitral or aortic valve regurgitation can be associated with up to 80% regurgitation (efficiency 20%). The forward flow then has to be five times greater than normal to allow for this leakage, and the chamber supplying the blood dilates accordingly. In aortic regurgitation, the left ventricle enlarges; in mitral regurgitation, the left atrium and left ventricle both enlarge greatly.

Acute regurgitation (such as mitral valve chordal rupture or aortic regurgitation from acute endocarditis), are badly tolerated, since the left ventricle and left atrium have not had time to increase in volume. The rapid increase in left ventricular diastolic pressure or left atrial pressure, has severe consequences for left ventricular perfusion and pulmonary capillary pressure.

Combined valve lesions

The combined effect of even mild stenosis with regurgitation is potentially catastrophic. Since the forward flow with as little as 50% regurgitation is twice normal, even a 50% stenosis becomes highly significant. This is shown in Table 12.13, where it can be seen that with a combined lesion, the regurgitation greatly potentiates the effect of the stenosis. This is particularly true of the mitral valve, where pressures need to rise much less before producing symptoms.

Table 12.13 Relationship between valve area, blood velocity and pressure gradient

Condition of valve	Area (cm^2)	Velocity (m/s)	Pressure gradient (mmHg)
Stenosis alone			
Normal	3	1	4
Mild stenosis	1.5	2	16
Severe stenosis	0.6	5	100
Stenosis and regurgitation			
Normal area, no regurgitation	3	1	4
Normal area, 50% regurgitation	3	2	16
Mild stenosis, 50% regurgitation	1.5	4	64
Mild stenosis, 66% regurgitation	1.5	6	144

The Bernoulli equation ($P = 4V^2$), relating blood flow velocity (V) to pressure gradient (P) across a valve, shows the effects of regurgitation on the pressure gradient if the forward stroke volume is maintained. The figures are chosen for simplicity. With 50% regurgitation, the forward stroke volume and (theoretically) the flow velocity doubles; with 66% regurgitation, they increase three-fold. In practice, the flow time also increases.

MITRAL STENOSIS

Aetiology

Mitral stenosis is almost always a consequence of rheumatic heart disease, and is the commonest valvular manifestation of the disease. A rare congenital form exists. The two valve cusps become adherent along their commissures, producing progressive stenosis with a 'fish mouth' orifice. Initially the cusps remain fairly pliable, but they become increasingly rigid with time and eventually calcify. The increasing degree of stenosis produces a rise in left atrial pressure and left atrial dilatation. The raised pulmonary venous pressure leads to left heart failure and can lead to progressive pulmonary hypertension.

Clinical features

Mitral stenosis, which is commoner in women, may remain asymptomatic for many years with little limitation of exercise tolerance. However, an additional load on the heart such as pregnancy, exertion, emotional stress or intercurrent chest infection (which is more common in patients with mitral valve disease because of the pulmonary vascular congestion) may produce the first symptoms of left heart failure. The onset of fast AF in middle-age is a common presentation, often leading to left heart failure, and thrombus formation with the risk of embolism. Right heart failure eventually develops as a consequence of pulmonary hypertension.

Symptoms

Of left heart failure

The symptoms of left heart failure (p. 343) are shortness of breath on exertion, orthopnoea, paroxysmal nocturnal dyspnoea, pulmonary oedema, and haemoptysis of fresh blood occurring from rupture of a congested bronchial or pulmonary vein (uncommon with other causes of left heart failure). Haemoptysis may be due to pulmonary infarction, which is more common in mitral valve disease.

Due to atrial fibrillation

The raised left atrial pressure may lead to AF, sometimes paroxysmal at first, but then stable. The loss of atrial filling and the shortened diastolic filling period can change an asymptomatic patient into one severely disabled by breathlessness, and may convert a quiescent stenosis into a life-threatening condition.

Systemic embolism. Thrombus can form in the enlarged left atrium and give rise to systemic emboli. A hemiplegia may occur and embolism to other sites is frequent. The patient in sinus rhythm is also at risk from embolism but

to a lesser extent. The greatest risk is in the patient who, having been in AF, reverts to sinus rhythm, as the return of coordinated atrial contraction can dislodge clot.

Due to a raised left atrial pressure

Massive enlargement of the left atrium can lead to hoarseness from pressure on the recurrent laryngeal nerve, dysphagia from oesophageal compression, and bronchiectasis from distortion of the left main bronchus. Longstanding raised left atrial pressure often leads to constriction of pulmonary arterioles and thickening of the capillary basement membranes. There is increased resistance to flow through the lungs and, thus, pulmonary hypertension.

Right ventricular hypertrophy compensates for the increased load on the right ventricle. When pulmonary hypertension is severe, right ventricular failure follows, usually, but not always, associated with left heart failure. The typical facial appearance of a patient with mitral valve disease – ruddy complexion, with red or vaguely cyanosed cheeks – is secondary to pulmonary hypertension (*mitral facies*).

Signs

The main signs of mitral stenosis are illustrated in Figure 12.40. Pure mitral stenosis in sinus rhythm without pulmonary hypertension is relatively uncommon. The signs are then purely auscultatory, as

Summary 4 Symptoms and signs of mitral stenosis	
Symptoms	
Of left heart failure	Shortness of breath, orthopnoea, paroxysmal nocturnal dyspnoea, haemoptysis
Of atrial fibrillation	Palpitations and syncope (at onset)
	May precipitate left heart failure
	Systemic embolism to CNS, limbs, gut and kidneys
Of pulmonary hypertension	Weight loss and cachexia
	Right heart failure
Signs	
Uncomplicated (auscultatory only)	Opening snap
	Mitral diastolic murmur
	Presystolic murmur
With atrial fibrillation	Irregular pulse
With pulmonary hypertension	Parasternal lift (RVH)
	Loud P2
	Tapping apex
If very severe	Mitral facies
	Cardiac cachexia

cardiac output is maintained and there is no significant right ventricular hypertrophy. The auscultatory signs are:

- *An opening snap*, best heard halfway between the apex and the left sternal edge. It occurs close to the aortic second sound in severe stenosis, but is more separated from it in mild stenosis.
- *A rumbling diastolic murmur*. This commences with the opening snap and fades rapidly in mild stenosis, but is full length and runs into the presystolic murmur in severe stenosis.
- *The presystolic murmur* coincides with atrial systolic flow through the valve. It is of the same character as the mid-diastolic murmur and is sometimes heard when the latter cannot be heard. It is absent in AF.
- *A loud first heart sound*. In the mobile stenotic valve, the cusps are still fully open as systole starts, so they close with a louder sound than normal. This is an unreliable sign.

Later signs are AF and pulmonary hypertension. These patients also have signs of a low cardiac output, mitral facies, small stroke volume with small volume pulse, a raised JVP, right ventricular hypertrophy, and a mid-diastolic murmur following the opening snap. When the cardiac output is very low the mitral murmur may be virtually inaudible, especially if the patient is in heart failure – so-called *silent mitral stenosis*.

Investigation

In sinus rhythm, the ECG may show P mitrale. Severe pulmonary hypertension may produce right ventricular hypertrophy or 'strain', but this aspect of the ECG is often unhelpful.

Chest X-ray. The chest X-ray may show enlargement of the left atrium (Fig. 12.40), redistribution of flow to the upper zones, left heart failure and enlargement of the right side of the heart if there is coincident pulmonary hypertension. A penetrated lateral X-ray will show a calcified valve in most patients over the age of 50.

Echocardiography. The echocardiogram shows thickening of the cusps (Fig. 12.40), which are fused together so that the posterior cusp moves anteriorly in diastole with the anterior cusp. The severity of the stenosis is assessed by the rate of ventricular filling, direct assessment of the valve area from 2D echo. The echo is extremely useful for examining the size of the left atrium and, thus, the risk of thrombus formation and embolism. Occasionally, clot can be demonstrated in the left atrium with 2D echo.

Doppler ultrasound demonstrates the blood velocity and, by calculation, can give a fair approximation of the pressure gradient across the valve non-invasively. It can also detect mitral regurgitation. Where there is doubt as to whether a patient's symptoms are from mitral valve disease or left ventricular disease and trivial mitral stenosis, cardiac catheterisation is still used to measure

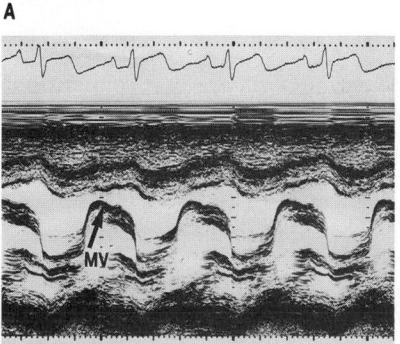

A

B

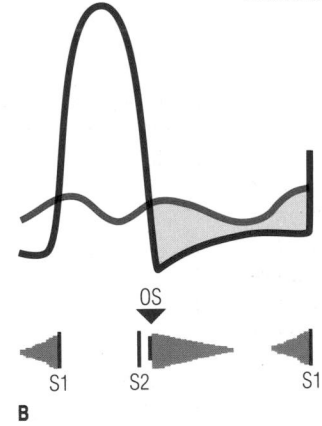

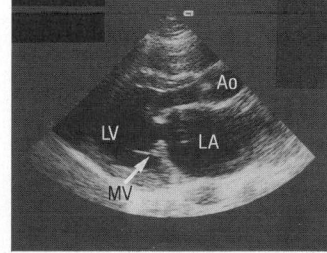

C

D

Fig. 12.40 Features of mitral stenosis. A. Chest X-ray showing cardiomegaly with gross left atrial enlargement. **B.** Diagrammatic illustration of the pressures in left atrium (red) and left ventricle (black), showing a diastolic pressure gradient (shaded pink). The timing of an opening snap (OS) and diastolic murmur is shown. S1 and S2 = first and second heart sounds. **C.** Typical M mode. The mitral valve (arrowed) movement is abnormal (compare with Fig. 12.17B). **D.** 2D echocardiographic appearance in mitral stenosis. Thickened mitral valve (MV), dilated left atrium (LA) and the LV cavity (LV) are shown.

the valve gradient and left ventricular function, and to examine the state of the coronary circulation.

Management

Management of mitral stenosis consists of three phases:

- *Monitoring* the asymptomatic patient with mild disease who does not require any treatment, with eventual decision on anticoagulation.
- *Medical* management of the symptomatic patient with a decision on surgery.
- *Surgical* management of the patient with more severe disease.

Medical

In the asymptomatic patient in sinus rhythm, no treatment is necessary, but the patient should be advised about prophylaxis against infective endocarditis (p. 418) and carefully assessed during pregnancy (p. 422). The onset of AF may lead to the development of symptoms. Even asymptomatic patients in sinus rhythm with moderate stenosis are at risk from thromboembolism from the left atrium, so the relative risks of anticoagulation have to be weighed against the benefits in each case. The indications for anticoagulation in mitral stenosis are listed in Table 12.14.

In the symptomatic patient, the aim of medical management should be to control the symptoms of left heart failure with diuretics. In AF, the ventricular rate should be controlled with digoxin, either alone or in combination with (or substituted by) a beta-blocker or verapamil (p. 360). The risk of thromboembolic episodes should be reduced by anticoagulation.

Surgical

Closed valvotomy and balloon valvotomy

Closed mitral valvotomy is an extremely effective operation. The valve cusps are separated where they are adherent along the commissures. The closed valvotomy does not require cardiac bypass and has been performed during the second trimester of pregnancy without much hazard to the fetus. A limited thoracotomy allows the

Table 12.14 Indications for anticoagulation in mitral stenosis

- Moderate or severe stenosis
- Enlarged left atrium
- Atrial fibrillation
- Sinus rhythm with recurrent palpitations
- Any symptoms suggestive of arterial embolism

atrium to be opened through the atrial appendage (which is usually amputated as it is the seat of clot formation), and a mechanical dilator is passed through a stab incision at the apex of the left ventricle to the mitral orifice, where it is opened and splits the valve. Increasingly a balloon introduced by cardiac catheter is used to split the valve. Hospital stay is only 2–3 days and results are comparable.

Open valvotomy

Open valvotomy through a midline sternal incision, with the patient on cardiac bypass, is necessary if there is doubt about the applicability of valvotomy. It allows direct inspection of the valve, and, should regurgitation result from splitting the valve, it can be replaced or even repaired. Valve replacement is essential if there is significant regurgitation or if the valve is heavily calcified.

Prognosis

Mitral valvotomy can dramatically improve the symptoms of the patient with mitral stenosis. With time, however, the valve tends to become more rigid and calcify, becoming restenotic even if there is no fusion of the commissures. Often, a degree of regurgitation develops and, occasionally, other heart valves affected by rheumatic heart disease start to cause problems.

MITRAL REGURGITATION

Aetiology

The percentage of valves coming to surgery which are rheumatic is now below 50% in many series. Regurgitation can result from:

- dilatation of the valve ring
- damage, retraction or perforation of the valve cusps
- damage to the subvalvular apparatus (chordae, papillary muscle, or the ventricular muscle to which the papillary muscles attach).

Non-rheumatic causes of mitral regulation are:

Heart failure

Dilatation of the left ventricle will produce 'functional mitral regurgitation' due to dilatation of the valve ring and a shift in the attachments of the chordae tendinae. This may disappear as the ventricle shrinks with treatment, but may become a permanent feature.

Myocardial infarction

Papillary muscle *dysfunction* can arise due to inferior myocardial infarction, producing a characteristic type of mitral regurgitation which is usually not severe. In contrast, infarction complicated by rupture of the papillary muscle produces catastrophic regurgitation and is usually fatal unless repaired urgently.

Degenerative changes

Degenerative changes are often seen in mitral valves at surgery. The pathogenesis is not fully understood, as degenerative changes can occur in rheumatic valves or others known to be mildly incompetent for a long period.

Rupture of the smaller chordae tendinae can occur slowly and progressively, causing increasing mitral regurgitation. Acute chordal rupture of a major trunk causes sudden severe mitral regurgitation.

Other causes

In *mitral valve prolapse* there is prolapse of a mitral valve cusp late in systole, often from a degree of 'redundancy' in the length of the chordae tendinae. It may be a feature of Marfan's syndrome and osteogenesis imperfecta. Elderly patients often develop a minor degree of mitral regurgitation from *calcification of the valve ring*. This produces a characteristic wheezy systolic murmur. *Endocarditis* may make even a trivial degree of regurgitation more severe, and acute endocarditis can rapidly destroy a normal valve. There is a degree of mitral regurgitation in most cases of *hypertrophic obstructive cardiomyopathy* (p. 411).

Congenital forms of mitral regurgitation include cleft cusps in AV canal defects and endocardial cushion defects in association with ostium primum atrial septal defects (p. 388).

Sharp (stabbing) and blunt (steering wheel injury) trauma to the precordium, acromegaly and Libman-Sacks endocarditis in systemic lupus erythematosus (SLE) are other rare causes.

Clinical features

Symptoms and pathophysiology

Chronic

The symptoms of chronic mitral regurgitation are essentially the same as those of mitral stenosis, but severe pulmonary hypertension is less common with pure mitral regurgitation. The slowly progressive regurgitation is accommodated by a gradual increase in size of the left ventricle, which ejects the blood into a slowly enlarging and compliant left atrium and pulmonary venous vasculature. Up to 80% of the left ventricular stroke volume may be regurgitant in severe cases, and the left ventricular stroke volume can exceed 250 ml. Symptoms in chronic mitral regurgitation usually develop when the left ventricle dilates sufficiently for there to be a significant rise in its filling pressure. Usually, systolic function and ejection fraction are well maintained, because the left ventricle is ejecting largely into a low impedance outflow. The symptoms of left heart failure, AF and pulmonary hypertension are the same as for mitral stenosis (p. 370).

Acute

In acute mitral regurgitation, e.g. due to rupture of chordae tendinae, a small left ventricle is regurgitating into a small uncompliant left atrium (high impedance), with a resultant very high pressure pulse or *v* wave in the left atrium which may reach 60 mmHg. Left atrial pressure rapidly exceeds that needed to produce pulmonary oedema. The low forward output may precipitate tachycardia, which makes the regurgitation worse. Acute mitral regurgitation thus usually presents with severe left heart failure or pulmonary oedema.

Signs

Uncomplicated pure mitral regurgitation, if trivial, has only auscultatory signs (Fig. 12.41). However, if the regurgitation is more severe, the left ventricular volume load becomes clinically evident by a hyperactive left ventricle with displacement of the cardiac apex down and laterally. Enlargement of the left atrium in systole may be felt as a parasternal heave. In severe regurgitation, the pulse may become small and rather jerky from a shortened ejection time. Severe regurgitation is evident on auscultation by the presence of a third heart sound and short mid-diastolic murmur, produced by the greatly enhanced forward flow through the mitral valve during diastole.

The pansystolic murmur of rheumatic mitral regurgitation, or other types of regurgitation with a central jet, is best heard at the apex of the heart and may be louder with the patient tipped to the left. Other types of mitral regurgitation – including the late systolic murmur of the floppy valve syndrome – may be best heard at the left sternal edge, and are often not pansystolic in character. Differential diagnosis from trivial aortic stenosis and ventricular septal defect can therefore be difficult, and requires non-invasive tests such as echocardiography and Doppler ultrasound or even cardiac catheterisation.

Mitral valve prolapse

Mitral valve prolapse (also known as floppy mitral valve, or Barlow's syndrome) varies in severity from a trivial abnormality picked up on echocardiography which has little or no consequence to the patient, to severe mitral regurgitation and heart failure. In its mild form there are

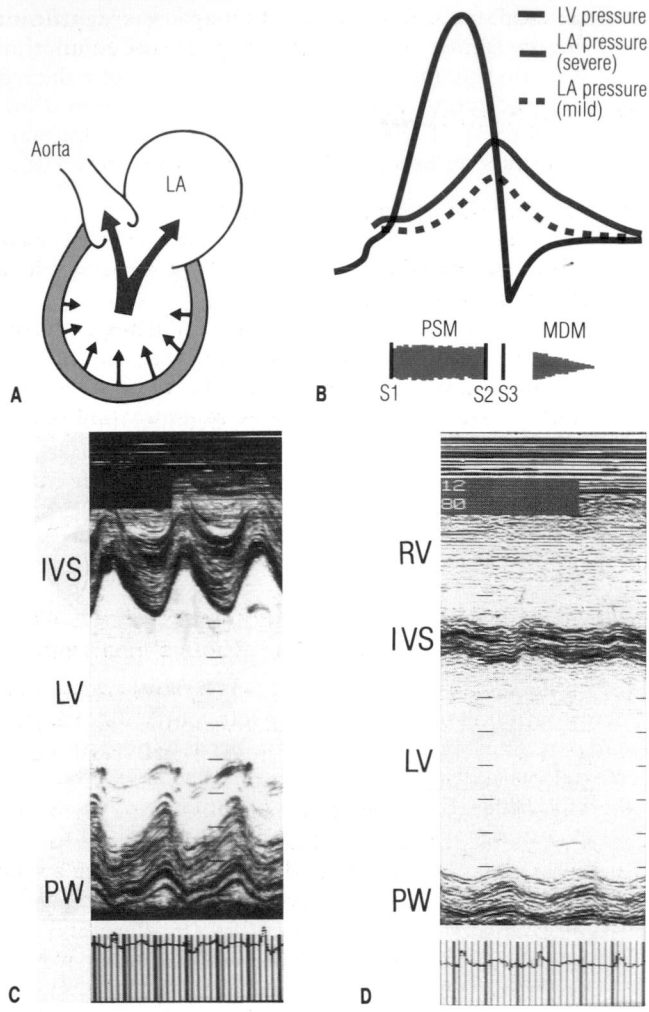

Fig. 12.41 Features of mitral regurgitation. A. Illustrates diversion of blood into the left atrium. **B.** Shows the pressures in the left ventricle and left atrium in both mild and severe cases and the accompanying murmurs. PSM = pansystolic murmur; MDM = mid-diastolic murmur. **C.** M mode echocardiogram through the left ventricle (LV) in a case of severe mitral regurgitation due to valvular disease. The ventricle is dilated and hyperkinetic. **D.** M mode echocardiogram at the same level in a patient with mitral regurgitation due to poor LV function. The LV is dilated and hypokinetic. IVS = interventricular septum; PW = posterior wall.

single or multiple systolic clicks in the mitral area, which may be associated with a late systolic murmur of mild mitral regurgitation. There may be a tendency to supraventricular arrhythmia and atypical chest pain and associated mild skeletal abnormalities, commonly a straight back (loss of thoracic kyphosis).

The underlying abnormality consists of redundancy in the chordae tendinae allowing posterior prolapse of one or other mitral cusp in late systole. More severe degeneration of the subvalvular apparatus is seen in certain patients, particularly those with Marfan's syndrome (Ch. 5, p. 78), although severely floppy mitral valves may

occur in isolation. Isolated mitral regurgitation, even if severe, can be tolerated for long periods if its development is gradual. It is uncertain whether patients with the mild 'click-murmur' syndrome suffer a significant number of complications, but systemic embolisation, arrhythmia and endocarditis are potential risks. Treatment of severe regurgitation is surgical.

Investigation of mitral regurgitation

ECG. The ECG is of little value in indicating the severity of the regurgitation. There may be P mitrale and left ventricular hypertrophy, but very severe regurgitation can exist in the presence of an almost normal ECG.

Chest X-ray may show enlargement of the left ventricle as well as the left atrium. There may be evidence of raised pulmonary venous pressure.

M mode echocardiography is useful in demonstrating the volume load on the left ventricle and the size of the left atrium. It is seldom capable of showing the presence of, or the cause of, mitral regurgitation, but will show a rheumatic thickened mitral valve, mitral valve prolapse or flail cusp. 2D echocardiography will often show lack of co-aptation of the mitral valve cusps in rheumatic mitral regurgitation.

Doppler ultrasound demonstrates mitral regurgitation and distinguishes it from aortic stenosis or a ventricular septal defect.

Cardiac catheterisation gives a direct measurement of the left ventricular filling pressure and left atrial pressure, which helps to distinguish left ventricular muscle pump failure from severe valvular regurgitation. *Angiography* shows the severity of the leak and often its mechanism.

Management

Trivial regurgitation is very well tolerated and requires only endocarditis prophylaxis (p. 418). Moderately severe mitral regurgitation can be well tolerated for years, but the patient may slowly come to accept a diminishing exercise tolerance. The timing of valve replacement can be difficult. Worsening left ventricular function is an indication, since the procedure carries more risk when left ventricular function is poor. Severe regurgitation and acute regurgitation merit early valve replacement.

MITRAL REGURGITATION WITH STENOSIS

The combination of mitral regurgitation with stenosis is almost invariably a result of rheumatic heart disease but occasionally arises in other conditions, such as Libman-Sacks endocarditis in SLE. Mixed mitral valve disease presents later than pure stenosis, and is very common after mitral valvotomy.

The physical signs are shown in Figures 12.40 and 12.41. AF is more likely than with pure stenosis, and severe pulmonary hypertension is less likely. Even a mild degree of regurgitation makes the effective degree of mitral stenosis much greater (p. 370). The predominant lesion can be difficult to assess in the presence of hypertension or aortic valve disease, which will also produce left ventricular hypertrophy. A pansystolic murmur alone may arise from coincident tricuspid regurgitation with pure mitral stenosis. The degree of mitral regurgitation can vary with the heart rate and the degree of left ventricular dilatation. What may appear to be severe regurgitation when the patient is in heart failure, may settle considerably as the patient improves. Management is as for mitral stenosis alone (p. 372).

Assessment of the mitral valve with Doppler ultrasound shows that minor degrees of mitral regurgitation are extremely common even when these cannot be detected clinically.

AORTIC STENOSIS

Aetiology

Outflow obstruction to the left ventricle can be at the valve itself (valvular), above it (supravalvular), or below (subvalvular). About 1% of cases of 'aortic stenosis' are supra- or subvalvular. Supravalvular stenosis is a congenital form of atresia of the ascending aorta, and is associated with a characteristic 'elfin' facies. Subvalvular stenosis is either a congenital ring lesion (which is amenable to surgery) or is a variable muscular obstruction produced by hypertrophic obstructive cardiomyopathy (p. 411).

Valvular aortic stenosis can result from:

- *Congenital* aortic stenosis, presenting in childhood, the valve having one, two or three cusps.
- *Bicuspid aortic valve* presenting in adulthood. About 1% of the population are born with two, instead of three, cusps. About one-third of these develop calcific aortic stenosis, one-third mixed aortic valve disease, and one-third have no significant valvular abnormality. The valve itself seems to be mechanically unsatisfactory and suffers mechanical stresses which lead to progressive damage.
- *Rheumatic heart disease.* This involves the aortic valve in about 50% of cases of rheumatic valvular disease, most frequently producing aortic regurgitation, often a mixed lesion but sometimes pure stenosis. As with mitral valve disease, stenosis with rheumatic heart disease seems more common in women, and regurgitation in men.
- *Senile aortic calcification.* Although calcification of the valve ring is commonly benign, it can invade the cusps and produce a calcified tricuspid valve as it renders the cusps immobile. This aetiology is more common over the age of 70. The valve cusps are not fused.

Pathophysiology

Outflow obstruction to the left ventricle leads to:

- *Concentric left ventricular hypertrophy.*
- *Compensatory enlargement of the coronary arterial circulation* as the metabolic demands of the hypertrophied left ventricle increase.
- *A relatively fixed cardiac output.* A resting pressure gradient of 100 mmHg would have to become 400 mmHg for the flow velocity through the valve to double. The heart is incapable of generating such a pressure, and is therefore near its limit at rest.

Clinical features

Symptoms

Aortic stenosis may remain asymptomatic until it is very severe and is then life-threatening. The symptoms are:

- *Left heart failure.* Shortness of breath on exertion may precede paroxysmal nocturnal dyspnoea and orthopnoea, or the patient may present with acute pulmonary oedema.
- *Angina.* The thickened myocardium is perfused by a lower than normal perfusion gradient due to low aortic diastolic pressure and a high left ventricular end diastolic pressure. For these reasons, angina can occur without any coronary atheroma. In the older age group, aortic stenosis may well coexist with coronary artery disease.
- *Syncope on exertion.* This is a sinister symptom which indicates a fixed cardiac output and presages sudden death. The mechanisms may be: skeletal muscle vasodilatation causing a drop in blood pressure; a rise in ventricular pressure producing reflex bradycardia and vasodilatation; myocardial ischaemia triggering ventricular arrhythmia.
- *Sudden death*, probably resulting from myocardial ischaemia and ventricular irritability, leading to a fatal arrhythmia. This may be provoked by exertion.

Summary 5 Symptoms of aortic stenosis

- Left heart failure – dyspnoea, orthopnoea, pulmonary oedema
- Angina
- Exertional syncope or near syncope
- Small cerebral emboli
- Right heart failure

- *Right heart failure*. Progressive myocardial ischaemia can lead to a 'myopathic heart', in which the most prominent symptom is oedema from right heart failure supervening on left.
- *Emboli from a heavily calcified valve*. These are usually fairly small and cause small strokes or visual disturbances.

Signs

The signs of pure aortic stenosis are shown in Figure 12.42. Although the systolic ejection murmur suggests the possible diagnosis, the most important physical sign is the slow-rising, poor volume pulse, best felt at the carotid where a systolic thrill may also be evident. The heart is not enlarged unless the patient has been in failure, but the left ventricular apex beat is powerful and 'pressure loaded'. Differential diagnosis from a 'flow murmur' is based on the single second sound (in calcific aortic stenosis), the pulse and the presence of left ventricular hypertrophy. The loudness of the murmur is a poor index of severity and the murmur may even be absent in heart failure. In congenital aortic stenosis, there may be an ejection click as the valve cusps tent as they tension.

Investigation

Electrocardiography

A normal ECG virtually rules out significant aortic stenosis, except in congenital disease when the trace may remain remarkably normal despite a large gradient. A number of ECG changes are seen in aortic stenosis:

- *Left ventricular hypertrophy*. Often widening of QRS and T wave changes of 'strain' predominate over voltage change. T wave inversion over LV leads may be the only feature. Loss of anterior R waves may occur.
- *Left axis deviation* and, eventually, *left bundle branch block* may occur either from severe hypertrophy or invasion of conduction system by calcium from the valve.
- *Left atrial hypertrophy* or '*P mitrale*'. A large negative component to the P wave in V1 indicates raised left ventricular filling pressure.
- *Complete heart block*.

Chest X-ray

The chest X-ray can be normal but may show a post-stenotic dilatation of the ascending aorta, prominence of the left ventricle and a calcified aortic valve on lateral chest X-ray. The latter suggests tight stenosis in a patient under 55; above this age, the valve may calcify even with an insignificant gradient. Significant enlargement of the left ventricle occurs with heart failure or coincident aortic regurgitation.

M mode echocardiography

M mode echocardiography can display thickening and calcification of the valve cusps, but is less useful in congenital stenosis. The compensatory hypertrophy of the left ventricular wall is well shown. 2D echocardiography may give a good view of the aortic valve orifice.

Doppler ultrasound

Doppler ultrasound measures the jet velocity and predicts the valve gradient. A high blood velocity (> 4 m/s) indicates a surgically significant gradient but, since jet velocities can be underestimated, a negative or low jet velocity record is of less significance.

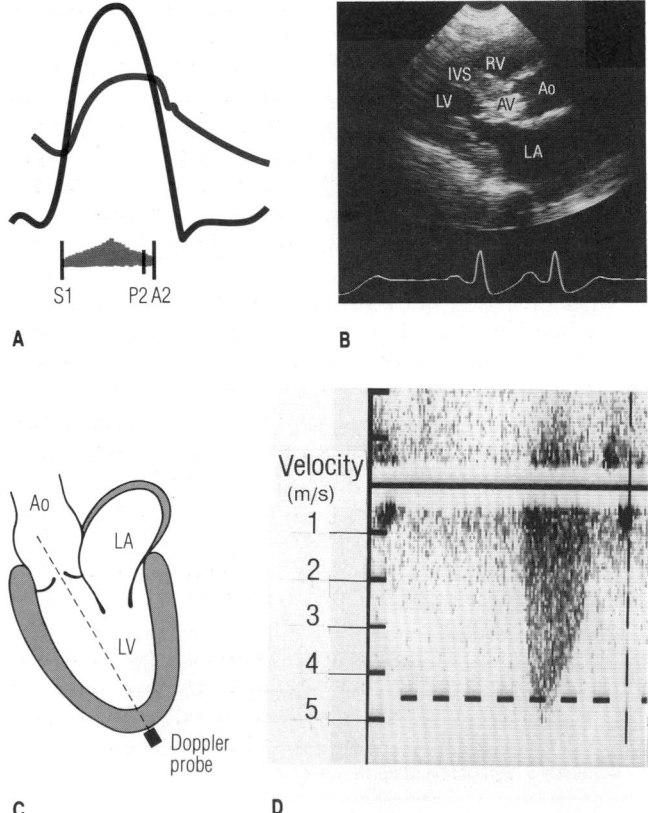

Fig. 12.42 Features of aortic stenosis. A. Pressures in the left ventricle (black) and aorta (red) showing a systolic pressure gradient due to aortic stenosis. The ejection systolic murmur is illustrated. **B.** 2D echocardiogram showing severe aortic valve (AV) thickening. Ao = aorta; LV = left ventricle; LA = left atrium; RV = right ventricle. **C.** Position of probe and direction of Doppler beam. **D.** Continuous wave Doppler record showing high velocity signals. Peak = 4.5 m/s (dotted line), predicting a gradient of 82 mmHg.

Cardiac catheterisation

Measurement of the valve gradient by cardiac catheterisation is not essential if the diagnosis is well established. Catheterisation is usually indicated where there is doubt about the site or degree of stenosis, a not infrequent occurrence in older patients who may be poor ultrasound subjects. It also allows analysis of ventricular function. Coronary angiography is now considered essential prior to operation in all but young women or the very elderly.

Management

Surgical

Tight aortic stenosis has such a poor prognosis that surgery should be offered to all patients. Valvuloplasty or valvotomy in children may gain sufficient time for them to reach a reasonable size before having aortic valve replacement. For adults, valve replacement is the only treatment. If the ventricle has already been badly damaged the results are less good, but in the asymptomatic patient with a normal ventricle, the left ventricular hypertrophy regresses fairly rapidly.

Lesser degrees of stenosis need serial follow-up, as the stenosis may become more significant with time.

Medical

Treatment of heart failure is along conventional lines (p. 348). Vasodilator agents are contraindicated, as reduction of systemic resistance can lead to a severe drop in blood pressure.

AORTIC REGURGITATION

Aetiology

The aortic valve cusps normally overlap on closure to the extent of about 25% of the cusp area. Aortic regurgitation can arise from:

- dilatation of the valve ring so that the cusps no longer meet adequately to prevent leakage
- damage to the cusps themselves
- in some diseases, a combination of these factors.

Dilatation of the valve ring occurs classically in syphilitic aortic regurgitation, but can also occur with hypertension and aortic dissection; less common causes include cystic medial necrosis in Marfan's syndrome, and osteogenesis imperfecta.

Damage to the valve cusps is a feature of rheumatic aortic regurgitation, infective endocarditis and less common conditions such as Libman-Sacks endocarditis, mucopolysaccharidoses and pseudoxanthoma elasticum.

The seronegative arthritides, ankylosing spondylitis, Reiter's disease and psoriatic arthritis can be associated with an aortitis and cusp damage, leading to aortic regurgitation. Rarely, rheumatoid arthritis is associated with a nodular cusp damage leading to aortic regurgitation.

Bicuspid aortic valve (found in 1% of the population) can lead to predominant aortic regurgitation (p. 375). There are other congenital forms of aortic regurgitation, e.g. that associated with a supracristal ventricular septal defect.

Clinical features

Symptoms and pathophysiology

Aortic regurgitation can be well tolerated for years if it develops slowly. Up to 80% regurgitation can be found in severe chronic aortic regurgitation, but acute regurgitation (such as follows aortic dissection or acute infective endocarditis) is poorly tolerated.

The severity of the regurgitation is normally indicated by a low diastolic blood pressure and wide pulse pressure. These may appear more 'normal' in heart failure as the stroke volume falls and the end diastolic pressure of the left ventricle rises. As aortic regurgitation progresses, the increasing leakage requires a larger and larger forward flow. This is usually achieved not by a tachycardia but by the left ventricular end diastolic size increasing with an increased stroke volume. Initially, the ejection fraction of the left ventricle is well maintained and exercise tolerance is excellent. However, after an unpredictable time, there is steady or sudden deterioration in left ventricular function, usually with a great increase in heart size and the development of symptoms of left ventricular failure. Eventually, right heart failure follows with the development of pulmonary hypertension. The development of heart failure indicates serious dilatation of the left ventricle and need for urgent consideration of valve surgery. Heart failure in aortic regurgitation is associated with rapidly worsening left ventricular function which may never recover even with valve replacement.

Angina can develop because the dilated left ventricle has increased oxygen requirements (as in congestive cardiomyopathy), but is usually associated with coronary artery disease. AF occurs in about 15% of cases, usually those with long-standing failure.

Physical signs

The physical signs of aortic regurgitation (Fig. 12.43) are related to the large stroke volume, the peripheral vasodilatation and the compensatory increase in size of the left ventricle. The pulse may be collapsing or bisferiens, or feel normal if there is heart failure. The blood

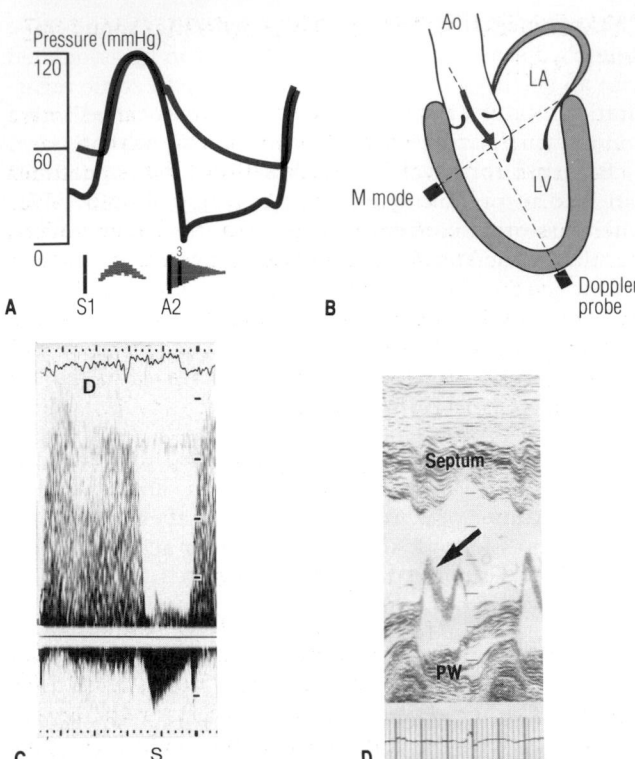

Fig. 12.43 Features of aortic regurgitation. A. Pressures in the aorta (red) and left ventricle (black) are illustrated with the accompanying murmurs (3 = third sound). **B.** Direction of regurgitant flow (arrow) and orientation of M mode and Doppler beams (dotted lines). **C.** Continuous wave Doppler signal showing a regurgitant jet throughout diastole with a maximal velocity of 4 m/s (upwards signal). The small downward signal excludes aortic stenosis. **D.** M mode echocardiogram showing flutter of the anterior mitral valve leaf (arrowed), which may close prematurely in severe aortic regurgitation causing early first heart sound.

pressure indicates the large pulse pressure and low diastolic pressure. If the diastolic pressure is well maintained in the presence of severe aortic regurgitation, coincident hypertension should be suspected. The left ventricle is very active and, in severe cases, the apex beat is displaced.

The increased forward flow is often accompanied by a systolic flow murmur which, of itself, does not indicate coincident stenosis. The early diastolic murmur is notoriously difficult to hear. The murmur is best heard with the diaphragm of the stethoscope, with the patient sitting forward having breathed out. It may be best heard at the left sternal edge, nearer the apex or the aortic area depending on the direction of the jet. Typically, valve ring dilatation regurgitation is better heard in the third right interspace rather than the third left.

An *Austin Flint murmur* may be associated with aortic regurgitation. This is an apical diastolic murmur, similar to that of mitral stenosis, arising from the anterior cusp of

---

Summary 6 Clinical features of aortic regurgitation

Symptoms
Left heart failure: breathlessness
Myocardial ischaemia, angina
Atrial fibrillation (less frequently)

Physical signs
Large stroke volume with vasodilatation
   Collapsing pulse
   Wide pulse pressure
   Head nodding, capillary pulsation
Enlarged left ventricle with dynamic displaced apex
Auscultatory
   High-pitched early diastolic murmur
   Forward flow systolic murmur
   Premature first heart sound (in severe cases)
   Austin Flint murmur

---

the mitral valve which vibrates in the jet of aortic regurgitation. Because aortic regurgitation may be both difficult to hear and is a frequent lesion in infective endocarditis, a patient with a fever and steadily widening pulse pressure is regarded as having aortic regurgitation and endocarditis until proved otherwise.

Investigation

ECG shows left ventricular hypertrophy of the diastolic overload type, in that, initially at least, voltage changes with prominent Q waves over the lateral leads predominate over T wave changes. Later, the T waves invert.

Chest X-ray shows increasing size of the left ventricle and often some dilatation of the proximal aorta. Generalised cardiac enlargement may follow and, eventually, changes of raised pulmonary venous pressure.

Echocardiography. M mode shows the dilated left ventricle and its wall thickness. Calculation can be made of the stroke volume and ejection fraction, which are useful for following progress. In many cases, vibration of the anterior cusp of the mitral valve or the septum can be seen, confirming the diagnosis. *Doppler ultrasound* will confirm the diagnosis but cannot yet quantify the lesion.

Cardiac catheterisation is necessary to examine left ventricular function, severity of the aortic regurgitation and its anatomy, as well as looking for other pathology, such as mitral regurgitation and coronary artery disease.

Management

Surgery

Those in heart failure have been left too late to benefit from surgery, since a dilated 'myopathic' heart never returns to normal and is associated with a high risk of sudden death. The currently used criteria for surgery are based on echocardiographic dimensions; others are now being developed based on the use of isotope left ventricular angiography. A fall in the ejection fraction of the left ventricle on exercise has been suggested as a criterion for surgery, since the ejection fraction is normally well maintained or even increases. Acute aortic regurgitation requires very close attention and urgent valve replacement at the first sign of heart failure. Delay can result in catastrophic heart failure and death of the patient, as the degree of regurgitation and size of the heart rapidly increase.

Medical

Medical management of chronic regurgitation consists of treatment of heart failure and control of other problems, such as arrhythmias and endocarditis prophylaxis (p. 418).

MIXED AORTIC VALVE DISEASE

About one-third of patients with aortic valve disease have a combined lesion with significant regurgitation and stenosis. As previously described, regurgitation makes a great difference to the valve gradient (p. 369, Table 12.13), and a stenotic valve with a gradient of 16 mmHg in systole would have a gradient of over 60 mmHg if twice the flow is accommodated, because of 50% regurgitation. The physical signs of the combined lesion are distinctive, with a large volume sustained or bisferiens pulse, a markedly hypertrophied left ventricle which is both pressure and volume loaded, and both systolic ejection and early diastolic murmurs. The second sound is single. A combined lesion cannot be caused by syphilis or other pathologies that primarily dilate the aortic root.

Investigation and management

Assessment of combined lesions has been greatly helped by Doppler ultrasound and echocardiography. The gradient measured by Doppler ultrasound may appear much greater than the pull-back pressure gradient measured at cardiac catheterisation.

Surgery for combined lesions is based on the same criteria as for single lesions. Onset of symptoms means that there is severe left ventricular hypertrophy and probably fibrosis, with consequent poor left ventricular function. Surgery is therefore ideally timed to anticipate symptoms and allow the left ventricular hypertrophy to regress. A gradient of over 50 mmHg, the development of a left ventricular strain pattern on ECG, left ventricular dilatation and any evidence of heart failure are all considered indications for aortic valve replacement.

COMBINED MITRAL AND AORTIC VALVE DISEASE

Over 50% of patients with rheumatic mitral valve disease will eventually develop evidence of aortic valve disease, most commonly aortic regurgitation, but sometimes stenosis as well. The presence of disease of both valves makes assessment of the severity of the individual lesions more difficult. Mitral valve disease, in particular, tends to reduce cardiac output and stroke volume, which may make the physical signs of aortic valve disease, such as the carotid pulse, far less evident. Aortic regurgitation and mitral regurgitation both cause a volume load on the left ventricle, so the contribution of each lesion to this is difficult to assess. The auscultatory signs may also be far more difficult to elicit, particularly if the patient is in heart failure.

Investigation and management

The presence of aortic valve disease should be suspected in every patient with rheumatic mitral valve disease, particularly if they have ECG evidence of left ventricular hypertrophy, or a slightly sustained carotid pulse. Fortunately, echocardiography and, in particular, Doppler ultrasound enable the valves to be individually examined for evidence of stenosis and regurgitation. This is far more accurate than inspection of the valves at surgery. If a patient is being considered for mitral valve replacement in the presence of aortic valve disease, it is unwise for the surgeon to leave anything but trivial aortic valve disease. What may seem a trivial degree of aortic regurgitation or stenosis at presentation, may become clinically important with replacement of the mitral valve.

TRICUSPID REGURGITATION

Tricuspid regurgitation most commonly arises as a result of dilatation of the valve ring secondary to right heart failure with pulmonary hypertension. Less common causes are actual rheumatic involvement of the tricuspid valve leaflets producing 'organic tricuspid disease', and right-sided endocarditis, which is rare in anyone other than intravenous drug addicts. Floppy tricuspid valve may be associated with floppy mitral valve and some congenital heart disease is associated with tricuspid regurgitation either as a primary phenomenon or secondary to right heart enlargement (e.g. atrial septal defect). Endomyocardial fibrosis, a disease occurring in the tropics, especially Africa, causes mitral and tricuspid regurgitation.

Doppler ultrasound has shown that a right-sided cardiac enlargement in rheumatic heart disease is almost invariably associated with a regurgitant jet through the tricuspid valve, very often in the absence of any physical signs. Similarly, it may be the cause of an 'innocent systolic murmur'.

Clinical features

Pathophysiology and symptoms

The leakage of a small percentage of the right ventricular stroke volume is easily accommodated by the right atrium. As the volume of regurgitation increases, there is increasing enlargement of the right atrium and right ventricle, and the movement of the interventricular septum becomes dominated by the right ventricle and so 'paradoxical'. The large systolic pressure pulse in the right atrium leads to stagnation and, eventually, reversal of flow of the blood in the great veins; the liver becomes distended and pulsatile (Fig. 12.44). The high hepatic venous pressure leads to cardiac cirrhosis and this may occasionally lead to secondary portal hypertension and splenomegaly.

The poor venous return, high venous pressures and poor hepatic function are associated, in most patients, with a degree of cardiac cachexia, poor wound-healing and difficulties with haemostasis.

Tricuspid regurgitation due to disease of the valve is much better tolerated, as the regurgitation is at a much lower pressure than when it is secondary to pulmonary hypertension.

The principal symptoms are those of right heart failure, with low cardiac output, fatigue, oedema and pain from hepatic congestion which may arise on exercise – so-called 'hepatic angina', i.e. epigastric or right-sided subcostal pain arising on exercise and gradually (more gradually than 'true' angina) disappearing with cessation of exercise.

Signs

The patient may have AF and is often slightly jaundiced. In moderate to severe cases, there is a highly pulsatile jugular vein with a big v wave and rapid y descent. The height of the v wave peak may be as much as 15 cm above the sternal angle and, in these circumstances, the jugular vein is palpably pulsatile and can be confused with an arterial pulse by a novice. The right ventricle is very active and gives rise to a right parasternal impulse. A pansystolic murmur is heard at the left sternal edge, or even at the cardiac apex, which may be formed by the right ventricle under these circumstances. The murmur is often of lower pitch than a mitral murmur. There can be a right ventricular third heart sound.

Abdominal examination reveals a pulsatile liver which is often visible, but is best felt bimanually.

Investigation

ECG may be unhelpful and is usually dominated by other factors associated with the underlying cardiac disease.

Chest X-ray shows right-sided cardiac enlargement, and there may be a fullness in the region of the distended superior vena cava.

Echocardiography shows an enlarged right ventricle with paradoxical movement of the interventricular septum suggesting 'volume load' of the right ventricle. The tricuspid valve leaflets are more easily seen with an enlarged right heart.

Doppler ultrasound will confirm a regurgitant jet through the tricuspid valve. The jet velocity will give an indication of the gradient across the valve, and hence the right ventricular pressure and the severity of the pulmonary hypertension (if any).

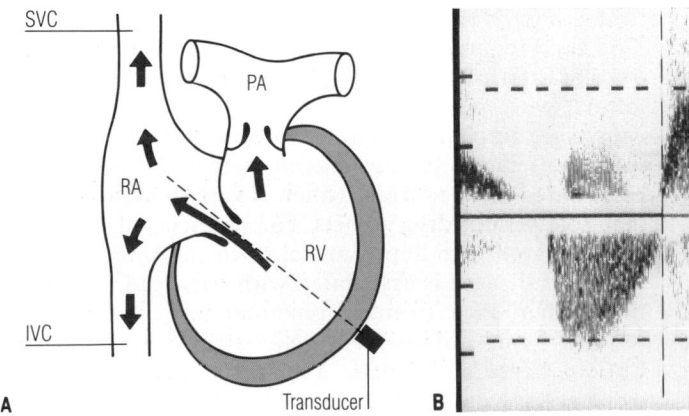
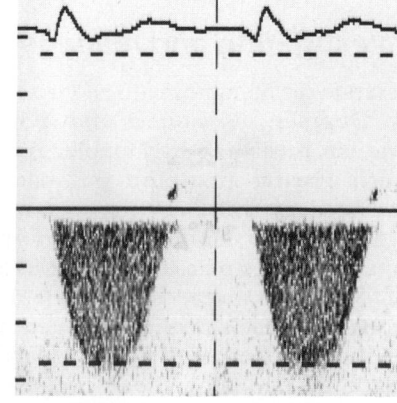

Fig. 12.44 Features of tricuspid regurgitation. A. Illustration of regurgitant flow and direction of Doppler beam (dotted line). PA = pulmonary artery; SVC and IVC = superior and inferior vena cava. **B.** and **C.** Continuous wave Doppler signals, both showing tricuspid regurgitation (downwards signal). In **B** there is severe (organic) regurgitation with normal pulmonary artery pressure and increased triscupid forward flow. In **C** there is pulmonary hypertension with a high velocity regurgitant jet through the triscupid valve.

Management

As tricuspid regurgitation is often secondary to pulmonary hypertension, the treatment is frequently that of the underlying cause. Bedrest and diuretics will be effective in many cases, with the murmur and pulsatile jugular veins disappearing. Intravenous diuretics may be required, as the oral drugs may be poorly absorbed. Organic tricuspid valve disease may require surgical treatment by replacement or annuloplasty at the same time as other cardiac surgery.

TRICUSPID STENOSIS

Tricuspid stenosis is a very uncommon manifestation of rheumatic heart disease. It mimics mitral stenosis, but produces right heart failure rather than left. It almost always complicates rheumatic involvement of the mitral and aortic valves, and should be suspected if there is a high venous pressure with a slow *y* descent in the JVP. The diastolic murmur is reputedly enhanced on inspiration and is heard best at the left sternal edge. There can be a tricuspid opening snap and often coincident tricuspid regurgitation.

Investigation and management

The diagnosis can be confirmed by echocardiogram which will show the thickened cusps. Doppler ultrasound can be used to measure the jet velocity and thus calculate the diastolic gradient. Cardiac catheterisation with a double lumen catheter is needed to measure the rather small valve gradient. Treatment is by valve replacement.

PULMONARY REGURGITATION

Pulmonary regurgitation is usually caused by dilatation of the pulmonary valve ring in pulmonary hypertension. It may also follow pulmonary valvotomy or valvuloplasty. In severe cases, the right ventricle is hyperactive from volume loading, and the murmur is difficult to distinguish from that of aortic regurgitation, being an early diastolic murmur at the left sternal edge starting immediately after the pulmonary component of the second sound. It may have a slightly lower pitch and be more obvious on inspiration, but the two can easily be confused. The Graham Steell murmur of pulmonary regurgitation in mitral valve disease is far more frequently due to aortic regurgitation than was formerly believed.

Pulmonary regurgitation is usually well tolerated but can be one reason why the heart size remains enlarged after surgical correction of Fallot's tetralogy.

PULMONARY STENOSIS

Pulmonary stenosis is the second most common form of congenital heart disease in adults; it is commoner in women. Mild cases, with gradients of less than 50 mmHg, are common. Stenosis may occur at valvular or subvalvular level, or even in the pulmonary arteries. There is a raised pressure in the right ventricle and, in severe cases, reduced lung blood flow and poor effort tolerance.

Clinical features

Most cases are asymptomatic. With gradients of over 80 mmHg, the most common symptom is dyspnoea on exertion. In very severe stenosis, symptoms of exertional syncope and angina become prominent, similar to those associated with aortic stenosis. In children and young adults, pulmonary stenosis may present with severe right heart failure.

The physical signs are of a small volume pulse, a large *a* wave in the JVP, a right ventricular substernal heave and a harsh systolic murmur in the pulmonary area. The latter appears very long and drowns the heart sounds in severe cases of infundibular stenosis, but can be a short ejection murmur in mild cases. The timing of pulmonary valve closure, which is delayed in severe cases, is a useful indication of severity.

Investigation and management

ECG shows right ventricular hypertrophy. The chest X-ray shows oligaemic lung fields; a large poststenotic dilatation with dilatation of the pulmonary conus is common in valvular, but not infundibular stenosis. The right ventricle is not significantly enlarged unless it has failed.

Doppler ultrasound assesses the valve gradient. Echocardiography will show the hypertrophy of the right ventricle and the site of the obstruction.

Surgical valvotomy has been largely replaced as a treatment of pulmonary stenosis by balloon valvuloplasty (see below).

SURGICAL MANAGEMENT OF ACQUIRED HEART VALVE DISEASE

The choices in surgical management of heart valve disease have recently become more complex, with closed valvotomy, open valvotomy and balloon valvuloplasty all being possible approaches.

Cardiac bypass

In the technique of cardiac bypass the circulation is arrested and there is extracorporeal circulation from a roller pump and external oxygenator. The brain is perfused at relatively low pressure, and the oxygenator and perfusion system introduce microemboli into the arterial circulation. There is therefore a morbidity associated with prolonged cardiac bypass. Most of the morbidity seems to be reversible (e.g. intellectual impairment) but patients with cerebrovascular disease, such as carotid stenosis, are at particularly high risk from cerebral infarction.

Balloon valvuloplasty

In balloon valvuloplasty, a balloon catheter is inserted through the valve orifice and then dilated to split open the valve. The aortic valve can be dilated in children, and balloon valvuloplasty has been especially successful for pulmonary and mitral stenosis. If torrential regurgitation is produced during mitral valvulopasty, valve replacement is essential.

Valve repair and replacement

Plastic surgical repair to a damaged valve uses pericardial or other tissue to repair defects in the valve cusps, or suturing of the valve ring to a prosthetic former to correct a grossly dilated valve ring. The latter is commonly performed in severe tricuspid regurgitation. The procedures are time-consuming and technically demanding and have had a history of variable results.

Prosthetic and biological valves

The type of valve used in valve replacement depends very often on local preference and expertise. Mechanical valves require permanent oral anticoagulation with warfarin. Biological valves do not, but are prone to early failure and calcification. The original prosthetic Starr-Edwards valve – essentially a ball in a cage – was built for durability, but early models formed thrombus on the struts and were also rather noisy. Numerous attempts have been made to improve on this valve, but many of these have developed mechanical problems and the Starr valve remains the most durable prosthesis currently available.

In order to avoid the anticoagulation essential with mechanical valves, various attempts have been made to use biological valves. Fresh human homografts have been used very successfully in the aorta, but availability has been a problem. The most widely used biological valves are pig xenografts. Porcine or bovine tissue is usually mounted on a ring or stent and they have the advantage of not requiring long-term anticoagulation, nor producing the loud prosthetic clicks of mechanical valves. Their disadvantages are that they have an unpredictable lifespan and can calcify and become stenosed

very rapidly in young patients. However, most of them last at least five years. One has been used in women of child-bearing age who wish to have a family without the risks of long-term anticoagulation. Such patients must be prepared to face the subsequent re-operation for valve replacement when the biological valve fails. Under current legislation in the UK, a heavy goods or public service vehicle licence holder cannot drive if he is on anticoagulants, so these patients may have to opt for biological valves if they wish to maintain their occupation.

CONGENITAL HEART DISEASE

Incidence and aetiology

Congenital heart abnormalities are present in about 8–12 per 1000 live births (excluding bicuspid aortic valve and floppy mitral valve). The simpler abnormalities are commonest with ventricular septal defect (VSD) accounting for 25–30% of cases and patent ductus arteriosus 10% (Table 12.15). Pulmonary stenosis, atrial septal defect (ASD), coarctation of the aorta, aortic stenosis and tetralogy of Fallot together account for another 35% of cases. Of the complex lesions, transposition of the arteries, AV septal defects and the hypoplastic left heart syndrome are the most frequently seen. The fetal circulation is shown in Figure 12.45.

Only a minority of these patients (10–15%) would survive to adolescence and adulthood without the help of

Table 12.15 Relative frequency of types of congenital heart disease

Congenital defect	Frequency (%)
Live births	
Atrial septal defect	30
Pulmonary stenosis	25
Tetralogy of Fallot	10
Ventricular septal defect	9
Eisenmenger syndrome	7
Patent ductus arteriosus	7
Coarctation of the aorta	5
Other	7
Stillbirths	
Ventricular septal defect	35
Univentricular heart (with tricuspid and mitral atresia)	13
Atrial septal defect	10
Coarctation of the aorta	9
Complete transposition	9
Atrioventricular septal defects	9
Hypoplastic left heart	6
Tetralogy of Fallot	3
Other	6

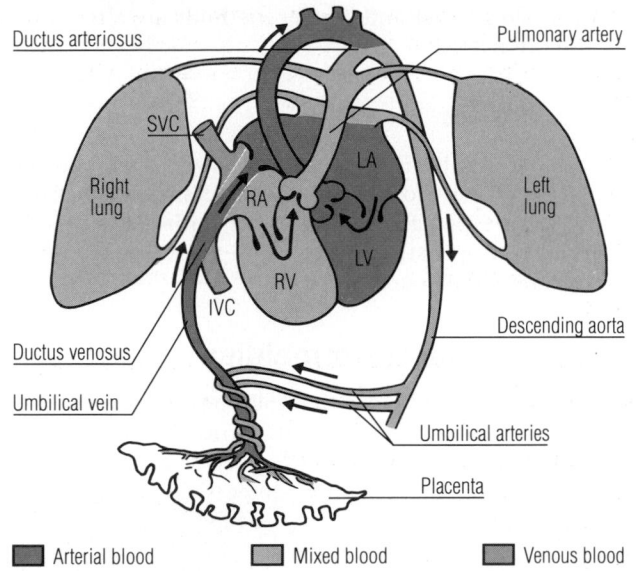

Ductus arteriosus
Pulmonary artery
SVC
LA
Right lung
RA
Left lung
LV
RV
IVC
Ductus venosus
Descending aorta
Umbilical vein
Umbilical arteries
Placenta

■ Arterial blood   ■ Mixed blood   ■ Venous blood

Fig. 12.45 Diagram of the fetal circulation. SVC and IVC = superior and inferior vena cava.

Table 12.16 Causes of congenital heart disease

Cause	Defect
Rubella	Patent ductus, atrial septal defect, pulmonary stenosis
Drugs	
Alcohol	Ventricular septal defect
Lithium	Ebstein's anomaly
	Tricuspid atresia
Thalidomide	Multiple defects
Inherited disease	
Connective tissue disorders	
Marfan's	Aortic dilatation and incompetence; mitral incompetence
Ehlers-Danlos	Mitral regurgitation; arterial dilatation
Inborn metabolic errors	
Mucopolysaccharidoses	Valve disease, cardiomyopathy
Homocystinuria	Aortic and pulmonary dilatation
Pompe's disease	Glycogen deposition in myocardium
Chromosomal abnormalities	
Down's syndrome	Atrial and ventricular septal defect; Fallot's tetralogy; endocardial cushion defect
Trisomy 13 and 18	Ventricular septal defect; right ventricular anomalies; pulmonary stenosis
Turner's syndrome	Coarctation of aorta, bicuspid aortic valve; pulmonary stenosis
Other inherited syndromes	
Di George	Fallot's tetralogy; aortic arch anomalies
Friedreich's ataxia	Cardiomyopathy
Holt-Oram	Atrial septal defect
Kartagener	Dextrocardia
Tuberous sclerosis	Cardiomyopathy

cardiac surgery and interventional cardiology. Over the last 15–20 years babies have survived who would previously have died, so that cardiologists and physicians are now more likely to see adult patients with medically or surgically corrected lesions than diagnose a congenital defect for the first time in adult life.

The relative frequency of different lesions at different ages depends on the compatibility of the lesion with longevity. ASD, for example, can present in the patient's seventies, but congenital aortic stenosis or coarctation of the aorta presents much earlier, either to the physician or as a cause of sudden death.

As the cohort of patients with surgically palliated or corrected hearts reaches maturity so special issues arise involving counselling, the advisability of pregnancy, the likelihood of inheritance in the next generation and the timing of heart or heart and lung transplantation in the disabled or deteriorating patient.

The commonest forms of congenital heart disease seen after birth are shown in Table 12.15. Spontaneously aborted fetuses have a much higher incidence of severe congenital heart disease than do normal term infants. Congenital heart defects may occur as part of more complex syndromes; there are often associated minor thoracic abnormalities.

Most cases of congenital heart disease remain unexplained. Some causes are listed in Table 12.16. Most lesions develop in the first trimester of pregnancy, many at about the seventh week. Many involve 'mistakes' in the complex embryological processes of flexing, twisting and formation of septa and the formation and closure of foramina (Fig. 12.45). The formation of a *patent ductus*

arteriosus (more correctly a *persistent* ductus arteriosus) and coarctation of the aorta appear to be due to physiological mechanisms that go wrong after birth.

Maternal viral illnesses

Viral infection in early pregnancy, typically rubella, appears to be the cause of some congenital heart defects. Rubella produces a characteristic association of defects including deafness, cataract and often persistent ductus arteriosus, although other lesions may occur. Although rubella is the best documented viral agent, mumps and influenza epidemics have been shown to increase the risk of congenital defects if the mother has the illness early in pregnancy. Other agents, e.g. cytomegalovirus, herpes simplex and coxsackie, have also been implicated. About 5% of cases of congenital heart disease can be explained by viral illness.

12 Cardiovascular Disease

Maternal illness and drug effects

Maternal illness, especially SLE, may predispose to congenital AV block. Drugs taken by the mother can be teratogenic, and drugs now associated with congenital heart disease include alcohol, lithium, amphetamines, phenytoin, oestrogen/progesterone and trimethadione.

Counselling, pregnancy and contraception

A mother who has congenital heart disease herself, or who has one affected child, can usually be counselled that subsequent pregnancy carries a low risk (1–5%) of congenital heart disease. Concordance rates for identical twins are between 15 and 20%, and for non-identical twins between 3 and 5%, suggesting environmental as well as genetic factor(s) in the development of congenital heart disease.

In families with affected first-degree relatives the risk to the fetus increases to 50% when there are three affected relatives. When both spouses have congenital heart disease risks may be up to 15%. In all these instances professional help from clinical geneticists is invaluable. Fetal echocardiography can be used to screen high-risk pregnancies. Mendelian dominant inheritance is seen in Marfan's syndrome and some families with hypertrophic cardiomyopathy; both conditions present in adulthood.

Pregnancy in cyanotic congenital heart disease carries a high risk of complications and accelerated deterioration, and frequently ends in spontaneous abortion. At particular risk are women with haemoglobin above 17 g/dl and those with pulmonary hypertension or the Eisenmenger reaction (p. 385). Patients with lesser degrees of cyanosis and polycythaemia may occasionally be brought through successful pregnancies, by a combination of rest and prevention of thrombosis, infection or prolonged labour.

Sterilisation is usually recommended for high-risk (Eisenmenger) women. Even this relatively minor surgical procedure can be dangerous, but is less so than pregnancy. High-oestrogen-containing contraceptive pills increase an already high risk of thrombosis and embolisation; it is not clear if the low-oestrogen pills are any safer in this group of women. The potential associated infective risk prevents the use of intrauterine devices. Vasectomy for the male partner and barrier methods are alternatives, but too unreliable.

Endocarditis

Only patients with ligated PDA, repaired ASD and VSD can be exempted from prophylaxis against endocarditis. There is an especially high risk for patients with aortic valve disease, prosthetic valves, L to R shunts, mitral regurgitation and coarctation.

Chromosomal abnormalities

Chromosomal abnormalities can be accompanied by congenital heart disease. Down's syndrome (Mongolism or trisomy 21, see Ch. 5, p. 73) is associated with endocardial cushion or AV canal defects (ASD mitral and tricuspid regurgitation), but VSDs and pulmonary stenosis also have an increased incidence. Turner's syndrome (XO) – characterised by stunted growth, web neck, female sexual stunting and cubitus valgus – has a greatly increased incidence of coarctation of the aorta and pulmonary stenosis.

CYANOTIC CONGENITAL HEART DISEASE

Central cyanosis occurs with an arterial oxygen saturation of < 85%. Milder degrees of cyanosis may not be evident at rest but are readily precipitated by mild exertion at the bedside. A degree of shunting through the ductus arteriosus occurs for several hours, or even days, after birth and this may persist. More commonly, right-to-left shunting occurs through persisting embryonic defects or through the foramen ovale (Fig. 12.46). The persistence of central cyanosis after birth, or its later onset, depends on a left-to-right communication and on the resistance to outflow from the right heart being higher than that of the left.

High resistance to outflow of the right heart is usually caused by congenital pulmonary stenosis (valvular or muscular) or by acquired pulmonary hypertension due to

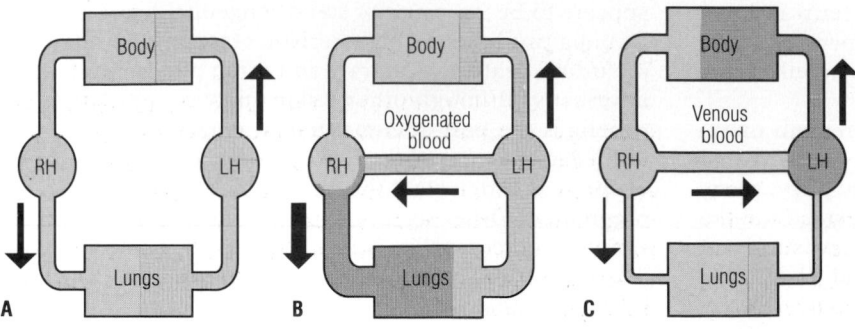

Fig. 12.46 Diagrammatic representation of blood flow in the systemic and pulmonary circulation. A. Normal. **B.** Left-to-right shunt. **C.** Right-to-left shunt; the pulmonary blood flow is reduced as a result of development of high resistance. RH = right heart; LH = left heart.

constriction of the pulmonary resistance vessels. Acquired pulmonary hypertension occurs with high flow through the lungs, so a left-to-right shunt can eventually reverse and become right-to-left with cyanosis (the *Eisenmenger reaction*).

Cyanotic heart disease produces a characteristic appearance with central cyanosis which may vary with activity, clubbing, impaired growth and intellectual development (if severe) and marked polycythaemia after the first year of life. Complications of the right-to-left shunt include cerebral abscess and paradoxical emboli, in which embolism from clot in peripheral veins gains access to the systemic circulation through the shunt. The severe polycythaemia can lead to thrombosis and infarction. Polycythaemia is proportional to the degree of desaturation. Regular venesection may be needed to maintain haemoglobin levels of 16–18 g/dl. Pulmonary hypertension can be complicated by recurrent haemoptysis.

FALLOT'S TETRALOGY

Fallot's tetralogy is the commonest form of cyanotic congenital heart disease seen after the age of 1 year. The four main features of this abnormality (Fig. 12.47) are:

- *a ventricular septal defect* (through which the shunting occurs)
- *pulmonary stenosis*, which may be muscular or valvular and acts as the obstruction which leads to the right-to-left flow
- *an overriding aorta*. The aorta is positioned above the VSD
- *right ventricular hypertrophy*, due to the pressure and volume load to which the RV is subjected.

Incomplete forms of the condition exist in which not all the features are present and the child may be acyanotic.

Clinical features

The child may be deeply cyanosed at rest and is subject to cyanotic and exertional syncopal episodes which appear to be related to changes in the degree of shunting. The physical signs are cyanosis, clubbing, right ventricular hypertrophy, a harsh systolic murmur at the upper left sternal edge (often with a thrill) and a single second heart sound.

Investigation

The characteristic features of Fallot's tetralogy on investigation are illustrated in Figure 12.47. Chest X-ray shows a characteristic cardiac silhouette of severe right ventricular hypertrophy which lifts the cardiac apex (*coeur en sabot*) and oligaemic lung fields. ECG shows right ventricular hypertrophy. Echocardiogram shows the overriding

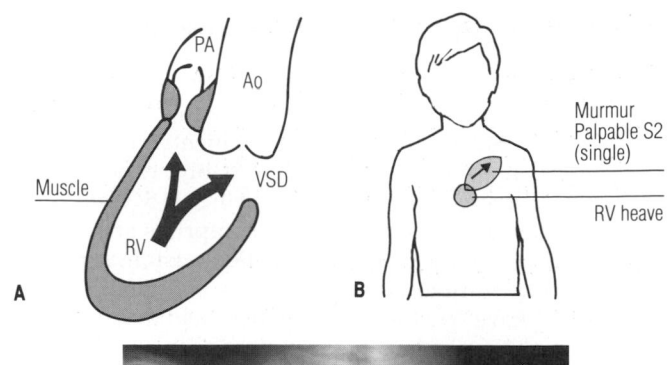
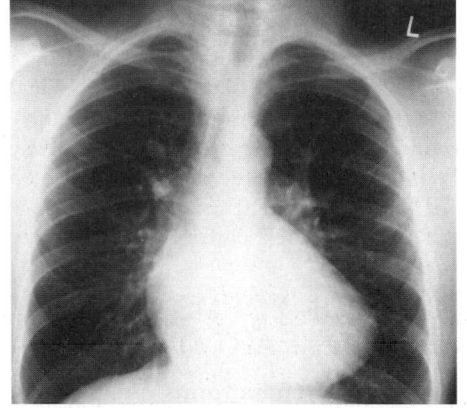
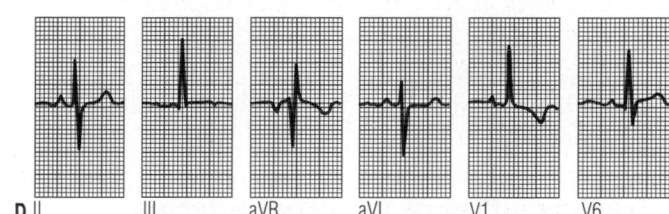

Fig. 12.47 Features of Fallot's tetralogy. A. Diagram of abnormality. VSD = ventricular septal defect; PA = pulmonary artery; Ao = aorta. **B.** Physical signs. **C.** Chest X-ray showing right ventricular hypertrophy, typical 'coeur en sabot'. **D.** ECG showing right atrial and ventricular hypertrophy and right axis deviation.

aorta and VSD and, with Doppler, can demonstrate the pulmonary stenosis, the right ventricular pressure and, sometimes, the flow through the VSD. Cardiac catheterisation can be used to measure the pressures and show the severity of the outflow tract obstruction.

Surgical treatment

Total surgical correction is now often attempted at an early age, but palliative operations to increase the lung blood flow were common in the past and are sometimes required now to encourage growth of the pulmonary vasculature, prior to complete intracardiac repair. The palliative shunts included the Blalock-Taussig anastomosis (subclavian to pulmonary artery) and aortic to pulmonary shunts.

Prognosis and clinical features after surgery

Without correction, less than 5% survive to adult life; 90% survive with surgery. In future, adult patients will have had a total repair at an earlier age, probably without prior palliative surgery. Late mortality, 10 to 15 years after repair, is low at 2–7% and mainly comprises arrhythmia including complete heart block. The vast majority of patients have normal exercise capacity and those that do not often have residual ventricular septal defects or pulmonary hypertension. These patients virtually all have a crescendo-decrescendo murmur. Many have a decrescendo murmur of pulmonary incompetence and signs of a residual VSD are somewhat less common. The chest X-ray can be normal but often shows cardiomegaly, and right bundle branch block on the ECG is almost always seen.

After palliative surgery the radial pulse may be weak on the side of the shunt and arterial collaterals may develop. The shunt may produce a continuous murmur.

LESS COMMON FORMS OF CYANOTIC CONGENITAL HEART DISEASE

Some of the less common forms of cyanotic congenital heart disease are important causes of neonatal and infant death; however, they can be diagnosed accurately with modern imaging techniques and treated surgically. Even in neonates, cardiac transplantation and heart lung transplantation may make some formerly inoperable conditions amenable to surgery.

Transposition of the great arteries

Complete transposition

In this uncommon abnormality the atria and ventricles are in normal relationship to each other but the great arteries arise from the wrong ventricles (transposed). The pulmonary and systemic circulations are therefore operating in parallel rather than in series, which is incompatible with life unless there is some communication between the two circuits.

About half the neonates have an intact ventricular septum and death ensues as the patent ductus arteriosus naturally closes. Survival is dramatically improved by a catheter method of producing an ASD (Rashkind procedure).

The other half of the group have large VSDs allowing bidirectional shunting and mixing of the bloodstream; 20% have a single ventricle, usually the right ventricle, now classified as double outlet right ventricle (DORV). Double outlet left ventricle (DOLV) is very rare. The natural history of this group is very variable with some individuals surviving to adulthood. Children who survive

due to the Rashkind procedure have few physical signs but remain cyanosed.

Corrective surgery

The 'Mustard' procedure produces an intra-atrial repair using a pericardial baffle to redirect flow in the atria to the appropriate ventricle. Results have been excellent with return to normal saturations, although arrhythmias may be a problem in later life.

Concern over the ability of the right ventricle to function in later life has led to the development of an arterial switch operation and the Rastelli procedure, where a valved conduit connects the right ventricle to the pulmonary artery. It is not yet clear whether these two demanding operations will improve on the results achieved with intra-atrial repairs.

Congenitally corrected transposition

Here the great arteries are transposed but blood flows correctly since the left and right ventricles are inverted. Thus, blood flows from the right atrium through a bicuspid mitral valve into a morphological left ventricle and into the pulmonary artery. From the left atrium a tricuspid valve leads to the right ventricle and the aortic valve.

Survival without surgery is common and the clinical features are dominated by associated abnormalities and problems (these include VSD, single ventricle (DORV or DOLV) and pulmonary stenosis or pulmonary vascular disease).

Abnormalities of venous return

The systemic veins may drain into the left atrium producing cyanosis with exercise. Both situations are rare on their own and are associated with other serious congenital defects.

Total anomalous pulmonary venous drainage (TAPVD) into the right atrium or left innominate vein is associated with right to left shunting across an ASD or patent foramen ovale. The physical features are those of an ASD with central cyanosis. Operations to re-route the veins and close the ASD produce excellent long-term results although the adults are susceptible to atrial arrhythmia.

Tricuspid atresia

Unoperated adults with this condition do exist although survival through childhood is unusual without surgical intervention. Blood flows from the right atrium to the left, through the mitral valve into the left ventricle and via a VSD through to a not uncommonly stenosed right ventricular outflow tract. The clinical signs are dominated by pulmonary stenosis and VSD murmurs. Cyanosis is variable and depends on the size of the VSD and degree of pulmonary stenosis. Surgical correction is by a Blalock-Taussig shunt or connection of the right atrium to the right ventricle, more commonly by Fontan's procedure where the right atrium is connected to the pulmonary artery.

Ebstein's anomaly of the tricuspid valve

This condition is often acyanotic. The septal and posterior leaflets of the tricuspid valve are attached to the right ventricular wall so that a large part of the right ventricle becomes atrialised. The right ventricle is small, but the right atrium becomes enormous. There is often some tricuspid regurgitation, and occasionally the abnormal valve obstructs filling, or even emptying, of the right ventricle. There is a high incidence of patent foramen ovale or ASD, and supraventricular arrhythmias are very common. The condition often presents in adult life. It may remain asymptomatic for years and present with an abnormal chest X-ray or ECG. The patient may, on the other hand, present with right heart failure, dyspnoea on exertion and, sometimes, mild cyanosis and clubbing.

Clinically, the heart is large and inactive. There is often a murmur of tricuspid regurgitation and a cV wave in the neck. ECG shows small voltages, right atrial hypertrophy and right bundle branch block. A Wolff-Parkinson-White configuration (p. 365) is common. Chest X-ray shows a globular or flask-shaped heart with a prominent convex right atrial border. Echocardiogram and cardiac catheterisation findings are characteristic.

Cardiomegaly alone is not an indication for surgical treatment since arrythmia and heart failure respond well to conventional medical therapy.

ACYANOTIC CONGENITAL HEART DISEASE

Conditions where blood is shunted from left to right may initially be without cyanosis, but, if undetected, high flows through the pulmonary vascular bed will eventually lead to a reversal of the blood flow and cyanosis, the Eisenmenger reaction. Thus some acyanotic lesions may later produce cyanosis.

ATRIAL SEPTAL DEFECT

ASDs can be of three types – secundum, primum or sinus venosus defect (Fig. 12.48). In adult cardiology, they occur in the above order of decreasing frequency. The foramen ovale only acts as an ASD if right-sided pressures exceed left, e.g. in pulmonary embolism. ASD constitutes 10% of congenital heart disease.

Pathogenesis

Blood flows from the left to right atrium, thence to the right ventricle and lungs. Because the lungs have a low impedance to flow, shunting is considerable. The patient has a limited exercise capacity, as a maximal systemic cardiac output cannot be achieved on exercise. The right ventricle hypertrophies and the lung blood flow is increased, which seems to increase the likelihood of pulmonary infections. Symptoms are usually not prominent until middle-age and include dyspnoea, fatigue (low exercise cardiac output) and, quite frequently, palpitations caused by atrial arrhythmias. Heart failure, when it occurs, is usually both right- and left-sided, since any rise in atrial pressure on one side of the septum will shunt the blood to the other side.

After middle-age, the pulmonary vascular resistance may rise, with the development of massive pulmonary arteries (visible on chest X-ray) and, occasionally, reversal of the shunt.

Secundum atrial septal defect

Clinical features

Secundum ASD (Fig. 12.49) is usually uncomplicated. The physical signs are the result of right ventricular hypertrophy and increased flow through the right side of the heart; this causes pulmonary and tricuspid flow murmurs and delayed closure of the pulmonary valve. The associated signs are wide, fixed splitting of the second sound and pulmonary systolic murmur; a tricuspid diastolic murmur is usually heard if shunting is significant.

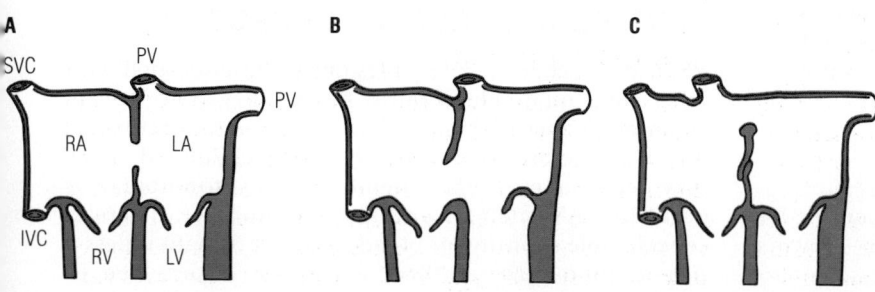

Fig. 12.48 Sites of atrial septal defect. A. Ostium secundum. **B.** Ostium primum (or atrioventricular canal defect). The septal leaflet of the mitral valve is often involved, allowing a communication between the left ventricle (LV) and both atria. **C.** Sinus venosus defect, where the abnormality involves anomalous pulmonary venous drainage. SVC and IVC = superior and inferior vena cava. PV = pulmonary vein.

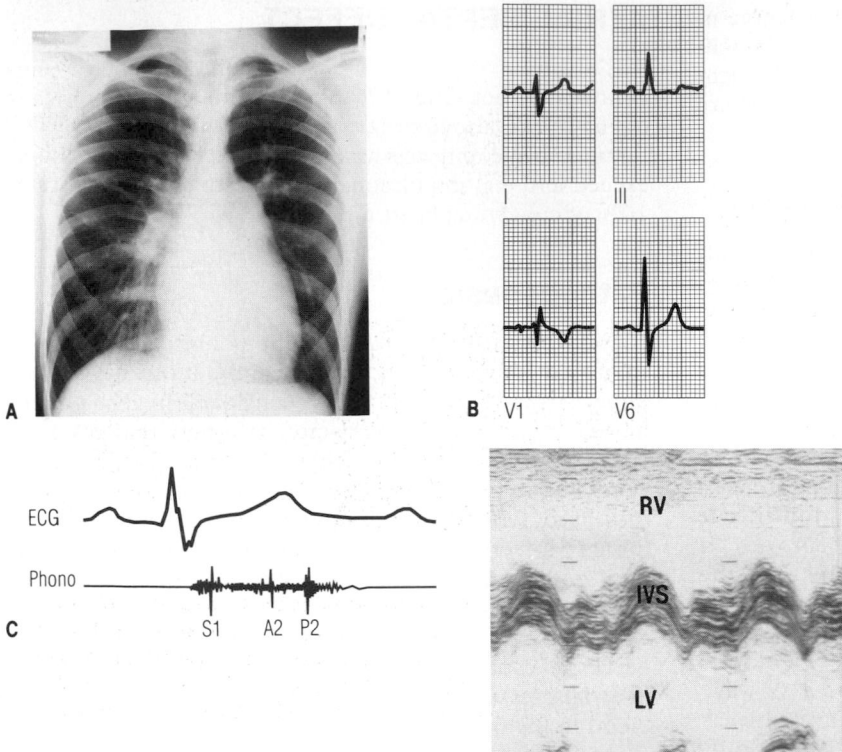

Fig. 12.49 Features of atrial septal defect. A. Chest X-ray showing enlarged pulmonary arteries, pulmonary plethora and relatively small aortic knuckle. **B.** ECG showing a vertical axis (normal) and partial right bundle branch block. **C.** Phonocardiogram demonstrating wide splitting of second heart sound. **D.** M mode echocardiogram at the ventricular level shows a volume overload RV with paradoxical movement of the interventricular septum (IVS) which is out of phase with the posterior wall (PW) of the left ventricle.

Investigation and management

Chest X-ray (Fig. 12.49) shows enlargement of the heart, prominent pulmonary arteries, pulmonary plethora and, usually, a small aortic knuckle. ECG shows right bundle branch block in most cases, with right axis deviation. Echocardiography shows dilated RV with a 'volume load' of the RV. The shunt can be demonstrated by contrast injection or with colour Doppler.

Cardiac catheterisation can demonstrate the size of the shunt. Blood samples taken in the different cardiac chambers show a step-up in oxygen content of the blood occurring at the lower right atrium. The shunt size can be calculated from the oxygen content of the pulmonary artery blood and left-sided samples. Angiography demonstrates the type of ASD and any associated mitral regurgitation.

Surgical closure is usually advised if the defect is associated with a shunt which gives a pulmonary flow greater than 1.5 times systemic flow.

Primum atrial septal defect

This is a much less common form of ASD, accounting for 10% of ASDs, but is relatively common in Down's syndrome.

Clinical features, investigation and treatment

The clinical features are similar to those of secundum ASD, but may be dominated by an associated mitral regurgitation and the ECG usually shows a left axis deviation. A left ventricular angiogram shows the defect. Surgical correction is more complex than for a secundum defect, and may involve mitral valve repair or replacement.

Sinus venosus defect

This is usually a high right atrial defect near the junction with the SVC. It is often associated with anomalous pulmonary venous drainage into the right atrium.

VENTRICULAR SEPTAL DEFECT

VSDs may occur as isolated lesions or be associated with other congenital defects of the heart. They are relatively common (Table 12.15) and have an equal sex incidence. About 50% close spontaneously during childhood. They may occur as muscular, membranous, infundibular or posterior (AV) defects and may be multiple. There is considerable shunting of blood from left to right unless a rise in pulmonary outflow resistance occurs due to vascular disease caused by the high pulmonary flow. In extreme cases, the flow reverses causing cyanosis and the Eisenmenger syndrome.

Small ventricular septal defects

Small VSDs are common and are asymptomatic. There is a loud systolic murmur with a thrill at the left sternal edge (Maladie de Roger), with no associated cardiomegaly and minimal, if any, changes of pulmonary plethora on chest X-ray. The ECG is usually normal. Differential diagnosis is from mitral regurgitation and is simply accomplished with Doppler ultrasound.

The only complication of a small VSD is the risk of *endocarditis*, and antibiotic prophylaxis is essential. Although the surgical mortality and morbidity for closure of small defects is low, surgery is not usually necessary.

Moderate and large-sized ventricular septal defects

With larger VSDs, systemic cardiac output is limited on exercise and can produce symptoms of fatigue and dyspnoea. As they are both volume loaded, both ventricles enlarge with displacement of the cardiac apex. The pansystolic murmur and thrill typical of Maladie de Roger may be softer in these patients, as the jet velocity of the VSD and the pressure gradient between the ventricles becomes smaller the larger the defect. As pulmonary hypertension becomes prominent, the murmur may almost disappear as the pressures in the two ventricles balance.

Investigation and management

The features of VSDs on investigation are illustrated in Figure 12.50. ECG shows biventricular hypertrophy, and there is increasing right ventricular hypertrophy with pulmonary hypertension. Chest X-ray shows pulmonary plethora, and cardiomegaly with both right and left ventricular hypertrophy. As pulmonary hypertension develops, the central pulmonary arteries increase in size and the peripheral vessels become pruned.

Echocardiography and Doppler ultrasound can show the location of the VSD, and can be used to calculate right ventricular pressure. Magnetic resonance scanning can demonstrate the defect and measure the shunt.

Surgical closure is advised unless pulmonary artery pressure has risen too high.

COARCTATION OF THE AORTA

Coarctation of the aorta is a narrowing, or even complete interruption, of the aorta distal to the aortic arch, with

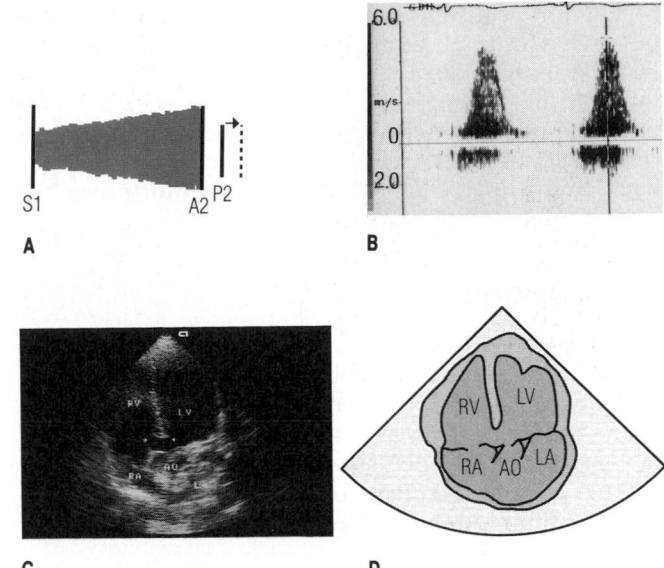

Fig. 12.50 Features of ventricular septal defect. A. The characteristic systolic murmur associated with a widely split second heart sound with a premature aortic second sound (A2) and maintained mobility of P2 with respiration (dashed line on inspiration). **B.** Doppler ultrasound showing high velocity jet (6 m/s). **C** and **D.** 2D echocardiogram showing the septal defect (VSD). IVS = interventricular septum.

blood flow to the lower body augmented by flow carried through collateral vessels. Coarctation represents about 5% of adult congenital heart disease, and is seen in males three times as frequently as females. The condition leads to upper body hypertension and an increased risk of aortic dissection. There is often a bicuspid aortic valve, which can become stenotic (or is congenitally stenosed). Other congenital defects are sometimes associated. There is also an associated risk of subarachnoid haemorrhage from berry aneurysm of the circle of Willis. These are presumed to be an associated congenital anomaly.

The coarctation is nearly always at the aortic isthmus distal to the left subclavian artery, but can, rarely, occur proximal to it. It may be due to ductal tissue in the wall of the aorta leading to progressive stenosis of the aorta, as in ductal closure. The degree of stenosis becomes comparatively more severe as the child grows. The coarctation is followed by a poststenotic dilatation in most cases; however, if there is complete interruption of the aorta, there may be some atresia of the descending aorta.

Clinical features

Presenting complaints include left ventricular failure, subarachnoid haemorrhage and aortic dissection; however, most cases should be identified in childhood. The coarctation itself may become the site of an endocarditis, as may the bicuspid valve.

The physical signs are hypertension, a large volume pulse in the arms and carotids, and weak, delayed, femoral pulses. Occasionally, the left subclavian is involved in the coarctation, producing weak left arm pulses. There is often palpable left ventricular hypertrophy, a systolic murmur over the precordium and in the back, and palpable collateral arteries running over the medial aspects of the scapulae.

Investigation

Diagnosis is confirmed by Doppler ultrasound, demonstrating a lower systolic blood pressure in the ankles than in the brachial artery. The chest X-ray often shows the characteristic '3' sign over the aortic knuckle, with the upper half being the left subclavian artery and the lower half the poststenotic dilatation of the aorta. Rib-notching is seen in most adults with coarctation, and is caused by the collateral arteries.

Visualisation of the coarctation is sometimes possible using 2D echocardiography, and the jet can often be located with Doppler ultrasound. Angiography of the aorta is not always needed, but cardiac catheterisation is often performed to look for associated lesions and to confirm the length of the narrow segment.

Management and prognosis

Significant coarctation should always be corrected in children, either surgically or by balloon catheter. In adults, surgical management is more difficult and carries a high morbidity and mortality, due to established hypertension with changes in the aortic wall. Reversal of hypertension does not occur if the correction is performed late. The associated aortic valve lesions may progress and subarachnoid haemorrhage may occur. Endocarditis prophylaxis is necessary.

PERSISTENT DUCTUS ARTERIOSUS

Persistent ductus arteriosus (PDA) is a congenital abnormality caused by failure of the ductus arteriosus to close and form the ligamentum arteriosum. The result is a shunt of blood from the aorta into the pulmonary circulation. The shunt is from the aorta just distal to the left subclavian artery, and so an increased flow occurs through the left heart and pulmonary circulation but not the right heart.

The ductus arteriosus remains patent for a variable time after birth, and failure to close can be associated with congenital abnormalities other than PDA. The isolated lesion is usually diagnosed in childhood from the presence of a continuous or 'machinery murmur' at the upper left sternal edge.

Clinical features

Overload of the left heart can lead to heart failure in older patients. The increased lung blood flow in infants can present with the consequences of increased pulmonary vascular resistance: extremely rarely, reversal of the flow through the ductus with cyanotic blood passing to the distal aorta occurs, producing clubbing of the toes but not the fingers. Rarely, the ductus may be the site of endocarditis.

Investigation and management

Diagnosis is based on the physical findings of the characteristic murmur, a collapsing pulse and a chest X-ray which usually shows a prominent pulmonary conus and increased lung blood flow.

Echocardiography and Doppler ultrasound are extremely useful in demonstrating both the lesion and the volume load on the left ventricle. Cardiac catheterisation with aortography is not usually necessary in the uncomplicated case, but it may be useful in differentiating the much less common aorto-pulmonary window, which requires much more complex surgery.

The simple case requires ligation and transection of the PDA.

COR TRIATRIATUM

In cor triatriatum the left atrium is divided by a diaphragm above the mitral valve which gives rise to obstruction to pulmonary venous return to the left heart. There is a variable size orifice (or none at all) which is easily opened surgically. The condition is thus eminently treatable.

DEXTROCARDIA

Dextrocardia – in which there is a mirror image of the normal heart – is usually quite benign if associated with situs inversus (stomach bubble also on the right); however, it may be associated with other congenital abnormalities and can be confused with dextroversion, in which the heart is rotated rather than being a mirror image.

ISCHAEMIC HEART DISEASE

Ischaemic heart disease (IHD) can be considered virtually synonymous with coronary artery disease. Atheromatous disease outweighs all other causes, but coronary arteritis and embolism can cause ischaemia. Demand also exceeds supply in very hypertrophied ventricles, especially in aortic valve disease.

THE CORONARY CIRCULATION

Flow in normal and abnormal coronary arteries

Flow through the coronary arteries is regulated, with mean flow maintained through wide changes in mean arterial pressure (Fig. 12.51). However, coronary vascular resistance is greatly affected by extrinsic compression during cardiac muscle contraction. Compression of the intramyocardial vessels during systole means that flow occurs in diastole (Fig. 12.51). This is particularly marked for the left coronary artery. Myocardial vessels are innervated and respond to neural, humoral and local metabolites.

The heart has little capacity for anaerobic metabolism, and cannot tolerate an oxygen debt. It is therefore dependent on increased perfusion to cope with an increased oxygen demand. Myocardial oxygen extraction is not increased with increasing demand, which must be met by increased coronary flow due to coronary vasodilatation. The coronary vascular resistance will fall to 20–25% of its basal state in response to maximal demand during exercise. This ability to lower the resistance to flow explains why it is possible to maintain normal flow at rest, even when there is an 80% reduction in the diameter of a large coronary artery. The relationship between changes in perfusion pressure and resistances of coronary arteries and flow is shown in Figure 12.52.

Coronary anatomy

The anatomy of the coronary circulation is shown in Figure 12.53. Three major coronary arteries provide the heart with its blood supply. Major anatomical variations

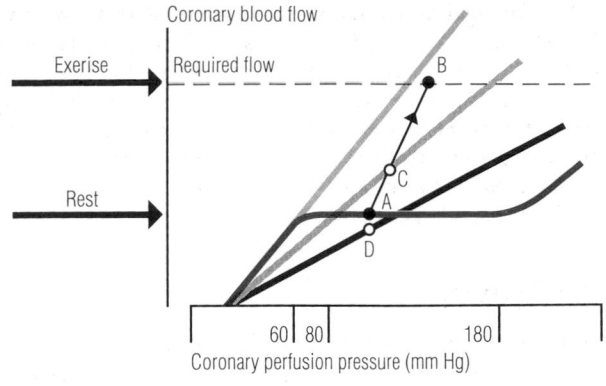

Normal coronary pressure - flow relationship

Maximally vasodilated artery, pressure flow relationship:
Normal artery
Moderately stenosed
Critically stenosed

Fig. 12.52 Effect of mean coronary arterial pressure on flow. Coronary blood flow (red line) is maintained constant despite variations in perfusion pressure. At perfusion levels below 60 mmHg coronary blood flow falls because the limit of coronary vasodilation is reached. A maximally vasodilated coronary artery has a linear pressure-flow relationship as shown (pink line). Stenoses of varying severity will alter the pressure-flow relationship of the dilated artery as shown by the grey and black straight lines. At rest an individual might have an artery flow at point A (a perfusion pressure approximately 100 mmHg), with exercise the demand rises (dashed line) and flow increases to point B, within the capacity of a normal vessel to dilate. If the individual's coronary had a moderate stenosis, only point C could have been reached, which is less than the flow required, so ischaemia (angina) is produced. A critical stenosis may interfere with the delivery of the necessary resting flow (D) so ischaemia at rest ensues.

are rare. The main stems of the left coronary artery (LCA) and right coronary artery (RCA) arise from the aorta at the sinuses of Valsalva. The main stem of the LCA is a relatively short vessel. It divides into the left anterior descending artery (LAD) – which is responsible for the blood supply to the major part of the left ventricle and the interventricular septum – and the circumflex

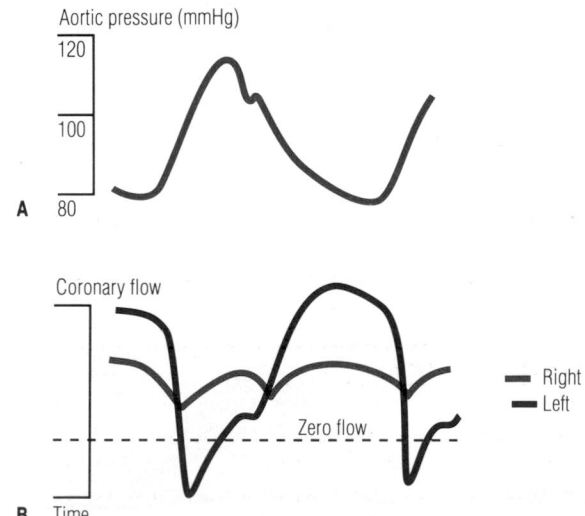

Fig. 12.51 Coronary arterial flow. A. Aortic pressure. **B.** Flow in the left and right coronary arteries. Note the abrupt fall in left coronary flow with the onset of systole.

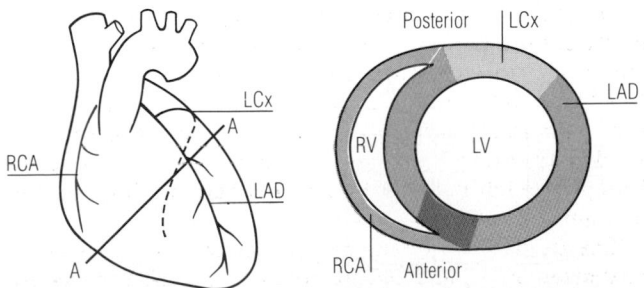

Fig. 12.53 Anatomy of the coronary circulation. LAD = left anterior descending, LCx = left circumflex (dotted line represents position of LCx at the back of the heart), RCA = right coronary artery. Section across heart (A–A) shows the approximate distribution of blood supply.

artery (Cx, usually the smaller branch of the left main stem), which supplies the posterior and variable amounts of the inferior walls of the left ventricle. The RCA supplies the right ventricle and inferior left ventricle. In some individuals, variable amounts of the left ventricular apex, septum and posterior wall may be supplied by the RCA. This artery usually (60% of cases) provides the SA and AV nodes with their blood supply.

The myocardium has a very rich capillary network which appears to be regulated by precapillary resistance vessels. In addition, there is the potential for a network of collateral vessels connecting coronary arterial networks to each other. When developed, these collaterals become important in coronary artery disease.

ATHEROMA OF THE CORONARY ARTERIES

The commonest cause of changes in the luminal diameter of the epicardial coronary arteries is the presence of atheromatous plaques (Fig. 12.54). The lesions may encircle an artery or be eccentric; they may be discrete and localised or involve the greater length of the vessel. The eccentricity of some plaques may be important when vasospasm is the cause of angina; the normal arterial wall opposite the plaque maintains its ability to contract, producing a very marked reduction in cross-sectional area even if the smooth muscle contraction is modest in degree and the atheromatous plaque small.

Acute changes in the plaques may account for unstable angina, myocardial infarction and sudden death. A fissure develops, breaching the thin endothelium which covers a lipid-rich plaque. The subsequent process is shown in Figure 12.54. These events appear to account for many of the more acute forms of coronary disease, and have renewed interest in the role of thrombosis in acute cardiac ischaemia. This has led to the successful use of fibrinolytic agents and aspirin in the treatment of infarction (p. 403).

Under some circumstances atheromatous plaques may regress. This has been achieved by drugs which lower LDL cholesterol and triglyceride and increase HDL cholesterol.

Clinical features

Symptoms

The cardinal symptom is angina pectoris. This is a chest discomfort precipitated by exertion and relieved by rest. It is often described as a pressing or constricting feeling and, less often, as a pain. It remains remarkably constant within each individual, even though its precipitants may vary significantly from day to day. The patient may hold a clenched fist in front of the sternum to indicate the squeezing nature of the pain, and may describe radiating discomfort in the arm (left more often than right), the jaw or even a choking sensation in the throat. Dyspnoea frequently accompanies angina. There is usually rapid relief of the symptom with sublingual, or spray, glyceryl trinitrate.

The pain of myocardial infarction may be similar, but generally begins at rest, does not respond so well to nitrates, lasts longer than 20 min and is often associated with feelings of impending death, nausea, sweating and collapse.

Unfortunately, in many patients with IHD, the first manifestation of the disease may be sudden death. Prevention of atheroma is necessary to reduce this, although out-of-hospital resuscitation may improve the survival of the few fortunate enough to collapse within reach of a person competent in basic life support.

Signs

There are few physical findings in uncomplicated IHD. An underlying cause such as aortic stenosis may give characteristic signs. There may be evidence of hypertension or hyperlipidaemia. Cardiac dilatation, hypertrophy and failure are all late features and are non-specific.

Some individuals undoubtedly have significant ischaemic episodes without symptoms. This may be discovered

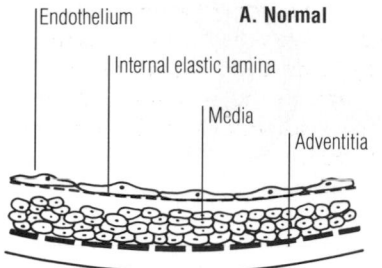
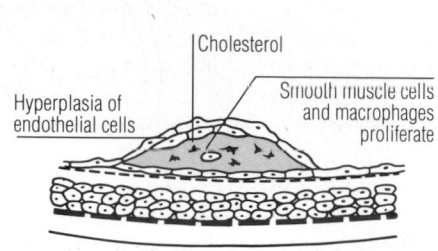
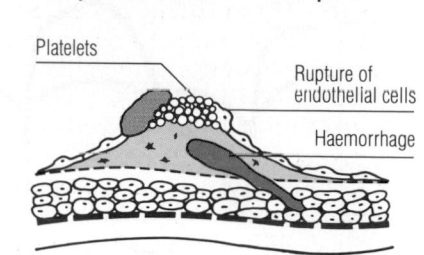

Fig. 12.54 Progression of atheromatous lesion. A and B. Normal endothelium and structure of atheromatous plaque. **C.** Acute expansion of the lesion occurs when the endothelial cells rupture, allowing haemorrhage into the plaque and platelet aggregation on the endothelial surface.

by routine ECG, when pathological Q waves may be found with no history of any antecedent chest pains. Investigations of patients with ambulatory recorders have also shown some individuals to have changes in the ST segments usually associated with ischaemia, despite a total lack of symptoms. Even patients with known angina may have episodes of ST segment change which appear to be clinically silent. Patients with known coronary disease who have silent ischaemia fare worse than those without this finding.

Other anginal syndromes

The above is a description of typical stable atheromatous coronary artery disease. Several other anginal syndromes occur which are less common but which often have implications for management.

Crescendo angina and unstable angina

Both crescendo and unstable angina may represent states of preinfarction. In *crescendo angina*, a history of increasingly frequent attacks of angina with ever-diminishing levels of exertion is obtained. *Unstable angina* includes situations where episodes of pain are frequent, may occur without obvious cause and at rest, and where acute infarction has been excluded. *Decubitus angina* is angina occurring at rest in bed.

Vasospastic angina

Some degree of arterial spasm is probably present in most episodes of angina, but spasm occurring in an otherwise normal coronary artery has also been observed. It can be severe enough to cause infarction, but is very rare. In *Prinzmetal's syndrome*, rest pain is frequent and is associated with acute ST segment elevation which resolves to normal with cessation of pain. This condition is rare and almost certainly involves coronary vasospasm.

Differential diagnosis of angina

Valve disease. Angina is a common symptom in aortic stenosis (p. 375) and aortic regurgitation (p. 377), particularly when the valve lesions are severe or acute. In cases of aortic regurgitation due to syphilis, chest pains may be due to severe aortic reflux, but coronary ostial stenosis may also occur. In hypertrophic cardiomyopathy, hypertrophy may lead to angina.

Aortic dissection and pulmonary embolism. These are discussed on pages 438 and 496.

Pericarditis. Chest pain may be severe with acute pericarditis and is exacerbated by movement, deep respiration or coughing. It is often relieved by sitting forward and

by non-steroidal anti-inflammatory drugs (NSAIDs). The clinical sign of pericardial friction rub may come and go.

Oesophageal spasm. The pain of oesophageal spasm may be severe and, since it occurs at rest and can be associated with T wave changes on the ECG, it may cause considerable confusion and be diagnosed as unstable angina in some patients.

Hiatus hernia with oesophagitis can cause chest pain. This can be demonstrated by infusions of mild acidic mixtures into the oesophagus of affected individuals. Radiological and endoscopic methods will demonstrate the abnormalities. IHD may coexist in the same individual.

Acute cholecystitis and peptic ulceration can produce severe pains in the lower chest and xiphisternal areas and may, infrequently, be mistaken for acute myocardial infarction. Non-specific T wave changes on the ECG have been observed during these acute illnesses.

Da Costa's syndrome (also known by several other names, e.g. neurocirculatory asthenia) has a long history and is characterised by sharp transient chest pains which occur with relaxation, may disappear with exertion and are associated with easy fatigue.

Mitral valve prolapse. Atypical (for IHD) chest pains may occur in patients with mitral valve prolapse of mild degree.

Hyperventilation. Patients who hyperventilate may produce symptoms indistinguishable from angina, and may have an abnormal resting and exercise ECG to accompany their symptoms.

So-called *Syndrome X* is characterised by typical angina in association with radiologically normal coronary arteries but a positive exercise test. It may be due to microvascular disease.

Tietze's syndrome may cause diagnostic confusion until the painful costal cartilage is palpated.

Investigation

The aim of investigations is to confirm that the clinical history is due to significant coronary artery disease, to determine at how much risk of infarction or progression the patient may be, and whether any remediable risk factors may be present. Once coronary artery disease has been confirmed using non-invasive tests, an assessment of ventricular function may be necessary and, finally, coronary angiography performed if surgery or angioplasty are being considered. (Investigation of myocardial infarction is considered on pp. 399–402.)

ECG

The resting ECG may be normal in IHD, even when it is severe. Signs of ischaemia characteristically involve the ST segments, with depression in the leads corresponding

12 Cardiovascular Disease

to the myocardial territory involved (Fig. 12.55). The associated T waves may be flattened or biphasic. These ECG signs are not specific, however; they may be found in some normal individuals and may be produced by hyperventilation or change in posture.

Exercise test

The exercise test has been described on page 336. Exercise will induce ischaemia with coronary stenoses of 70% or more (Fig. 12.55). If a population of asymptomatic individuals is subjected to an exercise test there will be an incidence of false positive tests of 10–20%. It is therefore not a good screening test for coronary artery disease in the population.

The exercise ECG has several uses:

- to detect IHD in patients with suspicious symptoms
- to gauge severity of coronary artery disease, although accurate anatomical localisation is not possible
- to identify patients at high risk of further infarction or death early after myocardial infarction
- to assess functional capacity and adequecy of treatment.

Although changes in the ST segment are the most characteristic features of a positive exercise test (Fig. 12.55), the development of angina and the workload performed up to the development of symptoms or ECG change also aid interpretation. A normal blood pressure response consists of a rise in systolic pressure by at least 20 mmHg. Diastolic pressure falls with exercise, but is so difficult to measure under these circumstances that it is not routinely taken. The gravest prognostic indicator in exercise testing is a failure of systolic pressure to rise, or even a fall. The appearance of multiple ventricular ectopic beats is also associated with severe disease.

Radionuclide studies

Radionuclide techniques (p. 341) are complementary to the other non-invasive methods used in assessing IHD. Information on ventricular wall motion abnormalities (MUGA scan) and regional perfusion (^{201}Tl scan) can be obtained.

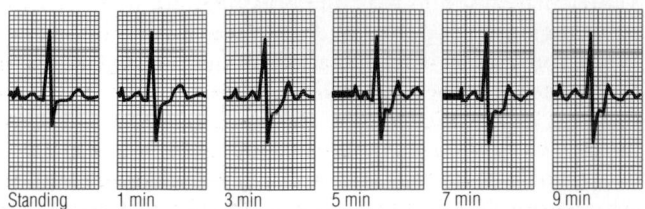

Standing   1 min   3 min   5 min   7 min   9 min

Fig. 12.55 Exercise ECG showing typical and severe down-sloping ST segment depression.

Echocardiography and Doppler ultrasound

Echocardiography (p. 339) may be useful to assess ventricular function and wall motion abnormalities, as well as excluding non-coronary causes of ischaemia such as aortic stenosis or hypertrophic cardiomyopathy.

Ambulatory ECG (Holter) monitoring

Ambulatory ECG monitoring (p. 351) is generally used to detect arrhythmias, but may also detect episodes of ST segment change during normal activities. Some of these episodes may not be accompanied by symptoms of angina (*silent ischaemia*). In the patient with known coronary disease, frequent episodes of silent ischaemia are associated with a high risk of infarction. In the patient with few or no symptoms the implications of this finding are not at all clear. The role of routine 24-hour ECG recording for ST segment analysis in IHD is not established, since it remains to be proven that the information gained is any more useful than the exercise test.

Left ventricular and coronary angiography

The aim of these investigations is to establish the functional state of the left ventricle, to exclude valve lesions which might account for the symptoms (such as occult aortic stenosis), and to obtain detailed pictures of the coronary arteries.

A global left ventricular ejection fraction (EF) of 50–70% is normal, and end diastolic pressure is usually below 12 mmHg. Subjective assessment is often sufficient to describe left ventricular wall motion abnormalities without recourse to the numerical estimation of EF.

The coronary arteries are selectively intubated and cine-angiograms taken in several projections. A 70% reduction in the diameter of an artery is generally considered to be a clinically significant stenosis.

Cardiac catheterisation provides unambiguous information on the location of coronary artery stenoses. However, the clinical significance of stenoses is sometimes difficult to judge; the exercise test and thallium scan may provide complementary information. Cardiac catheterisation is indicated in all patients in whom coronary angioplasty or coronary bypass surgery is being contemplated. In some patients with troublesome symptoms and a low likelihood of IHD, this examination is performed to finally exclude the possibility of coronary artery disease. This group may comprise between 10 and 20% of all patients undergoing cardiac catheterisation.

The invasive nature of catheterisation is necessarily associated with a morbidity ($<1.0\%$) and mortality ($<0.1\%$). This means that angiography cannot assume the role of a screening test for coronary disease.

MANAGEMENT OF CHRONIC STABLE ANGINA

Once the diagnosis is established, treatment should be aimed at restoring a normal exercise capacity. Investigations should establish the individual's risk, and contributory risk factors reduced as far as possible. A flow diagram of the management of angina is shown in Figure 12.56.

General measures

All patients should be advised to stop smoking, achieve their ideal weight and have raised blood pressure controlled. Lipid measurements should be made in patients below 50 years of age; those with severe abnormalities (total cholesterol >7.1 mmol/1; HDL/LDL <20%; triglyceride >2.0 mmol/1) should be given an appropriate diet (p. 119) until repeat estimations are within the normal ranges. Family members and children of young patients with IHD should have their lipid levels measured. The benefit of these measures in those over 50 years of age is debatable.

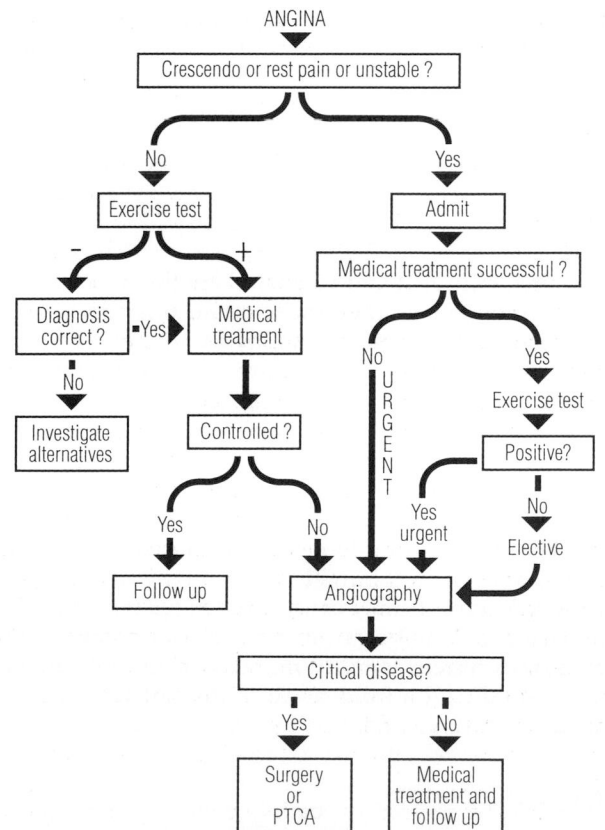

Fig. 12.56 Flow diagram of management of angina. PTCA = percutaneous transarterial coronary angioplasty.

The patient with angina of effort, a normal resting ECG and chest X-ray, and whose symptoms are well-controlled on simple treatment can probably be managed adequately without further investigation. The prognosis in IHD is dependent on the severity of the stenoses, the number of coronary arteries involved and on left ventricular function. This information can only be obtained accurately at cardiac catheterisation, which should be offered to patients below 40 years of age, whose risk is highest. The risk of death is approximately 4% per year in other patients, but increases to between 7 and 9% if there are associated abnormalities in the resting ECG. In many (up to 33%), angina may spontaneously resolve. Thus, although a resting ECG may be sufficient investigation for many patients, further determination of the risk to the individual is obtained by non-invasive tests, especially the exercise test. Catheterisation may then be required for those with a positive test at low workloads, or those in whom medical treatment is not being successful.

Drug treatment

The drugs commonly used in the treatment of angina are listed in Table 12.17.

Aspirin

Although not a symptomatic treatment, all patients should be given 75–150 mg of aspirin per day as an antithrombotic agent.

Nitrates

Therapy begins with sublingual or aerosol spray nitrates. These are used to treat an anginal episode and can be successfully used in prophylaxis by patients with predictable symptoms. The aerosol spray has the advantage of a long storage life compared with glyceryl trinitrate tablets, which deteriorate rapidly in their container. The onset of action is very rapid (within 1–2 min) and its duration can be up to 20 minutes. With all nitrates, troublesome headache can prevent their use in certain susceptible individuals, although this side-effect usually stops after a few days of treatment.

Longer-acting nitrate preparations include glyceryl trinitrate given via the skin, using small sustained-release plasters or patches. Isosorbide dinitrate is absorbed from the gut and metabolised by the liver to the active mononitrates. The duration of action is longer, but 6–8-hourly doses are needed to maintain blood levels. Mononitrates are absorbed in the gut and do not require hepatic conversion; thus, some variability in effectiveness due to liver metabolism is avoided. Their duration of action is longer, so one or two daily doses are adequate.

12 Cardiovascular Disease

Table 12.17 Drugs commonly used in the treatment of angina

Drug	Route	Dose	Frequency
Nitrates			
Glyceryl trinitrate (GTN)			
Tablets	Sublingual	0.3–0.6 mg	PRN and prophylaxis
Spray	Oral	0.4 mg/spray	PRN and prophylaxis
Patches	Skin	5–10 mg	Daily (omit for 8–12 hours)
Isosorbide dinitrate (ISDN)	Various types oral sustained release	20–80 mg	8-hourly
Isosorbide mononitrate	Oral	20–120 mg	12-hourly
Parenteral preparations			
GTN	i.v.	0.6–12 mg/h	Infusion
ISDN	i.v.	1–12 mg/h	Infusion
Beta-blockers. Many alternatives, including:			
Atenolol (beta-1 selective)	Oral	50–100 mg/day	Daily
Propranolol (non-selective)	Oral	30–360 mg/day	6-hourly
Calcium antagonists			
Nifedipine	Oral	10–20 mg	8-hourly (12–24-hourly for sustained release)
Diltiazem	Oral	60–120 mg	8-hourly (12- or 24-hourly for sustained release)
Verapamil	Oral	80–120 mg	8-hourly (12-hourly for sustained release form)

Tolerance

Tolerance to nitrates develops as sulphydryl (SH) groups on the vessel walls become oxidised by constant exposure to nitrates; this prevents the production of nitric oxide and stimulation of guanidylate cyclase, which is believed to be fundamental to the smooth muscle relaxation produced by these drugs. A nitrate-free period of 6 hours is sufficient to allow recovery of SH groups when longer-acting preparations are used.

Beta-blocking drugs

Beta-adrenoreceptor blockade has become established as a cornerstone in the treatment of angina. Although many beta-blocking drugs with varying pharmacological properties are available, there is no overwhelming evidence to suggest one drug is any better than the others. They are specifically contraindicated in patients with obstructive airways disease and severe ventricular dysfunction, and relatively contraindicated in diabetes and in those with peripheral vascular disease, bradycardia or heart block. Some patients find they are unpleasant due to a mild 'sedative' action and an interference with exercise capacity.

In angina, these drugs achieve their benefit by a reduction in myocardial oxygen demand consequent on the fall in heart rate, blood pressure and myocardial contractility that is produced.

Calcium antagonists

Nifedipine, diltiazem and verapamil are the three types of calcium antagonists; they vary in their pharmacological properties so their indications may be different. Calcium antagonists are certainly effective in angina, achieving their effect by smooth muscle relaxation in the coronary arteries and peripheral circulation, increasing myocardial supply and reducing myocardial work. The manner in which this is achieved varies with the three drugs, all of which inhibit cellular calcium entry, but differ in their tissue specificity. Nifedipine acts primarily by arteriolar vasodilatation with minimal effects on the SA node and the myocardium. It may cause a reflex tachycardia, so is often used in combination with a beta-blocker. The action of diltiazem is more marked on the SA and AV nodes, producing a mild bradycardia but less negative inotropy than verapamil.

Other compounds

Amiodarone is an effective antianginal preparation but has such potentially toxic side-effects (Table 12.6) that its use is limited to the treatment of potentially lethal arrhythmia.

Perhexilene alters the metabolism of cardiac muscle from FFA to glucose and can be effective in refractory angina. However in certain indentifiable genotypes, it can have serious side-effects, including hepatotoxicity and peripheral neuropathy.

Drug combinations in angina

There is a progression in therapy before medical treatment can really be said to have failed. Most patients begin treatment with nitrates and a beta-blocker or a calcium antagonist. Elderly patients may well be adequately controlled with nitrates and a reduction in activity, and many find that beta-blockers induce unpleasant lethargy. Younger patients may not wish to reduce their activity, and find the prophylactic action of beta-blockers or calcium antagonists a considerable advantage. Verapamil and diltiazem may produce profound bradycardia or heart block when used with a beta-blocker, so these combinations should be used cautiously. Patients with severe disease commonly require 'triple therapy' to control their symptoms.

Surgical treatment of angina

Effective surgical treatment has had a marked effect on the management of IHD in the developed world. Coronary artery bypass grafting can now be performed with an overall operative mortality of under 1%. Symptoms can be eradicated in 80–90% of patients and improved considerably in a further 5–10%; a few are no better or, indeed, are worse following surgery. It might therefore be asked why this form of therapy, which aims to 'revascularise' the heart, is not offered to all patients with angina. Several factors are responsible, including:

- finite morbidity from opening the chest
- deterioration of grafts
- survival advantage for surgical treatment has been proven for only high risk subgroups of patients
- benefit in symptoms has to outweigh the cost in well-being for up to 12 weeks post-operatively.

Deterioration of grafts

Saphenous vein bypass grafts have an appreciable rate of deterioration; more than 90% are patent immediately after surgery, but then occlude at a rate of approximately 2% of grafts per year between 5 and 10 years and at 4% per year thereafter. About 60% of grafts are patent after 10 years. This implies surgery is not a permanent cure, merely another method of symptom control in these patients.

Improvements in early vein patency rates have been achieved by the use of antithrombotic agents, such as aspirin. Even more significant has been the use of the internal mammary artery (gastroepiploic or internal thoracic artery) as a graft. The use of this vessel is slightly more demanding technically, but has been shown to provide greater than 90% patency rates at 10 years. Unfortunately, complete cardiac revascularisation is not often possible even when both internal mammary arteries are used.

Survival advantage

Survival is improved by surgery (Table 12.18) in those with left main stem disease and those with three vessel coronary disease and impaired left ventricular function. It is very likely to improve survival in patients with severe angina, three vessel coronary disease and normal ventricular function. The situation is less clear for patients with less marked symptoms and those with little in the way of symptoms but with a positive exercise test, although evidence is mounting that this group of patients also benefit from surgery.

Surgery appears to be a more effective treatment for patients with continued symptoms not controlled by drugs. There is a diminution in fatal heart attacks, but probably not in non-fatal events. Randomised studies have failed to show any differences between medical and surgical treatment in the numbers of patients who return to work, or in the amount of recreational activity they take up. However, the sociological measures may not reflect the changes in perceived quality of life in the two groups of patients.

Thus, in general, patients are considered for coronary artery surgery if medical therapy fails to control adequately their symptoms, or if they fall into the above high-risk groups. These broad guidelines conceal a large number of patients in a rather grey area, in whom individual assessments must be made. These might include young patients with severe stenoses causing highly positive exercise tests, in whom the consequences of occlusion might be a disabling infarction and in whom an internal mammary graft might be expected to be highly successful treatment.

Table 12.18 Indications for coronary artery surgery in angina

Indication	Comment
Left main stem stenosis	Proven survival benefit of surgery
Symptoms uncontrolled despite maximal medical treatment	Improved survival with surgery in some subgroups of patients
Impaired LV function especially with three vessel coronary artery disease	Improved survival with surgery
Proximal stenosis in left anterior descending coronary artery *with* positive exercise test at low workload	Likely improved survival with surgery (but debatable)

Patients with extensive left ventricular aneurysm may often improve, in terms of heart failure control and anginal symptoms, with plication or resection of the aneurysmal area.

Percutaneous transarterial coronary angioplasty

The indications for percutaneous transarterial coronary angioplasty (PTCA), first introduced in 1977, are

Table 12.19 Indications for coronary angioplasty

Indication	Comment
All indications for surgery (except left main stem stenosis) where coronary lesions suitable*	Single and double vessel PTCA. Low risk, high efficacy
Symptomatic single vessel coronary disease	PTCA is as good and safe as surgery but patients face a higher incidence of recurrence
Coronary disease where surgery impossible ('salvage PTCA')	Uncommon, but a suitable approach in the very elderly or infirm
In AMI especially if thrombolysis contraindicated	A survival advantage over medical treatment has been suggested

*Suitable coronary lesions: Proximal, discrete, not involving major branches, recent onset, non-calcified, circumferential lesions.

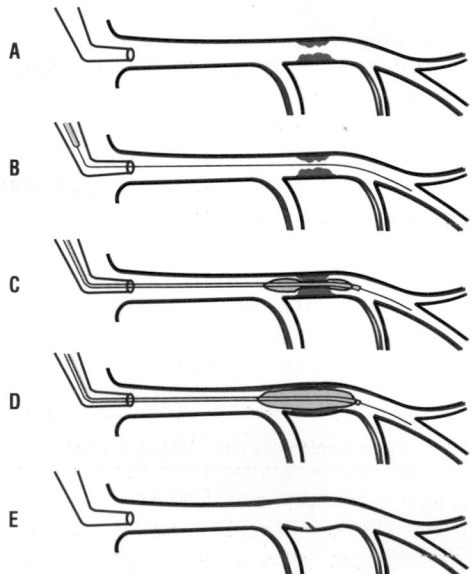

Fig. 12.57 Technique of coronary angioplasty. A. The guide catheter is introduced into the coronary ostium. **B.** A steerable guide wire is advanced across the lesion. **C.** The balloon catheter is advanced from the guiding catheter over the guide wire and positioned so that the balloon straddles the narrowing. **D.** Balloon inflation splits and compresses the atheromatous plaque. **E.** After deflation, the balloon and wire are removed and the arterial wall shows only mild irregularity at the site of the narrowing.

changing with experience (Table 12.19). The technique of PTCA is illustrated in Figure 12.57. In general, the patients treated are the same as those that would be selected for surgery. In most centres, one or two stenoses are tackled by angioplasty, and patients with severe three vessel coronary disease are not generally considered. Patients with left main stem disease are also not considered for PTCA, unless surgery is impossible for technical reasons or due to coincidental disease.

Recurrence rate. This varies from 15 to 30% of successful dilatations. Virtually all recurrences occur within 3 months of the first dilatation. The vast majority of these can be redilated, and 70–80% remain patent. The cause of recurrence is unknown, but most patients are given antithrombotic treatment with aspirin and/or dipyridamole, and antivasospastic medication with calcium antagonists and/or nitrates.

Immediate complications. Occlusion of the vessel being dilated may occur, causing myocardial infarction in 3–4% of patients, and precipitating urgent coronary artery surgery in 3–4% and death in 1–3%. Most operators use nitrates, aspirin, calcium antagonists and anticoagulation but it is not clear which of these, if any, is able to prevent complications.

Newer techniques

So-called interventional cardiology is a rapidly evolving field. In order to extend the principles of PTCA to more demanding lesions, various devices have been developed. These include laser-assisted PTCA (mostly for occlusions on calcified lesions); atherectomy devices; implantable coronary stents and catheters capable of delivering drugs or other therapies directly to the lesion. Their precise roles remain to be defined.

UNSTABLE ANGINA

Management

The diagnosis relies on the clinical history of crescendo angina (p. 393) or rest pain, which is not due to infarction. The patient should be admitted into a coronary care unit where complete bed rest is imposed. Light sedation is helpful.

Medical therapy includes increasing inspired oxygen, low-dose aspirin (75 mg orally) to reduce platelet aggregability and intravenous heparin to minimise thrombus formation. Nitrates (buccal or IV) should be given as a first-line anti-anginal therapy. Isosorbide dinitrate infusion is recommended, but if glyceryl trinitrate is given then the anticoagulation status should be monitored as glyceryl trinitrate is more likely to render heparinisation less effective. Close monitoring of blood pressure is required during nitrate infusion, and the systolic pressure should not be reduced by more than 20%. Beta-blockers and calcium antagonists may be added whenever appropriate. Routine use of thrombolytics in unstable angina has not been established. Opiates should be used if pain is persistent.

If medical treatment fails to control symptoms, coronary angiography should be undertaken. Suitable lesions may be dealt with by intracoronary thrombolysis, angioplasty or bypass surgery. If there is delay in performing these interventions, insertion of intra-aortic balloon counter-pulsation (balloon inflated during diastole in descending aorta, thereby increasing coronary perfusion pressure, and deflated during systole, thereby decreasing the afterload during left ventricular ejection) may be required to alleviate ischaemia.

MYOCARDIAL INFARCTION

About 200 000 people suffer a myocardial infarction each year in the UK. Half die from the infarction, and of these, half do so before they reach hospital (Fig. 12.58). Most of this group suffer an arrhythmia and death occurs instantaneously or within 1 hour of the first symptom. Clearly, these deaths will only be avoided by measures which prevent the development of coronary disease, although pre-hospital and community resuscitation schemes can make an impact.

Hospital admissions for infarction total 70–80 000 per year in the UK, with an overall in-hospital mortality around 10% and a 10% mortality in the first year.

The acute mortality varies with the type of infarct, from 3–6% for the patient with an uncomplicated infarction injuring only a limited amount of myocardium, to 50–80% with massive myocardial necrosis and shock (Table 12.20). The amount of muscle damaged determines both early and late outcomes from infarction.

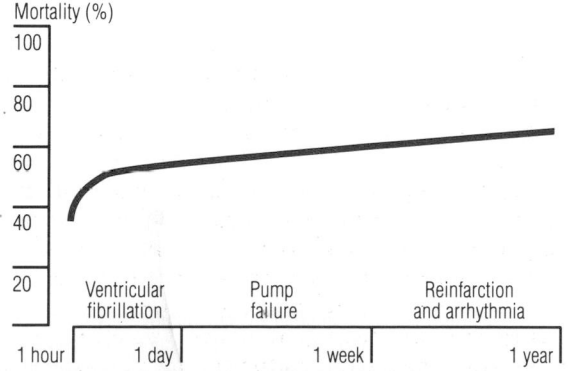

Fig. 12.58 Mortality following onset of acute myocardial infarction. A high proportion of patients die of ventricular fibrillation within 1 hour of onset.

Table 12.20 Mortality from acute myocardial infarction

Class	Definition	Admissions (%)	Mortality (%)
I	Uncomplicated, without clinical signs of LV failure	33	6
II	Generally asymptomatic, but manifesting a ventricular third sound, basal crackles or raised venous pressure	38	17
III	Clinical evidence of pulmonary oedema	10	38
IV	Cardiogenic shock indicated by a systolic EP below 90 mmHg and at least one of: oliguria (<20 ml/h), low skin temperature, or mental confusion	19	81

Data from: Killip and Kimball 1969 A M J Cardiol 20:457–467.

The advent of coronary care units (CCU) has led to a reduction in acute mortality, which has fallen from over 20% to 10% from 1966–67 to 1981–84.

DIAGNOSIS OF MYOCARDIAL INFARCTION

The clinical syndrome is less precise than the pathological definition, but a working diagnosis includes two of the following:

- a typical history
- the evolution of characteristic ECG change ending with Q wave formation
- a significant elevation and subsequent fall in creatine phosphokinase, preferably the MB isoenzyme fraction, aspartate transaminase, hydroxybutyrate dehydrogenase, or cardiac troponin-T.

CLINICAL FEATURES

History

A squeezing or tight chest or epigastric pain, with its onset at rest is reported by 80% of patients, a large proportion (40%) of whom may have an antecedent history of angina. The pain lasts longer than angina, typically more than 20 min, and is resistant to treatment with sublingual or buccal nitrates. Associated symptoms are sweating, nausea, vomiting, breathlessness and collapse. Like angina, the pain may radiate to the arms, throat and jaw. Many patients believe they are suffering from indigestion and consume antacids. With the advent of thrombolytic therapy, it has become even more important to be aware of possible differential diagnoses in the patient with acute chest pain (p. 393).

12 Cardiovascular Disease

Examination

There are no specific features that accompany myocardial infarction. During the acute phase, patients vary a great deal in their appearance, and the physical signs are largely those associated with pain and fear and are initially dominated by autonomic nervous activity. With *acute anterior infarction*, there is a tendency for sympathetic activity to dominate, with a tachycardia, cool pale periphery and a normal, or even slightly raised, blood pressure in the early minutes. This contrasts with *acute inferior infarction*, which is commonly associated with massive vagal discharge, producing a cold sweaty periphery, bradycardia, hypotension, nausea and vomiting.

The blood pressure tends to fall to lower than normal levels for the patient within a few hours of infarction but some may have a hypertensive reaction. The venous pressure is generally normal in the early stages unless there has been extensive right ventricular involvement, which may occur with an inferior or posterior infarction. In left ventricular infarction, heart failure may develop and the pulmonary venous pressure will rise signifying severe myocardial damage. Auscultation commonly reveals a fourth heart sound and a third sound over the apex in those patients in incipient left ventricular failure. The left ventricular impulse may be anterior and dyskinetic when a large segment of left ventricular wall is moving paradoxically; this is particularly marked later in those individuals who develop an aneurysm. Orthopnoea and basal crackles are present in patients developing pulmonary oedema.

A pyrexia develops within 12 hours in patients who suffer significant myocardial injury; it may persist for up to a week and is associated with a polymorphonuclear leucocytosis. Pericardial friction rubs are occasionally encountered soon after infarction, and signify a large loss of myocardium extending to the epicardium. This finding is distinct from the pericarditis and pneumonitis of Dressler's syndrome which usually, but not always, occurs during the first 6 weeks after a myocardial infarction and has an immunological basis (p. 409).

Other physical signs in myocardial infarction are due to the mechanical complications of the condition and are discussed individually below.

INVESTIGATION

ECG changes in acute infarction

The ECG changes of acute infarction may take some hours to develop and, occasionally, are absent completely. Treatment of acute infarction must often begin before there is any objective evidence confirming the diagnosis (a rise in plasma enzyme levels also takes some hours to occur).

ST segment elevation

The most characteristic feature of infarction on the ECG is the development of ST segment elevation, with a convex upward pattern in the leads facing the area of ventricle infarcted. The diastolic isoelectric line is depressed, so accentuating the ST elevation that follows it (Fig. 12.59). Reciprocal ST depression is often seen in leads opposite the infarction; this is usually indicative of severe multiple vessel coronary disease, but may on occasion represent a purely electrical phenomenon.

ST elevation (the *current of injury*) is produced by ischaemia, and can occur in the absence of infarcted tissue. Thus, such ST changes can be associated with anginal pain due to coronary vasospasm (Prinzmetal's angina) and resolve rapidly and completely when spasm is relieved and ischaemia reversed. ST elevation during acute infarction lasts for some days but may persist longer. If it is still present some weeks after infarction, left ventricular aneurysm or extensive dyskinesia is likely.

T wave inversion

The terminal portion of the T wave begins to invert within hours of infarction and produces symmetrical

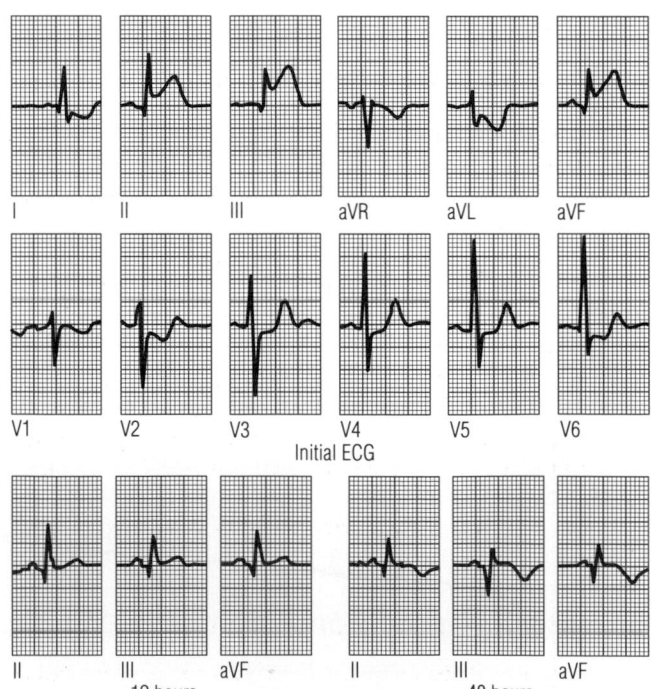

Fig. 12.59 Evolution of ECG change in an acute inferior infarction. Initially, there is marked ST segment elevation in II, III, aVF and reciprocal depression in V2–V4. At 12 hours, a Q-wave is developing in II, III and aVF and the ST segment has returned to the baseline. At 48 hours the Q wave has deepened and broadened and there is T wave inversion.

inversion after a few days (Fig. 12.59). This appearance persists for weeks or months and, occasionally, is a permanent feature of the ECG. In some patients at the very earliest stage of infarction, the only ECG change may be in the T waves, which become very prominent, peaked and symmetrical. This appearance is sometimes called the *hyperacute pattern* of infarction. Symmetrical T inversion alone, without Q wave formation, may indicate a limited infarction in some patients (see non-Q wave infarction, below) and this has important implications for their management.

Q wave formation

Q waves are often the latest change to be seen on ECG. They are often permanent and are sometimes considered the definitive ECG change of infarction. They must have a depth of at least 25% of the succeeding R wave height (or greater than 3 mV) and last longer than 40 ms (one small square at 25 mm/s). They may appear within 24 hours of infarction and are associated with loss in R wave height of the corresponding leads.

Alternative patterns

Ideally, ECG proof of infarction should include successive traces showing the presence and resolution of ST segment elevation, T wave inversion and pathological Q wave formation (Fig. 12.59). Often, such a classical progression is missing and the diagnosis may rest on a slightly deeper than normal Q wave in V4, loss of R wave height or the absence of the small *q* waves of initial septal depolarisation in I, aVL, V5 and V6; this may occur in septal infarction, but is also produced by incomplete left bundle branch block.

In the presence of bundle branch block, the ECG changes due to infarction may be difficult to detect or be absent. With right bundle branch block septal depolarisation occurs normally. Changes in ST segments and T waves may appear, but the ECG diagnosis of infarction often cannot be made with certainty. Bundle branch block patterns may precede infarction or be a consequence of it.

The posterior infarction (see below) may cause difficulty.

Localisation of infarction from the ECG

Although myocardial infarction can be endocardial, epicardial or involve the whole thickness of the ventricular wall, these distinctions cannot reliably be made by ECG. Localisation to an approximate region of the left ventricle is possible, however. The precordial leads give most information in this respect. If they have been correctly positioned, leads V1 and V2 face the right ventricle, although

an extra lead (V4R, at the level of V4 on the right of the sternum below V1) is better; V3 faces the interventricular septum; V4 the anterior and lateral borders; and V6 the postero-lateral wall of the left ventricle (this is because the apex faces backwards).

Inferior infarction

In inferior infarction, changes are seen in leads III, aVF and II, with reciprocal change in I, aVL and the anterior leads. Infero-lateral infarction extends to involve lead V6. The right coronary and its posterior descending branch account for most of these cases (Fig. 12.59).

Anterior infarction

Anterior infarction is extensive when leads V2 to V6 are involved with changes in I, aVL and II. There may be reciprocal changes in the inferior leads III and aVF. Anterior infarction implies involvement of the LAD coronary artery. Infarction may be antero-septal when the ECG changes are limited to leads V3 and V2. Antero-lateral infarction may present with changes in I, aVL and V5 with some involvement in V4 and V6 (Fig. 12.60).

Posterior infarction

The true posterior infarction is usually caused by occlusion in the circumflex coronary artery, and its hallmark on the ECG is a tall R wave in V1. There is often associated ST depression in leads V2 and V3, with subsequent peaking of T waves in V1–3.

Non-Q wave infarction

Non-Q wave infarction is a rather imprecise term used to identify patients who have suffered a relatively minor

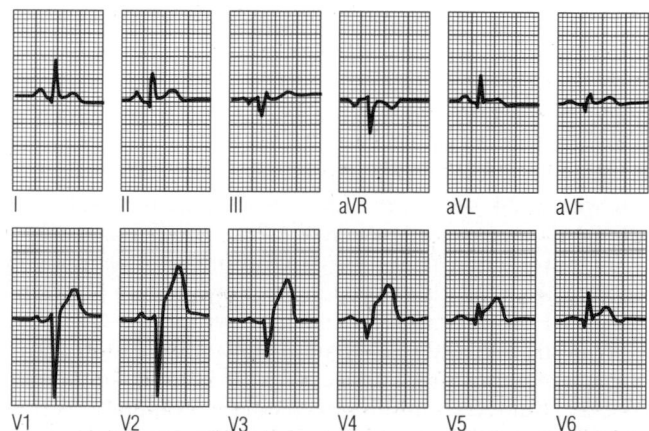

Fig. 12.60 ECG of acute anterior infarction. ST segment elevation in V1–V6 and Q waves in V2–V4 are shown.

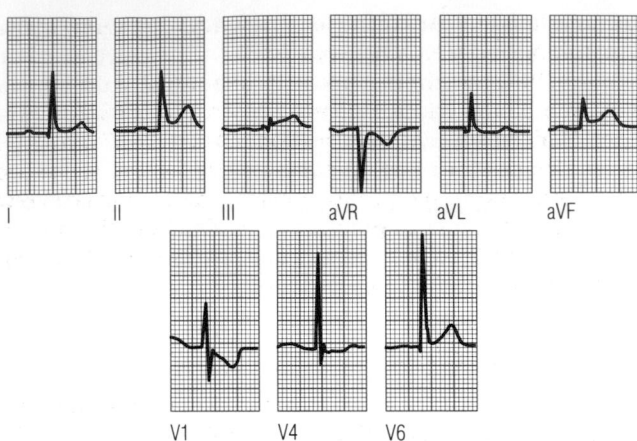

Fig. 12.61 ECG of acute posterior infarction. Inferior ST elevation (in II, III, aVF) and a tall R wave in V1 (mirror of the Q wave) are shown.

infarction. The interest in identifying these patients is that they appear to have a very high (40–60%) chance of developing a full-thickness, or Q wave, infarction in the weeks and months after presentation. Their mortality is also 20–30% higher than that for hospital survivors of infarction, presumably because some patients suffer sudden death as the next manifestation of their IHD. Previously, the term sub-endocardial infarction was used for these patients, but this implies a rather more accurate anatomical localisation than is warranted from the ECG and other clinical findings.

The features of non-Q wave infarction are a typical history with or without a modest enzyme rise, and often with T wave changes alone on the ECG. Management is along the lines followed for all high-risk postinfarction patients.

Laboratory tests

Infarction causes the release of intracellular enzymes into the circulation. These may be used to estimate the size of the infarction. The most specific enzyme available is an isoenzyme of CPK called the MB fraction (hence, CPK-MB). It is a better indicator than CPK itself, which is released into the blood with any skeletal muscle trauma. CPK and CPK-MB rise within hours of infarction, and fall within 24–48 hours. The absolute peak of CPK or CPK-MB gives a crude estimate of the size of infarction.

Lactate dehydrogenase (or its more cardiac-specific isoenzyme LDH_1) is assayed as hydroxybutyrate dehydrogenase (HBD); it appears in blood within 12–24 hours after infarction and may remain elevated for some days. Aspartate aminotransferase (AST) is relatively non-specific, but rises with an intermediate temporal position to CPK and HBD.

A raised polymorphonuclear leucocyte count, and an elevated erythrocyte sedimentation rate (ESR) are non-specific accompaniments of acute infarction. A very high ESR in the early stages of infarction raises the possibility of infarction being secondary to a giant cell arteritis or immunological disease such as polyarteritis nodosa.

Imaging techniques

Radionuclide studies may be used to measure ventricular function (MUGA scan, p. 341) or document areas of potentially reversible ischaemia (^{201}Tl scan, p. 341). The echocardiogram can be used to assess ventricular function and localise areas of infarction and dyskinesia.

DIFFERENTIAL DIAGNOSIS

Acute chest pain syndromes can pose diagnostic difficulties in acute myocardial infarction (p. 393), particularly as there are no specific physical signs in acute infarction and the diagnostic tests may be normal in the initial hours of the attack. With the advent of thrombolysis and acute beta-adrenoreceptor blockade used early in the management of acute infarction, diagnostic accuracy has become even more important.

The symptoms of *aortic dissection* (p. 438) may be very similar. Pain indistinguishable from acute cardiac ischaemia can be produced by the sudden increase in right ventricular work associated with an *acute massive pulmonary embolism*. Syncope is often the first manifestation of the embolism, which is associated with the marked dyspnoea, tachypnoea and cyanosis. *Acute pericarditis* (p. 425) produces chest pain, often accompanied by a fever and a friction rub.

MANAGEMENT OF ACUTE INFARCTION

The aims of management are pain relief, treatment of arrhythmic and mechanical complications, and infarct limitation. Management is subsequently directed to defining the relatively small proportion of patients at a greater than normal risk in the postinfarction period, and to rehabilitation and secondary prevention.

Analgesia and oxygen

Fear and pain exacerbate some of the ill effects of sympathetic hyperactivity. Analgesia and sedation is achieved with opiates, preferably diamorphine (2.5–5.0 mg i.v.) or morphine sulphate (4–8 mg i.m.). These drugs combine sedation with an advantageous vasodilatory action which improves haemodynamics. Respiratory depression is rare in the setting of acute infarction. The relief of pain itself may help raise blood pressure and reduce the heart rate. Associated nausea is treated using metoclopramide (10 mg i.v.) or prochlorperazine (12.5–25 mg i.m.). An inhaled mixture of nitrous oxide and oxygen (Entonox) provides pain relief prior to arrival in hospital.

Oxygen by mask is frequently given to patients with acute infarction to counteract the hypoxaemic effects of pulmonary oedema. However, many patients are not hypoxaemic and in these, oxygen delivery to the tissues will not be improved by this treatment.

Acute beta-adrenoreceptor blockade

Acute intravenous beta blockade can be given safely to many acute infarction patients. Large-scale trials have shown a small rate of reduction in early deaths caused by reinfarction and cardiac rupture. An additional effect is a reduction in pain. Acute intravenous beta blockade would have to be given to 200 patients to prevent one death, one reinfarction and one cardiac arrest. Chronic therapy after infarction saves two lives for every 100 patients treated for 1 year.

Limitation of infarct size

Six hours is the time limit within which it is possible that measures to restore blood supply will salvage ischaemic muscle. If collateral channels are poor, this time limit may be considerably less.

Thrombolysis

In approximately 80% of patients, a myocardial infarction is caused by thrombotic occlusion of a vessel, usually superimposed on an atherosclerotic plaque.

Intravenous infusion of streptokinase (1.2×10^6 units over 1 hour) has been shown to be nearly as effective as intracoronary treatment infusion, with a 60–70% restoration of patency. A large-scale trial has shown a reduction in acute mortality for patients treated with a single injection of streptokinase (SK) within 24 hours.

Haemorrhagic complications occur, though sufficiently rarely not to interfere with the overall beneficial effect of therapy. Patients with clotting disorders, a previous history of stroke or peptic ulceration, and those with severe hypertension or any injuries are excluded from this treatment. It is important to exclude aortic dissection, as fibrinolytic treatment can prove catastrophic. This may sometimes be difficult. Other relative contraindications are a known hypersensitivity to the drug, recent streptococcal infection, survivors from cardiac arrest who have had cardiac massage and those with heart block who may need a temporary pacemaker.

Unresolved problems with this undoubtedly effective treatment include managing the 15% of patients who suffer a reocclusion of the artery within a few days of treatment. Newer agents with less immunological side-effects, and a tendency to be more clot-specific, include

tissue plasminogen activator, now manufactured using recombinant DNA technology (rtPA).

Benefit from thrombolysis is increased if it is given within 6 hours, and preferably 3 hours, of the first symptom. This has led to a suggestion that newer fibrinolytic agents be produced which can be administered at the site of the presenting symptoms either by the ambulance crew or the family general practitioners. The benefit appears equal for the 3 commonly used agents, SK, rtPA and an acylated form of SK (anistreplase).

Aspirin and heparin

Aspirin alone reduces mortality by 25%, and, with streptokinase, a combined reduction of 45%. Continuous infusion of heparin after thrombolysis and after coronary angioplasty is routine in many centres, but formal proof that it keeps vessels patent or improves the prognosis in infarction is not yet available. Patients with large infarctions suffer fewer systemic emboli from ventricular clot if treated with heparin. Bleeding complications and stroke are slightly more common.

Angioplasty and surgery

Early revascularisation during acute infarction is possible. However, the cost of providing a 24-hour service for these complex, labour-intensive techniques is considerable. Individual cases will continue to be so treated in centres where angioplasty or surgical suites are closely linked to the acute admission wards. See also page 398.

Nitrates and calcium antagonist drugs

Nitrates by intravenous infusion (2–10 mg/h for isosorbide, 5–10 µg/min for nitroglycerin) are frequently used in the acute phase of infarction, where persistent pain is a problem; their use is associated with a modest reduction in mortality. They have the advantage of causing reduction in preload and afterload, which may relieve left heart failure (see p. 347). Hypotension can be a problem, particularly in patients who are dependent on a high right heart filling pressure to maintain stroke volume, such as patients with right ventricular infarction.

Cutaneous therapy is best reserved for the less acute stages of infarction, when converting patients from intravenous infusion to maintenance therapy. Calcium antagonist drugs are effective in improving ischaemic cardiac pain, but their use has not been associated with any improvement in infarction mortality. Nitrates and calcium antagonists are particularly useful if coronary vasospasm is contributing to the production of pain, such as in Prinzmetal's angina. Calcium antagonists can be used when there are contraindications to beta-blockade, or when adjunctive treatment is necessary.

Bed rest, mobilisation and rehabilitation

Prolonged bed rest is unnecessary and, indeed, harmful in myocardial infarction. Mobilisation can begin within 24 hours in uncomplicated infarction. Patients can generally be discharged on the tenth day, having demonstrated their ability to walk and manage a flight of stairs before returning home. Mobilisation should be slowed if there is a return of chest discomfort, a heart rate below 50 bpm or above 120 bpm, the return of ischaemic ST elevation on the ECG or an increase of more than 15 mmHg in systolic pressure with gentle ambulation.

Individual advice is required when patients are discharged. Many centres now issue booklets with advice on activity, work, diet and risk factor modification. Many patients, however, benefit from a more formal approach with a structured and supervised course of rehabilitation following a predischarge exercise test. This exercise test serves the purpose of identifying high-risk patients, and can be reassuring to the patient, illustrating the degree of exertion which can be undertaken with safety at home.

Rehabilitation programmes

Rehabilitation programmes with supervised exercise training, and usually associated relaxation therapy, counselling and educational sessions, have been taken up with variable enthusiasm. The results suggest a benefit in survival of between 25 and 35%, with an additional decrease in other coronary events. The risks in exercising postmyocardial infarction patients are small. Indices of general well-being and psychological status have been shown to improve, but it appears that the return to work is not always hastened by exercise programmes.

Ventricular function and, possibly, myocardial perfusion improve with prolonged exercise training. Most centres encourage the continued use of beta-blockers throughout exercise programmes. The amount and duration of exercise training that is required to produce benefit is 20 min of exercise at 75–80% of the maximal heart rate achieved on exercise testing, 2–3 days per week. Training effects may be seen after 6–12 weeks of this degree of effort.

Drug therapy in myocardial infarction survivors

Beta-blockers

The most successful agents in secondary prevention of further coronary events following myocardial infarction are the beta-blocking drugs. Despite differences in the pharmacology of different agents, it is likely that this effect is common to the whole class of drugs, the only exceptions being those with high intrinsic sympathomimetic activity such as oxprenolol. Sudden death and reinfarction appear to be successfully prevented. Data from all the randomised trials suggest a 10–25% reduction in mortality. Most events occur within the first 6–12 weeks of infarction. Treatment with beta-blockers is therefore recommended for at least 3 months, and, in high-risk individuals, for a year. Patients at very low risk of reinfarction or death may not require this form of treatment.

Antithrombotics

Aspirin is a safe antithrombotic. It is economical and well tolerated in the absence of peptic ulcer disease. Its role after infarction is not well established, and the precise dosage is contentious. A very small dose of 75 mg dissolved in 100 mls of water every day, or even alternate days, may have advantages over larger doses, since the desired antiplatelet activity is then achieved without the unwanted inhibition of endothelial wall prostacyclin activity. Two other antiplatelet drugs, *sulphinpyrazone* and *dipyridamole*, have no demonstrated advantage over aspirin alone.

Anticoagulants

Anticoagulation with *warfarin* following myocardial infarction has been a topic for controversy for many years. Although a small benefit in survival is apparent, particularly for a small subgroup of compliant elderly patients, there are considerable problems associated with its safe usage over many years. Where warfarin has been compared with aspirin, the benefits are equivalent and side-effects are equally common, although different. However, aspirin therapy requires much less supervision, and hence is preferable for patients and physicians alike.

Patients with extensive anterior infarction, with demonstrable intraventricular clot (shown by echocardiography) and with evidence of systemic embolisation, can have the risk of further emboli reduced by warfarin anticoagulation. The risks of emboli are highest in the first few weeks; hence, treatment may only be required for 3–4 months.

COMPLICATIONS OF MYOCARDIAL INFARCTION

ARRHYTHMIAS

Arrhythmias are a common complication of myocardial infarction.

Tachycardias

Sinus tachycardia

Sinus tachycardia (heart rate greater than 100 bpm) is associated with a poor prognosis if it persists, despite control of pain, anxiety and cardiac failure. It requires no specific therapy in most instances. Beta-blockers will reduce its incidence but cannot be given to patients with severe impairment of ventricular function.

Ventricular fibrillation

VF is a lethal arrhythmia which can complicate acute myocardial infarction from the moment of coronary occlusion. It is the cause of most cases of sudden death due to IHD. Its peak incidence is in the first few hours of the attack when it is termed primary VF and, if successfully dealt with in an otherwise uncomplicated infarction, has a good prognosis. Secondary VF occurs several days or weeks after infarction, usually in patients who have suffered extensive muscle damage and heart failure. Its prognosis is then very poor. Treatment is by DC defibrillation. The earlier it is used, the more likely is a successful outcome. The procedure itself is described fully on page 367.

Lignocaine is also given after successful defibrillation to prevent further episodes. Limitations on the use of lignocaine include its narrow therapeutic margin, with central nervous system side-effects being the most common. Doses have to be reduced in the elderly and in those with poor hepatic function. The use of lignocaine to prevent VF is controversial.

Many episodes of VF are preceded by multiple or frequent ventricular ectopic beats or early ectopics falling on the vulnerable period of the ECG – the *R on T phenomenon*. Warning arrhythmias give frequent false positive and false negative associations and their treatment does not reduce the incidence of VF.

Ventricular ectopic beats

At an early stage (6–72 hours) in an acute myocardial infarction, frequent ventricular ectopic (VE) beats (>10 VE/h) are seen in 70% of patients. Ectopy then diminishes so that only 10% of patients have frequent VEs at the time of discharge. Frequent VEs at the time of discharge from hospital carries an increased (two- to three-fold) risk of death in the first year. This association appears to be independent of ventricular function. Although drugs to effectively inhibit ectopic activity are available, controlled trials have not shown any benefit and indeed some worsening survival associated with treatment of frequent or complex VE.

Treatment of frequent VEs is indicated if their occurrence cause symptoms due to an effective bradycardia or diminished output.

Ventricular tachycardia

Haemodynamic disturbance and degeneration to VF is common with sustained VT in acute infarction. DC shock therapy is indicated in almost all cases, to be followed by intravenous or oral therapy (p. 363). Lignocaine is usually used in the acute situation, followed by other Vaughan-Williams class I drugs and amiodarone. Although drug therapy may suppress the arrhythmia the effect on survival is less certain.

Patients with non-sustained VT should probably be monitored carefully, receive a predischarge exercise test and oral antiarrhythmic therapy for the first few weeks after infarction. The risk of death is increased if VT is present at discharge.

Accelerated idioventricular rhythm

On occasion, a ventricular rhythm at a rate of 60–90 bpm can arise. It generally has broad complexes, but they may be narrow if the origin is high in the bundle of His. This rhythm rarely requires specific treatment, but may be an indication of profound sinus and AV nodal suppression which may respond to atropine (0.6–1.2 mg).

Supraventricular tachycardia

Atrial fibrillation (AF) is the commonest supraventricular tachycardia seen in acute infarction, atrial flutter being relatively uncommon. Tachycardias causing severe haemodynamic disturbance are usually best dealt with by DC cardioversion. In *atrial flutter*, this is generally the treatment of choice, as low energies are often required to convert to sinus rhythm. In AF, digoxin is given by oral loading (p. 360) (0.5–1.0 mg a.d.) followed by 0.125–0.25 mg o.d. Control of AF rate may require the concurrent administration of another drug (p. 360). Beta-blockers are often used, and verapamil or diltiazem are also effective.

Paroxysmal atrial tachycardia may complicate acute infarction; if hypotension is severe, DC cardioversion is the therapy of first choice. Intravenous adenosine or verapamil is effective in terminating many of these episodes, and intravenous beta blockade (atenolol 5 mg or metoprolol 5–15 mg) may be an alternative. If the first-choice drug fails to produce a satisfactory slowing of the rhythm or conversion to sinus rhythm, it is best to use DC cardioversion to avoid additive negative inotropic effects of antiarrhythmic drugs.

An alternative therapy for atrial flutter and atrial tachycardia is overdrive pacing; this has the advantage of avoiding negatively inotropic drugs, but requires a temporary transvenous pacemaker placed in the right atrium.

12 Cardiovascular Disease

Bradycardia

Bradycardia is often transient and requires no treatment. When bradycardia produces symptoms or impairs the haemodynamics, treatment with a pacemaker or drugs is required.

Sinus bradycardia

Up to 80% of patients with acute inferior infarction develop a heart rate less than 60 bpm in the very early stages of the condition. This usually responds to atropine (0.5–1.0 mg i.v.), but if symptomatic bradycardia persists a temporary pacemaker is required.

Heart block

First degree heart block

The lengthening of the PR interval may be seen during the evolution of an infarction, particularly inferior infarction. When pre-existing it requires no action. However, lengthening PR intervals deserve observation, as this implies interference with AV node function, and progression to higher grades of block may occur.

Second degree heart block

Both Mobitz types I and II (p. 353) require very careful observation. Progression to complete heart block and sudden death is uncommon with inferior infarction, where Mobitz type I is a frequent, though transient, complication (about 15% of cases). In anterior infarction with extensive involvement of the interventricular septum, Mobitz type II block may be seen and carries a poor prognosis (80% mortality), which owes more to the associated large mass of muscle loss than to conduction disturbance itself.

Temporary pacemakers should be used in all cases where second degree block produces symptoms (e.g. syncope) or haemodynamic disturbance, or when antiarrhythmic drugs are to be given. A permanent pacemaker should be considered for survivors of anterior infarction with persistent block.

Third degree or complete heart block

Complete heart block is a common complication of inferior infarction (about 10% of cases), when treatment is along the same lines as for second degree block. It needs no specific treatment if well tolerated, but temporary cardiac pacing should be employed if heart failure, or rates less than 50 bpm, occur. In anterior infarction, complete block (incidence approximately 5% of cases) may occur suddenly or be preceded by bifascicular block (see below). It generally occurs in large infarctions involving the septal tissue where the conducting tissue is concentrated, and always requires treatment with a permanent pacemaker. This may not always improve survival but management is eased considerably.

Complete heart block rarely persists, but if it does persist beyond 7–14 days after infarction a permanent pacemaker is required.

Bifascicular and trifascicular heart block

Interruption of conduction through the right bundle and either fascicle of the left bundle constitutes bifascicular block. When the anterior fascicle is involved (*left anterior hemiblock*, LAH) the QRS axis is greater than −30° with small r waves in II, III and aVF and absent initial q waves in V5 and V6. Posterior fascicular block (*left posterior hemiblock*, LPH) produces a rightward axis shift (greater than +100°) with an S wave in I and Q in III. Trifascicular block is any combination of bifascicular block associated with a long PR interval.

The association of right bundle branch block with LPH in anterior infarction indicates considerable ischaemic damage, and its appearance is an indication for prophylactic use of a temporary pacemaker, since progression to complete block may be sudden. Right bundle branch block with left anterior hemiblock does not carry such a poor prognosis, and is a slightly less powerful indication for pacing.

Temporary transvenous cardiac pacemakers

The indications for implanting a pacemaker in acute infarction are summarised in Table 12.21. There are various methods by which pacing can be achieved but, in general, transvenous routes are the most stable and can be maintained for the few days that are required. The methods require the insertion of a bipolar electrode into the right ventricular apex, usually under radiological control. Pacing thresholds of under 1 V at 2 ms pulse width duration should be established, since the threshold tends to rise after implantation. To achieve this, it may be necessary to try various positions in the right ventricular apex. The pacemaker is an external box which is always set in the demand mode; this ensures the patient's ventricular activity is sensed and pacing only begun when the intrinsic heart rate falls below a pre-set rate (usually between 70 and 90 bpm). A stable position of the temporary electrode is confirmed by establishing pacing at an output of 1 V, and ensuring ventricular capture is not lost during maximal inspiration, coughing or sniffing. There should be sufficient slack in the electrode to accommodate these movements of the thorax without displacing the tip of the electrode. Once the electrode position is finalised it

Table 12.21 Indications for temporary pacemaker in acute myocardial infarction (MI)

A. Indicated regardless of MI site	B. Indicated in anterior MI	C. Not indicated

Symptomatic and drug-resistant bradycardia due to:
  Sinus bradycardia, sinus arrest, SA block
  Second degree heart block
  Third degree heart block
Sick sinus syndrome with bradycardia-tachycardia
Drug-resistant tachycardia
DC shock-resistant tachycardia
Ventricular standstill
Alternating LBBB with RBBB
	All indications in **A**
	RBBB + LPHB
	RBBB + LAHB
	Trifascicular block:
	  Long PR + LBBB
	  Long PR, RBBB + LPHB or LAHB
	Second degree heart block, especially if Mobitz type II
		First degree heart block alone
		Asymptomatic Mobitz type I
		Asymptomatic bradycardia or junctional rhythm
		LAHB
		LBBB } in
		RBBB } isolation
		LPHB

is secured to the skin under a sterile dressing. Except in an emergency, it is rarely justified to manipulate a temporary pacemaker after it has been inserted for some time, since sterility cannot be ensured. If displacement has occurred, a replacement pacemaker will be required. Threshold measurements should be checked daily or more frequently if the patient is pacemaker-dependent. The pacemaker settings are adjusted to provide a voltage output of at least three to four times threshold. A threshold of over 2 V is an indication to replace the electrode.

Atrial and dual-chamber pacing

Although pacing via a ventricular electrode is sufficient in most instances, there are circumstances where atrial pacing or dual-chamber pacing are required. The former can be used to treat atrial flutter or bradycardia-dependent rhythms when AV nodal conduction is intact. Electrode positioning is more difficult and stability can be a problem.

In dual-chamber or physiological pacing, sequential pacing of first the atria followed, after a suitable pause, by the ventricles, offers a near physiological system maintaining the atrial contribution to cardiac filling. This can be very important in severe ventricular impairment, right ventricular infarction or when there is associated valvular disease, such as aortic stenosis. The technique requires suitable dual-chamber pacemakers and the expertise to implant atrial as well as ventricular electrodes; availability is thus likely to be limited to specialised cardiac centres.

CARDIAC FAILURE

Dyspnoea, basal crepitations and the radiographic signs associated with pulmonary oedema (p. 346) are frequently encountered in the early stages of infarction.

Management

Prompt treatment with intravenous loop diuretics (frusemide 20–40 mg or bumetanide 1–2 mg) has been the mainstay of treatment. Larger initial doses are often given, but are rarely necessary and may produce hypoten-

sion, worsening the patient's overall condition. Diamorphine 2.5–5.0 mg i.v. is also helpful, and oxygen, given by a close-fitting, low dead-space mask (e.g. MC mask at 4 l/min) is indicated. The preferred treatment is now with vasodilatation using intravenous nitrates, reducing preload. Patients with low blood pressure and heart failure are best managed using arterial and indirect left atrial pressure measurement. The latter is obtained with a Swan-Ganz catheter placed in a pulmonary arterial branch (see below). The aim of treatment should be to decrease the indirect left atrial pressure (or pulmonary capillary wedge pressure) to less than 20 mmHg, whilst maintaining systolic blood pressure above 100 mmHg and diastolic pressure over 60 mmHg. Nitrates with inotropes (dobutamine ± dopamine) may be better than diuretics in these difficult cases. A week after infarction, introduction of ACE inhibitors has been shown to improve prognosis.

CARDIOGENIC SHOCK

Cardiogenic shock in myocardial infarction is defined as hypotension with a systolic pressure under 100 mmHg; it is invariably accompanied by ventricular failure, peripheral vasoconstriction and oliguria (< 20 ml/h of urine) and usually arterial hypoxaemia, mental confusion and metabolic acidosis. Remediable causes, such as uncontrolled pain, arrhythmia or excesses of negatively inotropic or vasodilating drugs (e.g. beta-adrenoreceptor blockers or calcium antagonists and diamorphine) should be excluded and treated specifically.

Shock is caused by damage affecting 30–40% of ventricular muscle mass and, if untreated, carries an 80–100% acute mortality. Treatment may reduce early mortality but it remains high (approximately 50–60% at 1 month).

Right ventricular infarction may produce cardiogenic shock, as defined above, but carries a very much better prognosis. The findings are a lower than expected indirect left atrial pressure and a relatively high right atrial pressure. The ECG shows changes of inferior or posterior infarction, and lead V4R may reveal the infarction clearly. Treatment consists of maintenance of a high right-sided filling pressure which may have been inadvertently lowered by diuretics given to treat the seemingly high venous pressure. The cardiac output and systemic pressure may respond to infusion with colloid. Inotropes and diuretics may thus be avoided altogether in these patients.

Management

Pressure monitoring, including indirect left atrial pressure, systemic arterial pressure and a facility for measuring cardiac output, are the minimum requirements for managing patients with shock. Therapy consists of inotropic agents, diuretics and, very rarely, mechanical support of respiration by ventilation and of the circulation with intra-aortic balloon counterpulsation (see below).

Inotropic agents are required to maintain the systolic pressure to perfuse the tissues, but are arrhythmogenic and may increase oxygen requirement. Diuretics are used to relieve pulmonary oedema, but adequate ventricular filling pressures must be maintained or else cardiac output falls. The inotropic agents of choice are dopamine, dobutamine and phosphodiesterase inhibitors (milrinone, enoximone and amrinone).

Dopamine

Dopamine has three important actions which appear at increasing dose ranges. Low-dose dopamine infusion (0.5–2.5 μg/kg/min) primarily produces renal and mesenteric vessel dilatation, and is frequently used at this dose as a renal protector during times of systemic hypotension. Medium-dose dopamine infusion (5.0–10 μg/kg/min) has a direct myocardial inotropic action and at high doses (>10 μg/kg/min), the drug produces peripheral vasoconstriction (alpha-adrenoreceptor-mediated) so raising systemic pressure at the cost of vasoconstriction in tissue beds, including renal. The drug must be infused through a large central vein and, at medium to high infusion rates, may precipitate cardiac arrhythmias.

Dobutamine

Dobutamine is a synthetic dopamine analogue which directly stimulates beta$_1$ receptors; unlike dopamine, it does not release noradrenaline, and hence is less affected by the reduction in cardiac stores of this hormone in chronic heart failure. Dobutamine can be used via a peripheral vein and the dose is usually between 2.5 and 40 μg/kg/min. Its action is primarily inotropic, and hence improves cardiac output whilst at the same time reducing ventricular filling pressures.

Combination therapy

Dopamine in low dose to promote renal bed vasodilatation and dobutamine in doses to achieve an improved cardiac output are often used in combination in cardiogenic shock; thus, lower doses of each can be used. Filling pressures (measured via a Swan-Ganz catheter) are titrated against systemic pressure, and the drug dosages adjusted every 10 min to achieve an optimal cardiac output and sufficient perfusion pressure to maintain renal, cerebral and myocardial function, whilst avoiding excessive heart rates and pulmonary oedema. Ideally, therefore, the dose of dobutamine is adjusted each 10 min until the cardiac output reaches a plateau. Dopamine is adjusted to achieve a reasonable urinary output (>60 ml/h); this may require support with intermittent bolus doses of loop diuretics. Left atrial pressure is maintained between 15 and 20 mmHg (below the threshold to produce pulmonary oedema and above the level which begins to impair cardiac output). The right atrial pressure is maintained at a level high enough to support the cardiac output and left atrial pressure. The heart rate is kept between 100 and 120 bpm and systolic blood pressure between 110 and 120 mmHg with a diastolic pressure near 80 mmHg. The patient should be comfortable in this state, with near normal arterial oxygen saturation and no acidosis.

Mechanical support

Mechanical support of the circulation can be achieved using intra-aortic balloon pump counterpulsation. Mechanical ventilation of patients in cardiogenic shock is justified if the patient is to be offered more definitive therapy. Coronary angioplasty improves the outlook in these patients. This technique involves passing a balloon catheter into the descending aorta, by percutaneous techniques allied to cardiac catheterisation. The balloon is then inflated with helium and deflated, triggered to the ECG. This produces an enhanced aortic diastolic pressure.

ACUTE VENTRICULAR SEPTAL RUPTURE AND RUPTURED PAPILLARY MUSCLE

Acute ventricular septal rupture and ruptured papillary muscle are uncommon and very severe complications of acute myocardial infarction. They tend to occur 2–10 days after the acute event and produce sudden deterioration with acute heart failure, shock and the development of a new systolic murmur. It may be impossible to differentiate the two conditions clinically, although echocardiography and Doppler ultrasound can do so in most cases.

Treatment is early surgery in both instances, although mortality remains high. There may be an advantage to allow tissues to 'heal' before closure of a VSD, but, unfortunately, most patients will succumb before sufficient time elapses. There are some conspicuous successes with early surgery and, when possible, circulatory support prior to operation may be life-saving.

CARDIAC RUPTURE

Cardiac rupture is a much commoner cause of sudden death in hospital than has previously been recognised (10–20% of in-hospital deaths). It typically occurs several days after the acute infarction and appears to be commoner in men, in those with higher blood pressures and in those who suffer anterior infarction. Acute beta blockade protects from this complication which is manifested clinically by the sudden onset of severe pain followed rapidly by cardiovascular collapse. Resuscitation from this event is unusual; the clinical picture is of electro-mechanical dissociation (EMD), where an ECG rhythm is present but no output ensues.

VENTRICULAR ANEURYSM

Ventricular aneurysm is a late complication of myocardial infarction in 10–15% of patients. *True aneurysms* cause thinning and paradoxical motion of portions of ventricular wall. Recurrent arrhythmia, refractory heart failure, embolisation and rupture are the complications of true aneurysms, which are manifest clinically by paradoxical precordial pulsation, persistent ST elevation on the ECG and an abnormal LV border contour on the chest X-ray. *False aneurysms* are limited cardiac ruptures whose structure has become organised and stabilised; the main complications include those of true aneurysms as well as a greater tendency for late and fatal rupture.

Surgery is the treatment of choice for all false aneurysms and symptomatic true aneurysms. Antiarrhythmic therapy may be necessary and anticoagulation for true aneurysms is wise since 60–70% of them contain thrombus.

DRESSLER'S OR POSTMYOCARDIAL INFARCTION SYNDROME

Dressler's syndrome is an immunological syndrome of pleuro-pericarditis which may occur in 1–4% of patients, 2–12 weeks after infarction (or open heart surgery). Antibodies directed against the sarcolemma and subsarcolemma of myocytes may be found. The clinical syndrome is similar to acute pericarditis (p. 425), with pain, fever, leucocytosis, a high ESR and a 'pericarditic' ECG in 50% of cases. It must be differentiated from extension of myocardial infarction, pulmonary embolism or pneumonia.

Treatment usually consists of NSAIDs, although steroids may be required for severe and recurrent episodes. The prognosis is good.

DISEASES OF HEART MUSCLE

MYOCARDITIS

The causes of myocarditis are shown in Table 12.22. In the Western World the commonest causes are viral, of which the most important are Coxsackie B and echovirus infections. Toxoplasmosis affects the myocardium in the neonate. *Trypanosoma cruzi* is the major cause of infective heart muscle disease in South America and is discussed on pages 297–8.

Acute viral myocarditis may complicate many severe viral infections and has been described with almost all common viral diseases. Clinically important myocarditis is uncommon, but ECG changes possibly due to myocarditis are more frequent.

Clinical features

A febrile illness followed by acute unexplained heart failure, cardiac arrhythmias and chest pain are the main presenting features of myocarditis. Chest pain usually results from a myopericarditis. An arrhythmia, such as frequent ventricular ectopic beats, is probably the most frequent manifestation of a mild attack of myocarditis, and is often seen after any viral infection.

The physical signs may include gallop rhythm and heart failure with cardiac enlargement.

DIAGNOSIS AND INVESTIGATION

Diagnosis is made on the basis of the history and an ECG which may show a variety of arrhythmias, conduction defects, and myocardial injury with ST and T wave abnormalities. An echocardiogram is helpful in diagnosis and shows reduced ventricular contractility. Endomyocardial biopsy is occasionally necessary to make the diagnosis. This technique is used to obtain a small piece of myocardium for histological examination. In acute

Table 12.22 Causes of myocarditis

Cause	Example
Viral	Coxsackie B, but a wide range of enteroviruses echoviruses, adenoviruses, polio, influenza
Rickettsiae	Chlamydia and Coxiella (Q fever)
Toxoplasma	Infants and immune-compromised adults
Trypanosomiasis	*T. cruzi* (Chagas' disease of S. America)
Bacteria	Often toxin-mediated, e.g. diphtheria
Physical	Radiation, severe hypothermia
Drugs and poisons	Emetine, carbon monoxide

myocarditis, there is a marked lymphocytic and inflammatory cell infiltrate. Necrosis of myocytes is seen and, often, interstitial fibrosis. Later in the disease, the histological appearances become less marked and merge into those of congestive (dilated) cardiomyopathy (see below).

Management

Strict rest is advised until symptoms and signs and ECG abnormalities have resolved. Strenuous exercise is prohibited during this period. Cardiac arrhythmias are treated. Anticoagulants should be considered since intraventricular clots are common. Although most patients make an apparently full recovery, about 15% have a poor prognosis with continuing evidence of cardiac enlargement and, in some cases, of progressive heart failure. These patients may only be saved by cardiac transplantation. It seems likely that some patients will progress to a dilated cardiomyopathy. Immunosuppressive therapy may be helpful in the more severe cases.

CARDIOMYOPATHIES

Cardiomyopathy is the term used to describe heart muscle disease, and is usually only used when hypertension and coronary artery disease have been excluded. Cardiomyopathy is more frequent in people of African origin – not only in Africa and the Caribbean, but also in the UK. The reasons for this are still unknown.

Cardiomyopathies are now classified into three main groups, shown in Table 12.23.

Dilated cardiomyopathy

Dilated cardiomyopathies (DCM, also called congestive cardiomyopathy–COCM) comprise half or more of patients diagnosed with cardiomyopathy. The aetiology is usually not identifiable since an identical clinical histological and pathological picture can arise after damage to the heart from many causes, including toxins (such as cobalt), drugs (such as adriamycin), or following an attack of acute myocarditis. Chronic alcoholism is associated with DCM, and, since alcohol has a direct suppressant effect on the heart, it is thought to be an aetiological agent in many cases. Other causes are given in Table 12.23.

Clinical features

Presymptomatic DCM may be present for several years without coming to the notice of a doctor unless there is a routine chest X-ray. There may, at this stage, be some diminution in maximum effort tolerance, but unless the subject concerned is an athlete, this usually goes unnoticed or is ascribed to normal ageing.

Later on, symptoms are dominated by heart failure in severe cases, with both left- and right-sided failure being eventually intractable. AF and thromboembolism are frequent complications and 10% of patients have recurrent chest pain or angina on effort, despite normal coronary arteries.

The clinical picture is of a dilated heart that contracts very poorly, with a markedly reduced ejection fraction and a high filling pressure. Physical examination usually reveals cardiomegaly, with a gallop rhythm. Both mitral and tricuspid regurgitation are common when the patient presents in heart failure, and are secondary to the ventricular dilatation.

Investigation

Chest X-ray reveals the cardiomegaly, which often involves all the chambers of the heart. The ECG is non-specific, and may show features of ventricular hypertrophy, Q waves and widespread T wave inversion.

Echocardiography can be used to exclude a pericardial effusion and haemodynamically significant valve disease. The distinction between cardiomyopathy with mitral regurgitation and heart failure due to valvular disease is

Table 12.23 Types of cardiomyopathy*

Type	Features	Causes
Dilated cardiomyopathy (DCM)	Large cavity, poor contraction. AV valve regurgitation. Low ejection fraction	High percentage unknown (idiopathic) Following myocarditis of any cause Alcohol, cobalt, adriamycin, daunorubicin Systemic illness: amyloid; sarcoid; haemochromatosis
Hypertrophic (obstructive) cardiomyopathy (HCM or HOCM)	Idiopathic ventricular wall thickening, often asymmetric. Small cavity. High ejection fraction	Usually familial, may be sporadic. Similar picture may arise in the elderly, secondary to hypertension/aortic stenosis
Restrictive cardiomyopathy	Thick-walled ventricle or fibrosed endocardium restricts filling, but systolic function (ejection fraction) maintained. Much less common	Endomyocardial fibrosis and Löffler's endocarditis. Amyloid; sarcoid; haemochromatosis

*Some patients may have features of more than one type of cardiomyopathy, e.g dilated and restrictive, and individual diseases, such as haemochromatosis, may commonly have features of both.

important and can be made by echocardiography, which shows vigorous LV contraction when the valvular disease is primary.

Management and prognosis

When these patients present with heart failure, the prognosis is poor, with a 50% mortality in the following 2 years. Treatable causes of heart failure such as heart valve disease must be excluded, and endomyocardial biopsy may be necessary in the young patient to exclude an active myocarditis. Heart failure is treated conventionally (p. 344). Anticoagulation is advised if a high risk of thromboembolism exists.

Hypertrophic cardiomyopathy

Hypertrophic cardiomyopathy (HCM) is characterised by marked left ventricular wall thickening with a small left ventricular cavity. Usually, the wall thickening is asymmetric and predominantly affects the interventricular septum; this is known as *asymmetrical septal hypertrophy* (ASH). The hypertrophy can lead to left ventricular outflow obstruction with abnormal systolic anterior motion (SAM) of the mitral valve; when this occurs, there is almost always a variable degree of mitral regurgitation. The condition is then known as *hypertrophic obstructive cardiomyopathy* (HOCM). Similar processes can occur, but less frequently, on the right side of the heart, and sometimes both sides of the heart are involved.

Aetiology and pathology

There is a familial incidence of HCM. It is inherited as an autosomal dominant, but sporadic examples account for most cases. The condition may be mild and show only on echocardiographic examination. Some cases have associated 'triggers' for left ventricular hypertrophy, such as hypertension or aortic valve disease, but there is usually no obvious cause.

On microscopy, the muscle fibres are thickened and appear to be arranged haphazardly. The appearances are not specific. One theory suggests that the geometrical arrangement of the fibres is such that they pull antagonistically during systole, and that this results in myofibrillar hypertrophy and disruption.

Recently single point mutations on chromosome 14, coding for myosin have been identified as the genetic markers of the disease. One mutation loads to HCM with a very high risk of premature death, whilst others are associated with a more benign form of the disease. When confirmed, these findings will have fundamental implications for managing the disease and for the screening of affected families.

Clinical features

Syncope and palpitations from a variety of arrhythmias are common and sudden death may occur. Angina can develop without coronary artery disease. The thickened myocardium can produce an inflow obstruction and lead to heart failure from a raised filling pressure. In later stages, there is an enlarged heart and a risk of systemic embolism.

The physical signs depend on whether there is outflow obstruction. In its absence, there may only be third or fourth heart sounds and a rather muscular feel to the left ventricular impulse. In the presence of outflow obstruction, systolic ejection is shortened, there is a jerky carotid pulse (compared with a sustained and weak pulse in aortic stenosis) and the apex beat has a characteristic presystolic lift. Outflow obstruction produces a harsh late systolic murmur which may be masked by a pansystolic murmur of coincidental mitral regurgitation.

The presence of exertional angina, exertional syncope and a systolic murmur with left ventricular hypertrophy can easily lead to a mistaken diagnosis of aortic stenosis. Although the physical signs differ from those of true aortic stenosis, echocardiography has proved invaluable in establishing the correct diagnoses.

A significant number of sporadic cases are discovered at autopsy in young people, not infrequently having collapsed during physical activity or sport.

Investigation

Chest X-ray is often unremarkable in the absence of heart failure. The ECG is non-specific, showing left ventricular hypertrophy and, occasionally, Q waves. Echocardiography demonstrates the left ventricular wall thickening, particularly ASH, and, with obstruction, shows SAM of the mitral valve (see above). Two-dimensional echocardiography shows that the septal hypertrophy can be a localised bulge, and also the high ejection fraction. Doppler ultrasound will demonstrate the mitral regurgitation, as well as the high velocity jet in late systole that develops in the outflow tract of the left ventricle in the presence of obstruction.

Cardiac catheterisation and angiography are necessary to confirm normal coronary arteries, to judge the degree of mitral regurgitation and to measure the apex-to-base pressure gradient in the left ventricle.

Management

Sudden death is a continuing hazard even with antiarrhythmic therapy, and various agents are used to control symptoms of palpitations without apparently preventing sudden death. Beta-blockers can abolish outflow obstruction, and may help in the management of heart failure. Calcium antagonists, such as verapamil, have been used to reduce ventricular hypertrophy with variable results. Both types of drug slow the heart rate and aid diastolic function.

Surgical intervention has been used quite extensively, with mitral valve replacement and outflow tract myomectomy being used to abolish outflow tract obstruction. There is a high surgical mortality and, unless the myomectomy is radical, outflow tract obstruction can recur. The role of surgery therefore remains controversial.

Screening of siblings of those affected reveals a high incidence of mild degrees of asymptomatic asymmetrical hypertrophy. Investigation and monitoring of these subjects may eventually enable the mortality and morbidity of this condition to be reduced, but may also cause great anxiety in an asymptomatic individual.

Restrictive cardiomyopathies

There is a small subgroup of heart muscle disorders characterised by a very high filling pressure to the ventricles resulting from rigidity of the walls due to infiltration with abnormal tissue. Reasonable systolic function is usually maintained. Clinically, such restrictive cardiomyopathies present with very similar features to constrictive pericarditis, with evidence of severe heart failure and a relatively small heart.

Cardiac amyloid

Cardiac amyloid is the commonest cause of death in primary amyloidosis (p. 1101). The gastrointestinal tract and tongue are often also involved, as are the nerves and skin. Presentation is either with heart failure secondary to poor systolic function (like a DCM) or with severe right heart failure secondary to a restrictive pattern.

There may be evidence of tricuspid and mitral regurgitation with a loud gallop rhythm, and echocardiography shows thickening of the ventricular walls with a small left ventricular cavity. Characteristically, the ventricular walls, infiltrated by amyloid, have a very bright echo appearance, and there may be conduction abnormalities which may require a pacemaker. The diagnosis may be confirmed by rectal or gingival biopsy or, sometimes, by cardiac biopsy. There is no specific treatment for these patients, who fortunately present late in life.

Haemochromatosis and transfusion haemosiderosis

Overload of the body with iron can damage the heart. Haemochromatosis is a genetic disease in which iron overload occurs (see Ch. 16, p. 642). Transfusion haemosiderosis, in which repeated blood transfusion (usually more than 100 units) for chronic anaemias, such as thalassaemia, causes similar tissue loading with iron. The iron damages the liver, heart, gonads and pancreas causing hepatomegaly, heart failure, gonadal dysfunction and diabetes. There is a characteristic dusky skin pigmentation.

Cardiac manifestations are found in about 30% of patients. Cardiac involvement does not necessarily parallel other organ involvement, although cardiac failure is always associated with high levels of iron in the heart. There is usually myocardial thickening and dilatation, so the patient presents with features of both a dilated and restrictive cardiomyopathy. The diagnosis is based on demonstration of excessive iron in the body with the serum ferritin being particularly high.

Cardiac findings are of heart failure and arrhythmias – both supraventricular and ventricular – with disorders of conduction. There may be a low voltage ECG.

The main aim of management should be to reduce body iron levels by chelation or, in the case of haemochromatosis, by repeated venesection.

Cardiac carcinoid

In the carcinoid syndrome, where a carcinoid tumour (usually ileal) has metastasised widely, over 50% of patients have cardiac involvement consisting of endocardial plaques of fibrous tissue. This is almost always on the right side of the heart and involves the tricuspid and pulmonary valves, the vena cava and the coronary sinus, producing distortion and valvular stenosis. Serotonin and kinin peptides produced by the tumour are normally inactivated in the liver and lung; thus the left side of the heart is protected.

Clinically, the patient has the systemic manifestations of carcinoid syndrome – flushing, diarrhoea and, sometimes, bronchoconstriction. In addition, there are symptoms and signs of right heart failure, often with pulmonary stenosis and tricuspid regurgitation. The circulating vasodilators may also produce a hyperkinetic circulation with high output heart failure.

Sarcoidosis

Between 20% and 30% of autopsied cases of generalised sarcoid show cardiac involvement, although clinical manifestations are present in only about 5% of patients. Presentation may be with a cardiomyopathic picture of either the dilated or restrictive type, although it can also present with conduction abnormalities, heart block and sudden death. Heart block in a young patient may be the first manifestation of sarcoid.

Diagnosis and management

In the presence of the classical pulmonary findings, diagnosis does not require myocardial biopsy, but where there is doubt a biopsy can be extremely helpful. Isotope and magnetic resonance imaging may show infiltration.

Treatment is on the whole unsatisfactory. Pacing may reduce the risk of sudden death in patients with conduction system damage, and large doses of corticosteroids are usually advocated in an attempt to prevent progressive myocardial infiltration.

Endomyocardial fibrosis

Endomyocardial fibrosis is relatively common in regions of Africa, particulary Nigeria and Uganda, where it accounts for more than 20% of cardiac deaths. It is also found in other tropical areas and, occasionally, in Europeans who have been resident in endemic areas. Pathologically, there is gross fibrous thickening of the endocardium of one or both ventricles, usually associated with severe AV valve regurgitation. It commonly presents in young people of both sexes, often from low income groups.

Clinical features

The clinical presentation of endomyocardial fibrosis depends on whether one or both ventricles are involved. The disease may be heralded by fever, but usually presents with severe heart failure and sometimes arrhythmias. The heart is not usually markedly enlarged, although pericardial effusion is not uncommon. Clinical signs of valvular regurgitation and heart failure predominate. Systemic and pulmonary emboli may complicate the clinical course. Echocardiography, particularly 2D scanning, may demonstrate the thickened endocardium, which can obliterate parts of the ventricular cavity. Intraventricular clot may also be shown.

Surgical excision of the thickened endocardium with tricuspid and mitral valve replacement has given some encouraging results in a disease that appears to have, for most, a relentless progression.

Endocardial fibroelastosis

Endocardial fibroelastosis is a condition of infancy in which there is gross thickening of the endocardium with subsequent heart failure. It may present as a primary condition or follow aortic stenosis, other left-sided heart conditions or cardiac surgery in which endocardial perfusion may have been at risk.

Löffler's endocarditis

Löffler's endocarditis – a syndrome of prolonged eosinophilia with associated localised or widespread eosinophilic infiltrates – involves the heart in over 90% of cases. The hypereosinophilic syndrome is most commonly idiopathic, but may occur with eosinophilic leukaemia or secondarily with Hodgkin's disease, polyarteritis nodosa, tumours and parasitic infestation.

The clinical picture is of a severe progressive cardiomyopathy with a restrictive picture, often with systemic embolism, in a patient with a wasting disease and marked eosinophilia.

The disease process starts as an eosinophilic myocarditis, and progresses with the formation of multiple endocardial thrombi. In the third stage, there is fibrosis and a hyaline membrane forms over the endocardium. The disease thus has some similarities to endomyocardial fibrosis. The clinical course of the disease can be from a few months to 12 years.

INFECTIVE ENDOCARDITIS

Infective endocarditis is a multisystem disease due to infection of the heart valves or adjacent endocardium. It is characterised by prolonged fever, weight loss, embolic phenomena and renal failure.

Classification

Until recently, it was usual to divide the disease into two groups:

- subacute bacterial endocarditis
- acute bacterial endocarditis.

Subacute bacterial endocarditis (SBE) affects relatively young patients with an identifiable pre-existing cardiac abnormality, usually rheumatic valvular heart disease or a congenital abnormality of the heart associated with a jet lesion. The heart valves become infected with an organism of normally low virulence which slowly forms vegetations on the damaged valve and produces progressive valvular regurgitation. This is accompanied by intracardiac abscesses, embolic episodes and a slow, wasting fever, often associated with evidence of formation of immune complexes leading to glomerulonephritis.

Acute bacterial endocarditis occurs in immune-compromised patients or those suffering from a staphylococcal septicaemia. Apparently normal mitral or aortic valves are rapidly destroyed in the course of 24–48 hours, resulting in torrential regurgitation and death from heart failure. This usually occurs in someone with a pre-existing severe disease.

Over the last two decades, the clinical spectrum of infective endocarditis has changed greatly. This is due to the gradual decline in the numbers of patients with rheumatic heart disease, an increase in the number of patients who have had cardiac surgery, invasive investigation being used in elderly patients, and the epidemic of intravenous drug abuse.

Nowadays, infective endocarditis occurs quite frequently in elderly patients with degenerative disease of the heart valves and in whom there is no evidence of either rheumatic or congenital heart disease. Furthermore, infective endocarditis is not easily divided into the subacute and acute forms. There are a wide range of infective agents of different virulence, and the same organism, such as *Staphylococcus aureus*, can behave quite differently on different occasions depending on the patient's host defences and the particular strain of organism.

The intravenous drug abuser may develop infective endocarditis with a variety of unusual organisms, sometimes on apparently normal valves and quite commonly on the tricuspid valve. Bacteria are not the only causes of infective endocarditis. Fungal and rickettsial infections, as well as viral infective endocarditis, can occur. For these reasons, the more general term *infective endocarditis* is preferred to the earlier classification.

Pathogenesis

Pre-existing cardiac lesions

Endocarditis usually develops in congenitally abnormal or rheumatic hearts in which there is a 'jet' lesion. The altered flow of blood allows bacteria to impact directly on the endocardial surface. Previous damage to the endothelium (e.g. as a result of rheumatic heart disease) facilitates colonisation by bacteria present in the bloodstream, which stick to the endocardial lesion and multiply. A chronic lesion, such as one produced by a jet of blood impinging on the endocardium, remains susceptible. However, transient lesions, such as those produced by passing a cardiac catheter or cannula through the heart valves for as little as 15 min, heal rapidly and, as a result, rarely become infected.

Bacteraemia

Transient bacteraemia is common with trauma to the mouth and teeth; the organism most commonly present, *Streptococcus viridans*, is also very likely to stick to an endocardial lesion and colonise it. Gram-negative bacilli, which can be grown from the blood in Gram-negative infections and at the time of urogenital manipulation and surgery, are less likely to cause endocarditis and stick less readily to endocardial lesions.

In practice, any surgical procedure involving manipulation of any organ or part of the body not normally bacteria-free should be regarded as a potential cause of bacteraemia.

Infective endocarditis may occur following a chest or urinary infection or septicaemia. It can also occur following a variety of operative and investigative procedures, but the risk of these procedures producing a bacteraemia is variable. Minor medical procedures which may provoke bacteraemia include the following:

- *Dental extraction and manipulation.* Transient bacteraemia with streptococci and some enterococci lasts from 15 min to several hours. Chewing can cause bacteraemia even in edentulous individuals.
- *Oropharynx.* Tonsillectomy, rigid bronchoscopy, orotracheal intubation and nasopharyngeal suction.
- *Gastrointestinal tract.* Barium enema, sigmoidoscopy and colonoscopy.
- *Urogenital tract.* Urinary catheterisation, prostatectomy and prostatic massage have all been found to produce a bacteraemia, but normal vaginal parturition only does so occasionally.
- *Intravenous cannulae.* These are a potential source of bacteraemia and should not be used unnecessarily in patients at risk.

Growth of the vegetation

The vegetation grows as a concretion of bacteria and the reaction of the blood to their presence. The bacteria become covered in platelets and layers of fibrin. The exuberance of the vegetation depends on the organism. Fungal infections with Candida produce large vegetations which can even occlude the orifice of prosthetic valves. Other organisms may provoke so little reaction that the vegetations are too small to be demonstrated by echocardiography (which has a maximum resolution of a few millimetres).

Infection can perforate the valve cusps, and track into the adjacent myocardium and valve ring, causing abscesses and a variety of complications depending on the site. These include fistula formation, bundle branch block, complete heart block, infective pericarditis and papillary muscle and chordal rupture.

Embolism and immune complex manifestations

Embolism of fragments of infective vegetation can produce embolic abscesses in the spleen, kidneys, brain and elsewhere, with 'mycotic' aneurysm of the arterial wall which may result in rupture and sudden haemorrhage. Embolic episodes result in cerebral and peripheral ischaemic attacks, transient haematuria, splenic infarcts and coronary occlusion.

Long-standing infection leads to the formation of immune complexes which may themselves complicate the presentation and course of the disease. These complexes are probably responsible for the glomerulonephritis which may accompany infective endocarditis, and for the skin lesions.

Valve involvement

The frequency of involvement of the four cardiac valves is in direct relationship to the mechanical loading on the valves, i.e. mitral, aortic, tricuspid and pulmonary in descending order of frequency. This is related to the much higher jet velocities usually found on the left side of the heart, although the very low incidence of involvement of the pulmonary valve in pulmonary stenosis remains unexplained. Untreated infective endocarditis of the aortic valve may rapidly lead to infection of the mitral valve, as the regurgitant jet of blood through the aortic valve most commonly strikes the anterior cusp of the mitral valve. Tricuspid valve endocarditis leads to a picture of recurrent lung 'pneumonitis' of a patchy nature due to embolism of vegetation and organisms into the lung.

Infecting organisms

Streptococci

About 50% of cases of infective endocarditis are caused by alpha haemolytic streptococci from the mouth and oropharynx, formerly classified as *Strep. viridans* but now subdivided into many organisms, e.g. *Strep. mitior* and *Strep. sanguis*. These organisms are most likely to reach the bloodstream after dental extraction or manipulation, bronchoscopy and tonsillectomy and adenoidectomy.

The *Enterococci* of Group D streptococci have become more frequent causes and can be found in the gastro-intestinal tract, genitourinary tract and periodontal tissue. Accurate identification is sometimes difficult, and the prognosis is worse than for *Strep. viridans* infection. *Strep. bovis*, a non-enterococcal organism from Group D, is an increasingly common finding in infective endocarditis, and the disease in these cases is very similar to that caused by *Strep. viridans*.

Strep. pneumoniae is a less common agent but still causes some cases of acute infective endocarditis; the infection may be complicated by meningitis.

Anaerobic streptococci, organisms which are initially difficult to grow, are found increasingly frequently but necessitate anaerobic cultures. The discovery of *Strep. faecalis* should lead to investigation of the gut, since colonic carcinoma may be an underlying cause.

Staphylococci

A staphylococcal septicaemia with *Staph. aureus* often involves the heart valves; if several positive cultures are obtained, a prolonged course of antistaphylococcal therapy is indicated even without definite evidence of cardiac pathology. Acute endocarditis can damage apparently normal valves very quickly. The same organism can produce a subacute picture. It is a frequent finding in intravenous drug abusers and diabetics with endocarditis.

Staph. epidermidis (*albus*) may be grown as a contaminant of blood cultures, but repeated positive cultures are significant since it is a common cause of infective endocarditis both in patients with prosthetic valves and in intravenous drug abusers. It is occasionally found in patients with indwelling subcutaneous intravenous lines. Many months may pass between the introduction of the infection and the presentation with endocarditis.

Other organisms

Neisseria gonorrhoea and Gram-negative bacilli are relatively uncommon causes of infective endocarditis, but *Pseudomonas* is becoming more frequent.

Q fever endocarditis is uncommon and is diagnosed by finding a rising titre of antibodies in the blood. *Fungal* endocarditis occurs with prosthetic valves and in patients who have had prolonged periods of antibiotic or corticosteroids, or who are intravenous drug abusers.

Clinical features

The clinical features of infective endocarditis can be divided into several categories.

Features of chronic infection

The features of chronic infection include a remittent pyrexia, myalgia, arthralgia and general fatigue. These symptoms are accompanied by anaemia, anorexia and weight loss. Splenomegaly may be present but is usually not marked. Splenic infarction can lead to pain and a friction rub over the spleen. A splenic abscess can delay resolution of the fever. In long-standing cases, cachexia and mild finger-clubbing may occur.

Cardiac manifestations

Heart murmurs are present in over 85% of cases but may easily be missed, especially in the presence of heart failure. Early diastolic murmurs are notoriously difficult to hear, and a wide pulse pressure is often the first clue that aortic regurgitation is present. Changing heart murmurs are uncommon but, when present, are very suggestive of the diagnosis. Cardiac arrhythmias and conduction abnormalities may follow the spread of infection from the valve ring to form myocardial abscesses.

Heart failure can be a presenting symptom. Its presence signifies a poor prognosis and is an indication for early surgery. Sudden heart failure can occur with rupture of a valve cusp or chordae tendinae, or sinus of Valsalva aneurysm.

12 Cardiovascular Disease

Systemic embolism

Embolism is a prominent feature of infective endocarditis and the presentation may be with a cerebrovascular event (e.g. a dense hemiplegia), an ischaemic limb, mesenteric embolus or haematuria from renal infarction. Over 50% of cases exhibit embolic phenomena; fungal endocarditis with large friable vegetations is notorious for producing large emboli. Right-sided endocarditis usually presents with recurrent patchy consolidation (pneumonitis).

Immunological phenomena

Renal

A diffuse glomerulonephritis is present in many patients and is due to the deposition of immune complexes. The renal disease is shown by proteinuria and microscopic haematuria. In untreated endocarditis the blood urea begins to rise, but renal failure develops in less than 10% of cases. Even when advanced, renal failure recovers with adequate treatment of the infective endocarditis.

Skin and mucous membranes

Typical skin manifestations of infective endocarditis were much more common in the preantibiotic era, but are now seen in only 20–40% of cases. Thorough examination of the patient's skin, mucosae of the oropharynx, conjunctivae and retinae should be repeated during the course of the disease, to check for new lesions.

Petechial haemorrhages. Examination of the soft palate, pharynx, conjunctivae, hands, feet and anterior body wall may reveal *petechial haemorrhages*, often with a pale centre.

Subungual or *'splinter haemorrhages'* are usually seen as a faint dark line away from the nail margin in the fingers and, occasionally, toes. They may also be seen in patients who are debilitated for other reasons, or after trauma. When present, they occur in 'bursts' and indicate activity of the disease.

Osler nodes are painful, nodular, red to purple lesions that usually form on the fingertips but can also occur on the backs of the toes, soles of the feet, the thenar and hypothenar eminences and, occasionally, elsewhere. Formerly common, they are now seen in less than a fifth of cases. The lesions can last a few hours to a few days.

Janeway lesions are painless, 1–4 mm erythematous macules which are most common on the thenar and hypothenar eminences and the soles of the feet, and blanch on pressure.

Retinal lesions. The *Roth spot* is a 'cotton-wool exudate' consisting of a perivascular collection of lymphocytes. It is not specific to infective endocarditis. Boat-shaped haemorrhages with a pale centre and white spots have also been described.

All of these retinal and cutaneous lesions have been ascribed to 'septic emboli', but are now thought to be immunological manifestations of the disease.

Diagnosis

Infective endocarditis is a possible diagnosis in any patient with a fever and a heart murmur, and is established by taking blood cultures.

A patient with a heart murmur may have an intercurrent viral infection or some other cause for fever. Where the source of the fever is not clear, it is essential to take blood cultures before starting antibiotics should they be considered necessary. This is especially important when a patient at risk of endocarditis develops a fever following a procedure which has not been covered with antibiotic prophylaxis.

Any febrile patient who has had open heart surgery (other than coronary bypass grafting) should be considered at risk fom infective endocarditis, even if no murmur is evident. In the elderly patient, endocarditis can exist without significant fever. Other signs of chronic infection, such as unexplained anaemia and high ESR in a patient with a heart murmur, should arouse suspicion and lead to blood cultures being taken.

Blood cultures

Blood cultures should be taken on six to eight occasions, over the first 48 hours. It is not necessary to wait for peaks of fever. Anaerobic cultures should be taken and although a higher percentage of positive cultures has been claimed for arterial blood culture venous sampling is usually sufficient.

Close liaison with the laboratory is essential so that *any* organism that grows is kept in subcultures and not discarded. Appropriate culture techniques can then be instituted for poorly growing organisms.

Where the clinical evidence of the disease is overwhelming, especially if there is evidence of deteriorating valve function, antibiotic therapy may be started as soon as four to six cultures have been taken and before positive cultures are reported by the laboratory. There is, however, an inevitable risk that this may interfere with identification of the organism if the initial cultures are negative.

Where infective endocarditis is a high probability, and particularly if *Strep. viridans* is grown from blood culture, a dental opinion on possible septic foci in the mouth should be obtained. It is then possible to time any dental extraction or other dental work to follow by 1 hour or so the initiation of antibiotic therapy. This then removes the possibility of septic foci in the mouth harbouring antibiotic resistant organisms, which can then superinfect the heart after the initial organisms have been eradicated.

Culture-negative endocarditis

In 20% of cases, no organisms are grown despite many other features of the disease being present. This may occur because the patient has been treated with an antibiotic (which may render cultures negative for days or weeks after stopping treatment), because the organism involved is present in very small numbers, or because it is difficult to culture. Even in average cases of endocarditis, there may be only 100 organisms per ml of blood and, particularly in long-standing cases with renal failure, the patient's antibodies may render the blood almost sterile, despite the presence of organisms in large vegetations. Repeated blood culture samples of 10 ml should be inoculated into 100 ml of culture broth and incubated aerobically and anaerobically. The organisms may require special nutrients and may not grow for several days, or, in a few cases, for several weeks. If repeated cultures are negative, or the patient's condition is deteriorating, it may be necessary to embark on treatment without positive cultures.

This course of action must only be followed after close consultation with a microbiologist, who may suggest unusual sampling techniques (occasionally bone marrow or urine are positive when blood is not), and after blood has been taken for fungal and rickettsial antibodies.

Management

Successful treatment of infective endocarditis should involve close cooperation between physician and microbiologist. In the uncomplicated case, 4–6 weeks of bactericidal antibiotic therapy is required with serum levels of antibiotic sufficient to penetrate the vegetations and abscesses and eradicate the organism. Bacteriostatic antibiotics and bacteriostatic levels of bactericidal antibiotics are not sufficient, even with the host's natural defences to eradicate the organism.

Antibiotic therapy

Although oral antibiotic therapy can be used for sensitive *Strep. viridans* infection, the intravenous route is preferred for initiating therapy, and while awaiting 'back titrations'. For intravenous therapy, a central venous catheter may overcome the problems of superficial venous cannulae. All cannulae must be inserted under strict aseptic conditions and kept scrupulously clean to prevent the risk of superinfection with fungi. They should be changed at least every third day.

After culture and identification of the organism, its antibiotic sensitivity must be urgently assessed. The bacteriology laboratory assists by monitoring the patient's blood levels of antibiotic and titrating to determine what serum dilutions are bactericidal to the organism in culture. A level of 1 in 8 is considered satisfactory.

It is essential that the antibiotic regime for an acute septicaemic endocarditis includes antistaphylococcal antibiotics. Where a subacute infection is being treated, it is usual to use wide-spectrum antibiotics, such as gentamicin and ampicillin. The response to treatment is then monitored and the treatment changed or continued, depending on whether it appears to be controlling the infection. Culture-negative endocarditis, particularly with large vegetations or other indication of severe valvular involvement, may be an additional criterion for early surgical intervention, particularly if potentially hazardous antibiotics are being used.

Monitoring treatment

Successful antibiotic treatment ideally results in disappearance of the fever within a few days, a fall in the ESR, rise in the haemoglobin and an increase in the patient's weight and well-being. Measurement of C-reactive protein may give a more reliable guide to response than

Table 12.24 Endocarditis prophylaxis

Procedure	Recommendation
1. Dental procedure under local anaesthetic	A Penicillin allergy – B or C
2. Dental procedure under general anaesthetic	D or E or F
3. High risk – *Refer to hospital*	
• Patients with prosthetic valves	G Penicillin allergy – H
• Patients allergic to penicillin or who have had penicillin more than once in the previous month	H
• Patients who have had a previous attack of endocarditis	G Penicillin allergy – H
4. Surgery - upper respiratory tract	As 1 and 2 above Any postoperative antibiotic may have to be given intramuscularly or intravenously if swallowing painful
5. Surgery - genitourinary	Sterile urine, as 1 and 2 Infected urine - prophylaxis should also cover pathogens involved
6. Obstetrics and gynaecological patients	Cover only for patients with prosthetic valves - D or H
7. Gastrointestinal procedures	Cover only for patients with prosthetic valves - D or H

A: *Oral amoxycillin*
3 g single dose taken under supervision 1 hour before procedure
Children under 10 - ½ dose
Children under 5 - ½ dose

B: *Oral erythromycin*
1.5 g under supervision 1-2 hours before procedure
Children under 10 - ½ dose
Children under 5 - ¼ dose

C: *Oral clindamycin*
600 mg single dose taken under supervision 1 hour before procedure
Children under 10 - 6 mg/kg body weight single dose taken under supervision 1 hour before procedure

D: *Intramuscular amoxycillin*
1 g in 2.5 ml 1% llgnocaine hydrochioride lust before induction plus 0.5 by mouth 6 hours later
Children under 10 - ½ dose

E: *Oral amoxycillin*
3 g dose 4 hours before anaesthesia followed by a further 3 g by month as soon as possible after operation
Children under 10 - ½ dose
Children under 5 - ¼ dose

F: *Oral amoxycillin and probenacid*
Amoxycillin 3 g together with probenacid 1 g 4 hours before operation

G: *Intravenous amoxycillin and gentamicin*
1 g amoxycillin plus 120 mg gentamicin intravenously just before induction, then
0.5 g amoxycillin orally 5 hours later
Children under 10 - amoxycillin ½ dose gentamicin 2 mg/kg body weight

H: *Intravenous vancomycin*
1 g slow infusion over 1 hour followed by gentamicin 120 mg intravenously just before induction mins before procedure
Children under 10 - vancomycin 20 mg/kg gentamicin 2 mg/kg

the ESR. Evidence of microemboli, such as fresh splinter haemorrhages and microscopic haematuria, take longer to go, and large vegetations take several weeks to regress. Occasionally, the fever and high ESR do not settle although repeated blood cultures remain negative. If other causes for persistent fever (e.g. splenic abscess or superinfection) are eliminated, then the fever may be antibiotic-induced and disappear with cessation of antibiotic treatment.

Surgery

Severe valve failure and uncontrolled infection may require emergency valve replacement. If the patient presents with heart failure, early surgery is essential as, even with rapid successful antibiotic treatment of endocarditis, damaged valves shrink and fibrose with progressive increase in the degree of valve regurgitation and the heart failure may become irreversible. Prosthetic valve endocarditis almost invariably requires valve replacement for the infection to be eliminated.

A few days of antibiotic therapy prior to surgery reduces the risk of valve dehiscence from sewing the new valve into an infected valve ring, and reduces the risk of prosthetic valve endocarditis. A heavily infected valve with large vegetations may be electively replaced where there is risk of major embolism, or where the patient cannot be given effective bactericidal therapy. Tricuspid valve endocarditis with large vegetations can be treated by excision of the tricuspid valve without replacement, while the course of antibiotics is given. The prosthetic valve can then be sewn into a sterile ring.

Apart from valve replacement, surgical closure of intracardiac fistulae, such as aortic-to-right-atrial shunts, and limited thoracotomy for epicardial pacing for heart block are occasionally required.

Prophylaxis

The recommended regimens for endocarditis prophylaxis vary slightly, but all are based on the use of a bactericidal antibiotic to cover a procedure likely to produce bacteraemia. If a general anaesthetic is involved, the antibiotic is given intravenously or intramuscularly. If no general anaesthetic is involved, oral preparations are given if possible. Regimens are shown in Table 12.24.

A safe general rule is that prophylaxis should be given for all dental work where the teeth are manipulated, all pelvic, colonic and bladder instrumentation and surgery. Normal parturition does not need routine cover unless the bladder is catheterised or forceps used.

SYPHILITIC ENDOCARDITIS

Pathogenesis

Syphilis is now much less common as a cause of heart disease. Cardiac involvement is a manifestation of the tertiary stage of the disease, which often follows a prolonged quiescent period. An endarteritis obliterans of the vasa vasorum of the aorta weakens the media, which undergoes a slow necrosis and causes thickening and scar formation in the intima. The changes are irregular, and complicated by fibrosis and calcification. Dilatation of the aorta occurs and can be localised, giving a fusiform or saccular aneurysm; it often also involves the valve ring, causing progressive, and often severe, aortic regurgitation. There may be damage to the aortic valve cusps leading to retraction, but never stenosis. Intimal scarring of the aorta can lead to coronary ostial stenosis. The changes do not always lead to overt heart disease. There is a higher percentage of cases of aortic regurgitation and aortic aneurysms in manual labourers with aortitis, compared with sedentary men and women with necropsy evidence of aortitis. Thus, it may be that physical activity produces additional loads on the aorta which induce these changes.

Clinical features

The patient is usually a man (there is a 3:1 sex ratio for uncomplicated aortitis, but this rises to 10:1 for aortic aneurysm) in late middle-age.

Aortic regurgitation

The presentation may be with pure aortic regurgitation with evidence (best shown echocardiographically) of a dilated aortic valve ring, and serological proof of previous *Treponema pallidum* infection. If untreated, the regurgitation tends to be progressive and severe; indeed, the classical 19th century physical signs described for aortic regurgitation are almost all based on patients with severe syphilitic aortic regurgitation (water hammer pulse, head rocking, etc.). With a dilated aortic root, the early diastolic murmur is louder in the third right interspace than the third left interspace. If there is coronary ostial stenosis, severe angina is usually present, often leading to status anginosus (continuous pain), heart failure and death unless there is early surgical intervention.

Aortic aneurysm

Aortic aneurysm is much less common than regurgitation. It usually occurs in the ascending aorta or arch rather than the descending aorta, where aneurysms are much more likely to be arteriosclerotic. The clinical features depend on the position of the aneurysm. Classically, the ascending aortic aneurysm produces signs of aortic regurgitation, the arch aneurysm symptoms, such as dysphagia, cough, pain, dyspnoea, and the descending aneurysm pain from erosion of the spine.

Diagnosis and investigation

Serological proof of previous spirochaetal infection is usually followed by CSF examination, because of the close association with neurosyphilis. Positive serology cannot be taken as proof of syphilitic infection in patients with yaws scars, who often have persistent positive serology even after treatment. However, the combination of aortic dilatation and positive serology would be taken as confirmatory. Arteriosclerotic aneurysms, cystic medial necrosis of the aorta and aortic dissection are now common differential diagnoses.

Aortic regurgitation is investigated with particular emphasis on excluding coronary ostial stenosis. Aortic aneurysm is now often investigated by CT scanning. There is often laminated clot in the aneurysm, and classically, in aortitis, there is calcium seen in the ascending aorta. The treatment of syphilis is described on page 275. The Herxheimer reaction is particularly dangerous in aortic regurgitation with coronary ostial stenosis. The regurgitation may progress after effective penicillin treatment, due to further fibrosis. Surgical treatment is as for other causes of aortic regurgitation or aortic aneurysm, after effective chemotherapy.

NON-INFECTIVE ENDOCARDITIS

RHEUMATIC FEVER AND RHEUMATIC HEART DISEASE

Rheumatic heart disease is now uncommon in Western Europe and North America, but is an important historical cause of what was once the bulk of valvular heart disease. It is still important in the Third World as a disease of childhood and a major cause of heart disease. Its decline in Western countries started before the widespread use of antibiotics, and probably reflects increased standards of nutrition and hygiene and, possibly, a decline in the virulence and prevalence of Lancefield Group A haemolytic streptococci.

Rheumatic fever and chorea are the exclusive causes of chronic rheumatic heart disease, in which there is interstitial muscle fibrosis as well as the heart valve disease. However, some 50% of patients with chronic rheumatic heart disease give no history of either condition.

Rheumatic fever develops in about 3% of young people exposed to an epidemic strain of beta haemolytic Lancefield Group A streptococcus. These patients usually have pharyngitis, but may have scarlet fever. After apparent recovery, they develop fever, sweats, skin rashes, arthritis and, sometimes, cardiac involvement from what appears to be an autoimmune disease starting 2–4 weeks after the initial sore throat and lasting 6–8 weeks, but occasionally as much as 26 weeks. Some patients give no definite history of an antecedent sore throat.

Following the attack of rheumatic fever, some 70% of the patients will eventually have evidence of rheumatic valvular heart disease, although the time interval can be as long as 50 years. On the other hand, the valve disease may become manifest during the attack of rheumatic fever, especially where regurgitation develops. Rheumatic fever may be recurrent, and the chances of valve disease increase with the number of attacks.

Pathology

Although rheumatic fever follows a streptococcal infection, no bacteria are found in the lesions; however, they may still be present in the pharynx. There is an acute inflammatory reaction, with oedema in the affected tissues, and then granulomatous lesions develop in the myocardium (Aschoff nodules). Oedema of the valve cusps is followed by verrucous fibrin deposits developing along the lines of apposition of the valve cusps, which eventually adhere at the commissures. In the acute illness, there is an acute non-bacterial synovitis in the joints, and granulomata may develop subcutaneously on extensor surfaces of the limbs and over the Achilles tendons (rheumatic nodules). There is usually a high anti-streptolysin O titre, and other antistreptococcal titres may also be high. It is thought that cross-reactivity between the streptococcal antigens and host tissue antigens leads to an autoimmune inflammatory process.

Clinical features and diagnosis

The diagnosis of rheumatic fever depends on criteria proposed by Duckett-Jones (Table 12.25); two major criteria, or one major and two minor criteria, establish a high probability for the diagnosis.

The patient is almost always between the ages of 3 and 30 years (usually 5–15 years); drenching sweats and a prolonged feverish illness occur, with extremely painful arthritis that moves from joint to joint (usually involving large joints such as the knee and elbow) which become hot, red, swollen and extremely painful for a few days and then recover fully. The flitting arthritis is characteristic, as is the classical skin rash, erythema marginatum. Subcutaneous nodules may develop after several weeks, usually over the elbows.

Carditis may be pericarditis, myocarditis or, more importantly for the eventual appearance of valve disease, endocarditis. All may occur at once as *pancarditis*. The pericarditis is similar to any acute pericarditis (p. 426), with precordial pain, ECG changes (raised ST segments) and often an increase in cardiac silhouette on chest X-ray. Myocarditis is manifest by a tachycardia disproportionate for the degree of pyrexia, gallop rhythm, heart failure; there are also ECG changes, such as prolonged PR interval or greater degrees of AV block and T wave flattening or inversion, and raised serum creatine phosphokinase AV. Death occasionally occurs from myocarditis.

Endocarditis is indicated by transient or changing murmurs. The classical murmur, which is specific for the condition, is the Carey-Coombs murmur; this is a short rumbling diastolic murmur indicating mitral valvulitis.

Sydenham's chorea

Sydenham's chorea (St Vitus' dance) is usually a separate disease entity but, like rheumatic fever, appears to be related to recent beta haemolytic streptococcal infection and an autoimmune process; occasionally, it accompanies the rheumatic fever, although it may follow some weeks later. It is characterised by sudden, jerky, purposeless movements of the face and limbs such that the child is thought to be clumsy and grimacing. Pure chorea, even when unaccompanied by other evidence of rheumatic fever, is followed by a high incidence of rheumatic valve disease, indistinguishable from that following conventional rheumatic fever.

Investigation

Laboratory investigations show a raised ESR, C-reactive protein and anti-streptolysin O titre. Blood cultures are negative. Throat swab may be positive for beta haemolytic streptococcus, if the preceding pharyngitis has not been treated with antibiotic.

Differential diagnosis

Since there is no absolute diagnostic test, it is extremely common to find patients who have been diagnosed as having rheumatic fever on weak evidence, such as a childhood fever with a few aches and pains and the presence of

Table 12.25 Criteria for the diagnosis of rheumatic fever

Major criteria	Minor criteria
● Polyarthritis	● Fever
● Carditis	● Arthralgia
● Subcutaneous nodules	● Prolonged PR interval on ECG
● Chorea	● Raised ESR
● Erythema marginatum	● Raised white blood count or C-reactive protein
	● Preceding beta-haemolytic streptococcus infection
	● Previous rheumatic fever or inactive heart disease

a systolic murmur. In one study, some 50% of patients with mild congenital heart disease claimed to have had rheumatic fever, suggesting that a child with a heart murmur alone is very likely to be diagnosed as having rheumatic fever during the course of a febrile illness.

Management

Aspirin is traditionally used to control the arthritis and fever; it is used in maximum doses. Where the patient is extremely ill, corticosteroids are commonly used, but there is no evidence that these reduce the incidence of endocarditis or subsequent development of rheumatic valvular disease.

Prophylaxis

Anyone who has had acute rheumatic fever is at risk from a recurrence and is usually maintained on phenoxy-methylpenicillin (250 mg orally daily or an i.m. depot preparation of benzathine penicillin) or, if allergic to penicillin, oral sulphonamide, either until the age of 21 or for 5 years after the last attack of rheumatic fever, whichever comes later.

LIBMAN-SACKS ENDOCARDITIS

SLE (p. 1023) may lead to heart failure from hypertension and a myopathic process affecting the left ventricle. Involvement of the heart valves by a verrucous endocarditis is described as involving a significant proportion of postmortem specimens; however, valve disease is a clinical problem in only a few long-standing cases of SLE. The warty outgrowths occur at, and away from, the free edges of the valve cusps and over the mural endocardium. They involve the mitral valve in particular, and may lead to thickening of the chordae and subvalvular apparatus. Mitral regurgitation and aortic regurgitation are said to be the commonest lesions, but mixed valve lesions occur. Aortic stenosis has also been described in SLE. Libman-Sacks endocarditis may become the site of infective endocarditis and, if haemodynamically important, is treated by prosthetic valve replacement.

RHEUMATOID ARTHRITIS

A small percentage of patients with very active rheumatoid arthritis develop mitral and aortic valve disease, with exuberant nodular granulomatous lesions on the valve cusps and at other sites throughout the body. These lesions only occasionally cause significant valve disease but, very occasionally, may cause significant stenosis or regurgitation in a patient who has very exuberant and severe rheumatoid arthritis.

REITER'S DISEASE AND ANKYLOSING SPONDYLITIS

Reiter's disease and ankylosing spondylitis (p. 1005) can produce a degree of aortitis and aortic root dilatation and cusp retraction similar to that seen in syphilitic aortitis. There may be associated conduction abnormalities as well as aortic regurgitation, and, occasionally, these patients require aortic valve replacement and cardiac pacemakers.

CARDIAC TUMOURS

Cardiac tumours (Table 12.26) are rare. They can present a variety of clinical features and mimic many other cardiac and systemic diseases. Benign tumours comprise 75% of primary cardiac tumours.

MYXOMAS

The origin of myxomas is controversial. They appear as a gelatinous pedunculated mass usually arising from the fossa ovalis in the atria; 75% occur on the left, but occasionally the tumour invades both atria. About 75% are found in women. There is a slight familial tendency, and current theory suggests that myxomas arise from embryonic cells in the septum. Clinical presentation is in late middle-age, when they reach sufficient size. The clinical features are haemodynamic obstruction, embolisation and constitutional symptoms.

Left atrial myxoma

In left atrial myxoma, the large gelatinous mass obstructs the mitral valve and simulates mitral stenosis, producing left heart failure. A ball-valve mechanism can produce recurrent pulmonary oedema or syncope, which can lead to sudden death. Pulmonary hypertension with subsequent right heart failure mimics mitral valve disease. In one-third of patients, there are systemic emboli, with the

Table 12.26 Most frequent cardiac tumours

Tumour	Frequency (%)	Prognosis
Myxoma	30	Benign
Lipoma	10	Benign
Papillary fibroelastoma	10	Benign
Rhabdomyoma	8.5	Benign
Angiosarcoma	9	Malignant
Rhabdomyosarcoma	6	Malignant
Other (including secondary)	26.5	–

brain the most frequent site. Systemic symptoms are found in 90% of patients and mimic those of a collagen disease or infective endocarditis, with fever, anorexia, weight loss, myalgia, arthritis, Raynaud's phenomenon, petechiae and finger-clubbing. These features are thought to result from immunological reactions to necrosing tumour.

Physical signs can mimic those of mitral stenosis, with a diastolic murmur in about 20% of patients. More common is a systolic murmur of mitral regurgitation and, classically, there is a 'tumour plop' instead of the opening snap of mitral stenosis. However, the tumour can be silent or give only intermittent auscultatory findings.

Right atrial myxoma

Right atrial myxomas are less common than those on the left side; they can cause severe right heart failure with oedema, hepatomegaly, ascites and pleural effusion. Syncope and sudden death are also recorded, and recurrent emboli can lead to severe pulmonary hypertension and a paradoxical embolisation to the left side through a patent foramen ovale. Constitutional symptoms are as common as on the left. Physical signs are more frequent than on the left side, with systolic and diastolic murmurs being audible in over 80%, and endocardial friction rub audible in 20%.

Myxomas may arise in the ventricles, but these are less common. As with atrial myxomas, they are likely to embolise and cause obstruction.

Investigation

Echocardiography has revolutionised the diagnosis of myxoma. The tumour can often be visualised popping backwards and forwards through the valve orifice. However, the tumour can be missed, and a study from several windows may be needed to show small tumours and, particularly, right atrial myxomas. If satisfactory echo pictures are available, there is now nothing to be gained from cardiac catheterisation, which runs the risk of dislodging tumour and causing systemic emboli.

Laboratory tests are frequently abnormal, especially in patients with systemic symptoms. Haemoglobin is low (with normochromic normocytic film), but may, occasionally, be high with right atrial myxoma, severe pulmonary hypertension and right-to-left shunting through a patent foramen ovale. A neutrophil leucocytosis occurs. The ESR is often raised, with an increase in plasma gamma globulins.

Management

Surgical excision of the tumour is essential but carries some risk of tumour embolisation and recurrence, both from the site of excision, if incomplete, and from other sites in the heart. The tumour is therefore excised with its atrial attachment, and the atrial septum then patched. Many surgeons now inspect all four cardiac chambers, because of the high incidence of local recurrence and the occasional multiple tumour.

Atrial myxomas are relatively easily treated and should be suspected wherever there is unexplained systemic embolism, particularly if there are features of a 'collagen disease', if a case of 'infective endocarditis' is persistently culture negative, and if features of mitral valve disease are accompanied by syncopal episodes. Right atrial myxoma should be suspected in unexplained right heart failure and recurrent pulmonary emboli.

CARDIAC DISEASE AND PREGNANCY

Pregnancy places a sustained load on the heart which increases throughout the pregnancy and then peaks with labour. There is a considerable increase in cardiac output (30–50%), blood volume (40–50%) and extracellular volume (about 7 litres), with an increase in heart rate of about 10 bpm and a slight fall in mean blood pressure.

The circulation of the pregnant woman is as if she were vasodilated, with warm peripheries and an increase of up to 30% in resting oxygen uptake. The increase in cardiac output is accomplished by an increase in heart rate, stroke volume and ejection fraction. Venous pressure of the upper body increases marginally, if at all, whereas there can be an increase in lower body venous pressure when supine or standing, due in part to pressure of the gravid uterus on the inferior vena cava. This pressure increase, and the increase of up to 8.5 litres in total body water, often leads to oedema of the ankles. The increase in plasma volume occurs earlier than a compensatory increase in total red blood cell volume, so that an apparent anaemia ensues.

Diagnosis

Pregnancy makes the diagnosis of heart disease more difficult. The pregnancy may produce symptoms of fatigue, shortness of breath, ankle oedema and syncope. Physical examination may reveal flow murmurs, a mammary souffle, venous hum, a third heart sound, a raised *a* wave in the jugular venous pulse, displacement of the cardiac apex (by the elevated diaphragm) and basal rales (which clear on coughing) for the same reason, all of which may be taken to indicate heart disease.

The above confounding symptoms and signs are unfortunate because of the increased risk posed by heart disease to both the mother and the fetus. Another reason for establishing if heart disease is present, even if it appears to be asymptomatic, is the small risk of puerperal endocarditis. The murmur of pregnancy (*Still's murmur*) is a low-pitched, often vibratory murmur heard at the left sternal edge but usually loudest in the pulmonary area. It is extremely common, mid-systolic and unaccompanied by any other signs of heart disease. High-pitched systolic murmurs, and all diastolic murmurs, indicate heart disease. The use of echocardiography and Doppler ultrasound will often be of great value in these cases. Chest X-ray is relatively contraindicated. If essential, the fetus can be shielded. The risk to the fetus late in pregancy is much smaller than first thought.

The ECG is usually normal but the axis may shift to the left, with T wave inversion in lead 3, a small Q wave and sometimes even ST and T wave inversion in the limb and precordial leads; these ECG changes revert to normal at the end of pregnancy and recur in later pregnancies.

Management

If the pregnant mother is known to have heart disease and is in functional class 3 or worse of the New York Heart Association classification (p. 325, Table 12.1), it is hazardous for the pregnancy to continue. Certain types of heart disease, e.g. coarctation of the aorta, severe hypertension, severe aortic or mitral stenosis or cardiomyopathy, present particular hazards. Cyanotic congenital heart disease poses great risk to the mother if pulmonary hypertension is severe. Spontaneous abortion is frequent.

Surgery during pregnancy may offer a solution to the mother who is anxious to continue with the pregnancy; closed mitral valvotomy, or open valvotomy and valve replacement under cardiac bypass, have been performed with a low maternal mortality and acceptable fetal risk.

If valvular disease or a jet lesion (VSD, etc.) is diagnosed, appropriate antibiotic cover is given at the time of labour, particularly if instrumentation (e.g. urinary catheterisation) is used at the time of delivery.

Anticoagulants

A particular problem may be the need for anticoagulants. Discontinuation of anticoagulants is dangerous for a mother with a prosthetic heart valve, and possibly also for a mother who has had a pulmonary embolus. Warfarin is avoided during the first trimester, because of an increased risk of fetal abnormality. For a planned pregnancy, heparin can be given during the first trimester. Warfarin is then given until heparin is used to cover delivery by Caesarean section.

Peripartum cardiomyopathy

Pregnancy and labour may make occult heart disease manifest. Occasionally, catastrophic heart failure super-

venes and appears to be associated with a progressive cardiomyopathy.

Hypertension

Hypertension in pregnancy and pre-eclamptic toxaemia and eclampsia are discussed on page 431.

SECONDARY HEART DISEASE

A wide variety of pathological conditions may also increase cardiac output and produce heart failure. These include thyrotoxicosis, anaemia, cor pulmonale, beriberi, arteriovenous fistulae, generalised Paget's disease of bone and exfoliative dermatitis.

Thyrotoxicosis

Thyrotoxicosis dramatically increases metabolic rate, but the thyroid hormones also have a stimulant effect on the autonomic nervous system and the heart itself. There is usually a sinus tachycardia which is indicative of the severity of the disease, but in 15% of cases, thyrotoxicosis triggers a supraventricular arrhythmia, most frequently AF. Pulse pressure and blood pressure rise slightly and the heart contracts more vigorously in thyrotoxicosis.

Anaemia

Severe anaemia makes a two-fold demand on the heart. In order to supply the oxygen requirements of the body, the heart has to increase cardiac output, despite itself being perfused with anaemic blood. Mild anaemia is of marginal importance, but life-threatening anaemia may lead to cardiac dilatation and severe heart failure, with pathological changes in the myocardium of 'fatty heart'. As the myocardium extracts virtually all the oxygen from the blood in the coronary circulation, autoregulation of flow demands a dramatic increase in coronary flow to compensate for the extra myocardial work of severe anaemia. This cannot be accommodated if there is coronary disease of any severity, and continuous angina and heart failure may result.

Beriberi

Beriberi is uncommon outside Asia, but minor forms may occur in some alcoholics and food faddists. Severe thiamine deficiency (classically due to subsistence on polished rice) results in autonomic and other nervous system damage, with profound vasodilatation and a high cardiac output. In its fulminant form, the patient may die from pulmonary oedema within 48 hours of the onset of symptoms. Response to conventional heart failure therapy without thiamine is poor. Thiamine is given as soon as the diagnosis is suspected, and should be given to alcoholics in heart failure and in all cases of resistant heart failure where the nutritional background of the patient is doubtful.

Arteriovenous fistulae, Paget's disease of bone, exfoliative dermatitis

If they are severe enough, arteriovenous fistulae, Paget's disease of bone and exfoliative dermatitis may all cause a considerable reduction in peripheral resistance leading to a large increase in resting cardiac output. The patient has a bounding pulse and hyperkinetic circulation, often with a third heart sound and systolic murmur. Heart failure may supervene if the heart is already damaged or if the stress is severe enough. Treatment of the condition will alleviate the strain on the heart.

Inborn errors of metabolism and connective tissue disorders

Heart disease may complicate or be part of many other medical conditions (Tables 12.27–12.30).

Table 12.27 Inherited connective tissue diseases and the heart

Condition	Cardiac condition	General features
Cutis laxa	Peripheral pulmonary stenosis	General skin laxity, disrupted elastic fibres
Ehlers-Danlos	Mitral regurgitation Arterial rupture	Hypermobile joints Hyperelastic skin
Marfan's	Aortic dilatation, dissection, aortic and mitral regurgitation	Gracile habitus arachnodactyly, lens subluxation, sternal abnormalities
Osteogenesis imperfecta	Aortic regurgitation	Fragile bones, blue sclera
Pseudoxanthoma elasticum	Peripheral and coronary artery disease	Degeneration of elastin fibres leading to yellow pseudo-xanthomas of skin, retinal angioid streaks, hypertension

Table 12.28 Inborn errors of metabolism and the heart

Condition	Cardiac condition
Pompe's disease	Glycogen storage disease involving the heart muscle
Homocystinuria	Aortic and pulmonary artery dilatation
Mucopolysaccharidoses: Hurler's and Hunter's syndromes (mental deficiency)	Multivalvular disease, coronary artery disease and cardiomyopathy
Morquio's disease	Aortic regurgitation

Table 12.29 Chromosomal abnormalities and the heart

Chromosomal defect	Cardiac abnormality
Trisomy 21 (Down's syndrome)	Endocardial cushion defects, ASD, VSD, pulmonary stenosis
Trisomy 13	VSD, double-outlet right ventricle
Trisomy 18	VSD, persistent ductus arteriosus, pulmonary stenosis
Cri du chat (short arm deletion 5)	VSD
XO (Turner's syndrome)	Coarctation
XXXY and XXXXX	Persistent ductus arteriosus

ASD = atrial septal defect; VSD = ventricular septal defect

Table 12.30 Skeletal syndromes and the heart

Syndrome	Cardiac abnormality	Skeletal syndrome
Ellis von Creveld	Single atrium or ASD	Chondrodystrophic dwarfism
TAR	ASD or tetralogy of Fallot	Absent radius, thrombocytopenia
Holt Oram	ASD (and others)	Upper limb deformity, hypoplasia of clavicles
Laurence Moon-Biedl Bardet	Variable	Polydactyly, obesity
Noonan	Pulmonary valve dysplasia	Pectus excavatum
Tuberous sclerosis	Cardiomyopathy	Bone lesions
Leopard	Pulmonary stenosis	Broad facies, ribs abnormal
Cockayne	Accelerated atherosclerosis	Cachectic dwarfism
Progeria	Accelerated atherosclerosis	Skeletal hypoplasia
Apert	VSD	Craniosynostosis syndactyly

ASD = atrial septal defect; VSD = ventricular septal defect

Athlete's heart

Endurance athletes often have hearts which exceed 50% of the transverse diameter of the chest on chest X-ray, and they may have clinical cardiac enlargement as well. Associated with the cardiac enlargement is a slow resting heart rate and an increased stroke volume. The degree of enlargement seems to vary with the extent of the resting bradycardia, which can be as low as 35 bpm in extreme cases, but is more usually between 45 and 60 bpm. Exercise training appears to promote the bradycardia, which has both a vagal component and a component which appears to arise from withdrawal of the heart to chronotropic sympathetic drive. Elite endurance athletes with extremely slow resting heart rates and a large stroke volume can generate very high cardiac outputs, since their maximum exercising heart rate is the same as the normal (180–210 bpm). The high cardiac output enables them to maintain a superior oxygen uptake, and thus a superior work rate and endurance performance. A variety of ECG changes have been described in young athletes, some resulting from marked vagal tone, others from both right and left ventricular hypertrophy. The increased stroke volume can result in a soft systolic murmur, and third and fourth heart sounds are sometimes faintly audible with subjects who have marked bradycardia.

Diagnosis

Extreme examples of this condition can easily be confused with cardiomyopathy, and it is essential not to arrive at an erroneous pathological diagnosis. Fortunately, invasive investigation is not usually required. The assessment is based on exercise testing to measure aerobic capacity and echocardiography, which usually show superior performance of the heart.

An athlete with symptoms suggestive of heart disease should be rapidly investigated. They are not immune from heart disease, and superior athletic performance is compatible with several forms of cardiac pathology, some of which are potentially lethal. However, an athlete in strict training can lose form very rapidly if prevented from training. It is unfortunate for both the athlete and the credibility of the doctor concerned if training is interrupted for investigation of a suspected abnormality which is only part of the 'athletic heart syndrome'.

Sternal depression and straight back syndrome

Abnormalities of the shape of the thorax are a common cause of systolic murmurs; they may also give rise to musculoskeletal chest pains, an abnormal X-ray appearance of the heart and, in severe cases, ECG changes. Sternal depression and an abnormally vertical dorsal spine (straight back syndrome) both allow very little room for the heart in the anterior-posterior axis; this is well shown on the lateral chest X-ray. There is often a systolic murmur arising from the distorted great vessels; respiratory function may be impaired because of restricted chest wall expansion on inspiration, giving rise to a poor effort tolerance; and there may be associated mitral valve prolapse as a congenital anomaly. The ECG commonly shows right bundle branch block, and there may be anterior T wave inversion in the V leads in the most severe cases.

Assessment includes careful clinical examination to exclude primary cardiac pathology, and echocardiography and Doppler ultrasound where doubt exists as to whether there is more than a 'flow murmur'. Mild forms of this condition are commonly seen in pregnancy, when the patients are referred because of the murmur. Reassurance often helps the chest pains, which usually have a musculo-skeletal basis and become worse when the possibility of heart disease is raised. Simple back exercises may also help.

PERICARDIAL DISEASE

The pericardium is a fibrous bag which supports and invests the heart. Like the pleura, it may be the site of inflammation, neoplastic infiltration and calcification, and may also be the site of fluid collection with or without inflammation.

Aetiology

The causes of pericardial disease are shown in Table 12.31. All of these conditions can produce the clinical features of pericarditis with effusion. Heart failure can also cause a pericardial effusion, but these are small asymptomatic effusions, often discovered at routine echocardiography.

Acute viral pericarditis

The commonest viral causes are Coxsackie virus A or B, varicella, herpes simplex, influenza virus and echovirus (type 8). Frequently, a definite viral cause cannot be established. Typically, it occurs in young adults 1 or 2 weeks after an upper respiratory infection. The patient then develops fever, pericardial pain and malaise which may persist for a few weeks. Unfortunately, recurrences occur in about 25% of cases, possibly from an autoimmune mechanism. Tamponade is unusual.

Table 12.31 Causes of pericardial disease

Infections	Autoimmune
Viral, e.g. Coxsackie, influenza	Collagen disease, rheumatoid
Bacterial; pyogenic and tuberculosis	arthritis, SLE
Fungal	Postpericardiotomy and post-infarction
	(Dressler's) syndromes
Metabolic	Serum sickness and drug reactions
Uraemia	Idiopathic (benign recurrent viral)
Hypothyroidism	relapsing pericarditis
	Rheumatic fever
Neoplastic	
Carcinoma of the bronchus	**Haemopericardium**
Lymphomas	Cardiac rupture
	Aortic dissection
Myocardial infarction	Trauma and surgery
Radiotherapy	

Acute pyogenic pericarditis

Acute pyogenic pericarditis can follow pneumonia or a septicaemia and is treated with the appropriate antibiotics and repeated drainage, which may require surgical intervention. *Staphylococcus* and *Haemophilus* are the most common organisms involved. It may also occur in immunosuppressed patients and following cardiac surgery.

Tuberculous pericarditis

Tuberculous pericarditis may be asymptomatic until it presents as pericardial constriction (see below). It may present as a large pericardial effusion with enlargement of the cardiac silhouette on chest X-ray, or as a low-grade fever with weight loss, fatigue and features of pericarditis. Pericardial aspiration may reveal the organisms but occasionally (as with pleural effusions), culture of the fluid or pericardial biopsy may be required before the diagnosis is established.

Malignant pericarditis

Pericardial effusion fluid should always be sent for cytology, as malignancy may present with a pericardial effusion. The clinical features are similar to other types of pericarditis, but may be complicated by direct tumour extension into the pericardium with a degree of constriction. Lung cancer is the commonest cause.

Uraemic pericarditis

Uraemic pericarditis develops with severe untreated uraemia and disappears with dialysis. It appears to be directly related to the blood urea level.

Other types

In most other types of pericarditis, such as in autoimmune disease, pericardial involvement is an incidental finding, but occasionally may lead to constrictive pericarditis.

Clinical features

The principal symptoms of pericarditis are pericardial pain, breathlessness (if the effusion becomes large enough) and, eventually, tamponade. There may be systemic symptoms related to infection, such as fever, rigors, weight loss and symptoms of the underlying cause (lung cancer, tuberculosis, etc.).

Pericardial pain

Pericardial pain is a mediastinal pain that can be very similar to that of myocardial ischaemia, but differs in that it is more commonly referred to the shoulder and back and is often influenced by posture and mediastinal movements, such as coughing, sneezing and, particularly, swallowing. It is often relieved by leaning forwards. The diagnosis may be difficult because of the occurrence of pericardial pain following myocardial infarction. There can also be a pleural element to the pain.

Pericardial rub

Pericardial rub – the main physical sign of pericarditis – is very variable and often absent. It is a rough scratching sound which seems nearer to the observer than the stethoscope headpiece. Typically, it has three components – systolic, diastolic and atrial-systolic. However, the atrial-systolic and diastolic components may not be present, and a purely systolic scratchy murmur may have other causes. The noise can sometimes be accentuated by leaning the patient forward or, if conditions allow, by putting the patient in the knee-elbow position. The sound comes and goes and does not necessarily disappear with the formation of an effusion; indeed, it may be found in up to 70% of patients with pericarditis and effusion.

Pericardial effusion

Pericardial effusion does not usually cause symptoms unless it is large, when there may be some breathlessness and, eventually, features of tamponade (see below). The clinical signs of an effusion without tamponade (soft heart sounds, increased cardiac dullness, etc.) are not as helpful as chest X-ray and ultrasound.

Cardiac tamponade

If the pericardial cavity fills with blood or pericardial fluid, the pericardial pressure may rise sufficiently to embarrass filling of the heart and lead to a form of cardiogenic shock (*cardiac* or *pericardial tamponade*) with very low cardiac output, cerebral confusion, and severe hypotension proceeding to death, if the pericardium continues to fill.

The pericardium is visco-elastic and can therefore stretch slowly to accept as much as 2 litres of fluid over a period of time without the development of tamponade, but much smaller amounts of fluid can be fatal if they accumulate quickly.

Aetiology

Tamponade is usually caused by bleeding or effusion into the pericardial space. It can complicate aortic dissection and myocardial infarction with rupture into the pericardium. Bleeding can also follow surgery or trauma to the heart and mediastinum, and may follow perforation of the heart at cardiac catheterisation, or injury after pericardial aspiration. Malignant disease is a common cause, but tamponade is an uncommon complication of other causes of pericardial effusion.

Clinical features

Severe hypotension with impalpable or very weak peripheral pulses may be present. Classically, careful palpation of the arterial pulses reveals *pulsus paradoxus*, in which the pulse pressure drops considerably on inspiration and the pulse may even become impalpable. The paradox is not that the pulse volume diminishes with inspiration (which happens normally to a small extent), but that the stroke volume of the left ventricle declines markedly whilst – paradoxically – the heart seems to be beating normally. The mechanism of pulsus paradoxus is related to the pericardial tamponade dictating a small fixed volume to the heart. Normally, right ventricular filling is aided by inspiration but with tamponade (or pericardial constriction), this right-sided mechanism inhibits filling of the constricted left ventricle, whose stroke volume falls.

The jugular venous pressure is usually markedly raised, may show a marked systolic drop (prominent *x* descent) and, sometimes, rises with inspiration (*Kussmaul's sign*). Chronic tamponade can mimic constriction, with hepatic enlargement and oedema. The heart sounds may be faint and there can be a pericardial rub.

Investigation of pericarditis

The ECG changes of acute pericarditis are shown in Fig. 12.62. The ST elevation remains concave upwards and is followed later by widespread T wave inversion, probably indicating a degree of epicardial myocarditis. A large effusion can produce a diminution of ECG voltages;

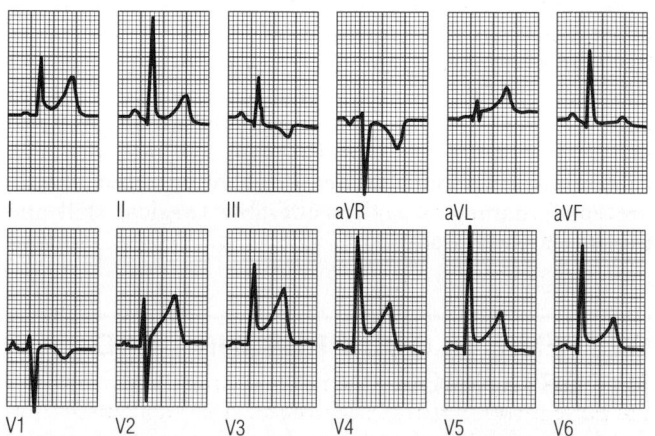

I   II   III   aVR   aVL   aVF

V1   V2   V3   V4   V5   V6

Fig. 12.62 ECG of acute pericarditis illustrating widespread concave ST segment elevation.

in extremely large effusions, there can be 'electrical alternans', with the voltage being influenced by the heart swinging backwards and forwards in the effusion.

Chest X-ray (if there is an effusion) shows increased cardiac silhouette, with a globular appearance to the heart but no evidence of raised pulmonary venous pressure. This appearance is not specific.

Echocardiogram is the technique of choice in demonstrating a pericardial effusion, preferably with a 2D scan. A small effusion can be localised, and may be missed unless the operator is experienced. With a large effusion, echocardiography will show the heart surrounded by a large bag of fluid which is seen as an 'echo-free' space.

Pericardial aspiration is described below. The fluid should be sent for bacteriological and cytological examination.

Management

Pericardial pain often responds to anti-inflammatory agents. Infective pericarditis demands prompt diagnostic aspiration and identification of the infective agent, with appropriate chemotherapy. In viral pericarditis anti-inflammatories alone are used, but where there is an autoimmune element, such as in postinfarction syndrome and recurrent 'viral' pericarditis, corticosteroids may help. A large effusion is drained as described below. If the patient suffers repeated attacks, a pericardial window can be made into the pleural space at operation.

Pericardial aspiration

Pericardial aspiration can be both diagnostic and therapeutic. In an emergency, e.g. after a road traffic accident with trauma to the chest, if a patient is moribund with features suggesting tamponade (i.e. very high venous pressure), then aspiration from the apex of the heart with a needle of adequate length should not be delayed. Removal of even 50–100 ml of blood from the pericardium may reverse the state of shock.

Elective aspiration is best performed in a coronary care unit with ECG, blood pressure and echo monitoring and a cardiac defibrillator available. After local analgesia of the chest wall, the pericardium is punctured either at the cardiac apex (which is free of major coronary vessels) or by a subxiphoid approach. The ECG monitor shows ventricular ectopics if the ventricles are touched. Using a metal needle connected to an ECG V-lead, a current of injury (raised ST segment) is produced as soon as the myocardium is touched and, hopefully, before the ventricle is pierced. Ideally, a cannula, rather than a needle, is left in the pericardium, and aspiration or drainage follows. If the fluid looks like blood, pericardial blood from a haemopericardium can be distinguished from ventricular blood by the fact that it is defibrinated and will not clot. It also has a lower haemoglobin and haematocrit than venous blood, since it is almost always diluted with serous pericardial fluid.

Diagnostic aspiration of a large effusion without subsequent drainage can lead to pericardial fluid draining into the pleural cavity. Drainage of a large effusion can take several hours, and recurrent effusion (e.g. in malignant disease) may require fenestration of the pericardium or insertion of a pericardioperitoneal drain by a cardiothoracic surgeon.

CONSTRICTIVE PERICARDITIS

Constrictive pericarditis results from thickening and fibrosis of the pericardium with, in some cases, extensive calcification.

Aetiology

There may be an antecedent history of acute pericarditis or radiotherapy. Tuberculous pericarditis is now rare in Western countries, but is the classic cause of calcific constrictive pericarditis.

Pathogenesis

The heart is effectively encased in a rigid box, which eventually prevents the heart from filling. Haemodynamically, the diastolic pressures or filling pressures of the two sides of the heart become the same as the intrapericardial pressure; as this rises, the patient goes into bilateral heart failure, in which features of right-sided failure predominate. Sometimes the constriction is selective so that the left or the right side, inflow or even outflow can be compromised most.

Clinical features

Symptoms

The major symptom is of severe oedema, often with ascites, liver engorgement and progressive weight loss secondary to hepatic engorgement and low cardiac output. Patients with long-standing disease look cachectic, and with the liver enlargement and a degree of jaundice are easily thought to have carcinomatosis or cirrhosis of the liver. The absence of significant left-sided heart failure symptoms is characteristic. The patient can often lie flat without problems and does not have a history of paroxysmal nocturnal dyspnoea, but will always have a limited exercise tolerance and dyspnoea on exertion. Constriction may arise with no previous history of pericarditis. A previous history of pericarditis is a valuable clue to the diagnosis.

Signs

A very high venous pressure is invariable, as the end diastolic pressure in both ventricles is about 25 mmHg. The high venous pressure is interrupted by a rapid x and y descent or *systolic collapse* of the venous pressure. The pulse exhibits pulsus paradoxus, but this is not invariable and the presence of AF in about 30% of cases makes the sign difficult to elicit. The pulse will, in any case, be of small volume. The heart is not clinically enlarged and the rigid pericardium may impede palpation of the cardiac impulse. The heart sounds may be faint with a loud additional sound, the *pericardial knock*. This is a loud early third heart sound, resulting from the rapid filling of the ventricles being suddenly impeded by the rigid pericardium. Murmurs are uncommon.

Investigation

The ECG is non-specific, showing low voltages and, usually, T wave inversion; other changes may reflect epicardial myocardial damage resulting from pericardial impingement on the epicardial coronary arteries.

Chest X-ray shows a normal-sized or slightly enlarged heart, often with an abnormal contour due to flattening of the atria. Calcification may be seen in the A-V groove on a lateral film. Depending on the sites of constriction, there may be signs of left or right atrial hypertension. Pleural effusions are common. Screening of the heart reveals a typical 'diastolic shock', with lack of pulsatility of the atria.

Echocardiography may demonstrate thickening of the pericardium. The ventricles fill rapidly in early diastole, but the differential diagnosis from constrictive cardiomyopathy is not easy.

Management

The only effective treatment is surgical decompression of the heart by removing enough of the pericardium to allow the heart to fill effectively. This means removing the adherent pericardium from around the great veins and atria, which are extremely thin-walled. Where the pericardium is adherent to the ventricles the coronary arteries are easily damaged, so considerable surgical skill and patience are required.

SYSTEMIC BLOOD PRESSURE AND HYPERTENSION

Cardiac performance and vascular resistance form part of an integrated system which controls arterial pressure and blood flow to the tissues. Despite our knowledge of many of the component mechanisms of pressure and flow control, many aspects remain unclear, both in health and disease.

CONTROL OF BLOOD PRESSURE

Neurosympathetic blood pressure control

Activation of preganglionic sympathetic neurones to the heart produces an increased heart rate and increased strength of contraction. Vasomotor sympathetic outflow constricts vascular smooth muscle, producing arterial vasoconstriction. The supply to the veins is richer and more sensitive than to the arterial system.

Increased vagal activity reduces the heart rate, but, with the exception of the coronary and salivary gland vascular beds, there is no parasympathetic control of the blood vessels.

Moment-to-moment reflex control of the circulation is via the arterial baroreceptors in the wall of the aorta and in the carotid arteries. The speed of this pressure-controlling mechanism is illustrated by its important role in maintaining systemic pressure during abrupt changes in posture.

Neurosympathetic influences on blood pressure and the circulation are rapid but tend to be transient; this is partly due to a tendency for the reflexes themselves to undergo accommodation, and partly because peripheral autoregulatory mechanisms may overcome neural constrictor effects.

Renin and angiotensin

The renin-angiotensin-aldosterone system (Fig. 12.24) plays a major part in the control of blood pressure, regional blood flow and blood volume, via its control of sodium balance. Renin secretion from granules in the juxtaglomerular apparatus is stimulated by a fall in plasma volume, a drop in blood pressure and sodium depletion. The consequent rise in angiotensin I I production and aldosterone secretion leads to sodium and water retention, and hence restoration of sodium balance and plasma volume. Under conditions of plasma volume reduction and sodium depletion (< 50 mmol Na^+/day), angiotensin II contributes to the maintenance of blood pressure by both vasoconstriction and interaction with the sympathetic nervous system. In the kidney, angiotensin II has a preferential constrictor effect on efferent (postglomerular) arterioles, and thus maintains glomerular filtration pressure when the overall arterial pressure is diminished.

The renin-angiotensin system plays a crucial role in the increased blood pressure seen with renal arterial constriction; the latter causes a rapid release of renin and angiotensin II and hence a rise in blood pressure. Angiotensin II causes changes in intrarenal flow patterns and stimulates aldosterone release. The combination of haemodynamic and direct effects on the renal tubules increases sodium reabsorption.

BLOOD PRESSURE MEASUREMENT

Korotkoff defined the auscultatory features (Korotkoff sounds) over the brachial pulse as pressure was released from an inflatable cuff. Systolic pressure correlates with the first sound (K_1) and diastolic pressure is usually within a few mmHg of sound muffling (K_4). Sound disappearance (K_5) is used to define diastolic pressure in many major trials of blood pressure treatment. In some individuals, K_5 cannot be defined when peripheral vascular resistance is low, as sounds carry on to zero cuff pressure. The anauscultatory gap (K_2–K_3) is particularly prominent in the elderly; this is important, as mistaken identification of K_3 as K_1 might lead to a serious underestimation of systolic pressure – by up to 15–20 mmHg in some cases. Its presence is accentuated by venous distension distal to the cuff.

Accurate blood pressure measurement requires a cuff of adequate size; a small cuff will seriously overestimate pressures. The subject should be seated with the manometer reservoir at the level of the sternal angle. The cuff bladder is arranged medially to overlap comfortably the medial aspect of the upper arm. Pressure in the cuff is inflated rapidly to 20–30 mmHg above that required to occlude the brachial or radial pulse. Pressure is then reduced slowly from the cuff whilst listening with a stethoscope over the previously located brachial pulse. The rate of pressure drop should not exceed 5 mmHg per second, and the line of sight should be such as to avoid parallax errors when reading the falling column of mercury.

SYSTEMIC HYPERTENSION

Definitions

Blood pressure varies considerably, rising during exertion, and is subject to a circadian variation which may not be completely activity-related. Ambient temperature and the degree of emotional or physical arousal will also affect systemic pressure levels. Systolic blood pressure rises with age in developed countries (Fig. 12.63). Within a community, blood pressure (systolic and diastolic) has a normal or Gaussian distribution, a factor which becomes very important when definitions of abnormalities of blood pressure are considered (Fig. 12.63).

Insurance companies were amongst the first to note that a reduced lifespan was associated with recordings of elevated blood pressure. It was clear from their data that no cut-off pressure level could be identified at which no increased risk of premature death was present. Hypertension could therefore be defined as a blood pressure above a particular value, e.g. 160/90 mmHg.

12 Cardiovascular Disease

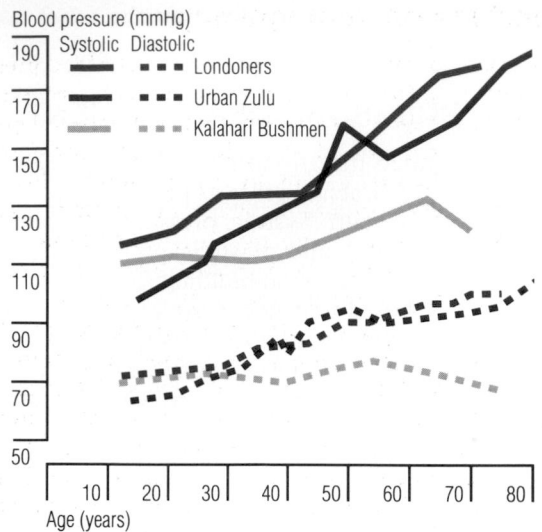

Fig. 12.63 Changes in blood pressure with age in three different communities: Londoners, urban Zulu and Kalahari Bushmen.

A more flexible definition – able to take into account new information derived from the results of therapeutic trials – might be preferable, for example, 'the level of blood pressure above which investigation and treatment do more good than harm.' Figure 12.64 illustrates how successive treatment trials (the Veterans Administration in 1965, compared with the Medical Research Council in 1985) have lowered the blood pressure at which treatment has been shown to have benefits.

Risk stratification

A small number of individuals have very high blood pressure and are at very high risk of complications of the

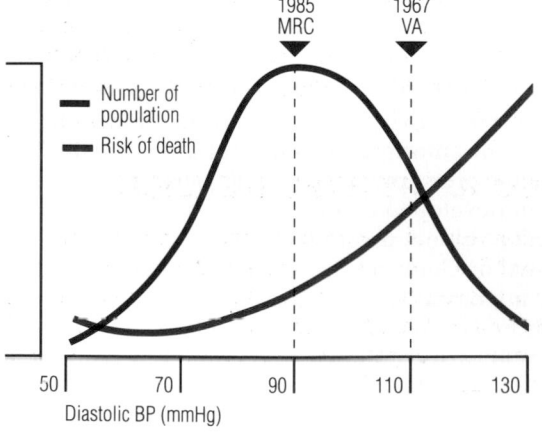

Fig. 12.64 Distribution of diastolic blood pressure in a Western population (black line). Risk of death is shown by the red line. The diastolic blood pressure levels are indicated at which treatment reduced mortality in two large trials (see text). VA = Veterans Administration; MRC = Medical Research Council.

disease, and death. At lower levels, the risk attributable to blood pressure is relatively less for the individual, but that low risk is shared by so many people that the associated complications and premature mortality pose a significant burden on the community.

Blood pressure is not the only risk factor in these calculations. Since drug treatment of great numbers of the population tends to carry unwanted financial and medical consequences (due to the requirement for life-long therapy), it is very important to pay attention to other contributing risk factors as well.

Hypertension in special groups in the community

There is a tendency to a high systolic blood pressure in old age and this carries with it the risks associated with hypertension at any age. Therapy is possible in older patients, and has been shown to reduce the risk of stroke and myocardial infarction.

Urban black populations have a higher incidence of hypertension than their white neighbours. Both environmental and genetic factors are likely to be responsible. Hypertension is rare in some rural African communities but a very major problem in others. Stroke is the most common complication amongst black hypertensives, and myocardial infarction is relatively rare; the opposite is the case for white hypertensives. The effectiveness of treatment is similar amongst blacks and whites; however, there are minor differences in the response to certain drugs, with a slight resistance to the effects of beta-adrenoreceptor blocking drugs being shown by black patients.

PRIMARY HYPERTENSION

Borderline and labile hypertension

About one-third of patients found to have an abnormal blood pressure at their first visit to the doctor will have lower blood pressure on subsequent visits. This border-line group may subsequently develop established hypertension. Some individuals appear to have wide swings in blood pressure, and have been called *labile hypertensives*. It seems likely that they do not form a pathologically distinct group, but manifest an accentuation of normal variability. As a group, they have a higher mortality than consistently normotensive individuals.

Isolated systolic hypertension

Due to arteriosclerotic changes in the major vessels of the elderly, the pulse pressure widens, with a greater rise in systolic compared with diastolic pressure. Thus, isolated systolic hypertension may be observed. Even in isolation, systolic hypertension is associated with an excess risk of morbidity through stroke, myocardial infarction and congestive cardiac failure. Unequivocal evidence of benefit of treatment in such cases is not yet available, but it seems reasonable to aim for a systolic pressure reduction to 140–160 mmHg, as long as treatment is well tolerated.

Benign or essential hypertension

Hypertension is never 'essential' and rarely benign; nevertheless these terms have the justification of common usage. This is the disease which affects the vast majority of those suffering from high blood pressure – possibly as much as 20% of the middle-aged population of the UK. The diagnosis depends on an established elevated systemic pressure in the absence of changes in the ocular fundi and of proteinuria, and where no identifiable cause of pressure elevation has been demonstrated. Essential hypertension can affect any age group and can, when untreated, lead to many complications, including malignant and accelerated-phase hypertension.

Malignant and accelerated-phase hypertension

Malignant or accelerated-phase hypertension is associated with vascular fibrinoid necrosis and loss of precapillary arteriolar autoregulation. The consequence is capillary vessel rupture and tissue necrosis through haemorrhage and ischaemia. The brunt of the damage is borne by renal, adrenal, cerebral, retinal, pancreatic and mesenteric vessels, for reasons that remain unclear. The clinical findings are elevated levels of blood pressure (which may be severe), associated with haemorrhages and exudates visible on the retina. Proteinuria due to similar vascular changes in the kidney is usual. Papilloedema (when present) reflects cerebral oedema and was previously used to differentiate malignant hypertension, where it was present, from accelerated-phase hypertension, where it was not. This differentiation has no clinical or prognostic value as the conditions are identical, with an untreated mortality of about 80%. Patients may have a past history of hypertension, but in most this is the first manifestation of their disease. It is one of the few occasions that hypertension is associated with symptoms, which include visual disturbance, headache and breathlessness due to pulmonary oedema; with severe degrees of cerebral oedema, blunting of consciousness, coma and epileptic seizures also occur. It is usually easy to treat and therapy is undoubtedly life-saving.

Many factors have been implicated in the genesis of malignant hypertension. The rate of rise of pressure may be more important than absolute levels of hypertension and there may be associations with other factors which damage blood vessels, such as cigarette smoking.

Hypertension in pregnancy

During pregnancy cardiac output rises, but blood pressure normally falls due to a decrease in vascular resistance. Obstetricians regard as abnormal a blood pressure greater than 140/90 (measured using Korotkoff 4 for diastolic pressure) in the first half of pregnancy, and by this criterion nearly one-quarter of the pregnant population will be hypertensive. About 2% will have a blood pressure greater than 160/105. *Pre-eclampsia* and *eclampsia* are placental syndromes, which are limited to the duration of pregnancy, and of which elevated blood pressure is just one manifestation. Pre-eclampsia was previously defined as hypertension with proteinuria (>0.5 g/l per 24 hours) and oedema. However, the latter is a frequent finding in normal pregnancies and often absent in pre-eclampsia, so that it is no longer included as a diagnostic criterion. Proteinuria is a late manifestation of pre-eclamptic renal impairment. Impaired uric acid clearance, which occurs much earlier in the disease process, is more useful diagnostically. Evidence of disseminated intravascular coagulation occurs late in the disease. Eclampsia is defined as the development of convulsions in the above setting.

The diagnosis of pre-eclampsia thus depends on the observations of an abnormal rise in blood pressure between the first and second halves of pregnancy of $\geqslant 30/20$ mmHg, associated with abnormal urate levels (>0.35 mmol/l at 32 weeks or >0.4 mmol/l thereafter); proteinuria, impaired renal function and clotting disorders confirm the diagnosis, but occur very late in the disease.

The consequences of pre-eclampsia are placental ischaemia and infarction and, in severe cases, maternal cerebral haemorrhage. Treatment is elective delivery, which confirms the diagnosis by effecting a rapid and complete cure. Medical management may reduce blood pressure but has not been shown to ameliorate other features of pre-eclampsia, which continues until delivery is effected.

Pre-existing hypertension, low social class and the first pregnancy with a particular partner are risk factors for pre-eclampsia; interestingly, it appears to be less common in smokers.

SECONDARY HYPERTENSION

The causes of secondary hypertension are given in Table 12.32. As a general rule, the younger the patient with hypertension, the greater is the likelihood that a cause will be found. In an adult hypertensive population, less than 5% of patients will have a discernible cause for their elevated blood pressure.

Renal disease

The precise cause of high blood pressure in chronic renal failure is not clear. Adequate management of hyperten-

Table 12.32 Causes of secondary hypertension

Type of cause	Examples
Renal	
Parenchymal disease	Chronic renal failure of any cause
	Acute and chronic glomerulonephritis
	Polycystic disease
	Pyelonephritis
	Tumours, e.g. haemangiopericytoma;
	Wilm's tumour
	Diabetes
Arterial disease	Arteriosclerotic disease
	Fibromuscular dysplasia
	Embolism
	Polyarteritis nodosa
Endocrine disease	
Adrenal cortical overactivity	Cushing's syndrome
	Conn's syndrome, adrenal hyperplasia
	Enzyme defects, e.g. congenital adrenal hyperplasia
Adrenal medullary overactivity	Phaeochromocytoma
Drug-induced	Contraceptive pill
	Liquorice-containing compounds
	Steroids
	Withdrawal of antihypertensives, esp. clonidine
	Cheese ingestion in patients taking monoamine oxidase inhibitors
	Sympathomimetic decongestant nasal sprays/appetite suppressants
Congenital defects	Coarctation of the aorta
Miscellaneous	Porphyria (during acute attacks)
	Lead poisoning (during acute phase)
	Raised intracranial pressure

sion is important to prevent vascular complication due to hypertension and prevent further deterioration of renal function. There is no justification for surgical removal of kidneys in unilateral renal disease, since medical treatment of hypertension is now likely to be more effective.

Renal arterial stenosis activates the renin-angiotensin system, and restoration of the normal vascular supply may potentially cure the associated hypertension. Atheromatous disease is the commonest form of renovascular disease; it mainly affects middle-aged male smokers, and is often part of a generalised degenerative disease of the arteries. Angioplasty may be useful, but the disease in smaller arteries limits the overall prognosis. In fibromuscular dysplasia (a disease of younger age-groups), surgical reconstruction of renal arteries may be very effective.

The importance of diagnosing renovascular hypertension has increased in recent years with the introduction of ACE inhibitors. These are to be avoided in renovascular hypertensives, as these drugs can precipitate renal failure due to the importance of angiotensin II in maintaining intrarenal haemodynamics in the underperfused kidney.

Endocrine disease

Hypertension, which may be severe, usually accompanies Cushing's syndrome (p. 702).

Hyperaldosteronism

Overproduction of aldosterone may be due to single or multiple autonomous adrenal adenomas (Conn's syndrome) or bilateral micronodular hyperplasia of the zona glomerulosa. Clinical suspicion of primary hyperaldosteronism is raised when untreated hypertension is associated with hypokalaemia ($K^+ < 3.5$ mmol/l), alkalosis ($HCO_3^- > 30$ mmol/l), and a serum sodium which is high or at the upper limit of normality ($Na^+ \geqslant 145$ mmol/l).

Investigation of *primary hyperaldosteronism* is aimed at differentiating adenomas from adrenal hyperplasia, as the former may be removed surgically. Radionucleotide adrenal scanning with labelled cholesterol, CT scanning and adrenal vein catheterisation to measure the production of aldosterone offer the best methods of diagnosis. Explorative surgery may be necessary in some instances. Hyperplasia is treated successfully with antialdosterone drugs, such as spironolactone or amiloride.

Phaeochromocytomas

Phaeochromocytomas are tumours, usually found in the adrenal, which secrete a mixture of catecholamines. They are responsible for clinical syndromes where hypertension may be episodic and alternate with episodes of postural hypotension. Paroxysms of hypertension are often associated with a constellation of symptoms, including headache, sweating, palpitations, feelings of apprehension and tremor. These symptoms are more sensitive in making the diagnosis than are most biochemical tests. The majority (90%) of the tumours are benign, and 10% arise outside the adrenals, most commonly at the bifurcation of the abdominal aorta. There are associated phaeochromocytomas in Sipple's syndrome (often a familial disorder with the combination of medullary carcinoma of thyroid and parathyroid adenoma) and in neurofibromatosis or von Recklinghausen's disease (p. 1154).

Investigation and management

Confirmation of the diagnosis is made by the detection of increased amounts of catecholamines and their breakdown products – normetadrenaline, metadrenaline and vanylmandelic acid (VMA) – in urine or plasma. Localisation of the tumours is by CT scanning and radionucleotide scans with MIBG (^{131}I meta-iodobenzylguanidine).

Treatment is surgical when possible, but can be hazardous due to surges of catecholamine secretion during tumour manipulation. Preliminary treatment with alpha-

and beta-blockade is essential, as are agents to raise blood pressure and prevent vascular collapse when the levels of these hormones fall rapidly as the tumour is removed.

Drug-induced hypertension

Mineralocorticoid-induced hypertension with hypokalaemia and alkalosis accompany the use of steroids, and may occur with carbenoxolone and excessive liquorice consumption. Hypertension induced by the contraceptive pill is generally mild and reversible on cessation of therapy, although this may take several months.

Coarctation of the aorta

In coarctation of the aorta, children or young adults present with asymptomatic upper limb hypertension and are noted on physical examination to have characteristically late and low-volume femoral pulses compared with the radial pulses (*radio-femoral delay*).

Hypertension may be difficult to treat medically and, if left until the patient is a teenager, is often only partially helped by surgical repairs of the narrowed aortic segment. Those operated on late (after 20 years of age) frequently suffer the complications of uncontrolled hypertension, and about 12% may die in their thirties of cerebral haemorrhage or ruptured aortic aneurysm. Surgery is now recommended before the age of 6, but balloon angioplasty has recently been successfully used in this condition and may be used more frequently in the future if initial good results are maintained.

The hypertension of coarctation is not fully explained, but renal hypoperfusion, aortic baroreceptor activity and mechanical effects of aortic obstruction may all play a part.

CLINICAL FEATURES OF HYPERTENSION

Until complications appear, essential hypertension has no symptoms and, by definition, no associated physical signs save for the elevated blood pressure. Headaches (once widely regarded as indicators of hypertension) are no more common in hypertension than in the general population, although very severe hypertension, associated with cerebral oedema, does produce headache. Breathlessness may be present, due to elevated left ventricular and end-diastolic pressure and pulmonary venous congestion produced by left ventricular hypertrophy.

Once the complications of essential hypertension are present, they are reflected in the symptoms and physical signs. Ventricular hypertrophy may lead to breathlessness, orthopnoea and frank cardiac failure; coronary disease to angina pectoris or myocardial infarction; cerebrovascular disease to stroke and dementia; and renal disease to all its associated symptoms.

The presence of some symptoms (e.g. those associated with phaeochromocytoma) will suggest a secondary cause. Symptoms of renal impairment (e.g. nocturia and polyuria) may reflect the consequence of long-standing hypertension rather than its cause.

Certain points in the examination of the hypertensive deserve emphasis, and require careful observation at diagnosis and during follow-up.

Pulse

Rate and rhythm. Atrial fibrillation is a late consequence of hypertension. A resting tachycardia might imply cardiac decompensation or a secondary cause, such as phaeochromocytoma or hyperthyroidism.

Arterial wall. If thickened arteries are palpated in an under 50-year-old, aggressive treatment of blood pressure and other risk factors would be justifiable.

Peripheral pulses. Radio-femoral delay is a sign of aortic coarctation, which may be a cause of hypertension in young patients. In older patients, atherosclerotic disease may cause peripheral vascular bruits and absent distal pulses.

Apex beat

A displaced and thrusting apex beat indicates left ventricular hypertrophy (LVH) and therefore hypertension worthy of aggressive treatment. The absence of this sign does not exclude LVH.

Abdomen

Palpable kidneys might be found with polycystic renal disease. A systolic and diastolic abdominal or flank bruit raises the possibility of renal arterial stenosis.

Optic fundus

Haemorrhage, exudates and papilloedema (grades 3 and 4) are all signs of accelerated or malignant hypertension. Early signs of arterial wall thickening are narrowing of the arterial lumen (grade 1, which is difficult to identify) and arteriovenous nipping (grade 2).

General aspects

Other important general signs include:

- signs of risk factors for vascular disease (xanthomata), which might tip the balance in favour of treatment because of the increase in vascular risk
- signs suggesting Cushing's syndrome or neurofibromatosis (associated with phaeochromocytoma)
- indications of congestive cardiac failure.

12 Cardiovascular Disease

INVESTIGATION

The extent to which patients with elevated blood pressure are investigated depends on the outcome of the history and clinical examination. Biochemical, radiological and cardiac investigations have two aims:

- to determine the effect that elevated blood pressure has already had on various organ systems, in particular the kidneys and the heart
- to identify a cause of the hypertension.

Numerically, the latter is far less rewarding since only about 5% of all cases of hypertension have an identifiable cause. This proportion is higher in young adults, all of whom should be investigated accordingly.

Urine testing

Even though the yield of abnormal results by dip-stick testing is not high, this simple test is essential in all cases. Persistent proteinuria requires detailed testing of renal function (p. 792). The discovery of haematuria should be followed by tests for inflammatory and neoplastic disease of the kidney.

A 24-hour urine collection is required to quantitate protein excretion; this may be helpful in hyperaldosteronism, Cushing's disease and phaeochromocytoma.

Blood tests

Routine haematological and biochemical tests are seldom rewarding. However, it is usual to obtain a full blood count and biochemical profile, which may occasionally provide useful information, for example:

- an indication of renal function (urea and creatinine)
- electrolyte disturbances (low K^+, raised HCO_3^- and Na^+) that might indicate hyperaldosteronism
- other associated risk factors, such as hyperuricaemia or hyperlipidaemia
- anaemia due to chronic renal disease, or polycythaemia secondary to renal disease.

ECG

An initial ECG may be helpful as a baseline for future changes, as well as in deciding whether to offer treatment. Features to be documented are signs of left atrial enlargement ('P mitrale', p. 332) and, with more severe levels of hypertension, evidence of LVH (Fig. 12.65) possibly associated with abnormalities in the ST segments and T waves that denote the 'strain' pattern. With effective blood pressure reduction these changes usually resolve.

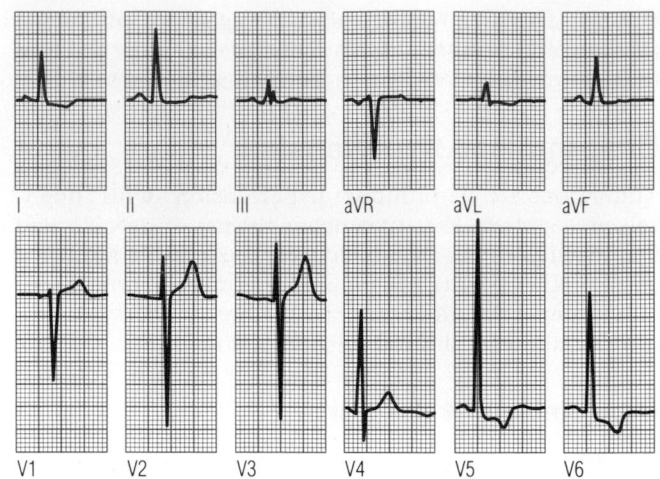

Fig. 12.65 Typical ECG in severe hypertension showing left ventricular hypertrophy.

Chest X-ray

The chest X-ray is helpful in establishing cardiac size and may reveal cardiac failure. In most Caucasian patients it is normal, but cardiac enlargement is common in hypertensives of African descent. In young hypertensives, signs of a coarctation (p. 389) may be found.

Ultrasound techniques

The echocardiogram can accurately measure ventricular hypertrophy and estimate function, while the abdominal examination shows kidney size, ureteric anatomy and some information on the renal substance. Both tests should be reserved for patients whose initial investigations reveal a problem requiring further definition.

Nuclear medicine techniques

Nuclear medicine techniques are used to measure dynamic aspects of kidney and cardiac function. These specialised methods should be reserved for those in whom a specific problem has been identified.

Intravenous urography

Intravenous urography may be helpful in assessing renal size and function and to exclude obstruction in patients with probable renal disease.

COMPLICATIONS OF HYPERTENSION

The development of LVH in hypertension is an adaptive response, but the effects on diastolic function may give rise to pulmonary venous congestion and, with increasing hypertrophy, inner layers of myocardium become ischaemic. The associated acceleration of atheromatous coronary disease contributes to the progression to left ventricular dysfunction and cardiac failure.

Atheroma deposition is accelerated by hypertension, and causes the most numerous of the complications of coronary artery disease; it also is responsible for most of the cases of stroke. Aortic dissection is a consequence of vessel wall degeneration and cystic medial necrosis.

A pathologically distinct process affects smaller vessels, particularly of the renal and cerebral circulations; this consists of medial and intimal proliferation. Renal impairment may follow, although renal failure is usually a complication of the fibrinoid necrosis of the resistance vessels, which characterises malignant or accelerated phase hypertension.

SUITABILITY FOR TREATMENT

At the highest levels of blood pressure (diastolic pressure greater than 115 mmHg) the risks to the individual patient are so high that treatment is mandatory. However, confirming that it is beneficial to treat patients with diastolic pressures between 90 and 114 mmHg has been more difficult. The combined results of randomised trials suggest that treatment has decreased the odds of stroke significantly, by about 40%. Treatment only managed to reduce the risk of heart attack by 10%. These large trials have provided no evidence to favour any one particular drug regimen over any other.

Patients with diastolic blood pressures above 105 mmHg are recommended for treatment, particularly if they demonstrate any ventricular hypertrophy or renal impairment. For the 10–15% of the middle-aged population with diastolic pressures between 90 and 104 mmHg, a more complex strategy is necessary. This is because halving the annual risk of a stroke, from 0.1 to 0.05%, in an asymptomatic middle-aged man may not be worthwhile, particularly when set against the requirement for lifelong treatment. However if the individual has already suffered a complication, such as a transient ischaemic attack, halving the annual stroke risk from 20 to 10% is a worthwhile goal.

A strategy for patients with diastolic blood pressure between 90 and 104 mmHg should aim to identify those individuals with the highest risk of complications. Treatment begins with measures to reduce associated risk factors, such as smoking, high blood lipids and obesity. Drug therapy of mild hypertension should therefore be reserved for those in whom all other measures have failed and those who carry the greatest risk of progression to severer forms of blood pressure or cardiovascular complications.

Systolic hypertension

Although epidemiological studies have shown that systolic blood pressure is at least as good a predictor of subsequent complications as diastolic pressure, there is less information on the levels of systolic pressure which should be treated. In most cases, systolic and diastolic pressures follow each other closely. However, difficulties arise in elderly patients, where isolated systolic hypertension is more common. Precise guidelines are not available, but the fears that treatment might reduce cerebral blood flow and worsen cerebrovascular risks have not been borne out. Reduction of high systolic pressures (greater than 180 mmHg) might therefore be expected to accrue benefits by reducing the stroke rate, and this indeed has been the finding in the few studies of elderly hypertensive patients.

METHODS OF TREATMENT

The importance of attention to associated risk factors, such as smoking and hyperlipidaemia, has already been emphasised, and is an important part of all treatment strategies. Blood-pressure-lowering drugs may not be needed if other methods are successful.

Non-pharmacological methods

Drug withdrawal. Withdrawal of drugs which may contribute to hypertension, e.g. NSAIDs, steroids and oestrogen-containing compounds such as the oral contraceptive pill, should be considered where possible.

Dietary measures. For each kilogram loss of weight, blood pressure can be expected to fall by 2.5–3.0 mmHg systolic and 1.5–2.3 mmHg diastolic. In general, salt restriction has not been found to be an effective treatment for hypertension at the levels of intake achievable with a tolerable Western diet. However, high salt intakes can negate the effectiveness of the thiazide diuretics used in treatment, so that it is important to ensure patients moderate their intake.

Relaxation. Teaching patients to relax – using formal programmes administered by non-medical personnel in general practices and continued at home by the patient – has been shown to produce a modest sustained blood pressure reduction.

Exercise. Aerobic exercise maintained for some 15–20 min will lower subsequent blood pressure readings by 5–10 mmHg for about 12 hours. Exercise may also improve associated cardiac risk factors, including obesity.

Drug treatment of essential hypertension

Principles of drug treatment of hypertension are theoretically simple. Therapy with a single drug given once a day is the ideal, but combination treatment is frequently necessary. A step-by-step approach is frequently used, starting with a first-line preparation alone, then in combination with another, before third- and fourth-line drugs are used (Table 12.33).

Diuretics

The long-acting thiazide diuretics such as chlorothiazide and bendrofluazide are effective, although symptomatic side-effects such as impotence and gout can occur. They are less powerful in renal failure, when loop diuretics such as frusemide and bumetanide have an advantage.

Thiazide diuretics cause biochemical changes which have given concern about their long-term safety. In particular, mild hypokalaemia is common, and may be associated with a risk of cardiac arrhythmias. Hyperuricaemia may produce symptomatic gout and, in conjunction with glucose intolerance and increases in cholesterol and triglyceride concentration, an overall worsening of the cardiovascular 'risk factor profile' is produced by these drugs. It is not at all clear whether these concerns are justified, although the lack of improvement in the incidence of myocardial infarction in the vast majority of hypertension treatment trials has been attributed in part to these unwanted biochemical effects of the thiazide diuretics.

Beta-adrenoreceptor blockers

Chance clinical observations led to the recognition that the beta-adrenoreceptor blockers are effective antihypertensives. These drugs are specifically contraindicated in obstructive airways disease, due to the production of asthma even by drugs with supposed cardiac selectivity. Other troublesome side-effects are related to the beta-receptor blocking action, with bradycardia, tiredness, claudication and cold limbs being prominent. The demonstration of their protective effect following myocardial infarction, as well as their antiarrhythmic and antianginal actions, make beta-blockers a rational choice when IHD complicates hypertension. They have to be used with great caution, if at all, in heart failure. Plasma lipids are altered with beta-blockade, potentially worsening the cardiovascular risk. However whether these alterations are deleterious in the long term has not been clarified.

Beta-blockers with diuretics have become established as the mainstays of the management of hypertension.

Table 12.33 Indications for specific antihypertensive drugs and their common side-effects

Type of drug	Indication	Advantages	Symptomatic side-effects	Other side-effects
Diuretics				
Long-acting thiazides	First line or adjunct to beta-blockers or Ca antagonists	Effective, cheap, usually once-daily treatment	Gout, impotence	Hypokalaemia Glucose intolerance ↑ Lipids
Spironolactone Amiloride	First line in Conn's or adrenal hyperplasia	Potassium-sparing	Gastrointestinal upset	Hyperkalaemia in renal impairment
Loop	In renal disease	Powerful diuretics	–	As for thiazides
Beta-adrenoreceptor blockers	First line	Antianginal and antiarrhythmic	Asthma in some subjects, tiredness, claudication and cold hands/feet	? lipid effect ↑ LDL ↓ HDL
Calcium antagonists	First or second line	Antianginal and antiarrhythmic	Flushing, oedema, gastrointestinal upset	Heart block and negative inotropy with some examples
Angiotensin-converting enzyme inhibitors	First line in renal disease First line in heart failure	Well tolerated and very powerful; useful in heart failure	Cough, postural hypotension	Profound hypotension Renal impairment in renovascular disease
Others				
Methyldopa/clonidine	Second/third line Methyldopa in pregnancy	Can be used alone effectively	Sedation, impotence	Haemolytic anaemia
Hydralazine	Third line	Largely superseded by Ca antagonists and ACE inhibitors	Headache	SLE-type reactions
Prazocln/indoramin	Third line	Largely superseded by Ca antagonists and ACE inhibitors	Postural hypotension	–
Diazoxide	Third line	Largely superseded by Ca antagonists and ACE inhibitors	Oedema	Glucose intolerance
Minoxidil	Third and fourth line	Extremely powerful vasodilator	Hirsutism, oedema	Fluid retention
Bethanidine/guanethidine	Fourth line	Rarely indicated	Postural hypotension/impotence	Hypotensive infarction

There are many examples of these drugs. In the UK, atenolol, metoprolol, propranolol, bisoprolol and pindolol are commonly used examples.

Calcium antagonists

The antihypertensive effectiveness of calcium antagonists is related to the fall in peripheral vascular resistance that follows resistance vessel vasodilatation. Side-effects of nifedipine can be attributed to its vasodilator activity and include flushing, headache and oedema; in contrast, verapamil has more gastrointestinal side-effects, and ought not to be combined with beta-blockade due to its propensity to produce heart block and impair ventricular contractility. Diltiazem fills an intermediate position with fewer peripheral effects and more cardiac effects than nifedipine, but less myocardial effects than verapamil. Although these drugs have not been subjected to close analysis in large trials, there is no doubt of their efficacy and popularity, even as a first-line therapy.

Angiotensin-converting enzyme inhibitors

The ACE inhibitors were specifically manufactured to inhibit the renin-angiotensin system, by blocking the conversion of angiotensin I to its active form, angiotensin II. These drugs are subjectively very well tolerated, and their associated efficacy, in all but the groups of patients with renal arterial stenoses, has led to their adoption as the first of the second-line treatments to be used in the severer degrees of hypertension. Cough is a common (>10%) side-effect of ACE inhibitors but at higher doses severe neutropenia, rashes and taste disturbance have been seen with captopril. Their hypotensive effect may be severe in relatively hypovolaemic patients and in those with hyponatraemia (which might occur in those taking diuretics). ACE inhibitors will cause a deterioration in function or renal failure in renal arterial stenosis.

Methyldopa

In pregnancy, methyldopa still maintains a place in the treatment of hypertension, but the associated CNS side-effects have made it less popular now that less sedative preparations are available.

Sympathetic ganglion blocking drugs

In the past, the sympathetic ganglion blocking drugs (guanethidine and bethanidine) were important as early effective treatments, but their use is now limited by their troublesome postural hypotensive effects, lack of supine blood pressure control and the sexual dysfunction that they produce in men.

Drug treatment of hypertension in pregnancy

Pre-eclampsia

The treatment of pre-eclampsia (p. 431) requires delivery of the fetus. Nevertheless, drugs may be needed to control the blood pressure before delivery can be achieved. Methyldopa (250–500 mg, 6-hourly by mouth) is used and, if necessary, can be given parenterally. It has the advantage of being effective and harmless to the fetus, although its sedative side-effects can confuse neurological assessment and its onset of action is slow (1 hour). Hydralazine, orally (<300 mg daily), by intramuscular injection (10–20 mg, 3–6-hourly) and by constant infusion (5–10 mg/h) is a suitable alternative, although flushing, tachycardia and vomiting may be side-effects at the higher doses. Given intravenously, it has a rapid onset of action which can be maintained by a constant infusion. Beta-adrenoreceptor blockers and calcium antagonists have been found to be effective in the acute situation, although experience with these drugs and follow-up of the delivered neonates has been shorter than for methyldopa and hydralazine. Diuretics are used only when cardiac failure complicates the picture.

Chronic hypertension in pregnancy

Due to its known lack of effects on the fetus, methyldopa is the drug of choice; hydralazine is the usual alternative, although beta-adrenoreceptor blockers are being used increasingly without undue hazard. Mothers who are known moderate hypertensives may be advised to cease treatment at the time of conception, although no teratogenicity has been associated with any of the commonly used antihypertensive drugs.

Drug treatment of hypertensive emergencies

Accelerated or malignant phase hypertension

This previously rapidly fatal condition is now managed by bed rest with admission to hospital and oral treatment. Parenteral treatment is avoided unless coma, fits or severe heart failure are present. Under these circumstances, an effective treatment is an intravenous infusion of labetalol starting at 25 mg/hour and increasing to 120 mg/hour with additional diuretic treatment for pulmonary oedema. Intravenous nitrates are also effective in this situation. Hydralazine given intramuscularly has been a popular treatment, but the 20 min delay in onset of action may lead to additional doses or drugs being given, resulting in hypotension some hours later. Methyldopa, even when given intravenously, is also too slow to be used effectively.

For cases due to phaeochromocytoma, phentolamine (2.5–10 mg i.v. bolus or 1 mg/min by i.v. infusion) produces a rapid pressure reduction by alpha-adrenoreceptor blockade, but such a response is not limited to this disease.

Oral treatment is optimal in most cases of malignant and accelerated hypertension, and any of the usual antihypertensive drugs can be used successfully. Recent observations show that sublingual nifedipine (10–20 mg) produces a smooth blood pressure reduction beginning within 10 min, although the reflex tachycardia it produces may require treatment with a beta-adrenoreceptor blocker. Additional diuretic treatment is often given.

The degree and rapidity of blood pressure reduction is important. In chronic hypertensives, cerebral autoregulation is lost at mean blood pressures above 150–175 mmHg and below 90–120 mmHg. Treatment should reduce mean blood pressure to 100–120 mmHg and no lower. This should be achieved over a 12–36 hour period to allow time for the relatively slow process of re-establishing normal cerebral autoregulation.

Aortic dissection

Aortic dissection is an emergency requiring prompt reduction of mean blood pressure to 100–110 mmHg; this is usually achieved with an infusion of sodium nitroprusside, starting at 12.5 mg/min and titrating the dose against blood pressure every 2–3 min. Infusion should not continue beyond 24 hours, but the resulting thiocyanate accumulation can be diminished by concomitant use of hydroxycobalamine by injection. There may be an advantage in reducing the systolic rate of change in aortic pressure as well as mean pressure. This can be achieved with beta-adrenoreceptor blockade, so that labetalol infusion with its mixed, though predominantly beta-receptor, effects has been advocated for use in dissection.

Hypertension in chronic renal failure

A proportion of patients with chronic renal failure have hypertension; in these, blood pressure may be controlled by dietary sodium restriction and fluid removal at haemodialysis. Drug treatment is necessary in some cases, and the excretory metabolism must be taken into account when dosages are calculated. Treatment is generally similar to that in essential hypertension.

Hypertension in phaeochromocytoma

Hypertensive crises in phaeochromocytoma can be treated conventionally, but it is important to avoid beta adrenoreceptor blockade before full alpha-adrenoreceptor blockade has been achieved, in order to avoid unopposed alpha effects exacerbating hypertension. Parenteral phentolamine can be used acutely, and longer-term control gained with phenoxybenazamine (10–30 mg t.d.s.) with the later addition of small doses of a beta-blocker, such as propranolol (40 mg t.d.s.). If a surgical cure cannot be effected, long-term treatment with alpha-methyl-tyrosine can be used, although side-effects are often troublesome.

Adrenocortical hyperplasia and Conn's syndrome

Surgical removal of the adenomas in Conn's syndrome may not always cure the electrolyte disturbances and hypertension. In these circumstances, as in idiopathic hyperplasia, treatment with amiloride (20–70 mg daily) or spironolactone (200–400 mg daily) is effective.

VASCULAR DISEASE

DISSECTING AORTIC ANEURYSM

Dissection occurs when there is haemorrhage into the wall of the aorta causing the media to separate from the other layers (Fig. 12.66). Most dissections are seen in middle-aged or elderly men with arteriosclerosis and hypertension. More than 50% of patients who present with dissection die within 24 hours. It is a particular complication of Marfan's syndrome, where cystic medial necrosis is common.

Dissections can be clinically classified according to the part of the aorta that is affected. When the ascending aorta is involved, it is termed a *type A* dissection (De Bakey types I and II), whereas those where only the aorta

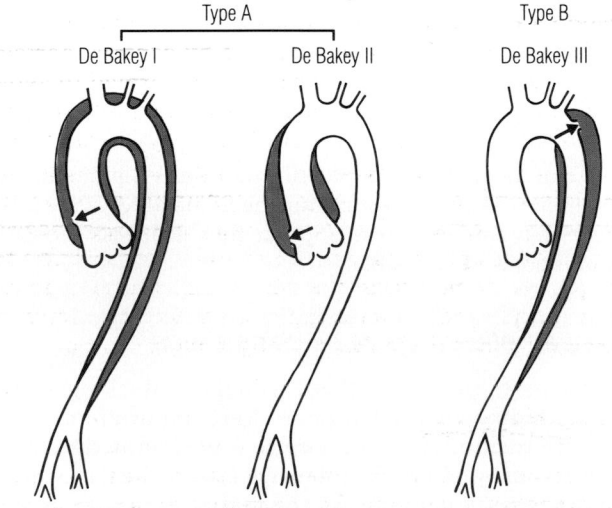

Fig. 12.66 Sites of dissection in aortic aneurysm.

beyond the left subclavian origin is involved are called *type B* dissections (De Bakey type III).

Clinical features

The most prominent symptom is a very sudden onset of excruciating pain, often described as tearing in nature. Unlike infarction pain, the pain is often totally unheralded and at its worst initially, but may uncommonly develop to a pulsating discomfort that persists. The pain may radiate through to the back and, in type B dissection, to the left shoulder. Typical myocardial infarction pain may also coexist if the coronary arteries are involved by the dissection.

Diagnosis and investigation

The diagnosis can be difficult, and its importance has considerably increased with the emphasis on early acute treatment of myocardial infarction with thrombolytic drugs. Clearly, these may have terrible consequences in dissection. The patients are frequently hypertensive or have a history of hypertension, which may or may not have been treated. Patients with Marfan's syndrome are usually easy to identify but form only a small proportion of cases. In about 10% of patients, a difference in blood pressure (20 mmHg or more) in the two arms may be found and, in some, a prominent pulsation is visible at the root of the neck. Auscultation may reveal aortic regurgitation in type A dissection, which is typically more obvious at the right sternal edge.

The ECG may be normal except in those cases with associated coronary artery involvement. In some individuals, the chest X-ray provides the first clue to the diagnosis, with mediastinal widening, left-sided pleural effusions and expansion of the aortic knuckle border beyond a calcified rim of endothelium. The diagnosis is confirmed at cardial catheterisation by contrast aortography. Coronary angiography is also performed to allow surgical repair. CT is helpful and less invasive, often being performed prior to catheterisation but rarely supplanting it totally. MRI is rapidly replacing CT. Echocardiography by the standard methods may demonstrate a proximal ascending aortic dissection, but transoesophageal echocardiography is the only ultrasound method able to adequately demonstrate the descending thoracic aorta. Transoesophageal colour Doppler is particularly useful, as the flow patterns make the intimal tear more obvious.

Complications

Complications of the dissection include occlusion of arterial branches, including the coronary arteries, head and neck vessels and indeed all distal arterial branches.

Stretching of the aortic annulus in type A dissection is responsible for aortic regurgitation, which may be severe and lead to left ventricular failure and shock. Progressive dilatation of the aorta may obstruct the airways or oesophagus. Finally, rupture of the aortic wall may occur, producing pericardial or pleural effusion and, occasionally, intrabronchial haemorrhage. This complication frequently, but not always, causes death.

Management

Treatment is usually surgical for type A dissection and many cases of type B. However, acute management includes blood pressure reduction by parenteral treatment, preferably with drugs reducing the inotropic force of the heart, such as labetalol by infusion. Pain control and sedation are also very important in this very distressing condition, where the outlook is often very poor.

ARTERITIS

Arteritis is an inflammatory process involving the artery wall. It can occur in vessels of various sizes. If these are small, the condition is called necrotising vasculitis and is found in a large number of 'autoimmune' conditions (discussed in Chapter 23, p. 1030). Involvement of large arteries is much less common and occurs principally in Kawasaki's disease, Takayasu's (or pulseless) disease and giant cell (or temporal) arteritis.

KAWASAKI'S DISEASE

Kawasaki's disease is a disease of children described originally in Japan but now reported from other parts of the world. The aetiological agent is unknown, but, as the disease occurs in cyclical epidemics, an infective agent is suspected. It was originally called 'mucocutaneous lymph node syndrome' because of the prolonged fever, skin rash and marked cervical lymphadenopathy. Later it was realised that there is a high incidence of coronary artery aneurysms, occlusions and myocardial infarction, which, because many of the patients are infants, were originally missed. Diagnosis of these lesions can often be made noninvasively by ECG and 2D echocardiography. Management is based on the use of antithrombotic agents and steroids, but aspirin alone has been found to result in a lower incidence of coronary artery complications than some other regimens.

TAKAYASU'S ARTERITIS

Takayasu's arteritis – a disease which predominantly affects Oriental women – was first described by an ophthalmologist whose first case was a young woman with cataracts and unusual arteriovenous anastomoses around the optic papillae. It was later realised that similar ophthalmic findings were seen in patients with absent radial pulses, hence its alternative name, 'pulseless disease'.

The disease can be classified into three types:

- Type I involves the aortic arch and its branches, producing diminished or absent pulses over the upper body (so-called 'reversed coarctation').
- Type II involves the descending aorta, particularly the renal arteries and vessels supplying the abdominal viscera.
- Type III is a combination of I and II.

Takayasu's arteritis has also been implicated in the development of primary pulmonary hypertension.

The aetiology is unknown but the disease commonly starts in female teenagers, with a sex ratio of 8:1.

Clinical features

There is often a systemic illness with fever, arthralgia and fatigue. There may be pain and tenderness over the affected arteries. This systemic phase passes and is followed by a latent period. Some time later, these patients, and others who had no systemic prodrome, present with the typical features of weak or absent pulses, low or unrecordable upper body blood pressure, hypertension, heart failure and ocular damage.

The hypertension is produced by an increased aortic impedance secondary to major vessel occlusion or narrowing, and also from renal artery stenoses causing renal hypertension. Bruits over affected vessels are common.

Heart failure is usually secondary to hypertension, but coronary artery ostial stenoses can occur, causing angina; aortic regurgitation has also been described.

Management and prognosis

The acute systemic illness is alleviated by corticosteroids, which may reduce the incidence of sequelae. Antiplatelet agents, such as aspirin and dipyridamole, and warfarin have been used to reduce the frequency of cerebral transient ischaemic attacks and possibly retard the progression of arterial lesions.

Morbidity is chiefly from heart failure and cerebrovascular events. Surgical treatment of severe vascular stenoses may become necessary.

GIANT CELL (TEMPORAL) ARTERITIS

Although predominantly affecting the cranial arteries, giant cell arteritis can, like Takayasu's arteritis, involve the aorta and its proximal branches. The disease is described more fully in Chapter 23, page 1032. Where major vessel arteritis occurs, it may complicate the more common presentation with cranial arteritis and polymyalgia rheumatica, or may occur alone. Symptoms are similar to Takayasu's arteritis, including angina and exercise-related ischaemia of upper and lower limbs. Aortic regurgitation, aneurysm and dissection can complicate giant cell arteritis of the aorta. Treatment, as for the commoner forms of the disease, is with corticosteroids.

PERIPHERAL VASCULAR DISEASE

ARTERIAL DISEASE

Thoracic outlet syndromes

In the past, the thoracic outlet syndromes were thought to be principally due to arterial compression of the subclavian artery, but it is now appreciated that many of the symptoms are due to compression of the brachial plexus as well. This is from an anomalous fibrous band stretching from a cervical rib to the first rib and, in doing so, compressing the neurovascular bundle. The patient has symptoms in the hand, which appear promptly when the arm is abducted to 90° and externally rotated. A bruit can then be found over the supraclavicular fossa. These features disappear when the arm is returned to a relaxed position.

Aneurysm of, and embolism from, the subclavian artery is a comparatively rare complication of this condition, which can lead to digital gangrene.

Peripheral arterial disease and arteriosclerosis

Arteriosclerotic arterial disease can be from atheroma, focal calcific sclerosis (Monckeberg's arteriosclerosis) or arteriosclerosis. Monckeberg's sclerosis leads to calcification of the media without any narrowing of the vessels, but is often associated with arteriosclerosis and luminal narrowing.

Most symptomatic disease is due to atheromatous plaque formation, with subsequent stenosis, occlusion or embolisation of the vessel. Haemorrhage into an atheromatous plaque may precipitate a sudden vessel occlusion. Emboli may arise from atheromatous plaques (as occurs frequently from the carotid); however, major emboli are more frequently from the heart, in such conditions as mitral valve disease, left ventricular aneurysm, mural thrombus following myocardial infarction, left atrial myxoma, endocarditis and from any enlarged heart, particularly if there is atrial fibrillation.

The sites of predilection for the atheroma are not fully explained, and any one patient may have principally coronary, cerebrovascular or peripheral vascular symptoms, with very similar risk factors to another patient whose symptoms are quite different. Atheroma tends to develop in the abdominal aorta and at the origins of major branches. These may be sites of mechanical stress or low shear.

Intermittent claudication

Ischaemia of the lower limbs is usually accompanied by effort-related cramp in the calves, thighs and buttocks, which disappears with rest. The site of claudication indicates the probable site of stenosis or occlusion – the higher the claudication the higher the atheroma is likely to be found. The walking distance on the flat is usually remarkably repeatable. Claudication is often accompanied by profound weakness as well as cramp in the affected muscles which have become acidotic from anaerobic exercise.

The combination of hip and thigh claudication with impotence in males (the *Leriche syndrome*) is due to severe atheromatous occlusion of the lower end of the aorta.

More severe ischaemia produces a continuous pain at rest, particularly in bed. The pain is most frequently in the toes or foot, with some paraesthesia. The foot is often hung over the edge of the bed and may be subject to ulceration and gangrene.

In diabetics with peripheral neuropathy, there may be no pain but only ulceration and gangrene.

Diagnosis and investigation

Peripheral vascular disease is assessed by a careful history and clinical examination for signs of ischaemia, absent pulses, audible bruits over the proximal arteries, poor skin nutrition, low skin temperature and loss of hair, and then by blood pressure measurement. This is usually done using Doppler ultrasound on the ankle arteries with a proximal cuff.

The normal ankle systolic pressure is usually higher than brachial (by about 20%) and should be maintained after exercise. The ischaemic leg often has an ankle pressure of about 50% of brachial at rest, which becomes unrecordable after exercise when the blood is diverted to areas of vasodilatation elsewhere. The severity of the hypotension is related to the degree of arterial disease.

Take Nr ~ 1
Claud ~ 0.5   GCSO·?
RP ~ 0.3

Management

Most patients with claudication benefit from medical measures such as weight reduction, complete cessation of smoking and an energetic training regime which increases the claudication distance. Vasodilators and viscosity reducing drugs have a limited role. Surgical intervention after angiography now includes angioplasty, as well as endarterectomy and bypass grafting. It is reserved for more severe cases.

Gangrene

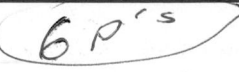
6 P's

Sudden ischaemia of a limb (from trauma, arterial thrombosis or embolism) leads to pain, pallor, coldness and then numbness of the limb distal to the occlusion. If perfusion is not restored, sensation is severely diminished in an hour; within 6 hours ischaemic contracture of the muscles has started. This is followed by subcutaneous haemorrhage and focal gangrene. Fixed staining of the skin indicates death of the underlying tissues. Persistent pain and numbness without loss of sensation indicate a collateral flow.

Management

Treatment is an emergency and is surgical, by embolectomy, emergency bypass grafting or eventual amputation. Embolectomy under local anaesthetic can often save a limb. Heparin is used to prevent further clotting, particularly if there is an obvious embolic source.

Buerger's disease

Buerger's disease was previously thought to be a distinct disease, but is now considered to be an accelerated form of atheroma affecting young men of 20–40 years of age who smoke (or chew) tobacco heavily. It affects the small arteries of the hands and feet, with an intense inflammatory response, and often involves the veins as well. Hand and instep claudication may occur, with loss of ankle and wrist pulses and gangrene of the toes and fingers. There is often an associated Raynaud's phenomenon (see below) and a migratory nodular phlebitis. Cessation of smoking or chewing tobacco is imperative.

Prognosis

For patients with symptoms of limb ischaemia, the rate of limb loss is about 2% per year for non-diabetics and 7% per year for diabetics.

Raynaud's syndrome and phenomenon

Raynaud's syndrome and phenomenon are vasospastic conditions affecting mainly the hands; they are often precipitated by cold and sometimes by motion, although random spontaneous attacks are common. Attacks are characterised by episodes of arteriolar spasm; these produce cold pale fingers and hands, progressing over minutes or hours to cyanosis and ending with a red flushing phase. When the condition is not associated with any underlying disorders, it is termed Raynaud's syndrome and skin changes are not seen. This is commoner in young women. Raynaud's phenomenon occurs

cold/pale → cyanosis → flushing.

secondary to underlying systemic conditions, the most common being scleroderma. Other collagen diseases may be associated with Raynaud's phenomenon, as may thoracic outlet compression, arteriosclerotic vascular disease, vibration trauma in pneumatic drill users and serum protein abnormalities.

Mesenteric ischaemia

Mesenteric (or small bowel) ischaemia is described in Chapter 15, page 584.

VENOUS DISEASE

Varicose veins are the commonest vascular disorder affecting the legs, and venous thrombosis is a frequent complication of many medical and surgical conditions.

Varicose veins

Varicose veins are dilated and tortuous veins, varying in size from large palpable bunches to mere discoloured superficial spider bursts on the skin. They arise either through primary abnormalities in the venous wall leading to dilatation and incompetence of the valves, or secondarily after damage caused by previous thrombosis. In either case, factors which impede venous flow or increase venous pressure in the legs contribute to their development, as does the prolonged standing required in certain occupations.

Many patients suffer no symptoms but they can be responsible for discomfort, usually described as heaviness or pulling. Oedema may occur and, in chronic severe disease, pigmentation of the skin, a disfiguring dermatitis, ulceration or, at its severest, gangrene may follow. These complications are more prominent in the areas subject to the highest venous pressures, where skin nutrition is consequently poorest, namely in the lower third of the leg, often more marked medially.

Management

Elastic stocking support, injection of sclerosants and surgical removal (or stripping) of the veins are used to treat the varicose veins. Relief of exacerbating factors, such as obesity, ascites and right heart failure, is also important. Ulcers often heal slowly, and must be kept clean and uninfected. Elevation of the limb aids healing.

Venous thrombosis

Occlusion of veins by thrombus is very common. It leads to considerable morbidity and, when the deep veins of the leg and pelvis are involved, to the risk of serious illness or death through pulmonary embolism.

Superficial venous thrombosis

Superficial venous thrombosis causes pain and swelling over the affected vessel, which is often palpable as a tender cord or small nodule. Unless complicated by progression to deep vein thrombosis (DVT), superficial venous thromboses are essentially benign and require only symptomatic treatment. NSAIDs, such as indomethacin or aspirin, plus local applied heat, are of help.

Deep venous thrombosis

Pelvic mass pregnancy test.

DVT is a frequent postoperative complication. The factors predisposing to thrombus formation within the veins are abnormalities in the vein wall, venous stasis and hypercoagulability of the blood. Certain operations are more frequently associated with DVT than others. These include orthopaedic procedures, particularly on the hip, and prostate surgery, although any condition leading to immobility is a potential cause of DVT. Congestive cardiac failure, malignant disease, pelvic masses and marked obesity are also recognised as conditions where DVT may occur. In most instances, it is the deep veins of the calf, thigh and pelvis which are involved and are the source of potentially lethal pulmonary emboli (PE). DVT of the axillary vein is much less common and rarely gives rise to significant PE.

Clinical features and diagnosis

The diagnosis of DVT is often difficult. The main features are pain and swelling of the affected limb. The symptoms vary with the extent and type of vein involved and are often absent. Dorsiflexion of the foot may produce calf tenderness (Homan's sign) in the extended leg, but this sign is often not very helpful. The most useful diagnostic test is the venogram, which, when technically adequate, will usually establish the presence and extent of any thrombus. Doppler ultrasound velocity profiles can be useful, although only for DVT affecting veins above the knee.

The major conditions which may mimic DVT include muscle trauma, rupture of a popliteal (Baker's) cyst (which resembles calf vein DVT) and sciatic nerve irritation.

Complications

cellulitis.

The most serious complication in DVT is PE (Ch. 13, p. 496). This is usually a complication of thrombus above the knee, but sometimes occurs with calf vein thrombosis.

Other complications include vein wall and valve damage leading to long-term venous insufficiency.

↑ varicose veins.

Management

Treatment of DVT is by intravenous heparin bolus (5000 U) followed by a constant infusion (24 000–48 000 U/24 h) sufficient to maintain a partial thromboplastin time two to three times normal. Oral anticoagulation with warfarin is then instituted after several days, with the heparin being discontinued once a prothrombin ratio of 2.5–3.0 is achieved. Oral anticoagulation is continued for some months unless recurrent DVT is a problem, when lifelong anticoagulation may be considered. Massive venous thrombosis (e.g. common iliac vein) is often treated by fibrinolysis in order to reduce the ensuing morbidity.

It has become clear that prophylactic treatment with relatively low doses of anticoagulants (heparin by subcutaneous or intramuscular injection: 5000 U 8-hourly) can prevent DVT, and hence PE, in patients at risk, such as those on prolonged bed rest after major surgery.

FURTHER READING

Bennett D H 1989 Cardiac arrhythmias: practical notes on interpretation and treatment, 3rd edn. Wright, Bristol. *An excellent discussion with good examples.*

Braunwald E (ed) 1991 Heart disease: a textbook of cardiovascular medicine, 4th edn. W B Saunders, London. *The outstanding reference work in cardiology.*

Fiegenbaum H 1986 Echocardiography, 4th edn. Lea & Febiger, Philadelphia. *Still one of the best books on the topic, with exhaustive discussion and reasonably good examples.*

Julian, D G, Camm A J, Fox K M, Hall RJC and Poole-Wilson PA 1989. Diseases of the heart. Ballière Tindall, London. *Somewhat more approachable than Braunwald with a distinctly British approach.*

Opie L H et al 1990 Drugs for the heart, 3rd edn. W B Saunders, London. *A small and excellent book with a comprehensive discussion of all aspects of therapy in cardiac disease. An excellent buy.*

Roberts W C 1986 Adult congenital heart disease. Davis, Philadelphia. *The best reference text concerning this increasingly important field of cardiology.*

Schamroth L 1990 An introduction to electrocardiography, 7th edn. Blackwell Scientific, Oxford. *Still the best introduction to understanding ECGs.*

Swanton R H 1993 Pocket consultant in cardiology, 3rd edn. Blackwell Scientific, Oxford. *Comprehensive manual small enough to be carried in the white-coat pocket. An excellent buy.*

13
Respiratory Disease

John Moxham and John F Costello

Respiratory diseases are responsible for a large proportion of premature mortality and serious morbidity among the population, and at the same time, for a large amount of minor illness. In 1989 in England and Wales respiratory diseases (including lung cancer) accounted for 20% of all male deaths and 15% of all female deaths. They are the second most common cause of death after cardiovascular disease.

STRUCTURE AND FUNCTION OF THE RESPIRATORY SYSTEM

Respiration can be defined as those processes concerned with gas exchange between an organism and its environment. In man respiration begins with the uptake of O_2 and ends with the elimination of CO_2. The adequacy of gas exchange by the lungs depends on four closely integrated processes:

- ventilation
- diffusion of gases
- pulmonary capillary blood flow
- the carriage of gases by the blood.

In addition, breathing is regulated in accordance with the constantly changing metabolic needs of the body by an intricate control system.

The anatomical organisation of the human lung is eminently suited to its role as an exchanger of O_2 and CO_2. A series of branching airways conduct air into and out of the alveolar spaces. Similarly, the pulmonary circulation delivers blood to, and drains blood from, the pulmonary capillaries. Ninety per cent of the alveolar surface (80 m^2 in an adult lung) is covered with capillaries, providing a thin but large film of blood for exposure to the gases in the alveolar spaces.

The lung has other functions besides gas exchange:

- It provides O_2 and substrates for its own metabolic needs.
- Its blood vessels serve as a reservoir for the left side of the heart.
- It modifies the pharmacological properties of a variety of drugs.
- It provides an elaborate defence mechanism that protects the body against inhaled pathogenic micro-organisms and toxic chemicals.
- The upper airways filter and humidify inspired air.

Ventilation

Ventilation is the cyclical movement of ambient air into and out of the lungs, and the distribution and mixing of that air within the lungs. This cycle is accomplished by contraction and relaxation of the respiratory muscles and the elastic recoil of the lungs. During normal quiet breathing, about two-thirds of the inspired gas reaches perfused alveoli; this fraction is known as alveolar ventilation (V_A). The rest of the inspired gas fills the conducting airways and alveoli that may not be well perfused and is known as physiological dead space (V_D) or 'wasted ventilation'. Therefore, total ventilation (usually in litres/min) = $V_A + V_D$.

The commonly measured static lung volumes are shown in Figure 13.1. The static volumes depend on the distensibility (i.e. compliance) of both the lung and chest wall. The distensibility or compliance of the lung is affected by the elastic recoil due to the connective tissue elements in the parenchyma and the surfactant that lines the alveolar surface. Thus the compliance of the lung is decreased in diffuse pulmonary fibrosis (tissue changes) and neonatal respiratory distress syndrome (reduced surfactant), and increased in emphysema.

Diffusion of gases

The term 'diffusion' describes the passive movement of O_2 and CO_2 between alveolar gas and pulmonary capillary blood (Fig. 13.2). It depends on three major factors:

- the matching of ventilation and blood flow (V/Q)
- the diffusion of gas from the alveolus to the red blood cell

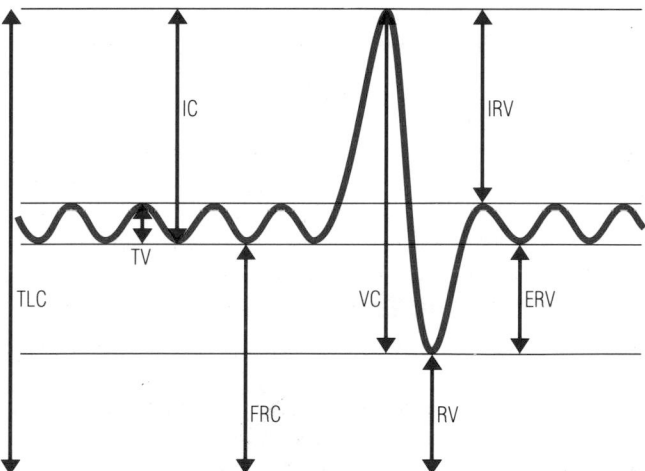

	Vital capacity (l)	Residual volume (l)	Total lung capacity (l)
Age 20 – 39			
Male	3.4 – 5.9	1.1 – 2.3	4.8 – 7.9
Female	2.4 – 4.3	1.0 – 2.0	3.6 – 6.1
Age 40 – 59			
Male	2.7 – 5.3	1.4 – 2.6	4.5 – 7.6
Female	2.0 – 4.0	1.1 – 2.2	3.4 – 6.0
Age 60+			
Male	2.4 – 4.7	1.7 – 2.7	4.3 – 7.3
Female	1.9 – 3.6	1.3 – 2.4	3.3 – 5.8

Fig. 13.1 The subdivisions of lung volume. Functional residual capacity (FRC) is the resting expiratory level. (TLC = total lung capacity; TV = tidal volume; IC = inspiratory capacity; VC = vital capacity; RV = residual volume; IRV = inspiratory reserve volume; ERV = expiratory reserve volume.) Normal values are also shown.

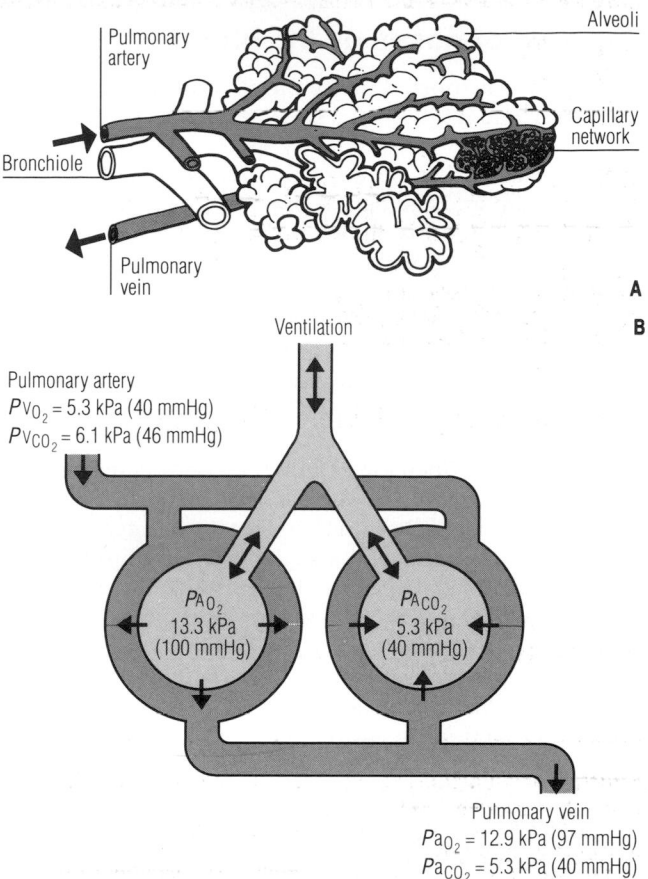

Fig. 13.2 The terminal respiratory unit. In the terminal respiratory unit (**A**) blood from the pulmonary artery is in close proximity to alveolar gas, facilitating gas exchange (**B**) and thus the uptake of O_2 and the elimination of CO_2.

- the availability of haemoglobin and the chemical reactions within the red blood cell.

Although O_2 is the physiological gas that is most likely to be affected by abnormalities of diffusion, the diffusion capacity of the lung is usually measured with a non-physiological gas, carbon monoxide (TLCO or transfer factor). If the haemoglobin concentration is normal, a decreased transfer factor means either a change in the alveolar–capillary surface available for diffusion (thickening or loss of membrane), or obstruction or destruction of capillaries (decrease in capillary blood volume).

Pulmonary capillary blood flow

The adequacy of pulmonary capillary blood flow depends upon the volume and distribution of right ventricular output. Because distribution is gravity-dependent, in the upright position there is more blood flow to the bases than to the apices of the lung; in addition local mechanisms exist to divert blood from poorly ventilated regions of the lung.

Carriage of gases by the blood

Oxygen is transported in the blood mainly in combination with haemoglobin; a small amount is present in solution.

The relationship between the per cent saturation of haemoglobin and the partial pressure (or tension) of O_2 (P_{O_2}) in the blood is shown in Figure 13.3. The shape of the curve is important: blood is nearly fully saturated when the P_{O_2} is greater than 8 kPa (60 mmHg), as it usually is in arterial blood; furthermore, when the prevailing P_{O_2} is low, 5.3 kPa (40 mmHg), as it is in the tissues, haemoglobin readily gives up its O_2, which is then available for metabolic activities. The position of the curve is not fixed, and shifts occur to the right (decreased affinity) and left (increased affinity) in many common clinical conditions. Shifts of the curve to the right, resulting from an increase in P_{CO_2}, H^+ concentration, temperature and organic phosphates (particularly 2,3-diphosphoglycerate) are beneficial because they facilitate O_2 transfer to the tissues and thus serve to maintain tissue oxygenation (See also p. 1049).

Carbon dioxide is transported in the blood as HCO_3^- in solution, or in combination with haemoglobin. The chemical reactions are reversed as blood flows through pulmonary capillaries, thus allowing CO_2 to evolve into alveolar gas. Carbon dioxide forms carbonic acid in the blood by the reaction:

$$CO_2 + H_2O \rightarrow H_2CO_3$$

catalysed by carbonic anhydrase, and the carbonic acid then dissociates by the reaction:

$$H_2CO_3 \rightleftharpoons H^+ + HCO_3^-$$

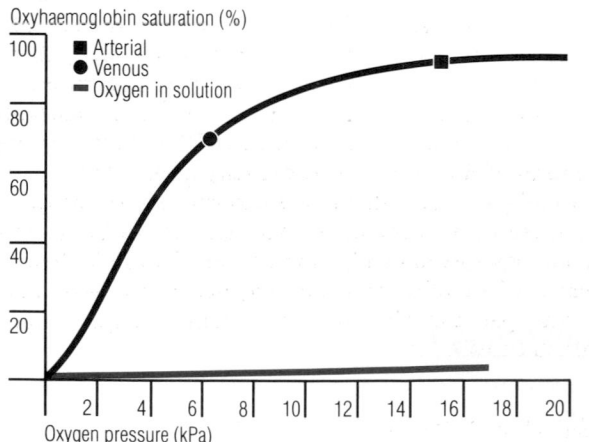

Fig. 13.3 Oxygen dissociation curve. In normal subjects a large fall in arterial oxygen tension causes a small reduction in oxyhaemoglobin saturation (and oxygen carriage). In a hypoxic patient (for example, with a Pa_{O_2} of 6 kPa/45 mmHg) a small fall in oxygen tension causes marked desaturation.

Accordingly, a rise in arterial P_{CO_2} tends to increase H^+ and decrease pH; this mechanism is of fundamental importance in acid–base balance and the regulation of ventilation (p. 855).

Control of ventilation

The rhythmic pattern of breathing is driven by the spontaneous discharge of neurons chiefly located in the medulla. The activity of these cells is modulated by signals from the pons, hypothalamus and cortex, and from central chemoreceptors and receptors in the lung. Although the physiological mechanisms involved are largely unknown, there is a remarkable matching of metabolic activities and ventilation.

PATHOPHYSIOLOGY

It is convenient to consider generalised lung disorders under the headings:

- airflow obstruction
- restrictive lung disease
- abnormalities of diffusion
- abnormalities of pulmonary blood vessels.

These functional categories often show considerable overlap and, of course, do not account for localised abnormalities such as those caused by tumours, pneumonia or pulmonary infarction.

Airflow obstruction

The all-embracing terms 'chronic obstructive lung disease' or 'chronic airflow limitation' are often used as diagnoses for patients who have chronic bronchitis, emphysema, asthma or even bronchiectasis. The disorders are grouped together because they share the common physiological abnormality of expiratory airflow limitation, because some of the symptoms and signs are similar, and because the disorders sometimes co-exist.

Determinants of bronchial calibre

The cross-sectional area of the tracheobronchial tree progressively increases as each generation of airways branches because the sum of diameters of the daughter branches exceeds that of the parent branch. Therefore, resistance to airflow, which depends on cross-sectional area, is greatest in the large or central airways and least in the small or peripheral airways. Airway calibre is influenced by the tone of bronchial smooth muscle, which, in turn, is regulated by a variety of neurohumoral mechanisms. Normally, there is a small amount of resting tone because parasympathetic-bronchoconstrictor impulses predominate over sympathetic-bronchodilator impulses. In addition to bronchoconstriction, airway calibre may be decreased by mucosal oedema, muscle hyperplasia, bronchial secretions and loss of elastic recoil. Bronchial calibre will also be reduced by external compression or intralumenal tumour.

Tests of airflow obstruction

There are simple tests to assess the severity of airflow obstruction that can be performed at the bedside, doctor's surgery or in the laboratory. Most commonly used are the *forced expiratory volume in 1 second* (FEV_1) (Fig. 13.4A) and the *peak expiratory flow rate* (PEFR).

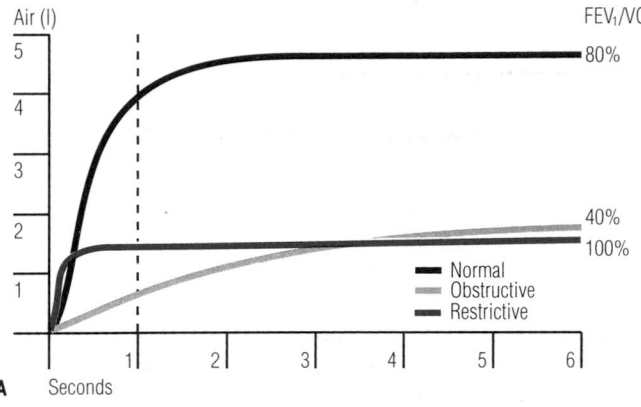

A

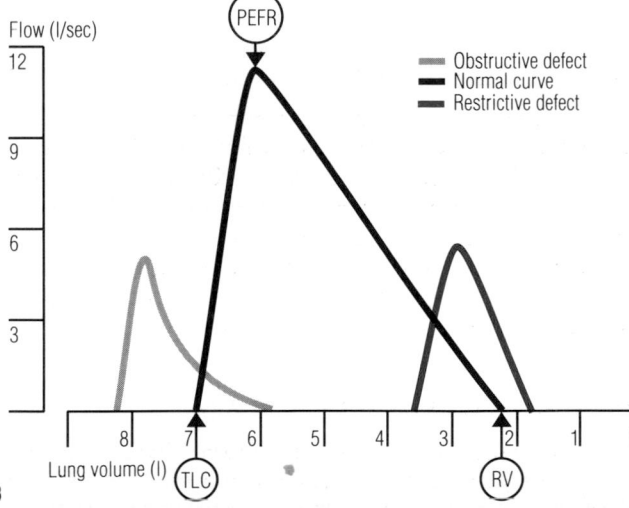

B

Fig. 13.4 A. Forced expiratory spirogram. Starting from a full inspiration, the volume expired during a forced expiration (forced vital capacity, FVC) is reduced in both obstructive and restrictive pulmonary disease. However, the volume expired in 1 second (FEV_1) is disproportionately reduced in patients with airways obstruction, but not in those with restriction. **B. Expiratory flow–volume curves.** In patients with airways obstruction expiratory flow is strikingly reduced as residual volume is approached. In restrictive disorders the shape of the flow–volume curve (although not the magnitude) is normal. (TLC = total lung capacity; RV = residual volume; PEFR = peak expiratory flow rate.)

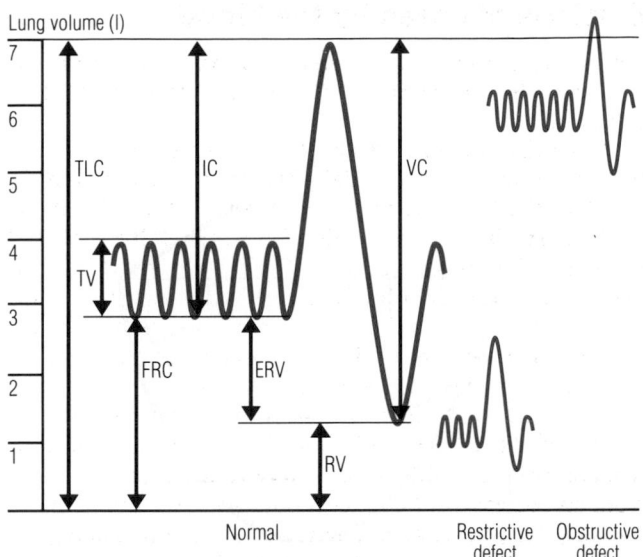

Fig. 13.5 The effect of obstructive and restrictive disorders on lung volumes. Both obstruction and restriction reduce vital capacity (VC). With obstruction, residual volume (RV) and functional residual capacity (FRC) increase due to airway narrowing and closure and the patient becomes 'hyperinflated'. With restrictive disorders total lung capacity (TLC) and FRC are reduced due to reduced compliance. (TV = tidal volume; IC = inspiratory capacity; ERV = expiratory reserve volume.)

Both depend on patient co-operation and effort and predominantly reflect the function of larger airways. Additional useful information can be obtained by recording flow against volume during a forced expiratory manoeuvre, producing a maximal expiratory flow–volume curve (Fig. 13.4B). The earliest changes of several important diseases (e.g. chronic bronchitis and asthma) are in airways less than 2 mm in diameter, and because these airways contribute only 15–20% of total airways resistance, simple tests of airways obstruction, such as FEV_1, or PEFR, are not sensitive enough to detect early disease. Hyperinflation of the lung, an important feature of airways obstruction, can be demonstrated in the laboratory as an increase in residual volume (RV) and an increase in the ratio of RV to total lung capacity (Fig. 13.5).

In all patients with airways obstruction, reversibility in response to an inhaled β_2 agonist should be assessed. Rapid improvement after inhalation of bronchodilators is characteristic of asthma and may occur to a lesser degree in some patients with chronic bronchitis, emphysema and bronchiectasis.

Upper airways obstruction

This may be caused, for example, by tumours of the larynx or trachea, by post-tracheostomy strictures or by inhaled foreign bodies. Clinically, it can be difficult to distinguish upper airway obstruction from other causes of airflow limi-

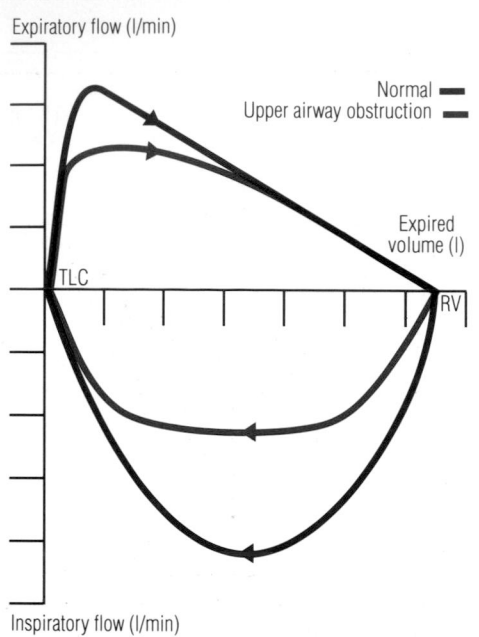

Expiratory flow (l/min)

Normal ■
Upper airway obstruction ■

Expired volume (l)

TLC

RV

Inspiratory flow (l/min)

Fig. 13.6 Flow–volume curves with upper airways obstruction. With obstruction of the upper airways (e.g. tracheal tumour) maximal flow rates are reduced, resulting in the characteristic shape of the flow–volume curve. When breathing out from full inspiration (total lung capacity: TLC), peak expiratory flow rate (PEFR) is reduced. Typically PEFR is reduced to a greater extent than the forced expiratory volume during the first second (FEV_1). (RV = residual volume.)

tation. The flow–volume loop is characteristic (Fig. 13.6). In patients with asthma or chronic bronchitis expiratory flow is most limited; when upper airway obstruction is present, inspiratory flow may also be markedly reduced.

Restrictive lung disease

Limitation of expansion of the lung can result from diseases of the bony ribcage, respiratory muscles, pleura or lung parenchyma. A restrictive defect is therefore a feature of disorders as diverse as kyphoscoliosis, the pneumoconioses and polyneuritis. Pleural thickening or effusion also limits expansion of the lungs. The most common causes of restrictive lung disease, however, are diffuse infiltrative processes within the lung, such as pulmonary fibrosis or extensive sarcoidosis. Regardless of the underlying cause, pulmonary function tests show small lung volumes (Figs 13.4 and 13.5) and, if there is destruction of the pulmonary capillary bed, a reduced transfer factor. Airways resistance is not increased and the ratio of FEV_1 to vital capacity (VC) is not reduced. As would be expected, lung compliance is reduced in diffuse pulmonary fibrosis.

Abnormalities of diffusion

Abnormality of any of the parameters that determine diffusion will reduce TLCO. Tests of diffusing capacity

are sensitive to the concentration of haemoglobin; thus TLCO is low in patients with anaemia and high in those with polycythaemia. When corrected for changes in haemoglobin concentration, decreased TLCO values are found in patients with destruction or obliteration of pulmonary capillaries (emphysema, pulmonary vascular disease, interstitial infiltrative diseases). Increased TLCO values are not common but are found in patients with left-to-right intracardiac shunts, polycythaemia, early left heart failure, pulmonary haemorrhage and asthma. Transfer factor may be expressed as the carbon monoxide transfer coefficient (KCO), which is the TLCO per litre of alveolar volume. When lung volume is reduced (e.g. pneumonectomy) but the remaining lung is normal, TLCO is reduced but KCO is normal. When lung volume is small due to an inability to expand the thorax (e.g. weakness) TLCO is low but KCO is normal or increased.

Abnormalities of pulmonary blood vessels

The function of the pulmonary vascular system is to expose mixed venous blood to adequately ventilated alveoli. Local mechanisms divert blood flow from poorly ventilated to better-ventilated regions. Conversely, if blood flow to part of the lung is compromised, ventilation of that region is reduced. Both these compensatory mechanisms tend to preserve the normal balance between blood flow and ventilation that is essential for efficient gas exchange.

The most common disorder of the pulmonary circulation is pulmonary embolism. Chronic obliterative disease of pulmonary arteries may cause severe dyspnoea on exertion but is difficult to diagnose at an early stage because physical examination, chest X-rays and spirometry show no abnormalities. In such disorders, gas transfer is reduced and hypoxaemia intensifies, or may only be apparent, on exercise.

Abnormalities of arterial blood gases and pH

Arterial blood gases and pH are also discussed in Chapter 21. The prime function of the lung is to add O_2 and remove CO_2 from blood. Thus the ultimate test of the adequacy of ventilation, diffusion, pulmonary capillary blood flow, and control of ventilation is measurement of P_{O_2}, P_{CO_2} and pH of arterial, or arterialised ear lobe, blood.

Arterial P_{O_2}

Arterial oxygen tension (P_{aO_2}) is normally between 11.3 and 13.3 kPa (85 and 100 mmHg) in healthy adults. Arterial hypoxaemia is a decrease in circulating O_2 (O_2 content), which depends on the amount of haemoglobin available for combining with O_2, as well as Pa_{O_2}. The causes of arterial hypoxia are listed in Table 13.1. A low inspired P_{O_2} is usually due to high altitude; of the remaining causes, abnormalities of diffusion seldom cause hypoxia at rest but may be important during exercise. Hypoventilation can be recognised by an increase in arterial P_{CO_2}.

Patients may have significant arterial hypoxia without symptoms. Central cyanosis only occurs when the saturation of arterial blood is less than 85%. Thus the clinical signs and symptoms of mild to moderate, but nevertheless important, arterial hypoxia are unreliable, and the diagnosis must be made by analysis of arterial blood gases. With chronic hypoxia patients develop secondary polycythaemia and pulmonary hypertension.

Arterial P_{CO_2}

The arterial CO_2 tension (Pa_{CO_2}) at rest is 4.6–6.0 kPa (35–45 mmHg). Regulation of arterial P_{CO_2} is determined according to the equation:

$$\text{Arterial } P_{CO_2} = K \times \frac{CO_2 \text{ production}}{\text{Alveolar ventilation}}$$

Only two variables, CO_2 production and alveolar ventilation, are involved. Deviation from normal values of arterial P_{CO_2} can be viewed as a failure of alveolar ventilation to increase or decrease in accordance with metabolic changes. Hyperventilation, an increase in ventilation in excess of metabolism so that arterial P_{CO_2} decreases, occurs in patients with a variety of common lung diseases (asthma, pneumonia, pulmonary embolism), presumably from reflexes arising from the chest wall or within the diseased lung. Hyperventilation also results from stimulation of the central nervous system by drugs (aspirin), irritative lesions (cerebral tumours, infections) or anxiety. When Pa_{CO_2} falls below about 20 mmHg, there may be sudden onset of dramatic symptoms such as paraesthe-

Table 13.1 Causes of hypoxia

Arterial hypoxia
Ventilation–perfusion abnormalities
Hypoventilation
Impaired diffusion
Right-to-left shunts
Reduced PO_2 in inspired air
Anaemic hypoxia
Insufficient haemoglobin for O_2 carriage
Stagnant hypoxia
Poor tissue perfusion
Histotoxic hypoxia
Respiratory chain enzyme abnormalities, poisoning of tissue enzymes, e.g. by cyanide

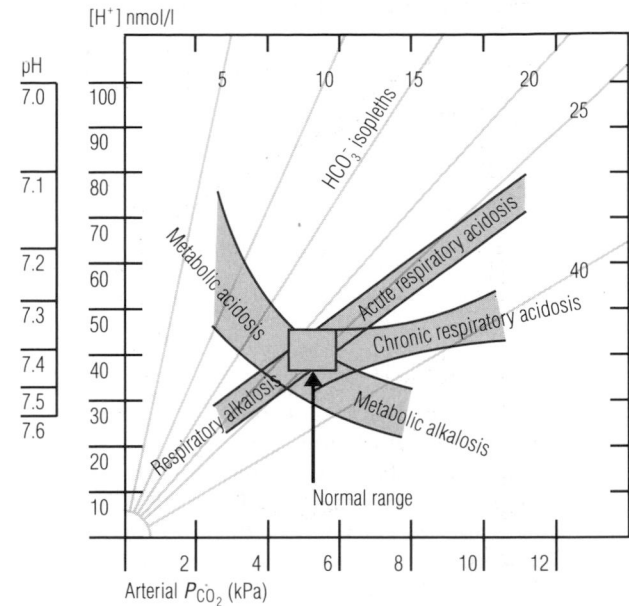

Fig. 13.7 Acid–base diagram. The relationship of arterial pH [H^+] P_{CO_2} and bicarbonate with disturbances of acid–base balance. For example, acute ventilatory failure leads to a raised arterial P_{CO_2} and a reduction in pH; compensatory renal mechanisms then increase bicarbonate and restore pH to normal. (Modified from Flenley D C 1971 Another non-logarithmic acid–base diagram? Lancet 1961.)

siae, blackouts and chest pain (due to vasoconstriction and increased nervous irritability). Such attacks are almost invariably misattributed by both the patient and the attending doctors to serious organic disease. Correct early recognition, treatment of the initiating disorders, and reassurance are helpful. Inappropriate breathlessness may be a separate syndrome which is often, but not invariably, associated with excessive breathing and hypocapnia during exercise. The causes are obscure but about one-third of such patients are depressed. There are few management strategies and response to treatment is poor. Hypoventilation can result from disorders that involve the airways (chronic bronchitis), lung parenchyma (advanced diffuse interstitial fibrosis), chest wall (kyphoscoliosis), respiratory muscles (myasthenia gravis) or central nervous system (sedative drugs).

Like arterial hypoxia, mild to moderate changes in arterial P_{CO_2} produce no or few signs and symptoms. Thus, analysis of arterial blood gases is required to determine the presence and severity of disturbances in P_{CO_2}.

Arterial pH

The arterial pH (Fig. 13.7) at rest is 7.38. It can also be expressed as H^+ content, and the normal value for this is 35–45 nmol/1. The arterial pH value represents the net effects of both respiratory and non-respiratory factors that regulate P_{CO_2} and HCO_3^- (and other buffers). When venti-

13 Respiratory Disease

Table 13.2 Patterns of abnormality in lung function tests

Feature	Asthma	Chronic bronchitis	Emphysema	Pulmonary fibrosis	Chest wall abnormalities*
Airflow obstruction	Yes	Yes	Yes	No	No
Reversibility	Yes	Slight	Slight	No	No
Hyperinflation	Yes	Yes	Yes	No	No
Reduction of lung volumes	No	No	No	Yes	Yes
TLCO	Normal or increased	Normal	Reduced	Reduced	Normal or reduced†
Compliance	Normal	Normal	Increased	Reduced	Normal or reduced

*e.g. kyphoscoliosis, muscle weakness.
†(see p. 448).

lation increases acutely, $P\text{CO}_2$ decreases and pH increases; conversely, when ventilation decreases acutely, $P\text{CO}_2$ increases and pH decreases. If the ventilatory changes persist, pH gradually returns towards normal values as the kidney makes appropriate adjustments in concentration of HCO_3^- in blood. Thus the pH value depends on both the magnitude of the change in $P\text{CO}_2$ and whether or not compensation has had time to occur.

Lung function testing

Patterns of lung function abnormality are easily identified (Table 13.2). Airflow limitation without reversibility and with a normal TLCO is compatible with chronic obstructive bronchitis; if emphysema is present, however, TLCO and KCO will be reduced. A more than 15% improvement in FEV_1 or peak flow after inhaled bronchodilator is suggestive of asthma. Restrictive lung disease due to pulmonary fibrosis will show low lung volumes with a normal or high FEV_1/VC ratio and a reduced TLCO, whereas if the restriction is due to chest wall disease the TLCO may be normal or slightly reduced, and the KCO raised.

A *treadmill exercise test* can help quantify the extent of ventilatory impairment and demonstrate any exercise-induced hypoxia.

SYMPTOMS AND SIGNS OF RESPIRATORY DISEASE

The most important symptoms of respiratory disease are:

- cough
- sputum
- haemoptysis
- breathlessness
- wheeze
- chest pain.

Cough

Cough is initiated when irritant receptors in the mucous membrane of the respiratory tract are stimulated. Cough is by far the most common respiratory symptom, and is characteristic in heavy smokers. Frequently, cough is triggered by the presence of sputum in the respiratory tract, and is useful in helping to clear infection from the bronchial tree. A wide variety of inhaled irritants in addition to cigarette smoke (e.g. noxious gases or cold air) may stimulate coughing, and this is more likely if the airways are already irritable because of inflammation as a consequence of infection. Similarly the irritant receptors in the bronchial tree may be stimulated by tumours, inhaled foreign bodies, allergens and the asthmatic response, pulmonary oedema and external compression by lymph nodes. With neurological disease laryngeal function may be impaired or oesophageal motility abnormal (e.g. achalasia), and cough may be due to repeated aspiration. Drugs can cause cough, by damaging the lung (p. 510) or causing asthma (p. 479). A characteristic persistent dry cough can occur with ACE inhibitors. Cough after drinking can also indicate an oesophago-bronchial fistula. In some patients cough is worse at night, particularly in asthma or pulmonary oedema. Prolonged coughing reduces venous return, causes a transient fall in cardiac output and cerebral oxygenation, and leads to cough syncope. Damage to the recurrent laryngeal nerve, commonly at the left hilum due to bronchial carcinoma, leads to vocal cord paralysis and an inability to produce a normal explosive cough, which becomes 'bovine'.

Sputum

In healthy subjects the bronchial tree produces approximately 100 ml of mucus each day; this is carried upwards by ciliary action and is then unconsciously swallowed. This ciliary mucus escalator is a normal part of the mechanism for clearing debris and pathogens from the bronchial tree. In disease processes causing the production of excess mucus, irritant receptors are stimulated and sputum is coughed up.

Sputum is not reliably described by patients and it is always best to inspect it. Sputum may be clear, white or mucoid, as in chronic bronchitis, or purulent, in which case pus is mixed with mucus and the sputum is yellow or green. Sputum may contain blood, which may be bright red (e.g. pulmonary infarction), a rusty colour (acute pneumonia) or pink (pulmonary oedema due to left heart failure). In asthma, the sputum may contain mucus plugs. Microscopically, sputum may contain bacteria, pus cells, eosinophils (as in asthma and pulmonary eosinophilia) or malignant cells. It is helpful to know the volume of sputum produced each day, and this can be particularly large: greater than 20 ml in bronchiectasis, cystic fibrosis, and lung abscess when there is a bronchopulmonary fistula. Clinical progress can be monitored by documentation of sputum volume. Occasionally patients with alveolar cell carcinoma produce very large volumes of clear watery sputum (bronchorrhoea). Anaerobic infection results in foul-smelling sputum.

Haemoptysis

Patients may have difficulty in being sure that blood has been coughed rather than vomited. Coughed blood may be from a lesion of the nose, nasopharynx and vocal cords. When infection causes haemoptysis, blood will be mixed with purulent sputum, whereas in non-infective causes (e.g. pulmonary infarction) there is usually frank blood and no sputum. In patients with chronic bronchitis it is common for the sputum to contain occasional specks of blood but more substantial haemoptysis is unusual (Table 13.3).

A cause for haemoptysis should be carefully sought in all cases, but a definite diagnosis is only achieved in 60–70%. Occasionally haemoptysis can be severe and life-threatening. This occurs most frequently in cavitating tuberculosis and bronchial carcinoma. In those patients in whom no definite cause for haemoptysis is found, careful follow-up is necessary, with repeated chest X-rays.

Breathlessness

Breathlessness is an unpleasant awareness of the effort of breathing. The history should document severity: How far can the patient walk on the flat? How many steps can the patient climb without stopping? Breathlessness may have characteristic features: in left heart failure breathlessness is worse when lying flat; in asthma it is frequently episodic, worse at night. With psychogenic breathlessness the patient complains of difficulty in taking air in, difficulty in fully filling the lungs with air and an inability to take a deep breath. These patients are often breathless at rest but not on exercise. Such 'behavioural breathlessness' causes a low arterial CO_2 and symptoms of the hyperventilation syndrome (e.g. faintness, chest pains) can be reproduced by asking patients to breathe deeply for 20–30 seconds. The time period over which breathlessness has developed is of great importance (Table 13.4).

Most causes of breathlessness are relatively easily diagnosed by history, physical examination, chest X-ray, blood gas analysis and lung function tests. In difficult cases observation of the patient during an exercise test may be helpful.

Although orthopnoea and paroxysmal nocturnal dyspnoea suggest left heart failure, many patients with asthma are worse at night and many patients with severe airways

Table 13.3 Important causes of haemoptysis

Pulmonary infections	**Pulmonary haemorrhage**
Bronchiectasis (particularly upper lobe bronchiectasis from past pulmonary tuberculosis)	Goodpasture's syndrome
	Idiopathic pulmonary haemosiderosis
	Systemic lupus erythematosus
Lung abscess	Pulmonary vasculitis
Pneumonia	
Tuberculosis	**Trauma**
Aspergilloma	Needle biopsy
Pulmonary infarction	Transbronchial biopsy
	Pulmonary contusion
Tumours	**Vascular abnormalities**
Carcinoma	Arterio-venous malformation
Adenoma	Hereditary haemorrhagic
(Haemoptysis is unusual with pulmonary metastases)	telangiectasia
	Bleeding disorders
Pulmonary oedema	Usually severe thrombocytopenia
Particularly due to mitral stenosis	from any cause
Disorders of the upper airways	
Epistaxis	
Tumours	

Table 13.4 Time course for the development of breathlessness

Immediate	**Weeks**
Pneumothorax	Pleural effusion
Pulmonary oedema due to cardiac arrhythmias	Anaemia
	Muscle weakness
Pulmonary embolism	
Inhalation of foreign body	**Months**
	Tumours
Hours	Pulmonary fibrosis
Asthma	Thyrotoxicosis
Left heart failure	Muscle weakness
Pneumonia	
Laryngeal oedema	**Years**
	Muscle weakness
Days	Chronic airways obstruction
Pneumonia	Pulmonary fibrosis
Adult respiratory distress syndrome	Primary pulmonary hypertension
Left heart failure	Chest wall disorders

obstruction are more comfortable sleeping with many pillows. Diaphragm weakness can cause profound orthopnoea.

Wheeze

Patients with airways obstruction frequently complain of wheeze which is predominantly expiratory in asthma, chronic bronchitis and emphysema. Patients may notice that a wheeze is inspiratory, indicating narrowing of the larynx, trachea or main bronchi, and occasionally they will remark that the wheezing sound is from only one side of the chest, as when a tumour narrows a major bronchus. Diffuse expiratory wheezes can occur in left heart failure.

Chest pain

The many causes of chest pain can usually be distinguished by careful history-taking, paying particular attention to the duration of the pain, its site and radiation, and the relationship to movement, breathing and exercise (see Ch. 12, p. 324). The quality of pain is also diagnostically important, especially if it is pleuritic in nature. Diseases within the lung are usually painless since there are no pain receptors within lung tissue.

Pleural pain

This usually indicates involvement of the parietal pleura by inflammation or malignancy but is also a feature of pneumothorax. Inflammation of pleura can be caused by:

- pneumonia
- pulmonary infarction
- lung abscess
- tuberculosis
- rheumatoid arthritis
- systemic lupus erythematosus
- uraemia.

Pleural pain is sharp, often well localised, worse on breathing, particularly deep inspiration, and causes the patient to catch his breath. Pain from inflammation of the central diaphragm is referred to the shoulder; pain from inflammation of the lateral diaphragm is referred to the lower lateral chest wall and upper abdomen.

Mediastinal pain

Central chest pain may occur with primary carcinoma of the lung, particularly when there is involvement of mediastinal structures including lymph nodes. Adenopathy due to other disorders, such as sarcoidosis, can cause pain. The differential diagnosis will include angina, oesophagitis and bone pain. Severe sudden central chest pain can occur with pulmonary embolism (p. 498).

Chest wall pain

With rib fractures there is local pain and tenderness. Occasionally coughing leads to fracture, particularly of the middle ribs posterolaterally. Osteoporotic ribs and those involved by tumour fracture easily. Perichondritis causes pain and swelling of the costochondral junction, often of the second ribs bilaterally (Tietze's syndrome). Pain within the distribution of thoracic nerves occurs with herpes zoster, the pain frequently preceding the vesicular rash. Nerve root pain, often described as burning, also occurs with an intervertebral disc or malignant and inflammatory diseases of the spine. Local pain and tenderness of the muscles of the chest wall is caused by coxsackie B viral infections (Bornholm's disease) which may sometimes involve the diaphragm. Rib pain occurs in sickle cell crisis. Localised muscle pain without any important underlying pathological process is common in breathless, coughing patients.

EXAMINATION OF THE RESPIRATORY SYSTEM

In thoracic medicine the *history*, *physical examination*, *chest X-ray* and *pulmonary function tests* all contribute to diagnosis and assessment in a complementary manner. The chest X-ray gives accurate information on thoracic anatomy, whereas clinical examination is much more useful in assessing pathophysiology.

Before the clinical examination, many relevant observations will have been made while talking to the patient concerning breathlessness, pain, cough and general appearance. In addition, the history will have served to focus attention on particular diagnostic probabilities and possibilities which subsequent examination will confirm or refute. If already available, the information from the chest X-ray will similarly direct the physician's examination of the patient.

Examination of the hands

Examination of the hands may give valuable information:

- *Finger and toe clubbing* (Fig. 13.8) is an important physical sign. The four criteria for documenting finger clubbing are: increased sponginess of the nail bed; loss of the usual acute angle between the nail and the nail bed; increased nail curvature; and increased bulk of the soft tissues over the terminal phalanges. The majority of patients with clubbing have pulmonary

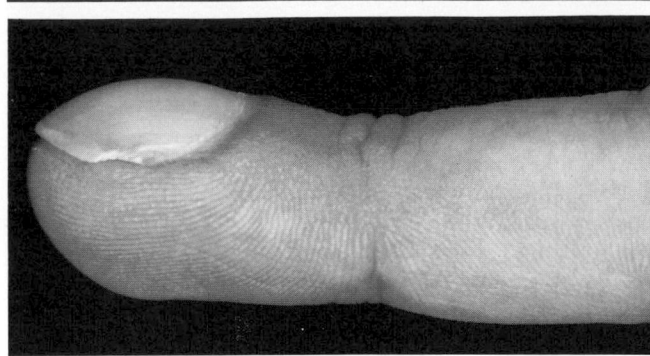

Fig. 13.8 Finger clubbing.

disease (Table 13.5). Clubbing is occasionally familial in otherwise normal subjects. It can develop very rapidly, within a few weeks (e.g. with an empyema), but its onset is usually gradual. The mechanism of clubbing is not understood. The bones of the fingers and toes are normal. If the underlying cause is successfully treated clubbing usually resolves.

- *Hypertrophic pulmonary osteo-arthropathy (HPOA).* Virtually all patients with this unusual condition have clubbing, but only a few patients with clubbing have HPOA. There is arthralgia and joint swelling affecting particularly the wrists and ankles. X-rays show subperiosteal new bone formation in the long bones of the lower limbs and forearm, the bone scan demonstrates increased activity, and often the serum alkaline phosphatase is raised. Ninety per cent of cases are associated with bronchogenic carcinoma, particularly peripheral squamous cell tumours.

- *Examination of the nails.* This may show that some or all of them are thickened and yellow or greenish in appearance. This occurs in the *yellow nail syndrome* which is associated with lymphoedema, exudative pleural effusions, bronchiectasis and sinusitis.

- *Carbon dioxide retention.* When there is carbon dioxide retention, peripheral vascular dilatation greatly enhances blood flow and the hands are strikingly warm. With severe and acute carbon dioxide retention, there may also be an irregular flapping tremor of the outstretched hands. The fingers may be blue

Table 13.5 Important causes of clubbing

Bronchial carcinoma (particularly squamous cell)	Cyanotic congenital heart disease
	Bacterial endocarditis
Mesothelioma	Atrial myxoma
Benign intrathoracic tumours	
Pulmonary arteriovenous fistula	Cirrhosis
Lung abscess	
Empyema	
Bronchiectasis	Ulcerative colitis
Fibrosing alveolitis	Crohn's disease
Asbestosis	
Advanced pulmonary fibrosis of any cause	Familial

(peripheral cyanosis), and if the limb is warm this is likely to reflect central cyanosis rather than poor peripheral perfusion.

Cyanosis

In patients with a normal haemoglobin concentration, oxygen saturation must fall to 85%, corresponding to an arterial oxygen tension of 7–8 kPa (approximately 55–60 mmHg), before cyanosis can be clinically detected. As a consequence of the sigmoid shape of the oxygen dissociation curve (Fig. 13.3), further small falls in oxygen tension then produce large, dangerous falls in saturation. In anaemia, severe hypoxia is required to produce the quantity of reduced haemoglobin (about 1.5 g/dl) necessary to cause cyanosis, whereas patients with polycythaemia become cyanosed at higher arterial oxygen tensions.

The bluish colour of central cyanosis is best appreciated by examination of the tongue in adequate daylight. Cyanosis is a difficult physical sign, and estimates of severity are so unreliable that measurement of the arterial oxygen tension is the next logical step. Cyanosis cannot be reliably detected in many black and Asian patients in whom severe hypoxaemia may go undetected.

In most cases central cyanosis is due to lung disease. Right-to-left shunts within the heart or within the lungs (arteriovenous malformation) cause central cyanosis, as do pulmonary shunts in advanced cirrhosis. Rarely patients appear cyanosed due to methaemoglobinaemia or sulphaemoglobinaemia, most commonly caused by drugs.

Pulsus paradoxus

The curious term 'pulsus paradoxus' is used to describe a greater than normal fall in blood pressure during inspiration. In normal subjects the systolic blood pressure falls by a few mmHg during inspiration. This fall is greater (not paradoxical) when venous return to the right heart is impaired, e.g. in patients with hypovolaemia, cardiac tamponade or massive pulmonary embolism. In respiratory disorders pulsus paradoxus is seen when there are large pressure swings within the thorax during the respiratory cycle. This is particularly likely to occur in severe acute asthma, when systolic blood pressure may fall by 40 mmHg on inspiration. The degree of paradox is best documented using a sphygmomanometer: as the pressure of the cuff is reduced, the systolic sound is initially only audible on expiration, but with a further reduction in cuff pressure it becomes audible throughout inspiration too. The pressure difference between the measurement taken when the systolic sound is first detected and the measurement taken when it is present throughout the breathing cycle is termed the *degree of paradox* (recorded in mmHg). In asthma paradox is dependent on respiratory muscle contraction and is reduced with exhaustion as well as with improvement in airways obstruction.

Jugular venous pressure

The jugular venous pressure is raised in right heart failure, which is itself frequently due to pulmonary disorders such as chronic bronchitis. The venous pressure is also elevated if the resting pressure in the thorax is raised, as with a tension pneumothorax or the hyperinflation of severe asthma. When there is severe airways obstruction the pressure swings within the thorax are large; intrathoracic pressure is positive during expiration, elevating the jugular venous pressure, which then falls during inspiration. Thus, interpretation of the jugular venous pressure in the tachypnoeic patient, particularly with severe airways obstruction, is difficult.

The jugular venous pressure is raised and not pulsatile in superior vena cava obstruction, most commonly due to malignant nodes or a tumour mass compressing the vein. The most common cause is an extending bronchial carcinoma but lymphoma, thymic tumours and metastases can all cause compression. Very rarely non-malignant lesions are responsible, e.g. mediastinal fibrosis or aortic root aneurysm or dissection. Superior vena caval obstruction produces drowsiness, a sense of fullness in the head, swelling and cyanosis of the face, neck and arms, and sometimes papilloedema.

Peripheral oedema

Peripheral oedema associated with severe pulmonary disease (cor pulmonale) is common, and is most often seen with chronic bronchitis in which there is hypercapnia as well as hypoxia. Patients with hypoxic normocapnic respiratory failure seldom have oedema. In some patients with oedema the jugular venous pressure is not elevated, the cardiac output is normal and fluid accumulation is related to factors other than right heart failure, perhaps mediated through the action of hypoxia and hypercapnia on renal blood flow and function.

Examination of the chest

Examination of the chest (Table 13.6) may reveal that the chest wall shows an abnormality of shape (kyphoscoliosis, a barrel chest or pectus deformity) or an abnormality of symmetry (a reduction in the volume of one hemithorax reflecting underlying chronic fibrosis, or perhaps an increase in volume reflecting a pneumothorax). Much can be learned about respiratory function by observing the patient's breathing pattern. An increase in respiratory rate is a sensitive index of cardiorespiratory disorders and is not sustained above 14–20 breaths per minute in normal adults. Disorders that cause widespread functional impairment, such as asthma, pulmonary fibrosis and pulmonary oedema, invariably increase respiratory rate. Conversely, respiratory rate is reduced by central nervous system injury or central depressant drugs.

Visible or palpable contraction of the accessory muscles is abnormal. Sternomastoid activity is particularly obvious in severely hyperinflated patients, whereas in patients who are not overinflated, accessory muscle activity is an indication of a greatly increased respiratory effort. In severely breathless patients abdominal muscle activity is vigorous.

Chest wall movements

Both sides of the thorax should be seen to expand equally during tidal and full inspiration. Hands placed flat on either side of the sternum can appreciate the predominantly forward movement of the sternum and upper ribs, whereas hands placed around the lower thorax can best detect the normal outward and upward movements of the mid- and lower ribs.

Overall movement of the ribcage is reduced by hyperinflation (e.g. emphysema), reduced pulmonary compliance (e.g. fibrosis), reduced chest wall compliance (e.g. ankylosing spondylitis) and weak inspiratory muscles (e.g. myasthenia gravis). Local chest wall movement is reduced in pleural effusion, pleural thickening, pulmonary collapse, and to a lesser degree in consolidation and pneumothorax.

The pattern of breathing is altered by disease. For example, patients with stiff lungs, a poorly compliant ribcage or weak respiratory muscles breathe rapidly and shallowly. It must be stressed that clinical assessment of the depth of respiration is notoriously inaccurate. Patients

Table 13.6 Signs in respiratory disease

	Mediastinal shift	Chest wall movement	Percussion note	Tactile fremitus; vocal resonance	Breath sounds	Added sounds
Collapse	Yes (towards collapse)	Reduced	Reduced	Reduced	Reduced	No
Effusion	Yes (away from effusion)	Reduced	Reduced	Reduced	Reduced	Occasional (rub)
Consolidation	No	Normal or reduced	Reduced	Increased	Increased (bronchial)	Crackles
Pneumothorax	Yes (with tension)	Reduced	Increased	Reduced	Reduced	Occasional (click)
Pleural thickening	No	Reduced	Reduced	Reduced	Reduced	No

with airflow obstruction have a prolonged expiratory phase and patients with left heart failure may have marked periodic respiration. With severe weakness or paralysis of the diaphragm the anterior abdominal wall moves paradoxically inwards during inspiration when supine (Fig. 13.68).

Trachea and apex beat

The trachea is an important anatomical landmark indicating the position of the upper mediastinum. It is best palpated by one finger gently placed in the suprasternal notch. Loss of volume in one hemithorax, as with pulmonary fibrosis, pulls the trachea to the same side. Expansion of a hemithorax (as with tension pneumothorax) or local masses (e.g. an enlarged thyroid) pushes the trachea towards the opposite side. When examining the trachea, the distance between the suprasternal notch and the cricoid cartilage is noted and is normally 3–4 fingers, and a reduction in this distance is a reliable sign of hyperinflation. Assessment of tracheal shift is difficult in patients with hyperinflation. A shift of the lower mediastinum displaces the cardiac apex. However, a displaced apex must be interpreted with caution because ventricular enlargement also moves the apex beat. In some patients the apex beat is not palpable, usually due to obesity or hyperinflation of the lungs. Less commonly the apex is difficult to palpate because of pericardial disease or poor left ventricular function, and the apex will be located on the right side with dextrocardia. Palpation at the left sternal edge may elicit the heave of right ventricular hypertrophy, common in patients with severe pulmonary disease causing pulmonary hypertension. In patients with hyperinflation heart sounds are much reduced at the apex, but well heard over the lower sternum in the midline.

Percussion

When percussing the chest comparison should be made between identical areas on both sides in an attempt to detect differences in percussion note. The percussion note is resonant over aerated lung, and hyper-resonant with emphysema, large bullae or pneumothorax. Percussion is dull over solid organs such as the liver and heart (except with hyperinflation when the aerated lung covers the heart). In the normal subject the upper level of liver dullness when supine is at the sixth rib in the mid-clavicular line.

The percussion note becomes dull when there is fluid in the pleural space, when there is collapse of a lobe or lung and when there is extensive consolidation. Less marked dullness occurs with pulmonary fibrosis, pleural thickening and large peripheral tumours. Basal dullness as a consequence of diaphragm elevation is easily confused with pleural fluid. Tactile fremitus and vocal resonance are both crude physical signs which are increased with pulmonary consolidation and decreased by pleural fluid.

Auscultation

Listening to the chest is of the greatest clinical importance. At the bedside the breathing of patients with airways obstruction is noisy, and this correlates well with the degree of obstruction documented by pulmonary function tests. This noisy breathing is particularly prominent in chronic bronchitis and asthma, but is less marked in emphysema. On auscultation breath sounds are noted to be generally reduced in patients with airways obstruction, particularly emphysema, and there may be local areas of greatly reduced breath sounds over bullae, a pneumothorax, pleural effusions and when a lobe or lung are poorly ventilated, as when there is substantial bronchial obstruction due to tumour. Expiratory breath sounds are prolonged with airways obstruction whereas expiration is rapid in patients with severe restrictive disease. Bronchial breathing is when the breath sounds become harsh and high-pitched due to enhanced transmission of sound through the abnormal lung. Whispered sounds are then easily heard as high-pitched 'whispering pectoriloquy'. Bronchial breathing is most commonly heard over areas of consolidated lung or over large peripheral cavities.

In addition to alteration of the normal ('vesicular') breath sounds the stethoscope may detect additional sounds:

- crackles
- wheezes
- pleural rub
- clicks.

Crackles

Crackles (crepitations or rales) are short explosive sounds thought to represent the equalisation of intraluminal pressure as collapsed small airways open during inspiration. Crackles therefore occur in disease processes causing small airway closure whether due to airway damage

Summary 1 Common causes of crackles
● Bronchiectasis
● Pneumonia
● Alveolitis
● Left heart failure
● Adult respiratory distress syndrome
● Pulmonary fibrosis
● Chronic bronchitis and emphysema
● Bronchiolitis

Table 13.7 Causes of wheeze

Generalised	Localised
Asthma	Tumour
Chronic bronchitis	Extrinsic compression
Emphysema	Foreign body
Pulmonary oedema	Bronchial secretions

(chronic bronchitis) or increased interstitial volume (pulmonary oedema, pulmonary fibrosis). With diffuse disease the effect of gravity makes crackles more prominent in dependent parts of the lungs. The crackles of chronic bronchitis and emphysema are characteristically early in inspiration, and are transmitted to the patient's mouth where they can be easily heard by the unaided ear. In bronchiectasis the crackles are maximum in mid-inspiration, and in pulmonary fibrosis or oedema they occur during mid- and late inspiration; in both circumstances the crackles are not transmitted to the mouth.

Wheezes

Wheezes are musical sounds reflecting airway narrowing such that the airway oscillates between being open and closed like the reed of an oboe. In asthma, chronic bronchitis and emphysema, multiple polyphonic wheezes are heard in expiration. A localised area of narrowing due to tumour or foreign body produces a single monophonic wheeze. Narrowing of the upper airway (larynx and trachea) causes a wheeze in inspiration as well as expiration, which may be audible at the bedside and is then described as stridor. The causes of wheeze are listed in Table 13.7.

Pleural rub

A pleural rub is always pathological and is the sound produced when the two layers of pleura move over one another in a jerking motion, generating a creaking sound similar to that produced by bending stiff leather.

Summary 2 Clinical examination: points to note

- Hands
- Cyanosis
- Respiratory rate
- Peripheral oedema
- Trachea and apex beat
- Jugular venous pressure
- Chest wall structure and movements
- Percussion notes
- Breath sounds

Clicks

A clicking sound with each heart-beat is occasionally heard with a left pneumothorax.

IMAGING THE THORAX

THE CHEST X-RAY

In thoracic medicine, the chest X-ray is of fundamental importance in demonstrating anatomy and is a direct extension of the physical examination of the chest.

Chest X-rays should be of good quality. Underexposure of films is a much greater problem than overexposure because it cannot be compensated for by any viewing conditions. All available films should be studied in sequence; past films are frequently the most important in understanding the patient's clinical problems. The chest X-ray should be taken with the patient properly centred and the medial end of the clavicles equidistant from the spinus processes. The film should be taken in full inspiration, in which case the dome of the diaphragm will normally be at the level of the sixth rib anteriorly and the tenth rib posteriorly in the mid-clavicular line.

Viewing the chest X-ray

A normal chest X-ray is illustrated in Figure 13.9. The following points should be considered.

Trachea

The translucent tracheal air column is readily seen in the neck and superior mediastinum; it is placed centrally or slightly to the right. The tracheal air column may be narrowed by intraluminal disease (e.g. tumour), external compression (e.g. enlarged thyroid) or displaced to the right or left (e.g. upper lobe collapse or fibrosis). The paratracheal regions of the superior mediastinum are

---

Summary 3 Viewing the chest X-ray

Points to consider

• Trachea	• Horizontal (minor) fissure
• Diaphragm	• Vessels
• Costophrenic angle	• Lymphatics
• Cardiophrenic angle	• The lung fields
• Subdiaphragmatic region	• Clavicle and lung apex
• Cardiac silhouette	• Pleura
• Behind the heart	• Ribcage
• Hilar shadows	• Soft tissues

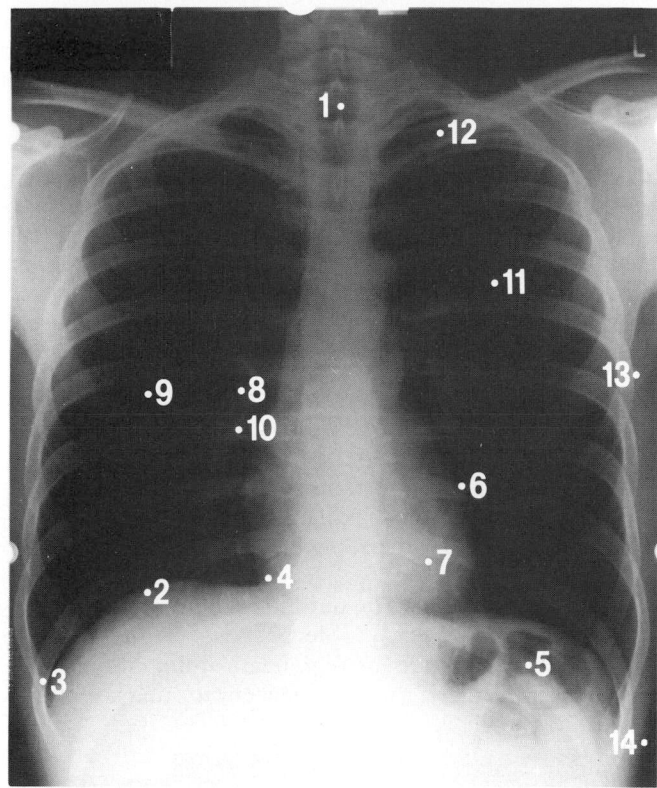

Fig. 13.9 Normal chest X-ray. Careful inspection will include: 1. Trachea; 2. Diaphragm; 3. Costophrenic angle; 4. Cardiophrenic angle; 5. Subdiaphragmatic region; 6. Cardiac silhouette; 7. Behind the heart; 8. Hilar shadows; 9. Horizontal (minor) fissure; 10. Vessels; 11. Lung fields; 12. Clavicle and lung apex; 13. Ribcage (Fig. 13.58); 14. Soft tissues (Fig. 13.58).

common sites of pathology (e.g. lymphadenopathy, apical pulmonary tumours).

Diaphragm

Downward displacement of the diaphragm indicates large-volume lungs (e.g. emphysema); upward displacement suggests small-volume lungs (e.g. pulmonary fibrosis), diaphragm dysfunction (commonly unilateral) or abdominal pathology. Both hemidiaphragms have a curved shape and a clear edge, and can be seen throughout their length. The right hemidiaphragm is 2 cm higher than the left. The level of the left hemidiaphragm, however, is influenced by the volume of gas in the bowel beneath it. The diaphragm becomes flattened by hyperinflation, best appreciated on the lateral chest X-ray.

Costophrenic angle

This sharp angle is obliterated and the lateral aspect of the diaphragm obscured by small pleural effusions.

Chronic pleural abnormalities (e.g. from past infection) also blunt the costophrenic angle.

Cardiophrenic angle

The cardiophrenic angle is blunted by pleural effusion or thickening and also obscured by pericardial fat pads.

Subdiaphragmatic region

Posteriorly, the lung extends below the level of the diaphragm as viewed on the PA film, and pathology in this recess is easily missed; inspection of this area is best on the lateral chest X-ray. On the left, gas in the stomach is commonly seen immediately below the diaphragm and provides some indication of the position of the diaphragm even when it is obscured by pleural or pulmonary pathology. Perforation of an abdominal viscus causes free gas below the diaphragm, as may abdominal surgery.

Cardiac silhouette

The mediastinum requires careful inspection to confirm that it is centrally placed and that the cardiac silhouette is of normal configuration and size (Fig. 12.15, p. 337). The heart may be displaced by pleural effusions, collapse of a lung or lobe, extensive fibrosis or pneumothorax. The heart is displaced to the left by a depressed sternum. Many disorders alter the configuration of the heart and mediastinum (e.g. cardiac disease, aortic disease, mediastinal tumour and lymphadenopathy) and the cardiac silhouette may be enlarged due to a pericardial effusion as well as dilatation of cardiac chambers. The cardiac diameter is usually less than 50% of the transthoracic diameter, but this is a crude measure and absolute measurements are more valuable; the cardiac diameter is less than 14.5 cm in females and less than 15.5 cm in males, and a change in diameter of greater than 1.5 cm between two X-rays is significant. Emergency chest X-rays taken in the AP plane magnify the cardiac silhouette, as do supine films.

Behind the heart

This is a notorious blind spot on the PA chest X-ray, particularly if the film is underpenetrated. The retrocardiac space is well seen on the lateral chest X-ray. A retrocardiac shadow can be caused by a hiatus hernia, which may contain a fluid level.

Hilar shadows

The left hilum is always higher than the right. The hilar shadows are vascular and the midpoint (the 'hilar point') is where the upper lobe veins cross the basal pulmonary artery. The lateral border of the hilum is concave. Both hila are of similar size, shape and density. Adenopathy (e.g. tumour) is a common cause of hilar enlargement, with increased density and convexity of the lateral border. Volume loss in the lung (e.g. fibrotic shrinkage) distorts the hilum and moves the hilar point towards the loss of volume. Any rotation of the chest X-ray will make the hila asymmetrical.

Horizontal (minor) fissure

This fissure is visible in 60% of normal chest X-rays, running from the centre of the right hilum, laterally and horizontally, to meet the sixth rib in the mid-axilla. The fissure is more easily visible when there is increased pleural fluid (e.g. cardiac failure), and encysted pleural fluid, within any fissure, can mimic a mass lesion. Localised volume loss in the right lung (e.g. collapse of the right upper lobe) moves the fissure from its normal position and the position of the fissure is therefore an important landmark when assessing the chest X-ray for possible obstructing lesions in the right bronchial tree.

Vessels

On the X-ray of normal lungs virtually all pulmonary shadows, apart from a few central bronchi, are vascular. Arteries can be traced back to the hilum but this is more difficult with pulmonary veins. As expected, vessels branch asymmetrically and taper towards the periphery. In the erect posture blood flow to the base of the lungs is greater than to the upper zones, and vessels at the bases are therefore larger. Vessels in the second intercostal space are usually less than 3 mm in diameter. The right basal artery measures approximately 15 mm. If vessels are enlarged, this implies that either pressure or flow is increased.

Loss of vascularity (e.g. in emphysema) makes the affected area of lung abnormally transradiant. Following lobar collapse the remaining lobes of the lung enlarge, the vessels per unit volume of lung are reduced, and the chest X-ray shows increased transradiancy. The vascular pattern of the lung is therefore an excellent index of localised volume loss. It is not possible to see any vessels in a large bulla, cyst or pneumothorax (Fig. 13.33).

Lymphatics

These are not normally visible on the chest X-ray but when distended by fluid and surrounded by oedema (left heart failure) or infiltrated by tumour (lymphangitis carcinomatosa, see Fig. 13.57) they are seen as linear shadows. In left heart failure the distended lymphatics are seen as 1–2 cm horizontal shadows extending inwards from the pleura, best seen just above the costophrenic angle (termed Kerley B lines or septal lines). On the lateral film, septal lines are best seen immediately behind the sternum.

The lung fields

Pathological processes within the lung increase its density (with the exception of pulmonary embolism, emphysema and bullous disease). The abnormality may be localised (e.g. tumour mass, pneumonic consolidation) or generalised (e.g. diffuse fibrosis, pulmonary oedema). Abnormal shadowing is often characteristic of a particular condition or group of disorders, e.g. the bilateral apical shadowing with cavitation characteristic of pulmonary tuberculosis. Two particularly important radiological signs arise from increased pulmonary shadowing: the air bronchogram and the silhouette sign.

- *Air bronchogram.* An air bronchogram (Fig. 13.10) is visible when alveoli are filled with exudate, transudate or other substance and the bronchi remain patent and filled with air. Important causes of an air bronchogram are pneumonia, cardiogenic pulmonary oedema, adult respiratory distress syndrome and alveolar cell carcinoma.
- *The silhouette sign.* The outline of many structures on the chest X-ray is visible because of an interface between opaque tissue (e.g. heart or diaphragm) and air in the lung. If the lung adjacent to such structures

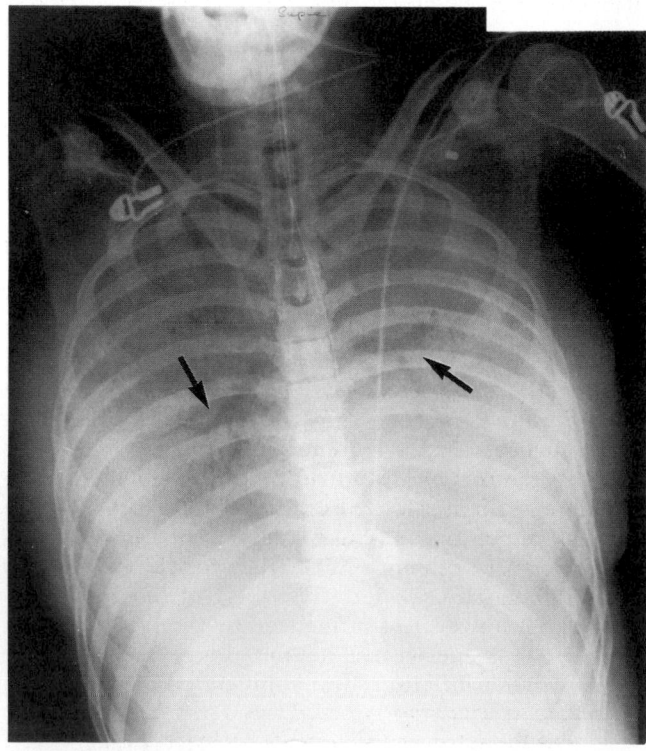

Fig. 13.10 Air bronchogram. The chest X-ray shows bilateral air-space consolidation in a patient with pneumocystis pneumonia and the adult respiratory distress syndrome. Note that the major airways (arrowed) are seen as an 'air bronchogram' against the background pulmonary shadowing.

also becomes opaque the 'silhouette' is lost (Fig. 13.11). Thus, collapse of the left lower lobe obscures the left hemidiaphragm and collapse of the lingula or right middle lobe obscures the left and right heart borders.

Clavicle and lung apex

The lung apex is an important site for pulmonary tumours and tuberculosis. If necessary, an apical view should be taken.

Pleura

Pleural effusions usually obliterate the costophrenic angle, but loculated effusions and pleural thickening (e.g. mesothelioma, Fig. 13.67) are easily missed unless care is taken to look all around the inner aspect of the thoracic cage. In some cases the pleura may calcify (asbestos plaques, tuberculosis, past empyema). With pneumothorax the line of the visceral pleura is seen.

Ribcage

The ribcage should be symmetrical. All bones should be inspected, particularly looking for fractures and destructive processes (Fig. 13.58). Destruction of ribs in the axillary line is easily missed unless care is taken to follow the curve of each bone, the 'skyline', down the outer aspect of both sides of the thoracic cage.

Soft tissues

Inspection of the soft tissues not uncommonly provides valuable information which is helpful to the interpretation of lung field abnormalities. Thus, a mastectomy may be noted in a patient with a pleural effusion.

The lateral chest X-ray

A lateral chest X-ray is necessary in all patients with cardiorespiratory problems in whom a comprehensive assessment of thoracic structure is required. On the lateral film some areas are better seen than on the PA view, and three-dimensional localisation of pathology is possible (Fig. 13.12).

Retrosternal area

This area is transradiant and should be of the same density as the retrocardiac area. With hyperinflation (e.g. emphysema) there is an increase in the size and transradiancy of the retrosternal space. Conversely, there is increased retrosternal shadowing with anterior mediastinal masses (see Figure 13.63).

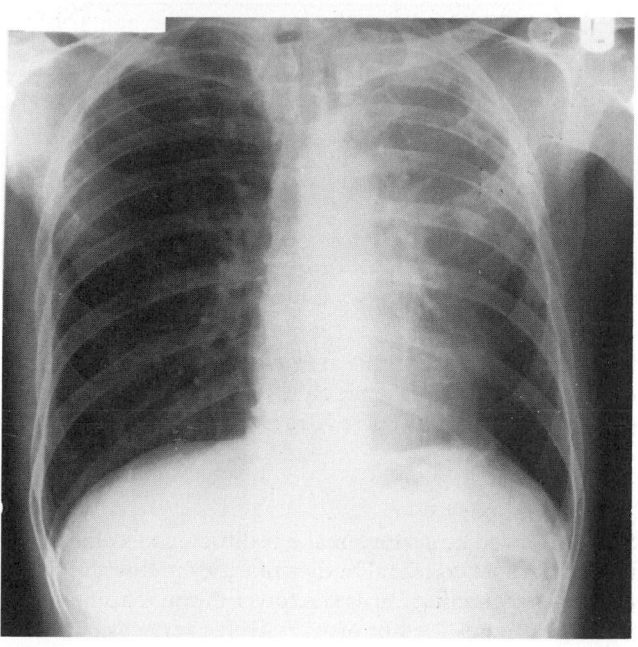

Fig. 13.11 Silhouette sign. On the normal chest X-ray (Fig. 13.9) there is a clear silhouette of the structures making up the left mediastinum. Collapse of the left upper lobe (including the lingular division) causes an opacity adjacent to the mediastinum and the silhouette is lost. Note the volume loss of the left lung and shift to the left of the trachea.

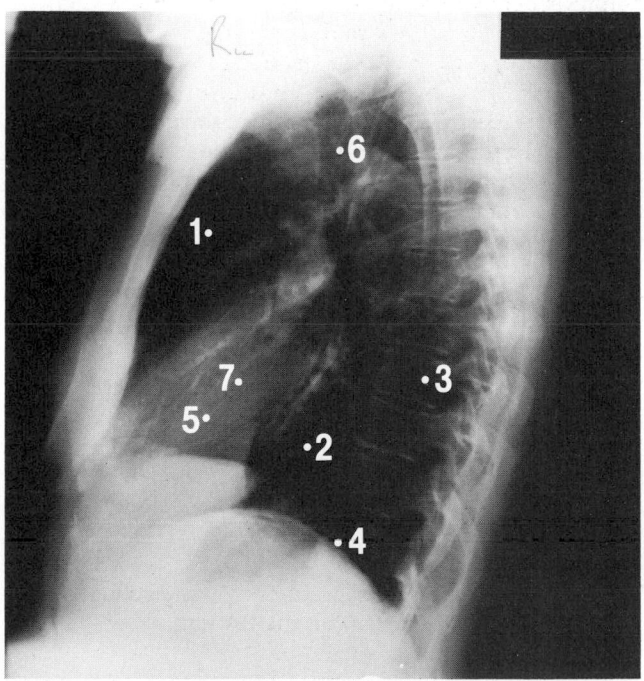

Fig. 13.12 Lateral chest X-ray. 1. Retrosternal area; 2. Retrocardiac area; 3. Vertebral bodies; 4. Diaphragm; 5. Greater (oblique) fissure; 6. Trachea; 7. Cardiac silhouette.

Retrocardiac area

Careful inspection of this area, which should be transradiant, is useful because much of the retrocardiac space is not visible on the PA chest X-ray.

Vertebral bodies

Superimposed structures make it difficult to visualise the upper thoracic vertebral bodies but they are progressively more clearly seen towards the lower thoracic spine. If the vertebral bodies are not progressively more easily viewed this suggests that there is pathology (e.g. consolidation or tumour) overlying the spine (Fig. 13.65).

Diaphragm

Both hemidiaphragms should be visible. The gastric gas bubble is beneath the left hemidiaphragm (Fig. 13.65).

Greater (oblique) fissure

The greater fissure passes from where the anterior quarter of the diaphragm meets the posterior three-quarters, through the hilum, and up to the level of the fourth thoracic vertebral body. Displacement of the fissure is an important sign of volume changes within the lobes of the lungs.

Horizontal fissure

The horizontal fissure between the right upper and middle lobes passes anteriorly and horizontally from the level of the hilum. Its position is altered by volume loss, particularly of the right upper and middle lobes.

Trachea

The tracheal air column is frequently better visualised on the lateral chest X-ray than on the PA film.

Cardiac silhouette

Intracardiac, aortic and pericardial calcification is best seen on the lateral chest X-ray.

Supplementary radiological examination of the chest

Films taken in expiration are useful for demonstrating small pneumothoraces not easily visible on the PA film at full inspiration and gas trapping in bullous disease or severe airways obstruction.

Screening of diaphragm movement can detect paralysis (p. 531).

For the differential diagnosis of pleural effusion from pleural thickening it can be useful to request a chest X-ray taken in the lateral decubitus position, in which free fluid will run along the lateral wall of the thorax.

Tomograms

Conventional tomograms visualise a slice of the thorax. The technique has, in large measure, been superseded by computed tomography (CT). Tomograms are useful for more precisely defining masses, demonstrating cavities, examining hilar structure (Fig. 13.13), detecting calcification, and visualising the lumen of the trachea and larger bronchi.

Computed tomographic scanning

Most patients with cardiorespiratory disorders can be satisfactorily investigated with simple radiological techniques. However, CT scans of the thorax can provide remarkably detailed information of thoracic anatomy (Figs 13.14, 13.25, 13.62, 13.67). CT scanning is particularly useful for imaging the mediastinum and demonstrating pleural and chest wall disease. For many patients with bronchogenic carcinoma CT scanning is necessary

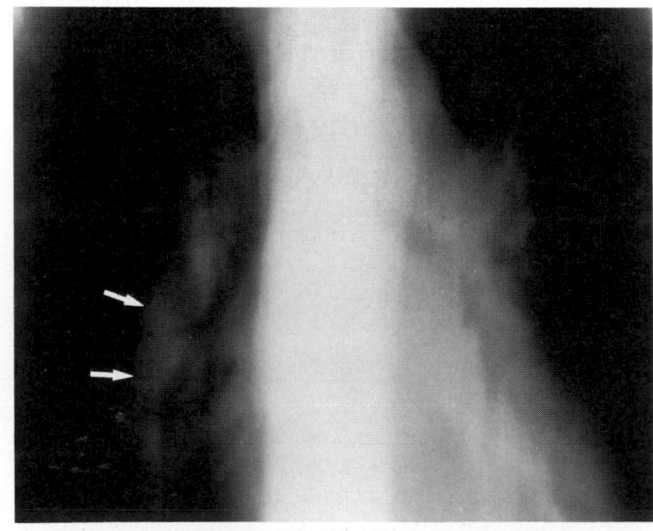

Fig. 13.13 Tomography. Conventional tomogram of hilar structures demonstrating marked right-sided adenopathy due to sarcoidosis (arrows).

A

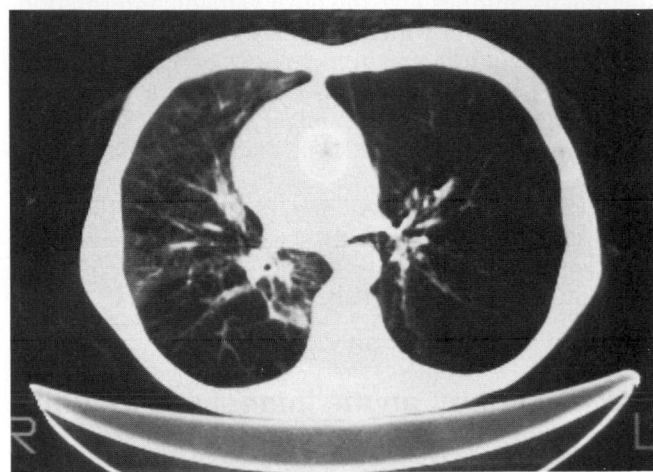

B

Fig. 13.14 CT scans of the thorax. A. Scan demonstrating the normal pulmonary vascular pattern. **B**. CT scan in alpha-1-antitrypsin deficiency. Bullous air spaces occupy most of the left lung and much of the right posteriorly: the peripheral vascular markings are lost and the mediastinum is shifted to the right.

to stage the disease adequately, particularly when surgery is being considered. Scanning is also valuable in the diagnosis and assessment of emphysema, bullous disease, bronchiectasis, lymphangitis carcinomatosis, alveolar proteinosis and pulmonary fibrosis.

Magnetic resonance scans are particularly good for demonstrating lesions of bone and for detecting lymphadenopathy.

Ultrasound

Ultrasound is not a suitable technique for visualising the lung but it is a good method for imaging pleural disease, both pleural fluid and pleural thickening, sub-diaphragmatic regions (particularly when investigating a subphrenic abscess), and assessing diaphragm movement.

BRONCHOSCOPY AND LUNG BIOPSY

Fibre-optic bronchoscopy

Fibre-optic bronchoscopy is an invaluable technique for diagnosis, assessment and therapy in thoracic medicine. For most patients the procedure is undertaken using local anaesthesia and on a day-case basis. As skills in the technique have increased, so the risks have become small and the indications for fibre-optic bronchoscopy have widened (Table 13.8). Fibre-optic bronchoscopy is of great value in many patients with seemingly inexplicable respiratory problems.

Bronchogenic carcinoma

Bronchogenic carcinoma is commonly visible as an obvious endobronchial tumour mass, in which case bronchial biopsy will confirm the diagnosis in 90% of cases. The flushing of saline over the surface of tumours and the subsequent aspiration of this fluid, or the brushing of the surface of tumours, provide cells for cytological examination, and these investigations have a diagnostic yield of 60–80% for visible endobronchial disease.

In assessing the extent of malignant disease, fibre-optic bronchoscopy is of great importance, allowing visualisation of the proximal spread of the tumour which determines the feasibility and likely extent of any surgical resection.

In selected patients endobronchial tumour can be destroyed by a laser, transmitted through a fibre passed down the biopsy channel of a fibre-optic bronchoscope. In patients with large central tumours causing breathlessness or haemoptysis that have not responded to radiotherapy, such palliative therapy can be of substantial benefit.

Haemoptysis

All patients with haemoptysis who are at risk of carcinoma of the bronchus should be bronchoscoped; approximately 10% of patients with a chest X-ray which does not obviously suggest tumour will nevertheless have malig-

Table 13.8 Major indications for fibre-optic bronchoscopy

Investigation of symptoms, signs or radiological appearances suggesting pulmonary tumour (e.g. haemoptysis, hoarseness, mass, persistent consolidation, or volume loss on chest X-ray)
Diagnosis of pneumonias, tuberculosis and pulmonary shadowing in the immunocompromised host
Removal of mucus, pus and aspirated material from the bronchial tree (frequently on the intensive care unit)
Diagnosis and assessment of activity in diffuse interstitial lung disease (e.g. sarcoidosis)

nancy. When bleeding is not due to tumour (for example, in bronchiectasis) bronchoscopy is useful to determine the site of bleeding, which is important should bleeding become a serious problem and bronchial arterial embolisation or thoracic surgery be considered.

Interstitial lung disease

Sarcoidosis is the most common cause of interstitial lung disease and in the majority of cases the diagnosis is easily confirmed by bronchoscopy. Overall, a bronchoscopic transbronchial biopsy has a positive yield of 90% (p. 501). With the technique of transbronchial biopsy (TBB) a small fragment of lung tissue is obtained when the forceps remove the bronchial wall of the carina of two small peripheral bronchi (Fig. 13.15). In pulmonary fibrosis, including cryptogenic fibrosing alveolitis (p. 509), TBB is less helpful. The small samples obtained are often not representative and if histological confirmation of the diagnosis is required, an open lung biopsy is preferable. TBB can be diagnostic in the uncommon conditions of alveolar proteinosis, histiocytosis X and pulmonary disease due to inorganic dusts.

Broncho-alveolar lavage

At fibre-optic bronchoscopy saline is instilled into the periphery of the lung, with the tip of the bronchoscope wedged in the segmental or subsegmental bronchus, and the fluid is subsequently gently aspirated. The lavage fluid contains thousands of cells (macrophages, lymphocytes, neutrophils and eosinophils), the numbers of which, and their differential count, give information on the nature of the interstitial lung disease. In occasional circumstances, broncho-alveolar lavage (BAL) can be diagnostic, as in alveolar proteinosis, pulmonary haemosiderosis and histiocytosis X.

Pulmonary infections

Some patients with pneumonia fail to show an adequate response to chemotherapy, yet do not have sputum for microbiological analysis. In such patients, BAL provides helpful information, although in patients already receiving antibiotics, bacterial culture is frequently negative and staining techniques give the most valuable information. Similarly, patients with pulmonary tuberculosis do not always have sputum and in these cases bronchoscopy and lavage of the affected lobes is an efficient technique for confirming the diagnosis. In miliary tuberculosis, BAL is commonly positive and TBB will confirm the diagnosis in virtually all cases.

Bronchoscopy with BAL and TBB is of great value in the investigation of pulmonary shadowing in the immunocompromised host (p. 468). The importance of these techniques has become greater since the advent of AIDS (p. 469).

Bronchoscopy on the intensive care unit

Many patients on the intensive care unit, as well as other ill patients often in the immediate postoperative period, develop sputum retention, basal atelectasis or pulmonary collapse. Bronchoscopy and BAL are effective at removing impacted secretions. BAL is frequently superior to conventional catheter suction in the diagnosis of intensive care unit pneumonias. Bronchoscopy is also valuable for the inspection of the bronchial tree, particularly the trachea, for catheter or endotracheal tube trauma, or stenosis.

Rigid bronchoscopy

As a diagnostic technique, rigid bronchoscopy, which requires a general anaesthetic, has been largely superseded by fibre-optic bronchoscopy. Rigid bronchoscopy remains of great value in the following situations:

- in the bronchoscopy of smaller children
- in patients who have a foreign body impacted in the bronchial tree
- for the biopsy of vascular tumours, particularly adenomas
- for obtaining a large biopsy sample to confirm sub-mucosal malignancy not demonstrated by the small

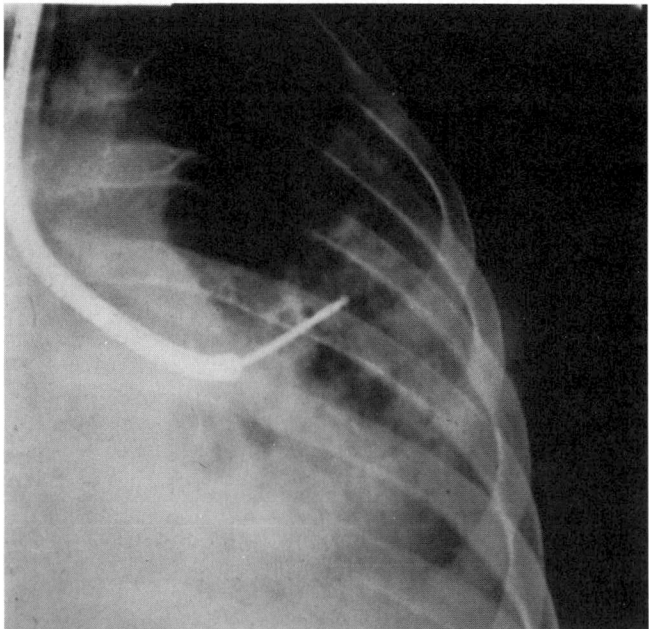

Fig. 13.15 Bronchoscopy. Using the flexible fibre-optic bronchoscope, biopsy forceps can be passed into peripheral bronchi and samples of lung obtained by transbronchial biopsy.

superficial biopsies that can be taken using the fibre-optic bronchoscope.

Transthoracic needle biopsy

Several techniques are available to biopsy the lung and diagnose pathological processes, most commonly tumours, within it. The usual technique is fine needle aspiration or biopsy under radiological control. If it is performed using local anaesthesia, patients seldom experience pain and major complications are rare. A small pneumothorax is common (30%), particularly in patients with emphysema, and a few patients will require tube drainage (5%). The overall mortality is very low and the technique is now extensively used in the investigation of pulmonary disease. In practice, the most common indication is to provide confirmation of malignancy for tumours which are not visible at fibre-optic bronchoscopy. With experience and expert laboratory support a yield of 90% or more is obtained in malignant disease. A further important use of the technique is in the investigation of pulmonary infections not diagnosed by more conventional techniques, particularly fungal, protozoal and mycobacterial infections in the immunocompromised host.

Open lung biopsy

Open lung biopsy is most commonly undertaken for diffuse interstitial lung disease, atypical tumours, and occasionally, serious pulmonary infections. A limited submammary thoracotomy allows biopsy of the anterior segments of all lobes as well as inspection of the pleura and mediastinum. Complications (approximately 5%) include infection and chronic pneumothorax and there is a small mortality (less than 4%) reflecting for the most part the serious nature of the underlying illness in many of the patients.

Mediastinoscopy, mediastinotomy and thoracoscopy

These techniques are mainly used to diagnose and stage bronchogenic carcinoma but occasionally are required to confirm other malignancies (e.g. lymphoma) or causes of adenopathy (e.g. sarcoidosis or tuberculosis). At *mediastinoscopy* an incision is made above the suprasternal notch, the tissues anterior to the trachea are dissected and the mediastinoscope inserted. Hilar, subcarinal and paratracheal nodes can be inspected, biopsied or removed. The involvement of mediastinal nodes in bronchogenic carcinoma is common (40% of all cases) and a positive diagnosis is achieved in sarcoidosis in more than 80% of cases. *Mediastinotomy* is occasionally required to evaluate areas of the mediastinum not accessible at mediastinoscopy, particularly the subaortic fossa on the left

side, and most commonly the surgeon gains access through the second left costal cartilage.

The insertion of a *thoracoscope* into the pleural space allows the pleural surface and underlying lung to be inspected and biopsied. The technique is most useful when investigating the cause of unexplained pleural effusion.

The development of CT scanning has reduced the need for mediastinoscopy and mediastinotomy. In carcinoma of the bronchus a CT scan which demonstrates a normal mediastinum obviates the need for surgical evaluation prior to thoracotomy. However, if the CT scan demonstrates adenopathy, such an evaluation may be still required to confirm that the nodes are involved by tumour and are not enlarged due to reactive hyperplasia.

RESPIRATORY INFECTIONS

UPPER RESPIRATORY TRACT INFECTIONS

Most upper respiratory tract infections (URTIs) are viral and the majority of these are the results of infection with picornaviruses of the rhinovirus group. However, adenoviruses, coronaviruses, coxsackie viruses, echoviruses, influenza viruses, para-influenza viruses and the respiratory syncytial virus (RSV) can all cause upper respiratory tract infections. URTIs represent the most common of all illnesses and are responsible for approximately half of all time lost from work.

In addition to URTI the influenza viruses, para-influenza viruses I and II, adenoviruses and RSV can cause acute infection of the larynx, trachea and major bronchi, and are causes of croup. URTIs are most common in the late winter months and early spring. The most frequent manifestation of these viral infections is the *common cold* (acute coryza), which may be complicated by secondary bacterial infection and subsequently by sinusitis, otitis media, obstruction to the Eustachian tubes and infection of the lower respiratory tract. *Viral laryngotracheobronchitis*, particularly in children, may be complicated by severe laryngeal oedema and life-threatening *croup*. Croup is also a feature of acute *epiglottitis* in children and occasionally adults, which is most commonly due to *Haemophilus influenzae* type B infection. The swelling of the epiglottis and surrounding soft tissues can rapidly produce respiratory distress. Unlike laryngitis, the voice is not hoarse. The epiglottis is hugely swollen and attempts to examine the throat can precipitate total upper airway obstruction.

In most patients with URTI the illness is self-limiting and symptoms subside after a few days. Antibiotics are not generally required unless there is acute epiglottitis due to *H. influenzae*. However, in patients in whom secondary bacterial infection is both likely and potentially serious (e.g. in chronic bronchitis and emphysema) immediate treatment with antibiotics is justified. The development of stridor requires careful observation in hospital with anaesthetic support for possible emergency intubation. Patients with stridor, particularly children with croup, adopt the posture that facilitates adequate ventilation and they should be allowed to do so. Inhalation of warm, humidified air is helpful. Given early, high-dose steroids reduce the need for intubation and, in those who are intubated, they shorten the time for which a tube is necessary.

Sinusitis

Sinusitis (infection of the paranasal sinuses) is a common complication of URTI and the bacteria most frequently involved are *H. influenzae* and *Streptococcus pneumoniae*. Facial pain and tenderness, headache, nasal discharge and a postnasal drip are the usual features. Radiology may demonstrate fluid levels within the maxillary sinuses or show sinus mucosal thickening. Sinusitis may complicate the nasal obstruction of allergic rhinitis, in which case topical steroid therapy is useful, in addition to antibiotics. Persistent or recurrent sinusitis may require surgical drainage. Sinusitis is a common feature of patients with bronchiectasis (occasionally, both are manifestations of the immotile cilia syndromes) and it is equally important to control infection at both sites.

LOWER RESPIRATORY TRACT INFECTIONS

Acute bronchitis

Acute bronchitis is common in smokers and in patients with chronic bronchitis and emphysema. However, it also occurs in otherwise healthy individuals and in both groups the bacteria most often incriminated are *Strep. pneumoniae* or *H. influenzae*. These infections cause an acute inflammation of the trachea and major airways, and as a consequence of this there is chest pain, commonly experienced as a raw feeling maximal on deep inspiration, as well as chest tightness. The patients may wheeze. In patients with pre-existing, chronic airflow limitation the development of acute bronchitis can cause severe breathlessness. Acute bronchitis causes an irritating, persistent, dry cough although after one or two days patients produce small amounts of mucoid thick sputum which subsequently becomes more plentiful and purulent. Appropriate antibiotic therapy is amoxycillin, tetracycline or co-trimoxazole. In patients with chronic airflow limitation, aggressive therapy with bronchodilators is important since acute bronchitis can precipitate a worsening of respiratory failure.

PNEUMONIA

Pneumonia remains an important clinical problem, causing many more deaths than any other infectious

Table 13.9 Differential diagnosis of a presumed pneumonia

Pulmonary infarction
Pulmonary eosinophilia
Allergic alveolitis
Pulmonary drug reaction
Radiation injury
Pulmonary vasculitis or haemorrhage
Alveolar cell carcinoma
Leukaemia, lymphoma, Kaposi's sarcoma and other pulmonary tumours
Empyema
Bronchial obstruction with distal collapse/consolidation

disease in the UK, both in the community and in hospitals. In recent years the aetiology of the pneumonias has changed with, for example, an increased incidence of legionella infection and opportunistic pneumonias in the immunocompromised host, particularly patients with HIV infection.

Although pneumonia is the most common cause of fever and pulmonary shadowing other conditions must be considered in the differential diagnosis (Table 13.9).

Having arrived at a clinical diagnosis of pneumonia, the next decision is what therapy to institute. For the adult patient, the clinical background of the pneumonia serves to reduce the range of possible pathogens. The most useful classification of the pneumonias is therefore a clinical one.

Community acquired pneumonia

Community acquired pneumonia is commonly due to a limited and predictable group of pathogens (Table 13.10).

Patients with pneumonia commonly have fever, cough, breathlessness, abnormal chest signs and X-ray shad-

Summary 5 Classification of pneumonia

- Community acquired pneumonia
- Hospital acquired (nosocomial) pneumonia
- Recurrent pneumonia
- Aspiration pneumonia
- Pneumonia in the immunocompromised host
- Unusual pneumonias

Table 13.10 Important causes of community acquired pneumonia

Streptococcus pneumoniae	*Legionella pneumophilia*
Mycoplasma pneumoniae	Viruses
Haemophilus influenzae	*Mycobacterium tuberculosis*
Staphylococcus aureus	

owing. Specific pneumonias may have additional features and *Mycobacterium tuberculosis* remains an important pathogen (p. 472).

Pneumococcal pneumonia

Pneumococcal pneumonia is more common in the winter months and upper respiratory tract viral infections are a predisposing factor. Fever is often high and there may be rigors. Pleurisy is common and the cough, which is initially dry and painful, subsequently becomes productive of rusty sputum. Altered blood from the congested lung tissue gives the sputum its characteristic colour. Labial herpes simplex is common (30% of cases). In some cases the onset of symptoms in pneumococcal pneumonia can be very rapid and patients may be critically ill within a few hours. In the usual case clinical examination demonstrates crackles more than classical signs of consolidation, and a pleural rub is common. The chest X-ray shows hazy shadowing, often with an air bronchogram, in any lobe, although lower lobes are the most frequently involved. In the majority of cases the consolidation does not involve the whole lobe.

Mildly or moderately ill patients can be managed adequately at home and are satisfactorily treated with oral amoxycillin, erythromycin or co-trimoxazole. Severely ill patients should be transferred to hospital for the adequate treatment of pain, dehydration and hypoxaemia. A Gram stain of the sputum will show typical Gram-positive diplococci and blood cultures will be positive in 25–40% of untreated cases. Pneumococcal antigen can be demonstrated in both blood and sputum. If the specific diagnosis is established, benzylpenicillin is the treatment of choice, but patients also do well with amoxycillin.

Recovery from pneumococcal pneumonia is usually rapid, although the X-ray may take several weeks to return to normal, as is the case with most pneumonias. In those patients who are more severely ill, and who are bacteraemic, mortality may be as high as 25%. Of all pneumonias, pleural effusion is most common in association with pneumococcal infection. Empyema complicating the pleural effusion is now relatively rare and occurs in 3% of cases with positive blood cultures. In such blood culture-positive patients pneumococcal pneumonia can be complicated by pericarditis, endocarditis, septic arthritis, peritonitis, cellulitis and, on rare occasions, meningitis.

Haemophilus influenzae *pneumonia*

It is unusual for *H. influenzae* to cause pneumonia in previously fit individuals. However, it is probably the most common cause of infection in patients with pre-existing lung disease, particularly in those with chronic bronchitis and emphysema. It is the organism most often responsible for the exacerbations that occur in chronic bronchitis, sometimes complicating an initial viral infection. The chest X-ray distinguishes haemophilus bronchopneumonia from simple infective bronchitis by showing shadowing, usually as nodules 0.5–3.0 cm in diameter at both bases, and on examination there may be bronchial breathing. The same picture of bronchopneumonia is sometimes seen with staphylococcal and pneumococcal infection.

Bronchopneumonia is very common. Patients are often wheezy and progressively more breathless. There is usually fever but in elderly and debilitated patients the temperature can be normal. Cough and purulent sputum are prominent features. As a consequence of diffuse airway inflammation and intraluminal sputum, patients with chronic bronchitis are frequently precipitated into respiratory failure and cor pulmonale. The first-line treatment of *H. influenzae* bronchopneumonia is amoxycillin.

Staphylococcal pneumonia

Staphylococcal infection causes more necrosis than other organisms responsible for pneumonia and there is a high incidence of abscess formation. In the community staphylococcal pneumonia is not common (about 1% of cases), but it is an important and serious complication of influenza and is therefore more common during influenza epidemics and during the winter months. Staphyllococcal lobar pneumonia can be fulminant and rapidly fatal. In most cases, the clinical picture is similar to pneumococcal pneumonia, but haemoptysis is more common. Cavitation is unusual in community acquired pneumonias, with the exception of staphylococcal or particularly virulent serotype 3 pneumococcal infections. The chest X-ray typically shows bilateral consolidation, usually basal, with abscesses that are thin-walled and cyst-like. Staphylococcal lung abscesses may rupture into the pleural cavity, resulting in pneumothorax or pyopneumothorax.

In the community, the development of pneumonia as a complication of influenza should be treated with flucloxacillin in addition to amoxycillin. Following admission to hospital, Gram stain of the sputum is helpful in confirming the diagnosis and blood cultures are frequently positive. With a definite diagnosis treatment should be with flucloxacillin and fucidic acid. Although the majority of patients make a good recovery from staphylococcal pneumonia, the combination of influenza A infection and staphylococcal pneumonia still carries an appreciable mortality. Important complications include the haematogenous spread of infection to brain, bone and other organs and occasionally patients can develop acute bacterial endocarditis.

Legionella pneumonia

Legionella pneumonia was first recognised in 1976 after an outbreak of pneumonia with a high mortality at a

13 Respiratory Disease

Legionnaires conference in Philadelphia. The pathogen is now known as *Legionella pneumophilia*, a small Gram-negative coccobacilliary organism. Infection is acquired from contaminated water, usually in air-conditioning systems and showers in hotels and hospitals, and transmission does not occur from person to person. Most cases have been in middle-aged or elderly males and have occurred in the summer months. Legionella is a cause of opportunistic chest infection in immunocompromised patients. Clinically, legionella pneumonia resembles viral or mycoplasma infection. There is a cough but little sputum, which is mucoid, not purulent. Patients are frequently severely ill with high fever, rigors, confusion, myalgia, abdominal pain, vomiting and diarrhoea. Hyponatraemia, hypo-albuminaemia and haematuria (50% of cases) are common. The white cell count may be normal or modestly elevated but seldom above $15\,000 \times 10^6/1$. Gram stain of the mucoid sputum reveals no organisms. The chest X-ray most commonly shows patchy shadowing which can be bilateral and which progresses to lobar consolidation.

Diagnosis is usually retrospective and based on a greater than fourfold increase in the indirect fluorescent antibody titre. The organism can be isolated from lung tissue, pleural fluid and blood. Treatment is with erythromycin (500 mg six-hourly) for a period of 3 weeks. In patients who fail to respond, rifampicin should be added. Ciprofloxacin may also be effective. The overall mortality is 15%, some patients dying despite appropriate antibiotic therapy.

Viral and viral-like pneumonia

Viral and viral-like pneumonias (Table 13.11) are characterised by fever, systemic symptoms (e.g. myalgia, headache) and a normal or near-normal white cell count.

Respiratory syncytial virus infection is important in children. Influenza and measles are frequently complicated by serious bacterial infection, particularly staphylococcal. Cytomegalovirus is a cause of pneumonia in the immunocompromised host (p. 468). Of the remaining causes, *Mycoplasma pneumoniae*, *Chlamydia psittaci* and *Coxiella burneti* are the most important.

Table 13.11 Organisms causing viral and viral-like pneumonias

Mycoplasma pneumoniae	Para-influenza virus
Respiratory syncytial virus	Rhinovirus
Influenza	Varicella (chickenpox)
Measles	*Coxiella burneti* (Q fever)
Cytomegalovirus	Chlamydial pneumonias
Adenoviruses	(psittacosis, ornithosis)

Mycoplasma pneumonia

M. pneumoniae is the most important agent causing the so-called 'atypical' pneumonias. In the past, this organism was the cause of major outbreaks of pneumonias in the armed forces; many cases still occur in clusters, and epidemics typically occur every 3 or 4 years. Infection is caused by an organism of the mycoplasmata group, the smallest known free-living organism. Most patients are aged between 15 and 30 years. After an incubation period of between 1 and 3 weeks the patient develops symptoms suggestive of viral pneumonia with systemic upset, arthralgia and myalgia being particularly common. Typically, the white cell count is not raised. The appearances on chest X-ray are very variable and although segmental and subsegmental shadows are most common, a lobar pattern can also be seen.

In mycoplasma pneumonia cold agglutinins are present in approximately 50% of cases and serological investigations demonstrate antibodies to mycoplasma in most instances. Mycoplasma titres may be raised for several years following infection.

The most effective therapy for mycoplasma infection is erythromycin or tetracycline. Complications can include a haemolytic anaemia and renal failure, due to the presence of cold agglutinins, as well as meningism, central nervous system involvement and myocarditis. For most patients the prognosis is excellent.

Psittacosis and ornithosis

Chlamydial infection is transmitted from parrots to man (psittacosis) or from other birds to man (ornithosis). The organism (intermediate between a virus and a rickettsial organism) is in the dust derived from excreta and feathers. The birds do not always appear to be ill. There is usually a history of close contact with birds (e.g. pigeon racers). The ensuing illness is rather like influenza. There is a cough, mucoid sputum and sometimes haemoptysis. The chest X-ray shows patchy consolidation. A complicating bacterial pneumonia is common. Diagnosis is best made by a rising titre for chlamydia antibodies and effective treatment is tetracycline or erythromycin.

Rickettsial pneumonia (Q fever)

The rickettsial organism (*Coxiella burneti*) is transmitted from animals (most commonly cattle and sheep) to man by dust inhalation. Slaughterhouse workers are most often infected. There is an abrupt onset of a viral-like illness with headache and meningism. Respiratory symptoms are less prominent. The chest X-ray shows patchy consolidation. Diagnosis is confirmed by a rising antibody titre. A prolonged course of tetracycline (or erythromycin) is effective, as is chloramphenicol. Rickettsia can cause endocarditis (p. 413).

Treatment of community acquired pneumonia

Because of the likely pathogens, most patients respond well to amoxycillin. For patients with features of an 'atypical' pneumonia, or legionella, erythromycin should be added, and in patients with a recent influenza-like illness, flucloxacillin.

Hospital acquired (nosocomial) pneumonia

Up to 5% of patients admitted to hospital for other causes subsequently develop a pneumonia; the mechanisms of infection are depicted in Figue 13.16. Particularly important predisposing factors are cigarette-smoking, chronic lung disease, obesity, the effects of anaesthesia and surgery, and prior use of broad-spectrum antibiotics.

The causative organisms for hospital acquired pneumonias are different from those responsible for community acquired pneumonia and, in particular, Gram-negative organisms are responsible for 50% of cases. Anaerobic infections are also important (Table 13.12).

The prior use of broad-spectrum antibiotics and the consequent colonisation of the oropharynx with Gram-negative bacilli reduces the value of sputum culture and makes it difficult to find the cause of hospital acquired pneumonia. The management of these pneumonias involves close collaboration between clinical staff and microbiologist. Gram stain of the sputum may be more useful than culture. Blood cultures will be positive in up

Table 13.12 Organisms responsible for hospital acquired pneumonia

Organism	% of cases
Gram-negative bacteria (especially *Klebsiella* spp. and *Pseudomonas* spp.)	50
Staphylococcus aureus	15
Anaerobes	9
Streptococcus pneumoniae	6
Others (legionella, fungi, etc.)	20

to 25% of cases. For potentially serious pneumonias clinical management is helped by a precise diagnosis and invasive techniques are appropriate. Bronchoscopy can yield useful information. The wide range of potential pathogens demands the use of broad-spectrum antibiotics, including good Gram-negative cover, in the initial therapy of hospital acquired pneumonia. An amoxycillin/ceftazidine or ureido penicillin/aminoglycoside combination is usually effective. Metronidazole should be added if anaerobic infection is likely.

Recurrent pneumonia

Prior to making a diagnosis of recurrent pneumonia, the possibility of a non-infective cause of recurrent pulmonary problems should be considered. Alternative diagnoses will include pulmonary infarction, pulmonary eosinophilia (including bronchopulmonary aspergillosis) and asthma. Recurrent pneumonia is unusual without a predisposing factor (Table 13.13).

Any cause of obstruction to a bronchus can result in recurrent or persistent pneumonia, but malignant tumours are most important (p. 514).

Aspiration pneumonia

Many patients with aspiration pneumonia have dental sepsis, a predisposition to aspiration, or both (Table 13.14). Infection is usually with anaerobic organisms derived from the upper respiratory tract. Aspiration pneumonia may be acute, extensive and progressive or it may

Table 13.13 Important causes of recurrent pneumonia

Diffuse bronchopulmonary disease	Local bronchial obstruction
Bronchiectasis	Tumour (benign or malignant)
Cystic fibrosis	Adenopathy
Chronic bronchitis, emphysema and chronic asthma	Foreign body
Immotile cilia syndrome	**Local bronchopulmonary disease**
	Bronchiectasis
Immune deficiency states	Congenital abnormalities
HIV infection	(sequestration)
Hypogammaglobulinaemia	
Myeloma	

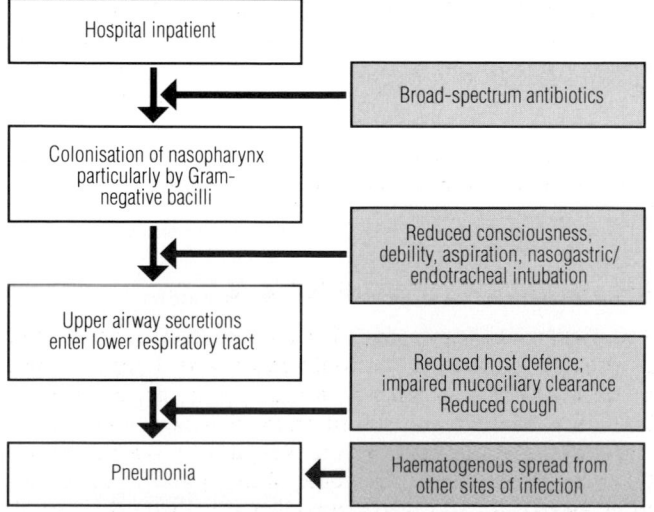

Fig. 13.16 Factors predisposing to hospital acquired pneumonia.

Table 13.14 Factors predisposing to aspiration pneumonia

Altered consciousness	Neurological disorders
Drug overdose	Pseudobulbar palsy
Anaesthesia	Myasthenia gravis, etc.
Epilepsy	
Cerebrovascular accident	**Nasogastric tubes**
Alcoholism	
	Severe dental and upper
Dysphagia and oesophageal disease	**airways sepsis**
Stricture	
Achalasia	**Terminal illness**
Oesophageal pouch	
Fistula	
Hiatus hernia	
Reflux	

run a more subacute course and progress to lung abscess formation.

When cavitating anaerobic pneumonias communicate with the bronchial tree the sputum is both copious and foul-smelling. The site of the pneumonia or lung abscess will depend on the position of the patient at the time of aspiration. Aspirated material enters the right lung more easily than the left, and will enter the lower lobes when the subject is standing, and the apical segment of the lower lobes or the posterior segment of the upper lobes when supine.

An important cause of anaerobic pneumonias and lung abscess is bronchial obstruction (e.g. with bronchogenic carcinoma), and if the diagnosis of aspiration is in doubt bronchoscopy is indicated. Barium swallow will frequently be a rewarding investigation. Anaerobic infection causes considerable tissue destruction with abscess formation, and empyema and metastatic abscesses can also occur. Prompt treatment avoids such problems. Most anaerobes are sensitive to penicillin. Early aspiration pneumonias are adequately treated with amoxycillin but more severe infections and lung abscesses require parenteral penicillin plus metronidazole for penicillin-resistant organisms. Postural drainage is important and antibiotic therapy should be continued for 6 weeks or more to minimise lung destruction.

Inhalation pneumonias

Aspiration pneumonia is the term used to denote aspiration of organisms into the lower respiratory tract (usually anaerobes); inhalational pneumonias refer to the consequences of inhaling non-infected particulate matter, fluids and irritant gases.

The inhalation of gastric contents during anaesthesia or other causes of reduced consciousness, or childbirth (Mendelson's syndrome) produces a chemical pneumonitis and respiratory distress. When severe, the features are of the adult respiratory distress syndrome

(p. 511). Management includes antibiotics, and metronidazole provides good cover for anaerobic organisms, but corticosteroids are not helpful.

Inhalation of food produces the clinical picture of a chronic, often recurrent pneumonia. The inflammatory infiltrate in the lung may progress to fibrosis. Lipoid pneumonia follows the aspiration of liquid paraffin laxatives, oily nosedrops or oily seawater. The lung pathology shows a foreign body giant cell reaction and fibrosis. Chronic pneumonias due to inhalation may mimic lung tumours and the diagnosis may only become evident following surgical resection. Repeated inhalation may eventually produce bilateral fibrosis and bronchiectasis. Hot smoke inhalation causes respiratory burns. There is oedema of the upper airways and bronchial tree, causing wheeze and croup. Severe injury is unlikely if there is no blistering of the mouth. Several hours or days after inhalation, pulmonary oedema may develop. Early corticosteroid therapy may be beneficial. Patients may progress to develop the adult respiratory distress syndrome (p. 511).

Pneumonia in the immunocompromised host

The increased use of immunosuppressive agents and the emergence of HIV infection has greatly increased the prevalence of pneumonia in the immunocompromised host, so-called 'opportunistic' infections. These infections are particularly common in certain well-recognised groups (Table 13.15).

In patients who are immunosuppressed, particularly following organ transplantation or cytotoxic therapy for malignancy, the development of fever and pulmonary infiltrates is not always due to infection (Table 13.16).

Occasionally bleeding into the lung occurs in patients who are thrombocytopenic. Radiation pneumonitis is most intense between 4 and 6 weeks after treatment. In a small number of patients a non-specific pneumonitis develops for which no cause is found, even when these patients are submitted to open lung biopsy.

Table 13.15 Groups at risk of opportunistic pneumonias

Primary immunodeficiency	Secondary immunodeficiency
B cell deficiency (agammaglobulinaemia)	HIV infection (AIDS)
T cell deficiency (Di George syndrome)	Leukaemias and lymphomas
T cell and B cell deficiency (combined immunodeficiency)	Corticosteroid therapy
	Cytotoxic agents (particularly following organ transplantation and the treatment of haematological malignancies)
	Malnutrition, general debility, uraemia, liver failure, etc.

Table 13.16 Fever and pulmonary infiltrates in immunocompromised patients

Infection	Malignant infiltration (e.g. leukaemia, Kaposi's sarcoma)
Pulmonary oedema	
	Pulmonary emboli
Pulmonary haemorrhage	
	Non-specific pneumonitis
Drug-induced pneumonitis	
Radiation pneumonitis	

Infection can be due to a wide variety of agents. Immunodeficiency facilitates infection with organisms seldom encountered in immunocompetent individuals and the clinical picture is often of a rapid, extensive and life-threatening pneumonia (Table 13.17).

Management of pneumonia in the immunocompromised patient

Pneumonia in the immunocompromised host requires immediate investigation and treatment. All patients should have blood cultures and appropriate serological investigations for likely pathogens. The chest X-ray is of limited value, with the exception of pneumocystis pneumonia in patients with HIV infection. Any pleural fluid should be sampled. Localised shadows are more common in bacterial infection; diffuse infiltration suggests an opportunistic organism. In all patients the likely value (and the risks) of invasive techniques to establish a definite cause for pneumonia must be considered.

Most patients with diffuse pulmonary infiltration do not have sputum and invasive investigations are therefore required to demonstrate the infective agent. Transtracheal aspiration, percutaneous needle aspiration biopsy, bronchoscopy and open lung biopsy can all yield useful information. Bronchoscopy is the most widely available technique. BAL is a valuable technique for diagnosing pneumocystis and cytomegalovirus infection and is safe in patients with thrombocytopenia and bleeding diatheses. TBB, although effective, can produce dangerous haemor-

Table 13.17 Important causes of pneumonia in the immunocompromised patient

Bacterial	Viral
Gram-negative organisms as well as Gram-positive	Cytomegalovirus
	Herpes simplex
Nocardia	
Mycobacteria	**Fungal**
Legionella	Candida
Mycoplasma	Aspergillus
Chlamydia	Cryptococcus
	Protozoal
	Pneumocystis

rhage in patients with bleeding problems (uraemic patients are particularly prone to haemorrhage) and pneumothorax is a complication, particularly hazardous in patients receiving positive pressure ventilation.

Specific pneumonias in immunocompromised patients

Gram-negative pneumonias

Bacterial pneumonias, particularly Gram-negative infections, are common in neutropenic patients (e.g. following bone marrow transplantation or chemotherapy for leukaemia), particularly if the granulocyte count is less than $500 \times 10^6/l$, and may be associated with life-threatening septicaemia. The chest X-ray usually shows localised shadowing, rather than diffuse infiltration. Following blood cultures empirical therapy should be started. Common organisms are *Pseudomonas aeruginosa*, *Escherichia coli*, *Klebsiella*, *Enterobacter* and *Serratia* spp. The use of broad-spectrum antibiotics favours the emergence of resistant organisms and also the development of fungal infections. Treatment of Gram-negative infections commonly requires aminoglycosides, cephalosporins and anti-pseudomonal pencillins.

Klebsiella pneumonia

The most common clinical setting for this Gram-negative pneumonia is the elderly male patient, often with chronic lung disease, whose 'immunosuppression' is due to general debility, associated with chronic illnesses such as diabetes or alcoholism. The illness can be severe (mortality 20–50%) with high fever, rigors and pleuritic pain, and haemoptysis occurs more often than in most bacterial pneumonias. The upper lobes are commonly involved with considerable necrosis and cavitation, often bilateral and with bulging of the fissure adjacent to the consolidated lung. There may be diagnostic confusion with tuberculosis.

Patients with Klebsiella pneumonia can develop empyema. Treatment is most effective with gentamicin plus cefuroxime but resolution is often slow and substantial residual pulmonary damage is not uncommon.

Pneumocystis carinii pneumonia (PCP)

Pneumocystis pneumonia occurs in patients receiving steroids and other immunosuppressive agents, and is particularly common in AIDS. The clinical picture is of fever, a dry cough and progressive breathlessness. On auscultation the lungs often sound remarkably normal. The chest X-ray is often clear when symptoms first develop, but there is progressive bilateral pulmonary infiltration, commencing in the perihilar regions, without effusions or adenopathy (Fig. 13.17). Untreated, all patients become

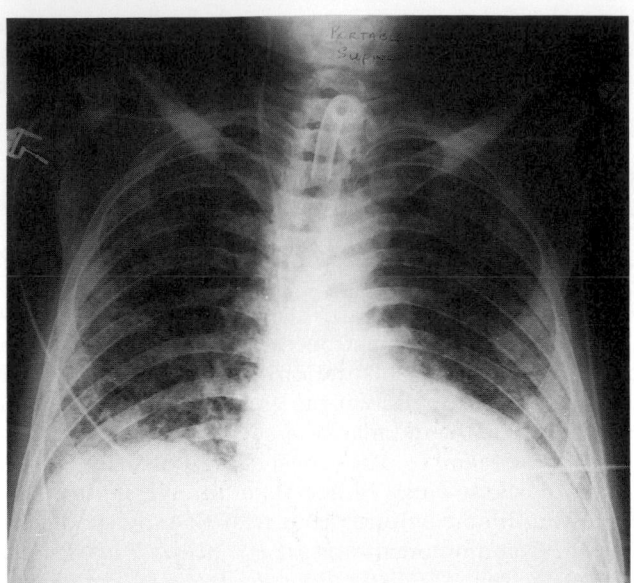

Fig. 13.17 Pneumocystis pneumonia (PCP). Note that the diffuse hazy consolidation is bilateral and maximal in the mid- and lower zones.

incapacitated by dyspnoea and die of hypoxaemia. In patients with AIDS, pneumocystis pneumonia characteristically evolves over several weeks, whereas in other patients at risk, the time course is more rapid. In AIDS, pneumocystis is the most common cause of diffuse pulmonary shadowing. Since pneumocystis pneumonia is so common in this group it is appropriate in some circumstances to initiate empirical therapy. Whenever there is doubt about the correct diagnosis, or if response to treatment for presumed pneumocystis infection is slow, a definite diagnosis is required; for this, bronchoscopy with BAL and, if lavage is negative, TBB, has a very high diagnostic yield. The diagnosis can also be achieved by inducing sputum production by nebulising hypertonic saline.

When treated early, pneumocystis pneumonia responds well to therapy with high dose co-trimoxazole given for 3 weeks. Mortality has fallen from 30% to 5% in the last decade. Trimethoprim and dapsone is an effective combination, whereas pentamidine, although effective, is a more toxic drug. Unfortunately, recurrence is common. Co-trimoxazole and inhaled pentamidine provide effective prophylaxis. Since PCP is unusual in HIV until the CD4 lymphocyte count is less than 250, it is usual to initiate primary prophylaxis at that level. In AIDS patients with severe pneumocystis pneumonia and respiratory failure, steroids, given early, improve survival.

Aspergillus pneumonia

Aspergillus fumigatus is a rare cause of pneumonia and patients usually have severe granulocytopenia or are on corticosteroid therapy, and have frequently received broad-spectrum antibiotics. Patients receiving therapy for leukaemia are particularly at risk. The clinical picture is of fever, dyspnoea, pulmonary infiltrates that resemble pulmonary infarction, sometimes with cavitation, and pleural involvement. There is frequently evidence of aspergillus infection at other sites, notably the brain, bones and endocardium. Diagnosis is most reliably achieved by open lung biopsy or TBB. BAL in immunosuppressed patients frequently demonstrates aspergillus, but biopsy material is required to confirm invasive pulmonary infection. Treatment is with intravenous amphotericin but mortality is high.

Candida albicans is an unusual cause of pneumonia, occurring in the same high-risk patient group as those who develop aspergillus pneumonia and presenting a similar clinical picture. Blood cultures are more frequently positive. Treatment is with amphotericin and flucytosine.

Nocardia pneumonia

Nocardia asteroides can rarely cause a chronic suppurative pneumonia in otherwise normal individuals but more commonly it is a cause of an acute pneumonia in the immunocompromised host. In addition to lung involvement, in which there may be a single lesion or extensive consolidation with cavitation, pleural disease, empyema and metastatic spread also occur. The sputum shows Gram-positive hyphae which are acid-fast and grow rapidly on aerobic culture. The treatment of choice is a sulphonamide in high dose.

Unusual pneumonias

A number of unusual infections (bacterial, viral, fungal and protozoal) can cause pneumonia and are particularly important in certain parts of the world (Table 13.18). They are described in Chapter 11.

Table 13.18 Unusual causes of pneumonia

Bacterial	Viral
Salmonella typhi and *paratyphi* (typhoid)	Varicella (chickenpox)
Brucella abortus and *melitensis* (brucellosis)	Herpes zoster
Pasteurella pestis (plague)	Epstein-Barr virus (infectious mononucleosis)
Pasteurella tularensis (tularaemia)	
Bacillus anthracis (anthrax)	**Protozoal, yeast and fungal**
Leptospira icterohaemorrhagicae (leptospirosis)	*Actinomyces israelii* (actinomycosis)
	Coccidioides immitis (coccidioidomycosis)
Rickettsial	*Histoplasma capsulatum* (histoplasmosis)
Typhus	

TUBERCULOSIS

Epidemiology

In 19th-century England one person in five died of *Myco-bacterium tuberculosis* infection. The dramatic decline in notifications (Fig. 13.18) and deaths (Fig. 1.6, p. 13) reflects one of the great medical advances of the century. However, tuberculosis remains a common cause of death in the developing world, in which there are approximately 10 000 000 infectious cases. There are well-recognised 'at risk' population groups in the UK and these include the elderly, immigrants from the Indian subcontinent and Far East, those of poor social circumstances, alcoholics, immunosuppressed patients and hospital employees. Tuberculosis is a common complication of HIV infection, and as a consequence, the incidence of TB has substantially increased in some areas of the world.

*Mycobacterium bovi*s was once a common cause of human infection but has now been eradicated in developed countries by inoculation of cattle and pasteurisation of milk.

Mycobacteria other than *M. tuberculosis* or *M. bovis* may cause infection in humans, including *M. kansasii, M. xenopi, M. avium* and *M. intracellulare*. The source of infection, unlike the droplet route of *M. tuberculosis*, is generally thought to be exposure of susceptible individuals to organisms in water, soil, dust and animals (particularly pigs, chickens, birds and monkeys). The organisms are not transmitted between humans.

Infectivity, immunology and pathology

The response to a primary infection is shown in Figure 13.19. The usual end result of this is a small subpleural lesion which heals with fibrosis; the glandular lesion also heals, and within about 18 months both may calcify. However, some lesions, especially in children, may

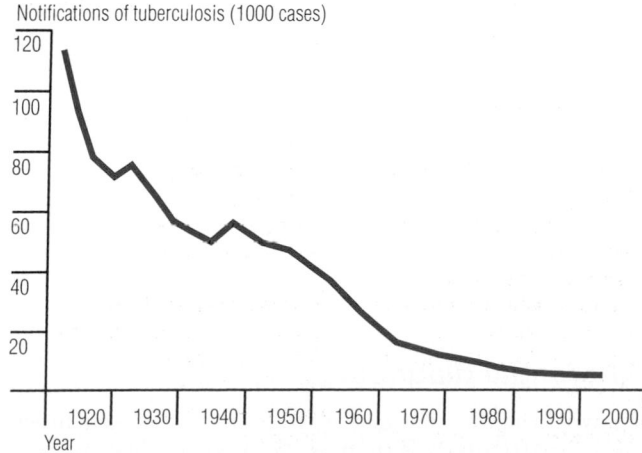

Notifications of tuberculosis (1000 cases)

Fig. 13.18 The decline in tuberculosis in England and Wales.

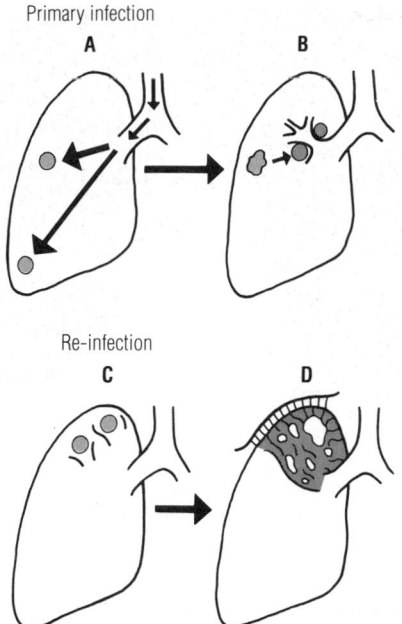

Fig. 13.19 Primary and postprimary (re-infection) tuberculosis. In primary tuberculosis there is pneumonic consolidation (Ghon focus) which is usually subpleural and affects the mid- or lower zones (**A**). Subsequently, infection involves the draining hilar nodes (**B**), which may cause bronchial compression. Re-infection tuberculosis (**C**) is usually apical and progresses to cavitation, fibrosis, volume loss and pleural thickening (**D**).

erode a blood vessel (Fig. 13.20) and progress to 'miliary' tuberculosis, so named because of the 'millet'-sized lesions on the chest X-ray. Alternatively the lung lesion may progress, and cavitate or involve the pleura causing a pleural effusion. Finally the lymph node involvement may progress, especially in Asians and negroes, and occasionally compress, obstruct or erode a bronchus, particularly that of the right middle lobe. Of those that heal, some develop postprimary tuberculosis (Fig. 13.19), sometimes referred to as re-infection adult tuberculosis. Whether the patients become re-infected exogenously or whether their existing lesions become active again is often not clear. Postprimary tuberculosis is usually apical and may have a variety of sequelae, including bronchiectasis and, most seriously, tuberculosis bronchopneumonia.

Clinical features

Some patients are asymptomatic, their disease being noted on routine chest X-ray. Many patients have fever and weight loss plus symptoms suggesting pulmonary infection. Tuberculosis may present insidiously in the elderly.

Investigation

Tuberculin testing, either with the Mantoux technique or the multiple puncture Heaf or Tine tests, is useful in

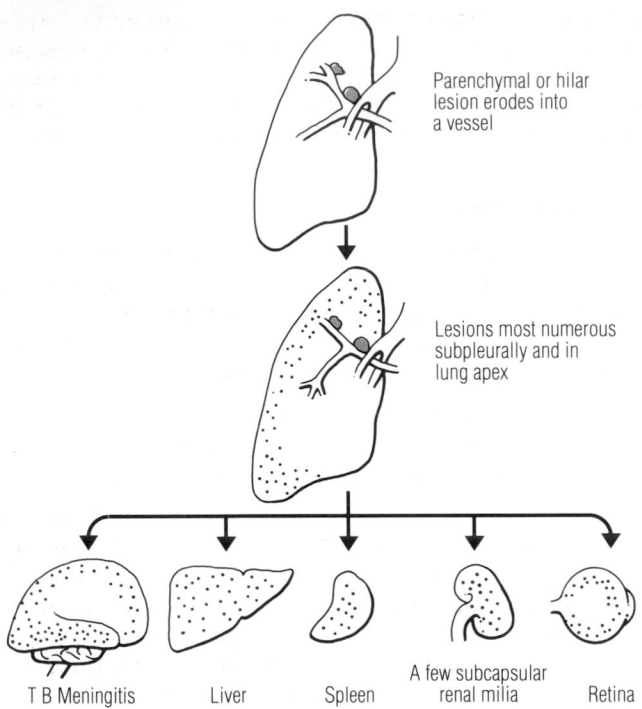

Parenchymal or hilar lesion erodes into a vessel

Lesions most numerous subpleurally and in lung apex

T B Meningitis   Liver   Spleen   A few subcapsular renal milia   Retina

Fig. 13.20 Miliary tuberculosis. In miliary tuberculosis multiple organs are involved. The diagnosis is most commonly suggested by the chest X-ray. Meningitis is relatively common.

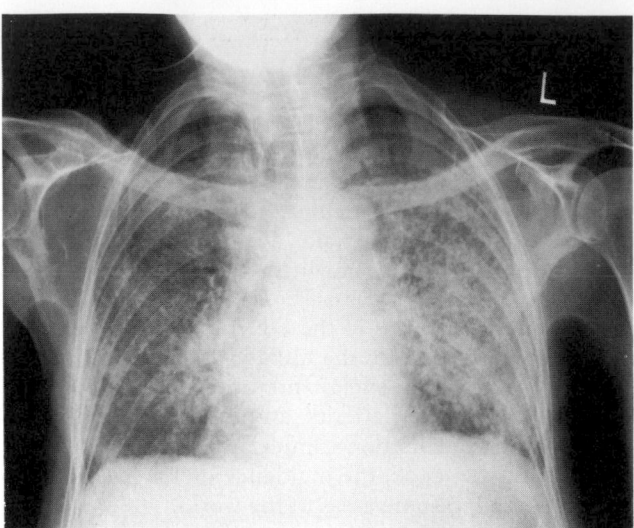

Fig. 13.21 Miliary tuberculosis. Thousands of small nodules, 'millet-size', all of similar size and distributed throughout the lungs.

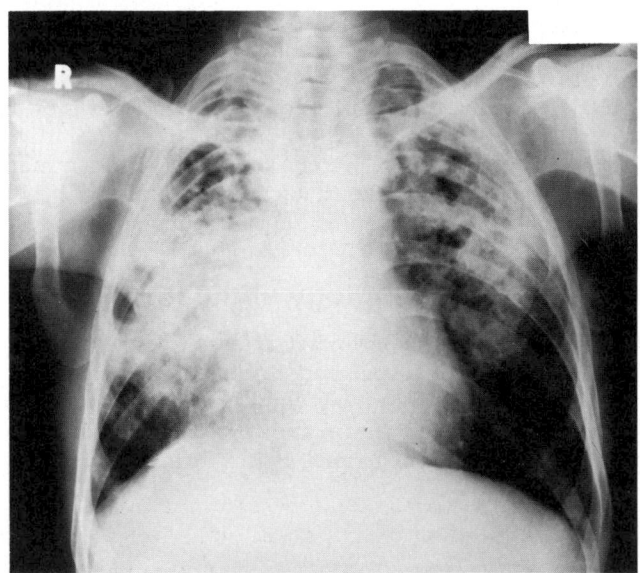

Fig. 13.22 Postprimary (re-infection) tuberculosis. The widespread tuberculous consolidation is predominantly involving the upper and mid-zones. The translucent areas in the upper zones are cavities. There is calcification in the right upper zone and the right hemidiaphragm, suggesting that the patient has re-activation of old disease.

assessing contacts and in children before BCG vaccination. A positive Mantoux should show 5 mm of induration using up to 10 tuberculin units. When performed correctly, a negative tuberculin test almost excludes active tuberculosis infection except in the very ill or in the presence of tuberculin anergy. A normal chest X-ray is rare in active pulmonary tuberculosis. Characteristic appearances include:

● primary tuberculosis with hilar gland enlargement
● miliary tuberculosis (Fig. 13.21)
● postprimary (re-infection) tuberculosis with cavitation (Fig. 13.22)
● tuberculosis bronchopneumonia.

Fluorescent techniques are usually used to screen sputum, and the Ziehl-Neelsen stain to confirm that bacilli are present. Routine culture of the organism takes 4–8 weeks, and is important for excluding atypical mycobacteria and determining drug sensitivities. If the patient has no sputum, fibre-optic bronchoscopy with bronchial lavage is a useful diagnostic tool. In adults gastric washings or laryngeal swabs are seldom necessary when bronchoscopy is available. The sedimentation rate is usually raised, and in advanced disease there may be an anaemia with a raised white cell count, occasionally with a lymphocytosis. Liver function tests may be abnormal.

Extrapulmonary tuberculosis can involve most organ systems (Table 13.19).

Differential diagnosis

In any febrile illness it may be relevant to consider tuberculosis, particularly if there is chest X-ray shadowing or lymph gland enlargement. It must be distinguished from

Table 13.19 Diagnosis of extrapulmonary tuberculosis*

Three early morning urine specimens
Liver biopsy
Lymph node biopsy
Bone marrow aspiration and trephine biopsy
Lumbar puncture
Laparoscopy and biopsy
Joint aspiration
Bone biopsy
Stool specimens in immunosuppressed patients

*All specimens should be cultured.

simple pneumonia, and in such cases the usual clinical feature which raises suspicion of tuberculosis is the indolent nature of the illness.

Complications

These may be due to dissemination of the disease, extensive lung damage or non-specific metabolic disturbances.

- *Dissemination (Extrapulmonary tuberculosis)*. Tuberculosis may involve lymph nodes, pleura, bones, joints, kidneys, adrenals, liver, peritoneum, bowel, epididymis, meninges and brain.
- *Extensive lung damage*. This may result in massive haemoptysis, bronchiectasis, breathlessness and eventually respiratory failure with cor pulmonale.
- *Associated metabolic conditions*. These can include hypokalaemia, hyponatraemia, hypercalcaemia and hypo-albuminaemia.

Mycobacterial infection in HIV/AIDS

Patients with the acquired immunodeficiency syndrome (AIDS) are frequently infected with mycobacteria, either typical *M. tuberculosis* or atypical mycobacteria, commonly *Mycobacterium avium*. Infection may result in pulmonary or extrapulmonary disease, and unusual clinical presentations may occur. Although *M. tuberculosis* infection is usually a reactivation of previous tuberculosis, typical upper lobe disease is not so common in patients with AIDS. *M. tuberculosis* in AIDS is usually responsive to conventional antituberculous treatment.

Prevention of tuberculosis is possible with isoniazid prophylaxis, and this should be considered in HIV positive patients who also have a positive PPD skin test.

Mycobacterium avium infection in AIDS

Infection with *Mycobacterium avium* complex is the commonest atypical mycobacterial complication of AIDS. Identification of the organism is best achieved from blood, bone marrow, liver and bronchi. Patients have advanced HIV disease and the mycobacterial infection is usually disseminated. The organism is resistant to pyrazinamide and isoniazid and treatment is difficult. Recommended drugs include combinations of clofazimine, ethambutol, rifampicin, amikacin and quinolones. Prognosis is poor, most patients dying within a few months.

Management

Organisms in the walls of pulmonary cavities, exposed to a high oxygen tension, tend to replicate rapidly, whereas those in caseous areas or within macrophages, in which the pH is low, divide relatively slowly. There are therefore three populations of organisms to be treated:

- the rapidly dividing extracellular organisms
- the slowly dividing extracellular organisms
- the slowly dividing intracellular organisms.

The immediate target for chemotherapy is to kill the large numbers of organisms in the 'rapidly dividing' group and to prevent survival of 'mutant' strains. The slow-growing intracellular and extracellular organisms will be completely eliminated only by a prolonged course of effective drugs, and if there are 'persisters' from these two groups they will cause late relapse of the disease.

Antituberculous drugs and treatment regimes

The four most commonly used drugs in developed countries are listed in Table 13.20. Cure can be achieved by the combination of isoniazid plus streptomycin, but the isoniazid must be continued for 18 months if relapse due to persisters is to be prevented.

With the use of isoniazid and rifampicin, both of which have activity against intracellular organisms, tuberculous lesions should be sterilised much more quickly. Effective chemotherapy of pulmonary tuberculosis is 6 months' isoniazid and rifampicin, plus pyrazinamide or ethambutol given for the first 2 months.

In patients with liver disease, standard therapy with rifampicin, isoniazid and pyrazinamide can be given but liver function should be closely monitored. In renal failure treatment of tuberculosis is with rifampicin, isoniazid and pyrazinamide, but if ethambutol or streptomycin is used the dosage should be reduced and drug levels monitored. Dialysis can greatly affect drug clearance. Rifampicin, isoniazid, pyrazinamide and ethambutol are safe in pregnancy but streptomycin should be avoided. Rifampicin reduces the effectiveness of the combined oral contraceptive and approximately halves the pharmacological effect of concurrent oral prednisolone.

Drug resistance

Drug resistance is due either to primary natural resistance of the organism or to infection with an organism from an ineffectively treated patient. Resistance to rifampicin and pyrazinamide is rare, but in the Far East and Africa initial resistance to isoniazid or streptomycin, or both, is high. In patients with resistant strains the use of 'second-line' drugs (e.g. streptomycin, capreomycin, cycloserine, prothionamide), particularly in the first 2–4 months of treatment, may be necessary. Four or even five drugs may be required in this initial period and to achieve cure a more prolonged, 18–24 month, regime is necessary.

Drug side-effects

Short-course regimes are relatively non-toxic (Table 13.20) and side-effects are unusual in patients under 35 years.

Cost

Rifampicin is an expensive drug and pyrazinamide is also costly. Cost limits their use in developing countries.

Patient non-compliance with treatment

The treatment of tuberculosis requires disciplined drug-taking, usually on a daily basis, for 6–9 months in most drug regimes. This may be difficult to achieve, particularly in the rural populations of developing countries and in the vagrant populations of the inner cities of Western countries. For this reason supervised twice-weekly regimes, ultra-short courses which accept less than 100% cure, or even supervision in a residential hostel, may have to be considered. Supervision can include direct observation of pill-taking, urine tests for isoniazid and urine inspection for the red discoloration of rifampicin. The advantage of combination tablets of rifampicin and isoniazid is that red urine or a positive urine test for isoniazid confirms that both drugs are being taken.

Table 13.20 'First-line' drugs for tuberculosis

Drug	Daily dose	Side-effects
Rifampicin	10 mg/kg usually 450–600 mg	Hepatitis, nausea, vomiting, fevers, thrombocytopenia, renal failure (on intermittent therapy), drug interactions (e.g. oestrogens)
Isoniazid (prescribed with pyridoxine 10 mg daily)	Children 6 mg/kg Adults usually 300 mg	Peripheral neuropathy, hepatotoxicity, hypersensitivity reactions
Pyrazinamide	20–30 mg/kg usually 1–2 g	Hepatotoxicity, hyperuricaemia, arthralgia
Ethambutol	15–25 mg/kg	Optic neuritis, rashes

Treatment of extrapulmonary tuberculosis

Treatment of renal, bone and joint, lymph node, liver, peritoneum and bowel tuberculosis is in general similar to that of pulmonary tuberculosis. The treatment of tuberculous meningitis deserves special mention, since treatment failure may be lethal. Treatment should include isoniazid, pyrazinamide and rifampicin in conventional doses. A fourth drug is controversial, but streptomycin is considered useful by some physicians. Intrathecal drugs are rarely given. Treatment should be given for 12 months.

The use of corticosteroids in tuberculosis

The administration of corticosteroids, in addition to anti-tuberculous drugs, may sometimes be beneficial. Their use should be considered in the very wasted patient, tuberculous meningitis and intracerebral tuberculomata, as well as pleural and pericardial effusions. Where a patient develops hypersensitivity to a drug that is essential and irreplaceable in a treatment regime, steroids may allow drug therapy to continue.

Prevention

The dramatic decline in tuberculosis in developed countries is due to several factors. Of great importance is the control of infection from human sources by effective chemotherapy. Isolation of infectious patients (those with smear-positive sputum) for a few days is helpful, although prolonged periods of barrier nursing, disposable cutlery and so on are not essential. Often, the simplest method is to get the patient to wear a face-mask when people come into the room. Contact tracing is crucial and immediate contacts, especially children, should have a tuberculin test and chest X-ray. Host defences are improved by better housing and social conditions and the use of Bacille Calmette Guérin (BCG) vaccination. This vaccine, using an attenuated strain of tubercle bacillus, gives a harmless primary infection and therefore a large measure of immunity. It is given to teenage children in developed countries and to infants elsewhere. However, with the decline in the incidence of the disease, routine use of the BCG in Caucasian children who are not otherwise at risk is questionable. Chemoprophylaxis with isoniazid is used in children with a positive skin test and a normal chest X-ray.

In many developing countries the incidence of TB is rising due to HIV infection, and this poses a formidable public health problem.

LUNG ABSCESS

Lung abscess can be defined as an infected, cavitated lesion within the lung parenchyma. Abscesses can occur

Table 13.21 Causes of lung abscess

Necrotising infection	**Pulmonary infarction**
Pyogenic bacteria (*Staphylococcus aureus, Klebsiella*, anaerobes, *Pseudomonas aeruginosa*)	Pulmonary thrombo-embolism
	Pulmonary foreign body embolism (e.g. i.v. drug abusers)
Mycobacteria (*M. tuberculosis* or atypical mycobacteria)	Septic pulmonary embolism
Fungi (*Histoplasma capsulatum, Coccidioides immitis*)	**Cavitation in malignant tumour**
	Bronchogenic carcinoma (esp. squamous cell)
Parasites (*Entamoeba histolytica, Paragonium westermani*)	Metastases
	Lymphoma
Secondary to bronchial occlusion	
Bronchial carcinoma or adenoma	**Others**
Foreign body aspiration	Wegener's granulomatosis
Bronchial stenosis	Infected cysts, bullae, sequestrations
	Pneumoconiosis (silica, coal)

as a result of primary infection, or secondary to other conditions (Table 13.21). The two factors critical to the pathogenesis of lung abscesses are necrotic tissue and infection. Apart from septic emboli, infection is via the tracheobronchial tree and seeds in an area of necrotic lung tissue. This leads to further breakdown of lung tissue and communication with a bronchus.

The presentation will vary with the cause: patients with acute lung abscesses secondary to bacterial pneumonia (e.g. *Klebsiella*) are acutely unwell, febrile and coughing foul, blood-stained sputum, whereas the presentation of a tuberculous abscess will be much more indolent. The patient's breath and sputum may smell faeculent in the presence of anaerobes. There may be finger clubbing.

Lung abscesses are more common in alcoholics and elderly debilitated patients, who are prone to aspiration, and in intravenous drug abusers. Lung abscess may follow the aspiration of infected material in patients with dental sepsis and sinusitis, and may complicate bronchiectasis.

The chest X-ray initially shows a rounded homogeneous opacity, and only when bronchial drainage is established does an air–fluid level appear (Fig. 13.23). Sputum should be sent for Gram stain, culture and sensitivity and examined for acid-fast bacilli. Fibre-optic bronchoscopy will provide useful information both for bacteriology (especially the isolation of anaerobes) and in identifying neoplasms or foreign bodies.

Patients with staphylococcal or *Klebsiella* pneumonias tend to develop abscesses. The commonest radiological appearances with staphylococcus are of multiple, thin-walled, cystic spaces with little fluid. Anaerobic abscesses due to *Entamoeba histolytica* usually involve the liver as well as the lung. The patients may have haemoptysis or cough up 'anchovy paste' or 'chocolate sauce' sputum.

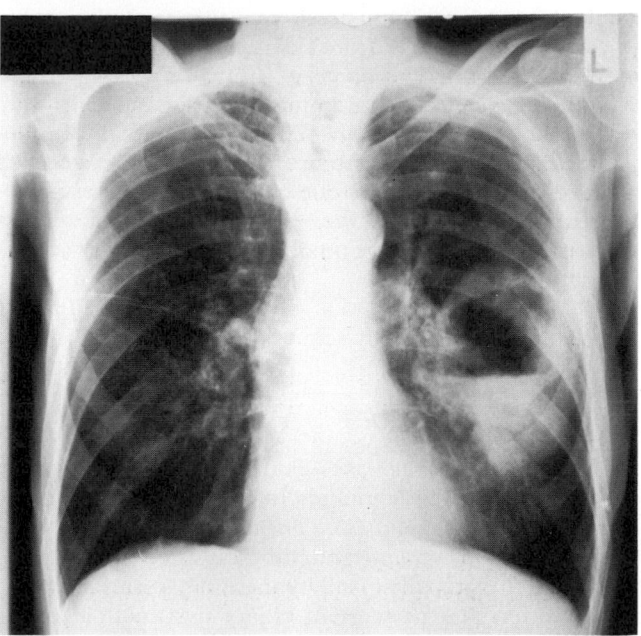

Fig. 13.23 Cavitating lung abscess. The abscess is in the lingular segment of the left upper lobe. The patient had a cough productive of large volumes of purulent sputum from the abscess cavity; note the fluid level.

The treatment of lung abscess depends on the cause. Foreign bodies and some cavitating tumours can be surgically removed. When there is no surgically resectable lesion, treatment centres on frequent physiotherapy and appropriate antibiotics, guided by the bacteriology of sputum, blood and bronchial washings, and given for 6 weeks or more. Needle aspiration to obtain samples of pus for microbiology may be helpful and percutaneous catheter drainage can facilitate resolution. Surgical resection is occasionally necessary.

BRONCHIECTASIS

Bronchiectasis is defined as chronic dilatation of bronchi, usually associated with deficient local clearance mechanisms. The disease may be localised to a lobe or segment or may be generalised throughout the bronchial tree. Clinically, bronchiectasis presents with intermittent or constant cough and sputum with or without haemoptysis.

Aetiology

Congenital factors

- *Cystic fibrosis* (p. 477). This multisystem disorder is associated with bronchial obstruction due to inspissated mucus and thus recurrent infection, the consequence of which is bronchiectasis.

- *Immune deficiency syndromes.* Bronchiectasis is particularly frequent in hypogammaglobulinaemia.
- *Kartagener's syndrome.* This is the triad of dextrocardia, sinusitis and bronchiectasis. The sinusitis and bronchiectasis are due to disorders of ciliary function. *The Chandra-Khetarpal syndrome* is similar, but with laevocardia and no demonstrable ciliary abnormality.
- *Pulmonary sequestration.* Bronchiectasis frequently occurs in congenitally sequestrated lung tissue.

Inflammatory factors

A variety of *infective* processes in the lung may produce bronchiectasis. These include infection with necrotising organisms such as *Klebsiella pneumoniae*, staphylococci, *Pseudomonas aeruginosa* and tuberculosis. The damage caused to the bronchial wall by these organisms may lead to dilatation and permanent ciliary dysfunction. Some viral infections, particularly adenovirus and influenza virus, may predispose to bronchiectasis, as may an episode of bronchiolitis or whooping cough in childhood. MacLeod's syndrome is a unilateral emphysema-like condition which follows early childhood infections and may be associated with bronchiectasis.

The other major inflammatory process predisposing to bronchiectasis is *immunological*. This may be important in bronchiectasis of any aetiology but the classical example is allergic bronchopulmonary aspergillosis (p. 485). It is likely that antigen/antibody complexes in the bronchial wall fix complement, causing an inflammatory reaction, tissue damage and bronchiectasis, characteristically in proximal large airways.

Bronchial obstruction and retraction

Proximal obstruction of an airway by foreign body, tumour, enlarged lymph gland or mucus plug causes secretions to accumulate distally; these then become infected, causing bronchial wall damage. The result of this process is often an area of bronchiectasis localised to a segment or lobe, which may be amenable to surgical resection.

Retraction of lung tissue can occur with healing of tuberculosis or with extensive pulmonary fibrosis, causing distortion and widening of adjacent bronchi.

Idiopathic

Probably the largest single group of patients are those in whom a cause is never found. They usually have bilateral lower lobe disease.

Clinical features

The usual presentation is with cough and sputum. In the advanced stage of the disease patients may produce up to 40–50 ml of sputum per day, most of it in the morning. Haemoptysis is common, usually as blood-streaking of the sputum. Massive haemoptysis does occur, often in association with a recurrence of infection, and is occasionally fatal. With widespread disease the patient is breathless, with malaise, weight loss and recurrent fevers.

The physical signs depend on the extent and stage of the disease. In the patient with severe, widespread bronchiectasis general health may be poor, finger clubbing is common, there are coarse crackles and wheezes and there may be central cyanosis and cor pulmonale. Complications of bronchiectasis include pneumonia, lung abscess, pleural effusion, empyema, brain abscess and amyloidosis. With effective antibiotic therapy these complications are unusual.

Investigation

The chest X-ray may be normal. However, the more characteristic radiographic changes (Fig. 13.24) include ring, line and parallel ('tramline') shadows – the appearances of thickened bronchial walls seen end on or laterally. Thin section CT scanning is a sensitive technique for demonstrating dilated bronchi (Fig. 13.25). If the disease is largely peripheral it usually has a cystic appearance, whereas when the major bronchi are affected they take on a fusiform or saccular appearance. Broncho-

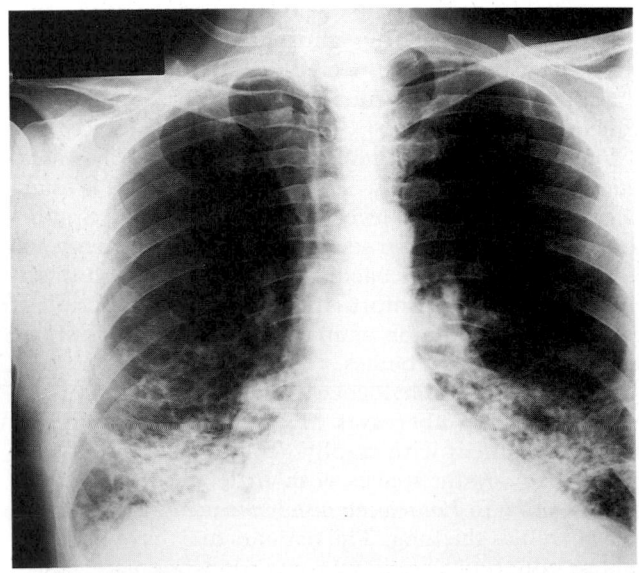

Fig. 13.24 Extensive bilateral basal bronchiectasis.

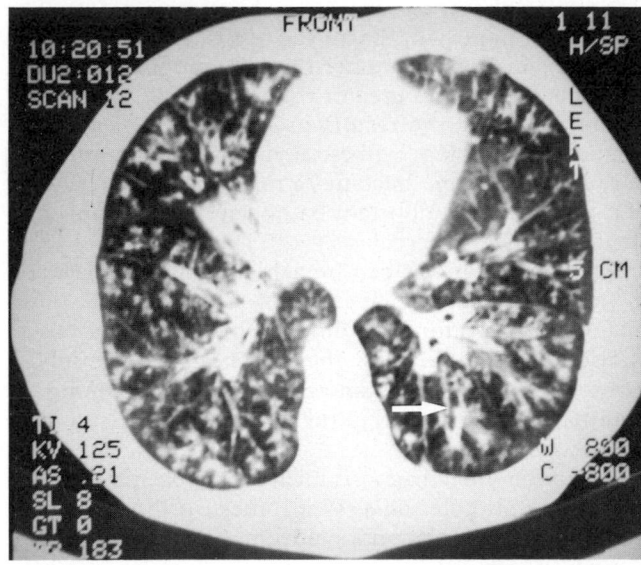

Fig. 13.25 Bronchiectasis: CT scan. There is extensive disease, with bronchial wall thickening and airway dilatation, easily seen in the left lower lobe (arrow).

graphy is only indicated for the diagnosis of minor disease not demonstrated by other techniques (Fig. 13.26).

The most common infecting organism is *H. influenzae*, but pneumococcus is also a frequent pathogen. Colonisation with *Ps. aeruginosa* is not uncommon.

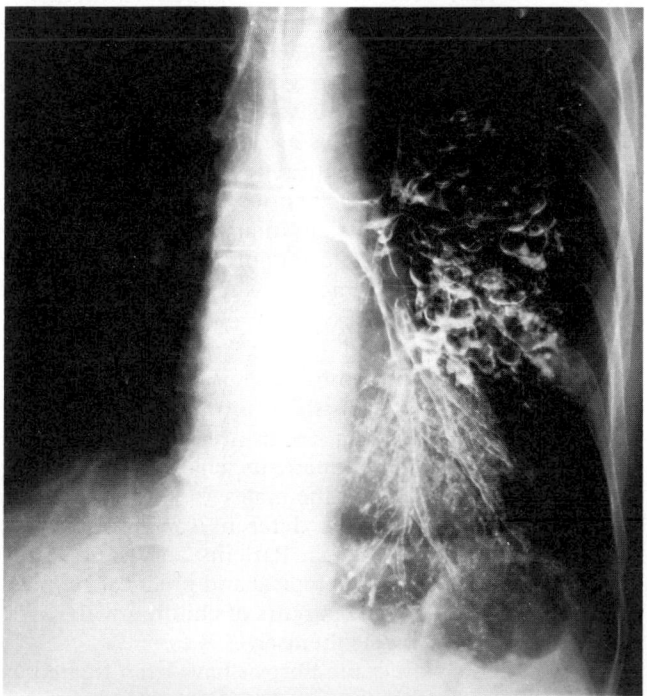

Fig. 13.26 Cystic bronchiectasis. Bronchogram demonstrating severe cystic bronchiectasis of the lingula.

Lung function tests reflect the extent and severity of disease. As the condition worsens a mixed obstructive/restrictive defect develops, with variable response to bronchodilators. Younger bronchiectatic patients require a sweat test to exclude cystic fibrosis and all patients should have a routine estimation of their serum immunoglobulins. A blood eosinophilia is common in allergic bronchopulmonary aspergillus. Ciliary function may require investigation, including a nasal mucosal biopsy with motility studies.

Management

The long-term management of bronchiectasis includes regular, effective physiotherapy. The patients and their relatives are taught postural drainage. In the majority of patients continuous long-term antibiotics are not appropriate and predispose to colonisation with *Ps. aeruginosa*. Prompt treatment of intercurrent and symptomatic infection with appropriate antibiotics is essential. Regular inhaled antibiotics may be helpful (e.g. gentamicin, piperacillin, colomycin), especially in patients with cystic fibrosis.

Inhaled β agonists are useful in those patients with airways obstruction. Oral steroids are required in bronchopulmonary aspergillosis and can be helpful in some other bronchiectatic patients in whom bronchial damage is immunologically mediated. In severe cases patients eventually develop cor pulmonale and require diuretic and domiciliary oxygen therapy. A proportion of patients with cystic fibrosis have been successfully treated by heart–lung transplantation.

Surgical resection for bronchiectasis is indicated in only a small number of cases, usually for localised disease caused by previous bronchial occlusion or lobar pneumonia. It may also be necessary to resect bronchiectatic lung for massive haemoptysis. Haemoptysis can sometimes be successfully treated by embolisation of a branch of the bronchial artery with foam.

With the exception of patients with generalised disorders, such as cystic fibrosis or immune deficiency, the long-term outlook for the majority of patients with bronchiectasis is good.

CYSTIC FIBROSIS

Cystic fibrosis (formerly called mucoviscidosis or fibrocystic disease of the pancreas) is the most common potentially lethal genetic disease in Caucasians. It is an autosomal recessive gene which is carried by one in 20–25 of the Caucasian population and its incidence is about one in 2000–2500 live births. The incidence amongst Caucasians varies a little from country to country, but it is rare in Asians and negroes.

Mucus in cystic fibrosis patients is no more viscid than in chronic bronchitis; however, mucus-secreting glands throughout the body show morphological changes, and the ducts of mucus glands are obstructed. Pathological changes are seen in the lung, pancreas, bowel, liver and genital tract. The cystic fibrosis gene was isolated in 1989. It is located on the long (q) arm of chromosome 7. The abnormality is a subtle one within the DNA molecule. Activity of the gene is expressed in cells in the respiratory tract, the digestive system (including the pancreas) and the male genital ducts. The cystic fibrosis gene encodes for a regulation protein (sometimes called the cystic fibrosis transmembrane conductance regulator). It controls ion and water flux across cell membranes, causing high sodium and chloride levels in the sweat ducts, a high transepithelial potential difference in the respiratory tract and elevated chloride and low water content in pancreatic secretions. The epithelial cells of the respiratory tract and sweat ducts are relatively impermeable to chloride ions with a secondary increase in sodium transport; chloride transport in other cells, such as erythrocytes, is normal. The ion transport abnormality leads to impaired local defence mechanisms in the respiratory tract and abnormal pancreatic secretions. The defect in the lung causes bacterial colonisation, damage to the bronchial wall and bronchiectasis. The defective pancreatic secretions cause a malabsorption syndrome and blockage of the ducts with autodigestion of the pancreas results in diabetes mellitus in 10–20% of adult patients (p. 743).

Clinical features and diagnosis

The clinical presentation differs between neonates, and older children and young adults (Table 13.22). Clinical examination of adolescents and adults usually shows finger clubbing secondary to chronic respiratory infection, retarded growth and development and a hyperinflated chest with coarse crackles and wheezes. Gynaecomastia is occasionally seen and there may be hepatosplenomegaly and other signs of chronic liver disease.

The chest X-ray shows hyperinflated lungs and widespread bronchiectasis (parallel line and ring shadows, with multiple nodular opacities, mainly in the mid- and upper zones; the hila are usually prominent). Lung function testing shows a progressive obstructive defect. The single most important diagnostic test is the sweat sodium which is consistently greater than 70 mmol/l in children with the disease and greater than 90 mmol/l in affected adults, although the results in adults are less reliable. Sputum bacteriology will often yield *S. aureus*, and later in life *Ps. aeruginosa* becomes a major problem. Haemophilus may be an important pathogen and patients occasionally develop tuberculosis.

Prenatal diagnosis can be achieved by the measurement of elevated levels of enzymes such as alkaline phosphatase in the amniotic fluid or by DNA analysis of chorionic villus biopsies; these techniques are only of value for 'at risk' pregnancies. Neonatal screening for immunoreactive trypsin in the blood is simple and inexpensive.

The differential diagnosis includes hypogammaglobulinaemia, immobile cilia syndromes, asthma, coeliac disease and Shwackman's syndrome (pancreatic insufficiency, neutropenia, metaphyseal chondrodysplasia, growth retardation and frequent infections).

Management

The outlook for patients with cystic fibrosis has improved and average survival is now about 30 years.

The corner-stone of treatment of respiratory disease is regular chest physiotherapy, particularly postural drainage. In the first year of life prophylactic antistaphylococcal drugs may be helpful. Severe infective exacerbations require intravenous antibiotics, usually antipseudomonal agents (e.g. gentamicin, ceftazidime, piperacillin, ciprofloxacin). As the disease progresses regular nebulised antibiotics are of value. To facilitate home care, some patients with repeated flare-up of infection have indwelling central venous lines and administer their own antibiotics. Bronchodilators and occasionally oral corticosteroids may be useful in patients with airflow obstruction. Pneumothoraces are not uncommon and should be treated conservatively whenever possible. Malabsorption is treated by oral pancreatic enzyme supplements. Abdominal emergencies occur, including adult meconium ileus equivalent, intussusception, acute pancreatitis and bleeding from oesophageal varices. Diabetes is common. Adult patients will need counselling about fertility since 98% of the males are infertile (due to maldevelopment of the vas deferens) and for females pregnancy can be hazardous. Patients and their family need constant moral, psychological and practical support. Genetic counselling of the parents of children with cystic fibrosis and of the patients themselves is essential.

Some patients with cystic fibrosis have been treated by transplantation. For the future, drug therapy may modify the effects of the gene defect and eventually gene replacement therapy may be possible.

Table 13.22 Clinical consequences of cystic fibrosis

Neonates	Older children and young adults
Meconium ileus	Bronchiectasis
Rectal prolapse	Malabsorption
Failure to thrive	Meconium ileus equivalent
Recurrent bronchopulmonary	Infertility
infections	Cirrhosis and portal hypertension

ASTHMA

Bronchial asthma has been recognised since ancient times. Despite recent improved understanding of its pathogenesis and consequent new treatments, morbidity and mortality from the condition remain a substantial clinical problem.

Definition

The American Thoracic Society defines asthma as 'a disease characterized by increased responsiveness of the bronchi to various stimuli, manifested by widespread narrowing of the airways that changes in severity either spontaneously or as a result of treatment'. Asthmatics may be said to have 'twitchy' airways, and it is an essential feature of the resulting bronchoconstriction that it is usually reversible, at least in part, with administration of inhaled bronchodilators. Most asthmatics can be classified as either 'extrinsic' or 'intrinsic' (Table 13.23). There are a number of non-specific trigger factors that can start an attack (Table 13.24).

Some late-onset asthmatics who have smoked may also have chronic bronchitis and are therefore difficult to classify, falling into the untidy category of 'asthmatic bronchitis'.

Asthma caused by sensitising chemicals and industrial agents is increasingly recognised (Table 13.25).

Table 13.23 The classification of extrinsic and intrinsic asthma

Extrinsic	Intrinsic
History of allergy (e.g. hay fever, eczema)	No allergic history
Skin tests positive	Skin tests negative
Early onset	Late onset
Family history of atopy	Family history of asthma only
Intermittent attacks, often seasonal	Persisting asthma, perennial
Elevated IgE	Normal IgE
Marked blood and sputum eosinophilia	Variable eosinophilia
Not aspirin-sensitive, occasional polyps	Aspirin-sensitive, nasal polyps
Good response to beta agonists	Variable response to beta agonists
Good response to disodium cromoglycate	Poor response to disodium cromoglycate

Table 13.24 Non-specific 'trigger' factors in asthma

Upper respiratory tract infection	Irritants: smoke, paint or chemical fumes
Exercise	Drugs, e.g. beta-blockers
Cold air	Industrial causes
Laughter	

Table 13.25 Sensitising chemicals and industrial agents as a cause of asthma

Material	Industry
Toluene di-isocyonate (TDI)	Polyurethane industry
Soldering flux	Electrical, engineering industry
Cotton dust (byssinosis)	Textiles
Urine, serum, danders of animals	Veterinary, agricultural and laboratory workers
Flour, grain	Bakers, millers
Wood dust	Carpenters
Sulphur dioxide, ozone, chloride	Chemical industry

Epidemiology

Asthma is common, affecting up to 5% of children and 2% of adults in the UK. The peak age of onset is under 5 years, and in this age group it is more common in boys by a ratio of 3 to 2; above 5 years there is an equal sex ratio. There is an allergic component in one-third to one-half of all cases. About 2000 patients die from asthma in the UK each year, and it is likely that many of these deaths are preventable. Asthma is a world-wide problem and in some countries the incidence is rising.

Pathogenesis

Bronchial 'hyper-reactivity' appears to be the key to the asthmatic reaction. It is the unique property of asthmatic airways to react, by bronchoconstriction, inflammation and mucus production, to stimuli that would not elicit this reaction in normal airways. Possible mechanisms for bronchial hyper-reactivity are listed in Table 13.26.

There can be little doubt that immunological mechanisms (Ch. 6) play an important part in the asthmatic reaction. Both immediate and delayed responses are involved and these can be demonstrated by the technique of bronchial provocation challenge testing. This is a method of provoking an asthmatic reaction in susceptible subjects by inhalation of antigens or chemicals. The immediate hypersensitivity reaction is mediated by degranulation of mast cells (Fig. 13.27). The mast cell degranulation is produced by the union of antigen with IgE antibody which is bound to the mast cell surface. Degranulation liberates a variety of substances including preformed mediators and newly formed metabolites of arachidonic acid from the cell membrane (prostaglandins, leukotrienes, etc. – see below).

Table 13.26 Mechanisms of bronchial hyper-reactivity

Inflammation, immunological liberation of bronchoconstrictor mediators
Alterations in autonomic nervous control
Abnormalities of Ca^{2+} flux
Damage to epithelial 'tight junction'

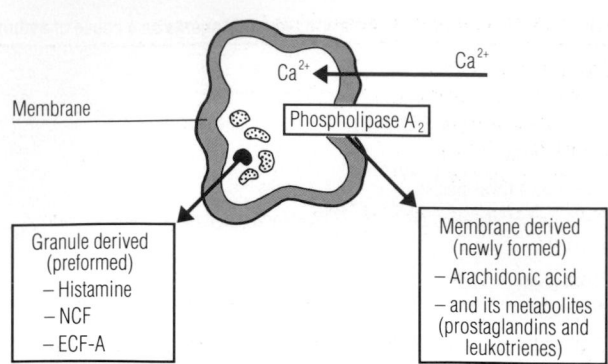

Fig. 13.27 Mast cell mediators. The release of preformed and newly formed mediators from mast cells involves calcium flux across the cell membrane, and in the case of the newly formed mediators, phospholipase A_2 activation.

When asthmatic subjects are challenged with appropriate inhaled antigen and lung function is measured, they may show an immediate bronchoconstriction response within a few minutes. Lung function then returns toward baseline but a further apparently unprovoked fall may occur 4–6 hours later.

The early response is thought, in the main, to be due to the acute effect of histamine release from mast cells. The late response is more complex, mediated through the actions of inflammatory mediators such as leukotrienes and platelet activating factor and the recruitment and activation of inflammatory cells. This highly complex pathogenic mechanism is the focus of much research, since it may represent a model for the ongoing inflammatory reaction in asthma and therefore be the target for anti-inflammatory prophylactic drugs.

Bronchial smooth muscle and secretions are regulated by neural mechanisms (Fig. 13.28). The balance of autonomic nervous control is important. The cholinergic vagal impulses have bronchoconstrictor and secretory actions. These effects are opposed by β_2 adrenergic receptors which are bronchodilator and antisecretory. The β adrenergic mechanism is supported by circulating catecholamines. In patients with asthma, vagal reflexes may play an important part in bronchial hyper-reactivity, particularly to stimuli such as cold air and exercise.

Other mechanisms may play a part in bronchial hyper-reactivity. Calcium flux across cell membranes is important for smooth muscle contraction and for mast cell degranulation, and agents which block this flux may prove to be useful in treatment. Finally, there is some evidence that the 'tight junction' between epithelial cells on the surface of the bronchial epithelium may be abnormally 'leaky', allowing antigen readier access to the mast cells underneath.

It is therefore clear that no single mediator or mechanism is responsible for the asthmatic reaction, and research continues to elucidate this highly complex process.

Pathology and pathophysiology

The pathogenic mechanisms involved in asthma result in the histological changes shown in Figure 13.29. These changes can be acute or chronic. The sputum of asthmatics is often yellow and tenacious and contains many eosinophils, epithelial cells and bronchiolar casts ('plugs'). At post-mortem in patients who die of acute asthma, many plugs are found in large and small airways.

Clinical features

Asthma is episodic. Between attacks, patients, especially younger ones, may be asymptomatic and have no

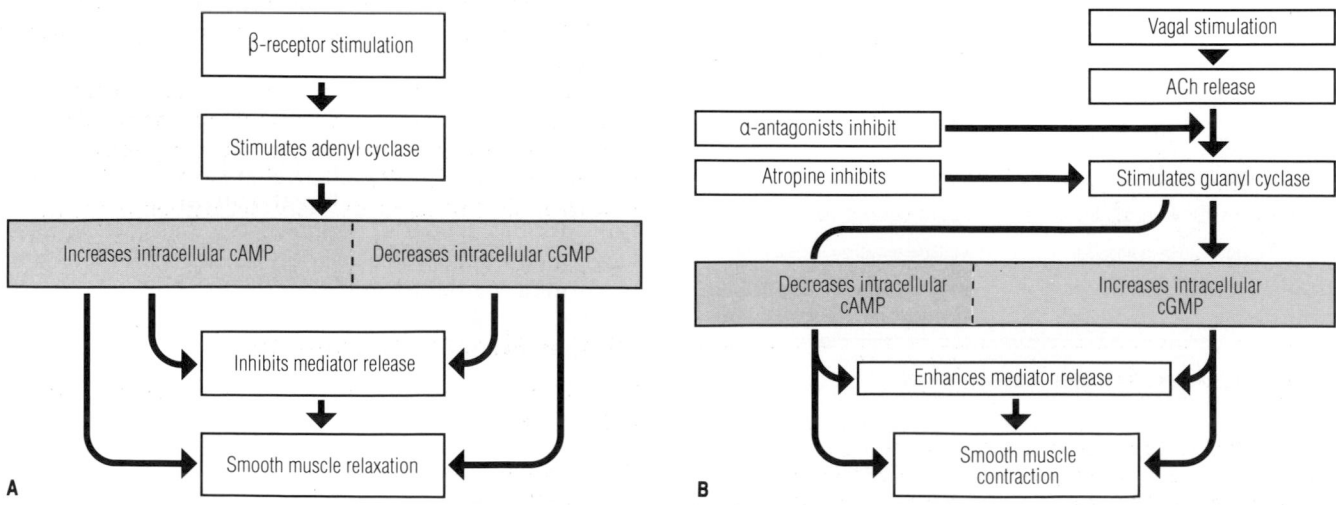

Fig. 13.28 The control of airway calibre. The balance of bronchodilatation from sympathomimetic β-receptor stimulation (**A**), and bronchoconstriction from parasympathetic vagal activity (**B**), is an important determinant of airway calibre.

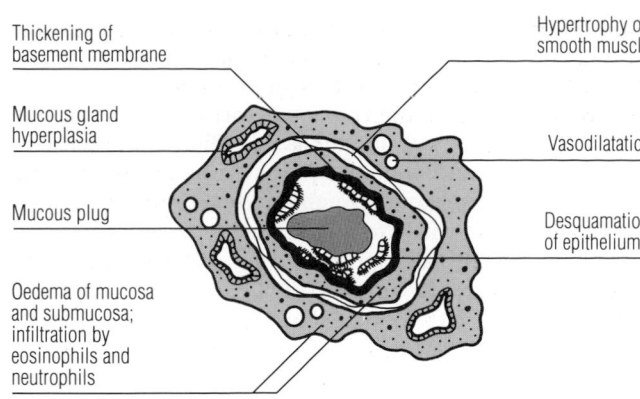

Thickening of
basement membrane

Mucous gland
hyperplasia

Mucous plug

Oedema of mucosa
and submucosa;
infiltration by
eosinophils and
neutrophils

Hypertrophy of
smooth muscle

Vasodilatation

Desquamation
of epithelium

Fig. 13.29 The pathology of asthma. Intense inflammation, with oedema and intralumenal mucous plugs, is the striking pathology of asthma.

abnormal physical signs. The common symptoms of an asthma attack are cough, wheeze and breathlessness. Cough may be the only symptom, especially in children. Almost all asthmatics are worse at night and most will feel 'tight' in the morning. The fall in peak flow rate in the early hours of the morning is referred to as 'morning dipping' (Fig. 13.30). Acute asthma and sudden asthma deaths occur most frequently in the early hours of the morning. There is a personal or family history of allergy (rhinitis, conjunctivitis, eczema or urticaria) in up to 50% of patients.

In chronic asthma, particularly that which has persisted from childhood, there may be chest wall deformity. When asthma is severe the patient is distressed and vigorously contracting the accessory muscles of respiration. When the condition progresses despite active treat-

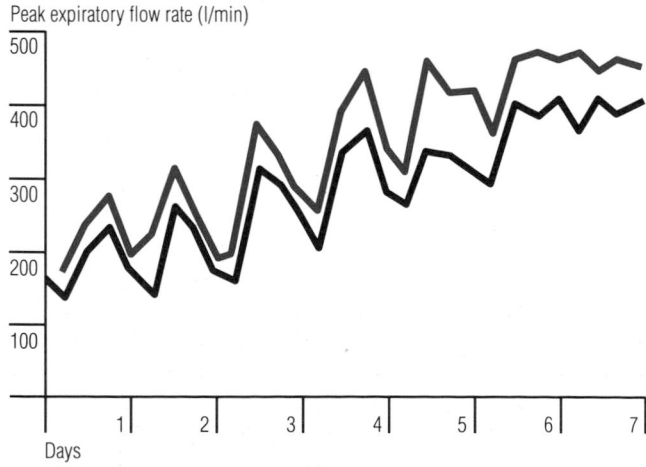

Peak expiratory flow rate (l/min)

Fig. 13.30 Peak expiratory flow rate (PEFR) in asthma. The measurement of peak flow is essential for the management of asthma. PEFR is variable in asthmatics; it is lower in the early hours of the morning and on wakening ('morning dipping') and increases with β_2 agonists (e.g. salbutamol). The chart is typical of a patient recovering from an episode of moderately severe asthma.

Table 13.27 Clinical syndromes associated with asthma

Eosinophilic syndromes
Allergic bronchopulmonary aspergillosis
Idiopathic pulmonary eosinophilia
Tropical eosinophilia
Churg-Strauss syndrome
Aspirin sensitivity and nasal polyposis
Pericarditis
Carcinoid syndrome

ment, the patient is then said to have '*acute severe asthma*' (p. 483).

A number of clinical conditions are associated with asthma (Table 13.27). *Allergic bronchopulmonary aspergillosis* and other eosinophilic syndromes are discussed on page 484.

Investigation

X-ray findings

Most asthmatics have normal or hyperinflated lungs on chest X-ray. Mucus plugs can cause focal or segmental atelectasis, and sometimes collapse of a lobe or lung. Transient infiltrates are seen in association with eosinophilia. Spontaneous pneumothorax can complicate asthma in the acute phase.

Other investigations

Blood eosinophilia is common; it is usually greater in atopic asthma. Skin prick tests to common allergens may occasionally reveal an unsuspected source of allergy.

Lung function tests may be normal between attacks. During episodes of asthma the PEFR, FEV_1 and FEV_1/VC ratio will be reduced and airways resistance increased.

In addition to airflow obstruction the patient with acute or chronic asthma will have laboratory evidence of *hyperinflation* with increased total lung capacity (TLC), residual volume (RV), and ratio of RV to TLC. The *transfer factor* (diffusing capacity) for carbon monoxide is normal or increased in uncomplicated asthma. Hypoxaemia is common.

Diagnosis and management

The four principles of diagnosis and management of asthma are:

- recognition
- supervision
- education
- treatment.

13 Respiratory Disease

Recognition of asthma is not always straightforward. It is often not recognised in children who present with episodes of cough, wheeze and dyspnoea. Such 'wheezy bronchitis' in childhood is almost always asthma. The differential diagnosis of chronic asthma includes: 'asthmatic' bronchitis, left heart failure, centrally obstructing tumour or foreign body and recurrent pulmonary emboli. It may be difficult or impossible to distinguish late-onset asthma from chronic obstructive bronchitis in the elderly smoker. Many of them respond well to bronchodilators and have a better prognosis than patients with fixed airways obstruction.

Supervision of chronic asthma is as important as in any serious chronic condition. Some hospitals run a very effective 'open door' policy for asthmatics, allowing them to obtain immediate specialist advice whenever their asthma is severe.

Education about the nature of the disease, the use of drugs and delivery systems, the avoidance of allergens and the recognition of deteriorating asthma are all important. Asthma can seldom be 'cured'. Long-term therapy is usually required, for prophylaxis or control, and it is critically important that this simple truth is appreciated by both the patient and the physician.

Treatment

Treatment regimes (Table 13.28) can be broadly classified as *long-term prophylactic treatment* and *treatment of exacerbations and acute severe asthma*.

Hyposensitisation therapy (desensitisation immunotherapy) is discouraged in the UK but widely practised throughout the world despite little evidence of efficacy.

Drugs of proven benefit

Sympathomimetics

Beta agonists exert their action by stimulating the enzyme adenyl cyclase which catalyses the formation of cyclic-AMP within the bronchial smooth muscle cell. All available β_2 agonists can be given by inhalation, which is the preferred route, and some by oral, i.v. and subcutaneous administration. Salbutamol and terbutaline are the two most commonly prescribed. Salbutamol is available in a metered dose inhaler (100 μg per dose), as a dry powder for inhalation ('Rotacap') for patients whose co-ordination is poor or for children, and as tablets, slow-release tablets, i.v. injection, a nebuliser solution and a syrup. Terbutaline is available in similar forms. Inhaler spacer devices can improve drug inhalation efficiency in patients unable to manage a conventional inhaler. With both drugs, muscle tremor and tachycardia commonly occur, but tend to settle with prolonged usage.

Longer acting β_2 agonists (e.g. salmeterol) have recently been introduced.

Methyl xanthine derivatives (aminophylline and theophylline)

Oral use is preferred in routine treatment and intravenous use for acute asthma. When used in a daily dose of 10 mg/kg body weight, divided doses of slow-release theophyllines are effective and safe bronchodilators. These sustained-release formulations are useful when given at night for the prevention of nocturnal asthma and 'morning tightness'. The therapeutic serum theophylline concentration is 10–20 mg/1. If excessive doses are given, or occasionally even when blood levels are in the therapeutic range, side-effects may occur. These include nausea, abdominal pain, headache, tremor, insomnia and palpitations, convulsions and cardiac arrhythmia. The dose administered should be reduced in elderly patients, those with liver disease, and those taking other drugs that increase theophylline blood levels (e.g. erythromycin).

Anticholinergics

Anticholinergic agents have proved to be of some value, particularly in older patients with late-onset asthma or 'asthmatic bronchitis'. Atropine can be delivered by inhalation in its methonitrate form from a nebuliser, although it is more convenient to administer the newer anticholinergics, ipratropium and oxitropium, as a metered-dose aerosol. For patients optimally treated with inhaled β_2 agonists the additional benefit of anticholinergic drugs is seldom important.

Disodium cromoglycate

It has been suggested (but it is by no means certain) that cromoglycate acts by 'stabilising' the mast cell and preventing mediator release. It is only effective when used on a regular prophylactic basis and it has no intrinsic bronchodilator activity. Younger extrinsic asthmatics tend to benefit most from its regular use and it can also be used to 'block' exercise-induced asthma when administered about 20 minutes before planned exertion. It is administered in the form of 'spincaps' which deliver a dry powder for inhalation, and a metered-dose inhaler is also available. Useful nasal and ophthalmic preparations are available for the treatment of hay fever. The drug has no

Table 13.28 Treatment of asthma

Proven benefit	Dubious benefit	Potential benefit
Sympathomimetics	Antihistamines	Calcium antagonists
Theophylline, aminophylline	Expectorants	Prostaglandin
Anticholinergics	Cough suppressants	analogues/antagonists
Disodium cromoglycate	Mucolytics	Leukotriene
Corticosteroids	Hyposensitisation	antagonists

serious side-effects. Nedocromil sodium is a recent, similar, preparation.

Corticosteroids

Corticosteroids, probably by their anti-inflammatory action, are the most powerful drugs available for the treatment of asthma. Attitudes towards, and use of, corticocosteroids for the long-term management of asthma have been dramatically changed by the introduction of powerful, topically active fluorinated corticosteroids for use by the inhaled route. Beclomethasone diproprionate and budesonide are most often prescribed. They enable asthmatics to be treated with low-dose inhaled corticosteroids, which are not absorbed in sufficient quantities to cause adrenal suppression or iatrogenic Cushing's syndrome, and are highly effective when used on a regular basis in the prophylaxis of asthma. However, high doses of inhaled steroids for prolonged periods can cause side-effects, including osteoporosis. In some patients inhaled steroids predispose to oral candida infection but this can usually be easily controlled.

If long-term oral corticosteroids are essential for the control of asthma, patients should also be on maximum doses of inhaled steroids, thereby permitting the oral prednisolone dosage to be reduced by as much as 10 mg daily.

Nebuliser therapy

Nebulisers can deliver β_2 agonists, anti-cholinergic drugs and, occasionally, corticosteroids to the airways. They are increasingly used at home by patients with chronic airflow obstruction, but, in view of the large doses of drug used (particularly β agonists), such treatment requires careful assessment and supervision. It is important to document that nebulised bronchodilators confer a genuine advantage over *maximal* treatment with metered dose inhalers.

Summary of routine treatment of asthma

Figure 13.31 illustrates the treatment strategy for asthma. Oral steroids are prescribed only when maximum therapy with all other drugs fails to control the disease. Selected patients with severe chronic asthma may be helped by immunosuppressive therapy (e.g. methotrexate).

Treatment of acute severe asthma

The patient with acute severe asthma is distressed, dyspnoeic and using accessory respiratory muscles; there are widespread inspiratory and expiratory wheezes and the chest is hyperinflated. When airways obstruction and bronchial plugging is severe and widespread, the flow of

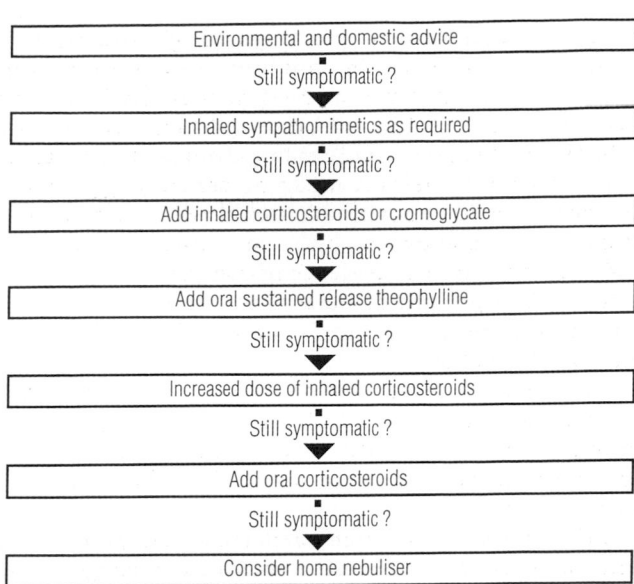

Fig. 13.31 Treatment strategy in asthma. Note the central importance of inhaled steroids in the treatment of moderate or severe asthma. Treatments are usually added, not substituted, as disease severity increases.

air through bronchi is greatly decreased, and wheezing becomes less obvious, eventually resulting in the ominous 'silent chest' of advanced acute severe asthma. As the condition progresses, cyanosis, dehydration, exhaustion and ventilatory failure ensue. Indices of the severity of acute asthma are listed in Table 13.29. In the accident and emergency department PEFR, heart rate and pulsus paradoxus (p. 453) are all related to asthma severity and should be documented with particular care. Arterial blood gas tensions should be measured in all patients whose asthma is sufficiently severe to require hospital assessment.

Acute asthma requires immediate evaluation and treatment. Oxygen is necessary, and in almost all circumstances can be liberally administered without fear of CO_2 narcosis. Salbutamol solution in a dose of 2.5–5.0 mg can be given via a nebuliser and is usually very effective. This

Table 13.29 Indications of severe asthma

Low PEFR (<150 l/min, poor bronchodilator response)
Associated with (one or more of):
Vigorous accessory muscle activity
Heart rate greater than 130
Pulsus paradoxus
Arterial P_{O_2} less than 8 kPa (60 mmHg)
Arterial P_{CO_2} greater than 5.5 kPa (41 mmHg)
Gross over-inflation (X-ray)
Central cyanosis
Disturbances of consciousness
ECG abnormalities
Pneumothorax/pneumomediastinum

can be repeated 3–6-hourly as required. Alternatively (or in very severe episodes, in addition), aminophylline is given in a dose of 5 mg/kg body weight intravenously over 20 minutes, to be followed by an infusion of 0.5 mg/kg per hour. In patients already taking theophyllines an infusion of aminophylline (0.5 mg/kg per hour) can be started and the blood theophylline level checked. The dose of aminophylline is reduced if the patient is more than 55 years old, or if there is evidence of liver disease or cardiac failure. A theophylline blood level should be measured 18 hours after starting the infusion and the dose adjusted to remain within the therapeutic range of 10–20 mg/l. If there are problems with venous access, subcutaneous terbutaline (0.25–0.5 mg) is helpful.

Systemic corticosteroids must be given to all patients whose asthma is of sufficient severity to warrant hospital admission, and also many less severe cases satisfactorily controlled in the emergency department. It is probably immaterial how corticosteroids are given; it may be as an i.v. bolus of hydrocortisone 3–6 mg/kg body weight followed by an infusion of 3–6 mg/kg 6-hourly, or alternatively 60 mg of oral prednisolone for the average-sized adult.

Supportive measures are also important. Patients with acute asthma become dehydrated. Physiotherapy is not helpful. Reassurance helps, but the best reassurance is improvement of the asthma. Sedatives should *never* be used unless intubation and mechanical ventilation are being contemplated. Antibiotics are prescribed if there is evidence of bacterial infection.

Some patients fail to respond to treatment and become progressively more hypoxic. At the onset of an asthma attack patients hyperventilate and therefore have an acute respiratory alkalosis. As airways obstruction increases, exhaustion supervenes, ventilatory pump failure occurs, alveolar ventilation diminishes, CO_2 rises and pH falls, leading to an acute respiratory acidosis. At this point the patient may require intubation and mechanical ventilation.

Small tidal volumes should be used, and most asthmatics who need mechanical ventilation will need at least 48 hours on the ventilator to allow their asthma to respond to therapy. Bronchodilator and steroid therapy should be continued while the patient is being ventilated.

Prognosis

About 50% of children 'grow out of' their asthma in early adult life. Late-onset asthma is almost always chronic, tends to be more severe, and usually needs more aggressive, treatment. About 30% of asthma deaths occur within 2 hours of the onset of the acute attack and these may be difficult to prevent. However, many of the remaining 70% of the 2000 deaths that occur annually in the UK should be preventable, by appropriate long-term therapy and the early recognition of deteriorating asthma.

ALLERGIC RHINITIS

Allergic rhinitis (commonly known as 'hay fever', although it is not related to hay and there is no fever) is a condition characterised by rhinorrhoea, nasal obstruction, sneezing, conjunctivitis, lacrimation, and nasal and pharyngeal itching. It is usually seasonal, with tree pollens being the allergen in the spring months and grass pollen in the summer. A perennial form occurs in those patients sensitive to allergens such as house dust, which are in the air all year round. Food allergy is an often quoted but clinically rare cause of rhinitis.

Pathologically the mucosa of the nose is oedematous and inflamed, and the secretions are rich in eosinophils. Nasal polyps and sinus infection may be present, especially in the perennial type. The conjunctivae are congested and oedematous. The diagnosis is made by taking a careful history. Skin prick testing for a battery of common allergens is helpful. Serum IgE is usually elevated, and occasionally a radio-allergo-immunosorbent test will help to define the allergen. The major differential diagnosis is from vasomotor rhinitis, which is a similar syndrome but with no documented allergic basis. Other conditions which may present in a similar fashion include exposure to irritants and repeated upper respiratory tract infections.

Management

Although the symptoms of allergic rhinitis tend to get better as the subjects get older, they can, when active, be severe. Most of the relevant allergens are ubiquitous and therefore unavoidable. The first line of treatment is topical; nasal sprays or drops containing corticosteroids such as beclomethasone or budesonide, or disodium cromoglycate, are useful when used on a regular basis. Disodium cromoglycate eye drops are also helpful for the conjunctivitis. These drugs can be supplemented by a non-sedating anti-histamine by mouth, such as terfenadine or astemizole. The place of hyposensitisation is debatable, and is usually reserved for isolated grass pollen allergy. Hyposensitisation can be complicated by anaphylactic shock and should only be undertaken where resuscitation facilities are available. Occasionally a small dose of oral corticosteroids, e.g. prednisolone (10–15 mg/day), or one or two injections of a depot corticosteroid during the season may be necessary.

PULMONARY EOSINOPHILIA

Pulmonary eosinophilia may be defined as transient pulmonary infiltrates associated with an elevated blood eosinophil count. A cause can only be identified in some cases (Table 13.30). The blood eosinophil count is

Table 13.30 Classification of pulmonary eosinophilia

Known causes	Drugs and toxins
Fungal allergy	Sulphonamides (including
Aspergillus fumigatus	sulphasalazine)
Candida albicans	Nitrofurantoin
Stemphylium canugenosum	Sodium aminosalicylate
Dresclera lawaiiensis	Penicillin
Curvularia lunata	Tetracycline
Helminosporium	Chlorpropamide
	'Spanish toxic oil' syndrome
Helminthic infections	Inorganic chemicals (e.g. nickel)
Ascaris lumbricoides (Loeffler's	
syndrome)	Lymphangiography
Strongyloides	
Filaria ('tropical pulmonary	Blood transfusion
eosinophilia')	
Ankylostoma	

Unknown causes
Cryptogenic pulmonary eosinophilia
Allergic argiitis and granulomatosis (Churg-Strauss syndrome)

elevated above its normal upper level of 400/mm^3 and may in some circumstances be as high as 50 000/mm^3. The serum IgE level is usually elevated in those conditions with an identifiable cause, especially in the allergic mycoses. Asthma is almost always present in cases of allergic bronchopulmonary aspergillosis, occurs in about half the patients with cryptogenic pulmonary eosinophilia, and is unusual with helminth infections apart from filariasis.

Pathogenesis

The eosinophil has cytotoxic and anti-inflammatory properties. The cytotoxic properties act against parasites but may also damage host tissues. The pathological response to the various identifiable causes of pulmonary eosinophilia depends on the route by which they reach the lungs; if inhaled (e.g. allergic mycoses) the response is in the airways (bronchocentric), whereas if delivered to the lung via the pulmonary circulation the response is in the blood vessels (angiocentric).

Allergic bronchopulmonary mycoses

By far the commonest cause is allergic bronchopulmonary aspergillosis (ABPA). This is due to sensitivity to the ubiquitous fungus *Aspergillus fumigatus*. This fungus thrives in warm, wet conditions, and symptoms therefore tend to occur in the autumn. The bronchial tree provides an ideal environment for colonisation. When the fungus is inhaled there is an immediate hypersensitivity reaction with eosinophils drawn into the area. There may be several responses thereafter:

- a simple asthmatic reaction with an eosinophilia but no radiological change
- pulmonary eosinophilic infiltrates with consolidation and chest X-ray shadowing
- mucus impaction with distal collapse and progressive airway damage due to the release of tissue-damaging factors; this in time may lead to a characteristic proximal bronchiectasis and upper zone fibrosis, sometimes making it difficult to differentiate ABPA from old tuberculosis.

Clinically, ABPA presents, often in early adult life, as worsening asthma. The patient may complain of coughing up rubbery brown or green plugs, and exacerbations of asthma are often accompanied by fever and fleeting pulmonary infiltrates. Almost all patients have a positive immediate-type hypersensitivity to *Aspergillus fumigatus* on skin prick testing and about 90% have precipitating antibody.

Treatment with oral prednisolone (30–40 mg/day) leads to rapid symptomatic and radiological improvement; whether or not it affects the long-term outcome is uncertain. Physiotherapy and occasionally bronchoscopy help to remove troublesome plugs, and the asthma responds to conventional treatment, usually including inhaled steroid. Many patients require a small maintenance dose of oral prednisolone to prevent relapse.

Drugs and toxins

There are a wide variety of drugs and toxins which can cause a pulmonary eosinophilic syndrome (Table 13.30). The drug reaches the lung via the pulmonary circulation and sets up an allergic reaction in the vessel wall. There is frequently an associated skin reaction. Patients may present with a pneumonia-like illness, with dyspnoea, cough, fever and pleuritic pain, or as a pulmonary vasculitis. Rarely, if the subject is exposed over a prolonged period, a type of fibrosing alveolitis develops. Whatever the progression, fleeting chest X-ray shadows and blood eosinophilia will be present. Almost all cases improve if the offending agent is stopped and oral corticosteroids help speed recovery.

Helminthic infections

Some helminths (*Ascaris, Strongyloides, Toxocara*) are borne to the lungs via the circulation, where they are attacked by eosinophils. During this phase the patient may be febrile and have pulmonary infiltrates, and the dying parasite may initiate an allergic response and thus an asthmatic attack. Filarial infection (due to infection with *Wuchereria bancrofti*) may cause asthma and patients can also develop diffuse fibrosis and pulmonary hypertension. The chest X-ray in helminthic infections shows widespread nodular infiltrates which are at first transient but may become persistent. The diagnosis is confirmed by appropriate complement fixation tests and by finding ova in the stools (see also Ch. 11).

Unknown causes

There is a spectrum of conditions of unknown aetiology which cause fleeting eosinophilic infiltrates in the lung and a blood eosinophilia. Pathologically, these range from a localised or generalised pulmonary eosinophilia to eosinophilic syndromes with vasculitis and granuloma formation. Classification is difficult; the most important distinction is between the clinical syndrome of cryptogenic pulmonary eosinophilia and those syndromes associated with vasculitis and granuloma formation.

Cryptogenic pulmonary eosinophilia (eosinophilic pneumonia)

Cryptogenic pulmonary eosinophilia is a syndrome of fever, weight loss, cough and breathlessness with widespread, mainly peripheral, pulmonary infiltrates (Fig. 13.32) and a marked blood eosinophilia. The patients are usually non-atopic but 10% have previous asthma. No cause can be identified. Some patients progress to the vasculitic/granulomatous type of disease. There is a rapid response to oral corticosteroids; treatment should be carefully tailed off as recurrences are

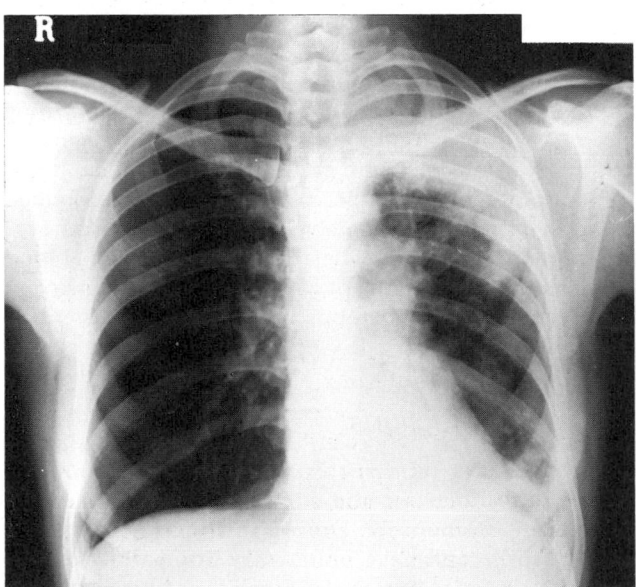

Fig. 13.32 Pulmonary eosinophilia. Extensive, ill-defined peripheral consolidation in the left upper zone and less marked consolidation in the left lower zone in a patient with cryptogenic pulmonary eosinophilia. Characteristically, new shadows appear and previous ones spontaneously resolve.

common, and usually corticosteroid treatment for up to 2 years is required.

Allergic angiitis and granulomatosis

This is a rare group of conditions in which asthmatic patients present with symptoms similar to cryptogenic pulmonary eosinophilia. Radiologically, they may show extensive transient pulmonary infiltrates, nodules, cavities and occasionally pleural and pericardial effusions. There is a blood eosinophilia and a raised erythrocyte sedimentation rate (ESR). Lung biopsy shows a vasculitis and if there is an allergic granulomatous reaction this is known as the *Churg-Strauss syndrome*, although there is probably a broad spectrum of pathological overlap in these syndromes. In many ways the syndrome is similar to polyarteritis nodosa, although lung involvement in typical polyarteritis nodosa is rare. Other organs such as liver, spleen, heart, skin and central nervous system may be affected by the vasculitis but, unlike polyarteritis nodosa, renal involvement is uncommon. Treatment with prednisolone in high doses, with or without azathioprine or cyclophosphamide, significantly reduces mortality although infective or cardiac complications may still be fatal.

CHRONIC BRONCHITIS AND EMPHYSEMA

Chronic bronchitis

Chronic bronchitis is a clinical diagnosis in which there is cough productive of sputum on most days for 3 months of the year for 2 or more years, which is not due to a specific respiratory disease such as bronchiectasis. The disorder is characterised by excess mucus secretion. Pathologically there is hyperplasia and hypertrophy of the tracheal and bronchial mucus glands and an increase in the glandular elements of the bronchial wall. The increase in intraluminal mucus and thickening of the bronchial wall produces airways narrowing and increased airways resistance, the fall in FEV_1 correlating with the increase in mucous membrane thickness.

Emphysema

Emphysema is defined by its pathology and is characterised by destruction of respiratory tissue and permanent enlargement of the unit of the lung distal to the terminal bronchiole (the acinus). Lung destruction causes loss of alveolar capillary bed and elastic recoil.

In the past much importance has been placed on the distinction between chronic bronchitis and emphysema. In the majority of patients both conditions co-exist, usually in heavy cigarette smokers, and the physician therefore makes a clinical diagnosis of chronic bronchitis *and* emphysema.

Aetiology and prevalence

Chronic bronchitis and emphysema are responsible for the personal disability and misery of tens of thousands of patients and impose a huge social and economic burden on society. Respiratory disorders are an important cause of death in the UK and of these chronic bronchitis and emphysema constitute a large proportion (p. 14). In the UK 10% of absence from work is caused by chronic bronchitis and emphysema and approximately 10% of occupancy of acute general medical hospital beds is the result of these diseases.

Atmospheric pollution and occupational dust exposure are minor aetiological factors in chronic bronchitis and the dominant causal agent is cigarette smoke. Smoking also causes emphysema, probably damaging the lung by the release of proteolytic enzymes. Smoke-affected pulmonary alveolar macrophages, present in greater numbers than usual, release neutrophil chemotactic factor and the attracted neutrophils are damaged by smoke and release proteolytic enzymes, especially elastase, capable of lysing elastin, collagen and basement membranes. The effectiveness of α_1-antitrypsin is impaired by smoking and the unchecked proteolysis results in centrilobular emphysema. This process is particularly rapid in patients who are deficient in α_1-antitrypsin.

Alpha$_1$-antitrypsin deficiency

This genetic disorder affects one in 5000 people, is equally common in men and women, and predisposes to the early development of emphysema often before the age of 40. The emphysema is panlobular and basal (Fig. 13.14) and lung destruction is accelerated by cigarette smoke. Non-smoking heterozygotes do not have emphysema but it is possible that smoking heterozygotes develop emphysema more readily than smoking normals. The feasibility and clinical value of α_1-antitrypsin replacement therapy is under investigation. Some patients with advanced disease have been managed by lung transplantation.

Mechanism of airflow obstruction

In chronic bronchitis and emphysema the fundamental cause of reduced ventilatory capacity and breathlessness is the limitation of expiratory airflow (p. 447). Secondary to expiratory limitation, residual volume is increased, the thorax is hyperinflated and inspiratory capacity is markedly impaired, in part due to the compromised function of the inspiratory muscles. In chronic bronchitis airways resistance is increased and expiratory airflow reduced by the thickening of the bronchial wall and

excessive intraluminal mucus. In emphysema a more important mechanism is the narrowing and collapse of airways during expiration as a consequence of loss of the lung elastic recoil which normally keeps airways open.

Clinical features

Chronic bronchitis and emphysema develop over many years and patients are rarely symptomatic before middle age. Symptoms are initially minor, perhaps a morning cough productive of a little sputum. In some patients chronic bronchitis can remain a trivial problem but in many, smoking-related airways obstruction co-exists and the patients then develop breathlessness. Initially breathlessness is on exertion but exercise capacity progressively and slowly deteriorates and eventually patients become respiratory cripples distressed by dyspnoea even at rest. Patients with predominant bronchitis are prone to periodic infections. Often the infective process remains confined to the bronchial tree but sometimes infection involves the surrounding lung with consequent pneumonia; thus, although some patients may have radiological changes of pneumonia in association with an infective exacerbation, the majority show no change on chest X-ray. Eventually patients with chronic bronchitis develop severe hypoxaemia, hypercapnia and peripheral oedema–cor pulmonale (the so-called '*blue bloater*'). Patients with substantial emphysema tend to be very breathless, ventilating sufficiently to maintain normal arterial carbon dioxide and near-normal oxygen tensions. The development of cor pulmonale is a late and terminal event in these '*pink puffers*'. These two clinical extremes overlap; many patients with a normal arterial carbon dioxide tension eventually become cyanosed, but the broad clinical distinction between the 'pink puffer' and the 'blue bloater' is useful. Oxygen therapy is much more difficult in the hypercapnic blue and bloated patient, sedation is more hazardous, and general anaesthesia poses greater risks due to postoperative sputum retention and difficulty in weaning such patients from assisted ventilation. Some patients have bronchial hyper-reactivity and exposure to cold air, acute temperature changes, dusts and cigarette smoke causes increasing breathlessness, respiratory distress and wheeze.

The development of cor pulmonale indicates a poor prognosis with a 30% 5-year survival. In association with severe hypoxia and hypercapnia, pulmonary arterial hypertension develops and some patients also have an elevated jugular venous pressure. However, in many patients cor pulmonale is not simple cardiac failure since cardiac output is frequently normal and there can be peripheral oedema without elevation of the jugular venous pressure. The mechanism of cor pulmonale remains obscure but in part it reflects an increase in blood volume perhaps due to hypercapnia and hypoxia causing sodium retention by the kidney. Cor pulmonale is unusual in the absence of hypercapnia. There is evidence that optimum therapy and careful follow-up of patients with cor pulmonale can produce good results.

Physical signs

In predominantly emphysematous patients, inspiratory airways resistance is not increased and inspiration is therefore quiet, whereas patients with predominantly chronic bronchitis have noisy breathing. To control airways collapse on expiration, patients with emphysema apply a positive pressure to the bronchial tree by the technique of purse-lipped breathing. As the diseases progress the physical signs may eventually include those of severe airways obstruction, hypoxia, hypercapnia and cor pulmonale. Patients with chronic airflow limitation often have early inspiratory crackles which can be heard at the patient's mouth by the examining physician. Weight loss is common with advanced emphysema.

Patients with emphysema have translucent lungs on the chest X-ray with few vascular markings, and bullae may also be present (Fig. 13.33). Patients with predominantly chronic bronchitis may show bronchial wall thickening. Hyperinflation is more severe in emphysema.

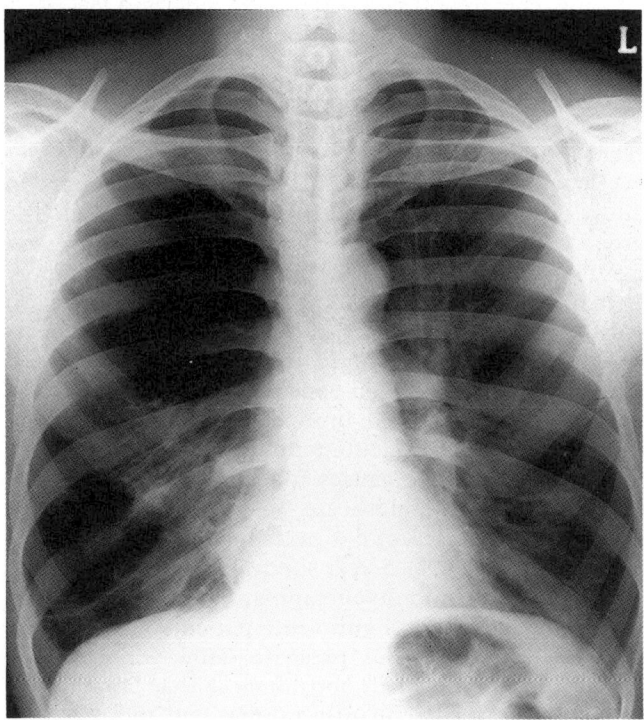

Fig. 13.33 Bullous emphysema. The large bullae (right upper zone, right lower zone peripherally) display no vascular markings. Elsewhere the lung markings appear obvious, partly due to increased blood flow through relatively normal lung and partly because bullae compress adjacent lung tissue.

Commonly, radiological abnormality is most striking in the upper zones but in α_1-antitrypsin deficiency disease is predominantly basal.

Respiratory function

In patients with chronic bronchitis and emphysema the FEV_1 is reduced and the $FEV_1/VC\%$ is low, indicating expiratory flow limitation (p. 447). VC for a relaxed manoeuvre is usually greater than for a forced effort. The PEFR, although low, is a less sensitive measure of the severity of airways obstruction. Hyperinflation is confirmed by the increase in RV and TLC. Gas transfer is more dramatically reduced in the 'pink puffer' with a substantial element of emphysema. In the 'blue bloater' there is severe hypoxaemia, hypercapnia and secondary polycythaemia.

Management

Restoration of normal function is not possible in chronic bronchitis and emphysema. The aim of therapy must therefore be to reduce disability by tackling the interrelated problems of airways obstruction, recurrent infections, breathlessness, hypoxia and poor exercise tolerance. Factors aggravating chronic bronchitis, particularly cigarette smoking, must be withdrawn.

Airways obstruction

Conventionally the airways obstruction of chronic bronchitis and emphysema is regarded as being irreversible. However, the majority of patients show some improvement in lung function with therapy directed at relaxing bronchial smooth muscle and, although small, this improvement can have an important impact on the disability of these patients. Prognosis in patients who respond well to bronchodilators is considerably better than for those with completely fixed obstruction. The most important bronchodilator agents are the selective β_2 adrenergic agonists (e.g. salbutamol and terbutaline), which are best administered by inhalation. For some patients, maximal bronchodilatation requires a large drug dose and may be best administered by nebuliser (e.g. salbutamol 2.5–5 mg).

Inhaled atropine analogues (ipratropium bromide) can be helpful, but provided optimum doses of β_2 agonists are administered, ipratropium bromide confers little additional benefit.

Oral theophyllines available in slow-release formulation are of marginal usefulness in chronic bronchitis and emphysema. It has been claimed that theophylline improves respiratory muscle contractility but recent studies have not confirmed this effect.

Patients with severe airways obstruction should have a therapeutic trial of steroids – for example, oral prednisolone (30 mg daily) for a period of 2–3 weeks – provided there are no contra-indications. Long-term oral steroids will not be indicated in most patients, but when prescribed require regular assessment and dosage should seldom exceed 7.5–10 mg daily, thereby minimising drug complications. Mucolytic agents (e.g. bromhexine) are of unproven value in chronic bronchitis, but occasional patients report substantial benefits, and when sputum retention is a major problem, a therapeutic trial is justified.

Infection

In acute exacerbations of chronic bronchitis an infective viral or bacterial pathogen is isolated in less than 50% of cases. Viral infections are frequently complicated by bacterial overgrowth and the majority of patients develop purulent sputum. Severe exacerbations have a mortality of up to 25%, and prompt antibacterial therapy is of the greatest importance. Common infective organisms are *Strep. pneumoniae* and *H. influenzae*, and suitable antibiotics are amoxycillin, erythromycin, co-trimoxazole and the cephalosporins. For most patients long-term chemoprophylaxis is not helpful but if intermittent treatment fails, a trial of continuous rotating antibiotic therapy is appropriate.

Oxygen therapy

During acute exacerbation of chronic bronchitis and emphysema, oxygen therapy is necessary to avoid death from hypoxia. In patients with hypercapnia oxygen must be given at low and controlled concentrations (usually 24% or 28% O_2). A more contentious question is the value of long-term domiciliary oxygen therapy. Studies suggest that long-term controlled oxygen therapy can benefit patients with severe airways obstruction who have severe hypoxia and who refrain from smoking cigarettes. It is necessary to administer oxygen virtually continuously, including during sleep (Fig. 13.34).

The administration of continuous oxygen presents considerable practical and financial difficulties. Oxygen may be supplied in cylinders, as liquid oxygen or, preferably, generated by an oxygen concentrator. This therapy should be reserved for patients with severe disease who are well motivated. Oxygen therapy requires careful pretreatment assessment and long-term supervision.

In practice much oxygen used by patients in their homes is for a few minutes only and the main purpose is to relieve breathlessness. Oxygen is also available in small portable cylinders and some patients find this helpful in reducing breathlessness on exercise, improving exercise capacity, and permitting excursions from the home. Many

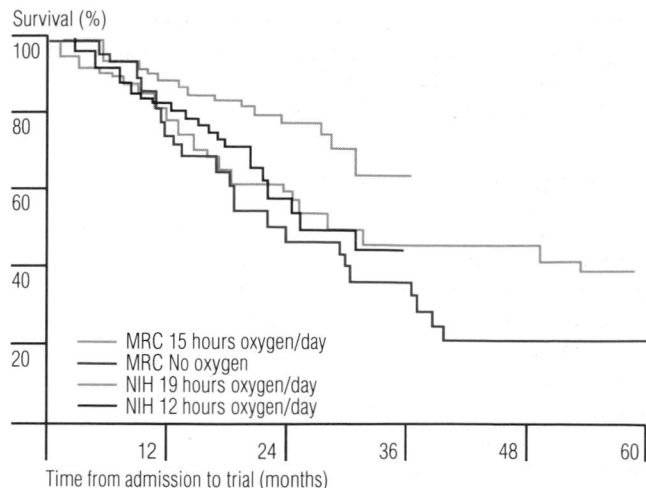

Fig. 13.34 Long-term domiciliary oxygen therapy. Effect of therapy on survival in patients with severe respiratory failure, due to chronic bronchitis and emphysema (MRC = Medical Research Council; NIH = National Institutes of Health, USA).

different techniques of delivering oxygen, including transtracheal catheters, are under evaluation.

Patients with severe chronic bronchitis and associated hypoxia, hypercapnia, pulmonary hypertension and cor pulmonale have profound nocturnal hypoxaemia (Fig. 13.35). This hypoxaemia is much more a feature of the 'blue bloater' than the 'pink puffer'. Much of the hypoxia is caused by hypoventilation and irregular breathing patterns during rapid eye movement (REM)

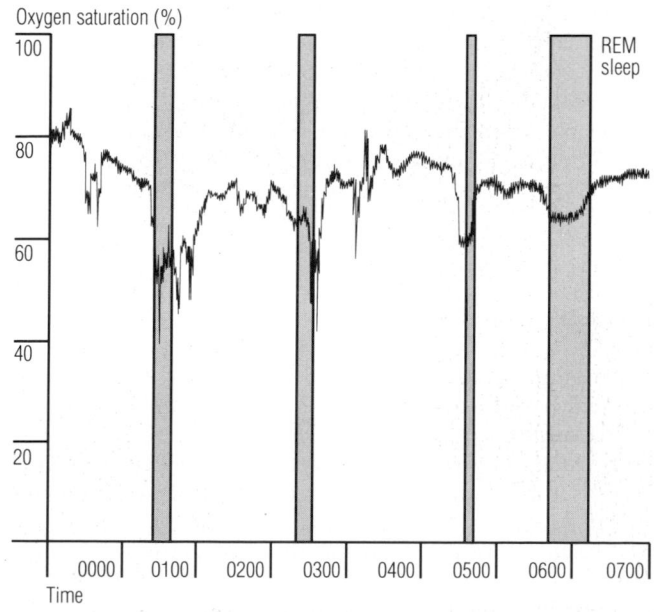

Fig. 13.35 Oxygen saturation during sleep in severe chronic bronchitis. Patients who are already hypoxic can markedly desaturate during sleep, particularly REM sleep (vertical bars).

sleep and is not due to obstructive sleep apnoea (p. 491). Oxygen therapy during the night (2 l/min by nasal cannulae) can alleviate hypoxaemia and make hypoxic periods less severe. The return of normal breathing patterns following REM sleep is impaired by sedatives and these should therefore be avoided in patients with chronic bronchitis. The non-sedative tricyclic drug protriptyline reduces time spent in REM sleep and can improve nocturnal hypoxaemia in some patients.

Drug therapy for breathlessness

In patients with airways obstruction it is the 'pink puffers' with normal CO_2 values and mild or moderate hypoxia who are most breathless. In some patients, reducing ventilation with diazepam, promethazine and dihydrocodeine can reduce breathlessness and in patients without carbon dioxide retention a careful trial of such therapy is justified when symptoms are severe. For the devastating dyspnoea which is frequently a feature of terminal respiratory failure, diamorphine is helpful whatever the cause.

Secondary polycythaemia

Polycythaemia produces symptoms attributable to hyperviscosity, including somnolence, lethargy, poor concentration and headache. Venesection reduces these symptoms but does not affect lung function or blood gases. Venesection also improves cerebral blood flow, pulmonary hypertension and exercise tolerance. Patients with a haematocrit of 0.60 or greater should benefit and the haematocrit should be reduced to 0.50. This can be achieved either by simple venesection, exchange transfusion with dextran or plasma, or erythropheresis. Continuous oxygen therapy for 6 weeks will also reduce the haematocrit. Whenever possible the first-line therapy for secondary polycythaemia is to improve lung function.

Chest physiotherapy

There have been few scientific studies of the long-term effect of chest physiotherapy techniques aimed at improving breathing patterns in patients with chronic bronchitis and emphysema; no benefit has been proven.

Postural drainage is of undoubted benefit in patients with excessive bronchial secretions. Its effectiveness is increased by coughing or forced expiratory manoeuvres ('huffs'). Postural drainage has little place if patients do not have sputum. Vigorous physiotherapy, especially forced expiratory manoeuvres, can increase bronchoconstriction in asthma.

During acute exacerbations of bronchitis and pneumonia several studies have, rather surprisingly, shown no benefit from physiotherapy. In the absence of excessive secretions physiotherapy is not justified in these patients. Mucociliary clearance is decreased and basal collapse is more common following general anaesthesia and surgery, particularly of the upper abdomen. The case for routine preoperative physiotherapy in chronic bronchitis patients is, however, not proven except for very high risk patients.

Assisted ventilation in chronic bronchitis

Patients with severe progressive chronic bronchitis and emphysema eventually die of intractable ventilatory failure, having been breathless at rest and confined to their homes in the months before death. The poor quality of life precludes such patients from being treated with mechanical ventilation to delay the inevitable outcome. Difficult decisions are posed by the less severely disabled, who require mechanical ventilation if they are not to die during an acute exacerbation of bronchitis. Many of these patients are difficult to wean from ventilation, particularly those with pre-existing hypercapnia and blunted ventilatory response to CO_2. Before embarking on mechanical ventilation, every effort must be made to establish the background severity of respiratory disability, exercise tolerance and quality of life. For selected patients, non-invasive nasal positive pressure ventilation is useful (p. 534).

Cessation of cigarette smoking

Tobacco smoke damages the bronchial tree and produces airflow limitation by a number of different actions. Smoke impairs mucociliary clearance and causes bronchial smooth muscle to contract by stimulating receptors and provoking the release of inflammatory mediators. In addition, smoke increases mucus production and causes mucous gland hypertrophy. Smokers are predisposed to bronchial infection and consequent inflammation; the increase in elastase and the impairment of α_1-antitrypsin, as well as impaired surfactant production, contribute to emphysema. It is therefore not surprising that chronic bronchitis and emphysema are found in 15% of middle-aged males who smoke moderately or heavily but are rare in non-smokers, and that deaths from bronchitis increase with the amount smoked.

If patients with chronic bronchitis and emphysema stop smoking, the rate of decline in pulmonary function is reduced to that of non-smokers (Fig. 13.36). Indeed, if patients stop smoking early in their disease there is improvement in pulmonary function. However severe the disease, stopping smoking will reduce cough.

Patients with chronic bronchitis and emphysema have smoked for many years and have great difficulty in abstaining. Stopping smoking is particularly difficult if a spouse or cohabitant smokes. In patients who are determined to stop smoking, nicotine replacement therapy can

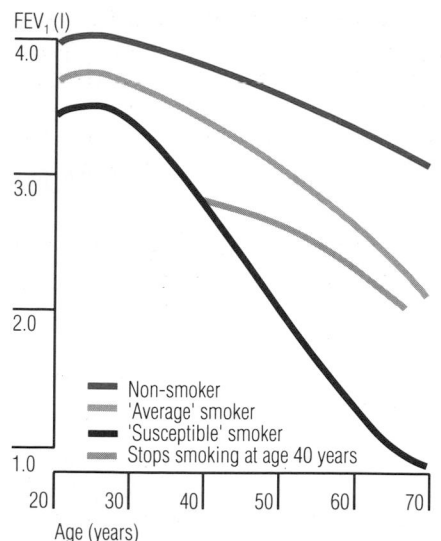

Fig. 13.36 Airflow limitation and smoking. FEV_1 declines with age. In smokers this decline is more marked, particularly in 'susceptible' smokers. Such patients, therefore, become breathless in middle or old age. When smokers stop the habit, the rate of decline in FEV_1 is markedly slowed. (From Fletcher C M Peto R 1977 The British Medical Journal Vol 1 p.1645)

be helpful, but in general the firm advice of the patient's physician (and other medical staff) is as effective as any other measure and is most likely to work when the patient is unwell. Cigarette smokers who change to smoking a pipe or cigars inhale the smoke and this change is therefore not helpful. If patients are unable to stop smoking completely, they should smoke as few cigarettes as possible, move to low-tar brands, reduce the number of puffs, and smoke less of each cigarette.

RESPIRATION DURING SLEEP

SLEEP APNOEA SYNDROMES

Apnoea is defined as no gas flow at the nose or mouth for 10 seconds, and a sleep apnoea syndrome is diagnosed if more than 30 such episodes occur during the night. Apnoea may be central, when there is no airflow and no chest wall movement; obstructive, when there is no airflow despite chest wall movement because of upper airways obstruction; or the apnoea may result from both mechanisms.

Obstructive sleep apnoea

Obstructive sleep apnoea is more common than central apnoea, perhaps occurring to some degree in up to 1% of the adult male population. The typical features are hyper-

Summary 6 Features of obstructive sleep apnoea

- Snoring
- Disturbed sleep
- Witnessed apnoeas
- Cardiac arrhythmias
- Excessive daytime sleepiness
- Morning headache
- Intellectual deterioration
- Systemic hypertension
- Pulmonary hypertension
- Right heart failure
- Obesity
- Small oropharynx

somnolence by day and upper airways obstruction during sleep. Many, but not all, patients are obese and have thick necks; hypertension is common. In severe cases there is chronic alveolar hypoventilation at night, daytime hypoxia, secondary polycythaemia and cor pulmonale. Patients often have loud, persistent snoring, and the frequent arousals from apnoeic episodes greatly disturb sleep (although the patient may be unaware of this). Patients fall asleep by day and may have road and other accidents. There is difficulty in concentrating, particularly in the morning, intellectual impairment, personality change and irritability. Abnormal limb and body movements during arousals following apnoea (thrashing around in bed), sexual dysfunction and morning headaches are important features. During apnoea there are cardiovascular disturbances, particularly bradycardia.

In many patients the upper airway is abnormally narrow (e.g. hypertrophy of tonsils and adenoids), but in some cases no anatomical abnormality is found. However, during obstruction the posterior and lateral walls of the pharynx collapse, occluding the oropharynx. The collapse of the upper airway is probably due to a failure to activate the upper airway musculature sufficiently during inspiration, and the negative pressures generated in the upper airway by the contraction of the respiratory muscles suck in the soft tissues of the oropharynx (Fig. 13.37). This negative pressure will be greater if the upper airway is narrowed, and nasal obstruction can be a contributory factor.

Central sleep apnoea

In central apnoea, the patients snore less, are seldom obese, and complain of night-time wakening. The central drive to breathing is abnormal and inspiration may fail to be initiated. The syndrome may be primary or secondary to organic lesions of the brainstem..

To document sleep apnoea, to determine whether it is central or obstructive and to assess the severity of nocturnal hypoxaemia, a formal sleep study in a specialist laboratory is required (Fig. 13.38). In patients with obvious obstructive sleep apnoea the assessment of

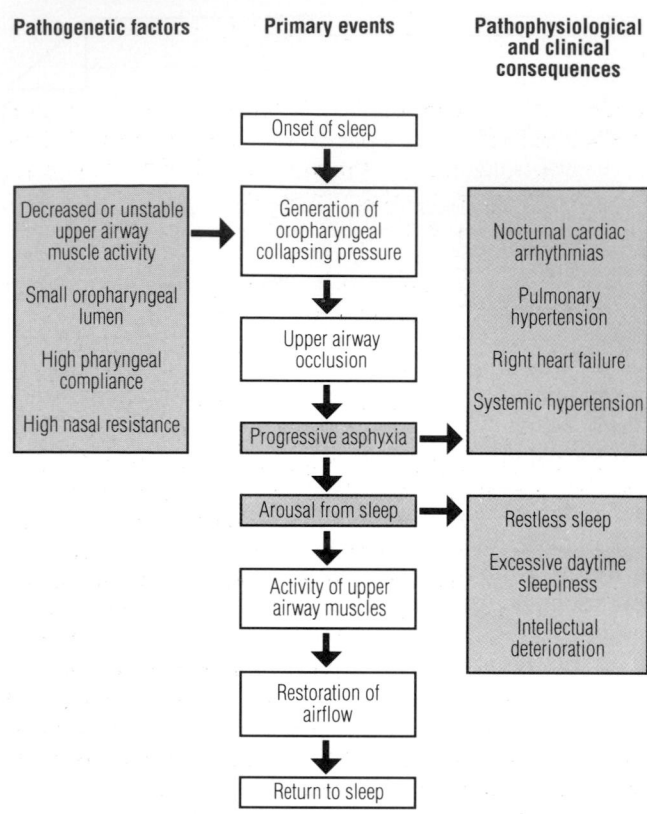

Fig. 13.37 **The mechanism of obstructive sleep apnoea (OSA).** In severe cases, since sleep stops ventilation, sleep is grossly disturbed and daytime somnolence is very striking. (From Strading J R and Philipson E A 1986 Breathing disorders during sleep. Q J Med (New Series) 58: 3–18.)

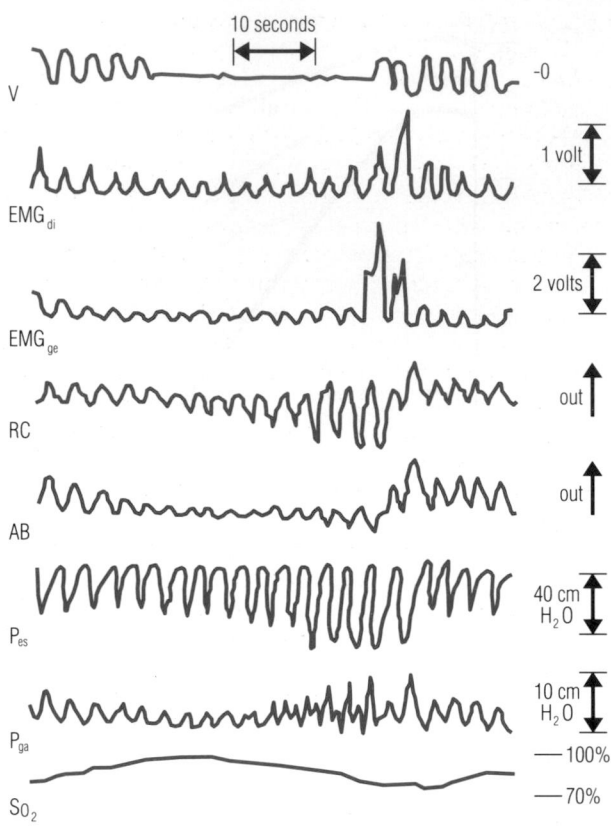

Fig. 13.38 **Sleep study in obstructive sleep apnoea.** The record shows a period when ventilation is obstructed and there is no airflow (V). At this time the diaphragm continues to contract (EMG_{di}); oesophageal (P_{es}) and gastric (P_{ga}) pressure swings occur, and there is ribcage and abdominal movement (RC and AB). As obstruction continues arterial oxygen saturation (So_2) falls. Eventually the activity of the upper airway muscles, including genioglossus (EMG_{ge}), increases, the upper airway becomes patent, and airflow is restored. Patients can have hundreds of similar episodes during the night. (From Onal *et al.* 1982 Am Rev Respir Dis. 125: 167–74.)

nocturnal hypoxaemia by oximetry may be all that is necessary.

Sleep in other respiratory disorders

Patients with airways obstruction and hypercapnia may become profoundly hypoxic at night as a result of hypoventilation (Fig. 13.35) (p. 489). Nocturnal hypoxaemia is also a clinical problem in patients with advanced kyphoscoliosis or severe respiratory muscle weakness (p. 531).

Treatment of apnoea syndromes

In the management of obstructive sleep apnoea weight reduction is helpful but difficult to achieve. Tracheostomy is effective but presents management difficulties, and many patients are resistant to this line of therapy. Nasal continuous positive airway pressure (CPAP) is very effective and remarkably well tolerated, although the technique is rather cumbersome. Palatopharyngoplasty (PPP), surgical reconstruction of the pharynx, can also be effective, but the site of obstruction may not be relieved

in some patients and the long-term effects of surgery are not yet known. Drugs may sometimes be helpful, particularly protriptyline (a non-sedative tricyclic antidepressant); this reduces REM, during which, as a consequence of reduced activity of upper airways musculature, obstruction is most likely. For many patients, weight reduction and perhaps protriptyline are worthy of trial before considering CPAP or PPP. Troublesome snoring, without desaturation, can be treated by minor palatal surgery in selected cases.

RESPIRATORY FAILURE

Definition

There is no precise clinical definition of respiratory failure; the diagnosis rests on the interpretation of arterial blood gas measurements. A patient can be said to be in respiratory failure if the arterial oxygen tension (Pa_{O_2}) falls below 8.0 kPa/60 mmHg (normal range 11.3–13.3 kPa or 85–100 mmHg) or if the arterial carbon dioxide tension (Pa_{CO_2}) rises above 6.6 kPa/50 mmHg (normal range 4.6–6.0 kPa or 35–45 mmHg), when the subject is at sea level, awake and breathing air. The condition may be acute or chronic; if the patient has arterial hypoxaemia with a normal or low Pa_{CO_2} then he or she is said to have *type I* respiratory failure; and if the Pa_{CO_2} is elevated, *type II* respiratory failure. Arterial hypoxaemia does not always imply respiratory failure: a low inspired O_2 at altitude or an anatomical right-to-left shunt, as in congenital heart disease or arteriovenous malformation, can cause hypoxaemia despite normal lung function. The causes of types I and II respiratory failure are shown in Table 13.31. Chronic respiratory failure in the UK is most commonly due to chronic bronchitis and emphysema (p. 486).

Measurement of the alveolar–arterial (A–a) gradient is useful in hypoxic patients, and may help to decide, for instance, whether the patient's hypoxaemia is secondary to central hypoventilation or to intrinsic lung disease. The A–a gradient indicates the contribution of venous admixture (i.e. true shunt or $\dot{V}\dot{Q}$ abnormality) to hypoxaemia. It can be calculated by using the concept of 'ideal alveolar air' (Pa_{O_2}):

$$Pa_{O_2} = \frac{FiO_2 - Pa_{CO_2}}{0.8}$$

where FiO_2 = inspired P_{O_2} (20 kPa on room air) and 0.8 = respiratory exchange ratio. Thus the normal alveolar oxygen tension is approximately 14 kPa, the normal arterial oxygen tension approximately 12.5 kPa, and the normal A–a gradient is therefore 1–2 kPa (see Ch. 14, p. 541).

In the management of the hypoxic patient it should be remembered that tissue O_2 delivery depends not just on Pa_{O_2} but also on the haemoglobin concentration and cardiac output. The most useful index of tissue oxygenation is the mixed venous (pulmonary arterial)/arterial O_2 content difference. The normal oxygen combining capacity is 1.4 ml O_2/g haemoglobin (approximately 0.06 mmol/g). The oxygen content of blood is the oxygen combining capacity × haemoglobin concentration × saturation (plus a small amount of dissolved oxygen in plasma, which is negligible at normal atmospheric pressure). Assuming the haemoglobin concentration is 15 g/100 ml, and the oxygen content of arterial blood is 1.4 × 15 × 0.95 = 20.58 ml/100 ml, and the oxygen content of mixed venous blood is 1.4 × 15 × 0.75 = 15.75, the arterial/mixed venous oxygen content difference is 4.83 ml/100 ml. If oxygen delivery is reduced (e.g. reduced cardiac output) the arterial/venous content difference widens.

Type II hypercapnic ventilatory failure represents inadequacy of the respiratory muscle 'pump'. The concept of 'pump' failure leading to hypercapnia is a useful one, focusing attention on the importance of CNS output, neuromuscular function and chest wall movement in the maintenance of adequate ventilation (p. 530), although severe impairment of gas exchange can contribute to an elevated CO_2.

Clinical features

Acute hypoxaemia or hypercapnia is less well tolerated than chronic gradual alteration in blood gases. Virtually all patients with respiratory failure, with the exception of some patients with CNS dysfunction (e.g. drug overdose), are breathless. Acute hypoxaemia causes restlessness, confusion and sweating, with a tachycardia, poor peripheral perfusion and central cyanosis.

Patients with acute severe hypercapnic ventilatory failure are breathless and cyanosed, and in addition may have confusion, flapping tremor of the hands, warm peripheries, bounding pulse and occasionally papilloedema. The mental state is probably the best clinical index to follow, since increasing confusion and restlessness often parallel a rising Pa_{CO_2}. When patients (for instance, those with advanced chronic bronchitis) progress to severe chronic respiratory failure, with a compensated respiratory acidosis, symptoms may also include sleep distur-

Table 13.31 Causes of types I and II respiratory failure

Type I (hypoxaemic)
Acute asthma
Pulmonary oedema
Pneumonia
Pulmonary fibrosis
Chronic bronchitis
Emphysema
Pulmonary vascular disease
Miscellaneous: lymphangitis, radiation pneumonitis, etc.

Type II (ventilatory)

CNS	Thoracic cage and pleura
Trauma	Crushed chest
Cerebral tumour	Kyphoscoliosis
Raised intracranial pressure	Extensive thoracic surgery
Drugs	(thoracoplasty)
Hypoventilation syndromes	Ankylosing spondylitis (rare)
Neuromuscular	Lung and airways
Cervical cord lesion	Severe acute asthma, pneumonia
Guillain-Barré syndrome	Upper airway obstruction,
Motor neurone disease	including obstructive sleep
Poliomyelitis	apnoea
Muscular dystrophies and myopathies	Chronic airflow limitation: chronic
Botulism	bronchitis, emphysema,
Myasthenia gravis	bronchiectasis
Muscle relaxant drugs	
Organophosphorus poisoning	
Status epilepticus	

bance with early morning headache and personality change. Such patients develop polycythaemia, pulmonary hypertension and cor pulmonale.

Chronic hypercapnic respiratory failure can occur despite normal lung function. Sleep apnoea syndromes, for example (p. 491), may be severe enough to produce pulmonary hypertension and cor pulmonale. Patients with neuromuscular disorders (e.g. myasthenia gravis or the Guillain-Barré syndrome) may also have life-threatening ventilatory failure despite normal lungs (p. 530).

Management

Acute respiratory failure

The general principles for the management of acute respiratory failure are those of any other respiratory emergency. The airway should be kept clear of sputum and protected. Oxygen should be given in sufficient concentration to ensure a Pa_{O_2} of 8 kPa (60 mmHg). This can be delivered via a Venturi mask which will give a fixed inspired oxygen concentration of 24, 28 or 35%, or a Hudson or MC mask which will deliver variable, but higher, inspired oxygen concentrations. In practice it is difficult to administer more than 40% O_2 by conventional face masks. Higher concentrations can be given using a tight-fitting face mask; this also permits the application of continuous positive airway pressure (CPAP), which further increases Pa_{O_2}. If identifiable, the underlying cause should be treated: for example, antibiotics for acute bacterial pneumonias, or bronchodilators and corticosteroids for acute asthma. If the patient's condition is worsening, with deepening cyanosis, disturbance of consciousness, a rising Pa_{CO_2}, and progressive acidosis, then a decision to intubate and employ assisted mechanical ventilation must be made. This decision is based on a number of considerations, including the previous exercise capacity, the possibility of treating the underlying cause, the overall clinical state of the patient and serial arterial blood gas measurements.

Chronic respiratory failure

Patients with chronic respiratory disease who develop additional acute problems require a rather different pattern of management. Patients with long-standing hypoxaemia and hypercapnia are dependent on hypoxaemia to maintain ventilatory drive. High concentrations of inspired oxygen reduce respiratory drive and ventilation, resulting in a rise in Pa_{CO_2} and a worsening respiratory acidosis. Oxygen must therefore be given in a controlled fashion, starting with an inspired concentration of 24% and with repeated monitoring of arterial blood gases. It should be emphasised that it is not necessary to raise the Pa_{O_2} into the physiological range; a Pa_{O_2} of more than 6kPa (45

mmHg) is usually sufficient to maintain the patient in a reasonable clinical state. Although it is correct to exercise caution when administering oxygen to hypercapnic patients, it should be remembered that severe hypoxaemia, Pa_{O_2} less than 5 kPa (38 mmHg), is life-threatening and must be relieved, and hypoxaemic patients without CO_2 retention (a common situation in fibrotic lung disease, for example) can receive high inspired oxygen concentrations without developing hypercapnia.

If, with the proper use of oxygen supplements, the Pa_{CO_2} continues to rise, a respiratory stimulant, such as doxapram, may, in the short term, occasionally be helpful. This may allow the use of a higher inspired oxygen concentration without precipitating a rise in Pa_{CO_2}. However, some patients will continue to deteriorate and the point may come when a decision will have to be made about whether to offer assisted mechanical ventilation. In this group of patients, above all, their background in terms of respiratory function, exercise tolerance, and when they were last reasonably well, must be taken into consideration. Discussions should involve the patient's family and, very often, the patient.

For selected patients, many with chest wall disorder (e.g. kyphoscoliosis) and some with chronic bronchitis, the technique of non-invasive intermittent nasal positive pressure ventilation may obviate the need for intubation.

LUNG TRANSPLANTATION

Improvements in surgical technique, combined with the development of immunosuppressive therapy, has led to heart–lung, single lung, and double lung transplantation becoming established procedures in the management of selected patients with severe respiratory disease (Table 13.32). (Cardiac transplantation is discussed on p. 350.) In general, heart–lung transplantation is preferred for patients with diffuse bronchiectasis (e.g. cystic fibrosis) or pulmonary vascular disease; and single lung transplantation is best for patients with pulmonary fibrosis. Emphysema (usually due to α_1-antitrypsin deficiency) can be treated by heart–lung transplantation, but single or double lung transplantation may also be suc-

Table 13.32 Suitability for lung transplantation

- Severe and progressive disease (but not moribund) with a poor prognosis (less than 2 years)

- Age less than 50 years for heart–lung transplantation, less than 60 years for single lung transplantation

- No significant renal, hepatic or other progressive systemic disease (no significant coronary artery disease in patients undergoing lung transplantation)

- Psychologically stable

Table 13.33 Classification of pulmonary hypertension

Passive pulmonary hypertension	Increased pulmonary vascular resistance
Left heart failure	Vasoconstrictive
Mitral stenosis	e.g. response to hypoxia
LVF	
Hyperkinetic pulmonary hypertension	**Obstructive**
Increased pulmonary blood flow	Pulmonary emboli
ASD	Veno-occlusive disease
VSD	
Patent ductus	**Obliterative**
	Polyarteritis nodosa
	Systemic lupus erythematosus
	Systemic sclerosis
	Schistosomiasis
	Chronic bronchitis and emphysema
	Primary pulmonary hypertension

cessful. The prognosis following lung transplantation has improved and is now similar to cardiac transplantation, with a 50% 3-year survival. The availability of donor organs remains a major problem.

PULMONARY HYPERTENSION

The normal resting pulmonary artery pressure is approximately 25/8 mmHg; values greater than 30/15 mmHg indicate pulmonary hypertension (Table 13.33).

More than one factor may operate in any particular patient; for example, patients with ventricular septal defects have increased pulmonary blood flow but eventually develop secondary obstructive and obliterative changes.

Clinical features

Pulmonary hypertension eventually leads to right ventricular hypertrophy and failure, low cardiac output, syncope, fatigue and breathlessness. Physical signs include a prominent 'a' wave in the jugular venous pulse, right ventricular hypertrophy and a loud pulmonary sound. The ECG confirms right atrial and right ventricular hypertrophy. The chest X-ray shows large central pulmonary arteries. Patients may also have signs of the particular underlying cause of pulmonary hypertension (e.g. airways obstruction, Fig. 13.39).

The most important causes of pulmonary hypertension are listed in Table 13.34.

Pulmonary hypertension due to diffuse lung disease

Chronic bronchitis is the commonest cause of pulmonary hypertension, but it also occurs in severe tuberculosis, bronchiectasis, cystic fibrosis, cryptogenic fibrosing alve-

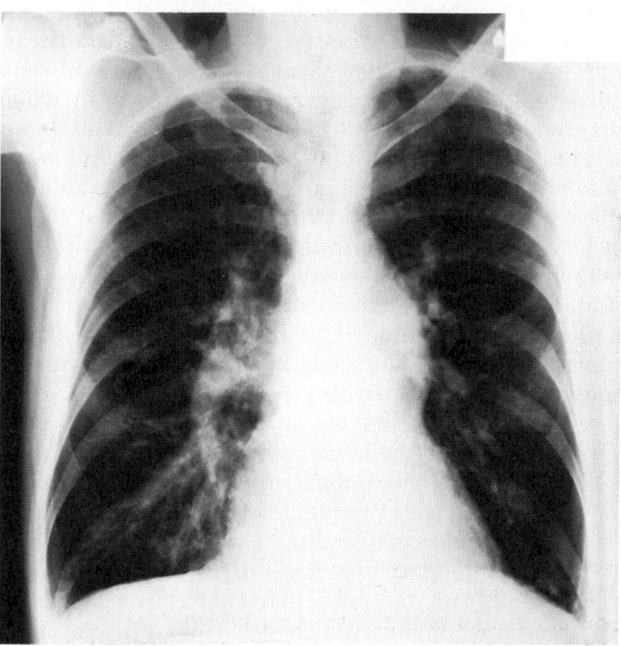

Fig. 13.39 Severe chronic bronchitis with marked hypoxaemia and pulmonary hypertension. In keeping with airways obstruction the lungs are of large volume. The main pulmonary artery (see below the aortic knuckle) is massively enlarged, as are the branches of the left and right pulmonary arteries.

olitis and other respiratory diseases causing widespread lung destruction and hypoxaemia. Pulmonary hypertension is due to destruction of the capillary bed, a secondary arteritis, and also hypoxic vasoconstriction. In patients with airways obstruction continuous oxygen therapy can reduce pulmonary arterial hypertension and improve prognosis.

Primary pulmonary hypertension

This diagnosis includes classical primary pulmonary hypertension in which the pulmonary arteries are diseased, and also a disorder localised to the pulmonary veins, pulmonary veno-occlusive disease. Both conditions are rare. In the differential diagnosis it is important to consider silent recurrent thromboembolic disease, systemic lupus erythematosus and lupus-like syndromes.

Primary pulmonary hypertension is of unknown cause and is seen most often in young adult females. Pulmonary

Table 13.34 Important causes of pulmonary hypertension

Diffuse lung disease
Recurrent pulmonary embolism (p. 499)
Chest wall abnormalities (p. 533)
Sleep apnoea syndromes (p. 491)
Mitral stenosis and congenital heart disease
Primary pulmonary hypertension (Ch. 12)

function shows hypoxia due to ventilation–perfusion mismatch, and reduced gas transfer. Patients become increasingly breathless, have syncopal episodes, develop right ventricular hypertrophy and eventually right ventricular failure. There is peripheral cyanosis with a small-volume peripheral pulse and cold, blue hands. Central cyanosis is a late development. The jugular venous pulse has a giant 'a' wave and on auscultation there is a right atrial gallop, tricuspid regurgitant murmur, a pulmonary systolic ejection click, closely split second sound with a loud pulmonary component and a murmur (Graham Steell) of pulmonary regurgitation. The chest X-ray shows a dilated pulmonary artery. The signs are similar in pulmonary veno-occlusive disease, with the important difference that there is pulmonary oedema and therefore more severe hypoxia as well as shadowing on the chest X-ray. The diagnosis of primary pulmonary hypertension is by exclusion of other causes of pulmonary hypertension and the diagnosis of veno-occlusive disease requires a lung biopsy. In primary pulmonary hypertension, no therapy has been demonstrated to be particularly effective, although pulmonary vasodilators (e.g. hydralazine, prostacycline) may be of some value. In veno-occlusive disease anticoagulants and possibly azathioprine may be helpful. Patients with primary pulmonary hypertension have been successfully treated by heart–lung transplantation.

PULMONARY THROMBO-EMBOLISM

Tumour, fat, amniotic fluid, parasites, air and injected material can all embolise to the lung but most emboli are from venous thrombosis, particularly in the lower limbs and pelvis (p. 442). Although massive pulmonary embolism is an important cause of death, few patients with such large emboli survive to reach hospital. Most commonly, the clinical picture is of less serious pulmonary emboli and pulmonary infarction. There is often a recent history of illness, trauma, anaesthesia or other factors known to predispose to deep venous thrombosis.

PULMONARY EMBOLISM AND INFARCTION

Pulmonary infarction follows embolisation to the peripheral branches of the pulmonary arteries. Emboli are frequently multiple, involving the lower zones more frequently than the upper part of the lungs and only some cause infarction. In many instances of pulmonary embolism without infarction the distal lung remains viable because of adequate oxygenation via the bronchial arterial blood supply and the airways. Pulmonary infarction is much more likely to occur when there is disease affecting the airways or bronchial circulation. Pathologically, the lesions of pulmonary infarction are markedly haemorrhagic and involve the visceral pleural surface.

Clinical features

The characteristic symptom of pulmonary embolism is sudden breathlessness. Indeed, relatively few processes cause such a sudden dyspnoea (p. 451). Lateral, usually basal, pleuritic chest pain and haemoptysis develop some time after the onset of breathlessness and are only clinical features if infarction has occurred. The haemoptysis consists of frank red blood without sputum. In addition to respiratory symptoms, there may be pain or swelling of a leg suggesting deep vein thrombosis, or a history indicating an increased risk of thrombosis.

On examination, there may be signs of deep vein thrombosis. The respiratory rate is usually raised and if infarction has taken place, there may be a pleural rub and a small pleural effusion. If embolisation has been extensive there will be cyanosis and signs of cardiovascular stress. The most important cardiovascular sign is a tachycardia. With extensive embolism, patients may have signs of pulmonary hypertension and occasionally a systolic murmur can be heard over the lung fields, as a consequence of turbulent pulmonary blood flow past partial pulmonary arterial occlusion. Within a few hours of pulmonary infarction fever is the rule.

Arterial blood gas analysis usually demonstrates hypoxaemia. However, not all patients are hypoxaemic and hypoxaemia is in itself a very non-specific abnormality. As a consequence of hyperventilation, there is hypocapnia. Patients with pulmonary embolic disease are frequently anxious as well as breathless and their hypocapnia is not uncommonly taken to reflect anxiety. However, anxiety hyperventilation syndromes produce hyperoxaemia. Immediately following embolisation, there is often bronchoconstriction, there may even be wheeze, and later, a reduction in surfactant in the affected lung is a contributory factor to atelectasis.

Diagnosis

The clinical diagnosis (Fig. 13.40) of pulmonary embolism is difficult and clinical criteria alone are seldom sufficient. Accurate diagnosis is important, since without specific therapy there may be further, fatal, embolisation. Furthermore, the institution of anticoagulation therapy has important consequences for the patient and is not justifiable without sound evidence. Important clinical factors in the diagnosis are a history of predisposing factors, a clinically obvious deep vein thrombosis, haemoptysis and a pleural rub.

The chest X-ray in pulmonary embolic disease is frequently normal. When pulmonary infarction occurs, radiological changes develop over the following 24 hours

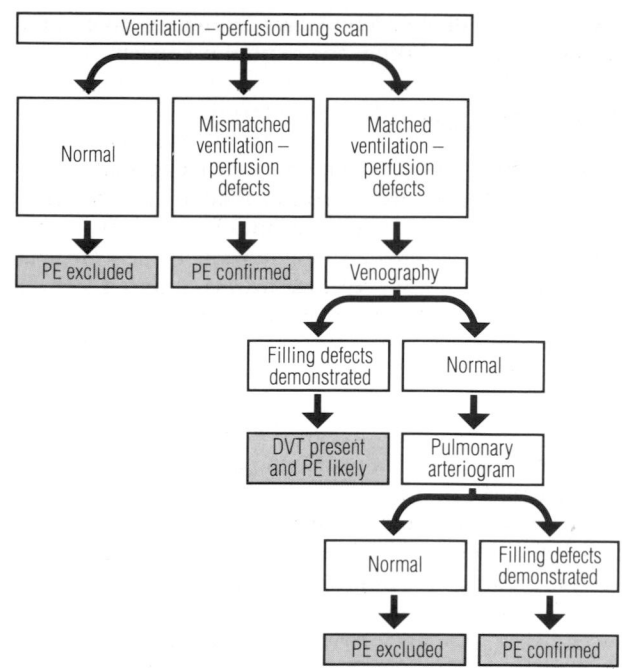

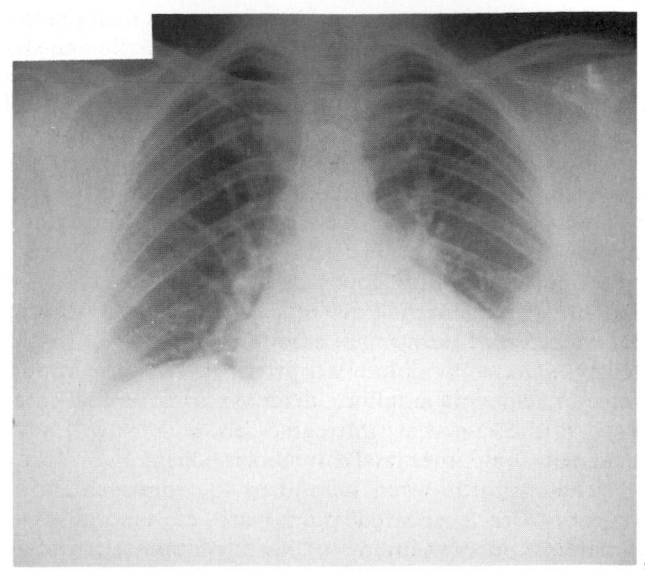

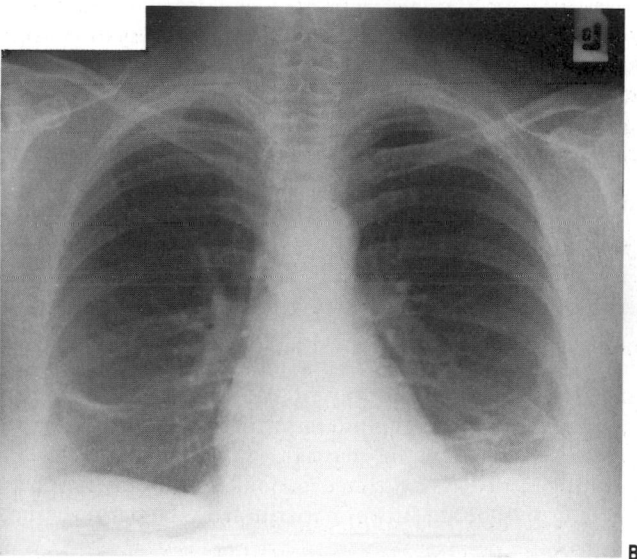

Fig. 13.40 Strategy for the diagnosis of pulmonary emboli (PE). The indication for venography to investigate patients with a matched ventilation–perfusion defect will depend on the degree of clinical suspicion of embolic disease. The same argument applies to a subsequent pulmonary arteriogram when venography is normal.

and may include peripheral shadows adjacent to the pleura, most often basal and frequently multiple, an elevated hemidiaphragm, some segmental or lobar volume loss, and small pleural effusions (Fig. 13.41A). If pleural fluid is aspirated it is found to be an exudate and is frequently haemorrhagic. Secondary infection of infarcted lung causes cavitation. With resolution, the linear shadows of pulmonary infarction are characteristic and usually have a pleural component (Fig. 13.41B).

The ECG is rarely helpful, except in the diagnosis of myocardial infarction or pericarditis, which may require consideration in the differential diagnosis of pulmonary embolic disease. Occasionally, the ECG changes are suggestive of pulmonary embolism in that they demonstrate right axis deviation, right bundle branch block or an S wave in lead I, a Q wave and inverted T wave in lead III. However, non-specific abnormalities, particularly T wave changes, are much more common. Severe or recurrent pulmonary emboli may be associated with pulmonary hypertension and the ECG changes of right ventricular and right atrial hypertrophy.

Isotope lung scans are the investigation of choice in most patients with pulmonary embolic disease, with the exception of a few patients with massive pulmonary embolism, in whom it may be more appropriate to proceed directly to pulmonary angiography. A normal perfusion lung scan largely excludes pulmonary embolic disease

Fig. 13.41 Pulmonary infarction: chest X-rays. A. Early changes. There is consolidation at both bases, particularly the left. The left hemidiaphragm is elevated. The patient has made a poor inspiratory effort due to pleuritic pain. **B.** Resolving infarction. Linear basal shadows are characteristic.

but an abnormal scan is non-specific. Although an abnormal scan in conjunction with a normal chest X-ray may be taken to suggest pulmonary embolism, perfusion scans may be markedly abnormal in some pulmonary disorders associated with a clear radiograph, as, for example, in asthma. Furthermore, pulmonary angiography demonstrates emboli in only 50% of patients with an abnormal perfusion lung scan and a normal chest X-ray. Thus, for many patients the confirmation of pulmonary emboli, rather than the exclusion of this diagnosis, necessitates a ventilation as well as a perfusion lung scan. Characteristically, the perfusion scan demonstrates a filling defect due to vascular obstruction, whereas ventilation to the affected area is relatively normal (Fig. 13.42). In doubtful cases, serial scans, during which the perfusion defects of pulmonary emboli resolve, are diagnostically helpful.

Large or multiple ventilation–perfusion mismatched areas are highly likely to be due to pulmonary emboli (80–90% of cases). In a minority of patients, perhaps up to 20% of cases, matched defects can be due to pulmonary embolism confirmed angiographically. For patients with a matched defect and a normal chest X-ray the diagnosis of pulmonary embolism can only be confidently excluded by pulmonary arteriography. The importance of achieving a definite diagnosis in equivocal cases rests on the fact that, untreated, about 50% will have recurrent, sometimes fatal thromboembolism.

Venography is often helpful in the management of patients with suspected pulmonary embolic disease. In patients documented to have pulmonary emboli angiographically, 70% will have deep vein thrombosis and therefore the demonstration or exclusion of deep vein thrombosis, by venography, plethysmography or isotopic techniques, is helpful in determining the likelihood of pulmonary emboli. However, a negative venogram occurs in up to 30% of patients with documented pulmonary emboli.

Management

The purpose of therapy is to halt the propagation of peripheral thrombus and avoid further pulmonary embolism, thereby allowing time for natural thrombolysis. The treatment of acute pulmonary embolism is intravenous heparin. Massive pulmonary embolism may require additional therapy (p. 499). The most effective heparin treatment regime is probably a continuous infusion such that the partial thromboplastin time is prolonged to 1.5–2.0 times normal, commonly requiring 30 000 to 40 000 units of heparin daily. Heparin require-

ments tend to fall after 2 or 3 days. If heparin treatment is complicated by bleeding, the action of heparin is rapidly reversed by the administration of protamine sulphate. Heparin therapy should be undertaken for 7–10 days. Thrombolytic therapy, most commonly used with massive pulmonary embolism (see below), is occasionally necessary when heparin treatment is inadequate, including cases with severe or extensive venous thrombosis, particularly when involving the inferior vena cava. Long-term anticoagulant therapy with warfarin is initiated 3–4 days before heparin therapy is stopped, and is continued for 3–6 months unless a chronic predisposing factor for deep venous thrombosis (e.g. chronic venous insufficiency of the legs) indicates the need for prolonged therapy. If bleeding complicates warfarin therapy, treatment is with vitamin K_1. In pregnancy, and in patients in whom intravenous heparin therapy is particularly hazardous, subcutaneous heparin administered 12-hourly is the treatment of choice.

The resolution of pulmonary emboli is rapid, usually within 2–4 weeks. Heparin therapy is highly effective in preventing further thromboembolism.

MASSIVE PULMONARY EMBOLISM

Massive pulmonary embolism is a relatively rare hospital emergency since most patients with fatal pulmonary emboli die within 2 hours, frequently before reaching medical help. For those who survive beyond 2 hours, the outlook is good in most cases, provided they receive appropriate medical treatment. Surgical intervention is only rarely required.

Clinical features

The clinical features of massive pulmonary embolism reflect the haemodynamic consequences of obstruction to a large proportion of the pulmonary arterial tree; more

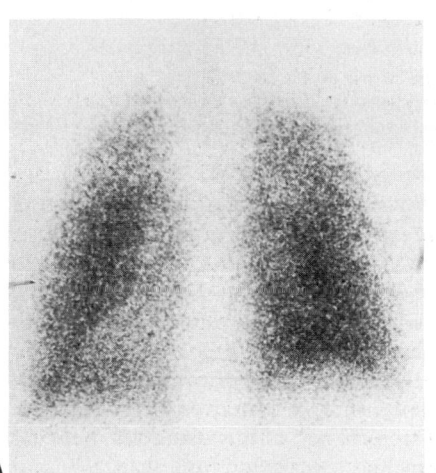
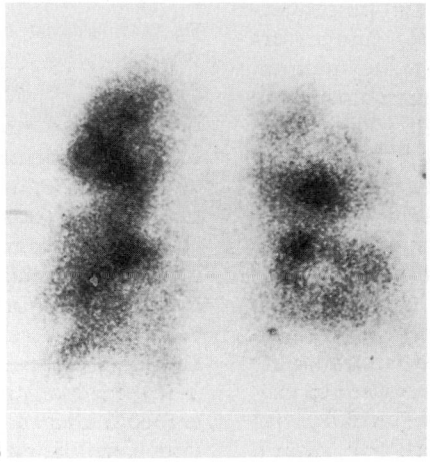

A   B

Fig. 13.42 Pulmonary embolic disease: ventilation and perfusion lung scans. Posterior scans demonstrate normal ventilation (**A**), and numerous, mainly peripheral, defects of perfusion (**B**), characteristic of multiple pulmonary emboli. Such changes usually resolve over a period of several weeks.

than 60% obstruction is necessary to produce serious consequences in a previously healthy individual. Less extensive embolism will be life-threatening in patients with severe pre-existing cardiorespiratory disease. Following embolism, some of the increase in pulmonary vascular resistance may be due to vasoconstriction, secondary to the release of agents such as serotonin from thrombus. The dominant symptom of massive embolism is severe breathlessness. In some patients, there is central chest pain due to myocardial ischaemia, reflecting the combination of a massive increase in right ventricular oxygen requirements and reduction in coronary artery blood flow. Hypotension may cause syncope. Examination shows tachypnoea, tachycardia, hypotension and poor peripheral perfusion. Signs of pulmonary hypertension and right ventricular strain are not always present. The ECG is frequently unhelpful, with the most common abnormality, other than a tachycardia, being T wave changes. The main importance of the ECG is in the differential diagnosis from massive myocardial infarction. The chest X-ray is frequently normal or non-specifically abnormal. Oligaemia of the lung fields is helpful when present but can seldom be appreciated on emergency supine chest X-ray films.

Diagnosis and treatment

Therapy is urgent and potentially life-saving. If the diagnosis of massive pulmonary embolism is probable and the ECG does not suggest myocardial infarction, urgent investigations are required but immediate treatment with intravenous heparin (15 000 units) is reasonable. When hypotension is severe, inotropic support to the right ventricle is needed. In patients who have collapsed with massive pulmonary embolism, external cardiac massage can move clot peripherally and restore part of the pulmonary circulation. Patients have and require high right heart filling pressures, and treatment with diuretics and vasodilators, including morphine, is deleterious. If the patient is capable of co-operation and facilities are immediately available, a ventilation–perfusion scan is performed. Indeed, a perfusion scan alone will be grossly abnormal and strongly support the diagnosis, provided the chest X-ray is clear. Patients who, for whatever reason, are unable to have isotope lung scans, require a pulmonary arteriogram, as do all patients for whom surgery is being considered. Pulmonary arteriograms normally demonstrate large central filling defects (Fig. 13.43).

Most patients who survive long enough to reach hospital, and who are then treated with intravenous heparin and inotropic support, rapidly improve. Following confirmation of the diagnosis some are best treated with thrombolytic agents, which achieve more rapid, and possibly more complete, resolution than intravenous heparin. Bleeding complications are, however, twice as likely than with heparin and thrombolytics should not be given if

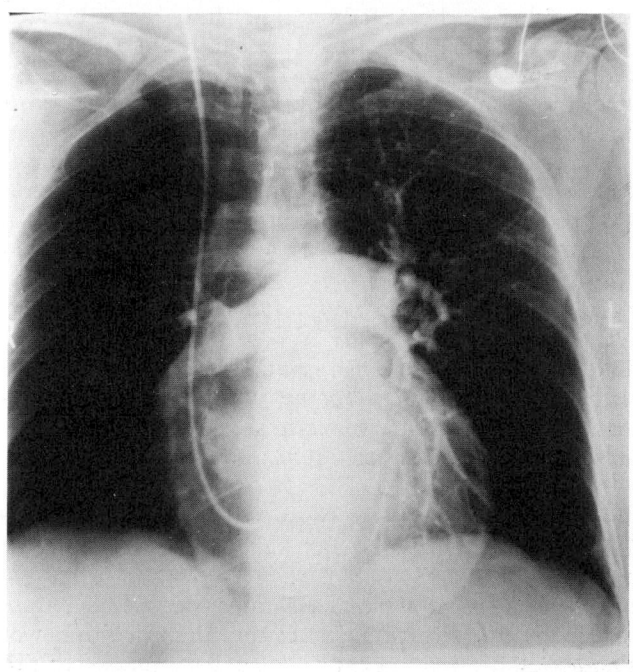

Fig. 13.43 Massive pulmonary embolism. The pulmonary arteriogram shows a large filling defect in the right pulmonary artery, with almost no perfusion of the right lung, and little perfusion of the left lower lobe peripherally.

patients have active haemorrhage, a history of a recent cerebrovascular accident or recent surgery, organ biopsy or childbirth. Streptokinase is the thrombolytic agent most commonly used, but is antigenic. Urokinase is less antigenic but more costly. Thrombolytic agents are usually infused directly into the pulmonary artery.

A small number of patients with severe haemodynamic disturbance fail to improve on medical therapy and require embolectomy. Surgery is performed with the patients on cardiac bypass. It is critically important that the definitive diagnosis of massive pulmonary embolism has been substantiated prior to surgery and, if so, the operative results are good (75% survival).

RECURRENT PULMONARY EMBOLISM

With adequate anticoagulation therapy recurrent pulmonary emboli are uncommon. Rarely anticoagulants are absolutely contra-indicated and in such patients, and those with recurrent emboli despite full anticoagulant therapy, inferior vena caval sieves can be used. Such surgical procedures are not always effective; the inserted devices may become dislodged, blocked or infected and, indeed, may become a source of future emboli.

Repeated, often silent, pulmonary emboli can gradually obstruct a large proportion of the pulmonary vasculature and lead to pulmonary hypertension. Such patients may have a chronic low cardiac output state and intractable right heart failure. They have severe breathlessness, the cause for which is frequently not appreciated at first presentation. Any possibility of recurrent pulmonary emboli warrants comprehensive investigations including angiography. Anticoagulant therapy can prevent progression of the disease. When angiography demonstrates central filling defects, some cardiothoracic centres have produced benefit to patients by surgical removal of organised clot.

Prevention of venous thrombo-embolism

The prevention of pulmonary embolism is possible if high-risk patients for the development of deep vein thrombosis and therefore pulmonary emboli are recognised and suitable prophylaxis undertaken (Ch. 12, p. 443).

SARCOIDOSIS

Sarcoidosis is a disease of unknown aetiology characterised by the involvement of more than one organ or tissue by non-caseating epithelioid cell granulomas which proceed either to resolution or to fibrosis.

Prevalence and distribution

Sarcoidosis is now recognised to be a worldwide disease which may present to all specialities and is relatively common. Worldwide, the prevalence is approximately 20 in 100 000. It is more common in temperate climates, American negroes, and West Indian and Irish immigrants to the UK, and is less common in Chinese and peoples of the Indian subcontinent. However, differences in incidence may reflect a difference in the awareness of the disease and the availability of diagnostic facilities, particularly radiology, and in many parts of the world the disorder has been frequently misdiagnosed as tuberculosis. Sarcoidosis is unusual in children and in the elderly and is most common between the ages of 20 and 40, with a slight female preponderance. In general, the disease is more florid in blacks than Caucasians.

Aetiology

The cause of sarcoidosis is not known. It is postulated that an as yet unidentified agent interacts with the host and produces a disease in which immunological factors are important (Fig. 13.44).

Inhalation is the most likely route for the causal agent and the sequence of events is probably one of alveolar injury and an influx of immune effector cells, followed by an inflammatory alveolitis. The alveolitis of sarcoidosis is predominantly lymphocytic (as shown by examination of lung tissue and bronchoalveolar lavage fluid), mostly activated T lymphocytes, with a reduction in circulating blood T lymphocytes. The increased lymphocytes in the lung are mostly T helper cells which are relatively

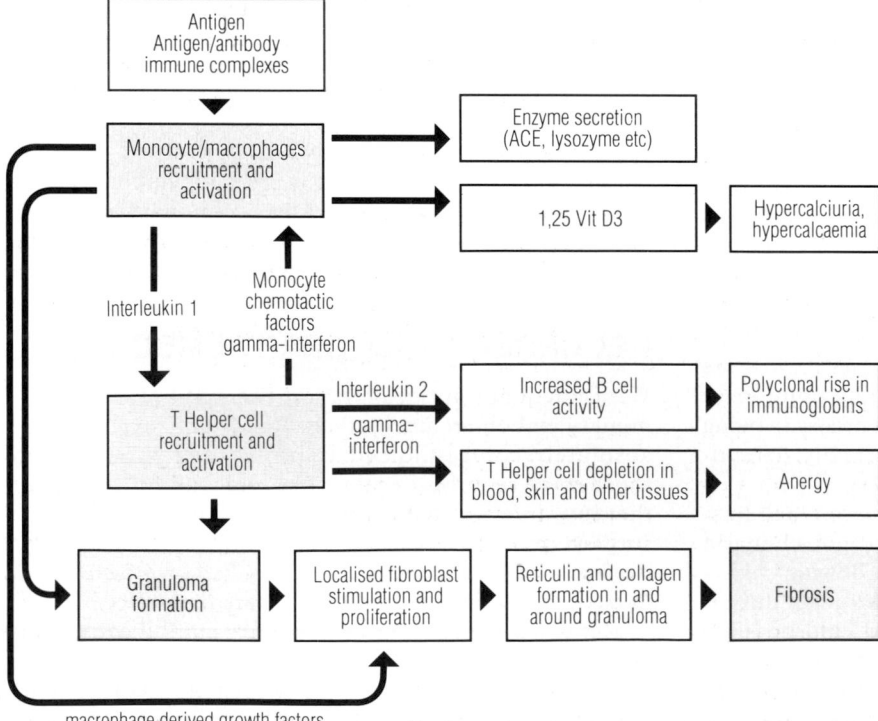

Fig. 13.44 Pathogenesis of sarcoidosis.

Table 13.35 Causes of non-caseating granulomata

Sarcoidosis	Berylliosis
Tuberculosis	Foreign body reactions
Primary biliary cirrhosis	Cat scratch disease
Leprosy	Hypersensitivity pneumonitis
Tertiary syphilis	Granulomatous arteritides
Brucellosis	Lymphomas
Hypogammaglobulinaemia	Carcinoma (regional lymph node)
Fungal infection	Crohn's disease

Table 13.36 Clinical spectrum of sarcoidosis in the UK

Clinical feature	% of cases
Liver biopsy positive with bilateral hilar adenopathy	80–90
Abnormal chest X-ray (lung involvement ± hilar or mediastinal adenopathy)	>85
Erythema nodosum	20–30
Lymphadenopathy	10–15
Palpable splenomegaly	6
Eye involvement	15–25
Skin sarcoid	5–20
Enlargement of parotid/lachrymal/other salivary glands	5–20
Symptomatic nervous system involvement	5
Bone cysts	3–8
Symptomatic heart disease	<5
Symptomatic myopathy	<1

depleted in peripheral blood. These changes may be responsible for the alveolitis, and partly explain the peripheral anergy of delayed type hypersensitivity of sarcoidosis.

Activated T lymphocytes secrete monocyte chemotactic factor, recruiting circulating monocytes and macrophages into the alveolitis, leading to granuloma formation. Lymphocytes also activate macrophages to form the epithelioid and giant cells of granulomata. The metabolic activity of macrophages is associated with increased levels of angiotensin converting enzyme (ACE) in lung tissue, bronchoalveolar lavage fluid and serum. Whether the granulomata resolve or progress to fibrosis may be determined by the intensity of the alveolitis.

The increase in T cell activity stimulates B lymphocytes, which results in raised serum immunoglobulins, circulating antibodies and immune complexes. Heredity may play a part in the predisposition to sarcoidosis and the condition is more common with some HLA groups.

The characteristic pathological finding of sarcoidosis is therefore granulomata that consist of collections of large histiocytes (epithelioid cells) with occasional multi-nucleated giant cells, and, more peripherally, lymphocytes (CD8-suppressor cells). There is no central necrosis, a point of contrast to many cases of tuberculosis, and the reticulin between the histiocytes is, therefore, intact. Non-caseating granulomata are not specific for sarcoidosis and can occur in other disorders (Table 13.35). Sarcoid granulomata are dynamic entities developing, ageing and resolving. In chronic cases the granulomata are replaced by hyalinisation and fibrosis.

Clinical features

Since sarcoidosis can affect virtually all organs and tissues of the body, with the probable exception of the adrenal glands, the clinical features of this disorder are varied (Table 13.36). The lungs, liver, eye and skin are most frequently involved, with more than 85% having some degree of pulmonary involvement, and many cases are diagnosed following a routine chest X-ray. Extensive sarcoidosis causes fever. Eye involvement can cause blindness. Respiratory, cardiac and renal failure are occasionally fatal.

Thoracic sarcoidosis

The chest X-ray is abnormal in more than 85% of cases and the radiological appearances form the basis for the classification of thoracic sarcoid (Table 13.37).

Stage I

Hilar adenopathy is usually bilateral and symmetrical, but can be unilateral. Adenopathy is the commonest manifestation of thoracic sarcoidosis and more than half of patients have no symptoms. In addition to enlargement of hilar glands, the right paratracheal gland is frequently enlarged (Fig. 13.45). Bilateral hilar adenopathy can also occur in other disorders (Table 13.38).

Table 13.37 Classification of thoracic sarcoid

Stage	Description of chest X-ray	Stage at presentation (%)	Elevated ACE levels (%)	Positive transbronchial lung biopsy (%)	Positive Kveim test (%)	Positive liver biopsy (%)
0	Normal	8	30	–	50	–
I	Hilar adenopathy	51	56	65–80	70	85
II	Hilar adenopathy plus parenchymal infiltrate	29	71	75–100	80	65
III	Parenchymal infiltrate ± fibrosis	12	56	75–85	40	60

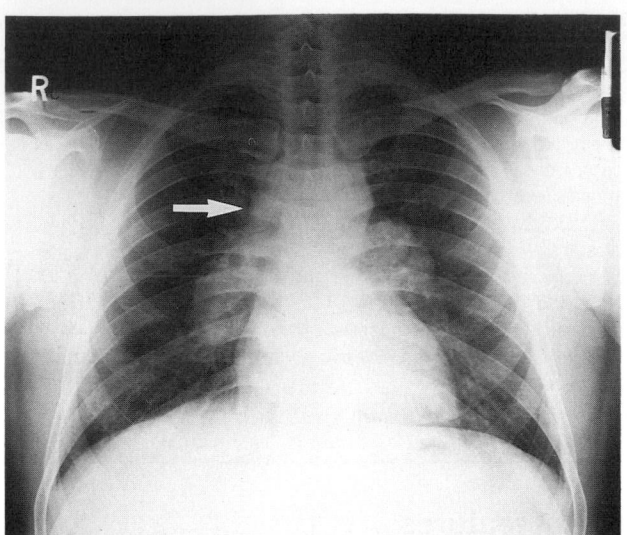

Fig. 13.45 Stage I sarcoidosis. There is bilateral hilar lymphadenopathy (BHL) and also enlargement of the right paratracheal nodes (arrow), characteristic of sarcoidosis.

Table 13.38 Differential diagnosis of bilateral hilar adenopathy

Sarcoidosis*	Beryllium disease
Tuberculosis	Hypogammaglobulinaemia
Lymphoma	Histoplasmosis
Leukaemia	Coccidioidomycosis
Metastatic malignant disease	Enlargement of pulmonary arteries

*Compared with sarcoidosis, all other causes of bilateral hilar adenopathy are uncommon.

In up to 40% of stage I cases there is also erythema nodosum, and in the UK 80% of cases of erythema nodosum in young adults are due to sarcoidosis. In association with bilateral hilar adenopathy and erythema nodosum there is commonly low-grade fever, polyarthralgia and a raised ESR.

Although few patients have severe symptoms with stage I sarcoidosis a minority have cough and chest pain due to adenopathy. Bilateral hilar adenopathy, with and without erythema nodosum, is usually benign, with 80% of cases resolving in less than 12 months and 90% by 2 years. In 10% of cases, glandular enlargement persists and eggshell calcification may develop, or patients may develop pulmonary opacities. Patients with bilateral hilar lymphadenopathy without erythema nodosum probably do rather less well, with up to 20% developing a pulmonary infiltrate.

Stage II

Pulmonary infiltrates co-exist with adenopathy in about 30% of patients (Fig. 13.46). More severely affected

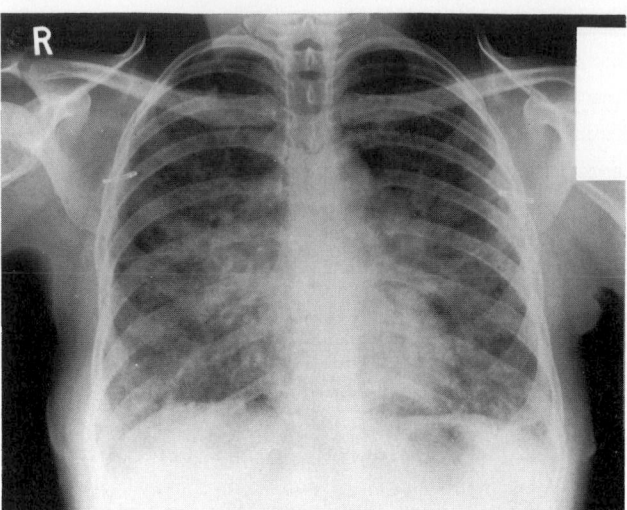

Fig. 13.46 Stage II sarcoidosis. The X-ray shows florid stage II sarcoidosis, with bilateral hilar lymphadenopathy (BHL) and extensive pulmonary infiltrates. Pleural abnormalities in sarcoidosis are rare.

patients have a restrictive ventilatory defect with exertional breathlessness and a reduction in gas transfer. The chest X-ray appearances correlate poorly with physiological disturbances, the patient being frequently asymptomatic, despite widespread pulmonary shadowing. The prognosis for stage II sarcoidosis is less good than for stage I. Although 50% resolve spontaneously within 2 years, some take longer, 30–40% require steroid therapy and in 10–15% long-term steroid therapy is required, despite which a small number develop progressive pulmonary fibrosis. The differential diagnosis of stage II and stage III sarcoidosis is shown in Table 13.39.

Stage III

With the development of pulmonary fibrosis, patients become breathless, hypoxic and ultimately develop cor pulmonale. Pulmonary function tests demonstrate a severe restrictive ventilatory defect. In addition to fibrosis, which is characteristically most marked in the mid- and upper zones, the chest X-ray may also show cavitation and bullae formation. As would be expected, the prognosis for stage III sarcoidosis is less good, with about 30% showing significant improvement with steroid therapy.

Table 13.39 Differential diagnosis of stage II and stage III sarcoidosis

Cryptogenic fibrosing alveolitis	Bronchopulmonary aspergillosis
Pulmonary tuberculosis	Ankylosing spondylitis
Extrinsic allergic alveolitis	Berylliosis
Carcinoma	Histocytosis X
Pneumoconiosis	*Pneumocystis carinii* pneumonia

Extrathoracic sarcoidosis

Skin

Erythema nodosum is the most common skin abnormality, and is associated with acute, usually stage I, sarcoidosis. When there is erythema nodosum and BHL in a young adult, a clinical diagnosis of sarcoidosis can be firmly made without resort to tissue biopsy. Erythema nodosum is an immunological response associated with sarcoidosis and skin biopsy demonstrates a characteristic histology, which is the same as for other causes of erythema nodosum (p. 1142). Sarcoid tissue itself can also infiltrate the skin, and biopsy shows typical non-caseating granulomata. Small papules, plaques and subcutaneous nodules are common, and the skin of the nose may be involved (lupus pernio), as are scars and keloid tissue. When there is lupus pernio the upper respiratory tract is frequently involved by the disease and nasal mucosal biopsy is positive. Skin sarcoid more commonly affects females and is more common, extensive and florid in blacks.

Eyes

Eye involvement is both common (up to 25% of cases) and potentially serious. Early eye involvement may be asymptomatic and all patients should be examined by an ophthalmologist. Uveitis, conjunctivitis and retinal involvement can all occur. Dry eyes (keratoconjunctivitis sicca) occurs in a Sjögren-like syndrome when the salivary glands are involved. The lachrymal, salivary and parotid glands may be enlarged. Eye involvement is an indication for steroid therapy, usually systemic.

Hypercalciuria

Hypercalciuria has, in the past, been reported in up to 60% of patients with sarcoidosis, of which as many as 11% have been reported to have hypercalcaemia. However, more recent series have suggested that these disorders of calcium metabolism (p. 729) are less common.

Lymphadenopathy

Enlarged lymph nodes are present in 10–15% of patients and splenomegaly occurs in 6%, both abnormalities being more common in blacks. Occasionally, the spleen is very large and associated with anaemia, neutropenia and thrombocytopenia, which may improve following splenectomy.

Cardiac sarcoid

Involvement of the myocardium by granulomatous infiltration may be relatively common and is discussed on page 412.

Nervous system

Sarcoid affecting the nervous system is discussed on page 974. Sarcoid involvement of muscle is usually asymptomatic but occasionally patients have myopathic symptoms.

Bone sarcoidosis

Arthritis, acute and transient, is common with BHL and erythema nodosum, but chronic skeletal problems are unusual (3%), characteristically affecting hands and feet in patients with skin sarcoidosis. Bone cysts, especially of the terminal phalanges, are most typical. Steroids have little effect and bone lesions are usually confined to cases of chronic sarcoidosis.

Diagnosis

Chest X-ray and TBB give the diagnosis in the majority of patients. Biopsy of any clinically involved tissue will confirm the diagnosis and a liver biopsy will be positive in 85% of patients. Frequently, the most important differential diagnosis is between sarcoidosis and tuberculosis and tissue should, therefore, be stained for acid-fast bacilli and cultured for *M. tuberculosis*. In cases where biopsy is relatively difficult (e.g. hilar adenopathy) or negative, a diagnosis of sarcoidosis can be substantiated by the Kveim test (Table 13.37). A suspension of particulate human sarcoid tissue is injected intradermally and in patients with active sarcoidosis epithelioid cell granulomata gradually develop and can be demonstrated following skin biopsy of the purplish red nodule at 4 weeks. A positive Kveim test strongly suggests a diagnosis of sarcoidosis (false positives 1–2%). However, the Kveim test is not always positive in sarcoidosis and there is a relatively high false negative rate in chronic fibrotic disease.

Depression of delayed type hypersensitivity in sarcoidosis reduces tuberculin reactivity. Two-thirds of patients do not react to 100 tuberculin units and more than 90% fail to react to 10 tuberculin units. A depressed tuberculin reaction persists for many years, long after clinical resolution of sarcoidosis. In the differential diagnosis of sarcoidosis and tuberculosis, the tuberculin test is of considerable value.

Management

Assessment of the severity and activity of disease

Although symptoms and signs are the main guide to management, further investigations are necessary and helpful in decision-making.

Radiology

Chest X-rays provide a crude index of the extent of thoracic sarcoidosis and the correlation between radiological findings and functional impairment is poor. However, serial chest X-rays over months and years remain indispensable for documenting qualitative changes that occur either spontaneously or in response to therapy.

Serum angiotensin converting enzyme

Serum angiotensin converting enzyme (SACE) levels are high with acute granulomatous disease and correlate with chest X-ray abnormalities. However, not all patients with sarcoidosis have raised SACE levels and conversely, some patients without sarcoid (perhaps up to 20%) can have high levels. SACE is most useful in monitoring granulomatous activity and the response to steroid therapy.

Broncho-alveolar lavage

In normal subjects, BAL usually shows less than 10% lymphocytes, whereas in sarcoidosis, average figures for lymphocyte counts are 30% with up to 50–60% in florid, acute disease. However, there is an overlap of the cell count in sarcoidosis with those in normal subjects, particularly smokers, as well as in patients with extrinsic allergic alveolitis, lymphomas and cryptogenic fibrosing alveolitis. BAL is not necessary for the management of most cases.

Lung function tests

The correlation between chest X-ray appearances and pulmonary function is poor. Pulmonary sarcoidosis leads to a restrictive ventilatory defect with a reduction in lung volumes, pulmonary compliance and gas transfer. The most sensitive index of impaired pulmonary function is abnormal gas transfer, which may be reduced even in stage I disease. Some patients with sarcoidosis have an obstructive defect due to endobronchial disease (confirmed by bronchoscopy and bronchial biopsy and improved by steroid therapy) or to airway distortion from fibrosis. With moderate or severe disease, patients may be hypoxic at rest and in mild disease there is hypoxia on exertion. Pulmonary function testing is essential in the assessment of sarcoidosis and repeated measurements are of great value in long-term management.

Treatment

The known effects of steroids on immunological mechanisms suggest that these drugs should be helpful in sup-

Table 13.40 Indications for steroid treatment in sarcoidosis

Eye involvement
Severe chest X-ray changes (stage II and stage III disease) associated with a high serum angiotensin converting enzyme
Intense alveolitis on broncho-alveolar lavage
Breathlessness
Hypercalcaemia and hypercalciuria
Severe skin infiltration
Severe involvement of the upper respiratory tract
Cardiac involvement
Nervous system involvement
Salivary gland involvement

pressing the immunologically mediated alveolitis of sarcoidosis and, indeed, patients with acute florid disease appear to respond rapidly. In most patients the short-term effect of steroids is to improve symptoms, suppress inflammation and granuloma production and lower SACE levels. Prednisolone at a dosage of 30–40 mg daily, with a gradual reduction towards the minimum dose that controls disease activity, frequently 7.5–10.0mg daily, is normally prescribed. Treatment with steroids is indicated whenever vital organs are severely involved or when there is substantial systemic disturbance (Table 13.40).

Alternative immunosuppressive agents (i.e. methotrexate, azathioprine or cyclosporin) may be used for chronic disease, particularly chronic skin infiltration, but there is no evidence that these agents are superior to oral steroids.

Prognosis

Approximately 60% of all patients with thoracic sarcoidosis resolve spontaneously, and have a normal chest X-ray, mostly within 2 years. A further 20% will resolve with steroid therapy which can then be discontinued. These patients have an acute or subacute type of the disease, clearly associated with a good prognosis. For the minority 10–20% with chronic disease, resolution, even with steroid therapy, is less likely, with radiographic clearing in about 50% who have stage II and 20% who have stage III disease. Patients with chronic pulmonary sarcoidosis may eventually develop pulmonary fibrosis and respiratory failure. Although only a small percentage of patients with sarcoidosis (2%) die of the condition, most of these deaths are from pulmonary fibrosis and respiratory failure. Chronic extrathoracic sarcoidosis often responds poorly to treatment. Central nervous system involvement is particularly chronic and poorly responsive to steroid therapy.

CONNECTIVE TISSUE DISEASES AND THE LUNG

Systemic lupus erythematosus (SLE)

Pleurisy is common in SLE, affecting 50% of patients, with effusions in approximately 30%. An acute pulmonary vasculitis can cause widespread pneumonitis in about 10% of cases, sometimes leaving a residual basal atelectasis. Interstitial fibrosis is unusual. Patients may develop small-volume lungs, the cause of which is unknown and which, in most cases, is not due to diaphragm weakness. In patients with the SLE-like syndrome characterised by the presence of anti-cardiolipin antibodies, thrombotic obliteration of the pulmonary vasculature can lead to pulmonary hypertension and severe breathlessness.

Mixed connective tissue disease

Mixed connective tissue disease (MCTD) is a syndrome composed of features of SLE, polymyositis, rheumatoid arthritis and scleroderma; it is not infrequently complicated by pulmonary involvement including pleurisy, pulmonary fibrosis and pulmonary hypertension secondary to vascular involvement.

Rheumatoid arthritis

The pulmonary manifestations of rheumatoid arthritis are described in Chapter 23, page 998.

Systemic sclerosis

The most common pulmonary manifestation of systemic sclerosis is pulmonary fibrosis, and pleurisy is unusual. Occasionally, pulmonary vascular disease occurs in the absence of parenchymal abnormalities, leading to pulmonary hypertension. Aspiration, with consequent pneumonitis, infection and bronchiectasis, is not uncommon in systemic sclerosis.

Pneumonitis and fibrosing alveolitis can occur in Sjögren's syndrome and dermatomyositis. In dermatomyositis muscle weakness can be a major factor contributing to breathlessness and ventilatory failure.

VASCULITIDES AND THE LUNG

Wegener's granulomatosis

In Wegener's granulomatosis, described by Wegener in 1936, the characteristic pathology is a necrotising granulamatous arteritis of the upper and lower respiratory tract and also of the kidney, where it causes a focal and segmental glomerulonephritis. Upper respiratory tract manifestations, particularly sinusitis, ulceration of the nasal mucosa and bleeding from the nose are a common presentation, but unlike midline granulomatous disease there is no facial ulceration. In Wegener's, middle-aged males are most frequently affected. Increasing breathlessness, haemoptysis and pleurisy occur with pulmonary involvement, which is present in 95% of cases. In most cases, there is a low-grade pyrexia. In contrast to polyarteritis nodosa, hypertension is unusual. Wegener's granulomatosis is a multisystem disease and the widespread vasculitis may affect eyes, skin, joints, heart and the nervous system. In most instances it is the renal involvement, present in 85% of cases, that is critical. The chest X-ray shows nodules or masses which are commonly bilateral (Fig. 13.47), and which may be large and cavitate. Mediastinal or hilar adenopathy is rare. Endobronchial disease may be visible at bronchoscopy.

In Wegener's, the ESR is usually raised and the platelet count may also be elevated. Eosinophilia is not a feature. The diagnosis is a clinical one (suggested by disease of the upper as well as the lower respiratory tract and by renal involvement), supported by tissue biopsy demonstrating characteristic histology. Open lung biopsy gives the highest diagnostic yield but the diagnosis is often possible by biopsy of more accessible structures such as the skin or upper airway mucosa. Renal biopsy confirms kidney involvement but the tissue obtained is commonly not diagnostic of Wegener's. A positive antineutrophil

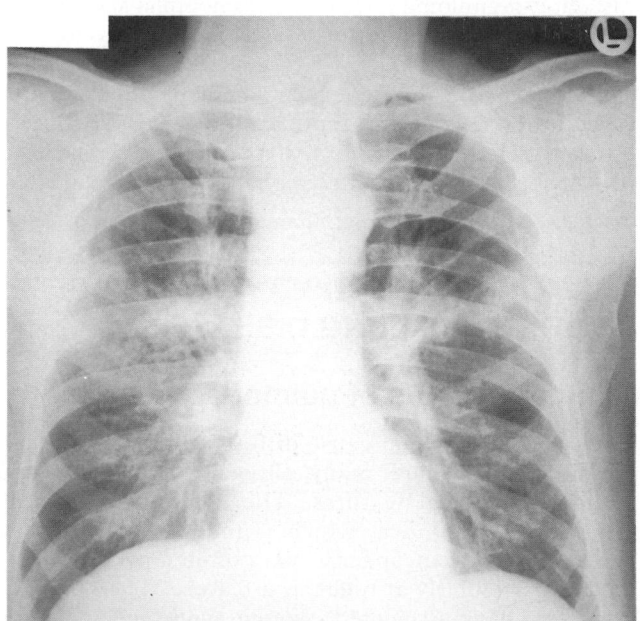

Fig. 13.47 Wegener's granulomatosis. There are large, irregular, central nodular shadows in both mid-zones, rather characteristic of Wegener's. Lesions commonly cavitate.

cytoplasmic antibody test (ANCA) strongly supports the diagnosis. Without treatment 80% of patients die within one year, the advancing renal disease being the major determinant of survival. Treatment with cyclophosphamide (1–2 mg/kg per day), initially combined with steroids (prednisolone, 60 mg daily), is often remarkably effective. Long-term remission is achieved by such therapy in up to 90% of patients, and in some cases with severe chronic renal impairment successful renal transplantation has been undertaken.

Midline granuloma

This is a rare disease, now thought to be a T cell lymphoma, in which there is destruction of the tissues of the nose and upper respiratory tract. The characteristic pathology is of granulomata; patients are most often middle-aged females. Nasal involvement is the most striking feature, with the development of septal perforation and saddle nose deformity. The disease is localised (unlike Wegener's) and there is no arteritis. Without treatment the disease is fatal. The treatment of choice is local radiotherapy and steroids are not helpful.

Polyarteritis nodosa

Pulmonary involvement in classical polyarteritis nodosa is unusual, but is a feature of the variant of polyarteritis known as allergic granulomatosis or the Churg-Strauss syndrome (p. 486), characterised by a necrotising vasculitis, granuloma formation, eosinophilia and asthma. Treatment is with high-dose steroids, and cyclophosphamide if necessary.

Pulmonary involvement occurs in many other systemic vasculitides including giant cell arteritis, Behçet's, Henoch-Schönlein purpura, hypersensitivity vasculitis (usually drug-induced) and lymphatoid granulomatosis.

PULMONARY FIBROSIS AND DIFFUSE INTERSTITIAL LUNG DISEASE

Clinical features of pulmonary fibrosis

The conditions which cause diffuse pulmonary fibrosis (Table 13.41) share many clinical, radiological and pathophysiological features. The common presenting symptom is dyspnoea, which is mild at first but can progress to total incapacity. Very often a persistent dry cough, particularly at night, is a feature. There may be symptoms of an associated systemic syndrome, including fever and weight loss during the acute phase. On examination, the patient may have few physical signs outside the chest. However, when fibrosis is widespread there

Table 13.41 Causes of pulmonary fibrosis

Inhalation of dust or chemicals
Organic dusts (e.g. avian proteins, moulds)
Mineral dusts (e.g. asbestos, silica, coal dust)
Chemicals (e.g. nitrogen dioxide, chlorine)

Unknown causes
Cryptogenic fibrosing alveolitis (syn. diffuse pulmonary fibrosis, idiopathic pulmonary fibrosis, usual or organising interstitial pneumonia)
Sarcoidosis
Idiopathic haemosiderosis
Histiocytosis X (Letterer-Siwe disease, Hand-Schuller-Christian disease, eosinophilic granuloma)

Iatrogenic and poisoning
Drugs (e.g. bleomycin, hydralazine, busulphan, amiodarone)
Paraquat
Radiation pneumonitis
Oxygen toxicity

Pulmonary involvement in systemic disease
Rheumatoid arthritis
Ankylosing spondylitis
Systemic sclerosis
Sjögren's syndrome
Dermatomyositis

Congenital
Niemann-Pick disease
Gaucher's disease
Tuberous sclerosis
Neurofibromatosis

may be tachypnoea, cyanosis and, at a late stage, cor pulmonale. There may be finger clubbing, especially in patients with cryptogenic fibrosing alveolitis and asbestosis. Auscultation of the chest usually reveals predominantly basal inspiratory crackles but there are exceptions (see below). The chest X-ray in the early stages shows a hazy, nodular infiltrate. As the lungs become more fibrotic, cystic spaces become evident and a 'honeycomb' pattern, sometimes with large bullae, develops.

Lung function tests show a restrictive ventilatory defect (p. 448), reduced transfer factor and hypoxaemia.

OCCUPATIONAL LUNG DISEASE

The lung can be injured by the inhalation of dusts, fumes or other noxious substances at work in certain specific occupations. There are strict criteria for the diagnosis of these conditions and, in the UK, for determining the level of compensation.

Pulmonary damage can occur in several ways:

- *mechanical effects of dust retention*
- *fibrogenesis* (e.g. coal dust, silica)
- *granulomatous reactions* (e.g. berylliosis)
- *toxicity* (e.g. mercury vapour)

- *irritation of air passages* (e.g. chlorine)
- *promotion of bronchial hyper-reactivity* (e.g. occupational asthma in laboratory workers who become hypersensitive to animal fur or urine).

Important occupational lung diseases include those due to *inorganic dusts* (e.g. silica, talc, asbestos, tin, iron); those due to *organic dusts* (e.g. cotton dust, maple bark dust) and those due to *gases and fumes* (e.g. chlorine, ammonia). Occupational exposure can also cause asthma, and lung and pleural malignancy.

Pneumoconioses due to inorganic dust inhalation

The common pneumoconioses are listed in Table 13.42.

Coal miners' pneumoconiosis

Inhalation of coal dust over a prolonged period damages the lung. The incidence varies with the type of coal being mined, occurring in about 12% of all miners but up to 50% in those who have mined anthracite for more than 20 years. For certification for compensation the diagnosis is radiological, not clinical. In the disease's early form, these radiological changes consist of small nodules less than 1.5 mm in diameter; this early form is termed *simple pneumoconiosis*. In a proportion of cases the nodules grow up to 10 mm in size, are irregular, and coalesce to form large masses which may cavitate, commonly in the upper lobes: this is referred to as *complicated pneumoconiosis* or *progressive massive fibrosis*.

About 15% of patients have positive antinuclear factor and in a small number, active rheumatoid arthritis is present. This is *Caplan's syndrome* and the chest X-ray shows rounded peripheral nodules in the lung fields 0.5–5.0 cm in diameter. First described in coal miners, the same appearances have since been seen in other forms of pneumoconiosis.

Silicosis

Although now less common as a result of protective measures, silicosis is still a major occupational hazard because of the ubiquitous distribution of free silica. Silicosis results from the inhalation of fine particles of silicon dioxide crystals or quartz particles. Those involved in mining, quarrying, metal casting, sandblasting and the pottery industry are at risk. Inhalation can cause an acute febrile illness with rapidly progressive dyspnoea and cyanosis which can occur after a short exposure and lead to death in a few weeks. This acute syndrome is rare. The more common chronic form of the disease is due to the highly fibrogenic potential of silica and presents as slowly progressive dyspnoea and cough, occasionally with haemoptysis. Co-existing tuberculosis is not uncommon. The disease may progress even after exposure ceases. The radiological appearances are of upper zone fibrosis with characteristic hilar 'eggshell' calcification.

Asbestos-related disease

Asbestos is the generic name for several silicates including chrysolite (90% of all world asbestos), crocidolite (blue asbestos), osmosite and anthopyllate. Fibres persist in the lung long after inhalation and cause characteristic pathological changes. Those at high risk include demolition workers, pipe laggers, brake lining industry workers and boiler makers. The respiratory effects of asbestos are a progressive pulmonary fibrosis (asbestosis), pleural plaques, and malignancy of the lung and pleura.

Asbestosis presents as progressive dyspnoea and cough, with finger clubbing and basal crackles. Like the other pneumoconioses it may progress to respiratory failure. Asbestos fibres are inhaled and phagocytosed, causing damage to cell membranes and the release of lysosomal enzymes. Radiologically there may be basal linear and irregular shadows which in the later stages progress to 'honeycombing' throughout the lung fields with the

Table 13.42 The common pneumoconioses

Disease	Occupation	Cause	Pathology
Coal miners' pneumoconiosis	Coal mining	Coal dust	Nodular and progressive massive fibrosis
Silicosis	Mining, quarrying, metal grinding, stone dressing, etc.	Silica	Focal fibrosis, centrilobular emphysema, progressive massive fibrosis, associated tuberculosis
Asbestosis	Demolition workers, shipbreaking, lagging and brake lining manufacture, etc.	Asbestos	Focal fibrosis, pleural calcification, bronchial carcinoma, pleural and peritoneal mesothelioma
Berylliosis	Electronics, atomic energy reactors, aero-engines	Beryllium	Granulomata and interstitial fibrosis
Talcosis	Rubber industry	Magnesium silicate	Focal fibrosis
Stannosis	Smelting	Tin oxide	Mineral deposition
Siderosis	Arc welding	Iron oxide	Mineral deposition

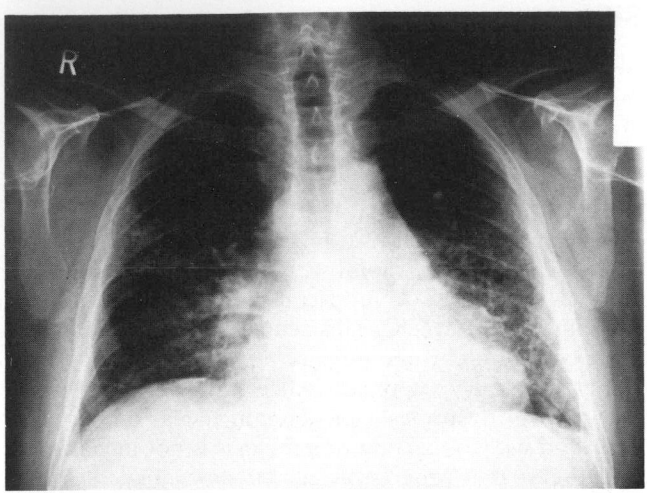

Fig. 13.48 Asbestosis. Bilateral pulmonary fibrosis of asbestosis. There is also pleural thickening, best seen adjacent to the lateral chest wall on the left and diaphragmatic pleural calcification on the right.

Berylliosis

Berylliosis differs from other pneumoconioses in that the initial pathological response to inhaling beryllium is a granulomatous one, which progresses to fibrosis. Histologically it may be difficult to distinguish from sarcoidosis. It can occasionally cause an acute pneumonic type of illness. Those at risk include workers in the atomic power and aero-engine industry.

Other inorganic dusts

Other inorganic dusts vary in their ability to generate fibrosis; iron and iron oxides in arc welding and silver finishing (siderosis) and tin oxide in smelting (stannosis) are relatively non-fibrogenic, whereas magnesium silicate in the rubber industry (talcosis) can be a potent cause of fibrosis. Other dusts cause mucus hypersecretion and airway irritation with or without pneumonitis, e.g. cement, graphite, cadmium and many others.

EXTRINSIC ALLERGIC ALVEOLITIS

This group of conditions is caused by the inhalation of organic dusts (Table 13.43). Chronic exposure to dusts which contain antigen sensitises the individual, a precipitating antibody is produced, and granulomata appear in the lung. These granulomata heal by fibrosis.

Clinically, the patient may present with an acute illness 6–8 hours after heavy antigen exposure, with fever, 'flu-like' symptoms, cough, dyspnoea and crackles. These resolve spontaneously in 24–48 hours if there is no further antigen exposure. The clinical features reflect the pathogenic mechanism, which is primarily an IgG-mediated 'late' type III hypersensitivity or Arthus' reaction to the antigen, although there is probably also a cell-mediated response. The result of repeated exposure is granuloma formation and eventually extensive fibrosis. More commonly the presentation is with established fibrosis,

cardiac silhouette becoming indistinct (Fig. 13.48). Lung function tests show a restrictive defect with reduced transfer factor. There are usually 'asbestos bodies' in the sputum or bronchial washings.

Pleural plaques are an indication of previous exposure to asbestos. They do not indicate lung disease or any increased risk over similarly exposed subjects of developing a tumour. They are usually basal or diaphragmatic and frequently calcify. CT scanning of the thorax is very useful in picking up early lesions, demonstrating the extent of pleural involvement, and distinguishing pleural from parenchymal disease.

Bronchogenic carcinoma is the most common tumour caused by asbestos exposure; cigarette smoking in asbestos workers greatly increases the risk, exerting a multiplicative rather than an additive effect. The tumours are usually adeno- or squamous cell carcinomas. Mesotheliomas of pleura and peritoneum are associated with asbestos exposure (p. 530).

Table 13.43 Some causes of extrinsic allergic alveolitis

Type	Disease	Source	Antigen
From fungi	Farmer's lung	Mouldy hay	*Micropolyspora faeni* *Thermoactinomycetes vulgaris* *Thermoactinomycetes sacherii*
	Mushroom worker's lung	Mushroom compost	
	Bagassosis	Mouldy bagasse	
	Ventilator pneumonitis	Air conditioning and hot air systems	
	Malt worker's lung	Mouldy barley	*Aspergillus clavatus*
	Maple bark stripper's lung	Mouldy maple bark	*Cryptostroma (coniosporium corticale)*
From birds	Bird fancier's lung	Pigeon/budgerigar/hen/parrot droppings	Avian serum proteins in droppings
From mammals	Pituitary snuff taker's lung	Porcine pituitary powder	Serum protein/pituitary antigens
	Rat handler's lung	Rat droppings	Rat serum protein

with dyspnoea and dry cough. Finger clubbing is uncommon, in marked contrast to cryptogenic fibrosing alveolitis. Inspiratory crackles and squeaks are characteristic. Radiologically, the changes are predominantly upper zone, with nodular and linear shadows and volume loss. Lung function tests show reduction in lung volumes and transfer factor. Precipitating antibodies are present in the blood, and intradermal skin tests, read at 6 hours, are available for some of the causes and are especially useful in the diagnosis of bird fancier's lung. Bronchial challenge tests, with measurement of temperature, lung volumes and gas transfer, are occasionally valuable.

The treatment of these conditions is firstly to stop exposure to the antigen. For the acute type of allergic alveolitis this is usually sufficient. However, when chronic exposure has led to granulomatous change in the lung, treatment with corticosteroids is required. In advanced fibrotic disease, as with all end-stage fibrotic lung diseases, there is little that can be done apart from considering lung transplantation.

CRYPTOGENIC FIBROSING ALVEOLITIS

Cryptogenic fibrosing alveolitis (CFA), a disorder of unknown aetiology, is characterised pathologically by migration of large mononuclear cells into the alveolar spaces with later thickening of alveolar walls, with fibrosis. The mononuclear cellular response is associated with acute symptoms, whereas the alveolar thickening and fibrosis is responsible for the more chronic clinical picture.

The pathogenesis of the condition is poorly understood. It is considered to be an altered state of host-responsiveness to an as yet unknown stimulus. An alteration of cell-mediated immunity has been proposed, since stimulated T lymphocytes increase fibroblastic activity. Activation of complement with consequent leucocyte aggregation may play a part. The pathological picture that emerges is, at first, an intra-alveolar inflammatory response, with many mononuclear cells and an increase in reticulin, collagen and elastin. As the disease progresses, there is fibrosis and destruction of lung architecture, with formation of cystic spaces.

Characteristically, CFA is a disease of late middle age, which affects males twice as frequently as females. The acute variant of the disease may present with rapidly progressive dyspnoea and cough, widespread crackles and progressive respiratory failure within a few months. The chronic (and much more common) form presents with dyspnoea and dry cough, and in approximately 20% of cases, polyarthralgia. About two-thirds of the patients have finger clubbing and almost all have basal crackles. The condition may be associated with a variety of systemic diseases: rheumatoid arthritis, Sjögren's syndrome

and systemic sclerosis. Other known causes of pulmonary fibrosis, such as the pneumoconioses or sarcoidosis, should be excluded, but with end-stage pulmonary fibrosis it is often difficult, even at post-mortem, to determine the aetiology.

The chest X-ray shows fine nodular and irregular shadowing (Fig. 13.49) and eventually 'honeycombing'. Lung function tests show a restrictive pattern with reduced transfer factor. Antinuclear antibodies are present in 45% of patients and rheumatoid factor in 20–25%. BAL usually yields a predominantly polymorphonuclear leucocyte pattern. To make a definitive diagnosis an open lung biopsy may be necessary. Patients who have a very active cellular histology respond better to treatment than those with established fibrosis.

Treatment

The usual treatment is with oral corticosteroids and the response is variable, with only 10% improving substantially. Treatment may need to be continued over several years. Cyclophosphamide or azathioprine may be used as steroid-sparing agents. It is unlikely that treatment substantially affects the long-term prognosis. The progression of CFA is variable; some patients with very acute, severe disease (the 'Hamman-Rich' syndrome) may die within months. Overall approximately 50% survive for 5 years and 25% for 10 years. There is a tenfold increase in the incidence of bronchogenic carcinoma. In some patients fibrosing alveolitis has been successfully treated by lung transplantation.

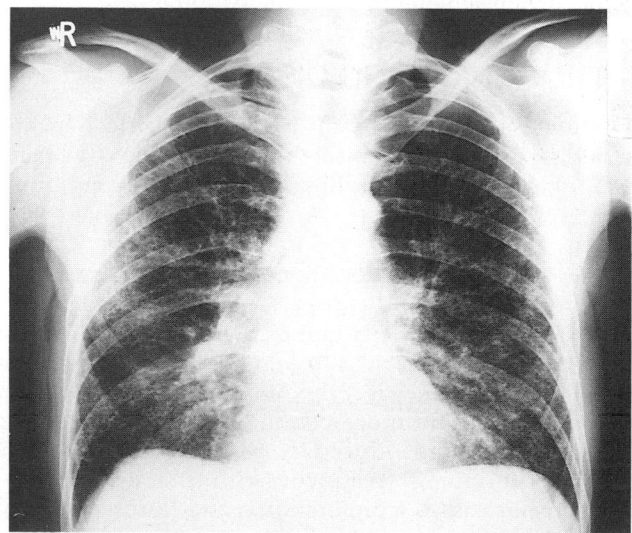

Fig. 13.49 Cryptogenic fibrosing alveolitis (CFA). Diffuse pulmonary fibrosis, with linear and nodular opacities throughout both lungs. In less severe CFA the radiological abnormalities are commonly maximal at the bases, with differential volume loss of the lower lobes.

13 Respiratory Disease

Honeycomb lung

This is a radiological description of a group of conditions that cause widespread cystic or 'honeycomb' appearances on chest X-ray. A 'honeycomb' appearance can be seen as the end stage of pulmonary fibrosis of any cause. Rare causes include Letterer-Siwe disease, tuberous sclerosis, Hand-Schuller-Christian disease, neurofibromatosis and eosinophilic granuloma. Patients with honeycomb lung tend to develop pneumothoraces. The long-term prognosis is poor, with respiratory and cardiac failure supervening.

Idiopathic pulmonary haemosiderosis

Idiopathic pulmonary haemosiderosis is a rare condition of unknown aetiology, characterised by recurrent episodes of intrapulmonary haemorrhage, pyrexia, haemoptysis and a secondary iron deficiency anaemia. Most cases occur in childhood; patients may die during an acute episode, but more commonly recurrent episodes eventually cause severe pulmonary fibrosis and respiratory failure. Some authorities consider that there is an association with Goodpasture's syndrome (p. 823). During acute episodes there may be crackles at the lung bases and occasionally hepatosplenomegaly. Chest X-ray during episodes of haemoptysis may show patchy, usually bilateral, shadowing in the middle zones. Management consists of treatment of the iron deficiency and corticosteroids and/or azathioprine during acute episodes, although their value is as yet unproven. At 3 years from diagnosis one-third of patients will have died, one-third will have active symptomatic disease and one-third will be symptom-free.

IATROGENIC LUNG DISEASE

There are a wide variety of drugs and physical agents, including oxygen and ionising radiation, which can cause temporary or permanent lung damage. The drugs most commonly responsible are cytotoxic agents (Table 13.44) (see also p. 139).

Bleomycin toxicity is commonest, occurring in 3–6% of patients treated with the drug; it is dose-dependent and there is increased toxicity in the elderly and in those who have received thoracic radiotherapy or combination chemotherapy. Likewise, the pulmonary side-effects of the *nitrosoureas* are more common in the elderly. The changes in the lung induced by *methotrexate* may resolve despite continuing treatment with the drug. *Cyclophosphamide* causes a pneumonitis and fibrosis that can respond remarkably well to corticosteroid therapy.

There are also a large number of non-cytotoxic drugs which can cause pulmonary toxicity (Table 13.45). The largest single group is antibiotics and the most common of these is nitrofurantoin. The antiarrhythmic agent amio-

Table 13.44 Cytotoxic drugs causing pulmonary toxicity

Drug	Toxic effects
Bleomycin	Interstitial pneumonitis Pulmonary fibrosis
Nitrosoureas	Interstitial fibrosis
Mitomycin	Pneumonitis and fibrosis
Busulphan	Diffuse pulmonary fibrosis
Methotrexate	Pneumonitis Blood eosinophilia
Cyclophosphamide	Interstitial fibrosis
Procarbazine	Pneumonitis Pleural effusion Blood eosinophilia
Chlorambucil	Pulmonary fibrosis
Melphalan	Pneumonitis Pulmonary fibrosis

Table 13.45 Non-cytotoxic drugs which cause pulmonary toxicity

Amiodarone	Neomycin
Nitrofurantoin	Ethionamide
Penicillin	Isoniazid
Erythromycin	Sulphonamides
Tetracycline	ACE inhibitors
Streptomycin	

darone is an important cause of pulmonary fibrosis. ACE inhibitors can cause a chronic dry cough.

Some antibiotics (e.g. penicillin, erythromycin, etc.) can cause acute asthma. Pulmonary eosinophilia is associated with drugs such as isoniazid and sulphonamides.

Radiation injury

Patients who receive radiation treatment to the thorax may sustain long-term lung injury. The acute injury is characterised pathologically by pulmonary vascular congestion, alveolar oedema and the formation of hyaline membranes. Patients become symptomatic at 4–8 weeks. This may progress, over a period of 6–12 months, to pulmonary fibrosis. Clinically, these processes cause a dry cough, chest wall pain and, depending on the extent of the damage, breathlessness. Radiation injury occurs most frequently in patients receiving treatment for carcinoma of the breast, lymphomas and carcinoma of the bronchus. The chest X-ray in the acute pneumonitis stage shows localised infiltration of the lung in the path of the radiation beam; when fibrosis has developed there is dense shadowing and volume loss. Symptoms and radiological appearances are poorly correlated; some patients with minor infiltrates may be severely dyspnoeic whilst others with widespread X-ray changes may be asymptomatic. Treatment with cortisteroids may be useful in the acute phase, but once fibrosis is established no treatment is effective.

Oxygen toxicity

The use of high levels of inspired oxygen causes lung injury indistinguishable from the adult respiratory distress syndrome (ARDS). The injury is related to both the inspired oxygen fraction (FiO$_2$) and the duration of exposure; a safe level has not yet been established but an FiO$_2$ of more than 0.7 over a period of more than several days may be associated with X-ray infiltrates and histological change. Toxic oxygen radicals (in particular superoxide anion, O$_2^-$) are thought to be important in oxygen-induced lung injury (see also ARDS below).

THE ADULT RESPIRATORY DISTRESS SYNDROME

The term adult respiratory distress syndrome (ARDS) is used to describe a pulmonary condition characterised by progressive hypoxaemia, chest X-ray infiltrates and reduced lung compliance in the presence of a normal left atrial pressure. In many respects the clinical presentation resembles the respiratory distress syndrome of the newborn, hence the name, but in view of its pathogenesis, 'non-cardiogenic pulmonary oedema' might be a more accurate and descriptive title. The condition occurs in

Table 13.46 Conditions associated with the adult respiratory distress syndrome

Shock (traumatic, septic, etc.)
Infection
Pneumonias (viral, bacterial, pneumocystis carinii)
Gram-negative sepsis
Trauma (fat emboli, head injuries, lung contusion)
Aspiration (gastric contents, fresh or salt water)
Drug overdose (narcotics, barbiturates)
Metabolic disorders (pancreatitis, uraemia)
Inhaled toxins (O$_2$, smoke, corrosives)
Blood disorders (disseminated intravascular coagulation, massive blood transfusion)
Miscellaneous
Paraquat ingestion
Radiation
Eclampsia
Raised intracranial pressure
Seizures
High altitude

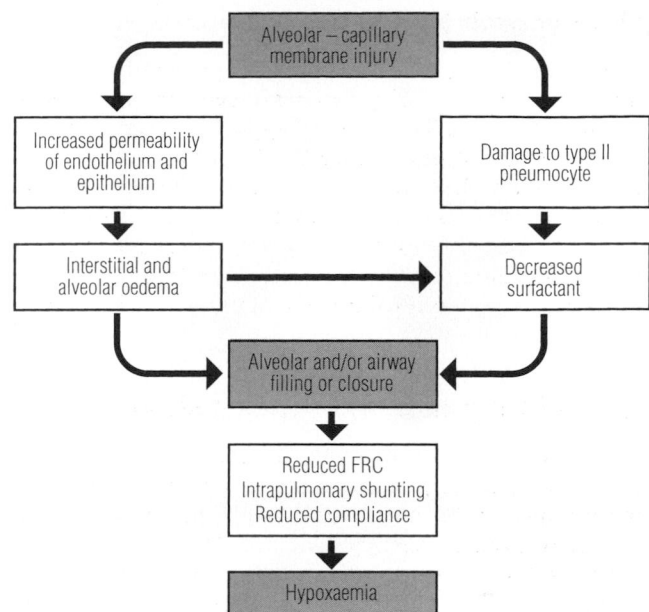

Fig. 13.50 Pathogenesis of the adult respiratory distress syndrome (ARDS). The many causes of ARDS have in common the damage of the alveolar–capillary membrane. The pathological changes that follow cause profound hypoxaemia (FRC = functional residual capacity).

response to a wide and seemingly unrelated variety of initiating events (Table 13.46).

The pathogenic mechanisms which produce the syndrome (Fig. 13.50) are due to diffuse damage to the pulmonary capillary endothelium, which results in increased 'leakiness' across the endothelial/epithelial barrier, resulting in the passage of plasma and red blood cells into the interstitial space, and thence into the alveoli, causing alveolar flooding. The mechanisms responsible for the capillary endothelial damage are poorly understood. Activation of complement with leucocytosis and release of lysosomal enzymes, and interactions between mediators such as leukotrienes, prostaglandins, neuropeptides and superoxides, are all considered to contribute. Damage is therefore due to a complex series of events involving cellular, chemical, neural and vascular responses, all combining to produce the clinical syndrome.

The clinical features are outlined in Table 13.47. A typical radiographic progression is shown in Figure 13.51.

Table 13.47 Clinical features of the adult respiratory distress syndrome

Initiating event	'Stiff lungs'
Dyspnoea and cough	Normal left heart pressures
Crackles over lung fields	With progression
Progressive hypoxaemia	Sepsis
	Failure of other organs
Chest X-ray infiltrates	(kidneys, liver, etc.)

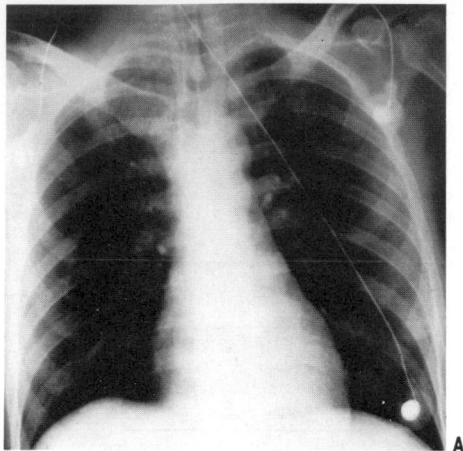

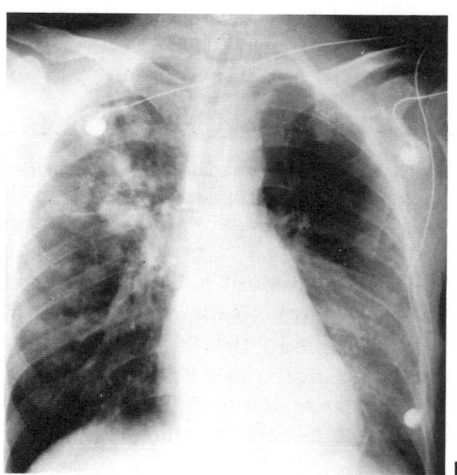

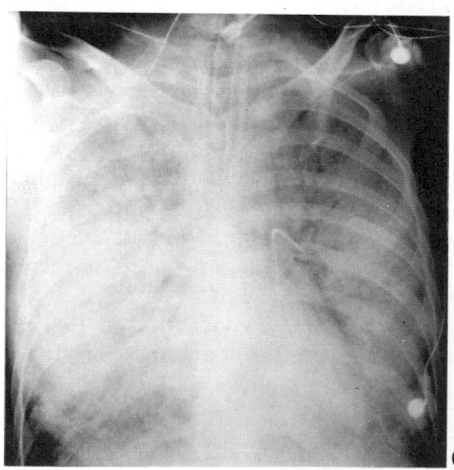

Fig. 13.51 Adult respiratory distress syndrome. The X-rays are of a young man who had sustained severe trauma and blood loss in a road traffic accident; the films cover a period of 5 days from a relatively normal X-ray (**A**), to bilateral infiltrates (**B**), to bilateral 'white-out' (**C**), accompanied by severe hypoxaemia. A Swan-Ganz catheter for measurement of pulmonary artery 'wedge' pressure (as a reflection of left atrial pressure) can be seen *in situ* on X-ray C. The patient died shortly after the last film.

Management

There are, as yet, no definite predictors as to which patients with the conditions listed in Table 13.46 will develop ARDS. However, the warning signs are *deteriorating gas exchange, worsening chest X-ray*, and, if the patient is being mechanically ventilated, *increasing inflation pressures* as the lungs become more 'stiff'. Early diagnosis and effective treatment can shorten the course, minimise the long-term sequelae and improve the prognosis of ARDS. Unfortunately, early treatment cannot salvage all patients, many of whom die despite vigorous therapy.

As measurements of pulmonary artery pressure, pulmonary artery wedge pressure and mixed venous O_2 content are critical, a Swan-Ganz catheter should be passed into the pulmonary artery (p. 536). For the diagnosis of ARDS to be secure, the clinical features of the disorder are combined with a normal pulmonary artery wedge pressure (normal PAWP = 8–12 cm H_2O).

Once the diagnosis of ARDS has been made the patient is usually so hypoxic that endotracheal intubation and mechanical ventilation is required.

The following aspects of the patient's therapy should be considered:

- fluid balance
- oxygenation
- drug therapy.

Fluid balance

Fluid balance is illustrated in Figure 13.52. The physician treating the patient with ARDS is faced with a dilemma. Excessive fluid administration may increase the pul-

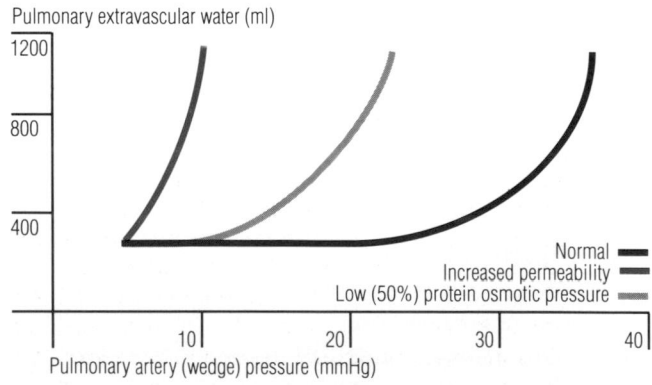

Fig. 13.52 The relationship of pulmonary extravascular water and pulmonary capillary pressure. In normal circumstances an increase in pulmonary extravascular water (and pulmonary oedema) does not occur until pulmonary artery 'wedge' pressure exceeds 3.3 kPa (25 mmHg). However, increased permeability (as in ARDS), and hypoalbuminaemia (common in intensive care unit patients) can cause pulmonary oedema at normal wedge pressures. (From Hopewell P C and Murray J F 1976 The adult respiratory distress syndrome. Annual Review of Medicine 27: 243–356.)

monary capillary hydrostatic pressure and thus cause further leakage of fluid into the lung interstitium and alveoli; if the patient is allowed to become fluid-depleted, however, systemic and pulmonary perfusion may be inadequate, causing renal and other organ damage. A reasonable approach is to administer sufficient fluid to maintain a PAWP of 6–8 cm H_2O, and if further circulatory support is required, to administer an inotropic agent such as dobutamine or isoprenaline. Fluid can be given in the form of 5% dextrose solution, or as a crystalloid, and if the patient is severely hypoalbuminaemic, intravenous salt-free albumin should be administered.

Oxygenation

The first step in improving arterial hypoxaemia is to add supplementary O_2. Very high concentrations of O_2 may be used initially (up to 100%) but these levels should not be sustained, as they may of themselves cause pulmonary damage. Steps must also be taken to minimise atelectasis, including:

- efficient removal of secretions by endotracheal suction and physical therapy
- the use of high tidal volumes on the ventilator (15 ml/kg body weight)
- occasional hyperinflation with 'sighs' may be of some value
- positive end expiratory pressure (PEEP).

PEEP has gained widespread acceptance as an effective method of ventilating patients with ARDS. Positive pressure (usually 5–15 cm H_2O) is applied at the end of expiration, thus preventing airway closure, limiting areas of atelectasis and reducing right-to-left shunting of blood through underventilated areas of lung. The net result of PEEP is usually an increase in PaO_2 without increasing the inspired O_2 concentration. However, PEEP is not without problems (see Ch. 14, p. 550). By increasing intrathoracic pressure it may reduce venous return to the heart and impair cardiac output. Inotropic support may be necessary, as is careful maintenance and monitoring of intravascular fluid volume. The higher the level of PEEP administered, the greater the risk of inducing barotrauma to the lung and pneumothorax. The optimum level of PEEP for individual patients can be determined by starting at low levels, say 5 cm H_2O, and working upwards in small increments, measuring at each level the effect of PEEP on gas exchange, lung compliance, cardiac output and mixed venous–arterial oxygen content difference (see p. 494).

Drug therapy

Sepsis, not respiratory failure, is now the commonest cause of death in patients with ARDS. Pulmonary and abdominal sepsis is particularly common. Steroids have little role in the treatment of ARDS and in some instances, particularly in septicaemic patients, they may be harmful.

Extracorporeal membrane oxygenation (ECMO) is a technique by which blood is continuously removed from the circulation, passed through a membrane oxygenator, and then returned. The results of controlled studies to date of ECMO in ARDS are discouraging and further technical advances are necessary before this can be considered a realistic option for treatment, except in a small number of selected patients.

The outlook for patients with ARDS remains poor. There is a 50–70% mortality, and if failure of an organ in addition to the lungs (e.g. the kidneys) supervenes, almost 100% of patients die. Of those who survive, most recover normal lung function; only a small proportion, usually those who have required ventilatory support for many weeks, develop bronchiectasis or pulmonary fibrosis.

LUNG TUMOURS

Carcinoma of the bronchus is one of the major causes of death in Western countries. In addition the lungs and mediastinum are common sites for metastatic malignant disease, with about 30% of cancer patients developing lung secondaries, in half of whom metastases are limited to the lungs. Intrathoracic disease is relatively common in Kaposi's sarcoma. By far the commonest primary lung tumour is bronchial carcinoma (Table 13.48).

BRONCHIAL CARCINOMA

In the 19th century bronchial carcinoma was unusual; by the mid-20th century, associated with the widespread habit of cigarette smoking, it reached epidemic proportions. In the UK, carcinoma of the bronchus is the commonest malignancy in males and is approaching the importance of breast cancer in females; in all, 35 000 patients die each year from this disease (p. 124).

The UK has a higher death rate from bronchial carcinoma than any other country in the world (p. 123). In America the incidence of the disease has reached a

Table 13.48 Relative frequency of primary pulmonary tumours

Tumour	%
Bronchial carcinoma	95
Alveolar carcinoma	1–2
Bronchial adenoma	1–2
Hamartoma	1
Other tumours	1

plateau; in the UK a plateau has been reached for males, but the number of female cases continues to rise.

Aetiology

Atmospheric pollution and industrial exposure to dusts, particularly asbestos, increase the incidence of lung cancer, but the dominant causative agent is tobacco smoke, which is responsible for 90% of cases. The disease is unusual in non-smokers and the increased incidence in smokers is related to the number of cigarettes consumed (Table 1.1, p. 4). The incidence in ex-smokers rapidly falls towards that of non-smokers. Passive smoking causes lung cancer in non-smokers and, in the UK, is responsible for approximately 300 deaths each year.

Pathology

Bronchial carcinomas are conventionally classified into four main histological groups (Table 13.49).

Squamous cell carcinoma

Squamous cell carcinomas are most common. The neoplastic epithelial cells produce keratin and frequently arise from major bronchi. The tumours are thought to originate in areas of squamous metaplasia which progress to carcinoma in situ and then to invasive carcinoma. Squamous tumours frequently cavitate; when peripheral they often invade the chest wall.

Adenocarcinomas

Adenocarcinomas arise both centrally and peripherally, from the bronchial epithelium or submucosal glands. They do not cavitate and their histology is characterised by tubules and gland-like structures, often producing mucin. Adenocarcinomas are related to cigarette consumption but also occur in non-smokers. There can be diagnostic diffi-

culty since an apparent primary tumour may prove to be a metastasis from a tumour of the gastrointestinal tract, kidney, ovary, pancreas, thyroid or breast.

Small cell carcinoma

Small cell carcinomas (oat cell) show differentiation into cells with amine-precursor uptake and decarboxylation (APUD) characteristics. Electron microscopy frequently shows neurosecretory granules. The malignant cells are small with little cytoplasm and dark, often oval nuclei. The tumours are usually central, highly invasive and disseminate rapidly. They secrete a wide range of hormones, particularly ADH and ACTH.

Large cell (undifferentiated) carcinoma

Large cell undifferentiated tumours constitute a heterogeneous group including giant-cell and clear-cell carcinomas, the cells of which show no evidence of maturation. They frequently arise centrally, invade the mediastinum and disseminate widely.

Studies of the natural history of bronchial carcinoma and analysis of the time taken for tumours to double in size suggest that by the time a tumour can be diagnosed it may have been present for many years, and has frequently metastasised (Table 13.49).

Clinical features

Symptoms of local disease

Bronchial carcinomas frequently arise in major bronchi, and therefore common problems include cough, haemoptysis, breathlessness, wheeze and stridor. Some patients have diffuse, poorly localised chest pain, and many have chest infections. Of these symptoms, haemoptysis, progressive breathlessness and persistent respiratory infection are the most important.

Haemoptysis

There are many causes of haemoptysis (Table 13.3, p. 451), but in a middle-aged or elderly smoker, carcinoma must always be excluded. A normal chest X-ray is unusual in bronchial carcinoma, but does not exclude a tumour.

Breathlessness

This is common in smokers who have developed generalised airways obstruction but progression is usually gradual and accelerated breathlessness commonly occurs as a tumour narrows a major airway. Such narrowing may produce a localised wheeze and occasionally stridor if the trachea or major bronchi are affected. Breathlessness may

Table 13.49 Natural history of untreated lung cancer*

Histology	%	Doubling time (days)	Years from malignant change to:		
			Earliest dignosis (1 cm)	Usual dignosis (3 cm)	Death (10 cm)
Squamous	35	88	7.2	8.4	9.6
Adenocarcinoma	21	161	13.2	15.4	17.6
Large cell undifferentiated	19	86	7.1	8.2	9.4
Small (oat) cell	25	29	2.4	2.8	3.2

*From Geddes D M 1979 The natural history of lung cancer: a review based on rates of tumour growth. Br. J. Dis. Chest. 73: 1–17.

also be due to the accumulation of a malignant pleural effusion or the development of lymphangitis.

Chest infections

These are not uncommon in chronic heavy smokers and usually resolve quickly when treated with antibiotics. When infection occurs distal to a tumour, however, it frequently persists or relapses. For this reason failure of a pneumonia to resolve is a common presentation of bronchial carcinoma.

Symptoms due to intrathoracic infiltration

The common sites of local infiltration and associated clinical problems are shown in Figure 13.53.

Extrathoracic metastasis

In bronchial carcinoma general symptoms such as lethargy, anorexia and weight loss frequently signify disseminated disease. The most important sites of secondary spread are liver, bone and brain, but virtually all parts of the body can be affected. In small cell carcinoma the bone marrow is involved in 10–20% of patients presenting with advanced disease and can produce a leuco-erythroblastic anaemia, but in most patients any anaemia is due to the non-specific effects of malignancy (Fig. 24.16, p. 1070).

Non-metastatic manifestations

Endocrine and metabolic changes occur in 10–15% of cases but cause symptoms much less frequently.

Hypercalcaemia

Hypercalcaemia (p. 729) occurs in 6–7% of tumours. In some cases of squamous carcinoma this is due to the production of parathyroid hormone-related peptide elab-

orated by the tumour. In most patients hypercalcaemia is due to extensive bone metastases.

Hyponatraemia

The secretion of ADH-like peptides is nearly always associated with small cell cancer, and is a feature in 10% of such tumours (p. 847). It results in a dilutional hyponatraemia.

Cushing's syndrome

The ectopic production of ACTH-like peptides by small cell tumours is common but only occasionally causes symptoms (1% of all cases) (p. 702).

Clubbing

Clubbing (Fig. 13.8, p. 452) is most frequently seen with squamous cell carcinoma (more than 50%) and is unusual in small cell tumours. Occasionally clubbed patients have hypertrophic pulmonary osteoarthropathy (HPOA) (p. 7).

Neurological manifestations

These are not common (less than 2%) and most frequently complicate small cell carcinoma. They are described on page 977. Neurological manifestations can predate any obvious tumour. They may remit spontaneously but usually progress and, except for rare cases, are little affected by treatment of the associated tumour.

Diagnosis

Carcinoma of the bronchus is so common and has such a variety of symptoms and signs that it should be considered in most heavy smokers presenting to a general physician. Diagnosis is usually straightforward and the first important investigation is a chest X-ray. Indeed, 5% of cases are discovered when a chest X-ray has been taken for unrelated reasons. In a smoker, clubbing, haemo-

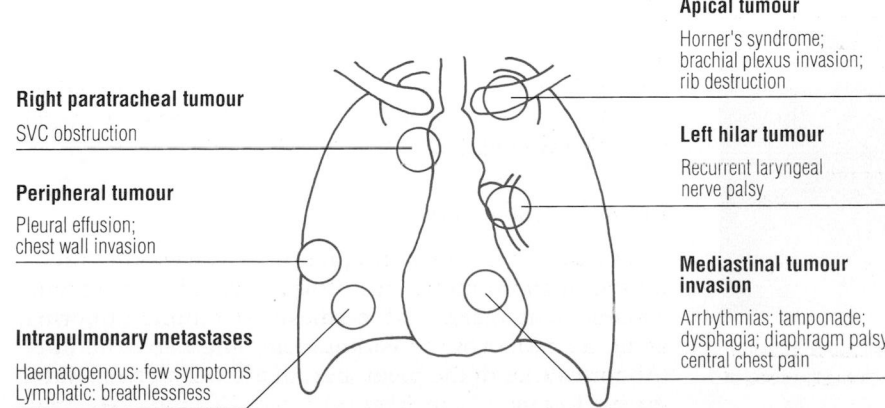

Fig. 13.53 Symptoms and signs of intrathoracic tumour invasion and metastases.

ptysis, persistent chest infection or weight loss demand an immediate X-ray of the chest.

Common radiological abnormalities

Unilateral hilar enlargement

Unilateral hilar enlargement (Fig. 13.54) is due to tumour and, frequently, involved lymph nodes. The hilum appears more dense than the opposite side, and the outer border of the hilum is frequently convex. Phrenic nerve invasion produces unilateral elevation of the diaphragm, and left recurrent laryngeal nerve involvement produces vocal cord paralysis with hoarseness.

Peripheral solid tumour mass

The tumour may be seen as a nodule, a large rounded mass or an irregular density (Fig. 13.55). Streaky shadows often extend into the surrounding lung, particularly towards the hilum, which may be abnormally bulky due to lymphadenopathy.

Peripheral cavitating tumour mass

A peripheral cavitating tumour mass is characteristic of squamous cell carcinomas. The cavitation is due to

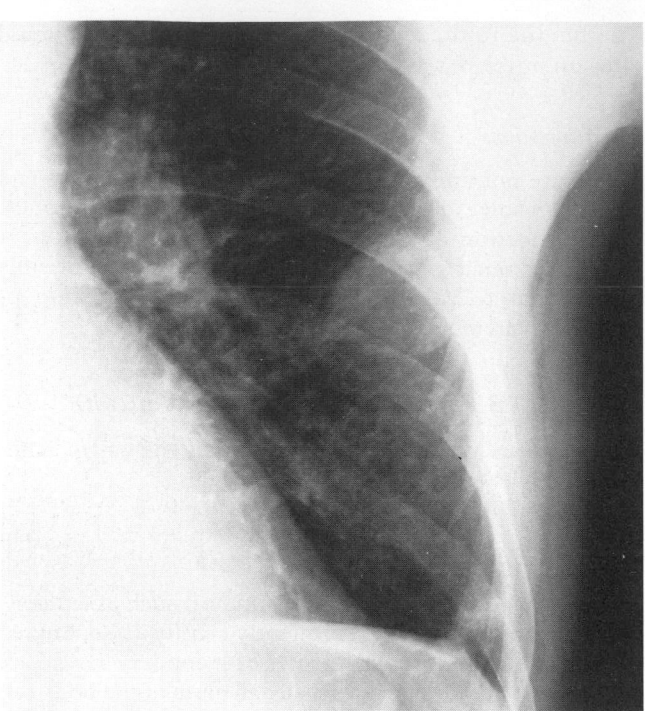

Fig. 13.55 Carcinoma of the bronchus: peripheral (squamous cell) carcinoma. The left hilum is enlarged due to adenopathy. Most pulmonary mass lesions more than 4 cm diameter are malignant tumours.

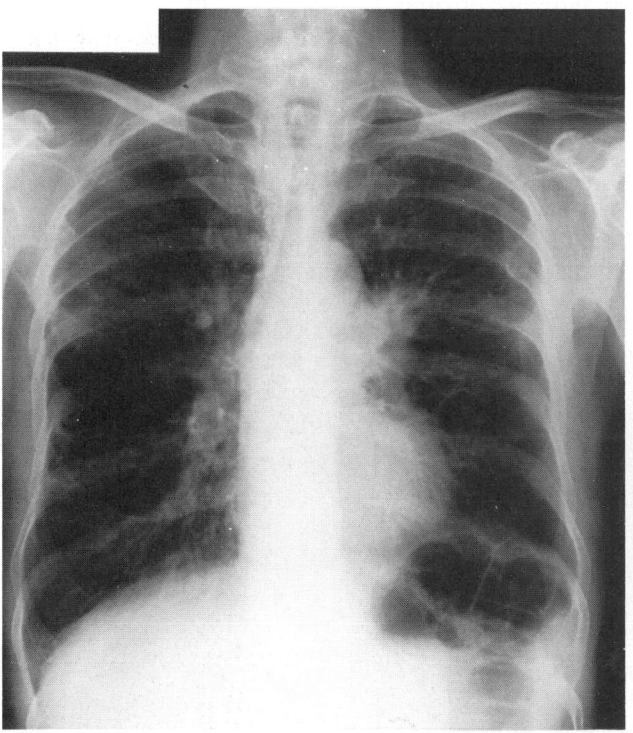

Fig. 13.54 Carcinoma of the bronchus. The left hilum is enlarged and more dense than the right. There are strands radiating from the hilum and this spiculated appearance is typical of tumour.

necrosis within the tumour and the cavity wall is irregular and thick. However, a certain diagnosis is not possible on radiological criteria alone, and the differential diagnosis can include tuberculosis, lung abscess (Fig. 13.23), pulmonary infarction complicated by infection, vasculitic lesions and a rheumatoid nodule. Sometimes cavitation occurs in the consolidated lung distal to an obstructing tumour.

Volume loss/collapse

Bronchial carcinoma frequently arises in a major bronchus and gradually narrows the airway, leading to volume loss in a lung or lobe on the chest X-ray. Volume loss is therefore a critically important radiological sign, particularly if progressive. Eventually the tumour causes collapse of a lobe or lung, producing an opacity on the chest X-ray (Fig. 13.11).

Abnormal mediastinum

Bronchial carcinoma frequently involves the mediastinum, and tumour infiltration as well as lymph node enlargement makes the mediastinal outline abnormal (Fig. 13.56). This is common in small cell tumours. Abnormalities of the mediastinum are well demonstrated by a CT scan.

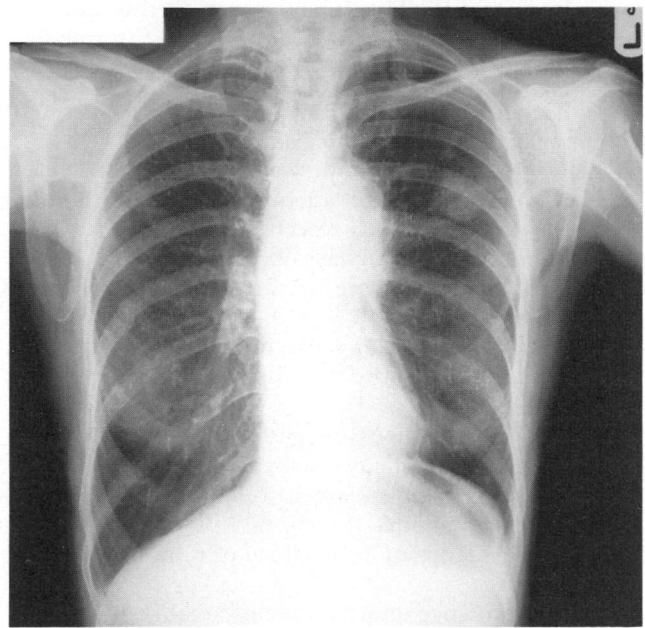

Fig. 13.56 Carcinoma of the bronchus. Central (small cell) carcinoma, lateral and inferior to the aortic knuckle. The usual outline of the aortic knuckle and configuration of the left hilar structures are lost. There is a secondary deposit in the left mid-zone.

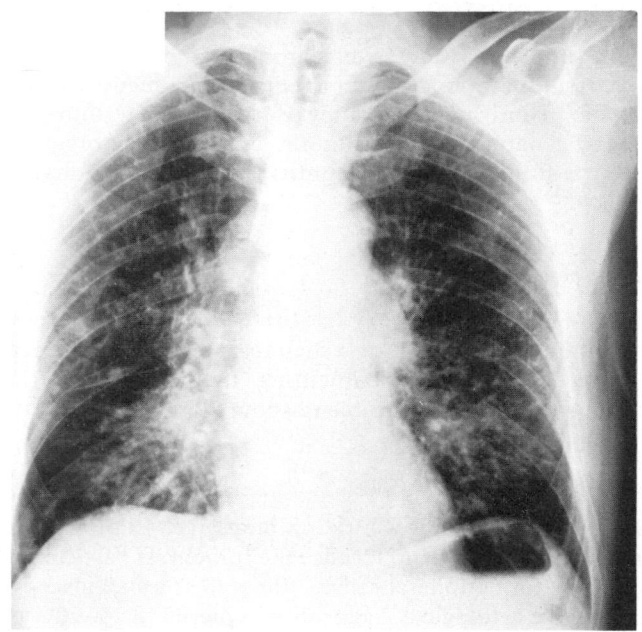

Fig. 13.57 Carcinoma of the bronchus: lymphangitis carcinomatosa. There are widespread linear and nodular opacities due to lymphatic infiltration. Basal septal lines are radiologically similar to those seen in left heart failure. Patients with lymphangitis usually have severe breathlessness.

Lymphatic invasion

The widespread involvement of the pulmonary lymphatics by tumour produces lymphangitis carcinomatosa (Fig. 13.57). This also occurs in malignant tumours of the stomach, pancreas and breast. Lymphatic invasion is well demonstrated by CT scans.

Apical (Pancoast) tumour

Apical tumours frequently invade the ribs, sympathetic chain (Horner's syndrome, p. 868), brachial plexus and chest wall (Fig. 13.58). Apical tumours are well seen on CT scans or MRI.

Pleural effusion

A common radiological manifestation of bronchial carcinoma at presentation is a pleural effusion, usually of large volume, which rapidly re-accumulates following aspiration, is commonly blood-stained and often contains malignant cells.

Confirmation of diagnosis

In addition to confirming the diagnosis, a knowledge of tumour cell type affects treatment; chemotherapy is frequently appropriate in small cell cancer but seldom useful in non-small cell disease.

Summary 7 Common radiological abnormalities in bronchial carcinoma

- Unilateral hilar enlargement
- Peripheral solid tumour mass
- Peripheral cavitating tumour mass
- Volume loss/collapse affecting a lobe or lung
- Abnormal mediastinum
- Lymphatic invasion
- Apical (Pancoast) tumour
- Pleural effusion

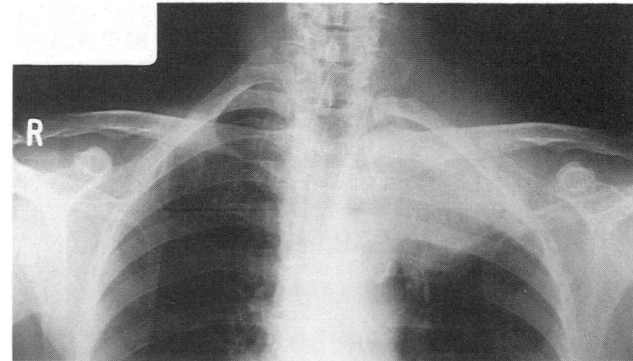

Fig. 13.58 Carcinoma of the bronchus: apical (Pancoast) tumour. The left first rib has been destroyed and there is a soft-tissue mass, due to metastatic nodes, in the supraclavicular fossa.

Sputum cytology

This simple, non-invasive technique can produce a positive result in up to 40% of patients. Sometimes the investigation confirms malignancy, but fails to determine the specific nature of the tumour. Similarly, cytology of pleural fluid will usually confirm a diagnosis of malignancy.

Bronchoscopy

Fibre-optic bronchoscopy (p. 461) is the most important technique for confirming a diagnosis of bronchial carcinoma (as well as documenting the location of the tumour). A tumour is visible in about 70% of cases.

Needle aspiration lung biopsy

Percutaneous needle aspiration biopsy (p. 463), with X-ray or CT screening to localise the tumour, is particularly effective for peripheral lesions not seen at bronchoscopy. A positive cytological diagnosis is achieved in 75–90% of patients with tumours.

Surgical biopsy

In a small number of patients, surgical biopsy is necessary to establish a diagnosis. Mediastinoscopy and mediastinotomy allow biopsy of tumour within the mediastinum (see p. 463), and thoracotomy gives access for lung and pleural biopsy. The pleura can also be inspected and tumour biopsied under direct vision using a thoracoscope.

Staging notation for lung cancer

Following diagnosis, patients can be staged according to the extent of their disease (Table 8.6, p. 131). In general, only patients with stage I disease are suitable for surgery.

The tumour, node, metastasis (TNM) system is surgically based and is useful for non-small cell lung cancer. In small cell carcinoma a categorisation into 'limited' disease (disease confined to one hemithorax) and extensive disease is made.

Management of lung cancer

Surgery

The overall results of surgery are not good, with a 5-year survival of about 25%, but surgery represents almost the only possibility of cure in non-small cell lung cancer. The critical question to be asked for each new patient with bronchial carcinoma is, 'Can this patient be cured by surgery?' The final answer to this question depends in turn on the answer to several intermediate questions:

1. Is the patient's general health good?
   Coronary artery disease is common.
   Elderly patients seldom do well.
2. Is pulmonary function adequate to cope with major surgery and pulmonary resection?
   Most patients have airways obstruction.
   An FEV_1 of less than 1.5 litres usually precludes pneumonectomy.
   How much 'useful' lung is to be resected?
3. What is the site of the tumour: is surgery technically feasible?
4. What is the tumour histology?
   Small cell carcinoma is usually disseminated.
   Most favourable histology is well differentiated squamous cell carcinoma.
5. Is there evidence of local spread of tumour within the thorax?
6. Is there evidence of distant metastases?

Patients with pulmonary hypertension, hypoxia and hypercapnia should not be operated upon, and those with excessive sputum production often develop postoperative chest infections. Static lung function can be misleading and information on exercise tolerance is helpful. For most cases this information is as easily obtained by the physician walking up the stairs with the patient as by formal exercise testing.

In addition to pulmonary function tests the contribution of the lung that will be resected can be obtained by perfusion and ventilation lung scans, and the postoperative FEV_1 and VC can be predicted from such information.

Recurrent laryngeal nerve invasion, malignant pleural effusion, chest wall involvement, superior vena caval obstruction, pericardial involvement, mediastinal lymph node spread and metastasis to the contralateral lung all preclude surgery. In considering surgery, assessment for mediastinal spread is critical. CT scanning can be helpful; a negative scan usually indicates that the mediastinum is clear, but a scan may demonstrate enlarged nodes that are subsequently found to be due to reactive hyperplasia rather than tumour. These cases may require surgical assessment of the mediastinum.

The relatively poor results of surgery in bronchial carcinoma reflect the widespread and early metastases so common in this disease. Prior to surgery, biochemical tests may reveal abnormal liver function, and liver secondaries can be confirmed by ultrasound or CT scan. Unfortunately, available tests for detecting metastases, particularly those in the liver, frequently fail to pick up tumour deposits. A raised alkaline phosphatase may reflect bone secondaries which can be confirmed by bone scan. CNS symptoms or signs indicate the need for a CT brain scan to exclude cerebral metastases.

Results of surgical therapy

Extent of disease, size of tumour, cell type, age of patient and the operation performed all affect the results from surgery (Fig. 13.59). Although the overall survival rates with surgery of 25% at 5 years and 17% at 10 years are poor, some patient groups do relatively well. Young, fit patients who have a lobectomy for stage I squamous cell carcinoma have a 5-year survival of 55–60%.

Chemotherapy

The results of chemotherapy for non-small cell tumours not suitable for surgery are very poor and chemotherapy is largely reserved for the treatment of small cell lung cancer. Small cell tumours can respond dramatically to multiple drug chemotherapy. The drugs in common use include ifosfamide, cyclophosphamide, vincristine, adriamycin and etoposide.

Treatment is given at 3–4 weekly intervals over a period of several months. A complete response to therapy with a return to normal of the chest X-ray and disappearance of tumour at bronchoscopy can be achieved in 25–50% of patients. Small cell tumours are rarely completely eradicated, however, and the tumours rapidly relapse. Chemotherapy increases the overall median survival from approximately 4 months without drug therapy, to 11 months with treatment (Fig. 8.11, p. 132). Approximately 10% of those patients with limited disease will continue symptom- and disease-free for 2 or 3 years. In general patients with least tumour bulk and good general health have the best prognosis. The great reduction of tumour mass following treatment can produce dramatic symptomatic improvement, often following only

two or three courses of drugs. Therapy can relieve breathlessness due to airways obstruction by tumour, bone pain due to metastatic disease, superior vena caval obstruction and haemoptysis.

Chemotherapy is well tolerated by most patients, but avoiding the problems of nausea and infection due to marrow suppression requires careful attention to detail. A few more patients may achieve long-term survival if radiotherapy is combined with chemotherapy. However, the outlook for small cell carcinoma remains poor and is unlikely to be substantially improved until better chemotherapeutic agents become available.

Radiotherapy

In bronchial carcinoma the principal purpose of radiotherapy is to produce symptomatic relief. Radiotherapy is particularly good at controlling bone pain, haemoptysis, superior vena caval obstruction and breathlessness due to narrowing of major airways. Following complete collapse of a lobe or lung, radiotherapy is less effective. Cerebral metastases often respond, albeit temporarily, to radiotherapy, with concomitant steroid therapy to control cerebral oedema. In carefully selected patients, radiotherapy can produce impressive results. For small, localised, well differentiated, particularly squamous cell, tumours in generally fit patients who are frequently not suitable for surgery because of poor lung function, it is possible to achieve a 5-year survival of up to 17% following radical high-dose radiotherapy. Survival in localised small cell carcinoma is not greatly extended by radiotherapy alone, but tumour bulk can be dramatically reduced with consequent excellent control of symptoms. In patients with small cell carcinoma who respond well to chemotherapy, prophylactic cranial irradiation can largely prevent the distressing development of symptomatic cerebral metastases.

Endobronchial therapy

In carefully selected patients with obstruction of major airways, not amendable to chemotherapy or external irradiation, symptomatic relief can be achieved by a variety of endobronchial therapies; including endoscopic laser destruction of tumour, endobronchial radiotherapy and tracheobronchial stenting.

Advanced bronchogenic carcinoma

As with all malignant disease, patients with advanced bronchogenic carcinoma which is no longer responding to treatment require much medical nursing and social support during their last months of life. Support of the patient's family is also important. The large

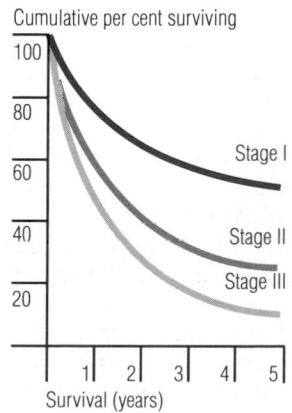

Fig. 13.59 Survival following surgical resection for non-small cell carcinoma of the bronchus.

number of patients dying of lung cancer represents an important challenge to hospitals, general practice, community terminal care teams and hospices. The future burden of lung cancer in countries that have only relatively recently adopted high levels of cigarette smoking will become a huge health care problem.

Pain is a particularly troublesome symptom and radiotherapy may be required for its control. Pain may also require regular analgesics, particularly oral morphine. For intractable pain peripheral nerve blockade may be necessary. Morphine helps reduce the sensation of breathlessness. Poor appetite and lethargy can temporarily be alleviated by steroids, which may also improve the symptoms from cerebral secondaries for a few weeks or months. Weakness, immobility, poor food intake and analgesics all contribute to constipation. In the last weeks of life, pain, constipation, anxiety, breathlessness and weakness can greatly reduce the quality of life. Frequent assessment of the patient's needs is necessary. In this respect the family doctor's contribution is of great importance and the domiciliary terminal care team are able to provide a regular assessment in the patient's home.

ALVEOLAR CARCINOMA

This is an unusual tumour with distinctive pathological and clinical features. It constitutes 1–2% of primary pulmonary tumours. The sexes are equally affected and the tumour occurs in all races. Alveolar carcinoma is most common in patients above the age of 50, and is not related to smoking tobacco.

Pathology

Alveolar carcinoma often arises within a damaged area of lung. Histologically the characteristic feature is malignant cells growing along the alveolar walls. On light microscopy it may be difficult to distinguish alveolar cell from primary or secondary adenocarcinoma. The good prognosis for resection of early single nodule disease suggests that in most cases multinodular disease represents spread of tumour rather than simultaneous multiple foci.

Clinical features

The presenting symptoms of alveolar carcinoma are similar to other tumours although, because the tumour is not endobronchial, haemoptysis, bronchial obstruction and distal infection are less common. When the tumour mass is large or affecting both lungs, patients become very breathless. In a few cases patients produce large volumes of clear, watery sputum (bronchorrhoea). The chest X-ray usually shows a single, irregular peripheral shadow sometimes resembling pneumonic consolidation, fre-

quently with an air bronchogram within the tumour opacity. Cavitation is uncommon, but effusions occur. Multiple tumour opacities develop, initially within one, and then within both lungs (Fig. 13.60).

Diagnosis

Malignant cells can be detected in the sputum in some cases, but the distinction from adenocarcinoma is frequently not possible. Bronchscopy and bronchial biopsy are usually negative although transbronchial biopsy can provide a diagnosis. Diagnosis can be achieved by needle aspiration biopsy or more frequently by surgical biopsy at thoracotomy. Diffuse and multiple lesions are often initially thought to be infective but failure to respond to antibiotic therapy raises suspicion of the true diagnosis.

Management

Alveolar carcinoma is often relatively slow growing, and disseminated metastatic disease is less common than in other pulmonary tumours. Surgical resection is therefore the treatment of choice whenever possible, and good results can be achieved with a 5-year survival of 50% for localised disease. More extensive disease has a poor prognosis and is difficult to treat, the tumour being resistant to chemotherapy and radiotherapy.

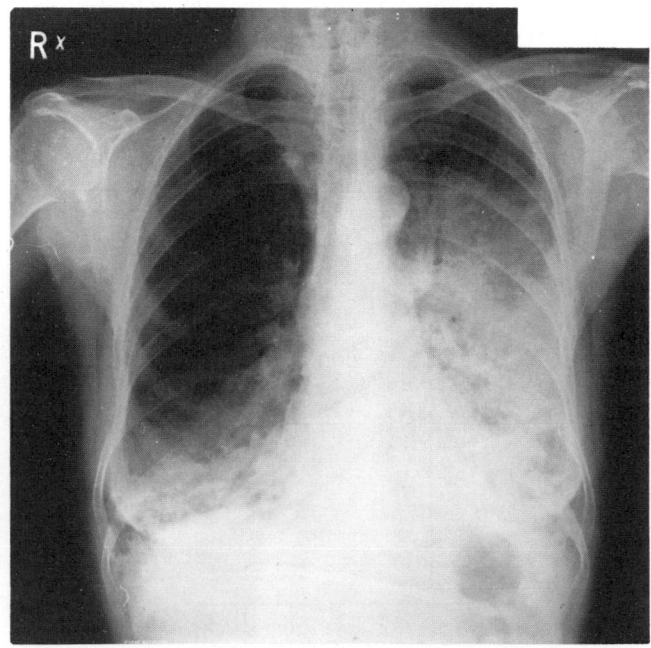

Fig. 13.60 Alveolar cell carcinoma of the lung. The appearances of 'consolidation' are common with this carcinoma. Bilateral disease is also common.

BRONCHIAL ADENOMA

The term 'adenoma' covers a variety of tumours, approximately 90% of which are carcinoid tumours arising from cells of the APUD series. The diagnosis is often made in young adults and the sexes are equally affected. These tumours are endobronchial, usually arising in larger airways, causing airway narrowing, volume loss, collapse and distal infection. Common clinical features are cough, haemoptysis, breathlessness, unilateral wheeze and recurrent infections. Most tumours are of low-grade malignancy and symptoms may be present for a long period before a diagnosis is made. Wheezing dyspnoea may lead to a mistaken diagnosis of asthma. Some tumours become malignant and occasionally (2% of cases) the patients develop the carcinoid syndrome (p. 585). It is important to note that tumour is not usually visible on the chest X-ray and the most common radiological abnormality is volume loss or lobar collapse. Diagnosis is frequently made at bronchoscopy, where 90% of these tumours are visible. The tumour is vascular and bleeds easily and profusely. Rigid bronchoscopy for biopsy is sensible if at fibre-optic bronchoscopy the appearances suggest an adenoma. The best treatment whenever possible is surgical resection, and the prognosis for these tumours is good unless there has been malignant change.

HAMARTOMA

Hamartomas are tumour-like malformations of disorganised tissue; in some the predominant tissue is cartilage, and in others smooth muscle. Unlike carcinoid tumours, hamartomas usually present over the age of 50. Males are three times more likely to be affected than females. Hamartomas are usually peripheral within the lung parenchyma and seldom within the bronchus. They grow slowly and are benign. Most hamartomas are asymptomatic and are incidental findings on chest X-ray. The mass of the hamartoma is usually small, less than 4 cm in diameter, rounded, well defined and sometimes calcified (Fig. 13.61). Cavitation is rare. In most cases in the absence of typical calcification, and without the benefit of past chest X-rays, a malignant bronchial carcinoma will be part of the differential diagnosis and the correct treatment will be surgical excision. At surgery the hamartoma is felt to be hard, can be removed without resecting lung, and the prognosis is excellent.

THE SOLITARY PULMONARY NODULE

A common diagnostic and management problem arises when the chest X-ray, frequently a 'routine' investigation, shows a solitary pulmonary nodule (Table 13.50 and Fig. 13.62). The larger the lesion, the more likely it is to be malignant; lesions greater than 4 cm in diameter

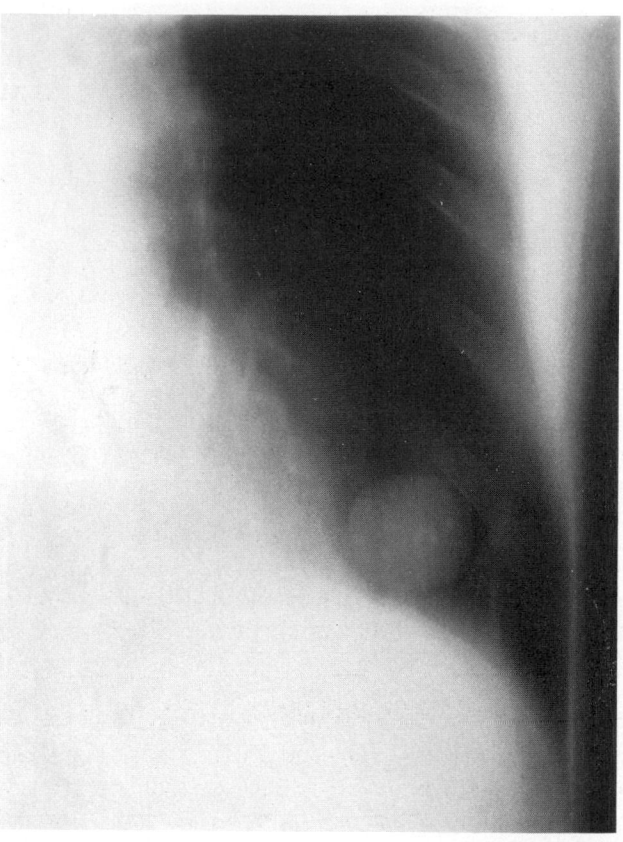

Fig. 13.61 Pulmonary hamartoma. Tomogram of a hamartoma in the left lower lobe; note the smooth rounded appearance and flecks of calcification.

Table 13.50 Causes of a solitary pulmonary nodule

Malignant (40%)	
Bronchogenic carcinoma	(25%)
Alveolar carcinoma	(3%)
Bronchial adenoma	(2%)
Metastasis	(10%)
Benign (60%)	
Infectious granuloma	(50%)
Non-infective granuloma	(2%)
Benign tumour	(2%)
Other rare causes	(6%)

are usually malignant; those less than 8 mm are usually benign.

Management

Resection of a single malignant nodule results in surgical cure for more than 60% of patients. Because 40% of all nodules are malignant, surgery should be considered in all patients who are fit for tumour resection, unless there is compelling evidence that the nodule is non-malignant.

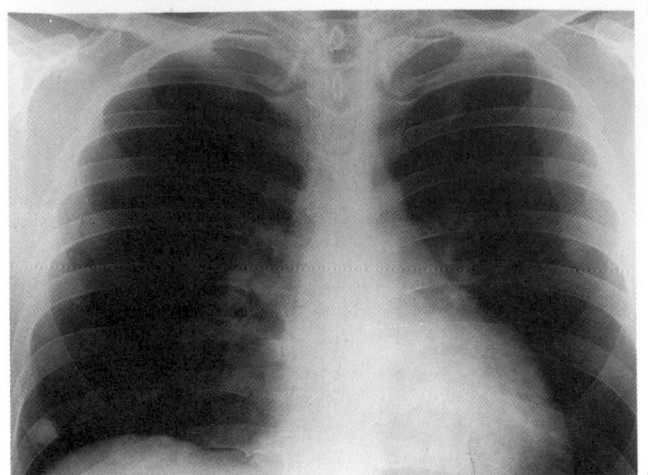

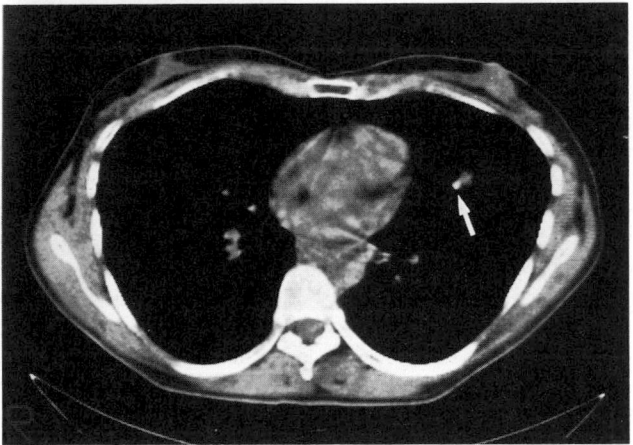

Fig. 13.62 The 'solitary pulmonary nodule'. A. Small peripheral 'solitary pulmonary nodule' in the right lower lobe. **B.** When there is doubt, calcification is best demonstrated by CT scan.

Nodules that have not grown in size for 2 years or which show calcification (especially central, diffuse or speckled) within the nodule are likely to be benign. Solitary nodules in patients below the age of 35, especially non-smokers, are likely to be benign. The search for past X-rays is often the most rewarding investigation in these patients. Tomography may show calcification more easily. A CT scan may demonstrate multiple pulmonary metastases. Fibre-optic bronchoscopy is seldom helpful because the lesion cannot be seen endoscopically. Needle aspiration biopsy is much more useful, confirming malignancy in 75–90% of tumours. For some tumours and most benign lesions, the precise diagnosis is only revealed by surgical removal.

MEDIASTINAL TUMOURS

Mediastinal tumours are illustrated in Figure 13.63. *Metastatic malignant disease* is the most common cause of

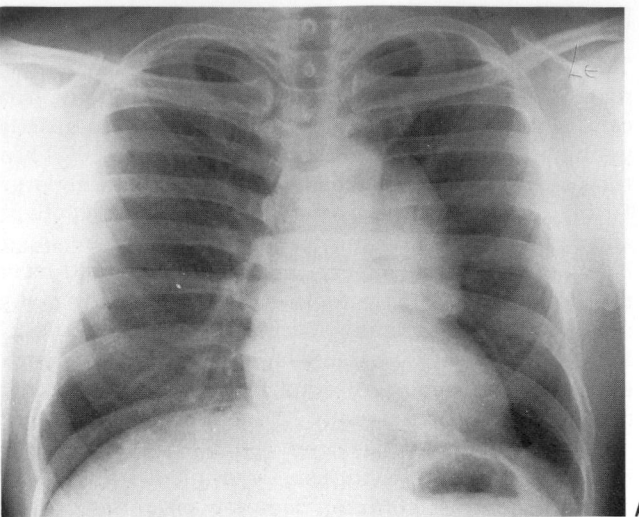

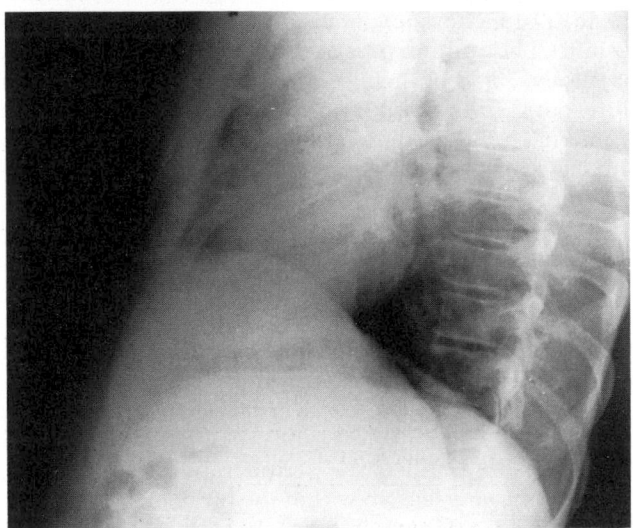

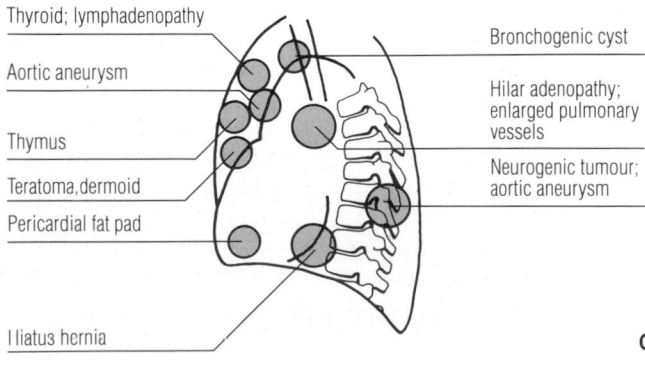

Thyroid; lymphadenopathy

Aortic aneurysm

Thymus

Teratoma, dermoid

Pericardial fat pad

Hiatus hernia

Bronchogenic cyst

Hilar adenopathy; enlarged pulmonary vessels

Neurogenic tumour; aortic aneurysm

Fig. 13.63 Mediastinal mass lesions. A. The chest X-ray demonstrates a mediastinal mass: the preservation of the silhouette of the descending aorta suggests that the mass is placed anteriorly. **B.** This is confirmed by the lateral chest X-ray: the retrosternal space, which is normally translucent, is opaque. The mass was a malignant thymoma. **C.** Location of the more common mediastinal masses.

a mediastinal mass, most frequently at the hilum. Lymphoma and sarcoidosis are common, with anterior mediastinal adenopathy favouring the former. In addition to the lateral chest X-ray, CT scanning is helpful in elucidating the nature of mediastinal masses; contrast studies demonstrate vascular lesions, and cystic lesions (usually benign) can be identified. Thyroid isotope scans confirm a retrosternal goitre. Solid, non-vascular lesions usually require biopsy for diagnosis (for example, the differential diagnosis of carcinoma, lymphoma and sarcoidosis) by needle aspiration biopsy, mediastinoscopy, mediastinotomy, or thoracotomy.

Neurogenic tumours are the most common cause of a posterior mediastinal mass. Symptoms arise from compression of local structures, a small proportion are malignant and treatment is surgical. Occasionally, a neurofibroma is associated with Von Recklinghausen's disease. *Dermoid cysts* arise from ectodermal tissue, whereas *teratomas* are germ cell tumours that contain ectodermal, mesodermal and endodermal tissue. These teratodermoid tumours arise in the anterior mediastinum, commonly of young adults. Dermoids are usually cystic and benign whereas teratomas are usually solid and malignant. Treatment is surgery to remove all or as much as possible of the tissue. In malignant cases, radiotherapy and chemotherapy may be necessary. *Thymomas* can be benign or malignant (about 25% of cases). Whereas many patients with thymoma have myasthenia gravis, only a minority of patients with myasthenia have a thymic tumour. Treatment of all thymomas is surgical excision and, for malignant cases, postoperative radiotherapy.

PLEURAL DISEASE

The visceral pleura, composed of a layer of mesothelial cells supported on connective tissue rich in lymphatics and blood vessels, covers the lung. The parietal pleura lines the thoracic cavity, covers the diaphragm and meets the visceral pleura at the hilum. The visceral pleura has no pain fibres, whereas irritation of the parietal pleura induces the pain characteristic of pleurisy. Normally, the two pleural layers are adjacent to one another, separated by a thin film of fluid, continually formed at the parietal and drained at the visceral pleural surface. As a consequence of the elastic property of the lung, the pressure within the pleural space is negative, approximately −5 cm H$_2$O at resting end-expiration.

PLEURAL EFFUSION

Water and electrolytes from the pleural space are taken up by the visceral pleura and cleared by the pulmonary and systemic (bronchial) circulation, whereas the proteins of pleural fluid are mainly cleared via the lower mediastinal lymphatics. Excess fluid accumulates within the pleural space when visceral or parietal pleural capillary pressure is raised (e.g. left or right heart failure); when capillary permeability is increased (e.g. infection); and when lymphatic drainage is decreased (e.g. lymphatic invasion by tumour). The turnover of pleural water and electrolytes is rapid, even when a large effusion is present, hence the rapid response to diuretics of effusions due to cardiac failure. Protein turnover is less rapid, contributing to the slow clearance of effusions with high protein content. The accumulation of pleural fluid reduces the volume of the underlying lung, causing a restrictive ventilatory defect. Large effusions will lead to breathlessness, particularly if they develop rapidly, and, when unilateral, cause mediastinal shift.

Radiology

The history and particularly the clinical examination may suggest pleural fluid but the most helpful, simple investigation is a chest X-ray (Fig. 13.64). Radiology may suggest fluid but cannot determine its nature (e.g. a clear transudate, pus or blood). When there is doubt about pleural fluid a film taken in the lateral decubitus position will demonstrate pleural fluid adjacent to the lateral chest wall. Very small effusions are clearly seen on CT scanning. On occasions, pleural fluid becomes loculated and ultrasound is a simple technique for confirming that fluid is present and locating its position. The collection of fluid in the pleural space beneath the inferior surface of the lung (subpulmonic effusion) can mimic an elevated hemidiaphragm. A lateral decubitus X-ray or ultrasound examination confirms the diagnosis of a subpulmonic effusion.

Differential diagnosis

There are many causes of pleural effusion (Table 13.51). The accumulated fluid may be a *transudate*, as a consequence of alteration in the pressure relationships of the pleural space (as in cardiac failure); or it may be an *exudate*, as a result of increased capillary permeability (as in infection).

Transudates have a protein content of less than 3 g/dl, are clear or light yellow, and often bilateral. Exudates have more than 3 g/dl of protein, are dark yellow or orange in colour, often slightly cloudy, may clot on standing and are usually unilateral.

Transudates

Left heart failure, right heart failure, or a combination of both, are common causes of pleural effusion. Initially, the fluid may be unilateral, usually right-sided; when bilateral,

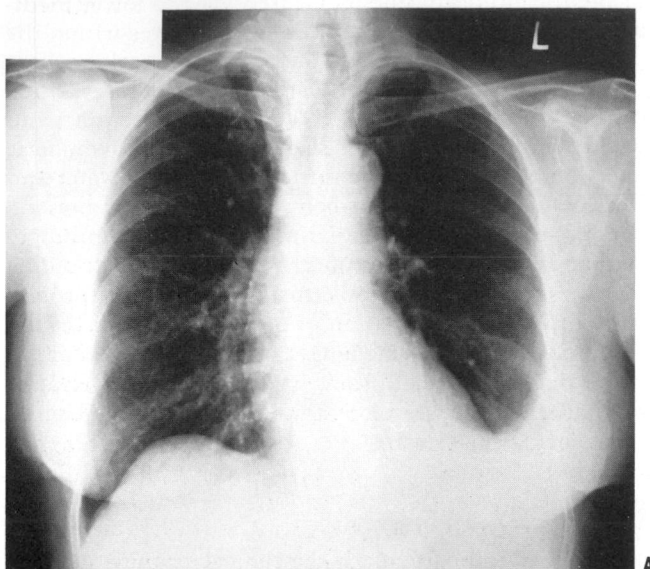

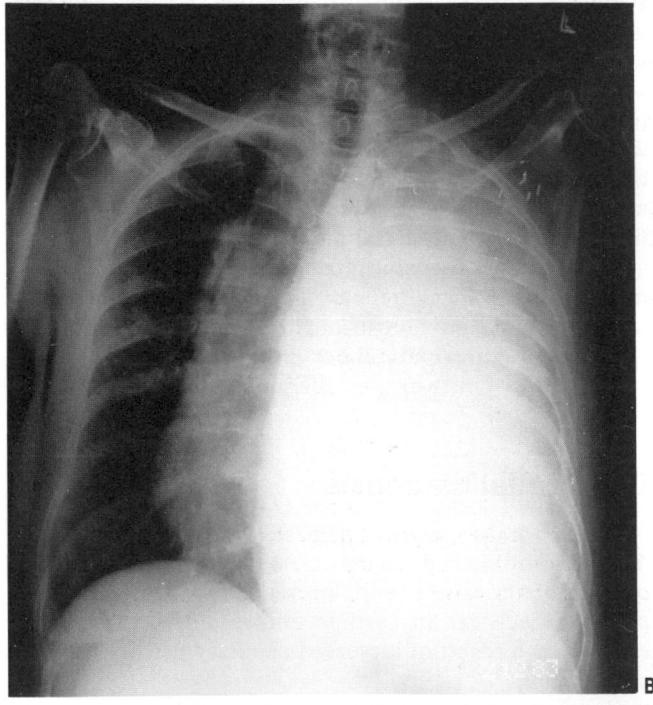

Fig. 13.64 Pleural effusion. A. Small left effusion. The left hemidiaphragm cannot be visualised and the fluid appears to rise laterally and medially: on a lateral chest X-ray it rises anteriorly and posteriorly. (The patient had the yellow nail syndrome.) **B.** Large effusion. Pleural fluid is homogeneous and without vascular markings or air bronchogram. The mediastinum is shifted to the right. Note the surgical clips in the left axilla. (The patient had metastatic pleural disease from breast carcinoma.)

the right effusion is usually larger than the left. In *constrictive pericarditis* the pleural effusions are less significant than the ascites. Any cause of *hypoalbuminaemia* may cause pleural effusion plus oedema and ascites; the nephrotic

Table 13.51 Causes of pleural effusion

Transudates (hydrothorax)
Cardiac failure
Hypoproteinaemia
Constrictive pericarditis
Myxoedema*

Peritoneal dialysis and ascites
(including Meigs' syndrome)
Superior vena cava obstruction

Exudates
Infections
Malignancy
Pulmonary infarction
Rheumatoid arthritis
Systemic lupus erythematosus
Acute rheumatic fever
Polyarteritis nodosa*
Scleroderma*
Dermatomyositis*
Postmyocardial infarction syndrome
Ovarian hyperstimulation

Pancreatitis
Subphrenic abscess
Asbestosis*
Familial Mediterranean fever
Hepatic and pulmonary hydatid
disease
Hepatic amoebiasis
Trauma
Drugs
Sarcoidosis*
Yellow nail syndrome
Radiotherapy*

Chylous effusion

Haemothorax

Iatrogenic
(e.g. misplaced subclavian infusion line)

* Denotes that it is unusual for that disease.

syndrome is often the cause. In *Meigs' syndrome* the pleural effusion is associated with ascites due to an ovarian tumour (usually a benign fibroma, occasionally malignant disease), and resolution occurs if the tumours are removed. Effusions can occur with *peritoneal dialysis* and *ascites*. The mechanism of the hydrothorax is the direct passage of fluid through the diaphragm into the pleural space. Small communications have been observed at postmortem in patients with hydrothorax and cirrhosis.

Exudates

Postinfective pleural effusions are most common with bacterial infections, particularly pneumococcal, and, if inadequately treated, may progress to an empyema. Even when not obviously purulent the fluid contains many polymorphonuclear leucocytes and is often associated with persistence of fever and leucocytosis.

Mycoplasma is rarely responsible. Effusions following *viral infections* occasionally occur, particularly as part of the pleuropericardial involvement of coxsackie B infections. Effusions have been described in glandular fever. Rarely, actinomycosis and other fungal infections can cause a pleural effusion. *Tuberculosis*, once a common cause of effusion, is now relatively unusual in the UK. An important aspect of diagnosis is pleural biopsy for histological examination and culture of the mycobacterium.

Malignant pleural effusion may be due to *primary pleural tumours*, most commonly mesothelioma (see below) and rarely a benign pleural fibroma. However, the most common cause is *metastatic pleural malignancy* from carcinoma of the bronchus, as well as breast, ovary and other extrathoracic tumours. Effusions, usually bilateral, may complicate *lymphangitis carcinomatosa* (p. 517). Occasionally, *lymphomas* involve the pleura. Involvement of ribs and adjacent parietal pleura by *myeloma* may produce a pleural effusion. It is characteristic of malignant effusions that they develop rapidly and recur quickly after aspiration; they are also commonly, though not invariably, blood-stained.

A pleural effusion is an important clinical feature of *pulmonary infarction* (p. 496).

Pleural effusion is relatively common in some of the *collagen vascular disorders* (p. 505). In SLE and MCTD pleurisy and pericarditis are not uncommon, particularly in young and middle-aged females. Aspirated fluid contains lymphocytes, occasionally lupus erythematosus cells and more often antinuclear factor and rheumatoid factor. In active *rheumatoid arthritis* 5% of patients have a pleural effusion (p. 998). Pleural effusions are rather uncommon in *polyarteritis nodosa, systemic sclerosis* and *dermatomyositis*. Acute *rheumatic fever* is complicated by pleural effusions, usually small, in 10% of cases, most of which also have pericarditis.

In the *postmyocardial infarction syndrome* pericarditis and fever develop several days or weeks after acute infarction, and occasionally there is also a pleural effusion. *Sarcoidosis* is a rare cause of pleural effusions. Recurrent, self-limiting effusions can be a feature of *familial Mediterranean fever* (familial paroxysmal polyserositis). In the *yellow nail syndrome* effusions are associated with a yellow discoloration of nails, plus lymphoedema and occasionally bronchiectasis and sinusitis. Lymphatic hypoplasia underlies the disorder and this is thought to explain the effusions. *Drugs* can cause pleurisy with effusions: hydralazine (as part of a lupus syndrome), nitrofurantoin, sulphonamides, PAS, methotrexate, practolol and methysergide have all been incriminated. *Radiotherapy* to the lung can produce a radiation pneumonitis and small bilateral effusions. Following *chest trauma* and *pulmonary contusion* a pleural effusion occasionally collects. However, a haemothorax must first be excluded.

Pathological processes below the diaphragm can cause pleural effusions, a common complication of *acute pancreatitis* when it is usually painless, left-sided and haemorrhagic. The pleural fluid has a high amylase concentration, higher than in the blood. Occasionally similar effusions are seen in patients with chronic pancreatitis or pancreatic pseudocysts.

Subphrenic abscess is frequently accompanied by a pleural effusion, most often on the right, with low lateral chest and shoulder pain as a consequence of diaphragm inflammation. On chest X-ray, in addition to the effusion, there may be elevation of the hemidiaphragm below which there is sometimes a fluid level. If treatment is delayed, an empyema develops. Prior antibiotic therapy may produce a chronic clinical picture.

Investigation of pleural fluid

Whenever there is doubt about the cause of an effusion, aspiration should be performed. Loculated or small effusions are best aspirated with ultrasound localisation.

Blood-stained effusions, rather than the frank blood of a haemothorax, are most common with malignancy but also occur in pulmonary infarction and following chest trauma. Rare causes of a bloody effusion include cirrhosis, tuberculosis and leukaemia. *Infected* pleural fluid is turbid and with advanced empyema becomes purulent. With a *chylous* effusion the fluid is a milky white colour.

Analysis of pleural fluid *protein* concentration broadly separates transudates (less than 3 g/dl) from exudates (more than 3 g/dl) but in a large number of cases borderline, unhelpful values are obtained.

Cytology is a key investigation, not simply for malignant cells. The presence of numerous polymorphonuclear leucocytes suggests bacterial infection; lymphocytes predominate in tuberculosis but are also common in any chronic effusion; *eosinophils* are numerous in the effusions of pulmonary eosinophilia, polyarteritis nodosa and Hodgkin's disease. Eosinophils can be the prominent cells following pulmonary infarction and may also accumulate following bleeding into the pleural space from any cause. Pneumonias and rheumatoid arthritis are less usual causes for an eosinophilic effusion. *Malignant* cells are identified in up to half of patients with tumour involving the pleura. *Bacteria* may be demonstrated in postpneumonic effusions, particularly in those progressing to empyema. In tuberculosis acid-fast bacilli are only occasionally identified but culture of pleural fluid for the mycobacteria is often useful.

In rheumatoid arthritis, the pleural fluid contains a characteristically very low concentration of glucose.

When pleural aspiration is not diagnostic; pleural biopsy should be performed. Biopsy is particularly helpful in malignant disease of the pleura and in tuberculosis.

Pleural biopsy

An Abrams' biopsy needle is most commonly used and the investigation should not normally be undertaken when there is no fluid present lest the biopsy needle puncture the visceral pleura. If the pleura is much thickened, biopsy with a cutting needle is safe even in the absence of fluid. Occasionally, diagnosis may require a large biopsy sample; for example, in mesothelioma a surgical biopsy is often indicated. Multiple biopsies increase the diagnostic yield and one of the biopsy samples should be sent to the laboratory for culture if a diagnosis of tuberculosis is possible.

Management

Infected pleural fluid should be promptly and completely drained; in many cases this is best done with an intercostal tube. Any pleural effusion causing breathlessness requires drainage. Malignant effusions may be large and recurrent and therefore require pleurodesis. Re-expansion pulmonary oedema is rare providing large volumes of fluid are not rapidly aspirated; passive drainage seldom causes problems. A variety of sclerosing agents can be introduced into the pleural space in an attempt to fuse the visceral and parietal layers, thereby avoiding the re-accumulation of fluid. *Corynebacterium parvum*, tetracycline and bleomycin can all produce satisfactory results.

If a large pleural effusion reaccumulates despite attempts at medical pleurodesis, surgical pleurodesis or pleurectomy should be considered. Medical pleurodesis is successful in approximately 50% of patients whereas surgery is effective in virtually all cases.

CHYLOTHORAX

Chylothorax most frequently follows rupture of the thoracic duct following trauma, particularly during intrathoracic surgery. Damage to the thoracic duct in the lower half of the mediastinum causes a right-sided chylothorax, whereas damage to the duct in the upper mediastinum produces a left chylothorax. When not due to trauma, malignancy involving the thoracic duct is the most common cause, particularly metastatic disease from carcinoma of the stomach, and lymphoma. Rarely chylothorax can complicate chylous ascites.

Patients with chylothorax present with symptoms and signs of a large pleural effusion and the diagnosis is only apparent following aspiration. Fluid rapidly reaccumulates and repeated drainage soon leads to severe wasting, hypoproteinaemia and lymphopenia.

In up to 50% of patients with chylothorax there is spontaneous healing of the fistula, but if this does not occur, the prognosis is poor unless the leak of chyle can be stopped. Following diagnosis a lymphangiogram is useful to determine the site of the fistula, and if the leak is demonstrated the patient should be submitted to thoracotomy and ligation of the thoracic duct below the leak. If no leak can be demonstrated at lymphangiography, repeated aspiration is performed and the patient is supported by parenteral feeding, in the hope that the fistula will heal spontaneously. When healing does not take place, pleural drainage combined with pleurodesis is sometimes successful.

HAEMOTHORAX

Haemothorax is usually the result of a penetrating injury or blunt trauma to the chest. Occasionally, a haemothorax develops without trauma. Such a *spontaneous haemothorax*, almost always left-sided, may occur with acute aortic dissection. Bleeding can occur with a pneumothorax, from the rupture of vessels within pleural adhesions, and in some cases the air may have been absorbed by the time of presentation. Bleeding disorders, heparin therapy, vascular pleural metastases and pleural endometriosis are rare causes of haemothorax. Haemothoraces, unless small and stable, should be drained by a wide-bore intercostal tube introduced in the mid-axilla connected to an underwater seal. If bleeding continues, the patient requires a thoracotomy. If blood is not removed from the pleural space, infection progressing to empyema can be a complication. In the long term an intense fibrous reaction to undrained blood can occasionally lead to a grossly thickened pleura and an encased lung which then requires decortication if there is not to be substantial ventilatory impairment.

EMPYEMA

Empyema refers to infected pleural fluid, whether a turbid effusion or frank pus. In many cases, the diagnosis only becomes apparent on aspiration of the fluid. Most commonly, an acute empyema complicates a bacterial penumonia, particularly pneumococcal, but other causes require consideration (Table 13.52).

Staphylococcal pneumonia is an important cause in children. Anaerobic infection is sometimes difficult to diagnose and it is likely that anaerobes are responsible for many 'sterile' empyemas. Tuberculous empyema is now unusual. It is not uncommon for empyema fluid to contain more than one organism. Empyema following thoracic surgery, and those associated with abdominal sepsis are frequently due to Gram-negative organisms. Amoebic liver abscess can rarely perforate the diaphragm and enter the pleural space, as can actinomycosis and hydatid disease. The empyema that occasionally complicates the mediastinitis of oesophageal rupture is usually left-sided.

The clinical features of acute empyema include fever, night sweats and chest pain, with signs of a pleural effusion. The most common clinical setting is that of a pneumonia that has failed to respond to therapy. The white cell count is elevated (15 000–20 000) with a polymorphonuclear leucocytosis. Pleural fluid aspiration is essen-

Table 13.52 Causes of acute empyema

Pneumonias	Thoracic surgery
Lung abscess	Penetrating chest injuries
Bronchiectasis	Subdiaphragmatic infection
Oesophageal perforation	Haematogenous spread of infection
Pulmonary infarction	

tial and diagnostic; the fluid may be turbid with numerous polymorphs or frank pus. Empyemas are usually posterior and lateral above the diaphragm. Initially, the pleural fluid moves freely in the pleural space and the chest X-ray demonstrates the appearances of a simple effusion, but the infected fluid rapidly becomes loculated and the chest X-ray then shows localised collections of fluid (Fig. 13.65).

An acute empyema can breach the lung and enter a bronchus, and thereby produce a bronchopleural fistula. Patients then cough large volumes of purulent sputum and on X-ray the empyema has fluid levels. Untreated, an empyema may discharge through the chest wall (empyema necessitatis). Empyema, particularly when due to staphylococcal infection, can be complicated by a pneumothorax (pyopneumothorax).

Management

Antibiotic therapy will depend on the bacteriology of aspirated fluid and regimes will often require metronidazole to cover anaerobic organisms. The pleural fluid must be completely drained as soon as possible. With early infection and freely moving fluid, needle aspiration can be successful. However, in most cases, a large-bore intercostal drain should be inserted. If such treatment fails to produce rapid resolution of symptoms and complete drainage of the empyema, surgery is required. At surgery, the empyema is evacuated and the lung is decorticated so

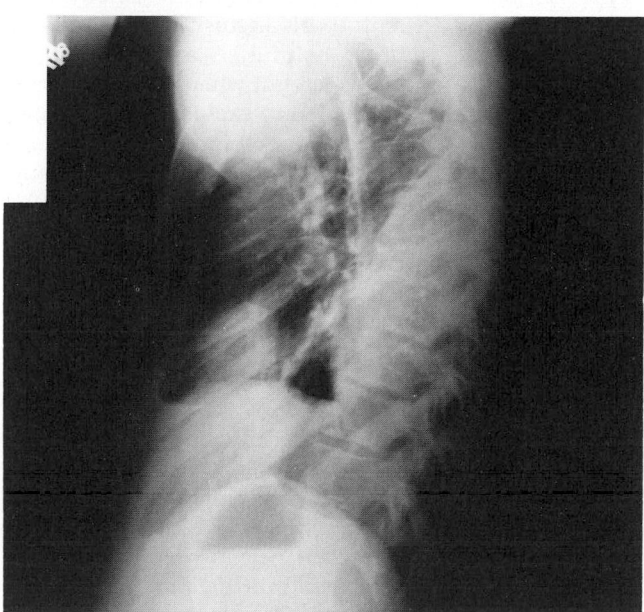

Fig. 13.65 Empyema. On the lateral chest X-ray the configuration of the posterior loculated pleural fluid is typical of empyema. The left hemidiaphragm is well seen, with the gastric bubble beneath it. The posterior curve of the right hemidiaphragm is obscured by the empyema.

that it may fully expand and thereby obliterate the pleural space.

Chronic empyema

Occasionally, the diagnosis of acute empyema is missed or the condition is inadequately treated and a stable chronic empyema develops. Infection is particularly likely to persist when there is an associated bronchogenic carcinoma or a bronchopleural fistula. Patients are usually not acutely ill. Fever is low-grade and there is likely to be clubbing, weight loss, anaemia and the clinical signs of extensive pleural thickening. The chest X-ray shows dense pleural shadowing, perhaps fluid levels and occasionally periosteal reaction in overlying ribs. A later radiological development is pleural calcification and a late clinical development is secondary amyloidosis. The treatment of chronic empyema is surgical, but in patients too frail for surgery, drainage by a wide-bore drain, progressively shortened as the empyema cavity reduces, can produce satisfactory resolution.

DRY PLEURISY

A variety of disorders can cause pleuritic chest pain, often with a pleural rub, but without a pleural effusion. Some of these conditions remain 'dry' but in others fluid may accumulate, and therefore many of the causes of a pleural effusion must be considered in the differential diagnosis of dry pleurisy. The most important causes of pleurisy without fluid are listed in Table 13.53.

Pleuritic pain is common feature of many radiologically obvious pneumonias but can also occur with minor bacterial and viral pulmonary infections, not radiologically apparent. Epidemic myalgia (Bornholm disease), most commonly due to the coxsackie B virus, is primarily an infection of intercostal muscle but occasionally the pleura is involved. The intercostal muscles are tender. There may be associated pericarditis, myocarditis or orchitis. Pain may relapse and remit several times before finally settling. Dry pleurisy is not unusual in

Table 13.53 Important causes of dry pleurisy

Pneumonia (particularly pneumococcal pneumonia)	Uraemia
	Coxsackie B virus (Bornholm disease)
Pulmonary infarction	Familial Mediterranean fever
Bronchogenic carcinoma	Trauma
Lung abscess	Asbestos pleural disease, including mesothelioma
Bronchiectasis	
Tuberculosis	
Rheumatoid arthritis	
Systemic lupus erythematosus	

rheumatoid arthritis and is a feature of systemic lupus erythematosus.

PNEUMOTHORAX

Pneumothorax is air in the pleural space, as a consequence of which there is partial or complete collapse of the lung. Due to the recoil of the chest wall and the lung, the pressure within the pleural space is normally negative. When the pleural membrane (visceral or parietal) is breached, air is therefore sucked into the pleural cavity and the lung collapses. When the defect in the pleura seals, the pneumothorax is *closed* and there is no movement of air in or out of the pleural cavity. When there is a persistent defect in the pleura the pneumothorax is *open*. When this defect is of the visceral pleura there is then a bronchopleural fistula, and air moves in and out of the pleural space during breathing. Occasionally, the damaged visceral pleura acts as a valve permitting air to enter the pleural space on inspiration but not to leave the space on expiration, leading to a *tension* pneumothorax.

A pneumothorax may be spontaneous, secondary to chest trauma, mechanical ventilation or ruptured oesophagus, or induced artificially. Causes of traumatic pneumothorax include blunt trauma to the chest, commonly external cardiac massage, and penetrating chest injuries (e.g. stab wounds or needle aspiration biopsies that breach the visceral pleura from without) and transbronchial biopsy and positive pressure ventilation that breach the visceral pleura from within. A spontaneous pneumothorax may be primary, in which case the patients are otherwise healthy, or may be secondary to some other disorder (Table 13.54). Of these, airways obstruction, particularly when due to bullous emphysema, is the most common predisposing cause.

Clinical features

Most commonly, spontaneous pneumothorax develops in an otherwise fit person as a result of the rupture of a small apical pleural bleb, probably congenital in origin. Young adult males are most frequently affected and are often of tall and slim build. Characteristically, there is sudden onset of chest pain, laterally, sometimes radiating to the shoulder. With substantial collapse of the lung there is associated breathlessness, and a dry, irritating cough is common. Sometimes the patient is aware of the partially collapsed lung flopping about within the thorax. On examination, the most striking findings are of reduced breath sounds and hyper–resonant percussion. A small left-sided pneumothorax may be associated with a clicking noise with each heart-beat noted by the patient and on occasions loud enough to be heard by others. A large pneumothorax in a normal person causes breathlessness, and in the presence of pre-existing pulmonary disease a small one may cause severe respiratory distress.

Tension pneumothorax is a medical emergency. The valve action of the pleural tear results in a progressive increase in the size and pressure of the pneumothorax. The underlying lung is totally collapsed. The mediastinum is shifted to the contralateral side, compromising the function of the opposite lung, and the high intrathoracic pressure elevates the jugular venous pressure, reduces venous return and causes tachycardia, low cardiac output and eventually circulatory collapse and death.

With the exception of a tension pneumothorax, when action may be required immediately, a chest X-ray is necessary in all patients in whom the diagnosis of pneumothorax is a possibility. Small apical pneumothoraces may be difficult to see and an expiratory chest X-ray, which enhances the contrast between lung tissue and air in the pleural space, is helpful. The X-ray allows an assessment of the size and position of the pneumothorax (the air may be loculated if there are pleural adhesions), any abnormality in the underlying lung and the presence of mediastinal or subcutaneous air. A loculated pneumothorax can be difficult to distinguish from a bulla, in which case a CT scan is helpful. A small volume of pleural fluid is commonly seen but when there is a larger collection it should be sampled to exclude bleeding and, occasionally, infection (pyopneumothorax).

Recurrence of pneumothorax is common; a young person with spontaneous pneumothorax has a 20–30% chance of a second one, usually on the same side; with each pneumothorax the probability of further episodes increases. The longer the time that elapses following a pneumothorax, the less chance there is of a recurrence.

Management

Any pneumothorax sufficient to cause or increase breathlessness requires drainage. Many patients, particularly young, otherwise fit males, present with a small or moderate pneumothorax and whatever breathlessness was experienced acutely has settled. Such closed pneumothoraces do not require therapy and the patient can be monitored as an outpatient, provided he is instructed to seek medical advice if breathlessness returns. A 20–30% collapse of a lung normally takes several weeks to expand fully. Simple aspiration is an effective treatment of many pneumothoraces. If aspiration is not effective (because of

Table 13.54 Conditions predisposing to pneumothorax

Chronic bronchitis and emphysema	Marfan's syndrome, Ehlers-Danlos syndrome
Asthma	Congenital cysts
Cystic fibrosis	Honeycomb lung
Tuberculosis	

a bronchopleural fistula) an intercostal drain is required. In a tension pneumothorax, if necessary, prior to the insertion of an intercostal drain, tension can be released by inserting an intravenous cannula into the pleural space in the second interspace in the mid-clavicular line. Unless a pneumothorax is loculated, the best site for a drain is in the mid-axilla at the level of the sixth intercostal space.

When the catheter is connected to the underwater seal drainage bottle, any pleural air under positive pressure bubbles out. Careful and regular inspection of the level and movement of the water meniscus of the draining tube provides important information in the management of a pneumothorax (Fig. 13.66). In a closed pneumothorax, coughing or other manoeuvres that produce a positive intrathoracic pressure drain the air and the pneumothorax rapidly resolves. When there is a large defect in the visceral pleura, producing an open pneumothorax and a bronchopleural fistula, any manoeuvre producing positive intrathoracic pressure causes much bubbling, but since the pleural defect remains the pneumothorax does not resolve. The chest drain is kept *in situ* in the hope that the pleural defect will close and the pneumothorax will convert from an open to a closed type and will then resolve. If resolution does not occur within a few days, it is common practice to apply suction to the pneumothorax. In practice, only a minority of open pneumothoraces, usually those in which the pleural leak is small, can be treated in this way. Frequently, the application of suction simply serves to hold the pleural defect open.

When air no longer bubbles from the catheter even when the patient coughs, a chest X-ray should be taken to confirm that the lung has fully expanded. If this is the case, the drain should be clamped for several hours and if the lung remains fully inflated the drain can be removed. Where a drain has been inserted for a recurrent pneumothorax a medical pleurodesis should be undertaken prior to removal of the catheter. If an open pneumothorax persists for a week despite a period of suction the patient should be referred for thoracotomy, closure of the bronchopleural fistula and parietal pleural abrasion or pleurectomy.

Mediastinal emphysema (pneumomediastinum)

Air can enter the mediastinum following penetrating neck injuries, and oesophageal and bronchial rupture, but the most common cause is rupture of alveoli. Air enters the interstitial tissues and tracks to the mediastinum. High intrapulmonary pressures due, for example, to vomiting are frequently the cause. In asthma, gas trapping, alveolar distension and high intrapulmonary pressures during coughing make mediastinal emphysema a relatively common complication. Positive pressure mechanical ventilation can produce mediastinal emphysema as well as pneumothorax. Mediastinal emphysema is usually asymptomatic but can cause chest pain which may be worse on swallowing or breathing. There may also be a crunching sound coincident with each heart-beat. Radiology may show air in the upper mediastinum, around the heart, within the soft tissues of the neck and, in 30% of cases, an associated pneumothorax. Treatment is of the predisposing cause, following which the mediastinal emphysema rapidly resolves. Resolution can be hastened by breathing a high inspiratory oxygen concentration, during which the more soluble oxygen replaces the insoluble nitrogen and is taken up by the pulmonary circulation.

TUMOURS OF THE PLEURA

The pleura can be the primary site of benign or malignant tumours or, more commonly, the site of metastatic malignant disease.

Fibroma

The pleura, usually the visceral surface, may be the site of a single benign fibrous tumour (localised fibrous mesothelioma). The tumour, which is well encapsulated and often pedunculated, is frequently first noted as a peripheral pleural mass on routine chest X-ray. A pleural effusion is not common. These tumours are not associated with asbestos exposure. Fibromas can become large and thereby cause breathlessness as well as chest pain. Patients are generally middle-aged or elderly and clubbing, as well as hypertrophic pulmonary osteoarthropathy, is a frequent association. A definite diagnosis is seldom possible

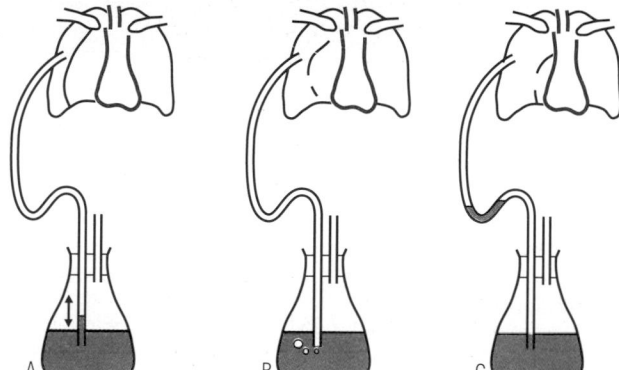

Fig. 13.66 Pneumothorax. A. In a closed pneumothorax, the meniscus in the drain rises and falls with breathing and at resting end expiration the small negative intrathoracic pressure supports a column of water. **B.** In an open pneumothorax air bubbles into the drainage bottle, with each breath, during active expiration. **C.** If pleural fluid blocks the drainage tube the bubbling of air ceases and there is little movement of the meniscus with breathing. This situation can, therefore, mimic that of a resolved pneumothorax.

without thoracotomy and biopsy, and surgical resection is the correct management. If left untreated, these tumours may eventually become locally invasive.

Diffuse mesothelioma

Diffuse mesothelioma, a highly malignant tumour, is related to asbestos exposure in most, perhaps all, cases. The patient's exposure to asbestos is, on average, 30 years prior to the malignancy becoming apparent. Most commonly, exposure to asbestos is in the shipbuilding, construction and demolition industries. Crocidolite (blue asbestos) is most commonly incriminated. In the UK 300–400 patients each year are diagnosed as having malignant mesothelioma. The tumour spreads over the pleural surface, causing great thickening of the pleura by malignant tissue, and the lung becomes encased. The tumour spreads into the mediastinum, through the diaphragm to involve the peritoneum, and invades the chest wall. An effusion is characteristic and is often blood-stained. Distant metastases occur, although relatively infrequently, and cause major clinical problems. The histology is pleomorphic and a definite diagnosis, particularly the distinction from secondary adenocarcinoma, is often difficult on a small biopsy sample.

Patients with malignant mesothelioma present at an average age of 60, most commonly with persistent dull chest pain. There is progressive breathlessness because of pleural thickening and the accumulation of fluid. Finger clubbing is relatively unusual. The chest X-ray commonly shows a large effusion with the pleural tumour often only apparent following aspiration. CT scanning clearly demonstrates the extent of pleural disease, and when pleural calcification is also present, the appearances are highly suggestive of the diagnosis (Fig. 13.67). Although cytology of aspirated fluid may demonstrate malignant cells and Abrams' or cutting needle pleural biopsy may also show malignancy, a large surgical biopsy is sometimes needed to confirm the diagnosis. However, surgical biopsy is not infrequently followed by additional chronic pain and infiltration of the thoracotomy scar by tumour. No therapy, whether surgery, cytotoxic drugs or radiotherapy, has been demonstrated to prolong life. Life expectancy is 1–2 years following presentation. In the UK patients with a history of asbestos exposure are eligible for industrial injuries benefit.

Metastatic malignant pleural disease

Pleural metastases with an associated effusion are very common, particularly with bronchial carcinoma. The effusion is usually painless but causes breathlessness and may require pleurodesis (p. 526). Pleural involvement is also common following malignant disease of the breast and ovary. Less commonly, pleural involvement occurs in

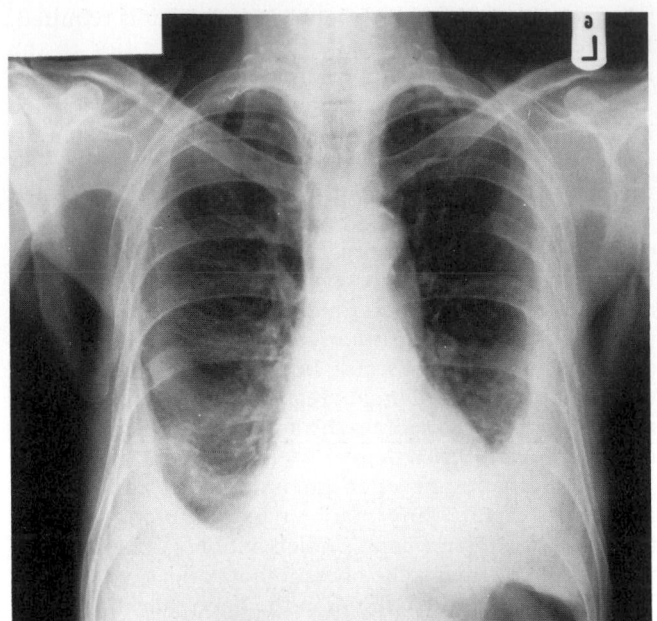

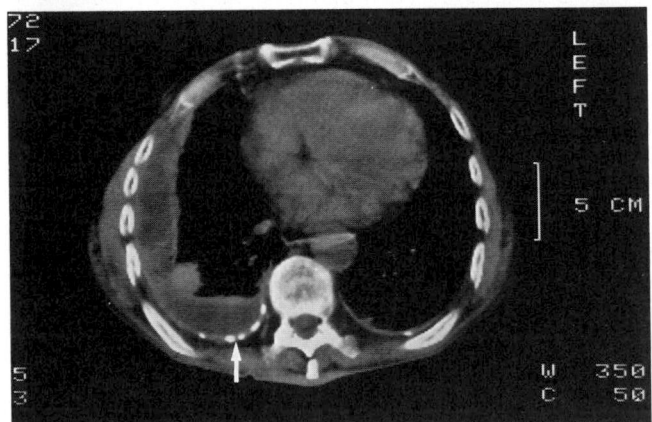

Fig. 13.67 Mesothelioma. A. The chest X-ray shows bilateral pleural thickening and fluid. **B.** The CT scan shows extensive pleural thickening, plus fluid, and pleural calcification posteriorly on the right (arrow).

other carcinomas, lymphangitis carcinomatosa, multiple myeloma, malignant lymphoma (particularly Hodgkin's disease), Kaposi's sarcoma and Waldenström's macroglobulinaemia.

NEUROMUSCULAR AND SKELETAL DISORDERS

NEUROMUSCULAR DISORDERS

Ventilation depends on adequate central respiratory drive and depression of central nervous system function can

Table 13.55 Neuromuscular disorders which cause respiratory muscle weakness

Neurogenic	Myopathic
Motor neurone disease	Muscular dystrophy/atrophy
Surgical trauma of phrenic nerves	Inflammatory myopathies
Polyneuropathy	Myotonic dystrophy
Neuralgic amyotrophy	Acid maltase deficiency
Poliomyelitis	Thyroid myopathy
Multiple sclerosis	Metabolic disturbance
Traumatic tetraplegia	(e.g. hypophosphataemia)
Acute porphyria	
Charcot-Marie-Tooth disease	
Neuromuscular junction	
Myasthenia gravis	
Lambert-Eaton syndrome	

therefore cause ventilatory failure. In such patients the diagnosis is usually self-evident and the resulting hypercapnia easily documented. Central nervous system dysfunction may also cause sleep apnoea syndromes (p. 491). In addition to these patients a wide range of neurological and muscular disorders can cause ventilatory impairment on the basis of respiratory muscle weakness (Table 13.55).

The respiratory muscles

In normal man, at rest, inspiration is active whereas expiration is a passive process; most of the respiratory muscles are therefore inspiratory in their action.

The *diaphragm* is the principal muscle of inspiration and is responsible for 80% of ventilation at rest. Diaphragm contraction causes descent of the diaphragmatic dome, anterior displacement of the abdominal wall, elevation of the lower ribs and expansion of the lower thorax. At resting lung volume (functional residual capacity) the *external intercostal muscles* are inspiratory and the *internal intercostal muscles* are expiratory. The *abdominal muscles* are the most powerful muscles of expiration. These muscles also return the diaphragm to its optimal resting length prior to inspiration. The *accessory muscles* of respiration are conventionally considered to be the sternomastoid, scalene and pectoral muscles, which act mainly to fix or elevate the upper ribcage. However, many of other muscles contract vigorously during maximum respiratory efforts.

The respiratory muscles in neuromuscular disease

Clinical assessment

Isolated involvement of the respiratory muscles by neuromuscular disease is unusual, and most patients will have evidence of more widespread involvement, with, for example, weakness of other muscle groups, bulbar problems and impaired cough, as well as breathlessness. On examination, there may be muscle wasting, weakness and fasciculation. Patients with bilateral severe diaphragm weakness or complete diaphragm paralysis present an unusual and striking clinical picture (Fig. 13.68).

Severe weakness of the inspiratory muscles reduces the lung volume on the chest radiograph, but this can be an unreliable sign; unless the radiologist is already aware of the diagnosis, it is likely that it will be assumed that the patient has chosen not to take a full inspiration rather than that he or she is incapable of doing so.

Diaphragm paralysis elevates the hemidiaphragm involved. Radiological screening, which should be performed with the patient supine, will demonstrate the upward movement of a paralysed hemidiaphragm during a sharp sniff. Diaphragm movement can be assessed by ultrasound.

Lung function

Respiratory muscle weakness reduces both inspiratory and expiratory capacity (Fig. 13.69). Total lung capacity is reduced, residual volume (RV) is increased and both of these changes decrease vital capacity (VC); this simple measurement is therefore an excellent one for the detection of respiratory muscle weakness. VC is an ideal measurement in the follow-up of patients with weakness and in muscular dystrophy, for example, the VC correlates well with both the clinical staging of disease and the assessment of prognosis. In neuromuscular disorders that can cause rapid profound weakness (e.g. Guillain-Barré syndrome) large falls in VC warn that assisted ventilation may be required. The measurement of VC is particularly

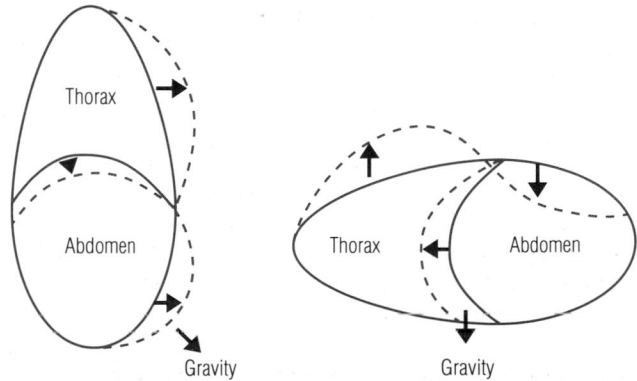

Fig. 13.68 Paralysis or severe weakness of the diaphragm. When upright the thorax is expanded by contraction of the intercostal muscles. The abdominal muscles relax, the diaphragm passively descends, and the anterior abdominal wall moves outwards. When supine the contraction of the intercostal muscles lowers intrathoracic pressure, sucks the diaphragm into the chest and the anterior abdominal wall moves inwards. Patients with diaphragm paralysis therefore have severe orthopnoea.

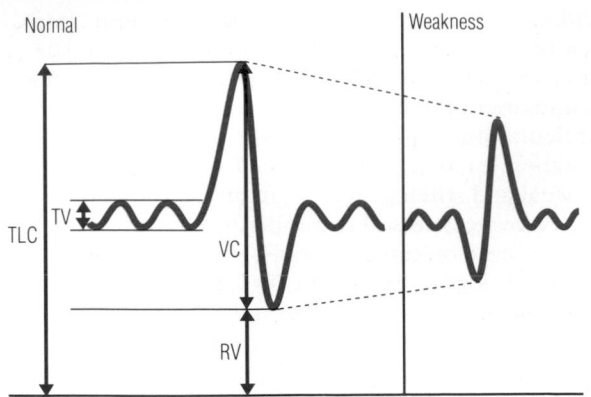

Fig. 13.69 The effect of respiratory muscle weakness on lung volumes. The principal effect of substantial weakness is to reduce vital capacity. (TLC = total lung capacity; TV = tidal volume; VC = vital capacity; RV = residual volume.)

useful when assessing diaphragm weakness. In the upright posture, VC is reduced, but when the patient lies flat there is a further marked fall in VC, characteristically by 50% with total paralysis of the diaphragm. Lung function in patients with respiratory muscle weakness shows no evidence of airways obstruction and the ratio of FEV_1 to FVC is normal. Although overall gas transfer may be reduced, when corrected for the reduction in lung volume, gas transfer coefficient (KCO) is normal or raised. With the progression of neuromuscular disease, patients gradually develop hypoxaemia, but hypercapnia is a late development associated with a poor prognosis. Hypercapnic ventilatory failure is unusual before the VC has fallen to below 50% of normal. With generalised respiratory muscle weakness, particularly when the diaphragm is severely involved, ventilatory failure is more pronounced when supine, and may be particularly severe during sleep.

Respiratory pressure

A normal supine VC excludes severe inspiratory muscle weakness, but a reduced VC is not specific for weakness and must be assessed in the context of possible co-existing lung disease. A more specific and sensitive index of global respiratory muscle strength is provided by measurement of maximum static mouth pressures. Pressures are measured by a transducer or gauge; expiratory mouth pressures are recorded during a maximum expiratory effort at TLC against an obstructed airway, and inspiratory mouth pressures are measured during a maximum inspiratory effort from RV.

In patients with generalised neuromuscular diseases, respiratory pressures are commonly reduced to 50% of normal, even though patients are often not particularly breathless. Hypercapnia is unusual unless inspiratory mouth pressures are reduced to below 30% of normal.

Diaphragm weakness

The phrenic nerves are commonly invaded by tumour, particularly carcinoma of the bronchus. Viral infections, including herpes zoster, can cause a phrenic neuropathy, as can the neurological disorders of motor neurone disease, poliomyelitis, Charcot-Marie-Tooth disease and many peripheral neuropathies. Trauma, particularly surgical, is important, and phrenic nerve dysfunction is quite common following cardiac surgery. In the past, phrenic crush and phrenic avulsion for the treatment of tuberculosis was a common cause of phrenic neuropathy. Unilateral phrenic nerve palsy causes a 20% reduction in ventilatory capacity and a reduction in maximum transdiaphragmatic pressures, but patients have few symptoms: perhaps transient breathlessness, in the absence of additional pathology. Bilateral phrenic nerve paresis, on the other hand, causes shortness of breath on exertion and severe orthopnoea; indeed, patients are quite unable to remain flat for more than a few seconds. Many patients sleep propped up or on their sides to assist ventilation (Fig. 13.67).

Diaphragm strength can be specifically and accurately measured by recording transdiaphragmatic pressure with oesophageal and gastric balloon catheters for a maximum sniff manoeuvre.

Management

Respiratory muscle weakness due to neuromuscular disease may spontaneously improve as in the Guillain-Barré syndrome, or may respond to appropriate therapy, as in myasthenia gravis. Prior to improvement, some patients may require a period of mechanical ventilation. In most patients, however, deterioration is relentless, particularly in those with muscular dystrophy or motor neurone disease, and these patients die of respiratory infection and ventilatory failure. In a few patients deterioration may be very slow or a plateau may be reached, with respiratory muscle weakness causing ventilatory failure and disabling breathlessness. For a small number of carefully selected patients, assisted ventilation may be appropriate, particularly at night. Positive pressure ventilation (via tracheostomy or nasal mask) and negative pressure ventilation (with tank ventilators, cuirasses and jackets) can both be used, usually in the patient's home, and long-term survival and quality of life can make this treatment worthwhile.

In patients with quadriplegia from high cervical cord lesions, the diaphragm and other respiratory muscles are paralysed and the patient is dependent on mechanical ventilation. If the phrenic nerves are intact, as shown by adequate diaphragm contraction with percutaneous phrenic nerve stimulation, diaphragm pacing via the phrenic nerves can sustain ventilation and mechanical ventilation is no longer required.

Metabolic disorders causing weakness

Acidosis impairs the contractility of both skeletal and cardiac muscle. Hypercapnia, perhaps mediated through acidosis, adversely affects muscle function and it is probable that the interaction of hypercapnic acidosis and hypoventilation contributes to the rapid deterioration of patients with ventilatory failure and a low pH. Hypophosphataemia is a well-recognised cause of ventilatory failure due to respiratory muscle weakness and is an important factor on the intensive care unit. Reversible weakness of the respiratory muscles also occurs with thyroid disease, hypokalaemia and disorders of magnesium and calcium metabolism.

Weight loss and muscle weakness

Patients with a wide variety of medical and surgical illnesses have profound weight loss and muscle atrophy with consequent weakness. This loss of muscle bulk involves the respiratory muscles, which therefore also become weak. Adequate nutrition (p. 547), particularly in hospitalised patients, can minimise wasting, as will the reversal of catabolic factors such as sepsis, fever, protein-losing states and steroid therapy. Immobilisation leads to rapid atrophy of skeletal muscle, and it is possible that prolonged mechanical ventilation causes disuse atrophy of the respiratory muscles.

Respiratory muscle function in patients with airways obstruction

Chronic bronchitis, emphysema and asthma cause airways obstruction and hyperinflation, both of which require the patient to generate greater than normal pressures during tidal breathing. The capacity of the respiratory muscles to produce the required large negative intrapleural pressure is compromised by muscle shortening, decreased diaphragm curvature, increased velocity of shortening and abnormal ribcage geometry. Respiratory muscle contractility may also be impaired by reduced oxygen delivery to the muscle, as a consequence of hypoxaemia and cardiovascular disease, and also by the respiratory acidosis associated with acute hypercapnia. The increased work of breathing combined with the reduced capacity of the respiratory muscles to generate tensions limits ventilatory reserve, causes breathlessness and may predispose to the development of respiratory muscle fatigue and hypercapnic ventilatory failure as, for example, in severe acute asthma. Patients with airflow limitation require a high respiratory centre output to maintain ventilation, and depression of neural output (for example, by sedatives) can markedly impair breathing. The work of breathing is reduced and the function of the respiratory muscles improved by therapy that reduces airflow limitation and lung volume.

In patients with chronic lung diseases, specific respiratory muscle training has been undertaken with a view to improving both the strength and endurance of the respiratory muscles. Although some studies have reported a modest benefit from training, the overall value of such training programmes remains a matter of debate. Attempts have also been made to improve respiratory muscle contractility with drugs. It has been postulated that theophylline may have a very small inotropic effect but it is doubtful whether under most circumstances this is of any clinical importance.

Respiratory muscle fatigue

All skeletal muscles fatigue when subjected to sufficiently high load, and the respiratory muscles are no exception. Careful studies of the stressed respiratory muscles of normal subjects have demonstrated fatigue in terms of electromyographic changes, slowing of relaxation rate and reduced contractile response to electrical stimulation. However, these complex techniques have not easily been applied to patients with ventilatory failure and the clinical importance of respiratory muscle fatigue remains to be established. Data from patients on ICU failing to wean from mechanical ventilation indicate that muscle fatigue may play a part. Some authorities, particularly in North America, advocate the 'resting' of the respiratory muscles by assisted ventilation to allow respiratory muscle fatigue to resolve. More clinical studies on the detection of respiratory muscle fatigue and its clinical importance are necessary before widespread use of this approach could be advocated.

THORACIC DEFORMITY

Adequate ventilation requires that the thoracic cage is of adequate volume, rigidity and mobility. Many of the disorders causing thoracic deformity are now rare (for example, rickets) and the most common problems are flail chest (a surgical and anaesthetic emergency), ankylosing spondylitis, scoliosis, thoracoplasty and fibrothorax.

Ankylosing spondylitis

Ankylosis of the ribs is characteristic of ankylosing spondylitis (p. 1005) and chest expansion is frequently reduced. Respiratory problems occur relatively late in the course of the disease and most patients are 50–70 years old before developing symptoms. In addition to the classical radiological changes affecting the spine (p. 1005), patients can also develop upper zone pulmonary fibrosis with cavitation and occasionally an aspergillus fungal ball (mycetoma). Despite the reduced expansion of the ribcage, ventilation is relatively little impaired because of good diaphragm function and, in the absence of co-existing

Table 13.56 Disorders causing chronic scoliosis

Idiopathic
Disorders of bone (e.g. osteogenesis imperfecta)
Neurological diseases (e.g. cerebral palsy, poliomyelitis)
Muscle disease (e.g. muscular dystrophy)
Connective tissue disorders (e.g. Marfan's syndrome, Ehlers-Danlos syndrome)
Thoracic surgery (e.g. pneumonectomy, thoracoplasty)
Chronic infection (e.g. empyema)

severe cardio-respiratory disease, ventilatory failure does not occur. As a consequence of the importance of diaphragm function, patients tolerate badly upper abdominal surgery or any other factors impairing diaphragm function.

Scoliosis

Scoliosis refers to a lateral curve of the spine and in most cases, perhaps three-quarters, it has no known cause. A wide variety of disorders are responsible for the remaining cases (Table 13.56). Although a congenital vertebral abnormality produces scoliosis in childhood, most scolioses develop in adolescence during the rapid growth spurt. Congenital heart disease is common in scoliotic patients. Scoliosis makes the thoracic cage stiff. The deformity also reduces the volume of the lungs and adversely affects the mechanical advantage of the respiratory muscles. Lung function tests show a restrictive ventilatory defect, the severity of which is related to the angle of scoliosis, with high thoracic curves causing the greatest impairment. Patients with moderate or severe scoliosis are breathless and with more severe deformity they eventually develop hypoxaemia, hypercapnia, pulmonary hypertension and cor pulmonale. Patients with scoliosis secondary to neurological disorders are frequently the most severely affected, particularly if diaphragm function is impaired. Ventilatory failure first becomes apparent during the night, particularly as a consequence of the hypoventilation associated with REM sleep. With the onset of ventilatory failure, the patients require assisted ventilation using negative pressure devices such as a purpose-built cuirass, a Tunnicliffe jacket, pneumosuit or body wrap. Positive pressure ventilation, via a nasal mask, is also very effective. Such domiciliary ventilation is usually only needed at night and can produce remarkable long-term well-being with control of respiratory failure by day, reversal of pulmonary hypertension and resolution of cor pulmonale. During acute episodes of deterioration, more prolonged ventilatory support may be required. From a respiratory point of view, the role of surgery to straighten a scoliosis is controversial. Most surgery is undertaken in adolescence with the aim of avoiding deterioration of the curvature and ventilatory function that otherwise occurs at this time.

Thoracoplasty, surgical collapse of the ribcage to compress the cavities of tuberculosis, was a relatively common surgical procedure in the treatment of pulmonary tuberculosis prior to modern drug management. It produces a similar ventilatory defect to scoliosis. Many patients with thoracoplasty develop breathlessness and eventually ventilatory failure in later life. Some of these patients have been treated with nocturnal domiciliary ventilation with excellent long-term results comparable to those for scoliosis. Such is the success of assisted ventilation programmes that all patients with severe or progressive chest wall deformity (and some patients with neuromuscular disease) require careful specialist long-term follow-up.

FURTHER READING

Brewis R A L, Gibson G J, Geddes D M 1990 Respiratory medicine. Baillière Tindale, London. *An up-to-date authoritative multi-author British textbook.*

Clark T J H, Godfrey S, Lee T H (eds) 1992 Asthma. 3rd edn. Chapman & Hall, London. *A comprehensive clinical account of all aspects of asthma.*

Fraser R G, Paré J A P, Pare P D, Fraser R S, Genereux GP 1989 Diagnosis of diseases of the chest. 3rd edn. W B Saunders Company, Philadelphia. *Splendid comprehensive textbook based on the radiology of chest disease.*

Murray J F 1986 The normal lung. 2nd edn. W B Saunders Company, Philadelphia. *A comprehensive, well-illustrated account of the structure and function of the respiratory system.*

Murray J F, Nadel J A (eds) 1988 Textbook of respiratory medicine. W B Saunders Company, Philadelphia. *Up-to-date, comprehensive and detailed American text of all aspects of respiratory disease.*

Seaton A, Seaton D, Leitch A G 1989 Crofton and Douglas's respiratory diseases. 4th edn. Blackwell Scientific, Oxford. *The most established British textbook of respiratory medicine.*

14
Critical Care Medicine

John Goldstone and John Moxham

Critical care medicine has its origins in the treatment of failing organ systems; it began with respiratory support, using techniques developed in anaesthesia, and was accelerated in the 1950s by the need to ventilate large numbers of patients with paralytic polio. Patients are now admitted to the intensive care unit (ICU) not only to receive mechanical ventilation, but also for the management of a wide variety of severe illnesses. The role of the 'intensivist' commonly involves the diagnosis of those who are obtunded as well as the management of those in organ failure. The skills required are extensive and the work demands the expertise of a team of medical and nursing staff. This team functions most effectively when led by an enthusiastic and committed critical care specialist.

By necessity, the ICU concentrates facilities in one area, with an array of technology. Facilities are available for immediate resuscitation. Many physiological variables are monitored continuously with the aid of electronic monitors at each bedside (Fig. 14.1). Infusions and fluid balance can be measured over time periods of minutes, hours or days. Routine laboratory investigations are often performed on the ward itself, enabling sequential analysis of arterial blood gases, electrolytes and other biochemical data. Central to this process of monitoring and adjustment of the patient's physiology is the intensive care nurse, usually allocated to the care of a single patient.

The most common causes for admission to the ICU are listed in Table 14.1.

CARDIOVASCULAR PROBLEMS

Patients admitted to the ICU frequently require assessment, monitoring and therapy directed at the cardiovascular system (CVS). Cardiovascular failure may be

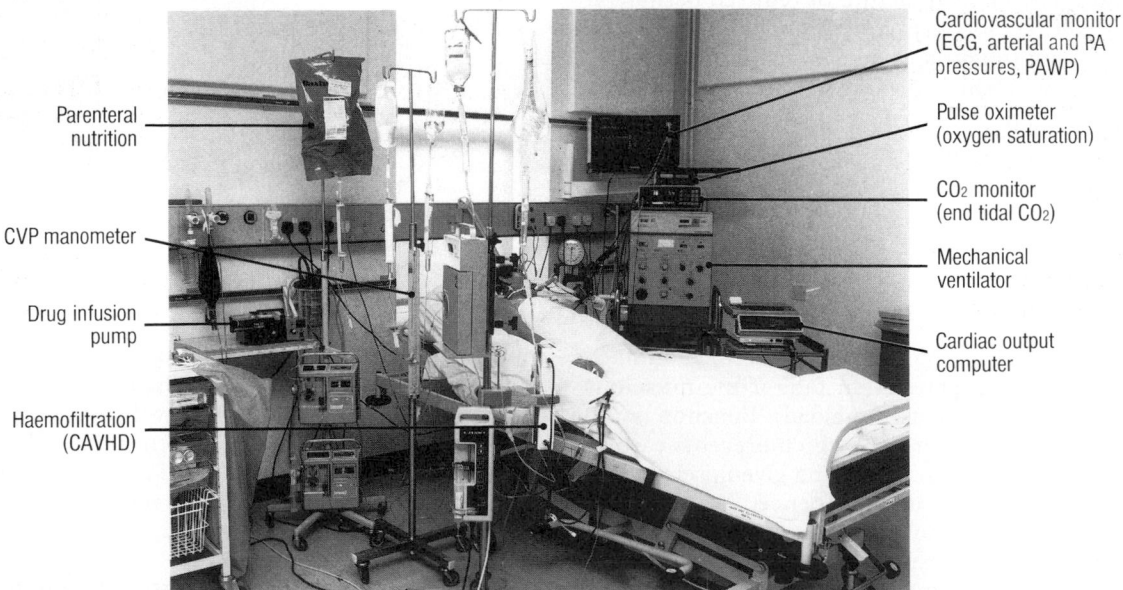

Fig. 14.1 Patient on the intensive care unit. Physiological monitoring is crucial to the management of failing organ systems. This patient is supported by mechanical ventilation, haemofiltration and parenteral nutrition. Clinical examination is as important as physiological measurement and is easily deterred by the array of equipment. (CVP = central venous pressure; CAVHD = continuous arterio-venous haemodialysis; PA = pulmonary artery; PAWP = pulmonary artery wedge pressure).

Parenteral nutrition

CVP manometer

Drug infusion pump

Haemofiltration (CAVHD)

Cardiovascular monitor (ECG, arterial and PA pressures, PAWP)

Pulse oximeter (oxygen saturation)

CO2 monitor (end tidal CO2)

Mechanical ventilator

Cardiac output computer

Table 14.1 Common causes for admission to the ICU

- Postoperative care (cardiac, major vascular and abdominal surgery)
- Major trauma, including head injury
- Respiratory failure
- Post-cardiopulmonary resuscitation
- Drug overdose

due primarily to a cardiac event, e.g. myocardial infarction, or secondary to other organ failure. The function of the heart is to deliver oxygenated blood and nutrients to peripheral organs and tissues, and when perfusion is reduced, secondary effects such as renal failure ensue. The aim of management is to determine the nature of the cardiovascular problem, monitor the effect of treatment and make adjustments to therapy as appropriate.

ASSESSMENT

Whether assessment is by clinical examination or complex monitoring, the approach to the CVS should involve an evaluation of cardiac output, peripheral perfusion and filling pressure. The normalization of cardiac output and peripheral perfusion may be urgent, to avoid organ damage. The maintenance of perfusion to vital organs enhances prognosis. In uncomplicated cases that respond rapidly to treatment, invasive measurements may not be required, but in many patients the need for physiological information to guide treatment requires invasive techniques. Traditionally, disorders characterised by hypotension are termed shock (hypovolaemic, cardiogenic or septicaemic). The clinical picture of reduced peripheral perfusion (cold, vasoconstricted limbs), reduced vital organ blood flow (oliguria or anuria, mental confusion) and compensatory tachycardia due to sympathetic overactivity are common to cardiogenic and hypovolaemic shock. In septicaemia, peripheral vasodilatation causes warm limbs with bounding pulses, making the clinical assessment misleading. Hypotension and poor perfusion cause oliguria, and further assessment is then required (Fig. 14.2).

Filling pressures

The force of contraction of cardiac muscle is determined by its length; tension generation falls if the muscle is excessively stretched (increased preload). Function is also impaired by excessive afterload, which prevents cardiac muscle shortening (see Ch.12). For a given preload and afterload, contractility is also influenced by ionic and hormonal factors (e.g. acidosis).

It is not possible to measure fibre length directly on the ICU, but it is possible to measure pressure within the heart during cardiac filling. During diastole, atrial pressure is related to fibre length, and the filling pressures rise

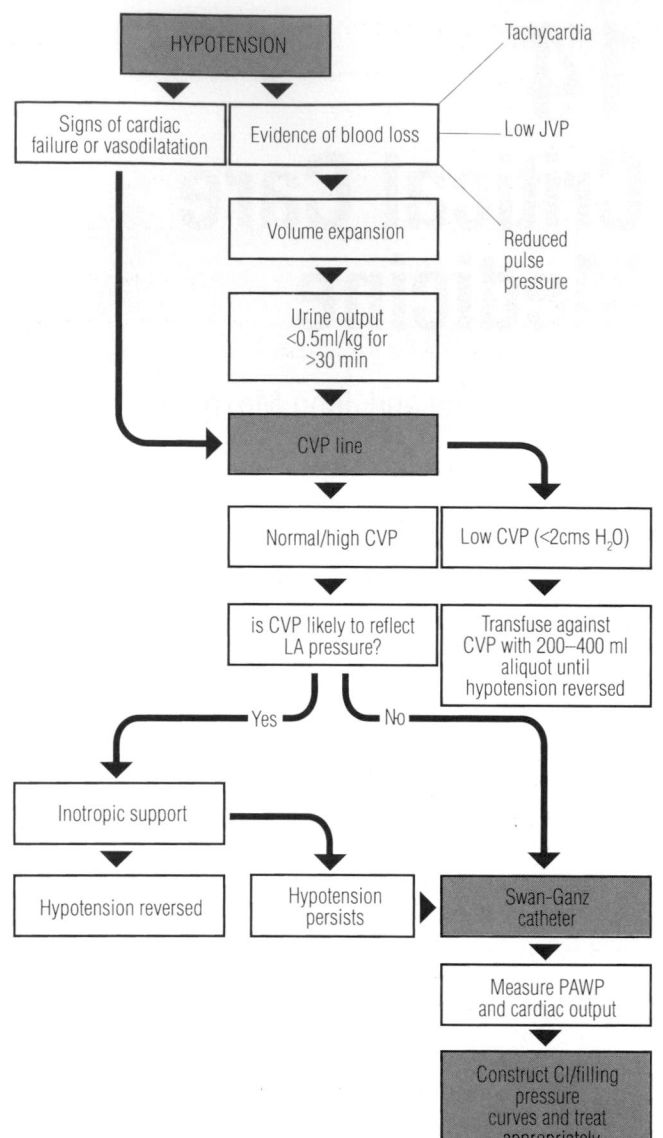

Fig. 14.2 Management of hypotension.

as the heart muscle fibres stretch. Initially the response to raising filling pressure (increased preload) is an increased stroke volume, but excessive pressures result in a fall in output. Pressures in the right atrium can be measured simply with a manometer; the height of the column of water is measured above the level of the right atrium, taken at the mid-axillary line when supine. Electromanometers convert the pressure signal into electricity, and this can be visualised on the bedside monitor. Requirements for accurate measurement of central venous pressure (CVP) are shown in Table 14.2.

CVP is influenced by circulating blood volume and in the hypovolaemic patient filling pressures may be *initially* maintained by an increase in smooth muscle tone

Table 14.2 Requirements for accurate measurement of CVP

- Freely falling meniscus when connected to the patient
- Meniscus has fallen to steady baseline
- Meniscus swings with respiration/ventilation
- Reference point and body position is standardised between measurements

Table 14.3 Common circumstances where left- and right-sided filling pressures do not agree

- Valvular heart disease (e.g. mitral stenosis)
- Myocardial infarction
- Pulmonary hypertension (e.g. secondary to lung disease, pulmonary embolus)

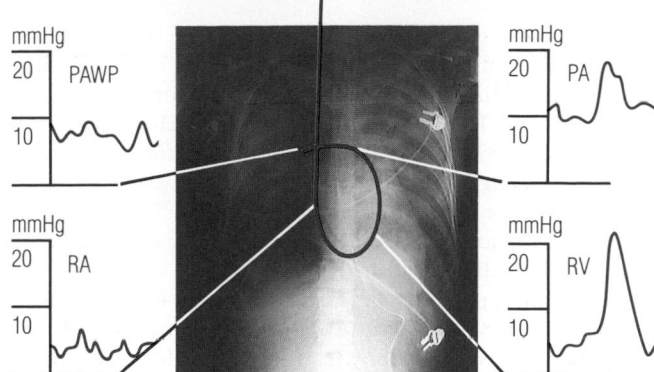

Fig. 14.3 Pulmonary artery (Swan-Ganz) catheter in position in a patient with severe pneumonia. As the catheter is advanced through the great veins into the right atrium (RA), right ventricle (RV) and pulmonary artery (PA), the characteristic pressure waves are displayed. The catheter is sited in the PA, and when measurement of pulmonary artery wedge pressure (PAWP) is required, the balloon at the tip of the catheter is inflated.

within the venous circulation. Under these circumstances the measurement of a normal CVP may be misleading. Further blood loss or vasodilation (eg administration of opiates) will lead to low filling pressures and hypotension. In health, right and left atrial pressures change in parallel, allowing assessment of left ventricular function from right-sided filling pressures. This relationship may be altered in disease (Table 14.3), requiring the more direct assessment of left atrial pressures. Left heart filling pressure can be measured by the insertion of a pulmonary artery catheter (see below), which can also be used to determine cardiac output and therefore the construction of filling pressure/cardiac output curves.

Pulmonary artery catheters

Pulmonary artery catheters are introduced via a great vein and advanced into the right atrium. Passage of the catheter into the right ventricle and out through the pulmonary valve into the pulmonary artery is enhanced by an air-filled balloon at the tip of the catheter. The flow of blood into the right atrium and out into the pulmonary artery carries the catheter into smaller arteries until it becomes wedged in a narrow vessel. When the balloon is deflated, the catheter recoils proximally, restoring perfusion to the distal lung segment.

Running through the catheter is a lumen that emerges at the tip. The pressure at the catheter tip is displayed continuously, and as the right catheter is advanced the characteristic pressures of the right atrium, right ventricle and pulmonary artery are observed (Fig. 14.3). The occluded pressure is termed the pulmonary artery wedge pressure (PAWP) and is related to the filling pressure of the left side of the heart. Pulmonary artery catheters commonly have several lumens so that cardiac output can be measured. Specialised fibre-optic catheters measure oxygen saturation at the tip, giving a continuous output of mixed venous oxygen saturation (Svo_2).

Cardiac output

Cardiac output can be determined in patients on the ICU by measuring the rate of disappearance of a dye introduced into the right atrium (dye dilution technique). The 'dye' conventionally used is cold saline and the fall and recovery in temperature is sensed at the tip of the catheter (in the pulmonary artery) by a miniature temperature gauge. In patients with a low cardiac output, the rate of disappearance of the 'dye' is slow, and the resultant curve of dye concentration against time is low and flat. If the cardiac output is high, dye is quickly washed away from the heart, and the curve is peaked and narrow.

Disorders of the circulation can be considered by constructing a graph of filling pressure versus cardiac output (Fig. 14.4). To allow for differing size of patients, cardiac output is normalised by dividing by the body

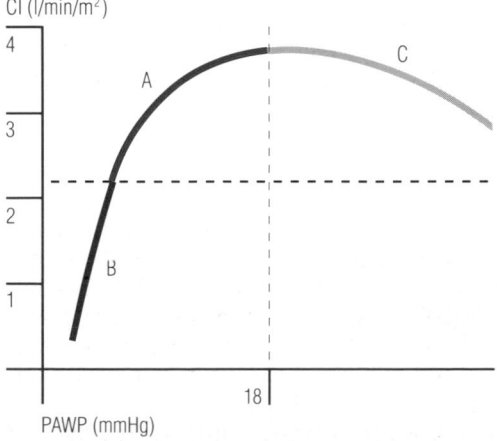

Fig. 14.4 The relationship between cardiac index (CI) and filling pressure (PAWP) for the normal heart. Patients are normally on the curve within square A; square B corresponds to decreased filling pressure; and square C to fluid overload.

surface area, producing a cardiac index (CI) which is expressed in litres/minute/m^2. The normal heart responds to a raised filling pressure (increased preload) by a rapid increase in CI. At the upper limits, further stretch or dilatation of the heart results in a reduction in cardiac output. When cardiovascular function is abnormal, the position of the curve is shifted (Fig. 14.5). The graph can be used to define the problem, monitor the effect of treatment and predict outcome.

The filling pressure of the heart can be reduced either by a reduction in circulating blood volume due to haemorrhage or severe dehydration, or by loss of venous return if the circulation is suddenly vasodilated. Baroreceptors detect the fall in filling pressure stimulating the release of catecholamines from the adrenal gland and sympathetic nervous system. Catecholamines act on the myocardium to increase the heart rate and force of contraction (positive inotropic effect) and on the peripheral vessels to maintain venous return by venoconstriction and blood pressure by vasoconstriction (increased systemic vascular resistance). Other neurohormonal reflexes are stimulated. Fluid loss from the kidney falls initially because of a reduction in glomerular filtration rate (GFR). Aldosterone is released, salt and water reabsorbed further decreasing urinary losses.

The vital signs in haemorrhage may be surprisingly normal in young fit patients, who can maintain blood pressure despite hypovolaemia. In these patients tachycardia helps to maintain cardiac output. Peripheral blood flow is reduced by the release of catecholamines and the skin is therefore pale, cold and clammy. The underperfused tissues respire anaerobically, producing lactic acid. With severe volume depletion, the patient may be confused, agitated and hyperventilating.

The important observation is that the filling pressure is low. The urine output is reduced and concentrated, with a high osmolality, and little filtered sodium is excreted. The skin is cold with a marked gradient between skin and central temperature.

Fluid replacement

Restoration of blood volume should be rapid to avoid organ damage. The speed of transfusion is often inadequate, especially in the elderly where there is a fear of precipitating heart failure. As a guide to the adequacy of fluid replacement, a fluid challenge via repeated aliquots of 200–400 ml of colloid can be monitored by serial measurement of the CVP. In the hypovolaemic patient the response to fluid challenge is a transient rise in pressure, falling back to the baseline value in 10–15 minutes. As fluid replacement continues, further volume challenges result in more gradual rises and falls in filling pressure until the point is reached where an increase in filling pressure is sustained. At this stage fluid replacement is adequate.

Choice of replacement fluid

The choice of replacement fluid depends on the cause of the decreased filling pressure. In haemorrhage, replacement with blood is essential, although blood substitutes may be used until blood is available. Severe dehydration requires predominantly salt and water replacement. Reduction in filling pressure due to vasodilatation can be corrected with a plasma substitute. If the circulation is restored quickly, the metabolic effects of an inadequate circulation will reverse spontaneously, but acidosis, hyperkalaemia and hyperglycaemia require careful management in patients in whom hypovolaemia has been prolonged.

Crystalloid solutions are readily available, but they rapidly redistribute away from the circulation and into the interstitial space. Only one-quarter of the volume transfused stays in the circulation. Large volumes are therefore needed to restore a deficit, and excess fluid in the interstitial space contributes to oedema. Oedema is worsened by the dilution of plasma albumin, and other osmotically active components of blood. Subsequent excretion of the excess volume load is often impaired in the critically ill.

Several fluids are available that contain osmotically active constituents. Gelatin solutions (Haemaccel) are maintained within the circulation for 2–3 hours, are stable in solution and have a long shelf-life at room temperature and are therefore immediately available. Starch polymers (hydroxyethyl starch) have a longer half-life (6–9 hours) and are less allergenic than the gelatins. Neither solution carries oxygen nor replaces clotting factors lost during haemorrhage. Their main value is in the maintenance of filling pressure during resuscitation prior to the availability of blood. The sodium content of these infusions is high, has to be cleared by the patient, and can contribute to oedema formation.

Human albumin in solution is available and in the iso-osmotic form (4.5%) is ideal for volume replacement, especially in the critically ill. It is pasteurised, avoiding the risk of infection, has a long shelf-life and, although more expensive than the other polymer solutions, is better retained in the circulation. It does not contain clotting factors.

Cross-matched blood may be available within 20 minutes. Blood is a living tissue; when stored, metabolites gradually accumulate and clotting factors become rapidly depleted. The amount of damaged cells and debris progressively increases, as well as the acidity and K$^+$ content. Blood is stored at a low temperature, and rapid transfusion will cool the recipient. Blood is commonly plasma reduced, and the packed units therefore have a high haemoglobin concentration.

The separated constituents of whole blood are available as plasma which is frozen to prevent degradation of the clotting factors (FFP). FFP is scarce and expensive, and should not be given routinely as volume replacement.

Fluid overload

Critically ill patients often retain fluid because of renal dysfunction, excess antidiuretic hormone (ADH) secretion or drug therapy (e.g. steroids). Volume overload may occur by injudicious intravenous fluid therapy in patients who cannot produce a compensatory diuresis. The filling pressure is raised, stretching cardiac muscle to the point where contractility declines, at the plateau of the PAWP/CI graph (square C, Fig. 14.4). The clinical signs can be similar to those of the poorly contracting ventricle (see below), both right- and left-sided filling pressures being raised. Treatment is to reduce filling pressures rather than infuse inotropes. Diuretic therapy reduces the volume of the circulation and promptly relieves oedema. If filling pressures are critically high, vasodilator therapy can reduce them acutely. Diuretic therapy will only be successful if cardiac output is sufficient to perfuse the kidneys and renal function is not impaired. If renal function is inadequate, volume reduction can be achieved by haemofiltration or veno-venous dialysis (p. 810).

Poor contractility

The relationship between filling pressure and CI when left ventricular function is depressed is shown in Figure 14.5. As filling pressure rises, the response of the ventricle is reduced and the CI is low. This typically occurs after myocardial infarction (cardiogenic shock). The crucial point is that rises in the filling pressure do not improve the CI. Pulmonary oedema occurs when the filling pressure is raised (square D, Fig. 14.5). The pressure at which fluid extravasates into the lung is determined by the balance of forces driving the fluid out of the circulation (hydrostatic pressure) and the osmotic pressure of the plasma, acting to retain fluid within the vasculature. As the filling pressures rise, this point is exceeded

and oedema fluid develops (p. 512, Fig. 13.52). Oedema develops at low pressure if plasma proteins are reduced or capillary permeability is increased.

Patients with pump failure have a low-volume pulse, raised jugular venous pressure, third heart sound and sometimes signs of pulmonary oedema. As a result of the low CI, urine output may be reduced. In such patients, monitoring of the circulation is, of necessity, invasive. Continuous monitoring of arterial pressure requires a cannula inserted into a peripheral artery. A pulmonary artery catheter is used to monitor left and right ventricular function, cardiac output, and pulmonary and systemic vascular resistances. A urinary catheter is necessary to measure urine output as an index of renal perfusion.

Management

In pump failure, the aim of management is to increase the output of the heart for a given filling pressure, thereby altering the slope of the PAWP/CI curve.

Positive inotropic agents

The naturally occurring inotropic agents are adrenaline, secreted by the adrenal medulla, and noradrenaline, produced by the sympathetic nervous system. Other inotropic drugs include the adrenaline precursor dopamine and the synthetic dobutamine. These drugs increase the force of cardiac contraction by stimulation of beta receptors. A further category of drugs, the phosphodiesterase inhibitors (enoximone and milrinone) produce an inotropic response by increasing intracellular cyclic AMP. These drugs are also vasodilators, leading to reduction in peripheral vascular resistance. These newer agents are more expensive, and unlike the catecholamines, their half-life is measured in hours, making it difficult to finely adjust their effect. Positive inotropes are detailed in Table 14.4.

Preload reduction with vasodilators is most effective when the filling pressure/cardiac output curve is flat, and changes in filling pressure produce reversal of pulmonary oedema without large decreases in the CI. Careful monitoring of the circulation is essential, as slight alterations in vasodilating dose may produce large reductions in cardiac output. All vasoactive drugs should be given by volumetric pumps, and the shorter-acting drugs are an advantage. Alteration in peripheral vascular resistance can be particularly effective if combined with inotropic support, improving forward flow while maintaining myocardial perfusion pressure.

Negative inotropes

The force of contraction of the myocardium is depressed by acidosis, hypokalaemia, hypoxaemia and hypercapnia.

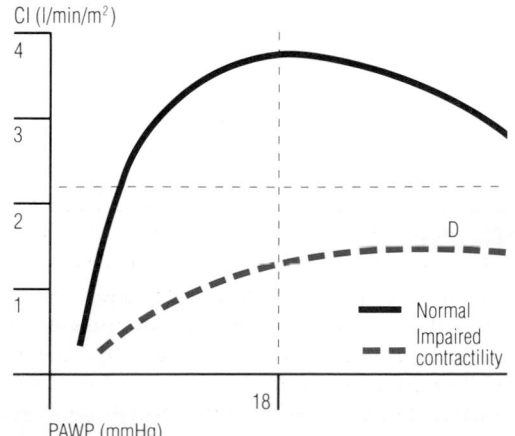

Fig. 14.5 Poor contractility. Compared with normal, the PAWP/CI curve (dashed line) is almost horizontal over a wide range of filling pressures.

Table 14.4 Positive inotropes (dosages shown are an initial guide)

Agent	Receptors	Dose range (μg/kg/min)	Actions	Comments
Dobutamine	Beta	1–10	HR and contractility increased	Preferred initially as vasodilatation enhances cardiac output
Adrenaline	Alpha and beta	1–10	Low dose: HR ++, contractility ++ Increasing dose: vasoconstriction, SVR ++	Useful alternative to dobutamine, but vasoconstriction may reduce peripheral perfusion
Noradrenaline	Alpha	0.1–4.0	Vasoconstriction ++	Increases blood pressure at expense of perfusion
Isoprenaline	Beta	1–10	HR ++, contractility ++	Improves contractility but increases myocardial O_2 consumption
Dopamine	Dopaminergic, beta, alphanergic	3 (low dose) 5–10 (intermediate) 10–40 (high dose)	Low dose: renal and mesenteric vasodilation Intermediate dose: HR and contractility raised High dose: vasoconstriction	Used to promote renal perfusion. Often used in conjunction with dobutamine

These negative inotropes, particularly acidosis, offset the effectiveness of treatment. The dose response of catecholamines is adversely affected by acidosis. Correction of these disturbances may depend on restoration of peripheral circulation, although in the short term, reversal of acidosis by hyperventilation (in patients receiving mechanical ventilation) and bicarbonate may be necessary.

The major determinant of oxygen delivery to heart muscle is coronary blood flow, which, if reduced, impairs contractility. Myocardial blood flow, especially to the subendocardial layer, is reduced by an increase in ventricular wall tension. This is the case in the dilated heart and in one contracting against a raised peripheral vascular resistance. Flow to all layers of the myocardium is crucially dependent on diastolic pressure and duration, and both are reduced by tachycardia. Improvement of coronary circulation can be effected by a reduction in afterload (reducing ventricular wall tension), if it is achieved without markedly decreasing diastolic pressure or causing a tachycardia.

Summary 1 Factors that reduce O_2 delivery to the myocardium

- Diastolic pressure <60 mmHg
- Overdistension of ventricles
- Tachycardia
- Vasoconstriction

Mechanical support

Myocardial function may remain depressed despite conventional therapy. Mechanical devices have been developed to enhance heart action by decreasing left ventricular work and improving coronary blood flow. One device is the intra-aortic balloon pump (IABP). The pump is connected to a sausage-shaped balloon that is introduced percutaneously into the femoral artery and placed in the descending aorta. The gas-filled balloon is inflated during diastole, and blood flow in the aorta away from the heart is reversed, increasing coronary blood flow. The balloon collapses at the start of systole, decreasing peripheral vascular resistance. The IABP therefore reduces afterload but maintains coronary perfusion. It has had considerable success in the management of pump failure following cardiac surgery, but much less success in patients with a low CI after, for example, myocardial infarction. New techniques, including artificial hearts, may in the future allow time to prepare selected patients for cardiac transplantation.

With severe pulmonary oedema, the work of breathing is greatly increased. Overall oxygen consumption (and myocardial work) is reduced by mechanical ventilation. Although mechanical ventilation may depress the CI when patients are hypovolaemic, positive pressure breaths may enhance cardiac function in the failing heart. Improvements in cardiac function may also occur by controlling pulmonary oedema, reducing the work of breathing and allowing for a stable period during which other therapies can be pursued.

SEPTIC SHOCK

Hypotension as a complication of septicaemia is an important development, indicating the progression of a frequently fatal illness despite antibiotics. Vasodilating fragments and mediators (Fig. 14.6) cause a fall in peripheral vascular resistance, leading to hypotension despite maintenance of a normal or raised CI. Peripheral blood flow is diverted to the skin and muscle, with poor perfusion of vital organs. In addition, substances released

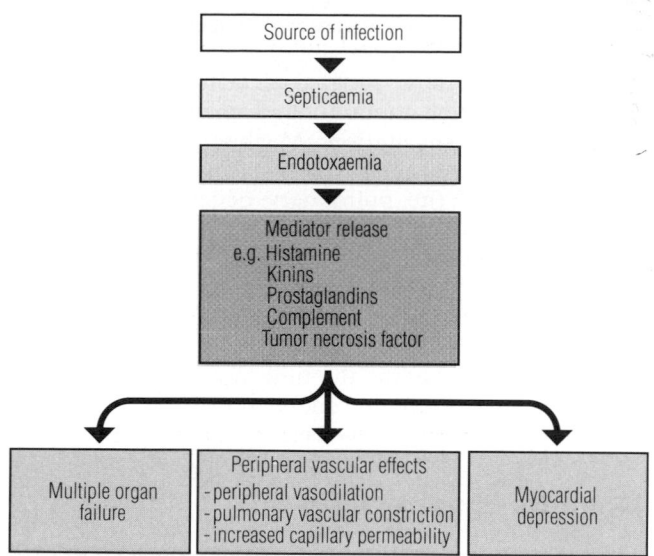

Fig. 14.6 Septic shock.

during acute endotoxaemia depress myocardial function. This mediator release rapidly becomes a cascade phenomenon involving interleukins and other cytokines, resulting in further tissue breakdown. Although research has focused in blockade of this inflammatory response, no beneficial treatment regime has so far emerged.

The patient is vasodilated, with warm peripheries and bounding, high-volume pulses. Pyrexia is usual, but less commonly the temperature may be depressed. To maintain a high CI, in order to perfuse vital organs, filling pressures are monitored and plasma substitutes (PPF) given, often in large volumes. Despite adequate filling pressures, inotropic support may be required to maintain the CI. Vasoconstricting drugs (alpha agonists) may worsen peripheral perfusion, but may occasionally be of value in intractable hypotension and may increase urine output.

RESPIRATORY PROBLEMS

Respiratory failure has many causes (p. 493, Table 13.31). Severe hypoxaemia with or without hypercapnia is a common indication for transferring a patient to the ICU for monitoring and, where necessary, mechanical ventilation.

Assessment of ventilation and tissue oxygen delivery

During steady-state conditions, when the amount of CO_2 from the tissue is constant, arterial CO_2 tension is dependent on alveolar ventilation. The adequacy of ventilation can therefore be judged by Pa_{CO_2}. As ventilation becomes inadequate, CO_2 is retained and eventually the patient becomes acidotic. Over many weeks acclimatisation to

hypercapnia may occur, and the respiratory acidosis is compensated for by a metabolic alkalosis (p. 856). Despite the undoubted value of CO_2 measurements in the assessment of ventilation, it should be emphasised that in some patients (e.g. those with severe asthma) there can be acute respiratory distress with CO_2 levels that are normal or reduced.

Adequacy of oxygenation is more difficult to assess. Arterial oxygen tension should be judged against the added oxygen the patient is breathing. In disease, as gas exchange deteriorates, so the difference between the inspired oxygen tension and that of arterial blood increases (the $A–aO_2$ gradient (p. 493) widens). The size of the $A–aO_2$ difference indicates the failure of the lung to perform gas exchange (see Table 14.5). An indication of this deficit is easily assessed by calculating the PaO_2/FiO_2 ratio. In health, this number is greater than 450 (e.g. $100/0.21 = 476$), and severe disease is indicated when the ratio is less than 150 (e.g. $70/0.5 = 140$). This may be due to impaired diffusion or ventilation–perfusion (V/Q) mismatch, and added oxygen can correct these defects. However, if the hypoxaemia is due to blood bypassing ventilated alveoli (physiological shunt), then increasing the oxygen fraction will not dramatically improve blood gases. Both the level of added oxygen that is required, and the rate at which it is necessary to increase this fraction, reflect the severity and progression of disease.

Table 14.5 Assessment of oxygen uptake by the lung

The difference between alveolar and arterial oxygen tension is normally small. The extent of the alveolar–arterial ($A–aO_2$) gradient provides a useful measure of the severity of respiratory failure.

Alveolar–arterial gradient (A–a) = oxygen tension in alveolar air (PAO_2) minus oxygen tension in arterial blood:

$$A – aO_2 = PAO_2 – PaO_2$$

The oxygen tension in alveolar air (PAO_2) = oxygen tension in inspired air (PIO_2) minus the arterial CO_2 tension (Pa_{CO_2})/Respiratory Quotient (R):

$$PAO_2 = PIO_2 – Pa_{CO_2}/R$$

Thus in a *normal subject*:

PAO_2 = $[0.21 \times (760 – 47)^*] – 40/0.8$
= 100 mmHg
$A – aO_2$ = 100 – 98 = 2 mmHg

(normal gradient is small, rising with age, and is less than 15 mmHg; 2 kPa)

For a *patient with severe respiratory failure* on the ICU, ventilated with 50% oxygen who has an arterial PaO_2 of 80 mmHg, the results could be:

PAO_2 = $[0.5 \times (760 – 47) – (48/0.8)]$
= 297 mmHg
$A – aO_2$ = 297 – 80 = 217 mmHg

Serial measurement of the A–a gradient provides excellent information on oxygenation.

*Water vapour pressure.

Summary 2 Tissue oxygenation

- Oxygen carriage in blood – Pao_2, Sao_2, Hb
- Tissue perfusion – cardiac output
- Tissue uptake of oxygen – mixed venous oxygen tension and saturation

Arterial blood gases provide a single respiratory assessment of the patient, and can be misleading when the patient's circumstances are changing rapidly. Repeated samples are often preferable and require the insertion of an arterial cannula. The clinical context of the arterial sample (e.g. FiO_2, ventilator settings) should always be documented. Oximeters that continuously and non-invasively measure oxygen saturation (SaO_2) are very useful.

O_2 must be delivered to the tissues, and therefore the state of oxygen transport and uptake from the circulation are important. Transport of oxygen depends on the amount of haemoglobin and its ability to take up oxygen (O_2 dissociation curve, p. 446). The cardiac output and state of the peripheral microcirculation then determine the delivery of oxygen to the respiring cells.

The tissues extract oxygen from the blood and in health the amount of oxygen delivered to the tissues each minute is much greater than is needed. In the critically ill, this may not be the case, and the level of oxygen in the venous blood may be reduced, indicating that not enough oxygen is being supplied. The cause may be failure of the lung to perform gas exchange, or inadequate tissue perfusion. The average O_2 tension in venous blood (mixed venous oxygen) provides useful information and can be measured from samples taken from the pulmonary artery or continuously by a fibre-optic catheter.

Indications for mechanical ventilation

Intubation and ventilation are easier to undertake as a considered manoeuvre rather than as an emergency event. The entire clinical situation is relevant, and ventilation is seldom indicated solely on blood gas results. An increasing demand for oxygen over a few hours, failure adequately to oxygenate the patient with a facemask or mental deterioration indicate the likely need for mechanical support. Patients who are distressed initially often have a normal or slightly lowered $Paco_2$, with rapid shallow respirations. Further distress, an increase in the respiratory rate or increasing sympathetic activity (tachycardia, hypertension) indicate greater difficulty in eliminating CO_2, and exhaustion, with associated hypercapnia, is a common end-point prior to ventilation.

The clearance of secretions by the patient is dependent on the ability to cough vigorously, and sputum retention may worsen or precipitate respiratory failure. Endotracheal intubation allows efficient removal of secretions by suction and also protects the upper airway from aspiration.

Many postoperative patients are ventilated electively to provide a period of stabilisation. Some patients are intubated during resuscitation. Mechanical ventilation is sometimes required to provide a stable setting during the management of the pulmonary oedema of left heart failure.

For artificial ventilation to be initiated, the patient must be anaesthetised and intubated. Patients may already be critically ill; if so, the cardiovascular effects of the anaesthetic agents, lack of reflexes guarding the larynx, mechanical problems in passing the tube and effects of positive intrathoracic pressure on venous return make intubation and ventilation a potentially dangerous procedure.

Methods of ventilation

The ventilator provides the motive power to drive oxygen-enriched air into the patient's lungs. This may need to be done at high pressure, as, for example, when ventilating an asthmatic with severe bronchoconstriction. With modern ventilators it is possible to determine the respiratory rate, tidal volume, driving pressure, and the timing and waveform of the inspiratory cycle. Many patients on the ICU are deeply sedated and sometimes paralysed. All the ventilatory requirements of such patients are provided by the mechanical ventilator: this is termed controlled mandatory ventilation (CMV). Other patients often require partial support from the ventilator, and may breathe spontaneously between machine breaths. In order to avoid a machine breath coinciding with spontaneous exhalation the inspiratory cycle of the ventilator is synchronised to the patient's own inspiratory effort. The patient's inspiratory effort is sensed at the start of each breath, and the inspiratory cycle of the machine is initiated. The machine rate and tidal volume are set to provide adequate alveolar ventilation; this is termed synchronised intermittent mandatory ventilation (SIMV). Newer ventilators can now assist each spontaneous breath, the level of assistance ranging from partial support to full ventilation. This is performed by providing a constant, positive pressure to the patient with each spontaneous breath (inspiratory pressure support, IPS). The amount of IPS can be adjusted up and down. However, this form of respiratory support is critically dependent on the patient's spontaneous effort, and will provide no support if the patient becomes apnoeic (i.e. during sleep).

A further feature of ventilators is the capacity to add a positive (greater than atmospheric) pressure throughout the expiratory phase of the respiratory cycle. The purpose of such positive end-expiratory pressure (PEEP) is to prevent collapse of peripheral airways and subsequent atelectasis, thereby improving gas exchange. The addition of PEEP, commonly 5–10 cmH_2O, usually improves arterial oxygen tension, but impedes venous return and can reduce the CI. Oxygen delivery to the tissues may therefore be decreased despite an improvement in Pa_{O_2}. PEEP may also increase pressure damage to the lung. The optimum level of PEEP for a particular patient is that which maximises tissue oxygen delivery.

Complications of ventilation

There is significant morbidity and occasional mortality associated with mechanical ventilation.

Pressure damage to the lung is termed barotrauma, and the incidence is increased when high airway pressures are required to ventilate the lungs. Pneumothorax is not uncommon and may present as gas in the pleural space, mediastinum or soft tissues (surgical emphysema). A tension pneumothorax can occur. When drained, the pleural leak may persist (bronchopleural fistula), and, if severe, the volume of gas escaping from the leak may exceed the capacity of the ventilator, leading to hypoventilation. Selective ventilation of each lung (differential ventilation) can isolate the side with the leak. High levels of oxygen produce lung damage, and cause or exacerbate the adult respiratory distress syndrome (ARDS, p. 511). Patients on ventilators are often deeply sedated and therefore totally dependent on the correct functioning of the equipment. They are also dependent on a supply of humidified, oxygen-enriched air. Constant nursing care is crucial. Secretions in the respiratory tract must be aspirated by the ICU staff, and airway collapse and atelectasis are common complications. The artificial airway is a portal for the entry of pathogens.

Patients can be ventilated via an endotracheal tube for several weeks, but because the tube is a constant source of irritation to the mouth, a tracheostomy is often performed when it is likely that an artificial airway will be required for a prolonged period (Table 14.6).

Withdrawal of mechanical ventilation

As patients on the ICU recover, the aim is to withdraw mechanical ventilation. For this to be feasible, the patient's CVS must be stable, with good peripheral perfusion. Gas exchange must be good, with satisfactory oxygenation and an inspired oxygen concentration of less than 50%. The patient should not be septic. There should be no gross acid–base or electrolyte abnormality.

Table 14.6 Major indications for tracheostomy

- Provision of prolonged positive pressure ventilation
- Control of secretions
- To prevent aspiration
- To bypass upper airway obstruction

In patients where the period of ventilation has been short (hours), the withdrawal of assisted ventilation usually poses few problems. Sedation is withdrawn, the patient wakes up and breathes spontaneously from a source of oxygen, and is then extubated. In patients who have been ventilated for a number of days, it is often not possible to withdraw ventilation suddenly, and a period of gradual withdrawal, or weaning, is necessary. Successful weaning requires careful consideration of the following interrelated questions:

- Is central drive optimal?
- Is the respiratory muscle pump as effective as possible?
- Has the load on the respiratory muscle pump been reduced to the minimum?
- Given the capacity of the respiratory muscle pump (Fig. 14.7), can the ventilatory load be sustained or is fatigue likely?

Opinions differ as to the best method of weaning. Gradual reduction in the number of machine breaths by using SIMV allows the patient to breathe spontaneously, with a background of support from the ventilator. Alternatively, inspiratory pressure support (IPS) can be gradually reduced so that the patient progressively takes over the work of breathing. Another approach is to allow the patient to breathe spontaneously and unaided for successively longer periods of time, alternating with machine ventilation. In some patients the work of breathing can be reduced and weaning facilitated by continuous positive airway pressure (CPAP), which can be continued post-extubation via a face or nasal mask. Some patients can be weaned by using non-invasive nasal ventilation (nasal intermittent positive pressure ventilation, NIPPV).

During weaning it is important to optimise the function of the respiratory muscle pump. Any metabolic disturbances known to reduce the contractility of the

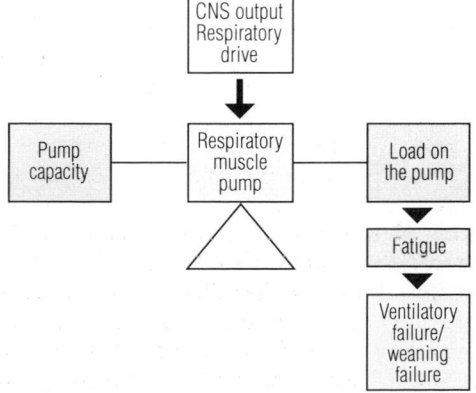

Fig. 14.7 The respiratory muscle pump. When assessing the likelihood of successful weaning from mechanical ventilation the key factors are ventilatory load, drive and capacity. If the demands made of the pump exceed capacity, weaning will fail.

Table 14.7 Metabolic abnormalities that impair respiratory muscle contractility

- Acidosis
- Hypophosphataemia
- Hypomagnesaemia
- Hypokalaemia
- Hyper- and hypothyroidism
- Steroid therapy
- Other drugs (e.g. drug-induced myasthenic syndromes)
- Hypoxia
- Hypercapnia

respiratory muscles should be corrected (Table 14.7). In patients with airways obstruction, bronchodilatation is helpful in reducing hyperinflation and improving muscle efficiency, as well as reducing ventilatory load. Treatment of pulmonary oedema also reduces the work of breathing. The effort of breathing through the tubing, ventilator and endotracheal tube should be minimised and the airway made as comfortable as possible. The patient should be sitting upright, preferably in a chair, and the abdomen should be free to allow the diaphragm to descend. During weaning, nutritional support must be maintained.

Several factors distinguish patients who will sustain spontaneous ventilation from those that are ventilator dependent (Table 14.8). Despite this, it is possible for seemingly weak patients to wean when the load applied to the muscles is low. If such patients are assessed by a measurement of respiratory muscle strength alone, weaning would erroneously not be attempted. An assessment of the balance between strength, load and drive is more likely to accurately predict weaning outcome than any single test.

The patient should not be allowed to become distressed off the ventilator. The sensation of breathlessness is terrifying, especially since the patient has difficulty with communication. Much psychological support is needed. In the early stages of weaning the patient should receive full ventilation during the night, and the benefit of a full

Table 14.8 Factors favourable to successful weaning

- Adequate Pao_2 on <40% inspired oxygen (Fio_2<0.4)
- Maximum voluntary ventilation greater than twice resting ventilation
- Respiratory rate <25 breaths/minute breathing spontaneously
- Minute ventilation <10 litres/minute
- Vital capacity >20 ml/kg
- Maximum static inspiratory pressure >30 cmH$_2$O
- Frequency (breaths/min): Tidal volume (litres) ratio <105 breathing spontaneously

night's sleep. Sedative drugs are in general best avoided, but may be required if the patient is sleep-deprived.

CENTRAL NERVOUS SYSTEM PROBLEMS

ICU therapy is directed towards ventilation, supportive care and control of intracranial pressure (ICP).

Pathophysiology

The brain is enclosed in a rigid box. In addition to brain substance, the cranium contains blood and cerebrospinal fluid (CSF). The ability of the box to accommodate a swollen brain or a space-occupying lesion is, of necessity, dependent on a parallel reduction in the volume of either CSF or blood. This compensation continues until a further increase in the contents of the box produces a sharp and rapid rise in pressure. Initially the change in pressure during the accommodating process is slight, but the response to a small volume of fluid added to the box shows how compliance is falling. At the beginning of the curve illustrated in Figure 14.8, the addition of aliquots of fluid to the box (in this case via a ventricular catheter) produces a slight and transient rise in ICP. Further along the curve, although the baseline pressure has only risen slightly, the rise in pressure with the added volume is substantial. Such fluid challenges demonstrate the seriousness of cerebral oedema with greater sensitivity than absolute ICP measurements.

Sudden rises in pressure reduce brain perfusion. The mean pressure in the cerebral arteries is opposed by the ICP, and the balance is the pressure available to perfuse the brain. As ICP rises, so the flow of blood to the brain

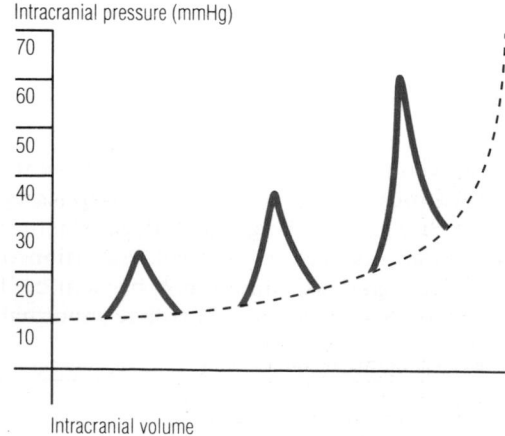

Intracranial pressure (mmHg)

Intracranial volume

Fig. 14.8 Relationship between intracranial volume and pressure. Initially, increased volume has little effect on pressure but eventually further small increases cause a dramatic rise in ICP. The location of a patient on the curve can be determined by volume challenge (red lines) (see text).

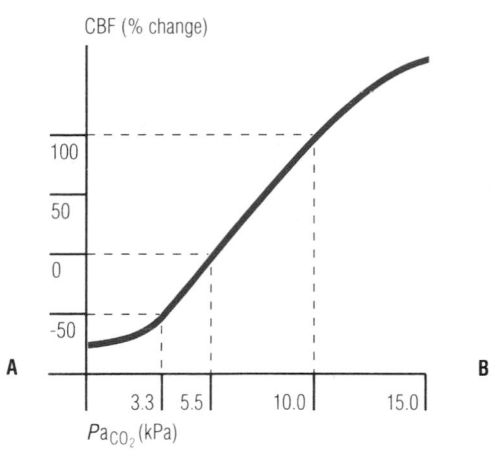

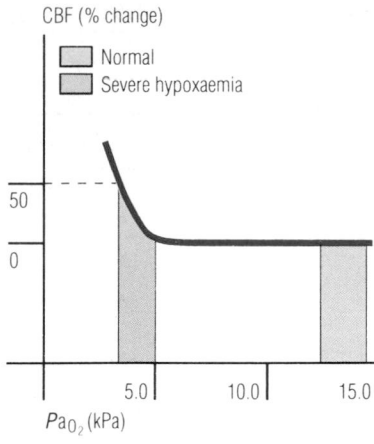

Fig. 14.9 Cerebral blood flow. A. Effect of arterial CO_2 tension (Pa_{CO_2}) on cerebral blood flow (CBF). Hypercapnia markedly increases CBF (whereas hypocapnia reduces CBF). **B.** Effect of arterial O_2 tension (Pa_{O_2}) on cerebral blood flow. Severe hypoxaemia substantially increases CBF.

decreases, and the consequent ischaemia worsens the insult to partially damaged tissue surrounding the damaged centre.

Many other factors can raise the pressure within the closed box. Cerebral blood volume can be increased by dilating the cerebral arteries, the calibre of which is greatly affected by CO_2 and O_2 tensions (Fig. 14.9). Increases in CO_2 have a particularly deleterious effect, doubling blood flow to the brain. Whilst decreasing CO_2 tension reduces flow and therefore lowers pressure in the brain, this is not sustained indefinitely. Severe hypoxaemia increases cerebral blood flow and ICP therefore rises.

Assessment and management

Conscious level is determined by grading the patient's response in terms of best verbal response, best motor response and ability of the patient to speak, according to the Glasgow Coma Scale score (p. 859). The pupillary reflexes, focal neurological signs, blood pressure and pulse are checked and recorded sequentially. The coma score on admission to the ICU and subsequent changes

in the score are useful indicators of progress and prognosis (Fig. 14.10). Patients admitted after head trauma may also have other injuries that can easily be overlooked.

Initial therapy for patients with a head injury should include the administration of oxygen, as many patients are hypoxaemic. Crystalloid therapy exacerbates oedema, both in the head and lung. Cardiovascular resuscitation is important, as hypotension may further damage the brain, especially if the ICP is raised. Facilities to reduce or control raised ICP should be available.

The initial treatment of patients with severe head injury usually precedes a definitive diagnosis, as diagnostic facilities, particularly CT scanning, are rarely available immediately. Mechanical ventilation may be necessary to reverse hypercapnia and reduce ICP.

Therapy to reduce ICP

Therapy may be initiated on the assumption that the ICP is raised, or following ICP measurement. Reduction in pressure can be achieved by reducing the volume of the brain and reducing cerebral blood volume by controlling cerebral blood flow. Therapy is also aimed at decreasing the oxygen requirement of the brain, by reducing cerebral metabolism, and maintaining the perfusion of brain cells.

Reduction in brain size

Decreasing brain water can be achieved by diuretics, most commonly the osmotic diuretic mannitol. Over-vigorous treatment can cause severe fluid depletion.

Control of cerebral blood volume

Cerebral blood volume is related to the flow of blood to the enclosed box. The lowering of CO_2 and the reversal of hypoxaemia reduce cerebral blood volume and ICP.

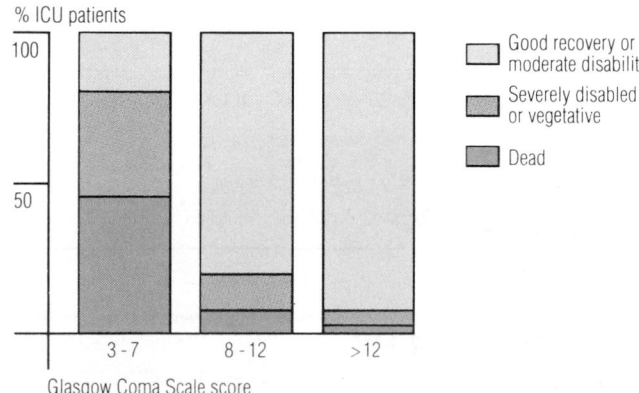

Fig. 14.10 Prognosis following head injury related to Glasgow Coma Scale score.

Mechanical ventilation may be necessary for the close control of blood gases.

Reduction in venous drainage transmits pressure retrogradely, raising ICP. A disadvantage of mechanical ventilation is that the positive pressure in the chest raises the venous pressure in the head. Ventilation must be adjusted to ensure that the pressure in the chest is kept as low as practicable.

Cerebral metabolic rate

Damage to surviving neurones occurs due to a reduction in local capillary blood flow. By reducing the requirement for oxygen (by lowering the cerebral metabolic rate), the survival of brain cells is enhanced. Sudden rises in cellular metabolism, during which the consumption of oxygen outstrips supply, must be avoided. Sedative drugs reduce cerebral oxygen consumption. The prevention of convulsions, which dramatically raise cerebral metabolic rate, is essential.

General care

Intracranial pressure may rise transiently during many manoeuvres on ICU, decreasing cerebral perfusion pressure.

The general care of patients includes:

- avoiding painful stimuli
- avoiding overtransfusion of crystalloid solutions
- moderate fluid restriction
- maintaining a head-up position to enhance venous drainage.

Monitoring

During appropriate treatment of raised ICP the use of sedation and mechanical ventilation removes many clinical signs that would otherwise indicate changes in the patient's cerebral status. Pupillary and cardiovascular reflexes may be the only signs preserved. Invasive monitoring of ICP is therefore important if changes in the patient's status are to be detected. ICP can be measured by several techniques, including a simple manometer system introduced into the cerebral ventricles, or the measurement of pressure at the surface of the brain via intra- or extradural probes. Both absolute pressure and response to therapeutic manoeuvres are of great help in management.

The detection of grand mal seizures is difficult if the patient is paralysed. However, the electrical activity during fitting is increased, and this can be detected by measuring the electrical activity of the cerebral hemispheres (cerebral function monitor).

Table 14.9 Suitable organ donors

- Age 0–70 years
- Patient has suffered irreversible brainstem death
- Ventilator-dependent
- No malignancy (except primary brain tumour)
- No systemic sepsis
- Hepatitis and HIV negative
- ABO compatibility

Brainstem death and organ transplantation

Irrecoverable damage to the brain may occur after massive global insults such as prolonged hypoxaemia, trauma and cerebrovascular events. In the absence of conditions that invalidate testing (neuromuscular blockade, drug overdosage, uncertain diagnosis, hypothermia) assessment of the brainstem involves two independent observers of senior status and a repeated investigation, typically after 24 hours. Brainstem death implies a deeply comatose patient with no response to peripheral and central painful stimuli, the absence of deep reflexes (corneal, gag and tracheal), no eye movement in response to ice-cold water irrigation to the external ear and no respiratory efforts when hypercapnic.

Such patients may be suitable for organ transplantation (Table 14.9), which could include cornea, heart, lung, liver and kidneys. Under the circumstances of bereavement, which is often sudden and unexpected, the subject of donation requires understanding and compassion. In the UK, advice is available from the regional donor transplant coordinator, who will organise the transplantation of any or all suitable organs.

Summary 3 Brainstem death

- Absence of corneal reflexes
- No light or consensual reflex
- No eye response to ice-cold saline slowly infused into the external auditory meatus (n.b. tympanic membrane intact)
- No gag or response to tracheal suction
- No ventilatory response to a CO_2 challenge
- No motor response to painful peripheral stimulation

RENAL PROBLEMS

The development of renal failure is a common and serious complication in the critically ill, associated with high mortality. Whilst the major insult to the kidney may have occurred prior to admission, rapid and effective resuscitation may prevent further deterioration of renal function. Incipient or established renal failure are discussed in Chapter 20. Sepsis, sometimes occult, is a common cause of renal failure on the ICU.

Commonly, the first indication of renal dysfunction is reduced urinary volume. Assessment and manipulation of the CVS are often important. Despite hypovolaemia, the blood pressure may be normal due to intensive vasoconstriction. Renal ultrasound is of value in excluding obstructive lesions.

Once an adequate circulation has been established, urinary output may be enhanced by low-dose dopamine (<5 μg/kg/minute). A further reduction in urine output is likely to herald established renal failure; although output may be enhanced by high-dose frusemide, this may only postpone eventual anuria. Filtration will be depressed by severe acidosis.

Fluid intake should be adjusted to the falling urine output. The multiplicity of intravenous infusions makes volume overload a possible error. Drug dosages should be reviewed in the light of the patient's renal function, and nephrotoxic drugs avoided (e.g. aminoglycoside antibiotics, NSAIDS, frusemide).

Indications for dialysis include the control of extracellular volume, electrolyte imbalance and acidosis, and uraemia. Intermittent haemodialysis or peritoneal dialysis can be difficult in the seriously ill. New techniques have revolutionised the management of renal failure. Haemofiltration filters can be perfused with blood and require only a small driving pressure to produce a urine-like filtrate. Whilst this continuous filtration can control extracellular volume, the clearance of urea and electrolytes requires high volumes of filtrate per day and, without skill, fluid imbalance can lead to circulatory collapse. By passing a solution across the membrane against the direction of blood flow, dialysis of urea and other molecules occurs by diffusion and convection gradients. This low-volume continuous arteriovenous haemodialysis (CAVHD) can be enhanced by using a pump to control the flow of dialysis fluid past the filter.

MULTIPLE ORGAN FAILURE

The syndrome of progressive multiple organ failure is not uncommon on the ICU and mortality is very high. The syndrome is characterised by an alteration in tissue blood flow, local release of mediators that are cytotoxic, and an inability of peripheral tissue to use oxygen at a mitochondrial level. It is not always associated with sepsis, but failing organs demand a careful and systematic search for infection. Frequent samples of blood and body fluid should be cultured. Repeated pelvic and abdominal ultrasound examination, echocardiography and CT scanning

may be needed. Despite appropriate antibiotic therapy, mortality remains high if any source of infection is not eradicated. In the presence of sepsis, antibiotic therapy should be started immediately. Choice of antibiotics can be made based on the following criteria:

- the site of infection
- whether the infection is hospital or community acquired
- whether the patient has had recent surgery
- the immunocompetence of the patient
- the presence of Gram-negative bacilli in infected material.

Treatment with a single agent with a narrow spectrum of activity against a known organism is preferable, but in a severe life-threatening situation multiple antibiotic therapy is difficult to avoid. (Antibiotic therapy is discussed further in Chapter 11.)

As organs fail, progressive hypoxaemia is common. There is a general increase in capillary permeability, and in the lungs the leak of osmotically active fluid at normal or low filling pressures causes pulmonary oedema. This pattern of non-cardiogenic pulmonary oedema is termed the adult respiratory distress syndrome (ARDS, p. 511).

Renal perfusion is decreased by episodes of systemic hypotension. Perfusion may also be reduced by local vasoconstriction and filtration impaired by fibrin deposition. Local disturbances of coagulation or disseminated intravascular coagulation (DIC) may occur. Jaundice develops as hepatic function deteriorates.

NUTRITION

In normal man there is a limited reserve of rapidly available energy substrates (glucose and glycogen), which is depleted within 24–36 hours of starvation. Prolonged fasting leads to the production of glucose from protein catabolism via gluconeogenesis, and metabolism is shifted towards the utilisation of fats. In starvation the metabolic rate is decreased and nitrogen loss (from protein breakdown) is reduced, with the result that previously well-nourished patients can fast for several weeks. In the severely ill, not only is protein catabolised to glucose at a faster rate, but calorie requirements are also raised, by as much as 125% in those with extensive burns (Fig. 14.11). Many patients are compromised by a degree of malnutrition prior to admission to the ICU.

Nutritional failure is associated with increased morbidity and mortality. Synthetic capability is reduced, one of the consequences of which is decreased immunocompetence and increased susceptibility to infection.

Nutritional status requires careful assessment in the critically ill, and the history and length of illness should be noted. Precise measurement of nutritional status and

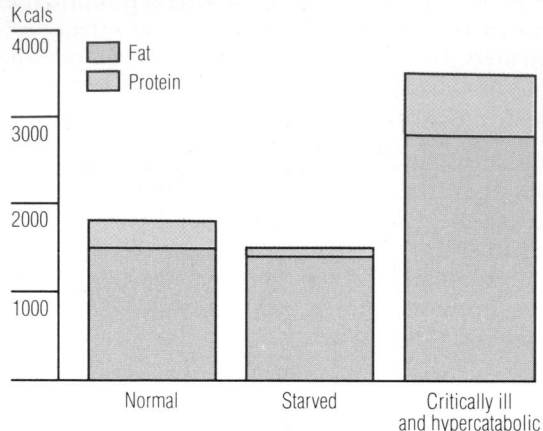

Fig. 14.11 Calorie requirements in normal individuals compared with those starved or critically ill and hypercatabolic.

requirements is difficult. Easily available measurements of synthetic capacity (albumin, total protein) are rather variable and discriminate poorly between nutritional states. (Nutrition is fully discussed in Chapter 7.)

If possible, feeding should be continuous and controlled using a fine-bore nasogastric tube. This route is simple, economical and less likely to lead to infection. The incidence of gastric erosions is reduced in the enterally fed. However, absorption is often decreased by gastric stasis, or the volume that can be given limited by diarrhoea. Parenteral administration is then necessary (p. 118), which involves the placement of a dedicated intravenous line. Patients often tolerate high fluid loads poorly and feeding therefore requires concentrated solutions which may only be administered via a central vein. The constituents of intravenous feeding are ideal culture media and there is always a risk of infection. The volume of fluid, even when made up of highly calorific fats and concentrated glucose solutions, can precipitate volume overload. Careful attention to detail is required to provide appropriate quantities of trace elements and vitamins.

During cellular respiration, fats and carbohydrates, when metabolised, produce differing amounts of CO_2, to be excreted mainly by the lungs. High carbohydrate feeds increase CO_2 production and can contribute to CO_2 retention and breathlessness in patients with marginal ventilatory function.

GENERAL CARE OF THE CRITICALLY ILL

Care on the ICU must be total as well as intensive. The patient who recovers from serious illness may have decades of life ahead and any residual handicap will be important. Attendant injuries, especially peripheral limb injuries, can be overlooked in the initial effort to resuscitate the patient, but may result in significant disability once the drama of intensive care is over. The maintenance of limb mobility and the prevention of contractures are important in bed-bound supine patients. Skin and pressure area care is crucial. Poor peripheral perfusion commonly contributes to skin breakdown. Healing is enhanced when pressure is relieved, and this can be facilitated by air beds. Reflexes are lost during paralysis and sedation. The eyes and mouth are vulnerable. If the patient is ventilated the artificial airway must be kept clear and clean.

There is no ideal sedative drug for patients on the ICU. The administration of sedation does not imply unconsciousness, and levels of sedation can be difficult to judge if the patient is receiving neuromuscular blocking drugs. For this reason local anaesthesia should always be used during painful procedures. Discussions around the bedside should be conducted as if the patient were aware.

Patients are often mentally obtunded, or may experience hallucinations and paranoia, causing severe agitation. A night-time sleeping regime is of great help in the care of the longer-term patient on the ICU, especially when weaning from mechanical ventilation.

The morale of patients and staff is central to the success of an intensive care unit. The sustaining of morale, along with high standards of patient care, is a great challenge for the critical care specialist.

OUTCOME

The outcome of patients admitted to the ICU can be assessed in different ways (Table 14.10). Survival is, in general, related to the severity of the presenting illness and the response to therapy. Patients with multiple organ failure have a particularly poor prognosis. Great care should be taken, however, when judging the prognosis of

Table 14.10 Outcome

Outcome from a single treatment technique for a defined disease

- IPPV for severe asthma: >80% of patients discharged from hospital
- IPPV for poisoning: >80% of patients discharged from hospital
- IPPV for pneumonia or non-traumatic coma: <35% of patients discharged from hospital

Outcome for organ system failure (e.g. cardiac, respiratory or renal failure)

- Failure of one organ system for more than one day: mortality approximately 35%
- Failure of two organ systems for more than one day: mortality approximately 60%
- Failure of three or more organ systems for more than three days: mortality approximately 90%

an individual patient, and the application of scoring systems to assess prognosis for a particular case has limited value. All staff on intensive care units have seen occasional patients survive against massive odds.

FURTHER READING

Bradley R D 1977 Studies in acute heart failure. Edward Arnold, London. *Essential monograph of disorders of the circulation*

Ledingham I McA, 1988 Recent advances in critical care medicine-3. Churchill Livingstone, Edinburgh. *Contains good accounts of many of the important topics in critical care medicine*

Tinker J, Zapol W M, 1991 Care of the critically ill patient. 2nd edn. Springer Verlag, Berlin. *Comprehensive textbook of critical care medicine*

Tobin M J, State of the art: Respiration monitoring in the intensive care unit. American Review of Respiratory Disease 1988, 138: 1625–1624. *An execellent review of all aspects of respiratory monitoring.*

Yang K L, Tobin M J. A prospective study of indexes predicting the outcome of trials of weaning from mechanical ventilation. The New England Journal of Medicine. 1991, 324:1445-50. *An up-to-date assessment of weaning from mechanical ventilation.*

15

Gastrointestinal Disease

Richard G Long and Brian T Cooper

INTRODUCTION

Diseases of the gastrointestinal tract are a major cause of morbidity and mortality throughout the world. In the UK, gastrointestinal disorders are responsible for one in 10 of all deaths and one in six of all admissions to general hospitals. The gastrointestinal tract is the commonest site for cancer. In British General Practice, one in 10 of all consultations are for indigestion, and one in 14 for diarrhoea. Worldwide, gastrointestinal disease is a vast cause of ill health and it has been estimated that on any one day, two hundred million people suffer from diarrhoea.

CLINICAL FEATURES OF GASTRO-INTESTINAL DISEASE

Typical symptoms of gastrointestinal disease are shown in Table 15.1. General symptoms are useful in assessing the state of health of many patients with gastrointestinal symptoms. Patients commonly complain of non-specific symptoms, but these are rarely associated with serious disease. Dyspepsia and indigestion are non-specific terms which describe a variety of different symptoms related to eating. It is important that patients define precisely what they mean. Proctalgia fugax is a transient shooting pain in the rectum. Tenesmus, an uncomfortable desire to defaecate often when there is no stool in the rectum, may be associated with rectal inflammation and the irritable bowel syndrome.

Abnormal signs in patients with gastrointestinal disease are summarised in Table 15.2. Diseases of the gut can result in malnutrition, while a failure of fluid intake or increased loss due to vomiting or diarrhoea results in dehydration. Peripheral oedema and ascites occur because of hypoproteinaemia due to protein loss, malabsorption or malnutrition. Vitamin D and calcium malabsorption result in hypocalcaemia and osteomalacia (Ch. 18). Finger clubbing can be associated with inflammatory bowel disease and coeliac disease, leuconychia (white nails) with hypoalbuminaemia, and koilonychia (spoon-shaped nails) with chronic iron deficiency anaemia. Aphthous ulcers occur in patients with coeliac disease, and more indolent mouth ulcers in Crohn's

Table 15.1 Symptoms of gut disease

General symptoms	**Small intestinal symptoms**
Anorexia	Diarrhoea
Weight loss	Steatorrhoea
Nausea and vomiting	Symptoms of anaemia
Malaise and lethargy	Abdominal colic
	Abdominal distension
Non-specific symptoms	
Flatulence	**Large intestinal symptoms**
Abdominal bloating	Symptoms of anaemia
Poorly or variably localised pain	Diarrhoea
	Constipation
Oesophageal symptoms	Abdominal colic
Dysphagia	Blood and mucus per rectum
Heartburn	Tenesmus
Regurgitation	Proctalgia
Retrosternal pain	Incontinence
Painful swallowing (odynophagia)	
Gastroduodenal symptoms	
Upper abdominal pain/discomfort	
Early satiety	
Haematemesis	

Table 15.2 **Signs of gut disease**

General	**Gastroduodenal**
Malnutrition	Epigastric tenderness
Dehydration	Epigastric mass
Anaemia	Succussion splash
Oedema	
Bone tenderness ⎤	**Small intestinal**
Chvostek's sign ⎬ Hypocalcaemia	Diarrhoea
Trousseau's sign ⎦	Steatorrhoea
Nail clubbing	Mass
Leuconychia	Abdominal distension
Koilonychia	Intestinal obstruction
Oral	**Colonic**
Aphthous ulcers	Mass
Other oral ulcers	Obstruction
Angular cheilitis	Distension
Stomatitis	
Glossitis	**Anorectal**
Telangiectasia	Anal fissures, tags,
	haemorrhoids
	Rectal examination: mass,
	blood, mucopus
	Sigmoidoscopy: proctitis,
	ulcers, tumours, melanosis,
	haemorrhoids

disease. Angular cheilitis, stomatitis and glossitis occur in patients with iron and water-soluble vitamin deficiencies. Facial and oral telangiectasia are associated with telangiectasia lower in the gut and these may bleed.

INVESTIGATION OF GASTROINTESTINAL DISEASE

Haematological and biochemical abnormalities

Iron and folate are absorbed from the upper small intestine, and malabsorption of either results in characteristic haematological changes (Table 15.3). In some patients with upper intestinal malabsorption (especially coeliac disease), a mixed folate and iron deficiency may be seen (dimorphic anaemia). Dietary iron deficiency can occur in patients with diets low in meat, and is particularly common in the elderly and in vegans. Blood loss can occur throughout the gut with consequent iron deficiency and anaemia. Gastric surgery can cause iron deficiency by reduced acid secretion impairing absorption, by bypassing the upper small intestinal mucosa, and by intestinal hurry. Folate is present in large amounts in green vegetables and liver but dietary deficiency may occur if the diet is inadequate.

Vitamin B_{12} is bound to intrinsic factor in the stomach and is absorbed specifically in the terminal ileum (as are bile acids). Intrinsic factor deficiency can be congenital or secondary to pernicious anaemia or gastrectomy. Malabsorption of the B_{12}–intrinsic factor complex is generally due to terminal ileal resection or disease (usually Crohn's disease). However, it can also occur (rarely) secondary to

Table 15.3 **Haematological abnormalities in gut disease**

Abnormality	Laboratory changes	Causes

Iron deficiency anaemia	Blood film: hypochromic microcytic red cells
	Low mean cell volume (MCV)
	Low serum iron and high total iron binding capacity
		Dietary
		Blood loss
		Malabsorption
		    Postgastrectomy
		    Upper small bowel disease

Folate deficiency anaemia	Blood film: macrocytic red cells High MCV Low red cell folate	Dietary Upper small bowel disease Drugs (e.g. sulphasalazine)
B_{12} deficiency anaemia	Blood film: macrocytic red cells High MCV Low serum B_{12}	Pernicious anaemia Terminal ileal disease Postgastrectomy Chronic pancreatic disease Fish tapeworm (*Diphyllobothrium latum*)
Hyposplenism	Howell-Jolly bodies Giant platelets	Coeliac disease Tropical sprue Crohn's disease
Neutrophil leucocytosis and high ESR		Chronic inflammation ± e.g. inflammatory bowel disease, abscess, etc.)

infestation with the fish tapeworm (*Diphyllobothrium latum*), to intestinal fistulas and blind loops, or with chronic pancreatitis (p. 610). The double isotope Schilling test (p. 1055) is used to determine whether B_{12} deficiency is due to lack of intrinsic factor or to malabsorption of the intrinsic factor–B_{12} complex.

Hyposplenism is a feature of some bowel disorders, particularly coeliac disease. The typical finding on a blood film is of Howell-Jolly bodies (red cells containing small nuclear fragments). It also occurs in some patients with inflammatory bowel disease.

Neutrophil leucocytosis and raised acute phase reactants (e.g. ESR, serum orosomucoids or C-reactive protein) are useful non-specific markers of intra-abdominal inflammation, particularly inflammatory bowel disease, and sepsis.

A low serum albumin is commonly seen in patients with bowel disease (Table 15.4) and reflects protein leakage into the gut, decreased dietary intake, reduced absorption and, rarely, decreased synthesis. Albumin has a plasma half-life of about 23 days. Proteins such as transferrin and pre-albumin have a shorter half-life and plasma levels consequently fall earlier.

Electrolytes may be deranged. In patients with gastric outflow obstruction (pyloric stenosis), a hypochloraemic hypokalaemic alkalosis may occur. Diarrhoea may result in dehydration and electrolyte loss, particularly potassium.

Postgastrectomy patients and patients with severe small bowel disease causing malabsorption may have a *low serum calcium* and osteomalacia. These patients develop secondary hyperparathyroidism, hyperphosphaturia and thus hypophosphataemia. Elderly patients with small bowel disease can develop osteoporosis.

Table 15.4 Gastrointestinal causes of a low serum albumin

Increased loss (protein-losing enteropathy)	Decreased intake
	Anorexia
Stomach	Protein deficient diet
Ménétrièr's disease (giant rugae)	
Multiple gastric ulcers	**Decreased synthesis**
Gastric tumours	
	Associated liver disease (as can
Small intestine	occur in inflammatory bowel disease)
Coeliac disease	
Crohn's disease	**Decreased absorption**
Tropical sprue	
Lymphoma	Coeliac disease
Lymphangiectasia	Crohn's disease
Large intestine	
Crohn's disease	
Ulcerative colitis	
Colonic tumours	

Endoscopy

The development of flexible fibre-optic endoscopes in the 1970s revolutionised the gastroenterologist's view of the gut. Endoscopy is generally superior to radiology as an investigative technique, as it provides a direct mucosal view, enables biopsies to be taken for histological and biochemical analysis, and permits therapeutic manoeuvres.

Endoscopes are used in the upper gut to examine the pharynx, oesophagus, stomach and duodenum. Oesophageal strictures can be dilated using bougies, and prosthetic tubes can be put through strictures (usually malignant). Bleeding lesions can be cauterised by electric current or lasers. The ampulla of Vater can be cannulated and contrast medium injected to reveal the anatomy of the pancreatic ducts and biliary tree (endoscopic retrograde cholangiopancreatography (ERCP)). If there are stones in the biliary tree, a sphincterotomy can be performed to allow them to fall out or be extracted by baskets or balloons. Malignant strictures in the biliary tree can be bypassed by teflon or metal stents passed endoscopically, or percutaneously, through the liver.

The lower rectum can be examined by a rigid proctoscope, which is particularly useful for demonstrating haemorrhoids, and the rectum and lower sigmoid colon by a 25 cm rigid sigmoidoscope. A flexible fibre-optic sigmoidoscope can be used for the distal colon and rectum, and may be advanced to the splenic flexure (Fig. 15.1). Colonoscopes can be passed to the caecum and thence, via the ileocaecal valve, into the terminal ileum. As well as biopsies of suspicious lesions, polypoid lesions can be snared by excision diathermy and abnormal colonic blood vessels (angiodysplasia) can be cauterised. The small bowel mucosa from the end of the second part of the duodenum to the terminal ileum cannot normally be viewed endoscopically except by the little-used enteroscope; at laparotomy, however, it is possible to make an enterotomy and inspect the whole small bowel endoscopically.

Biopsy

Diffuse mucosal disorders and focal lesions can be diagnosed by histological examination of tissue biopsies. Biopsies of stomach, duodenum and colon are taken via the appropriate endoscope. A proximal small bowel biopsy is essential in suspected small bowel disease (e.g. coeliac disease). In the past, proximal small bowel biopsies were taken from the jejunum with a swallowed capsule but now such biopsies are usually taken from the distal duodenum via a fibre-optic endoscope. All gastrointestinal biopsies should be correctly orientated on card. This is helpful with small bowel biopsies so the villous pattern can be assessed with a hand lens or dissecting microscope before being processed for histological exami-

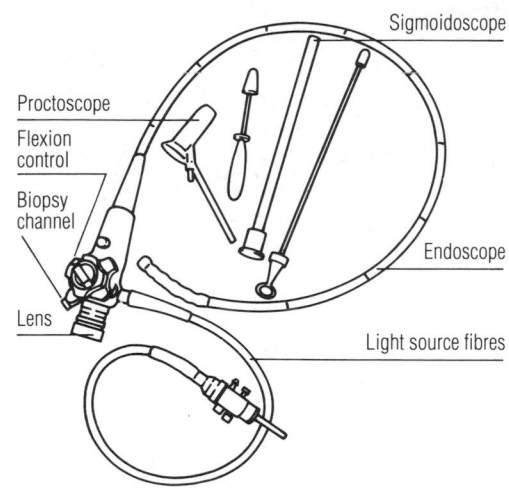

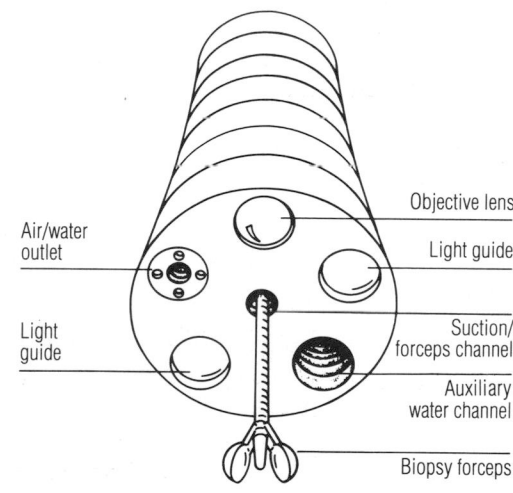

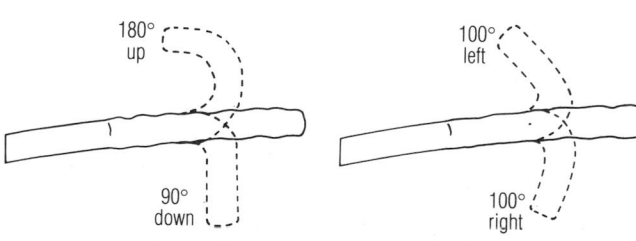

Fig. 15.1 Endoscopic instruments. A. A rigid proctoscope and sigmoidoscope with their respective trocars removed are seen centrally. They are surrounded by a diagram of a typical fibre-optic gastroscope. **B.** Diagram of the distal end of a typical fibre-optic gastroscope. Light is provided by the guides and the image is transmitted via the objective lens to the operator. The air and water outlets allow insufflation of the gut with air and cleansing of the lens with water. Gastric contents and secretions can be removed via the suction channel and biopsy forceps and cytology brushes can also be passed by this route. **C.** Diagram of the movements which the tip of a typical fibre-optic endoscope can achieve.

nation. Some disorders show a predilection for the distal ileum (e.g. Crohn's disease), and this can be biopsied via a colonoscope passed through the ileocaecal valve.

Barium studies

If a patient has difficulty with swallowing (dysphagia), a barium swallow can be used before endoscopy to outline the anatomy and to avoid possible endoscopic perforation. A barium swallow on video is very helpful in elucidating motor problems of the oesophagus, such as bulbar palsy, spasm and achalasia. In the investigation of gastroduodenal symptoms, upper gastrointestinal endoscopy is preferred to a barium meal as it is more accurate and allows biopsy and cytology specimens to be obtained.

The small intestine can be examined by a small bowel meal, in which barium is swallowed and its progress followed to the terminal ileum. For better views of the distal small bowel and focal lesions, a small bowel enema, in which contrast medium is placed directly into the upper jejunum via a nasal tube, is performed (Fig. 15.2).

Double-contrast enemas with air and barium are useful in demonstrating colonic lesions such as carcinomas, polyps and inflammatory bowel disease. Barium enema should be delayed for at least one week after rectal biopsy to avoid the risk of perforation. Colonoscopy should be performed if there is doubt about the barium appearances, if angiodysplasia is suspected and if lesions requiring polypectomy are present.

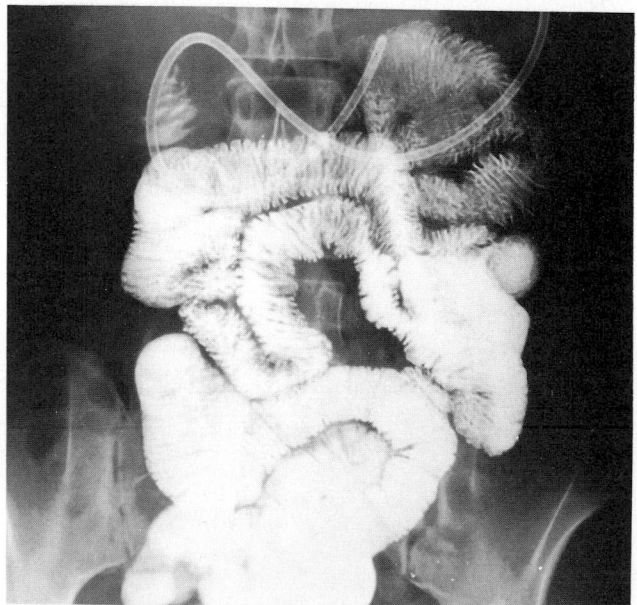

Fig. 15.2 A normal small bowel enema, showing jejunum and ileum in the upper and lower parts of the picture respectively.

15 Gastrointestinal Disease

Imaging techniques

Ultrasound, computed tomography (CT scanning) and nuclear magnetic resonance (NMR) are all useful in imaging the liver, biliary tree, spleen, pancreas, pelvis and retroperitoneal structures. They are helpful in demonstrating tumours, abscesses and stones, but are of little help in outlining the bowel.

Isotopic techniques can be used to investigate gut disease. Technetium^{-99m} sulphur colloid can be used to monitor the liquid and solid phase of gastric emptying (in general, liquids empty faster) and to measure the time taken by nutrients to pass through the small bowel (small bowel transit). Red cells can be radiolabelled with chromium^{-51} to demonstrate active gastrointestinal blood loss, especially when this cannot be demonstrated by conventional endoscopic and radiological means. White cells can be radiolabelled to demonstrate abscesses and areas of active inflammatory bowel disease. Meckel's diverticula often contain gastric epithelium and can be localised by radiolabelled pertechnate, which is secreted by the parietal cells.

Arteriography outlines the coeliac axis and superior and inferior mesenteric arteries and can define stenosis or occlusion of these arteries in patients with pain after eating (mesenteric angina) and sites of active bleeding (e.g. tumours and angiodysplasia).

Gut regulatory peptides

Three classes of regulatory peptides have been defined.

- *Hormones,* such as secretin and gastrin, are released as a result of food in the gut and have effects at distant sites.
- *Paracrine regulatory peptides,* discovered in the gut mucosa, are released locally and have profound effects on neighbouring cells.
- *Neurotransmitters.* Immunocytochemistry has demonstrated some peptides in the nerves of the gut, e.g. somatostatin, vasoactive intestinal polypeptide (VIP) and substance P, which are thought to act as non-adrenergic non-cholinergic neurotransmitters (neuropeptides).

The site of origin, mechanism of action and main physiological effects of the best documented regulatory peptides are summarised in Table 15.5. Clinically, the most important aspects of these hormones are their use in diagnostic tests (e.g. the pentagastrin test for gastric acid secretion and the secretin-cholecystokinin test for pancreatic function) and their role in tumour syndromes (p. 614). Measurement of the peptides in plasma or tissue can be performed by radioimmunoassay. The following abnormal results may have a role in diagnosis:

- In untreated coeliac disease, which is a proximal enteropathy, meal-stimulated plasma levels of the upper small intestinal hormones (secretin, cholecystokinin and gastric inhibitory polypeptide) are low. The terminal ileal hormones (neurotensin and enteroglucagon) are increased.
- In chronic pancreatitis with steatorrhoea, levels of meal-stimulated plasma pancreatic polypeptide are reduced.
- In neuropathic diseases of the gut, such as Hirschsprung's disease and Chagas' disease, tissue neuropeptide levels are reduced.

Table 15.5 Origin and action of some gastrointestinal regulatory peptides

Regulatory peptide	Site of origin	Mechanism of action	Main physiological effect
Gastrin	Gastric antrum	Hormone	Stimulates gastric acid secretion
Secretin	Duodenum	Hormone	Stimulates pancreatic bicarbonate secretion
Cholecystokinin	Duodenum	Hormone	Stimulates pancreatic enzyme secretion and gallbladder contraction
Motilin	Upper small bowel	Hormone	Increases gastric emptying and gut motility
Gastric inhibitory polypeptide (GIP)	Upper small bowel	Hormone	Stimulates insulin secretion
Enteroglucagon	Terminal ileum and colon	Hormone	Delays gastric emptying; trophic effects on gut mucosa
Neurotensin	Terminal ileum	Hormone	Delays gastric emptying
Pancreatic polypeptide	Pancreas	Hormone	Decreases pancreatic and biliary secretion
Somatostatin	Pancreas and all the gut	Hormone Paracrine ? Neurotransmitter	Reduces hormonal and intestinal secretions
Vasoactive intestinal polypeptide (VIP)	Pancreas and all the gut	Neurotransmitter	Increases intestinal secretion

Tests of function

Motility

Normal gut motility promotes the passage of food and food residue along the lumen at a rate that allows the appropriate physiological processes to take place. Well-regulated 'brakes' occur at the gastro-oesophageal junction, the pylorus, the ileocaecal valve and the rectum. Control of gut motility is thought to be mainly neural but hormones, in particular motilin, may also play a role. The stomach plays a major role in grinding food to small particles and in controlling the exit of contents into the duodenum, which may take up to five hours after a large meal.

Oesophageal motility can be investigated by a barium swallow on video, by static or 24-hour ambulatory manometric pressure studies and by radionuclide transit studies. A pH probe in the lower oesophagus can assess gastro-oesophageal reflux. Gastric emptying can be investigated by labelling the solid or the liquid phase with an isotope. Small intestinal motility can be assessed by the time taken for isotopes to reach the caecum, or by demonstrating a peak of breath hydrogen excretion liberated from bacterial breakdown of a carbohydrate load when a test meal reaches the distal ileum and caecum. Mouth to anus motility can be assessed by marker beads or by non-absorbable dyes.

A variety of clinical syndromes give rise to abnormal motility (Table 15.6). This usually causes a delay in transit, but gastric and other surgery can result in excessively rapid transit.

Gastrointestinal secretion

The salivary glands, stomach, pancreas, biliary tree and intestine all produce a large volume of secretions; these

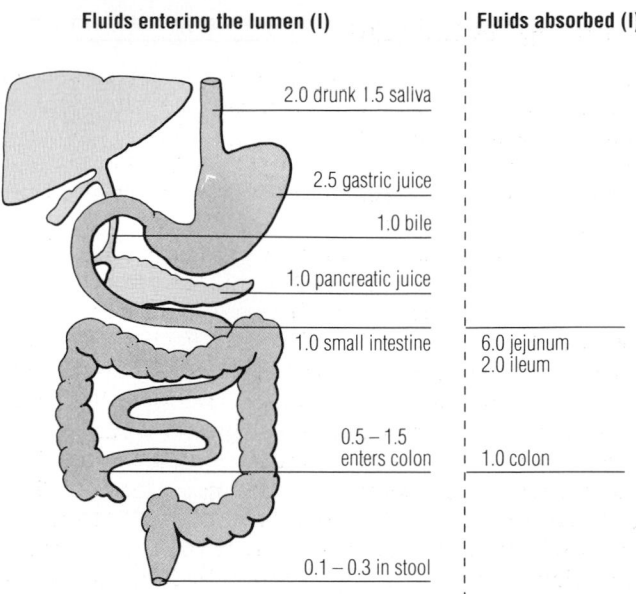

Fluids entering the lumen (l)   Fluids absorbed (l)

2.0 drunk 1.5 saliva

2.5 gastric juice

1.0 bile

1.0 pancreatic juice

1.0 small intestine   6.0 jejunum 2.0 ileum

0.5 – 1.5 enters colon   1.0 colon

0.1 – 0.3 in stool

Fig. 15.3 The typical daily fluid intake, secretions and absorption in a healthy person.

change the pH and produce enzymes which allow digestion of food and thus absorption of nutrients (Fig. 15.3). The secretions are controlled by vagal nerves including non-cholinergic non-adrenergic fibres, by local paracrine substances and by classical hormones.

Modes of investigation and abnormalities of secretion are shown in Table 15.7. In general, meal tests are more physiological than hormonal tests, e.g. the pentagastrin and secretin-cholecystokinin tests, where pharmacological doses of hormones are given intravenously. The triple lumen tube can be passed perorally into the intestine and various solutions containing a non-absorbable marker

Table 15.6 Disorders of gut motility

Oesophagus	Stomach	Small bowel	Colon
Anatomical			
Tumours ↓	Tumours ↓	Tumours ↓	Tumours ↓
Inflammatory stricture (e.g. acid and acid/alkali burns) ↓	Pyloric stenosis ↓	Inflammatory stricture (e.g. Crohn''s disease and tuberculosis) ↓	Inflammatory strictures (e.g. Crohn's disease) and ischaemic colon ↓
	Post-gastrectomy ↓↑	Post-surgical resection ↑	Post-surgical resection ↑
Neuropathic			
Achalasia ↓	Postvagotomy ↓	Diabetes mellitus ↓	Hirschsprung's and Chagas' diseases ↓
Systemic sclerosis ↓	Diabetes mellitus ↓	Systemic sclerosis ↓	
Functional			
Globus hystericus	Non-ulcer dyspepsia Vomiting Aerophagy	Irritable bowel syndrome ↑	Irritable bowel syndrome ↑↓ Simple constipation ↓

↑ increased motility   ↓ decreased motility

15 Gastrointestinal Disease

Table 15.7 Investigation and examples of important hyper- and hyposecretion syndromes

Type of secretion	Modes of investigation	Examples of increased secretion	Examples of reduced secretion
Salivary glands	Volume, pH and amylase levels, with or without local oral stimulant	Sialorrhoea	Sjögren's disease
Stomach	Pentagastrin and meal-stimulated acid output	Duodenal ulcer Gastrinoma	Carcinoma of stomach Atrophic gastritis
Pancreas	Lundh test meal and secretin-cholecystokinin stimulation		Chronic pancreatitis with exocrine insufficiency
Small intestine	Triple lumen tube and assessment of secretion/absorption over given length of intestine	VIP-secreting tumours Cholera Phenolphthalein	
Large intestine	Triple lumen tube	VIP-secreting tumours Dihydroxy bile acids Long chain fatty acids	

may then be perfused. By sampling at the end of the tube, the amount of secretion or absorption can be assessed.

Gastric acid studies

Gastric acid secretion can be assessed by collecting gastric juice via a nasogastric tube in the fasting state, measuring basal acid output and, after stimulation with a gastrin analogue, pentagastrin, assessing maximal acid output. Very high levels of basal acid outputs are seen in patients with gastrin-secreting tumours (gastrinomas), and high maximal acid outputs often occur in patients with duodenal ulcers. Twenty-four-hour acid secretion can also be monitored, to assess the effects of drugs which reduce acid secretion. Insulin hypoglycaemia stimulates gastric acid secretion via the vagus and can therefore be used postoperatively to assess the efficacy of surgical vagotomy. pH probes can also be placed in the oesophagus to monitor acid reflux, and in the stomach to monitor the effects of treatment.

Intestinal digestion and absorption

The stomach secretes acid and pepsin and, by physical churning and mixing, breaks down food into proportions which allow pancreatic and small intestinal brush border enzymes to digest it ready for absorption. Fat and fat soluble vitamins require bile acids, lipase and micellar formation to permit absorption. Proteins require gastric pepsin, pancreatic trypsin and brush border peptidases to break down proteins to absorbable single amino acids or 2–4 amino acid peptides. Carbohydrates require pancreatic amylase, and then brush border disaccharidases, to form monosaccharides which can be absorbed (Fig. 15.4). Calcium, iron and folic acid are absorbed in the duodenum and upper jejunum, while vitamin B_{12} and bile acids are absorbed in the terminal ileum; all other

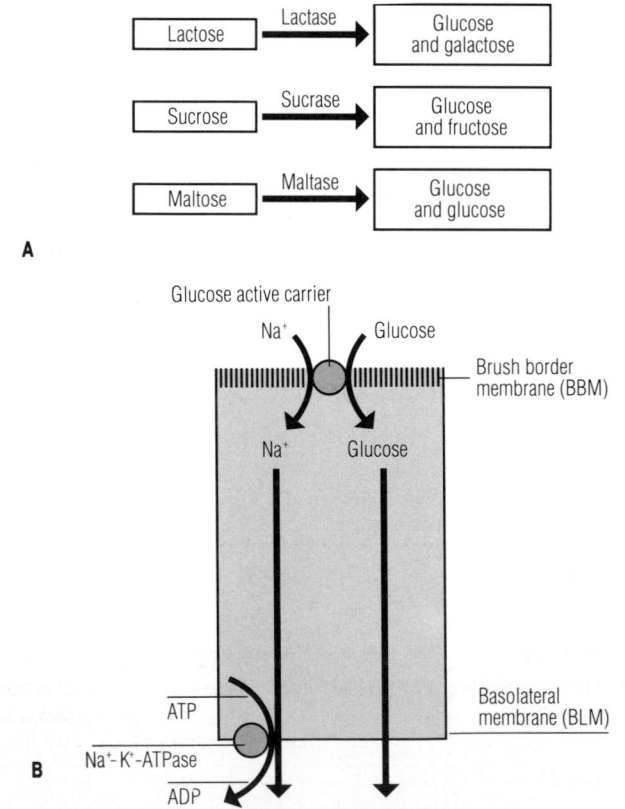

Fig. 15.4 Intestinal digestion and absorption. A. Enzyme activity allowing the conversion of major unabsorbable disaccharides to monosaccharides, which the enterocyte then can absorb. **B.** Glucose is transported by an active carrier with sodium at the brush border membrane. The gradient of sodium across the enterocyte is maintained by the Na^+-K^+-ATPase at the basolateral membrane, which allows sodium to pass out of the cell in exchange for potassium. Glucose leaves the cell at the basolateral membrane by a Na^+-independent carrier.

nutrients are absorbed throughout the small intestine. Small intestinal absorption requires active or passive transport across the brush border membrane, transport through the cell (often in Golgi or mitochondria) and then extrusion through the cell's basolateral membrane.

The most important test of small bowel function is the measurement of fat absorption because most diffuse disorders of the small intestine can cause fat malabsorption. Specific tests of carbohydrate digestion and absorption are available; brush border disaccharidase activity (e.g. lactase) can be measured in small bowel biopsies, and digestion and absorption of specific disaccharides can be assessed by measuring blood sugar levels after oral ingestion of the test sugar or by specific breath hydrogen tests. Protein absorption is assessed rarely although faecal nitrogen excretion and faecal protein loss can be measured. Terminal ileal function is assessed by B_{12} absorption (e.g. Schilling) tests or bile salt absorption tests (e.g. ^{75}Se-labelled homocholic acid conjugated with taurine (^{75}SeHCAT)). The integrity of the small bowel mucosa can be assessed by measuring the permeability of the mucosa to small inert hydrophilic non-metabolised molecules of varying molecular sizes (e.g. L-rhamnose, mannitol, lactulose, cellobiose, EDTA). Exocrine pancreatic function can be assessed by faecal fat measurement and specific pancreatic function tests (p. 606).

The colon is primarily involved in the absorption of water and electrolytes. Normally, up to 1500 ml of fluid passes through the ileocaecal valve daily, and this is concentrated to a 100 g formed stool. Specific colonic function tests are of research interest only.

THE MOUTH

Normal and abnormal function

The importance of the mouth, tongue, teeth and salivary gland secretions in starting the digestive process is often overlooked. Mastication and lubrication of the food bolus is desirable to facilitate its painless progression. Once swallowing has been voluntarily initiated, the rest of the act is automatic. Coordination of the soft palate rising to occlude the nasopharynx, the epiglottis tilting backwards to occlude the larynx, and the temporary cessation of respiration, is under complex neurological control, principally by the brainstem. Afferent pathways from taste and olfactory receptors initiate the cephalic phase of vagally mediated gastric secretion. Saliva contains two digestive enzymes – an amylase and a lipase. Lingual lipase may be important in patients with chronic pancreatic insufficiency.

Xerostomia (dry mouth) can be severe enough to cause problems in initiating swallowing. Lack of saliva may predispose to ascending bacterial infections of the salivary glands (sialadenitis), especially the parotid glands (paro-

titis). Saliva also contributes to the prevention of dental caries, the pathogenesis of which involves the facultative anaerobe, *Streptococcus mutans*, together with carbohydrate (mainly sucrose) and the formation of dental plaque.

Both the edentulous and patients with ill-fitting or painful dentures may limit their food intake, often unconsciously, and thus lose weight. Other painful lesions of the mouth or tongue may have a similar effect but, being more obvious, come readily to medical attention.

Diseases of the mouth

Disease of the mouth may be of import because:

- The disease, although confined to the mouth, may give rise to unpleasant symptoms and disordered function (Table 15.8).
- It may represent mucous membrane involvement of a generalised dermatological condition (Table 15.9).
- Involvement of the mouth may be part of a systemic disease (Table 15.10).
- The condition may be iatrogenic (Table 15.11).

ORAL ULCERATION

Recurrent aphthous ulcers

There are many possible causes of oral ulceration (Tables 15.8–15.11) but the commonest is *idiopathic aphthous*

Table 15.8 Diseases confined to the mouth

Ulceration	Plaques
Herpes simplex (HSV1)	Candida
Recurrent herpes labialis	Leucoplakia
Primary gingivostomatitis	Carcinoma
Acute ulcerative gingivitis	
(Vincent's angina, caused by	
Fusobacterium fusiformis and	
Borrelia vincenti)	
Cancrum oris	
Coxsackie A	
Herpangina	
Hand, foot and mouth disease	
Recurrent aphthous ulcers	
Minor	
Major	
Denture gingivitis	

Table 15.9 Dermatological conditions involving the mouth

Ulceration (burst bullae)	Plaques
Pemphigus vulgaris	Lichen planus
Pemphigoid	Psoriasis
Erythema multiforme	
Lichen planus	

Table 15.10 Mouth involvement in systemic disorders

Mouth involvement	Systemic disorder
Mucocutaneous pigmentation of lips	Peutz-Jegher's syndrome
Telangiectasia (lips)	Scleroderma (CRST syndrome) Hereditary haemorrhagic telangiectasia (Osler Weber Rendu syndrome)
Buccal pigmentation	Addison's disease ACTH-producing tumour
Macroglossia	Hypothyroidism Acromegaly Amyloid
Glossitis	Iron deficiency (also angular cheilitis) Folate and vitamin B_{12} deficiency
Gingival hypertrophy	Acute leukaemia Amyloid
Gingivitis (with or without bleeding)	Acute leukaemia Scurvy Thrombocytopenia Agranulocytosis
Oral ulceration	Behçet's disease Reiter's syndrome Crohn's disease Coeliac disease Wegener's granulomatosis Systemic lupus erythematosus Tuberculosis Syphilis Glandular fever

Table 15.11 Iatrogenic disorders of the mouth

Iatrogenic disorder	Cause
Xerostomia	Atropine-like drugs Tricyclic antidepressants
Gingival hyperplasia	Phenytoin, primidone, phenobarbitone, cyclosporin
Gingival pigmentation	Bismuth, mercury, lead, arsenic, silver
Ulceration	Sulphonamides, barbiturates, penicillin (cause erythema multiforme) Gold Penicillamine Cytotoxics Drugs causing agranulocytosis, e.g. carbimazole, sulphasalazine

ulceration. This occurs in up to 20% of patients seen in hospital and 10% in general practice. It often begins in late childhood or the early teens and frequently recurs. In about 80% of cases the condition (though still unpleasant) is regarded as minor with up to five ulcers, less than 1 cm diameter, affecting lips, cheeks and tongue and healing within a week. Major ulcers are larger, often more numerous, and may involve the pharynx and palate. Cervical lymph node enlargement may occur, and healing may be delayed for several weeks, leaving scarring. The aetiology of aphthous ulcers is unknown. The preponderance of the disease in females, its onset at the menarche, relationship to menstruation and improvement in pregnancy have led to the postulation of hormonal factors. A proportion of patients with coeliac disease present in this way and appropriate tests, including small bowel biopsy, are indicated.

Herpes simplex

The commonest manifestation of *Herpes simplex* (HSV1) is of recurrent herpes labialis or cold sore. The virus lies dormant in the trigeminal ganglion. Antiviral therapy with local idoxuridine or acycloguanosine (acyclovir) is probably only necessary in the immunocompromised patient.

A rarer, more severe and usually non-recurrent infection is primary herpetic gingivostomatitis. It occurs primarily in childhood and the sore mouth and gums, with vesicles preceding ulceration, is accompanied by fever and regional lymphadenitis. Treatment is analgesia and antibiotic to prevent secondary bacterial infection.

Acute ulcerative gingivitis

Acute ulcerative gingivitis (Vincent's angina) is thought to be due to bacterial infection; *Fusobacterium fusiformis* and *Borrelia vincenti* are the currently incriminated organisms. This disease affects young adults and the immunosuppressed, and is again accompanied by fever and lymphadenitis. The painful gums may bleed. Vincent's angina may be distinguished from herpes by the foul fetor and absence of vesicles. Penicillin or metronidazole are usually effective treatments.

Crohn's disease

Oral lesions are relatively common, particularly if there is colonic involvement (p. 592). The lesions include aphthous ulceration and cobblestoned or fissured epithelium. They can be the sole presenting feature of the disease and may be painful. Biopsies of the lesions may show typical non-caseating granulomata.

Other causes of ulceration

Oral ulceration may predominate in Behçet's disease, Reiter's syndrome and erythema multiforme. In all three conditions, ocular and genital lesions may be present. Although many cases of erythema multiforme have no apparent cause, some are induced by Herpes simplex and drugs, such as sulphonamides, barbiturates and penicillin.

Bullous disorders of mucous membranes result in their rupture to form ulcers in the mouth. As at other sites, differentiating the intraepithelial bullae of pemphigus from the subepithelial bullae of pemphigoid may be difficult (p. 1145). Lichen planus may also present with erosion of vesicles causing ulceration and, in a significant number of patients, the mouth may be the only site of the disease (p. 1147).

PLAQUE LESIONS

Candida

Candidiasis usually arises as a result of a defect in immunity, since the causative fungus is a common commensal. Candidiasis may complicate HIV infection and is common in poorly controlled diabetics (see Ch. 11, p. 279 and Ch. 25, pp. 1129–30).

Leucoplakia

Leucoplakia is a serious condition because of its propensity for malignant transformation in about 5% of cases. The white patches can occur anywhere within the oral cavity. Biopsy, which must be repeated regularly to detect atypia or early cancer, confirms the diagnosis by showing epithelial keratosis and hyperplasia. The aetiology is multifactorial, but idiopathic cases do occur. There is no specific treatment other than excision and avoiding the presumed causative factors. These include smoking, local friction and chronic infection, e.g. chronic candidiasis or tertiary syphilis; the latter has a worse prognosis regarding malignant change. Leucoplakia is an important manifestation of HIV infection (p. 243).

Carcinoma

Squamous carcinoma of the oral cavity may affect the lips, tongue or any other part of the mouth, and may present as a nodular or ulcerating lesion. As with leucoplakia, its incidence appears to be declining, emphasising the important association between the two conditions. Pipe and cigar smoking are strongly associated with oral cavity carcinoma, as is the chewing of tobacco or betel nut.

OTHER LESIONS

Other disorders of the mouth are listed in Tables 15.8 to 15.11. Minor abnormalities of the tongue may, because easily seen by the patient, give rise to considerable anxiety.

Geographic tongue (benign migratory glossitis) is caused by shifting areas of desquamation of short duration in any

one location. It is invariably symptomless and the patient should be reassured of this.

Fissure tongue may be associated with symptomatic glossitis but, if symptomless, the patient can be reassured.

Black hairy tongue is asymptomatic but may cause anxiety. Tripotassium dicitrate bismuthate (Denol) in liquid form is an obvious cause and the disorder may also follow antibiotics, but the aetiology is usually unknown. Reassurance is required.

THE OESOPHAGUS

Normal swallowing involves coordinated action of the oropharynx, relaxation of the cricopharyngeus, peristalsis down the oesophageal body (upper one-third striated muscle, lower two-thirds non-striated muscle) and relaxation of the lower oesophageal sphincter.

Clinical features of oesophageal pathology

Dysphagia

Difficulty with swallowing (dysphagia or 'food sticking') is a most important symptom. Some of the causes are shown in Table 15.12. When there are obstructive lesions such as carcinoma, dysphagia is initially for large boluses of food, but then progresses to less solid food and finally to liquids ('total dysphagia'). Most of the causes can be elucidated by a good history, examination, barium swallow and then endoscopy. Patients with central and peripheral nervous diseases, and primary muscle disorders, usually have other neuromuscular symptoms and

Table 15.12 Causes of dysphagia

- Local oropharyngeal problems, e.g. infections, tumours
- Central nervous system disorders affecting oropharyngeal function, e.g. brainstem lesions associated with multiple sclerosis, cerebrovascular disease, Parkinson's disease, Huntington's chorea and motor neurone disease
- Malignant and benign oesophageal strictures
- Other local oesophageal problems, e.g. reflux oesophagitis, infections, web, diverticulum
- Disorders affecting oesophageal unstriated muscle, e.g. achalasia, chronic alcoholism, diabetes mellitus
- Generalised striated muscle diseases, e.g. myasthenia gravis, dystrophia myotonica
- Extrinsic compression (e.g. mediastinal tumour)
- Psychiatric, i.e. globus hystericus

15 Gastrointestinal Disease

signs. Hysterical dysphagia is a diagnosis of exclusion and usually occurs in psychiatrically disturbed patients.

Other symptoms

Painful swallowing and retrosternal pain are important symptoms. On occasions, it may be difficult to differentiate oesophageal and cardiac pain and there is evidence that gastro-oesophageal reflux may lower the threshold for angina. Regurgitation of gastric juice into the lower oesophagus and the back of the mouth may cause heartburn and is due to an incompetent lower oesophageal sphincter; this is commonly precipitated by raising the intra-abdominal pressure (lifting, pregnancy). If food accumulates in the oesophagus, nausea, vomiting and weight loss may occur. The oesophagus is also a site of bleeding from varices, ulcers and inflammatory lesions (oesophagitis).

Signs

Abnormal physical signs are unusual in patients with oesophageal disease, but epigastric tenderness may indicate oesophagitis, peptic ulceration or a carcinoma. Neurological examination of palatal movement and the gag reflex are important when dysphagia could be due to a neurological cause. An epigastric mass or palpable supraclavicular lymph nodes suggests a neoplasm. Decreased oesophageal clearance of solids and fluids (especially in patients with achalasia and carcinomas) may cause pulmonary aspiration.

Summary 1 The main symptoms, signs and investigations of oesophageal disease

Symptoms
Difficulty with swallowing (dysphagia)
Painful swallowing (odynophagia)
Retrosternal pain
Heartburn
Regurgitation
Vomiting
Weight loss
Gastrointestinal bleeding

Signs
Epigastric tenderness or mass
Abnormal palatal movement
Supraclavicular lymphadenopathy
Chest signs due to aspiration

Investigations
Full blood count
Barium swallow
Chest X-ray
Endoscopy
Manometry
pH monitoring

Investigation of oesophageal pathology

A barium swallow outlines the oropharyngeal and oesophageal anatomy, and a video recording can be taken to look for disordered motility. A chest X-ray helps to assess oesophageal dilatation. If a patient has dysphagia, a barium swallow is carried out before endoscopy; this is because patients' symptoms alone cannot always localise the site of the lesion and, if the endoscopist is unprepared for the abnormal anatomy, perforation of an oesophageal carcinoma or diverticulum may occur. Manometry is useful to assess the oesophagus and lower oesophageal sphincter in achalasia and other motility disorders. Reflux can be monitored by a pH-sensitive probe in the distal oesophagus (24-hour ambulatory oesophageal monitoring).

GASTRO-OESOPHAGEAL REFLUX

Normally, gastro-oesophageal reflux is prevented by the lower oesophageal sphincter, aided by the diaphragm. In patients with reflux, there are repeated episodes of significant quantities of acid, bile and food regurgitating into the lower oesophagus. This can lead to inflammatory change (reflux oesophagitis), which is associated with decreased oesophageal clearance of liquids and solids.

Aetiology

The main cause of gastro-oesophageal reflux (Table 15.13) is the failure of lower oesophageal sphincter tone and of secondary peristalsis in the oesophageal body. Pregnancy is commonly associated with reflux, due partly to sex hormones lowering the gastro-oesophageal sphincter pressure, and partly to pressure from the intra-abdominal mass. Smoking, eating fat and chocolate, drinking coffee, tea and alcohol, and certain drugs (e.g.

Table 15.13 Factors predisposing to gastro-oesophageal reflux

Cause	Example
Disordered anatomy	Hiatus hernia
	Obesity
	Post-surgical treatment of achalasia
	Presence of tube for treating carcinoma
Myogenic	Systemic sclerosis
	Reflux oesophagitis
Hormonal	Pregnancy
	Menstruation
External influences	Smoking
	Eating fat/chocolate
	Coffee/tea
	Large meals
	Alcohol
	Drugs

calcium antagonists and β_2 agonists) act by reducing the lower oesophageal sphincter pressure. The presence of a hiatus hernia is not necessary for reflux but is often an associated finding.

Clinical features

The typical symptoms of gastro-oesophageal reflux are heartburn and regurgitation; chest pain may also occur. They are often aggravated by lying down, bending or raising intra-abdominal pressure (e.g. by lifting). If reflux is complicated by oesophagitis or stricture formation, vomiting, haemorrhage, anaemia, dysphagia and pulmonary aspiration may occur.

Investigation

Gastro-oesophageal reflux with typical symptoms requires little investigation. However, if the symptoms are less typical, severe, or include gastrointestinal bleeding or dysphagia, further investigation is indicated. Endoscopy is preferred, as this allows more accurate visualisation of associated lesions (oesophagitis, ulcers, stricture formation, etc.) and permits biopsies of inflamed, ulcerated or questionably malignant areas. However, endoscopy does not permit satisfactory demonstration of reflux itself; this can be achieved by a barium swallow or ingestion of a radioisotope. The most objective assessment of reflux can be obtained by placing a pH probe in the lower oesophagus and measuring falls in pH due to acid regurgitation over a 24-hour period. Manometry is useful in distinguishing other conditions where symptoms can be similar, such as achalasia, systemic sclerosis and diffuse oesophageal spasm.

REFLUX OESOPHAGITIS

Reflux oesophagitis is an inflammatory response secondary to gastro-oesophageal reflux. It can be graded into four stages.

1. *Mild.* Single or non-confluent areas of superficial mucosal erosions and erythema.
2. *Moderate.* Confluent erosions not including the whole circumference of the oesophagus.
3. *Severe.* Confluent erosions including the whole oesophageal circumference.
4. *Complicated.* Oesophagitis with additional complications, e.g. peptic ulcers, strictures.

Management

Medical

Obesity is frequently a major causal factor. Raising the head of the bed on blocks by 20 cm or more discourages nocturnal acid regurgitation, and is more satisfactory than increasing the number of pillows. The avoidance of big meals before going to bed and precipitating foods and drinks also often helps. In mild cases, a mixture of alginic acid and a simple antacid is effective. In patients with troublesome symptoms (especially if there is coexistent oesophagitis), a six-week course of metoclopramide before meals, full dose H_2-receptor antagonists (taken twice daily or all at night), and an alginic acid antacid mixture is usually effective. Metoclopramide increases lower oesophageal sphincter tone and gastric emptying, and the H_2-receptor antagonist reduces gastric acid secretion. In refractory severe oesophagitis or cases resistant to the above therapy, the parietal cell proton pump inhibitors (e.g. omeprazole) are the treatment of choice. Relapse after stopping treatment is a problem in 30–80% of patients who may require a maintenance H_2-blocker or proton pump therapy.

Surgical

Surgery is indicated in patients with severe symptoms of reflux unresponsive to all medical treatment. Selected patients should preferably be non-obese, free of other serious medical problems and under 70 years of age.

Summary 2 Treatment of gastro-oesophageal reflux and oesophagitis

- Simple measures
  - Lose weight
  - Raise head of bed on blocks
  - Avoid bending

- Avoid possible aetiological factors which reduce lower oesophageal sphincter pressure
  - Smoking
  - Eating fat/chocolate
  - Coffee/tea
  - Alcohol

- Drugs to reduce gastric acid secretion
  - H_2-receptor antagonists
  - Proton pump inhibitors

- Drugs to increase gastric emptying
  - Metoclopramide
  - Domperidone
  - Cisapride

- Drugs to protect mucosal lining
  - Alginic acid containing antacid
  - Carbenoxolone

- Drugs to neutralise gastric acid
  - Simple antacids

- Surgery

Patients under 50 whose symptoms can only controlled by proton pump inhibitors should also be considered. Surgery involves an antireflux procedure (e.g. fundoplication). The long-term results of antireflux surgery are sometimes disappointing.

HIATUS HERNIA

Hiatus hernias can be congenital, in which case they usually present, and are treated, during childhood. Acquired hiatus hernias are often of the sliding type and result in varying lengths of the stomach being in the chest (Fig. 15.5). The rolling or para-oesophageal type is less common, and occurs when a portion of the fundus of the stomach lies anterior to the oesophagus.

Clinical features

Sliding hiatus hernias may be asymptomatic or associated with symptoms of gastro-oesophageal reflux. Difficulty with swallowing suggests the presence of a complicating stricture.

The symptoms of rolling hiatus hernias do not include reflux and are commonly very non-specific, such as vague upper abdominal discomfort, nausea and fullness after eating. Complications include bleeding from gastritis or a gastric ulcer (sometimes presenting as an iron deficiency anaemia), gastric volvulus and hernial strangulation.

Investigation

If a sliding hiatus hernia is large, it may be seen on a chest X-ray as a retrocardiac shadow with a fluid level. Endoscopy is the diagnostic procedure of choice, allowing direct assessment of hernial size, oesophagitis and stricture formation, the taking of diagnostic biopsies and the passage of dilating bougies to treat a stricture. Alterna-

tively, a barium swallow can be used to assess hernia size and the development of complications.

Management

A sliding hiatus hernia does not require treatment but its complications, such as reflux, oesophagitis and stricture formation, do. Surgery is sometimes indicated to reduce a large rolling hernia in view of the risk of strangulation. However, as rolling hernias are often found in the very elderly, surgery may be postponed until a major complication occurs.

BARRETT'S OESOPHAGUS

Barrett's oesophagus is a complication of long-standing gastro-oesophageal reflux whereby a portion of the lower oesophagus is lined by metaplastic columnar epithelium instead of normal squamous epithelium. It presents as reflux or its complications and is thought to be premalignant, giving rise to an adenocarcinoma of the lower one-third. The disorder therefore requires regular endoscopic evaluation.

PEPTIC OESOPHAGEAL STRICTURE

Peptic oesophageal strictures are fibrous strictures which occur at the lower end of the oesophagus as a result of persistent gastro-oesophageal reflux. The main symptom is intermittent and then progressive dysphagia, first for solids and then for liquids. Patients become frightened to eat, regurgitate meals, develop increasing pain and sometimes aspiration and, as a result, become anorexic and lose weight.

Treatment is by passage of dilators with the aid of an endoscope. Treatment can be repeated if symptoms recur, but many patients only require it once or every few years. Oesophageal perforation is rare. Surgery is indicated in younger individuals requiring frequent dilatation.

CORROSIVE AND FOREIGN BODY INGESTION

In certain parts of the world (e.g. India and South America), strong acid or alkali solutions are commonly taken with suicidal intent. These cause severe inflammation, most commonly affecting the oesophagus, though the stomach and duodenum can also be damaged. In some patients, oesophageal perforation requires urgent surgery. In patients without perforation, conservative treatment with neutralising lavage can be successful without long-term complications, but in others a stricture develops. Gastric or duodenal strictures usually require surgical intervention.

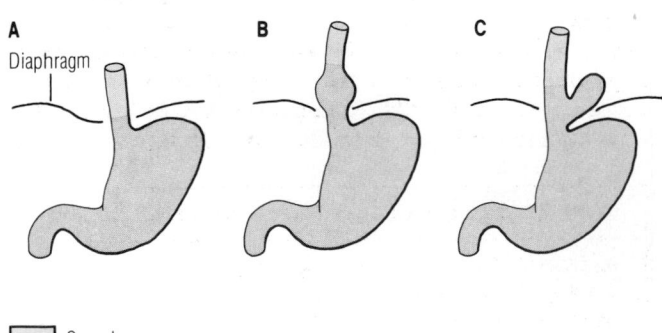

Oesophagus

Gastric mucosa

Fig. 15.5 Diagram of (A) normal anatomy, (B) sliding hiatus hernia and (C) rolling hiatus hernia.

Table 15.14 Basic classification of oesophageal tumours

Class	Example
Malignant	Squamous cell carcinoma
	Adenocarcinoma
	Melanoma
	Sarcoma (usually leiomyosarcoma)
Benign	Leiomyoma
	Adenoma
	Cysts

Foreign bodies (e.g. fish bones, coins) may stick in the the oesophagus and cause dysphagia. Small articles can be extracted endoscopically. A bolus of food often obstructs the oesophagus of patients with benign or malignant strictures, and this can usually be treated by using the endoscope to push the bolus distal to the obstruction. When larger solid articles are swallowed and are thought likely to obstruct the bowel or cause perforation, a laparotomy should be considered.

OESOPHAGEAL TUMOURS

A basic classification of oesophageal tumours is shown in Table 15.14. Benign tumours are rare. Malignant tumours occur in the upper third of the oesophagus (about 15%) but are more common in the middle (about 40%) and lower third (45%). The majority of oesophageal tumours are squamous cell in origin (if adenocarcinomas which arise in the stomach and invade upwards are excluded). The tumours spread early by local invasion and lymphatic and blood-borne metastases.

The incidence of oesophageal cancer varies greatly in different regions of the world, with a high incidence in Central Asia, the Far East and Transkei (Fig. 15.6). The age-specific incidence is shown in Figure 15.7. There are also racial differences: squamous carcinoma is commoner in North American blacks than whites.

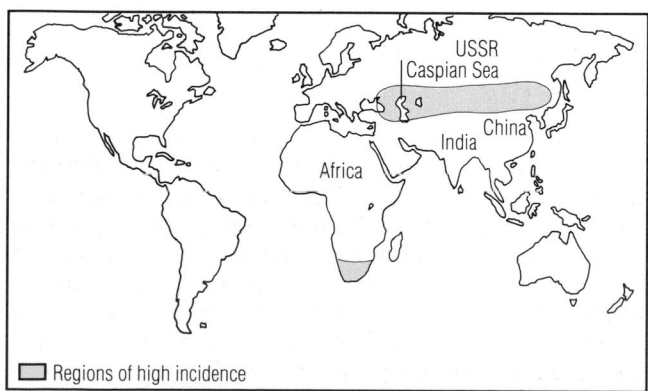

Fig. 15.6 Areas of high incidence of oesophageal carcinoma worldwide.

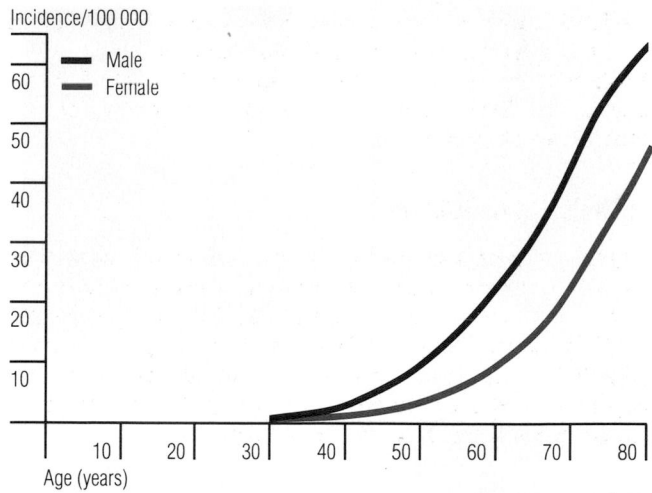

Fig. 15.7 Age-specific incidence of carcinoma of the oesophagus in the UK.

Aetiology

Possible aetiological factors in squamous cell carcinomas of the oesophagus are cigarette smoking, high alcohol intake, coeliac disease, radiation, achalasia, ingestion of strong acids and alkalis, environmental carcinogens and, possibly, reflux oesophagitis. Squamous carcinoma is rarely preceded by histological dysplasia, which can be detected by endoscopic biopsies. Barrett's oesophagus predisposes to the development of adenocarcinomas and premalignant dysplasia may be seen. The Plummer-Vinson syndrome, which occurs in long-standing iron deficiency anaemia is, rarely, associated with postcricoid squamous carcinoma. A rare inherited syndrome of palmar hyperkeratosis (tylosis palmaris) is associated with squamous oesophageal cancer.

Clinical features

Dysphagia is the main symptom of oesophageal carcinomas, and is rapidly progressive. Pain is usually retrosternal and is due to invasion into the mediastinum. A productive cough may reflect aspiration or a broncho-oesophageal fistula. On examination, weight loss is often obvious. Anaemia usually reflects bleeding. Lymph node

Summary 3 Symptoms and signs of oesophageal carcinoma

Symptoms	Signs
Dysphagia (initially solids, then liquids, then complete)	Weight loss
	Anaemia
Pain	Enlarged cervical lymph nodes
Weight loss	Hepatomegaly
Cough	
Acute gastrointestinal bleeding	

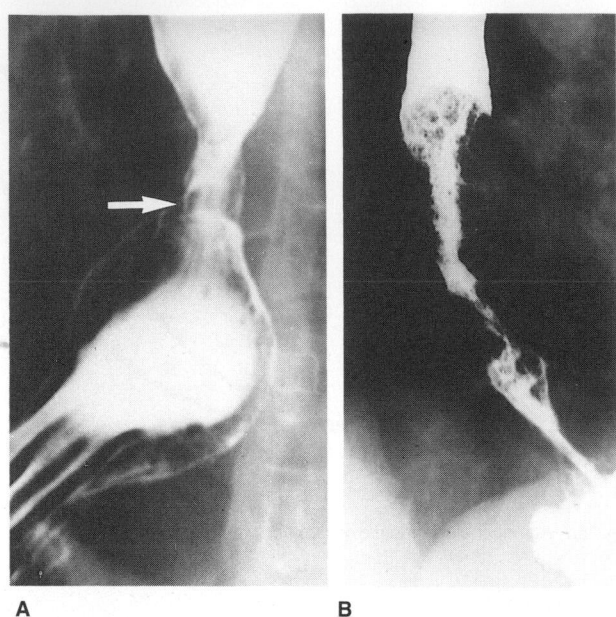

Fig. 15.8 Barium swallow examinations. A. A smooth benign oesophageal stricture (white arrow) above a hiatus hernia. **B.** A typical carcinoma with a long irregular stricture narrowing the oesophageal lumen.

enlargement and hepatomegaly due to distant spread are late signs.

Investigation

Patients who present with dysphagia often localise the point where food sticks, but this does not always correlate with the anatomical site of obstruction. The first investigation is a barium swallow (Fig. 15.8) or an endoscopy with biopsy to ascertain cell type. A chest X-ray is performed to assess mediastinal spread, and liver function tests and ultrasound are performed to detect metastases. If curative surgery is contemplated, a CT scan of the chest is necessary to define the degree of local infiltration.

Management

The management of squamous oesophageal carcinoma (Table 15.15) is controversial because the tumours are radiosensitive and the best results after radical radiotherapy may be as good as after surgery. Surgery or radical radiotherapy may be effective in patients who are fit, with no involved nodes or metastases, but these patients make up only about 10% of those presenting with the disease.

In the upper third, radiotherapy may be the preferred treatment as radical surgical treatments are technically difficult. Surgery involves total oesophagectomy and colonic interposition. In the middle and lower thirds, surgery is preferred to radiotherapy if the patient is fit enough. The stomach is mobilised and anastomosed to the oesophagus in the chest. Radiation may be complicated by oesophagitis and stricture, and surgery by stricture, mediastinitis and anastomotic leaks. Overall survival with either treatment is probably no better than 5% but some surgical series report 30% survival at 5 years.

Malignant stricture formation can be palliated by repeated endoscopic dilatations; when these are needed more than once every six weeks, it is useful to insert a tube to keep the lumen open and to allow liquidised food to pass. The tube can be placed using a fibre-optic endoscope under local or general anaesthesia, and is also useful for sealing off fistulas with bronchi or the trachea. Tubes can be replaced as necessary; if they become blocked by food, fizzy drinks can be tried first, and then endoscopic procedures. Repeated endoscopic laser treatments or absolute alcohol injections are alternative approaches. Adenocarcinomas are not radiosensitive and few are amenable to curative surgery, with less than 5% five-year survival.

ACHALASIA

Achalasia is a functional obstruction at the level of the lower oesophageal sphincter due to a failure of relaxation. It results in progressive dilatation of the oesophagus prox-

Table 15.15 Treatment of squamous carcinoma of the oesophagus

Aim	Treatment modality	Criteria	Result
'Curative'	Radical surgery (with or without pre- or postoperative radiotherapy)	Tumour localised to oesophagus	Less than 40% five-year survival for squamous cell carcinoma
	Radical radiotherapy	Tumour localised to oesophagus	Less good than surgery, usually reserved for elderly and infirm
Palliative	Radiotherapy Endoscopic dilatation Endoscopic intubation Endoscopic laser therapy Pain relief and general nutritional support	Widespread local tumour; distant metastases; other medical conditions preclude surgery or radical radiotherapy	Good palliation, but few survive more than six months

imal to the 'obstruction'. Achalasia is caused by degeneration of ganglion cells in the muscle of the mid and lower oesophagus. In the West, the aetiology is obscure although the disease is sometimes familial. In South America, a similar problem occurs as a late result of destruction of the ganglion cells by the protozoon *Trypanosoma cruzi* (Chagas' disease; see p. 297).

Clinical features and investigation

Presentation is usually with intermittent but slowly progressive dysphagia for both solids and liquids. There may be associated pain and regurgitation of food swallowed some hours before may occur; heartburn is unusual. Anorexia and weight loss may also occur and some patients develop symptoms of pulmonary aspiration.

The diagnosis is best made radiologically. A barium swallow reveals a failure of the lower oesophageal sphincter to relax, and sometimes proximal dilatation with food and fluid in the lumen (Fig. 15.9). Manometry confirms the diagnosis, with an elevated lower oeso-

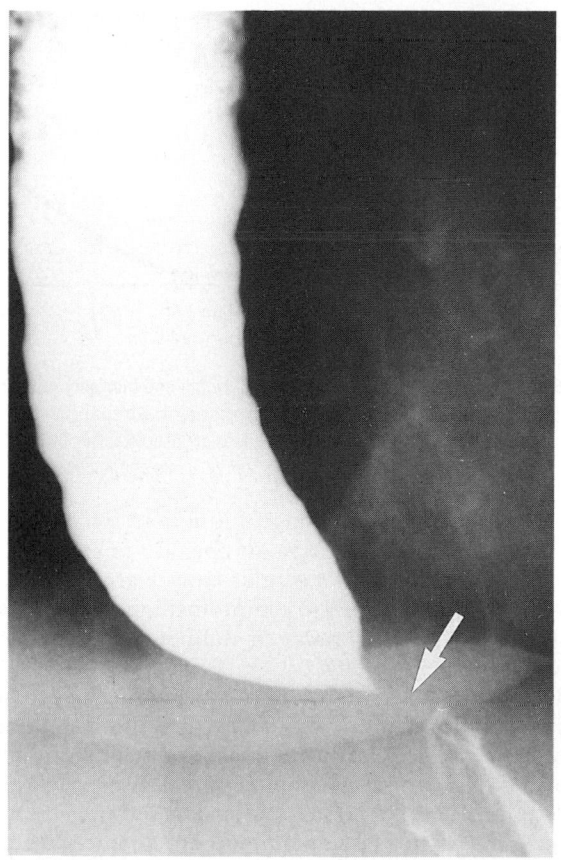

Fig. 15.9 Barium swallow examination showing oesophageal achalasia. There is hold-up of barium at the level of the gastro-oesophageal junction (arrow) and oesophageal dilation and lack of contractions above. Advanced cases also have a fluid level which may be seen on a chest X-ray.

phageal sphincter pressure and weak contractions of the oesophagus above. Upper gastrointestinal endoscopy excludes mechanical obstruction at the cardia and often reveals food in the oesophagus despite a prolonged fast.

Management

Achalasia is treated with either pneumatic balloon dilatation under endoscopic control or oesophageal myotomy (Heller's operation). Both these treatments are effective, but balloon dilatation has the advantage of being less invasive. Carcinoma of the oesophagus is a rare complication of achalasia.

OESOPHAGEAL SPASM

Diffuse oesophageal spasm is usually seen in the elderly and presents with retrosternal chest pain and/or dysphagia. A barium swallow shows a normal oesophagus, but the oesophagus may undergo diffuse spasm during the investigation to produce a corkscrew configuration. Manometry shows intermediate bursts of high amplitude contractions often unrelated to swallowing. Angina is a major differential diagnosis, but oesophageal spasm is not precipitated by exertion and stress.

Treatment is also similar to angina since glyceryl trinitrate sublingually (as necessary) and regular isosorbide dinitrate or nifedipine often help. In resistant cases, balloon dilatation or myotomy can be considered, but the results are not as good as for achalasia.

SYSTEMIC SCLEROSIS

Systemic sclerosis causes loss of oesophageal contractions (which may also occur in patients with Raynaud's phenomenon, systemic lupus erythematosus and polymyositis). Dysphagia and heartburn may occur. A barium swallow shows lack of peristalsis, and thus failure of the barium to move if the patient lies flat. The gastro-oesophageal sphincter may become incompetent, with consequent risk of reflux, oesophagitis and peptic stricture.

ANATOMICAL ABNORMALITIES

Oesophageal diverticula are outpouchings of the oesophageal wall that can occur at any position in the oesophagus. Dysphagia and regurgitation are both typical symptoms. If symptoms become severe, corrective surgery may be necessary.

Oesophageal webs are thin structures impinging a few millimetres into the lumen and consisting of mucosa and submucosa. They occur throughout the oesophagus and can be multiple. An association with chronic iron deficiency is now rare; treatment of the latter may prevent an associated postcricoid carcinoma. Dilatation helps if dysphagia occurs.

Oesophageal rings occur at the lower end of the oesophagus and contain muscle as well as mucosa and submucosa. They can be asymptomatic or present with intermittent dysphagia, which may become more common as the years pass. If symptoms are serious, endoscopic dilatation usually relieves them.

OESOPHAGEAL INFECTIONS

The most important oesophageal infections are candidiasis and *Herpes simplex*. Both occur in patients who are immunosuppressed, e.g. in patients who are receiving corticosteroids or cytotoxic drugs, or who have AIDS or diabetes. Antibiotic treatment predisposes to candidal infections.

Patients with oesophageal infections usually present with dysphagia and odynophagia. Diagnosis of candidiasis is by endoscopic demonstration of the creamy exudates on the oesophageal wall (the mouth and pharynx are often also involved) and by demonstration of the typical yeast hyphae on biopsy. *Herpes simplex* appears similar at endoscopy, but can be confirmed by histological demonstration of inclusion bodies in epithelial cells and by viral culture.

The treatment of oesophageal Candidal infection is initially with nystatin or amphotericin in the form of lozenges. Herpes simplex is treated symptomatically with local anaesthetic drinks, although acyclovir is necessary in severely immunosuppressed patients. Candidiasis responds quickly to adequate treatment unless there is severe immune suppression, in which case ketoconazole or fluconazole is helpful; herpes usually settles over one to two weeks.

GASTROINTESTINAL BLEEDING

ACUTE GASTROINTESTINAL BLEEDING

Upper gastrointestinal bleeding presenting with haematemesis (vomiting blood or altered 'coffee ground' material) and/or melaena (the passage of black tarry faeces) is a common medical emergency. In the UK, it has an annual prevalence of about 50 cases per 100 000 population. The different sites of gastrointestinal bleeding and approximate mortality rates in the UK are shown in Figure 15.10.

Aetiology

The causes of gastrointestinal bleeding are shown in Table 15.16. Peptic ulcers, gastritis, Mallory-Weiss tears, varices and tumours account for the majority of cases. Bleeding may be provoked by ingestion of alcohol, aspirin, corticosteroids and non-steroidal anti-inflammatory drugs (NSAIDs). A Mallory-Weiss tear is a small

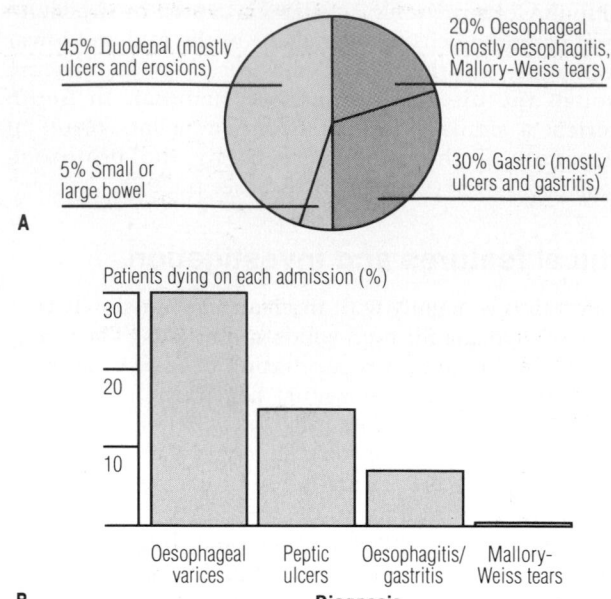

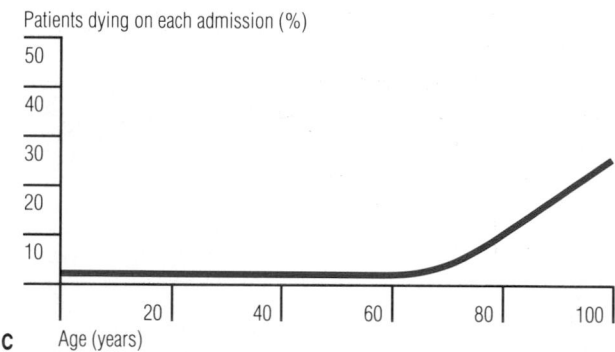

Fig. 15.10 Gastrointestinal bleeding: sites of origin and mortality rates in the UK. A. Typical values for the site of origin of gastrointestinal bleeding. **B.** Approximate mortality rates for different causes of gastrointestinal bleeding. **C.** Mortality rates related to age showing a rise from 60 years of age onwards.

lesion at the gastro-oesophageal junction, which usually follows vomiting and causes an episode of self-limiting bleeding. Systemic and vascular causes are rare. Occasionally, patients invent the symptoms, ingest blood from outside (e.g. from animals) or deliberately break their mucosa to cause bleeding.

Haematemesis is usually from a bleeding site proximal to the distal duodenum. If there is rapid intestinal transit and very severe haemorrhage, fresh blood per rectum may be passed from upper gastrointestinal lesions. Melaena is altered, partially digested blood passed per rectum. Meckel's diverticula are uncommon developmental abnormalities in the distal ileum; these frequently contain gastric acid-secreting cells, and usually present with recurrent melaena before adolescence. Angiodysplasia is increasingly recognised as a cause of melaena. In this condition, there

Table 15.16 Causes of gastrointestinal bleeding (parentheses indicate a rare cause)

Causes of haematemesis

Oesophagus	Systemic causes
Carcinoma	Chronic renal failure
Oesophagitis	(Thrombocytopenia)
Peptic ulcer	(Clotting factor deficiency)
Varices	(Anticoagulant therapy)
Stomach	Vascular causes
Peptic ulcer	(Mesenteric ischaemia)
Acute erosions	(Hereditary telangiectasia)
Carcinoma	(Systemic vasculitis)
Acute gastritis	
Mallory-Weiss tear	Swallowed blood
(Varices)	from oropharynx, nose and
(Other tumours)	respiratory tract
(Angiodysplasia)	
Duodenum	(Munchausen's syndrome)
Peptic ulcer	– symptom invented
Duodenitis	– ingested blood
(Tumours)	– self-induced

Causes of melaena

Causes of haematemesis (see above)

Jejunum and ileum
  (Meckel's diverticulum)
  (Angiodysplasia)
  (Tumours)
  (Crohn's disease)
  (Infarction of bowel)

Colon
  Right-sided tumours
  Angiodysplasia
  Inflammatory bowel disease

Causes of blood intermixed with stool

Colon
  Left-sided colonic tumours
  Inflammatory bowel disease
  Diverticular disease
  Infective colitis
  Angiodysplasia
  Ischaemic colitis

Causes of fresh blood per rectum

Anus and rectum
  Haemorrhoids
  Proctitis of any cause
  Carcinoma of anus or rectum
  Crohn's disease of anus

---

are leashes of dilated mucosal vessels which usually occur in the ileum and right side of the colon, although any part of the gastrointestinal tract may be involved.

Clinical features

The history is important in diagnosis, particularly with regard to previous symptoms (e.g. pain, vomiting, weight loss), past medical history (e.g. previous episodes, ulcers, liver disease) and ingestion of alcohol, aspirin, steroids and NSAIDs.

Frank gastrointestinal bleeding may present with haematemesis and melaena. With severe bleeding there will be signs of shock, with a tachycardia and hypotension (particularly a postural drop in blood pressure). Anaemia suggests either acute bleeding over several days with time for haemodilution, or an underlying chronic disease which has been causing blood loss over weeks or months. Spooning of the nails (koilonychia) infers long-standing iron deficiency. Signs of chronic liver disease suggest varices as a possible aetiology. Vascular malformations on the face and mucous membranes of the lips or mouth suggest hereditary telangiectasia.

Investigation

The most precise investigation for finding the cause of upper gastrointestinal bleeding is endoscopy. The patient should be resuscitated and endoscoped as soon as practicable. At this stage, most Mallory-Weiss tears, acute ulcers and areas of acute inflammation are obvious and the bleeding point may be identified. Perendoscopic thermal coagulation, laser therapy or injection with adrenaline and sclerosants may be used on any bleeding vessels seen.

The small intestine, beyond the distal duodenum and proximal to the distal terminal ileum, can only be reached by an endoscope during a laparotomy. Small intestinal bleeding may, however, be identified preoperatively by arteriography. Colonic bleeding may be identified by sigmoidoscopy or colonoscopy, or by arteriography if the bleeding is sufficiently profuse.

Management

A joint medical and surgical approach to acute gastrointestinal bleeding is important. Before investigation, if there are signs of shock, a central venous pressure line is essential. Blood should be given if the haemoglobin is less than 10 g/dl or if there is a tachycardia or hypotension. H_2-receptor antagonist drugs are widely used, but there is little evidence that they reduce operation rates or mortality. Tranexamic acid (which inhibits fibrinolysis) and somatostatin (which reduces acid secretion and splanchnic blood flow) may have a role in controlling bleeding. Vasopressin, which also reduces splanchnic blood flow, is usually reserved for variceal bleeding (Ch. 16, p. 647).

Surgery is indicated if the bleeding is life-threatening, restarts after apparently stopping or is persistent despite receiving three or more litres of blood, especially if the patient is over 60 years of age. Early surgery is indicated if there is a visible vessel at the base of an ulcer or if an operable carcinoma is present. Surgery is best avoided in self-limiting conditions, such as Mallory-Weiss tear, and in clotting disorders or varices (Ch. 16, p. 647).

The overall mortality of acute gastrointestinal bleeding is 5–10% with each episode. However, this relatively high mortality is mostly due to deaths in patients aged over 65 (Fig. 15.10) because of associated disorders (such as vascular, pulmonary or renal diseases), rather than exsanguination.

CHRONIC GASTROINTESTINAL BLEEDING

Aetiology and clinical features

A microcytic hypochromic anaemia is a common presentation of chronic gut blood loss. The commonest causes are shown in Table 15.17. Patients usually present with symptoms of anaemia – malaise, dyspnoea and angina. Clinical examination usually shows signs of anaemia, but the classical signs of iron deficiency (glossitis, cheilitis and koilonychia) are often not present.

Investigation

The purpose of investigations is to identify the site of the bleeding. Positive faecal occult blood testing suggests gastrointestinal blood loss, but bleeding may be spasmodic so false negatives can occur. False positives may occur with meat ingestion and bleeding gums. Other causes of blood loss (e.g. the genital and urinary tracts) must be considered.

In the presence of upper gastrointestinal symptoms, or if there are no specific symptoms and signs, upper gut endoscopy is usually performed first. This may be combined with duodenal biopsy if there is a possibility of

Table 15.17 Causes of chronic occult gastrointestinal bleeding in the UK (in approximate order of frequency)

- Colonic neoplasm
- Duodenal ulcer
- Reflux oesophagitis/oesophageal ulcer
- Gastric ulcer
- NSAID-induced erosions and gastritis
- Gastric carcinoma
- Meckel's diverticulum
- Angiodysplasia

Note: Hookworm is the commonest worldwide cause

underlying iron malabsorption. If no abnormality is found in the upper gut, sigmoidoscopy and double contrast air and barium enema are the next investigations. If still no cause is evident, colonoscopy and investigation of the small bowel (e.g. small bowel enema, Meckel scan (p. 554) or arteriography) must be considered.

Management

Wherever possible, the primary cause of the bleeding is treated. The iron stores are replenished by giving oral iron in the form of ferrous sulphate, fumarate or gluconate. Oral iron can cause nausea, dyspepsia and altered bowel habit. If these side-effects develop, a lower dose or a different preparation should be tried. If the patient is unable to tolerate oral iron, a total dose infusion of intravenous iron dextran, or intramuscular doses of smaller amounts of iron sorbitol, can be used (p. 1053). Severe symptomatic anaemia may require blood transfusion; this is especially likely to occur if the primary cause cannot be found or treated successfully. If no cause is found, the patient is followed carefully and reinvestigated if the problem recurs.

THE STOMACH AND DUODENUM

Anatomy and physiology

The lower end of the oesophagus and the fundus of the stomach are separated by the gastro-oesophageal sphincter, which prevents reflux and allows the downward passage of food. The stomach is divided into three parts: fundus, body and antrum. The pyloric sphincter controls passage of gastric contents into the first part of the duodenum. Parietal cells in the fundus and body of the stomach synthesise hydrochloric acid; gastrin is synthesised in the antral G-cells. Pepsinogens are produced by the chief cells in the crypts.

The stomach has three main functions.

- *The secretion of HCl*, which converts pepsinogen to pepsin to initiate protein digestion into polypeptides and protects the small intestine from bacteria. The pH is kept at around 2. In man, HCl secretion is mainly stimulated by the hormone gastrin, which is released in response to dietary protein, gastric distension and vagal stimulation. At the level of the parietal cell, the final common pathway of HCl synthesis is K^+-H^+-ATPase which pumps H^+ ions into the lumen of the stomach. The interrelationships of these stimuli are shown in Figure 15.11.
- *Acting as a reservoir*. The stomach constantly churns food into small particles. Gastric emptying proceeds slowly so that the small bowel can digest and absorb

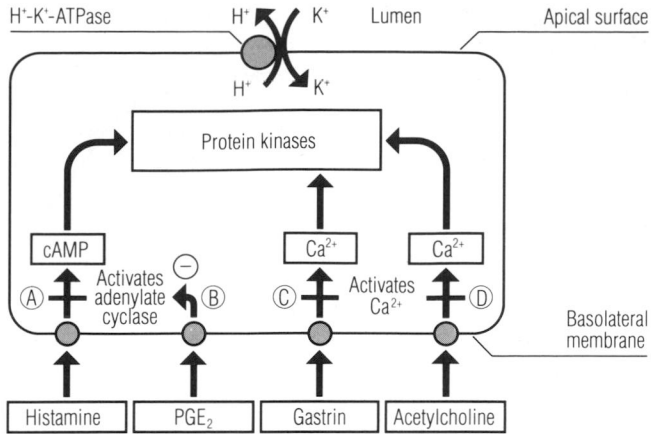

Fig. 15.11 Diagram showing secretion of H⁺ by a gastric parietal cell. There are receptors on the basolateral membrane for histamine (H₂), gastrin and acetylcholine, all of which can mediate the activation of second messengers. A complex series of metabolic events then occurs with the result that H⁺-K⁺-ATPase at the apical surface pumps H⁺ into the gastric lumen in exchange for K⁺. Antagonists exist for each of the three basolateral receptors (e.g. cimetidine (A), proglumide (C) and pirenzipine (D) and for H⁺,K⁺, ATPase (omeprazole). The prostaglandin E₂ receptor inhibits the stimulatory effect of histamine on cAMP; misoprostol (B) is a PGE₂ analogue.

maximally. Gastric emptying is a complex process, dependent on duodenal receptors; it is, for example, slower for fats than protein. Control is partly vagal and partly hormonal (motilin accelerates the process, while enteroglucagon and neurotensin slow it down).

- *Secretion of intrinsic factor,* by the parietal cells.

The duodenum is largely retroperitoneal and is divided into first, second, third and fourth parts. The pH is lowest in the first part and nearly all duodenal ulcers are sited here. The medial border of the second part of the duodenum receives alkaline biliary and pancreatic secretions. The duodenum contains Brunner's glands, which secrete bicarbonate and help bring pH towards neutral. Villi are present throughout the duodenum and increase in size down its length. Both enzyme digestion and absorption of small molecules not needing digestion (e.g. calcium, iron, folic acid) occur in the duodenum.

Clinical features of gastroduodenal pathology

The site of gastroduodenal pain is usually epigastric, but may radiate through to the back and to the right and left hypochondria. Duodenal ulcer pain is typically relieved by food and simple antacids. Functional dyspepsia usually occurs at the time of maximal stress. Nausea, vomiting, anorexia and weight loss raise the possibility of luminal obstruction or a carcinoma. Bleeding can cause haematemesis and melaena.

Summary 4 The main symptoms, signs and investigations in the diagnosis of gastroduodenal disease

Symptoms	*Signs*
Pain or discomfort	Tenderness
Site	Presence of an epigastric mass
Relationship with food, drugs	Succussion splash
stress	Supraclavicular lymphadenopathy
Nausea and vomiting	Hepatomegaly
Haematemesis and melaena	
Anorexia	
Weight loss	
Heartburn	
Early satiety	

Investigations
Endoscopy
Barium meal
Gastric acid secretory studies
Plasma gastrin
Full blood count
Liver function tests

Epigastric tenderness may be present on superficial or deep palpation. An epigastric mass may be palpable, and can be difficult to distinguish from the liver. With gastric carcinoma, metastatic supraclavicular nodes and the liver may be palpable. A succussion splash, present three or more hours after the last drink or meal, suggests delayed gastric emptying commonly due to pyloric obstruction. It is elicited by shaking the patient's upper abdomen while listening over the epigastrium.

Investigation of gastroduodenal pathology

Endoscopy is the preferred method of investigation. A barium meal is reserved for patients who are frail, have poor lung function, refuse endoscopy or cannot swallow the endoscope. The clinical indications for measuring gastric acid secretion are to exclude a gastrinoma (when the basal acid secretion is very high) and to confirm that parietal cell innervation has been lost after a surgical vagotomy (if successful, insulin-induced hypoglycaemia no longer causes acid secretion).

PEPTIC ULCERS

Peptic ulcers can occur in the oesophagus (usually in association with gastro-oesophageal reflux), the stomach, the pyloric canal and the duodenum. An erosion is present when the mucosal surface is broken; ulcers are present when the muscularis mucosae is penetrated. In practice, it may be difficult to tell the difference at endoscopy. Lesions may vary in size from 1 mm to several centimetres in diameter.

Aetiology

The aetiological factors in peptic ulceration are shown in Table 15.18. The aphorism 'no acid: no ulcer' is true for benign peptic ulcers. Gastric ulcers, however, are usually associated with normal or low acid outputs, although this may partly reflect duodenogastric reflux of alkaline juice. The bacterium *Helicobacter pylori* is present in the gastric antrum of more than 90% of duodenal ulcer patients and its continued presence is related to a high rate of recurrence (90% of patients treated with H_2 receptor antagonists in the first year after stopping treatment). *H. pylori* may also have an aetiological role in gastric ulcers. Duodenogastric reflux of alkaline juice, bile and pancreatic enzymes is thought to be important for gastric ulcers. NSAIDs, corticosteroids and aspirin are associated with an increased incidence of peptic ulcers and of the complications of bleeding and perforation. Smoking plays a role in pathogenesis and delays healing of duodenal ulcers. The objective evidence that ordinary stress causes ulcers is poor, but severe head injuries (Cushing's ulcer) and burns (Curling's ulcer) are associated with the development of acute ulcers. Duodenal ulcers are often familial and are associated with blood group O. The factors involved in mucosal cell resistance or liability to ulceration are not understood. Other possibly important factors are gastric mucus, and gastric and duodenal bicarbonate secretion which may have protective roles. An additional, and rare, cause of peptic ulceration is gastrinoma (p. 573).

Duodenal ulcers are approximately four times as common as gastric ulcer. Whereas there appears to be a tendency for spontaneous remission with duodenal ulcers, the prevalence of gastric ulcer progressively increases with age (Fig. 15.12).

Clinical features

The symptoms and signs of ulcer disease are non-specific for each type of ulcer and commonly overlap those found

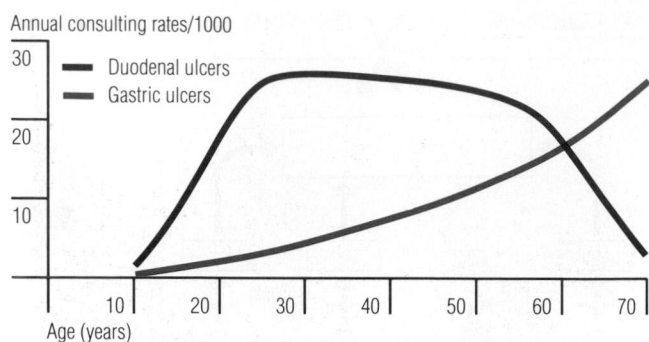

Fig. 15.12 Incidence of peptic ulcer related to age, in the UK.

in patients with cholelithiasis, oesophagitis, pancreatitis and no demonstrable organic disease (non-ulcer dyspepsia). Duodenal ulcer patients tend to have epigastric pain which is worse with fasting, better with antacids and food, and wakes them at 2–4 am. Gastric ulcer patients' epigastric pain is sometimes worse with food and relieved by vomiting. Nausea and vomiting are relatively unusual and imply outlet obstruction. Anorexia and weight loss can occur with both gastric and duodenal ulcers. Ulcers may be asymptomatic.

In an uncomplicated peptic ulcer patient, epigastric tenderness is usually the only abnormal sign, and even this is often absent. If there is gastric outflow obstruction, a succussion splash may be present.

Investigation

Endoscopy is more accurate than barium studies in the diagnosis of peptic ulcers (Table 15.19 and Fig. 15.13). *H. pylori* contains the enzyme urease and can be diagnosed by culture of an antral biopsy in urea-containing broth or by a urea breath test. Antibiotic sensitivities can also be assessed. It also enables accurate histological diagnosis of malignancy, and treatment with electrocautery

Table 15.18 Aetiological factors in peptic ulceration

Causal factor	Gastric ulcer	Duodenal ulcer
Helicobacter pylori	Important	Very important
NSAIDs and steroids	Small role	Small role
Acid	Normal or low acid output	High or normal acid output
Smoking	Important	Important
Stress	Evidence for head injuries and burns only	
Family history	Uncommon	Common

Table 15.19 Relative merits of endoscopy and barium studies in diagnosis of peptic ulcer

Merit	Endoscopy	Barium study
Accuracy	Almost 100%	Lower, especially for superficial lesions
Ability to obtain biopsies and brush cytology	Yes	No
Enables other treatments (e.g. diathermy, lasers)	Yes	No
Detection of bleeding	Good	Poor
Assessment of healing	Good	Poor for duodenal ulcers
Complications	Very few	Very few

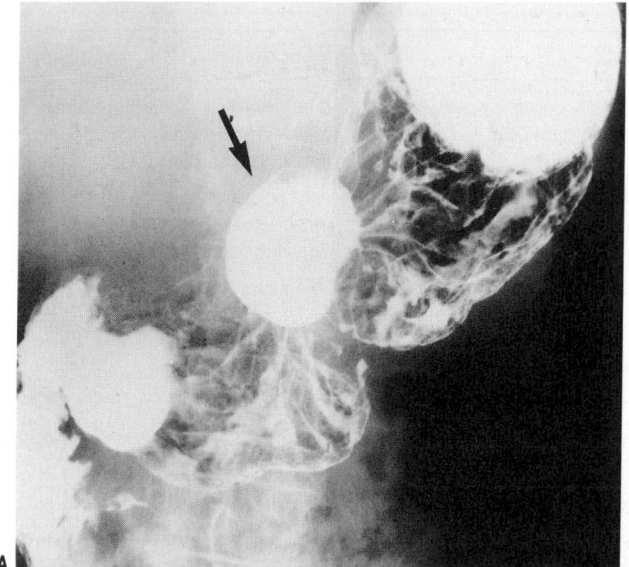

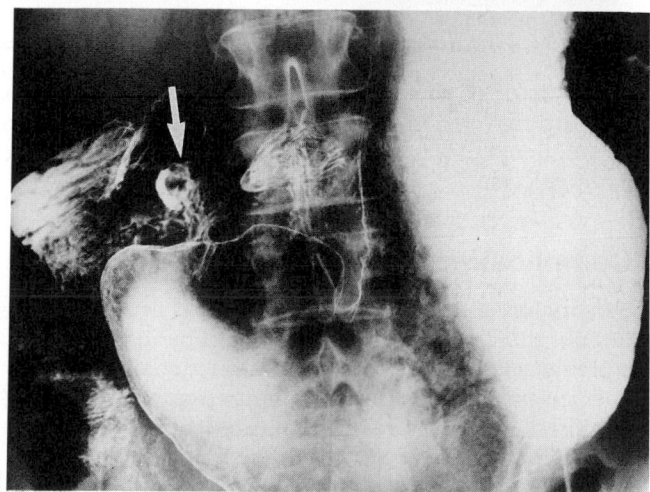

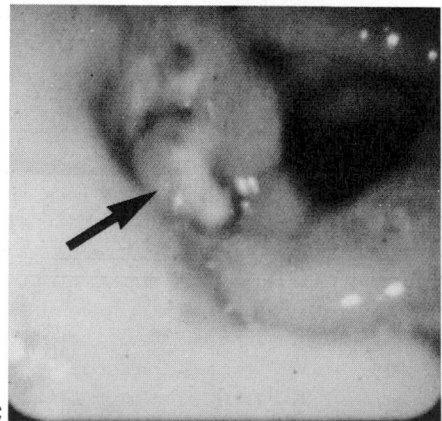

Fig. 15.13 Barium studies and endoscopy in diagnosis of peptic ulcer. A. Barium meal demonstrating a large gastric ulcer filled with barium. **B.** Typical duodenal ulcer with pyloric stenosis. **C.** Endoscopic appearance of a chronic prepyloric ulcer.

and lasers as necessary. Endoscopic complications are rare, but bleeding and perforation can occur.

Complications

There are three main complications of peptic ulcers:

- *Gastrointestinal bleeding* (p. 566) is the first symptom of a peptic ulcer in a small proportion of patients, but usually there is a variable period of preceding dyspepsia.
- *Perforation* of an ulcer usually presents with acute severe upper abdominal pain, and circulatory collapse may rapidly develop. Specific symptoms may be minimal or absent in the elderly and in patients on corticosteroid therapy. After resuscitation, surgery should be performed to clean the peritoneum and oversew the ulcer; a procedure may also be performed to prevent further ulcers, e.g. a vagotomy with or without a drainage procedure. Rarely, surgery may be contraindicated by high anaesthetic risks. Under these circumstances, the perforation will sometimes heal with conservative management.
- *Gastric outflow obstruction* (pyloric stenosis) usually follows long-standing duodenal ulcer or pyloric channel ulcer and/or oedema. Patients complain of vomiting food eaten many hours before. The failure of gastric emptying results in postprandial fullness, anorexia and weight loss. A succussion splash may be heard many hours after the last meal. If there is an active ulcer with oedema, pyloric stenosis may respond to medical treatment. Otherwise, surgery is necessary although, in a medically very sick patient, endoscopic dilatation with a balloon can be considered.

Management

Medical

Before a definite diagnosis is made, patients can be treated by simple antacids. In standard doses these are effective symptomatically, but rarely heal significant ulcers. When a diagnosis is made, patients should be encouraged to give up smoking as this will improve their chance of healing and reduce relapse rate. Minimisation of alcohol intake should also be encouraged.

Many effective medical treatments are now available (Table 15.20). In *H. pylori* positive duodenal ulcer patients, the organism should be eradicated. A current regime, which eradicates *H. pylori* in 80–90% of patients, is a two-week course of colloidal bismuth, oxytetracycline and metronidazole. If the bacterium is eradicated, ulcer recurrence is rare. More effective treatments with higher eradication rates are sought. *H. pylori* should also be eradicated when present in patients with gastric ulcers but the rates of relapse are also low on the treatment with H$_2$-

15 Gastrointestinal Disease

Table 15.20 Main drugs used in treatment of peptic ulcers

Drug	Mode of action	Efficacy	Main side-effects
Colloidal bismuth and antibiotics	Eradication of *H. pylori*	Good (80% long-term healing with reduced relapse rate)	Colloidal bismuth – unpleasant taste common, black tongue Antibiotics – diarrhoea
Cimetidine	H_2-receptor antagonist	Good (80% healing)	Anti-androgenic effects (e.g. impotence, gynaecomastia) Enzyme induction
Ranitidine	H_2-receptor antagonist	Good (80% healing)	Mild rashes
Omeprazole	Proton pump inhibitor	Good (>95% healing)	Gastric carcinoid tumours in animals
Aluminium hydroxide	Simple antacid	Good for symptoms; poor for healing	Constipation
Magnesium trisilicate	Simple antacid	Good for symptoms; poor for healing	Diarrhoea
Carbenoxolone	Mucosal protection	Good	Sodium retention leading to heart failure, hypertension and potassium loss
Sucralfate	Mucosal protection	Good	Constipation
Misoprostol	Prostaglandin E_2 analogues; mucosal protection; acid and gastrin reduction	Good	Diarrhoea Abortion
Pirenzipine	Anticholinergic	Good	Dry mouth

receptor antagonists or proton pump inhibitors. The H_2-receptor antagonists are widely used and heal about 80% of ulcers within six weeks. Acid secretion at night is particularly damaging and so taking all the tablets at bedtime is as effective as splitting them during the day. Proton pump inhibitors are even more effective for peptic ulcer healing but are reserved for resistant cases. Other drugs are probably as effective as H_2-receptor blocking drugs but tend to have more side-effects. Gastric ulcers should be followed up by endoscopy at six weeks to check healing, and by rebiopsy to exclude a tumour if unhealed; repeat endoscopy is less important in duodenal ulcers but is helpful in some patients.

Surgical

The indications for surgery for peptic ulcers are shown in Table 15.21. Severe haemorrhage and perforation are indications for surgery unless the patient is thought unfit for a general anaesthetic. Gastric outflow obstruction also usually requires surgery, although occasionally medical

Table 15.21 Indications for surgery for peptic ulcers

- Failure of healing on medical treatment
- Repeated relapses despite treatment
- Non-compliance to medical treatment
- Severe haemorrhage
- Perforation
- Gastric outflow obstruction
- Patient unwilling to take maintenance treatment

treatment of an active ulcer may improve symptoms. The best current operations may be highly selective vagotomy for duodenal ulcers and Bilroth I partial gastrectomy for gastric ulcers.

Complications of gastric surgery

Surgery for gastric and duodenal ulcers is usually successful, but the ulcer may recur in 10% of patients who have a highly selective vagotomy for a duodenal ulcer. Postoperative weight loss is a common symptom but usually stabilises. If a partial gastrectomy is performed, bile reflux may result and cause gastritis in the remnant.

Following gastric surgery, gastric emptying into the small intestine may become very rapid. Hyperosmolar contents cause fluid to be secreted into the jejunum, the plasma compartment contracts and the haematocrit rises. This results in 'early dumping', and the patient complains about 30 minutes after a meal of sweating, palpitations, faintness and abdominal distension. These symptoms may be mediated in part by the vasomotor peptides, neurotensin and vasoactive intestinal polypeptide (VIP, p. 554). The rapid emptying also results in increased early insulin secretion, so that reactive hypoglycaemia may occur 3–4 hours after a meal ('late dumping'). As a result of the rapid gastric emptying, there may be small bowel malabsorption, causing diarrhoea associated with raised faecal fat excretion (steatorrhoea). All these problems can be improved by small, regular and relatively iso-osmolar meals.

After partial and total gastrectomy, some patients become iron, vitamin B_{12}, calcium and vitamin D deficient. A full blood count and plasma calcium, phosphate and alkaline phosphatase should be checked regularly, and life-long supplementary treatment initiated as necessary.

Carcinoma of the stomach is more common after partial gastrectomy, particularly after 20 years.

GASTRINOMA

Rarely, tumours secreting gastrin stimulate gastric acid secretion, resulting in severe duodenal and upper small bowel ulceration. The primary tumours are usually in the pancreas or duodenum. The tumours may be malignant, and 50% have metastasised at the time of diagnosis. The gastrinoma syndrome (originally described by Zollinger and Ellison in 1955) is characterised by severe peptic ulceration but 40% of patients may have diarrhoea, occasionally associated with malabsorption. The duodenal ulcers are often multiple and may be associated with perforation, bleeding and pyloric stenosis. The acid may also reflux into the oesophagus and cause oesophagitis and oesophageal strictures. About a third of the patients have a functioning parathyroid tumour causing hypercalcaemia, and adenomas also occur in the pituitary, adrenal and thyroid (multiple endocrine neoplasia type 1, see p. 613). Diagnosis is by demonstrating gastric hyperacidity and a high fasting plasma gastrin. Localisation of the tumour(s) is by CT scanning, arteriography and, if there is still doubt, portal venous sampling for gastrin.

The tumours are usually slowly progressive, and should only be resected if they are thought to be single and non-metastatic. The acid hypersecretion is best controlled by proton pump inhibitors (Table 15.20).

GASTRITIS

In gastritis, there are areas of inflamed red oedematous mucosa and the diagnosis can be confirmed by biopsy.

Acute

Acute gastritis is commonly associated with infections, NSAIDs, alcohol or iron intake, and renal failure. It may cause dyspepsia and can present with gastric bleeding. It can be diagnosed by direct vision with an endoscope, but not by a barium meal. Treatment is by removing the cause, together with simple antacids. Patients with renal disease have a poor prognosis if they bleed so prophylactic H_2-receptor antagonists are therefore used in those with dyspeptic symptoms on inflammatory changes on endoscopy.

Chronic

Chronic gastritis may not give rise to symptoms although occasionally it may be associated with dyspepsia. There are two types: chronic superficial and chronic atrophic. The former may be associated with *H. pylori* colonisation of the stomach and the latter may lead to vitamin B_{12} malabsorption. There is an increased incidence of gastric adenocarcinoma if atrophy or metaplasia are present.

MÉNÉTRIÈR'S DISEASE

Ménétrièr's disease is a rare condition, where the normal gastric rugae are increased in height to 1–2 cm. The aetiology is unknown. The main problem is gastric protein loss leading to peripheral oedema (Table 15.4). Reduced acid secretion and iron and vitamin B_{12} deficiency occur; occasionally, a gastric ulcer develops.

In some patients, the condition may improve with a high protein diet and antacids. There is a tendency to spontaneous remission. In some patients, however, only total gastrectomy relieves the problem. There is an increased risk of developing gastric adenocarcinoma.

DUODENITIS

In duodenitis, the mucosa appears inflamed, reddened and sometimes haemorrhagic. It may be seen in isolation or around ulcer craters and may follow or precede the development of duodenal ulcers. When no break in the mucosa (i.e. ulcer) is present, histology shows acute and chronic inflammation. The relationship of duodenitis to symptoms is variable; sometimes patients are asymptomatic and sometimes they have typical ulcer symptoms.

Treatment is by avoiding potential aetiological factors such as smoking, alcohol and NSAIDs, and with simple antacids. If symptoms are severe, H_2-receptor antagonists may help.

MALIGNANT TUMOURS OF THE STOMACH: ADENOCARCINOMA

There are marked geographic variations in the incidence of adenocarcinoma (Fig. 15.14). In the UK, the incidence is 30 per 100 000 for men and 20 per 100 000 for women. As in other Western countries, there has been a gradual decline in death rate in the last 20 years.

Aetiology and pathology

Gastric carcinoma is five times more common in patients with pernicious anaemia. *H. pylori* is also found more frequently. Other risk factors include achlorhydria, previous partial gastrectomy, gastric adenomatous polyps and blood group A. It has been postulated that gastric atrophy leads to a fall in acid production which allows colonisation of the stomach with bacteria. The result of bacterial growth may be to convert dietary nitrates to

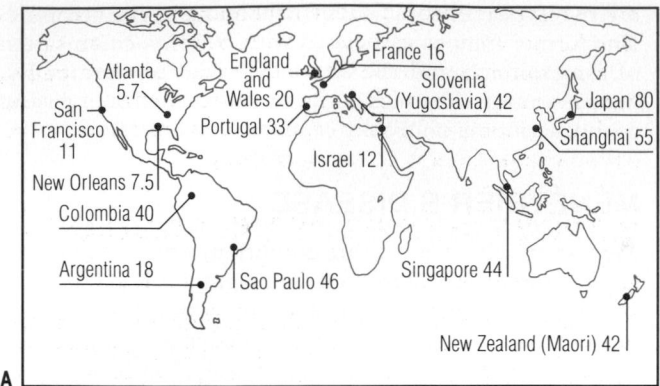

A

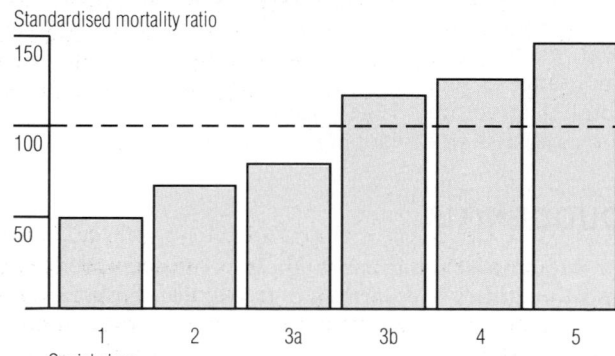

B

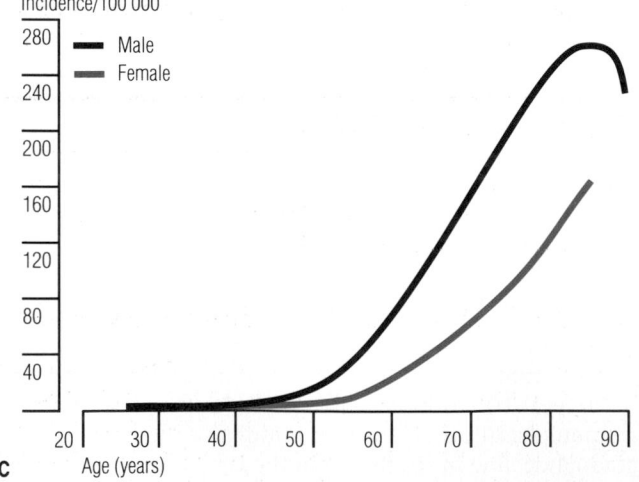

C

Fig. 15.14 Gastric adenocarcinoma: incidence and mortality. A. Worldwide incidence per 100 000. **B.** Gastric adenocarcinoma mortality related to social class. Figures are for men aged 15–64 in England and Wales in 1970–72 (OPCS data, 1978). Values for each social class are in proportion to 100 which represents all social classes combined. **C.** Age adjusted incidence of gastric carcinoma in England.

nitrites which then react with amino acids in food to form N-nitroso compounds. These have been shown to be carcinogens in animals.

The typical tumour is a diffuse infiltrating carcinoma of variable size with a rolled edge and a central ulcer. It spreads through the gastric wall, invades lymph nodes and metastasises to the liver via the bloodstream. It may also seed into the peritoneal cavity giving rise to abdominal and pelvic tumours and ascites. Less commonly, the tumour infiltrates diffusely through the stomach wall (linitis plastica or 'leather bottle stomach'). Microscopically, the carcinomas may resemble intestinal cells or may be diffusely infiltrating tumours. The 'intestinal' type of tumour has a better prognosis and is more frequent in areas of high incidence such as Japan. In Japan, screening for gastric carcinoma has led to the detection of early stage tumours limited to the mucosa or submucosa; such tumours have a good prognosis.

Clinical features

Gastric carcinoma is commonest in 55–65 year olds and is rare at less than 30 years of age. Typically, the patient presents with anorexia, nausea, early satiety and vague abdominal discomfort. More severe epigastric pain may develop later. Bleeding is common, leading to iron deficiency and, occasionally, frank haematemesis or melaena. There may be dysphagia if the tumour involves the gastro-oesophageal junction, and vomiting if there is outflow obstruction. Non-metastatic, paraneoplastic manifestations (p. 130) are unusual and include acanthosis nigricans (of which it is the commonest cause), venous thrombosis and dermatomyositis. Physical examination may reveal evidence of weight loss, anaemia and an epigastric mass. Enlarged lymph nodes may be palpable in the supraclavicular region.

Investigation

The diagnosis should be suspected when dyspepsia appears for the first time in later life and is usually made at endoscopy when an ulcer is found. It is safest to assume that every gastric ulcer is malignant until proved otherwise. Diffusely infiltrating tumours of the *linitis plastica* type may be more easily diagnosed on a barium meal, when the stomach appears contracted and non-distensible. On barium meal, the ulcerative neoplasms appear as an ulcer with irregular borders and disruption of the normal mucosal folds (Fig. 15.15). If there are no clinically evident metastases, and surgery is a possible treatment, it is essential to stage the tumour further. This will include chest X-ray, liver enzyme measurement and liver ultrasound. Tumour markers are not helpful in diagnosis or management.

Management

Surgical resection is the only curative treatment for adenocarcinoma and a total or partial gastrectomy is performed. The prognosis is directly related to stage,

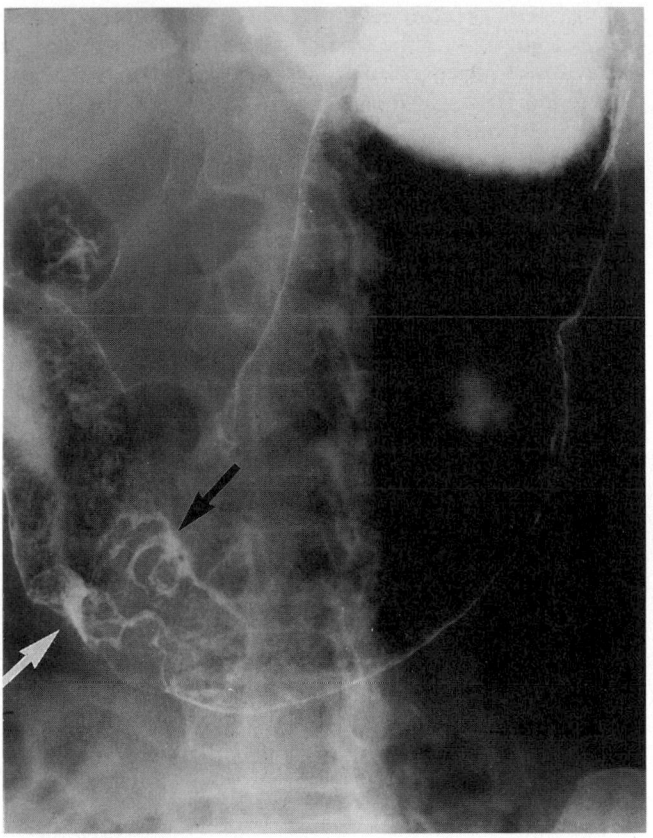

Fig. 15.15 Barium meal examination showing typical gastric carcinoma.

being good (five year survival, 55%) when the tumour is confined to the mucosa or submucosa. Only 2.5% of tumours are in this category. If the tumour has spread through the stomach wall (but no further), the survival falls to 25%; if the lymph nodes are involved few patients will survive five years. Overall, only 60% of patients undergoing surgery have resectable tumours and of these, only 20% will live five years.

Chemotherapy may sometimes be helpful in palliating symptoms of metastatic disease. Radiotherapy may be helpful in palliation of symptoms resulting from local recurrence.

MALIGNANT TUMOURS OF THE STOMACH: GASTRIC LYMPHOMA

Although uncommon (less than 3% of neoplasms) gastric lymphoma is of interest because it remains localised for a considerable period and the prognosis is much better than with gastric carcinoma. It typically presents with upper abdominal discomfort, nausea or gastrointestinal bleeding, and an ulcer is found endoscopically. The histological appearances may be misinterpreted as inflammatory infiltrate and the diagnosis established only later when the

disease is more florid. Gastric lymphoma is a tumour of B lymphocytes (centrocytes and centroblasts, see Ch. 24).

Surgical resection may be curative in the early stages, but the prognosis with surgery alone is worse if local nodes are involved. These patients should receive combination chemotherapy following surgery.

BENIGN TUMOURS OF THE STOMACH

Gastric leiomyomas

Gastric leiomyomas are benign submucosal tumours which rarely become sarcomatous. They arise from the muscularis mucosae. The aetiology is unknown. In many patients they are asymptomatic but, in others, may present with non-specific features such as epigastric pain. The centre of the tumour often ulcerates and patients can present with haematemesis and melaena. In this situation, surgical resection is indicated.

Gastric polyps

Gastric polyps should be biopsied endoscopically. Hyperplastic polyps are not known to be associated with specific symptoms, have no malignant potential and can therefore be ignored. Adenomatous polyps may be premalignant and should be removed endoscopically or surgically. They are usually asymptomatic but can be associated with dyspepsia, gastrointestinal bleeding or gastric outflow obstruction.

THE SMALL INTESTINE

The small intestine is the prime site of nutrient digestion and absorption. It is also a site of water and electrolyte secretion and consequent marked fluid fluxes.

Clinical features of small bowel disease

The most common symptom of small intestinal disease is loose stools, which may be steatorrhoeic due to malabsorption of fat, or watery due to increased secretion or osmosis of water. Pain is usually colicky and a feature of obstruction. Malabsorption of folic acid, iron and vitamin B_{12} results in anaemia. Fat-soluble vitamin deficiency and hypokalaemia also occur. The faeces must be examined for colour, consistency and amount, and a sigmoidoscopy performed to exclude rectal disease.

Investigation of small bowel disease

Investigation of systemic effects

The haemoglobin, blood film and serum vitamin B_{12}, folate and iron assess haematinic deficiency and hyposplenism. A raised white cell count, C-reactive protein or ESR is a non-specific indicator of underlying inflammation. The albumin is measured to look for protein-losing enteropathy and nitrogen deficiency. The plasma urea and electrolytes are measured to assess renal function and hypokalaemia. A low plasma calcium usually indicates calcium deficiency which is due in part to malabsorption of vitamin D which is fat-soluble. This may be associated with low plasma 25-hydroxy and 1, 25-dihydroxy vitamin D levels. As a consequence, there may be increased parathyroid hormone secretion (secondary hyperparathyroidism) resulting in hypophosphataemia and a rise in the plasma bone alkaline phosphatase. Abnormal liver function tests are associated with the hepatic complications of Crohn's disease. With steatorrhoea, malabsorption of the other fat-soluble vitamins (A, E and K) may lead to a low plasma vitamin A and the prothrombin time may be prolonged due to vitamin K deficiency. Water-soluble vitamin deficiencies are rare; thiamine can be assessed by the red cell transketolase level. Faecal weight and fat can be measured in a three-day collection. Small intestinal function tests are discussed on page 557.

Radiology

The small bowel can be visualised by a small bowel meal (patient drinks barium) or a tube small bowel enema (dilute barium is infused directly into the upper jejunum via a peroral tube). The former is adequate for diagnosing most diffuse mucosal disorders but the latter is superior for demonstrating focal lesions and examining the terminal ileum. Arteriography is used to assess ischaemia and demonstrate bleeding sites. The small bowel cannot be satisfactorily imaged by ultrasound, CT or NMR.

Radioisotopes

Radiolabelled albumin is used to assess protein-losing enteropathy and radiolabelled (e.g. indium) white cells are used to indicate the site of active inflammation in patients with Crohn's disease. Chromium^{-51} labelled red cells can be used to indicate the site of small intestinal bleeding, if this is more than 1 ml blood per minute. Bile acid and vitamin B_{12} absorption can also be measured by the use of radionuclides (p. 557).

MALABSORPTION

A simple classification of small intestinal malabsorption is shown in Table 15.22. Osmotic diarrhoea occurs when the luminal contents are osmotically active and draw excessive amounts of water into the small bowel. Secretory diarrhoea occurs when small intestinal water and electrolyte secretion is increased and overcomes absorptive capacity. A number of drugs can cause malabsorption.

The most severe steatorrhoea (more than 100 g fat/24 hours) is seen in patients with very short small intestines or in pancreatic exocrine failure. The amount of fat malabsorption in most patients with small intestinal malabsorption is less than 40 g/24 hours. Steatorrhoea is minimal or absent in patients with osmotic or secretory diarrhoea.

Large volumes of stool (more than 1 kg/24 hours) are usually seen in patients with secretary diarrhoea, and occasionally in patients with osmotic diarrhoea and in those with substantially reduced lengths of functional small intestine.

COELIAC DISEASE

Coeliac disease is also known as gluten-sensitive enteropathy and non-tropical sprue. The disorder results in abnormal small bowel mucosa, with loss of villi, crypt hyperplasia and infiltration with chronic inflammatory cells. The clinical syndrome and small bowel histology improve with removal of dietary gluten and return if gluten is eaten again.

Aetiology

The aetiology of coeliac disease became clear at the end of World War II when it was realised that Dutch coeliac chil-

Table 15.22 Classification of small intestinal diarrhoea

Abnormality	Causes	Steatorrhoea	Watery stool	Other results
Upper small bowel disease	Coeliac disease Giardia etc.	+	+	Iron ↓ Folate ↓ Calcium ↓
Osmotic diarrhoea	Disaccharidase deficiencies Magnesium salts	–	++	
Secretory diarrhoea	Cholera VIP Phenolphthalein	–	+++	Dehydration Hypokalaemia
Rapid transit	Postgastrectomy Thyrotoxicosis	+	+	
Short gut	Surgery Fistula	++	++	
Lower small bowel disease	Crohn's disease Tuberculosis etc.	+	+	Vitamin B$_{12}$ ↓ Bile acids ↓
Drug-induced	Neomycin Cholestyramine Alcohol	+	±	

dren improved when wheat was unavailable (they subsisted on tulips and sugar-beet) but deteriorated when wheat was reintroduced into their diets. Wheat, rye, barley and sometimes oat gluten are toxic. During milling, bran is separated from flour. Gluten is contained in the water-insoluble portion of flour; the toxic moiety is present in an alcohol-soluble portion of gluten, known as gliadin. Digestion of gliadin with pepsin and trypsin results in smaller toxic subunits. The mode of gluten's toxicity is uncertain but there are three main hypotheses:

1. *Immunogenetic.* The strong association of coeliac disease with the HLA B8-DRW3 haplotype links it with many of the autoimmune diseases (see p. 96–7) and suggests a possible immunological origin. This is consistent with the finding of a predominantly TR lymphocyte infiltration of the mucosal lesions, and the local production of antigluten antibody. However, neither humoral nor cellular tests show any consistent changes to distinguish coeliac disease from other inflammatory bowel conditions. Recent evidence suggests abnormal expression of the Class II HLA antigens, DR, DP and DQ on coeliac enterocytes, converting them into antigen presenting cells.
2. *Peptidase deficiency.* It has been suggested that coeliac disease is due to a lack of an intestinal peptidase, leading to accumulation of gliadin and gluten which are directly toxic to small intestinal mucosal cells. The discordance of 30% among identical twins does not support the inherited enzymatic deficiency theory. No missing peptidase has ever been found.
3. *Enterocyte membrane defect.* This hypothesis suggests that there is a defect in the glycoprotein structure of

the brush border membrane which allows gluten to bind to it and cause cell damage and death.

The highest recorded incidence of coeliac disease is in the west of Ireland where it is one in 300. In the UK, the incidence is about one in 2000. The disease is very unusual in Negroes and Japanese. There is evidence that the incidence in children is falling in the UK and this may reflect the fact that most infant feeds are now gluten-free. There is a modest female preponderance. About 10% of asymptomatic first degree relatives have the disorder, but the mode of inheritance is unknown.

Clinical features

Coeliac disease can present at any age, but there are peaks between one and five years of age and in the third and fourth decades. Typically, the disease is now diagnosed in patients found to be iron or folate deficient when being investigated for non-specific symptoms. The extreme case of a cachectic, oedematous, clubbed, pigmented, dying patient with multiple vitamin deficiencies is now rare.

The main symptoms and signs are shown in Table 15.23. In children, the symptoms are often non-specific, with failure to thrive in infancy or growth retardation. Presentation in adolescence is unusual. Diarrhoea is more common in adults than children. Diarrhoea is not universal and coeliacs may, rarely, present with constipation. Abdominal pain is usually mild. About 30% of patients have aphthous ulcers which are usually severe and recurrent but respond to a gluten-free diet. Dermatitis herpetiformis is an itchy vesicular rash which is usually

Table 15.23 Clinical manifestations of coeliac disease

Symptom/sign	Mechanism
History	
Non-specific, e.g. malaise, anorexia	Iron, folate or calcium deficiency
Diarrhoea and steatorrhoea	Water, electrolyte and fat malabsorption
Weight loss	Fat and carbohydrate malabsorption
Abdominal pain and bloating	Distended bowel loops
Aphthous ulcers	
Nausea and vomiting	
Itchy spots on extensor surfaces (dermatitis herpetiformis)	
Positive family history	
Irish background	
Oedema	Hypoproteinaemia
Pigmentation	
Tetany	Vitamin D and calcium deficiency
Bone pains; muscle weakness	Vitamin D and calcium deficiency
Bleeding tendency	Vitamin K deficiency
Night blindness	Vitamin A deficiency
In children	
Failure to thrive	
Irritability	Malabsorption
Growth failure	Malabsorption
Delayed puberty	
Examination	
Anaemia	Iron and folate (and, rarely, vitamin B_{12}) deficiency
Weight loss	Malabsorption
Pigmentation	Unknown
Glossitis	Iron and folate deficiency
Angular cheilitis	Iron and folate deficiency
Aphthous ulcers	Gluten sensitivity and/or vitamin deficiency
Koilonychia	Iron deficiency
Clubbing	Unknown
Oedema	Hypoproteinaemia
Bruising	Vitamin K deficiency
Abdominal distension	Distended bowel loops
Positive Chvostek's and Trousseau's signs	Hypocalcaemia
Bone tenderness; proximal myopathy	Osteomalacia
Reduced light adaptation	Vitamin A deficiency
Dermatitis herpetiformis	

predominant on extensor surfaces such as the elbows and knees (p. 579).

Examination is often non-contributory, with mild anaemia, weight loss, abdominal distension and diarrhoea or steatorrhoea on rectal examination being the most common physical signs. Hypocalcaemia may develop relatively quickly, but bone tenderness and proximal myopathy imply long-standing hypocalcaemia with osteomalacia.

Investigations

Small bowel histology

The diagnosis is made by demonstrating the characteristic small bowel biopsy changes which improve on gluten withdrawal. The villi may be totally or, less commonly, partially lost (subtotal or partial villous atrophy, see Fig. 15.16). The duodenum and jejunum are predominantly affected but, in severe cases, villous abnormalities may also be seen in the ileum.

Subtotal villous atrophy usually indicates coeliac disease. However, in the absence of a response to a gluten-free diet and with lesser degrees of villous atrophy, conditions such as giardiasis, tropical sprue, small bowel ischaemia and gastrinoma must also be considered. Transient gluten intolerance with subtotal villous atrophy can be seen in children.

Haematology

The most common haematological abnormality is anaemia due to iron and/or folate deficiency as a consequence of malabsorption. Folate deficiency is most reliably characterised by a low red blood cell folate which reflects long-standing folate deficiency. Serum B_{12} levels are quite often low, often secondary to a defect in mucosal absorption as a result of folate deficiency. Hyposplenism is present in many patients, and Howell-Jolly bodies may be seen on the blood film. The ESR is raised in a minority of patients. Sideroblastic anaemia may occur due to vitamin B_6 deficiency. If there is severe malabsorption of vitamin K, the prothrombin time may be prolonged.

Biochemistry

Hypoalbuminaemia is relatively common and is due to protein loss from the small intestine and peptide malabsorption. Faecal fat levels are usually raised. Hypocalcaemia due to malabsorption of calcium is common, with consequent secondary hyperparathyroidism. In chronic hypocalcaemia, the serum bone alkaline phosphatase rises. Some patients are vitamin D deficient and this is best demonstrated by a low serum 25-hydroxy vitamin D. Serum vitamin A and magnesium levels may also be low. Zinc deficiency is rare.

Absorption tests

Absorption tests are not specific for coeliac disease. Radiosotopic fat tests can be used to screen for fat absorption and are less unpleasant for laboratory personnel, but less

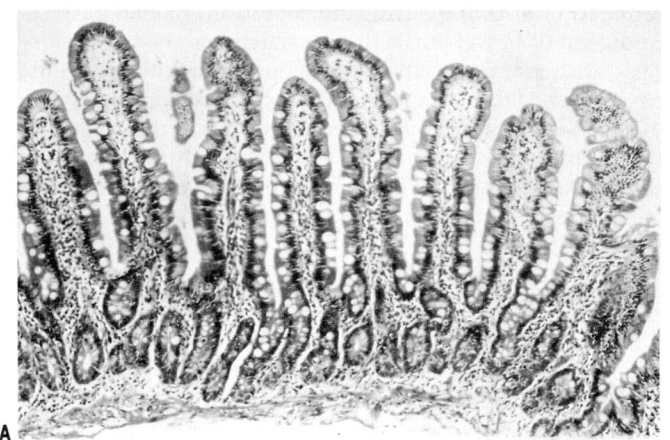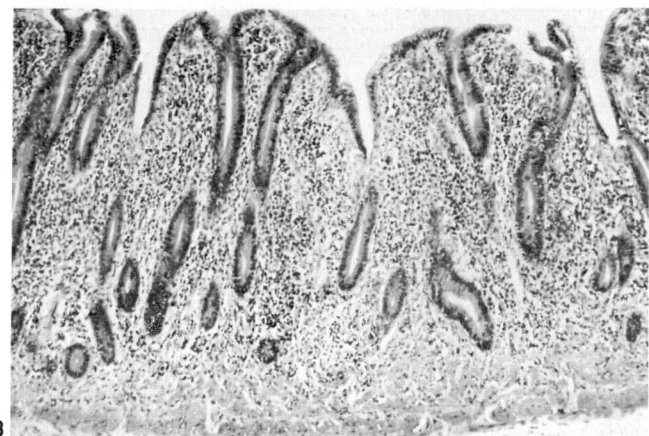

Fig. 15.16 Comparison of normal small bowel histology with that of a patient with coeliac disease. A. Photomicrograph of normal small intestinal finger-like villi with columnar surface cells. **B.** Photomicrograph of small bowel biopsy in a patient with coeliac disease. There is total villous atrophy with complete loss of the villi, cuboidal surface cells, crypt hyperplasia and an increased number of lymphocytes.

accurate, than faecal fat estimation. Small bowel permeability tests are abnormal (p. 557).

Radiology

Small bowel radiology may show non-specific jejunal dilatation and flocculation of barium; its main value is to exclude anatomical abnormalities and inflammatory disorders (e.g. Crohn's disease). Bone radiology may show signs of osteomalacia (bone thinning and pseudofractures) and secondary hyperparathyroidism (subperiosteal erosions; see Ch. 18).

Management

Management is with a strict gluten-free diet, avoiding flour from wheat, rye, barley and occasionally, oats. This means the avoidance of most bread, cakes and biscuits as well as foods where flour has been used as a thickening agent (e.g. gravy). Rice and maize can be used as substitutes. In the UK, gluten-free foods can be obtained on prescription. Such a diet allows the small bowel mucosa to return almost to normal in all children and most adults. A strict diet is essential in most patients but in the newly diagnosed elderly patient with minor symptoms, strict adherence to diet is less essential. In the UK, membership of the Coeliac Society should be encouraged.

Supplements of folic acid, iron, vitamin B_{12}, calcium, vitamin D, etc. should be given to correct deficiency states. Most patients make a good response to the diet and nutritional supplements. Rarely, corticosteroids are indicated in patients who have a poor response to a gluten-free diet.

Small bowel biopsies are repeated after three to six months of a gluten-free diet in all patients. Biopsy after a gluten challenge is required to confirm the diagnosis in children but is rarely needed in adults. For adults stable on a gluten-free diet, an annual review is useful to check the patient's weight and exclude deficiency states. In children, more frequent follow-up is necessary to monitor growth and development.

Development of malignancy

There is a greatly increased risk of developing lymphoma, which is thought to be a tumour of T lymphocytes in most cases. It is usually multifocal throughout the small bowel and responds poorly to chemotherapy. There is also a higher incidence of adenocarcinoma of the small bowel and squamous cell carcinomas of the oesophagus and pharynx. Recent evidence suggests that a gluten-free diet may reduce the risk of lymphoma.

DERMATITIS HERPETIFORMIS

Dermatitis herpetiformis is a blistering and pruritic skin eruption which particularly affects the extensor surface of the knees and elbows (p. 1146). Most patients have associated small intestinal villous atrophy identical to that of coeliac disease, and may also develop other complications of coeliac disease. Histology of the skin lesions shows blister cavities, while immunofluorescence shows IgA deposits at and just below the dermo-epidermal junction (p. 1146, Fig. 25.25). The rash and intestinal lesion improve with gluten withdrawal. The rash is also helped by treatment with oral dapsone.

BACTERIAL OVERGROWTH
Aetiology

Under normal circumstances, the stomach and upper intestine have a low concentration of bacteria, due to gastric acid secretion and normal small bowel motility. Greater numbers of bacteria, intermediate in amount between the jejunum and the colon, are found in the ileum. Bacterial overgrowth of the upper small bowel is associated with jejunal diverticular disease (Fig. 15.17A),

reduced or absent gastric acid secretion, partial gastrectomy, small bowel stasis due to strictures, systemic sclerosis, diabetic neuropathy, adhesions and fistulas from the small to the large bowel. It can also occur spontaneously in the elderly. Bacterial deconjugation and dehydroxylation of bile acids is thought to be the main mechanism of the steatorrhoea, but there is also some damage to the small intestinal mucosa.

Clinical features and investigation

Patients present with weight loss, anorexia, nausea, diarrhoea (but sometimes constipation) and increased flatulence. Steatorrhoea and B_{12} malabsorption (resulting in red cell macrocytosis) are the commonest laboratory abnormalities. Deficiencies of iron, protein and calcium may occur. The red cell folate levels can be high because of bacterial synthesis of folic acid.

The diagnosis can be confirmed by demonstrating increased numbers of bacteria in upper small bowel aspirates. This is technically difficult, however, and instead the ^{14}C-glycocholate breath test is often used to demonstrate early deconjugation of bile acids by bacteria (Fig. 15.17B). The diagnosis is supported by finding a high fasting breath hydrogen. It is also important to demonstrate the cause of the overgrowth. This may be obvious from the history (such as a partial gastrectomy) or may require a small bowel enema (e.g. to show diverticular disease, systemic sclerosis or fistula formation).

Management

If feasible, the underlying cause is treated, e.g. surgical correction of adhesions, fistulae and blind loops. Noncorrectable upper small bowel abnormalities, such as multiple diverticula and systemic sclerosis, have to be treated medically with broad-spectrum or anaerobe-directed antibiotics. Tetracycline, ampicillin or metronidazole may be effective. There is a tendency for the problem to recur and, if one antibiotic is ineffective, another should be tried but there is little evidence that bacterial aspirate sensitivities help in the choice of antibiotics. Deficiencies, particularly of vitamin B_{12}, should be corrected. In severe cases, there must be careful attention to nutrition with the avoidance of dietary fats and their substitution with mid-chain triglycerides.

GIARDIASIS

Giardia lamblia is a protozoon which colonises the bowel, especially the upper small intestine causing diarrhoea and malabsorption; it is discussed in Chapter 11 (p. 282).

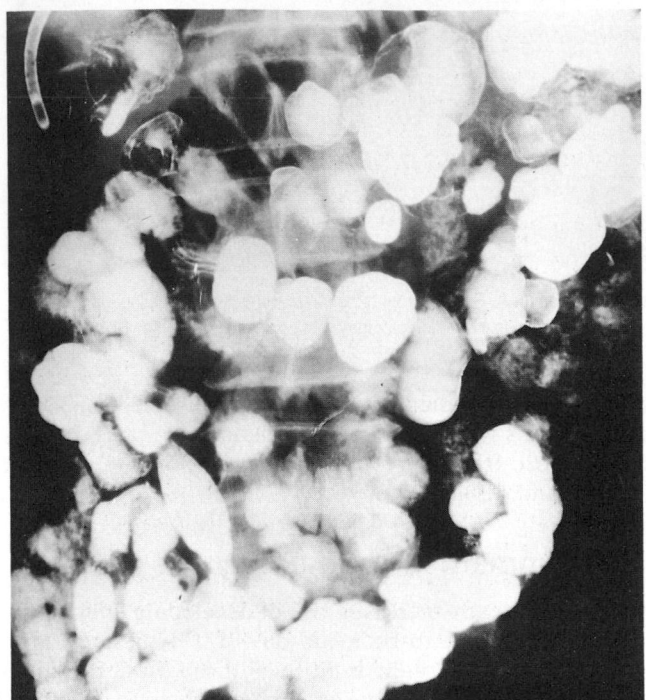

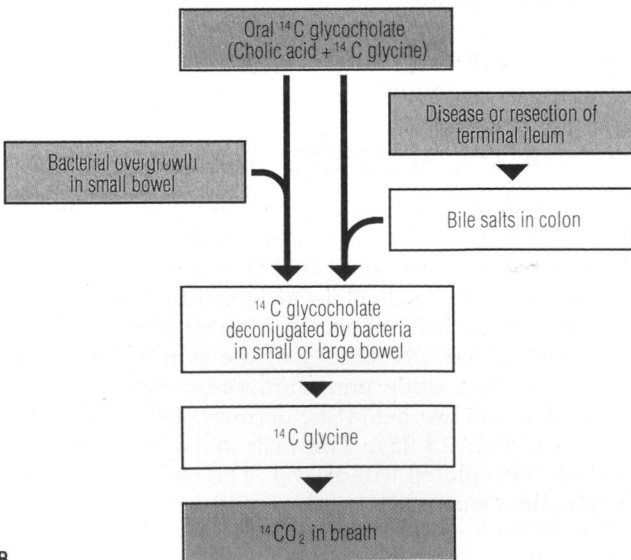

Fig. 15.17 Diagnostic findings in bacterial overgrowth. A. Small bowel enema showing multiple small bowel diverticula. **B.** In the normal ^{14}C glycocholate breath test, little $^{14}CO_2$ appears in the breath until 4–5 hours after ingestion. In the presence of small bowel bacterial overgrowth, there is early cleavage of glycine and thus an early peak of $^{14}CO_2$ at 1–2 hours.

TROPICAL SPRUE

Tropical sprue is a chronic malabsorption disorder which occurs in patients who live, or have lived, in the tropics (in particular, India, South-East Asia and the Caribbean). The aetiology is unknown, although viruses or toxin-forming coliform bacteria have been implicated in some patients. Tropical sprue results in intestinal partial villous atrophy.

Clinical features, investigation and management

Symptoms include diarrhoea, steatorrhoea, weight loss, abdominal distension, oral ulceration and also those of nutritional deficiency and hypoproteinaemia.

The diagnosis is made by demonstrating villous atrophy and malabsorption of more than one nutrient in a patient from an endemic area. If subtotal villous atrophy is present, coeliac disease must be considered.

Many patients are cured by a one-month course of oxytetracycline with folic acid and vitamin B_{12} supplements; any other deficiencies should be treated as necessary. The diarrhoea may be treated symptomatically with codeine phosphate or loperamide. There is a tendency to spontaneous remissions and relapses.

WHIPPLE'S DISEASE

Whipple's disease is a rare multisystem disease. The small intestine is characterised by large, foamy periodic acid Schiff (PAS)-positive macrophages containing glycoprotein within the lamina propria. The overlying villi are distorted and upper small bowel radiology shows thickened and oedematous mucosa. The patients are often iron or folate deficient. Whipple's disease is thought to be due to a bacterial infection, as rods are often seen in affected tissue; the precise organism is unknown.

Clinical features, investigation and management

The disease usually affects middle-aged men. Early symptoms are arthritis, fever, malaise, recurrent cough, pleuritic chest pain and lymphadenopathy. Intestinal symptoms such as diarrhoea, steatorrhoea, weight loss and abdominal pain occur 1–10 years later. Small bowel biopsy is diagnostic even before intestinal symptoms develop. Associated features are nail-clubbing, cutaneous pigmentation, cardiac complications (such as pericarditis, myocarditis and left-sided valvular lesions) and central nervous system complications, such as depression, dementia and fits.

Broad-spectrum antibiotics are rapidly effective in abolishing all the problems and are life-saving. It is generally suggested that intramuscular penicillin and strepto-mycin are used for two weeks and then replaced by tetracycline continued for one year. About 30% of patients subsequently relapse, and so long-term follow-up is recommended.

LYMPHANGIECTASIA

Primary lymphangiectasia is a rare idiopathic condition of children and young adults, associated with dilated lacteals in the villi due to hypoplasia of the lymphatics. Secondary lymphangiectasia may result from intra-abdominal malignancy or constrictive pericarditis.

Clinical features, investigation and management

The most common symptom is peripheral oedema secondary to hypoproteinaemia due to protein-losing enteropathy. Diarrhoea, steatorrhoea, abdominal pain, hypocalcaemia and growth retardation occur. Protein loss leads to immunodeficiency.

Diagnosis is by small bowel biopsy which shows dilated lymphatics throughout the villi. A small bowel enema shows large intestinal folds, mucosa nodularity and contrast flocculation.

The idiopathic variant should be treated with a low fat diet and possibly substitution of dietary fat by mid-chain triglycerides. Occasionally, only a small segment of bowel is involved and this can be excised. Pericardectomy may result in complete resolution of the syndrome if constrictive pericarditis is the problem.

ABETALIPOPROTEINAEMIA

Abetalipoproteinaemia is a rare disorder, inherited as an autosomal recessive and usually presenting in childhood. Plasma betalipoproteins are absent and plasma cholesterol, triglycerides and phospholipid are low. The defect appears to be a failure of synthesis of apoprotein B, with defective transport of triglyceride from the liver and gut. The red cells are spiked acanthocytes. The patients initially have mild diarrhoea and steatorrhoea but, by 20 years of age, most have developed progressive neurological deficits with peripheral neuropathy and cerebellar ataxia. A small bowel biopsy shows cytoplasmic fatty vacuolation of the enterocytes at the apex of the villi.

No treatment is known to affect the underlying problem but a low fat or medium chain triglyceride diet is usually given and deficiencies of fat-soluble vitamin deficiencies are corrected.

SYSTEMIC SCLEROSIS

Systemic sclerosis (p. 1028) may affect the small bowel causing poor motility, duodenal dilatation and a distended jejunum with prominent folds. Histology shows submucosal collagen and muscle atrophy. Bacterial overgrowth often occurs. Weight loss, nausea, abdominal distension, diarrhoea and steatorrhoea occur, and colonic involvement may result in constipation.

Treatment is of the nutritional deficiencies and bacterial overgrowth with antibiotics. No treatment influences the underlying gastrointestinal process.

RADIATION ENTERITIS

Radiation enteritis usually occurs in the small intestine of patients who have undergone abdominal and pelvic irradiation. In the early phases of treatment, there is cell necrosis and shortening of the villi; with increasing dose, polymorphs become prominent. Oedema, collagen formation and telangiectatic blood vessels develop as long-term sequelae.

During treatment, patients develop anorexia, nausea and diarrhoea; this usually settles when treatment stops. Chronic complications are unusual and may follow years later. They include diarrhoea, steatorrhoea, intestinal obstruction from stricture formation, intestinal ulceration with haemorrhage or perforation, bleeding from telangiectatic vessels, fistula formation or infarction.

Medical treatment of the chronic diarrhoea is unsatisfactory, but attention to diet, cholestyramine, corticosteroids and broad-spectrum antibiotics may help. Some patients require surgery for strictures but this can be hazardous.

OSMOTIC DIARRHOEA

The two major causes of osmotic diarrhoea are brush border enzyme deficiencies and purgative abuse.

Brush border enzyme deficiencies

Primary lactase deficiency is the commonest cause of osmotic diarrhoea and is an inherited deficiency of the brush border membrane enzyme, lactase. It develops in late childhood. Lactose is not split into its constituent monosaccharides, galactose and glucose, is not absorbed and becomes osmotically active.

Clinical features

Eating dairy products (which are rich in lactose) results in loose stools, abdominal distension, borborygmi, colic and increased rectal flatus. The distension and flatus are due to colonic bacterial digestion of lactose.

Most Negroes and Asians have primary lactase deficiency and may suffer diarrhoea, bloating and flatulence if they eat lactose. The incidence of primary alactasia in the Caucasian population in Europe and North America is up to 20% (about 6% in the UK). Secondary lactase deficiency may also occur as a result of small bowel diseases (such as coeliac disease and Crohn's disease) and during and after bowel infections.

Investigation

In many patients, especially where the symptoms occur following an acute infection, a response to a low lactose diet allows a clinical diagnosis to be made. If definitive diagnosis is necessary, lactase activity is measured in a small bowel biopsy specimen. Bacterial breakdown of unabsorbed lactose in the colon results in abnormally high hydrogen excretion in the breath, so that measurement of exhaled hydrogen is an index of lactase deficiency.

Management

Lactose in the diet is reduced until symptoms resolve. An underlying cause should be sought if symptoms persist. The majority of patients with secondary hypolactasia can resume lactose some weeks after treatment.

Sucrase-isomaltase deficiency is a rare enzyme deficiency which results in diarrhoea when sucrose is introduced into the diet in infancy. It responds to elimination of sucrose, and tolerance may improve later in life. Very rarely, the small intestinal glucose and galactose transport system itself is ineffective; this results in an infant with watery motions and glucose in the faeces. Treatment is by avoidance of glucose- and galactose-containing foods.

Purgative abuse

The laxatives magnesium sulphate, magnesium hydroxide, magnesium carbonate and lactulose act by osmosis. Magnesium salts may be used for bowel preparation for surgery and colonoscopy, while lactulose (a synthetic disaccharide) is used for mild constipation and portosystemic encephalopathy. Patients may secretly take these drugs in excess (see also p. 605) to produce watery diarroea of unknown cause, but a diagnosis can be made by finding high faecal magnesium levels for the magnesium salts, and a low faecal pH for lactulose.

SECRETORY DIARRHOEA

Under normal circumstances, there is a daily flux of about 8 litres of water and electrolytes across the small intestinal mucosa, but only about 1000 ml of this passes through the ileocaecal valve.

Secretory diarrhoea is due to absorption being exceeded by active secretion, leading to profuse watery diarrhoea, often more than 1 kg per 24 hours. In the Western World, secretory diarrhoea is usually due to a vasoactive intestinal polypeptide (VIP)-secreting tumour (p. 614) or laxative abuse, especially phenolphthalein (p. 605). The enterotoxin of *Vibrio cholerae* (cholera) is also an important cause. Oral dehydration solutions at up to 800 ml/hour are the mainstay of cholera treatment. Intestinal glucose and sodium absorption are interdependent and the solutions drive sodium-dependent glucose and water absorption (see also Ch. 11, p. 250). Secretory diarrhoea may also occur with the carcinoid syndrome associated with small intestinal primary tumours, medullary carcinoma of the thyroid, and gastrinomas. Unabsorbed bile acids and long chain fatty acids can cause colonic secretion and diarrhoea.

Investigation

The presence of secretory diarrhoea is suggested by persistence of diarrhoea during fasting and a stool osmolarity similar to plasma. Confirmation of excess secretion is best obtained by placing a triple lumen tube in the small intestine, and measuring the absorptive and secretory response to various physiological solutions over a defined segment. Normally, there is water and electrolyte absorption but, under these circumstances, the solutions are further diluted by active intestinal secretion of water and electrolytes.

DIARRHOEA DUE TO RAPID TRANSIT

Diarrhoea may be caused by the rapid transit of food and secretions through the small intestine. Causes include rapid gastric emptying, short bowel syndrome, enteroenteric or enterocolonic fistulae, thyrotoxicosis and the irritable bowel syndrome.

SHORT GUT

Diarrhoea and malabsorption may follow small intestinal resection. This is most commonly due to Crohn's disease, ischaemia due to superior mesenteric artery infarction or radiation damage. The greatest problems with water and electrolyte handling occur with loss of the duodenum or upper small intestine.

Some patients can be managed by regular small meals, and isotonic glucose and electrolyte solutions. If the patient continues to produce several litres of stool daily and to lose weight, long-term total parenteral nutrition must be considered.

LOWER SMALL BOWEL DISEASE

The terminal ileum is the primary site of absorption of vitamin B_{12} and bile acids; it is part of the enterohepatic circulation (Ch. 16).

The commonest cause of terminal ileal disease in the Western World is Crohn's disease, while in parts of Asia it is tuberculosis. Rare causes include tumours and radiation damage. All of these lesions may require surgical resection which unfortunately perpetuates the problems of malabsorption.

Clinical features

B_{12} deficiency due to ileal disease is unresponsive to intrinsic factor in the Schilling test (Ch. 24, p. 1055). If there is malabsorption of bile acids, the following complications may arise:

- *Diarrhoea.* Excess bile acids in the intestinal lumen reduce the colonic absorption of water and electrolytes, and may induce net secretion.
- *Depletion of the bile acid pool.* This can result in small intestinal fat malabsorption and an increase in the cholesterol:bile acid ratio in the bile. Bile supersaturated with cholesterol increases the incidence of gallstones.
- *Oxalate renal stones.* The increased intracolonic bile acid concentration results in increased absorption of oxalic acid; this is excreted by the kidneys and may result in oxalate renal stones.

Management

Treatment is firstly of the causative disease process. Vitamin B_{12} deficiency is treated with an intramuscular loading dose of 1 mg daily for five days: thereafter, 1 mg at three-month intervals is adequate. Cholestyramine is an anion exchange resin which can alleviate bile acid-induced diarrhoea by binding bile acids and reducing intracolonic free bile acid concentrations. Unfortunately, this often fails to cure the diarrhoea and results in further depletion of the bile acid pool, and hence a greater tendency to cholelithiasis. Gallstones should be treated surgically. Hyperoxaluria should be treated with a low oxalate diet which includes avoiding fruits such as strawberries; surgical treatment may be necessary for renal stones.

Table 15.24 Examples of drugs causing diarrhoea and malabsorption

Drug	Mechanism of action	Result
Cholestyramine	Binds bile acids	Steatorrhoea Gallstones Malabsorption of fat-soluble vitamins
Colchicine and cytotoxic drugs	Arrest enterocyte mitosis	Diarrhoea
Neomycin	Causes partial villous atrophy and enzyme inhibition	Steatorrhoea Iron, vitamin B_{12} and glucose malabsorption
Methyldopa	Causes partial villous atrophy	Steatorrhoea
Ferrous sulphate	Binds with tetracycline	Malabsorption of both drugs
Ethanol	Damage to enterocyte subcellular organelles	Folate deficiency and steatorrhoea

DRUG-INDUCED MALABSORPTION

Numerous drugs have been implicated (Table 15.24); the effects are all dose-related and reversible.

SMALL BOWEL ISCHAEMIA

Aetiology

Aetiological factors in small intestinal ischaemia are shown in Table 15.25; experimentally, venous occlusion can cause infarction but it is not known whether this is the case in man.

Clinical features and management

Small bowel ischaemia may present acutely, with gut infarction following occlusion of the coeliac and superior mesenteric arteries, or chronically, with postprandial pain and weight loss.

Acute ischaemia

Acute ischaemia presents with pain, diarrhoea, vomiting and an acute abdomen. The patient should be resusci-

Table 15.25 Aetiology of small bowel ischaemia

- Arterial atheroma
- Arterial thrombosis
- Arterial emboli (usually from the heart)
- Vasculitis due to collagen disorders
- External compression of arteries (e.g. tumours, aneurysms)
- ? Venous thrombosis

tated with fluids and treated with antibiotics and urgent laparotomy performed. At operation, an attempt is made to restore patency to embolised or thrombosed major arteries and all non-viable bowel is resected. The mortality is high and, if a large proportion of the upper jejunum and/or duodenum is removed, the patient has severe malabsorption, often with profuse diarrhoea. Such patients may require long-term total parenteral nutrition.

Chronic ischaemia

Chronic ischaemia is usually due to atheroma and, if undiagnosed, may progress to acute ischaemia. The patient is usually middle-aged or elderly and complains of colicky abdominal pain after eating ('intestinal angina'). This may be relieved by analgesics or vasodilating drugs. Weight loss follows, mainly due to a fear of eating, but malabsorption may also occur. Examination is relatively unhelpful. Investigation is by arteriography which shows a localised narrowing at the origin of at least two of the major arteries off the aorta. Reconstruction of stenoses can help some patients.

SMALL BOWEL TUMOURS

Despite its long length, the small intestine is the site of less than 1% of all malignant tumours and less than 5% of gastrointestinal neoplasms. Malignant tumours occur more frequently in the duodenum and jejunum, and benign lesions, such as leiomyomas and adenomas, in the jejunum. Small bowel malignancy is more common in patients with coeliac disease, Crohn's disease and Gardner's syndrome (p. 589). The commonest tumours are adenocarcinomas (50%), carcinoid tumours (30%), lymphomas (15%) and sarcomas (5%).

Adenocarcinomas

Aetiology and pathology

The tumours usually occur in the upper small bowel and are more common in patients with coeliac and Crohn's disease. They present as ulcerating obstructing neoplasms and metastasise to regional lymph nodes and the liver.

Clinical features and investigation

Patients usually present with abdominal pain, and intussusception may occur. Chronic blood loss is frequent and there may be melaena. The diagnosis can sometimes be made by small bowel enema and, occasionally, endoscopically (if in the duodenum) or by colonoscopy (if in the terminal ileum).

Management

Surgical excision is the treatment of choice but only 70% are resectable. The regional lymph nodes are resected where possible. Metastatic lesions respond poorly to cytotoxic chemotherapy.

Carcinoid tumours

Gut carcinoid tumours are rare; their behaviour is to some extent dependent on the part of the gut from which they are embryologically derived (Table 15.26). Histology shows sheets of neuroendocrine cells which are usually of low-grade malignancy. Immunocytochemistry shows positive silver staining for amines, and mid-gut tumours are often also positive for gut regulatory peptides such as neurotensin. Foregut tumours usually originate in the stomach and predominantly secrete histamine. Appendiceal carcinoid tumours are commonly found in appendicectomy specimens but do not metastasise or cause clinical problems. Terminal ileal carcinoids are those most likely to metastasise. They cause the *carcinoid syndrome* and predominantly secrete 5-hydroxytryptamine. Hind-gut tumours do not produce the syndrome and behave similarly to colonic adenocarcinomas.

Carcinoid syndrome

Aetiology

The carcinoid syndrome only occurs when the liver is bypassed and cannot metabolise tumour products. Symptoms thus arise when there are hepatic metastases which drain direct into the hepatic vein. Symptoms can also be seen in the absence of hepatic metastases with primary pulmonary, testicular and ovarian tumours whose venous drainage is directly into the systemic circulation.

Clinical features

The most characteristic symptom of the carcinoid syndrome is a flush, usually of the face and upper trunk. Provoking agents include stress (via noradrenaline), alcohol and food (possibly via gastrin). Other symptoms

Table 15.27 Biochemical pathway for the synthesis and degradation of 5-hydroxytryptamine

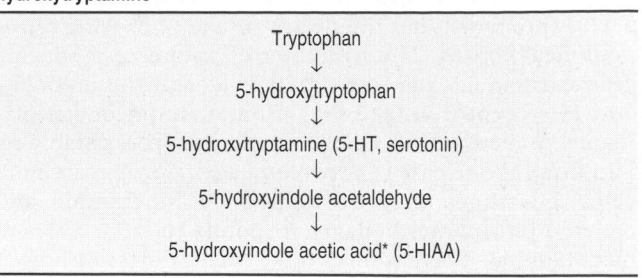

Tryptophan
↓
5-hydroxytryptophan
↓
5-hydroxytryptamine (5-HT, serotonin)
↓
5-hydroxyindole acetaldehyde
↓
5-hydroxyindole acetic acid* (5-HIAA)

* 24-hour urinary 5-HIAA levels are raised in mid-gut and foregut carcinoids.

include secretory diarrhoea, weight loss, wheezing, dyspnoea, pellagra and right hypochondrial pain. This is due to the marked hepatomegaly which is usually the main clinical sign. Fibrotic right heart valve signs (giving both stenosis and regurgitation) may be present.

Mid-gut carcinoid tumours produce large amounts of 5-hydroxytryptamine (5-HT, serotonin; see Table 15.27). This substance is thought to play a part in the pathogenesis of carcinoid syndrome symptoms such as flushing and diarrhoea. Foregut tumours may secrete histamine and 5-hydroxytryptophan, producing a pink, weal-like flush which may itch and migrate. Pellagra due to nicotinic acid deficiency (resulting from tryptophan consumption by the tumour) may occur. The cause of the right-sided cardiac fibrosis is unknown, but serotonin has been suggested as a possibility.

Investigation

Functioning carcinoid tumours can be diagnosed by demonstrating raised 24-hour urinary 5-HIAA levels or by whole blood 5-HT. If the diagnosis is confirmed by urine 5-HIAA, but no liver metastases are demonstrable, a bronchial carcinoid should be suspected.

Management

Surgical removal of primary tumours may be helpful, but is rarely so in patients with terminal ileal tumours, where the primaries are usually small and multiple. Symptoms

Table 15.26 Clinical features of gut carcinoids according to embryological origin

Embryological origin	Usual primary site	Principal active substance	Diagnosis	Treatment
Foregut	Stomach	Histamine 5-hydroxytryptophan	Normal or raised urinary 5-HIAA	Surgery H$_1$- and H$_2$-receptor antagonists
Mid-gut	Terminal ileum	5-hydroxytryptamine	Raised urinary 5-HIAA	Surgery Cyproheptadine, methysergide and somatostatin Embolisation of hepatic metastases
Hind-gut	Colon and rectum	None	Histology	Surgery only

of the carcinoid syndrome may be controlled by 5-HT antagonists such as cyproheptadine. Methysergide, also a 5-HT antagonist, has the disadvantage of causing retroperitoneal fibrosis. The symptoms of histamine-producing gastric carcinoids can be blocked by a combination of H_1- and H_2-receptor antagonists. Somatostatin or its analogues prevents flushing and diarrhoea, presumably by inhibiting the release of provoking agents from carcinoid cells. Diarrhoea may be helped by loperamide and codeine phosphate. Pellagra responds to large doses of nicotinamide. There is no definite role for cytotoxic drugs or radiotherapy, but hepatic arterial catheterisation and embolisation or surgical tumour debulking may help. In a carcinoid crisis, when the flushing is so severe that arterial hypotension develops, corticosteroids and plasma volume expansion may be necessary.

Lymphomas

Lymphomas are the commonest gut tumours in children and a rare small bowel tumour in adults.

Aetiology

In the West, most cases of primary lymphoma arise without any predisposing cause, but coeliac disease may be complicated by a diffuse ulcerating lymphoma. In the Middle East, an immune proliferative disease of the small intestine, of unknown aetiology, frequently develops into a non-Hodgkin's lymphoma of B lymphocytes, which secretes free α-heavy chains (Mediterranean lymphoma).

Most cases in the West are of non-Hodgkin's lymphoma and are B cell in origin. The histology usually shows diffuse infiltration of the bowel wall; nodular forms are rare. The lower small bowel is involved most frequently. The disease spreads early to involve local nodes but distant dissemination is late. Extraintestinal lymphoma can spread to involve the gut in the late stages of the disease.

Clinical features

Presentation is often with subacute intestinal obstruction. Bleeding may occur and is usually chronic. Perforation is not unusual. When extensive, the disease may present as a fever of unknown origin.

Management

The main treatment of primary Western lymphoma is surgical resection. Further treatment is not required if there is no evidence of spread, but involvement of nodes or distant spread are indications for intensive combination chemotherapy. Local recurrences may respond to radiotherapy. In childhood, the risk of CNS involvement is small, in contrast to other childhood lymphomas.

The prognosis of localised resected gut lymphoma is good, with over 60% of patients alive at five years. It is not yet clear what impact modern chemotherapy will have on survival in more advanced cases. Malignant lymphoma complicating coeliac disease has a poor prognosis.

COLORECTAL DISEASE

The colon and rectum act to reduce up to 1500 ml of fluid material per day passing through the ileocaecal valve to a formed stool of 50–200 g. Important symptoms of colorectal disease are constipation, diarrhoea, blood per rectum, tenesmus, colicky abdominal pain and the symptoms of iron deficiency anaemia. Important signs are abdominal masses and abnormalities on rectal examination. Radiologically, the rectum and colon can be visualised by the plain abdominal X-ray and double contrast barium enema. Endoscopically, the rigid sigmoidoscope, flexible fibre-optic sigmoidoscope and flexible fibre-optic colonoscope are used to view the mucosa directly and to take biopsies.

CONSTIPATION

The normal person opens his or her bowels with a frequency of from two to three times a day to once every two to three days. The normal daily stool weight in the West is 50–200 g, but 500 g is more usual in countries where a much higher fibre intake is consumed. Constipation can be considered to be present when a patient defaecates twice a week or less. Constipation is a common complaint in the Western World, and vast quantities of laxatives are purchased annually to treat the symptom.

Aetiology and diagnosis

Some of the many causes of constipation are listed in Table 15.28. Simple constipation is diagnosis of exclusion where there is no cause other than a low fibre diet. It is common in women and, in young women in good health on a low fibre diet, it is usually not necessary to search further. Constipation is common in old age, when impaired colonic muscle function may contribute to the problem. Anorectal problems are associated with constipation because the patients delay defaecating to avoid pain. Inflammatory proctitis may result in faecal loading proximal to the inflamed mucosa (best seen on plain abdominal X-ray); the patient usually complains of passing small amounts of faeces frequently. Hypothyroidism, hypopituitarism and hypercalcaemia may have constipation as one of their earliest features. A careful drug history should be

Table 15.28 Causes of constipation

Simple constipation	Drugs
	Anticholinergics
Colonic obstruction	Antidepressants
Tumours	Anticonvulsants
Encarceration in hernias	Antacids (aluminium and calcium salts)
Volvulus	Diuretics
	Opiate analgesics
	Iron
Abnormal muscle function	
Old age	**Metabolic and endocrine problems**
Irritable bowel syndrome	Diabetes
Diverticular disease	Hypothyroidism
Crohn's and ulcerative colitis	Hypercalcaemia
Ischaemic colitis	Pregnancy
Systemic sclerosis	Uraemia
Hirschsprung's disease	Fever
	Hypokalaemia
Anorectal problems	Porphyria
Ulcerative proctitis	Lead poisoning
Anal fissure	
Thrombosed haemorrhoid	**Proximal gastrointestinal disease**
	Gastric carcinoma
Neuro-psychiatric disorders	
Depression	
Spinal cord injury	
Cauda equina lesions	
Multiple sclerosis	
Parkinson's disease	
Cerebral tumours	
Cerebrovascular accidents	
Anorexia nervosa	

Table 15.29 Dietary fibre content of foods

Fibre content	g fibre/100 g food
High (more than 10 g/100 g food)	
Bran	44.0
Partially purified bran	26.7
Haricot and kidney beans	25.0
Dried apricots	24.0
Desiccated coconut	23.5
Almonds	14.3
Potato crisps	11.9
Lentils	11.7
Spaghetti, macaroni, lasagne	10.0
Medium (5–10 g/100 g food)	
Wholemeal bread	8.5
Peas	7.8
Peanuts	7.6
Raspberries	7.4
Muesli	7.4
Sultanas	7.0
Chestnuts	6.8
Spinach	6.0
Low (below 5 g/100 g food)	
Cornflakes	3.0
White bread	2.7
Boiled potato	2.4
White rice	2.4
Cauliflower	1.8
Lettuce	1.5
Jam	1.1
Grapes	0.9

taken. Peripheral and central nervous system diseases (apart from Hirschsprung's, which usually presents in early childhood) commonly have obvious manifestations before constipation develops. Constipation may be the presenting symptom of depression.

Management

Wherever possible, the underlying cause of constipation is treated. In simple constipation and where a low residue diet is being consumed, a high fibre diet should be recommended. Diet sheets and the advice of a dietician can be useful (Table 15.29). Bran is the best source of fibre as it absorbs a large amount of water and allows the passage of larger amounts of soft stool. Beans, dried fruits, some nuts and pasta also contain large amounts of fibre, and fruit and vegetables contain non-absorbable polysaccharides, such as cellulose and pectins, which are useful. Pharmacological preparations of agents such as methylcellulose, isphaghula husk, sterculia and, possibly, guar are helpful if patients cannot remedy the situation by diet alone. The osmotically active disaccharide lactulose can be used as a mild laxative. If possible, the stimulant laxatives which increase intestinal motility (e.g. senna, cascara, castor oil, bisacodyl, docusate sodium and

danthron) should be avoided, as it is thought they can cause ganglion degeneration and an acquired megacolon, thus perpetuating constipation. Stimulant laxatives also tend to cause abdominal colic and hypokalaemia. Faecal softeners (e.g. liquid paraffin and dioctyl sodium sulphosuccinate) have a short-term role in softening stool in the presence of anal disease. Cisapride is a prokinetic agent which shortens intestinal transit time and helps some patients.

NEUROPATHIC COLON

Neuropathic colon occurs as a result of a loss of Auerbach's and Meissner's plexuses along with the associated intrinsic neurones. This results in failure of colonic motility and constipation.

Hirschsprung's disease

The most common cause of neuropathic colon is Hirschsprung's disease, which usually presents in early childhood but has been reported in patients up to the age of 70. Constipation and abdominal distension are the usual symptoms. Barium enema shows a narrow aganglionic segment with grossly dilated proximal colon. The diagnosis can be confirmed by demonstrating lack of ganglia and neurones and high acetylcholinesterase activities in rectal biopsies. Treatment is by surgical resection.

Chagas' disease

Chagas' disease is endemic in South America and is due to infection with the protozoon *Trypanosoma cruzi* (p. 297). Chronic myocarditis, megaoesophagus and megacolon are late symptoms of the disease. Destruction of the ganglia produces a dilated and atonic colon. Treatment is with bulking agents and laxatives but, occasionally, panproctocolectomy and ileostomy may be necessary.

Other causes

Other cases of ganglionic destruction sometimes occur where the aetiology is uncertain. The possible role of stimulant laxatives, senna in particular, is controversial. Treatment is usually medical as for Chagas' disease but, on rare occasions, surgical resection may become necessary.

BENIGN TUMOURS OF THE LARGE BOWEL

Large bowel polyps

Some polyps may progress to carcinomas, and early diagnosis and removal therefore has the potential to prevent colonic carcinoma. Colonoscopes allow the passage of wire snares which can be pulled tight around the stalk of polyps; a diathermy current can then be passed through the polyp enabling its removal. Many laparotomies have been avoided by the use of this technique.

Classification

A classification of colonic polyps is shown in Table 15.30. Colonic carcinoid tumours are relatively rare and do not produce biologically active amines or peptides. Metaplastic polyps are usually small (<1 cm), whereas adenomas may grow to several centimetres in diameter. Small adenomatous and metaplastic polyps cannot be differentiated visually and, as subsequent management is different, all polyps must be assessed histologically. Inflammatory polyps are islands of regenerating mucosa which occur with severe ulcerative or Crohn's colitis. Hamartomas are heaped-up areas of normal tissue arranged in a disorganised way; they are commonest in children but may be seen in patients of any age. *Peutz-Jegher's syndrome* is a dominantly inherited disease associated with pigmentation of the skin and mucous membranes, and hamartomatous polyps in the stomach and small and large intestines. The polyps only rarely undergo malignant change.

Table 15.30 Histological classification of colonic polyps

Potentially malignant	No malignant potential
Adenomas	Metaplastic (hyperplastic polyps)
Tubular	
Villous	Connective tissue polyps
Tubulovillous	Lipomas
May be single or multiple	Fibromas
(e.g. Gardner's syndrome)	Leiomyomas
Carcinoid	
	Inflammatory
	Ulcerative colitis
	Crohn's disease
	Hamartomas
	Peutz-Jegher's
	Juvenile

Clinical features and investigation

Many polyps are asymptomatic. When symptoms do occur, the most common is the passage of blood per rectum; altered bowel habit, colicky abdominal pain and, rarely, anorexia and weight loss may also be seen. For non-malignant polyps, the only physical signs are anaemia due to blood loss or mucocutaneous pigmentation (in Peutz-Jegher's syndrome).

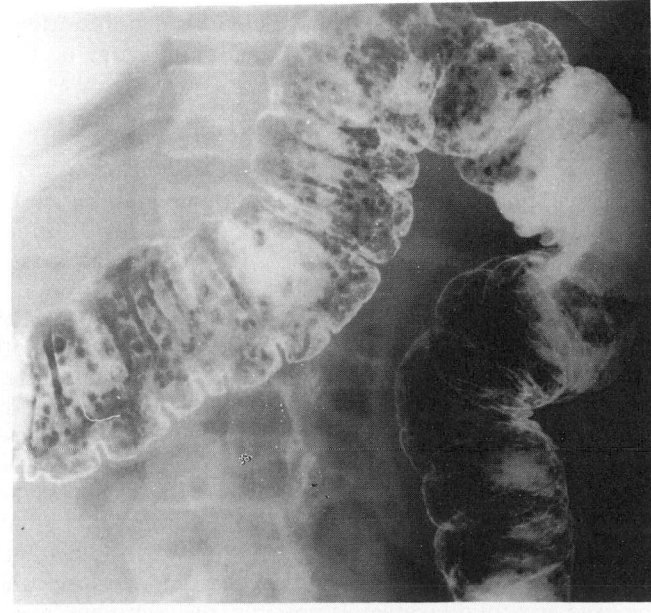

Fig. 15.18 Demonstration of colonic polyps. Double-contrast barium enema showing many small colonic polyps.

A double-contrast barium enema shows most polyps (Fig. 15.18). Colonoscopy is performed when the barium enema is equivocal and is also essential for biopsy and treatment. If potentially or frankly malignant polyps are removed, long-term colonoscopic follow-up is required.

Multiple polyposis coli

Familial adenomatous polyposis is a dominantly inherited condition where affected individuals develop multiple (usually more than 100) adenomatous colonic polyps. A variant of this condition, associated with epidermoid cysts and osteomas, is known as *Gardner's syndrome*. Most patients develop carcinomatous change in their polyps before the age of 40. Panproctocolectomy with ileostomy formation, or ileoanal anastomosis with a pelvic ileal pouch, is therefore recommended in affected individuals in their late teens. Family screening for affected siblings is essential. Some of the patients also develop adenomas of their small intestine and stomach and these may rarely become malignant.

CARCINOMA OF THE LARGE BOWEL

Colorectal carcinoma is primarily a disease of Western Europe, Australia and North America. In England and Wales, it accounts for approximately 17 000 deaths annually, and is thus second only to carcinoma of the bronchus as a cause of death from malignant disease. Carcinoma of the colon affects the sexes equally (Fig. 15.19) but carcinoma of the rectum has a higher incidence in men.

Aetiology

The aetiology is unknown although clearly there are factors associated with a Western lifestyle. For example, the incidence is low in Japan but higher in Japanese who have moved to the USA. Diet has been implicated in the aetiology with suggestions that high animal fat and low fibre intake are important. Altered colonic bacterial flora and changes in bile acid secretion may be important in pathogenesis. Genetic factors are important in familial polyposis and Gardner's syndrome, both of which are inherited as autosomal dominant traits. Adenomatous polyps and ulcerative and Crohn's colitis are well established precursors; the familial adenomatosis polyp gene is now known to reside on chromosome 5.

Pathology

The pathology is a malignant epithelial tumour of the rectum or colon. Macroscopically, there are three main appearances: polypoid, ulcerative and annular lesions. The primary site is most commonly the rectum, followed by the sigmoid colon and the right side of the colon. These tumours then spread outwards through the wall of the bowel and invade local tissues, lymphatics and the blood vessels. Staging of the tumour by Dukes' classification is important in predicting prognosis (Fig. 15.20). Microscopically, the tumour is nearly always an adenocarcinoma.

Clinical features

Many tumours are initially asymptomatic or their symptoms (rectal blood loss, constipation) are misinterpreted

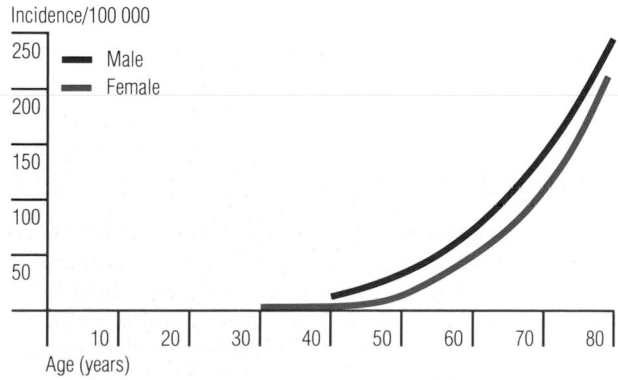

Fig. 15.19 Age-specific incidence of carcinoma of the large bowel in the Western World.

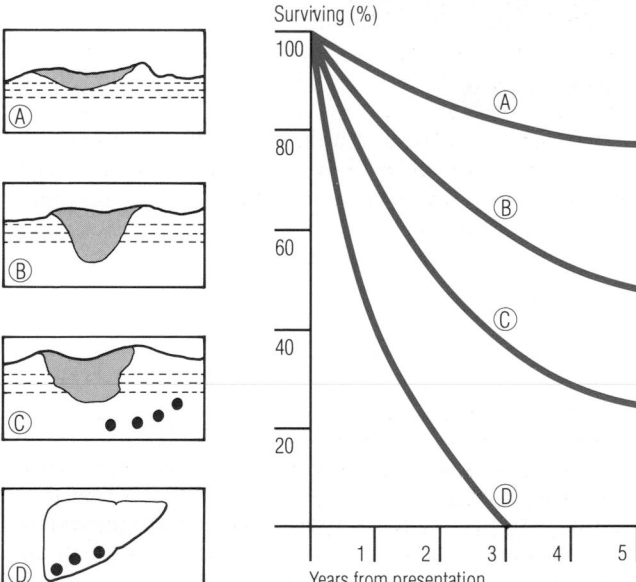

Fig. 15.20 Dukes' staging of carcinoma of the colon. (A) Tumour involves mucosa and submucosa only, good prognosis. (B) Tumour has penetrated muscle, moderate prognosis. (C) Tumour has spread to lymph nodes, poor prognosis. (D) Distant metastases are present. The corresponding five-year survival rates are also shown.

by the patient, resulting in a delay in diagnosis. The change in bowel habit may be constipation, diarrhoea or one alternating with the other. Colicky abdominal pain is usually associated with colonic obstruction, whilst a constant pain implies local invasion. Tenesmus suggests a rectal carcinoma, whilst anal pain suggests local invasion down towards the anus. Air and faeces being passed via the urethra or the vagina imply local invasion anteriorly from the rectum with fistula formation; posterior invasion may result in sacral pain.

Tumour bleeding may cause anaemia. Liver metastases may give rise to hepatomegaly, with jaundice as a late sign. Lymphatic spread is usually to para-aortic nodes and may cause extrahepatic biliary obstruction. Ascites may occur due to peritoneal carcinomatosis. The tumour may be palpable and, if it is obstructing the bowel lumen, there will be proximal faecal loading. Rectal examination and sigmoidoscopy are essential as part of the initial assessment. The fibre-optic sigmoidoscope can visualise the whole of the left side of the colon. Patients may present with large bowel obstruction or perforation in which case urgent surgery is required.

Investigation

If colorectal carcinoma is suspected, a double contrast barium enema is carried out. However, non-malignant lesions, particularly those due to inflammatory disease, can mimic tumour. In doubtful cases, colonoscopy is essential. Investigations are necessary to determine the extent of spread of the tumour.

Management

A laparotomy is indicated unless a carcinoma is localised within a resectable polyp. For right-sided tumours, a right hemicolectomy is performed, and a left hemicolectomy for left-sided tumours. Very low rectal tumours are usually treated with abdominoperineal resection of the tumour and rectum. There is some interest in treating very small rectal tumours by local diathermy or laser techniques. These techniques may also be used palliatively in advanced inoperable lesions causing obstruction or bleeding. For operable lesions, the role of pre- or postoperative radiotherapy is still being assessed. There is now evidence that adjuvant chemotherapy postoperatively improves the prognosis in patients with Duke's B or more advanced tumours. Embolisation of hepatic metastases can be helpful for pain, as can external beam irradiation.

The prognosis depends on the extent of spread at the time of surgery. The overall five-year survival rate in the UK is approximately 25% (80% for Dukes' stage A, 60% for stage B and 20% for stage C). Most patients with Dukes' stage D die within a year. Early diagnosis is therefore critical.

OTHER MALIGNANT COLORECTAL TUMOURS

Malignant colorectal tumours other than adenocarcinomas form less than 5% of primary malignant colorectal neoplasms. They behave in a similar way to adenocarcinomas, and include carcinoids, lymphomas, leiomyosarcomas, fibrosarcomas and melanomas. Squamous carcinoma of the anus may also invade the rectum and be clinically indistinguishable from a rectal adenocarcinoma.

DIVERTICULAR DISEASE (DIVERTICULOSIS)
Incidence and aetiology

Colonic diverticula are herniations of mucosa and submucosa through the wall of the large bowel, usually at the point where arteries pass through the submucosa. The most common site is the sigmoid colon, but colonic diverticula may occur throughout the large bowel and can be very numerous. They are rare before the age of 30 but occur in about 50% of people by the age of 70. They are uncommon in the Middle and Far East and in Africa.

Diverticula occur because of a weakness in the bowel wall and increased intracolonic pressure. The former is associated with an age-related reduction in strength of colonic connective tissue. The latter is thought to be due to reduced colonic contents resulting from a low fibre intake.

Clinical features

Uncomplicated diverticulosis may be asymptomatic or be associated with colonic symptoms similar to those of irritable bowel syndrome (p. 602). Symptoms may arise due to the complications of diverticular disease, the most important of which is an inflammatory mass (diverticulitis). This presents with abdominal pain, tenderness and fever and sometimes as an emergency with ileus, septicaemic shock, pericolic abscess or perforation. Diverticulitis can result in stricture formation. In diverticular disease, there may be profuse colonic bleeding or a chronic iron deficiency anaemia. The differential diagnosis will then include other causes of chronic blood loss, such as a carcinoma.

Investigation

Anaemia suggests blood loss, and a raised white cell count and ESR suggest inflammation. If patients are acutely unwell, a plain abdominal X-ray may show subdiaphragmatic gas due to perforation. When the problem is not acute, a double contrast barium enema is useful to show the extent of the diverticula (Fig. 15.21). If the patient is persistently unwell with a pyrexia, ultrasound should be performed to detect an abscess following a

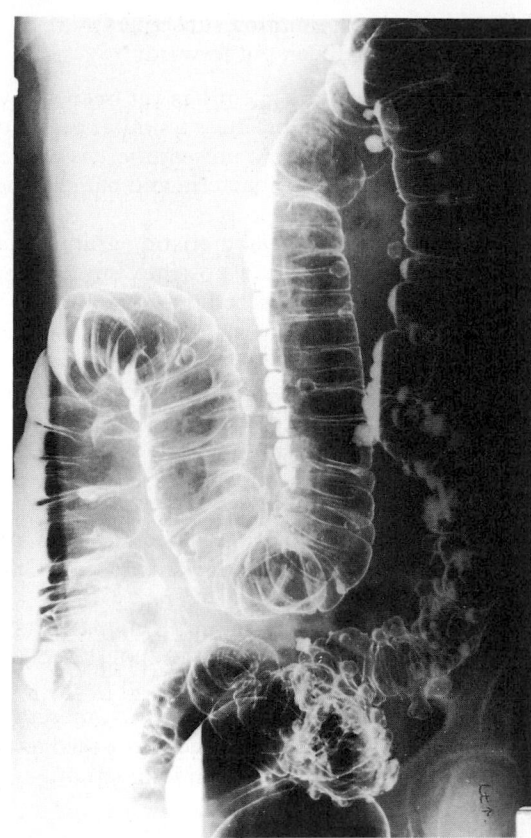

Fig. 15.21 Double contrast barium enema showing widespread diverticula, worst in the visible descending and sigmoid colon.

localised perforation. A difficult diagnostic problem is the presence of a carcinoma in a segment of colon affected by diverticular disease. If the barium enema is difficult to interpret, colonoscopy is indicated.

Management

There is no specific treatment for uncomplicated diverticular disease. A high fibre diet may prevent further diverticula developing. The patient should be reassured that complications are unlikely to develop. Antispasmodic drugs such as mebeverine may help some patients with colicky pains. Broad-spectrum antibiotics are indicated for diverticulitis.

Surgery is indicated for severe haemorrhage, local abscess, perforation and stricture causing obstruction.

PNEUMATOSIS COLI

Pneumatosis coli is a rare syndrome where cysts of gas up to 2 cm in diameter form in the submucosal and subserosal surfaces of the colon (and occasionally the small intestine). It can occur as a result of a peptic ulcer. In some patients there may be no evidence of a mucosal break, and most have chronic obstructive airways disease.

Most patients are asymptomatic, but symptoms can include bloody diarrhoea, lower abdominal pain and increased rectal flatus. The cysts may be palpable rectally and sigmoidoscopy usually shows them as multiple blue swellings. Biopsy causes deflation, and the biopsy specimen often floats on the surface of the formol saline fixative. Plain abdominal X-ray shows multiple translucent cysts along the course of the colon and may be used to follow progress.

Management

Treatment is symptomatic, but breathing high concentrations of oxygen accelerates resorption of the cysts. This is usually effective within five days but there is a tendency to relapse.

PRURITUS ANI

Itching around the anus is a common symptom and can have a number of causes (see Table 25.30, p. 1163). A careful history to identify an aetiological factor is followed by anal inspection, rectal examination and, if necessary, proctoscopy or sigmoidoscopy. In the UK, many patients use proprietary ointments and creams for their 'piles' and these treatments commonly produce contact dermatitis and pruritus. Unless there is a thrombosed pile or hygiene is poor, pruritus rarely complicates haemorrhoids.

Investigation of infections requires the laboratory examination of anal smears and, sometimes, faeces for threadworms and infections such as candida. Tight-fitting clothing and obesity cause local warmth and moisture, and predispose to skin infection and inflammation. In some patients, no cause can be identified; some of these have an obsessive and neurotic attitude which may be the primary problem.

Management

Treatment is directed at the underlying cause. The patient is reassured and encouraged to take a high fibre diet to avoid constipation. The anus is kept clean by washing twice daily without use of strong soaps, ointments, etc. If the problem is persistent and there is no obvious treatable cause, local 1% hydrocortisone and oral antihistamines may help.

INFLAMMATORY BOWEL DISEASE

Inflammatory bowel disease can be defined as chronic inflammatory disease of the gut of uncertain aetiology. It is divided into two types:

- *Crohn's disease,* which affects the gut from mouth to anus and is characterised pathologically by non-caseating giant cell granulomata
- *ulcerative colitis,* which affects only the large bowel.

In Crohn's disease, small aphthoid ulcers, larger ulcers and strictures are seen macroscopically. Histology shows the whole bowel wall to be infiltrated by lymphocytes and plasma cells. In contrast, ulcerative colitis (UC) is primarily a superficial mucosal inflammation. In both diseases, the large bowel may initially be the only site of involvement, and differentiation of the two is then of less importance, as the presentation, complications and management of the two types of colitis are very similar. It is possible that the two diseases are different responses to the same aetiological agent.

CROHN'S DISEASE

Crohn's disease is a granulomatous disease most commonly affecting the terminal ileum and right side of the colon. It is named after Dr Burrill Crohn of New York, who described 52 cases in 1932.

Crohn's disease is common in the Western World but rare in underdeveloped countries. The annual incidence of new cases appears to be rising in all countries studied (England, Wales, Scotland, Scandinavia and North America) and is currently 3–6 per 100 000 population (Fig. 15.22). It occurs equally in the sexes. The initial presentation can be at any age but is most common in early adult life.

Aetiology

The aetiology is unknown but evidence suggests that the cause is largely environmental. For example, when a population migrates from areas of low to high incidence, the incidence in that population subsequently rises. The following theories have been put forward:

- *Infection.* No infectious agent has yet been shown to transmit the disease or produce a similar granulomatous reaction in animals. At present there is interest in the possible role of mycobacteria and campylobacter species.
- *Immunological.* The characteristic granuloma of Crohn's disease suggests a possible immunological origin. Both food and bacterial antigens have been implicated, but there is no clear evidence for either. As with other inflammatory bowel diseases, minor, non-specific, immunological changes have been reported.
- *Dietary.* A high intake of refined sugars and a low intake of fibre have been suggested as aetiological factors, but the evidence that they are primary factors is weak.
- *Genetic.* There is a higher incidence of both Crohn's disease and UC in relatives of patients with Crohn's disease.
- *Smoking.* In direct contrast to UC, patients with Crohn's disease are more likely to be cigarette smokers than appropriate controls.
- *Others.* Oral contraceptives, detergents, mercury and psychological trauma have all been proposed as aetiological agents, but with little firm foundation.

Pathology

At laparotomy, Crohn's disease is seen as thickened bowel with associated enlarged lymph nodes. Microscopically, the inflammation is transmural, in contrast to ulcerative colitis where only the mucosa is usually involved. The other hallmark of Crohn's is the microscopic finding of non-caseating granulomas. As a result of transmural inflammation, there may be local abscesses or fistulae between two pieces of bowel (entero-entero or entero-colonic) or between the bowel and the skin (entero-cutaneous), usually in the anterior abdominal wall or around the anus. Fistulae may also form between the bowel and bladder or vagina.

Clinical features

The commonest initial presentation is with terminal ileal disease, often with coexistent oral and anal involvement. Less common initial presentations are acute right iliac fossa pain simulating acute appendicitis and acute colitis identical to UC.

General symptoms

When the disease is active the majority of patients have a mild fever and general malaise. Loss of appetite and

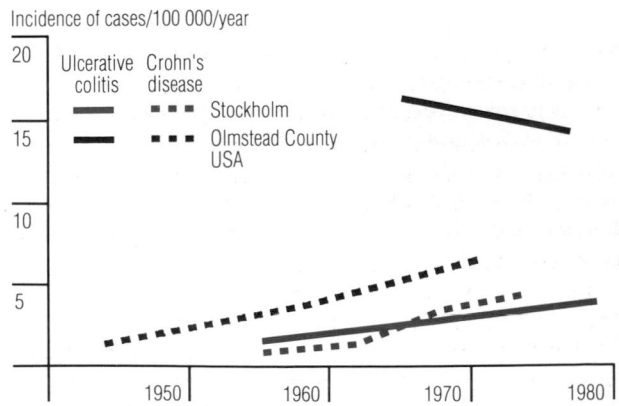

Fig. 15.22 Incidence of ulcerative colitis and Crohn's disease in two centres in Sweden and the USA.

malabsorption contribute to weight loss. In prepubertal and pubertal children, there may be no history of diarrhoea or abdominal pain. Children usually present with non-specific symptoms: failure to thrive, decreased growth velocity, delayed puberty and symptoms of anaemia.

Gastrointestinal symptoms

The gastrointestinal symptoms depend primarily on the site of disease. As a result of stricture formation, many patients with ileal disease complain of colicky abdominal pain, usually in the right iliac fossa. Diarrhoea, usually modest and containing excess fat, is usual. Disease in the right side of colon produces similar symptoms, although colonic disease alone does not cause steatorrhoea. It is often combined with ileal disease. Left-sided colonic disease results in diarrhoea without steatorrhoea but with blood per rectum.

Urinary frequency and dysuria may result from inflamed bowel adjacent to the urinary tract (especially the right ureter and bladder). Pneumaturia (air in the urine), and faeces via the urethra or vagina indicate a fistula from bowel to the genito-urinary tract.

Complications due to nutritional deficiency

The complications of nutritional deficiency may cause symptoms. Anaemia may be due to blood loss or reduced absorption of iron, folate and vitamin B_{12}. Oedema secondary to hypoproteinaemia is a consequence of both protein loss into the lumen of the gut (protein-losing enteropathy) and reduced dietary intake. Gallstones are due to terminal ileal bile acid malabsorption which results in cholesterol-supersaturated bile and causes cholesterol gallstones. Vitamin D and calcium malabsorption can result in hypocalcaemia (manifest as tetany) or, when long-standing, pseudofractures (Looser's zones) or fractures due to osteomalacia (p. 727). Night blindness and spontaneous bleeding may rarely occur due to vitamin A and K malabsorption. Angular cheilitis, glossitis and even scurvy can result from vitamin B and C deficiency. Hypokalaemia results in malaise and muscle weakness and hypomagnesaemia can cause tetany. Zinc deficiency can cause a rash similar to that seen in zinc-deficient children with acrodermatitis enteropathica.

Non-intestinal manifestations

Both Crohn's disease and UC may be associated with non-intestinal manifestations (Table 15.31). Acute large joint arthritis seen commonly affects the knees and ankles. Erythema nodosum and pyoderma gangrenosum usually affect the limbs, particularly the legs (p. 1142). If urticaria and erythema multiforme are seen, they should

Table 15.31 Non-intestinal manifestations of inflammatory bowel disease

Affected part	Manifestation
Reflecting acute illness	
Joints	Acute large joint arthritis
Skin	Pyoderma gangrenosum
	Erythema nodosum
	Vasculitis
Eyes	Conjunctivitis
	Episcleritis
	Uveitis
Venous thromboembolism	
Not reflecting acute illness	
Joints	Sacro-iliitis
	Ankylosing spondylitis
Liver	Fatty change
	Pericholangitis
	Primary sclerosing cholangitis
	Carcinoma of bile duct (cholangiocarcinoma)
	Autoimmune chronic active hepatitis

be assumed initially to be due to sulphasalazine. If there are ophthalmic symptoms, an assessment with a slit lamp is needed to exclude uveitis. Sacro-iliitis occurs in up to 10% of patients. The association with ankylosing spondylitis is rare. Abnormal liver function tests occur in about 10% of patients with colitis and are usually asymptomatic. The commonest lesions are pericholangitis and fatty infiltration. Primary sclerosing cholangitis (p. 635) is the most common clinically significant problem. Cholangiocarcinoma and autoimmune chronic active hepatitis are rare. Cholesterol gallstones, secondary to bile acid malabsorption, are common in patients with terminal ileitis or resection. Acute colitis is associated with an increased risk of venous thromboembolism.

Signs

Physical examination of a patient with Crohn's disease should start with a search for nail changes (including clubbing, leuconychia and koilonychia), anaemia, pyrexia, tachycardia and mouth ulcers. In the abdomen, there may be operation scars, evidence of fistulae and signs of intestinal obstruction with visible peristalsis. Palpation may reveal a mass, most commonly in the right iliac fossa, due to disease in the terminal ileum and the right side of the colon. Auscultation may suggest intestinal obstruction. Perianal inspection, sigmoidoscopy and rectal biopsy are essential. Sigmoidoscopy may show ulceration, a granular inflamed mucosa, spontaneous bleeding and increased mucus formation. Even in the absence of obvious inflammatory changes, the rectal biopsy may demonstrate diagnostic granulomas.

Summary 7 Clinical presentation of Crohn's disease

General
Fever
Malaise
Weight loss
Amenorrhoea
In children: failure to thrive, growth
retardation, delayed puberty

Terminal ileal disease
Abdominal pain
Diarrhoea (with or without steatorrhoea)
Right iliac fossa tenderness or mass
Signs of small intestinal obstruction

Colonic disease
Abdominal pain
Diarrhoea
Blood and mucus per rectum
Tenesmus
Abdominal tenderness

Anal disease
Skin tags, fissures and abscesses
Incontinence
Fistulae between anal canal and skin

Mouth
Cobblestone mucosa
Aphthous ulcers
Glossitis
Stomatitis

Fistula formation
Entero-enteric or entero-cutaneous
Urinary frequency, dysuria,
haematuria and pneumaturia
Faeces per vaginam and per
urethram

*Complications due to nutritional
deficiencies*
Anaemia
Oedema due to hypoproteinaemia
Gallstones
Tetany
Osteomalacia
Vitamins A and K deficiency
Water-soluble vitamin deficiency
Ion deficiencies (potassium,
magnesium and zinc)

Investigation

The diagnosis is confirmed by demonstrating the characteristic granulomatous histology, often by rectal biopsy. In the presence of active disease, the haemoglobin is usually low and the neutrophil count and acute phase reactants are raised. The serum albumin is low if there is widespread disease. Stool culture and microscopy should be performed; infections, particularly *Yersinia* (p. 600) and *Campylobacter* (p. 269) may mimic Crohn's disease.

A plain abdominal X-ray will determine if there is colonic dilatation. A chest X-ray may reveal tuberculosis, which may present with ileal disease similar to Crohn's disease. A small bowel enema or meal shows involvement of the small bowel, which is characterised by stricture formation, rose-thorn ulcers, proximal dilatation and fistula formation (Fig. 15.23A). The colon and caecum (and often the terminal ileum) are visualised by a double-contrast barium enema (Fig. 15.23B). Multiple aphthous ulcers, seen at colonoscopy or barium enema, are typical of early Crohn's colitis. Colonic changes include thickening of the wall, deep ulcers (rose-thorn and collar-stud ulcers) and skip lesions, with areas of normal bowel interspersed between diseased segments. Colonoscopy allows direct inspection and biopsy of the colon and terminal ileum.

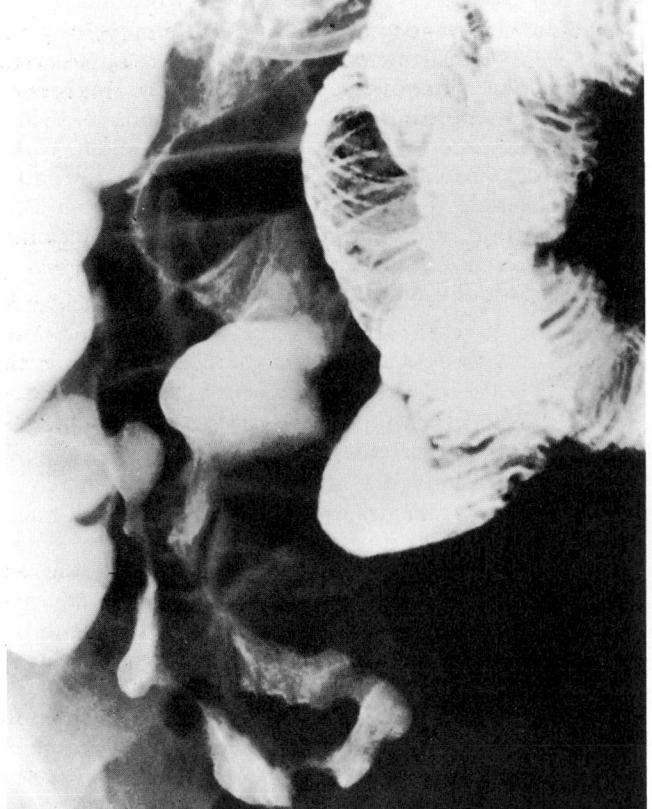

A

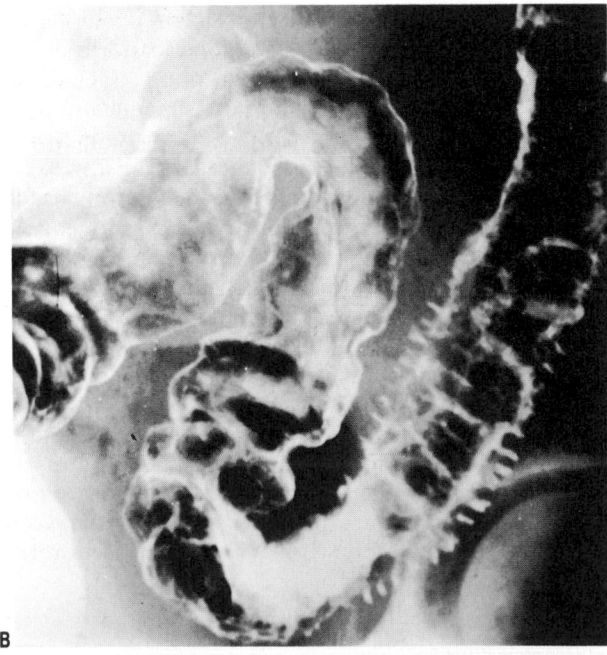

B

Fig. 15.23 Barium enemas demonstrating Crohn's ileitis and colitis. A. Small bowel enema showing stricture formation and ulceration of the terminal ileum, typical of Crohn's ileitis. **B.** Barium enema showing deep ulceration of the distal colon suggesting Crohn's colitis.

disease and hypopituitarism can also be present as weight loss and diarrhoea.

Summary 8 Investigation of Crohn's disease

- Sigmoidoscopy and rectal biopsy
- Stool culture and microscopy
- Abdominal and chest X-ray
  Small bowel enema or meal
  Barium enema
- Colonoscopy
  Upper gastrointestinal endoscopy (when indicated)
- Full blood count, ESR, CRP or orosomucoids
  Serum iron, iron binding capacity, folate and B_{12}
  Liver function tests including serum albumin
- Indium-labelled white blood cells (when indicated)

A potentially useful technique is to label the patient's white cells in vitro with an isotope such as indium[111]. After reinjecting them into the patient, the localisation and activity of the disease can be assessed by determining the site of migration using a gamma camera.

Differential diagnosis

The differential diagnosis of Crohn's disease is shown in Table 15.32. In many parts of the Middle and Far East, ileocaecal tuberculosis is quite common and Crohn's disease is rare. The barium radiological appearance is similar to that of Crohn's disease; however, in the case of tuberculosis, caseating granulomas are found on histology, acid-fast bacilli may be seen on microscopy, and mycobacteria are isolated on culture of the biopsy.

Yersinia can present with an acute ileitis in young people, but signs disappear within three months.

Some patients with Crohn's disease may be wrongly diagnosed and treated for anorexia nervosa. Addison's

Table 15.32 Differential diagnosis of Crohn's disease

Symptoms	Differential diagnosis
Terminal ileal disease	Tuberculosis Yersinia Tumours, especially lymphoma and primary carcinoid Irritable bowel disease
Colitis	Ulcerative colitis Infective colitis Ischaemic colitis Irritable bowel syndrome
Weight loss and diarrhoea	Carcinoma (especially of the large bowel in older people) Other causes of malabsorption, e.g. coeliac disease Hyperthyroidism Anorexia nervosa (with or without surreptitious purgative abuse) Addison's disease Hypopituitarism

Complications

- *Acute colonic (toxic) dilatation*, indistinguishable from that seen with UC and sometimes complicated by perforation and haemorrhage.
- *Subacute small bowel obstruction*, due to stricture formation and obstruction by a food bolus.
- *Fistula formation.*
- *Renal stones.* Oxalate stones due to increased urinary oxalate excretion is a complication of small bowel disease because increased bile or fatty acids in the colon enhance oxalate absorption.
- *Carcinoma of the colon* may complicate long-standing (usually more than 20 years) Crohn's colitis. Small intestinal carcinomas may complicate Crohn's disease.
- *Amyloid* may occur in the bowel and other organs and may regress with resection of diseased bowel.
- *Perforation* may occur in acute toxic megacolon or silently in acute disease during steroid therapy.
- *Severe colonic haemorrhage.*

Management

Crohn's disease can cause considerable morbidity but, with joint medical and surgical specialist care, the overall quality of life should be good. The mortality rate is about twice that of normal controls.

Medical

Management of patients with Crohn's disease depends on the site, severity and extent of disease (Table 15.33). In general, patients should be encouraged to take a balanced diet with an adequate amount of fibre. Dietary fibre should only be restricted when there is stricture formation, as it may then contribute to intestinal obstruction. Replacements are given if there is evidence of haematinic, fat-soluble vitamin or mineral deficiency.

Active ileitis and colitis

Active ileal disease causing diarrhoea, abdominal pain and a right iliac fossa mass is usually treated with a three-month course of oral prednisolone (starting at 30–40 mg/day). If the disease is resistant, azathioprine (2 mg/kg) may be used. Clinical trials have shown that 5-aminosalicylate preparations are of minor value when the disease is restricted to the ileum. An elemental diet (a solution of essential amino acids, carbohydrate, fat, vitamins and trace elements) may also be of value in the treatment of active ileal disease.

Table 15.33 Medical treatment of Crohn's disease

Symptoms	Treatment
Nutritional deficiencies	Good balanced diet
	Folic acid
	Vitamin B_{12}
	Iron
	Vitamins A, D, E and K
	Potassium, zinc and calcium
Ileal disease	Prednisolone
	Elemental diet
	Azathioprine
	5-aminosalicylate drugs
Colonic disease	Prednisolone
	Sulphasalazine
	Azathioprine
	5-aminosalicylate drugs
Severe active ileitis and/or colitis	Intravenous hydrocortisone
	Intravenous fluids or total parenteral nutrition
	Antibiotics
Anal disease and fistulae	Metronidazole
	Azathioprine
	Elemental diet/total parenteral nutrition and nil by mouth
Non-intestinal manifestations	Local measures
	Prednisolone (if acute illness)

Active colonic disease is also treated with prednisolone. Sulphasalazine, which is 5-aminosalicylic acid bound to a sulphonamide (sulphapyridine), may be of some use in Crohn's colitis although its main role is in the prevention of relapse in UC. However, because of the numerous and potentially serious side-effects (Table 15.34), mostly due to the sulphapyridine, 5-aminosalicylic acid preparations have been developed. One of the enteric coated preparations uses an acrylic-based resin outer coat (mesalazine) which, like the semi-permeable membrane of the slow-release preparation of sulphalazine, is pH-dependent and allows release of 5-aminosalicylic acid into the ileum and colon. Azodisalicylate consists of two molecules of 5-aminosalicylic acid bound by an azo bond which is split by lower intestinal bacteria. Another option is the use of 5-aminosalicylic acid enemas. The new 5-aminosalicylate preparations are as effective as sulphasalazine and are replacing it.

Patients with severe active ileitis and/or colitis have constitutional symptoms and require hospital admission. Intravenous hydrocortisone sodium succinate (usually 100 mg eight-hourly) is usually given for about five days and then oral prednisolone is substituted. Intravenous fluids are needed and, if the patient is malnourished, total parenteral nutrition should be undertaken. If there is a possibility of infection or abscess, the patient is treated with intravenous broad-spectrum antibiotics (e.g. ampicillin, gentamicin and metronidazole).

Anal disease

Anal disease with sinuses, abscesses or fistulae can be treated with metronidazole for several weeks, but the patient should be warned to report any symptoms suggestive of drug-induced peripheral neuropathy.

Resistant anal disease may respond to dietary measures or require surgical resection with formation of a stoma. In severe cases, an elemental diet will greatly reduce stool frequency and help healing. Entero-cutaneous and entero-enteric fistulae usually require surgery.

Non-intestinal manifestations

Disorders reflecting acute illness settle with removal of the affected bowel (usually colon) but those due to the chronic illness do not. Severe joint, skin or eye disease requires prednisolone. The treatment of sacro-iliitis and ankylosing spondylitis is described in Chapter 23, page 999.

Surgical

Surgery is required for a severe acute attack unresponsive to treatment, persisting active disease resistant to corticosteroids, symptomatic strictures, non-healing fistulae and complicating carcinoma. Most Crohn's patients will at some time require intestinal surgery. Limited resections and end-to-end anastomoses are performed as necessary, usually to relieve obstruction or fistula formation. Occasionally, panproctocolectomy with formation of an ileostomy is indicated for severe colitis. The complications of ileostomy are discussed on page 599.

ULCERATIVE COLITIS

Ulcerative colitis (UC) is a chronic inflammatory condition of unknown aetiology affecting the colon and rectum.

Table 15.34 Role and side-effects of salicylate drugs used in Crohn's disease and ulcerative colitis

Drug	Side-effects	Role
Sulphasalazine	Skin rashes	Prevention of relapse in UC
	Marrow suppression	Some use in ileal and
	Haemolysis	colonic Crohn's disease
	Male subfertility	
	Gastrointestinal symptoms	
	Orange urine	
5-aminosalicylic acid (mesalazine)	Headache	Alternative to sulphasalazine
	Diarrhoea	
	Nephrotoxicity	
Azodisalicylate (olsalazine)	Headache	Alternative to sulphasalazine
5-aminosalicylic acid enemas	Headache	Alternative to sulphasalazine enemas

Like Crohn's disease, it is most common in the Western World (Fig. 15.22). The incidence of UC appears to be stable. It is slightly more common in women than men. Most patients present in early adult life, but all ages can be affected.

Aetiology and pathology

Aetiological factors are similar to those for Crohn's disease (p. 592). There is recent evidence that relapses can be associated with stopping smoking cigarettes; the explanation for this is not known.

UC primarily involves the mucosa; only in very severe disease is the muscularis mucosae penetrated. Microscopy shows plasma cells and neutrophils, particularly in the crypts of Lieberkühn, which can break down to form 'crypt abscesses' communicating with the luminal surface. If the disease is confined to the rectum (proctitis), it is clinically less severe and there is no increased long-term risk of carcinomatous changes. The extent of disease varies from patient to patient but in almost all cases the rectum is involved.

Clinical features

Acute attack

The usual presenting symptom is the passage of frequent loose, small-volume, brown motions with fresh blood and mucus either on the surface of the stools or intermixed with them. Blood per rectum alone or diarrhoea alone are common first symptoms. Attacks can be usefully divided into mild, moderate and severe (Table 15.35). Patients with mild attacks open their bowels up to five times a day, with moderate attacks up to 10 times a day, and with severe attacks over 10 times a day. The faeces become increasingly soft with more severe relapses. Cramping abdominal pains are common in attacks of moderate severity, while rectal pain and a painful feeling of incomplete evacuation (tenesmus) are common in the more severe cases.

Fever and tachycardia indicate severe disease – usually widespread and active – rather than infection. Anaemia, if present, is usually hypochromic and microcytic and due to blood loss.

Sigmoidoscopy and rectal biopsy are essential for the assessment of proctocolitis. In proctitis, the mucosa becomes oedematous, diffusely reddened, and granular when it loses its normal 'wet' appearance. The blood vessels and mucosal folds are lost, and contact bleeding and spontaneous haemorrhages may be present. 'Pseudopolyps' are islands of residual mucosa around which mucosa has been lost. Sigmoidoscopy in active proctitis should be brief; no attempt should be made to insert the instrument far into the rectum and only a little air insufflated.

Colonic blood loss causes anaemia, while protein loss leads to hypoproteinaemia and peripheral oedema. With

Table 15.35 Ulcerative colitis: clinical features of mild, moderate and severe attacks

Clinical feature	Mild	Moderate	Severe
Diarrhoea	+	++	+++
Blood per rectum	+	++	+++
Mucus	+	++	+++
Abdominal pain	–	+	++
Tenesmus	±	+	++
Anorexia	–	+	++
Weight loss	±	+	++
Acute extracolonic manifestations	+	+	++
Fever	–	±	+
Tachycardia	–	±	+
Anaemia	±	+	++
Distended abdomen	–	±	+
Abdominal tenderness	–	±	+
Sigmoidoscopy	Fine granularity	Coarse granularity Spontaneous bleeding	Ulceration Pseudopolyps Mucopus
Abnormal plain abdominal X-ray	–	–	+
High ESR	±	+	++
High neutrophil count	±	+	++
Hypoproteinaemia	–	+	++

acute colonic dilatation, the patient becomes ill, febrile with abdominal tenderness and reduced bowel sounds. Signs of peritonitis (abdominal rigidity, extreme tenderness and absent bowel sounds) suggest colonic perforation, a complication with a mortality rate approaching 50%. Colectomy may therefore be necessary in acute colonic dilatation to avoid this complication.

Chronic ulcerative colitis

Following recovery from an acute attack, patients may return to a normal bowel habit. Acute exacerbations of varying severity usually occur intermittently. In some patients, these periods of remission may be very short so that treatment becomes almost continuous. Other patients have persistent symptoms which typically become worse when their prednisolone dose is reduced.

Development of malignant change

Patients with total colitis for more than 10 years are at an increased risk of developing carcinoma of the colon, hence the need for regular colonoscopic screening.

Non-intestinal manifestations

The non-intestinal manifestations of UC are similar to those of Crohn's disease (p. 593 and Table 15.31).

Table 15.36 Investigation of acute attack of presumed ulcerative colitis

- Rectal biopsy
- Haemoglobin, white cell count, acute phase reactants
- Liver function tests, plasma proteins
- Stool microscopy and culture
- Plain abdominal X-ray
- Barium enema or colonoscopy (delay until after acute attack)
- Radiolabelled white cell scan (selected cases)

Investigation

The relevant investigations in UC are shown in Table 15.36. Stool microscopy and culture are necessary to exclude infection. A plain abdominal X-ray may demonstrate colonic dilatation, usually best seen in the transverse colon (Fig. 15.24). Barium enemas or colonoscopies can precipitate toxic dilatation, and should therefore be avoided in acute disease. When used, they show loss of haustra, dilatation of the lumen and superficial ulceration.

Management

Acute attack

The most important treatment for acute episodes of colitis is corticosteroids. In mild attacks of distal disease, corticosteroid or 5-aminosalicylic acid enemas are usually effective. In mild but more extensive disease, oral 5-aminosalicylic acid preparations or prednisolone are effective. In moderately severe attacks, oral prednisolone (30–40 mg daily) is the usual therapy, with the dose then being tapered off over three months. In severe attacks, intravenous hydrocortisone (100 mg t.d.s.) is given. Antibiotics and total parenteral nutrition are indicated in sick toxic patients.

Sulphasalazine (1 g b.d.) or other 5-aminosalicylic acid compounds (e.g. mesalazine, 400 mg t.d.s.) reduce symptoms in patients with mild attacks. Some patients benefit from the exclusion of dietary milk products.

Maintenance treatment

Numerous studies have shown that 5-aminosalicylate preparations reduce the relapse rates of patients in remission (see Table 15.34). There is no indication for steroids in patients in remission.

Management in pregnancy

Most patients with inflammatory bowel disease improve during pregnancy, although a minority (about 20%) have relapses. There is no contraindication to the use of sulphasalazine and prednisolone in any trimester. Azathioprine and metronidazole, however, may adversely affect the fetus and should be avoided. Patients tend to relapse postpartum because of a fall in plasma steroid levels. Patients should be warned of this possibility and the disease treated vigorously if it occurs.

Management in childhood

Children should be treated actively in the same way as adults to maximise growth. Prednisolone should be used sparingly because, although it reduces disease activity, it tends to inhibit growth. Particular attention should be paid to diet. In medically resistant disease, a colectomy should be performed.

Surgery

The standard operation for UC is panproctocolectomy with ileostomy. However, subtotal colectomy is now often performed and, at a second operation, a pelvic pouch is constructed from the terminal ileum to act as a reservoir and anastomosed to the anus. Inflammation of the pouch ('pouchitis') is a complication. There are three major indications for surgery:

1. Patients with severe acute disease where the colon is dilated more than 6 cm on plain abdominal X-ray and the patient is toxic with a pyrexia and tachycardia. The operative mortality becomes much higher (50%) if patients perforate their colon and develop a faecal

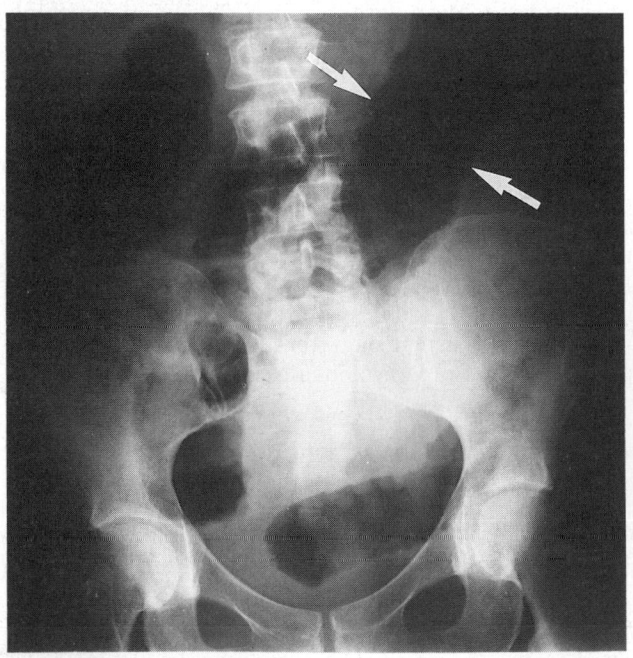

Fig. 15.24 Plain abdominal X-ray showing a dilated transverse colon outlined by air (arrowed) – the toxic megacolon of colitis.

peritonitis (compared with 3% for elective and 10% for urgent operations). Acute severe colonic bleeding is also an indication for surgery.

2. Patients with chronic severe extensive disease which persistently requires high dose corticosteroid treatment. Patients usually feel dramatically better after colectomy, which also avoids the development of further complications (apart from chronic liver disease).

3. In patients with total colitis for more than 10 years, there is a significant risk of carcinomatous change (Fig. 15.25). Carcinomas may be multifocal and are often preceded by the development of epithelial cell dysplasia. After 10 years' total colitis, regular colonoscopies are therefore indicated. Severe dysplasia or carcinoma are indications for total colectomy.

Complications of an ileostomy

Complications of ileostomy are usually minimal apart from minor problems with the abdominal wall around the stoma. There may be high fluid outputs (more than 1 litre/day), especially if there has been small bowel surgery or Crohn's disease. This can be helped by avoiding hyperosmolar food and by the use of drugs which slow intestinal motility (e.g. loperamide, codeine phosphate).

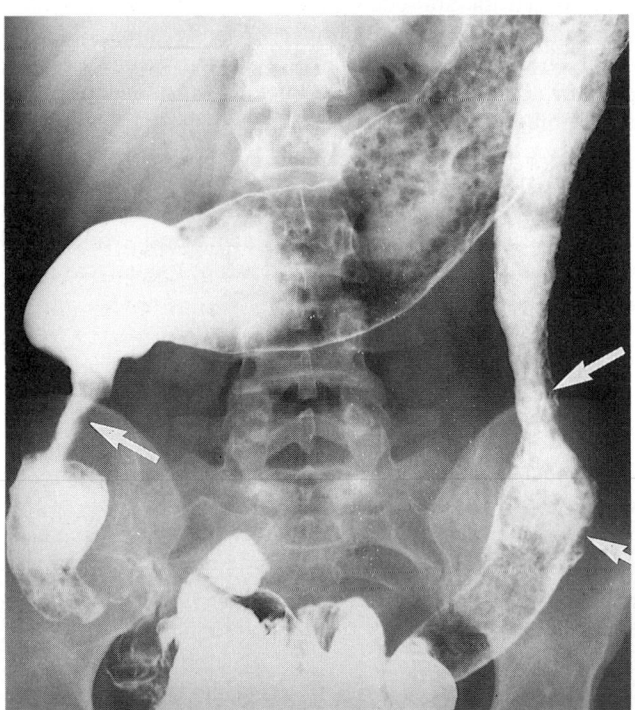

Fig. 15.25 Barium enema findings with pancolitis. Long-standing UC with disease throughout the colon, mucosal ulceration (white arrows at right-hand side) and loss of haustrations. There is an 'apple-core' lesion of the ascending colon (single white arrow) typical of carcinoma.

Impotence due to damage to the sacral nerves is unusual. Most patients with an ileostomy have excellent health.

Psychological problems can be severe and patients require sensitive counselling by medical and nursing staff. Many hospitals have full-time 'stoma nurses', who care for patients' equipment and basic medical and psychological needs both in and out of hospital. Many patients also find it helpful to meet other stoma patients. Colitis and stoma societies and self-help groups are of great value in helping patients to lead a normal life.

Prognosis

Less than 5% of patients suffering from UC die within a year of presentation. In contrast, after their first attack settles, 10% of patients will have at least 15 subsequent asymptomatic years. Up to 25% of patients require colectomy within 5–10 years of developing the disease. Deaths can be avoided by performing colectomies before advanced carcinomas develop. Overall, the mortality rate is about twice that of the normal population.

INFECTIVE, ISCHAEMIC AND RADIATION COLITIDES

PSEUDOMEMBRANOUS COLITIS

Pseudomembranous colitis is usually due to a toxin produced by *Clostridium difficile* and nearly always follows the use of broad-spectrum antibiotics, e.g. ampicillin. The symptoms develop four days to six weeks after starting the drugs.

Clinical features and investigation

The patients develop cramping abdominal pains and diarrhoea with mucus and, sometimes, blood. Sigmoidoscopy reveals diarrhoea, a proctitis and, sometimes, multiple yellow elevated plaques up to 20 mm in diameter. Investigations may demonstrate *C. difficile* toxin in the faeces. A rectal biopsy is usually diagnostic and shows necrotic foci with inflammatory cells migrating through to the lesion ('the summit lesion') and pseudomembranes.

Management

The treatment of choice is vancomycin but metronidazole is also effective. Cholestyramine, an anion-exchange resin, can be used to bind the toxin and reduce diarrhoea. Supportive measures, which often include intravenous fluids, are important. The prognosis is usually good, except in the elderly or if there is a delay in making the diagnosis. Relapse can occur.

YERSINIA

Yersinia enterocolitica and *pseudotuberculosis* are organisms which may cause an acute ulcerative inflammation of the ileum, appendix and colon. They may be associated with erythema nodosum and an acute arthritis. Barium studies show a swollen terminal ileum with tortuous folds and filling defects giving a cobblestone appearance or a colitis. Some patients may have a laparotomy because a mistaken diagnosis of acute appendicitis is made. The condition is self-limiting and resolves completely within three months. Tetracycline or cotrimoxazole are indicated in patients with severe systemic symptoms.

ABDOMINAL TUBERCULOSIS

This is rare in Western countries but relatively common in developing countries, particularly the Indian subcontinent. Tuberculosis can affect any part of the gastrointestinal tract, but is commonest in the ileocaecal area, proximal colon and peritoneum. Fifty per cent of patients have evidence of previous or active pulmonary tuberculosis.

Intestinal tuberculosis

Either the human or bovine form of *Mycobacterium tuberculosis* is ingested to cause disease. The affected bowel becomes ulcerated and may alternate with normal bowel (skip lesions). The radiological and macroscopic appearances can be very similar to those of Crohn's disease. Histology shows caseating granulomas, and acid fast bacilli may be seen.

Clinical features and investigations

There is gradual onset of abdominal pain, anorexia, weight loss, diarrhoea and fever. Intestinal obstruction, perforation and haemorrhage can occur and, if there is extensive small intestinal involvement, malabsorption can be a feature. In tuberculous colitis, there may be blood and mucus in the stool. Perianal tuberculosis may cause ulceration, fistula and abscess. Tuberculous intestinal lesions are shown on small bowel meal and/or barium enema. These are not specific so colonoscopy with biopsy or even laparotomy with biopsy is indicated to obtain a histological diagnosis. The differential diagnosis for small intestinal tuberculosis includes Crohn's disease, Yersiniosis and lymphoma, and for large bowel tuberculosis, Crohn's disease, ulcerative colitis, infective colitis and carcinoma.

Tuberculous peritonitis

Tuberculous peritonitis is usually due to haematogenous spread from pulmonary tuberculosis and is rarely associated with intestinal tuberculosis. It presents with progressive ascites accompanied later by anorexia, weight loss, fever and minor abdominal pain. Oedema, hepatosplenomegaly and generalised lymphadenopathy may appear late. A dry form of the disease can occur which presents with palpable abdominal masses due to multiple intraabdominal adhesions. Other causes of ascites, particularly malignancy and cirrhosis, must be considered in the differential diagnosis.

M. tuberculosis organisms are rarely seen in ascitic fluid (5%) which is an exudate and may contain numerous lymphocytes but culture is positive in about 80% of cases. Sometimes diagnosis is made by biopsy and culture of peritoneal tissue obtained at laparoscopy or laparotomy.

Management

Standard antituberculous chemotherapy (see p. 473) leads to complete resolution of abdominal tuberculosis and should be continued for 12 months. Occasionally, long-term problems are caused by intestinal strictures or intra-abdominal adhesions.

GAY BOWEL SYNDROME

Homosexuals have an increased incidence of diarrhoea from infections such as shigella, salmonella, campylobacter, giardia, amoeba and cryptosporidium. They also commonly develop perianal warts (condylomata acuminata). These patients may have a proctitis due to gonococcal or *Herpes simplex* type 2 infection and, occasionally, anal syphilis (see Ch. 11).

The acquired immune deficiency syndrome (AIDS) can be associated with fulminant bowel infections as well as the development of plaques of Kaposi sarcoma throughout the bowel (p. 245). Eating and swallowing may be painful due to oral and oesophageal candida infection.

ISCHAEMIC COLITIS

Aetiology and pathology

Ischaemic colitis usually affects the region of the splenic flexure or the rectosigmoid area. Rarely, ischaemia of the superior mesenteric artery may affect the ascending and proximal transverse colon. Atheroma is a more common cause than embolus; but aetiological factors are otherwise similar to those seen in small bowel ischaemia (p. 584).

Clinical features and investigation

The patients are usually elderly and present with bloody diarrhoea and abdominal pain. Examination shows mild peritonism and the rectal mucosa may be normal or show a non-specific proctitis. Sometimes, a plain abdominal X-ray shows a dilated colon with 'thumb printing', which is confirmed by a barium enema.

Management

In most patients, the symptoms resolve with analgesia and intravenous fluids. Perforation is rare. A late complication is stricture formation.

RADIATION COLITIS

Damage to the transverse colon may occur during upper abdominal radiotherapy and damage to the sigmoid colon and rectum during pelvic irradiation. In the acute phase (during or immediately after treatment) the symptoms are bloody diarrhoea, tenesmus and abdominal pain. These are treated with a low residue diet and rectal steroids if there is a proctitis. Later complications include the development of a chronic proctitis or colitis with telangiectatic lesions which may bleed, benign ulcers and stricture formation. The proctocolitis and ulcers may sometimes improve with rectal or systemic steroids.

FUNCTIONAL BOWEL DISORDERS

Incidence

In the UK, it is estimated that some 15% of the population have symptoms of a functional disorder of the bowel. These patients have abdominal symptoms without any evidence of underlying organic pathology. Many individuals do not seek medical advice, presumably because they understand the nature of their symptoms and may be able to attribute them to a particular cause; they thereby learn to avoid or live with them. Others will consult their general practitioner, sometimes because of the discomfort experienced but often out of fear that the symptoms might indicate more serious disease. Some will then be referred to a specialist. This may be because of the severity or intractability of the symptoms or because the presence of atypical features causes concern. More often, however, the referral will be made in order to reinforce the reassurance already given and, hopefully, to make treatment more effective. Specialists thus tend to see a selected sample of patients who will often form the basis of clinical studies.

Because the cause or causes are not known, and because the range of symptoms is wide and relates to the whole of the gastrointestinal tract, it is sensible to consider all the manifestations of functional bowel disorder as a single entity due to multiple factors. At different times, the same patient may experience either predominantly lower gastrointestinal symptoms (irritable bowel syndrome, IBS), or upper gastrointestinal symptoms (functional or non-ulcer dyspepsia).

Functional bowel disorders commonly present in the third and fourth decades with a slight predominance in women. In retrospect, many patients can recall intermittent symptoms in childhood, often at times of stress, to which various labels may have been applied, e.g. bilious vomiting, grumbling appendix, abdominal migraine. Symptoms first presenting in the mid-forties onwards should be regarded more seriously, and as possibly indicating organic disease. Many of these older patients will, nonetheless, be found to have sigmoid diverticular disease which has pathophysiological features in common with IBS. However, there is no convincing evidence that IBS of young adults progresses to diverticular disease in the middle-aged.

Surveys of the general population show that symptoms of IBS are common; 30% of such a sample of 301 apparently healthy people had either abdominal pain, constipation or diarrhoea. When 2000 new attenders at a gastroenterology outpatient clinic in Bristol were prospectively studied over a five-year period, about half turned out to have functional disorders. It is interesting to contrast these patients with the remainder found to have organic disease, as many of the organic conditions have to be considered in the differential diagnosis of functional bowel disorders (Table 15.37).

Aetiology

Many aetiological factors have been postulated for functional bowel disorders. Whether the bowel is inherently irritable or normal until irritated cannot be determined. Analogies might be drawn with duodenal ulcer where, though an individual may be born with a greater parietal cell mass of acid secretory cells than normal, an ulcer will only develop if certain environmental factors supervene. No clear pattern of inheritance of functional bowel disorders has been demonstrated; while it may sometimes appear to be familial, this can probably be explained by the similar environmental factors.

Motility disturbance

Hyperreactivity of the gut, both in the sense of provoking reflex contraction and of a lowering of the threshold to stimuli causing pain, has been demonstrated in many ways, including balloon distension studies. Pressure transducer studies have shown that some patients have increased frequency and strength of small intestine motility.

Previous gut infection

The postinfective variant of IBS may comprise up to a third of all patients. Damage to the epithelium by microor-

15 Gastrointestinal Disease

Table 15.37 Organic vs functional disorders in a sample of 2000 gastroenterology outpatients*

Diagnosis	Number of patients
Definite non-organic	888
Spastic colon	449
Painless diarrhoea	107
Painless constipation	39
Depression and pain	50
Anxiety and GI symptoms	24
Functional dyspepsia	77
Others	59
Definite organic	980
Peptic ulcer	197
(Duodenal ulcer)	(135)
(Gastric ulcer)	(62)
Oesophagitis	188
Carcinoma of stomach	13
Postgastrectomy	14
Inflammatory bowel disease	168
(Crohn's disease)	(57)
(Ulcerative colitis)	(111)
Coeliac disease	26
Infective diarrhoea	21
Carcinoma of colon	28
Gallstones	48
Hepatitis	11
Cirrhosis	21
Alcoholism	16
Other	229

* After Harvey, Salih and Read 1983. Lancet 1: 632–634. The study was based on 2000 new attenders at a gastroenterology outpatient clinic over a period of five years. Of these, 57 had a non-gastroenterological diagnosis and 75 remained undiagnosed.

ganisms, their toxins or bile acids may allow stimulation of mast cells or paracrine cells initiating the syndrome.

Dietary factors

Many patients with IBS have diets high in refined carbohydrates and low in dietary fibre. Food intolerance is often suspected by patients. In different studies, its estimated frequency varies between 6% and 60%. Although exclusion diets, with recurrence of symptoms when the suspected food is reintroduced, would seem to support this possibility, relatively few double blind studies have been undertaken. True allergy, in an immunological sense (using such criteria as a rapid reaction to small doses of antigen accompanied by raised IgE levels and positive skin prick tests) is exceedingly rare. The usually transient cows' milk intolerance of infants is the best-known example. Alternative non-immunological mechanisms have been postulated to account for some apparent reactions which require large amounts of the suspect food and come on so slowly that the offending food may not be

---

Summary 9 Contributory factors in functional bowel disorders

- Motility disturbance
- Altered sensory threshold
- Previous gut infections
- Altered gut flora
- Dietary
  Fibre deficiency
  Food intolerance – Immunological ('allergy')
  – Non-immunological
  Food additives
- Psychological
  Anxiety
  Depression

---

recognised. Prostaglandin release or alterations in gut hormone profiles seem unlikely. It has recently been suggested that changes in gut flora to give high counts of facultative anaerobes (analogous to changes produced by antibiotic therapy) may enhance the production of toxic metabolites from undigested food residues.

Psychological

The psychosomatic mechanisms postulated seem to be borne out by the frequently found evidence of stress and anxiety. Nonetheless, attempts to modify autonomic nervous activity pharmacologically have met with limited success, perhaps in part because the less accessible enteric nervous reflexes may be at fault.

Much remains unexplained. It is not known what determines which of the various symptom patterns will develop in an individual patient, nor what makes some individuals accept the situation without recourse to orthodox, or even complementary, medical advice. A study screening consecutive non-complaining blood donors showed that the psychoneurotic symptomatology in the non-complaining IBS subjects more closely matched that of IBS patients than that of the remaining blood donors. It is not clear whether the differences between patients and the normal population are quantitative or qualitative.

Clinical features

The descriptive names given to functional bowel disorders indicate many of the symptoms – spastic colon, mucous colitis (in fact, a misnomer as the colon is not inflamed), and functional dyspepsia. Globus hystericus is difficulty with swallowing which has non-organic basis. Most patients will experience alteration of bowel habit, many will have pain and bloating, and distension and excess flatus are common in the predominant lower gastrointestinal IBS.

Pain after food, with nausea, distension, belching and regurgitation, in patients who have had negative gastroscopy and gallbladder studies, are the hallmarks of functional dyspepsia, though the symptoms may overlap those of IBS. Unlike IBS, which does not progress to any other condition, up to 20% of patients with functional dyspepsia may subsequently develop demonstrable peptic ulceration or oesophagitis.

Pain

It has long been recognised that pain arising from the gut is not always localised to the midline. In addition to 'classical' subumbilical griping, pain in many other sites and radiations, sometimes extra-abdominal, can occur. This can lead to a wide differential diagnosis (Table 15.38). Although not feasible as a routine diagnostic procedure, it can be useful to perform studies in which a balloon attached to a colonoscope is inflated at different sites as it is withdrawn from the caecum. This not only confirms that colonic distension can produce pain at both conventional and unconventional sites, but may also exactly reproduce a patient's pain. Severity and quality of pain may vary considerably, even mimicking biliary colic and other acute abdominal emergencies. Palpable and tender bowel in the left iliac fossa is a relatively non-specific finding, but evidence of spasm (by feeling transmitted pressure waves in the reservoir bulb on sigmoidoscopy) or

Table 15.38 Differential diagnosis of typical and atypical IBS and functional dyspepsia

Functional bowel disorder	Differential diagnosis
Typical IBS	Inflammatory bowel disease (Crohn's>ulcerative colitis)
	Colorectal cancer
	Diverticular disease
	Infective diarrhoea
	Malabsorption (coeliac disease)
	Endocrinopathies
	Thyrotoxicosis
	Hypothyroidism
	Carcinoid syndrome
Atypical IBS	
Right iliac fossa pain	Appendicitis, Crohn's disease
Right hypochondrial pain	Gallstones
Left hypochondrial pain	Ischaemic heart disease, chronic pancreatitis
Back pain	Pancreatic disease
	Spinal osteoarthritis
Loin pain	Renal disease
Menstrual exacerbation	Endometriosis
Dyspareunia	Pelvic inflammatory disease
Functional dyspepsia	Peptic ulcer
	Oesophagitis
	Gastric cancer
	Ischaemic heart disease

reproduction of pain by the above procedure are particularly helpful in making a positive diagnosis. Proctalgia fugax is a transient shooting pain in the rectum; the cause is unknown.

Constipation

Constipation may be the predominant presenting symptom in functional bowel disorders, but often alternates with diarrhoea and may be associated with pain. The stools may be pellet- or ribbon-like and be commonly associated with the passage of mucus. Rectal bleeding must always be fully investigated, even if only to confirm that it is due to haemorrhoids. Although some patients may have large amounts of dry stool in the rectum with little awareness of its presence there, others, despite not having a bowel action for several days, may have an empty rectum with greatly delayed colonic transit. Constipation dating back to childhood commonly emerges in the history, when 'potty training' may have been at fault, the urge to defaecate repeatedly ignored, and purgatives regularly administered.

Diarrhoea

Diarrhoea is often a distressing symptom because of the uncertainty and anxiety which it may generate in an already anxious patient. The fear of faecal incontinence is a real one and, as the diarrhoea frequently occurs during the morning, the journey to work may be dreaded. The stool may vary between liquid and semi-formed. There is often much flatus and another uncertainty is thus whether the urge to pass wind may result in passage of diarrhoea and consequent soiling. The patient may be greatly relieved to be asked about this as he or she may be too embarrassed to volunteer the symptom. A sense of wanting to evacuate when there is nothing there (tenesmus) or of incomplete defecation is also particularly common. Although the patient may think large amounts are being passed, stool weights are in fact within the normal range. Diarrhoea occurs less commonly at other times of the day and, unlike inflammatory bowel disease or other organic diarrhoeas, does not usually disturb sleep. Rumbling and gurgling (borborygmi) accompany diarrhoea and flatus.

Dyspepsia

Functional dyspepsia may cause pain (mimicking an ulcer or oesophagitis), distension, flatulence with belching, and nausea. The symptoms are more clearly related to eating than in IBS. An important differential diagnosis is gastro-oesophageal reflux (p. 560) which may occur without a hiatus hernia or endoscopic evidence of oesophagitis.

15 Gastrointestinal Disease

Other symptoms

Other associated, non-specific symptoms may confuse the diagnosis. Sweating, tremor, hyper-reflexia and tachycardia in association with diarrhoea are usually due to anxiety rather than thyrotoxicosis; a marked sinus arrhythmia, indicating autonomic overactivity, is frequently present. Gynaecological symptoms, e.g. increased severity of pain premenstrually, low back pain and dyspareunia, are common and often lead to unnecessary gynaecological investigation.

Psychological symptoms are common, and underlying stress and disorders of mood and personality are frequently invoked as major factors in pathogenesis. Nonetheless, the results of formal studies have often been conflicting. The perennial problem of whether anxiety provokes symptoms or vice-versa cannot be clearly resolved, although the vicious circle of symptoms (anxiety – more symptoms – more anxiety) is real enough. Although depression may present with predominantly functional bowel symptoms (which regress with antidepressants), this is not as common as was once thought. Even if there were initially other reasons for a patient's anxiety, the symptoms frequently reinforce it. An important part in history-taking is to ask the patient what he or she considers the cause to be. Frequently, a fear of cancer, which the patient was reluctant to voice, will be revealed. Many will also be worried about inflammatory bowel disease, a worry perhaps reinforced by a previous vague diagnosis of mucous colitis or peptic ulcer.

Prognosis

Morbidity from functional bowel disorders can be considerable. There have been few long-term studies, but in one such study, of 77 of 91 patients recalled after six years, 29 had no bowel problems and many of the 44 who still had IBS symptoms found the condition easier to cope with. In view of the difficulties in making a positive diagnosis, it is of note that only four patients had a new diagnosis made, invariably prompted by a change in the clinical picture.

Investigation and management

The first problem that arises in the management of functional bowel disorder is the confidence with which one can make the diagnosis and the extent to which further investigation should be undertaken. The need for a full history and examination (including sigmoidoscopy) is self-evident; the history may be further supplemented at the follow-up appointment, which should be given to every patient. Many important psychological and social factors may then be disclosed to a doctor who has earned the patient's confidence. All investigations should be ordered at the first visit and the patient told that they are expected to be normal. To go on asking for 'just another test' counters the essential reassurance given by the doctor. In hospital practice, the stool should be examined for pathogens and parasites if the history is of recent diarrhoea, especially after foreign travel. A barium enema or colonoscopy, to exclude other colonic disease, is not necessary in all patients, particularly if they are young with typical symptoms. Sometimes, however, the patient will require this investigation for complete reassurance. The most important diagnoses to exclude are inflammatory bowel disease in young adults and colorectal tumours in older patients.

The less typical the clinical presentation the more the exclusion of other diseases may be necessary, but a positive diagnosis should be made rather than one arrived at purely by exclusion. Such a minimalist approach is therapeutically effective and safe with the proviso that fuller investigation or even reinvestigation is undertaken under the following circumstances:

- patients over 40 years of age presenting with symptoms for the first time
- any change in the pattern of symptoms or development of new symptoms which sound organic
- presence of additional symptoms which are not part of IBS, such as weight loss, rectal bleeding or fever.

At the end of the first consultation, the physician should be able to make a positive diagnosis and suggest an explanation for the cause of the symptoms. Even if the symptoms are bizarre, their existence should not be questioned. The patient should be asked what he or she feared might be the cause and then be reassured by pointing out how common the problem is and the generally good prognosis.

After identifying any provocative factors, the doctor should suggest modifications in the patient's lifestyle that might be beneficial. The constipated may need to increase dietary fibre and also ensure an adequate daily fluid intake. Smoking and excess alcohol consumption should be stopped and the effects of other medications reviewed. At a subsequent interview, the results of normal tests can be used to reinforce the fact that there is no serious underlying cause for the symptoms.

Medication

Drugs play only a minor role in management. When properly conducted, all drug trials in IBS and functional dyspepsia have shown very high rates of response to placebo (often over 50%).

Antispasmodics. Anticholinergic drugs may relieve pain but are limited in dosage by their side-effects. The directly acting smooth muscle relaxant mebeverine is widely used and, in some studies, has been shown to be superior to placebo. An old remedy, peppermint oil, in a new colonic release capsule is probably as effective.

Antidiarrhoeals. Disabling morning diarrhoea can be treated with codeine phosphate on rising and repeated if necessary. If not effective, loperamide can be substituted. Constipation should be avoided.

Laxatives and purgatives. Only bulking agents should be encouraged. Many constipated patients may have been using purgatives for many years and these should be stopped, despite the fears and reluctance of patients to abandon them. Simple suppositories, or even periodic enemas, may have to be given temporarily while attempts are made to re-educate the bowel.

Psychotropics. Long-term use of benzodiazepine or other tranquillisers must be avoided, but they may be necessary as a short-term measure to combat periods of stress. Antidepressants, usually given at night, should also only be considered if there are clear depressive symptoms.

Antinauseants. The postprandial distension and nausea of functional dyepepsia is often greatly helped by metoclopramide syrup or tablets before meals. If ineffective, or if the drug is not tolerated because of somnolence or dyskinetic movements, domperidone or cisapride should be substituted.

Antacids. These may be helpful in patients with dyspepsia.

SELF-INDUCED BOWEL DISEASE

Self-induced bowel disease may be a variant of the Munchausen syndrome, where patients deliberately invent symptoms (p. 193), or be a result of drug abuse. Both problems are rare, and tend to occur in young female patients. The diagnosis is often well disguised.

Invention of symptoms

The patient who is inventing symptoms most commonly presents with severe abdominal pain or with gastrointestinal bleeding (sometimes fictitious and sometimes simulated by the ingestion of animal blood). The history may be convincing but background information is vague. Examination often reveals an abdomen with multiple scars from when surgeons have been misled in the past. If this diagnosis is suspected, investigations should be minimal and the treatment is observation and reassurance. Psychiatric support rarely helps.

Laxative abuse

The patient abusing laxatives usually presents with profuse watery diarrhoea secondary to purgative abuse. There may be several litres of watery diarrhoea a day with consequent weight loss, dehydration and hypokalaemia. The diagnosis may be suggested by the appearance of pigment deposition in the rectal mucosa at sigmoidoscopy

(melanosis coli). It may be confirmed by chemical analysis that purgatives are present in the faeces or urine, or by finding the patient surreptitiously taking them. Confrontation should be avoided, and psychiatric treatment is often disappointing.

DISEASES OF THE PERITONEUM

Peritonitis

Acute bacterial peritonitis. This follows perforation of an abdominal viscus or abdominal diverticulum as a result of ulceration, inflammation, ischaemia, trauma or (rarely) malignancy, or follows infection in the female genital tract. The patient develops an acute abdomen with severe abdominal pain, nausea, vomiting, fever and tachycardia followed by shock. Septicaemia and multi-organ failure can occur. On examination in the early stages, there may be guarding, rebound tenderness and scanty bowel sounds. Later the abdomen becomes rigid and extremely tender with absent bowel sounds. There is often a neutrophil leukocytosis and there may be metabolic acidosis. A plain erect abdominal or chest X-ray shows free gas under the diaphragm. Treatment requires a laparotomy if there is a ruptured viscus. Preoperatively the patient will need nasogastric suction, intravenous fluid and electrolytes, oxygen, opiate analgesia and broad-spectrum antibiotic therapy including cover for anaerobic organisms.

Primary (spontaneous) peritonitis. This is acute or subacute bacterial inflammation of the peritoneum. It occurs in patients with cirrhotic or malignant ascites, immune deficiency states and in children with nephrotic syndrome or urinary tract infections. The commonest organism is *Streptococcus pneumoniae.*

Tuberculous peritonitis (see p. 600).

Chemical peritonitis develops when a sterile but irritant fluid, e.g. bile, blood or pancreatic secretions, leaks into the peritoneal cavity.

Granulomatous peritonitis can be caused by infections (tuberculosis, fungi, parasites), secondary adenocarcinoma, sarcoidosis, Crohn's disease or foreign bodies (e.g. starch).

Vasculitic peritonitis occurs when there is gut involvement in SLE, polyarteritis nodosa, systemic sclerosis, dermatomyositis or Henoch-Schönlein purpura.

Familial Mediterranean fever is characterised by recurrent episodes of acute self-limiting serositis, especially involving the peritoneum (see p. 1101).

Peritoneal malignancy

Secondary carcinoma is the commonest cause of peritoneal malignancy. Most cases result from adenocarcinoma of the stomach, colon, pancreas, ovary, lung or breast. Primary mesothelioma is rare, slightly more common in men and is usually associated with asbestos exposure. About 50% of patients have signs of asbestosis on chest X-ray.

Clinical features and investigations

The main symptoms are abdominal pain, nausea, vomiting, weight loss and abdominal swelling due to ascites. The ascitic fluid has a high protein content, may be blood-stained and contain malignant adenocarcinoma or mesothelial cells. Laparoscopy or laparotomy are sometimes necessary to make a diagnosis. Differential diagnosis includes tuberculosis peritonitis, cirrhosis and Budd-Chiari syndrome.

Management and prognosis

Prognosis is poor in secondary carcinoma and mesiothelioma. Radiotherapy or chemotherapy may sometimes help in palliation of secondary carcinoma. Patients' symptoms may be helped by regular paracentesis.

THE PANCREAS

The pancreas is a retroperitoneal organ which, along with the common bile duct, drains through the medial wall of the second part of the duodenum via the ampulla of Vater.

The pancreas has exocrine and endocrine functions. Duodenal release of the hormone secretin results in acinar bicarbonate secretion. The pancreatic enzymes trypsin and chymotrypsin break down proteins, lipase digests fats, and amylase acts on starch. These enzymes are released in response to cholecystokinin and activity of the parasympathetic nervous system. The endocrine cells of the pancreas are localised to the islets of Langerhans and make up about 1% by volume of the pancreas. The most numerous endocrine cells are the beta cells secreting insulin but also present are alpha cells secreting pancreatic glucagon, D cells secreting somatostatin and PP cells secreting pancreatic polypeptide. With disorders of the pancreas, exocrine function is usually lost before endocrine function.

Clinical features of pancreatic disease

The symptoms of pancreatic disease include pain (severe, epigastric or central abdominal, and often radiating through to the back), steatorrhoea (indicating lipase deficiency), weight loss, nausea, vomiting and those of hyperglycaemia. Patients with acute pancreatitis may present with an acute abdomen. Other features include anaemia,

jaundice due to common bile duct obstruction or associated liver disease, an abdominal mass, ascites and pleural effusion (usually left-sided).

Investigation of pancreatic disease

General

A full blood count is done primarily to look for an anaemia and for the white cell count (high in acute pancreatitis and abscesses, etc., low in the Shwachman syndrome; see p. 608). A serum amylase is only indicated if the diagnosis of acute pancreatitis or continuing pancreatic obstruction due to an abscess or pseudocyst is being considered. Pancreatic proteases play a role in making vitamin B_{12} available for absorption in the terminal ileum and a deficiency may result in megaloblastic anaemia. Three-day faecal fats are useful to assess the degree of steatorrhoea, and very high levels (more than 100 g fat per day) may be seen with pancreatic insufficiency.

Tube pancreatic function tests

Tube pancreatic function tests involve the passage of a thin catheter into the second part of the duodenum. The duodenal contents are then aspirated for measurement of bicarbonate and pancreatic enzymes, after an intravenous pharmacological dose of cholecystokinin and secretin, or a Lundh test meal which consists of a 500 ml standard mixture of fat, protein and carbohydrate.

Summary 10 Investigations of pancreatic disease

General

Full blood count
Liver function tests and serum proteins
Serum amylase
Blood glucose
Serum B_{12}
Three-day faecal fat excretion

Tube pancreatic function tests

Cholecystokinin-secretin test
Lundh meal

Tubeless pancreatic function tests

PABA test
Fluorescein dilaurate test

Imaging techniques

Plain abdominal X-ray
Ultrasound
CT scan
ERCP
Angiography

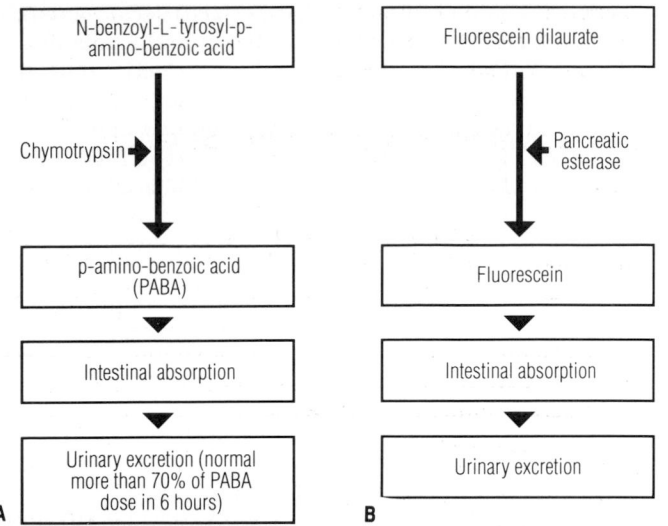

Fig. 15.26 Tubeless pancreatic function tests. A. The PABA test involves chymotrypsin cleavage of N-benzoyl-L-tyrosyl and the subsequent measurement of PABA in urine or plasma. **B.** The fluorescein test involves esterase cleavage and the subsequent measurement of fluorescein in urine. If either test is abnormal, the basic chemical (i.e. PABA and fluorescein) should be given on a separate day to exclude a problem with intestinal malabsorption.

Tubeless pancreatic function tests

Tube tests are uncomfortable for patients and oral tests (Fig. 15.26) are fortunately now available. In the PABA test, pancreatic chymotrypsin cleaves N-benzoyl-L-tyrosyl-p-amino-benzoic acid; the resulting para-amino-benzoic acid (PABA) is absorbed and the urinary PABA is measured in a six-hour collection. To exclude possible intestinal malabsorption, a trace dose of ^{14}C-PABA is given at the same time and urinary radioactivity measured. The test is invalidated by paracetamol and cotrimoxazole and is dependent on normal gastric emptying and renal function. A similar test involves the cleavage of fluorescein dilaurate by pancreatic esterase, and subsequent measurement of urinary fluorescein.

Imaging techniques

The pancreas is relatively difficult to image because of its retroperitoneal location. The plain abdominal X-ray is often unhelpful, but pancreatic calcification may be seen with chronic pancreatitis and a 'sentinel loop' of dilated proximal small intestine may be seen over the pancreas in acute pancreatitis. An ultrasound or CT scan is useful in delineating abnormal anatomy and can be used to direct needle biopsies. Endoscopic retrograde pancreatography (ERP) is usually combined with cholangiography (ERCP). ERP is particularly useful in demonstrating abnormalities due to chronic pancreatitis or carcinoma. Angiography may help to diagnose pancreatic tumours.

CONGENITAL PANCREATIC ANATOMICAL ABNORMALITIES

Embryologically, the pancreas is derived from an anterior and a posterior bud which normally fuse and drain into the medial wall of the duodenum. Developmental abnormalities include:

1. *Accessory pancreatic tissue*, which is separate from the body of the pancreas. This is found in about 10% of autopsies, with ectopic tissue most commonly located in the wall of the stomach and intestine. Rarely, it may ulcerate and cause gastrointestinal bleeding or be the site of carcinomatous change.
2. *Annular pancreas*, where the second part of the duodenum is encircled by pancreatic tissue. This is a rare abnormality which usually presents in the first months of life with duodenal obstruction; it requires a bypass gastrojejunostomy. Mild cases are asymptomatic, but the condition may present for the first time in adults with abdominal pain and vomiting, sometimes associated with peptic ulcer or obstructive jaundice.
3. *Pancreas divisum*, due to failure of the two pancreatic ducts to fuse. Most of the gland is drained through the accessory ampulla. It is associated with an increased incidence of acute pancreatitis. Sphincterotomy of the accessory ampulla may reduce the number of attacks.

CONGENITAL PANCREATIC FUNCTIONAL ABNORMALITIES

Cystic fibrosis

Cystic fibrosis is the most important congenital disease of the pancreas. The pancreatic and intestinal effects of the disease are summarised in Table 15.39. Other complications include cirrhosis of the liver (Ch. 16), pulmonary disease (Ch. 13) and male infertility due to atrophy or absence of the vas deferens, seminal vesicles and epididymis.

Table 15.39 Pancreatic and intestinal complications of cystic fibrosis

Effect	Complication
Pancreatic insufficiency	Enzyme deficiency
	Diabetes mellitus
Meconium ileus	Intestinal obstruction
	Volvulus
	Peritonitis following perforation
	Polyhydramnios in utero
Meconium ileus equivalent	Intussusception
	Intestinal obstruction

Cystic fibrosis is characterised by hyperviscous secretions containing mucus and protein from exocrine glands, which result in plugging of ducts leading to destruction of glandular tissue (Table 15.39).

Pancreatic insufficiency

The destruction of pancreatic exocrine acini is often rapid. The patient develops steatorrhoea and oedema secondary to hypoproteinaemia. A good response is seen with the introduction of pancreatic enzyme supplements taken with each meal, and H_2-receptor antagonists can help by raising duodenal pH to increase pancreatic enzyme activity. Supplements of vitamins A, D, E and K also have a role in the presence of steatorrhoea. With severe malnutrition, dietary supplements of easily absorbed medium-chain triglycerides and protein hydrolysates in the form of milk-shakes or cooking additives may be helpful.

Diabetes mellitus due to destruction of pancreatic endocrine tissue is a late event.

Meconium ileus

In cystic fibrosis, the meconium protein content at birth is about eight times the normal level. As a result, neonates with cystic fibrosis often present with intestinal obstruction which may be complicated by a volvulus or peritonitis due to a perforation. Treatment is with instillation of high osmolarity diatrizoate (e.g. Gastrografin) which causes shrinkage of the plug and allows its passage down the gut. If a perforation or volvulus has occurred, surgery is usually needed. Maternal polyhydramnios is due to fetal meconium ileus in utero.

Meconium ileus equivalent

'Meconium ileus equivalent' is, as the name suggests, a problem similar to meconium ileus, but it occurs later in life and is complicated by the presence of faeces. A high fibre diet to soften the stool, and laxatives are effective in mild cases. N-acetylcysteine can be used as a mucus-clearing agent. In severe cases, diatrizoate is usually effective in shrinking the faecal mass; surgery should be avoided if possible, because of the high mortality from intestinal and pulmonary complications.

Prognosis

The prognosis is variable, but many affected children are now surviving into their twenties and thirties.

Macroamylasaemia

Macroamylasaemia is a condition of unknown aetiology characterised by large molecular weight amylase in the serum. It accounts for 2.6% of elevated serum amylase levels. The amylase may be bound to immunoglobulins or glycoproteins and is too large to be excreted by the glomerulus like normal amylase. Consequently, very high serum amylase levels occur. The diagnosis can be confirmed by chromatography and by showing low urinary amylase and normal plasma trypsin and lipase levels. It is important to make the diagnosis to avoid mistaking the condition for acute pancreatitis. There is an association with coeliac disease.

No therapy, other than reassurance, is needed for macroamylasaemia.

Shwachman syndrome

Shwachman syndrome is the association of pancreatic enzyme deficiency, neutropenia, short stature, and metaphyseal dysostosis. Sometimes there is also an anaemia, thrombocytopenia and low intelligence. It is inherited as an autosomal recessive. The usual presentation is with steatorrhoea and failure to thrive in young children; a normal sweat sodium and chloride excludes cystic fibrosis.

The pancreatic insufficiency is treated with pancreatic enzyme supplements and possibly H_2-receptor antagonists. Infections should be treated aggressively in the presence of the neutropenia, which is associated with a deficiency of white cell precursors. The prognosis is usually good.

ACUTE PANCREATITIS

Acute pancreatitis is an acute inflammatory condition of the pancreas which results in necrosis of exocrine tissue. It causes abdominal pain and is associated with high plasma and urinary pancreatic enzyme levels.

The incidence is 10 per 100 000 per annum in the UK and North America and was 28.1 per 100 000 in people over the age of 20 in Copenhagen in 1970–80. The median age is 53 years, with an equal sex incidence.

Summary 11 Aetiology of acute pancreatitis

- Gallstones in common bile duct
- Alcoholism
- Iatrogenic – usually post-ERCP
- Trauma
- Viral – mumps and coxsackie B
- Pancreatic tumours
- Drugs, e.g. corticosteroids, oral contraceptives, thiazide diuretics
- Possibly hyperlipidaemia and primary hyperparathyroidism
- Idiopathic

GET SMASHD

Aetiology

Pancreatitis occurs as a result of pancreatic duct obstruction, bile and duodenal content reflux and direct action of toxins. In the UK, about 80% of cases are due to gallstones or alcohol abuse. In some parts of the world (e.g. South America), alcohol abuse is the most important factor. Gallstones are thought to block pancreatic enzyme outflow, but may be passed via the ampulla of Vater before investigations are undertaken. In this situation, gallstones are usually found in the gallbladder or in the common bile duct. The mechanism by which alcohol causes acute pancreatitis is controversial. It may be due to a rise in pancreatic duct pressure or to a direct action on acinar cell membranes.

ERCP may cause acute pancreatitis, possibly as a result of increased pressure in the pancreatic duct. Exploratory laparotomy, other intra-abdominal operations and translumbar aortography may also be complicated by acute pancreatitis. Patients with a Polya gastrectomy with a 'blind' duodenal loop are at increased long-term risk. Acute pancreatitis due to viral infection (e.g. mumps) is rare, and is caused by viral destruction of acinar cells. Pancreatic tumours may cause pancreatitis by ductular obstruction. Many drugs have been reported as possible causes. It is often stated that types I, IV and V hyperlipoproteinaemia and hypercalcaemia are causes of acute pancreatitis; however, recent studies have suggested that the associations are doubtful.

Clinical features

The main symptom of acute pancreatitis is severe abdominal pain. Its usual site is epigastric or hypochondrial, but it may occur around the umbilicus. In about half the patients, it radiates through to the back. The onset is usually sudden, such that the main differential diagnosis is intestinal perforation. The pain settles within 48 hours in most patients. The other common initial symptom is vomiting.

Examination reveals a patient in great pain with severe abdominal tenderness and often guarding and rigidity. Bowel sounds are usually reduced. Extra-abdominal signs may include fever, tachycardia and hypotension. In severe cases, complications (Table 15.40) may supervene.

Investigation

The diagnosis is made by finding a serum amylase at least four times the upper limit of normal. A smaller rise in serum amylase may be seen in patients with perforated peptic ulcers, intestinal obstruction, other intra-abdominal emergencies, diabetic ketoacidosis, after opiate analgesia, macroamylasaemia and renal and hepatic failure. If the serum amylase is less than four times the upper limit

Table 15.40 Complications of acute pancreatitis

Early complications

Clinical	Biochemical
Cardiac failure	Uraemia
Renal failure	Hypocalcaemia
Respiratory failure (ARDS)	Hypoalbuminaemia
Hyperglycaemia	Abnormal liver function
Anaemia	Hyperglycaemia
Jaundice	Metabolic acidosis
Disseminated intravascular coagulation	Hypoxaemia

Late complications

Pseudocyst
Abscess
Pancreatic duct stricture
Ascites/pleural effusion
Diabetes mellitus

of normal, or if it is thought that the high amylase may be due to macroamylasaemia, a high amylase:creatinine urinary excretion, serum lipase or serum trypsin may be used as confirmatory evidence of acute pancreatitis. A plain abdominal X-ray may show a 'sentinel loop' of air-filled small intestine lying over the pancreas. It may also show evidence of ascites or intestinal ileus, which may complicate acute pancreatitis. Ultrasound or CT scanning may demonstrate an oedematous enlarged gland, gallstones and complications such as pseudocysts.

The differential diagnosis of acute pancreatitis includes gastric or intestinal perforation, peptic ulcer disease, acute cholecystitis, intestinal obstruction, acute mesenteric ischaemia, ruptured aortic aneurysm and myocardial infarction.

Management

Acute pancreatitis may have a self-limiting short course, be associated with the development of late complications or be very severe and result in early death from circulatory collapse. In order to predict severity and prognosis, a number of indicators are helpful (Table 15.41); if more than three of these indicators are present there is a risk of early death or complications.

Table 15.41 Indicators of severe acute pancreatitis

- White blood cell count over 15×10^9/l
- Glucose over 10 mmol/l
- Urea over 16 mmol/l
- PaO$_2$ below 8.0 kPa
- Calcium below 2.0 mmol/l
- Albumin below 32 g/l
- LDH over 600 units/l
- AST over 100 units/l
- Over 55 years of age

NOT MORPHINE!

?CVP

Initial treatment is to restore fluid and electrolytes by intravenous infusion. A central venous pressure line is helpful to monitor fluid replacement. Analgesia should be maintained with pethidine or buprenorphine; morphine is contraindicated because it causes spasm of the sphincter of Oddi. A sedative such as diazepam may be helpful. Nasogastric suction is indicated initially, and should be continued until there is evidence that gastric emptying is normal and any intestinal ileus has resolved. Neither drugs such as cimetidine, anticholinergics, glucagon, aprotinin (a trypsin and kinin inhibitor), antibiotics and calcitonin, nor parenteral nutrition have been shown to have overall benefit when subjected to clinical trial. The roles of peritoneal lavage and somatostatin or its analogues are uncertain. Early endoscopic sphinctero-tomy may be helpful in severely ill patients with stones in the common bile duct.

Complications of acute pancreatitis

↓, DIC CCF ARF ARDS ↑GLUC ANAEMIA

The treatment of these severe problems (Table 15.40) is supportive (usually in an intensive care unit) with fluids, cardiac inotropes, oxygen, ventilation, dialysis, calcium and insulin as necessary. Pseudocysts are collections of pancreatic juice in the lesser sac, and may need surgical or endoscopic drainage into the stomach. Pancreatic abscesses are usually due to *E. coli* infection and require surgical drainage and antibiotics. Ascites and pleural effu-sions due to a fistula from the pancreatic duct system into the peritoneal or pleural spaces are characterised by very high amylase concentrations in the fluid aspirate. The effusions can often be treated with drainage via a cannula, but sometimes surgical closure is required.

The overall mortality rate is about 10% per attack; this rises with age and other indicators of severity. The mor-tality of initial attacks is more than 10 times higher than that of recurrent attacks, and is twice as high with gall-stones compared with alcoholism. The recurrence rate is greatly reduced by successful treatment of gallstones or alcoholism.

CHRONIC PANCREATITIS

Chronic pancreatitis is associated with destruction of pancreatic exocrine tissue which persists even when the underlying cause has been removed. Inflammation is followed by fibrosis and atrophy. Chronic relapsing pancreatitis is a variant in which symptoms, such as pain, are intermittent. The disease may be further classi-fied according to its aetiology and whether steatorrhoea or diabetes mellitus is present. Steatorrhoea implies loss of lipase due to advanced acinar damage; diabetes mellitus indicates severe loss of islet tissue and advanced disease.

In 1978–79 the prevalence of chronic pancreatitis in Copenhagen was 27.4 per 100 000 adult population per year. There was a 3:1 male preponderance. The median age at onset was 39. The annual incidence in Minnesota in 1960–69 was 3.5 per 100 000 population. The inci-dence rises in areas with high alcohol intakes.

Aetiology *ALCOHOL!*

Alcohol is by far the most important factor in those cases where a cause can be identified. Protein precipitates have been found in the pancreatic juice of alcoholics with chronic pancreatitis, and it is suggested that these form plugs which block the small pancreatic ducts and cause acinar damage. Gallstones are a common case of acute pancreatitis but a rare cause of the chronic form.

In the hereditary form of chronic pancreatitis, the chil-dren in affected families usually present in adolescence. It is inherited as an autosomal dominant but penetrance is variable. Pancreas divisum, which occurs when the ventral and dorsal embryological buds do not join, is a rare cause of chronic pancreatitis, as are hyperlipidaemia and hypercalcaemia. The disease may also occur in primary biliary cirrhosis, sclerosing cholangitis and with choledochal cysts. In a significant number of patients no cause can be found.

Summary 12 Aetiology of chronic pancreatitis	
• Alcohol	• Hyperlipidaemia
• Gallstones	• Hypercalcaemia
• Hereditary	• Idiopathic
• Pancreas divisum	

Clinical features

The main symptom of chronic pancreatitis is upper abdominal pain. This is usually severe and chronic, although, in about 10% of patients, pain is not a feature. Radiation to the back is common and sometimes the pain can be relieved by leaning forward. It may be exac-erbated by eating. Anorexia, nausea and vomiting may be prominent. Steatorrhoea occurs with very high faecal fat output, and is associated with weight loss despite a good appetite. After eight years of symptoms, about 70% of patients have steatorrhoea. If there is gross steatorrhoea, deficiencies of vitamin A, B_{12} (see p. 606), D, E and K may occur. Coexistent alcoholic cirrhosis, or thrombosis of the portal or splenic vein as a complication of pancre-atitis, may cause oesophageal or gastric varices. Gastric outflow obstruction due to swelling of the pancreatic head or a pseudocyst, and pancreatic ascites due to a

panc prob play role allow B_{12} ws↑

fistula from the pancreatic duct to the peritoneum, occasionally occur. About a third of patients develop diabetes.

Investigation

Biochemical

Serum amylase levels are not raised in chronic pancreatitis. Although faecal fat excretion may be very high (more than 100 g/24 hours), this is not diagnostic of pancreatic disease, as amounts approaching this level may be seen in patients with small bowel disease.

Low pancreatic enzyme and bicarbonate outputs can be measured by pancreatic function tests (p. 606). Mild abnormalities of liver function tests are common. Rarely, the head of the pancreas may swell and cause an obstruction to the lower end of the common bile duct; this results in jaundice and cholestatic liver function tests.

Radiological

Abdominal X-ray may show pancreatic calcification (Fig. 15.27A). Ultrasound and CT scanning may show swelling and dilatation of the main pancreatic duct. The diagnostic investigation of choice in chronic pancreatitis is ERCP (Fig. 15.27B).

Summary 13 Investigations for chronic pancreatitis	
Biochemical	*Radiological*
Faecal fat estimation and other tests for malabsorption	Plain abdominal X-ray
Secretin-cholecystokinin test	Ultrasound, possibly CT scanning
Lundh test	Endoscopic retrograde pancreatography (ERP)
PABA test	
Liver function tests	
Blood glucose	
Serum amylase (only useful in acute attacks)	

Management

It is important, whenever possible, to treat the underlying cause, although this may not prevent progression and pain. Mild analgesia is rarely effective. Codeine, pethidine or buprenorphine may control pain, and destruction of the coeliac ganglion with injection of 100% alcohol may give relief. Surgery in the form of total or subtotal pancreatectomy should be considered in patients with severe pain, preferably before addiction to opiates has developed. However, the results are variable and often poor if patients continue to abuse alcohol. A minority of patients require regular methadone.

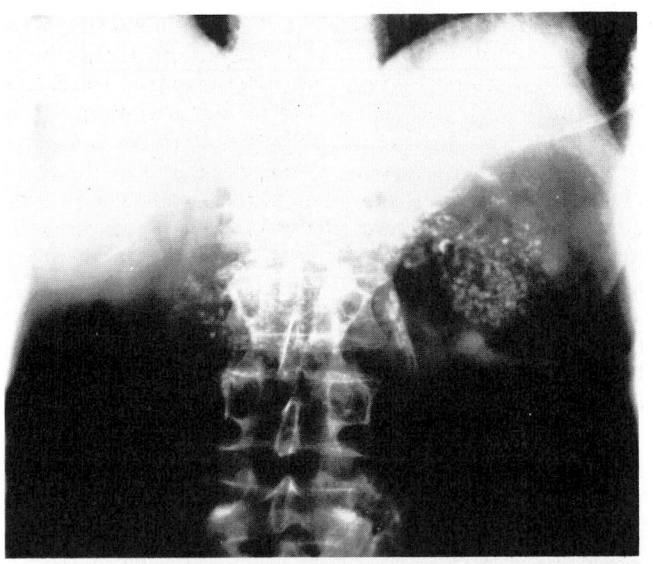
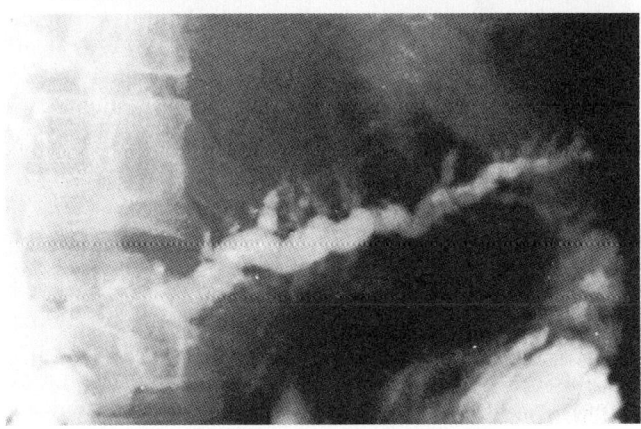

Fig. 15.27 Chronic pancreatitis. A. Plain X-ray showing pancreatic calcification. **B.** ERCP in chronic pancreatitis showing a dilated main pancreatic duct with associated dilated side branches.

Steatorrhoea and the resulting malnutrition may be helped by a low fat and high carbohydrate diet. Pancreatic enzyme supplements should be taken with food. H_2-receptor antagonists raise the intraduodenal pH which is otherwise pathologically low due to lack of bicarbonate. Food may be cooked in, or be supplemented by, mid-chain triglycerides (MCTs) as these can be absorbed directly without lipolysis. Supplements of vitamins A, D, E and K should be prescribed as necessary.

Diabetes mellitus requires standard treatment. A particular problem is variable absorption of carbohydrate due to exocrine deficiency or after surgical procedures, as this may result in poor control of blood glucose ('brittle diabetes'). Protein supplements may help raise plasma proteins, and parenteral vitamin B_{12} is occasionally required.

Summary 14 Treatment of chronic pancreatitis

- Treatment of aetiological problem. No alcohol.
- *Pain* – Simple analgesics
    - Avoid opiate analgesics (if possible)
    - Coeliac ganglion block
    - Surgery
- *Steatorrhoea* – Low fat/high carbohydrate diet
    - Enzyme supplements
    - H_2-receptor antagonists
    - MCTs/fat-soluble vitamins
- *Diabetes mellitus* – Diet
    - Oral hypoglycaemics
    - Insulin
- *Metabolic complications* – Protein supplements
    - Vitamin B_{12}

Prognosis

The prognosis, if not the quality of life, of patients with chronic pancreatitis is generally good. Patients rarely die directly of complications and most survive 20 years from the onset. Pain may settle spontaneously; this may reflect 'burning out' of the pancreas and be complicated by steatorrhoea and diabetes. Sometimes, patients whose pain is poorly controlled become dependent on narcotics.

TUMOURS OF THE EXOCRINE PANCREAS

The overall incidence of carcinoma of the pancreas is about 10 per 100 000 per year, but this rises to 100 per 100 000 in those over 65 years of age (Fig. 15.28). It accounts for 5.5% of cancer deaths and is the fourth most common cause of such deaths in men. The incidence is rising throughout the world, with particularly high rates seen in Afro-Americans and New Zealand Maoris.

Aetiology and pathology

The aetiology is unknown. The disease is twice as common in cigarette smokers and in females with diabetes mellitus; chemists and non-oven coke workers also have an increased incidence. There is no definite association with alcoholism, coffee drinking or acute or chronic pancreatitis (except of the rare familial chronic type). However, there may be an increased incidence in chronic calcific pancreatitis.

In those cases where a histological diagnosis is established, the tumour is almost always an adenocarcinoma. The carcinoma usually arises from the ductular epithelium. It may be mucin-producing. About 5% of tumours arise from the acinar cells and, rarely, sarcomas may occur. The tumour metastasises to local lymph nodes adjacent to the vascular supply and, by invasion of blood vessels, to the liver and distant sites. Sixty-five per cent of tumours occur in the head of the pancreas, 30% in the body and 5% in the tail. The tumour infiltrates locally into the duodenum and the retroperitoneal space. It may involve the portal vein, causing thrombosis and splenomegaly, and may also seed into the peritoneal cavity causing ascites.

Clinical features

Symptoms tend to occur late, and are often non-specific. Consequently, there may be a delay in diagnosis, and the majority of patients already have inoperable large tumours and/or metastases by the time the diagnosis is made. Jaundice and pruritus indicate obstruction to the common bile duct or multiple hepatic metastases. Vomiting may be due to gastric or duodenal invasion or peritoneal metastases. Haematemesis and melaena may also occur as a result of invasion of the stomach or intestine. Steatorrhoea may occur as a result of bile duct obstruction. The development of diabetes may predate all other symptoms. Hepatomegaly and/or jaundice are found in the majority of patients at presentation, and the coexistence of a palpable distended gallbladder suggests the presence of a carcinoma

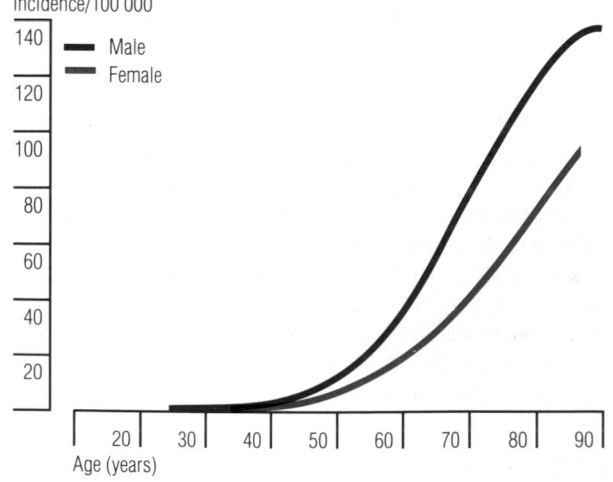

Fig. 15.28 Age-specific incidence of pancreatic carcinoma per 100 000 population in the UK. It is commoner in males and the incidence increases with age.

Summary 15 Symptoms and signs of carcinoma of the pancreas

Symptoms	Signs
Weight loss	Hepatomegaly
Abdominal pain	Jaundice
Jaundice	Palpable pancreatic mass
Vomiting	Palpable gallbladder
Steatorrhoea	Thrombophlebitis
Pruritus	Ascites
Diabetes	

obstructing the lower end of the common bile duct (Courvoisier's sign). This is, however, an unreliable sign as it can also occur with cholelithiasis and is often absent with pancreatic cancer. Thrombophlebitis at remote sites, or deep venous thrombosis, occur in about 10% of patients as a paraneoplastic syndrome (Ch. 8, p. 130).

Investigation

A full blood count and liver enzyme tests may show anaemia and an obstructive jaundice, but these are non-specific and do not help make the diagnosis. In experienced hands, ultrasonography can be diagnostic; it also allows the passage of an ultrasound-directed needle to biopsy from the tumour for histology. CT scanning (Fig. 15.29) has an equal or greater accuracy and is of great help if ultrasound is negative or equivocal. Endoscopy may allow a direct view and biopsy of ampullary lesions, while ERCP often demonstrates main duct lesions and gives information about the biliary tree. In the case of ductular lesions, pancreatic juice may be aspirated for cytology. Laparoscopy and biopsy under direct vision are helpful in some difficult cases. Selective angiography may help to make the diagnosis and is important in determining resectability.

Management

The surgical treatment of carcinoma of the pancreas is very unsatisfactory due to the organ's inaccessibility, the frequency of local spread and metastases. Radical surgery may be performed for localised tumours, especially of the ampulla, and a small number of patients are cured. However, even in operable cases, the five-year survival is less

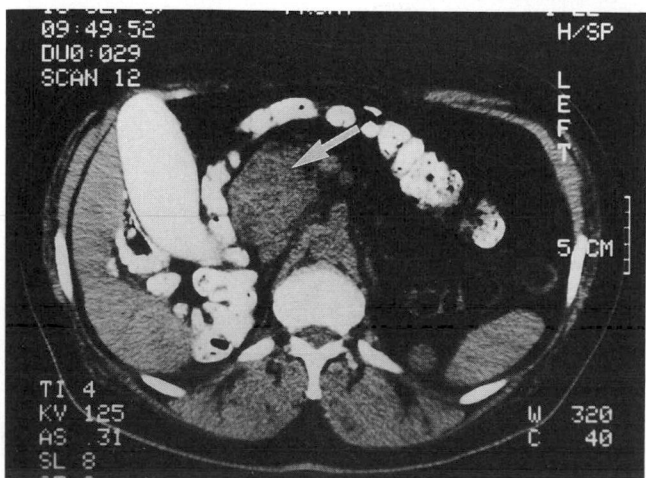

Fig. 15.29 CT scan of abdomen demonstrating a dilated gallbladder (filled with contrast medium following an ERCP) and a large tumour mass in the head of the pancreas (arrowed).

than 15%. If there is obstruction to the common bile duct, a palliative bypass procedure relieves jaundice and pruritus. Hepatic metastases and portal vein thrombosis are contraindications for surgery.

For most patients with carcinoma of the pancreas, treatment is directed to symptomatic relief. Analgesics and coeliac plexus block may be needed. There are few cytotoxic drugs which are effective in pancreatic carcinoma, although responses are sometimes seen with alkylating agents, nitrosoureas and 5-fluorouracil. If a blocked bile duct is causing jaundice and itching, a stent should be used to bypass the obstruction; this may be done from below via an endoscope, or from above by the percutaneous transhepatic route. Use of these techniques reduces the need for surgical bypass operations.

PANCREATIC ENDOCRINE TUMOURS

The pancreas is the primary site for a number of rare functioning endocrine tumours (Table 15.42) which may be benign or malignant and can produce characteristic syndromes. These tumours are important, because surgical cure by resection may be possible. The symptoms caused can be predicted by the known physiological action of the hormone produced, the exception being pancreatic polypeptide which is secreted by many of these tumours and can be used as a tumour marker. Multiple endocrine neoplasia type I (MEN Type I, or Wermer's syndrome) is inherited on an autosomal dominant basis, and is the association of hormone-synthesising parathyroid adenomas (parathyroid hormone), pituitary adenomas (prolactin, growth hormone) and pancreatic endocrine tumours. MEN Type II (or Sipple's syndrome) is similarly inherited, and is the association of hormone-synthesising parathyroid adenomas (parathyroid hormone), phaeochromocytomas (catecholamines) and medullary carcinoma of the thyroid (calcitonin).

Investigation

Diagnosis of these tumours is by demonstrating a high plasma level of the appropriate peptide by radioimmunoassay. The tumours can often be demonstrated by ultrasound or CT scanning. On occasions, it is necessary to sample blood along the portal vein and to demonstrate a peak of hormone secretion corresponding to the site of tumour venous drainage. Arteriography can also be used, and is helpful in demonstrating multiple primary tumours (common with gastrinomas) and hepatic metastases.

Management

Treatment is surgical resection if possible, and this often results in cure. In the presence of metastatic disease, the cytotoxic drugs streptozotocin and 5-fluorouracil can

Table 15.42 Pancreatic endocrine tumours

Peptide	Cellular source	Title	Clinical syndrome
Pancreatic glucagon	Alpha cell	Glucagonoma	Necrolytic migratory erythema Diabetes mellitus
Insulin	Beta cell	Insulinoma	Hypoglycaemia
Somatostatin	D cell	Somatostatinoma	Diabetes mellitus Steatorrhoea Cholelithiasis
Gastrin	G cell	Gastrinoma (Zollinger-Ellison syndrome)	Duodenal ulcers and malabsorption secondary to hyperacidity in the duodenum
Pancreatic polypeptide	Pancreatic polypeptide cell	PP-oma	None
Vasoactive intestinal polypeptide	Nerves	VIP-oma (Verner-Morrison syndrome)	Watery diarrhoea, hypokalaemia and achlorhydria (WDHA syndrome)
Adrenocorticotrophic hormone	Unknown	Cushing's syndrome	Cushing's syndrome (p.702)
Parathyroid hormone	Unknown	Ectopic hyperparathyroidism	Hypercalcaemia
Growth hormone releasing hormone	Unknown	Pituitary acidophil hyperplasia	Acromegaly

produce worthwhile remissions. The symptoms of most of the tumours may be helped by somatostatin therapy. The rash of the glucagonoma syndrome can be improved by zinc, and the hypoglycaemia of insulinomas by diazoxide. The symptoms of gastrinomas are helped by high dose H$_2$-receptor blocking agents or omeprazole, and the diarrhoea of VIP-omas by a variety of agents including corticosteroids, metoclopramide and trifluoperazine.

FURTHER READING

Allan R N, Keighley M R B, Alexander-Williams J, Hawkins C F 1991 Inflammatory bowel diseases. 2nd edn. Churchill Livingstone, Edinburgh and London. *The standard British textbook covering all aspects of diagnosis and management of these difficult and relatively common diseases*

Bouchier I A D, Allan R N, Hodgson H J F, Keighley M R B 1993 Textbook of gastroenterology. 2nd edn. Baillière Tindall, London. *The major British text, which is detailed and comprehensive*

Cotton P B, Williams C B 1990 Practical gastrointestinal endoscopy. 3rd edn. Blackwell, Oxford. *A comprehensive guide to investigative and therapeutic endoscopy*

Shearman D J C, Finlayson N D C 1989 Diseases of the gastrointestinal tract and liver. 2nd edn. Churchill Livingstone, Edinburgh and London. *A good basic postgraduate textbook, which contains a considerable amount of detail*

Sleisenger M H, Fordtran J S 1993 Gastrointestinal disease. 5th edn. W B Saunders, Philadelphia. *The best American textbook, which is particularly strong on the basic pathophysiology of gastrointestinal diseases*

16

Liver and Biliary Tract Disease

Adrian L W F Eddleston

INTRODUCTION

Liver disease occurs worldwide but the main causes are very different. Alcoholic liver disease and gallstones dominate in the West while viral hepatitis predominates in the Middle East, Far East and Africa. All the main hepatitis viruses have now been identified and characterised, and vaccines are available for two of the varieties. If the underdeveloped world can afford them, these vaccines could radically alter the pattern of liver disease in the world. Controlling excessive drinking is proving more difficult.

Liver transplantation is one of the most exciting advances in treatment for both adults and children. However, recurrent disease, particularly in liver cancer and hepatitis virus infection, limits its use to selected cases.

STRUCTURE AND FUNCTION

ANATOMY

Although there is a classical division into a large right lobe and smaller left lobe, this bears no relationship to the true functional division, on the basis of blood supply, into almost equal right and left lobes. The liver has a dual blood supply, from the hepatic artery, which is usually a branch of the coeliac axis, and from the portal vein, formed from the mesenteric vein and splenic vein (Fig. 16.1). The total liver blood flow is about 1300 ml/min, one-quarter of the resting cardiac output. The hepatic artery supplies about 25% of the total liver blood flow but 50% of the oxygen, while the remaining 75% of the volume and 50% of the oxygen comes from the relatively deoxygenated, low-pressure portal vein supply. Both vessels run in the free edge of the lesser omentum to the liver hilum before dividing into major right and left branches. The hepatic veins drain directly into the inferior vena cava, which runs in a groove along the back of the liver between the functional right and left

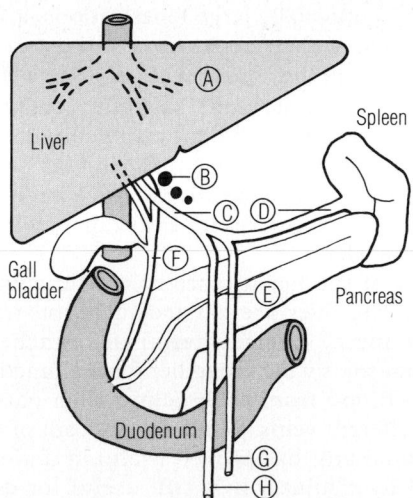

Fig. 16.1 A simplified view of the gross anatomy of the liver and its major relationships. Hepatic veins (A); hilar lymph nodes (B); portal vein (C); splenic vein (D); pancreatic duct (E); bile duct (F); inferior mesenteric vein (G); superior mesenteric vein (H).

lobes. Three large veins enter just below the diaphragm, but there are a number of smaller veins draining the posterior aspect of the right lobe which enter the vena cava directly. These assume importance in two clinical situations: they may be the only remaining draining vessels if there is thrombosis of the main hepatic veins (the Budd-Chiari syndrome), and they are particularly difficult to dissect during a right hemihepatectomy.

The biliary system collects bile, stores and concentrates it in the gall bladder, and delivers it to the duodenum when required. The main right and left hepatic ducts join in the hilum of the liver to form the common hepatic duct. The gall bladder lies on the under-surface of the right lobe of the liver with its fundus usually projecting slightly below the lower edge. The cystic duct runs upwards and backwards to join the common hepatic duct, and the resulting common bile duct then runs with the hepatic artery and portal vein in the free edge of the lesser omentum to pass behind the first part of the duodenum and the head of the pancreas before turning to the right to enter the duodenum. This part of the duct is often completely buried in the pancreas and it is here that it is susceptible to obstruction by pancreatic tumours. The pancreatic and bile ducts usually share a common channel for the last 2–7 mm which opens through a small papilla on the inner wall of the duodenum (the ampulla and papilla of Vater). In this part of the duct the choledochal muscle is thickened to form the sphincter of Oddi.

Micro-anatomy

At a micro-anatomical level, the liver essentially consists of a series of channels, or sinusoids, running between plates of hepatocytes. These are lined by endothelial cells which contain unusually large fenestrations, allowing the sinusoidal part of each hepatocyte surface to have free access to almost all the constituents in plasma (Fig. 16.2). Specialised phagocytic cells (Kupffer cells) are also present in the sinusoids. Biliary canaliculi form between the contiguous surfaces of hepatocytes, and here, and on the sinusoidal surface, there are extensive microvilli in the cell membrane to increase the capacity for trans-membrane transfer.

Branches of the hepatic artery, portal vein and bile duct within the liver are carried in portal tracts. The smallest of these, carrying terminal branches, supply groups of sinusoids which together form a functional unit, the acinus. Blood from each acinus then passes into a number of efferent veins. While the concept of the acinus as a functional unit has proved useful in understanding patterns of liver injury, it is still useful for descriptive purposes to refer to the lobule as the classical structural unit of the liver. Each lobule is centred on an efferent (or central) vein surrounded by radially orientated sinusoids and with five or six portal tracts at the periphery.

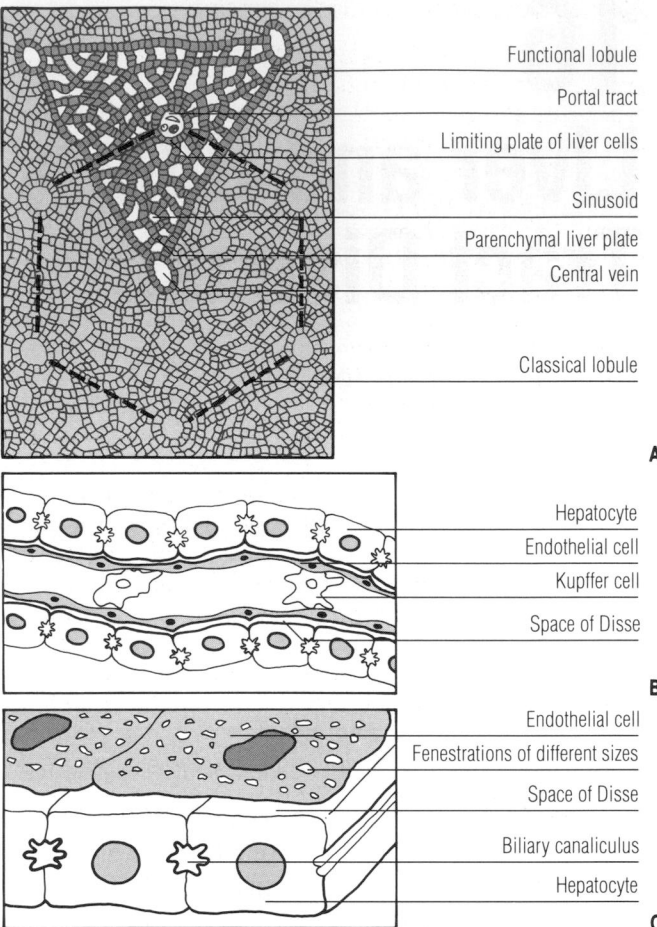

Fig. 16.2 **The micro-anatomy of the liver.** **A.** The classical liver lobule is centred on the central vein with the portal tracts at its periphery. The concept of the functional lobule emphasises the portal tracts as the points of entry of the arterial and portal venous blood, with the sinusoids then extending from there to the 'central veins'. **B.** A liver sinusoid with liver cell plates separated from the lining endothelial cells by the space of Disse. The Kupffer cells straddle the blood-filled centre of the sinusoid. **C.** The endothelial cells riddled with fenestrations allow macromolecules to pass between the blood and the hepatocytes. The biliary canaliculi run between the hepatocytes in the liver cell plates.

Physiology

Essentially the liver has four quite distinct functions:

- It supplies bile salts and bicarbonate to assist in digestion.
- It acts as a buffer between the gut and the systemic circulation, maintaining stable levels of amino acids and glucose.
- It synthesises a large number of specialised proteins, carbohydrates and lipids.
- It is a major excretory pathway for larger and more hydrophobic metabolites, foreign substances and drugs.

Bile acid metabolism and secretion

The primary bile acids, *cholic and chenodeoxycholic acid*, are synthesised from cholesterol in the liver, conjugated with taurine or glycine to form bile salts and then excreted by an active transport mechanism into the bile canaliculi, and eventually into the duodenum. In the distal ileum, there is another active transport system which ensures conservation of bile salts when they have fulfilled their digestive function (Fig. 16.3). This system of enterohepatic circulation is extremely efficient. The entire body pool of bile salts is circulated through the gut about twice in each main meal and only about 5% is newly synthesised in the liver. The small fraction reaching the colon is modified by bacteria, which perform 7-alpha-dehydroxylation, producing the secondary bile acids, *deoxycholic and lithocholic acid*. All bile salts are powerful detergents, solubilising lipids by enclosing them in bile salt aggregates called micelles. These are organised so that hydrophobic groups are orientated into the lipid-rich interior while the hydrophilic hydroxyl and carboxyl groups are on the outside. Cholesterol and lecithin in bile itself are carried in such micelles, and, if the concentration of these molecules rises too high relative to the concentration of bile salts, then the bile becomes supersaturated. Precipitation of cholesterol may then occur, particularly if a nidus for crystal formation is present. This is the pathophysiological basis for gallstone formation which is discussed further on page 633.

The active transport of bile salts is the main driving force for bile secretion, and its failure may be an impor-tant cause of intrahepatic cholestasis. Bile salts accumulate in cholestasis, whether due to mechanical obstruction or a defect in excretion, and deposition in the skin may account for the pruritus which is often a troublesome symptom. There is also a bile salt independent contribution to bile secretion which is probably driven by active sodium transport in the distal canaliculus. Bicarbonate is added in the small bile ductules and this process is stimulated by the hormone secretin. Cholecystokinin principally stimulates gall bladder contraction.

Protein metabolism

The liver receives amino acids from the gut and the muscles and regulates their levels in plasma by controlling the rate of gluconeogenesis and transamination. It also converts ammonia into urea by the urea cycle. Ammonia is produced intrahepatically by de-amination, in other tissues by nucleotide metabolism, and by bacterial action on proteins or urea in the colon. The liver is the major site of synthesis of almost all the plasma proteins, and, for many, is also the principal site of degradation.

In an average 70 kg adult, total body protein is about 12 kg, and turns over at a rate of about 250 g/day. There is a close relationship between the muscles, liver and gut with respect to amino acid fluxes (Fig. 16.4). Muscle contributes the biggest source of protein turnover, about 130 g/day, while dietary intake is about 90 g/day. Only 23% of amino acid nitrogen absorbed into the portal bloodstream after a meal is passed on to the peripheral tissues, and in exercising this gate function, the liver is responsible for extensively modifying the blood amino acid composition. The aromatic amino acids – phenylalanine, tyrosine and methionine – are preferentially processed to urea, while the branched chain amino acids – valine, leucine and isoleucine – are selectively passed to the periphery where they are predominantly metabolised by muscle. This selectivity is lost in severe liver disease and it is possible that the resulting change in the ratio of the plasma concentrations of these two groups of amino acids may alter cerebral neurotransmitter metabolism and contribute to the pathophysiology of portosystemic encephalopathy (p. 648).

Of the many proteins synthesised in the liver, *albumin* and *prothrombin* are of particular interest in relation to liver

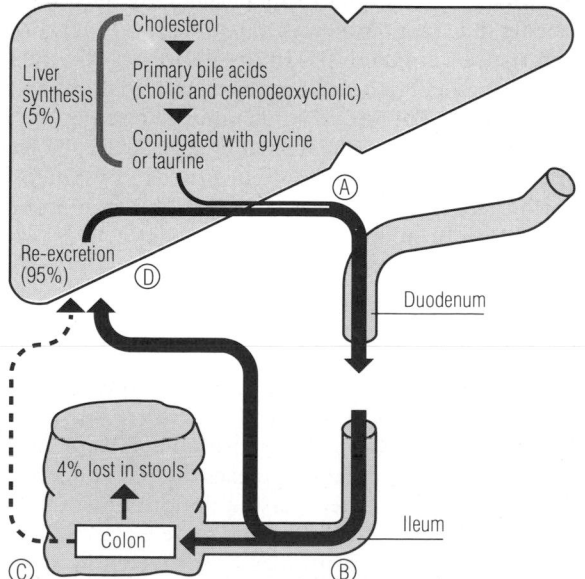

Fig. 16.3 Enterohepatic circulation of bile acids. Bile salts entering the duodenum via the bile duct (A); absorption of bile salts in the terminal ileum (B); secondary bile acids formed by bacterial degradation (C); uptake and re-excretion of bile salts by liver (D).

Summary 1 Liver physiology	
Normal function	*Consequence in disease*
Bile acid metabolism	Fat malabsorption
Glucose and amino acid homeostasis	Encephalopathy
Synthesis of plasma	Ascites, bleeding,
proteins, clotting factors, lipids	xanthalasmata
Metabolism/excretion of	Jaundice, encephalopathy,
bilirubin, ammonia/urea, drugs	drug toxicity

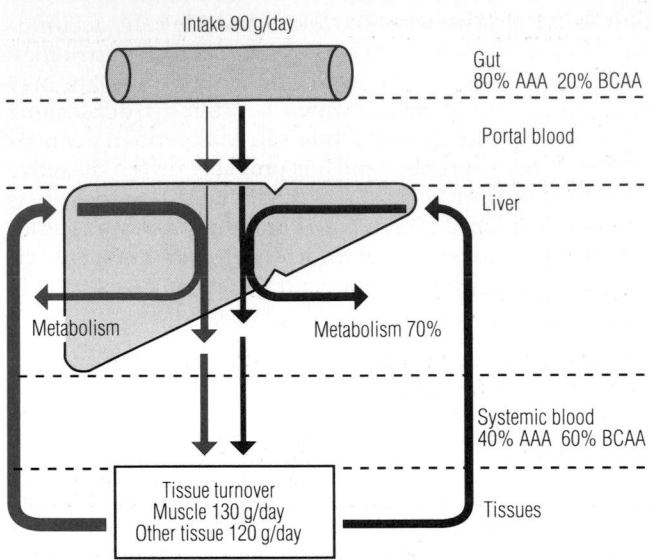

Fig. 16.4 Amino acid and protein metabolism in health. Branched chain amino acids (BCAA), marked in red, constitute only 20% of the dietary intake, while aromatic amino acids (AAA), marked in black, make up 80%. The liver preferentially metabolises AAA rather than BCAA which are passed to the tissues (particularly muscles). The thickness of the red and black lines represents the relative amounts of the amino acids in the different body compartments.

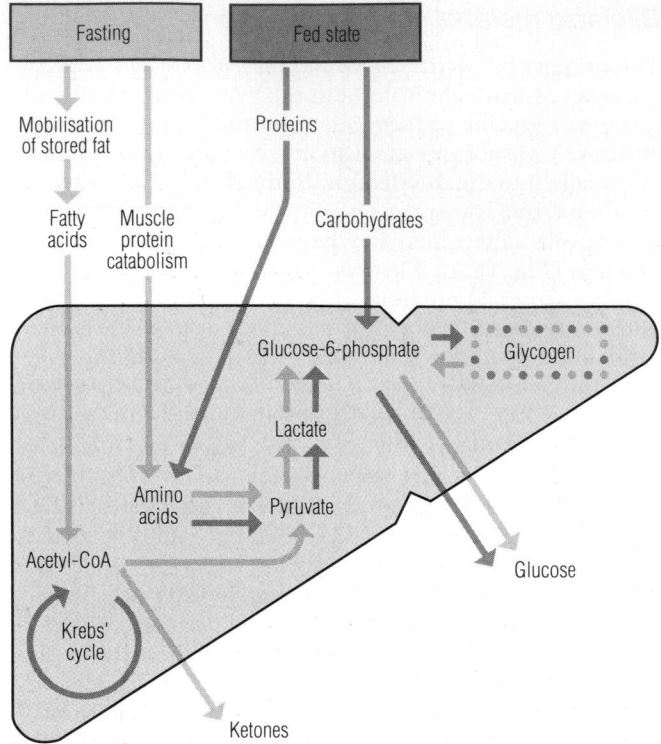

Fig. 16.5 The main routes of carbohydrate metabolism in the fed state and fasting.

disease and are discussed as liver function tests on page 619. Since albumin is also the most important mediator of the plasma colloid osmotic pressure, the fall in albumin concentration which accompanies chronic liver disease is of relevance to the pathophysiology of ascites, one of the frequent complications of cirrhosis (p. 645).

Carbohydrate metabolism

The liver acts as a gate for the large amounts of glucose delivered from the gut during digestion, by storing it as glycogen, and is also the main source of glucose during starvation. Initially, glycogenolysis is the principal metabolic pathway used, but, as the glycogen stores become depleted, gluconeogenesis assumes greater importance. The main substrates for this pathway are lactate, pyruvate, glucogenic amino acids (mainly alanine from muscle) and glycerol (from lipolysis in fat stores). In the fed state, about 160 g/day of glucose are needed for those tissues with an obligatory requirement for this substrate, principally the brain and haemopoietic tissues. During prolonged starvation, the brain adapts to ketone bodies as an alternative energy source, and the total body requirement for glucose drops to about 40 g/day. Although blood glucose levels may directly influence carbohydrate metabolism in the liver, the principal instruments for metabolic control are the hormones, insulin, glucagon, catecholamines and glucocorticoids (Fig. 16.5). The fall in

insulin levels during starvation releases glycogenolysis and gluconeogenesis from the inhibitory effects of this hormone, with glycogenolysis being particularly sensitive. The increasing glucagon and catecholamine levels act directly to stimulate glycogenolysis. In the periphery, the relative excess of glucocorticoids compared with insulin leads to increased release of amino acids into the circulation, and high glucagon levels stimulate alanine uptake by the liver.

In liver disease, the supply of glucose by gluconeogenesis is generally well preserved, and hypoglycaemia is only usually a problem in severe (fulminant) liver failure. Glucose intolerance is more common but rarely a clinical problem.

Lipid metabolism

The major plasma lipids, *cholesterol, cholesterol esters, phospholipids* and *triglycerides*, are highly insoluble in water and are carried in macromolecular complexes of lipid and a protein carrier (apoprotein) called plasma lipoproteins. Only the intestine and the liver synthesise and secrete plasma lipoproteins. There are four main classes, differing in size and density, and having different proportions of the main lipids:

- *Chylomicrons* are made in the mucosal cells of the small intestine during dietary fat absorption, and are the main carriers of triglyceride.

- *Very low density lipoproteins (VLDL)* are produced in the liver and intestine and have a core which contains 50–60% triglyceride. Their apoprotein content is low (about 10%).
- *Low density lipoproteins (LDL)* are formed in the plasma by catabolism of VLDL. They have a higher protein content (22%) and lower triglyceride proportion (10%) than VLDL.
- *High density lipoproteins (HDL)* are made to some extent within the plasma, but are also synthesised in the liver and intestine. They have the highest protein content (50%) and lowest triglyceride proportion (5%).

Hypercholesterolaemia is a feature of any liver disease in which there is obstruction to bile flow, whether this is intra- or extrahepatic. The increase is due to a rise in free cholesterol levels. Although total plasma phospholipids are often normal, lecithin levels are increased, due to regurgitation back into the blood from the obstructed biliary tree. Although the elevated free cholesterol levels may also be due to regurgitation, there is some evidence to suggest that the increased plasma lecithin stimulates hepatic cholesterol synthesis. A marked increase in LDL levels, and the appearance of an abnormal lipoprotein, lipoprotein X, are due to the lipids providing increased substrate drive. Among the clinical effects of these lipid changes are the yellowish plaques of cholesterol deposited in the skin (xanthomata) in long-standing biliary obstruction, and the appearance of 'target' red cells in the peripheral blood film, probably a reflection of altered membrane fluidity.

Drug metabolism

The liver is an important site for the clearance of many drugs. In general the more lipophilic and the higher the molecular weight, the more likely the drug is to be cleared by the liver rather than the kidney. Such hepatic clearance usually involves metabolic biotransformation with or without conjugation. In liver disease alteration of drug handling can have clinically important consequences (Ch. 2).

INVESTIGATIONS IN LIVER DISEASE

LIVER FUNCTION TESTS

Blood tests often described as 'standard' liver function tests are not true tests of liver function, but reflect present or previous liver cell damage and biliary obstruction. Although they are useful in differential diagnosis, and may be the first indication of liver disease, they are rarely of diagnostic value alone. Most of these tests are not specific indicators of liver damage and the influence of

Table 16.1 Non-hepatic causes of impaired liver function tests

Cause	Nature of abnormality
Haemolysis	Isolated hyperbilirubinaemia
Adolescence, Paget's disease, osteomalacia, bone tumours	Isolated elevation in (bone) alkaline phosphatase
Enzyme-inducing drugs (and alcohol)	Increased gamma glutamyl transpeptidase (GT) levels
Malnutrition, malabsorption, protein loss and chronic illness	Decreased serum albumin
Fat malabsorption, disseminated intravascular coagulation (DIC), warfarin therapy	Prolonged prothrombin time
Myocardial infarction, myositis	High serum aspartate aminotransferase (AST) levels

disease in other organs needs to be carefully considered when evaluating their significance (Table 16.1).

Serum bilirubin

The main source of bilirubin is the reticulo-endothelial system, where haemoglobin from effete red blood cells is split to haem, then bilirubin. This is lipophilic, and is carried in the plasma, tightly bound to albumin. Uptake into the hepatocytes is mediated by a carrier system in the liver cell membrane, and ligands in the cytosol (Fig. 16.6). Bilirubin is then converted to a water-soluble compound by conjugation with glucuronic acid, and excreted, as the diglucuronide, into bile. Conjugated bilirubin refluxing back into the blood can be excreted by the kidney, but the water-insoluble unconjugated bilirubin cannot. Hence jaundice without bilirubinuria indicating high serum levels of *unconjugated* bilirubin is a feature of haemolysis (increased formation), failure of bilirubin uptake or conjugation in the liver. Excess *conjugated* bilirubin in serum occurs with cholestasis. In hepatitis there is intrahepatic cholestasis in addition to liver cell injury but conjugated bilirubin is found in the plasma since conjugation is preserved even with severe liver damage.

Tests reflecting synthetic function

Serum albumin

Although low albumin levels may be due to malnutrition, malabsorption, increased loss and hypercatabolism, as well as decreased liver synthesis, serum levels can be useful as a guide to functioning liver cell mass. Its relatively long half-life (about 21 days) means that serum albumin is often normal in acute hepatitis, and is of most value in assessing the severity of chronic liver disease.

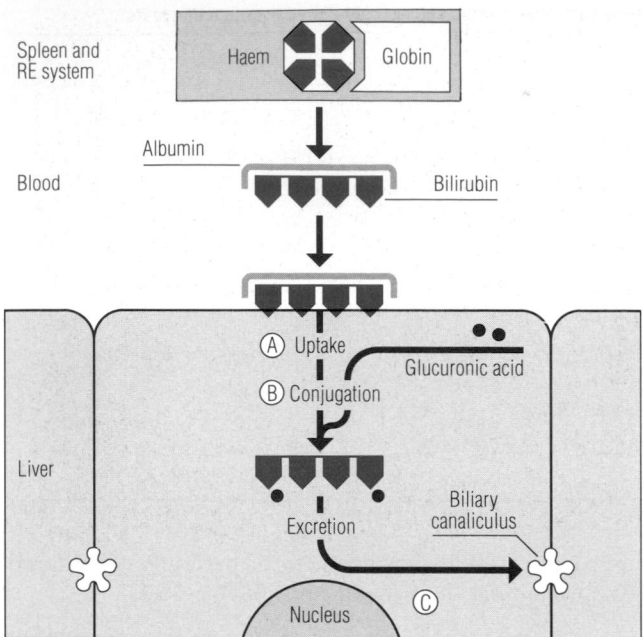

Fig. 16.6 The formation and metabolism of bilirubin. The main sites of congenital defects leading to jaundice are indicated. Failure of uptake into hepatocytes; probably the main abnormality in Gilbert's syndrome (A). Failure of conjugation; the main abnormality in more serious cases of unconjugated hyperbilirubinaemia in childhood (e.g. Crigler-Najjar syndrome) (B). Failure of excretion can occur in some rare congenital causes of conjugated hyperbilirubinaemia such as Dubin-Johnson syndrome (C).

Prothrombin time

The one-stage prothrombin time test is dependent on the function of several clotting factors, many of which are synthesised in the liver (Table 16.2). It is a relatively insensitive test of liver function, but because of the short half-life of many of the clotting factors, it is an early indicator of severe acute liver damage. In chronic liver disease, it tends to parallel changes in serum albumin levels. In cholestasis, the prothrombin time is often prolonged, even though synthetic liver function is intact. This is because several of the factors evaluated in the test are dependent for their activity on vitamin K, one of the fat-soluble vitamins which is poorly absorbed when bile salts are not reaching the intestine. Giving vitamin K parenterally (10 mg daily for 3 days) is, therefore, a clinically useful

Table 16.2 Clotting factors synthesised in the liver

Fibrinogen
Vitamin-K dependent factors (II, VII, IX and X)
Labile factors (V and VIII)
Contact factors (XI and XII)
Fibrin stabilising factor (XIII)

test of liver synthetic function. The prothrombin time corrects completely in cholestasis but remains abnormal in severe hepatitis or chronic liver disease.

Tests reflecting cholestasis

Serum alkaline phosphatase

Different isoenzymes are found in bone, liver, intestine and placenta, and serum electrophoresis can be useful to identify the source of elevated levels. The liver isoenzyme is located mainly in the bile canalicular region of the hepatocyte surface membrane, and high serum levels are a sensitive indicator of segmental or global biliary obstruction whether within or outside the liver. Much of the rise is due to increased production of the enzyme in areas of the liver proximal to an obstruction, together with reflux of a high molecular weight form of the liver type of isoenzyme, the 'biliary isoenzyme'. This is associated with vesicular structures which may be actual fragments of the canalicular membrane. Although high plasma bilirubin levels often accompany high alkaline phosphatase levels, bilirubin values can be normal in spite of markedly raised serum alkaline phosphatase levels. This usually indicates a patchy or incomplete obstructive lesion, with bilirubin being excreted by the non-obstructed areas. This pattern is a feature of space-occupying lesions in the liver, e.g. granulomata, cysts and abscesses, as well as secondary deposits.

Serum gamma-glutamyl transpeptidase

Serum gamma-glutamyl transpeptidase (gamma GT) is a more liver-specific enzyme than alkaline phosphatase and also reflects cholestasis. However, it is less sensitive to biliary obstruction, and an important clinical point is its sensitivity to enzyme-inducing drugs, such as phenytoin, and alcohol, both of which can cause quite marked elevations in serum levels in the absence of significant liver damage. A useful practical guide to interpretation is to compare the levels of gamma GT and alkaline phos-

---

Summary 2 Liver function tests

All non-specific – so consider disease in other organs
Synthesis
Albumin – long half-life, so slow response = chronic liver disease
Prothrombin time – short half-life, so fast response = acute and chronic liver disease
Excretion
Bilirubin – conjugated bilirubin elevated in liver disease, whatever the cause
Alkaline phosphatase – sensitive indicator of cholestasis
Gamma GT – not so sensitive, but elevated with enzyme induction including alcohol
Cell damage
AST/ALT – released from damaged liver cells = active liver inflammation

phatase in serum. In cholestasis, the alkaline phosphatase is usually higher than the gamma GT, while the reverse is usually true in alcoholic liver disease or in patients taking enzyme-inducing agents.

Tests reflecting liver cell injury

Serum aspartate aminotransferase

Serum aspartate aminotransferase (AST) is found in particularly high levels in liver and skeletal and cardiac muscle; serum levels can rise after injury to any of these tissues. High levels in liver disease are classically associated with liver cell necrosis in acute or chronic hepatitis, but membrane damage without cell death may also allow enzyme to leak out into the circulation. Thus, high levels of serum AST can occur in conditions like acute left ventricular failure and septicaemia, in which hypoperfusion and anoxia lead to transient liver cell injury. Correction of the circulatory disturbance often results in a very rapid fall in AST levels.

Serum alanine aminotransferase

Although more liver-specific, changes in serum levels of serum alanine aminotransferase (ALT) tend to parallel those of serum AST.

SPECIAL INVESTIGATIONS

Imaging techniques

Plain X-ray of the abdomen

Plain X-ray of the abdomen may allow an assessment of liver and spleen size, and show calcified gallstones and cysts, or gas in the biliary tree.

Ultrasound scanning

Ultrasound scanning is often the first specialised investigation in patients with liver disease. It enables a rapid assessment of liver and spleen size, vessel size and patency, and the calibre of bile ducts (Fig. 16.7) and cysts and tumours. It is particularly good at detecting gallstones, as they are so echogenic; it may, however, be less successful at detecting some tumours in the liver.

Liver scintiscanning

Liver scintiscanning can be obtained by gamma camera imaging of the upper abdomen after the intravenous injection of technetium-99m-labelled sulphur colloid which is taken up by Kupffer cells in liver sinusoids. Liver and spleen size can be accurately assessed and most

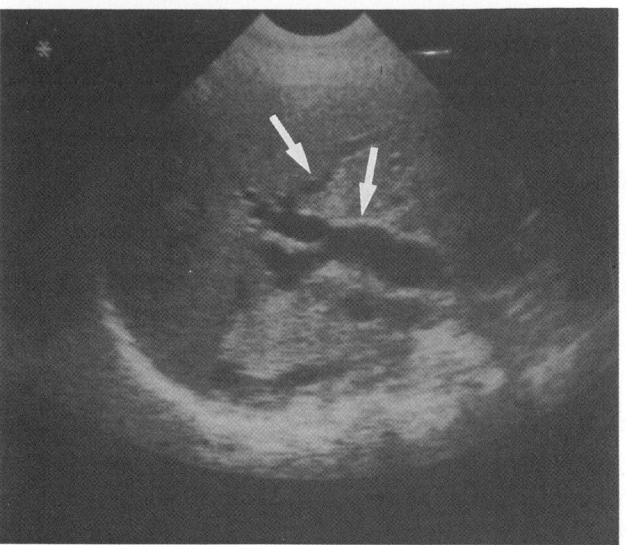

Fig. 16.7 Ultrasound of the liver demonstrating dilated intrahepatic and common bile duct.

space-occupying lesions larger than 2 cm in diameter located. In cirrhosis, effective hepatic (sinusoidal) blood flow is reduced, and other parts of the reticulo-endothelial system, notably the spleen and bone marrow, show markedly increased isotope uptake. Recent improvements in ultrasound imaging have reduced the diagnostic value of scintiscanning.

Computed tomography

Computed tomography (CT scanning) is capable of providing high-resolution sectional views of the liver and surrounding structures in the upper abdomen (Fig. 16.23B, p. 653). Contrast enhancement is of value in further defining the nature of abnormal areas. The technique is best used for cases where ultrasound has failed to provide the expected morphological information, and for examination of retroperitoneal structures.

Contrast radiology

Although ultrasound scanning is the best technique for detecting gallstones and dilated bile ducts, radiological contrast studies are of great value in further defining the morphology of the biliary tree. In some cases therapeutic procedures for long-term biliary drainage and treatment of bile duct tumours have been developed from these investigative techniques.

Oral cholecystography

Oral cholecystography may be used as a screening procedure in patients with suspected gall bladder disease, but ultrasound is usually preferred. Like all procedures which rely on excretion of contrast material by the liver, poor results are obtained in the presence of liver disease, particularly cholestasis.

Percutaneous transhepatic cholangiography

In percutaneous transhepatic cholangiography (PTC), a very fine flexible needle is introduced into the liver substance until a bile duct is punctured. Contrast medium is then injected to fill the biliary system. More widespread use of ERCP has meant that PTC is now not often used.

Endoscopic retrograde cholangiopancreatography

Endoscopic retrograde cholangiopancreatography (ERCP) involves cannulation of the ampulla of Vater via an endoscope, followed by the injection of contrast medium into the bile ducts. It allows excellent pictures of the biliary tree to be obtained (Fig. 16.8) and is the procedure of choice in most patients in whom biliary disease is suspected. Prophylactic broad-spectrum antibiotics are used immediately before the procedure in those with biliary obstruction to prevent ascending cholangitis.

If gallstones are discovered in the main bile duct they can often be removed by cutting the sphincter of Oddi in the ampulla with a diathermy attachment and then pulling the stone through.

Angiography

Clear views of the vascular anatomy of the liver can be obtained by selective catheterisation of the coeliac axis and hepatic artery. This is a useful part of the work-up for transplantation and is also used to detect the abnormal vascular supply to hepatic tumours. Visualisation of the hepatic veins by contrast medium injection after cannulation is one of the most reliable diagnostic techniques in Budd-Chiari syndrome (thrombosis of the hepatic veins).

Liver biopsy

Percutaneous needle biopsy of the liver has been increasingly accepted as part of the routine investigation of patients with liver disease. In experienced centres it is an extremely safe procedure, the overall mortality in one of the largest published series (79 381 liver biopsies) being 0.015%. Nevertheless it is an invasive procedure which needs to be approached with care.

Indications and contraindications

These are listed in Table 16.3. The patient must be able to understand the instructions, particularly to hold his or her

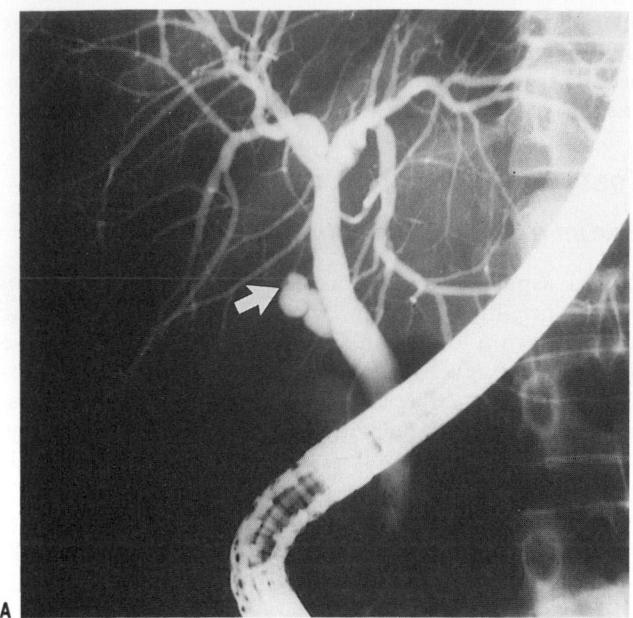

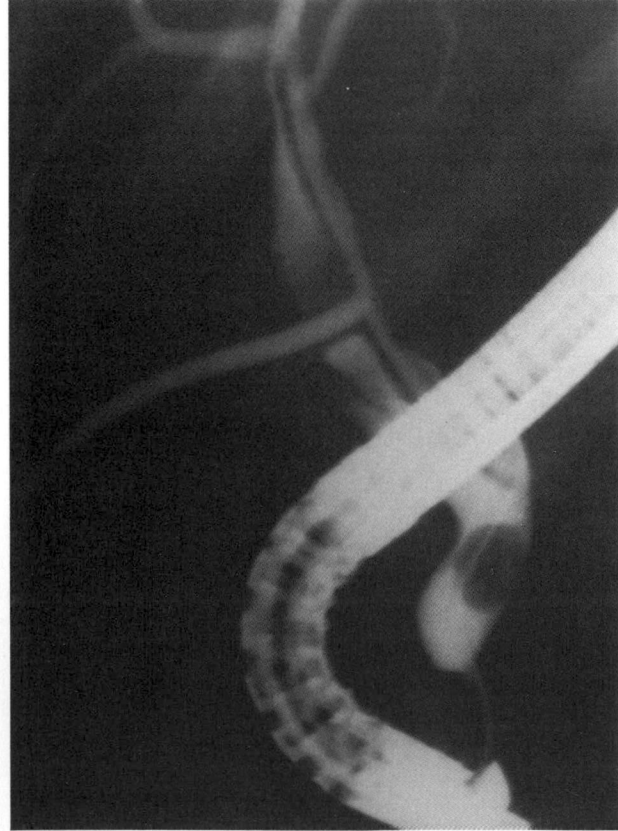

Fig. 16.8 Endoscopic retrograde cholangiopancreatography. A. ERCP demonstrating a normal duct system in a patient who has had a previous cholecystectomy (arrow). **B.** ERCP in a patient immediately following cholecystectomy (note T-tube). There is a stone at the lower end of the common bile duct which is dilated.

breath at the appropriate moment. Determination of the patient's blood group is a sensible precaution, with some serum being saved for cross-matching should transfusion be required. The contraindications (Table 16.3) are not absolute, but in the presence of any of these risk factors the chance of complications is considerably increased.

Technique

Sedation is rarely necessary, except in young children where general anaesthesia is often used. The lateral intercostal route is usually preferred, although an anterior approach can be useful in specific lesions in the left lobe, particularly when combined with ultrasound guidance. Two different types of needle are used: one in which the biopsy is aspirated into the lumen of a large-bore needle (the *Menghini needle*), and one where a core of liver tissue is cut out by a needle sheath sliding over a notched introducer (the *Tru Cut needle*). The latter is often preferred because of the good preservation of the integrity of the specimen in hard fibrotic or cirrhotic livers, although technically the Menghini is easier to use.

After the biopsy, the patient is advised to lie on the right side for 2 hours, and during this time quarter-hourly pulse and blood pressure measurements are recorded.

Complications

Bleeding at the site of liver puncture is inevitable and usually causes mild pain, either locally or at the right shoulder tip because of diaphragmatic irritation. Persistent bleeding into the peritoneum or biliary tree (*haemobilia*) is much rarer and more serious, and laparotomy is needed to secure haemostasis. *Sudden transient hypotension* immediately after the biopsy, probably due to vagal stimulation, is not uncommon. Occasionally it may be dramatic and lead to loss of consciousness but rapid recovery can be confidently anticipated. *Perforation* of the colon, or *puncture* of the kidney or pancreas, is rare, but can usually be managed conservatively. *Pneumothorax* may occur in patients with obstructive airways disease and hyperinflated lungs, and in those who have been unable to co-operate at the time of the biopsy. *Biliary peritonitis* can usually be avoided if biopsies are not performed in patients with biliary obstruction. It is a potentially very serious complication with a high mortality; early laparotomy is indicated. Introduction of a needle into an obstructed biliary tree also carries a high risk of *cholangitis* and *septicaemia*, another reason for avoiding biopsy in these patients.

Summary 3 Complications of liver biopsy

- Bleeding
- Sudden transient hypotension
- Perforation of colon/puncture of kidney or pancreas
- Pneumothorax
- Biliary peritonitis
- Cholangitis
- Septicaemia

THE JAUNDICED PATIENT

Differential diagnosis

Four broad categories of disease cause jaundice:

- prehepatic (unconjugated hyperbilirubinaemia)
- hepatitis
- intra- or extrahepatic obstructive jaundice
- chronic liver disease.

The initial aim should be to use the clinical history, physical examination, liver function tests and special investigations to establish a working diagnosis in terms of one of these broad groupings. This will then determine the next steps to be taken in establishing the final diagnosis and treatment. The organisation of this chapter reflects this clinical approach.

Clinical features

While the jaundice itself is often the dominant feature of the illness for the patient, it is important to explore the first symptoms in detail as these often contain the most reliable clues to the diagnosis. A prodromal 'flu-like' illness with anorexia and myalgia is characteristic of acute

Table 16.3 Indications and contraindications for liver biopsy

Indications

For diagnosis of
  Primary liver disease
  Multisystem disease commonly affecting the liver, e.g. sarcoidosis, lymphoma
  Pyrexia of unknown origin and disseminated infection, e.g. tuberculosis
  Malignant disease
  Metabolic disease, e.g. glycogen storage disease

For assessment of
  Progression of disease and response to treatment

Contraindications

Clotting defect
  Prothrombin ratio greater than 1.3 (not more than 4 seconds prolonged)
  Platelet count less than $50 \times 10^9/1$

Hydatid cyst
  Risk of dissemination

Haemangioma or amyloid
  Increased risk of bleeding

Biliary obstruction
  Risk of biliary leak, cholangitis and peritonitis

viral hepatitis and usually starts from a few days to 2 weeks before the onset of jaundice. A longer history of mild malaise and anorexia (often 3–6 months in duration), associated with weight loss of more than 3 kg, is common with carcinoma of the pancreas. Biliary colic with pain referred to the right scapula and shoulder a day or two before the jaundice suggests passage of a stone down the common bile duct.

Generalised itching is another symptom of considerable importance. It often precedes or parallels the jaundice in patients with biliary obstruction, but is usually absent or delayed in acute hepatitis, only becoming of major clinical importance in those with an unusually prolonged cholestatic phase during recovery. Important exceptions to this general rule are acute alcoholic hepatitis, where cholestasis is sometimes a dominant early feature, and hepatitis associated with some drugs and chemicals, in which the dominant feature is a disturbance of biliary secretion rather than hepatocellular damage.

Pale stools and dark urine are to be expected in jaundice due to obstruction, and in acute and chronic hepatitis. This finding is therefore of no help in differential diagnosis. In contrast, normal-coloured urine and stools in the presence of obvious jaundice strongly suggests a prehepatic cause.

In addition to these general features, specific risk factors should be identified, including homosexuality, drug addiction, foreign travel, contact with jaundiced patients and alcohol intake. It is essential to take a complete drug history. Drug-induced hepatitis can mimic a viral hepatitis, including a prodromal illness, or can present with all the features of a pure obstructive jaundice.

Physical examination

In contrast to the history, which may point strongly to the diagnosis, the physical examination usually gives less specific information. Tender hepatomegaly is often present in both acute hepatitis and obstructive jaundice, while minor splenomegaly is present in a small proportion of patients with viral hepatitis. The finding of a palpable gall bladder is well recognised as a classical sign of carcinoma of the head of the pancreas, but is not often present. If jaundice is due to hepatic metastases, hard, irregular and sometimes tender hepatomegaly is usually a prominent feature. Cutaneous stigmata of chronic liver disease, such as spider naevi, liver palms, leuchonychia and Dupuytren's contracture, should be looked for carefully, since these are important clues that an apparently acute episode may instead be a manifestation of chronic liver disease. Conversely, in acute alcoholic hepatitis there may be signs suggestive of chronic liver disease, including splenomegaly, ascites and florid cutaneous stigmata, but no histopathological features of cirrhosis. Patients that survive the acute episode and remain abstinent can be expected to make a complete clinical and biochemical recovery.

Liver function tests

While it is generally true that the ratio between the serum AST (or ALT) and alkaline phosphatase helps to distinguish between hepatitic (ratio high) and cholestatic (ratio low) types of jaundice, there is a large 'grey area', and the results of these tests are best regarded as an extension to evidence from the history and examination, rather than being diagnostic in their own right. A prolonged prothrombin time is an exception, the response to parenteral vitamin K clearly distinguishing between a hepatitic and cholestatic cause. In isolated hyperbilirubinaemia, the determination of conjugated and unconjugated serum bilirubin levels is of considerable value in confirming a diagnosis of prehepatic jaundice.

Special investigations

The most useful special test in the jaundiced patient is an ultrasound scan. The aim is to determine whether or not the intrahepatic biliary system is dilated, which is one of the most reliable indicators of extrahepatic obstruction. If duct dilatation is detected, it is usual to proceed to ERCP (p. 622). If the ducts are of normal calibre and the history is consistent with an acute hepatitis, then the specific diagnosis should be established with the appropriate virological tests. Liver biopsy is only indicated if there is real doubt as to the diagnosis, or if chronic liver disease is suspected.

UNCONJUGATED HYPERBILIRUBINAEMIA

The two principal diagnostic categories are haemolysis and congenital defects in bilirubin uptake or conjugation.

Haemolytic jaundice

The diagnostic features of haemolytic jaundice are acholuric jaundice (jaundice without bilirubinuria), unconjugated hyperbilirubinaemia and a raised reticulocyte count. The differential diagnosis, further investigation and treatment are discussed on page 1058.

Defects in bilirubin uptake or conjugation

The commonest defect in bilirubin uptake or conjugation (Fig 16.6) is *Gilbert's syndrome*, probably due to defective uptake of bilirubin into hepatocytes and secondary deficiency of hepatic glucuronyl transferase. The condition is of no functional significance, but is frequently the cause of much diagnostic confusion, with 'recurrent hepatitis' being the commonest misleading label. The finding of unconjugated hyperbilirubinaemia, rising further after a 48-hour fast, and a normal reticulocyte count, with no other abnormalities on the standard tests of liver function, is sufficient to make the diagnosis with confidence. A full explanation to the patient is all that is required for successful management. More serious congenital defects in bilirubin conjugation, such as the *Crigler-Najjar syndrome* (Fig. 16.6), can produce higher unconjugated bilirubin levels in the blood and kernicterus in infants, but are rare.

ACUTE HEPATITIS

The term 'viral hepatitis' is often used rather loosely to mean infection with one of the hepatotropic viruses, although jaundice can occur as part of a systemic infection with several other viruses (Table 16.4), or as a reaction to drugs or alcohol. The general features of hepatitis described earlier are similar whichever virus is responsible, but there are major differences in epidemiology and prognosis between the various hepatotropic viruses. Serological identification of the responsible agent is therefore of considerable help in management.

Treatment is generally supportive, and in controlled clinical trials neither bed rest nor low fat diets, which are often advised, have been shown to be of any value in speeding recovery. Similarly, although abstinence from alcohol is usually advised for about 6 months after recovery from the acute illness, there is no hard evidence that this makes any difference to the outcome. There is anecdotal evidence that vigorous exercise in the prodromal phase may increase the severity of the illness.

HEPATITIS A VIRUS

Virology

Hepatitis A virus (HAV) is an RNA virus whose major polypeptides are similar to the enterovirus group (Fig. 16.9). Serologically the diagnosis of acute HAV infection is usually made by testing for the presence of specific IgM anti-HAV antibodies which are present in serum for about 80 days after the acute illness.

Little is known of the mechanisms leading to cell necrosis. The virus is not cytopathic in tissue culture.

Epidemiology

HAV is transmitted by the faecal/oral route and rarely, if ever, parenterally. It may be endemic or sporadic and

Table 16.4 Viral causes of hepatitis

Virus	Features
Hepatotropic viruses	
Hepatitis A virus (HAV)	RNA virus; faecal/oral transmission; 1-month incubation
Hepatitis E virus (HEV)	RNA virus; faecal/oral transmission; 1–2 month incubation
Hepatitis B virus (HBV)	DNA virus; blood and sexual transmission; 3-month incubation
Hepatitis Delta virus (HDV)	RNA virus; blood (and sexual?) transmission; needs HBV
Hepatitis C virus (HCV)	RNA virus; blood and sexual transmission; 2-month incubation
Other viruses which can cause hepatitis	
Epstein-Barr virus (EBV) (infectious mononucleosis)	DNA herpes-type virus, close contact and aerosol transmission; liver function tests abnormal in most cases but jaundice in only 15%
Cytomegalovirus (CMV)	DNA herpes-type virus; blood and close contact transmission, behaves like EBV infection
Herpes simplex and H. zoster	Rarely involves the liver, but may cause severe liver damage in immunosuppressed patients
Lassa fever, Marburg virus and Ebola virus	Rare diseases; imported from Africa; severe organ damage, including liver

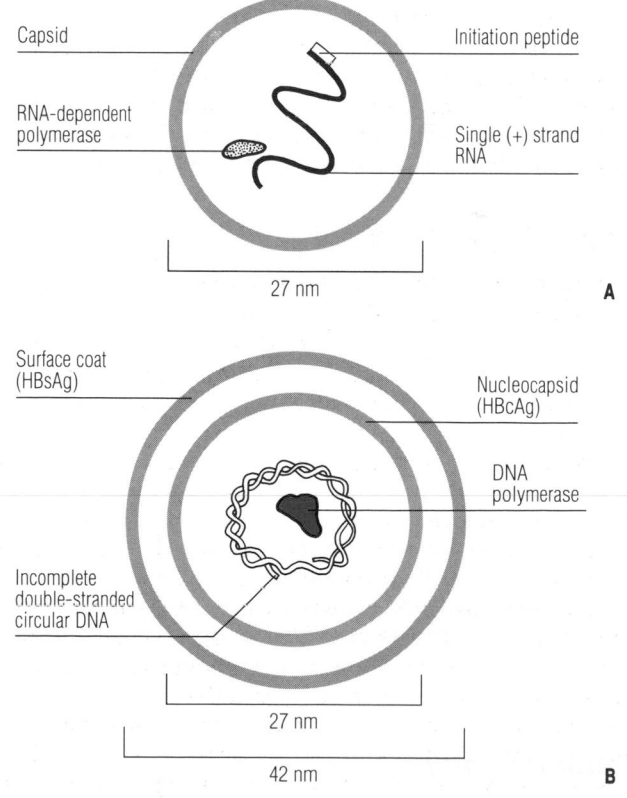

Fig. 16.9 The structure of the hepatitis viruses. A. Hepatitis A. **B.** Hepatitis B.

epidemics sometimes occur. Although direct contact, often during travel abroad, is the usual source of infection, asymptomatic cases are very common and a history of contact is often not obtained. Contaminated food, particularly fresh seafood, is a well-recognised source of infection. The incubation period is about 1 month (2–7 weeks). Carriers have not been detected.

Clinical features

Acute hepatitis A is usually a mild illness preceded by a typical prodrome. This may be so similar to 'flu', with prominent myalgia, that the patient does not connect the prodrome with the jaundice and should be asked about a preceding febrile illness. The patient is most infectious during the prodrome and less so during the first week of the clinical illness. Fulminant hepatic failure is a rare complication and progression to chronic liver disease does not occur. Aplastic anaemia, particularly in children, is a rare complication with a high mortality.

HEPATITIS B VIRUS

Virology

Hepatitis B virus (HBV) is a member of an unusual group, called the HepaDNA viruses. It has an outer and inner protein coat, with double-stranded DNA and a DNA polymerase in the nucleocapsid (Fig 16.9). The main antigenic protein of the outer coat, the hepatitis B surface antigen (HBsAg), is produced in excess during viral replication, and forms large numbers of smaller empty particles in the serum. The complete core protein coat reacts antigenically as hepatitis B core antigen (HBcAg). The core gene of the virus also makes a soluble protein having a different antigenic reactivity, the hepatitis B 'e' antigen (HBeAg), which is also found in excess in the serum. Thus, HBsAg and HBeAg found together in serum signifies active viral replication in the liver, and HBeAg is commonly used as a marker of infectivity.

Each of these antigens can elicit a corresponding antibody response (anti-HBs, anti-HBe and anti-HBc). In an acute HBV infection, the appearance of these antigens and antibodies in serum, and changes in serum AST levels, follow a well-defined pattern (Fig. 16.10). In most cases, HBV infection is detected by finding HBsAg in serum. The diagnosis of acute, as opposed to chronic, HBV infection is best made by testing serum for IgM-class anti-HBc antibodies.

Epidemiology

The main route for HBV infection is by parenteral inoculation, although direct blood transfusion is now very

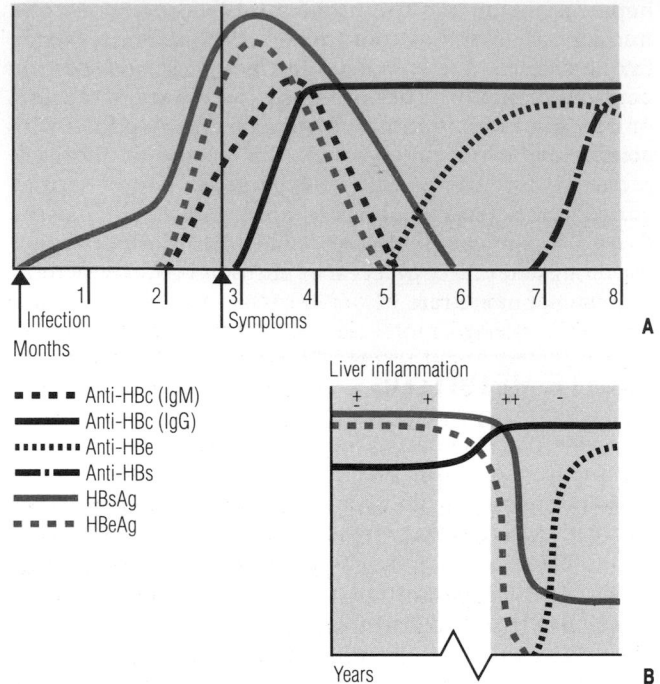

Anti-HBc (IgM)
Anti-HBc (IgG)
Anti-HBe
Anti-HBs
HBsAg
HBeAg

Fig. 16.10 The main serological changes in acute HBV (A) and chronic HBV (B) infection. The break in the x-axis of B has been used to indicate the very variable length of time which can elapse between the establishment of the chronic carrier state and the spontaneous cessation of viral replication.

uncommon following the development of sensitive serological tests to detect infectious material. The virus has a wide global distribution (Fig. 16.11). Chronic carriers are especially prevalent in the Middle and Far East and in sub-Saharan Africa, where they may constitute up to 30% of the population. In these areas vertical transmission from mothers to their children and horizontal spread in early childhood seem to be the principal modes of infec-

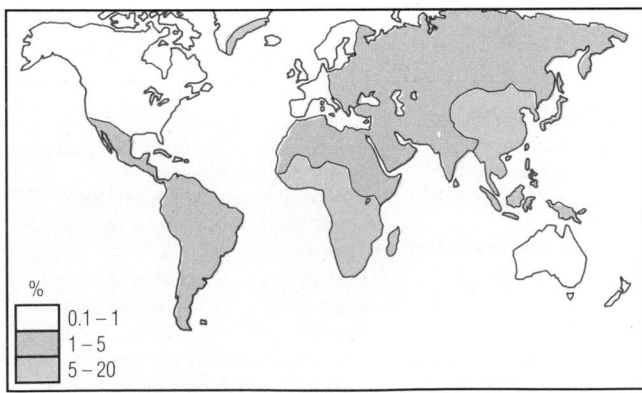

%
0.1 – 1
1 – 5
5 – 20

Fig. 16.11 The distribution of HBV infection in the world as judged by the prevalence of hepatitis B surface antigen in different populations.

tion. In northern Europe and the USA, where chronic carriers are less common and where the screening of blood donations is accepted practice, the main reservoirs for the virus are urban homosexual communities and intravenous drug abusers. The virus seems to be readily transmitted by rectal intercourse.

Immunopathology

Recent evidence suggests that the complete hepatitis B virion has an area of its surface protein coat that resembles the IgA molecule and that this can bind to IgA receptors on hepatocytes. This probably explains the hepatotropism of HBV. During replication of the virus, viral antigens, principally HBsAg and HBcAg, appear on the surface membrane of infected hepatocytes and trigger a cytotoxic T lymphocyte response (Fig 16.12). This is largely directed at HBcAg, and leads to cytolysis, seen clinically as acute liver damage (jaundice and AST elevation), and histologically as spotty necrosis of hepatocytes scattered throughout the liver lobules. Released virions are then neutralised by antibodies probably directed at the region responsible for hepatocyte binding. Complete recovery involves a co-ordinated T cell and antibody response to different viral antigens. Failure of these complex mechanisms results in about 5% of apparently normal adults not clearing the virus, and becoming chronic carriers (Fig. 16.10).

The carrier state is commoner in infancy and childhood, and in those with an associated immunodeficiency, whether this is congenital; due to drugs, as in immunosuppressed transplant recipients; or secondary to other diseases, such as immunosuppressive viral infections in promiscuous homosexuals. The human immunodeficiency virus (HIV) is the most dramatic of these associated virus infections, and AIDS and HBV infection

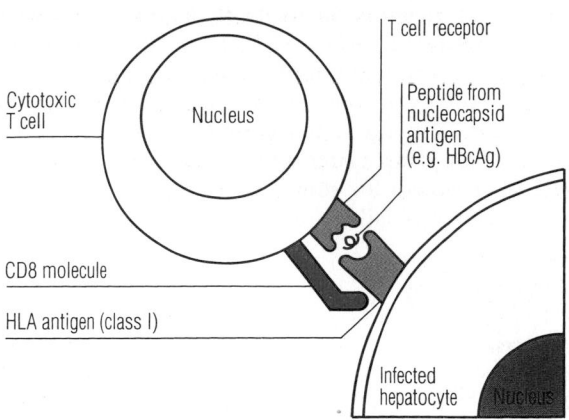

Fig. 16.12 The immunopathology of hepatitis B. Liver cell damage in HBV infection is due to an immune attack by T cells against viral antigens expressed on the surface of infected hepatocytes. The T cells recognise the foreign viral antigens as small peptides bound to class I histocompatibility antigens (HLA class I).

often co-exist in homosexuals. In both these conditions, a reduction in promiscuity is an important preventive measure. In the case of HBV, an effective vaccine made by purifying HBsAg from the plasma of carriers and a recombinant HBsAg vaccine are available for those at increased risk. These include sexual and family contacts of carriers, as well as healthcare workers and children born to carrier mothers.

Clinical features

The prodromal illness may be particularly severe, with arthralgia, urticaria and occasionally a full 'serum sickness' syndrome with associated glomerulonephritis. Fulminant hepatic failure is a rare complication, and the

Summary 4 Clinical aspects of viral hepatitis				
Type	Incubation period	Clinical features	Outcome	*Vaccines*
Faecal/oral spread				
A	4 weeks	Mild often subclinical	No chronic disease	First clinical trials successful
E (Enteric non-A, non-B)	6 weeks	High mortality in pregnancy	No chronic disease	None
Parenteral/sexual transmission				
C (Parenteral non-A, non-B)	8 weeks	Mild often subclinical	20–40% progress to chronic disease	None
B	12 weeks	Variable severity	Neonatal 90% carriers Childhood 10–40% carriers Adult 1–10% carriers	Widely available and in national programmes
D (Delta)	4–12 weeks	Severe in HBV carriers	Carrier on chronic HBV; Recovery in most co-infections	None

main clinical concern is the relatively high rate of progression to a chronic carrier state. The resulting liver lesions are described on page 640. Careful follow-up with repeated serological tests is an essential part of the management. While persistence of HBsAg for more than 6 months is the usual criterion for chronicity, persistence of HBeAg in serum for more than 8 weeks may give an earlier indication of failure to clear the virus normally.

DELTA VIRUS

Virology

This is a small RNA virus with a genome which does not code for its own protein coat; instead it borrows HBsAg provided by a concurrent HBV infection (Fig. 16.13). Serologically, Delta infection can be detected by testing for anti-Delta antibodies in serum. These appear early in the course of the infection but may not persist.

Epidemiology

Delta infection is absolutely dependent on a helper function of HBV, and so is only found in two settings: either there is a dual acute infection of HBV and Delta virus, or Delta virus infects an existing HBsAg carrier. Like HBV it is spread by the parenteral route or intimate contact. It is endemic in countries around the Mediterranean basin, and in northern Europe and the USA is mainly found in drug abusers.

Immunopathology

Clinical evidence and studies in primates suggest that the Delta virus is directly cytopathic to the cells it infects. The contribution of immune responses to cell damage and recovery is not known.

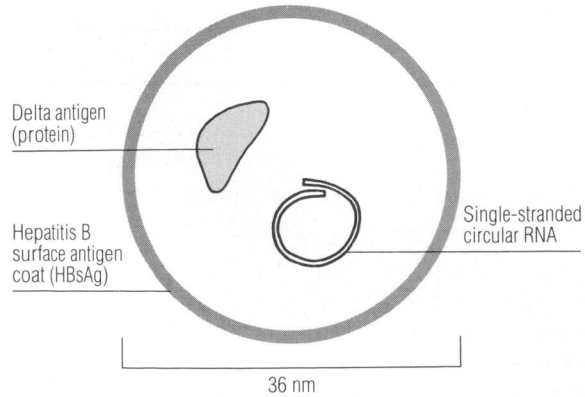

Fig. 16.13 The Delta virus. The Delta virus is a strange structure. It borrows its coat from the hepatitis B virus (HBsAg), so HBV must also be present in hepatocytes. The infective material of Delta is a small circular strand of RNA.

Clinical features

Coinfection produces an acute hepatitis, clinically indistinguishable from HBV infection alone, although there is some suggestion that the illness may be more severe. Recovery from the HBV infection is always associated with the disappearance of Delta. Infection in an HBsAg carrier can produce a severe acute hepatitis, and in some cases fulminant hepatic failure. Chronic Delta infection is also more likely to occur and has a bad prognosis (p. 640).

NON-A, NON-B VIRUSES

Virology

Until recently, when all known virus infections of the liver and possible hepatotoxins had been excluded, there remained a number of cases with clinical features typical of viral hepatitis. The presumed viral agents responsible were called 'non-A, non-B'. It is now known that at least two different viruses are present in this group; one, enterically transmitted, has been called hepatitis E virus, and the other, parenterally transmitted, is called hepatitis C virus.

Hepatitis E

This is an RNA virus which is spread by the faecal/oral route and first came to attention because of a major water-borne hepatitis epidemic in India, initially thought to be due to hepatitis A. It is common in the Indian subcontinent. The incubation period is about 6 weeks and the clinical illness it produces is in most respects like any viral hepatitis. However, there is an unusually high mortality amongst pregnant women who become infected. It does not produce chronic hepatitis. Diagnostic tests for the virus and antibodies to its antigenic components are still in the laboratory stage.

Hepatitis C

This is also an RNA virus. It belongs to the Flavivirus family and is quite common throughout the world. Although assays to detect antibodies to the main antigens of the virus are still being refined, the results of epidemiological studies suggest that the carrier rate varies from about 0.2% in Northern Europe through 1 or 2% in the Mediterranean to 5% or more in the Far East. It is an important cause of chronic liver disease, cirrhosis and hepatocellular carcinoma.

It is transmitted mainly by parenteral inoculation. Blood transfusion was one of the most important sources until the recent introduction of reliable blood tests for the detection of carriers. Drug abusers remain an important group at risk. Sporadic cases may follow travel abroad. Promiscuous homosexuality does not seem to be as important a risk factor as for hepatitis B, and neonatal transmission is also less frequent, possibly because of the relatively high doses of infectious materials required to transmit the infection.

Acute hepatitis leads to chronic carriage of the virus in more than 50% of cases, but the degree of liver damage is often very mild, and it may be many years before significant chronic liver disease is seen. This means that liver function tests alone are very unreliable in determining whether or not recovery has occurred. Serological tests, or detection of the viral RNA in serum, are better indicators of the outcome.

NON-HEPATOTROPIC VIRUSES

Epstein-Barr virus

Liver function tests are often abnormal in glandular fever, but jaundice occurs in less than 10% of cases. The Epstein-Barr virus (p. 231) does not seem to infect hepatocytes and liver cell necrosis is minimal. Recovery is almost always uneventful, although fatigue, as part of a postviral syndrome, can be troublesome for a few months.

Cytomegalovirus

In adults cytomegalovirus (p. 232) can produce an illness like glandular fever, with accompanying jaundice in some cases, but recovery is usually rapid. Liver biopsy, although not required to make the diagnosis (which is made serologically), may show the characteristic eosinophilic nuclear inclusions in infected hepatocytes.

Herpes simplex

Herpes simplex (p. 230) is a rare cause of severe acute hepatitis, usually affecting immunosuppressed patients. There is usually a local oral lesion, but the striking feature is disseminated infection with encephalitis or myocarditis, in addition to hepatitis.

DRUG-INDUCED JAUNDICE

The continued production of new drugs has been accompanied by an increasing problem with drug-induced liver damage (Table 16.5). It is generally stated that about 10% of cases of jaundice in hospital practice are due to medication. There are two main types of adverse reaction: *predictable or dose-dependent* (type A), and *idiosyncratic or dose-independent* (type B). In the former, liver damage is dose-dependent and relatively common, and can usually

Table 16.5 Drugs causing liver damage

Drug	Comments
Antituberculous	
Para-aminosalicylic acid (PAS)	Idiosyncratic type; 1% get drug hepatitis in first 2 months
Isoniazid (INAH)	Raised transaminases in 10%; 1% jaundice in first 2 months
Rifampicin	Up to 4% develop hepatitis; ?increases isoniazid toxicity
Pyrazinamide and ethionamide	Late-onset hepatitis in 1%
Other antibiotics	
Tetracycline	Microvesicular fatty liver
Sulphonamides including co-trimoxazole	Idiosyncratic; mimics viral hepatitis
Erythromycin	Cholestasis; especially estolate
Ketoconazole	Hepatitis in 0.1%
Nitrofurantoin	Cholestasis and chronic hepatitis
Psychotropic drugs	
Monoamine oxidase inhibitors	Viral hepatitis look-alike in 1–2% after about 4 months
Phenothiazines	Mixed cholestatic and hepatitic picture in 1–2% after 2–4 months; can persist
Tricyclic antidepressants	Rare cholestatic hepatitis
Analgesics	
Paracetamol	Predictable liver necrosis in overdose (more than 10 g); methionine/cysteamine antidote
Aspirin	Acute anicteric hepatitis, especially in children; may cause Reye's syndrome
Non-steroidal analgesics	Three withdrawn because of hepatotoxicity (benoxaprofen, ibufenac and aclofenac)
Steroid drugs and hormones	
17-alkyl/ethynyl substituted steroids (including contraceptive pill)	Predictable (dose/duration-dependent) cholestasis, especially the 19-nortestosterones; increased risk of adenoma
Anaesthetic agents	
Halothane	Commonly produces minor increase in transaminases, very rarely fatal hepatitis
Immunosuppressive drugs	
Azathioprine	Rare cholestasis
Methotrexate	Long continued treatment, as in psoriasis, may cause fibrosis and cirrhosis
Corticosteroids	Fatty infiltration
Cardiovascular drugs	
Methyldopa	Acute and chronic hepatitis starting after 2–5 months
Perhexilene	Rare hepatitic illness, looks like alcoholic liver damage
Thiazide diuretics	Cholestatic hepatitis; may be prolonged
Oral hypoglycaemic drugs	
Chlorpropamide	Cholestatic hepatitis in 5%, with granulomatous reaction

be reproduced in laboratory animals. Idiosyncratic cases are infrequent, not related to dose and not usually reproducible experimentally. Recognition of these cases is important for two main reasons: withdrawal of the drug usually leads to rapid recovery, and repeat prescription, which may be associated with a more severe reaction, can be avoided. Over the last 20 years reports to the Committee on Safety of Medicines (CMS) have indicated that between 10 and 24 adult patients have died each year from drug-induced liver disease.

The liver damage produced by drugs can mimic almost any acute or chronic hepatic or biliary disorder. In most cases, liver damage is predominantly hepatitic or cholestatic.

Drug-induced hepatitis

Paracetamol- and halothane-induced liver damage are two examples of drug-induced hepatitis; both are potentially fatal. Paracetamol is a predictable hepatotoxin, while the liver damage induced by halothane occurs idiosyncratically.

Paracetamol

Paracetamol is safe in normal therapeutic doses but produces a severe hepatitis if taken in overdose (more than 10 g or 20 tablets). Liver damage is due to the formation of highly reactive metabolites (Fig. 16.14). At normal dose levels these are inactivated by conjugation with glutathione. Insufficient glutathione is available for

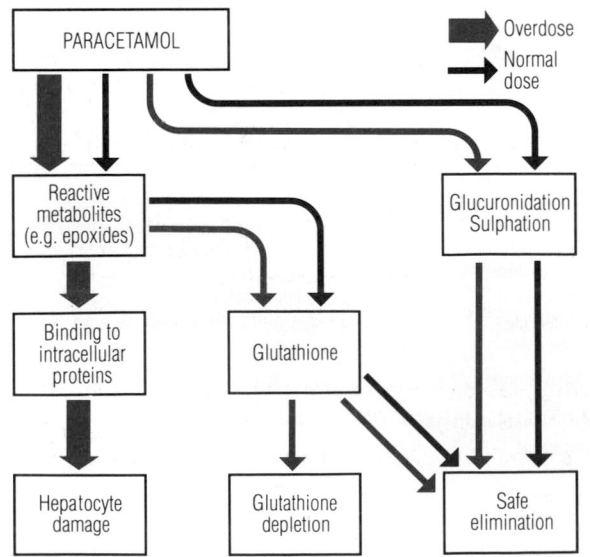

Fig. 16.14 Paracetamol overdose. Paracetamol is normally safe to take because the metabolites are inactivated by conjugation. After an overdose the conjugating material, particularly glutathione, is used up and reactive metabolites damage the liver cell proteins.

detoxification when a large amount of drug is taken, and the metabolites damage the cell by binding to cellular macromolecules. Compounds acting as -SH donors can prevent this process. The most effective and non-toxic of these is N-acetyl cysteine given intravenously (p. 47).

Halothane

Halothane is an example of an unpredictable (idiosyncratic) hepatotoxin. Significant liver damage is very rare (1 in 30 000 halothane anaesthetics), but when it occurs it is often fatal. It is more common after repeated halothane anaesthesia. The clinical picture is very similar to viral hepatitis, with a prodromal illness starting a few days after the surgical procedure. In about one-third of cases unexplained pyrexia has been noted following a previous halothane anaesthetic. Progression to fulminant hepatic failure is common, although the exact frequency of this complication is difficult to assess because of uncertainty about the diagnosis in mild cases. The mechanism of liver damage is thought to be immunological. A reactive metabolite, produced during oxidative metabolism of halothane, alters the normal antigens on the liver cell membrane. In patients with halothane hepatitis these new antigens have been shown to stimulate an immune response, which may produce the liver damage. The idiosyncrasy seems to be related to the ability of the immune system to recognise these subtle antigenic alterations.

Drug-induced cholestasis

The cholestatic jaundice induced by C17 substituted testosterone derivatives and chlorpromazine are examples of predictable and idiosyncratic hepatotoxicity.

C17 substituted testosterone derivatives

C17 substituted testosterone derivatives produce liver damage by direct hepatotoxicity. The agents include androgenic and anabolic steroids, progestogens and oestrogens. The cholestatic effect is dose-related. The obstructive jaundice resolves following cessation of treatment. Histologically, there is evidence of centrilobular cholestasis, without obvious hepatocellular damage. The exact mechanism is unknown.

Chlorpromazine

Chlorpromazine is a rather dramatic example of an idiosyncratic reaction. About 1–2% of those taking this drug develop a severe cholestasis, which may persist for weeks after the drug has been withdrawn. The reaction has been described following only one dose. The mechanism responsible for the cholestasis is unknown.

FULMINANT HEPATIC FAILURE

Pathophysiology

Rarely, liver damage in the course of acute hepatitis is very severe, and leads to secondary disturbance of function in other organ systems. This complex and potentially serious development is recognised clinically as fulminant hepatic failure. *Encephalopathy* is the commonest and most obvious complication. Although the exact cause is unknown, potential factors include release of toxins from the damaged liver, failure to detoxify metabolites and alterations in cerebral neurotransmitters due to amino acid imbalances (p. 648). *Renal failure* is also common and carries a particularly bad prognosis. It may be due to endotoxaemia or septicaemia.

Epidemiology

Fulminant hepatic failure is a rare complication of almost any of the causes of acute hepatitis. About half the cases in the UK are due to paracetamol poisoning, with most of the remainder being associated with a hepatitis virus infection (about one-third each of A, B and non-A, non-B). A small proportion are due to other drugs such as halothane, isoniazid and rifampicin. In France ingestion of the poisonous mushroom *Amanita phalloides* is an important cause.

Clinical features

Patients will develop the signs of fulminant hepatic failure within 8 weeks of the onset of the illness and have no previous history of liver disease. This distinguishes fulminant hepatic failure from rapidly progressive chronic liver disease. The first signs of the disease often relate to the encephalopathy with the appearance of mild confusion, irrational behaviour or even euphoria. A confusing early feature can be an agitated noisy phase, when the use of sedatives may seem necessary but must be avoided. A widely fluctuating but progressive deterioration in mental condition then follows, leading to coma. The usual grading of the level of coma is according to a four-stage model (Table 16.6). In some rapidly progressive cases, jaundice may never be apparent and the whole illness, from first symptoms to death, may last less than a week. Important signs on examination include fetor hepaticus (a rather sweet and sickly odour on the breath), a flapping tremor (asterixis), slurred speech, and difficulty in writing and copying simple diagrams (constructional apraxia). At this stage, serum aminotransferase (AST or ALT) is often elevated by 40-fold or more, and the prothrombin time is usually prolonged more than 20 seconds. In the early stages of grade IV coma, hyperventilation is common, and the pupils are dilated and react sluggishly to light. Hyper-

Table 16.6 Grades of coma in liver failure

Grade	Clinical features
I	Slowness of mentation and affect, fluctuant mild confusion; reversed sleep rhythm; slurred speech; alternating euphoria and depression; untidiness
II	Accentuation of Grade I; inappropriate behavior; drowsy
III	Marked confusion; sleeps most of the time but rousable; incoherent speech
IV	Unrousable; may or may not respond to noxious stimuli

tonia and grasp reflex are readily elicited, and in deep coma, decerebrate postures are seen. Terminally, the oculovestibular reflex is lost and hypotension, cardiac arrhythmias and respiratory arrest occur.

Complications and management

Complications and management of acute liver failure are listed in Table 16.7. Treatment consists of skilled supportive therapy based on a sound knowledge of the expected course of the disease and its complications. Admission to an intensive care area is essential. The encephalopathy is treated by withdrawal of dietary protein, emptying of the large bowel using a magnesium sulphate enema, and administration of lactulose orally. Intravenous nutritional support is with 10% dextrose. Serum sodium and potassium levels are measured daily and any abnormalities corrected. Hypoglycaemia and hypokalaemia are early life-threatening abnormalities which must be detected and corrected quickly. Erosive oesophagitis and gastritis leading to severe gastrointestinal haemorrhage used to be a major problem, but the prophylactic use of H_2-receptor

Table 16.7 Complications and management of acute liver failure

Problem	Treatment
Coma	Lactulose, neomycin and magnesium sulphate enemas to reduce gut ammonia load
Cerebral oedema	Mannitol infusions given promptly reverse pressure rises
Nutrition, fluid and electrolytes	10% dextrose into a central vein; extra potassium needed; low sodium is usually dilutional
Renal failure	Common problem; half have 'functional renal failure', others acute tubular necrosis. Attention to fluid balance may help, but dialysis may be needed
Gastrointestinal haemorrhage	H_2-receptor antagonists significantly reduce risk, and are given routinely
Respiratory failure	Common late complication. Intubate early to protect airway

antagonists has proved very effective. Renal failure is common, and haemodialysis may be needed. Coagulation disorders are also common, due to failure of synthesis of clotting factors and, in some cases, the occurrence of disseminated intravascular coagulation (p. 1113). Fresh frozen plasma is the usual treatment for the clotting disturbance. Cerebral oedema is an important cause of death, and mannitol infusions are useful in reducing increased intracranial pressure. Liver support systems based on charcoal haemoperfusion, with prostacyclin infusion to reduced platelet consumption and improve biocompatibility, are being developed but have not yet been evaluated in controlled clinical trials. Liver transplantation is an increasingly common treatment for the most severe cases.

The mortality of fulminant hepatic failure is high: greater than 80% in those who develop grade IV encephalopathy. However, survivors rarely develop cirrhosis or chronic liver disease, probably because of the remarkable regenerative capacity of the liver.

JAUNDICE IN PREGNANCY

Two causes of jaundice are peculiar to pregnancy.

Cholestasis of pregnancy

Cholestasis of pregnancy is a rare condition, in which pruritus, with or without painless jaundice, occurs in the last trimester of pregnancy. Some women taking the oral contraceptive pill seem to develop a similar condition, suggesting that it represents an unusual response to high oestrogen levels. The itching usually responds to cholestyramine. The symptoms disappear following the birth, and liver function tests return to normal. The cholestasis tends to recur with each pregnancy.

Acute fatty liver of pregnancy

Acute fatty liver of pregnancy is a serious but rare condition. It presents in the last trimester with a prodromal illness which is similar to acute viral hepatitis, and which starts about a week before the jaundice appears. The histological changes are quite distinct from viral hepatitis. There is a widespread, centrilobular, microvesicular fatty change in hepatocytes. The aetiology is unknown, although identical changes are rarely seen following tetracycline treatment. Serum transaminases are usually very high, and the prothrombin time is markedly prolonged. Maternal and fetal mortality is high, even with full intensive care support. Urgent delivery is recommended, as dramatic recovery can occur in some cases following the birth.

Neonatal hepatitis

Jaundice due to increased plasma levels of unconjugated bilirubin occurs in up to 90% of healthy newborn infants, and in most is due to a temporary inefficiency of hepatic excretion of bilirubin. Conjugated hyperbilirubinaemia in infancy is always pathological. Neonatal hepatitis, better called the hepatitis syndrome in infancy, is the commonest cause of elevated plasma levels of conjugated bilirubin. The standard liver function tests often show a rather mixed picture of obstruction and liver cell damage. There are many causes, including viral infections, metabolic disorders, bile duct abnormalities and vascular lesions.

ACUTE ALCOHOLIC HEPATITIS

Clinical features

The term 'alcoholic hepatitis' has two quite different meanings. To the histopathologist, it indicates certain specific features found in some patients with alcoholic liver disease, particularly perinuclear eosinophilic hyaline inclusion bodies (Mallory's hyaline) in hepatocytes in, or near to, areas of spotty parenchymal necrosis. An associated inflammatory infiltrate consists largely of polymorphonuclear leucocytes. There may or may not be associated fibrosis or cirrhosis. Although some patients with these changes on liver biopsy are entirely asymptomatic, the pathological features are important as they indicate a greatly increased chance of the development of cirrhosis. This progression occurs in 90% of patients with features of alcoholic hepatitis on liver biopsy if they continue to drink, while complete regression is the rule in 90% of those who subsequently remain abstinent.

To the clinician, the term 'alcoholic hepatitis' is also used to describe an acute illness associated with alcohol abuse, in which deep jaundice, abdominal pain, fever, marked polymorphonuclear leucocytosis, and elevated prothrombin time are the principal features. Cutaneous stigmata of chronic liver disease are common, even in the absence of cirrhosis. Cholestasis is often prominent and may lead to a mistaken diagnosis of extrahepatic obstructive jaundice, and possibly a laparotomy, which can be fatal. The mortality of the condition is high (30–60%).

Both the clinical illness and the pathological changes are commoner and more severe in women, and in people of northern European origin (including America). Although the histological changes can be found in southern European patients, the severe acute clinical illness is uncommon. There is no definite relation to the pattern of drinking or the type of alcoholic drink.

Management

Trials of specific drug treatments have proved disappointing, and abstinence remains the most effective therapy (p. 202).

OBSTRUCTIVE JAUNDICE

As with the diagnosis of acute hepatitis, a good history is the key to identification of obstructive jaundice. While pale stools and dark urine are common to both, the early appearance of itching and, more rarely, high fevers with rigor (ascending cholangitis) are general pointers to extrahepatic bile duct obstruction. The commonest causes are outlined in Table 16.8 and the specialised investigations which may be required to identify the site and cause of the obstruction are described on page 621. An essential early investigation is an ultrasound scan of the upper abdomen. The presence of dilated bile ducts is an almost certain indication of major duct obstruction. Gallstones, which are echo-dense, are also detected easily, but it can be more difficult to comment with certainty on the pancreas and other retroperitoneal structures. In some cases, a CT scan may be helpful. The final determination of the site of obstruction is best made by ERCP or PTC.

GALLSTONES

Pathophysiology

Mixed cholesterol stones

Mixed cholesterol stones are the commonest variety in the Western world, and consist largely of cholesterol crystals with a variable proportion of calcium salts. The main constituents of bile are cholesterol, phospholipids and bile salts. The ratio between cholesterol and the other constituents is crucial in maintaining cholesterol in solution. Bile supersaturated with cholesterol can develop because of an increased cholesterol concentration, or decreased bile salt content. These changes in the constituents can be due to altered rates of secretion, either congenital or acquired, or changes in the relative proportions during concentration and storage of bile in the gall bladder.

Pigment stones

Pigment stones consist of bilirubin and salts such as phosphates and carbonates. They are common in the Far East. Increased delivery of bilirubin in chronic haemolytic anaemias is a frequent cause in the UK, while in the Far East parasitic and bacterial infection of the bile is the usual causative factor. These organisms promote the

Table 16.8 Causes of obstructive jaundice

Intrahepatic	
Metabolic/unknown cause	Liver damage
Pregnancy	Primary biliary cirrhosis
Contraceptive pill;	Late viral hepatitis
Methyltestosterone	Alcoholic hepatitis
Parenteral nutrition	Biliary hypoplasia
Lymphoma	Secondary deposits
Benign recurrent	
intrahepatic, and post-	
operative cholestasis	

Extrahepatic	
Benign	Malignant
Gallstones in bile duct	Carcinoma of the gall bladder
Post-traumatic structure	Carcinoma of the bile duct
Sclerosing cholangitis	Hilar lymphadenopathy
Biliary atresia	Carcinoma of the ampulla of Vater
Choledochal cyst	Carcinoma of the pancreas
Acute and chronic	
pancreatitis	
Retroperitoneal fibrosis	
Ascending cholangitis	
Haemobilia	

formation of insoluble deconjugated bilirubin by the release of enzymes such as glucuronidase.

Epidemiology

The epidemiology of gallstone disease is changing. Cholesterol gallstones occur more often in women than in men (Fig. 16.15), and the prevalence increases with age, obesity and parity. Other suggested risk factors are diet (a vegetarian diet appears protective), a positive family history, low social class, and use of oral contraceptives. There are marked racial differences in prevalence, with American Indians being particularly susceptible. There is a predisposition to cholesterol stone formation in patients

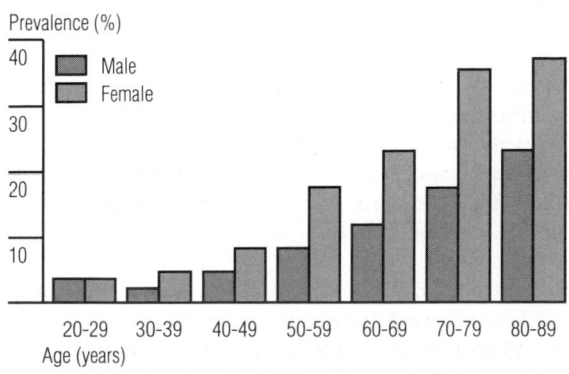

Fig. 16.15 The increasing prevalence of gallstones with age in both men and women.

with chronic liver disease where there is reduced excretion of bile salts, and also in patients with a resection or disease of the terminal ileum. In these cases there is reduced bile salt re-absorption from the gut and a consequent fall in bile salt excretion into the bile.

Detection

Only 10% of cholesterol gallstones contain enough calcium salts to be visualised on plain X-ray of the abdomen. Ultrasound is replacing oral cholecystography as the investigation of choice to detect stones in the gall bladder. Several studies have shown that, using ultrasound, stones can be detected with an accuracy of more than 95%.

Clinical features

Stones in the gall bladder are a common incidental finding and, if they remain there, may never give rise to symptoms. Stones in the biliary tree may cause biliary colic. Impaction in the cystic duct followed by infection produces acute cholecystitis, while passage down the common bile duct produces biliary colic, obstructive jaundice and cholangitis.

Acute cholecystitis

The presenting symptoms of acute cholecystitis are malaise, anorexia and pyrexia, with pain in the right hypochondrium sometimes radiating to the right shoulder. There is guarding and rigidity in the right upper quadrant. Tenderness on inspiration over the gall bladder area (Murphy's sign) is usually present. Jaundice suggests stones in the common bile duct.

A polymorphonuclear leucocytosis is usually present, but does not help in the differential diagnosis, which includes acute appendicitis and pancreatitis. Ultrasound is the best investigation to confirm the presence of gallstones.

There are two different approaches to treatment: either *early cholecystectomy* or initial *broad-spectrum antibiotic therapy* (e.g. cephalosporin with metronidazole), *fluid replacement* and *analgesia*, followed by elective cholecystectomy several weeks later. Exploration of the common bile duct, with operative cholangiography, should be undertaken if there is jaundice, dilatation of the duct or evidence on previous investigations of stones in the common bile duct.

Complications include empyema and perforation of the gall bladder, and liver abscesses following portal pyaemia. Perforation is particularly frequent in the elderly. The signs are those of generalised peritonitis, unless previous episodes of cholecystitis have led to dense adhesions, when a localised abscess may be produced.

Empyema results from infection of obstructed bile in the gall bladder, which fills with pus. There is a very tender mass in the right hypochondrium, with fever and sometimes Gram-negative septicaemia. Treatment is by emergency drainage of the biliary system under broad-spectrum antibiotic cover.

Stones in the common bile duct

Although the classical symptoms of biliary colic, followed by jaundice, might be expected to accompany the passage of a stone down the common bile duct, it is important to realise that a substantial proportion of patients with biliary obstruction due to gallstones may present with painless jaundice. Cholangitis and Gram-negative septicaemia are frequent and dangerous complications, and the diagnosis must be established quickly.

Ultrasound is again of great value in demonstrating a dilated biliary system, and may also show the stone in the common bile duct. It is usually necessary to proceed to cholangiography (PTC or ERCP, p. 622) to confirm the diagnosis, but antibiotics should be given first to minimise the risk of cholangitis.

Treatment is usually surgical, involving exploration of the duct, removal of stones and temporary T-tube drainage. It is best to start antibiotics, give intramuscular vitamin K, and correct fluid balance or electrolyte abnormalities before surgery. Many broad-spectrum antibiotics have been shown to be effective in this prophylactic setting, and cephalosporins with their low incidence of toxic reactions are usually favoured. Mannitol infusion has been shown to reduce the incidence of postoperative renal failure. In the elderly or bad-risk patients, endoscopic sphincterotomy, followed by removal of any remaining stones with a basket or balloon via the endoscope, is an alternative procedure and in some centres this is becoming the preferred treatment for all cases.

Acute cholangitis

In any patient with obstructive jaundice the biliary system can become infected, often with dramatic clinical consequences. Rigors usually accompany a high fever, and this in the presence of jaundice is sometimes known as *Charcot's intermittent biliary fever*, or more simply *ascending cholangitis*. Vascular collapse and renal failure are common complications, reflecting the high incidence of Gram-negative septicaemia. Urgent broad-spectrum antibiotic therapy, after taking blood cultures, is essential, and must be coupled with early relief of the biliary obstruction. A combination of antibiotics active against aerobic and anaerobic organisms is usually chosen. A suitable combination is gentamicin, ampicillin and metronidazole, although it is usually necessary to monitor the serum gentamicin levels carefully as renal impairment is common.

Chronic cholecystitis

Chronic inflammation of the gall bladder is usually found in association with gallstones, but whether or not this produces symptoms, and what these are, is a subject of continuing debate. The diagnosis of chronic cholecystitis is almost certainly made too frequently. The symptoms are often vague, with 'flatulent dyspepsia', fullness in the upper abdomen and excessive eructations (belching). In a sizeable minority of cases, treatment by cholecystectomy does not alter these complaints. Other conditions, like the irritable bowel syndrome (p. 601), can produce identical symptoms. Nausea is the commonest single symptom and is often triggered by fatty food. Gallstones are best detected by ultrasound or oral cholangiography, but are common in older women and should not be used as the sole criterion for making a diagnosis of chronic cholecystitis. Careful investigation of the upper gastrointestinal tract by endoscopy is often helpful. In the elderly, medical dissolution of gallstones with bile salts is an alternative to cholecystectomy, but the rate of dissolution is slow and the stones usually return after withdrawal of treatment.

BENIGN BILE DUCT STRICTURE

Benign bile duct stricture is almost always a consequence of prior surgical intervention. The bile duct may have been cut and repaired, or stenosis may develop after interference with its blood supply, or be secondary to local sepsis.

Clinical features

The usual history is of recurrent episodes of obstructive jaundice, fever and rigors, due to ascending cholangitis. After many months of recurrent symptoms progressive fibrosis and secondary biliary cirrhosis may develop.

Diagnosis and management

Good-quality cholangiography, often using a combination of PTC and ERCP, is essential for diagnosis and planning treatment. Antibiotic cover for these procedures is a sensible precaution. Surgical relief of the obstruction offers the best chance of long-term relief of symptoms, but it is often difficult to find suitable sites in the biliary tree for an adequate bypass anastomosis. Fat malabsorption is common, and should be treated with replacement of the fat-soluble vitamins A, D and K. Sequential use of antibiotics can reduce the number of disabling and potentially dangerous attacks of ascending cholangitis.

SCLEROSING CHOLANGITIS

In sclerosing cholangitis, short strictures form in the intrahepatic and extrahepatic biliary system. It is of unknown cause, although about 70% of cases have mild ulcerative colitis. Episodes of ascending cholangitis and jaundice are common. ERCP shows a characteristic beaded appearance of the bile ducts, and liver biopsy typically shows concentric, onion-skin fibrosis around the bile ducts. Drainage procedures are rarely possible. Corticosteroids and penicillamine have been tried, but are of no proven benefit. The disease is slowly progressive and secondary biliary cirrhosis usually develops. Liver transplantation is now a treatment option.

Carcinoma of the pancreas

A full discussion is included on page 612.

CANCER OF THE BILE DUCTS AND GALL BLADDER

Incidence and aetiology

Tumours of the bile duct and gall bladder have an equal sex incidence and occur most frequently over the age of 60 (Fig. 16.16), when they are commoner than hepatoma. Known aetiological factors include liver flukes (*Opisthorchis felineus* and *Clonorchia sinensis*) and gallstones. The risk of these tumours in patients with long-standing gallstones is about 2%. Bile duct cancer is more common in long-standing ulcerative colitis, occurring in about 1 in 200 of all cases.

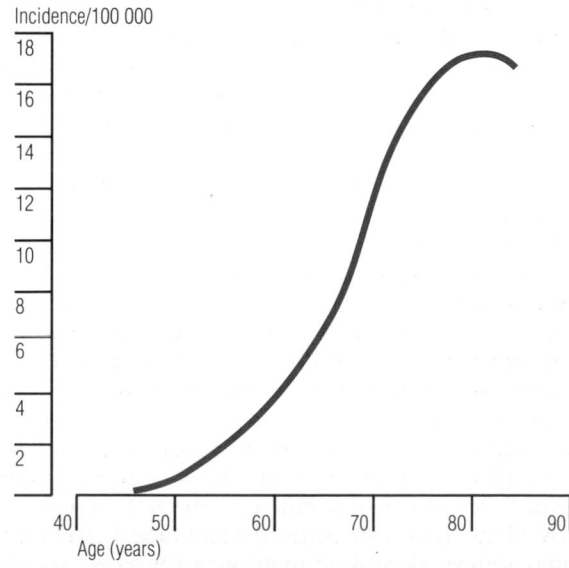

Fig. 16.16 The steep rise in the incidence of gall bladder cancer with age.

Pathology

In the biliary tree the distal common bile duct is the commonest site (50% of cases) and the ampulla of Vater is the most usual location. Of the remainder, 20% of cases arise from the small intrahepatic biliary ducts, and 30% from the proximal extrahepatic duct. Gall bladder cancers usually arise in the body (95% of cases).

Bile duct cancers are adenocarcinomas which usually provoke a fibrous reaction. In the liver they may be difficult to distinguish from hepatoma. Gall bladder cancers are usually adenocarcinomas (85%), with occasional squamous and anaplastic forms. The tumours infiltrate locally and metastasise to regional lymph nodes. They spread to involve the liver by both local infiltration and metastases.

Clinical features

Bile duct tumours grow slowly and cause obstructive jaundice with pruritus. The jaundice may fluctuate if the tumour sloughs and obstruction is temporarily diminished. The gall bladder may be distended if the tumour is distal to the junction of hepatic and cystic ducts. Intrahepatic tumours may not cause jaundice until they are very large. Right upper quadrant pain is common. Carcinoma of the gall bladder causes similar pain, with obstructive jaundice occurring later.

Diagnosis and investigation

The presentation with pain may lead to a diagnosis of gallstones. A palpable mass usually means the tumours are inoperable. With gall bladder cancer, ultrasound and CT scanning may show a mass, but the diagnosis is frequently made at laparotomy. With bile duct cancer, PTC is usually carried out before surgery and will show the dilated proximal ducts and the upper limit of the block. ERCP may be used to demonstrate the distal extent.

Management

Gall bladder cancer is often unresectable, and a biliary decompression operation is undertaken when technically possible. Resection may involve removal of part of the liver as well as the gall bladder. Only 20% of carcinomas of the biliary tree are operable, and major resections carry a high operative mortality (10–15%). Biliary bypass procedures are effective in palliation and may be accomplished during PTC or ERCP, with the passage of a cannula (stent) through the site of the obstruction. Radiotherapy can be used to reduce tumour size, and may relieve obstruction and pain for a considerable time.

Table 16.9 Classification and distribution of cirrhosis

Common causes	
Alcoholism	Primary biliary cirrhosis
The commonest cause in the Western world	Broad geographical spread, 90% female
Chronic active hepatitis	Schistosomiasis
Chronic virus infection (HBV, Delta, HCV)	Equatorial and in the Middle and Far East; fibrosis is usual, but cirrhosis is found in
The commonest cause in the Middle and Far East	*S. japanicum*
Autoimmune	
Almost restricted to north European caucasians	

Rare but potentially reversible causes	
Wilson's disease (hepatolenticular degeneration)	Drug-induced
Early copper chelation can reverse liver damage	Methotrexate, methyldopa, isoniazid, perhexiline
Haemochromatosis	Galactosaemia and fructosaemia
Venesection removes iron, improves liver function	Genetically determined metabolic disorders; diet can prevent cirrhosis
Constrictive pericarditis, congenital venous web	Biliary atresia
Two examples of chronic venous congestion, often completely reversible	Early proto-enterostomy can prevent cirrhosis

Rarities	
Secondary biliary cirrhosis	Sclerosing cholangitis
Cystic fibrosis	Neonatal hepatitis syndrome
Glycogen storage disease	Alpha-1-antitrypsin deficiency
Indian childhood cirrhosis	Veno-occlusive disease

CIRRHOSIS

Definition

Cirrhosis (Table 16.9) is an irreversible change in liver structure, the essential features being disorganisation of the lobular architecture, the presence of regeneration nodules and increased fibrosis. The size of the regeneration nodules can be smaller than the size of a normal liver lobule (micronodular cirrhosis) or embracing several portal tracts and central veins (macronodular cirrhosis). These are not separate varieties. The nodules tend to be small when there is active, continuing liver cell destruction, and larger when there is low-grade inflammation and necrosis. The most important pathological distinction is from portal fibrosis, which is a reversible increase in collagen deposition in and between portal tracts.

Classification

Table 16.9 gives a classification of cirrhosis based on aetiology. In the developed countries of the West, alcohol is the commonest cause of cirrhosis (about 80% of cases in the UK), but is relatively less frequent in Africa and Asia. Cirrhosis due to chronic viral infection dominates the picture in the Middle and Far East and in many places in Africa, while both these main causes are common in southern Europe. Whatever the cause, cirrhosis produces common complications (p. 645).

Presentation and general clinical features

If the process causing the cirrhotic transformation is inactive, presentation is usually delayed until portal hypertension and liver cell failure produce symptoms of ascites, haematemesis from bleeding varices, or encephalopathy. In older males, primary hepatocellular carcinoma (primary hepatoma) is a frequent complication, usually associated with an underlying inactive, macronodular cirrhosis. In some cases the disease is detected at an asymptomatic stage during routine physical examination or biochemical screening. Some of the causes of cirrhosis produce more florid liver damage, and may present with jaundice, pruritus or symptoms of other organ involvement before cirrhosis has become established.

On examination, cutaneous stigmata of chronic liver disease are usually prominent. Spider naevi are restricted to the upper half of the body. Possible causal mechanisms are inappropriate vasodilatation or high oestrogenic activity, which are normal features of pregnancy and sometimes found in females taking oral contraceptives. Leuconychia is a manifestation of low serum albumin levels and is not specific for liver disease. The term 'liver palms' refers to a blotchy erythema of the thenar and hypothenar eminences, and may be a visible manifestation of a widespread disturbance in vasomotor tone. Dupuytren's contracture is due to a thickening of the palmar fascia and is particularly common in alcoholic liver disease. A flapping tremor of the outstretched hands (asterixis), best seen when the wrists are extended, is a feature of hepatic encephalopathy. Feminisation in males, with gynaecomastia, testicular atrophy and loss of body hair, is particularly common in alcoholic liver disease and haemochromatosis. It is not due to high oestrogen levels alone but also to more complex gonadal and hypothalamic dysfunction. Female patients with cirrhosis may develop amenorrhoea. Examination of the abdomen usually reveals hepatosplenomegaly, although the liver may become very small in advanced cirrhosis. Ascites may be present, and striae may be a sign of previous abdominal distension. Patients with portal hypertension may have dilated veins on the abdominal wall.

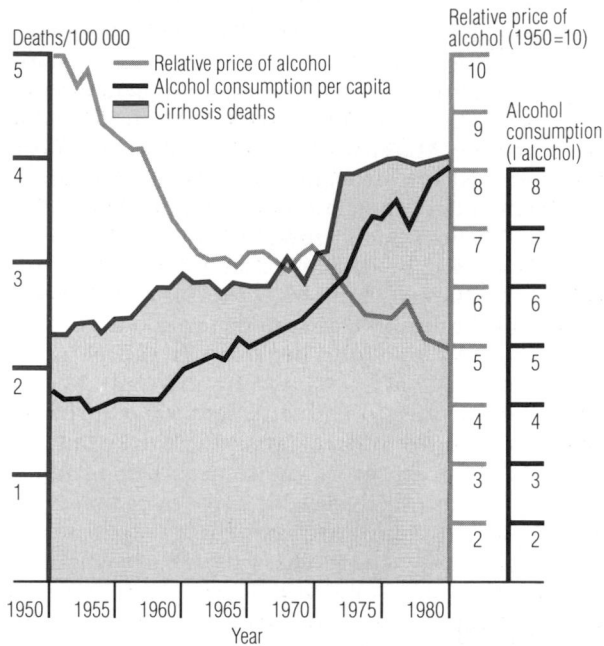

Fig. 16.17 Chronic alcoholic liver disease. The steady increase in alcohol consumption in the UK from 1950 to 1980 was accompanied by an increase in deaths from cirrhosis of the liver, and a fall in the relative price of alcohol as a fraction of average income.

CHRONIC ALCOHOLIC LIVER DISEASE

Epidemiology

Chronic alcoholic liver disease is the commonest cause of cirrhosis in Europe, and is increasing in prevalence in most countries (Fig. 16.17). In district general hospitals in Britain, 80% of all cases of cirrhosis are associated with alcohol abuse. In the USA, deaths from cirrhosis, mostly alcohol-related, increased by 72% between 1950 and 1974, making it the fourth commonest cause of death in white male adults.

Pathology

There is a striking range of histopathological changes produced by alcohol. The most consistent is increased fat deposition (steatosis), which is almost invariably present in those drinking more than 80 g (1 bottle of wine or 3 pints of beer – 6 units, p. 200) of alcohol per day. Although a large proportion of the cytoplasm of affected hepatocytes is occupied by a single large triglyceride inclusion, liver function is surprisingly normal. The fatty change is rapidly reversible during abstinence. In most cases, isolated steatosis does not progress to cirrhosis, although in some there may be slowly increasing fibrosis around central veins, leading to stellate scarring and incomplete septum formation. It is possible that this could eventually lead to cirrhosis. The particular histological changes seen in alcoholic hepatitis (p. 632) are thought to be of fundamental importance in determining progression to cirrhosis. The perinuclear eosinophilic inclusion bodies (Mallory's hyaline), one of the most obvious features, are probably condensed and disorganised fragments of the cytoskeletal framework of the hepatocyte. They are not specific to alcoholic liver disease, but may also be seen in Wilson's disease, primary biliary cirrhosis, Indian childhood cirrhosis and perhexiline-induced liver injury. Collagen deposition is another striking feature of alcoholic hepatitis. It can be pericellular, in the space of Disse, and around central veins (central hyaline sclerosis). This latter lesion is particularly associated with rapid progression to cirrhosis, and is commoner and more severe in women than in men. Collagen bridges eventually develop between central veins and portal tracts, isolating groups of hepatocytes which form the regeneration nodules characteristic of cirrhosis.

Pathogenesis

The metabolism of ethanol to acetaldehyde and acetate is normally dependent on the enzymes alcohol dehydrogenase and acetaldehyde dehydrogenase (Fig. 16.18). These oxidation reactions are associated with the formation of NADH from NAD and alter the redox state of the cell. This in turn has profound effects on lipid and carbohydrate metabolism, one of which results in steatosis. In habitual drinkers, a microsomal mixed function oxidase, the microsomal ethanol oxidising system (MEOS), is increased by enzyme induction, and is also responsible for the production of acetaldehyde. Breakdown of acetaldehyde may then become the rate-limiting step in ethanol

metabolism, and it is now thought that this toxic metabolite may be responsible for the liver cell injury.

The direct correlation, in populations, between alcohol intake and risk of cirrhosis obscures the wide individual variation in susceptibility, for which there is at present no satisfactory explanation. Retrospective analyses of lifetime alcohol consumption in patients with cirrhosis have shown that women develop cirrhosis about twice as fast as men, and that those individuals who have inherited the histocompatibility antigen HLA B8 have a much shorter history of heavy drinking. This particular HLA antigen is strongly associated with organ-specific autoimmunity, and there is other evidence suggesting that immune reactions against Mallory's hyaline, or against new antigens on the surface of hepatocytes, induced by acetaldehyde, could be responsible for liver cell damage.

Diagnosis

The presenting features of cirrhosis and alcoholic hepatitis have already been discussed. However, some cases with significant liver damage are asymptomatic, and liver biopsy is the only way reliably to assess the degree of liver injury. Recognition of alcohol abuse is crucial so that disease can be detected at a stage where abstinence can still lead to complete resolution of tissue damage. Important points in the history and examination are discussed on pages 200 and 624. A high mean corpuscular volume and serum gamma-GT are important clues from laboratory tests.

Management

Malnutrition is common in those with alcohol addiction, and should be treated with vitamin supplements and a high protein diet. Withdrawal from alcohol is best initiated in hospital, where appropriate physical support is available. Fits are best controlled with diazepam, and delirium tremens prevented and treated with chlormethiazole, either orally or by slow intravenous infusion. The drug should be gradually withdrawn over 2 or 3 weeks. Other causes of confusion and coma, such as Wernicke's syndrome, subdural haematoma, hypoglycaemia and hepatic encephalopathy, must be excluded.

Abstinence is the key to successful long-term management (p. 202). Ninety per cent of patients with alcoholic hepatitis alone will show complete regression of the liver damage, while those with cirrhosis who remain abstinent have a much better prognosis than those who continue to drink.

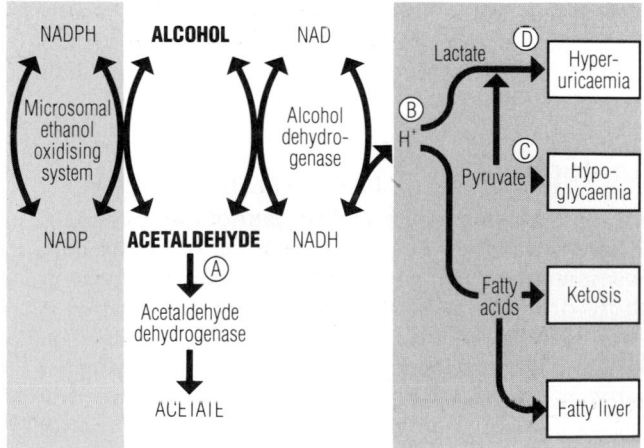

Fig. 16.18 The metabolism of ethanol. Ethanol metabolism largely takes place in the mitochondria. The main product is acetaldehyde (A) which may itself be damaging. Hydrogen ions (B) are an important by-product which can drive many metabolic reactions in the liver cell cytosol to create harmful effects (C, D).

CHRONIC ACTIVE HEPATITIS

Chronic active hepatitis is a syndrome consisting of several different diseases with similar histological appear-

Table 16.10 Classification of chronic active hepatitis

Type	Distribution	Features
Autoimmune		
Classical	Northern Europe, USA, Australia, South Africa	Female/male ratio 7:3; high titre antinuclear antibodies
LKM positive type	Europe	Female/male ratio 1:1; high titre liver/kidney microsomal antibodies
Chronic virus infection		
Hepatitis B	Mediterranean, Middle and Far East	Female/male ratio 1:9; low titre antinuclear antibodies
Delta hepatitis	Mediterranean and Middle East	Endemic in HBV carriers in Mediterranean; intravenous drug abusers in northern Europe
Hepatitis C	Wide distribution	Commonest post-transfusion hepatitis; also transmitted by blood products
Drug-induced	A phenomenon of the developed world	Examples are methyldopa, isoniazid, nitrofurantoin and dantrolene, usually like autoimmune chronic active hepatitis
Metabolic		
Wilson's disease	Wide distribution	Can mimic any liver disease, so easily missed
Haemo-chromatosis	Wide distribution, but note Brittany and Utah Mormons	Usually inactive fibrosis, but rarely resembles chronic active hepatitis, almost exclusively males affected
Alcohol	Wide distribution, but particularly the developed world	Controversial as a cause of chronic active hepatitis; may be in recovery phase of alcoholic hepatitis

ances on liver biopsy (Table 16.10). Portal tracts are enlarged, and contain a chronic inflammatory cell infiltrate of lymphocytes, plasma cells and macrophages. The cells extend beyond the edges of the portal tracts, through the limiting plate of periportal hepatocytes, and there is 'piecemeal necrosis' of liver cells in this part of the lobule. Collagen deposition is prominent in areas of liver cell damage, leading to formation of fibrous septa linking portal tracts to each other and to central veins. If the disease process continues unchecked, cirrhosis is an inevitable consequence.

AUTOIMMUNE

Aetiology and pathogenesis

Autoimmune chronic active hepatitis is the commonest cause of the syndrome in northern Europe and Australia, and was the first to be described. It is best considered as one of the organ-specific autoimmune diseases. There are two main subtypes. In the classical variety women are affected more commonly than men and antinuclear and/or smooth muscle antibodies are commonly found in the serum, while the other variety is characterised by the findings of a liver/kidney microsomal antibody in serum which reacts with one of the p450 microsomal liver enzymes. In both forms of the disease serum globulin and IgG levels are high, and there is evidence of both cellular and humoral liver-specific autoimmune reactions directed at normal antigens on the surface of hepatocytes. HLA B8 and DR3 antigens are found in a high proportion of cases.

Antibodies reacting with liver cell membrane components are almost always present, and probably damage hepatocytes in co-operation with cytotoxic lymphocytes bearing Fc receptors for the antibody molecules. There is a profound disturbance in immunoregulation associated with functionally abnormal suppressor T cells.

Clinical features

Two-thirds of patients present with an illness indistinguishable from acute viral hepatitis, although the causative agent is not usually identified. The remainder have symptoms due to an already established cirrhosis, such as ascites, haematemesis from bleeding varices, or encephalopathy. Half of those with an initial acute hepatitis remain jaundiced and have biochemical evidence of continued liver necrosis. The others appear to recover normally, but develop a second episode of jaundice some months later. Multisystem involvement is common, and includes arthralgia, ulcerative colitis, autoimmune thyroid disease and haemolytic anaemia. Cutaneous stigmata of chronic liver disease are often present, and more than 70% of patients already have cirrhosis when the diagnosis is first made.

Investigations

Liver function tests usually show a hepatitic picture with high serum transaminases. A marked elevation in the total globulin (more than 40 g/l), with a high IgG, is a useful pointer to this subgroup. The diagnosis is made on liver biopsy, while the presence of the appropriate non-organ-specific autoantibodies indicates the correct classification.

Management

The response to corticosteroids is excellent. The survival rate is greatly increased, with more than 60% alive at 10 years, although cirrhosis, if absent initially, may still develop. Azathioprine in a dose of 1–2 mg/kg is a useful adjunct to steroid therapy and may allow a lower dose of steroid to be used. This can be particularly important in older women who are prone to osteoporosis. Although serum transaminase levels are often used to monitor progress, liver biopsy is useful in establishing the activity of the disease during follow-up. If the disease has remained inactive for more than 2 years, steroid treatment can be cautiously withdrawn. However, relapse is very common (60–80%) and can be severe, necessitating prompt re-introduction of corticosteroids.

CHRONIC HEPATITIS B VIRUS INFECTION

Worldwide, HBV is the commonest type of chronic active hepatitis, being particularly prevalent in the Mediterranean, the Middle and Far East, and tropical Africa. The serology and structure of HBV have been described earlier (p. 626).

Clinical features

Many patients are asymptomatic, the chronic virus infection being detected on screening for blood donations or investigation of other diseases. When symptoms do occur, they are often mild and non-specific, malaise being the commonest; some progress from an acute HBV infection. There is a striking male preponderance. The incidence of multisystem disease is lower than that found in the autoimmune variety. The liver function tests usually show a relatively mild hepatitic picture, with only moderately raised levels of serum transaminase. Antinuclear antibodies are not usually present in serum, although smooth muscle antibodies may be detected in low titre.

Serological markers

There are two phases to the infection. Initially, there is active viral replication, with HBsAg, HBeAg, HBV DNA, and the DNA polymerase of the virus detectable in the serum. In this phase the histological features of chronic active hepatitis are most often present. After several years, there may be a rather abrupt cessation of viral replication, with loss of serum HBeAg, HBV DNA and DNA polymerase. This change is often preceded by a rise in the levels of serum aminotransferase, but is frequently followed by a striking decrease in the activity of the disease, with reduction in the extent of the inflammatory infiltrate in the liver. HBsAg levels in serum decrease because free viral DNA has been lost, but usually remain detectable in serum, probably because there has been integration of the viral genome into the hepatocyte DNA.

The defect responsible for the failure to clear the virus after the initial infection has not been identified. Antibodies reacting with whole virions are absent, which may allow continued viral penetration of uninfected hepatocytes. Cellular immunity to HBcAg on the surface of infected liver cells, which is probably responsible for liver cell necrosis in acute HBV infection, is present, and may be a component of the inflammatory liver lesion. On the other hand, factors must be present which interfere with effective clearance of infected cells. Autoimmune reactions to normal liver cell membrane antigens, similar to those found in 'autoimmune' chronic active hepatitis, can be demonstrated, which could explain the similarity of the periportal histological changes in two diseases with quite distinct aetiological backgrounds.

Management

Corticosteroids are of no benefit in the phase of active viral replication, and may be harmful. There is current interest in antiviral agents, particularly the alpha interferons, which appear to act by stimulating existing immune responses against the virus as well as by suppressing virus replication. Although immediate effects on viral replication can be convincingly demonstrated, only 20–40% of cases show long-lasting benefit. Treatment is particularly effective in those with pre-existing active liver inflammation.

CHRONIC DELTA VIRUS INFECTION

The histological changes of chronic active hepatitis are often present in chronic Delta virus infection (p. 639). The diagnosis is made by finding anti-Delta antibodies in serum or demonstrating Delta antigen in the nuclei of liver cells by immunofluorescence. Progression to cirrhosis seems to occur quite rapidly, and the prognosis is poor. Little is known about the mechanisms of tissue damage, and no specific treatment has been shown to be effective.

CHRONIC NON-A, NON-B VIRUS INFECTION

Since a specific serological test for one of these non-A, non-B viruses has only recently become available (p. 628), most of the information on the existence and natural history of this type of chronic active liver disease has come from follow-up of cases with acute non-A, non-B hepatitis acquired from blood transfusion or blood products. The clinical and immunological features are more like those of chronic HBV infection rather than the 'autoimmune' cases. Thus, smooth muscle antibodies may be present in low titre, but antinuclear antibodies are usually absent. The disease activity is usually mild, and seems to become less severe with time. In some cases, cirrhosis may not develop. Corticosteroids are of no benefit but low-dose alpha interferons suppress virus replication, and if continued for a year, may be of lasting benefit in some cases.

DRUG-INDUCED CHRONIC ACTIVE HEPATITIS

Although rare, these cases are important, as the disease almost always responds to drug withdrawal. All reported cases are examples of idiosyncratic reactions, which have not been reproduced experimentally. The drugs most frequently implicated are isoniazid, alpha methyldopa, nitrofurantoin and oxyphenisatin. In many cases, the disease is very similar to the 'autoimmune' type, with antinuclear and smooth muscle antibodies present in serum.

OTHER CAUSES

The most important of these is Wilson's disease (p. 643), which can mimic the changes seen in viral or autoimmune cases. Since long-term survival on D-penicillamine is possible, it is clearly of great importance to exclude this condition in all cases of chronic active hepatitis in children and young adults. The histological features of chronic active hepatitis can also be found in some cases of alpha-1 antitrypsin deficiency, and in alcoholic liver disease.

PRIMARY BILIARY CIRRHOSIS

Like chronic active hepatitis, primary biliary cirrhosis is a condition which is not necessarily associated with cirrhosis at presentation, although this frequently develops later in the course of the disease. The essence of the disease is a slowly progressive destruction of intrahepatic bile ducts, possibly due to immune-mediated injury.

Incidence and aetiology

In most series more than 90% of patients are women, with most being in middle age. In the UK the incidence is between 6 and 12 per million, with a prevalence of 40–80 per million. There is no definite HLA association but familial cases are well described. The antibodies in serum reacting with mitochondria, which are such a strong feature of the disease, are also found in family members, but in most cases there is no apparent liver or bile duct injury associated with this finding. There is one report of the disease developing in a daughter, her mother and a close friend who nursed the daughter, suggesting that environmental factors may play a role. This is supported by the finding that, in Sheffield, 90% of the patients came from an area of the city with only 4% of the population, and were supplied with water from one reservoir.

Pathology

Four stages in the histopathology of the disease have been described. They are not necessarily sequential, and there is considerable overlap between them.

1. *First stage.* There is focal damage to the larger intrahepatic bile ducts, with a surrounding chronic inflammatory infiltrate of lymphocytes, plasma cells, eosinophils and macrophages. In some areas the infiltrate may be organised into an epithelioid cell granuloma, lying close to a damaged duct.
2. *Second stage.* Some of the larger ducts are replaced by lymphoid aggregates, and there is proliferation of smaller ductules. Fibrosis is present.
3. *Third stage.* Fibrosis extends beyond the edges of the portal tracts. There is often periportal cholestasis and accumulation of copper-binding proteins.
4. *Final stage.* The features are those of an established cirrhosis. Ill-defined collections of lymphocytes and a paucity of bile ducts may be the only clues to the aetiology.

Immunopathogenesis

Antimitochondrial antibodies are directed at an antigen on the inner membrane of the mitochondrium, and are unlikely to be of pathogenetic importance. However, they are clearly an important feature of the disease. An attractive but unproven hypothesis is that they are cross-reactive antibodies generated by an immune response to an as yet unidentified bacterium which is in some way responsible for the bile duct destruction. This hypothesis has been reinforced by the finding that the antimitochondrial antibodies are directed at the pyruvate dehydrogenase complex and cross-react extensively with the corresponding bacterial enzyme complex in *E. coli*. Granulomas are usually indicative of a cellular immune reaction, but it is not clear what the antigenic stimulus could be. T cells sensitised to antigenic components in bile ducts may be responsible for their destruction. The disease in other organs may be an indication of a generalised disturbance in immunoregulation, but could also be due to an observed antigenic cross-reactivity between bile duct antigens and secretory duct epithelium in other organs.

Clinical features

The disease is much commoner (9:1) in females than males, and usually presents in the fifth and sixth decades. Pruritus is often the first symptom, and may lead to a dermatological consultation. Weight is usually well maintained and abdominal pain is unusual. Jaundice is a late feature. On examination there is often quite marked hepatosplenomegaly and skin pigmentation. Skin xanthomas are common.

With the increasing availability of automated biochemical profiles, and screening tests for non-organ-specific auto-antibodies in serum, asymptomatic cases are being seen more frequently. In these patients, minor hepatomegaly may be the only abnormality.

The most striking serological feature is the presence of antimitochondrial antibodies in serum. These are of considerable help in the differential diagnosis, as they are found in 95% of patients with primary biliary cirrhosis, but are usually absent in prolonged extrahepatic obstruction.

Associated diseases

Disease in other organs is very common, and includes one or more of the components of the CRST syndrome (calcinosis, Raynaud's phenomenon, sclerodactyly, telangiectasia), autoimmune thyroiditis, renal tubular acidosis, rheumatoid arthritis and the 'sicca complex' (dry eyes and dry mouth).

Course and management

In symptomatic cases, average survival is 6 years, but it is difficult to give an accurate prognosis in individual cases. The bile duct destruction is slowly progressive, but bilirubin levels usually remain stable for several years, before rising steadily in the last year or two of the illness. Steatorrhoea with malabsorption of fat-soluble vitamins can be a problem, and it is important to give supplements of calcium and vitamins D and K. Cholestyramine usually controls pruritus. Corticosteroids are not usually given because of the likely exacerbation of osteoporosis in postmenopausal women. D-penicillamine has several potentially useful effects, including chelation of copper, which slowly accumulates in chronic cholestasis, interference with collagen synthesis, and immunosuppression. However, controlled clinical trials have provided conflicting evidence of benefit, and side-effects such as skin rashes, nausea and vomiting, proteinuria and bone marrow suppression are common. Cyclosporin A is now being evaluated as a possible therapeutic agent. This is an immunosuppressive drug which acts by interfering with the production of interleukin 2, an important stimulator of lymphocyte proliferation. Colchicine and ursodeoxycholic acid also seem to be beneficial in controlled trials, and in advanced cases liver transplantation is a useful and successful treatment option.

An important finding is that asymptomatic cases often have an excellent prognosis. In some of these patients,

serial observations over several years have shown no evidence of deterioration.

HAEMOCHROMATOSIS

Increased iron deposition in hepatocytes is the hallmark of haemochromatosis. In idiopathic haemochromatosis this is due to a genetically determined increase in iron absorption. The inheritance is now known to be autosomal recessive and is associated with an increased frequency of HLA A3 (75% of patients, compared with 25% of controls). The exact mechanism of the defect in control of iron absorption is not understood.

Haemosiderosis, secondary iron overload, is usually due to a chronic haemolytic anaemia such as thalassaemia. The increased liver iron content is due to both increased iron release and repeated blood transfusions (p. 1075).

Clinical features

There is a striking male preponderance, almost certainly because menstruation in women prevents a significant rise in iron stores. The disease usually presents in middle age. 'Bronzed diabetes' is a useful reminder of two of the important clinical features. The pigmentation is due to *increased melanin* in the skin, and is often seen best over the shins where it gives a slate-grey appearance. Patients may present with *diabetes*, sometimes well before the liver disease becomes symptomatic. It is associated with iron deposition in the pancreas. An *arthritis*, particularly affecting the knees and metacarpophalangeal joints, can also be a presenting feature, and is associated with the deposition of calcium pyrophosphate crystals in the affected joints.

On examination, *gynaecomastia*, *testicular atrophy* and *loss of body hair* are often present, and seem to be due to a combination of partial testicular and pituitary failure, associated with iron deposition in these areas. *Hepatomegaly* is invariably present, but splenomegaly is uncommon. In younger patients, *congestive cardiomyopathy* can be an unusual but troublesome complication.

Diagnosis

Liver function tests can be entirely normal and haemochromatosis is a good example of a disease which must be considered before it can be diagnosed. Liver biopsy allows demonstration of the iron deposition in liver cells, usually in a periportal distribution. Extensive portal fibrosis develops before there is progression to a true cirrhosis, with regeneration nodules. Serum iron levels are high, with greater than 90% saturation of the total iron binding capacity. Serum ferritin levels are a good reflection of total body iron content, but do not correlate precisely with the concentration of liver iron.

Management and prognosis

Gradual depletion of the body iron stores is best achieved by regular venesection, initially 1 unit weekly. Serum ferritin and a repeat liver biopsy are the most useful markers of complete removal of the excessive iron deposits. The severity of the associated diabetes tends to decrease, and there is a general improvement in malaise and decrease in liver size. The changes of cirrhosis in the liver are not reversible, and one of the long-term risks is the development of primary hepatocellular carcinoma. Venesection is most effective when started early in the course of the disease, before the development of diabetes or cirrhosis, and investigation of the patient's relatives is an essential part of management. Undiagnosed cases may be detected by the combination of HLA A3 and a high serum ferritin. In 1935 the mean survival after diagnosis was 4.4 years, in 1969 the 5-year survival rate was 89%, and as more asymptomatic family members are picked up and treated, it is becoming clear that the disease can be prevented if excess iron is removed at an early stage and future accumulation of iron prevented.

WILSON'S DISEASE

In this disease, genetically determined accumulation of copper in the liver, basal ganglia, kidney and cornea can produce a wide variety of liver lesions with or without associated extrapyramidal dysfunction. It is an autosomal recessive condition with an incidence of about 1 in 50 000. Heterozygous individuals remain in virtually zero copper balance throughout their life and show no clinical features of the disease. Radiocopper studies indicate that the inherited defect in copper metabolism principally affects copper excretion from hepatic lysosomes to bile (Fig. 16.19). Pathologically and clinically the liver is the first organ to be affected. The appearance of lipid droplets in the liver cell cytoplasm is the first abnormality, followed by increasing fibrosis and cirrhosis.

Clinical features

Wilson's disease is a great mimic of many other liver diseases, and because of the excellent response to D-penicillamine in the early stages of the disease, must always be considered and excluded in any child or young adult with chronic liver disease. In some cases there is a combination of fatty change, Mallory's hyaline and fibrosis, which may be wrongly attributed to the effects of social drinking. In others, there is a mononuclear infiltrate in the portal tracts with piecemeal necrosis of periportal hepatocytes,

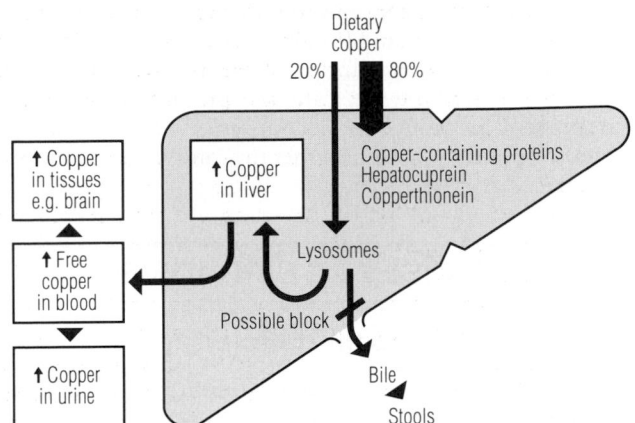

Fig. 16.19 Wilson's disease. The postulated block in copper metabolism in Wilson's disease is a failure to excrete copper from lysosomes into bile. This leads to a build-up of the toxic metal in the liver and other tissues, particularly the basal ganglia in the brain.

which can lead to a diagnosis of non-A, non-B or autoimmune chronic active hepatitis. In children, an 'acute hepatitis', sometimes progressing to fulminant hepatic failure, may be a presenting feature. This may be accompanied by acute haemolysis. At the other extreme, the disease may remain silent until a slowly progressive, inactive cirrhosis presents with haematemesis, ascites or encephalopathy. Neurological abnormalities may be absent in younger patients; when present, they are often subtle. They include deteriorating school performance, changes in personality, slurring of speech, clumsiness and difficulties with fine movements. In adults, dysarthria and bulbar palsy may accompany more classical extrapyramidal signs and symptoms.

Diagnosis

Brown deposits of copper in the margins of the cornea, called *Kayser-Fleischer rings*, are diagnostic. They are always present in patients with neurological symptoms, but can be absent in young patients presenting with liver disease. They are best seen on slit-lamp examination. Serum caeruloplasmin levels are typically low, but may also be decreased in chronic active hepatitis and fulminant liver failure as well as in about 10% of healthy heterozygotes. Urinary copper excretion is high, and rises dramatically after a test dose of D-penicillamine. Liver copper levels are between 1.5 and 25 times the upper limit of normal, but are also increased in some conditions with chronic cholestasis, such as primary biliary cirrhosis.

Management

The chelating agent, D-penicillamine, gradually depletes the copper stores, and is the mainstay of treatment. In cases picked up early, and in those with a relatively inactive well-compensated liver lesion, there is usually some improvement in liver function and no further progression of the liver disease. Patients who present with fulminant hepatic failure or decompensated cirrhosis show little response to chelation therapy, and have a poor prognosis.

OTHER CAUSES OF CIRRHOSIS

Alpha-1 antitrypsin deficiency

Alpha-1 antitrypsin, a protease inhibitor, is remarkably polymorphic, with more than 30 different variants now recognised. The inheritance of these alleles is autosomal and codominant, with the normal phenotype being designated MM. The clinically important variant is called Z. This codes for a defective protein core which has altered carbohydrate side chains, and cannot be excreted from hepatocytes. It can be seen in liver biopsies as diastase-resistant, PAS-positive granules in periportal hepatocytes. Heterozygotes, with an MZ phenotype, have about half the normal circulating levels of alpha-1 antitrypsin, while none can be detected in ZZ homozygotes. It is these ZZ individuals who are susceptible to the development of emphysema (p. 486) and cirrhosis, but the mechanisms responsible are not understood.

The liver disease usually presents in infancy, with symptoms of the neonatal hepatitis syndrome (conjugated hyperbilirubinaemia with pale stools, dark urine and hepatomegaly). At this stage, cirrhosis may already be present on liver biopsy, although varying degrees of hepatocellular damage and fibrosis are more usual. In those who survive, cirrhosis usually develops, and about a quarter will die in early childhood. The clinical course in the remainder may be relatively long, although decompensation can occur in adolescence or early adult life. There is no specific treatment. Some adults with alpha-1 antitrypsin deficiency can present with cirrhosis without a history of jaundice in infancy. In these patients, primary hepatoma is a recognised complication.

Cystic fibrosis

Cystic fibrosis is considered in detail in Chapter 13. There is a generalised disorder of exocrine secretory glands, whose ducts become blocked with viscid, tenacious secretions. The liver can be involved in this process, with mild focal biliary obstruction due to inspissated bile being found in almost all cases. In some, for unknown reasons, this process slowly progresses to a relatively inactive cirrhosis. This is present in about 10–15% of adolescents with cystic fibrosis, and can present with the complications of portal hypertension.

Secondary biliary cirrhosis

Secondary biliary cirrhosis can be a complication of any disease in which there is prolonged biliary obstruction. For example, it may arise as a long-term complication of biliary stricture due to operative damage to the bile duct, or in sclerosing cholangitis (p. 635). There is slowly progressive portal fibrosis, often for several years before the development of true cirrhosis. If adequate biliary drainage can be restored during the earlier stages there may be substantial regression of the portal fibrosis and a fall in portal pressure.

Hepatic venous congestion

'Cardiac cirrhosis' occurs in patients with chronic right heart failure. It is a progressive liver fibrosis due to chronic centrilobular congestion. An important cause is constrictive pericarditis. Treatment, by surgical removal of the pericardium, usually leads to resolution of the ascites and regression of the liver fibrosis. A congenital web in the inferior vena cava at, or above, the level of the diaphragm, is another rare but correctable cause.

A more dramatic cause of hepatic venous congestion is sudden occlusion of the main hepatic veins: the *Budd-Chiari syndrome*. The presenting features, of pain and tenderness over a large liver and tense ascites, are due to the marked elevation in portal pressure, the severe hepatic congestion and liver cell necrosis. In some cases the onset is more gradual, with refractory ascites being the dominant clinical feature. The occlusion of the hepatic veins is occasionally due to obstruction by tumour tissue extending up the vena cava from a hypernephroma, but is usually thrombotic. This may be initiated by trauma, or due to a thrombotic tendency in diseases such as polycythaemia rubra vera, primary thrombocythaemia, paroxysmal nocturnal haemoglobinuria and chronic myeloid leukaemia. A number of cases have been reported in young women taking the oral contraceptive pill, but since its oestrogen content has been reduced, this association seems to have become less frequent. A liver scintiscan can be helpful in establishing the diagnosis. The characteristic finding is reduced liver activity, except for a central area where uptake is well preserved. This is probably the caudate lobe, which often has a separate venous drainage. The patency of the main hepatic veins may be investigated by ultrasound, but radiological contrast studies are more definitive. Treatment is difficult, with control of the ascites being a particular problem. Cases with an acute onset have a high mortality. If the vena cava is patent, liver transplantation should be considered.

Childhood metabolic diseases

Type IV glycogen storage disease, galactosaemia, fructosaemia and tyrosinaemia are all rare causes of cirrhosis in infancy and childhood (see Ch. 19).

CONGENITAL HEPATIC FIBROSIS

Although this inherited condition is not a cause of cirrhosis, the presentation, with the symptoms and signs of portal hypertension, place it firmly in this context with respect to differential diagnosis. The basic hepatic architecture is preserved, but portal tracts are linked by broad bands of fibrous tissue. Increased numbers of bile ductules are seen in the portal areas, and some may appear cystic. The presentation is usually in childhood with hepatosplenomegaly, and haematemesis from bleeding oesophageal varices. Liver function tends to be well preserved, and a portosystemic shunt operation is usually performed to reduce portal vein pressure. The prognosis is good.

COMPLICATIONS OF CIRRHOSIS

Although there is no specific therapy for many types of cirrhosis, skilled management of the complications can often provide prolonged relief from disabling symptoms.

ASCITES

Pathophysiology

There are two main hypotheses which seek to explain the formation of ascitic fluid in cirrhosis (Fig. 16.20). The first, sometimes referred to as the '*underfill theory*', suggests that the reduction in plasma colloid osmotic pressure, due to a fall in serum albumin concentration together with raised portal pressure, leads to a net extravasation of capillary filtrate from the splanchnic circulation. This in turn reduces the circulating plasma volume, and promotes secondary hyperaldosteronism with retention of sodium and water in the kidneys. This theory predicts a normal or reduced cardiac output, decreased plasma volume and peripheral vasoconstriction. The observations that cardiac output is usually increased, that plasma volume is high and that there is peripheral vasodilatation in most patients with cirrhosis and ascites prompted the development of an alternative view, sometimes known as the '*overflow theory*'. This suggests that the primary abnormality is increased renin and aldosterone levels producing inappropriate sodium and water retention. The plasma volume and cardiac output are increased. Formation of oedema is a secondary event which is encouraged by the low colloid osmotic pressure in plasma, and tends to be localised to the ascitic compartment because of the portal hypertension. Although this theory fits better with the clinical measurements, it does not explain why there should be a primary increase in renin and aldosterone levels in some patients with

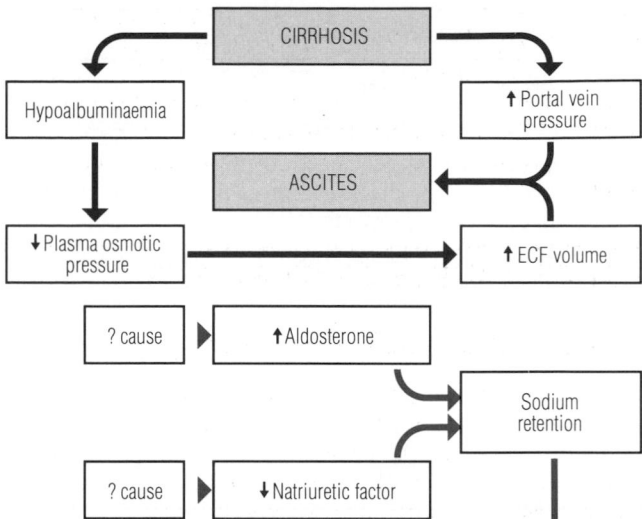

Fig. 16.20 **The pathophysiology of ascites formation in cirrhosis.** In addition to direct effects of the cirrhotic process leading to ascites, such as increased pressure in the portal vein and decreased albumin lowering the plasma osmotic pressure, there is also an aldosterone-driven increase in sodium retention.

cirrhosis. Renal haemodynamics are certainly altered, with a tendency for redistribution of blood flow from cortical to juxtamedullary nephrons, a tendency which is opposed in many patients by an increase in renal prostaglandin synthesis. However, the relationship between these changes and the liver disease is not clear.

Clinical features

Fullness in the flanks, with dullness on percussion which shifts with a change of position, is the earliest sign of ascites and is often asymptomatic. Ultrasound can reveal small amounts of fluid. Later the abdomen becomes tense and uncomfortable. At this stage, a fluid thrill is more useful than shifting dullness in confirming the presence of fluid. It can be difficult to palpate the liver and spleen, although ballotting through the fluid may reveal them. A pleural effusion, particularly on the right side, may be present, and peripheral oedema often develops.

Spontaneous bacterial peritonitis is a serious complication, with a high mortality. It can be asymptomatic, although fever, abdominal pain and a general deterioration in well-being, with encephalopathy and renal failure, may be accompanying features.

Management

A diagnostic paracentesis is first performed to exclude bacterial peritonitis. The fluid should be clear or straw-coloured and any cloudiness should lead to suspicions of infection. Bacterial culture may be negative, and the most frequent abnormal finding is a polymorph count of more

16 Liver and Biliary Tract Disease

than 500 per mm^3. The causative organisms are usually coliforms or streptococci, including anaerobes, and broad-spectrum antibiotics should be started as early as possible. Tuberculous peritonitis is rare, but should be considered, particularly in a malnourished alcoholic and when the ascitic leucocytes are predominately mononuclear.

Diuretics

Treatment of the ascites is only necessary if it is producing symptoms. *Diuretics* are the mainstay of treatment, but care is necessary since overdiuresis precipitates renal failure and encephalopathy, and must be avoided. Therapeutic paracentesis is possible but usually unnecessary. The diuretic of choice is the aldosterone antagonist spironolactone in a starting dose of 100 mg per day. In addition to being a logical choice to combat the high aldosterone levels, it is also potassium-sparing. Total body potassium levels are usually low, and hypokalaemia not only increases the risk of a cardiac arrhythmia, but also exacerbates encephalopathy. The rate of fluid loss is best assessed by changes in daily weight. A figure of 0.5 kg per day is ideal, as the maximum rate of transfer of fluid from the ascitic to the vascular compartment is only about 700 ml per day. If a satisfactory response is not forthcoming in a few days, the daily dose of spironolactone should be increased in 100 mg increments to a maximum of 600 mg per day. It is not usually necessary to add loop diuretics. If they are used, the rate of weight loss, renal function and plasma potassium levels must be carefully monitored. Measurement of urinary sodium concentration can be helpful in assessing the effectiveness of diuretic therapy. Strict control of sodium intake is not always necessary, but does allow lower doses of spironolactone to be effective.

Additional medications should be reviewed with care. The aim of the treatment is to relieve symptoms, not to remove all the ascitic fluid. Reduction of diuretics to maintenance doses should be started before the ascites has disappeared.

Further measures

Failure of response to these treatment measures is unusual. It often indicates severe liver disease and carries a poor prognosis. Hyponatraemia can be a problem, and is usually due to impaired renal free water clearance. Restriction of fluid intake is an appropriate therapeutic measure; sodium infusion simply increases fluid retention.

Direct removal of ascitic fluid is safe if decompression is gradual, electrolyte levels are monitored and corrected and albumin is given intravenously. Maintenance diuretic therapy can then be used to prevent re-accumulation of fluid. Alternatives include ascites re-infusion or a Le Veen peritoneal venous shunt. Both techniques have a high incidence of complications and should only be used if conventional therapy has been ineffective.

VARICEAL HAEMORRHAGE

Distortion of the lobular architecture in cirrhosis almost always produces raised portal venous pressure. Collateral veins develop between the portal and systemic systems. The most important clinically are those which run beneath the oesophageal mucosa, as these frequently rupture, producing life-threatening haematemesis (variceal haemorrhage).

Clinical features

Evidence of portal hypertension may be detected on examination. Splenomegaly is almost invariable. Dilated collateral veins may be seen in the abdominal wall, and may radiate outwards from the umbilicus. In rare cases these may be especially prominent, forming a caput medusa. The obliterated umbilical vein may recanalise, and flow through it sometimes produces a venous hum heard best in the epigastrium or around the umbilicus.

Management

Immediate measures

The first priority is resuscitation. Blood transfusion is usually necessary, often with large quantities. The next step is to establish the source of the bleeding. Peptic ulceration is common in cirrhosis, and acute erosive gastritis and oesophagitis are often present, particularly in alcoholics. Early endoscopy is therefore helpful in demonstrating the likely bleeding site. Most patients stop bleeding spontaneously after resuscitation. In those who do not, two immediate treatment options are available:

- *Vasopressin* (initially 0.4 units per minute intravenously for 1–2 hours) is a powerful vasoconstrictor of the splanchnic bed, which reduces portal vein pressure and flow through the portosystemic collateral veins. It also produces coronary vasoconstriction, and can trigger cardiac arrhythmias or precipitate myocardial infarction. Recently a glyceryl trinitrate infusion has been added to counteract the systemic vasoconstriction and appears to offer some benefit.

- A *Sengstaken-Blakemore tube* is an alternative. This has a long oesophageal balloon which can be inflated to compress the varices, and a gastric balloon which anchors the lower end in the fundus of the stomach, and which may assist in reducing variceal flow by compressing gastric varices. It is very effective, but skill is needed in its introduction and in maintaining it in position with safety.

The decision whether or not to give longer-term treatment is dependent on an assessment of the risk of early rebleeding. The Child's classification, a scoring system where points are given for adverse factors (Table 16.11), is useful. Almost all those with Child's grade A stop bleeding soon after admission and may not rebleed for many months, while the grade C patient is likely to have a serious rebleed during the same hospital admission. In these cases, mortality in the first admission due to variceal

Table 16.11 Child's classification of severity of cirrhosis

Feature	Points scored for increasing abnormalities		
	1	2	3
Encephalopathy (grade)	None	1 and 2	3 and 4
Ascites	None	Mild	Moderate/ severe
Plasma bilirubin (mol/l)	less than 25	25–40	more than 40
Plasma albumin (g/l)	more than 35	28–35	less than 28
Prothrombin time (secs prolonged)	1–4	4–6	more than 6

Total score: 5–6 = grade A; 7–9 = grade B; 10–15 = grade C

haemorrhage may be as high as 80%. Another important factor to be considered is the pattern of admissions in individual patients. Those with infrequent episodes usually retain this pattern and it may be worth adopting a conservative approach.

Longer-term management

If, after full assessment, further treatment is considered desirable, then there are again two main options:

- The varices can be obliterated by a direct approach
- The portal pressure can be reduced by some form of surgical portosystemic shunt.

The shunt approach is becoming less popular, as several controlled trials have shown no benefit for porto-caval shunting in terms of mortality at any stage. Reduced deaths from rebleeding were offset by an increased incidence of liver failure and encephalopathy, presumably due to the reduction in liver blood flow and increased amount of blood bypassing the liver after the shunt procedure.

The most successful form of direct variceal attack is by *endoscopic sclerotherapy*. Sclerosant solution is injected under direct vision into or around the varices at repeated endoscopy sessions until the varices have been obliterated. Recanalisation and formation of new collaterals does occur, and regular follow-up treatments are necessary. This is the only procedure to have been shown in controlled clinical trials to prolong survival significantly.

Extrahepatic portal vein obstruction

Although relatively uncommon, this is a condition with a good prognosis which often presents with variceal haemorrhage, and must be distinguished from cirrhosis. The cause of the portal vein obstruction is often not apparent and in many cases is thought to be due to portal vein thrombosis in infancy, possibly secondary to umbilical sepsis. Patients first present with haematemesis from bleeding oesophageal varices in childhood, adolescence or early adult life. Clinically, there are no cutaneous stigmata of chronic liver disease, and although splenomegaly is often marked, the liver is usually impalpable. Liver function tests are normal, and ascites does not occur. Liver biopsy is helpful in excluding cirrhosis, and ultrasound can often determine the patency of the portal vein. Direct confirmation of the diagnosis is best obtained from the venous phase of selective coeliac axis and superior mesenteric angiograms. These usually show a leash of collateral vessels in the porta hepatis where the portal vein would normally be seen. In adults portal vein thrombosis can be a complication of intra-abdominal sepsis or carcinoma of the pancreas.

Treatment is aided by the excellent liver function. Most patients stop bleeding after resuscitation. Portosystemic shunts can be technically difficult, although if successful the risk of encephalopathy is much less than in patients with cirrhosis because liver cell function is not impaired. Endoscopic sclerotherapy is a suitable alternative.

ENCEPHALOPATHY

This complication of cirrhosis is a sign of severe liver cell failure, and it usually has a poor prognosis. However, a treatable precipitating factor is often present, and its identification and correction is an important clinical objective.

Pathophysiology

A reduction in functioning liver cell mass, and diversion of portal blood past the liver via portosystemic collaterals, are the two important ingredients which predispose to the disturbance in cerebral function, but the precise mechanisms involved are not known. There are two main theories:

- Toxic substances normally detoxified by the liver are thought to gain access to the systemic circulation and thus the brain where they alter cerebral metabolism.
- An alteration in the balance between cerebral neurotransmitters is postulated with formation of false neurotransmitters, possibly because of altered amino acid levels in the circulation, which in turn alter the levels of these neurotransmitter substrates in the brain.

Possible candidates as toxins in the first theory include ammonia, mercaptans, amines and indoles. All can be shown to induce encephalopathy in experimental animals, but in concentrations higher than those found in hepatic encephalopathy. Increased serum levels of the aromatic amino acids, and decreased levels of branched chain amino acids, have promoted the concepts outlined in the second theory. There have been attempts to treat the encephalopathy by correcting the balance between the aromatic and branched chain amino acids, but the place of this therapy in clinical practice is not established.

Recently changes in the relative proportions of high and low affinity receptors for some of the cerebral neurotransmitters have been demonstrated in animal models of hepatic encephalopathy, and this seems to be a fruitful area for further research.

Clinical features

The main difference between the encephalopathy of chronic liver disease and that of fulminant hepatic failure is the relapsing acute-on-chronic course and the consequent emphasis on the search for, and correction of, precipitating factors. The prodromal phase of an acute-on-chronic episode may be very gradual. Impairment of judgment can be an early sign. Anorexia is common and the reversal of sleep pattern may be troublesome. Fatigue, withdrawal, apathy and slowness of response often precede a more profound disturbance in consciousness (Table 16.6). There may be spatial disorientation with confusion as to place, time and person, and a flapping tremor of the outstretched, extended hands.

Although not specific to liver disease, changes in the EEG can be helpful in identification and management. There is generalised slowing of the main components, with a resulting fall in the mean dominant frequency. Serial recordings are one objective way of following progress during treatment, although simple bedside tests for constructional apraxia, such as the copying of a five-pointed star, are sufficiently reliable and sensitive in practice.

Management

An important objective is to search carefully for a possible precipitating cause (Table 16.12).

Treatment of the encephalopathy is mainly directed at minimising the absorption of nitrogenous material, particularly ammonia, from the bowel. Protein is removed from the diet, the colon is emptied using a magnesium sulphate enema, and ammonia-producing colonic bacteria are reduced in number by giving oral neomycin and lactulose. Lactulose is a synthetic disaccharide which is broken down into its constituent monosaccharides by bacteria in the colon, and then into lactic acid. This not only acts as

Table 16.12 Factors precipitating encephalopathy in cirrhosis

Intercurrent infections
Urinary tract
Chest
Upper respiratory tract
Genito-urinary tract
Spontaneous bacterial peritonitis
Septicaemia

Dietary indiscretion
High protein meal
Alcohol binge

Gastrointestinal haemorrhage
Blood acts as protein load, and hypotension impairs liver function (may be occult; melaena on rectal examination)

Electrolyte imbalance
Hyponatraemia or hypokalaemia (possibly due to vomiting, reduced free water clearance or effect of diuretics)

Drugs
Usual candidates are sedatives (increased end-organ sensitivity and reduced clearance) and diuretics (electrolyte imbalance)

Primary hepatocellular carcinoma
Worsening of encephalopathy may be the first indication

a purgative, but also discourages the growth of ammonia-producing bacteria. Because of the change in pH, ammonia may also be fixed in the colon as ammonium ions.

HEPATOCELLULAR CARCINOMA

Often referred to as hepatoma, hepatocellular carcinoma arises from the hepatic parenchymal cells.

Incidence, epidemiology and aetiology

In Africa and the Far East, hepatocellular carcinoma is one of the commonest tumours, while it is unusual in Europe and the USA (Fig. 16.21).

Hepatocellular carcinoma usually arises in the cirrhotic liver, and in this setting is commoner in males than females. In Europe and North America, the peak in-

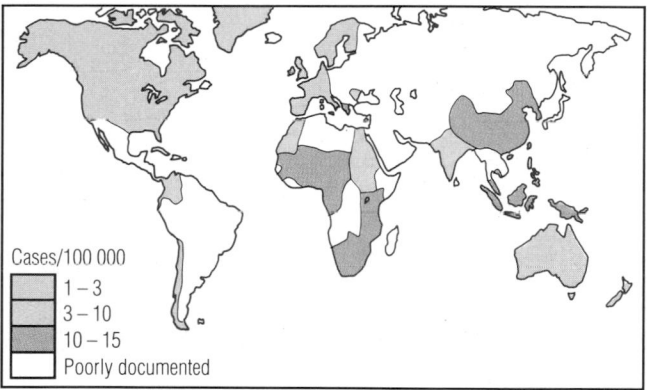

Fig. 16.21 The distribution of hepatocellular carcinoma in the world. It almost parallels the distribution of HBV infection (Fig. 16.11).

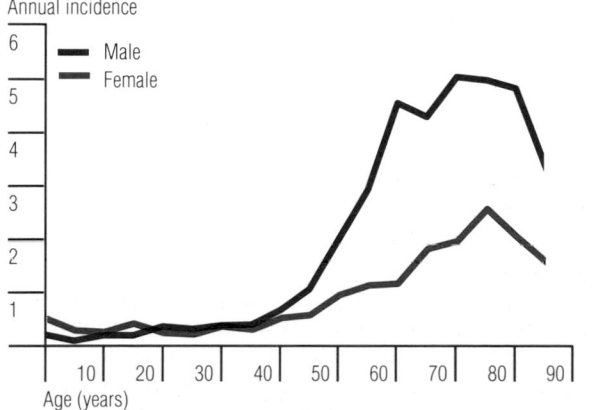

Fig. 16.22 Primary hepatocellular carcinoma. The average number of cases of primary hepatocellular carcinoma seen each year in the south-east of England between the years 1965 and 1984 in men and women by age group (per 100 000).

cidence is from 50 to 70 years of age (Fig. 16.22), but in high-incidence areas patients are often in their twenties or thirties. When there is no underlying cirrhosis, the sex ratio is equal, and the tumour usually presents in teenagers and young adults.

Chronic HBV infection is strongly associated with the development of the tumour, particularly in areas with a high HBsAg carrier rate. The finding of subgenomic fragments of HBV DNA in liver cell and tumour DNA, even in some patients without serological markers of previous HBV infection, has led to the suggestion that the virus may be directly oncogenic. However, the pattern of integration of viral DNA appears to be random and molecular mechanisms which could be responsible for oncogenesis have not yet been identified. Careful prospective studies of hepatoma development in patients with cirrhosis in the UK have shown that previous HBV infection, as detected serologically, is not a significant independent risk factor.

Aflatoxin, a product of the fungal mould *Aspergillus flavus*, can induce liver damage and hepatocellular carcinoma in animals, and is a food contaminant in many tropical countries. Very rarely, hepatocellular carcinoma has been described following prolonged use of the oral contraceptive pill, and in individuals exposed to Thorotrast, an early radioactive X-ray contrast material.

Pathology

The commonest microscopic pattern of hepatocellular carcinoma is the characteristic trabecular or sinusoidal pattern, which reproduces the normal relationship between clusters of liver cells and a flat endothelial cell covering (Fig. 16.2).

Fibrolamellar carcinoma is a distinct variant with a better prognosis, found in mainly young female non-cirrhotic patients. The tumour cells are large and polygonal and are arranged in trabeculae separated by parallel bundles of collagen which merge in places to form broader bands of fibrous tissue.

Clinical features

In the UK, there is usually a slow deterioration in well-being, with anorexia, weight loss and abdominal pain in a patient known to have cirrhosis. Rare, non-metastatic systemic manifestations can occur, and include hypercalcaemia, hypoglycaemia and porphyria cutanea tarda. There may be no specific signs on examination, but hepatomegaly is usually present and there may be an arterial bruit and a friction rub over the tumour. In high-incidence areas, the presentation is often more dramatic, with pain over the tumour, fever and weight loss. The deterioration in liver function is more profound in the patient with pre-existing cirrhosis.

Diagnosis

The most important biochemical marker of the tumour is alpha-fetoprotein (AFP). This is a glycoprotein, which can be thought of as a fetal albumin. It is synthesised by the fetal liver, but levels fall rapidly after birth. In adults it is present in serum in a concentration of less than 10 ng/ml. About 80% of patients with hepatocellular carcinoma arising in a cirrhotic liver, and 50% of those without an underlying cirrhosis, will show elevated AFP levels in serum. In a cirrhotic, levels above 1000 ng/ml are almost diagnostic of hepatocellular carcinoma. AFP is also greatly elevated in patients with germ cell tumours of the testis and ovary but this is not a diagnostic problem. Some patients with hepatic metastases can also have elevated AFP levels, but not as high as those found in hepatoma. In active cirrhosis, levels of AFP can, on occasions, rise above the normal adult range, probably reflecting increased liver cell regeneration, but a rapid, sustained rise in the serum levels on serial estimations is typical of hepatoma.

Ultrasound, CT and scintiscanning are all capable of visualising hepatocellular carcinoma. Selective hepatic arteriography is a very useful diagnostic technique, and also provides information on the distribution of the tumour within the liver. There is usually a well-defined tumour circulation, with new vessel formation. Although the definitive diagnosis can only be made by histological examination of tumour tissue, in practice liver biopsy may not always be possible because of a prolonged prothrombin time. In these cases a working diagnosis is established from a combination of elevated AFP levels in serum and the demonstration of a tumour circulation on arteriography.

Management

Hepatocellular carcinoma is usually a rapidly growing tumour which presents late. The prognosis is poor, with a mean survival of about 4 months. Resection is potentially curative but is only possible in those cases where tumour is limited to one lobe of the liver and where there is no underlying cirrhosis. The long-term outlook following successful resection is good, with local recurrence being much commoner than distant metastases. On this basis, it might be expected that liver transplantation would be another effective treatment, also applicable to those with cirrhosis. However, both tumour recurrence in the liver graft and distant metastases are commonly observed within 1–2 years of the procedure. It is not clear whether this is due to immunosuppressive therapy, or that the tumours are often more advanced than initially suspected.

The only cytotoxic drug to show any benefit so far is adriamycin (doxorubicin). About one-third of those treated show a response, but in most of these survival is only prolonged by a few months. Embolisation of the hepatic artery or the branches supplying the tumour with gelatin foam can give useful pain relief, and is often used before cytotoxic drug therapy to reduce tumour mass.

LIVER METASTASES

Many tumours metastasise to the liver, particularly those arising in the abdomen; in Western societies, this is the commonest cause of malignancy within the liver.

Clinical features

Although the primary tumour may have already been identified, in some cases the metastatic tumour may be the cause of the presentation. In these cases, malaise, weight loss, pain over the liver and abdominal distension are the likely symptoms. Examination often confirms substantial weight loss and usually demonstrates a hard, enlarged liver with an irregular surface and edge.

Investigations

The serum alkaline phosphatase is often elevated. Jaundice is usually a late occurrence, and has a poor prognosis. Ultrasound and scintiscans frequently confirm the presence of filling defects in the liver, and the definitive diagnosis can then be made on liver biopsy. Tumour tissue can be expected on liver biopsy in more than 70% of cases, and the success rate can be further enhanced by using ultrasound to indicate where the biopsy should be taken.

Differential diagnosis

Because of the importance of the diagnosis of metastatic liver cancer, it is usually necessary to obtain histological proof of malignancy. The conditions most likely to be misdiagnosed are cysts, abscesses and granulomas. In areas where hepatoma is common, the pain, fever and rapidly enlarging liver make amoebic abscess and hydatid disease important treatable conditions to be considered in the differential diagnosis.

Management

Treatment depends on the nature of the primary tumour. For certain tumours, such as small cell carcinoma of the lung, breast cancer and lymphoma, chemotherapy may be highly effective in producing regression of metastases and symptomatic improvement. With other tumours, such as metastatic gastrointestinal and pancreatic cancer, chemotherapy is usually ineffective, although infusion of cytotoxic drugs such as 5-fluorouracil into the hepatic artery occasionally relieves pain and produces regression. It is questionable whether this complex procedure is more effective than intravenous administration. Pain in the liver is usually controlled by analgesics, but severe pain may be helped by external irradiation and even hepatic artery ligation or tumour embolisation. Rarely, resection of an isolated metastasis may be feasible; carcinoid tumour (p. 585) is a slow-growing tumour where this approach may be valuable.

Symptoms of pain, nausea and anorexia are best treated by palliative measures including analgesics, anti-emetics such as metaclopramide, and corticosteroids.

LYMPHOMA

The liver is often directly involved with infiltration of lymphoma cells. Liver biopsy can therefore be helpful in diagnosis. Documenting liver involvement is also important in staging the disease before deciding on appropriate therapy. Serum alkaline phosphatase levels may be increased and jaundice can occur. In Hodgkin's disease a cholestatic jaundice may appear before there is obvious lymph node involvement, and occasionally in the absence of any evidence of direct hepatic involvement.

THE LIVER IN SYSTEMIC DISEASE

Rheumatoid arthritis

Increased serum alkaline phosphatase levels from the liver are frequently seen in rheumatoid arthritis. Histological changes on liver biopsy are often non-specific and unremarkable. Amyloidosis and primary biliary cirrhosis are well defined but infrequent associations. Nodular regenerative hyperplasia is sometimes found in Felty's syndrome (p. 986).

Systemic lupus erythematosus

The early finding of lupus erythematosus (LE) cells in about 10% of cases of autoimmune chronic active hepatitis, and the use of the term 'lupoid hepatitis' to describe these patients, created considerable confusion concerning the relationship between chronic active hepatitis and systemic lupus erythematosus (SLE). Although anti-DNA antibodies are frequently present in autoimmune chronic active hepatitis, it is now clear that the two conditions are quite distinct. In particular, clinically significant renal involvement, an important feature in SLE, is very rare in chronic active hepatitis. Furthermore, careful studies of liver involvement in SLE have in most cases shown only minor portal tract inflammation.

Polyarteritis nodosa

Chronic HBV infection has been reported in up to 40% of cases of polyarteritis nodosa, but this is not a consistent finding. The associated liver disease in these cases is usually very mild, with minor histological changes on liver biopsy. The appearance of characteristic arterial lesions in biopsy material can be of help in diagnosis.

Scleroderma

There is a well-recognised association between scleroderma and primary biliary cirrhosis (PBC). In some cases of PBC the associated sclerosis is truly systemic but in most it is limited to the skin of the terminal phalanges (sclerodactyly), and may be part of the CRST syndrome.

Amyloidosis

The liver is often involved in systemic amyloidosis (p. 1101) but this does not produce clinically significant liver disease. Rectal biopsy is safer than liver biopsy in establishing the diagnosis.

Porphyria

Porphyria cutanea tarda (Ch. 19) may be associated with alcoholic liver disease, and sometimes hepatoma; the accumulation of protoporphyrin in the liver in erythropoietic protoporphyria may eventually lead to cirrhosis and liver failure.

Granulomatous conditions

The finding of granulomata in liver biopsy specimens is relatively common. Although they are a feature of some primary liver diseases, particularly primary biliary cirrhosis, they are more often a reflection of a systemic condition (Table 16.13). In the UK the commonest causes are sarcoidosis, tuberculosis, and drug reactions. There is usually hepatomegaly, with a raised serum alkaline phosphatase but a normal serum bilirubin level. In up to 30% of cases the cause of the hepatic granulomata cannot be determined in spite of rigorous investigation. Occasionally portal hypertension may develop either because of a direct effect of the granulomata on liver blood flow or in association with increasing liver fibrosis. In these cases a trial of steroids is justified to try to halt the progress of the disease.

Granulomatous hepatitis denotes the presence of focal parenchymal liver damage in association with multiple granulomata. In some cases of unknown aetiology there may be quite striking symptoms of a systemic illness, including fever, malaise and weight loss. There is often a dramatic improvement on corticosteroid therapy.

Table 16.13 Causes of granulomatous liver disease

Infections	Drug-induced
Bacterial	Sulphonamides and derivatives
Usually chronic	Sulphonamide-containing antibiotics*
intracellular	and anti-diabetics like chlorpropamide*
infections	Others
Mycobacterial including	e.g. Phenylbutazone*
tuberculosis*	Allopurinol
Brucellosis*	Hydralazine
Leprosy	Carbamazepine
Listerosis	Quinidine
Fungal	
Histoplasmosis*	**Multisystem diseases**
Nocardia	Collagen-vascular disease
Candidiasis	Polymyalgia rheumatica*
Actinomycosis	Systemic lupus erythematosus
Parasitic	Others
Schistosomiasis*	Sarcoidosis*
Ascariasis	Whipple's disease
Toxacara	Wegener's granulomatosis
Amoebiasis	Granulomatous disease of childhood
Strongyloides	
Giardiasis	**Miscellaneous**
Viral	Primary biliary cirrhosis*
Cytomegalovirus	Crohn's disease*
Lymphogranuloma venereum	IV drug abusers
Infectious mononucleosis	Patients on haemodialysis
Other	Haemophilia
Syphilis	After ileal bypass surgery
Q fever	Erythema nodosum
Neoplasms	
Hodgkin's lymphoma*	
Adenocarcinoma	
Hepatocellular carcinoma	

*Common causes of liver granulomata

NON-VIRAL INFECTIONS INVOLVING THE LIVER

Schistosomiasis

Worldwide schistosomiasis (p. 312) is a common cause of chronic liver disease. Adult worms live in small veins of the colon (*Schistosoma mansoni*) and the small intestine and colon (*S. japonicum*). The liver damage is due to granulomatous reactions to eggs which have embolised in the liver, and impacted in presinusoidal branches of the portal vein. Resolution of granulomata leads to severe periportal fibrosis in patients with heavy infections. Portal hypertension usually accompanies the developing fibrosis, but liver cell function is well preserved unless there is co-existing cirrhosis from another cause. Patients often present with haematemesis from ruptured oesophageal varices; gross splenomegaly is common and ascites

occurs. The prognosis is fairly good. Diagnosis and management are discussed in Chapter 11.

Liver flukes

Fasciola hepatica is a flatworm which is common in sheep, and, to a lesser extent, cattle worldwide (p. 316). It lives in the biliary tree and sheds its ova into the stools. The liver damage is caused by worms in the biliary system. In severe infections there is intermittent obstructive jaundice with high fever, painful hepatomegaly and jaundice. Eosinophilia is common, and a complement fixation test is usually positive in high titre. The definitive diagnosis is made by finding ova in stool concentrates. The infection responds to treatment with praziquantel.

Clonorchis sinensis is found in the Far East (p. 314). The worms inhabit the biliary system. Symptoms are usually mild, except in heavy infections when there may be upper abdominal pain, tender hepatomegaly and diarrhoea. Praziquantel is an effective treatment. Late complications include obstructive jaundice, cholangitis, stones in the common bile duct and cholangiocarcinoma (p. 635).

Hydatid cysts

Hydatid cysts (p. 319) are cysts in the liver formed by the larval stages of two tapeworms, *Echinococcus granulosus* and *E. multilocularis*, which normally live in dogs and wild carnivores respectively.

Cysts may be asymptomatic or may present with pain in the right hypochondrium. If they are very large, they can cause abdominal distension and discomfort. Secondary infection in a cyst is a serious complication, presenting with fever and pain like other pyogenic liver abscesses.

Ultrasound and CT are the most useful investigations and can be diagnostic if 'daughter' cysts are identified (Fig. 16.23). Complement fixation and haemagglutination tests for antibodies to hydatid material can also be helpful in making a specific diagnosis, although negative results can occur, particularly in asymptomatic cases.

Mebendazole and, more recently, albendazole have been used for treatment and information is now available regarding the relationship between serum and cyst concentrations. Drug treatment may become the first line of therapy. Surgical removal of the cysts still offers the best chance of cure but great care must be taken to prevent rupturing of the cysts, which leads to dissemination of daughter cysts into the peritoneal cavity. This risk is minimised by injecting formalin, alcohol or hypertonic saline into the cyst before attempting removal. It is wise to leave asymptomatic cysts alone.

Amoebiasis

In some cases of amoebic colitis, and in others without bowel symptoms, the organisms reach the liver through

with myalgia and high fever. This may progress to prostration, jaundice and renal failure. Headache, confusion
and meningism are often present. Epistaxis, haematuria
and petechiae occur. There is often a prominent leucocytosis, and the urine contains red cells and albumin.
Identification of the causative organism in blood or urine
is the definitive diagnostic test although there is a rise in
serum IgM antibody at the end of the acute phase of the
disease. Although the jaundice may be deep, liver failure
does not occur, and general toxaemia and renal failure are
the usual problems in management. The organism is
sensitive to benzyl penicillin and large doses are usually
given. However, there is no convincing evidence that this
contributes to the resolution of the disease, and skilled
intensive care is essential. The reported mortality varies
from 4 to 40%.

Septicaemia

Cholestasis is not uncommon in severe sepsis. A rise in
serum bilirubin occurs in 25–50% of cases, but serum
aminotransferase and alkaline phosphatase are often
normal. The pathogenesis is not understood but there is
no evidence of gross liver damage and there is usually
rapid resolution with appropriate antibiotic therapy. In
jaundice due to staphylococcal sepsis, treatment with
fucidic acid should be avoided as this interferes with
bilirubin excretion.

PYOGENIC LIVER ABSCESS

The commonest cause of liver abscess worldwide is amoebiasis, but in the developed world pyogenic causes are of
increasing importance. In the past pyogenic liver abscess
was most commonly seen in children or young adults in
association with appendicitis. However, as antibiotics
have become more widely prescribed, the condition is
now most often seen in the elderly, due to incomplete
treatment of biliary tract disease or diverticulitis. In these
patients, the presenting symptoms are often non-specific
and the diagnosis is often delayed.

Aetiology

Possible causes of pyogenic liver abscess are listed in
Table 16.14. Infection in any site drained by the portal
vein can cause portal pyaemia which can then seed the
liver with abscesses. These are usually multiple and often
concentrated in the right lobe. The primary site, particularly in diverticular disease, may be relatively silent.
Direct spread of infection from the biliary tree is the
presumed route of entry of the bacteria in those cases
where abscess complicates biliary tract disease. Trauma
and hepatic malignancy are uncommon causes.

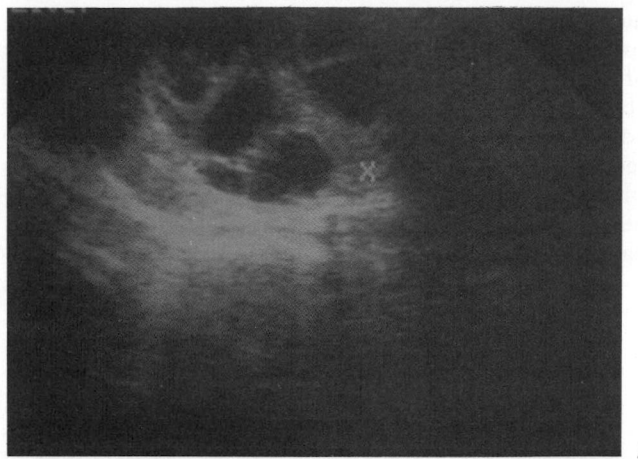

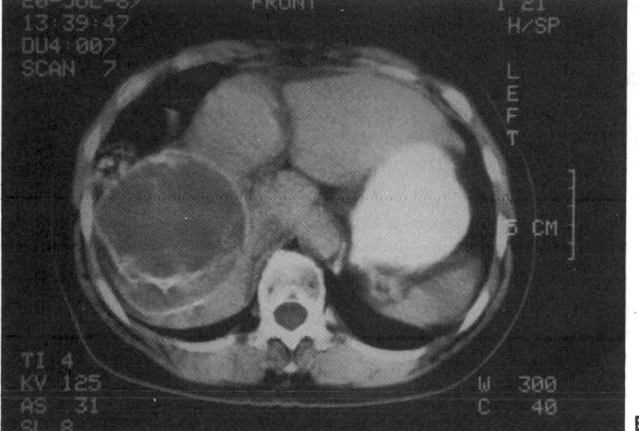

Fig. 16.23 Hydatid disease of the liver. A. Ultrasound scan demonstrating
multiple cysts. **B**. CT scan demonstrating 'daughter' cysts in the liver. There is
calcification within the cyst wall.

the portal venous system and form intrahepatic amoebic
abscesses. Pain in the right hypochondrium, with tender
hepatomegaly and fever, are the usual manifestations. A
right-sided pleural effusion can also occur if an abscess
has ruptured through the diaphragm. Ultrasound and CT
scans are very useful investigations, and antibody tests are
almost always positive. A week's course of metronidazole
is a very effective treatment and can be used as a therapeutic test of the diagnosis; however, anaerobic pyogenic
liver abscess will also respond.

Weil's disease

The spirochaete *Leptospira icterohaemorrhagica* can be
transmitted to man from infested rats' urine. Those in
contact with sewage and rat-infected water are at highest
risk. The incubation period is 1–2 weeks. At first the
illness may resemble a prodromal stage of viral hepatitis,
with mild fever and malaise, but it is often more severe,

Table 16.14 Causes of pyogenic liver abscess

Biliary tract disease
Ascending cholangitis is the commonest cause and may be a complication of any obstruction in the biliary tract; it can also follow cholecystitis

Portal phlebitis
Any primary septic focus within the abdomen (diverticulitis, appendicitis, infected haemorrhoids, etc.) can cause thrombophlebitis in the local branches of the portal vein, and infect the liver

Septicaemia
Severe generalised sepsis can infect the liver via the hepatic artery

Trauma
Secondary infection of a damaged area of liver or a haematoma can lead to abscess formation

Malignancy
Some tumours develop areas of central necrosis, and pyogenic infection can then follow

Extension of local infection
e.g. Subphrenic abscess and empyema of the gall bladder

Bacteriology

The dominant organism isolated from hepatic abscess has changed over the last few years. While aerobic Gram-negative organisms, especially *E. coli*, used to predominate, anaerobes, particularly *Streptococcus milleri*, are now found in up to 50% of abscesses. Mixed infections are identified in about one-third of cases.

Presentation

Classically there is upper abdominal pain, swinging pyrexia, anorexia, malaise and weight loss. However, in many older patients the symptoms and signs may be much less dramatic, and pain and hepatomegaly may not be present. This is one of the causes of pyrexia of unknown origin.

Investigations

A polymorphonuclear leucocytosis is usually present and the routine liver function tests often show a high serum alkaline phosphatase. The most useful investigation is an ultrasound scan. If there has been no previous antibiotic treatment, aerobic and anaerobic cultures of blood or direct aspirates of pus under ultrasound control will usually reveal the causative organism.

Management

Antibiotics are always needed and are best chosen according to the bacteriological findings. However, a combi-

nation of gentamicin (or a broad-spectrum cephalosporin), metronidazole and flucloxacillin will cover most of the likely organisms. In cases with very small multiple abscesses, appropriate antibiotic treatment alone may be adequate therapy but in most cases drainage is also required. In a solitary abscess or where the number is small, it may be possible to achieve satisfactory percutaneous drainage by repeated needle aspiration. In elderly patients the first line of treatment is usually closed aspiration combined with antibiotics instilled into the abscess cavity and given intravenously. When the abscesses are difficult to approach, open surgical drainage is used. Soft pliable drains are placed in the largest cavities and intensive broad-spectrum antibiotic treatment started. Whichever approach to drainage is used, the antibiotics need to be continued for 6 weeks to ensure resolution of infection.

Prognosis

Unfortunately the diagnosis of pyogenic liver abscess is often delayed, and under these circumstances the mortality may be as high as 80%. With a high index of suspicion and early diagnosis the mortality has been as low as 10% in some series. Co-existent biliary tract disease, old age and multiple abscesses are associated with a poor prognosis.

CONGENITAL BILIARY AND HEPATIC DISORDERS

Caroli's disease

Caroli's disease is a rare condition in which saccular dilations of the intrahepatic biliary tree predispose to ascending cholangitis. Symptoms usually begin in childhood or early adult life. Long-term antibiotic treatment reduces the frequency of attacks.

Choledochal cyst

Choledochal cyst is a gross dilatation or diverticulum of the common bile duct, which obstructs normal bile flow and presents as cholestatic jaundice in childhood. The diagnosis is made on ultrasound and cholangiography. Treatment is by surgical resection and drainage, usually via a Roux-en-Y anastomosis.

Biliary atresia

Originally thought to be a congenital anomaly, with failure of development of the extrahepatic biliary system, biliary atresia is now recognised as an acquired condition in many cases. There is gradual destruction of the common bile duct soon after birth, leading to deepening jaundice and secondary biliary cirrhosis. Early surgical intervention, with a bypass anastamosis high in the porta hepatis, has proved remarkably successful in some cases. More recently, liver transplantation has also produced promising results.

Polycystic disease of the liver

Polycystic disease of the liver may be a congenital anomaly related to biliary atresia, but rarely presents with jaundice. Large cysts, similar to those seen in polycystic kidney disease and often associated with them, may be found throughout the liver. Gross nodular hepatomegaly, often asymptomatic, is usual. Although pain, due to haemorrhage or infection in a cyst, can occur, the prognosis with respect to the liver lesions is excellent.

LIVER TRANSPLANTATION

Replacement of the liver by an orthotopic graft is a technically difficult procedure but one that is now accepted as a feasible and appropriate treatment for advanced liver disease.

Selection of suitable patients is difficult (Table 16.15). If the disease process is too advanced then the operative mortality will be unacceptably high. Survival figures (Fig. 16.24), although improving, are not as good as after

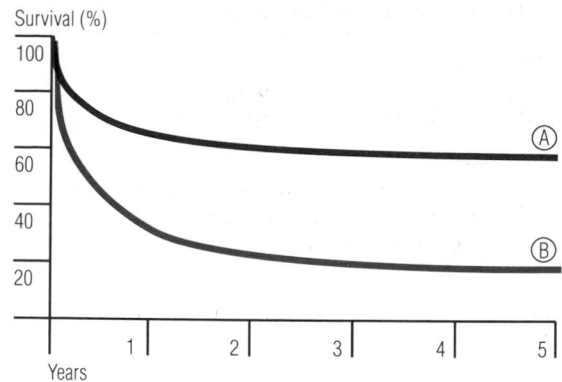

Fig. 16.24 Liver transplant survival rates. The dramatic improvement in the survival of liver transplants after 1978 (A) compared with before 1978 (B) is partly due to improved surgical techniques, but also better patient selection and better immunosuppression following the introduction of cyclosporin A. Many centres are now reporting results as good as those shown in curve A.

renal transplantation. Currently the best results are obtained in patients with advanced cirrhosis, either cryptogenic or due to chronic active hepatitis or primary biliary cirrhosis. Many of these patients have severe portal hypertension, with encephalopathy and bleeding varices, but these are not contraindications to the procedure. The reversal of encephalopathy is often dramatic, even in those in whom it has been present for many months. In acute liver failure there are difficulties in obtaining donor organs at an appropriate time, but patients with subacute hepatic necrosis and the Budd-Chiari syndrome have been successfully treated. In America, children with biliary atresia have been successfully treated by liver transplantation for many years. In the UK donors of a suitable age have only recently become more readily available, and the operation is proving useful in those cases presenting too late for a successful biliary drainage procedure.

The postoperative period

The immediate postoperative period is often remarkably uneventful in those patients who have received a well-preserved donor liver. In experimental animals the liver is rejected less vigorously than other organs and this also seems to be true in man. Cyclosporin A, a potent inhibitor of antigen-induced lymphocyte proliferation, has reduced the severity of rejection even further, although nephrotoxicity, its most important side-effect in man, is a continuing problem. Biliary obstruction and fistulae were important early problems, but changes in technique have led to some improvements in this area.

Overall, 1-year survival rates are now about 80% in most series, with about 70% surviving 5 years or more with an excellent quality of life.

Table 16.15 Common indications for liver transplantation

Cirrhosis	
Primary biliary cirrhosis	Increasing bilirubin a good indication of advanced disease; results excellent
Chronic active hepatitis	
Autoimmune	Good results; not so easy timing transplant
HBV	Frequent recurrence of HBV infection in transplant
Cryptogenic	Timing difficult; results good if not too advanced
Fulminant hepatic failure	Simple tests can indicate prognosis and need for transplant; urgent need for donor organ makes organisation difficult but results good
Biliary atresia	Transplantation of half a liver makes a wider range of donor organs available; early Kasai operation (porto-enterostomy) may make later transplant unnecessary

FURTHER READING

Schiff L, Schiff E R 1993 Diseases of the liver. 7th edn. J P Lippincott Co., Philadelphia. *A major US text. Heavy but complete.*

Sherlock S 1992 Diseases of the liver and biliary system. 9th edn. Blackwell Scientific Publications, Oxford. *The latest edition of the 'standard' liver text.*

Wright R, Millward-Sadler GH, Alberti K G M M, Kattin S J 1992 Liver and biliary disease. 3rd edn. Bailière-Tindall, London. *The modern British composite liver textbook. Readable, accurate and combining basic science with clinical medicine.*

17

Endocrine Diseases

David C Anderson

HISTORICAL INTRODUCTION

Endocrinology emerged as medical science in the 19th century. Berthold of Göttingen, in 1849, was the first to provide 'experimental proof' for the existence of an internal secretion, by demonstrating that transplantation of the testis to another part of the bird's body prevented atrophy of the cock's comb, known to be caused by castration. In 1855, Thomas Addison described the clinical picture which resulted from destruction of the adrenal glands in man. The first clear demonstration that an extract of a gland could correct a deficiency disease was provided by Murray and others, who showed that the administration of sheep thyroid extract would cure myxoedema and its childhood equivalent, cretinism, and the effects of thyroidectomy. In 1915 Kendall isolated the active principle and named it thyroxine. By then, the first demonstration of a hormone had been made in 1902, by Baylis and Starling, who extracted the hormone they termed secretin from the duodenum, and found that it promoted pancreatic enzyme secretion. Adrenaline was extracted from the adrenal glands at about the same time. By the mid-1930s, German chemists had isolated and later synthesised testosterone and the main oestrogen, oestradiol, followed in the 1940s by the adrenal glucocorticoids, cortisone and cortisol. Because of its unusual chemical structure and high potency, the main mineralocorticoid, aldosterone, was not discovered until the mid-1950s. The major pathways of steroid synthesis were not completely identified, nor the inborn errors of steroid production recognised, until this time.

From an early stage, clinical observation has had a major impact on the development of the science of endocrinology and the recognition of different hormones. This is particularly true of the pituitary gland and its subservient endocrine glands. Early this century, Harvey Cushing, the father of pituitary surgery, recognised that some features of pituitary disease were due to deficiencies, and others (for example in acromegaly) to hormone excess (in this case, growth hormone).

Geoffrey Harris, working in Cambridge, was responsible for the concept that the anterior pituitary gland was controlled by secretions coming to it through a portal blood supply from the hypothalamus. Since the late 1960s, we have seen the isolation and synthesis of several of these releasing factors and their entry into clinical practice.

Recently, the pace of development of our understanding of basic and clinical endocrinology has been truly staggering. Much has come from advances in methods for measuring the minute concentrations of hormones in body fluids. In many instances, the concentration of active hormones in the circulation is in the range of picograms (10^{-12}g) per ml. In the 1960s, initial bioassay and chemical methods gave way to protein-binding assays of which the most widely used have been radioimmunoassays. These depend upon developing highly specific antibodies to hormones, coupled if necessary (e.g. for steroids) to a protein. A further essential development was the capacity to make radiolabelled hormones. Such methods have demonstrated, amongst other phenomena, the episodic nature of release of certain hormones. Thus, administration of gonadotrophin-releasing hormone (GnRH) (initially to monkeys) showed the importance of pulsatile secretion of GnRH in transmitting the correct message. Continuous administration was found to switch off secretion of the hormones that it stimulates when given episodically.

Recently, very sensitive bioassay methods have been developed, such as those using isolated cells; these are especially important for polypeptide hormones. Furthermore, immunoradiometric assays for many polypeptide hormones have now become available, with even greater sensitivity and specificity than radioimmunoassays.

THE PHYSIOLOGY OF HORMONE ACTION

Hormone action through cell surface receptors

All receptors have a high affinity hormone-binding region: binding of the hormone to this site alters the conformation of the receptor. They also have a region which couples to an intracellular signalling mechanism which mediates the function of the hormone.

Actions mediated by adenylate cyclase

The first such effector mechanism to be recognised was the adenylate cyclase system which, when activated, generates cyclic-AMP (from ATP) as second messenger (Fig. 17.1). It is now recognised that hormones can either activate or inhibit this enzyme, depending upon whether they are linked to it via a stimulatory (Ns) or inhibitory (Ni) guanosine triphosphate (GTP)-containing coupling protein. The N (or G) protein consists of three subunits, α, β and γ. When the receptor is activated by the hormone, it associates with an Ns coupling protein; the α-subunit dissociates and activates adenylate cyclase. The α-subunit is also a guanosine triphosphatase (GTPase), and its activation leads to a simultaneous breakdown of GTP to GDP, switching-off adenylate cyclase.

Cyclic-AMP, in turn, binds to and activates certain intracellular protein kinases which then activate other enzymes and proteins by phosphorylation. The concen-tration of cyclic AMP is determined by the combined activity of adenylate cyclase and the enzyme that destroys cyclic-AMP, phosphodiesterase.

Hormones which act wholly or in part via the second messenger cyclic-AMP include many *polypeptide hormones* such as adrenocorticotrophic hormone (ACTH), luteinising hormone (LH), follicle stimulating hormone (FSH), thyroid stimulating hormone (TSH), parathyroid hormone, calcitonin and vasopressin. The effects of the catecholamine hormone adrenaline (also called epinephrine), mediated by the β-receptor, are also produced by activation of adenylate cyclase. On the other hand, its alpha-adrenergic effects are mediated, in part at least, by *inhibiting* adenylate cyclase (via the Ni coupling protein discussed above). This accounts in part for the mutually antagonistic α and β effects of adrenaline, at least in tissues that possess both types of receptors. Many of the effects of *prostaglandins*, which are not systemic hormones but do act via cell surface receptors, are also mediated by adenylate cyclase.

Actions mediated by phosphatidyl inositols and calcium transport

Many hormones act through cell surface receptors independently of adenylate cyclase. These include insulin and related growth factors, and some or all of the hypothalamic releasing hormones. Many such effects are due to transport or release of calcium and/or to cleavage of cell membrane phospholipids to generate two further second messengers, inositol 1,3,4 trisphosphate (IP$_3$) and diacylglycerol (DG) (Fig. 17.2).

IP$_3$ is believed to act principally by stimulating calcium release from the microsomal pool of calcium. A transient rise in intracellular calcium activates intracellular proteins, notably calmodulin, which has four binding sites for calcium. Activated calmodulin stimulates certain protein kinases which, using ATP as substrate, will then phosphorylate other proteins, thus activating them. Analogues of DG (the phorbol esters) will stimulate prolonged cell growth and proliferation and promote tumour growth.

Many hormones act through more than one of these mechanisms. There is a wide variety of possible combinations of different effects involving these simple organic compounds and calcium. An appreciation of the general structure of the system is of increasing importance not only in endocrinology, but also in our understanding of tumour growth and development.

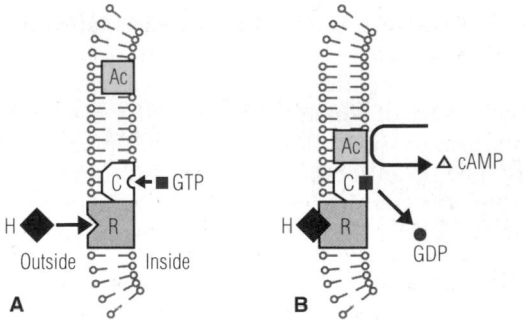

Fig. 17.1 Mechanism of action of hormones that activate adenylate cyclase.
A. The hormone (H) binds to the receptor (R) which alters the conformation of the coupling protein (C) allowing GTP to bond. **B**. The binding of GTP causes the coupling protein to bind and activate adenylate cyclase in the membrane generating cAMP. GTP breaks down to GDP and the activation then ceases.

Actions mediated by tyrosine kinase activity

The insulin receptor is now well characterised; it consists of four subunits, two α and two β. The β-subunit acts as

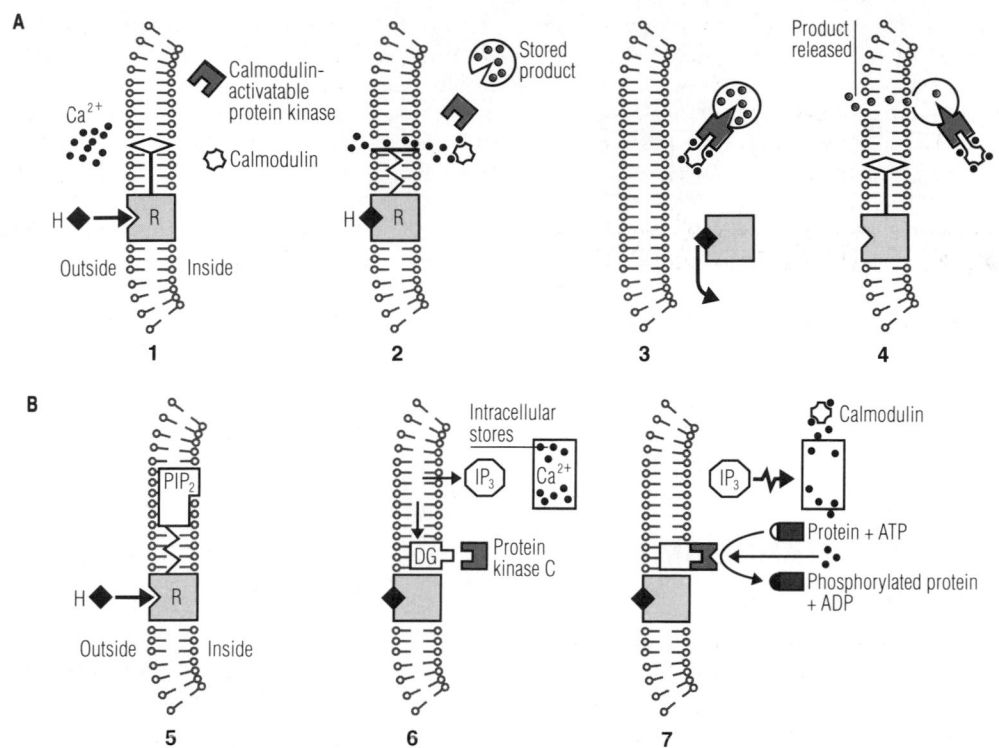

Fig. 17.2 Mechanisms of hormone actions mediated by calcium transport or release. A. Hormones that promote calcium transport into the cell. (1) Absence of hormone. (2) Hormone (H) binds to receptor (R) and opens up Ca^{2+} channel. (3) Ca^{2+} binds to calmodulin, which binds to secretory granule. (4) Secretory granule fuses with cell surface and releases product. **B.** Hormones that act via cleavage of phosphatidyl inositol bisphosphate (PIP2). (1) Hormone binds to receptor. (2) Receptor (activated) cleaves PIP_2 to diacylglycerol (DG) and inositol trisphosphate (IP_3). (3) IP_3 causes Ca^{2+} release from microsomes; Ca^{2+} binds to calmodulin. DG binds and activates protein kinase C (PKC). PKC action, potentiated by Ca^{2+}, phosphorylates protein.

a tyrosine kinase, which is capable of phosphorylating and thereby activating a number of intracellular enzymes (Fig. 17.3). These include serine kinases and serine/threonine phosphatases, which in turn activate their substrates. One of these substrates is the insulin-related growth factor II (IGF II) receptor, which cycles from the cell surface to microsomes and back again, carrying IGF II into the cell in the process. Insulin greatly reduces the amount of this receptor on the cell surface. It is probable

that phosphorylation and dephosphorylation of the IGF II receptor provides the driving force for this cycle of endocytosis and exocytosis. It seems likely that the action of insulin in promoting glucose uptake depends upon a similar effect of altering the phosphorylation state of the glucose transporter molecule.

Hormone action through intracellular receptors

Receptors for steroid hormones (including vitamin D) and thyroid hormones are located principally in the nucleus. In the presence of its ligand, the receptor binds with high affinity to specific promoter sites on DNA. Specific regions of DNA are then 'read' by the enzyme RNA polymerase, with synthesis of messenger RNA and specific important proteins (Fig. 17.4). Most of the actions of steroid hormones are believed to be mediated by such receptors, although at high concentrations, non-receptor-mediated effects may also operate.

Some hormones are made from conversion of less active precursors in target tissues. The clearest example of this is dihydrotestosterone, which is synthesised from

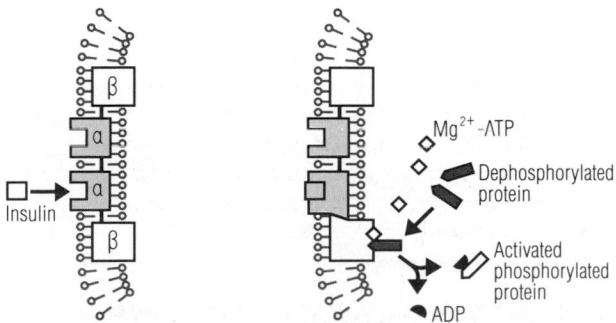

Fig. 17.3 Mechanism of action of insulin. Binding to subunit(s) alters conformation of the β subunit and switches on its protein kinase activity.

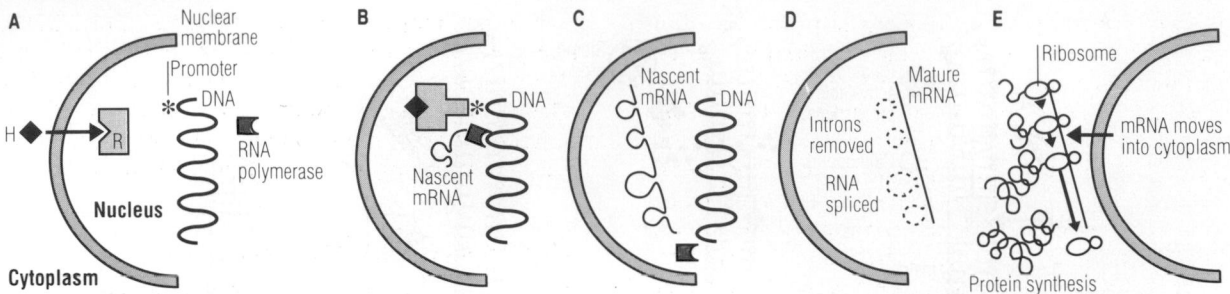

Fig. 17.4 Mechanism of action of steroid and thyroid hormones. A. Hormone (H) binds to nuclear receptor (R). **B.** Activated receptor now binds to specific promoter on DNA, allowing access of RNA polymerase. **C.** and **D.** RNA transcript is processed by removal of introns and splicing. **E.** Messenger RNA (mRNA) is translated in cytoplasm by ribosomes which synthesise proteins.

testosterone (the circulating form) by the enzyme 5-α-reductase. This transformation is essential for many of the actions of testosterone.

CIRCULATION AND METABOLISM OF HORMONES

Most polypeptide hormones have a relatively short half-life (minutes) in the circulation, before they are degraded by proteases in the liver, kidneys, lungs and elsewhere. As implied above, some of the hormone is also internalised in target tissues. Exceptions to the short half-life are the glycosylated peptides – TSH, LH, FSH and human chorionic gonadotrophin (HCG) – where a coating of sugar residues partially protects the protein from degradation, without apparently affecting its binding to the receptor. In some instances, such as FSH, the hormone is secreted episodically, but this is difficult to demonstrate because of its long half-life (several hours). LH, on the other hand, has a much shorter half-life, so episodic secretion is easily detected, with 'pulses' occurring up to once every 90–120 minutes.

The steroid and thyroid hormones are partially protected from degradation by the liver and from renal excretion by circulating binding proteins, the most important of which are corticosteroid binding globulin (CBG), sex-hormone globulin (SHBG), vitamin D-binding protein (DBP), and thyroxine binding globulin (TBG). These proteins are less specific than the receptors; indeed, no general rules can be made for the relation between the affinity of a compound for its binding protein and its biological activity except to say that these proteins generally bind biologically active compounds. In addition, a substantial fraction of many of these hormones bind to albumin and, in some cases, to other proteins with low affinity. Since the concentration of albumin is high, albumin binding is, in some cases (e.g. oestrogens), quantitatively important.

Hormone-binding proteins serve a damping role, reducing the fluctuations produced by episodic secretion of hormones, and reducing their rate of degradation. The small fraction (0.1–5%) of total hormone in free solution (unbound) is believed to be the 'biologically active' fraction, i.e. the amount available to activate cellular receptors. In the case of steroid hormones, it is probably also the unbound plasma steroid that is monitored as part of the feedback control mechanism. In the case of the IGFs there is a whole family of binding proteins, whose control is complex, but clearly has a major influence on the local availability and action of the growth factors.

INTERACTIONS BETWEEN DIFFERENT HORMONES

Two hormones acting together may transmit information differing both qualitatively and quantitatively from that conveyed by either separately. For example, glucocorticoids and adrenaline interact at the levels of both production and action. Glucocorticoids induce the last enzyme necessary for adrenaline synthesis; they also promote production of the β-adrenergic receptor and so enhance some target hormone responses to β-adrenergic agonists (Fig. 17.5). The two hormones together enhance fetal lung maturation at birth. This may have therapeutic importance in treating respiratory distress syndrome and, in later life, bronchial asthma, when analogues of glucocorticoids and adrenaline act synergistically.

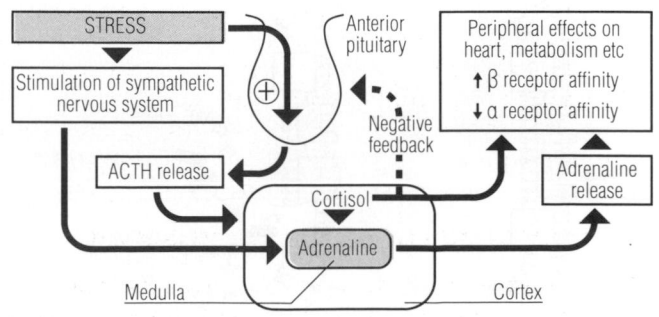

Fig. 17.5 Interactions between glucocorticoids and adrenaline at levels of production and action.

Many of the symptoms and signs of thyroid hormone excess result from an augmented sensitivity to adrenaline from enhanced responsiveness to β-adrenergic effects. The mechanism which enhances β (and probably diminishes α) agonist activity is not yet clear. Many of these effects (excess sweating, lid lag, tachycardia, and tremor) can be blocked acutely by administering a β-adrenergic blocking agent while the thyroid hormone excess persists.

A third example of hormone–hormone interaction is that between oestrogens and progestogens. One effect of oestradiol (and its synthetic counterparts) is to induce production of the progesterone receptor, without which progesterone has little if any effect. The presence of progesterone receptors in breast cancer is among the best available evidence that the tumour is oestrogen-dependent, and amenable to an antioestrogen, such as tamoxifen.

CLASSIFICATION OF ENDOCRINE DISEASES

Hyper-, hypo- and dysfunction

Although excess and deficiency diseases form the basis of endocrine practice, it is an oversimplification to think of endocrine disease simply in terms of 'too much or too little hormone'. It is true that with some systems, e.g. the thyroid gland, normal production of the hormone(s) is relatively steady and the concept of pure excess or deficiency approximates to the truth. However, in other systems, e.g. the adult female reproductive system, there is an inbuilt and complex rhythm. Each of the major components of this system (hypothalamus, pituitary and ovary) secretes hormones and responds to those produced by other components. The interactions depend on both the circulating levels of hormone (often more than one), and the very important dimension of time. Here, the capacity for responses to become out of phase with one another is considerable, and many of the syndromes that we see with this system have features which suggest dysfunction rather than simple hyper- or hypofunction. Since one abnormality may lead to another, with endocrine dysfunction we are in many instances still unable to dissect out the primary abnormality. Our only hope of doing so is to use the model of the normal system as a starting point.

Primary vs secondary abnormalities

It is essential to identify whether an abnormality of hormone production is primary or secondary. Adrenal or thyroid insufficiency, for example, may be due either to intrinsic disease of these glands, or to a failure of secretion of the trophic hormone (ACTH and TSH respectively) by the pituitary. Pituitary deficiency in turn may also be intrinsic, or due to damage to the hypothalamus. The distinction may be important from the point of view of treatment and in predicting and treating accompanying features, including other hormone deficiencies.

Target organ disease

There are many instances of 'target organ' endocrine diseases. This generally involves receptor proteins with a binding site for the hormone, linked to an effector system. Although major disorders due to problems at this level are rare they are well documented and minor problems are quite common. Only recently have methods become available for examining such defects.

THE AETIOLOGY OF ENDOCRINE DISEASES

Tumours

Neoplasms of endocrine tissue are extremely common; they are usually benign and may secrete one or more hormones or be apparently functionless. Such tumours cause problems for one of three reasons:

- They may present as a local space-occupying lesion. This is particularly true of tumours of the pituitary gland because there is very little room for expansion without producing pressure effects on important surrounding structures.
- By secreting a hormone, or hormones, they may produce the syndrome associated with excess of that hormone or of the gland that it controls.
- They may destroy or compress the normal gland and lead to underproduction of other hormones (again this applies almost exclusively to the pituitary gland).

Malignant tumours of endocrine tissue share many of the properties common to other cancers. With some (such as the pituitary) distant metastases are infrequent.

With endocrine tumours, hormone production may continue, or be abnormal; for example, carcinomas of the adrenal cortex may secrete the normal product cortisol, or precursor steroids, or no steroids at all. The control mechanisms of hormone secretion for malignant tumours are generally more disturbed than are those of benign tumours. Occasionally, the properties of the normal gland can be used to treat the tumour; thus, for example, the uptake of radioactive iodine by the tumour can be used very effectively to treat metastases in papillary and follicular carcinomas of the thyroid gland.

In some familiar syndromes, in which tumours occur in more than one endocrine gland (so-called multiple endocrine neoplasia syndrome, MEN), an underlying fundamental defect in cell regulation is suspected (p. 706).

Primary, secondary and tertiary hyperfunction

Primary, secondary and tertiary hyperfunction can be readily appreciated in the case of the parathyroid glands.

Primary hyperparathyroidism exists when excess secretion of parathyroid hormone, not apparently secondary to any other process, leads to hypercalcaemia and other metabolic changes. It may be due to parathyroid adenoma, or to 'primary hyperplasia'.

Secondary hyperparathyroidism is a physiological adaptation to hypocalcaemia. For example, in vitamin D deficiency, calcium malabsorption leads to hypocalcaemia and secondary increased parathyroid hormone (PTH) secretion. This exerts effects on kidneys and bone which restores the plasma calcium level to normal, while increasing phosphate excretion. In chronic renal failure, other factors make this a less efficient process (p. 805), and so the parathyroid hyperplasia and PTH excess tends to be more prolonged and more extreme.

If this secondary hyperparathyroidism leads to the development of an autonomous parathyroid tumour or tumours, *tertiary hyperparathyroidism* is said to have developed. After renal transplantation temporary hypercalcaemia is quite common; although often referred to as tertiary hyperparathyroidism, it is usually due to the increased bulk of hyperplastic parathyroid tissue which has developed during prolonged renal failure rather than to true autonomous tumour development.

Abnormalities of hormone biosynthesis and action

As the pathways of production and action of the major hormones have been defined, so defects in these pathways leading to specific clinical syndromes have been discovered. Often, logical and effective treatment of the condition has resulted. The defects may be inborn, due to single point mutations, or produced by pharmacologists developing new drugs.

Most inborn errors occur in the peripheral rather than the central (hypothalamus and pituitary) endocrine glands. A single example illustrates some general principles. The commonest inborn error of adrenal cortex function is 21-hydroxylase deficiency (Fig. 17.31, p. 701) which is inherited as an autosomal recessive condition. In its extreme (salt-losing) form, it is associated with blocks in the conversion of progesterone to aldosterone,

and 17-hydroxyprogesterone to cortisol, leading to mineralocorticoid and glucocorticoid deficiency. Clinical disease results in part from deficiencies of these two hormones, and in part from the build-up of precursors and their androgenic by-products. Finally, excess ACTH secretion (in response to cortisol deficiency) and excess renin and angiotensin secretion (in response to aldosterone deficiency) also result. These tend to restore a new steady state, but at the expense of marked adrenal hyperplasia and even greater secretion of androgenic by-products.

Recently, increasing numbers of 'target organ' endocrine diseases have been characterised, e.g. the androgen receptor defect (which causes testicular feminisation) and 5-α-reductase deficiency (which causes a particular form of male pseudohermaphroditism, see p. 715).

Autoimmune endocrine disease

In recent years, the role of the immune system in causing destruction and malfunction of parts of the endocrine system has become increasingly apparent. It is evident that both antibody-mediated and cell-mediated immunity may be involved, but the former is better understood. A wide range of antibodies may be involved, which may be directed at cell surface components, or at microsomes, mitochondria and other intracellular organelles. In many cases, it is not clear which, if any, of the antibodies cause tissue damage and which are produced in response to cell destruction.

The immune disturbance may lead to:

- *Destruction of the gland*, e.g. in autoimmune Addison's disease (where antiadrenal antibodies are generally present in plasma) or in primary autoimmune hypothyroidism.
- *Lymphocytic infiltration of the gland*, as in Hashimoto's thyroiditis (where a high titre of antimicrosomal and antithyroglobulin antibodies is invariably present).
- *Uncontrolled stimulation of the gland.* In thyrotoxic Graves' disease, antibodies are produced that mimic TSH sufficiently closely to bind to, and activate, the TSH receptor.
- *Blocking of the tropic hormone*, e.g. some cases of autoimmune hypothyroidism and Addison's disease.

Different individuals vary greatly in their inherited tendency to develop autoimmune endocrine disease. The full basis for individual susceptibility is not known, but one factor is the histocompatibility (HLA) antigen status of the individual. Certain HLA types, particularly those expressed normally only on lymphocytes (the so-called DR antigens) confer particular susceptibility (p. 684). One hypothesis is that, in autoimmune thyroid disease, certain DR antigens necessary for immune recognition are exposed on the external surface of the thyroid follicle cells and activate an immune response against the cells.

The term *organ-specific autoimmune disease* encompasses both endocrine and non-endocrine diseases, and includes autoimmune Addison's disease, Graves' disease, Hashimoto's disease, autoimmune hypothyroidism, myasthenia gravis, hypoparathyroidism, true autoimmune diabetes mellitus, pernicious anaemia, autoimmune ovarian failure and vitiligo (autoimmune skin depigmentation). As a general rule, individuals with one such disease are more likely than normal individuals to develop another.

SYSTEMIC EFFECTS OF ENDOCRINE DISORDERS

Central nervous system

Local expansion of pituitary tumours commonly causes headache (due probably to tension on the diaphragma sellae) and damage to adjacent structures. The optic nerves are particularly vulnerable to pressure, especially at the optic chiasm, and bitemporal hemianopia may result. Less frequently, pituitary or suprapituitary tumours may cause damage in the region of the fourth ventricle, resulting in a syndrome of recent memory loss similar to Korsakoff's psychosis (p. 979).

Both *hyper- and hypocalcaemia* may precipitate any psychosis to which that individual is predisposed or cause neuropsychiatric symptoms *de novo*. Hypocalcaemia may be associated with raised intracranial pressure, epileptic fits and, of course, tetany.

Hyperfunction of both the adrenal cortex and the adrenal medulla may present with *psychiatric manifestations*. In Cushing's syndrome, the individual may present with depression or with a schizophrenia-like syndrome. Excess cortisol secretion may occur in severe depression per se, so it can be very difficult to establish whether or not the patient has Cushing's syndrome. Many of the symptoms and signs of emotional or physical stress result from release of hormones, notably adrenaline, from the adrenal medulla. Tumours of the adrenal medulla (phaeochromocytomas) usually secrete predominantly noradrenaline, thus causing hypertension, but sweating and anxiety attacks are often an accompanying feature.

Thyroid disease may also be accompanied by a variety of neuropsychiatric features. Thyrotoxicosis may present as anxiety, depression or behavioural disturbance, although warm sweaty hands and a rapid pulse usually distinguish the condition from a simple anxiety state. Occasionally, the patient appears unduly apathetic.

Proximal muscle weakness is another common feature of thyrotoxicosis. Accompanying exophthalmos due to ocular muscle infiltration may cause diplopia. Hypothyroidism may also present with depression. Its other neurological manifestations include carpal tunnel syndrome, myotonia and cerebellar dysfunction.

Coma may be the presenting sign of a number of endocrine disorders. These (and other) manifestations of hyper- and hypoglycaemia are considered in Chapter 19. In profound hypothyroidism, coma is likely to be due to hypothermia. In severe hypopituitarism, stupor leading to coma commonly follows a relatively minor disturbance (such as a trivial accident or infection). It is due in part to profound cortisol deficiency, in part to hypothyroidism, and is usually associated with hyponatraemia due to excess secretion of antidiuretic hormone as a consequence of cortisol deficiency. In diabetes insipidus (DI), hypernatraemia may occur rapidly and produce convulsions or irreversible brain damage if access to water is restricted (e.g. post-operatively). Conversely, in the treated patient with DI, unlimited drinking may lead to cerebral dysfunction and fits from hyponatraemia (water intoxication).

Cardiovascular system

Hypotension, especially in the upright posture, commonly results from either glucocorticoid or mineralocorticoid deficiency, while hypertension, usually of mild degree, may result from mineralocorticoid excess. Endocrine diseases leading to electrolyte disturbances such as hyper- or hypocalcaemia or hypokalaemia may present with dysrhythmias and/or characteristic ECG abnormalities. Prolonged hypercalcaemia and prolonged glucocorticoid excess are associated with an increased incidence of arterial calcification. Patients with primary hypothyroidism have a high incidence of ischaemic heart disease, partly due to hypercholesterolaemia. Those with angina are particularly vulnerable to myocardial infarction when treated with thyroxine. In the elderly, thyrotoxicosis commonly leads to atrial fibrillation. Acromegaly is associated with cardiac enlargement, hypertension and a form of cardiomyopathy.

Skeletal system

Skeletal manifestations of endocrine disease are commonly caused by osteoporosis, as in Cushing's syndrome, sex hormone deficiency or prolonged hyperthyroidism. Primary hyperparathyroidism may lead to calcification of articular cartilage, and present with calcium pyrophosphate crystal arthropathy (pseudogout, see p. 1022). The classical bone disease of Von Recklinghausen, with giant cell tumours of bone due to primary hyperparathyroidism, is now exceptionally rare. Occasionally, autoimmune thyrotoxicosis is associated with finger clubbing and periosteal new bone growth (so-called thyroid acropachy). In mild acromegaly, peri-articular overgrowth of new bone and increased cartilage quite commonly lead to osteoarthritis. In severe acromegaly and gigantism, skeletal abnormalities may be gross.

Genito-urinary and reproductive systems

Conditions which affect sex hormone secretion in utero produce malformation of the external and internal genitalia (p. 715). Renal function may be disturbed by a number of metabolic disorders, some of which are of endocrine origin. For example, both hypercalcaemia and hypokalaemia may present with a form of (nephrogenic) diabetes insipidus and polyuria due to a water diuresis.

Integumentary system

Hirsutism and acne are common manifestations of androgen excess in the female. Mild hirsutism, skin atrophy, bruising and poor wound healing are features of Cushing's syndrome. Hyperpigmentation is common in Addison's disease. Vitiligo and mucocutaneous candidiasis occur in some autoimmune endocrine diseases. Of other endocrine disorders presenting with skin manifestations, the glucagonoma syndrome, which causes migratory necrolytic erythema, is probably the most striking (p. 613).

Alimentary system

Thyrotoxicosis commonly causes diarrhoea and sometimes malabsorption. Hypothyroidism causes constipation. Conditions such as Addison's disease, hypopituitarism and diabetic ketoacidosis may present as apparent upper abdominal emergencies with epigastric pain and rigidity. Hypercalcaemia commonly causes vomiting, constipation and abdominal pain.

ENDOCRINE FUNCTION TESTING

Endocrine function tests are used to establish or to refine the diagnosis, to monitor the response to treatment, to assess the prognosis, and to establish the pathogenesis of the condition. Clearly, it is important to understand both the underlying physiology on which the test is based and the limitations of the assay method. The minimum number of tests should be made to answer a particular question. Old tests are rapidly being superseded by new and better methods.

Basal measurements

Much can be learnt by *basal measurements* of so-called routine biochemistry (Table 17.1). Where endocrine disease involves hormones that control the electrolytes, these measurements are the mainstay. Thus, a parathyroid tumour is most unlikely unless the serum calcium level is raised, and a low serum phosphate further suggests the diagnosis. Aldosterone deficiency in Addison's disease is suggested by the finding of a high serum potassium level, usually associated with a low sodium and elevated urea, due to extracellular fluid depletion.

In assessing posterior pituitary function, the tests (fluid deprivation) depend upon assessing the renal response, mediated by vasopressin, to deliberate but controlled withholding of fluids. In most cases, and certainly to exclude diabetes insipidus, simple study of the relationships of fluid loss to serum and urine osmolality suffice, without the need for difficult assays of vasopressin.

Basal measurements of hormone levels or metabolites are most practical when they can be conducted on serum or urine samples collected at random. Nowadays, the widespread development and application of radioimmuno- and immunoradiometric assays has helped enormously, especially for hormones that are relatively stable in body fluids. This applies to the steroid hormones thyroid hormones and most of the pituitary hormones. In most cases, serum is preferred to plasma; clotted blood can be left for 1–2 hours before centrifugation, and serum stored indefinitely at −20°C. Economic and methodological considerations dictate that samples are assayed batch-

Table 17.1 'Routine' biochemical pointers in blood plasma to endocrine disorders

Pointers	Condition
Hyperkalaemia, hyponatraemia	Addison's disease
Hypokalaemia, metabolic alkalosis (high serum bicarbonate)	Conn's syndrome Cushing's syndrome (severe)
Hyponatraemia, hypochloraemia	Inappropriate ADH secretion Hypopituitarism Severe hypothyroidism
Hypernatraemia, hyperchloraemia	Diabetes insipidus
Hyperglycaemia, hyperchloraemia, metabolic acidosis (low serum bicarbonate)	Diabetic ketoacidosis
Hyperglycaemia, uraemia, hypernatraemia, hyperchloraemia	Diabetic-hyperosmolar
Hypercalcaemia, hypophosphataemia, hyperchloraemia	Primary hyperparathyroidism
Hypocalcaemia, hyperphosphataemia	Hypoparathyroidism

wise, so that the result is often not available at once. It may therefore be necessary to start treatment while the result is awaited. Urine sometimes has the advantage of reflecting integrated secretion and the 'free' (unbound) level (e.g. with cortisol). However, the major steroids in urine are metabolites several steps away from the biologically active compound.

Dynamic function tests

The static nature of information obtained by basal measurements has led to the development of a whole range of *dynamic function tests*, where the system under study is deliberately driven, usually by interrupting negative feedback or by stimulation at one or more levels. In testing anterior pituitary function, there is a bewildering array of possible tests, not all of which are useful. For example, stimulation tests for ACTH (and so cortisol) with insulin hypoglycaemia, glucagon, vasopressin and CRH have all been devised, in addition to direct adrenal stimulation with synthetic ACTH (synacthen). With TSH and the thyroid hormones, marked episodic and diurnal variation – a problem inherent in assessing the ACTH-cortisol axis – is missing and, especially with new sensitive TSH assays, dynamic testing with TRH is thus seldom needed. Sometimes, two or more tests can be carried out simultaneously, e.g. insulin, TRH and GnRH can all be given together to assess the extent of hypopituitarism. An example of a test used to monitor or predict response to treatment is the measurement of serum prolactin or growth hormone levels after a single dose of bromocriptine in patients with prolactinoma or acromegaly respectively. In complex endocrine systems such as the ovulatory cycle, repeated samples over the cycle of more than one hormone may be necessary, and may be much more useful than contrived 'dynamic function' tests (see Fig. 17.6).

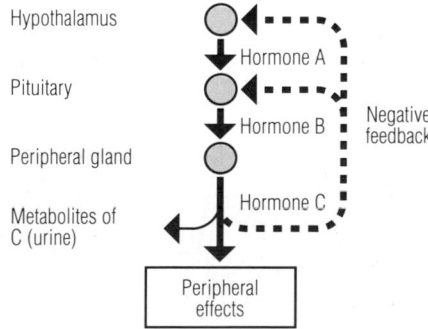

Fig. 17.6 Principles of dynamic endocrine function testing. Hypothalamic hormone A stimulates pituitary to produce pituitary hormone B which then stimulates peripheral gland to produce C. Hormone C (or a synthetic analogue) inhibits production of A and/or B by negative feedback.

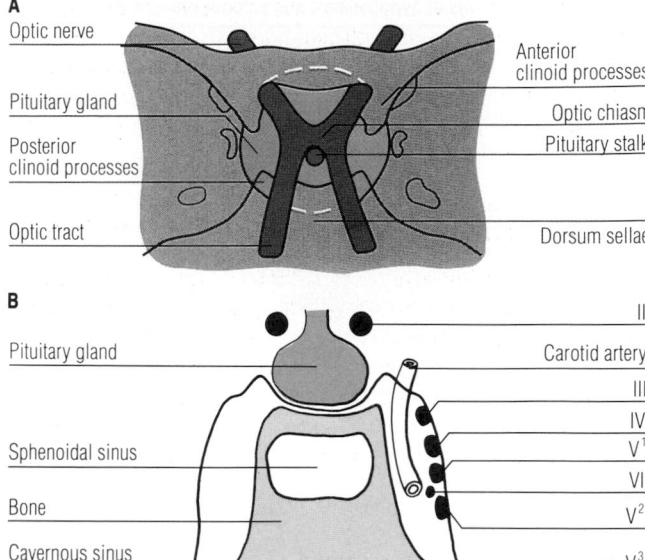

Fig. 17.7 Gross anatomy and relations of the pituitary gland. A. View of pituitary gland, anterior clinoids, dorsum sellae and optic chiasm from above. **B.** Coronal cross-section through pituitary gland to show relation to important structures nearby.

THE PITUITARY GLAND

The pituitary gland is composed of two functionally separate lobes, the anterior and the posterior (pars nervosa), with an intermediate lobe which is vestigial in man. The gland is derived from a down-growth from the floor of the third ventricle and from Rathke's pouch, which is formed by invagination of part of the roof of the primitive nasopharynx.

The pituitary gland is almost entirely enclosed in a bony box, the sella turcica; this has a floor and an anterior and posterior wall, the lateral extremities of which become the anterior and posterior clinoid processes. Immediately lateral to the pituitary gland are the two cavernous sinuses, with the IIIrd, IVth and Vth cranial nerves sandwiched between; the carotid syphon courses through the cavernous sinus (Fig. 17.7). Overlying the pituitary is a fibrous sheet, the diaphragma sellae, which is pierced by the pituitary stalk; this slender structure carries the nerve fibres to the posterior pituitary gland and the blood supply to both lobes including the portal blood vessels draining from the median eminence of the hypothalamus.

Terminology of hypothalamic and pituitary hormones

The terminology of hypothalamic and pituitary hormones is a complex subject, made more so by a wide range of acronyms and synonyms. Those peptides produced in the

Table 17.2 Terminology of hypothalamic and anterior pituitary hormones

Hypothalamic hormone	Effect (stimulation or inhibition)	Pituitary hormone
Gonadotrophin releasing hormone GnRH, LH-releasing hormone/factor, LH-FSH releasing hormone	+	Luteinising hormone (LH) Follicle stimulating hormone (FSH)
Corticotrophin-releasing hormone/factor (CRF)	+	Adrenocorticotrophic hormone (ACTH, corticotrophin)
Vasopressin (ADH)	+	
Somatostatin (growth hormone/somatotrophin release inhibiting hormone)	−	Growth hormone (GH, somatotrophin)
Growth hormone releasing hormone (GHRH)	+	
Thyrotrophin releasing hormone (TRH)	+	Thyroid stimulating hormone (TSH, thyrotrophin)
Dopamine (prolactin inhibiting factor, PIF)	−	Prolactin

hypothalamus which act locally on the pituitary gland are referred to interchangeably as 'factors' or 'hormones'. Some of the more important interchangeable terms are given in Table 17.2.

THE ANTERIOR PITUITARY GLAND

SYNTHESIS AND SECRETION OF THE MAIN HORMONES

Much is now known about how the synthesis and secretion of anterior pituitary hormones is controlled, and this is summarised in Table 17.3.

Table 17.3 Factors directly affecting anterior pituitary hormone synthesis and release

Pituitary hormone	Stimuli	Inhibitors
ACTH	CRF Vasopressin (ADH) Interleukin 1 (IL-1)*	Cortisol
GH	GHRH	Somatostatin Insulin-like growth factor I (IGF I) Cortisol
TSH	TRH	T3, T4
LH	GnRH Oestradiol (+ve feedback)	Oestradiol Progesterone Testosterone (male)
FSH	GnRH	Inhibin Oestradiol Progesterone Testosterone (male)
Prolactin	TRH Oestradiol**	Dopamine

*Effect probably via CRF
**Increases prolactin synthesis, produces lactotroph hyperplasia but inhibits milk secretion

Adrenocorticotrophic hormone

ACTH is synthesised in specific cells (the corticotrophs) from a large precursor molecule called pro-opiomelanocortin (POMC, Fig.17.8). It is produced in both the anterior and intermediate lobe of the pituitary, but the final processing differs in the two. Of the other ACTH-related peptides, β lipotrophin (LPH), β endorphin, and α melanocyte stimulating hormone (MSH) are important. LPH and β endorphin are synthesised and secreted with ACTH. Beta endorphin may have a role as an opiate in modifying the response to pain at times of stress.

The synthesis and release of ACTH is controlled by corticotrophin-releasing factor (CRF), which acts synergistically with vasopressin and possibly another hypothalamic factor. There are at least two basic rhythms of ACTH secretion; episodes of secretion every 1–3 hours and at meal times are superimposed on a 24-hour rhythm, with lowest levels during the earliest hours of sleep and peak secretion just before wakening (Fig. 17.9). At any time, exposure to sudden physical or mental stress will overcome this rhythm and lead to a pulse of ACTH secretion. The adrenal cortex responds in turn with a pulse of cortisol secretion within minutes, so that the 24-hour

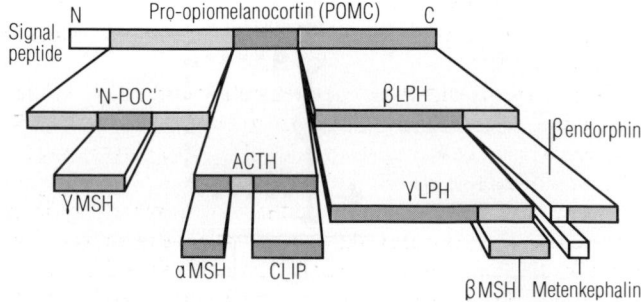

Fig. 17.8 Relationship between pro-opiomelanocortin (POMC) and the various intermediates and end-products of its processing in the pituitary gland. LPH = lipotrophin; N-POC = N-pro-opiomelanocortin; MSH = melanocyte stimulating hormone; CLIP = corticotrophin-like intermediate lobe peptide.

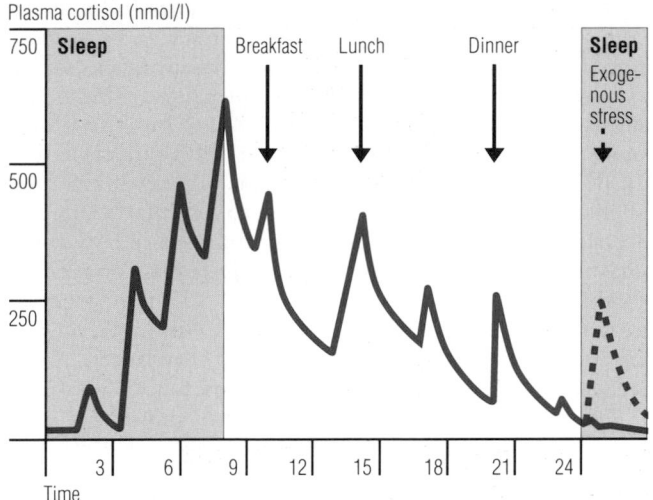

Fig. 17.9 Plasma cortisol levels through the 24-hour cycle to show circadian variation, pulsatile secretion and influence of meals and stress.

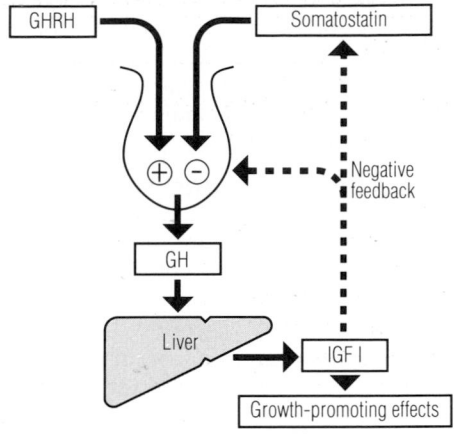

Fig. 17.10 Control of growth hormone and IGF I secretion.

plasma profile of cortisol is a somewhat dampened version of the 24-hour ACTH profile.

The most important role of ACTH is to control the synthesis and secretion of the glucocorticoid cortisol. As would be expected from its relationship to MSH (see Fig. 17.8), ACTH possesses MSH activity, and will directly stimulate the melanocytes of the skin and buccal mucosa when secreted in excessive amounts. This accounts for the increase in pigmentation to above normal (for that individual) seen in Addison's disease (p. 699) and Nelson's syndrome (pp. 678 and 704).

Growth hormone

Growth hormone (GH), human placental lactogen (HPL) and prolactin (PRL) belong to a family of polypeptide hormones. GH and HPL both contain 191 amino acids, and PRL 199. GH and HPL are closely homologous (with 85% identical residues) and probably arose by gene duplication relatively recently in evolution; their genes are located on chromosome 17. PRL is much less closely related.

GH is synthesised in specific cells (known as somatotrophs), where it is stored in granules and released episodically in response to peaks of hypothalamic secretion of GHRH (Fig. 17.10). The precise physiological interactions of GHRH with somatostatin, which inhibits its release, are complex. Much of the GH is secreted at night and episodically. Its secretion is inhibited by a rise in blood glucose (the basis of a useful suppression test) and stimulated by hypoglycaemic stress and by amino acids such as arginine (the basis of stimulation tests). GH controls the secretion of insulin-like growth factor I (IGF I, somatomedin C), which functions as a hormone con-

trolling the growth of cartilage and soft tissues. During puberty, secretion of sex hormones appears to increase the pituitary secretion of GH, which is probably important in promoting growth before the sex hormones lead to closure of the epiphyses. GH also acts directly on tissues to control local production of IGF I. The effects of IGF I are modulated by specific binding proteins, which are also under hormonal control.

Prolactin

PRL is produced in the lactotrophs, under stimulation by TRH and under tonic inhibition by dopamine. PRL has a basically nocturnal pattern of secretion and is also released in response to stress. Oestrogens probably act directly on the lactotrophs, increasing their number and activity. In pregnancy, PRL levels are high and so lead to hypertrophy of the breast epithelium (Table 17.4).

Table 17.4 Action of hormones on the human breast

Hormone	Action
Polypeptide hormones	
Prolactin	Milk protein synthesis and excretion in ducts and lobules
Oxytocin	Milk ejection. Contraction of myoepithelial cells
Human placental lactogen	Similar to prolactin
Growth hormone	'Permissive' effects
Insulin	'Permissive' effects
Steroid hormones	
Oestrogens	Increase duct and breast fat growth Inhibit prolactin-induced milk secretion
Progestogens	Inhibit lactation (effect requires oestrogen)
Cortisol	'Permissive' effects
Androgens	Inhibitory effects on ? stroma

However, high oestrogen and progesterone levels inhibit milk production until after delivery of the baby. During lactation, suckling stimulates secretion of PRL via a reflex arc. High PRL levels have a contraceptive effect, probably by inhibiting cyclical gonadotrophin release.

Luteinising hormone and follicle stimulating hormone

LH and FSH appear to be controlled by the same releasing hormone and are produced in the same cell type (the gonadotroph). They resemble TSH and HCG in being two-subunit polypeptides, and in possessing a sugar 'coat'. The α-subunits of these peptides differ very little, but the β-subunits differ greatly and confer the specificity. The ratio and absolute amount of LH and FSH secreted in response to a single pulse of GnRH varies greatly under different circumstances. In both sexes, it appears to be modified by age, sex hormone secretion by the gonads and the preceding pattern of discharge of GnRH. Low frequency discharge seems to favour FSH synthesis and release. In females, a rise in oestrogen level differentially reduces FSH and eventually promotes LH release ('positive feedback', see Fig. 17.35A). These interactions and their significance are discussed on page 711. The gonads also produce a polypeptide hormone (inhibin) which feeds back to the pituitary to switch off FSH synthesis and secretion selectively.

Thyroid stimulating hormone

TSH promotes the synthesis and secretion of thyroid hormones, and the growth of the thyroid gland. The principal hypothalamic control is from thyrotrophin releasing hormone (TRH), whose secretion, as with GnRH, is apparently pulsatile. The thyroid hormones feed back on both the hypothalamus, to regulate the synthesis of TRH, and on the pituitary gland, inhibiting TSH release.

ANTERIOR PITUITARY HYPOFUNCTION

Anterior pituitary hypofunction may develop rapidly or insidiously, and may affect all the pituitary hormones, a few or only one. We consider here those causes associated with partial or complete loss of all the anterior pituitary hormones, causing a state of so-called *(anterior) panhypopituitarism*. This will, in some cases, be associated with diabetes insipidus, where vasopressin secretion from the posterior pituitary is also impaired.

Aetiology

The causes of panhypopituitarism are listed in Table 17.5. The commonest *vascular* cause is Sheehan's syndrome, in which hypopituitarism occurs following a pregnancy complicated by a period of shock and hypotension, commonly due to postpartum haemorrhage. The pituitary normally enlarges during pregnancy under the action of oestrogens on the lactotrophs, but the blood supply does not; it is therefore particularly vulnerable to a fall in blood pressure. There are usually no symptoms (such as headache) directly related to the infarction, but lactation does not occur, and the symptoms of hypopituitarism soon follow. Menstrual periods do not return. Rarely, prolonged shock in other situations may precede the development of panhypopituitarism. Similarly, *meningitis* in pregnancy (tuberculous or otherwise) is more likely to be followed by pituitary deficiency.

Tumours, both within the pituitary and suprasellar (e.g. the craniopharyngioma, which develops from Rathke's pouch), are common causes of panhypopituitarism. The clinical features include pressure effects on surrounding structures, including the optic chiasm and the hypothalamus. In the case of *intrasellar* tumours, panhypopituitarism is usually a late development, since some normal pituitary tissue remains. If the tumour is functional, there may be additional features other than those from pressure on the remaining normal pituitary. A prolactinoma, for example, may cause hypopituitarism and hyperprolactinaemia. Suprasellar tumours are more likely to affect the pituitary stalk, and thereby the posterior pituitary gland. If a large pituitary tumour becomes infarcted, it will cause the syndrome of 'pituitary apoplexy' (severe headache, neck stiffness, vomiting), which may be followed by hypopituitarism if the normal tissue is compromised.

Granulomatous conditions that may occasionally be responsible include eosinophilic granuloma (histiocytosis X, p. 1096) and sarcoidosis. Carotid aneurysms may occasionally damage the pituitary. Panhypopituitarism may develop long after pituitary irradiation (e.g. for a growth-hormone secreting tumour). This is usually a consequence of hypothalamic damage, and commonly affects growth hormone and gonadotrophin secretion before other hormones.

In many cases of panhypopituitarism, the aetiology is obscure; some may be autoimmune. In some cases, there is an empty sella turcica and a defective diaphragma. It is still undecided whether the so-called 'empty sella syndrome' is a primary cause of hypopituitarism.

Local pressure effects of pituitary and suprasellar tumours

The principal pressure symptoms are headache, which may be severe and persistent, and visual field disturbances. Bitemporal hemianopia, which starts with loss of the upper quadrant (if the tumour is below the chiasm), is characteristic. The patient may notice loss of the lateral

Table 17.5 Causes of panhypopituitarism

Cause	Mechanism	Associated features
Developmental abnormalities	Failure of hypothalamic or pituitary development Perinatal asphyxia	Severe cranial abnormalities Midline facial abnormalities GH deficiency predominant
Infection Encephalitis Bacterial meningitis	Hypothalamus or stalk damage, or pituitary destruction	History of encephalitis or bacterial meningitis
Granulomata Eosinophilic granuloma Sarcoidosis	Infiltration of pituitary/hypothalamus	Eosinophilic granuloma Sarcoidosis (p. 500)
Vascular Infarction Haemorrhage Aneurysms	Hypotension, especially when the pituitary is enlarged, e.g. by pregnancy or tumour Pituitary apoplexy Subarachnoid haemorrhage Pressure	Sheehan's syndrome from antepartum or postpartum haemorrhage Hypotension (surgical or traumatic) Pituitary enlargement/tumour Cranial nerve lesions Apoplexy simulates subarachnoid Ballooning of pituitary fossa
Tumour Suprapituitary (craniopharyngioma) Pituitary	Pressure on stalk Pressure or invasion of normal gland	Pressure on optic chiasm or brainstem Suprasellar calcification (craniopharyngioma) Large pituitary fossa Hormone excess if tumour functional
Empty sella	Mechanism uncertain	Ballooning of pituitary fossa
Autoimmune	Antibodies to pituicytes	Other organ-specific autoimmune disease Anti-pituitary antibodies
Trauma	Severe head injury causing stalk damage	Brain and cranial nerve damage

part of the visual fields; the defect will not at first be detectable by confrontation, but can be shown by formal perimetry with a Bjerrum's screen, and may be most obvious if a red object is used. Fundoscopy may reveal bi- or unilateral optic atrophy. Other field defects are also quite common. More rarely, other cranial nerves (the IIIrd, IVth, Vth and VIth) are involved.

A syndrome reminiscent of Korsakoff's syndrome with recent memory loss may occur if there is pressure on the floor of the third ventricle. Disturbances of appetite (causing hyperphagia) and thirst may be seen. The latter causes particular problems if diabetes insipidus is also present, since the patient does not drink enough to prevent hyperosmolarity. The occurrence of pressure effects depends mainly on the size of the tumour; for example GH-secreting pituitary tumours (in acromegaly) are generally much larger than ACTH-secreting tumours (in Cushing's disease). Non-functioning tumours and prolactinomas are the two other intrasellar lesions which commonly cause pressure symptoms.

Clinical features of anterior pituitary hypofunction

The clinical features of anterior pituitary hypofunction depend in part upon the age of onset.

Childhood

If the onset of panhypopituitarism is before growth is completed, the patient will have the features of hypopituitary dwarfism, i.e. normal body proportions but failure to grow. The latter is detected and documented by careful measurements of height using a stadiometer recorded on standard growth charts (Fig.17.11). From serial measurements, growth velocity (cm/year) can be calculated and

---

Summary 1 Clinical features of hormone-producing pituitary tumours

- Local symptoms are headache and visual disturbance

- In acromegaly the tumour is usually large, but small in Cushing's disease.

- Incipient visual loss may merit an immediate trial of bromocriptine.

- Macroprolactinomas occur equally in men and women. Microprolactinomas in women only.

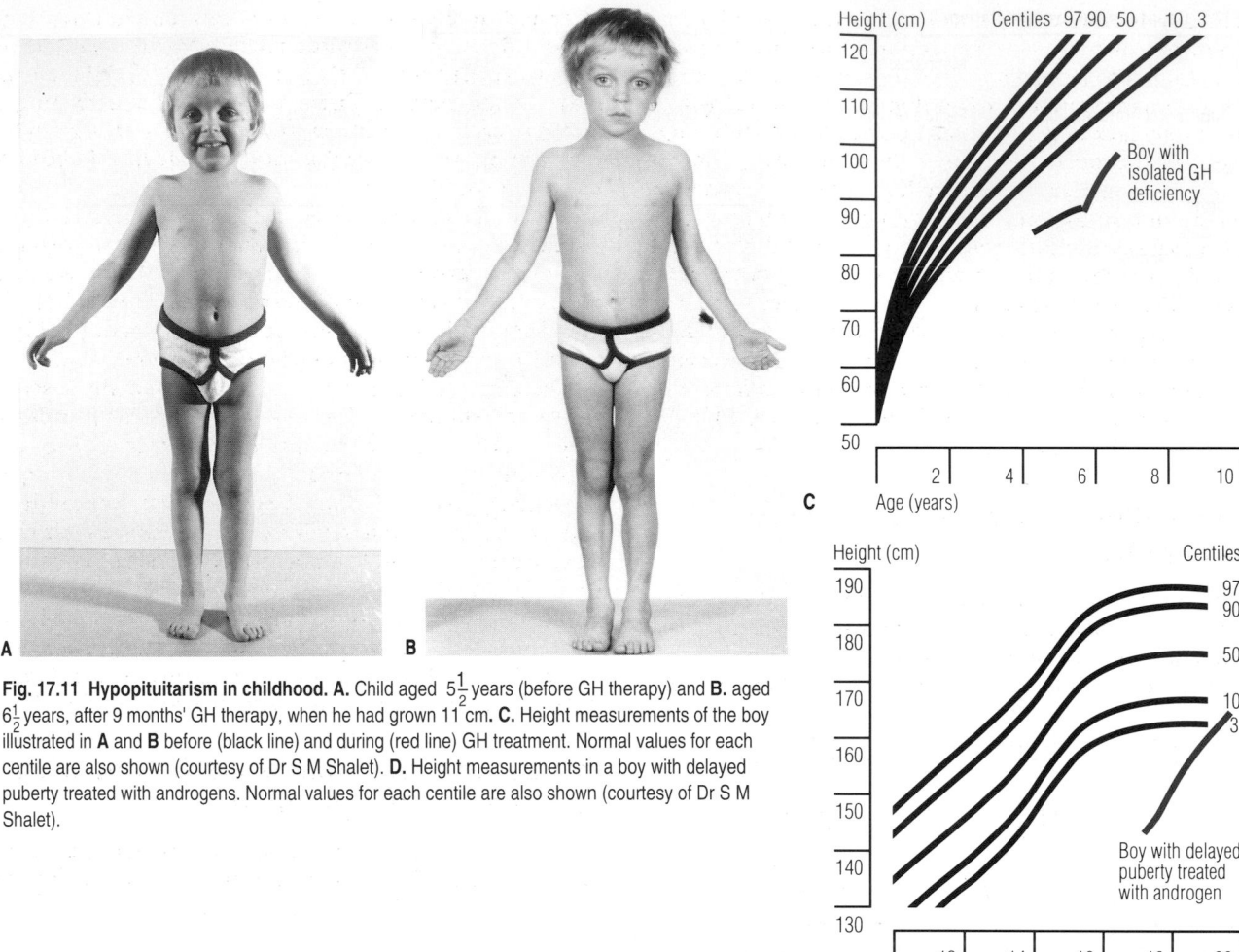

Fig. 17.11 Hypopituitarism in childhood. A. Child aged $5\frac{1}{2}$ years (before GH therapy) and **B.** aged $6\frac{1}{2}$ years, after 9 months' GH therapy, when he had grown 11 cm. **C.** Height measurements of the boy illustrated in **A** and **B** before (black line) and during (red line) GH treatment. Normal values for each centile are also shown (courtesy of Dr S M Shalet). **D.** Height measurements in a boy with delayed puberty treated with androgens. Normal values for each centile are also shown (courtesy of Dr S M Shalet).

related to standard rates of growth. Panhypopituitarism in childhood is also associated with failure of pubertal development.

Other common features of hypopituitarism in childhood include a tendency to hypoglycaemia and other general features discussed below.

Adult life

In panhypopituitarism developing in adult life, the patient usually feels unwell in a non-specific way. They appear pale without being anaemic and the skin has a 'waxen doll' appearance. They notice the cold, although features of hypothyroidism are often not as gross or obvious as in myxoedema. Women have amenorrhoea and men lose their sex drive and potency. Loss of secondary sexual hair and decline of other secondary sexual characteristics is a feature in both sexes. The patients may present with a 'hypopituitary crisis' when challenged by trivial stress, which would normally be met by increased secretion of ACTH and cortisol. Acute abdominal pain may mimic acute abdominal emergency. This syndrome responds rapidly to cortisol administration. Patients commonly develop hypoglycaemia but, because of an associated lack of adrenaline secretion (see Figure 17.5, p. 660), they do not develop symptoms of 'classical' hypoglycaemia, i.e. a sympathetic response to the low blood sugar. They may therefore present with coma due to hypoglycaemia. Coma may also be due to hyponatraemia, since there is commonly an excess of ADH secretion (cortisol inhibits this secretion and the renal response to ADH).

Manifestations of *growth hormone deficiency* include pallor, thin skin and hypoglycaemia. Those of *ACTH* (and thus cortisol) *deficiency* include malaise, somnolence, hyponatraemia, poor response to stress, hypoglycaemia, confusion, coma, hypotension and fever.

Effects of *sex hormone deficiency* include delayed puberty, sexual infantilism, amenorrhoea and lack of breast development. Men show abnormal 'puppy fat' distribution of body fat and lack of muscular development. Loss of secondary sexual hair is much more marked in panhypopituitarism than in conditions where there is only lack of gonadal sex hormones. As with other causes of androgen deficiency in men, the patient's partner may complain more than him. Loss of sex drive is also common in hypopituitary women. Features due to *TSH deficiency* include cold intolerance and dry skin, although hypothyroidism may be masked by other deficiencies. *Diabetes insipidus* is discussed on pages 681–682; its effects are often less marked when cortisol is also deficient, since the latter is necessary for a water diuresis in vasopressin deficiency. *PRL deficiency* leads to failure of milk production, which is of importance only to the woman who is breast feeding.

Investigation of suspected pituitary hypofunction

If hypopituitarism is suspected, a clotted blood sample is taken for hormone analysis and glucocorticoid treatment commenced at once, most conveniently by giving 100 mg hydrocortisone intravenously, followed by 50 mg 6 hours

later and then a normal regular replacement dose. If the patient does not have pituitary or adrenal insufficiency, such treatment is unlikely to be harmful, and if they do it may be life-saving. There is a risk of precipating an adrenal crisis with stress tests or by starting thyroid replacement first (since this increases the metabolic clearance of cortisol).

Much of value can be learnt from *basal measurements* of serum urea and electrolytes, LH and FSH, testosterone (in men), progesterone and oestradiol (in women), cortisol, thyroxine (T4) and tri-odothyronine (T3), GH and PRL. These measurements help considerably to establish the diagnosis and possibly its cause.

Dynamic hormone tests are conventionally used as the 'gold standard' for assessing pituitary function (Fig. 17.12). Insulin should be given in a low dose (0.15 units/kg) with close observation by a doctor throughout. An ECG should be done first, but not in the elderly or those with heart disease or epilepsy. In this situation, glucagon (1 mg) can be used as an alternative stimulus to ACTH and cortisol secretion. Glucose for intravenous injection, or glucagon, should be available, and given early rather than late. GH and cortisol measurements are made serially over 2 hours. For convenience, GnRH, TRH and insulin can be given simultaneously (Fig. 17.12).

Investigations to establish the underlying cause of hypopituitarism

The history and physical examination may point to a particular cause of hypopituitarism, such as previous infarction, meningitis or radiotherapy.

Imaging

Lateral and antero-posterior X-rays of the skull may reveal expansion of the pituitary fossa and erosion of the dorsum sellae and anterior or posterior clinoids (Fig. 17.13), although such changes do not indicate that the tumour responsible still exists – the fossa may be empty. For this reason, a CT or MR scan is essential (Fig. 17.14), and has now superseded more invasive studies with injection of contrast media such as metrizamide or air into the subarachnoid space. Angiography still has a role in defining the relationship of major blood vessels before surgery.

Plain X-rays may give specific diagnostic clues, e.g. suprasellar calcification suggests a craniopharyngioma. Rarer causes include eosinophilic granuloma, in which case 'punched out' bone lesions may be present in the skull or elsewhere and there may be a reticular lung pattern on the chest radiograph. The pituitary gland may be the site of a metastasis from a carcinoma, in which case the skull X-ray may show bone destruction. Where there is no evident cause, and no history to suggest

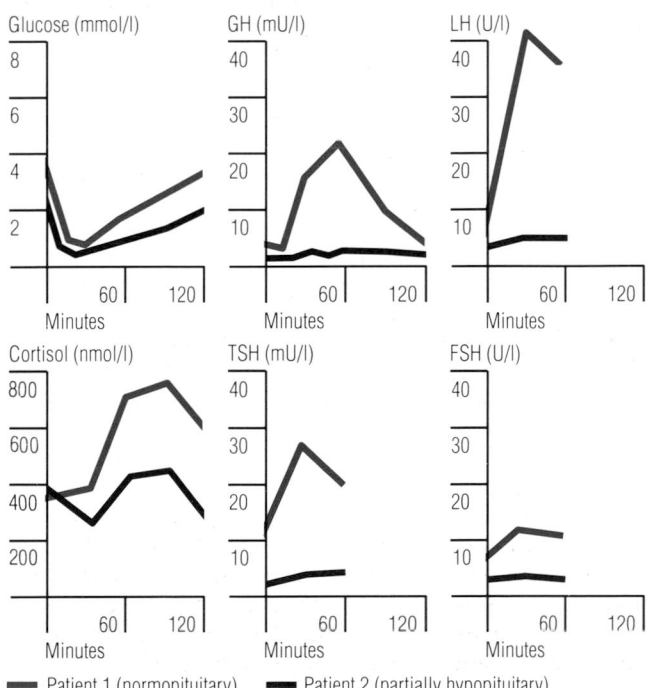

Fig. 17.12 Responses in two patients to combined pituitary stimulation with insulin (0.15 U/kg), GnRH (100 μg) and TRH (200 μg) given i.v. as a bolus at time 0. Patient 1 is a woman with amenorrhoea. She has normal responses despite previous operation for a functionless pituitary adenoma. Patient 2 is a man, also with a functionless pituitary tumour. He has absent responses for all except cortisol, which is blunted. The diagnosis is panhypopituitarism, requiring replacement therapy.

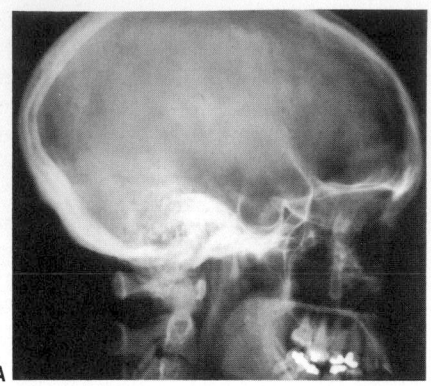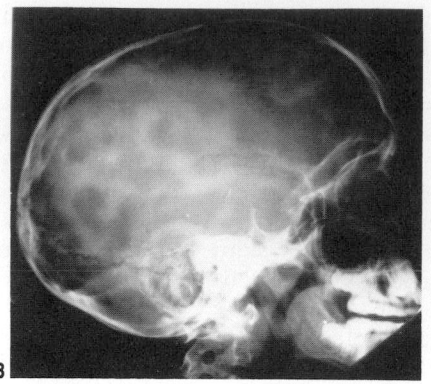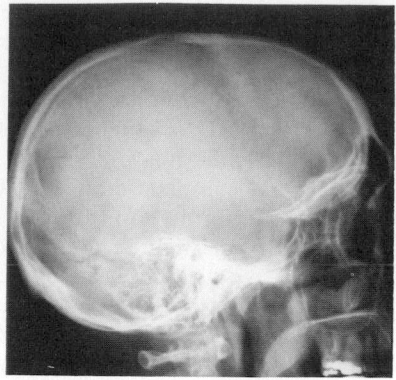

Fig. 17.13 Lateral X-rays of skulls of patients with pituitary tumours. A. Expansion of pituitary fossa and a 'double floor' due to asymmetrical enlargement. **B.** 'Copper-beaten' skull with expanded sutures due to obstructive hydrocephalus in a girl of 15 (Courtesy of Dr St Clair Forbes). **C.** Complete destruction of pituitary fossa and dorsum sellae.

Sheehan's syndrome or an infarcted pituitary tumour, the condition may be due to organ-specific autoimmune disease, with antibodies directed against the pituitary cells. The 'empty sella' syndrome, in which a CT scan shows an absent pituitary gland, is usually a diagnosis of exclusion after the relevant radiological studies. In some cases the syndrome follows infarction of a tumour, while others are possibly due to the transmission of cerebrospinal fluid pressure to the pituitary fossa as a result of a defective diaphragma sellae.

Hormone measurements

Hormone measurements (PRL, GH, gonadotrophins, TSH) will indicate the nature of a functioning pituitary

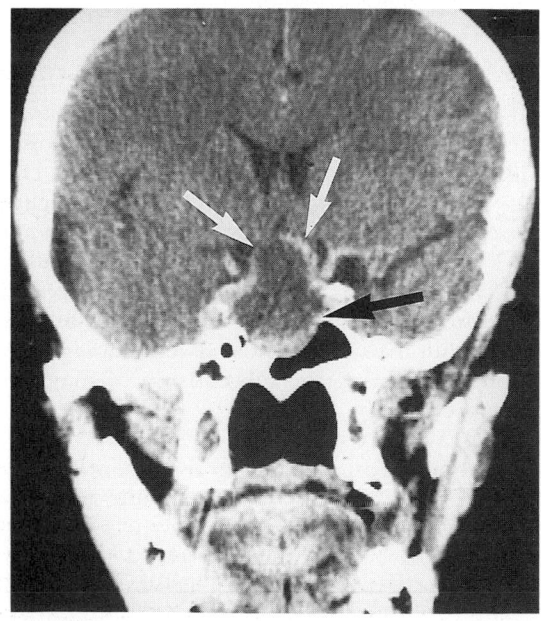

Fig. 17.14 CT scan of pituitary tumour eroding floor of fossa (black arrow), and expanding upwards (white arrows).

tumour, but there may still be major difficulties in diagnosis. For example, modest elevation of PRL may be due simply to stalk damage, and not to prolactinoma. Levels more than about 10 times the upper limit of normal are, however, always due to a prolactinoma. Similarly, gonadotrophin levels are normally elevated after the menopause. Raised TSH is most likely to be due to primary myxoedema rather than a TSH-producing pituitary tumour. In the former, serum T3 and T4 levels will be very low. ('Feedback tumours' secreting TSH are, however, a well recognised complication of long-standing untreated myxoedema; they will usually shrink with thyroid hormone replacement.)

Management of anterior hypopituitarism

Although patients with hypopituitarism may have been ACTH- (and therefore cortisol-) deficient for many months or years without severe illness, they are, nevertheless, extremely vulnerable to even minor stress. A minor infection, illness or trauma may precipitate acute glucocorticoid deficiency, as may ill-advised prior treatment of hypothyroidism.

Immediate

The patient with pituitary collapse or coma should be given intravenous hydrocortisone (100–200 mg repeated in 2–4 hours), which will generally lead to rapid improvement in the clinical condition, a rise in blood pressure and a fall in temperature. In some cases, volume expansion may be necessary and, if the serum sodium level is very low (below 115 mmol/l) because of inappropriate ADH secretion (p. 682), slow correction to around 120 mmol/l may be indicated by means of small amounts of hypertonic saline. Steroids should always be replaced before thyroid hormones, which can generally be given orally from the outset. Sex hormone replacement therapy, particularly (in men) testosterone therapy, should be considered and generally instituted without delay, since this will greatly hasten the return of strength and well-being.

Where occult posterior pituitary hormone deficiency coexists, it may be uncovered by glucocorticoid therapy. This should be suspected when there is marked and continuing water diuresis in the recovery phase, with low urine and rising serum osmolalities. It is best corrected with the synthetic ADH analogue, desmopressin (DDAVP, p. 682).

Long-term

Steroid therapy

There is no convenient way of mimicking the episodic secretion of glucocorticoids. Fortunately, however, this does not seem to matter, and oral treatment with hydrocortisone (cortisol) in a total daily dose of 20–40 mg given in two or three divided doses (to approximate the normal diurnal variation) is usually satisfactory. At least half the dose is given on waking in the morning (with reversal for anyone working on a night shift). Cortisone acetate is generally equally effective, since the acetate is hydrolysed and cortisone converted to cortisol by the liver. However, a possible disadvantage of cortisone over cortisol is that the plasma cortisol level rises to a peak more gradually on treatment with the former. In addition, some individuals, especially those with liver disease, have impaired conversion of cortisone to cortisol. Prednisolone is a suitable alternative (5 mg being roughly equivalent to 20 mg hydrocortisone), but dexamethasone – an even more potent halogenated glucocorticoid – should probably be avoided for long-term treatment because its much longer half-life means that glucocorticoid levels do not fall at night. Low levels then may be important to allow collagen repair.

Thyroid hormones

Thyroid hormones are best replaced as oral thyroxine (100–200 μg once daily). This is converted to the more active tri-iodothyronine in the liver.

Sex hormone replacement

In *men* testosterone is given in one of three ways, none of which is ideal. It may be implanted subcutaneously in the abdominal wall as fused pellets of testosterone (600–800 mg every 4–6 months). More commonly, but with wider fluctuation in plasma testosterone levels, it may be given as testosterone esters – Sustanon (mixed testosterone esters) or Primoteston depot (testosterone enanthate, 250 mg i.m. every 2–4 weeks). Finally, it may be given as the orally absorbed ester testosterone undecanoate (40–80

mg twice daily), but this has the disadvantage of high price, and the capsules may cause gastrointestinal symptoms, perhaps due to the oleic acid vehicle.

In *women*, where the uterus is present, oestrogen therapy is indicated combined with a cyclical progesterone to prevent endometrial hyperplasia (p. 714).

Restoration of fertility

In hypopituitary patients of either sex, restoration of fertility can usually be achieved by administering gonadotrophins. In men HCG (1500–2000 IU i.m. weekly) is given to stimulate Leydig cell testosterone production, and after some 3 months or more this is combined with three times weekly injections of 225 units of FSH (Pergonal). Spermatogenesis should be evident after 3 months, as indicated by increased testicular volume and the appearance of motile spermatozoa in the ejaculate. Gonadotrophin therapy in women is much more complex, since FSH must be given early in the cycle and the follicular response followed by ultrasound scanning and serum or urinary oestrogen measurements (p. 711). When one or two follicles have achieved a diameter of 2 cm, ovulation is produced by giving intramuscular HCG (5000 units). This treatment should only be undertaken in units with facilities for ultrasound and rapid oestrogen assays, and probably with access to egg retrieval and in vitro fertilisation. An alternative treatment, effective in some cases of isolated gonadotrophin deficiency, is to administer GnRH in a pulsatile fashion through a pump connected to a subcutaneous needle.

Posterior pituitary hormone replacement

Posterior pituitary hormone replacement is discussed on page 782.

ISOLATED GROWTH HORMONE DEFICIENCY AND RELATED SYNDROMES

GH deficiency only produces clinically obvious manifestations when it occurs in childhood. Although GH is secreted from early fetal life, it is not until infancy that its deficiency leads to impaired growth.

Aetiology

In most cases of isolated GH deficiency, the cause is unknown. There are, however, several familial syndromes inherited as autosomal recessive conditions with defective GH secretion. Recent evidence indicates that in one of these, pituitary somatotrophs synthesise GH but there is failure to respond to the releasing hormone, GHRH. In others, the abnormality appears to be a deletion of the GH gene. Patients in the latter group in particular may respond to injected GH as if it were a foreign protein and develop antibodies to it. In some cases of GH deficiency, it may become apparent after GH therapy is initiated that TSH synthesis is also impaired; it appears that GH therapy accelerates the metabolism of TSH.

Laron dwarfism is the term given to a syndrome which mimics GH deficiency, but in which GH levels are high and IGF I levels low (p. 667). It is apparently due to failure of target organ response to GH. Some cases of short stature may also be due to failure to respond to IGF I. In Pygmies, the short stature and other somatic features appear to be due in part to low levels of IGF I.

Clinical features

Abnormally low rates of overall growth, leading to short stature, are associated with typical somatic abnormalities. In particular, the face appears baby-like, with persistence of a small nose, poorly developed nasal bridge and small chin. The dentition may be delayed with later crowding of teeth. Muscle development is poor, with excess subcutaneous fat, thin hair and skin, small larynx and high-pitched voice. Puberty is typically delayed until 18–20 years when there is a small growth spurt. Even in patients with complete GH deficiency, longitudinal growth occurs, but at only about one-third of the normal rate. There is a tendency to hypoglycaemia, which may be the most obvious feature in the neonate. GH deficiency developing in adult life may be associated with increased mortality and the value of GH therapy is under investigation.

Management

The diagnosis of GH deficiency is established by a combination of clinical observation (including serial measurements of growth and assessment of growth velocity) and provocative testing with insulin injection or arginine infusion. GH therapy is then initiated. GH isolated from cadaver pituitaries was associated in some cases with Jakob–Creutzfeldt disease, leading to its withdrawal; biosynthetic GH is now available although expensive. Treatment is with 0.5 IU/kg/week as daily s.c. injections. Recent work indicates that the response can be improved in boys by addition of small doses of synthetic androgens. Biosynthetic IGF I is also effective and may be useful in Laron dwarfism.

The response is monitored by frequent measurements of height, and calculation of growth velocity (Fig. 17.11, p. 670). There is an initial 'catch-up' period, followed by more steady growth.

Growth retardation in other conditions

It is often difficult to distinguish partial idiopathic GH deficiency from other states in which GH or IGF I secretion is secondarily impaired. These states include psychological deprivation, growth failure due to inadequate nutrition (e.g. malabsorption due to coeliac disease) and chronic liver and kidney disease. Simple delayed puberty may also present with growth failure. In these cases, if GH secretion in response to insulin is low, the test will usually become normal when repeated after a short course of androgen (or oestrogen) replacement therapy. In teenage boys with delayed puberty and short stature, it is often justified to give a 3–6 month course of treatment with HCG or androgens. The resulting growth spurt results in part from the androgens and in part from the augmentation of (nocturnal) GH secretion that they cause.

GROWTH HORMONE EXCESS

The term *acromegaly* refers to the syndrome of GH excess when it develops in adult life. *Gigantism* is when its onset in childhood also leads to excessive height. At the turn of this century, Harvey Cushing recognised that acromegaly and gigantism were due to acidophil tumours of the pituitary gland that produce GH. He was the first clinician to recognise and distinguish features due to hyperpituitarism (hormone excess) from those due to hypopituitarism.

Clinical GH excess is almost always due to a pituitary tumour with two exceptions. Firstly, tall stature in boys may be linked to episodic high GH secretion without a tumour. Secondly, pancreatic tumours secreting GHRH may lead to acromegaly by stimulating the pituitary gland to produce GH. Indeed, it was recognition of this syndrome that led recently to the extraction and purification of pancreatic GHRH which was rapidly shown to be present in identical form in the hypothalamus.

Aetiology

The factors leading to the development of a GH-secreting adenoma are still uncertain. Most such tumours are benign and secrete GH alone, although occasional mixed tumours also synthesise and secrete PRL.

Normally GH release is stimulated by dopamine, probably acting via the hypothalamus. Paradoxically the dopaminergic agent bromocriptine usually has a modest, but significant, inhibitory effect on GH secretion. In some cases, especially in individuals with mixed GH and PRL-secreting tumours, this effect may lead to complete inhibition of secretion and be of therapeutic benefit. Somatostatin inhibits GH secretion, a phenomenon which has led to the use of the synthetic analogue octreotide.

Clinical features

The clinical features of acromegaly and gigantism are due to a combination of GH excess, a local space-occupying lesion and other hormone deficiencies. Except where the tumour is large and growing rapidly, the latter usually occur late in the disease as a result of attempted treatment (radiotherapy or surgery), especially transfrontal surgery.

Gigantism

Gigantism is the most obvious and serious consequence of GH excess in childhood and adolescence. Normally, GH secretion occurs at a low level throughout childhood, and increases with the rise in sex hormones at the time of puberty. With a GH-secreting tumour in childhood, however, inappropriate GH secretion occurs out of phase with the stage of puberty. The growth of cartilage at the epiphyseal plates is greatly stimulated due to the action of IGF I (p. 667). Normally, this effect is held in check by an inhibitory action of sex hormones on the epiphyseal cartilage stem cell, ultimately leading to epiphyseal closure.

The first feature of gigantism is therefore the onset of an inappropriate, continuing and excessive growth spurt, coupled with increased hand and foot size and general skeletal enlargement. Later, other features (increased skin and soft-tissue growth) become evident. The most devastating skeletal deformities affect the chest wall, and are probably due to the combination of GH excess and sex hormone deficiency which together predispose to osteoporosis. Severe kyphosis may result.

In childhood, as in adult life, the pituitary tumour is often large at the time of presentation, and may lead to local pressure effects. These include headache (thought to be due to pressure on the diaphragma sellae) and visual field defects due to pressure on the optic chiasm (pp. 665, 669).

If pubertal failure results, either as a direct effect of a large tumour or as a result of treatment, epiphyseal closure will be delayed and the ultimate height attained even more extreme.

Acromegaly

There is a highly variable time between the onset of symptoms and signs and the diagnosis of GH excess in adults. This is dependent, among other things, on chance and the index of suspicion of any doctor who encounters the patient. In general, the greater the experience of the doctor, the more likely he or she is to make a confident and correct diagnosis early. Clinical features due to the *local tumour* include headache and visual field defects (most commonly bitemporal hemianopia).

Features due to GH excess may occur in many organs, but the most obvious involve the soft tissues, skin, and skeleton. Together, these give the classical *acromegalic facies* (Fig. 17.15), with prominent orbital margins, large nose, prominence of the lower jaw (prognathism) and

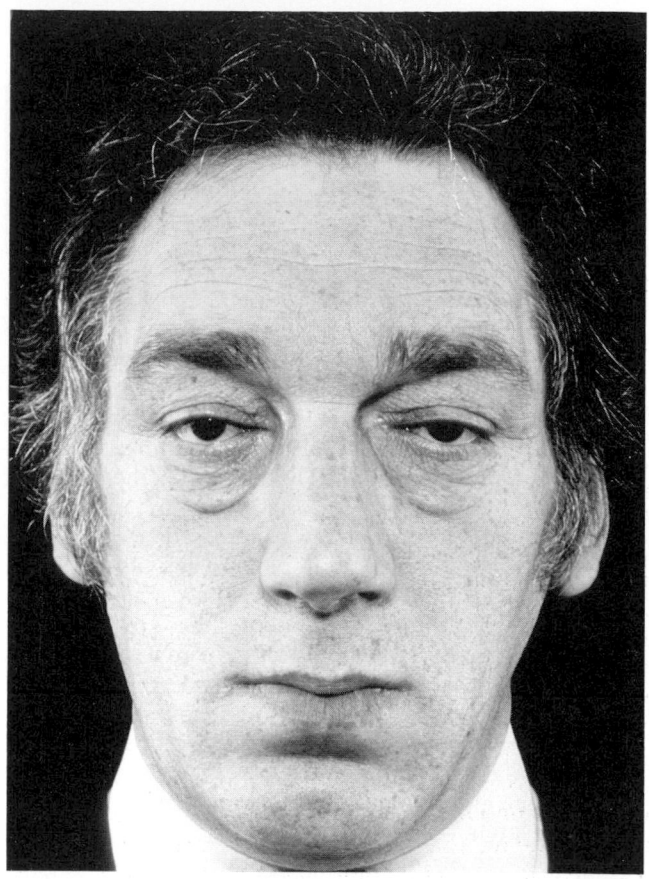

Fig. 17.15 Typical appearance of acromegaly.

thickening of the skin and soft tissues, including the lips and tongue. In men especially, there is often a typical rather rough vibrant voice, due to thickening of the vocal cords, enlargement of the sinuses and changes in other tissues in the nasopharynx and larynx. There is often dental malocclusion, with protrusion of the lower jaw, and the teeth may become more widely spaced or dentures may need to be changed.

There is obvious enlargement of the hands and feet. The wide 'spade-like' hands are due to increased thickness and volume of skin and soft tissues and growth of periarticular cartilage. Ring, glove, shoe and hat sizes increase. In longstanding and severe acromegaly, major skeletal deformities are common. Severe thoracic kyphosis and accompanying respiratory disease are common in acromegalic giants. In adult-onset acromegaly, growth of articular cartilage and soft tissues in and around a joint commonly leads to secondary osteoarthritis, which may be compounded by necrosis of articular cartilage.

Neurological problems include carpal tunnel syndrome and, in advanced gigantism, peripheral neuropathy. The age-related mortality rate of patients with untreated

Summary 2 Clinical features of acromegaly

- Symptoms and signs are due to local tumour, growth hormone excess and deficiency of other hormones.
- Prognathism, enlarged soft tissues, skeletal deformity, nerve entrapment occur.
- Hypertension and diabetes mellitus contribute to mortality.

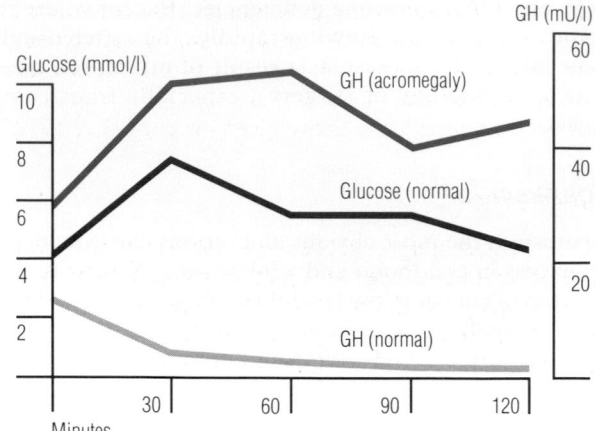

Fig. 17.16 GH respone to oral glucose load in a normal subject (suppression) and a man with acromegaly (no suppression or paradoxical rise)

acromegaly is probably twice normal, largely attributable to cardiovascular disease – hypertension, cardiac muscle hypertrophy, cardiomyopathy and ischaemic heart disease. The latter is particularly likely in acromegalics with diabetes mellitus. Overt diabetes probably occurs in about 10% of acromegalics, although insulin secretion is increased in most because GH antagonises the effects of insulin.

A common early complaint is increased sweating, due to an increase in both number and activity of sweat glands. About one-quarter of patients have a goitre, which is commonly multinodular. Together these features may lead to an erroneous diagnosis of thyrotoxicosis (which may coexist). Macroglossia may lead to sleep apnoea, due to obstruction of the airway at night, often presenting with daytime somnolence. Enlargement of the liver, spleen, pancreas and kidneys seldom causes problems, although the glomerular filtration rate may be increased due to the latter.

Patients with acromegaly have quite often been labelled as neurotic because many of the symptoms are rather vague. Impotence is a common complaint, which only rarely appears to be due to hypogonadism. Women commonly have menstrual irregularities, and some are hirsute. Galactorrhoea due to accompanying hyperprolactinaemia occurs in about one acromegalic woman in five. In some, this is due to a mixed PRL and GH-secreting tumour; in others, to damage to the pituitary stalk.

Investigation

Clearly, the association of classical clinical features with evidence of local pressure effects will lead to a confident and accurate diagnosis at the time of presentation. However, it is clearly preferable to make the diagnosis before it is grossly obvious clinically. Furthermore, there are cases where 'acromegaloid' features may occur without GH excess. In some of these, the primary abnormality may be excess production of IGF I (somatomedin C), which mediates many of the effects of GH.

GH suppression test. Baseline GH levels are of limited value in diagnosis because GH is normally secreted episodically. The best screening test in suspected cases remains the oral glucose load (50–75 g) with accompanying measurements of GH (Fig. 17.16). Normally, GH

suppresses to below 2 mU/l after 50 g oral glucose load, probably as an effect of central inhibition of GHRH secretion. In acromegaly, levels either fail to suppress or show a paradoxical rise. About 30–40% of cases also show a paradoxical rise of GH in response to TRH or GnRH given intravenously, presumably because the tumour possesses receptors for these hormones. Dopamine infusion in acromegaly often inhibits GH secretion, again in contrast to the normal response which is of stimulation. Bromocriptine suppresses GH in the majority of acromegalics, though it is only clinically useful in a minority. An indication of its potential usefulness in an individual case is obtained from measurement of GH hourly for 4–6 hours after 5 mg bromocriptine orally. Octreotide is now commonly used for GH suppression. A test dose (50–100 μg s.c.) with hourly GH measurement is a useful predictor of longer-term response.

IGF I assay. The normal response of GH to hypoglycaemia is for the level to rise acutely; this response is commonly absent in acromegaly. An important new development is the availability of reliable assays for circulating levels of IGF I. Levels in gigantism and acromegaly are almost always elevated, and the measurement may be particularly informative in cases with equivocal results to conventional tests, for example relatively low GH levels which nonetheless fail to suppress with oral glucose.

GHRH assay. In occasional cases with normal pituitary radiology or other atypical features, it is possible to measure circulating levels of GHRH which, if elevated, point to a rare extrahypothalamic GHRH-secreting tumour (e.g. in the pancreas). Injection of GHRH or somatostatin and measurement of the subsequent GH response appears to be of little practical value.

The rapidly growing tall child presents a particular problem, for whom a number of the above tests, perhaps combined with measurements of basal GH secretion, may be indicated. Recent evidence indicates that very tall children may secrete excess GH in a physiological but exaggerated way at night, and after initial suppression following food or glucose.

Radiological investigations are given on pages 671–672.

Management

The aim of treatment of GH excess is to arrest and, where possible, to reverse the local and systemic effects of the tumour. Except in the growing child, correction of GH excess is seldom urgent. Visual field defects, however, present an immediate and compelling indication for surgery.

Surgery

Surgery is now usually carried out through a midline, trans-sphenoidal route, approaching the pituitary gland through an incision in the mouth, and removing part of the nasal septum or deflecting it. Some surgeons approach the pituitary through the medial wall of the orbit and ethmoid sinuses. Even when there is a large suprasellar tumour, trans-sphenoidal surgery may relieve pressure on the optic chiasm and allow the suprasellar part of the tumour to fall into the fossa. The transfrontal approach, which almost inevitably causes hypopituitarism, is therefore seldom needed.

With small tumours, the best centres now achieve 70% cure rates by trans-sphenoidal resection, without causing hypopituitarism, although the balance between endocrine benefit and penalty shifts unfavourably with increasing tumour size.

Drug therapy

Bromocriptine causes tumour shrinkage in only a minority of cases of acromegaly, but is indicated when surgery is not thought desirable (e.g. in mild disease or the elderly) or when GH is effectively suppressed by the drug. Usual doses needed are 10–30 mg daily, in four doses, although additional benefit with higher doses has been reported. The clinical effect often exceeds the biochemical response, possibly because of a direct suppressive effect on IGF I secretion. The somatostatin analogue octreotide is expensive but usually effective in a dose of 50–100 μg s.c. three times daily. It is especially helpful for headache in acromegaly. Octreotide causes tumour shrinkage, usually of small degree, in about half the cases treated. A long-term complication is development of gallstones.

Radiotherapy

External radiotherapy can be used to produce tumour regression. It requires careful planning and megavoltage machinery. The treatment is remarkably safe but its effect is delayed, with a gradual and progressive benefit over 2–5 years. Interstitial radiotherapy by pituitary implantation of yttrium-90 has proved effective, and is more akin to surgery than radiotherapy in the rapidity of its effect. However, it is now practised by few centres, having been largely superseded by improved neurosurgery.

Complications of treatment

The complications of surgery and radiotherapy vary greatly with the skill and technique of the operator. After surgery by the trans-sphenoidal route, panhypopituitarism is quite rare, except where radical removal of a large tumour has been attempted. Postoperative diabetes insipidus is usually transient. If anterior hypopituitarism is suspected in the recovery period, full replacement therapy should be initiated and combined pituitary function tests conducted about 6 weeks postoperatively. After external radiotherapy, the onset of hypopituitarism should be suspected if the patient complains of lassitude, lethargy and/or impotence. If in doubt, pituitary function tests should be performed and replacement therapy initiated without delay. One should not wait for gross hormone deficiencies to develop.

ACTH DISORDERS

Physiology

ACTH is the most important hormone synthesised and secreted by the corticotrophic cells; these may appear basophilic on staining due to the glycoprotein nature of POMC, the ACTH precursor. Processing of POMC to produce the hormone ACTH (39 amino acid residues) occurs as a result of selective enzymatic cleavage within the cells' hormone-containing granules; the relationship of the principal cleavage products is shown in Figure 17.8 (p. 666). It will be apparent that ACTH, β LPH and β endorphin are secreted simultaneously in response to CRF and other 'physiological' stimulants, such as insulin-induced hypoglycaemia.

The principal hormonal action of ACTH is to stimulate cortisol secretion, particularly from the zona fasciculata. Its action is via cell surface receptors which act in part by activation of adenylate cyclase, but also by inducing changes in cell membrane phospholipids and consequent calcium fluxes into the cell (p. 659). ACTH secretion is under synergistic control from several hypothalamic factors, including corticotrophin-releasing hormone (CRF/CRH, a 41 amino acid neuropeptide), ADH and, possibly, bombesin. The factors that influence ACTH and hence cortisol secretion are shown in Fig. 17.9 (p. 667), and include circadian rhythm (which affects both pulse amplitude and frequency), stress and food.

Isolated ACTH deficiency

Isolated ACTH deficiency is uncommon and may be difficult to diagnose. Patients are usually middle-aged at time of presentation with weakness, lethargy, hypoglycaemia, and sometimes hyponatraemia. The diagnosis is confirmed by a low urinary free cortisol excretion, and low plasma ACTH and cortisol levels which do not rise normally in response to insulin hypoglycaemia. The defect may result either from CRF deficiency or from isolated failure of corticotroph function. Treatment is with glucocorticoid replacement.

ACTH excess

ACTH excess due to a hypothalamic defect or an ACTH-secreting microadenoma leads to pituitary-dependent Cushing's syndrome (p. 702). 'Physiological' ACTH excess occurs when the adrenal glands fail due either to an inborn error of secretion, or to destruction by disease. Under these circumstances, the normal episodic and circadian fluctuations in ACTH secretion occur at much higher than normal levels. Rarely, sustained stimulation of ACTH secretion may lead to development of a 'feedback tumour'.

Nelson's syndrome is the name given to hyperpigmentation, ACTH excess and pituitary expansion that may follow bilateral adrenalectomy for Cushing's syndrome due to a pituitary adenoma. It is presumed to result from removal of negative feedback inhibition of a semi-autonomous pituitary adenoma that was previously subject to some restraint by the high circulating levels of cortisol.

PROLACTIN DISORDERS

Physiology

PRL is a polypeptide hormone of 199 amino acid residues.

Secretion of prolactin

PRL is synthesised and secreted by cells of the pituitary (lactotrophs), which are mainly located laterally in the gland and are chromophobe in staining. There is little PRL stored in the pituitary. The lactotrophs secrete PRL in the absence of stimuli, and the predominant influence of the hypothalamus is to restrain this by secretion of dopamine. Besides causing TSH release, TRH also stimulates PRL secretion. PRL secretion is episodic and increases at night; in females, the level increases at the time of puberty. Androgens probably have a modest inhibitory effect, both on its secretion and on the response of the breast.

In pregnancy, PRL levels rise about five-fold. Oestrogens, probably together with progesterone, cause hyperplasia of the lactotrophs and enhance PRL secretion, while inhibiting its effect on the breast epithelium. The decline in sex hormones after delivery, coupled with the stimulus of suckling, is responsible for postpartum lactation. Postpartum breast-feeding causes a marked increase in PRL secretion, as a result of a reflex involving sensory fibres from the breast, the dorsal nerve roots and the hypothalamus. This is probably important in maintaining milk production for weeks and months after delivery, when baseline PRL levels have declined to normal. Another reflex arc is responsible for suckling-induced oxytocin secretion, which is important in stimulating myo-epithelial cells of the breast and so causing milk-ejection from the ducts.

Action of prolactin and other hormones on the breast

PRL has an action on the breast that is essential for lactation (Table 17.4 (p. 667)). Oestrogens promote ductal growth, while PRL and progesterone promote growth of the lobules and alveoli. Progesterone enhances the synthesis of β-lactalbumin, a non-catalytic subunit that converts the function of the enzyme galactose synthetase to lactose synthesis. Other hormones with important effects on the breast include insulin and cortisol (which are permissive or facilitatory), GH and placental lactogen. The decline in oestrogen and progesterone levels after delivery releases the brake on PRL-stimulated lobulo-alveolar milk production.

Pathology

PRL deficiency occurs in Sheehan's syndrome when pituitary infarction results from postpartum haemorrhage and consequent hypotension. It results in failure of lactation.

PRL excess. Hyperprolactinaemia and associated disorders are common, particularly in women. The low incidence in men is a reflection of the inhibitory effects of androgens both on the lactotrophs and on the breast. Unlike the situation in women, the occurrence of hyperprolactinaemia and/or galactorrhoea in men is almost always of pathological significance.

HYPERPROLACTINAEMIA

Aetiology

The causes of hyperprolactinaemia are best considered in relation to PRL physiology. Table 17.6 lists the principal causes, most of which lead to only mild to moderate hyperprolactinaemia (levels up to 5–10 times normal).

Table 17.6 Classification of causes of hyperprolactinaemia

Cause	Example
Pituitary lactotroph excess	
Physiological	Pregnancy
Drug-induced	Oestrogens
Pathological	Tumour – microprolactinoma
	– macroprolactinoma
	– mixed GH and prolactin tumour
Inhibition of dopamine secretion	
Neurogenic	Thoracic sensory nerve stimulation
	Chest wall burns/incisions
	Suckling/nipple stimulation
Pituitary stalk damage	Stalk section
	Stalk/hypothalamic tumour
Drug-induced	Methyldopa, reserpine, opiates, H_2-receptor blockers
Inhibition of dopamine action	
Neuroleptic drugs	Phenothiazines, e.g. chlorpromazine
	Butyrophenones, e.g. haloperidol
Anti-emetics	Metoclopramide
Endocrine disorders	TRH-mediated, e.g. primary hypothyroidism
	Miscellaneous, e.g. adrenal insufficiency
	Cushing's syndrome

Drugs that inhibit the secretion or action of dopamine are commonly implicated in hyperprolactinaemia. Oestrogens may stimulate lactotroph growth and (in those on the contraceptive pill, or during pregnancy) a modest elevation of PRL secretion. Primary *hypothyroidism* may cause modest hyperprolactinaemia, probably as a consequence of increased TRH secretion. *Cushing's syndrome* and adrenal insufficiency may both be associated with mild hyperprolactinaemia.

Pituitary tumours may lead to hyperprolactinaemia for one of two reasons – they may interfere with the pituitary stalk and so produce local dopamine deficiency, or they may secrete PRL. Pure *prolactinomas* are classified into two broad categories: the *microprolactinoma,* which is less than 1 cm in diameter, and is associated with mild to moderate hyperprolactinaemia and no pressure symptoms; and the *macroprolactinoma.* In many instances, the diagnosis of microprolactinoma is presumptive, based on exclusion of other causes. Some patients with *acromegaly* have coincident hyperprolactinaemia, in which case a mixed tumour containing GH- and PRL-secreting cells is suspected. Such cases usually respond well to bromocriptine, in terms of both GH and PRL suppression.

Clinical features and management

The unwanted *secretion of milk* (galactorrhoea) is common in women, but in only about one-third of cases is it due to PRL excess. If treatment is required, bromocriptine may be effective, even when PRL levels are normal. Increased secretion of PRL has an inhibitory effect on cyclical ovarian function, probably due to direct inhibition of GnRH secretion in hypothalamic neurones. Erratic and anovulatory cycles or amenorrhoea result. Treatment with a dopaminergic drug such as bromocriptine results in a drop in PRL and resumption of normal ovulatory cycles. It should be remembered that the commonest cause of hyperprolactinaemic amenorrhoea is, of course, pregnancy!

Microprolactinoma

Clinical features

Classical presentations of microprolactinoma are with erratic menstrual cycles or amenorrhoea, with or without galactorrhoea. In some patients, presentation is because of infertility, usually associated with amenorrhoea (primary or secondary). Frequently, presentation follows cessation of the pill (post-pill amenorrhoea) or pregnancy. Long-term, the amenorrhoea is associated with osteoporosis. Patients with microprolactinoma never present with visual field defects or other pressure effects. Indeed, the presence of these effects associated with modest PRL excess indicates dopamine deficiency due to a non-PRL secreting tumour in the pituitary stalk or above (e.g. a craniopharyngioma).

Investigation

Diagnosis depends upon demonstration, in several serum samples, of hyperprolactinaemia in the absence of other causes of PRL excess. Pituitary radiology is (by definition) normal or borderline abnormal. It is doubtful if the resolution power of CT or MR scans is yet adequate to allow a confident demonstration of micro-adenomas of any kind, and the issue is further confused by the high incidence of small pituitary adenomas (some of which stain for PRL) at autopsy in normal individuals.

Management

Treatment should generally be conservative, using bromocriptine or other dopaminergic agents such as pergolide or lisuride. Bromocriptine may initially cause nausea and postural hypotension, and should be started at a low dose (1.25 mg at night) with food, and increased gradually over 1–2 weeks to 2.5 mg three times daily with food. In most cases, this is highly effective both in suppressing PRL, and in resolving the amenorrhoea and galactorrhoea. If pregnancy is desired, it may be sensible to advise contraception for 6 months to allow reduction in adenoma size. In contrast to the situation with acromegaly, PRL-secreting tumours commonly shrink in size with bromocriptine. Although it may be safely continued, bromocriptine is usually stopped once the pregnancy test is positive. With a microprolactinoma, the risk of tumour expansion sufficient to cause visual field defects is probably negligible.

In many cases, mild hyperprolactinaemia continues without progression for years and may remit spontaneously. Surgery (trans-sphenoidal) or radiotherapy are probably seldom indicated, unless there is clear biochemical or radiological evidence of progression. It is as yet uncertain for how long dopaminergic therapy should be given in such cases. A reasonable policy, if pregnancy is not desired, is to treat for 1–2 years, and then to repeat PRL levels 1 week after stopping the drug. Sustained normal levels would suggest that the tumour has regressed and that treatment can be safely stopped and the patient observed.

If contraception is desired by a patient with microprolactinoma, bromocriptine may be combined safely with the contraceptive pill.

Macroprolactinoma

The definition of macroprolactinoma is arbitrary, but any non-pregnant patient with circulating PRL levels in excess of 10 times the upper limit of normal (over 5000 mU/l, 200 ng/ml) probably has a more aggressive prolactinoma which is potentially or actually large and expanding. Virtually all detected prolactinomas in men and about one-fifth of those in women fall into this category.

Clinical features

All features are likely to be more extreme than with a microprolactinoma. These include the endocrine consequences of PRL excess (galactorrhoea, amenorrhoea, and, in the case of men, impotence). The latter is principally due to gonadotrophin (and so testosterone) deficiency, suggested also by lethargy, depression and loss of secondary sexual hair. Rarely, presentation may be with infertility and oligo- or azoospermia. Local pressure effects – headache, visual field defects and other cranial nerve lesions – are often present at the time of diagnosis. As with other pituitary tumours, the occurrence of panhypopituitarism in the untreated patient indicates the presence of a large and destructive tumour. In the male, galactorrhoea may be present even in the absence of gynaecomastia.

Investigation

Radioimmunoassay measurement of serum PRL shows levels often 10–200 times normal. Plain X-ray of the pituitary gland will usually show enlargement, an apparent 'double floor', and erosion of the dorsum sellae (Fig. 17.13, p. 672). CT and MR scanning will show the full extent of the tumour, superseding more invasive methods of soft-tissue imaging.

Management

The urgency of treatment depends upon the severity of local pressure effects. Significant changes have taken place in recent years. Transfrontal surgery (which almost invariably causes hypopituitarism) is now seldom conducted, even when the tumour is expanding upwards; instead, decompression can often be achieved rapidly with either bromocriptine or trans-sphenoidal surgery. Most would agree that a therapeutic trial of bromocriptine (2.5–5 mg three times daily), with daily measurement of visual fields and acuity, is the initial treatment of choice, followed if necessary by trans-sphenoidal decompression. In macroprolactinomas, it is impossible to eradicate the tumour surgically, and external radiotherapy in a specialist unit is ultimately indicated in every case, regardless of whether or not an operation has been performed.

GONADOTROPHIN DISORDERS

Gonadotrophin disorders are considered in more detail under the section on gonads (pp.706–718). *Gonadotrophin secreting tumours* are rarely diagnosed. Most published cases have been FSH-secreting tumours. Some 'functionless' pituitary tumours stain for LH and FSH or their subunits, and so may be non-secreting gonadotrophinomas.

Ectopic secretion of gonadotrophins appears to be confined to HCG, which is a normal product of the placenta and a tumour marker for hydatiform mole and its malignant counterpart the choriocarcinoma (a tumour which can now be cured by intensive chemotherapy). Germ cell tumours of the testis and ovary often secrete HCG, as may some carcinomas (e.g. adenocarcinoma of the lung). This leads to excess testicular oestrogen secretion and gynaecomastia. In children, hepatoblastomas may produce pseudo-precocious puberty by HCG secretion.

TSH DISORDERS

TSH disorders are principally discussed under panhypopituitarism (p. 671) and thyroid disorders (pp. 682–694). Isolated TSH deficiency is a rare cause of secondary hypothyroidism.

Primary TSH excess due to a *thyrotrophinoma* is a rare cause of hyperthyroidism. Patients with long-standing severe primary hypothyroidism (myxoedema) often develop pituitary enlargement due to thyrotroph hyperplasia and, occasionally, TSH-secreting pituitary ('feedback') tumours. However, the latter usually shrink with thyroxine replacement therapy and probably do not become autonomous.

THE POSTERIOR PITUITARY GLAND

The posterior lobe of the pituitary gland consists principally of the secretory terminal extensions of neurones that arise in the pre-optic nucleus of the hypothalamus. Its blood supply is derived principally from the hypophyseal arteries, rather than from the hypothalamus-pituitary portal circulation.

SYNTHESIS AND SECRETION OF THE MAIN HORMONES

The posterior pituitary gland secretes two principal octa-peptide hormones, vasopressin and oxytocin. In man, the vasopressin produced is arginine vasopressin (AVP; also known as ADH). Both hormones are synthesised in specialised neurones in the pre-optic and ventromedial nuclei as part of a larger precursor which, in each case, also includes the sequence of another protein (a neurophysin). Axonal flow carries the normal precursors to the specialised nerve terminals in the posterior pituitary gland, where they are stored in cytoplasmic granules. Neuronal activation leads to the release of the hormone and its neurophysin into the hypophyseal capillaries and hence into the general circulation.

Control mechanisms

ADH secretion is stimulated by an increase in osmolality, and by 'stress' stimuli such as hypoglycaemia (Fig. 17.17).

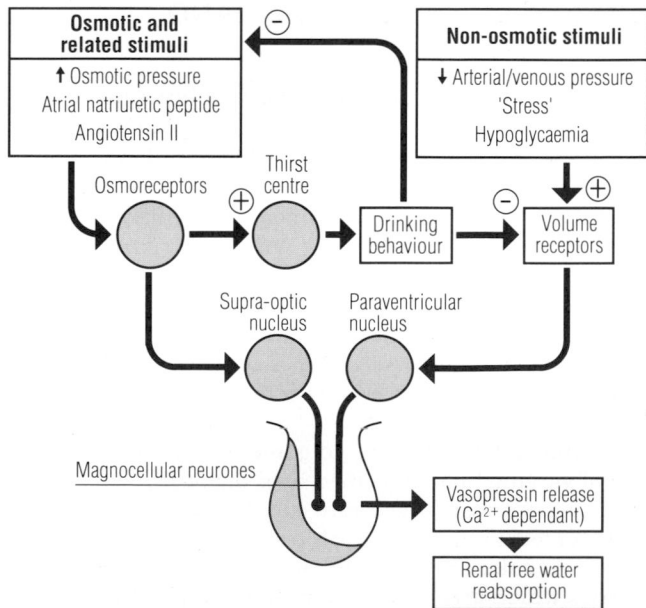

Fig. 17.17 Factors stimulating vasopressin secretion by osmotic and non-osmotic mechanisms. Osmoreceptors also activate the thirst centre to stimulate drinking.

Glucocorticoids exert an inhibitory effect on its release and also interact with ADH at the renal tubule so that, in the presence of glucocorticoid insufficiency, diabetes insipidus may be masked. ADH acts on two different kinds of receptors, those on the renal tubules (type I) and those on blood vessels (type II). The action on the former is mediated by cyclic-AMP; ADH opens up pores in the basolateral membrane for water and urea.

Oxytocin acts on the smooth muscle of the uterus and mammary ducts (to cause milk ejection). It also causes contraction of myo-epithelial cells of the seminiferous tubules.

ADH DEFICIENCY

Deficiency of ADH causes the syndrome of diabetes insipidus (see also Ch. 21, pp. 844–846).

Aetiology

ADH deficiency may be caused by trauma (head injury or neurosurgery); primary or secondary neoplasms of the pituitary, pituitary stalk or hypothalamus; inflammatory disorders such as sarcoidosis; and eosinophilic granuloma. It may be part of a familial syndrome of diabetes insipidus, diabetes mellitus, optic atrophy and nerve deafness (DIDMOAD). In addition, the condition may be simulated by disorders which lead to renal resistance to vasopressin. These include X-linked nephrogenic diabetes insipidus (confined to males), and hypercalcaemia and hypokalaemia, both of which lead to a water diuresis from resistance to ADH.

Clinical features

The principal symptom of ADH deficiency is thirst and incidental polyuria, since the patient is forced by the osmotic stimulus to drink large volumes of water or other fluids. It is not uncommon for patients to pass in excess of 10 litres of urine a day, of very low specific gravity (1.003 or less, osmolality less than 100 mosmol/kg). The serum sodium concentration is generally moderately raised, but seldom over 150 mmol/l provided the patient has free access to water. The major danger is when such access is denied, or when the patient is unconscious, e.g. due to an anaesthetic or head injury. Under these circumstances, the osmolality and sodium concentration climbs rapidly. A serum sodium concentration over 160–170 mmol/l may lead to severe and irreversible brain damage. As with hyponatraemia, correction should be gradual.

Investigation

The major differential diagnosis is from psychogenic polydipsia and from other causes of thirst and polyuria (Ch.

20, Table 20.10). The mainstay of diagnosis is measurement of serum and urine osmolality, serum sodium concentration (a more reliable measurement than the osmolality) and urine specific gravity (approximately 0.010 above that of water (1.00) for every 300 mosmol/l of urine solutes). Vasopressin assays are not widely available and seldom needed.

The formal water deprivation test is conducted once the serum sodium concentration and osmolality are known (and shown to be normal). Free access to water is allowed up to the start of the test at 8 am, when the patient is weighed and blood and urine samples taken for osmolality. Timed hourly urine collections, serum osmolality measurements and body weight recordings are made. For safety, the test is discontinued if 3% of body weight is lost or 3 litres of urine are passed. At the end of 8 hours, if urine concentration has not occurred, 1 μg of the analogue DDAVP is given i.v., and further samples taken; in true diabetes insipidus this leads to prompt urine concentration. Further details are given in Chapter 21, page 845.

Management of diabetes insipidus

A major advance in the treatment of diabetes insipidus came in the early 1970s, with the development of the long-acting vasopressin analogue, desamino-D-arginine vasopressin (DDAVP, desmopressin). This acts almost exclusively on the (type I) receptors of the renal tubule, and so does not cause hypertension and constriction of the splanchnic circulation. It is also resistant to enzyme degradation in the circulation or peripheral tissues and has a greatly prolonged half-life. DDAVP is given once or twice a day intranasally (10–20 μg) or, for the post-operative patient, intravenously (1–2 μg). With the introduction of desmopressin, diabetes insipidus is no longer a problem of management, provided the patient has an intact thirst centre and does not drink excessive volumes of water. Chlorpropamide enhances the renal response to ADH, but is now seldom used in its treatment.

'INAPPROPRIATE' SECRETION OF ADH

Aetiology

The syndrome of inappropriate secretion of ADH is frequently encountered in a variety of different conditions (Ch. 21, p. 847). These include acute and chronic pulmonary disease, congestive cardiac failure, small-cell carcinoma of bronchus, cerebral disease, hypoglycaemia, anterior hypopituitarism and hypothyroidism. ADH secretion is a transient accompaniment of surgery for 24–48 hours. Of the above conditions, only small-cell carcinoma of bronchus is ever associated with true ectopic tumour synthesis and secretion of vasopressin.

Even in this condition, however, hyponatraemia is often caused by excess hypothalamo-pituitary ADH secretion, rather than an ectopic source.

Clinical features, investigation and management

The hallmark is a low serum sodium concentration (usually below 125 mmol/l), and serum osmolality (below 270 mosmol/kg), associated with an inappropriately high urine osmolality (well in excess of 295 mosmol/kg), in a patient who is not clinically volume depleted. Volume depletion from any cause is a stimulus to ADH secretion, so these biochemical abnormalities would be appropriate in, for example, a patient overtreated with diuretics, a common cause of hyponatraemia in the elderly.

The major clinical features are confusion, coma and fits (water intoxication) if the serum sodium falls much below 120 mmol/l (osmolality below 250 mosmol/kg). Treatment is with fluid restriction and by correction of the underlying cause. If this is not possible, the patient can be treated with small volumes of hypertonic (1.8%) sodium chloride (in severe cases), or with the tetracyclic antibiotic demethylchlortetracycline which diminishes the renal response to ADH. For further details, see Chapter 21, page 848.

THE THYROID GLAND

EMBRYOLOGY, ANATOMY AND PHYSIOLOGY

The thyroid gland is derived in early embryonic life from an outpouching of the floor of the pharynx which becomes displaced caudally and fuses with the fourth pharyngeal pouch. During its caudal displacement, it leaves the thyroglossal duct, which usually becomes fragmented and resorbed, but may persist to form thyroglossal cysts. If migration is incomplete, ectopic thyroid tissue may lie at the base of the tongue. In adults, the thyroid gland weighs about 20 g and lies in front of the thyroid cartilage, its two lobes connected by a narrow isthmus. It moves upwards with the thyroid cartilage on swallowing.

Histologically, the thyroid gland is composed of follicles of varying diameter lined by a single-layered epithelium; these are arranged into lobules of 10–12 follicles, each served by a common blood supply. The gland is highly vascular, being supplied by two pairs of thyroid arteries which arise from external carotid (superior) and subclavian (inferior) arteries. There is a rich lymphatic drainage and adrenergic and cholinergic innervation. The gland also contains *parafollicular* or *C-cells*, which lie next to the follicle but do not abut the colloid. These cells, which arise from the last pair of pharyngeal pouches, secrete the calcium-lowering hormone calcitonin.

The glycoprotein thyroglobulin, which is rich in thyroxine residues, is the major constituent of colloid. The thyroid epithelial cells synthesise and secrete thyroglobulin into the colloid. Later, they resorb it, cleave the thyroid hormones from the glycoprotein backbone and secrete them into the circulation. Thyroglobulin is both an integral part of the process of thyroid hormone synthesis, and a major storage form of iodine and thyroid hormones within the thyroid.

Synthesis and secretion of thyroid hormones

The thyroid gland contains about 90% of the body's total iodine, mainly in organic form. The thyroid cells actively transport the iodide into the cells by a process which is competitively inhibited by other anions of similar size, such as perchlorate. Iodide is then oxidised to iodine and incorporated into mono- and di-iodotyrosine (MIT and DIT) residues on thyroglobulin. Favoured residues at particular sites on the thyroglobulin molecule are then converted to thyroxine (T4) and tri-iodothyronine (T3) residues (principally the former) either by interaction with other DIT and MIT residues, or by interaction with an oxidation product of DIT and MIT themselves. This process of 'organification' of iodine (which requires the action of a peroxidase) is believed to take place principally at the basal membrane of the thyroid cell, as thyroglobulin is being formed and secreted into the colloid (Fig. 17.18).

Iodination is most active when iodide levels are low. TSH is the principal active regulator, and exerts its action via a cell-surface receptor, at least in part via adenylate cyclase. TSH accelerates iodoprotein synthesis, and resorption of colloid by a phagocytic process, followed by fusion with lysosomes. Thyroglobulin is then hydrolysed, facilitated by reduction of disulphide bonds in the mole-

Thyroxine T4

3',3,5-tri-iodothyronine
T3 (active)

3',5',3-tri-iodothyronine
reverse T3 (inactive)

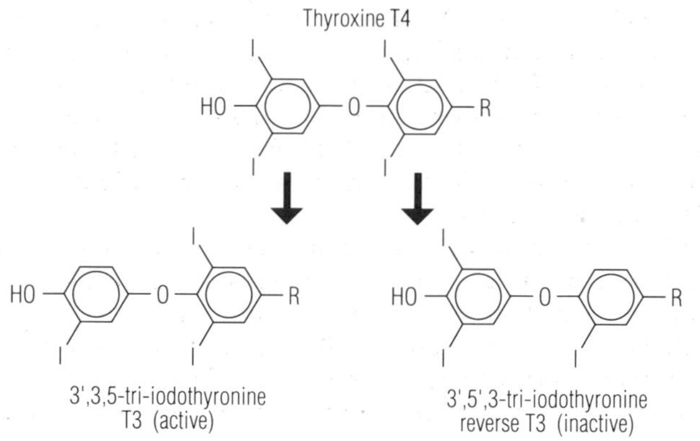

Fig. 17.19 Structures of T4, T3 and reverse T3. R is the alanine residue (–CH₂-CHNH₂-COOH).

cule. De-iodinases remove iodine from the iodotyrosine residues, and this iodine returns to the iodide pool for iodination of more thyronine residues.

Circulation, action and metabolism of thyroid hormones

T4 is the major form of thyroid hormone secreted by the thyroid; it is converted enzymatically to either T3 or reverse T3 (rT3) (Fig. 17.19), of which only the former is biologically active. Regulation of the activity of the relevant deiodinases, in the liver and in other tissues, appears to be important both in health and disease. Generally, the production of T3 and/or rT3 appears to be reciprocally controlled. T4 itself is probably largely active by virtue of its conversion to T3. It is, however, the principal circulating form of thyroid hormone and is more than 99% bound to three plasma proteins – thyroxine binding globulin (TBG), thyroxine binding prealbumin (TBPA) and albumin. TBG has the highest affinity but the lowest capacity, followed by TBPA. T3 binds with lower affinity to TBG, also binds to albumin, but not at all to TBPA. In their bound state(s), T3 and T4 are not biologically active. It is the concentration of unbound hormone which determines the level to which the target cells are exposed (the biologically active fraction).

The liver is the major site of degradation. Although much of the iodine is recycled, some is inevitably wasted, being excreted principally in the urine as iodinated degradation products and inorganic iodide. Under normal circumstances, this is matched by a daily intake of iodide of about 500 μg.

The normal circulating level of T4 (50–150 nmol/l) exceeds that of T3 (1–3 nmol/l) by 50-fold; the difference in their unbound concentrations is about 10 times less than this, because of both the lower binding of T3 to TBG, and its failure to bind to TBPA.

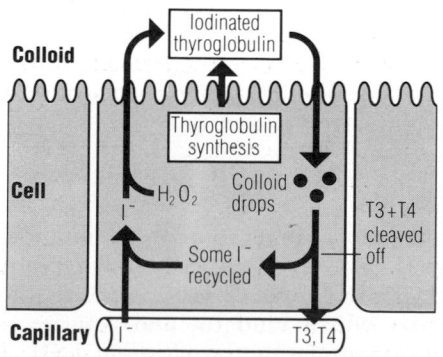

Fig. 17.18 Thyroid hormone synthesis and release (see text for details).

Physiological changes in thyroid hormones

Physiological changes in thyroid hormones are shown in Figure 17.20. The fetus derives little of its thyroid hormones and no TSH from the mother. During the second trimester, the fetal pituitary-thyroid axis becomes active, although it appears that hypothyroidism up to the time of birth does not greatly impair fetal development except for delayed appearance of some of the ossification centres. Although T4 is secreted in the fetus, very little T3 is produced before birth, rT3 being the major product. After birth there is an immediate switch of hepatic metabolism of T4 from rT3 to T3, so that levels of T3 rise briskly during the first week of life. This change may well be important in adaptation to postfetal life (in a way reminiscent of the critical role of thyroid hormones for the metamorphosis of amphibians). TBG levels in the fetus are low, and rise after birth. T3 levels throughout infancy and childhood tend to be higher than those of the adult.

In adults, a change occurs during pregnancy when total T4 and T3 levels rise passively in response to an oestrogen-induced rise in TBG. A similar change is produced by the oestrogen-containing oral contraceptive pill. In a wide variety of conditions of stress and ill-health, hepatic production of T3 declines and of rT3 increases. This decline in T3 production also occurs in old age. It is of uncertain biological significance, and conversion of T4 to T3 still occurs in some target tissues. Exposure to extreme cold is associated with reduced production of rT3 and increased production of T3.

PATHOLOGY OF THYROID DISEASE

The thyroid gland may be the subject of defective development, inborn biosynthetic errors, toxic or nutritional damage, autoimmune disease, and benign and malignant tumours. Many of these abnormalities give rise to enlargement of the gland and to the appearance of a *goitre* (thyroid enlargement). This may be focal (as in adenoma, cyst, or carcinoma) or generalised, in which case it may be either multinodular or diffuse and smooth. Clinical assessment alone will often allow an accurate assessment of the cause of the goitre.

Autoimmune disease and the thyroid

The thyroid is the endocrine gland most commonly affected by autoimmune disease. Immune mechanisms are involved in the pathogenesis of Graves' disease, Hashimoto's thyroiditis and primary myxoedema. For reasons that are as yet unclear, these disorders are about five times commoner in women than in men. Viral or other damage may result in the thyroid cell presenting HLA antigens on the external surface of the follicle; these may then set in motion an autoimmune response, which is partly humoral and partly cellular. In Graves' disease, the TSH receptor is an important antigen to which antibodies may be produced. These antibodies may bind to the receptor, causing stimulation. Growth-promoting antibodies may also be produced, as are antibodies to thyroid microsomes and thyroglobulin. The factors which determine what antibodies are produced in an individual case are uncertain.

Measurement of circulating levels of relevant antibodies may be of diagnostic value. In general, however, both the presence of antibody and its titre are disappointingly non-specific. The most commonly measured antibodies (which are of the IgG subclass) are those against thyroid cell microsomes, thyroglobulin (Tg) and the TSH receptor. Antibodies to microsomes, Tg or both are present in about 10% of apparently healthy individuals, usually women. In disease, they are most commonly detected against microsomes, being present in 85% or more of patients with autoimmune thyroid disease. Very high titres indicate the presence of foci of lymphocytic infiltration and Hashimoto's thyroiditis.

There is a significant association of autoimmune thyroid disease with certain HLA types, most strikingly DW3 and DR3. It has been suggested that the presence of this tissue type predicts a high chance of recurrence in a patient with Graves' disease (p.688).

Antibodies to the TSH receptor

Antibodies to the TSH receptor are of importance in the pathogenesis of Graves' disease and hypothyroidism. Thyrotoxicosis in Graves' disease is due to the presence of antibodies which bind to, and activate, the TSH receptor, thus simulating the action of TSH. These are now best detected in assays using purified porcine thyroid

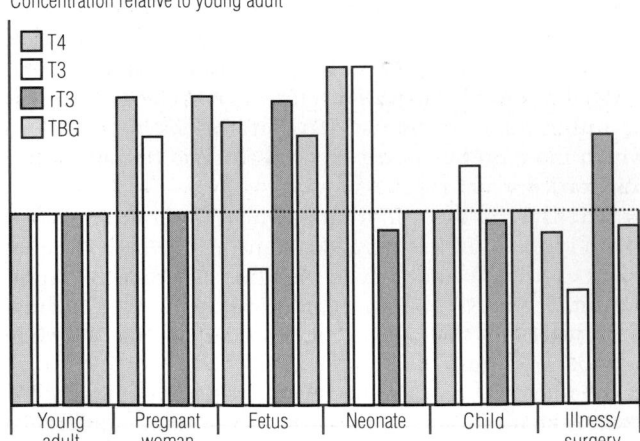

Concentration relative to young adult

Fig. 17.20 **Relative changes of serum T4, T3, reverse T3 and thyroxine binding globulin (TBG) in different physiological states and in illness.**

cell membranes and competition with labelled TSH, or by activation of adenylate cyclase. They were first detected as so-called long-acting thyroid stimulator (LATS) in a mouse bioassay. Other antibodies bind to the TSH receptor but do not activate it, and so cause hypothyroidism, often in the presence of a goitre. (In most cases of myxoedema, however, the thyroid dysfunction is due to the destructive effect of cell-mediated immunity and cytotoxic antibodies.)

Antibodies can cross the placenta and cause thyrotoxicosis in the newborn infant. Measurement of antireceptor antibody in the mother allows detection of babies at risk. Otherwise, there is a generally poor correlation between the circulating titre of thyroid-stimulating antibodies and the activity of Graves' thyrotoxicosis; this is probably because the antibodies are produced largely within the thyroid gland itself and spill over into the circulation.

Nutrition and thyroid disease

There is a wide geographical variation in the incidence of endemic goitre which is only partly understood. The major factors appear to be dietary iodine deficiency and ingestion of goitrogenic substances which interfere with either uptake or organification of iodine. For example, cassava, a root crop eaten extensively in Africa, is rich in goitrogens. Women are particularly susceptible to goitre because of the demands of the fetus for iodine. Endemic cretinism is a neurological disease which afflicts the offspring of goitrous mothers in parts of the world where iodine is deficient, especially in the mountainous regions of New Guinea. It appears to be due to fetal iodide deficiency at the stage of early brain development, rather than to thyroid hormone deficiency. It is completely prevented by providing the mother with iodised salt.

INVESTIGATION OF THYROID DISEASE

Examination of the thyroid gland

The thyroid should be carefully examined by observation from the front, and by palpation from behind while the patient swallows. The consistency of the gland should be assessed. In Graves' disease, the gland is typically either diffusely enlarged or slightly asymmetrical. The swelling is firmer with a carcinoma and associated with enlargement of local lymph nodes. A midline swelling that moves up with protrusion of the tongue is likely to be a thyroglossal cyst or ectopic thyroid. The gland, if enlarged, should be auscultated; a bruit, which when very loud may be heard in diastolic as well as in systolic, indicates a vascular gland and usually points to Graves' disease.

Laboratory assessment of hypo- and hyperthyroidism

Radioimmunoassay

The laboratory assessment of hypo- and hyperthyroidism is now extremely simple, thanks to specific radioimmunoassays for T3 and T4, to a specific and sensitive immunoradiometric assay for TSH, and (where relevant) to methods of assessing thyroid hormone binding. In most cases, clinical assessment combined with a single measurement of serum T3, T4 and TSH levels is sufficient.

In *primary hypothyroidism*, T4 and T3 levels are low and TSH rises markedly. In the early stages, or in patients who have had a subtotal thyroidectomy, T4 and T3 levels are normal, and TSH modestly raised. In most cases of symptomatic hypothyroidism, TSH will be more than five times the upper limit of normal. Serum T4 is more reliable for the assessment of early cases than T3, which may be low as a non-specific consequence of illness.

In *secondary (pituitary) hypothyroidism* one would expect TSH to be undetectable, but this is frequently not the case; T3 and T4 levels are low.

In *hyperthyroidism* serum T3 and T4 levels are elevated. In mild cases, serum T3 may be raised before T4 and so is a more reliable test for early detection of thyrotoxicosis. TSH levels are low but, until recently, assays were not sufficiently reliable to detect this. It was therefore necessary to inject thyrotrophic releasing hormone (TRH 200 μg i.v.), and to demonstrate an absent TSH response over the next 60 minutes. Highly sensitive two-site immunoradiometric assays allow subnormal TSH levels to be detected and so have largely eliminated the need for the TRH test.

Protein-binding tests

Tests of protein binding are widely used. TBG levels are generally reduced in hyperthyroidism, and increased in hypothyroidism. Oestrogens promote the hepatic synthesis of TBG along with other binding proteins; thus, the situation most commonly encountered where the T4 is raised and protein binding has to be taken into account is in a woman during pregnancy or while on the contraceptive pill. The test for long used to elucidate this problem is an in vitro thyroid hormone-uptake test, in which TBG in dilute serum and sephadex compete to bind radiolabelled T3 (Fig. 17.21).

Recently, a *direct free T4 assay* has become commercially available. This assay uses a synthetic ligand which binds to the T4 antibody but not to TBG, and thus allows assessment of the actual unbound T4. All tests, including this one, have pitfalls for the unwary and require expert assessment whenever the clinical features and biochemical results are conflicting.

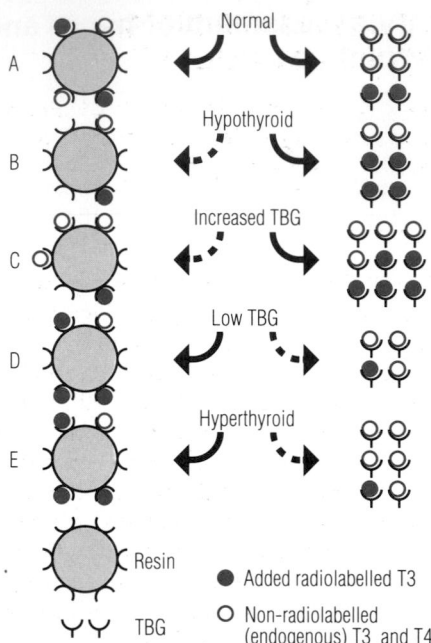

Fig. 17.21 Distribution of radiolabelled T3 between resin (left) and binding proteins (right), in different clinical states. Arrows indicate direction of distribution.

Radioactive uptake tests

Historically, ¹³¹I uptake was routinely carried out to confirm the diagnosis of hyper- and hypothyroidism. This test required serial measurements of uptake over 1–2 days, to allow a curve to be plotted. In thyrotoxicosis, both uptake and discharge are more rapid than normal so that the protein bound ¹³¹I level at 48 hours was perhaps the most reliable measurement. A major problem was the variable background concentration of circulating inorganic iodide.

Nowadays, virtually the only isotope to be used diagnostically is ⁹⁹ᵐTc (as radiolabelled pertechnetate, Fig. 17.22), a short-lived gamma-emitter with a half-life of 6 hours. Scans are of great value in assessing the distribution of uptake within the gland. Uptake may be confined to one area in a functioning autonomous adenoma, since uptake by the rest of the gland is suppressed; conversely, uptake is absent in an area occupied by a cyst or carcinoma. Even a well-differentiated carcinoma will seldom take up isotope in the presence of a normally functioning gland.

Ultrasound

Ultrasound is a useful technique, particularly for demonstrating the cystic nature of a lesion. Unfortunately, some tumours may also be cystic, so the test is not completely reliable.

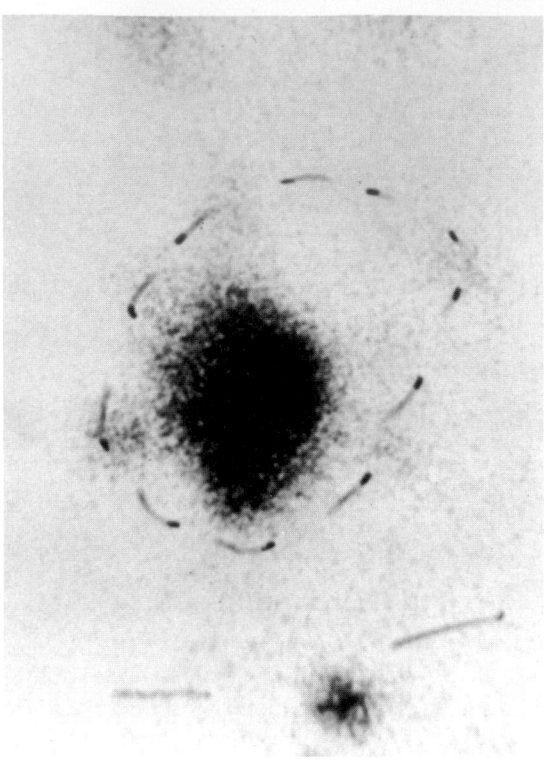

Fig. 17.22 ⁹⁹ᵐTc-labelled pertechnetate isotope scan showing asymmetrical uptake in the thyroid (dashed outline) with one particularly large 'hot' nodule. The dark spot below the thyroid is the suprasternal notch, marked with the isotope.

Needle aspiration

Needle aspiration of the thyroid is also a simple and useful technique for non-invasive diagnosis of thyroid masses. Interpretation requires a degree of expertise on the part of the histopathologist, particularly if there is a suspected carcinoma. However, once the technique is mastered, it greatly reduces the need for thyroid scans, and for surgery on benign nodules.

PRIMARY HYPOTHYROIDISM: CONGENITAL AND JUVENILE

Hypothyroidism may be present before birth (although it is probably not of great importance until immediately after birth) or may develop at any time thereafter.

Congenital hypothyroidism

The causes of congenital hypothyroidism are listed in Table 17.7. Endemic cretinism is a severe developmental disorder occurring in areas of endemic goitre in children born to goitrous and iodine-deficient mothers. Severe neurological defects (deaf mutism, spasticity and motor

Table 17.7 Causes of congenital hypothyroidism

Non-goitrous
Complete failure of thyroid development
Ectopic thyroid
Endemic cretinism
Pituitary or hypothalamic insufficiency

Goitrous
Maternal antithyroid drugs
Endemic cretinism
Iodine treatment of mother
Defects in thyroid hormone biosynthesis
Iodide transport, organic binding defects
Iodotyronine coupling defect
Iodotyronine dehydrogenase (iodine recycling) defect
Abnormal iodoprotein secretion
Thyroid hormone resistance

impairment) are associated with variable hypothyroidism and goitre. In non-goitrous areas, congenital hypothyroidism occurs with a frequency of around 1 in 5000 births, and is usually due to failure of normal development or to atrophy of the thyroid. It is usually not clinically apparent at birth, but may be diagnosed reliably within 1–2 weeks by TSH assay on a blood spot dried on filter paper.

Suggestive early features include postmaturity, hypothermia, enlargement of the posterior fontanelle, neonatal jaundice and delayed passage of meconium. Failure to diagnose and treat leads to retardation of physical growth and mental development, which becomes gross by late infancy. Early signs are feeding difficulty, failure to thrive, protuberant abdomen, dry skin and hair, and delayed eruption of teeth. The infant is slow to reach the usual milestones. Radiological abnormalities include delayed development and 'stippling' of the epiphyses. The longer treatment is delayed, the greater is the likelihood of permanent mental retardation; any delay is likely to result in a lower than maximum potential IQ.

Juvenile hypothyroidism

Hypothyroidism starting in childhood results in mental slowness but no permanent mental retardation. Features seen are less obvious than in the myxoedematous adult, but growth and sexual development are retarded, often markedly. Delay in body development principally affects the long bones and the bones of the face which therefore appears immature. Epiphyseal dysgenesis with 'stippling' of the epiphyses on X-ray is common, and epiphyseal closure is delayed. Puberty is usually delayed, although, paradoxically, precocious puberty may also occur. Replacement therapy results in some catch-up growth and in spontaneous puberty (if this was delayed).

PRIMARY HYPOTHYROIDISM DEVELOPING IN ADULT LIFE

Hypothyroidism with onset in adult life is almost always due to autoimmunity, unless it results from previous treatment of thyrotoxicosis.

Clinical features

The onset is usually gradual, and the symptoms are often attributed incorrectly to increasing age. Increasing lethargy, slowness, memory loss and depression are often coupled with increasing weight (without eating more) and cold intolerance. The skin becomes dry and the hair 'lifeless'. Puffiness below the eyes, especially in the morning, is frequently noted. Symptoms are referred to many systems; constipation is common, and may be associated with abdominal distension; in the nervous system, symptoms of carpal tunnel syndrome and a complaint of dizziness are common. Deafness is a frequent symptom due to fluid in the middle ear. The patient may have noticed a change in the voice with deepening or 'gruffness'. Rarely, the patient develops cerebellar ataxia. Myotonia is a rare complication.

Hypercholesterolaemia predisposes to vascular atheroma, and angina in the untreated patient is particularly important, as treatment may precipitate myocardial infarction. Effusions may occur into any serous cavity – pericardial, pleural, peritoneal or joint spaces. Mild anaemia of macrocytic type is quite common; megaloblastic anaemia suggests coincidental pernicious anaemia. Other organ-specific autoimmune diseases, such as vitiligo and Addison's disease, may be associated. Rheumatoid arthritis and polymyalgia rheumatica are also significantly associated with autoimmune thyroid disease. Menorrhagia and galactorrhoea (with elevated PRL) are common in young women. In severe myxoedema, the patient is grossly retarded and may become psychotic when treated; rarely, however, they paradoxically appear mentally hyperactive (myxoedema madness). Hypothyroidism predisposes to hypothermia; it may cause hyponatraemia, since hypothyroidism predisposes to inappropriate secretion of ADH. If hypothyroidism is suspected, a past history of thyrotoxicosis (with surgery or ^{131}I therapy) and a family history of thyroid disease should be sought.

With experience, a confident clinical diagnosis of hypothyroidism can often be made from the history and physical examination. However, the aim should be to make the diagnosis before it is clinically obvious, and serum T3, T4 and TSH estimation allows this to be done. Early signs are lethargy, depression, slowness in answering questions, a malar flush, puffy eyes, dry skin and delayed relaxation of the tendon reflexes (e.g. ankle jerks, if present, or biceps jerks). The voice may be husky or 'gruff'. There is usually a relative or absolute bradycardia. The patient may have gained weight.

Summary 3 Clinical features of myxoedema

- Symptoms include lethargy, increased weight, cold intolerance, mental slowing.
- Signs include dry skin, puffy face, gruff voice.
- Complications include serous effusions, vascular disease, psychosis.

The commonest conditions with which hypothyroidism is confused are obesity and depression. With good clinical practice, gross myxoedema should be a thing of the past. In doubtful cases, thyroid function tests (TSH and T4 will suffice) should be measured on a blood (serum) sample. The thyroid is usually impalpable, except where hypothyroidism is due to an enzyme deficiency or to TSH receptor-blocking antibodies, rather than destruction of the gland.

Investigation

T4 and T3 are low (the former being more reliable) and TSH greatly raised. Free T4 is reduced. Investigations to establish the aetiology depend on the clinical setting. In a child, a thyroid scan may demonstrate ectopic tissue and, if a goitre is present, a perchlorate discharge test may uncover an organification deficit. This test depends on the failure of iodide to be used in thyroxine synthesis; free (labelled) iodide can therefore be discharged from the gland when perchlorate is administered. Antithyroid antibodies, if present, point to an autoimmune aetiology.

It is important to carry out investigations to determine the extent of damage that has resulted from the hypothyroidism, such as X-rays of bones in a child and endocrine tests to assess pubertal stage. Juvenile hypothyroidism is commonly confused with panhypopituitarism, but TSH will be low in the latter and high in the former. Chest X-ray may reveal a pleural or pericardial effusion. An ECG is important in the elderly patient with possible ischaemic heart disease; T4 replacement should be started cautiously and under β-adrenergic blockade. Measurement of serum electrolyte levels may reveal hyponatraemia due to inappropriate ADH secretion.

Management

In treating hypothyroidism, it is important to be certain before commencing thyroid hormones that the patient is not hypopituitary or hypoadrenal. If in doubt, hydrocortisone replacement should also be given, until ACTH and/or cortisol deficiency have been excluded. In mild cases, the patient can be commenced forthwith on a full replacement dose of T4 (100–200 μg/daily). In an adult, the median dose required to suppress TSH to normal is about 125 μg/day. In severe cases, especially if there is ischaemic heart disease, replacement should be more cautious, with 5 μg b.d. of T3 or 25–50 μg of T4. Myxoedema coma and hypothermia carries a poor prognosis and requires rewarming, cardiovascular support, hydrocortisone, parenteral T3 (15–30 μg daily) and antibiotics if there is infection. There is no advantage to be gained long-term from giving T3 or T3–T4 mixtures.

Prevention

Thyroid failure cannot be prevented, but much can be done to ensure its early detection and treatment. Thyroid hormone replacement is the simplest form of therapy so, for practical purposes, prevention is by early detection. Patients with any form of autoimmune thyroid disease, such as Graves' disease, should be told that there is an increased chance of developing thyroid failure later, and that if there is clinical suspicion they should therefore ask for thyroid function tests to be performed. Patients who have had radioactive iodine therapy are at particular risk and should be told of this, as should previously thyrotoxic patients who have had subtotal thyroidectomy. The earliest biochemical change is a rise in serum TSH although, particularly after thyroid surgery, this may simply indicate a new steady state, with normal T3 and T4 being produced under modestly increased TSH drive. Borderline thyroid function tests may present a problem; in such cases, the tests can be repeated after an interval and, if thyroid failure is developing, TSH will rise progressively.

Once on T4, patients must be told to stay on it for life, advice that may easily be ignored, especially by the elderly and the confused. Sadly, many early cases of hypothyroidism are still missed by doctors each year, perhaps because they expect the patient to have 'textbook' myxoedema. The aim should be to diagnose hypothyroidism *before there are any physical signs*. A careful history and a high index of suspicion is the key. Thyroid function tests should be checked if there is any possibility of hypothyroidism. Thyrotoxic patients on antithyroid drugs should be monitored carefully both clinically and biochemically, since the dose needed varies considerably and a patient may develop a lower requirement with time.

Prevention of cretinism now depends upon TSH assays done on blood spots in the neonatal period as a screening test. High or borderline levels lead to more detailed clinical and biochemical screening.

HYPERTHYROIDISM

In areas where iodine is abundant, most patients with thyrotoxicosis have autoimmune thyroid disease (Graves' disease). Thyrotoxicosis due to multinodular goitre, or to a toxic adenoma, is less common.

There is a wide clinical spectrum of severity of thyroid hormone excess, of the systemic manifestations of the disease, the size and vascularity of the thyroid gland, and the extent to which other systems, notably the extraocular muscles and the skin, are involved in associated autoimmune disorders. The clinician should therefore consider separately those features which are directly or indirectly due to thyroid hormone excess, from associated abnormalities (such as some of the eye signs).

Toxic multinodular goitre usually develops after the age of 50 against a background of many years of non-toxic goitre. It is therefore much more common in areas of endemic goitre. For reasons that are not clear, diffuse or focal autonomous nodule formation develops in the enlarged thyroid (detected as areas of increased radio-iodine uptake), with associated thyrotoxicosis which is generally of a relatively mild degree and associated with suppressed TSH. This disorder is not associated with infiltrative ophthalmopathy.

In *toxic adenoma*, an autonomous nodule (follicular adenoma) develops and progressively enlarges. It secretes an increasing amount of thyroid hormone until TSH is switched off completely and (generally mild) thyrotoxicosis develops. This usually happens only when the nodule reaches 2.5 cm diameter or more.

In *Graves' disease*, antibodies to the TSH receptor stimulate the thyroid gland in ways analogous to the normal action of TSH. The disease presents most commonly in the third and fourth decades of life. As with many organ-specific autoimmune diseases, Graves' disease is much commoner in women than in men; this also applies to toxic multinodular goitre. Especially in the latter disorder, hyperthyroidism may be induced by high doses of iodine or iodine-containing drugs (the Jod-Basedow phenomenon). Hashimoto's disease, which is also of autoimmune aetiology, may also be associated with mild thyrotoxicosis in the early stages, as may sub-acute (viral) thyroiditis. Occasionally, thyrotoxicosis is due to exogenous hormone consumption.

Clinical features due to thyroid hormone excess

History

The history of the patient with thyroid hormone excess is variable. Typically, the patient develops weight loss, increased appetite, heat intolerance and sweating, and becomes anxious, nervous, restless, depressed, irritable and difficult to live with. A fine tremor is common, and proximal myopathy may cause muscle weakness, especially in the elderly. In women, menstrual disturbances such as oligomenorrhoea and menorrhagia are common. Increased gut motility may lead to diarrhoea. Palpitations are common and symptoms of heart failure are especially likely in the elderly, often precipitated by atrial fibrillation. A goitre may be noted, and complained of, especially if the gland is large and vascular. It rarely obstructs swallowing or breathing unless it is retrosternal. To assess the patient quickly when thyrotoxicosis is suspected, a clinical check-list is useful, such as that given in Table 17.8.

Examination

Most of the features of thyroid hormone excess are due to increased sensitivity to circulating catecholamines. Part of the levator palpebrae superioris is sympathetically innervated, and overactivity causes a staring appearance, lid lag, lid retraction, and infrequent blinking. This may be associated with feelings of anxiety, nervousness, tremor, sweating, tachycardia and supra-ventricular arrhythmias (notably atrial fibrillation).

Thyroid hormones also stimulate the metabolic rate, probably both directly by inducing a number of metabolic enzymes, and also indirectly, through catecholamine sensitivity. Heat intolerance and weight loss (in spite of increased appetite) result.

Features that may occur and are of uncertain pathogenesis include myopathy, cardiac failure, hypercal-

Table 17.8 Symptoms and signs of thyrotoxicosis (Graves' disease)

Mechanisms	Symptoms	Signs
Primary autoimmune process	Swelling, dysphagia, pain	Goitre, bruit
	Exophthalmos, discomfort	Exophthalmos, ocular palsies
	Diplopia, etc.	Congestion, papilloedema, etc.
	Itchy/painful rash on legs	Pretibial myxoedema (rare)
Thyroid hormone excess		
Combination of catecholamine sensitivity, thyroid hormone excess and hypermetabolism	Palpitations* Breathlessness	Resting tachycardia*, atrial fibrillation, other arrhythmias* Heart failure
	Heat intolerance* Sweating*	Warm and sweaty*
	Increased appetite	Increased bowel sounds
	Weight loss	Malabsorption
	Diarrhoea*	
	Weakness	Proximal myopathy
	Nervousness and irritability*	Inability to sit still Emotional lability* Tremor*
	'Staring' eyes*	Infrequent blinking* Lid lag* Lid retraction*

*Signs and associated symptoms (partially) blocked by beta-blockers caemia, raised alkaline phosphatase, low magnesium, gynaecomastia and female infertility. The hypercalcaemia is usually mild and does not always respond to rendering the patient euthyroid. Gynaecomastia probably results from metabolic alterations of androgen and oestrogen metabolism, and increased sex hormone binding globulin (SHBG) levels, which lead to an increased ratio of free oestradiol to testosterone.

Natural history of thyrotoxicosis

Graves' disease. While it is difficult to be certain, it seems likely that, before treatment became available, one-third to one-half of patients with Graves' disease had a spontaneous remission of their thyrotoxicosis. This applied particularly to thyrotoxic patients during pregnancy, possibly because of the weak glucocorticoid-like effect of progesterone. An uncertain proportion (perhaps 20%) of patients will spontaneously become hypothyroid if followed long enough. The reverse pattern – hypothy-roidism progressing to hyperthyroidism – is a rare but recognised presentation of Graves' disease. The prognosis for relapse after medical treatment is probably worst if there is a large vascular goitre.

Hashimoto's disease. In Hashimoto's disease, a similar percentage of patients to that seen in Graves' will go into remission spontaneously. In others, an early thyrotoxic phase is followed by progressive hypothyroidism.

Toxic adenoma. Occasionally, patients with toxic adenoma treat themselves by infarcting the tumour, a condition associated with sudden development of pain and swelling of a thyroid nodule. Usually, the condition gradually progresses until the patient becomes overtly toxic.

Dysthyroid eye disease

Dysthyroid eye disease (infiltrative ophthalmopathy) remains one of the more puzzling clinical features of endocrinology.

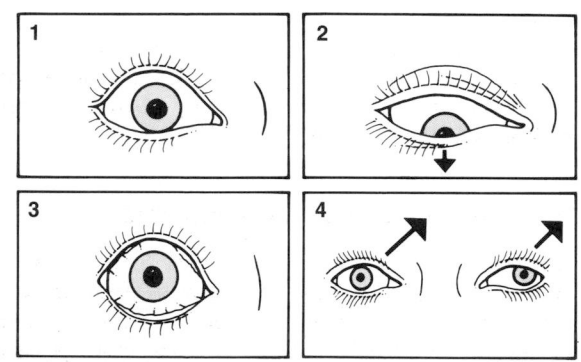

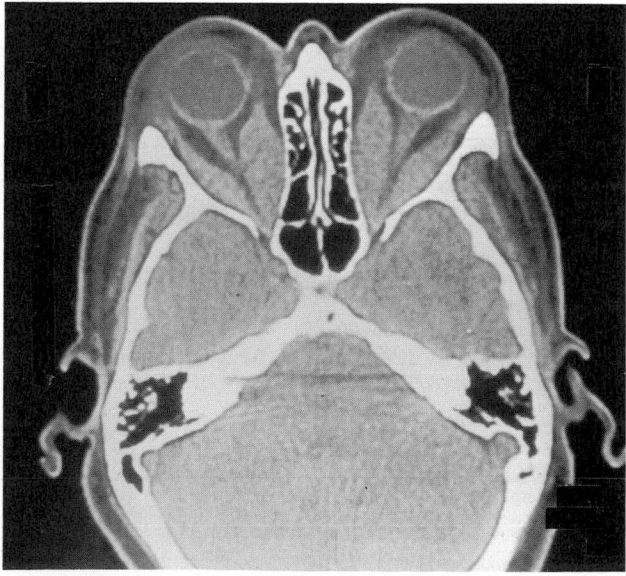

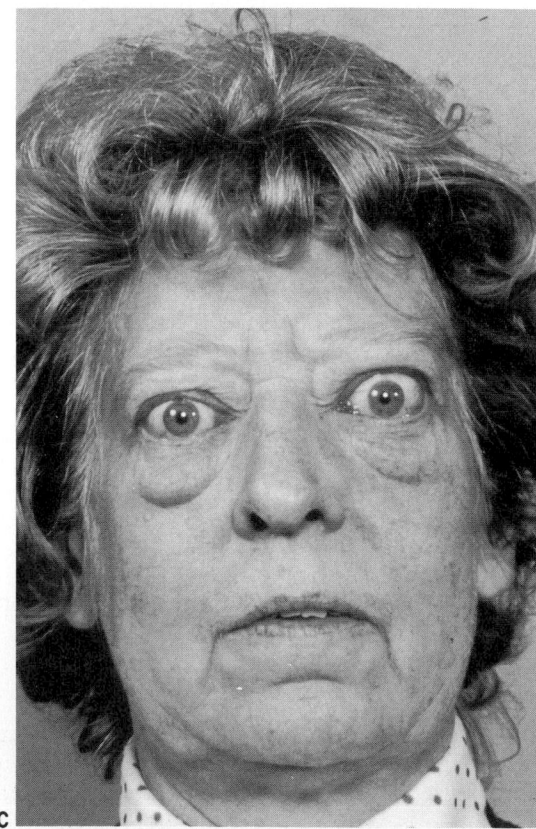

Fig. 17.23 Eye signs in thyrotoxicosis and dysthyroid eye disease. A. Eye signs in thyrotoxicosis: (1) lid retraction; (2) lid lag; (3) exophthalmos with conjunctival oedema; (4) strabismus with diplopia due to paralysis/tethering. Arrows indicate direction of gaze. **B.** CT scan through orbits in a case of exophthalmos. Note oedematous and enlarged extraocular muscles. **C.** Patient with typical features of dysthyroid eye disease with exophthalmos.

Aetiology

Dysthyroid eye disease occurs in Graves' disease but not in other causes of thyrotoxicosis. An autoimmune process involves the extraocular muscles and appears to be indirectly linked with that causing the thyroid disease. The eye muscles become infiltrated with lymphocytes, swollen and, in the later stages of the disease, fibrosed. Later, there is involvement of the retro-orbital fat in the inflammatory process.

Clinical features

The clinical features of dysthyroid eye disease are to be distinguished from those due to thyrotoxicosis, which become less marked on treatment with beta-adrenergic blockers (Table 17.8). Protrusion of the eyeball (Fig. 17.23) is most obvious if the orbits are shallow. It is usually, but not invariably, symmetrical. If marked, it leads to inability to close the eye fully, corneal damage (exposure keratitis) and a risk of secondary infection. Increased orbital pressure leads to suffusion of the ocular and orbital circulation with conjunctival oedema, retinal venous congestion, raised intraocular pressure (glaucoma) and papilloedema. Ocular muscle paresis is common and leads to troublesome diplopia. Ocular muscles frequently become tethered to surrounding soft tissues; this is particularly so for the inferior rectus muscles, so that diplopia is often most marked on looking upwards. Conjugate deviation may be impossible.

The symptoms of dysthyroid eye disease include discomfort, grittiness, swelling, redness and pain in the eyes which is often most marked on wakening (because of orbital congestion on recumbency and exposure of the cornea during sleep). The patient or relatives may have noticed the development of 'bulging eyes'. Occasionally, presentation may be with visual failure due to glaucoma or optic nerve damage (e.g. retinal vein thrombosis). The signs of a dangerous rise in ocular and orbital pressure are obvious conjunctival or periorbital oedema, painful eyes, exposure keratitis, retinal venous congestion and papilloedema. These should lead to urgent specialist referral.

Management

In 90% of cases, the eye condition will settle spontaneously. Local use of artificial tears at night is helpful if there is corneal exposure with the eyelids closed. Ocular congestion is an indication for use of diuretics to cause minimal sodium depletion and, in more severe cases, admission to hospital and treatment with systemic steroids in high dosage (e.g. prednisolone, 60–80 mg daily). In severe cases, if improvement does not occur, or if deterioration follows gradual reduction in dosage, orbital decompression may save vision. This involves removal of part of the wall or roof of the orbit. Later (but only after the condition has been stable for 6 months or more), ocular surgery may be indicated for diplopia that cannot be managed by refractive means (e.g. use of prismatic spectacles). It is important to avoid over-treatment of thyrotoxicosis, since treatment-induced hypothyroidism can lead to rapid deterioration in the eyes; this is probably because myxoedematous congestion is added to an already critical situation. In severe cases orbital radiotherapy may be helpful.

Pretibial myxoedema and thyroid acropachy

Pretibial myxoedema, a rare feature of Graves' disease, is purplish infiltration of the dermis of the skin over the anterolateral aspect of the lower legs. It is of unknown aetiology. In texture, the surface resembles the skin of an orange. Pathology shows deposition of mucin between collagen bundles. Pretibial myxoedema may present incidentally, for cosmetic reasons or because the lesion is itchy.

Thyroid acropachy is usually associated with pretibial myxoedema, and is the association of Graves' disease with extreme finger clubbing and periosteal reaction in the bones of the forearm.

Management of thyrotoxicosis

Traditionally, young patients have been treated with antithyroid drugs (carbimazole or propylthiouracil). If the condition relapses, they have been subjected to subtotal thyroidectomy, while patients over about 40 years of age have been given radioactive iodine therapy. Different strategies are used in different centres, some physicians prescribing ^{131}I as definitive treatment even for young patients, and others giving carbimazole long-term. As a general principle, surgery should not be undertaken, nor ^{131}I given, while the patient is grossly thyrotoxic. The patient should first be made euthyroid with antithyroid drugs because there is a risk of precipitating a thyrotoxic 'storm' with ^{131}I or surgery when the patient is still thyrotoxic.

Drug therapy

The major antithyroid drugs used are *thiourea compounds*, of which carbimazole is usually used in the UK and methimazole and propylthiouracil in the USA. They are generally well tolerated, with reversible leucopenia or skin rashes developing in only about 1% of cases, usually during the first 6 weeks of therapy. During this time, the white blood count should be checked every 2 weeks or if a sore throat develops. The drugs are usually given initially at high dosage. Thus, carbimazole is given at first in a dose of 30–60 mg daily, in three or four divided doses because of its short half-life. This is tapered off after 3–4 weeks to a maintenance dose of 5–30 mg daily. An alternative policy is to start straightaway with the likely maintenance dose (higher for gross thyrotoxicosis, with a large vascular gland) and to titrate this against the circulating T3 and T4 levels. On treatment, the ratio of T3 to T4 is higher than normal, because of preferential suppression of T4 formation, but this does not seem to matter clinically. It is important to realise that there is a lag of 1–2 weeks between the achievement of biochemical and that of clinical euthyroidism. It is easy to overtreat if this is not appreciated, and to have a patient who is biochemically hypothyroid yet still clinically thyrotoxic; such a patient will eventually and rapidly become clinically hypothyroid. It appears satisfactory to maintain patients on a daily dose of carbimazole. In some centres, a high dose of carbimazole is routinely combined with replacement doses of T4. Since most of the adverse effects of the thiourea drugs occur during the first few weeks of treatment, patients stabilised on a small dose but who relapse when taken off it can safely be maintained on the drug long-term.

Beta-adrenergic blocking drugs are useful for symptomatic treatment during the first 4–8 weeks until several weeks after biochemical euthyroidism is achieved. Usually, small doses (e.g. 20–40 mg of propranolol twice daily) are sufficient. In mild cases, beta-blockers alone may be used while the effect of ^{131}I therapy is awaited. If beta-blockers are contraindicated, calcium channel blockers such as diltiazem may be used instead.

Potassium perchlorate is now no longer used because of a high incidence of toxic reactions.

The optimal duration of antithyroid drug therapy is probably 12–18 months. The drugs may act in part by exerting an immunosuppressive effect within the thyroid, thereby preventing relapse, and this may be an argument for prolonging treatment. It has also been used as an argument for giving all patients high doses of carbimazole therapy, 'covered' with T4 (100–150 μg daily) to prevent the otherwise inevitable development of hypothyroidism.

Thyroid surgery

The indications for thyroid surgery are not clear-cut. Where patients are referred first to a surgeon, the operation rate tends to be high. In centres where radio-iodine therapy is given the frequency of surgery is lower. Patients should be rendered euthyroid medically for 3 months before surgery is undertaken (see above). Surgery should probably not be considered in Graves' disease before a proper trial of medical therapy (except in cases where thyrotoxicosis is excessively difficult to control). Other exceptions are where the goitre is unusually large or painful, or is causing tracheal obstruction.

Pre- and postoperative management

Potassium iodide is generally administered by mouth in a dose of at least 5 mg daily (many surgeons use much more) for 7–10 days before operation. This blocks the release of thyroid hormones but also, more importantly, leads to a marked accumulation of colloid in the thyroid follicles and, partly as a consequence of this, reduces the vascularity of the gland. Laryngoscopic examination of the cords is undertaken routinely before surgery. Most surgeons remove about seven-eighths of the gland, taking care to identify and preserve the parathyroid glands and, of course, the left recurrent laryngeal nerve. Nevertheless, there is a significant incidence (5–10%) of postoperative hypocalcaemia from hypoparathyroidism, as some vascular damage to these glands is probably inevitable. It is usually transient, however. Serum calcium levels should be checked 12 and 24 hours after surgery.

Radio-iodine treatment

It is impossible to judge accurately the optimum dose of ^{131}I to be given in radio-iodine treatment although, in general, large vascular glands are more resistant than small avascular glands. The usual dose for an adult is 15 mCi given by mouth. Antithyroid drugs should be stopped for a few days beforehand and can then be restarted 7–10 days afterwards. There is an acute effect in the first few weeks or months and a more prolonged effect thereafter. Any patient rendered euthyroid by ^{131}I is at long-term risk of developing hypothyroidism (sometimes as much as 20 years later). Patients should be told of this probability and reassured that it is easily treated. There does not appear to be any increased risk of thyroid or other cancer after ^{131}I therapy. The treatment is obviously contraindicated in pregnancy, or where there is a significant likelihood of pregnancy.

Follow-up of patients who have been thyrotoxic is important, regardless of the treatment used, as both recurrence and hypothyroidism are difficult to predict and best spotted early. After ^{131}I therapy, patients should have T3, T4 and TSH estimations at lengthening intervals; a rising TSH should warn of the likelihood of impending overt hypothyroidism. Once T4 therapy has been started, no special follow-up is needed.

Summary 4 Management of hyperthyroidism

- Carbimazole is usually the first treatment for patients of all ages.
- Beta-blockers are useful symptomatically for the first 1–2 months.
- Surgery is considered for failed medical treatment and large goitres.
- ^{131}I is considered for older patients and for toxic adenomas.

Management of thyrotoxicosis in the elderly

In the elderly, the same principles of management of thyrotoxicosis apply, except that surgery is rarely indicated. Where atrial fibrillation is present, it is advisable to anticoagulate the patient (if there is no contraindication). Atrial defibrillation may be undertaken if the patient is off digoxin and does not revert to sinus rhythm spontaneously.

Treatment of toxic adenoma is usually by surgical excision, although in the elderly or frail ^{131}I or long-term drug therapy may be used.

Thyrotoxicosis and pregnancy

A number of autoimmune conditions commonly improve during pregnancy, probably due in part to the high levels of progesterone (which has a mild glucocorticoid action) and in part to increased cortisol production. Thyrotoxicosis often enters remission during pregnancy, and relapses in the puerperium. It is important to avoid overtreatment with antithyroid drugs during pregnancy. In the fetus, these can cause hypothyroidism, increased TSH secretion and thyroid enlargement (which may cause respiratory obstruction in the newborn). It is therefore the rule to keep the mother on the minimum dose needed to maintain euthyroidism, and usually to discontinue the drug in the last 4 weeks or so of pregnancy.

If the titre of thyroid stimulating antibodies (which can cross the placenta) is high, this may lead to significant thyroid stimulation in the baby, and neonatal thyrotoxicosis. As the titre of antibodies (principally of the IgG subclass) declines, so does the thyrotoxicosis. The infant is treated with beta-blockers and carbimazole until the condition subsides spontaneously. Neonatal thyrotoxicosis can be predicted by measuring maternal TSH. The clinical manifestations do not occur until 1–2 weeks after birth, so prolonged hospital observation of the at-risk neonate is essential.

OTHER THYROID DISORDERS

Simple diffuse goitre

Simple diffuse goitre with euthyroidism is extremely common, especially in women, and seldom requires treatment. The aetiology is poorly understood but, since it usually develops at puberty, oestrogens may be partly responsible. It is TSH-dependent and generally diminishes on treatment with T4 in replacement doses. Pseudogoitre is also common. Here, a normal-sized gland is readily visible because it is high-lying, usually in a girl with a long neck.

Diffuse multinodular goitre

Diffuse multinodular goitre is common, but poorly understood. In Western countries, where salt is iodised, it is now seldom due to iodine deficiency. The high incidence in many underdeveloped parts of the world is almost certainly due to the ingestion of goitrogens, e.g. from the cassava root, which apparently interfere with the organification of iodine. In a goitrous area, there are also other factors (such as mild enzyme deficiencies and the iodine-drain of recurrent pregnancies) which predispose certain individuals (usually women) to gross degrees of goitre. Eventually, the nodules (which are initially TSH-dependent) may become autonomous. Sudden introduction of high levels of iodine in the diet in such communities has led to epidemics of thyrotoxicosis (the so-called Jod-Basedow phenomenon). This is due in part to unmasking cases of Graves' disease, and in part to cases of multinodular goitre.

Management of multinodular goitre

In the early stages, non-toxic goitre will respond either to suppression of TSH by giving exogenous thyroid hormones, or to removing the cause (goitrogens or iodine deficiency). Once autonomous nodules have developed, TSH suppression with T4 is much less effective, and iodine administration carries the risk of precipitating hyperthyroidism. The chances of successful response are highest if TSH levels are not completely suppressed.

Toxic multinodular goitre is usually treated with ^{131}I therapy, though it is often relatively resistant and repeated doses may be needed. Patients should generally be rendered euthyroid with carbimazole first. Where the goitre is large (Fig. 17.24) or causing severe obstructive symptoms (especially pressure on the trachea), surgery is the treatment of choice, especially since ^{131}I therapy may temporarily cause further thyroid enlargement. Tracheal compression is confirmed by soft tissue X-rays of the neck.

Familial goitre. There are a number of rare conditions where defects in thyroid hormone synthesis lead to goitre. Most are autosomal recessive. Pendred's syndrome is familial goitre and nerve deafness. The defect is in organification of iodine.

Riedel's thyroiditis

Riedel's thyroiditis is a peculiar condition of unknown aetiology associated with woody fibrous infiltration of the thyroid gland and surrounding tissues.

Viral thyroiditis

The condition of viral thyroiditis commonly presents with acute painful generalised swelling of the thyroid gland, fever, elevated protein-bound iodine (due to release of thyroglobulin) and mild transient hypothyroidism. Some cases appear to be due to Coxsackie B viruses.

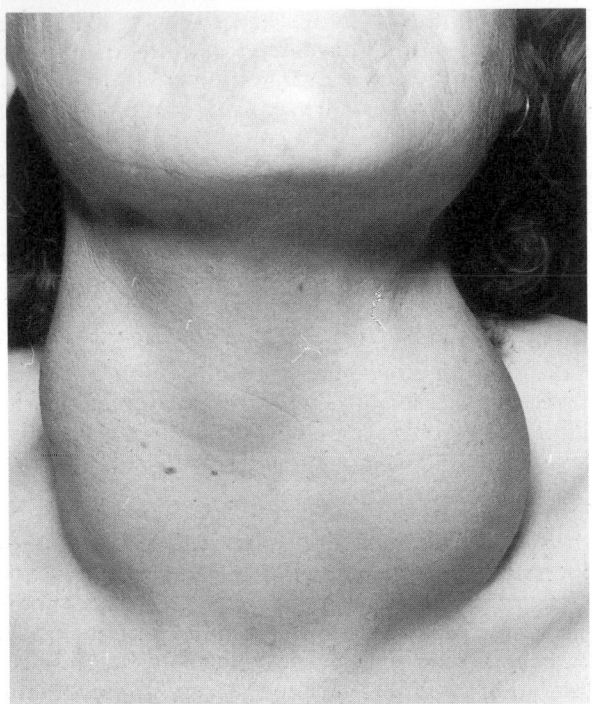

Fig. 17.24 Large multinodular goitre.

Localised thyroid swellings

The most important of the localised thyroid swellings is thyroid carcinoma which, however, only accounts for 1–2% of such lesions. Well-differentiated carcinomas may be papillary, follicular or mixed. Anaplastic carcinomas account for 15% of tumours and are commonest in the elderly. All these tumours are derived from the thyroid epithelial cell and, since they are less efficient than the surrounding normal gland at concentrating iodine, show on thyroid scans as 'cold' nodules. About 5% of thyroid carcinomas are of different origin, being derived from the calcitonin-secreting parafollicular C-cells. These are the medullary carcinomas, associated with high circulating levels of calcitonin. They are sometimes familial and associated with phaeochromocytomas, with or without neurofibromas in the mouth (multiple endocrine adenomatosis type II, see p. 706). Many thyroid adenomas are also cold on scan, but a 'hot' nodule (Fig. 17.22, p. 686) is virtually always benign. Here, the (autonomous) adenoma synthesises and secretes thyroid hormones without the need for TSH stimulation. TSH secretion is switched off, and so the rest of the gland becomes atrophic and inactive. Simple thyroid cysts are common, and also show up on a scan as a 'cold' nodule that is cystic on ultrasound. A cystic nodule is not, however, necessarily benign.

Thyroid scans, ultrasound and fine-needle aspiration with expert cytology are all useful techniques in the differential diagnosis of isolated thyroid swellings. If doubt remains, the nodule is removed surgically. 'Hot' nodules respond well to ^{131}I therapy (p. 693).

Management of thyroid cancer

Where possible, thyroid carcinomas are treated surgically. ^{131}I therapy is of value if the carcinoma takes up the isotope, and is required for patients with residual and metastatic disease. Uptake usually only occurs in papillary and follicular tumours. If the patient has had a subtotal thyroidectomy, the remaining normal thyroid is ablated with a high dose of ^{131}I. Replacement therapy is then started and continued for 6 weeks. It is then withdrawn to allow TSH levels to rise, following which an ablative dose of ^{131}I is given to treat metastatic or persistent local disease. This treatment can be repeated 3–4 monthly as long as isotope scans show persistent metastatic or local disease. Poorly differentiated cancers, and those which do not take up ^{131}I, are treated with radiotherapy to the local tumour. Results of treatment of metastatic disease with chemotherapy are disappointing.

THE ADRENAL GLANDS

ANATOMY AND PHYSIOLOGY

The gross anatomy of the adrenal glands is shown in Fig. 17.25. The adult adrenal glands weigh 4–5 g each, and are situated at the upper poles of the kidneys.

The adrenal cortex

The cortex, whose role is to secrete steroid hormones, consists of a capsule, a subcapsular layer (the zona glomerulosa), the middle zone (zona fasciculata) and a zona reticularis. The latter envelops the adrenal medulla. The blood supply runs from the cortex to the medulla. All the steroid-secreting cells appear to be of common origin. Cell division occurs between the zona glomerulosa and zona fasciculata, and cell cords loop up through the zona glomerulosa and then down through the zona fasciculata to the zona reticularis, cells changing function as they go. In utero, the glands are much larger, and the cortex is dominated by a large innermost (fetal) zone, which degenerates shortly after birth.

The zona glomerulosa synthesises and secretes mineralocorticoids, of which the most important is aldosterone. The zona fasciculata synthesises cortisol, and the reticularis and fetal zone the weak adrenal androgens, notably dehydroepiandrosterone (DHEA) and its sulphate. The fetal zone appears to develop as a consequence of the high levels of ACTH and oestrogen in utero. Oestrogens impair cortisol synthesis by inhibiting the action of the enzyme 3-β-hydroxysteroid dehydrogenase. A separate adrenal androgen-stimulating hormone seems unlikely.

The basic pathways of steroidogenesis in the adrenal cortex are set out in Figure 17.27. The functional differences between the three zones are due to the presence or absence of a few critical enzymes.

Physiological control of the adrenal cortex

Mineralocorticoids

Aldosterone is the most potent adrenal steroid; about 100 μg is secreted per day as compared with 10 mg for cortisol. Aldosterone acts on intranuclear mineralocorticoid receptors in the distal renal tubule to promote sodium uptake and potassium secretion. Interactions between this sodium retaining system and the secretion and action of the atrial natriuretic peptide (ANP) are still being elucidated.

The synthesis and secretion of aldosterone are relatively independent of ACTH secretion. The major control factors are angiotensin II and the extracellular sodium and potassium concentration (Ch. 20, Fig. 20.19). Angiotensin II acts through cell surface receptors, but not by activation of adenylate cyclase (p. 659), and principally stimulates enzymes late in the biosynthetic pathway. Renin is an enzyme secreted by the juxtaglomerular apparatus, which acts on a circulating substrate of hepatic origin to release the decapeptide angiotensin I. This is then converted to the active octapeptide angiotensin II in peripheral tissues, including lung, by angiotensin converting enzyme (ACE).

The kidney lowers plasma cortisol by converting it to cortisone so maintaining mineralocorticoid receptors free for aldosterone. Cortisone is 'shuttled' back to cortisol in the liver. Recently it has been shown that liquorice can inhibit this enzyme, and hence lead to excess mineralocorticoid action.

Glucocorticoids

Glucocorticoids, of which the main one in man is cortisol (hydrocortisone), have a wide range of actions on many different cells and tissues. They have a major influence on glucose homeostasis, with catabolic actions on muscle and enhanced hepatic gluconeogenesis. In their absence, the response to stress of any kind is greatly impaired. Glucocorticoids inhibit the immune system, repair processes and collagen synthesis in bone and soft tissues. They also modify the effect of many other hormones on a range of cell types. The endocrine actions of glucocorticoids are therefore very diverse. Glucocorticoids are secreted episodically with a very pronounced diurnal variation. It is probable that glucocorticoids facilitate the immediate requirements of daytime activity while inhibiting other processes, such as tissue repair, which then occur at night.

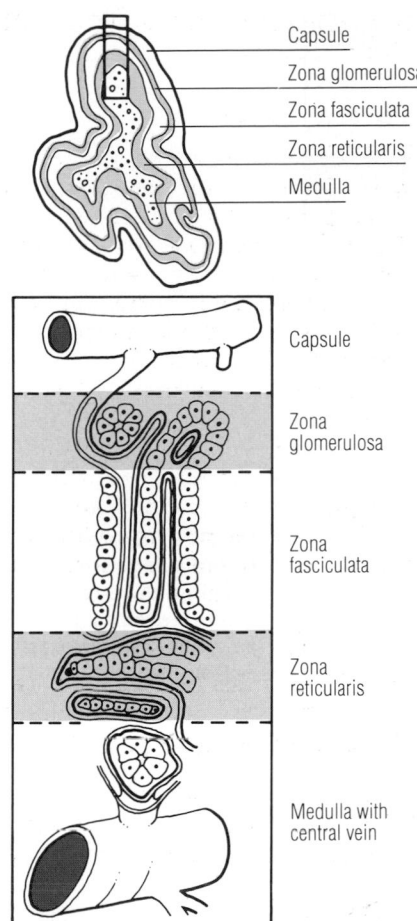

Fig. 17.25 Coronal section through the adrenal gland.

The two-dimensional structures of aldosterone, cortisol and dehydroepiandrosterone sulphate are shown in Figure 17.26.

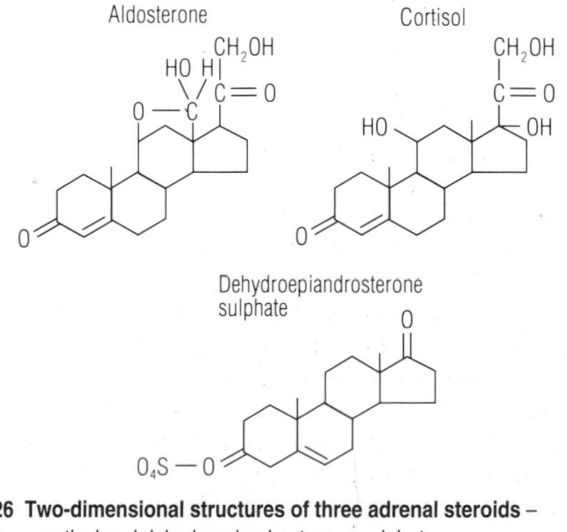

Fig. 17.26 Two-dimensional structures of three adrenal steroids – aldosterone, cortisol and dehydroepiandrosterone sulphate.

17 Endocrine Diseases

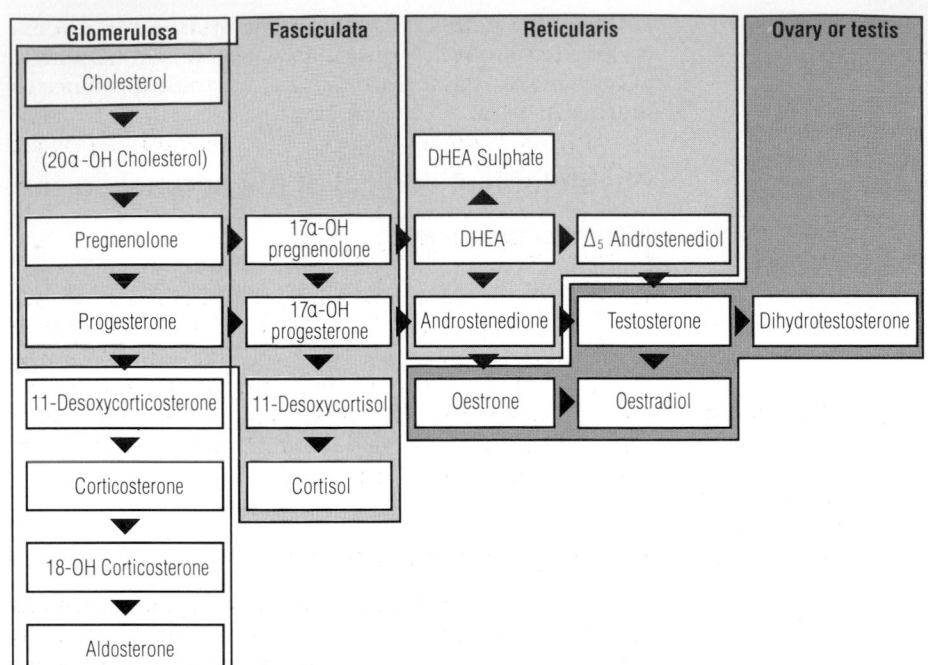

Fig. 17.27 The major steroid pathways in adrenal zona glomerulosa, fasciculata and reticularis, plus ovary or testis. The balance of steroids secreted is determined by the enzymes present (represented by arrows).

Adrenal androgens

Apart from their role as oestrogen precursors in utero, adrenal androgens appear to be of relatively trivial importance. Increased synthesis before puberty (the adrenarche) contributes to the development of secondary sexual hair. Their control is a matter of continuing controversy.

The adrenal medulla

The adrenal medulla receives a sympathetic nerve supply, which is responsible for initiating adrenaline (epinephrine) secretion in response to stress. Its blood supply comes largely from the adrenal cortex and is therefore very rich in cortisol. The pathway of adrenaline synthesis from phenylethanolamine is indicated in Figure 17.28. The last stage (the methylation of noradrenaline) is cortisol-dependent; cortisol appears to control the synthesis of the enzyme phenylalanine N-methyl transferase. As a result, pituitary ACTH and adrenal cortisol deficiency also leads to adrenaline deficiency. Glucocorticoids and adrenaline (particularly its α-receptor-mediated effects) also interact at target tissues, and in many conditions (e.g. bronchial asthma) synthetic analogues of these hormones are used together therapeutically.

Adrenal glands and the response to changes in trophic hormones

Chronic ACTH excess leads to hypertrophy of the adrenal cortex, particularly the zona fasciculata-reticularis, and to

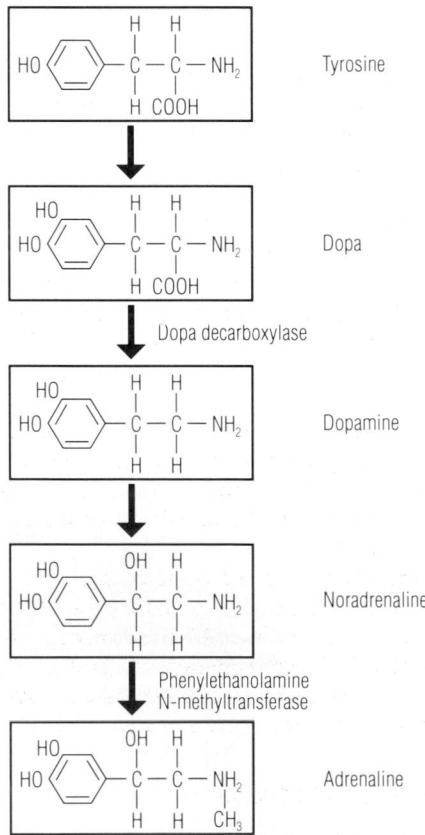

Fig. 17.28 Pathway for the biosynthesis of adrenal catecholamines.

alterations in the blood vessels. In some individuals, the chronic consequence appears to be multinodular hyperplasia, in which the nodules of hyperplastic tissue tend to become semi-autonomous; rarely, malignant tumours may develop in these nodules.

Chronic ACTH insufficiency leads to adrenal atrophy, particularly of the androgen-secreting zona reticularis. The zona glomerulosa continues to function under the trophic stimulation of angiotensin II, so that the picture is predominantly one of glucocorticoid (and adrenal androgen) deficiency, rather than of mineralocorticoid lack.

INVESTIGATION OF ADRENAL DISORDERS

Methods once considered essential have been supplanted by direct, simple, cheap and reliable techniques. For example, chemical methods for the analysis of steroid metabolites have now been largely replaced by radioimmunoassay of the levels of the steroids themselves. The clinical investigator should only use such tests as are necessary to answer a question (such as the existence of primary adrenal insufficiency) beyond reasonable doubt.

Cortisol assay

Cortisol assay is useful in many situations. Since direct radioimmunoassays are readily available, the older indirect methods of assessing metabolites (e.g. the urinary 17-hydroxycorticosteroids, and 17-oxogenic steroids) are not often used now. The urinary free cortisol excretion in 24 hours correlates very well with both the cortisol secretion rate (a tedious radioisotopic measurement) and the mean 24-hour free plasma cortisol level. It is more widely used to diagnose hyper- than hypocortisolism. Serum cortisol assays have the disadvantage that the hormone is normally secreted episodically, so that repeated measurements are usually needed for reliable interpretation. The 11 pm or midnight cortisol assay (often used in the investigation of Cushing's syndrome) has the disadvantage that stress can cause its elevation, even in normal individuals. Also, the patient has to be admitted to hospital, which makes it expensive.

Assays for precursors of cortisol are of use in diagnosing enzyme deficiencies or assessing drug-induced enzyme blocks; they include 17-hydroxyprogesterone (or its urinary metabolite pregnanetriol) and 11-desoxycortisol. The two-site immunoradiometric assay has made the plasma ACTH assay more sensitive and reliable.

Mineralocorticoid assays

Aldosterone can be measured by radioimmunoassay in serum or urine; plasma renin measurements are also reasonably reliable. Provided the patient is not on diuretics, and the electrolyte levels are known, renin and aldosterone measurements in lying and standing positions are very helpful in the investigation of suspected mineralocorticoid disorders, notably in the diagnosis of primary hyperaldosteronism.

Adrenal androgen assays

Urinary 17-oxosteroid levels may still be of use in investigating virilisation. High levels point to excess secretion of (weak) adrenal androgens and a possible adrenal tumour or enzyme defect. Plasma androstenedione and testosterone levels should also be assayed. The serum level of DHEA sulphate is also of value, high levels pointing to an adrenal source of androgen excess.

Use of dynamic function tests

Adrenal function is intrinsically dynamic, and much can be learnt from examining spontaneous changes in activity, e.g. by the serial measurement of serum cortisol levels and its diurnal changes. Several morning and evening samples will be helpful in diagnosing Cushing's syndrome, where there is loss of the diurnal rhythm and levels remain high in the evening. In contrast, there is little point in taking late evening samples in a patient with suspected cortisol deficiency, since cortisol levels are normally low at that time.

Suppression tests

The most useful suppression test involves the administration of dexamethasone (which does not cross-react in the cortisol assay), with subsequent measurement of serum and urinary cortisol. The *overnight dexamethasone suppression test* involves the patient taking 1–2 mg of dexamethasone orally at 11 pm, with a serum sample taken for cortisol assay the following morning. In a normal individual, dexamethasone suppresses the morning secretion of ACTH so that the morning serum cortisol value is low. This simple overnight test is a useful screening test for Cushing's syndrome. Failure to suppress indicates Cushing's syndrome or excess metabolism of dexamethasone due to enzyme induction by alcohol, or drugs such as phenytoin and carbamazepine. Traditionally, investigation of Cushing's syndrome involves the use of low dose (0.5 mg 6-hourly for 48 hours) and high dose (2 mg, 6-hourly for 48 hours) suppression with dexamethasone; urine and serum cortisol levels are assayed. In theory (but sometimes not in practice), there is partial suppression on the high dose in pituitary-dependent, but not in other forms of, Cushing's syndrome.

Stimulation tests

Insulin-induced hypoglycaemia is a potent stimulus to ACTH (and hence cortisol) release in normal individuals. Provided its use is not contraindicated, it is the final arbiter in diagnosing ACTH deficiency. A convincing rise in serum cortisol levels to above about 500 nmol/l in the presence of hypoglycaemia indicates that the hypothalamic-pituitary-adrenal axis is intact. Since the stimulus is also effective for testing GH secretion, this test is very useful.

Corticotrophin-releasing factor (CRF) can sometimes be of value in distinguishing pituitary-dependent ACTH secretion (where ACTH responds to CRF) from ectopic ACTH secretion.

The adrenal can be stimulated directly with ACTH – usually *synthetic ACTH* (synacthen) – and the response measured 30–60 minutes after an i.m. dose of 250 μg. For prolonged stimulation (which is rarely needed), ACTH gel should be used.

Metyrapone blocks the last stage in cortisol biosynthesis (Fig. 17.29); ACTH levels rise and the adrenal gland normally responds with increased production of the cortisol precursor 11-desoxycortisol. This in turn is metabolised and excreted as urinary 17-hydroxycorticosteroids. The response is exaggerated in pituitary-dependent Cushing's syndrome. The test can be refined by measurement of ACTH, serum or urine 11-desoxycortisol and cortisol. However, its diagnostic usefulness is limited and there is a serious risk of producing adrenal insufficiency in cases of primary adrenal tumour where ACTH levels do not rise and partly overcome the effect of the block. In specialist units ACTH can

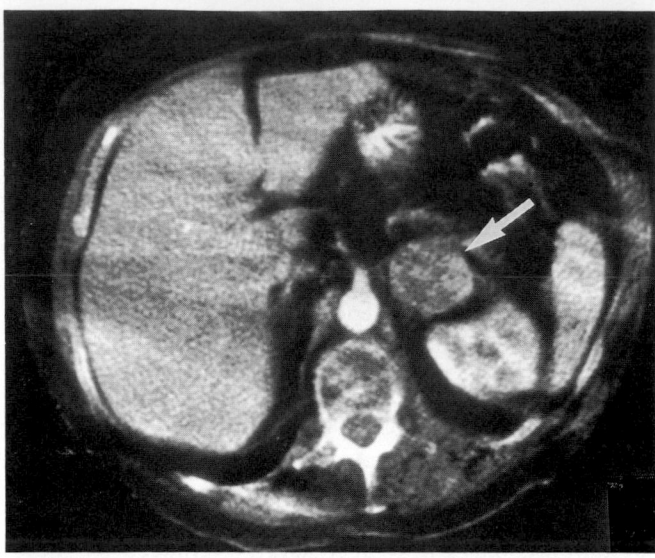

Fig. 17.30 CT scan of the adrenal glands. The scan shows a tumour (arrowed) in a patient with Cushing's syndrome.

be measured in the draining venous sinus after CRH stimulation.

Investigation of the adrenal medulla

The diagnosis of phaeochromocytoma is confirmed by one or more of a number of methods for measuring catecholamines or their metabolites. The simplest is the urinary excretion of vanyl mandelic acid, followed by urinary normetadrenaline. Serum assays for noradrenaline (by a radioenzymatic method) and adrenaline taken lying and standing are also of considerable diagnostic value.

Radiological methods

CT scanning is particularly useful for localising adrenal tumours of the cortex and medulla (Fig. 17.30). Radioisotope scans are sometimes of use; those for cortical tumours involve use of a selenium-labelled cholesterol derivative, while those for the medulla use labelled catecholamine precursors.

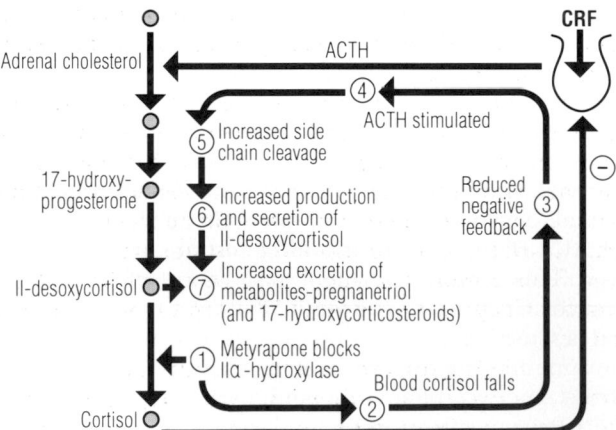

Fig. 17.29 Principles behind the metyrapone test. Metyrapone competitively blocks adrenal 11α-hydroxylase (1). In a normal individual, cortisol falls (2), ACTH rises (3–4) and increased production of precursors (5–7) leads to a rise in 11-desoxycortisol, and increased excretion of metabolites (17-hydroxycorticoids). In Cushing's due to adrenal tumour, no such increase occurs as ACTH is suppressed. In Cushing's disease, there is classically an exaggerated response to metyrapone as tumour-derived ACTH 'drives' the hyperplastic adrenal glands.

DISEASES OF THE ADRENAL CORTEX

ADRENO-CORTICAL INSUFFICIENCY

Aetiology

The major causes of adrenal insufficiency are shown in Table 17.9. It may be due to ACTH deficiency, congenital disorders (notably enzyme defects) or destruction of the adrenal glands, which can be destroyed rapidly or

Table 17.9 Causes of adrenocortical insufficiency

Primary (High ACTH)
Congenital/familial
Adrenal enzyme defects (usually 21-hydroxylase deficiency)
Congenital adrenal hypoplasia
Adrenal leucodystrophy

Acquired
Infections	–	tuberculosis†
	–	histoplasmosis
Autoimmune†		
Vascular	–	meningococcal septicaemia and haemorrhagic destruction
	–	thrombosis (adrenal vein catheterisation)
Neoplastic	–	secondary carcinoma
Degenerative	–	amyloid

Secondary (low ACTH)

Hypopituitarism
Isolated ACTH deficiency
Glucocorticoid therapy

Enhanced glucocorticoid metabolism

Drug-induced, e.g. rifampicin*, carbamazepine

*Important – may precipitate adrenal failure if already compromised, e.g. in tuberculosis. Accelerated hepatic steroid metabolism enhancer enhances steroid requirements.
†These commonly present as Addison's disease (chronic adrenal insufficiency with pigmentation).

slowly. Acute destruction occurs in septicaemia, particularly due to the meningococcus (the so-called Waterhouse-Friderichsen syndrome). Meningococcal septicaemia is associated with purpura and haemorrhage, including massive haemorrhagic destruction of the adrenals. Untreated, it leads rapidly to circulatory collapse and death. Chronic destruction of the adrenal glands is most commonly due to tuberculosis or autoimmune disease, leading to the clinical features of Addison's disease (see below).

Adrenal insufficiency should always be considered in any patient with circulatory collapse; the picture will vary somewhat depending on whether it is primary or secondary (p. 670). Other causes of adrenal insufficiency tend to be much more insidious. Tuberculosis leads to enlargement of the adrenals and, eventually, total destruction of the normal tissue and caseation. Possibly, the high cortisol levels within the adrenal make it difficult to mount the necessary cellular immune response to eradicate the bacteria. In Western countries, the decline in tuberculosis makes autoimmune destruction of the adrenals the commonest cause of chronic adrenal insufficiency.

Adrenal insufficiency is often familial, and associated with a high incidence of other organ-specific autoimmune disease, especially thyroid failure (Schmidt syndrome). There is an association with HLA-B8, which increases the relative risk of developing the disease about twelve-fold (see Ch. 6).

In the presence of chronic primary adrenocortical insufficiency, there is usually an increase in the individual's normal level of pigmentation, sodium and water depletion, postural hypotension and hyperkalaemia.

Secondary adrenal insufficiency due to hypopituitarism and isolated ACTH deficiency is discussed on page 670.

ADDISON'S DISEASE

Clinical features

This was first described by Thomas Addison in 1857. The speed of onset varies from insidious to sudden. When the onset is insidious, the early symptoms are often extreme and unaccustomed lassitude, somnolence and depression. Dizziness due to postural hypotension or fasting hypoglycaemia and nocturia due to failure to excrete a waterload in the daytime may occur. Frequently, the patient notices an increased pigmentation or simply retention of the summer suntan; as a result the patient may appear 'healthy' to relatives.

In its most dramatic form, the disease presents with Addisonian crisis which, in the absence of effective treatment, is also the terminal picture. The patient is ill and anorexic, with vomiting and abdominal pain, often with rigidity simulating an abdominal emergency. There is usually a fever, tachycardia, hypotension (with a marked postural drop in blood pressure), cramps and postural dizziness, and signs of sodium and water depletion. There is marked loss of skin turgor with loose skin like damp leather and sunken eyes. The blood urea rises because of poor renal perfusion, and the serum potassium concentration is raised. There may be hypercalcaemia, and there is commonly hypoglycaemia.

The features of the associated ACTH excess are variable, and consist of increased pigmentation of skin (especially exposed areas, pressure points, skin creases and recent scars), buccal mucous membrane and sometimes sclerae, and streaked pigmentation of the nail beds. These changes are due to stimulation of melanocytes by ACTH and related peptides, and may be absent when adrenal insufficiency is due to ACTH-receptor blocking antibodies.

The clinical features due to mineralocorticoid deficiency – principally sodium and water depletion, hyperkalaemia and hypercalcaemia – are unique to primary adrenal failure, and are absent or much less marked in secondary adrenal failure. The serum sodium concentration is usually low in both conditions, in part due to excessive secretion of ADH. Features due to glucocorticoid deficiency include hypoglycaemia (more marked in pituitary insufficiency since GH is also usually lacking), inability to respond to stress and infection, and also, in

Summary 5 Clinical features of Addison's disease

- Increased pigmentation in mouth, skin creases, pressure areas.

- Crises of hypotension, salt and water loss, hyperkalaemia, hypercalcaemia, hypoglycaemia.

- Associated vitiligo, myxoedema or pernicious anaemia.

part at least, hypotension and pyrexia. The white cell count is usually elevated, with a neutrophil leucocytosis and an elevated eosinophil count.

Other suggestive clinical features are the presence of other forms of organ-specific autoimmune disease (e.g. hypothyroidism, pernicious anaemia or vitiligo) or a history, or signs of, tuberculosis.

Investigation

A high index of suspicion is important in the diagnosis of Addison's disease. Once suspected, the appropriate blood samples should be taken for electrolyte and cortisol assay, and treatment instituted forthwith. Hyperkalaemia (with or without a low serum sodium concentration) in a patient with Addisonian-type pigmentation, hypotension and fluid depletion is suggestive of primary adrenal insufficiency. In pituitary insufficiency, aldosterone secretion generally persists, and so hyperkalaemia is not usually seen. Inappropriate ADH secretion is common in pituitary insufficiency, however, and leads to a low serum sodium concentration. In Addison's disease, circulatory collapse and unexplained pyrexia are common, as are non-specific T wave abnormalities on ECG.

Blood should be taken for a serum cortisol assay. If time permits, synacthen (250 mg i.m.) may be given and the sampling for cortisol assay repeated after 30–60 minutes. There will be a poor or absent response to this short synacthen test in both primary and secondary insufficiency since, in the latter, long-standing ACTH deficiency makes the gland slow to respond. Immediate treatment should be instituted (see below).

Further investigations include tests for adrenal (and other) auto-antibodies, plain X-ray of abdomen (to show adrenal calcification due to tuberculosis) and CT scanning of the adrenals (Fig. 17.30).

Management

Immediate treatment is with fluids, electrolytes and hydrocortisone (100–200 mg i.v., then 100 mg in 6 hours, with subsequent doses tapered down to replacement doses). Mineralocorticoid therapy is only required when the dose of hydrocortisone is being reduced to two to three times normal replacement doses (i.e. about 60 mg/day), and then only in primary adrenal insufficiency.

Long-term management of adrenal failure is generally simple if the patient is co-operative. Glucocorticoid and mineralocorticoid replacement are required. It is not possible to simulate precisely the normal episodic pattern of hormone secretion. Cortisol itself can be conveniently given as hydrocortisone in a split dose which, for an adult, is normally 20 mg on rising, and 10 mg at about 5 pm. Alternatively, cortisone acetate can be used (equivalent doses being 25 and 12.5 mg). The disadvantage is that, with this form of replacement, peak cortisol levels occur a little later, since the drug has to be converted to cortisol by the liver. The process may thus be disturbed in liver disease. There is little advantage in using synthetic glucocorticoids, such as prednisolone or dexamethasone.

Mineralocorticoid replacement is with the synthetic mineralocorticoid fludrocortisone (0.05–0.2 mg daily). The dose is adjusted empirically according to blood pressure and serum potassium levels. A minority of Addisonian patients do not need mineralocorticoid therapy, because zona glomerulosa function may be spared and replacement glucocorticoids have a weak mineralocorticoid effect.

Patients on long-term steroid replacement should be given a special card clearly stating the steroids that they are on, and keep it with them at all times. It is important that additional glucocorticoid is given in emergencies. If the patient has a gastrointestinal upset he or she should be given an increased dose parenterally.

Some drugs increase steroid requirements because they accelerate steroid metabolism; this occurs particularly with anticonvulsants and the antituberculous drug rifampicin, which is given as part of triple chemotherapy if tuberculosis is the cause of Addison's disease.

ADRENAL ENZYME DEFECTS

Adrenal enzyme defects are rare disorders which should be managed by the endocrine specialist. The pathways of steroidogenesis and the defects associated with them are discussed on pages 695–696. The principal defects affecting the adrenal glands exclusively are 21-hydroxylase and 11-hydroxylase deficiency (Fig. 17.31).

21-hydroxylase deficiency

21-hydroxylase deficiency is inherited as a recessive condition. It is due to a mutation or loss of the gene for 21-hydroxylase, which is located on chromosome 6, close to the HLA locus. The frequency of the defective gene is about 1 in 40, which gives a frequency of the disorder of $1/4 \times (1/40)^2$, or about 1 in 7400 births. Almost one-third of cases have a severe form and, if untreated, develop

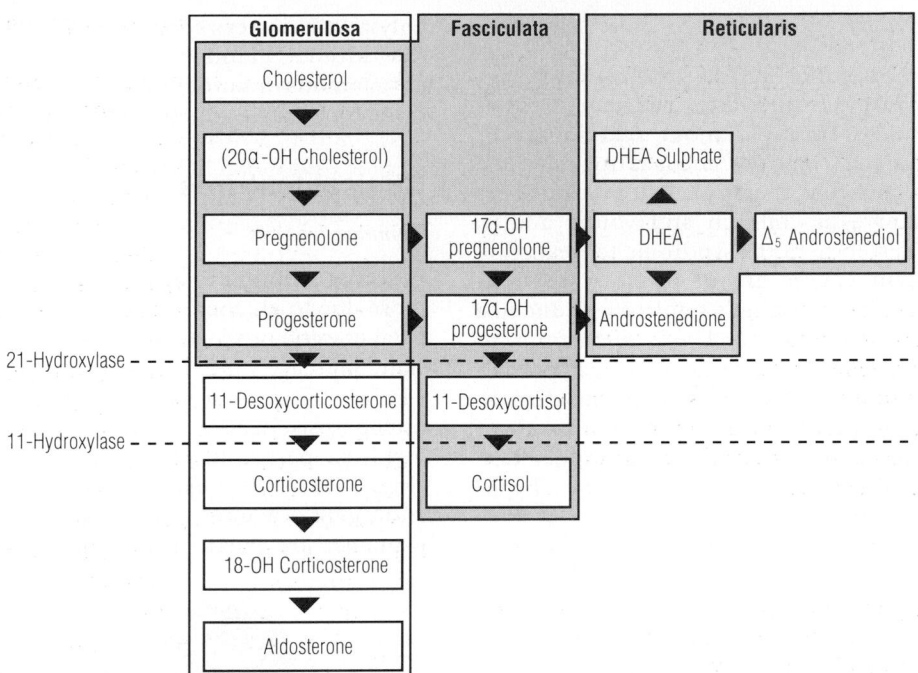

Fig. 17.31 Normal adrenal steroid pathways with sites of action of 21-hydroxylase and 11-hydroxylase, the two enzymes most commonly defective in congenital adrenal hyperplasia.

severe mineralocorticoid deficiency and salt loss. The remaining two-thirds are able to maintain adequate aldosterone secretion and generally present with the side-effects of androgen excess, or with glucocorticoid insufficiency in the face of stress.

Female infants with the condition are usually recognised at birth, because of their ambiguous (virilised) external genitalia, before salt deficiency can develop. Uncommonly, mildly affected females do not have any genital virilisation at birth, but develop it instead at puberty, when they present with hirsutism, amenorrhoea and clitoral enlargement.

Male infants appear normally virilised. Salt-losing males present with acute adrenal insufficiency and sodium and water depletion, usually within the first few weeks of life. The mortality is therefore much higher with male infants and the cause of death may not be recognised unless previous affected siblings have drawn attention to its likelihood. Non-salt-losing males will present with accelerated growth and sexual development but small testes (sexual precocity and pseudopuberty). Ultimate height is reduced and, if treatment with replacement glucocorticoids is delayed until the epiphyseal bone age has advanced to 11 years or more, affected males often undergo true precocious puberty.

Once suspected, the diagnosis is easily made by measurement of plasma, salivary or urinary levels of 17-hydroxyprogesterone or its urinary metabolite pregnanetriol, with or without ACTH stimulation.

The importance of early diagnosis in female infants is obvious, and corrective genital surgery is generally required in childhood and again later with the onset of sexual activity. Replacement therapy is with glucocorticoids and mineralocorticoids as for Addison's disease.

11-hydroxylase deficiency

Deficiency of 11-hydroxylase (Fig. 17.31) is less than a fifth as common as 21-hydroxylase deficiency. It also causes the 'adreno-genital syndrome', but the androgen excess is generally less marked and the picture is dominated instead by the presence of hypertension. This is due to ACTH-induced excessive secretion of 11-desoxycorticosterone (DOC). When glucocorticoid therapy is introduced, ACTH and DOC levels fall, and insufficiency of the zona glomerulosa is uncovered. The blood pressure falls and sodium depletion and potassium excess may result unless the condition is also treated with fludrocortisone.

ADRENO-CORTICAL EXCESS (CUSHING'S SYNDROME)

The diagnosis and treatment of the disorders which lead to adrenal glucocorticoid excess (Cushing's syndrome) remain problematic, and are therefore best conducted in specialist endocrinology units. The conditions are relatively rare, but very troublesome.

Aetiology

Cushing's syndrome is either ACTH-dependent or independent (Table 17.10). In the latter event, it is either caused by a steroid-secreting tumour (carcinoma or adenoma) of the adrenal cortex or else is iatrogenic (due to excessive glucocorticoid therapy). Adrenal tumours generally predominate in children and young adults; adenoma is the easiest form of the syndrome to treat.

ACTH-dependent causes are of pituitary or non-pituitary origin. Pituitary Cushing's syndrome is due to a pituitary basophil adenoma (*Cushing's disease*) or to hyperplasia. The latter may be due to intrinsic hypothalamic disease, chronic alcoholism or endogenous depression. Since depression is, in turn, a common result of ACTH excess, it can cause obvious diagnostic difficulties. Some rare cases are due to secretion of a CRF by a hypothalamic or extrahypothalamic tumour.

Ectopic ACTH syndrome is caused by ACTH secretion from a tumour outside the pituitary gland. The commonest types are carcinoid tumours of the bronchus, thymus and pancreas, small cell lung cancer and thymoma. Pancreatic carcinoma, medullary thyroid carcinoma and phaeochromocytoma are other rare causes (see Table 8.4, p. 130).

Multinodular adrenal hyperplasia is a rare variant of pituitary-dependent Cushing's syndrome in which, probably as a long-term consequence of high ACTH levels, the adrenal glands become hyperplastic with semi-autonomous or autonomous nodules. Occasionally, frank carcinoma may develop in one of the nodules.

Clinical features

Common features

Features common to all forms of Cushing's syndrome are those due to glucocorticoid excess. These include centripetal obesity, proximal muscle weakness and wasting, thin skin, increased sebaceous gland activity and acne (p. 1161), striae, poor wound healing, thin bones due to osteoporosis, hypertension, vascular calcification, diabetes mellitus, peptic ulceration, depression and psychosis (Fig. 17.32). Because they lack the protective effect of androgens, women (and especially postmenopausal women), are particularly susceptible to the catabolic

Table 17.10 Causes of Cushing's syndrome

Cause	Example
ACTH-driven	
Pituitary-dependent	Pituitary hyperplasia
	Pituitary adenoma*
	Pituitary carcinoma
	CRF-secreting tumour**
	Hypothalamic
	Ectopic
Ectopic ACTH secretion	Tumours
	Oat cell carcinoma
	Bronchial carcinoid
	Medullary thyroid carcinoma
	Pancreatic carcinoma
	Phaeochromocytoma
ACTH therapy	
Non-ACTH-driven	Adrenal adenoma
	Adrenal carcinoma
	Glucocorticoid therapy
Doubtful or mixed aetiology	Multinodular hyperplasia
	Alcohol-induced 'pseudo' Cushing's
	Cyclical Cushing's syndrome

*'Cushing's disease'
**Very rare

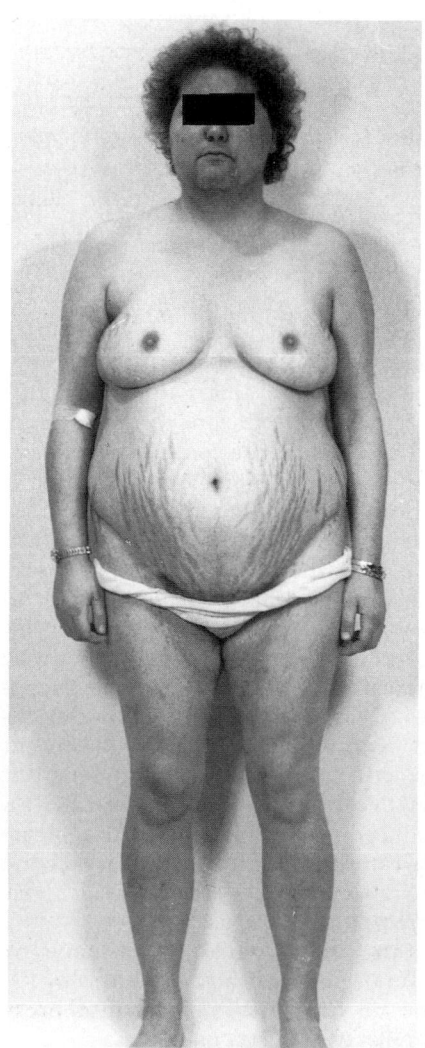

Fig. 17.32 Classical features of severe Cushing's syndrome.

Table 17.11 Investigation of suspected Cushing's syndrome

1.	**Clinical assessment**		
2.	**If suspicion:**	24-hour urine free cortisol Overnight dexamethasone suppression	
	If no suspicion:	No tests necessary	
3.	**If one or both abnormal:**	Plasma electrolytes Further 24-hour cortisol Circadian blood cortisol ACTH levels Formal dexamethasone suppression (2 mg/day)	
	If both normal:	Reassure	
4.	**If abnormal, find cause:**	Alcohol? – Withdraw and reassess Ectopic ACTH? – Adrenal tumour? –	 CXR and mediastinal CT Adrenal CT Steroid metabolites ACTH levels
		Pituitary dependent? –	High dose dexamethasone Pituitary CT Metyrapone test CRH test with petrosal sinus sampling
	If normal:	Reassure/observe	
5.	**Treat**		

effect of glucocorticoid excess. Mild hirsutism is common and is due to adrenal androgen as well as glucocorticoid excess. In men, LH and testosterone secretion may be inhibited, and libido consequently reduced.

Features unique to specific forms

Cushing's syndrome that disappears or diminishes under hospital scrutiny is commonly alcohol-induced. Some other forms of pituitary-dependent Cushing's syndrome may be cyclical. Addisonian-type pigmentation suggests marked ACTH excess, which is found most often with the ectopic ACTH syndrome (unless the adrenals have been removed, when it suggests Nelson's syndrome; see below and p. 678). The presence of profound hypokalaemia suggests the ectopic ACTH syndrome. Abnormalities on pituitary X-ray are extremely uncommon, even with a pituitary adenoma, except after bilateral adrenalectomy. The ectopic ACTH syndrome due to a small cell carcinoma of lung may not be attended by centripetal obesity, because of cachexia and rapid dissemination of the tumour.

Investigation

The investigation of suspected Cushing's syndrome is summarised in Table 17.11. The difficulties have been discussed under dynamic testing. The high 24-hour urinary free cortisol excretion and overnight low dose dexamethasone test (p. 697) are the mainstays of initial diagnosis. Adrenal radiology with a CT scan (Fig. 17.30, p. 698) is of great importance in diagnosis and localisation of adrenal tumours, as is the (suppressed) plasma ACTH level. Pituitary radiology – including high resolution CT scanning with i.v. injection of contrast medium – is often surprisingly unhelpful (and occasionally misleading) in the investigation of Cushing's syndrome. Pituitary tumours are usually small, and rarely cause any distortion of the pituitary fossa. CT scan of the thorax may reveal a small bronchial or thymic carcinoid which is the source of ectopic ACTH.

Management

Drug therapy

Drugs, such as metyrapone and aminoglutethimide, that inhibit adrenal steroidogenesis have a place in the preoperative, and occasionally also the long-term, management of Cushing's syndrome. Steroid production can readily be inhibited in patients with adrenal tumours by the 11-hydroxylase inhibitor metyrapone. Indeed, there is real risk of inducing adrenal insufficiency. The dose (250–750 mg every 4 hours, omitting 4 am dosage) should be titrated against the serum and urinary cortisol response. Before surgery, it is wise for the patient to be treated with metyrapone for several weeks to improve wound healing.

Palliative drug therapy in ectopic ACTH syndrome generally requires the simultaneous use of metyrapone and aminoglutethimide (or ketoconazole) to block biosynthesis of cortisol; the dose is titrated against cortisol secretion. The DDT analogue ortho, para, dichlorodiphenyl-dichlorophenazone (O'p'DDD) also has an established place in the management of adrenal carcinoma; it induces adrenal cell necrosis and may produce prolonged remissions. Cytotoxic chemotherapy is the treatment of choice for small cell lung cancer, but the prognosis of the disease is especially poor when accompanied by ectopic ACTH secretion.

Adrenal surgery

Surgery is clearly indicated for an adrenal adenoma or carcinoma, where operable. In a young person, and even when not totally resectable, removal of the bulk of a carcinoma may be indicated in order to maximise the efficacy of chemotherapy. Surgery is also the treatment of choice for carcinoid tumours causing ectopic ACTH secretion.

Bilateral adrenalectomy was formerly the preferred treatment for Cushing's disease. This has the advantage of eliminating the possibility of cortisol excess (provided no remnant is left behind). The disadvantages are that it involves major surgery, with a significant mortality, and also a significant (10–20%) risk of developing *Nelson's syndrome* (the condition of hyperpigmentation, increasing ACTH excess and an expanding pituitary tumour). The syndrome probably only develops where there is already a semi-autonomous ACTH-secreting pituitary tumour, previously kept under partial restraint by the high circulating cortisol levels. Many centres now combine bilateral adrenalectomy for Cushing's disease with external pituitary radiation, to minimise the risk of this unpleasant complication. Bilateral adrenalectomy is probably the treatment of choice in multinodular adrenal hyperplasia.

Pituitary surgery

Having excluded, as far as is possible, the ectopic ACTH syndrome and an adrenal tumour, most endocrinologists would now refer the patient with pituitary-dependent Cushing's syndrome (Cushing's disease) to an expert centre for surgery by the trans-sphenoidal route. If a tumour is present it is removed; if not, then as much as possible of the pituitary gland is resected. Hypopituitarism (with replacement therapy) is generally preferable to continuing active Cushing's syndrome.

Pituitary radiotherapy

Pituitary radiotherapy can be an effective treatment for Cushing's disease and may be given either by external irradiation or by pituitary implantation of radioactive seeds of yttrium-90. The latter is now rarely used. Radiotherapy may be particularly useful in the elderly or frail patient with moderately active disease, who has shown some hormonal response to drug therapy.

In summary, there is no single universally effective treatment, probably because Cushing's syndrome is not a single condition but a group of conditions.

TUMOURS OF THE ADRENAL CORTEX

Tumours of the adrenal cortex may be functioning or non-functioning; the latter secrete either no steroids, or weak steroids (e.g. pregnenolone) with little or no biological activity. The mode of presentation of the tumour generally depends on the nature and amount of steroid being produced. Recognised consequences are Cushing's syndrome (cortisol secretion), Conn's syndrome (mineralocorticoid), virilisation (usually weak adrenal androgens, but sometimes testosterone) and feminisation (oestrogens). With the exception of aldosterone-secreting tumours, the tumour is likely to be quite large by the time of presentation and readily detectable on an adrenal CT scan. Sometimes, other techniques are indicated to establish the diagnosis, such as scanning with radiolabelled cholesterol, or adrenal vein catheterisation and blood sampling for hormone assay. Treatment is by surgery, after appropriate medical treatment.

DISORDERS OF ALDOSTERONE SECRETION

The basic components (renin, angiotensin and aldosterone) of the mineralocorticoid system are discussed on page 695. In addition, the heart is also now known to be involved in salt and water homeostasis, through the recently discovered ANP. This peptide is produced by endocrine cells in the right atrium, and acts on the renal tubule to cause a sodium diuresis (Ch. 20, p. 789).

Hypoaldosteronism

Hypoaldosteronism may be a result of general adrenal insufficiency due to destruction of the adrenal glands (p. 699), or it may occur in the presence of normal secretion of other adrenal steroids. The disorder may be primary, due to a selective adrenal enzyme deficiency late in the aldosterone pathway, or secondary to isolated renin deficiency. This occurs quite commonly in long-standing diabetes mellitus, and may be a consequence of autonomic neuropathy, since beta-adrenergic stimulation is normally a stimulus to renin secretion from the juxtaglomerular apparatus. Aldosterone deficiency is manifested by a tendency to sodium depletion, hypotension and hyperkalaemia. Treatment is with fludrocortisone.

Hyperaldosteronism

Primary hyperaldosteronism (Conn's syndrome) is a rare cause of a generally mild hypertension and hypokalaemia. In Chinese especially it may present with hypokalaemic paralysis. It is caused either by an adrenal adenoma, or by zona glomerulosa hyperplasia. The diagnosis is confirmed by the finding of elevated serum aldosterone, and low renin levels, and by the clinical response to a therapeutic trial of spironolactone. Treatment is with spironolactone or (in the case of definite adenoma) adrenal surgery. Some cases respond to low doses of dexamethasone.

Secondary hyperaldosteronism is a common physiological adaptation seen in such disorders as congestive cardiac failure, accelerated hypertension, cirrhosis of the liver and nephrotic syndrome. Reduced renal perfusion is the major stimulus to increased renin secretion, angiotensin II production and aldosterone secretion, and thus to sodium retention and potassium excretion. Aldosterone antagonists, such as spironolactone, or drugs which act on the distal tubule sodium pump (such as amiloride) are commonly used in its treatment. Rarely, hyperaldosteronism is caused by a renin-secreting tumour of the kidney.

THE ADRENAL MEDULLA

Adrenaline (epinephrine) is the major product of the normal adrenal medulla; 90% of the adrenaline in the circulation arises from this gland; the remainder is produced in the central nervous system. The main pathways of adrenal catecholamine synthesis are shown in Fig. 17.28. It is of particular importance in the acute response to stress, causing increased alertness, tachycardia, nervousness, glucose and fat mobilisation and inhibition of insulin secretion.

Adrenal medullary insufficiency is of importance in the impairment of the response to hypoglycaemia in hypopituitarism and in generalised autonomic neuropathy (the Shy-Drager syndrome). It may play a part in so-called idiopathic hypoglycaemia of infancy.

ADRENAL MEDULLARY EXCESS

There is no doubt that the adrenal cortex and medulla are integrated in their response to stress. The stimulus is ACTH secretion for the cortex and neural activation for the adrenal medulla. Cortisol is necessary for adrenaline biosynthesis, and glucocorticoids and catecholamines interact at the target tissues, the former potentiating beta-adrenergic effects, for example. In thyrotoxicosis, many of the effects (symptoms and signs) are those of catecholamine excess. This is not because adrenaline secretion is increased (it is normal), but because thyroid hormones augment the target organ sensitivity to catecholamines, particularly their beta-adrenergic effects.

Phaeochromocytoma

Phaeochromocytomas are tumours of the adrenal medulla and are, fortunately, rare. The usual figure quoted is 1 per 1000 cases of hypertension; however, in a large autopsy series from the Mayo Clinic, three-quarters of the patients found to have had phaeochromocytoma were undiagnosed during life, so the true incidence may be considerably higher. Death in cases previously undiagnosed is commonly from cardiovascular disease or cerebral haemorrhage. The tumours are usually located in the adrenal medulla, with 10% being in extra-adrenal chromaffin tissue, usually in the sympathetic chain in the abdomen. Most predominantly secrete noradrenaline. Ten per cent of all phaeochromocytomas are malignant. They can occur at any age but present most commonly between 40 and 60 years of age. They may be associated with neurofibromatosis, tuberous sclerosis, and with the Sturge-Weber (p. 903) and von Hippel-Lindau (p. 903) syndromes. They may be multiple, and are a component of types II and III multiple endocrine neoplasia (see below).

Clinical features

The history is of 'attacks' of headache, sweating, palpitations, flushing and nervousness. The blood pressure is generally moderately raised and becomes grossly so during 'attacks', which may be precipitated by exercise or abdominal palpation. Because the hypertension is accompanied by secondary volume depletion, there is commonly a significant drop in blood pressure on standing; this is unusual in untreated hypertension from other causes.

Investigation

Diagnosis of phaeochromocytoma is made by measurement of plasma levels of noradrenaline, or its urinary precursors or metabolites – vanylmandelic acid (VMA) and normetadrenaline. When carried out in specialised laboratories these tests, particularly plasma noradrenaline, are very reliable. The paroxysmal nature of the secretion may lead to normal plasma levels being obtained at times and repeated blood and urine measurements may therefore be necessary. The tumour can be localised by adrenal CT scan. Occasionally, radioisotope scanning with a radiolabelled catecholamine precursor is helpful to demonstrate an ectopic site. Pharmacological tests using the α-adrenergic blocker phentolamine with blood pressure monitoring are seldom used, because the response to them is erratic and sometimes excessive.

Management

The principles of treatment of phaeochromocytoma are to start with pharmacological measures, namely adrenergic blockade (initially with the α-adrenoreceptor blocking agent phenoxybenzamine), followed a few days later by beta blockade (e.g. with propranolol). Seven to ten days should be allowed before surgery for volume repletion. During surgery, blood pressure is closely monitored and any elevation treated with an intravenous infusion of phentolamine (an α-adrenoreceptor antagonist).

Multiple endocrine neoplasia (MEN)

There are at least three different syndromes associated with multiple neoplasia of endocrine glands (Table 17.12); in each case, inheritance is autosomal dominant. The involved glands may be the subject of hyperplasia, adenoma or carcinoma development, and different glands may be involved in different individuals in the same family.

In MEN type I (Wermer's syndrome), hyperparathyroidism due to parathyroid hyperplasia is present in 95% of cases at the time of diagnosis. Major morbidity and mortality results from the development of pancreatic tumours, notably insulin-secreting islet cell tumours causing hypoglycaemia, and gastrinomas causing intractable peptic ulceration (Zollinger-Ellison syndrome). Pituitary tumours (prolactinomas, GH or ACTH-secreting) are also common, and carcinoid tumours too are recognised as part of the syndrome.

In both types II and III, the components include medullary cell thyroid carcinoma (calcitonin-secreting) and phaeochromocytoma. The former occurs in virtually all cases, and the latter in about half. MEN type III is similar to type II but is associated with mucosal neurinomas and with a body habitus similar to Marfan's syndrome (p. 78), but without the lens subluxation and cardiovascular problems.

Hyperparathyroidism occurs in MEN types I and II. Families with hypercalcaemic MEN types I or II should

be distinguished from familial hypocalciuric hypercalcaemia (p. 729); this condition is also inherited as an autosomal dominant but lacks the association with endocrine tumours.

The MEN syndromes appear to be related to deletions of a regulating gene or genes, such that a further mutation of its pair in an endocrine cell can lead to the cell's uncontrolled proliferation.

THE TESTES

ANATOMY AND PHYSIOLOGY

The testes have a crucial early role in the male fetus in determining that primary sex differentiation is male. After puberty, they serve the dual function of spermatogenesis and androgen (testosterone) production. The initial gonadotrophin stimulation in utero comes principally from the placental hormone human chorionic gonadotrophin (HCG). However, during and after puberty, the stimulation comes from the pituitary via its two gonadotrophins, FSH and LH.

The testes in utero: sex differentiation

After the primitive germ cells have been joined by steroid-producing cells, the primitive 'indifferent' gonads develop in fetuses of both sexes. Much of the current knowledge on the role of the testes was obtained more than 40 years ago, in pioneering experiments by the French biologist Alfred Jost on rabbit fetuses. The Y chromosome contains a testis-determining gene, recently cloned, controlling differentiation at 6 weeks into a testis. Shortly thereafter, two pairs of duct systems, the Müllerian and the Wolffian, extend from the region of the gonads to the genital groove. The basic pattern of sex differentiation, which requires no hormonal function for its persistence, is female. In the absence of testes, the Müllerian ducts persist and become the uterus and Fallopian tubes, and the Wolffian ducts disappear. The Sertoli cells of the developing testes produce a peptide hormone, the anti-Müllerian hormone, which causes the Müllerian ducts to disappear permanently.

The major pathway of steroidogenesis that leads to testosterone production occurs in the Leydig cells and is shown in Figure 17.27 (p. 696). At around 12 weeks, testosterone is secreted, under stimulation from HCG, and acts on the Wolffian ducts to ensure they persist to form the male internal genital ducts. If testosterone is absent at this time, the duct cells die.

The development of the external genitalia is also dictated by androgen secretion from the Leydig cells at around 12–14 weeks. Full virilisation involves fusion of

Table 17.12 Multiple endocrine neoplasia (MEN)

Type	Major glands/areas involved	Clinical features
I (Wermer) (Autosomal dominant)	Parathyroid	Hypercalcaemia
	Pancreas	Insulinoma
		Gastrinoma
		Glucagonoma
	Anterior pituitary	Prolactinoma
		Acromegaly
		Cushing's syndrome
	Bronchus, bowel	Carcinoid tumours
II (Sipple)* (Autosomal dominant)	Thyroid (C cell)	Medullary carcinoma
	Adrenal medulla	(high calcitonin)
	Parathyroid	Phaeochromocytoma
		Hypercalcaemia
III (mucosal neurinoma)** (Autosomal dominant)	Thyroid (C cell)	Medullary carcinoma
	Adrenal medulla	Phaeochromocytoma
	Tongue etc.	Mucosal neurinoma
		Marfanoid habitus

*Sometimes referred to as IIa
**Sometimes referred to as IIb

the labioscrotal folds to form a scrotum, enlargement of the genital tubercle (to become a penis) and incorporation into the latter of a penile urethra. Both these effects and development of the prostate require conversion of testosterone to 5-α-dihydrotestosterone; this occurs by local action of the enzyme 5-α-reductase in target tissues.

Later in utero, at around 20 weeks, pituitary secretion of LH and FSH commences. HCG secretion reaches a peak at around 12 weeks and subsequently declines.

The testes in infancy and childhood

Late in utero or shortly after birth the testes descend to the scrotum. During the first 6 months of extra-uterine life, there is a transient rise in plasma levels of LH and secretion of testosterone. Since levels of the plasma binding protein, sex hormone binding globulin (SHBG) also rise during the first week of life, plasma testosterone levels in early infancy are in the low adult male range (although free testosterone levels are lower). Gradually, activity of the hypothalamo-pituitary-testis axis subsides, and remains low throughout childhood.

The testes in puberty

The first endocrine event of puberty is the onset of pulsatile secretion of LH during sleep; this initiates pulsatile nocturnal secretion of testosterone (Table 17.13). FSH levels also rise, which, together with testosterone from the Leydig cells, stimulates spermatogenesis. During the course of puberty, the volume of the testes increases some 20-fold from about 1 ml to 15–25 ml each; 95% of the volume of the testes consists of the tubules and their contents. The interstitial (Leydig) cells are the sole source of *de novo* steroidogenesis, which occurs under stimulation of LH. The action of LH is via specific cell surface receptors, mediated principally by cyclic-AMP. FSH also acts via surface receptors and cyclic-AMP, but on the Sertoli cells. The Sertoli cells are now known to be crucial in the control of spermatogenesis. Beyond the stage of Type A spermatogonia, the

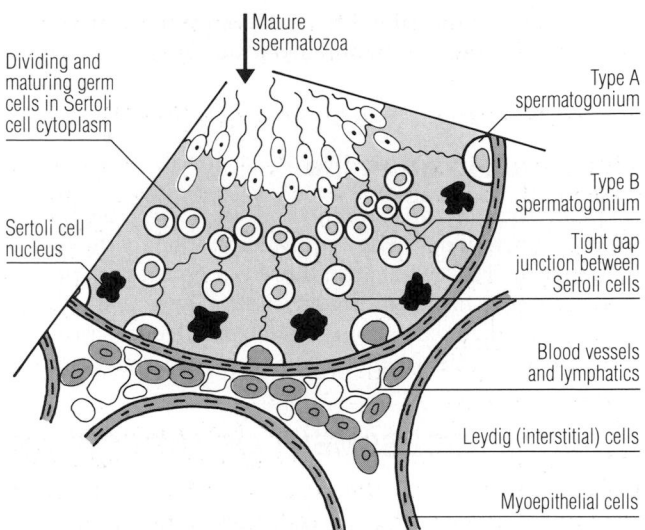

Fig. 17.33 Relationship between testicular tubules (cut in cross-section) and interstitial (Leydig) cells. Only type A spermatogonia lie outside the Sertoli cells (pink) and so outside the blood–testis barrier.

germ cells are enclosed in the cytoplasm of Sertoli cells (Fig. 17.33). Adjacent Sertoli cells form tight junctions which ensure that the germ cells and contents of the tubule are kept secluded by a very effective 'blood–testis barrier'.

During puberty, systemic secretion of testosterone initially occurs only at night-time, but later, as LH levels rise during the day, throughout the 24 hours. Testosterone and, in some tissues, dihydrotestosterone, leads to progressive development of secondary sexual characteristics. In man, these include: enlargement and development of external and internal genitalia; muscular development; growth of long bones followed by closure of the epiphyses; and male sex drive and sexual behaviour including nocturnal emissions and masturbation. There is no evidence that homosexuality is in any way related to abnormal sex hormone levels. Since oestradiol is also produced by conversion from testosterone, in amounts otherwise sufficient to cause breast development, there is strong evidence to suggest that testosterone is res-

Table 17.13 Actions of LH and FSH

Hormone	Effect on testis	Effect on ovary		
		Follicular phase	Midcycle	Luteal
LH	Stimulates Leydig cells to produce testosterone, which has local and general effects	Theca cell androgen secretion	Midcycle surge induces ovulation and luteinisation	Sustains corpus luteum until HCG from blastocyst takes over
FSH	Stimulates Sertoli cells. With local testosterone, regulates spermatogenesis	Stimulates next cohort of follicles, and growth of dominant follicle	Small midcycle surge possibly helps ovum maturation	FSH prepares next crop of follicles if no pregnancy

ponsible for inhibiting breast development in males. Plasma SHBG levels decline by about 50% during male puberty.

The testes in adult life

In men, there is no evidence of an abrupt decline in gonadal function in old age equivalent to that of the female menopause. This is because there is a constant supply of new germ cells from mitotic division of Type A spermatogonia; in women, the supply of oöcytes declines progressively even from before birth, and eventually none remain.

CLINICAL ASSESSMENT OF TESTICULAR FUNCTION

The clinical assessment of testicular function depends upon the age of the subject. A detailed history of sexual activity is important. For example, if a patient has normal nocturnal erections and ejaculation (wet dreams or masturbation), a complaint of lack of potency (erection or ejaculation) during intercourse is unlikely to be due to androgen deficiency. Assessment of testicular size can best be made by reference to an orchidometer – a series of ovoids of known volume. Small testes are usually a sign of damage to the seminiferous tubules. Examination of external genitalia will also determine if there has been any failure of intrauterine virilisation. Failure of normal pubertal development may be associated with a degree of growth failure or, conversely, with excessive growth of the long bones before epiphyses close so that span exceeds height. Female fat distribution, gynaecomastia and failure of development of secondary sexual hair are also features of failure of pubertal development, but the latter is most difficult to interpret in view of great inherited variability in potential for body hair.

Where the patient is normally virilised and the clinical problem is subfertility, examination for proper intrascrotal descent or previous damage (leading to a small testis or testes) and varicocele (which may depress the sperm count) is important. Phimosis should be specifically excluded.

DEFECTIVE TESTICULAR FUNCTION IN UTERO

Defective testicular function in utero leads to male pseudohermaphroditism. The major causes are listed in Table 17.14. The defects in testosterone and dihydrotestosterone biosynthesis are inherited as autosomal recessive disorders and are extremely rare. They are discussed below, under disorders of sex differentiation (p. 715).

Table 17.14 Causes of male pseudohermaphroditism

Pure XY gonadal dysgenesis
Testicular enzyme deficiencies
With adrenal enzyme deficiency
Cholesterol desmolase
Δ_5, 3β-hydroxysteroid dehydrogenase
17-hydroxylase
Without adrenal deficiency
17,20-desmolase
17-ketosteroid oxidoreductase
Target organ abnormalities
5-α-reductase deficiency
Androgen receptor defect – testicular feminisation, complete or partial

DEFECTIVE TESTICULAR FUNCTION IN ADULT LIFE

Male infertility without androgen deficiency

In at least one-third of couples presenting with infertility, the condition is attributable largely or entirely to abnormalities in the male, leading either to azoospermia, oligospermia or abnormal sperm. A general classification of causes is given in Table 17.15. Management is in most cases unsatisfactory and is beyond the scope of this book.

In general, if the serum level of FSH is elevated in a patient with azoospermia or severe oligospermia, severe irreversible testicular damage will be present on biopsy and no treatment will be effective. Recently, it has been recognised that, in many men with normal sperm counts but poor virility, there are antibodies in semen which are impairing fertility. Antibodies can also be detected in serum.

Androgen deficiency (male hypogonadism)

The presentation of testicular dysfunction with androgen deficiency may be at the time of puberty, or much later. A few men presenting with infertility have a mild degree of androgen deficiency and associated oligo- or azoospermia; most such men, and all who are severely androgen-deficient, are sexually inactive. The causes of androgen deficiency, classified according to whether the gonadotrophin levels are low (hypogonadotrophic) or high (hypergonadotrophic), are given in Table 17.16. In both groups, the severity of the androgen deficiency can vary considerably; it is usually least severe in Klinefelter's syndrome (which in most cases is associated with an XXY chromosomal constitution) and where the Leydig cells continue to function (although subnormally) despite severely

Table 17.15 Causes of male infertility

Level of dysfunction	Cause
Pituitary/ hypothalamic	Gonadotrophin deficiency 　Primary*† 　Secondary, e.g. tumour*†, radiation, etc. Gonadotrophin suppression 　Exogenous androgens (e.g. body builders)* 　Endogenous, e.g. 21-hydroxylase deficiency*
Testicular	Chromosomal defect, e.g. Klinefelter's syndrome† Germ cell damage, e.g. Sertoli cell only syndrome Undescended testes Radiotherapy† Drugs: cytotoxic, sulphasalazine* Temperature-induced damage: varicocele*, pyrexia* Castration† Anorchia†
Post-testicular	Absent or obstructed vasa Vasectomy* Epididymal damage Prostatitis, orchitis*
Ejaculatory failure	Erectile failure: psychogenic, vascular, neurogenic Retrograde ejaculation Spinal cord or cauda equina damage
Spermatozoal dysfunction	Infection* Antisperm antibodies Failure to penetrate mucus/poor viability Miscellaneous, e.g. defects in sperm structure

*Partially or totally treatable or reversible
†Associated with androgen deficiency and therefore also with infrequent or absent intercourse

Table 17.16 Causes of androgen deficiency in phenotypically normal adult men

Gonadotrophin levels	Cause of androgen deficiency
Low LH and FSH	Simple delayed puberty Illness and malnutrition Anorexia nervosa Isolated gonadotrophin/GnRH deficiency 　Normal sense of smell 　Anosmia (Kallman's syndrome) Panhypopituitarism 　Tumour　－ Suprapituitary 　　　　　　 (craniopharyngioma) 　　　　　 － pituitary 　Infarction 　Haemochromatosis Drugs – cyproterone acetate*
High LH and FSH	**Developmental** Klinefelter's syndrome (XXY and its variants) **Acquired** Trauma 　Castration 　Injury 　Torsion Anorchia (testicular degeneration) Viral orchitis (mumps) Radiation Drugs, e.g. cyclophosphamide Dystrophia myotonica
Variable LH and FSH	Prader-Willi syndrome Hyperprolactinaemia Noonan's syndrome Cirrhosis of liver Drugs, e.g. spironolactone, alcohol Cushing's syndrome

*Gonadotrophin suppression combined with androgen resistance

damaged tubules. In this condition, the testes are usually firm and pea-sized. Gynaecomastia may occur in any form of hypogonadism, due in part to increased oestrogen but mainly to reduced testosterone action on the breasts. If the condition dates from before puberty, the limbs continue to grow, so that the final height is increased, with long extremities ('eunuchoidal proportions', Fig. 17.34). Isolated gonadotrophin deficiency (due usually to GnRH deficiency) may be sporadic or familial (X-linked or X-limited). When associated with anosmia, it is termed Kallman's syndrome. The anosmia is due to failure of development of the amygdala. When hypogonadism develops after puberty, it is highly likely that a pituitary tumour or craniopharyngioma is responsible, a suspicion that can be confirmed by appropriate radiology and hormone assays.

A common clinical problem is of the teenage boy with delayed puberty. The differential diagnosis between simple delayed puberty and permanent isolated gonadotrophin deficiency may be impossible. It is usually advisable to boost puberty artificially with testosterone to avoid psychological problems, and review the diagnosis later.

Investigation of endocrine function of the testes

A great deal can be learned about the endocrine function of the testes from a single measurement of the serum or plasma level of testosterone, plus the gonadotrophins LH and FSH. A grossly raised prolactin points to a prolactinoma which, though rare in men, is important to diagnose as early as possible since such tumours are often rapidly growing. If gynaecomastia is present, serum oestradiol and SHBG levels should be included in the assessment. Stimulation tests can be carried out at the level of the pituitary (with GnRH 10–100 μg i.v.) or the testes (with HCG 1500–5000 IU i.m.), or oestrogen negative feedback can be assessed (with clomiphene citrate). These tests, especially the

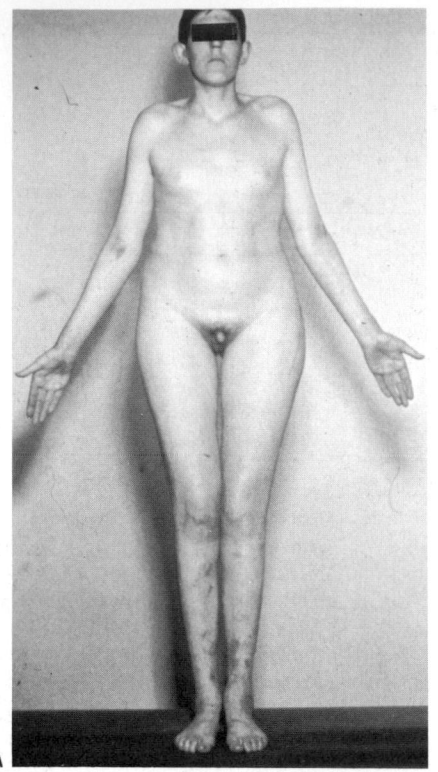 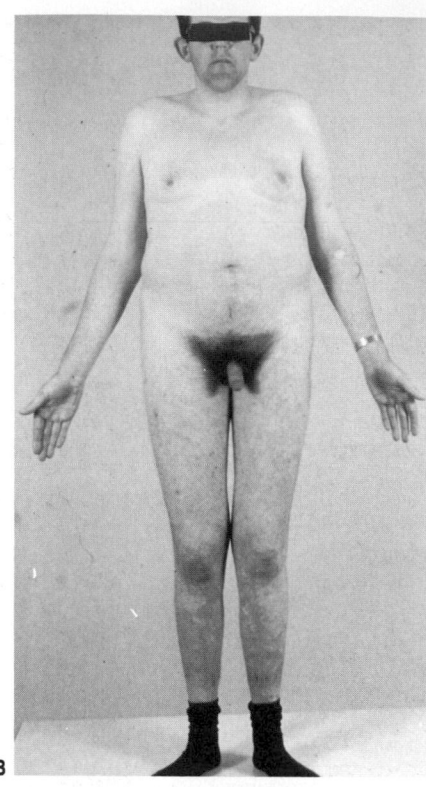 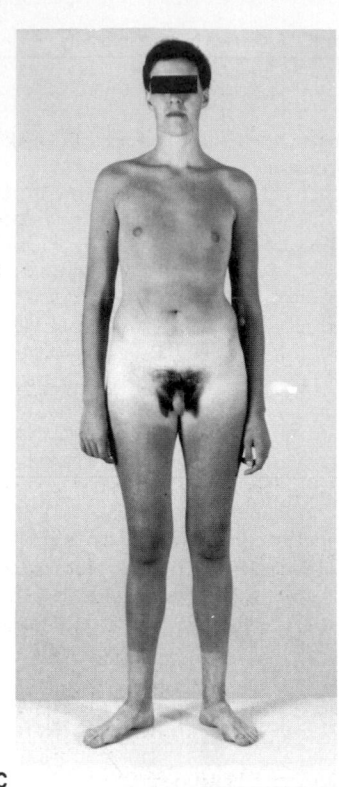

Fig. 17.34 Testicular dysfunction with androgen deficiency. Grossly eunuchoidal 31-year-old man with Kallman's syndrome **A.** before and **B.** after 2 years of androgen replacement. **C.** A 21-year-old man with Klinefelter's syndrome. Note partial virilisation and minimal gynaecomastia.

latter, are generally no more informative than basal hormone measurements.

Management

Male infertility

The principal treatable causes of male infertility (Table 17.15, p. 709) are oligospermia due to varicocele, or exposure of testes to high temperature (the scrotum keeps the normal testes at about 32°C and prolonged high temperature impairs spermatogenesis). Sulphasalazine-induced infertility in ulcerative colitis can be treated by transfer to aminosalicylic acid. Gonadotrophin deficiency from any cause may lead to some permanent testicular damage. In most such cases, adequate spermatogenesis can be stimulated by administering HCG with later addition of FSH. An adequate trial of therapy is 3–6 months, the response being followed by semen analysis (count and motility). An alternative therapy, also expensive, is to administer GnRH by subcutaneous pump in a pulsatile manner (15 μg every 90 minutes). Where gonadotrophin deficiency is caused by extratesticular androgens (as in congenital adrenal hyperplasia) the appropriate treatment is with replacement glucocorticoid therapy.

Androgen deficiency

When hypogonadotrophic, one option is to give HCG (1500–2000 IU twice a week, or 5000 IU once a week). Direct replacement is best made with testosterone. Implantation of fused pellets is made, under local anaesthetic, subcutaneously in the lower abdominal wall. This provides steady release of testosterone, in contrast to marked peaks and troughs from depot testosterone injections. Oral testosterone undecanoate is also effective and safe, but expensive. In an adult who has never been through puberty, dosage should be cautious at first (e.g. 40 mg b.d. of testosterone undecanoate), to avoid triggering undue aggression.

Impotence

Most patients presenting with impotence do not have an endocrine cause. In those who do, libido is also poor and androgen replacement is usually effective. When there is failure to achieve an erection (as in diabetic autonomic neuropathy and some young men with psychogenic impotence), self-injection of intracavernous papaverine or rogitine has been a major recent advance.

THE OVARIES

ANATOMY AND PHYSIOLOGY

The ovaries consist of germ cells surrounded by granulosa cells (the homologue of the Sertoli cell); these are surrounded in turn by stromal cells of the theca interna.

The ovaries have no role in female genital development, which simply requires the absence of testes. They secrete little steroid before birth so FSH and LH are higher in female fetuses. After birth and a transient surge in LH levels, the hypothalamic-pituitary ovarian axis becomes quiescent until puberty.

Changes during puberty

On average, puberty starts about 2 years earlier in girls than boys. The full complement of ovarian follicles (about half a million) is complete at birth, and their number declines progressively thereafter, until exhaustion at the time of the menopause. Crops of immature follicles advance to a certain stage and become atretic even before puberty. With the rise in FSH levels, these crops of follicles produce increasing amounts of oestrogen; at about 7 days before ovulation, one follicle becomes sensitive to FSH and LH (via increased numbers of receptors) and makes more oestradiol (Fig. 17.35A). This suppresses FSH and leads to atresia of the less advanced follicles in that cohort.

There is good evidence that the first cycles in girls are anovulatory, and they may be associated with erratic 'break-through' menstrual bleeding, due to oestrogenic stimulation of the endometrium. Eventually, however, conditions are right for the first ovulatory cycle.

Ovulation and the normal menstrual cycle

The biological purpose of ovulation is pregnancy. Menstruation may be thought of as biological failure, and the starting point of the next cycle, whose purpose is once again to achieve release of a single fertilisable ovum and to prepare the reproductive tract for pregnancy.

The cohort of follicles destined to develop in a particular cycle have been selected, by an unknown process, two cycles earlier. The menstrual cycle depends on inherent cyclicity within the ovary, the hypothalamus and the pituitary gland. Defects in this complex system are common.

Figure 17.35B shows the stylised profile of hormone levels obtained if blood samples are taken at daily intervals throughout a normal cycle. Oestradiol exerts predominantly negative and intermittently positive feedback. When follicular oestradiol secretion rises, this appears to switch the pituitary gonadotrophs from an FSH- to a mainly LH-

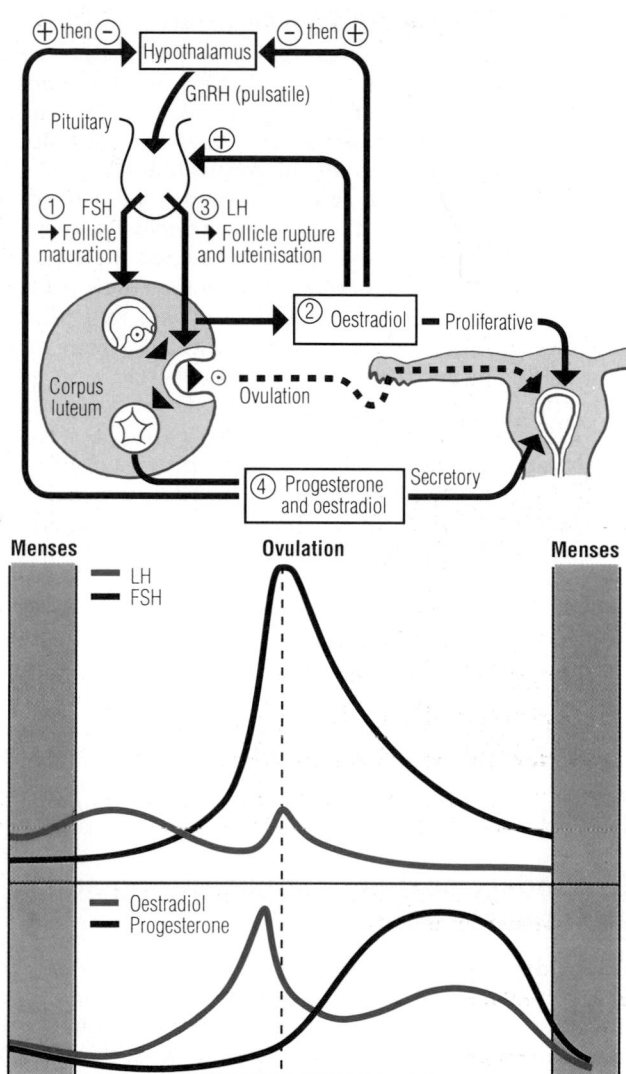

Fig. 17.35 The normal menstrual cycle. A. Diagram of the sequence of events of the normal menstrual cycle. (1) FSH leads to follicle maturation, and secretion of oestradiol which leads to proliferative endometrium and, with other factors, (2) feeds back on pituitary and hypothalamus. Mid-cycle positive feedback triggers LH surge (3) leading to follicle rupture and luteinisation. Corpus luteum (4) secretes progesterone and oestradiol, leading to a secretory endometrium. If conception occurs, implanted blastocyst secretes HCG, which maintains the corpus luteum and its secretions. **B.** Overall pattern of circulating hormone levels during a normal menstrual cycle.

secreting mode, and to reduce the pulse amplitude of GnRH secretion. Meanwhile, the gonadotrophs become more sensitive to GnRH. The signal for the preovulatory surge in LH secretion is a decline in oestradiol levels, together with the onset of progesterone secretion with attendant rise in GnRH pulse amplitude. The mid-cycle LH surge, characterised by 24–48 hours of high peaks of

LH secretion, is one of the turning points of the cycle. It arrives at the ovary when one follicle has reached a diameter of 2 cm, and its granulosa cells have proliferated and developed LH receptors sufficient to be induced to ovulate. The LH surge completes ovulation, and induces the granulosa cells to become the corpus luteum.

Postovulatory steroid secretion, which is still dependent on low concentrations of LH, comes principally from the corpus luteum, whose cells have developed the capacity for de novo steroid synthesis and secrete both progesterone and oestradiol. It should be noted that plasma oestradiol levels fluctuate 10-fold and progesterone more than 20-fold during the normal menstrual cycle.

In the uterus the changes are: firstly, *proliferative phase* development, due to the preovulatory oestradiol surge; and secondly, postovulatory progesterone and oestradiol conversion of this to the receptive *secretory phase* endometrium. Mucus secretion from the cervix is only conducive to sperm penetration during the late proliferative phase and mid-cycle; thereafter progesterone rapidly inhibits it. If fertilisation occurs, the blastocyst penetrates the endometrium and secretes its own LH-like hormone, HCG, which is absorbed into the circulation and maintains the corpus luteum. In the absence of HCG, the corpus luteum atrophies, progesterone secretion declines, the spiral arteries of the endometrium collapse and the surface layers of endometrium die, and are shed as menstruation.

Secondary sexual changes during and after female puberty

Breast development commences at around 9–11 years. Primary changes are caused by the action of oestradiol on the duct epithelium; this in turn probably stimulates stromal fat development (most of the bulk of the breast). Progesterone also acts on the oestrogen-primed breast epithelium, which is of importance in pregnancy to prepare for lactation. Progesterone is responsible for the increase in breast volume (about 20%) during the luteal phase.

Oestradiol, and ovarian and adrenal androgens are responsible for stimulation of female pubic and axillary hair. Changes in uterine size (myometrial and endometrial) are caused by the joint effects of oestrogen and progestogen.

Oestradiol is principally responsible for the pubertal growth spurt by a direct effect on epiphyseal cartilage, and an indirect effect on GH and gonadotrophin secretion. The earlier time of puberty and the potent effect of oestrogens on epiphyseal plates leads to the shorter final stature. Oestradiol has a major effect in increasing endosteal new bone formation and skeletal mass, but is less potent in this respect than testosterone. The increased muscle mass in males is probably also a factor

in increasing the bone density (cortical and trabecular) in men (see also p. 725).

Age-related changes in ovarian function and the menopause

The menopause is preceded by hormone changes over 10 years or more, which stem from the progressive depletion of follicles, causing deeper troughs in oestradiol levels and higher peaks of FSH. The role of the ovarian peptide hormone inhibin is still not entirely clear. High FSH levels stimulate premature development of the next crop of follicles. Luteinisation without ovulation is commonplace; bleeding becomes erratic and the woman subfertile long before the last menstrual period, which usually occurs at about 50 years of age.

The menopause is commonly attended by frequent disabling and embarrassing hot flushes – due to central sympathetic nervous discharge. The flushes coincide with discharge of LH and FSH, but are not due to them. Vaginal dryness, lack of libido, breast atrophy, urethritis and bone loss are all common symptoms of postmenopausal oestrogen deficiency.

OVARIAN DYSFUNCTION: AMENORRHOEA AND OLIGOMENORRHOEA

Ovarian dysfunction is usually associated with erratic and infrequent cycles (oligomenorrhoea) or absent periods (amenorrhoea). The presenting complaint may be of the menstrual disorder, infertility or accompanying problems such as breast discomfort, galactorrhoea or hirsutism.

Amenorrhoea or oligomenorrhoea may occur from the time of puberty (primary) or develop later (secondary). It is obviously always important to exclude pregnancy by a pregnancy test or ultrasound scan even in women who ovulate only occasionally. It is especially important in patients with primary amenorrhoea to try to determine whether the external and internal genitalia are those of a normal female.

Pituitary/hypothalamic causes

Gonadotrophin deficiency

Deficiency of GnRH is most commonly secondary to weight loss. Many teenage girls diet excessively and, as a consequence, develop amenorrhoea at a weight or lean body mass that varies between different individuals. In anorexia nervosa (Ch. 10, p. 193) circulating LH and FSH levels are low, as are those of oestradiol and progesterone. As a consequence there is, in addition to amenorrhoea, a degree of regression of secondary sexual characteristics towards a prepubertal state, with reduction in oestrogenisation of breasts and genital tract. A variable degree of osteoporosis will occur in the long term. A similar state can result from weight loss or starvation, or in athletes (especially long-distance runners) and ballet dancers: the periods usually, but not always, return if and when weight is regained.

Isolated gonadotrophin deficiency without weight loss (due almost certainly to GnRH deficiency) may occur as a lifelong selective hypothalamic defect in the female, as in the male. If associated with anosmia, it is called Kallman's syndrome (p. 709). It may also be seen in patients with craniopharyngioma, or after pituitary irradiation, in which case it is likely to be associated with other pituitary hormone deficiencies.

Prolactin excess

PRL excess from any cause is frequently associated with disordered ovarian function, with amenorrhoea occurring when the PRL level rises to more than two or three times above normal. A classification of the causes is given in Table 17.6 and the condition discussed on pages 678–680.

PRL excess is believed to exert a 'short loop feedback' effect at hypothalamic level, reducing the pulse frequency of GnRH secretion. Its effects can be overcome by gonadotrophin replacement or pump-induced GnRH administration, and so are probably not exerted on the gonads directly.

Ovarian causes

The ovarian causes of amenorrhoea and oligomenorrhoea are summarised in Table 17.17. In such cases, the circulating levels of LH and FSH are elevated.

Table 17.17 Ovarian causes of amenorrhoea or oligomenorrhoea

Failure of normal ovarian development

Pure XX gonadal dysgenesis
    Familial
    Sporadic
Turner's syndrome (XO)
Ovarian enzyme deficiencies (e.g. 17,20 desmolase)

Premature ovarian failure (follicular degeneration)

Idiopathic (low initial follicle number)
Autoimmune (antiovarian antibodies)
Infection (e.g. mumps oöphoritis)
Radiotherapy
Cytotoxic drugs (e.g. for Hodgkin's disease, leukaemia)
Surgical/traumatic

Ovarian dysfunction

Polycystic ovary syndrome (uncertain if ovarian in origin)
Resistant ovary syndrome

Premature menopause

Menopausal failure may be seen sometimes as early as the 20s, presumably as a consequence of starting with a greatly reduced number of follicles. Occasionally, the immune system may be implicated, with production of antiovarian antibodies (p. 662). An identical syndrome often results from irradiation of the ovaries or administration of chemotherapeutic agents, usually directed against Hodgkin's lymphoma or other malignancies (p. 138).

Gonadal dysgenesis

An important group comes under the general heading of *gonadal dysgenesis*. Here, the ovaries may either fail to develop or degenerate before puberty, often because of an abnormal X chromosome complement which leads to follicular death.

Turner's syndrome

Turner's syndrome (Fig. 5.13) is the commonest form. Primary amenorrhoea is associated with short stature and a variable number of skeletal and somatic abnormalities (Table 17.18; see also Ch. 5, p. 75). The condition is most commonly caused by a 45X (termed XO) chromosome constitution, which has resulted from the loss of an X or Y chromosome before the first mitotic division of the fertilised ovum. The features of this syndrome result in part from the existence of only one X chromosome (without a Y), and in part from the resulting sex hormone deficiency from the time of puberty onwards. The clinical features are given in Table 17.18.

Other forms of gonadal dysgenesis

Some patients with a classical 'Turner's' phenotype (Fig. 5.13) have a normal chromosome complement, but have part of an X chromosome missing. With XO/XY mosaicism and other variants, the patient normally has less severe skeletal abnormalities and may be of normal stature. Rare individuals have an apparently normal male genotype (46 XY), but normal female internal genitalia; in these instances, it is believed that the testes never develop (pure XY gonadal dysgenesis; see p. 715).

THE POLYCYSTIC OVARY SYNDROME (PCOS – the Stein-Leventhal syndrome)

This was originally described in 1935 as hirsutism, obesity and oligomenorrhoea associated with enlarged ovaries with a thickened and whitish-looking 'capsule' and multiple follicular cysts. There is persistent elevation of serum LH. At ovulation the levels are suppressed to

Table 17.18 Clinical features of 45XO Turner's syndrome

Type	Feature
Sexual	Streak ovaries
	Sexual infantilism
	Primary amenorrhoea
	High gonadotrophins
	Normal female genitalia
Skeletal	Short stature (<150 cm)
	Characteristic facies – micrognathia, epicanthic folds, low-set ears, fish-like mouth, high arched palate
	Shield-like chest
	Wide carrying angle
	Short neck, low hairline
	Short metacarpals
	Scoliosis
	Localised areas of rarefaction
	Osteoporosis
Soft tissues	Lymphoedema
	Webbing of neck
Cardiovascular	Coarctation of aorta
	Bicuspid aortic valve
	Aortic stenosis
Renal	Rotation of kidney
	Duplex ureters, etc.
	Hydronephrosis
Cutaneous	Small nipples
	Pigmented naevi
	Cheloid formation

normal but rise again when progesterone levels fall. There is a subgroup of patients that are obese, and here it is possible that increased production in adipose tissue of the oestrogen oestrone (from androstenedione) may trigger excessive pituitary LH secretion. Many cases are of normal weight, however. It is likely that the cause varies from hypothalamic, pituitary, ovarian and possibly even adrenal defects. About 20% of normal women have polycystic ovaries on ultrasound. The high LH levels are generally associated with increased ovarian secretion of androstenedione, which is converted in peripheral tissues to testosterone. Plasma oestradiol is relatively constant at levels seen in the mid-follicular phase of the cycle; levels of SHBG are reduced, and so the unbound testosterone level is modestly raised.

The extent of development of hirsutism and more marked virilisation in this syndrome is very variable, and depends both on the hormone abnormality (which can be measured) and on the capacity of target tissues to respond. Likewise, the ovulatory disturbance varies from slightly erratic cycles through to long-standing amenorrhoea (primary or secondary).

Summary 7 Polycystic ovary syndrome

- Erratic cycles or amenorrhoea
- Subfertility
- Variable obesity and hirsutism
- Polycystic ovaries on ultrasound
- Inappropriately high LH
- Modest increase in androgens
- Low sex hormone binding globulin

Management of amenorrhoea

The treatment of patients with erratic cycles depends on the underlying cause, the age of the patient and their requirements (e.g. for contraception, treatment of hirsutism or infertility). With PRL excess, restoring the PRL level to normal is usually sufficient to restore normal ovulation and fertility. If the latter is not desired, then the oral contraceptive pill can be given safely with bromocriptine.

With gonadal dysgenesis or ovarian failure, attempts to restore ovarian function and fertility are generally unsuccessful. These women are suitable candidates for natural ovarian hormone replacement and embryo implantation (donor eggs fertilised by husband's sperm). Sex hormone replacement is indicated in most cases, at least until the time of the menopause. This can be provided by low-dose oral contraceptive pills, most of which provide 20–30 μg daily of ethinyl oestradiol, and a progestogen (21 days out of 28). Alternatively, the treatment can be tailored to the patient's perceived needs. Where there is a history of deep vein thrombosis or hypertension, oestrogens can more safely be given as a subcutaneous implant in the lower abdominal wall of solid oestradiol (50 mg), periods being induced by administration of a progestogen for 10–14 days per month. Adhesive plastic patches containing oestradiol dissolved in ethanol (Estraderm), which are applied to the skin and from which the hormone is absorbed, are an alternative.

After the menopause, for most women, opinion increasingly favours hormone replacement therapy (HRT). There is little doubt that it protects the bones against osteoporosis and the genital tract against atrophy, and that many women feel much better on it. Oestrogens give protection against vascular disease. Cyclical progestogens prevent an increased risk of endometrial cancer. There is a small increase in breast cancer risk, offset by the greater reduction in vascular mortality.

Management of female infertility

With *hyperprolactinaemia*, restoring the PRL to normal usually restores both periods and fertility.

Gonadotrophin deficiency may be treated either by gonadotrophin administration, or by pulsatile administration of GnRH, which is safer. Gonadotrophin therapy consists usually of 3–7 days of injections of a preparation of human FSH. The dose is titrated by measuring blood or urine oestrogens and by ovarian ultrasound scanning. When the right amount of follicular development has occurred, ovulation is induced by an injection of HCG. This treatment is only given in specialised units where there is also an egg retrieval and fertilisation programme.

Polycystic ovaries. Treatment of the infertility is difficult and often unsatisfactory. About one-quarter of cases will ovulate on a low dose of glucocorticoid (such as prednisolone 7.5 mg daily). Clomiphene citrate (the antioestrogen) is often given, and induces ovulation in about half the cases. Some units are now treating patients by producing 'paradoxical' suppression of LH and FSH with a GnRH analogue, followed by conventional stimulation with FSH followed by HCG.

PREMENSTRUAL TENSION

Premenstrual tension is a common but rather poorly defined condition, in which a wide range of physical and emotional symptoms and signs are worst during the week or two preceding a menstrual period and generally improve with its onset. It is not primarily an endocrine disorder, but is probably best thought of as a cyclical disorder 'locked in' on the normal fluctuation in hormone levels that accompanies the menstrual cycle. It may, in many cases, be an exaggeration of the normal; in many women, however, it can be extremely disabling. Treatment may be directed at smoothing out or eliminating the normal hormone changes or at treating the symptoms, and few of the many treatments have a sound scientific basis.

DISORDERS OF SEX DIFFERENTIATION

The underlying mechanisms of primary sex differentiation are described on page 706. Where sex differentiation is evidently abnormal at birth, the problem is made particularly difficult by the urgency of determining the appropriate sex of rearing. Parents are under great pressure to declare the sex of the infant and to stick to it. They require very sensitive handling. Most cases of abnormal sex differentiation are cases of pseudo- (rather than true) hermaphroditism.

MALE PSEUDOHERMAPHRODITISM

The male pseudohermaphrodite is a *genetically male* infant who does not have completely normal male sexual char-

acteristics. In its mildest form, the infant has failure of development of the penile urethra (hypospadias); in its most severe form, the external genitalia appear to be those of a completely normal female. The causes are listed in Table 17.14 (p. 708).

Pure XY gonadal dysgenesis

Here, the individual is XY in sex chromosome constitution but testes never imposed maleness on the 'background' female phenotype. Apart from the absence of gonads, the patient is a completely normal female. The gonadal remnants (streak gonads) are at risk of developing tumours (dysgerminomas) at, or after, the age of puberty, and should therefore be removed. From puberty onwards, female sex hormone replacement should be given.

Testicular feminisation

Testicular feminisation occurs with a frequency of about 1 in 10 000 live births, and is inherited through an X-linked gene. XY individuals develop testes as normal, but are unable to respond to the androgen that these produce because they lack the androgen receptor. There are a variety of genetic defects responsible for the complete and partial forms of the syndrome. In the complete form, the external genitalia are those of a normal female, but with a very short blind vagina. There is no development either at or after puberty of even the normal female amount of pubic and axillary hair. The testes are in the inguinal canal. Presentation is often with inguinal herniae.

The correct sex of rearing for individuals with either the partial or complete form of the syndrome is undoubtedly female. It is generally felt to be advisable to leave the testes in situ until breast development has taken place at the normal age of puberty. Feminisation of the breasts is usually excellent, under the influence of normal levels of testicular oestradiol (unopposed by androgen action). Circulating levels of LH and FSH are usually somewhat elevated, and testosterone levels in the high adult male range (after puberty). The gonads should be removed in early adult life, as there is considerable risk of development of tumours (dysgerminomas) within them.

5-α-reductase deficiency

5-α-reductase deficiency is an autosomal recessive disorder, and is therefore most common where there has been intermarriage. The primary defect lies in the enzyme 5-α-reductase which is absent or of reduced activity. Production of 5-α-dihydrotestosterone (DHT) in androgen target tissues is reduced (Fig. 17.27, p. 696) and those effects that depend on DHT are therefore compromised. Females with the condition appear normal, but males have impairment of virilisation of the external genitalia. The phallus is small, and there is complete perineo-scrotal hypospadias, and incomplete fusion of the scrotum with a blind vaginal opening. The testes, epididymes, vasa and seminal vesicles are normal, while the prostate gland is, and remains, atrophic. Regardless of the sex of rearing, affected individuals generally insist that they are male, both at the time of puberty and beyond, and generally demonstrate male patterns of behaviour. After puberty, the voice deepens and normal male muscular development occurs but facial hair is absent or scanty.

FEMALE PSEUDOHERMAPHRODITISM

In female pseudohermaphroditism, a *genetic female* is partially or completely virilised. The most likely cause is excess androgen secretion in utero, generally as a result of the action of increased ACTH on the (abnormal) adrenal glands. The commonest cause is 21-hydroxylase deficiency (p. 700).

RARE DISORDERS OF STEROID BIOSYNTHESIS

Rare deficiencies of almost all the enzymes have been described, and the clinical picture can usually be understood by reference to these pathways and the normal physiology of the glands (Fig. 17.27, p. 696). Conditions that affect the testosterone pathway(s) lead to male pseudohermaphroditism; if they lie early on the pathway (which is shared with the adrenals) then adrenal insufficiency also occurs.

In addition to 21-hydroxylase deficiency (which is about five times commoner than the others put together), there are a number of other disorders of steroid biosynthesis which also lead to pseudohermaphroditism in affected females. These include 3-β-hydroxysteroid dehydrogenase deficiency, in which the weak Δ_5-androgens from the adrenals cause some virilisation of females (but males are inadequately virilised). Likewise, 11-hydroxylase deficiency is associated with a build-up of adrenal androgens; desoxycorticosterone is also overproduced, leading to hypertension.

DISORDERS OF MALE SECONDARY SEX DIFFERENTIATION

The physiological mechanisms that lead to male secondary sex differentiation are discussed on pages 706–707.

Gynaecomastia

Gynaecomastia (breast development in the male) is so common in puberty and old age as to be regarded as physiological. It also features in a wide range of disorders (Table 17.19). These are generally associated with an increase in oestrogen production, and/or a decline in testosterone production. Some drugs cause gynaecomastia, the most notable being the aldosterone antagonist, spironolactone. This compound also binds to androgen receptors and is an antiandrogen. It may also inhibit the secretion of androgen, but not that of oestrogen. Digitoxin and the main metabolite of cannabis cause gynaecomastia because of intrinsic oestrogenic activity.

Treatment may be directed at the underlying cause, but it is often not apparent. Danazol, a synthetic androgen, has been used to treat the condition, as have antioestrogens such as tamoxifen. Hypogonadism should be treated with testosterone replacement. This is probably best given either as oral testosterone undecanoate or by implant, rather than by injection of testosterone esters (Sustanon or Primoteston), which lead to high peaks of testosterone and oestradiol levels after injection.

Prostatic hyperplasia

Prostatic hyperplasia results from increased androgen effect (via dihydrotestosterone and its hydroxylated metabolites) on the ventral lobe of the prostate, and commonly causes urethral obstruction. It is usually treated by transurethral resection, although antiandrogenic progestogens have a significant effect in causing regression.

Prostatic cancer

Prostatic cancer is the commonest cancer in elderly males and is commonly androgen-dependent. A mainstay of treatment is thus suppression of androgen secretion and/or action. Surgery (subcapsular orchidectomy) is commonly used, as is medical therapy with the antiandrogenic progestogen, cyproterone acetate, or GnRH analogues to cause down-regulation of LH and so testosterone secretion.

DISORDERS OF FEMALE SECONDARY SEX DIFFERENTIATION

Hirsutism in women is the obverse of gynaecomastia in men and is almost equally common. The term *virilisation* is reserved for androgenisation associated with very high levels of testosterone in, or approaching, the adult male range. Only 1–2% of women with hirsutism in Britain have frank virilisation. This may be due to ovarian or adrenal tumours, or to the so-called late-onset form of congenital adrenal hyperplasia. Virilisation usually declares itself by a rapid development of hirsutism, with

Table 17.19 Causes and mechanisms of gynaecomastia

Cause	Low testosterone production	High oestrogen production	Direct oestrogenic effect	Direct anti-androgenic effect	Decreased androgen sensitivity
Physiological					
Neonatal	+	+	–	–	–
Pubertal*	+	+	–	–	–
Old age*	+	+	–	–	–
'Refeeding' (after starvation)	+	+	–	–	–
Pathological					
Hypogonadism	++	–	–	–	–
Steroid disorders					
17-ketosteroid reductase deficiency	+	+ (oestrone)	–	–	–
Testicular feminisation	–	+	–	–	++
Cirrhosis**	+	+	–	–	–
Thyrotoxicosis*	+ (increased clearance)	+	–	–	–
Tumours					
HCG-secreting	–	+	–	–	–
Leydig cell	+	++	–	–	–
Adrenal	+ (LH suppressed)	–	–	–	–
'Idiopathic'†	–	–	–	–	+?
Pharmacological					
Spironolactone	+	+	–	++	–
Digitalis	–	–	+	–	–
Cannabis	–	–	+	–	–
Cyproterone acetate	+ (LH suppressed)	–	–	++	–
Oestrogen ingestion*	+ (LH suppressed)	–	++	–	–
Alcohol	+	–	–	–	–

*Associated with elevated SHBG levels, which may have moderate amplifying effect
ˣ Fall in albumin selectively elevates free oestradiol
†Decreased androgen sensitivity and increased oestrogen sensitivity may be secondary to altered hormone production

other signs such as frontal balding, clitoral enlargement and deepening of the voice.

Hirsutism

Hirsutism is conventionally subdivided into:

- that due to *polycystic ovarian disease*, in which case menstruation is irregular or absent
- '*idiopathic*' hirsutism, in which the periods are regular. The latter was long thought not to be due to androgen excess, but to increased target organ sensitivity.

It is evident from the wide variation in the extent of facial and body hair in men, that the same genetic variability must also exist in women. Thus, some women with chronic anovulation, erratic cycles, polycystic ovaries and high levels of testosterone and androstenedione coming from the ovaries under the stimulation of LH show little or no hirsutism; while others, with a lesser endocrine defect, are severely hirsute. Another problem is to determine how much of the androgen excess is arising from the ovaries and how much from the adrenals. With the exception of 21-hydroxylase deficiency, the ovaries are probably usually the major source.

Prevention and management of hirsutism

Hirsutism develops over many years, and treatment should not be delayed until there is a serious clinical problem. Treatment may be hormonal or cosmetic and usually both are needed simultaneously.

Cosmetic treatment involves the use of creams, waxes (which root out the hairs), shaving or electrolysis. The latter is usually reserved for strong terminal hairs on the face and breasts, or other psychologically important areas, and should only be carried out by a trained electrologist. Contrary to popular belief, shaving does not make unwanted hair grow faster. At present no treatment is officially licenced for treating hirsutism.

Hormonal treatment involves the use of adrenal and/or ovarian suppression and antiandrogens. Adrenal androgens can generally be suppressed with doses of glucocorti-

---

> **Summary 8 Hormonal treatments for hirsutism**
>
> **Ovarian suppression**
>
> Contraceptive pill (e.g. ethinyl oestradiol 20–30 μg and low dose cyproterone acetate, 3 weeks out of 4)
>
> **Adrenal suppression**
>
> Prednisolone (up to 7.5 mg/day)
>
> **Antiandrogens**
>
> Spironolactone (50–200 mg/day)
> Cyproterone acetate 100 mg/day for 10 days per month with ethinyl oestradiol for 21 days

coid that are less than those required to suppress cortisol. In about one-third of cases with erratic cycles, ovulation becomes much more regular and ovarian androgen production also declines. Ovarian suppression is achieved by using a low-dose 'pill' that does not contain a virilising androgen, e.g. Marvelon, which combines ethinyl oestradiol with dydrogesterone. 'Pills' that contain androgens, such as norgestrel, should be avoided. The antiandrogens include cyproterone acetate which in low dosage is a component of a contraceptive pill (Dianette); much higher doses are needed for maximum antiandrogen effect. Spironolactone is sometimes remarkably effective, but it can lead in some cases to menstrual disturbance.

Psychological support is of great importance and must include reassurance that the woman is not losing her femininity, or 'turning into a man'. Sometimes minimal hirsutism is a focus for an anxiety state; conversely, some women react by refusing to accept that there is a problem, and avoid even elementary cosmetic measures. The duration of drug therapy for hirsutism can be open-ended, and determined by the severity of the problem and the response; the patient with erratic cycles will simply have the same problem (no worse) when treatment is stopped.

Where *pregnancy* is desired, a different strategy, designed to produce ovulation, is required. At its simplest, this involves low dose glucocorticoid therapy (if cycles are irregular) with or without clomiphene. In severe polycystic ovary disease, it may be necessary to induce ovulation with injections of FSH; this requires close monitoring of oestrogens and follicles on ultrasound and is a specialist procedure. Under no circumstances should cyproterone acetate be given on its own (i.e. without an oestrogen) to the premenopausal woman; there are serious consequences for sex differentiation in any male fetus if the woman conceives while on the drug.

SEX HORMONES AND BEHAVIOUR

Androgens, oestrogens and progestogens all affect the individual's behaviour either directly or indirectly. However, homosexuality, trans-sexualism and sexual deviation are not directly linked to androgen or oestrogen levels. It has been suggested that XYY men are more violent than normal men, in view of the finding of an increased number in penal institutions; however, the significance of this is uncertain.

Androgen-deficient men may develop protective mechanisms and become aggressive to compensate for the lack of physical development. If they are then abruptly put onto androgens at high doses, the aggression may become more overt. The transition to adult hormone levels (i.e. going through an endocrine adolescence, but very late) again requires medical guidance. Generally, hypogonadal men adapt very well to their new endocrine status and many go on to develop satisfactory heterosexual relationships.

FURTHER READING

Belchetz P E (ed) 1984 Management of pituitary disease. Chapman and Hall, London. *Comprehensive discussions of many aspects of pituitary disease.*

Edwards C R W (ed) 1986 Endocrinology. Integrated Clinical Science Series. Butterworth-Heinemann Medical, London. *A well-illustrated and clear account of the physiology and pathology of the endocrine system.*

Felig P, Baxter I D, Broadus A E, Frohman LA 1993 Endocrinology and metabolism, 3rd edn. McGraw Hill, New York. *A first class textbook of endocrinology and metabolism – highly recommended.*

Hadley Mac E 1992 Endocrinology, 3rd edn. Prentice Hall International, New York. *An excellent, up-to-date, single author text on endocrine biochemistry, physiology and pathophysiology.*

Knobil E, Neill J D (eds) 1988 The physiology of reproduction (2 vols). Raven Press, New York. *An enormous multi-author tome for the serious student who wishes to make an in-depth study of particular aspects of reproduction.*

Stanbury J B, Wynmgaarden D S, Frederikson, J L, Goldstein J L, Brown M S 1983 The metabolic basis of inherited disease, 5th edn. McGraw Hill, New York. *A valuable reference book on all inherited metabolic and endocrine disorders.*

Wilson J B, Foster D W 1991 Williams' textbook of endocrinology 8th edn. W B Saunders, Philadelphia. *A comprehensive textbook – for long considered the 'bible' of basic and clinical endocrinoogy.*

Yen S S C, Jaffe R B (eds) 1991 Reproductive endocrinology, physiology, pathophysiology and clinical management, 3rd edn. W B Saunders, Philadelphia. *A good book, edited and largely written by two of the foremost reproductive endocrinologists in the US.*

18

Metabolic Bone Disease and Mineral Metabolism

John Cunningham, David C Anderson and John P Monson

ANATOMY AND PHYSIOLOGY

The skeleton

- supports the soft tissues
- encases and protects certain organs such as the central nervous system (CNS) and
- acts as an enormous reservoir for minerals, in particular calcium, phosphorus, magnesium and sodium.

Although in health these functions are not in conflict, there are circumstances, for example, calcium deprivation, when the skeleton's contribution to chemical homeostasis may lead to progressive demineralisation and compromise its mechanical functions.

Distribution of mineral

The adult skeleton contains some 99% of total body calcium (Table 18.1), ranging from 1 to 2kg (25–50mol) depending on size, 88% of total body phosphorus, 80% of body carbonate, 50% of body magnesium and 35% of body sodium. Although calcium is distributed approximately equally between extracellular fluid (ECF) and intracellular fluid, the free calcium ion concentration in cell cytosol is approximately 10^{-7} to 10^{-6} molar, this being about three orders of magnitude less than the ECF free calcium ion concentration (10^{-4} molar, or 1 mM). Most of the intracellular calcium must therefore be sequestered in, or on, specific cell organelles. Calcium in blood plasma at 2.4 mM is present in three main forms (Table 18.1). The biological functions of ECF calcium are thought to be effected by the ionised fraction only.

Inorganic phosphate in plasma is only slightly protein-bound (approximately 12%), the rest being present as $HPO_4^{2-}/H_2PO_4^-$ (in the ratio 4:1 at physiological pH), as well as in the form of sodium, calcium and magnesium phosphates. Most of the intracellular phosphate is covalently bound to organic compounds or in the form of phospholipids. The free inorganic phosphate concentration in cells is probably less than 1 mM.

Bone composition

Bone consists of a calcified (mineralised) organic matrix. The organic matrix (osteoid) makes up about 30% of the total skeletal mass, and consists mainly of type I collagen and the vitamin K-dependent protein osteocalcin, with small amounts of other proteins. The mineral phase, which is deposited throughout the organic matrix, makes up the remaining 70% of skeletal mass and consists mainly of a complex crystalline salt of calcium and phosphate

Table 18.1 Distribution of body calcium

Compartment	Quantity/conc.
Whole body	
Skeleton	1 kg (25 mol)
Rapidly exchangeable-bone surface	8 g (200 mmol)
Extracellular fluid (ECF)	1 g (25 mmol)
Intracellular fluid (ICF)	1 g (25 mmol)
In plasma	
Free ionised Ca^{2+}	1.1 mmol/l
Protein-bound	
Albumin	0.75 mmol/l
Globulin	0.25 mmol/l
Ultrafiltrable bound (by bicarbonate citrate and phosphate)	0.3 mmol/l
Total in plasma	2.4 mmol/l

called hydroxyapatite ($Ca_{10}(PO_4)_6(OH)_2$). There are also smaller amounts of amorphous acid phosphate, carbonate, sodium and magnesium.

Bone is a dynamic living tissue, with continuous modelling and remodelling by bone cells which allows the skeleton to grow and adapt itself to prevailing mechanical needs. The result is an organ that is, for its weight, extremely rigid and strong, without being brittle. The skeletal adaptation provides for appropriate strength only where it is needed, thus avoiding excess weight.

At least three distinct cell types contribute to these processes (Fig. 18.1).

The osteoblast

The osteoblast is derived from mesenchymal precursor cells and is the main bone-forming cell. It synthesises organic matrix (osteoid) and probably also controls the subsequent mineralisation of the matrix. It has plentiful mitochondria and an extensive Golgi apparatus associated with rapid protein synthesis. It is rich in alkaline phosphatase. Cells of the osteoblast line possess specific receptors for parathyroid hormone (PTH) and 1,25-dihydroxyvitamin D ($1,25(OH)_2D$, calcitriol).

The osteocyte

Osteocytes are derived from osteoblasts that no longer have a major biosynthetic role and have become encased in bone, communicating with each other by extensions running through canaliculae in the bone. They are likely to be involved in the movement of mineral in the vicinity of the osteocyte lacunae and in detecting stresses in bone.

The osteoclast

Osteoclasts are multinucleated bone-resorbing cells derived from cells related to macrophages. When actively resorbing they have a deeply folded plasma membrane, creating a 'ruffled border' in close proximity to the bone surface. Although they are influenced by the calcium regulating hormones, PTH and $1,25(OH)_2D$, they do not apparently possess specific receptors for these hormones; it is therefore likely that hormonal control is exerted by way of communication with osteoblasts, or by effects of hormones on osteoclast precursors.

Osteoclasts may also be influenced by other hormones, including calcitonin, thyroxine, glucocorticoids and the sex steroids. The functions of osteoclasts and osteoblasts are closely linked, osteoclastic bone resorption being followed by an increase in osteoblastic bone formation. This coupling is probably effected by locally produced regulators.

Bone growth, modelling and remodelling

Longitudinal bone growth in childhood depends on proliferation of cartilage at the hypertrophic zone, which becomes mineralised and then formed into bone. Diameter is increased by periosteal bone formation. Once growth has ceased, coupled activity of osteoblasts and osteoclasts continues, although at a much slower rate, a process which allows alteration of bone architecture (without growth) in response to factors such as mechanical loading. As shown in Figure 18.2, skeletal mass peaks at about the age of 25, decreasing thereafter at a constant rate in males and with a transient acceleration after the menopause in females. This progressive decrease indicates that, throughout most of adult life, net bone resorption just exceeds net formation. In some individuals, bone mass may decrease to the point where clinically important mechanical weakening arises (osteoporosis), leading to fractures that may be spontaneous or follow minimal trauma.

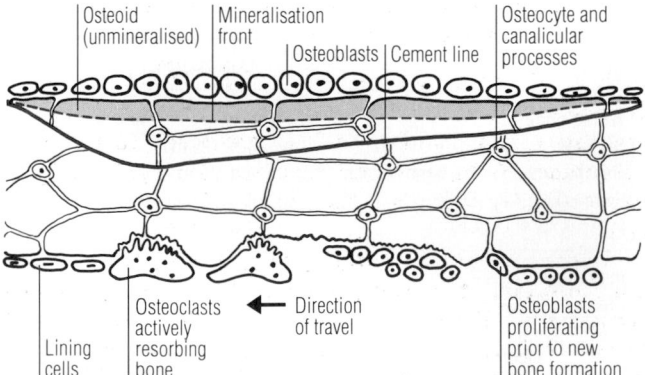

Fig. 18.1 Diagram of normal trabecular bone undergoing osteoclastic resorption followed by new bone formation by osteoblasts. The cement line is shown by a solid red line, and the mineralisation front by a broken red line. Unmineralised osteoid is shaded red.

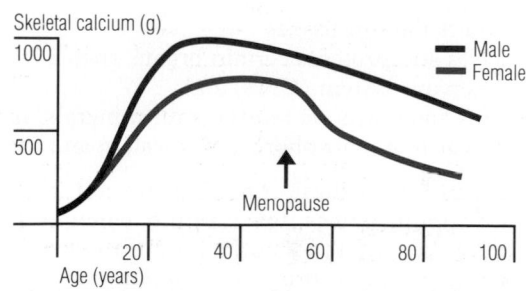

Fig. 18.2 Relationship between bone mass and age.

HORMONAL CONTROL OF BONE, CALCIUM AND PHOSPHORUS METABOLISM

The interrelationships between ECF calcium and inorganic phosphorus, and the skeletal reservoirs of these ions and their main entry and exit points (the intestine and the kidney respectively) are controlled by a hormonal system that is dominated by PTH and $1,25(OH)_2D$ (Fig. 18.3). The role of the third potential calcium regulating hormone, calcitonin, is more enigmatic.

Parathyroid hormone

PTH is an 84 amino acid peptide hormone manufactured, stored and released by the chief cells of the parathyroid glands. Two intracellular precursors have been identified, pre-pro PTH being cleaved successively to yield pro-PTH and, finally, PTH 1–84 itself. PTH release is highly responsive to the prevailing ionised calcium concentration in the ECF, particularly in and around the range of physiological calcaemia. Thus, modest hypocalcaemia triggers a substantial PTH response and modest hypercalcaemia almost completely suppresses the secretion of biologically active PTH.

As shown in Figure 18.3, PTH forms part of a feedback loop that is well suited to maintaining calcium homeostasis. The actions of PTH itself are directed towards the elevation of blood and ECF calcium concentration. These actions are:

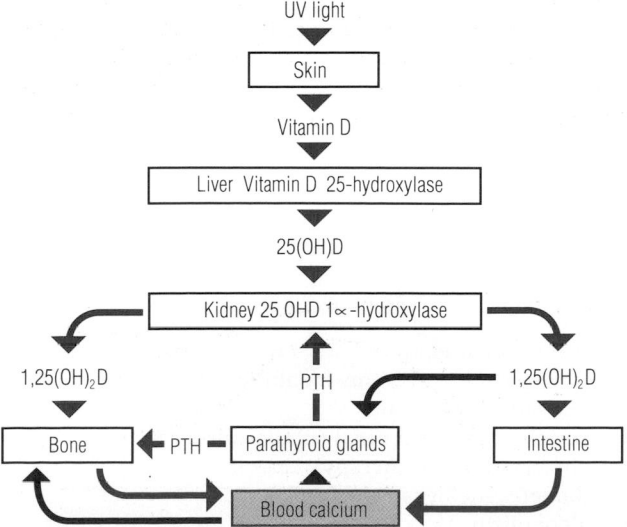

Fig. 18.3 Vitamin D metabolism and the hormonal regulation of calcium metabolism. Calcaemic processes are shown in red.

- to promote recruitment and activation of osteoclasts and so accelerate bone resorption (indirectly through osteoblasts)
- to *increase* the renal tubular resorption of calcium
- to *decrease* the renal tubular reabsorption of inorganic phosphate, thus promoting phosphaturia
- to stimulate the production of $1,25(OH)_2D$, thereby promoting intestinal calcium absorption.

1,25-dihydroxyvitamin D (1,25(OH)$_2$D, calcitriol)

The potent steroid hormone, 1,25-dihydroxyvitamin D, is produced almost uniquely in the kidney. It is the product of a series of chemical transformations that starts with the production of cholecalciferol (vitamin D_3) in the skin under the influence of ultraviolet light, or with the ingestion of ergocalciferol (vitamin D_2) added to the diet. Normally, very little comes from the latter source. Subsequently, the 25-hydroxylation of vitamin D in the liver and, finally, 1-hydroxylation of 25-hydroxyvitamin D in the kidney results in production of the active hormonal form of vitamin D, $1,25(OH)_2D_3$ (Fig. 18.3). Other hydroxylated metabolites of vitamin D are also produced by the kidney, but $1,25(OH)_2D$ is the only one with clearly defined biological actions. Like PTH, $1,25(OH)_2D$ is a calcaemic hormone; its known actions complement those of PTH. $1,25(OH)_2D$ has two major target organs, intestine and bone, and also reduces PTH release by a direct effect on parathyroids.

In the intestine, $1,25(OH)_2D$ increases the absorption of calcium and, to a lesser extent, phosphate by:

- increasing the permeability of the brush border to calcium
- promoting the synthesis of a high-affinity calcium-binding protein in the cell
- accelerating active extrusion of calcium across the basolateral membrane.

In bone, the main action of $1,25(OH)_2D$ is to increase resorption. This is probably by stimulating proliferation and differentiation of osteoclast precursors. In addition, osteoblasts (which possess receptors for $1,25(OH)_2D$) can probably modulate the function of nearby osteoclasts.

These actions of $1,25(OH)_2D$ favour elevation of the concentration of ionised calcium and inorganic phosphorus in blood. The extent to which bone formation, as well as resorption, is under the direct control of vitamin D metabolites is unclear, although indirectly the vitamin D system certainly influences bone formation by controlling calcium and phosphate concentrations in the ECF. Renal production of $1,25(OH)_2D$ is under tight control by PTH, hypocalcaemia and hypophosphataemia, all of which stimulate production of 1α-hydroxylase. The phosphaturic effect of PTH prevents the calcium × phosphate product rising when PTH rises and bone resorption increases.

Other hormones

Although many other hormones have demonstrable effects on bone metabolism under appropriate circumstances, their physiological role is uncertain.

Calcitonin

Calcitonin is a 32 amino acid peptide hormone secreted by the C-cells of the thyroid gland. Its best defined actions are on bone, where it binds to specific receptors in osteoclasts leading to decreased resorptive activity. Not surprisingly, this effect is most striking where bone turnover is high, such as in growing bone or in Paget's disease (p. 737). Even when given in pharmacological doses, the influence of calcitonin on calcium and bone metabolism in the normal adult is minimal.

Sex steroids

The acceleration of bone loss after the menopause and its amelioration by oestrogen therapy, together with the high prevalance of osteoporosis in women with untreated primary or secondary hypogonadism, has long suggested that oestrogens exert an important influence on bone metabolism. Recent evidence suggests a direct effect, mediated by oestrogen receptors on osteoblasts.

Androgens are responsible for the attainment of higher peak bone mass in males (Fig. 18.2) directly, or indirectly by increasing muscle bulk and strength. Androgens and oestrogens also act on growth cartilage, in concert with growth hormone, promoting growth and, later, epiphyseal closure.

Glucocorticoids

In physiological amounts, glucocorticoids are important regulators of bone growth, probably by actions on both bone-forming and bone-resorbing cells. Pharmacological doses of these steroids decrease bone mass, leading to osteoporosis.

Thyroxine

About one-third of patients with thyrotoxicosis have mild hypercalcaemia, hypercalciuria, or both, and neglected thyrotoxicosis may lead to osteoporosis. Conversely, hypothyroidism is associated with low bone turnover which may be restored to normal by physiological doses of thyroxine.

Local modulation of bone, calcium and phosphorus metabolism

A variety of local factors contribute to the delicate balance that exists between the actions of the different types of bone cells, although many of these have not yet been fully characterised.

Prostaglandins

Local production of prostaglandins, such as PGE_2, may influence bone metabolism directly, or by promoting the synthesis of other locally acting factors such as epidermal growth factor and platelet-derived growth factor. Inhibitors of prostaglandin synthesis have little if any effect on bone.

Cytokines

Interleukin-1 is a potent bone-resorbing agent derived from activated macrophages. Although its physiological role in bone is unclear, it has many interactions with other cytokines, such as gamma-interferon, consistent with local regulatory functions in bone. Tumour necrosis factors and transforming growth factor β also have effects, and some or all may be involved in bone cell coupling.

MAGNESIUM HOMEOSTASIS

Magnesium ions have a similar cellular/extracellular distribution to potassium, and parallel alterations in concentration of these cations are observed in a number of situations. However, the high content of magnesium found in bone results in important associations with calcium metabolism. In addition, magnesium is an effector of PTH secretion.

Hypomagnesaemia may occur with:

- severe malnutrition
- long-term intravenous feeding in the absence of magnesium supplements
- certain long-term renal tubular disorders
- chronic diuretic therapy
- diabetes mellitus
- alcoholism
- following surgical correction of hyperparathyroidism
- cytotoxic treatment with cisplatin.

Hypomagnesaemia is rarely severe but may, on occasions, give rise to symptoms and signs similar to hypocalcaemia, with tetany progressing to convulsions and cardiac arrhythmias, with or without associated hypocalcaemia. This may necessitate magnesium supplementation by oral magnesium salts (of which magnesium glycerophosphate is least likely to cause diarrhoea) or parenteral magnesium sulphate. Coexisting hypocalcaemia is refractory until the hypomagnesaemia has been corrected; this is due to impaired secretion of PTH and also to target organ resistance to circulating PTH during hypomagnesaemia.

Hypermagnesaemia may complicate renal impairment. It results in gastrointestinal disturbance and may, if severe, cause CNS depression. It is rarely of clinical significance.

INVESTIGATION OF BONE DISEASE

Investigations of bone disease fall into five groups:

- biochemical: blood and urine (Table 18.2)
- radiographic
- radionuclide studies
- measurement of bone mass
- histology.

Biochemistry

Blood calcium

Total calcium in plasma or serum is the usual measurement taken in clinical practice although, in some instances, direct measurement of the physiologically important ionised fraction is undertaken, using a calcium ion-selective electrode. The latter is likely to be employed with increasing frequency in the future, since it avoids the difficulties that may arise when abnormalities of plasma protein concentration or acid–base status alter the normal relationship between total and ionic calcium in blood. A reduced plasma protein concentration leads to a reduction in plasma total calcium concentration, even though free ionic calcium is normal. The error may be reduced by 'adjustment' of the observed calcium concentration, using the formula:

$$Ca \ (adjusted) = Ca^t + 0.02 \ (46 - alb)$$

where Ca^t is the observed concentration of total calcium in mmol/l and *alb* is the albumin concentration in g/l. As pH falls, so does calcium binding to plasma proteins. Thus, during severe acidosis, plasma total calcium may be low, with a normal free ionic calcium concentration.

Increases in blood calcium usually reflect accelerated entry into the ECF, either as a result of rapid bone resorption (primary hyperparathyroidism, vitamin D in-

Table 18.2 Biochemical investigation of bone disease

Measurements	Associated disease
Blood plasma	
Urea, creatinine	Renal disease
Na^+, K^+, Cl^-, HCO_3^-	Acid-base disturbance
Calcium	*Increased* in primary hyperparathyroidism, malignant disease, granulomatous disease, vitamin D intoxication
	Decreased in renal disease, osteomalacia, hypoparathyroidism
Phosphate	*Increased* in renal disease, hypoparathyroidism and pseudohypoparathyroidism
	Decreased in primary hyperparathyroidism, vitamin D deficiency, renal tubular disorders
Alkaline phosphatase	*Increased* in childhood, hyperparathyroidism, vitamin D deficiency, fracture, malignancy, Paget's disease
	Decreased in hypophosphatasia
Parathyroid hormone (PTH)	*Increased* in hyperparathyroidism and pseudohypoparathyroidism
	Decreased in hypoparathyroidism
25-hydroxyvitamin D	Vitamin D deficiency or intoxication
Urine	
Calcium	Hypercalciuria Familial hypocalciuric hypercalcaemia
Phosphate	*Decreased* tubular reabsorption in hyperparathyroidism
cAMP	*Increased* in hyperparathyroidism (provided kidneys normal)

toxication, osteolytic metastases), or of increased intestinal absorption (high dietary calcium intake, primary hyperparathyroidism, vitamin D intoxication, or milk alkali syndrome), or both processes acting together.

Decreases in blood calcium are due to diminished bone resorption and/or diminished intestinal absorption of calcium. Important causes are hypoparathyroidism, vitamin D deficiency with calcium malabsorption, and severe renal disease.

Urine calcium

Urine calcium ranges from 2.5 to 7.5 mmol/24 hours in adults and is increased in situations where calcium entry to the ECF is enhanced (leading to potential or actual hypercalcaemia), or where the renal tubular reabsorption of calcium is decreased ('renal leak' type of hypercalciuria), or both.

Plasma inorganic phosphate

Plasma phosphate is normally determined by the level of renal tubular reabsorption of phosphate, a process that is itself modulated by the dietary intake of phosphate and by PTH. Tubular reabsorption of phosphate is decreased by PTH and increased by low dietary intake of phosphate. A low plasma phosphate is found in association with primary hyperparathyroidism, vitamin D deficiency, certain renal tubular disorders (p. 728) and prolonged dietary phosphate deprivation. Serum phosphate is elevated in patients with substantial impairment of renal function and reduction of glomerular filtration rate (GFR) and, occasionally, in patients with greatly accelerated tissue catabolism (e.g. rhabdomyolysis, tumour necrosis).

Alkaline phosphatase

The enzyme alkaline phosphatase is produced by osteoblasts, and its release into the circulation increases as osteoblast numbers and/or activity increases. This is seen in normal children and also in generalised disorders characterised by high bone turnover (e.g. hyperparathyroidism) and in focal lesions (e.g. healing fractures, Paget's disease or bone metastases). Many other tissues also contain alkaline phosphatases which often differ slightly from one another (isoenzymes). To avoid diagnostic confusion, elevation of blood alkaline phosphatase must be interpreted in the clinical context and not in isolation. Measurement of specific isoenzymes is increasingly being undertaken to identify the tissue of origin.

Parathyroid hormone

Although measurement of PTH by radioimmunoassay is an important adjunct to the diagnosis of some metabolic bone disorders, interpretation of the results requires appreciation of the limitations of the methodology and of the relationships between PTH, calcium and the vitamin D endocrine system $(1,25(OH)_2D)$. PTH in plasma is present as intact PTH (84 amino acids) and also as several different peptide fragments. New assays use antibodies to two sites on the molecule and detect only the intact PTH. Elevated PTH is found in primary or secondary hyperparathyroidism, and in all patients with target organ resistance to the action of PTH (pseudohypoparathyroidism). PTH is undetectable in patients with hypoparathyroidism.

25-hydroxyvitamin D

Although 25-hydroxyvitamin D (25(OH)D) is the precursor of the active hormonal form of vitamin D (Fig. 18.3), measurements of 25(OH)D are the best guide to vitamin D status. 25(OH)D in plasma shows a seasonal variation, being high in summer and lower in winter. This reflects dependence of cutaneous production of vitamin D on ultraviolet light. Plasma levels are lower in vitamin D deficiency, due to lack of sunlight exposure and poor diet, normal in patients with renal disease, and elevated in patients with vitamin D intoxication. Measurement of $1,25(OH)_2D$ (the active hormonal form of vitamin D) has little clinical application.

Urinary cyclic-AMP

Most of the cyclic-AMP (cAMP) in urine is generated by PTH action on the kidney; urinary cAMP therefore provides a good measure of a biological effect of circulating PTH and theoretically avoids the difficulties inherent in the radioimmunoassay of PTH. As expected, urinary cAMP is elevated in primary hyperparathyroidism (p. 731) and secondary hyperparathyroidism due to intestinal disease, and is low in hypoparathyroid states (p. 733).

Radiography

Plain radiographs are of great value in the diagnosis of localised disorders of bone, e.g. developmental abnormalities, fractures, tumours and infections. In addition, some diseases affecting the entire skeleton may also be diagnosed in this way. For example, severe osteoporosis may lead to radiologically evident fractures, and hyperparathyroidism may be associated with visible subperiosteal erosions in the hands and elsewhere (Fig. 18.4). In these instances, local abnormalities are acting as markers for generalised disease.

Radionuclide studies

Bone-seeking radionuclides such as ^{99m}Tc methylene bisphosphonate may be given by intravenous injection, and the pattern of uptake assessed by external counting using

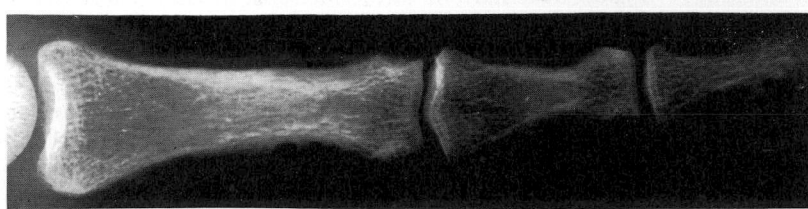

Fig. 18.4 X-ray showing subperiosteal erosions in the hands in a case of hyperparathyroidism.

a gamma camera. Uptake is largely determined by blood flow to bone and by the rate of bone turnover; the technique is therefore extremely good at detecting focal lesions, such as metastases, infections, Paget's disease or subtle fractures, that may not be visible on conventional radiographs.

Measurement of bone mass

The increasing proportion of elderly people in populations worldwide inevitably leads to an increase in the incidence of age-related diseases such as osteoporosis. The ability to measure bone mass with precision and accuracy, and in a simple and safe manner, is central to the identification, assessment and monitoring of patients with osteoporosis. Conventional radiography is imprecise and crude, and has little to offer apart from identification of fractures. Recently, dual x-ray absorptiometry has been developed, which has high precision for measuring bone and mineral content of the spine and femoral neck.

Histology

The technique of transiliac bone biopsy, whereby a cortex-to-cortex core of bone 5–8mm in diameter is taken from the ilium under local anaesthetic, is increasingly employed in the diagnosis and assessment of generalised metabolic bone disease. The specimens may yield useful information on the number and activity of osteoblasts and osteoclasts, and indicate whether organic matrix production is normal and being appropriately mineralised. A useful adjunct is the technique of tetracycline labelling. Here, tetracycline (600–900 mg of demeclocycline) is given twice, with a 10-day interval between; the biopsy is performed four or more days after the second label is taken. The drug is taken up at the mineralisation front in bone, and can be detected in the biopsy specimen by fluorescence under ultraviolet light. Uptake is poor or absent in osteomalacia (p. 728) and enhanced in states of high bone turnover (e.g. hyperparathyroidism and thyrotoxicosis).

OSTEOPOROSIS

The term osteoporosis denotes loss of bone mass per unit volume; bone composition is normal. It becomes clinically important when bone is so weak that pathological fractures result. Most examples of osteoporosis arise as a result of the progressive decrease in bone mass with age (Fig. 18.2); since this occurs to a greater or lesser extent in all individuals, the distinction between pathology and the normal ageing process is blurred.

Pathological changes in bone mass

Bone mass is governed by the balance between bone formation and resorption. Positive, neutral and negative bone balance are found at different ages. Thus, in infancy and again in adolescence, bone formation clearly exceeds resorption; in early adult life, the processes are approximately equal; and later, a disparity in favour of resorption results in a slow decline in total bone mass (Fig. 18.2). Whether or not this gives rise to clinical problems (fractures) depends to a large extent on the maximum bone mass achieved as an adult. This is greater in men than women and is also greater in blacks than whites.

Women are further disadvantaged by a more rapid decrease in bone mass in later adult life, and the net result is a much higher incidence of osteoporotic complications. On average, they also live for about five years longer than men. The reasons for the sex differences in rate of bone loss are probably multiple, but postmenopausal oestrogen deficiency is most strongly implicated. This condition may sensitise the skeleton to the bone-resorbing effects of PTH and possibly also impairs renal synthesis of $1,25(OH)_2D$. The resulting changes are subtle, but may lead to mild but chronic calcium malabsorption and consequent secondary hyperparathyroidism (pp. 727 and 733). In extreme old age bone loss in men catches up with that in women.

Idiopathic osteoporosis may occasionally occur in young people, especially during the adolescent growth spurt. It is usually self-limiting, but may be complicated by fractures.

Clinical features and investigation

Osteoporosis remains asymptomatic unless structural collapse or fracture of bone occurs. Damage is particularly likely to occur in the dorsal vertebrae, femoral neck and distal radius; precipitating trauma may be trivial.

There are usually no abnormalities on routine plasma biochemistry, except in those cases secondary to specific endocrine disorders (see below). In some patients, urinary calcium excretion may be elevated consistent with net bone resorption, and plasma calcium may be marginally elevated. This is particularly common when immobility is a contributory factor.

Plain radiographs demonstrate decreased bone density due to loss of trabeculae, and reduced cortical thickness of long bones, in severe cases. The dorsal vertebrae may show the classical 'wedge collapse' of osteoporotic crush fracture and herniation of the disc into the centre of the vertebra to give a 'codfish' vertebra, and exaggeration of the normal curvature of the thoracic spine (Fig. 18.5). Detection and assessment of osteoporosis is best achieved by measurements of bone mass by dual X-ray absorptiometry or CT scanning of the spine.

Normality of plasma calcium, phosphate and alkaline phosphatase helps to exclude osteomalacia but, in doubtful

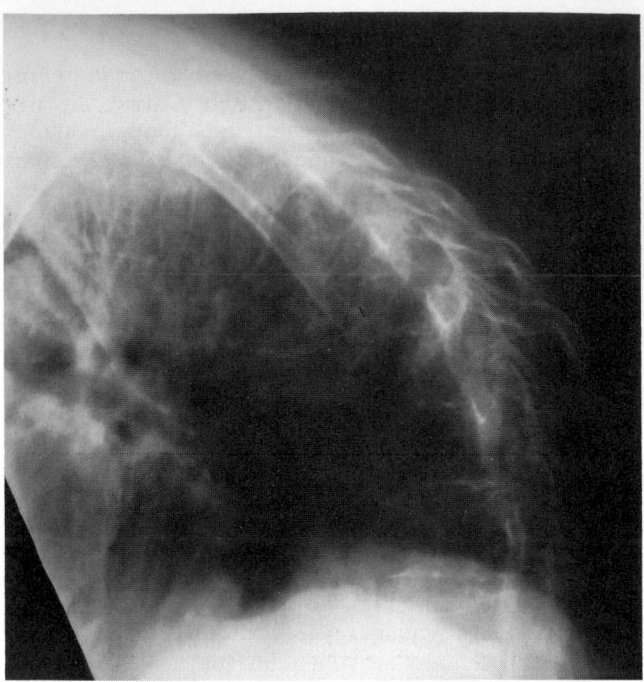

Fig. 18.5 X-ray of lateral thoracic spine of a 60-year-old woman with severe postmenopausal osteoporosis. Note gross loss of density, collapsed and 'codfish' vertebrae and kyphosis.

cases, further investigation may be necessary, including measurement of plasma 25-hydroxyvitamin D and transiliac bone biopsy.

In most instances, no specific underlying cause for osteoporosis will be found. However, careful consideration should be given to the causes outlined below, and further investigation initiated if the overall clinical picture so warrants.

Specific causes of osteoporosis

Osteoporosis is common in the elderly and it may be difficult to decide whether a vertebral collapse is due to osteoporosis or to another, coincidental, underlying disease such as secondary carcinoma. Cancer of the breast, lung, kidney and thyroid typically cause lytic lesions in bone. Prostatic cancer may also do so, though sclerosis is more common. Breast cancer in particular has a predilection for secondary spread to the axial skeleton. Myeloma (Ch. 24, p. 1078) may be accompanied by generalised thinning of bones and/or focal lytic areas. Physical examination will usually detect a primary breast cancer, but further investigation may be needed to exclude other forms of cancer and myeloma.

Chronic liver disease (especially primary biliary cirrhosis) may give rise to a mixed picture of osteoporosis and osteomalacia (see below). Hereditary abnormalities in bone formation are discussed on page 737.

The conditions which may be complicated by significant osteoporosis are listed in Table 18.3.

Management

Prevention

Prevention of the development of osteoporosis in individuals at risk is of the utmost importance. This is most obviously the case in females with primary or premature ovarian failure, who should be treated with oestrogens. Progestogen supplements should also be given cyclically or at low dose continuously (p. 714) to avoid unopposed endometrial stimulation with its risk of neoplastic change. However, the use of prophylactic oestrogen supplements after the physiological menopause is more controversial. Oestrogen undoubtedly reduces the rate of bone loss after the menopause (and even increases bone mass in many patients); despite earlier concerns, this is probably not associated with an increased risk of vascular pathology, at least at low dosage. Appropriate exercise, e.g. regular swimming, should be encouraged in patients with relative immobility, and regular non-strenuous exercise in the elderly.

Treatment

The treatment of established osteoporosis is, unfortunately, often unsatisfactory. With the exception of oestrogens and bisphosphonates, no form of therapy has been shown to have a consistent effect in reversing bone changes, although retardation of bone loss may be possible. Dietary calcium should be generous (at least 25–50

Table 18.3 Causes of generalised osteoporosis and their mechanisms*

Cause	Bone resorption	Bone formation
Common causes		
Corticosteriod excess	↑	↓
Early menopause	↑	Normal
Immobility	↑	↓
Multiple myeloma[†]	↑	↓
Rare causes		
Hypogonadism (primary or secondary)	Normal	↓
Thyrotoxicosis[†]	↑	↑
Type I diabetes mellitus	Normal	↓
Pregnancy	↑	↓
Primary hyperparathyroidism[†]	↑	↑

Primary liver disease is omitted since this is associated with a combination of osteoporosis and osteomalacia.
[†] Conditions in which the plasma calcium may be increased.

Summary 1 Prevention and management of osteoporosis

Prevention	Management
Physical activity (youth and throughout adulthood)	Physical exercise
	Weight gain if underweight
Non-smoking	Stop smoking
Good diet (generous calcium intake and avoiding excess alcohol)	Calcium supplements
	Oestrogen therapy
Early and effective treatment of predisposing conditions:	
Hypogonadism/premature menopause	Bisphosphonates or calcitonin
Thyrotoxicosis	Symptomatic therapy, e.g. lumbar supports
Cushing's syndrome	
Diabetes mellitus	
Hyperparathyroidism	

mmol per day); if this is not achieved, the diet may be supplemented with calcium carbonate tablets. The evidence that calcium supplements are of benefit is conflicting, but the therapy is easy and does no harm. There is strong evidence now that in the very old, calcium and vitamin D supplementation reduces hip fracture incidence. In selected patients, an argument may be made for oestrogen supplements, particularly where oestrogen deficiency has been present at an abnormally early stage in life.

Preparations of 'hydroxyapatite compound' are of no proven benefit above that of simple calcium salts, and anabolic steroids are of doubtful value. Other measures currently under investigation include the use of calcitonin, interval bisphosphonate therapy with calcium and vitamin D supplements, PTH, and sodium fluoride.

RICKETS AND OSTEOMALACIA

Rickets and osteomalacia are conditions characterised by pathological defects in bone matrix mineralisation. Rickets refers specifically to osteomalacia where the defect occurs in *growing* bone. The aetiological factors are diverse, but the end result is an increased quantity of unmineralised bone matrix (osteoid). Histologically this is characterised by widened osteoid seams, morphologically flat 'inactive' osteoblasts, and absence of tetracycline uptake indicating impairment of mineralisation. The increase in osteoid must be distinguished from that seen in thyrotoxic bone disease, Paget's disease or hyperparathyroidism. In all these conditions, there is high bone turnover with 'hyperosteoidosis'; mineralisation of matrix is normal or enhanced.

Aetiology

The aetiology of osteomalacia (or rickets) is shown in Table 18.4. The conditions may arise in three distinct situations:

- deficiency or abnormal metabolism of vitamin D
- phosphate depletion
- chronic metabolic acidosis.

Vitamin D deficiency is numerically by far the most important cause of osteomalacia (or rickets). It leads to combined deficiency of calcium and phosphorus. There is intestinal malabsorption of calcium and, to a lesser extent, phosphorus. *Secondary hyperparathyroidism* results, and the ensuing phosphaturia accelerates the phosphate deficiency. Lack of vitamin D is often due to a combination of poor exposure to sunlight together with dietary deficiency. The elderly population is particularly at risk. In the UK, there is a very high incidence of osteomalacia

Table 18.4 Causes of osteomalacia/rickets

Cause	Mechanism
Vitamin D deficiency	Defective intake/formation
	Lack of solar exposure (D_3) and lack of dietary intake or fat malabsorption (D_2)
	Severe chronic liver disease
	Increased/wasteful metabolism
	Liver-enzyme-inducing drugs, e.g. phenytoin, phenobarbitone, carbamazepine, rifampicin
	Failure of activation, $25(OH)D \rightarrow 1,25(OH)_2D$
	Chronic renal failure
	Hereditary vitamin D-dependent rickets type I
	Target organ defect
	Hereditary vitamin D-dependent rickets type II
Phosphate deficiency	Poor intake
	Aluminium hydroxide – excess binding of dietary phosphate
	Increased loss
	X-linked hypophosphataemia (vitamin D-resistant rickets)
	Fanconi's syndrome
	Renal tubular acidosis
	Ureterocolic anastamosis
	Tumour-associated
Chronic metabolic acidosis	Renal tubular acidosis (may be phosphate depletion also)
	Ureterocolic anastamosis
Osteoblast/ mineralisation defect	Hypophosphatasia
	Etidronate therapy
	Aluminium intoxication (in renal disease, see p. 809)

in the Asian immigrant population (p. 111). The reason for this is multifactorial and incompletely understood but dietary deficiency of vitamin D and calcium together with binding of calcium by the phytate contained in chapatti flour may contribute. In addition, deeply pigmented skin generates less vitamin D_3 in response to a given amount of ultraviolet exposure and this may be disadvantageous in temperate climates. Vitamin D deficiency may complicate fat malabsorption from any cause. Finally, calcium deficiency enhances the rate of degradation of 25(OH)D in the liver, further exacerbating the shortage of vitamin D and its metabolites.

Failure of 25-hydroxylation of vitamin D (p. 721, Fig. 18.3). This may be a feature of severe hepatocellular dysfunction. It may also result from hepatic enzyme induction consequent upon long-term anticonvulsant medication (leading to enhanced degradation).

Reduced 1-hydroxylation of 25-hydroxyvitamin D by the kidney occurs in chronic renal failure, and also as a rare recessively inherited condition in which levels of the 1-hydroxylase enzyme are low (vitamin D-dependent rickets type I). Failure to hydroxylate 25-hydroxyvitamin D also occurs in hypoparathyroidism and pseudohypoparathyroidism. Another rare form of rickets is associated with an abnormality of the 1,25(OH)$_2$D receptor in target tissues (vitamin D-dependent rickets type II).

Phosphate depletion is a less common cause of rickets than deficiency or altered metabolism of vitamin D. It arises as a result of a reduced maximal capacity for renal tubular phosphate reabsorption. This may either be inherited as an X-linked recessive characteristic (vitamin D-resistant rickets) or occur as part of Fanconi's syndrome – a more generalised hereditary or acquired renal tubular defect typified by aminoaciduria and glycosuria (p. 814). Rarely, excessive ingestion of antacids may restrict intestinal phosphate absorption to the point where clinically important phosphate depletion, and even osteomalacia or rickets, may appear.

Chronic metabolic acidosis, usually resulting from renal tubular disorders, may lead to rickets or osteomalacia. The bone lesions usually heal satisfactorily following treatment to correct the acidosis.

Oncogenic osteomalacia. Severe osteomalacia may rarely be a non-metastatic manifestation of tumours. The tumours are almost always sarcomas or connective tissue tumours of borderline malignancy (neurofibromatosis, haemangioendothelioma). The osteomalacia is cured by removal of the tumour.

Clinical features

In children, failure of bone mineralisation gives rise to classical bone deformities which include widening of the metaphyses, prominence of costochondral junctions (so-called 'rickety rosary') and varus or valgus abnormalities of the knee joints. The bones are painful and statural growth is reduced. In adults, bone pain and tenderness are the most prominent features. A characteristic proximal myopathy may develop, and is more common in cases due to vitamin D deficiency.

Investigation

Biochemical. In osteomalacia due to deficiency or abnormal metabolism of vitamin D, investigations typically demonstrate a low normal plasma calcium (leading to secondary hyperparathyroidism), a low plasma phosphate resulting from increased PTH-dependent phosphaturia, and a raised alkaline phosphatase indicating increased numbers of osteoblasts (Table 18.5). Vitamin D deficiency may be confirmed by measurement of 25-hydroxyvitamin D in plasma. X-linked hypophosphataemia, on the other hand, is characterised by normocalcaemia, hypophosphataemia and little or no alteration in plasma alkaline phosphatase level.

Radiological features of rickets include widening and irregularity of the metaphysis with an increased width of the growth plate. In osteomalacia, the bones appear less dense than normal and the long bones may show localised areas of decalcification on the concave surface, referred to as pseudofractures or Looser's zones (Fig. 18.6). Decreased strength of bone may result in biconcave deformity of the vertebrae. In hypophosphataemic rickets, there may be a paradoxical apparent increase in bone density.

Histological. Occasionally a bone biopsy may be needed (following double tetracycline labelling) to confirm a diagnosis of osteomalacia when biochemical investigations are equivocal. This is particularly the case when seeking possible treatable factors in elderly patients with decreased bone density.

Table 18.5 Plasma measurements in various causes of osteomalacia/rickets

Cause	Plasma measurements					
	Calcium	Phosphate	Alk. phos.	Urea	Creatinine	pH
Vitamin D deficiency	N or ↓	↓	↑	N	N	N
Familial hypophosphataemia	N	↓↓	N or ↑	N	N	N
Chronic renal failure	N or ↓	↑	N or ↑	↑	↑	↓
Renal tubular acidosis	N or ↓	N or ↓	N or ↑	N	N	↓↓

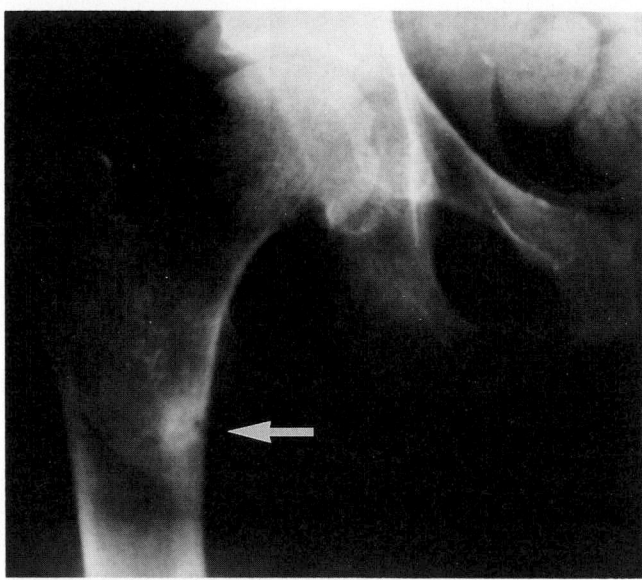

Fig. 18.6 Radiological features of osteomalacia. Arrow indicates Looser's zone.

Management

Dietary vitamin D deficiency is treated by oral replacement of vitamin D_2 or vitamin D_3 in physiological quantities (500–1000 units per day). This can conveniently be given as combined calcium with vitamin D tablets. Alternatively, a single i.m. dose of 150 000 IU of D_2 in oil is effective prophylaxis and treatment for at least six months. The possibility of intestinal malabsorption should be borne in mind, and appropriate investigation initiated if necessary. Osteomalacia associated with anticonvulsant therapy requires higher doses of vitamin D (3000–6000 units/day). Treatment of X-linked hypophosphataemia is generally unsatisfactory. The logical treatment is with oral phosphate supplements, but the doses needed are large and they may be poorly tolerated because of gastrointestinal side-effects. Oral phosphate works better when combined with pharmacological doses of vitamin D or (and probably best) in combination with $1,25(OH)_2D_3$. When $1,25(OH)_2D_3$ or $1\alpha OHD_3$ is given, great care must be taken to adjust the dose against the serum calcium as hypercalcaemia may easily be induced. The management of renal tubular acidosis and renal osteodystrophy is dealt with in Chapter 20, pages 814–816.

HYPERCALCAEMIA

Elevation of total plasma calcium is usually associated with a concomitant increase in ionised calcium concentration.

Causes

A large number of conditions may be associated with hypercalcaemia (Table 18.6). Improvements in our understanding of vitamin D and parathyroid physiology enable reasonably accurate classification of the condition according to basic mechanisms. In Table 18.6 they are classified according to the level of $1,25(OH)_2D$. When this hormone is elevated, it may be presumed to be causing hypercalcaemia by stimulating intestinal absorption of calcium and bone resorption. The details of pathophysiology are discussed in the subsequent section.

Clinical features

Mild hypercalcaemia is generally asymptomatic. Severe hypercalcaemia, however, leads to a life-threatening acute illness; its treatment constitutes a medical emergency. The principal symptoms and signs are renal, gastrointestinal and neurological.

Renal. Thirst and polyuria are early symptoms of nephrogenic diabetes insipidus. The increased ionised calcium level impairs the ADH-mediated mechanism of water reabsorption in the distal nephron. Sodium and potassium excretion are increased, leading to volume contraction, pre-renal reduction of GFR (Ch. 20, p. 788) and a further decrease in renal calcium excretion. The situation is compounded if the patient is ill and confined to bed, and so enters further negative skeletal calcium balance.

Table 18.6 Causes of hypercalcaemia

Elevated levels of $1,25(OH)_2D$	
With high levels of PTH	
Primary hyperparathyroidism	– Adenoma
	– Hyperplasia
	– Carcinoma
'Tertiary' hyperparathyroidism	
With low levels of PTH	
Increased vitamin D intake	
Increased extrarenal synthesis of $1,25(OH)_2D$	
– Lymphoma	
– Sarcoidosis	
– Tuberculosis	
– Glucocorticoid deficiency (Addison's disease)	
Tumour–induced with circulating PTH-related peptide (PTH-rp)	
– Squamous carcinoma	
– Adenocarcinoma of kidney	
Low or normal levels of $1,25(OH)_2D$	
Tumour-induced	
Osteolytic bone lesions	– carcinoma (breast, oesophagus, lung, thyroid)
	– Multiple myelomatosis
Cytokines	– Leukaemias
Milk alkali syndrome	
Familial hypocalciuric hypercalcaemia	

Gastrointestinal. Common early symptoms are anorexia and constipation. Later, particularly when pre-renal uraemia develops, the patient develops nausea and vomiting.

Neurological symptoms commonly include lassitude, anxiety and depression, or any psychosis to which that person may be otherwise predisposed. In severe hypercalcaemia (calcium levels above 4 mmol/l), confusion and drowsiness may be superseded by coma.

Regardless of cause, hypercalcaemia is liable to be complicated by ectopic calcification. This is particularly likely if the hypercalcaemia is of long standing as in primary hyperparathyroidism or sarcoidosis. The renal tract is particularly susceptible, and renal stones or nephrocalcinosis (Fig. 18.7) commonly occur. Frequently, there is calcification of blood vessels, especially the media of arteries. Calcification bands on the medial or lateral edge of the cornea may be visible (band keratopathy) and conjunctival inflammation may develop if hypercalcaemia is severe. Acute pancreatitis is an important complication, particularly if other factors, such as high alcohol intake, are also operating.

Finally, the cardiovascular system is also susceptible through the increased incidence of hypertension associated with chronic hypercalcaemia. The ECG shows shortening of the QT interval.

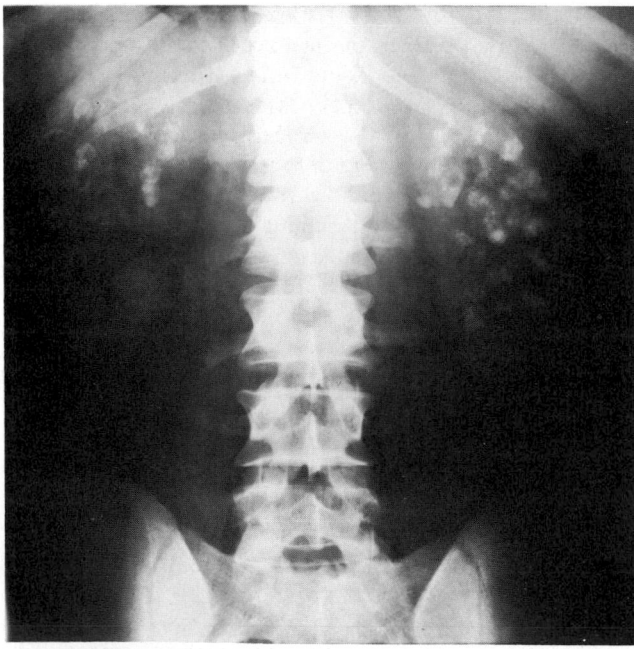

Fig. 18.7 Nephrocalcinosis in a patient with severe primary hyperparathyroidism.

Investigation

Potentially useful investigations in hypercalcaemia are listed in Table 18.7.

The *steroid suppression test* aims to identify those cases in which pharmacological doses of glucocorticoids reduce significantly the elevated plasma calcium. Hypercalcaemia due to extrarenal $1,25(OH)_2D$ synthesis usually suppresses fully, and this is likely to be the case with underlying granulomatous disease (e.g. sarcoidosis, tuberculosis), some malignancies (e.g. leukaemia, lymphoma) and glucocorticoid deficiency (Addison's disease). Prednisolone is given at 30 mg/day for 10 days, with measurement of plasma calcium before, after 5 days and after 10 days of treatment.

Management of symptomatic hypercalcaemia

Asymptomatic hypercalcaemia requires no therapy except appropriate management of the underlying condition.

Table 18.7 Diagnostic yield in hypercalcaemia

Investigation	Potential information
Full blood count	Anaemia suggests non-parathyroid aetiology if renal function normal
ESR	Usually over 80 in myeloma
Plasma chloride	Upper normal in hyperparathyroidism
Plasma bicarbonate	Low normal in hyperparathyroidism
Creatinine	Significantly raised in the tertiary autonomous hyperparathyroidism of renal failure. Moderately raised in renal impairment secondary to hypercalcaemia
Plasma protein electrophoresis	Monoclonal band suggests myeloma
Bradshaw's test and urinary immunoelectrophoresis	Presence of light chains suggests myeloma
Plasma phosphate	Low normal in primary hyperparathyroidism unless renal function impaired
Plasma PTH	Upper normal or raised in hyperparathyroidism. Suppressed with other causes of hypercalcaemia
Steroid suppression test	Sarcoid hypercalcaemia always suppresses; hyperparathyroid never; malignant causes occasionally
24 h urine calcium	Decreased in familial hypocalciuric hypercalcaemia
Chest X-ray	Look for primary neoplasm; metastases; hilar lymphadenopathy suggesting sarcoid
Isotope bone scan	'Hot spots' suggest metastatic malignant disease
X-ray hands	Subperiosteal erosions suggest hyperparathyroidism

General measures

Symptomatic hypercalcaemia requires measures directed towards rehydration and appropriate sodium and potassium repletion. A forced saline diuresis (normal saline given i.v. at 4–6 l/day) substantially and immediately augments the urinary excretion of calcium; a further increase in calciuria may be induced by the addition of frusemide (20 mg/hour), *provided that the saline infusion is fast enough to keep the patient volume-expanded.* With such treatment alone, the plasma calcium will usually come down to safe levels (3.5 mmol/l or less).

Specific measures

Specific treatment depends on the cause. Glucocorticoids are only effective for the hypercalcaemia of sarcoidosis, vitamin D intoxication, lymphomas and Addison's disease; for the first two, a high dose rapidly tapering down is used. Sodium phosphate infusion (10 mmol/hour for a maximum of 10 hours) is very effective in the short term, but is dangerous, as it lowers calcium principally by causing microscopic precipitation of calcium phosphate in soft tissues; this is particularly marked if initial plasma phosphate is high. For hypercalcaemia due to increased bone resorption, calcitonin at high dose is effective but very short-lived.

The treatment of choice in hypercalcaemia of malignancy is now the bisphosphonate pamidronate, which reliably restores calcium levels to normal within five days when infused at doses of 15 mg i.v. in saline over two hours daily for four days, or as a single dose of 60 mg over eight hours. Clodronate is equally effective and can be given orally as maintenance treatment. The drugs act by inhibiting osteoclastic bone resorption, but because of a delayed action (24–72 hours) saline diuresis remains an important part of early management. Calcitonin given at the same time accelerates the fall in calcium by up to 24 hours.

Summary 2 Treatment of severe hypercalcaemia

- Correct salt and water deficit with normal saline
- Begin forced saline diuresis + frusemide
- Give bisphosphonate, e.g. pamidronate, clodronate
- Treat underlying cause if possible

SPECIFIC CAUSES OF HYPERCALCAEMIA

PRIMARY HYPERPARATHYROIDISM

Primary overactivity of one or more parathyroid glands is common, especially in elderly women. In the UK, routine measurement of serum calcium in the hospital population reveals an incidence of at least 1%. Of these, approximately three-quarters are associated with a single adenoma; in the others, there is either more than one adenoma, or four-gland hyperplasia. In about 1% of cases, a parathyroid carcinoma underlies the disease. Adenoma or hyperplasia may be associated with one of the syndromes (I or II) of multiple endocrine neoplasia (p. 706).

In primary hyperparathyroidism, PTH is elevated, usually as a result of a parathyroid adenoma, and stimulates osteoclastic bone resorption, tubular reabsorption of calcium and the activity of 1-hydroxylase in the proximal renal tubular cells. This in turn promotes conversion of $25(OH)D$ to $1,25(OH)_2D$, which acts on the upper small intestine to increase active calcium transport. Since PTH also enhances renal phosphate excretion, the serum phosphate level falls.

Clinical features

The clinical features of primary hyperparathyroidism are variable. Patients commonly remain asymptomatic for long periods, and the finding of a mild elevation of serum calcium in an elderly asymptomatic patient requires no active intervention. In more severe cases, the symptoms may be those of *hypercalcaemia* (p. 729). Immobilisation is a potent precipitating factor, which may lead to a rapid rise in serum calcium.

Renal complications include renal calculi, which may present with renal colic and nephrocalcinosis (Fig. 18.7). This is particularly likely in warm climates, where insensible fluid and sodium loss are excessive and urine flow rate low. Hypertension is common, even in the absence of overt renal damage; there is debate as to whether it responds to surgical treatment of hyperparathyroidism.

The bone disease of hyperparathyroidism is characterised by high turnover due to excess osteoclasis. It is usually asymptomatic, although there may be osteoporosis, especially in postmenopausal women. Very infrequently, osteitis fibrosa cystica occurs, with the development of so-called 'brown tumours' of the mandible or long bones. Again, the finding of such a lesion is an indication to check the serum biochemistry. The typical radiological lesion is subperiosteal erosion in the phalanges of the hands (Fig. 18.4).

Management

The severity of the hypercalcaemia should be assessed, as well as the occurrence of complications. In cases with severe clinical hypercalcaemia, emergency treatment should be initiated along the lines outlined above. The only curative therapy is parathyroid surgery. Modern diagnostic techniques which may help to localise a tumour include technetium-thallium subtraction scanning of the neck and (rarely) catheterisation of the veins draining from the neck, for measurement of PTH in blood from different sites. High resolution CT scanning and ultrasound may also be of value.

Surgery

Ultimately, treatment falls to the surgeon, whose expertise in identifying all four parathyroids will determine the success of the operation. Adenomas of the lower parathyroids (derived from the upper pair of branchial arches) are sometimes retrosternal, but can be located at surgery by pulling up the thymus gland, with which they are closely associated. All four glands should be biopsied, and adenomatous tissue removed. With four-gland hyperplasia, the safe course is probably to remove all four, and then to maintain the hypoparathyroid patient on $1,25(OH)_2D_3$ or $1(OH)D_3$ (alfacalcidol), a synthetic precursor of $1,25(OH)_2D_3$. Pre- and postoperative treatment with $1,25(OH)_2D_3$ or $1(OH)D_3$ may be helpful in preventing postoperative hypocalcaemia.

Other measures

In some patients, surgical cure is not achieved. Failure to remove enough parathyroid tissue may leave the patient with 'incurable' hyperparathyroidism. Some patients refuse surgery and, because primary hyperparathyroidism is principally a disease of the elderly, some will be deemed unfit for surgery. Conservative management of these patients may entail observation only, with monitoring of plasma calcium concentration and checking for complications. More active measures include the use of oral phosphate supplements or the bisphosphonate pamidronate (p. 731). However, although both will alleviate hypercalciuria and hypercalcaemia in the short and medium term, surgery remains the preferred treatment in most younger and symptomatic older patients.

HYPERCALCAEMIA OF MALIGNANCY

Malignancy is an important cause of hypercalcaemia. There are several mechanisms:

- Direct invasion of bone and production of local factors, which either destroy bone directly or stimulate local osteoclasts to do so, leads to accelerated bone resorption. Breast cancer commonly causes hypercalcaemia by this mechanism. If calcium is elevated in a patient with breast cancer, it virtually always indicates that metastases are present.
- Haematological malignancies may produce lymphokines which act as osteoclast-activating factors; included in this group is multiple myeloma, which

may also cause a spurious elevation of (protein-bound) calcium, when the monoclonal immunoglobulin also binds calcium.
- Some haematological malignancies can produce excessive amounts of $1,25(OH)_2D$ although this is uncommon.
- Finally, some solid tumours (such as renal carcinomas and some squamous carcinomas) may cause hypercalcaemia by secreting PTH-related peptide (PTH-rp), a factor which activates bone resorption, and/or enhances renal tubular calcium reabsorption and the renal production of $1,25(OH)_2D$. This peptide has partial sequence homology with PTH (accounting for the hypercalcaemia) but is not detected by PTH immunoassays.

Clinical features

These are of hypercalcaemia normally associated with those of the underlying cancer. The hypercalcaemia is usually rapidly progressive and severe, with salt and water depletion and disturbance of renal and CNS function.

Management

This is as for hypercalcaemia generally (p. 731). Saline rehydration and diuresis and bisphosphonates are the main methods. The cancer is treated when possible.

MISCELLANEOUS HYPERCALCAEMIC SYNDROMES

In *sarcoidosis*, and some other granulomatous diseases, macrophages in the diseased tissue make $1,25(OH)_2D$ outside the kidneys in amounts that are sufficient to produce hypercalcaemia. Calcium is absorbed by the intestine in increased amounts, PTH is suppressed, and the normal feedback of the vitamin D-endocrine system is effectively sabotaged. The same mechanism occurs in some lymphomas and sarcomas.

Milk alkali syndrome, now rarely seen, is associated with excessive ingestion of milk and alkali, particularly if taken in the form of calcium carbonate, to relieve dyspepsia. The hypercalcaemia is accompanied by metabolic alkalosis and is due to a combination of increased intestinal calcium absorption and decreased renal calcium excretion.

Addison's disease may present with hypercalcaemia through extrarenal production of $1,25(OH)_2D$. Glucocorticoid replacement leads to a prompt response. In a patient with coincidental Addison's disease and hypoparathyroidism, the potential hypocalcaemia of the latter may be masked until glucocorticoids are given.

Thyrotoxicosis. Thyroid hormones increase bone turnover and, in excess, cause net efflux of calcium from bone. Some 30% of these patients display hypercalciuria and/or hypercalcaemia, although the latter is not severe. These abnormalities are corrected by treatment of the underlying thyrotoxicosis.

Familial hypocalciuric hypercalcaemia is a recently recognised syndrome that may be detected at any age. It is usually asymptomatic, and is not associated with renal damage (although it may cause pancreatitis). It is inherited as an autosomal dominant condition, and so can usually be excluded if both parents are available for blood sampling. It appears to be due to excessively avid renal tubular calcium reabsorption.

HYPOCALCAEMIA

Causes and pathophysiology

The principal causes of hypocalcaemia are listed in Table 18.8. Since the major calcium-binding protein in plasma is albumin, hypoalbuminaemia is associated with a proportionate fall in plasma total calcium (see correction formula on p. 723), though not in ionised calcium. The ionised calcium concentration is affected by the blood pH, since the avidity of albumin for calcium falls at acid pH and rises with alkalosis. Hence, respiratory alkalosis due to overbreathing can lead to depression of ionic calcium and tetany. Rarely, infusion of citrate (e.g. in repeated blood transfusions) leads to a serious fall in ionised calcium by complexing the ion.

In *hypoparathyroidism* (p. 734) the major abnormalities result from failure of PTH-dependent renal synthesis of l,25(OH)₂D, leading to a reduction of intestinal calcium absorption. This is compounded by failure of osteoclastic bone resorption, by enhanced (inappropriate) urine calci-

Table 18.8 Causes of hypocalcaemia

Cause	Comments
With low levels of PTH	
Hypoparathyroidism	Phosphate high
Post-surgical	Alkaline phosphatase and
Congenital	renal function normal
Idiopathic (autoimmune)	
With normal or high levels of PTH	
Rickets/osteomalacia	Phosphate low
Sunlight/dietary deficiency	Alkaline phosphatase high
Malabsorption	Calcium deficiency
Increased D metabolism	Drug-induced
Tumour-induced	
Chronic renal failure	Urea, creatinine, phosphate high
Pseudohypoparathyroidism	Phosphate high, somatic manifestations (type I only)

Table 18.9 Causes of secondary hyperparathyroidism

Cause	Example
Vitamin D deficiency	Lack of solar exposure
	Dietary deficiency
	Increased catabolism – drug-induced (e.g. anticonvulsants, rifampicin)
Dietary calcium deficiency	Low calcium intake
	High phytic acid intake (chapattis, wholemeal bread)
Gastrointestinal causes of low calcium or vitamin D intake	Gastric surgery
	Partial gastrectomy
	Gastroenterostomy
	Vagotomy and pyloroplasty
	Jejunal diverticulosis
	Crohn's disease
	Small bowel resection
Renal	Chronic renal failure
	Phosphate retention
	Reduced 1α-hydroxylation of 25(OH)D

um excretion and by hyperphosphataemia; all of these are due to loss of the normal effects of PTH on bone and kidney.

Secondary hyperparathyroidism is a consequence of hypocalcaemia (Table 18.9). In *chronic renal failure* (CRF), hypocalcaemia results from phosphate retention and loss of renal parenchyma with failure to produce normal amounts of 1,25(OH)₂D. A rise in serum phosphate from any cause depresses the serum calcium, partly by leading to microprecipitation of calcium phosphate in soft tissue. The associated bone disease is discussed on page 806. In CRF, metabolic acidosis is commonly present, and this diminishes the fall in ionised calcium. Tetany is rare in adults (but more common in children), at least until the acidosis is corrected. Hypocalcaemia in *vitamin D deficiency* is usually not severe, because secondary hyperparathyroidism enhances bone resorption and maintains the serum calcium level. The typical biochemical changes are borderline low serum calcium, a low phosphate, and elevated alkaline phosphatase level. If the parathyroid glands do not respond, or calcium intake is very low, hypocalcaemia may be more profound.

In CRF and vitamin D deficiency, and in other conditions (listed in Table 18.9), the parathyroid hypersecretion (secondary hyperparathyroidism) is an *appropriate* response to threatened or actual hypocalcaemia. In some patients, however, long-standing appropriate hypersecretion (secondary hyperparathyroidism) transforms to *inappropriate* autonomy and consequent hypercalcaemia. This is called tertiary hyperparathyroidism.

Pseudohypoparathyroidism is discussed on page 734.

Clinical features

The clinical manifestations of hypocalcaemia are principally in the nervous system. Tetany, painful cramps and tingling in the extremities may occur, and muscle spasm may lead to a characteristic position of the hand, the so-called 'main d'accoucheur'. These symptoms may be precipitated by exercise. Laryngeal spasm may lead to stridor and obstructed respiration. Hypocalcaemia lowers the epileptic seizure threshold, and fits may be the presenting symptom. The differential diagnosis is principally of tetany due to anxiety leading to hyperventilation and respiratory alkalosis, or hypokalaemic metabolic alkalosis. Hypocalcaemia, particularly when chronic, may present with psychiatric manifestations varying from general malaise to overt psychosis.

Differential diagnosis of hypocalcaemia

Correction for a low serum albumin concentration will allow the distinction between true (ionised) hypocalcaemia and the spurious fall due to hypoalbuminaemia. As with other calcium disorders, the combination of clinical context and routine biochemistry will usually establish the cause. Uraemia and elevated serum creatinine concentration point to CRF. *Hypoparathyroidism* and *pseudohypoparathyroidism* (see below) are associated with normal renal function and an elevated serum phosphate level. There may also be clinical pointers, e.g. recent thyroid or parathyroid surgery for the former, skeletal abnormalities for the latter.

Management

Hypocalcaemic tetany responds rapidly to the intravenous infusion of 10 ml of 10% calcium gluconate; the response, however, is short-lived. The underlying cause should be treated and, in the case of hypoparathyroidism, this has been greatly helped by the availability of $1,25(OH)_2D_3$ (calcitriol) or 1 hydroxyvitamin D_3 (alfacalcidol). The latter is then 25-hydroxylated in the liver to yield $1,25(OH)_2D_3$. By virtue of their high potency, rapid onset and short duration of action, these compounds have converted a very difficult therapeutic problem into an easy one. Hypocalcaemia in osteomalacia due to vitamin D deficiency is seldom marked; here, correct treatment is with vitamin D itself, rather than the active metabolite (p. 729).

SPECIFIC CAUSES OF HYPOCALCAEMIA

Hypoparathyroidism

There are three principal types of hypoparathyroidism, all of which are associated with hypocalcaemia and hyperphosphataemia despite normal renal function.

Postsurgical hypoparathyroidism

Postsurgical hypoparathyroidism is the commonest cause of hypocalcaemia and follows thyroid or parathyroid surgery. Estimates of its frequency vary from 0.2% to 22%, depending on diagnostic criteria and the length of follow-up after surgery. Vascular or mechanical trauma to the parathyroid glands may contribute to the subsequent parathyroid insufficiency.

Idiopathic hypoparathyroidism

This is usually acquired in adolescence or early adult life, and may be associated with autoantibodies to parathyroid tissue, and with other organ-specific autoimmune diseases such as Addison's disease and immune thyroiditis. Some cases are familial. An autoimmune aetiology has been postulated but not proven. Patients may suffer from widespread candida infections and dystrophic nails, alopecia, calcification in the basal ganglia and cataract, in addition to other symptoms and signs of hypocalcaemia.

PTH is undetectable despite hypocalcaemia, and the lack of its effect on the kidney is reflected by renal phosphate retention leading to hyperphosphataemia and low conversion of $25(OH)D$ to $1,25(OH)_2D$. Administration of PTH corrects all the biochemical abnormalities, indicating that target organ responsiveness to PTH remains normal in this condition. However, long-term treatment with PTH is impractical and management is with $1,25(OH)_2D_3$ or $1(OH)D_3$. Most cases respond well to 1–3 µg daily of either; there is, however, little margin for error and the dose should be titrated carefully against the serum calcium levels. Oral calcium supplements enhance the effect of any given dose.

Pseudohypoparathyroidism

Pseudohypoparathyroidism is a rare disorder thought to be due to a defect in the PTH receptor or its coupling to adenylate cyclase. The clinical and biochemical features of hypoparathyroidism are associated with characteristic somatic manifestations; these include short stature, mental deficiency, and unusually short fourth and fifth metacarpals and metatarsals. There is a partial or complete failure of response (urinary cAMP or phosphaturia) to PTH, and high serum PTH levels. As with true hypoparathyroidism, $1,25(OH)_2D$ levels are low. Some patients have the somatic manifestations without the hypocalcaemia (*pseudopseudohypoparathyroidism*). In some cases, the biochemical changes are associated, paradoxically, with hyperparathyroid bone disease, possibly reflecting isolated renal resistance with normal skeletal responsiveness to PTH.

Hypomagnesaemia

Hypomagnesaemia is a rare but important cause of hypocalcaemia. It is refractory to calcium, but responds to magnesium therapy (p. 722).

PAGET'S DISEASE OF BONE

In 1879, Sir James Paget described a bone disease which he named 'osteitis deformans'.

Paget's disease is common and its frequency increases with age. In the UK as many as 4% of the population over the age of 40 may have evidence of the disease, although most have no associated symptoms. It is a chronic focal disease, which may affect virtually any bone in the body. It varies widely in extent, with individual patients having anything from one to 20 or 30 bones affected. Even in a patient with extensive disease, the structure of unaffected bones appears to be quite normal. In general, the axial bones and large long bones are more commonly affected than the small bones of the hands or feet, or the ribs. Within an individual, the distribution appears to be random. In most patients, the majority of affected bones are asymptomatic; this does not necessarily mean that they will always remain so.

Aetiology and pathophysiology

The primary disease process in Paget's disease appears to be in the osteoclasts of affected bone, and there is much circumstantial evidence pointing to a viral aetiology. These osteoclasts are abnormal both in structure and function, being larger than normal with more nuclei, and resorbing bone apparently without regard to normal anatomical restraints. Affected osteoclasts contain numerous cytoplasmic and nuclear particles thought to be viral nucleocapsids. Immunological and other evidence from molecular biology techniques suggests that a virus similar to the measles virus, possibly canine distemper virus, may be responsible.

Residual osteoclasts in bone behind the leading edge of advancing disease remain abnormal in size and shape, and continue to resorb bone chaotically. Wherever it occurs, bone resorption is followed by bone formation which, after an initial lag, catches up and keeps pace with resorption. However, the new bone laid down follows the chaotic pattern of bone resorption, and the gross structure of the whole bone therefore becomes progressively distorted. Affected bones are greatly weakened and become expanded and bent – this is particularly so for the major long bones, such as tibia, femur, humerus and radius, which may develop partial fractures. The latter are unusual in extending from the inner cortex outwards, and being concentrated on the convexity of the bowing bone (Fig. 18.8). Vertebrae and the pelvis become distorted, and the skull

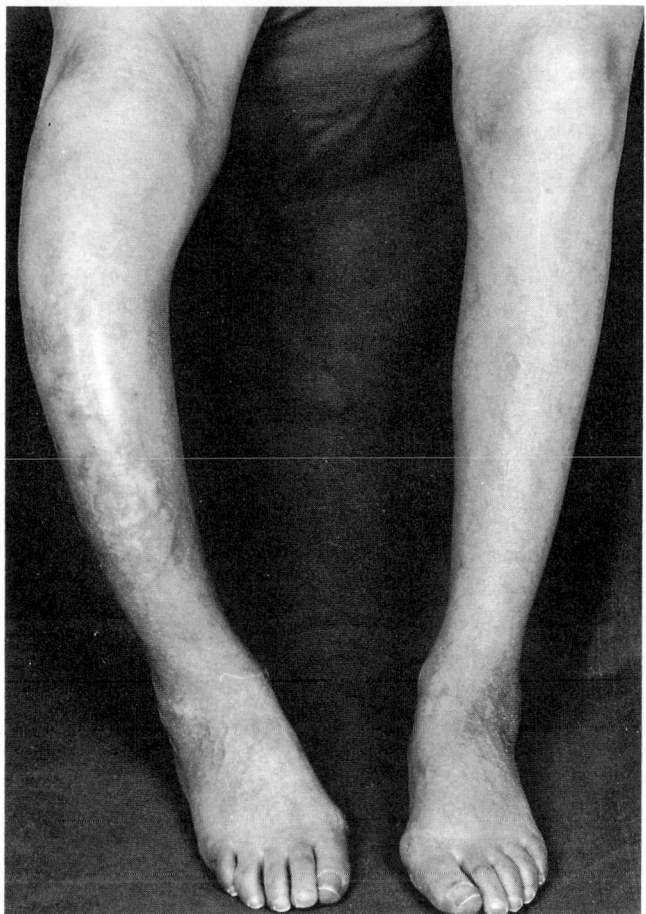

Fig. 18.8 Gross expansion and deformity of right tibia in long-standing Paget's disease.

thickens and its front and back sink, as the vertebral column selectively supports its centre. Secondary changes include osteoarthritis, e.g. of hips and knees.

Within an individual, the disease usually appears to be at the same stage of development at different sites, and unaffected bones remain so throughout the disease; this possibly reflects a single episode of widespread viral infection of blood-borne osteoclast precursors which were then carried into affected bones. Continuing viral replication within affected cells, combined with transfection by cell fusion (cell fusion being a normal property of the osteoclast), appears to explain why the disease is rampant in affected bones while initially unaffected bones generally seem to remain normal.

Clinical features

Since the natural time-course of Paget's disease is very long, and many patients have had it for 20–40 years or more before diagnosis, virtually nothing is known of the early clinical features of the disease, or whether there is an acute illness at the onset of the putative initial viral infection.

Many patients present fortuitously, either because a biochemical screen has revealed a high serum alkaline phosphatase level, or because an X-ray has revealed an affected bone. Typically, the disease starts in one or more specific areas, e.g. epiphysis of a long bone or skull base, and spreads through it with a lytic advancing edge at a rate of about 1 cm per year. In the skull, this gives rise to the picture of osteoporosis circumscripta, and in long bones to the 'blade of grass' appearance. This is the leading edge of 'vandal' osteoclasts which resorb bone in an uncontrolled way.

Bone pain is of at least four types:

- a deep boring dull pain, probably due to increased vascularity, which is present at rest and not relieved by analgesics
- a sharp pain, worse on movement or pressure, at the site of a partial or complete fracture
- the pain of secondary osteoarthritis
- pain due to pressure on nerve roots.

The patient may complain of deformity of an affected bone or bones, or enlargement and irregularity of the skull. There may be pressure effects, including cranial nerve lesions – of which tinnitus and deafness (nerve, as well as conductive) are very common – if the disease involves the skull. Occasionally, Paget's disease of the spine leads to paraparesis. Platybasia of the skull may lead to obstruction of the aqueduct and internal hydrocephalus.

Pagetic bone is highly vascular, and the patient is often aware of the warmth of an affected limb, especially of the tibia; the part is obviously hot to touch. Increased vascularity of the skull leads to prominence of the superficial temporal arteries and, occasionally, to distended external jugular veins. The cardiac output is modestly increased in extensive Paget's disease, as a result of vascular shunting of blood through diseased bone; this may occasionally lead to high output congestive cardiac failure. Patients with extensive Paget's disease commonly have generalised malaise and lethargy, which may improve with effective treatment.

An uncommon, but serious, complication of the condition is the development of bone sarcoma (usually osteogenic sarcoma), which is marked by expansion of the affected bone and further elevation of serum alkaline phosphatase activity. This complication may arise simultaneously at more than one Pagetic site and probably develops in less than 1% of cases.

Investigation

Bone resorption is reflected by increased excretion of collagen-derived hydroxyproline in urine (best measured as the fasting morning urine hydroxyproline/creatinine

ratio). Bone formation is reflected by the level of serum alkaline phosphatase. These two markers, which together provide a measure of bone turnover rate, are a function both of the extent of skeletal involvement and of the disease activity within affected bones.

In addition to these measurements, a bone scan is performed using ^{99m}Tc-labelled bisphosphonate (Fig. 18.9). This is followed by radiology of 'hot' bones. It is important to document the baseline state of disease before instituting therapy.

Management

Until the late 1960s, there was no effective treatment for Paget's disease. Although most patients have a mild condition which is rarely fatal, in some the disease is extremely disabling. Traditional criteria for instituting treatment, hitherto only for symptomatic disease, will change once an effective and simple treatment can be shown to arrest progress or cure the condition.

The bisphosphonates (diphosphonates)

The bisphosphonates are analogues of pyrophosphate that bind to hydroxyapatite, and are therefore taken up by newly laid down bone collagen matrix.

Pamidronate and *clodronate* are highly effective, especially parenterally. Figure 18.10 illustrates the dramatic response to a short course of intravenous infusions of pamidronate in severe Paget's disease. Remineralisation of lytic Paget's disease may be evident radiologically as

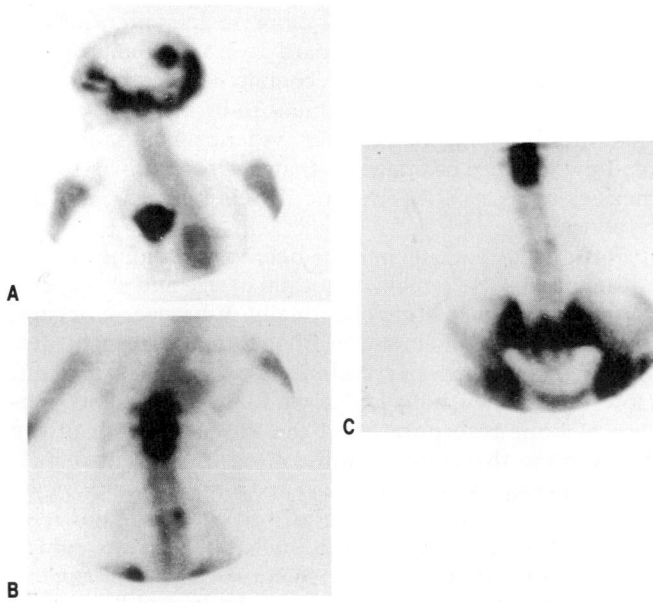

Fig. 18.9 Bone scan from a patient with extensive Paget's disease in skull (A), several dorsal vertebrae, sternum, left humerus (B), and the whole pelvis (C).

early as four months after the start of a three-month course of therapy and, in many cases, is followed by prolonged remission. In the early stages, pamidronate treatment is commonly followed by an increase in bone pain and by mild transient fever; however, this is quickly followed by symptomatic improvement and reduction in bone pain. These are now the preferred treatments for Paget's disease, although they are still not licensed as such. *Mithramycin*, although also quite effective, is much more toxic than pamidronate, and cannot now be generally recommended for the treatment of Paget's disease.

Calcitonin

Calcitonin given by repeated injection was the first treatment to have any beneficial effect, on bone pain or the course of the disease. The hormone inhibits osteoclasts. There is an abrupt reduction in bone resorption, while bone formation continues; thus the onset of treatment in a severely affected patient with extensive disease leads to a transient fall in serum calcium concentration. Synthetic salmon, or human, calcitonin is given in doses of 50–100 IU by subcutaneous injection three times a week. The hydroxyproline and plasma alkaline phosphatase levels fall, but rarely dramatically, and an improvement in bone structure and recalcification of affected bone occurs. Unfortunately, 'escape' is commonly seen within a year of treatment, usually as a result of antibody production. Side-effects are frequent and include flushing, palpitations, headache and malaise shortly after each injection. Calcitonin therapy is extremely expensive.

MISCELLANEOUS RARE BONE DISEASES

Hypophosphatasia

Hypophosphatasia is characterised by failure of mineralisation, possibly as a result of inhibition by increased concentrations of pyrophosphate. Its inheritance is autosomal recessive and it takes its name from the low levels of plasma alkaline phosphatase usually found. The fully expressed severe form of the disease may be lethal neonatally but later a clinical picture similar to that of severe rickets is found, with abnormal dentition and premature fusion of the cranial sutures. Urinary phosphoethanolamine excretion is increased but the mechanism is not known. There is no specific therapy.

Osteogenesis imperfecta

Osteogenesis imperfecta, which is also termed *fragilitas ossium* or *brittle bone disease,* is a collection of rare inherited disorders in which there appear to be specific defects

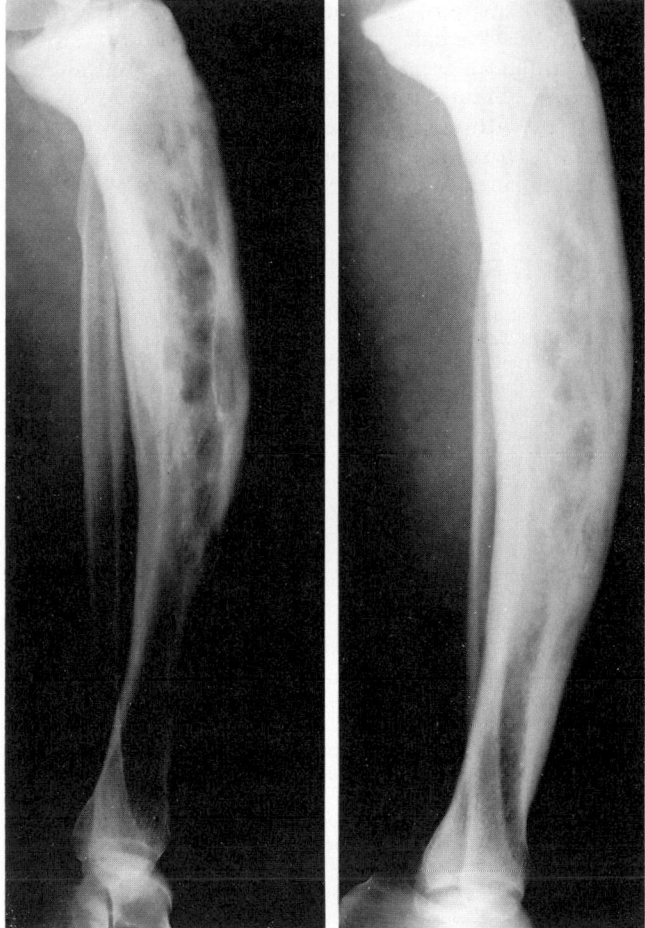

A

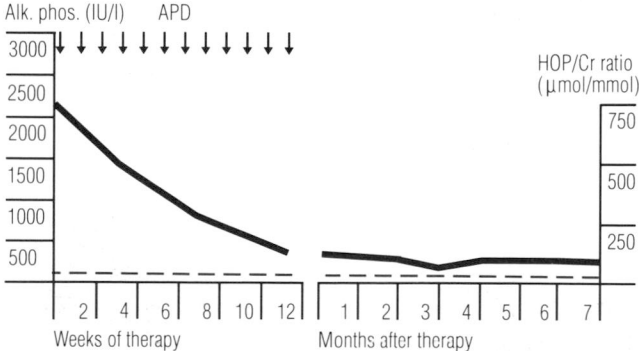

B

Fig. 18.10 Response to pamidronate treatment in Paget's disease. A. Paget's disease in a 71-year-old woman before (left) and nine months after a course of i.v. pamidronate (right). Note restoration of bone in areas of osteolysis. Bone distortion remains. **B.** Decline in alkaline phosphatase level (normal less than 130 IU/l) and hydroxyproline/creatinine (HOP/Cr) ratio (normal less than 20 μmol/mmol) during and after a single course of 12 weekly 30 mg infusions of i.v. pamidronate (APD). Note decline in activity. Upper limit of normal indicated by red dotted line.

in the formation of type I collagen, the predominant collagen in mature bone. There are four main forms:

- a dominantly inherited mild form in which structural abnormalities are unusual
- a dominant form with fragility and short stature
- a recessive form with early multiple fractures and skeletal deformity
- a severe, often lethal form due to new mutations in collagen genes.

Abnormal dentition may occur in all forms and the sclerae are often blue in forms 1, 3 and 4.

Treatment is directed towards prevention of trauma and correction of post-traumatic deformity. There is a suspicion that some patients with osteoporosis and a strong family history of the disease may in fact have mild forms of osteogenesis imperfecta.

Osteopetrosis (marble bone disease, Albers-Schoenberg disease)

The term osteopetrosis describes a number of very rare conditions characterised by *increased* bone mass throughout the skeleton. Of these, a dominantly inherited and relatively mild form, and a recessively inherited severe form, are numerically the most important. The increase in bone mass is thought to be due to a defect in osteoclast activity. Radiological appearances are characteristic, with patchily increased bone density throughout the skeleton. In severe disease, encroachment of bone on the marrow or neural canals may lead to bone marrow failure with leucoerythroblastic anaemia (which may be fatal) and to cranial nerve palsies respectively. Hepatosplenomegaly may be evident, indicating extramedullary haemopoiesis. The dominantly inherited mild disease is usually symptomless, but classical radiological changes are found, with increased bone density and alternating dense and lucent bands in the vertebral column.

Severe osteopetrosis is, predictably, associated with a markedly positive calcium balance, and some benefit has been claimed for treatment of severe disease by calcium restriction. Treatment by marrow transplantation has been tried with some success; transplanted osteoclast precursors, formed in the bone marrow, are able to re-establish normal bone resorption.

FURTHER READING

Altmann P, Cunningham J 1987 Post Grad Med J. 63:77, London. *A review of the treatment of severe hypercalcaemia.*

Cohen R D, Lewis B, Alberti KGMM, Derman AM, Eds, 1990 Metabolic and molecular basis of acquired disease. Ballière Tindall, London. *The bone disease section comprises detailed chapters on metabolic bone disease and hypercalcaemia.*

Kanis J A 1991 Pathophysiology and the treatment of Paget's disease of bone. Martin Dunitz, London. *A comprehensive and authoritative monograph on Paget's disease.*

Mallette L E 1991 The parathyroid polyhormones – new concepts in the spectrum of peptide hormone action. Endocrine Reviews, Vol 12: pp. 110–117. *A superb review of actions of PTH and PTH related peptide.*

Manolagas S C, Olefsky J M 1988 Metabolic bone and mineral disorders. Churchill Livingstone, Edinburgh. *A good review of important aspects of metabolic bone disorders.*

Mundy G R 1990 Calcium homeostasis: hypercalcaemia and hypocalcaemia, 2nd edn. Martin Dunitz, London. *An excellent simple, but comprehensive and up-to-date account from an acknowledged expert in the field.*

Nordin B E C 1993 Metabolic bone and stone disease, 2nd edn. Churchill Livingstone, Edinburgh. *A general review of metabolic bone disease.*

Riggs B, Melton L 1988 Osteoporosis: aetiology, diagnosis and management. Raven Press, New York. *A detailed and up-to-date account.*

Smith R 1987 Disorders of the skeleton. In: Weatherall D J, Ledingham J G G, Warrell D A (eds) Oxford textbook of medicine, 2nd edn., Oxford University Press, Oxford. *A general review of skeletal disorders.*

Woolf A D, Dixon A St J 1988 Osteoporosis: a clinical guide. Martin Dunitz, London. *A well-illustrated and authoritative account of many of the current issues relating to osteoporosis.*

19

Diabetes Mellitus and Disorders of Lipid and Intermediary Metabolism

Gareth Williams and John P Monson

REGULATION OF METABOLISM

An appreciation of metabolic processes is essential to understand the causes, effects and treatment of diabetes, which is a common, important and interesting disease. The following section is therefore a brief account of the normal control of metabolism.

Insulin

Synthesis and structure

Insulin is synthesised and secreted by the β cells which form the core of the islets of Langerhans. Translation of the insulin gene yields a precursor, preproinsulin, which is cleaved proteolytically to produce proinsulin. This is further split into equimolar amounts of insulin and C-peptide, which are released from the β cell by exocytosis of secretory vesicles (Fig. 19.1).

Insulin consists of A- and B-chains, linked by two disulphide bridges. Human insulin differs structurally from porcine insulin in a single amino acid residue, and both these species differ from bovine insulin in two additional residues (Fig. 19.2). Various point mutations in the molecule ('insulinopathies') have been identified, some of which cause glucose intolerance by interfering with the molecule's biological activity. Insulin belongs to a large family of structurally similar proteins, conserved during evolution, including the epidermal and insulin-like growth factors.

C-peptide is biologically inert. It is cleared more slowly than insulin and its circulating levels are therefore a more stable indicator of β-cell secretion than insulin itself. Subnormal C-peptide levels after stimulation by either glucagon (a powerful insulin secretagogue) or a high-carbohydrate meal can be used to identify diabetic patients who are sufficiently insulin-deficient as to need insulin replacement.

Insulin secretion

Some insulin is secreted all the time and is important in restraining glucose release from the liver and preventing triglyceride breakdown in fat. This 'basal' secretion occurs in regular 10- to 15-minute pulses, which may serve to maintain the sensitivity of insulin receptors on target tissues.

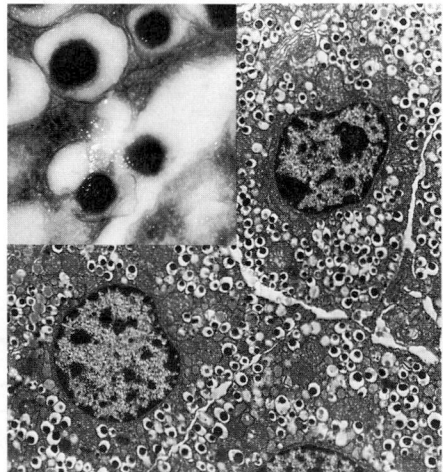

Fig. 19.1 Electron micrograph showing secretory granules containing insulin in β-cells. Higher magnification (inset) shows granules which are released from the cell surface by exocytosis.

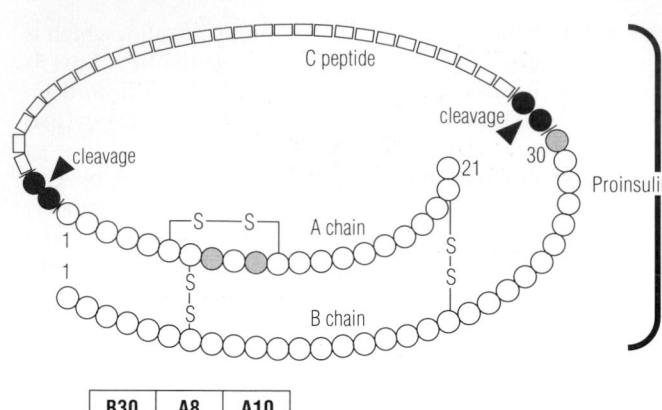

Fig. 19.2 Structure of insulin. Proinsulin is cleaved to produce insulin and the connecting C peptide. The amino acid residues which differ between human, porcine and bovine insulins are highlighted.

	B30	A8	A10
Human	Thr	Thr	Ile
Porcine	Ala	Thr	Ile
Bovine	Ala	Ala	Val

Eating induces an additional, rapid surge of insulin secretion, roughly proportional to the size of the meal; levels rise several-fold after an average breakfast (Fig.19.3). This is due mainly to the secretagogue actions of absorbed nutrients, and also to stimulation by humoral and autonomic nervous signals. Glucose is the main insulin secretagogue, and arginine and other amino acids are also active. Glucose is metabolised in the β cell and generates ATP. This closes a potassium efflux channel, causing a rise in intracellular potassium, followed by calcium influx. This in turn activates the microtubules which propel insulin-containing vesicles to the cell surface.

After an acute secretagogue challenge (e.g. an intravenous glucose bolus), the insulin secretory response can be resolved into an immediate *first phase* surge lasting a few minutes, followed by a slowly rising *second phase* which declines when the stimulus ends. This pattern is blurred after meals by the relatively sluggish absorption from the gut. Prandial insulin release is also stimulated by the vagal innervation of the islet and by the 'incretins', hormones secreted by the gut into the circulation after eating, such as gastric inhibitory peptide.

Insulin is secreted into the islet capillaries which drain into the pancreatic vein, a tributary of the portal vein. It is therefore delivered directly to the liver, where it exerts most of its metabolic effects. Insulin is cleared from the circulation within a few minutes, mostly being removed during its first pass through the liver.

Metabolic actions of insulin

Insulin is an exclusively anabolic hormone, promoting storage of carbohydrate, fat and protein. It causes glucose to be converted into glycogen (glycogenesis) in the liver and muscle, promotes the formation of triglyceride (lipogenesis) in fat, and stimulates protein synthesis in many tissues. It also inhibits the opposing catabolic processes of glycogenolysis, lipolysis and proteolysis. Basal insulin levels are enough to inhibit lipolysis and restrain glucose output by the liver, by inhibiting glycogenolysis and gluconeogenesis. The much higher levels occurring postprandially also stimulate the uptake of glucose into muscle and fat, by activating specific glucose transporter proteins in these tissues.

Insulin acts through specific receptors on its target cells. These consist of paired α-subunits lying extracellularly, each linked by disulphide bridges to a β-subunit which spans the cell membrane. Insulin binds to the α-subunit and triggers autophosphorylation of the intracellular part of the β-subunit. A few cases of congenital insulin resistance have been attributed to mutations

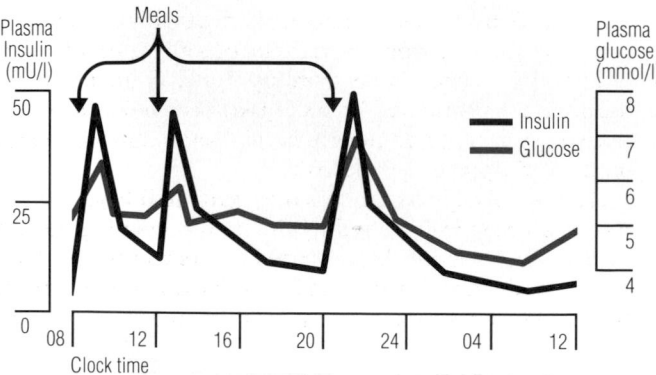

Fig. 19.3 Diurnal changes in plasma insulin and glucose concentrations in non-diabetic subjects. Insulin levels vary several-fold whereas plasma glucose is maintained between tight limits of 4–7 mmol/l.

Summary 1 Main metabolic effects of insulin

Carbohydrate
Promotes glycogen formation ⎫ reduces hepatic
Inhibits gluconeogenesis ⎬ glucose output*
Stimulates glucose uptake into muscle and fat
Lowers blood glucose concentration

Fat
Promotes triglyceride formation
Inhibits lipolysis and ketogenesis*

Protein
Promotes protein synthesis

*Actions occurring at low (basal) insulin concentrations

The counter-regulatory hormones (glucagon, catecholamines, growth hormone and cortisol) oppose these actions

---

affecting the insulin-binding or phosphorylation domains of the receptor.

Counter-regulatory hormones and somatostatin

Counter-regulatory hormones oppose the anabolic effects of insulin, either by direct catabolic actions or by making the tissues insensitive to insulin. *Glucagon*, secreted by the α cells in the islet periphery, powerfully stimulates glycogenolysis and gluconeogenesis in the liver; together, these actions rapidly increase hepatic glucose output and cause hyperglycaemia. Glucagon also stimulates keto-genesis. All these actions are accentuated by insulin deficiency, when glucagon also enhances lipolysis. *Catecholamines*, either circulating or released locally in tissue by activation of the sympathetic nervous system, cause glycogenolysis and gluconeogenesis in the liver and lipolysis in fat. *Cortisol* renders tissues insensitive to insulin and stimulates proteolysis, lipolysis and gluconeo-genesis. *Growth hormone* also reduces insulin sensitivity and stimulates lipolysis, but cooperates with insulin in promoting protein synthesis.

The counter-regulatory hormones are secreted during stress and assist glycaemic recovery from hypoglycaemia. Their secretion is also influenced by insulin and vice versa, e.g. glucagon potently stimulates insulin release. By contrast, insulin inhibits glucagon secretion; insulin defi-ciency therefore allows glucagon levels to rise, aggravating catabolism in diabetes.

Somatostatin, secreted by the δ cells of the islet, is not a counter-regulatory hormone, but strongly suppresses the release of both insulin and glucagon. It also inhibits the secretion of growth hormone, gastrin and many other peptides.

Carbohydrate, fat and protein metabolism

The three branches of metabolism – carbohydrate, fat and protein (Figs 19.4–19.7) – are all interlinked at various levels. Each is finely balanced between anabolism, largely mediated by insulin, and catabolism due to the counter-regulatory hormones and activation of the sympathetic nervous system.

Carbohydrate metabolism

Glucose is the body's main metabolic substrate and normally is the sole fuel for the brain, which uses about 50% of the 200 g of glucose produced by the liver each day. Glucose is supplied steadily to the brain and other tissues by maintaining blood levels between tight limits (4–7 mmol/l; see Fig. 19.3).

Between meals, blood glucose is determined mainly by how much glucose is released by the liver into the circula-

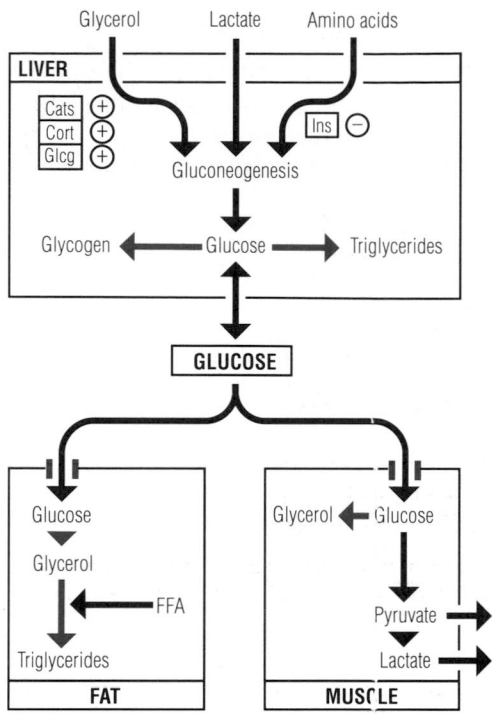

Fig. 19.4 Principal pathways of carbohydrate metabolism. Ins, insulin; cats, catecholamines; cort, cortisol; glcg, glucagon; FFA, free fatty acids; +,–, reactions stimulated, inhibited. Red indicates actions stimulated by insulin.

tion. The liver contains most of the body's glycogen, the glucose polymer which is the main storage form of carbo-hydrate. *Glycogenesis* is promoted by glycogen synthase, an enzyme which is stimulated by insulin and inhibited by glucagon. Conversely, *glycogenolysis* (under the action of phosphorylase) is inhibited by insulin and stimulated rapidly and powerfully by glucagon and the catechola-mines. Hepatic stores of glycogen are soon depleted. The liver also secretes glucose produced by *gluconeogenesis* from lactate, amino acids and glycerol, either formed within the liver or taken up from the circulation. Lactate is a product of glycolysis in muscle; amino acids, especially alanine and glutamine, derive from proteolysis or amination of pyru-vate; and glycerol results from lipolysis. Gluconeogenic enzymes are stimulated by glucagon, catecholamines and cortisol, and inhibited by insulin; glucagon also stimulates amino acid uptake into the liver.

After meals, glucose enters the circulation from the gut and its storage is favoured by the high prevailing insulin levels. Insulin stimulates glucose uptake into skeletal muscle and adipose tissue and its subsequent conversion into glycogen and triglyceride, respectively.

Fat metabolism and ketogenesis

Circulating triglyceride, either absorbed from the gut or secreted by the liver, is hydrolysed by lipoprotein lipase in

19　Diabetes Mellitus and Lipid Metabolism

the capillary endothelium of adipose tissue and skeletal muscle (Fig. 19.5). This *lipolysis* yields free (non-esterified) fatty acids (FFA, or NEFA) and glycerol, which are metabolised mainly in adipose tissue. Their recombination into triglyceride *(lipogenesis)* is stimulated by insulin. Subsequent lipolysis of triglyceride (mediated by triacylglyceride lipase) is inhibited by insulin at low concentrations and stimulated by catecholamines, growth hormone and, in severe insulin deficiency, by glucagon. Glycerol is exported and in the liver is a substrate for gluconeogenesis. FFA are also exported and are used as a fuel by skeletal muscle and many tissues. FFA taken up by the liver can either be used for lipogenesis or undergo oxidation to ketone bodies *(ketogenesis)*.

Ketogenesis (Fig. 19.6) takes place within the mitochondria of the hepatocytes, using fatty acyl-coenzyme A (CoA) derivatives formed in the cytoplasm by the reaction of FFA with CoA. These are carried inwards across the mitochondrial membrane by a 'shuttle' enzyme (carnitine palmitoyl transferase) and then undergo β-oxidation to acetyl-CoA and further conversion to acetoacetate. This and its derivatives, 3-hydroxybutyrate and acetone, are the ketone bodies. Ketogenesis is stimulated by glucagon and suppressed by insulin, which respectively enhance and inhibit the activity of the carnitine shuttle, the rate-limiting step of the pathway. Ketogenesis is also regulated by the supply of FFA and is therefore greatly increased by the combination of insulin deficiency and glucagon excess – as in untreated insulin-dependent diabetes mellitus (IDDM) – which releases the brake on lipolysis.

Normally, ketone bodies are exported from the liver and can be used by many tissues as metabolic fuels;

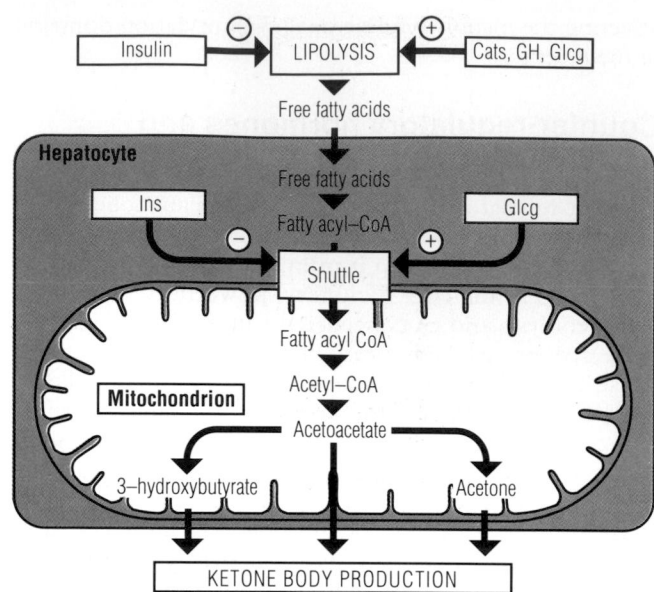

Fig. 19.6 Ketogenesis. Ketone body production is inhibited by insulin (ins) which reduces both the supply of FFA (from lipolysis) and indirectly the activity of the shuttle enzyme (carnitine palmitoyl transferase) which carries the precursor fatty acyl-CoA into the mitochondria. Glucagon (glcg), catecholamines (cats) and growth hormone (GH) stimulate ketogenesis by opposing these actions.

indeed, they are the main source of energy in prolonged starvation, when fat reserves are mobilised. In uncontrolled IDDM, however, their overproduction greatly exceeds their utilisation; 3-hydroxybutyrate and acetoacetate, and the accompanying hydrogen ions, accumulate to cause diabetic ketoacidosis.

Protein metabolism

Protein synthesis is promoted by insulin and growth hormone and normally balances proteolysis, which is stimulated especially by cortisol (Fig. 19.7). Circulating amino acids, either derived from proteolysis, amination of pyruvate or absorption of digested proteins, are taken up by the tissues. Alanine and glutamine are important substrates for gluconeogenesis in the liver, where their uptake is stimulated by glucagon.

Regulation of metabolism in health, starvation and stress

Fasting is characterised by low basal insulin levels, without rises in counter-regulatory hormones. This permits controlled glycogen breakdown, gluconeogenesis and glucose production by the liver and so maintains blood glucose levels. Lipolysis is not increased; FFA and ketone body levels remain low.

After eating, insulin release increases several-fold in step with the influx of glucose, triglycerides and amino

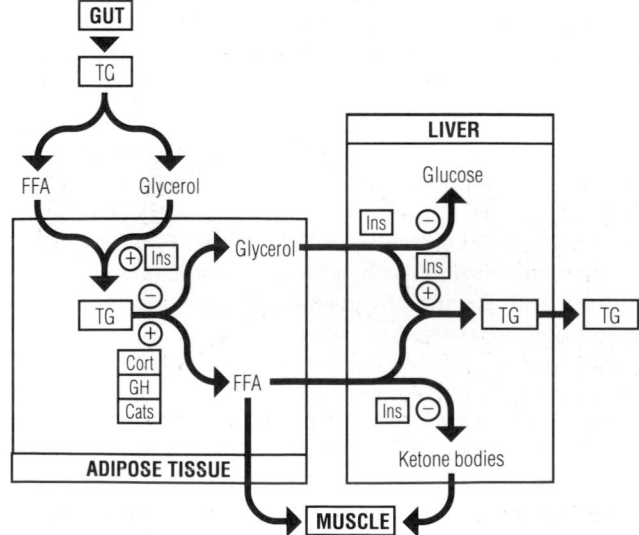

Fig. 19.5 Principal pathways of fat metabolism. TG, triglyceride; FFA, free fatty acids; cort, cortisol; ins, insulin; cats, catecholamines; GH, growth hormone; glcg, glucagon, +,–, reactions stimulated, inhibited (shown in one direction only).

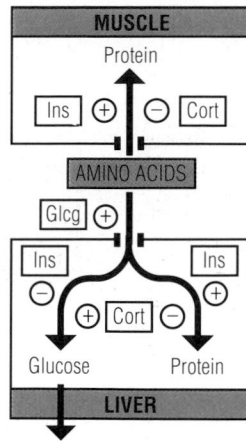

Fig. 19.7 Major pathways of protein metabolism. Ins, insulin, glcg, glucagon; cort, cortisol; +,–, reactions stimulated, inhibited (shown in one direction only).

acids from the gut, promoting the storage of nutrients not needed immediately. High insulin levels promptly suppress hepatic glucose secretion, and stimulate glucose uptake and storage in skeletal muscle (as glycogen) and adipose tissue (as triglyceride). This prevents postprandial hyperglycaemia, and lipogenesis and protein synthesis are encouraged.

In *prolonged starvation*, insulin levels fall below the threshold necessary to suppress lipolysis, ketogenesis and hepatic glucose production. These processes are enhanced by increased glucagon levels (stimulated by insulin deficiency itself) and by the other counter-regulatory hormones, whose secretion is increased by the stress of starvation. The result is controlled catabolism. Blood glucose levels are maintained initially by hepatic glycogenolysis and then, when this is exhausted, by gluconeogenesis, again predominantly in the liver. The body's fat reserves, its major energy store, are then mobilised by lipolysis and ketogenesis. Blood ketone levels increase greatly (the ketosis of starvation) and are used as fuels by most tissues – even the brain, after several days of starvation. Protein metabolism is defended until relatively late, possibly because ketone bodies inhibit proteolysis. Muscle and other proteins are ultimately broken down under the influence of increased cortisol concentrations to support gluconeogenesis.

Severe stress (e.g. sepsis, trauma or surgery) greatly increases counter-regulatory hormone secretion and leads to uncontrolled catabolism. Excess gluconeogenesis, lipolysis and proteolysis lead to rapid loss of body fat and muscle, the latter being exacerbated by impaired protein synthesis. The situation is even more precarious in diabetic patients who are insulin-deficient because they are untreated or inadequately treated; profound ketoacidosis and hyperglycaemia can develop with alarming speed.

DIABETES MELLITUS

The simple definition of diabetes mellitus as 'a state of chronic hyperglycaemia' belies the immense medical, scientific, social and economic implications of the disease. Because it is common and affects virtually every system in the body, every medical practitioner must be familiar with it. People with diabetes must learn to cope with a life-long disease which is treatable, but not curable, and which carries the threat of complications which may endanger the future quality of life and even life itself. Society as a whole has to shoulder a considerable burden from diabetes. In the UK, diabetes affects about 2% of the population (over 1 million people) and probably absorbs over 5% of health-care expenditure. Worldwide, there are probably 50 million people with diabetes. The problem of diabetes in the Third World is only now receiving the attention it deserves. Research and advances in clinical care are already making the disease easier to live with.

The diagnosis of diabetes

Blood glucose concentrations are normally remarkably constant: fasting concentrations in whole blood are 3.5–6.7 mmol/l and peak values after meals rarely exceed 8 mmol/l. Glycosuria therefore never occurs unless the renal threshold for glucose reabsorption is below the normal value of 10 mmol/l.

Diabetes is diagnosed by a fasting venous whole blood concentration of over 6.7 mmol/l, or a random value exceeding 10 mmol/l (Fig. 19.8). A single very high value (>15 mmol/l) in a symptomatic patient is diagnostic, but otherwise two separate estimations should be made. The values relate to venous whole blood; as red cells contain less glucose, the corresponding plasma values are about

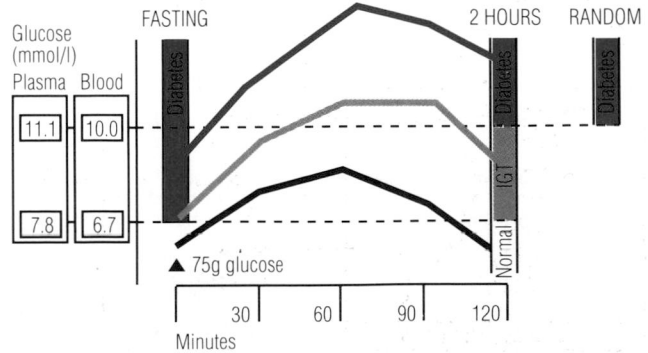

Fig. 19.8 Diagnostic criteria for diabetes. Diabetes is diagnosed by a fasting blood glucose level >6.7 mmol/l, or a random or 2-hour post-OGTT value >10.0 mmol/l. A 2-hour value of 6.7–10.0 mmol/l identifies impaired glucose tolerance. Corresponding plasma glucose values are 7.8 and 11.0 mmol/l. The 1-hour intermediate readings on OGTT are not used for diagnosis.

1.1 mmol/l higher. Because glucose is extracted by the tissues, arterial and capillary (e.g. fingerprick) blood levels are higher than those in venous blood.

In borderline cases and for research applications, the oral glucose tolerance test (OGTT) is used as recommended by the WHO Expert Committee on Diabetes. After an overnight fast, the subject drinks 75 g of glucose (dextrose) dissolved in water and blood glucose is measured before and 2 hours after glucose administration. The normal values and diagnostic criteria for diabetes and impaired glucose tolerance (IGT) are shown in Figure 19.8. A low renal threshold is diagnosed if glycaemia is normal but glycosuria occurs; urine should be collected during the test if this is suspected.

The diagnosis of diabetes carries considerable personal and social disadvantages and must be certain. Only laboratory measurements of blood glucose should be used for diagnostic purposes; test-strip readings, urinary glucose levels or glycosylated haemoglobin or fructosamine concentrations must *never* be used. OGTT results vary considerably between and within normal individuals and the test should be repeated if a marginal abnormality is found. Glucose tolerance is particularly sensitive to changes in nutritional state and is worsened in normal subjects by dieting during the preceding days. An adequate diet must therefore be taken for 3 days before an OGTT.

Classification of diabetes

Most cases of diabetes are 'primary', and relatively few are secondary to identifiable causes (Table 19.1). Primary diabetes is subdivided on clinical grounds into insulin-dependent and non-insulin-dependent diabetes mellitus (IDDM and NIDDM). The features distinguishing IDDM and NIDDM are shown in Table 19.2. The critical difference is the degree of insulin deficiency, which is so profound in IDDM that even the low insulin concentrations which normally prevent lipolysis and ketogenesis cannot be sustained; without insulin replacement, IDDM patients become ketotic and die. By contrast, NIDDM patients have enough endogenous insulin to prevent ketosis and will survive (albeit with hyperglycaemia)

Table 19.1 Classification of diabetes mellitus

Primary diabetes mellitus		
IDDM	~ 25%	of cases
NIDDM	~ 70%	in the UK
Secondary diabetes mellitus	~ 5%	
Malnutrition-related diabetes		
Pancreatic disease		
Endocrine diseases		
Gestational diabetes		
Drugs and toxins		
Rare other conditions		

Table 19.2 Features distinguishing IDDM from NIDDM

	IDDM	NIDDM
Metabolic features		
Insulin deficiency	Severe (C-peptide-negative)	Moderate, variable (C-peptide-positive)
Spontaneous ketosis	Yes	No
Need insulin to survive	Yes	No
Insulin insensitivity	Mild, variable	Severe, variable
Aetiology		
Genetic susceptibility	Moderate	Very strong
HLA markers	Yes (DR3/4)	None known
Autoimmune features	Yes	No
Environmental factors	? Viruses	? Overeating
Clinical features at presentation		
Age (not very useful)	Most <40 years (peak at 13 years)	Most >40 years (peak at 70 years)
Body weight	BMI* mostly <25; recent loss common	BMI mostly >25; recent loss sometimes
Microvascular complications	Rare	Sometimes present

*BMI = body mass index = weight (kg)/height (m)^2.

without insulin therapy. Many NIDDM patients are treated with insulin as this is the only available means to lower glycaemia effectively, but these insulin-*treated* patients can be distinguished from those who are truly insulin-*dependent* because they have measurable C-peptide levels and do not become ketotic if insulin is withdrawn.

The essentially clinical terms, IDDM and NIDDM, are generally used synonymously with 'type 1' and 'type 2' diabetes, respectively. The latter are distinguished aetiologically: type 1 diabetes is due to autoimmune destruction of β cells which usually results in severe insulin deficiency and therefore IDDM. IDDM and NIDDM have replaced the old terms, 'juvenile-onset' and 'maturity-onset' diabetes, as these are based on unhelpful generalisations regarding age of onset to which there are frequent exceptions (e.g. 10% of diabetic patients aged over 65 years are insulin-dependent).

INSULIN-DEPENDENT DIABETES MELLITUS (IDDM)

Epidemiology

In Britain, IDDM accounts for about 25% of all diabetic patients and perhaps 50% of those treated with insulin. The frequency of IDDM shows striking geographical variation: in Finland, it is some 35 times commoner than in Japan. Within the UK, the highest frequency is found in Scotland, where, as in several other countries, the incidence appears to have doubled within a decade. Incidence shows a pronounced seasonal variation, with most

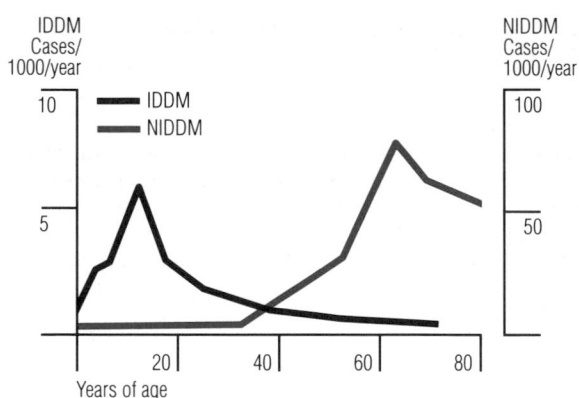

Fig. 19.9 Incidences of IDDM and NIDDM with age. Note that the scale for NIDDM is 10 times that for IDDM.

cases presenting in the autumn and winter. These observations all suggest that environmental factors are important in causing or precipitating the disease. Also unexplained is the age predilection of IDDM. Any age can be affected but most cases present before 20 years of age and the incidence peaks at 12 years (Fig. 19.9).

Aetiology and pathogenesis

It is now accepted that IDDM results from autoimmune destruction of the islet β cells, which is partly determined by heredity. The genetic markers for diabetes susceptibility are relatively common in Caucasian populations, whereas IDDM is relatively rare, again indicating that an additional factor, presumably environmental, is superimposed.

Genetic factors

The genetic component of IDDM is less important than in NIDDM, as shown by studies of identical twins of whom one becomes diabetic. In the case of IDDM, the chances of the unaffected twin developing the disease are about 50%, whereas the overall risk in NIDDM exceeds 95%.

Several genetic markers for IDDM have now been identified, notably specific HLA class II antigens whose genes lie on the short arm of chromosome 6. Possession of HLA antigens DR3 and DR4 increases the risks of developing IDDM by seven- and nine-fold respectively above the general population rate, and possession of both (DR3/4) increases the risk by 14-fold; over 90% of children with IDDM have DR3 and/or DR4, compared with 50% of the non-diabetic population. By contrast, possession of HLA-DR2 appears to protect against the development of IDDM, reducing the risk to one-eighth of that in the general population. How these class II HLA antigens might influence the course of autoimmune destruction of the β cells is not known.

Autoimmune phenomena in IDDM

An association of IDDM with organ-specific autoimmune diseases has long been recognised, e.g. with Schmidt's syndrome (adrenal and thyroid failure) in type 2 polyglandular endocrinopathy syndrome (p. 706). Studies in human IDDM and in rodents which develop spontaneous IDDM-like syndromes have documented convincing evidence of autoimmune disease. Furthermore, β-cell damage in animals and man, if detected early enough, can be limited by immunosuppressive drugs.

Like thyroid, adrenal and other tissues which are the target of autoimmune disease, the pancreatic islets of newly diagnosed IDDM patients are infiltrated with immunologically active cells (mostly cytotoxic/ suppressor T lymphocytes), an appearance termed 'insulitis'. With the passage of time, the intensity of the insulitis abates, but surviving islets are found to be specifically depleted of β cells, implying that these were the victims of the autoimmune attack. β cells may attract immune damage by their 'aberrant' expression of class II HLA antigens (which they do not normally express). The subsequent events thought to occur are shown in Fig. 19.10.

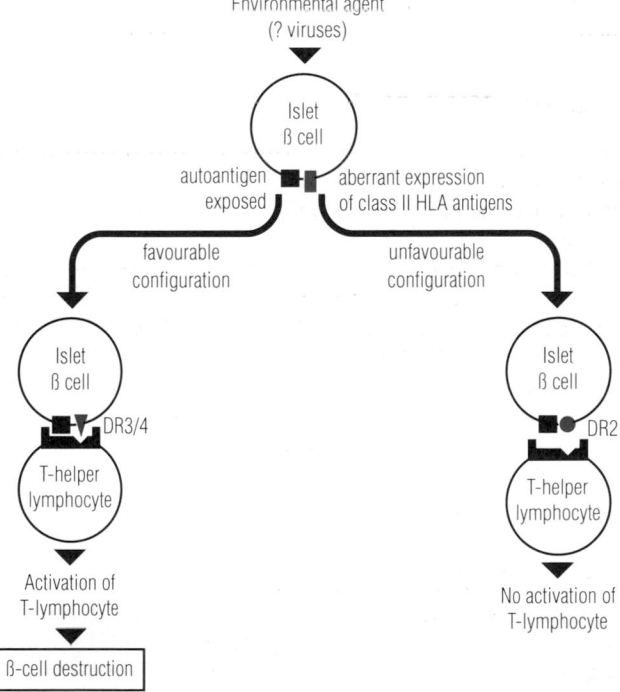

Fig. 19.10 Hypothetical scheme of autoimmune β-cell destruction in IDDM. Viruses or other agents could induce islet β cells to express class II antigens and to 'expose' autoantigens (viral antigens could be expressed on β cells, or a normal β-cell antigen could mimic viral antigens). The autoantigen (indicated in red), when coexpressed with HLA DR3 and/or 4, has a 'favourable' configuration which activates T-helper lymphocytes and triggers autoimmune damage. By contrast, HLA DR2 has an 'unfavourable' configuration which prevents this from happening.

As well as insulitis, newly diagnosed IDDM patients show other evidence of ongoing autoimmune processes, with activated T cells and autoantibodies directed against islet cells and insulin, in the circulation. Although most islet-cell antibodies (ICA) react with all islet cell types, some complement-fixing ICA may recognise the β cell membrane specifically. The crucial β-cell autoantigen is still unknown, although recent work has implicated the enzyme glutamate decarboxylase (GAD).

Viruses and environmental factors

Environmental factors must account for a large part of the susceptibility to IDDM. Many viruses target the pancreas and some selectively attack the β cells, where they could persist and alter the cells' activity or antigenicity.

In man, IDDM presents when seasonal viral infections are common, and some newly diagnosed IDDM patients have serological evidence of previous (sometimes recent) encounters with viruses such as mumps and the Coxsackie B series. Because IDDM has a long subclinical course, such infections may represent a final insult which tips the patient into critical insulin deficiency. IDDM develops in up to 20% of children with congenital rubella, but there is little evidence that rubella is diabetogenic if acquired after birth. Various chemical toxins destroy β cells and cause IDDM-like syndromes in animals (e.g. the cytotoxic agent, streptozotocin, in the rat) but few toxins seem relevant to man.

Natural history of IDDM

Long-term, prospective studies of subjects at high risk of developing IDDM (especially siblings of children with recently diagnosed IDDM) indicate that IDDM is the culmination of many years of low-level autoimmune damage, which is manifest clinically when a critical mass (>95%) of β cells has been destroyed. This is in striking contrast to the acute presentation of IDDM: symptoms are present in most patients for less than 4 weeks.

ICA and insulin autoantibodies appear during the *prodromal* phase, up to 10 years before IDDM presents. This is asymptomatic, as is the subsequent *prediabetic* phase in which subtle disturbances of insulin secretion (loss of first-phase release) can be identified. Later, the OGTT becomes abnormal and, finally, frank hyperglycaemia supervenes and symptoms appear. Interestingly, the process may abort without leading to IDDM in a proportion of susceptible subjects.

Biochemical disturbances of IDDM

Insulin deficiency, with the glucagon excess which it causes, results in hyperglycaemia due to unrestrained hepatic glucose output, lipolysis and proteolysis. These catabolic processes can be exacerbated by counter-regulatory responses to infection and other stresses. The insulin-dependent tissues, notably skeletal muscle and fat, 'starve in the midst of plenty' as lack of insulin decreases glucose entry, despite its very high extracellular concentrations. An osmotic diuresis, polyuria and dehydration occur when blood glucose levels exceed the renal reabsorption threshold (usually 10 mmol/l). Severe insulin deficiency greatly accelerates lipolysis which fuels ketogenesis (p. 742). Proteolysis causes muscle breakdown and wasting.

Clinical features of IDDM

Presentation

Young patients typically have a short history (a few days or weeks) of the classical symptoms of polyuria, thirst and polydipsia, and weight loss. Polyuria is due to an osmotic diuresis driven by high glucose and ketone body concentrations in the urine, and may reach several litres per day; sleep is disturbed by nocturia, and previously continent children may develop enuresis. Thirst is often intense. Weight is lost rapidly, often despite increased appetite, due to both dehydration and catabolism of muscle and fat. General tiredness and malaise are common.

Other features include blurred vision (due to osmotic disturbances in the lens), muscle cramps, infections (boils, urinary tract infections, or candidiasis causing balanitis or pruritis vulvae) and, especially in children, abdominal pain. Patients with impending ketoacidosis may display the nausea, acidotic breathing and other features described on page 761. Chronic diabetic complications (retinopathy, neuropathy) are exceedingly rare in newly diagnosed IDDM patients because significant hyperglycaemia is usually only a recent event, and very few cases are detected incidentally in asymptomatic subjects.

Many patients look tired and unwell, sometimes with clinically evident dehydration and loss of muscle and fat. The signs of ketosis are described on page 761. A full examination should be performed as it is important to

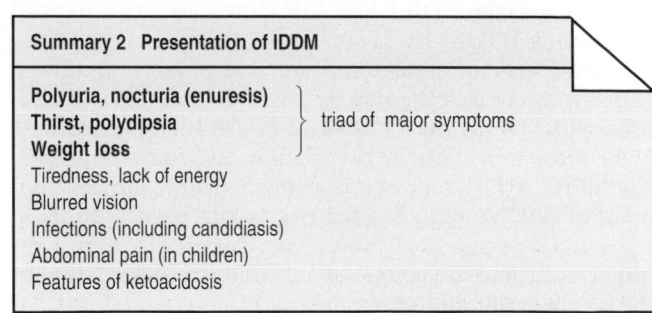

Summary 2   Presentation of IDDM

Polyuria, nocturia (enuresis)
Thirst, polydipsia   } triad of major symptoms
Weight loss
Tiredness, lack of energy
Blurred vision
Infections (including candidiasis)
Abdominal pain (in children)
Features of ketoacidosis

document the presence of any complications and to identify precipitating illnesses. Examination may be entirely unremarkable, which makes it mandatory to check the blood glucose concentration in any patient who is unwell.

Investigations and diagnosis

The diagnosis is confirmed by demonstrating hyperglycaemia (defined on p. 743). The urine must be tested for ketones. Routine blood biochemistry may show features of dehydration and ketoacidosis. Other tests should aim to identify any infection which could have precipitated diabetes (full blood counts, urine and blood cultures, chest X-ray) and, in older patients especially, any co-existent risk factors for diabetic complications, notably vascular disease (ECG, fasting lipid concentrations).

Management of IDDM

Insulin replacement is mandatory, but other aspects – diabetes education, blood glucose monitoring, diet and other lifestyle changes – are essential for the day-to-day and long-term management of IDDM.

Insulin treatment

Insulin was originally extracted from porcine and bovine pancreases. Insulin of human sequence can now be synthesised on an industrial scale by inserting a cloned synthetic gene into either bacteria or yeasts. Biosynthesis can either mimic the natural process, yielding proinsulin which can be cleaved in vitro, or produce A- and B-chains by separate fermentation reactions, which are then combined chemically. Human insulin 'emp' (enzymatically modified porcine) is made from porcine insulin by removing and substituting the single residue which differs between the two sequences (Fig. 19.2).

All insulins are now highly purified ('monocomponent') and therefore unlikely to provoke antibody formation. In the UK, many preparations of bovine insulins have been phased out and porcine insulins are becoming less popular; over 70% of patients now use human insulin. Human insulin preparations are absorbed slightly more rapidly and have somewhat shorter action profiles than the porcine equivalents, but these differences are unimportant in clinical practice. Human insulins are less antigenic than porcine and especially bovine insulins, and allergic reactions (see below) are very rare. The suggestion that human insulin is associated with decreased awareness of hypoglycaemia is unsubstantiated.

Insulin preparations in the UK, North America and most European countries contain a standard concentration of 100 U/ml.

Insulin preparations

Insulin replacement aims to reproduce the normal pattern of insulin secretion, with a background basal supply and additional peaks at mealtimes. Two basic types of insulin, short- and long-acting, are therefore required (see Table 19.3).

Table 19.3 Types of insulin preparation

Type	Examples	Approximate action profile (hours)*			Schedule
		Onset	Peak	Duration	
Soluble	Actrapid, Humulin S	0.5–1	2–4	5–8	30–40 minutes before eating
Intermediate Isophane (NPH)	Protaphane, Humulin I	2–4	6–10	12–24	b.d. with soluble insulin before meals *or* o.d. in the morning or evening
Lente (IZS)	Monotard, Humulin Zn				
'Long-acting' Ultralente	Ultratard (human)	3–4	12–18	≤24†	o.d. or b.d., as for intermediate
Biphasic Soluble 30:70 Isophane 50:50	Mixtard Humulin M5	0.5–1	2–10	12–18	b.d. or o.d., 30–40 minutes before meals

*Action profiles vary widely between and within individuals.
†Intermediate and even 'long-acting' insulins based on human insulin often last less than 24 hours, and twice-daily injections are needed in many cases.
NPH, neutral protamine Hagedorn; IZS, insulin-zinc suspension; o.d., b.d. = once, twice daily.

Short-acting (soluble) insulins (e.g. Actrapid, Humulin S) are simple solutions of unmodified insulin, which appear clear. When injected subcutaneously, they have a relatively short action profile, with a peak hypoglycaemic effect after 2–4 hours and a duration of 5–8 hours. Soluble insulins are therefore used to cover major meals, and are injected 30 minutes before eating so that their maximal effect coincides with the postprandial glycaemic peak. Soluble insulins are also used for intravenous infusion (e.g. in treating ketoacidosis) and in insulin pumps.

Prolonged-action insulins are chemically modified to delay absorption. These suspensions must be shaken gently before injection and appear cloudy. There are two main types:

- *Insulin–zinc suspensions* are complexed with excess zinc, to produce either large crystals which dissolve and are absorbed very slowly ('ultralente'), or amorphous material with a shorter action profile ('semi-lente'). These are combined in a 70:30 ratio to produce the commonly used 'Lente' insulins (e.g. Humulin Zn and Monotard).
- *Isophane insulins* (e.g. Humulin I, Protaphane) are combined with protamine, and are also known as NPH ('Neutral Protamine Hagedorn').

An ideal long-acting insulin would provide constant basal levels for 24 hours, so that a single daily injection would suffice. In practice, none of the available preparations – including the 'long-acting' human ultralente – reliably lasts a full day, and most severely insulin-deficient (C-peptide-negative) IDDM patients therefore require two daily injections of prolonged-action insulin. Their sluggish onset of action means that these insulins can be injected at any time of day, but for convenience they are usually injected before meals, together with any short-acting insulin. Lente insulins contain excess zinc, which combines with soluble insulin and retards its action. If the two are mixed in the same syringe, soluble insulin should be drawn up before lente to avoid contaminating the soluble bottle with zinc, and the mixture must be injected immediately.

Premixed (biphasic) insulins consist of isophane and soluble insulins mixed in 70:30 (Mixtard), 50:50 (Humulin M5) or other proportions. Their action profiles reflect both components.

Insulin injection regimens

The normal pancreas produces about 40 U of insulin each day. A diabetic patient needs less than this if some endogenous β-cell function remains (e.g. during the 'honeymoon' period of IDDM, described below), and more if insulin sensitivity is impaired by increased counter-regulatory hormone secretion during intercurrent illness, or by obesity in NIDDM.

If little endogenous insulin remains, insulin replacement must provide both the basal and the prandial components of normal insulin secretion. Most C-peptide-negative IDDM patients ultimately require twice-daily injections of prolonged-action insulin, together with soluble insulin before breakfast and the evening meal. Midday meals (if not large) are usually covered by the morning dose of prolonged-action insulin. About two-thirds of the total daily dose is usually given before breakfast and one-third in the evening, each dose consisting roughly of two-thirds of prolonged-action and one-third soluble insulin. Some patients can be controlled by premixed insulins (two-thirds of the daily requirement before breakfast and one-third before supper), whereas others prefer the flexibility of adjusting the soluble and prolonged-action components separately.

'Intensified' insulin regimens use more injections to try to achieve very close glycaemic control. Soluble insulin is injected 30 minutes before each meal, the dose being determined by the amount eaten and previous postprandial glucose measurements; for convenience, this is often given using a pen injection device (see below). The basal needs are covered by long-acting insulin injected once (before breakfast or at bedtime) or twice daily.

Patients with enough residual insulin will be able to fill in gaps in insulin replacement and can achieve good glycaemic control with fewer doses, such as one or two injections of prolonged-action insulin.

A flow-chart for determining insulin treatment is shown in Figure 19.11, and adjustment of insulin dosages on the basis of glycaemic monitoring is discussed on page 757.

Insulin injections, pen devices and pumps

Insulin injections are almost painless. Disposable plastic syringes are now in general use and can be reused several times, if kept socially clean. Insulin should be injected at an angle into a skin-fold raised between finger and thumb, to avoid intramuscular injection which can hasten absorption unpredictably. The skin does not need to be cleaned. Suitable injection areas are the abdomen (where absorption is fastest and most reliable), upper arm and thigh. Sites should be used in rotation to avoid lipoatrophy or lipohypertrophy.

'Pen' injection devices contain a prefilled vial of soluble or isophane insulin of which metered doses can be selected and injected by pressing a button. They are easily portable and popular with active and younger patients, especially for intensified injection regimens. These devices may encourage compliance in individual cases, but do not otherwise improve control.

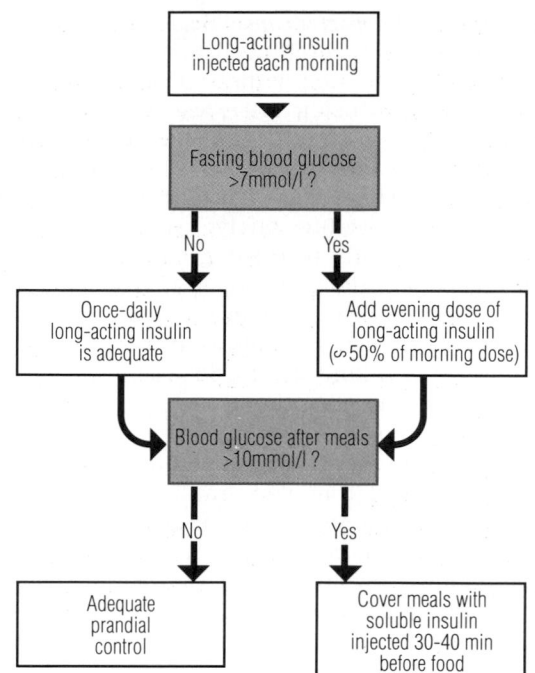

Fig. 19.11 Flow-chart for adjusting insulin treatment. Long-acting insulins provide background requirements; they generally do not last a full 24 hours and C-peptide-negative patients normally need two daily injections. Short-acting insulins are designed to limit hyperglycaemia after meals.

Insulin infusion devices

Insulin pumps are a form of intensified therapy which provides constant background insulin delivery on which extra doses are superimposed to cover meals.

Continuous subcutaneous insulin infusion (CSII) is delivered by a miniaturised battery-driven pump. Insulin in a prefilled cartridge is infused continuously through a butterfly cannula implanted subcutaneously in the abdomen; the infusion site is changed daily. The basal rate can be varied and is often reduced at night, when insulin requirements fall. Prandial boluses, judged according to the size of the meal, are given about 30 minutes before eating, by pressing a button on the pump.

CSII can achieve essentially normal blood glucose levels in selected patients, including some who are poorly controlled by other regimens. However, the technique is accepted by relatively few patients, and requires great commitment from the patient and the diabetes care team. Pump failure is rare, but interruption of insulin delivery, e.g. by blockage or disconnection of the cannula, can rapidly precipitate hyperglycaemia and ketoacidosis because the subcutaneous insulin depot is small. Other problems include infection at infusion sites and the transient deterioration in retinopathy which can accompany any rapid tightening of glycaemic control (p. 765). CSII is currently seldom used in the UK and is usually reserved

for short-term improvement of diabetic control, e.g. before and during pregnancy and for acute painful neuropathy.

Insulin may also be infused intraperitoneally using a pump implanted subcutaneously. Intraperitoneal insulin is absorbed into the portal system and can achieve good control, even in some cases when CSII has failed.

Problems with insulin treatment

Hypoglycaemia

Most insulin-treated IDDM patients suffer occasional hypoglycaemia and, each year, about one in seven patients will have an episode severe enough to require help. Fear of hypoglycaemia probably prevents many patients from trying to achieve tight control. Hypoglycaemia is a recorded cause of death in young IDDM patients, but the chances of a patient dying during a hypoglycaemic episode, even if profound, are very low. The threat of hypoglycaemia can be greatly reduced by education of the patient and his or her family.

Causes of insulin-induced hypoglycaemia. Hypoglycaemia occurs when circulating insulin levels are too high and are insufficiently antagonised by counter-regulatory hormones. Contributory factors are:

- Too much circulating insulin: wrong dose (errors in drawing up and injecting insulin are surprisingly common) or timing (e.g. injection given too long before next meal).
- Not enough food: delayed, missed or inadequate meals.
- Exercise: this hastens absorption of insulin injected into the limbs and increases glucose uptake into muscle; the latter effect continues for several hours after acute strenuous exercise in order to replenish muscle glycogen, and may cause hypoglycaemia the following day.
- Alcohol: this is a potent cause of hypoglycaemia. Ethanol directly inhibits gluconeogenesis and glucose output by the liver.

The widely variable absorption of insulin probably contributes to the many episodes which cannot be explained. Episodes recurring at the same time of day may be due to basic mismatching of the insulin, dietary and exercise regimens. Other possible causes of severe and repeated hypoglycaemia include loss of counter-regulatory hormones (especially in hypothyroidism and Addison's disease), alcohol abuse, the loss of awareness of hypoglycaemia which affects patients with long-standing IDDM, and factitious hypoglycaemia (see below). Patients with diabetic nephropathy clear insulin more slowly from the circulation and so are prone to hypoglycaemia.

Clinical features of hypoglycaemia. Hypoglycaemia triggers a sympathetic discharge and counter-regulatory hormone secretion. This corrects hypoglycaemia by

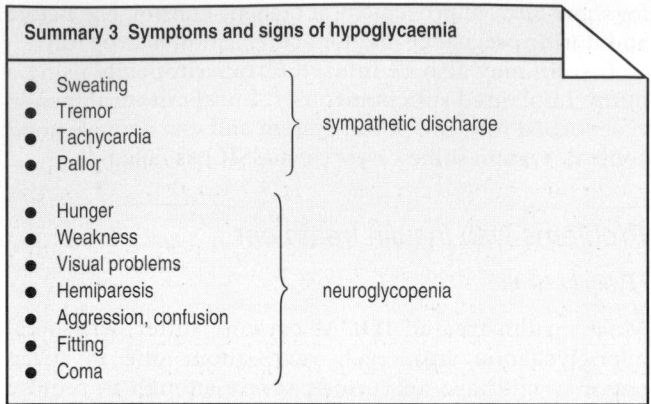

Summary 3 Symptoms and signs of hypoglycaemia

- Sweating
- Tremor — sympathetic discharge
- Tachycardia
- Pallor

- Hunger
- Weakness
- Visual problems
- Hemiparesis — neuroglycopenia
- Aggression, confusion
- Fitting
- Coma

reducing insulin sensitivity in its target tissues; glucagon and adrenaline also stimulate gluconeogenesis, glycogen breakdown and hepatic glucose production. If this response fails to correct the hypoglycaemia, neuroglycopenia may follow.

The main symptoms of hypoglycaemia are attributed to either sympathetic stimulation (sweating, tremor, tachycardia and pallor) or neuroglycopenia, whose many features include hunger and weakness; irritability, confusion and aggression; clumsiness; blurred vision and diplopia; aphasia and hemiparesis. Profound neuroglycopenia can cause fitting, coma and finally death. Repeated, severe hypoglycaemia may cause intellectual impairment. Nocturnal hypoglycaemia may not wake the patient but may be suggested by sweating and restlessness (often apparent to the patient's partner), nightmares and a 'hung-over' feeling with headache the following morning.

Patients with long-standing IDDM (>10 years' duration) may lose their perception of hypoglycaemic symptoms and suddenly develop neuroglycopenia (confusion, fitting, coma) without warning. Most long-standing patients also display blunted glucagon and noradrenaline responses to hypoglycaemia.

Diagnosis of hypoglycemia. After a few episodes, most patients claim to be able to recognise hypoglycaemia. However, some tolerate very low glycaemia without symptoms. Insulin-treated patients must therefore be educated to check their blood glucose levels immediately if they feel unwell in any way, and their relatives should also be able to do this if the patient becomes confused or unconscious or behaves atypically. Patients with possible nocturnal hypoglycaemia (see below) should test themselves during the night (especially at 2–4 a.m.).

Using test-strips, patients can diagnose hypoglycaemia quickly. Test-strip readings on fingerprick samples of <2.5 mmol/l require treatment. If severe features are present, treatment should be started immediately and levels checked as soon as possible afterwards, as they will remain low for some minutes.

Management of hypoglycaemia. Because of the small but significant risks of cerebral damage and death, all episodes must be treated without delay. Most features, including fitting (which is often resistant to anticonvulsants) and coma, are rapidly reversible when glycaemia is normalised.

Mild episodes, where the patient is conscious, cooperative and able to swallow safely, are treated with oral carbohydrate. Twenty to thirty grams of carbohydrate should be taken initially and again if glycaemia has not started to rise after 10–15 minutes.

Severe hypoglycaemia requires intravenous glucose (dextrose). Fifty millilitres of a 50% solution should be given over a minute into a large vein; small veins will be painfully thrombosed by the hypertonic solution. The patient may improve immediately but the intravenous cannula should be left in place until glycaemic and clinical recovery are complete. An alternative is glucagon (1 mg; 0.5 mg in children), which mobilises liver glycogen and acts within a few minutes after intravenous injection. Glucagon injected i.m. or s.c. produces recovery within 10–15 minutes. It is suitable for emergency use outside hospital, and the technique should be taught to the relatives of hypoglycaemia-prone patients.

Patients should always carry easily swallowed carbohydrate, glucose test-strips and documentation that they are receiving insulin (e.g. a clinic or shared-care cooperation card, MedicAlert bracelet or necklace). All episodes should be recorded in the patient's self-monitoring diary and discussed with the diabetes care team.

Summary 4 Management of hypoglycaemia

- Check blood glucose to confirm hypoglycaemia and recovery
- Mild episode (patient able to swallow):
  - Oral carbohydrate (20 g)
- Severe episode (patient unconscious or uncooperative):
  - Glucagon 1 mg i.m. or s.c. or
  - Glucose 50 ml of 50% solution i.v. (use a large vein)
  - Admit to hospital if recovery is not immediate

Injection-site problems

Minor bleeding or bruising after injection sometimes worry the patient but are unimportant. *Lipoatrophy*, pitting of the skin due to loss of subcutaneous tissue, is apparently an allergic response to injected insulin and is uncommon with the use of highly purified human insulin. *Lipohypertrophy* is local thickening of subcutaneous tissue, possibly due to the lipogenic and growth-promoting effects of high ambient insulin concentrations, which may form prominent lumps. Both conditions can be unsightly and may impair the absorption of insulin injected into lesions. They are commoner at frequently used injection sites and can be avoided by using several sites in rotation.

Insulin allergies

Allergic reactions to insulin are now rare. Allergy can cause *local inflammation*, either acute or delayed. *Anaphylaxis*, mediated by IgE antibodies, is rare. *Immune insulin resistance* is due to absorbed insulin combining with IgG antibodies, forming large immune complexes which are cleared rapidly from the circulation by the reticuloendothelial system. Daily insulin requirements of several thousands of units have been recorded.

Insulin allergy may be side-stepped by changing to an unrelated species of insulin (e.g. human, tunafish), and may respond to immunosuppressive drugs or desensitisation with repeated small doses of the allergenic species.

Summary 5 Side-effects of insulin treatment

- Hypoglycaemia
- Injection-site lipoatrophy and lipohypertrophy
- Allergies (rare with highly-purified insulin)
    local inflammation
    anaphylaxis
    immune insulin resistance

Specific problems with insulin treatment

Starting insulin treatment

If the patient is clinically well, insulin therapy can be started at home by the diabetes specialist nurse. Newly diagnosed IDDM patients can be given one or two daily injections of prolonged-action insulin, and soluble insulin can then be added if postprandial glucose levels (90 minutes after eating) are unacceptably high (see Fig. 19.11). Initial insulin doses should be low (e.g. 8–12 U) to avoid severe hypoglycaemia, which can demoralise the newly presenting patient. Except for young children, the elderly and the partially sighted, patients should be encouraged to give their own injections as soon as possible.

After starting insulin treatment, many IDDM patients enjoy a period of high-quality glycaemic control, achieved relatively easily with low insulin requirements; dosages may fall to a few units per day and very rare patients can manage without insulin. This 'honeymoon period' is due to transient recovery of insulin secretion following correction of hyperglycaemia; this ultimately ends because remaining β cells are destroyed by continuing autoimmune disease. Both the 'honeymoon period' and its end have to be anticipated and explained to the patient, as failure to reduce insulin dosages can cause hypogly-

caemia, while at the end, worsening control and increasing dosages can be demoralising.

Poor glycaemic control overnight

Many IDDM patients have fasting early morning hyperglycaemia, sometimes preceded by nocturnal hypoglycaemia. The '*dawn phenomenon*' is a rise in glycaemia during the 2–4 hours before waking. It is apparently due to delayed insulin insensitivity of the tissues, caused by surges of growth hormone secreted after falling asleep, which are accentuated in IDDM. Rebound hyperglycaemia may also occur after hypoglycaemia, and is attributed to discharge of counter-regulatory hormones.

Nocturnal hypoglycaemia followed by fasting hyperglycaemia is often due to the time-course of prolonged-action insulin. When injected in the early evening, its hypoglycaemic action often peaks at 2–4 a.m., but fades thereafter. Simply increasing the evening dose of long-acting insulin may worsen nocturnal hypoglycaemia; the insulin does not last longer, so fasting hyperglycaemia may not improve. Both problems can be improved by delaying the evening injection of long-acting insulin until just before bedtime, so that its peak hypoglycaemic effect is postponed and helps to cancel out the hyperglycaemia of the dawn phenomenon. This regimen requires an extra injection, as short-acting insulin is still needed to cover the evening meal.

Erratic control and 'brittle' diabetes

Few patients enjoy continuously good glycaemic control. This is not surprising, as subcutaneous insulin absorption is extremely variable, both between and within individuals, and because the short-acting preparations act too slowly and for too long, whereas long-acting insulins do not last long enough (Table 19.3).

Patients whose metabolic control is so unstable as to prevent them from living a normal lifestyle (so-called '*brittle*' *diabetes*) are fortunately rare. Unpredictable glycaemic swings are sometimes due to intercurrent infection, endocrine disease (e.g. hypopituitarism) and poor education or treatment regimens. When identifiable causes are excluded, most of the remaining patients are young women who are typically obese and apparently have high insulin requirements. They suffer recurrent ketoacidosis and/or hypoglycaemia. The causes of brittleness in these patients are unknown, but some deliberately manipulate their own treatment (e.g. by omitting insulin) to induce poor control. Management is extremely difficult. They should be admitted to exclude known causes of unstable control and for intensive education and evaluation of control while following a strictly supervised intensive regimen. CSII may be useful in some cases. Sympathetic counselling and psychotherapy of the patient and her family may also help.

Insulin resistance

Most IDDM patients need less than 1 U/kg/day of insulin, but obese NIDDM patients are insulin insensitive and often need more. Clinically, *insulin resistance* has been arbitrarily defined as a daily requirement of >200 U. Causes include excess counter-regulatory hormones (e.g. in septicaemia and glucocorticoid treatment), immune resistance due to insulin antibodies, and defects of the insulin receptor or postreceptor sites. The latter are either inherited (type A syndromes) or acquired (type B syndromes, due to autoantibodies to the receptor). Both syndromes are associated with acanthosis nigricans (p. 739).

Intercurrent illness

The stress of intercurrent illness stimulates secretion of counter-regulatory hormones. Basal insulin requirements therefore increase and the total daily insulin dosage will tend to rise, even if the patient is unable or unwilling to eat. Failure to increase insulin dosage therefore causes hyperglycaemia and ketoacidosis. Some patients reduce or even stop their insulin when they fall ill, mainly because they fear hypoglycaemia while not eating normally. This basic mistake, all too often endorsed by doctors, still causes avoidable deaths in the UK each year. Vomiting is particularly worrying as it may herald ketoacidosis. Patients must be given clear rules stating what to do if they become ill.

Exercise

Regular exercise should be part of the diabetic person's normal lifestyle. Exercise increases glucose uptake into muscle, so favouring hypoglycaemia. Insulin-treated patients can help to avoid hypoglycaemia by reducing insulin dosages before exercise, by checking blood glucose levels before and at intervals during exercise, and by taking carbohydrate (e.g. a small chocolate bar) if glycaemia is <5 mmol/l. They must be told that delayed hypoglycaemia may occur up to a day after strenuous exertion.

Dietary management of IDDM

Food eaten by IDDM patients must balance insulin injections and exercise so as to limit both hyper- and hypoglycaemia.

Total calorie intake. This can be calculated from a person's sex, body weight and level of activity. Most IDDM patients are not obese, and caloric restriction is not needed, although it is in NIDDM. Indeed, some patients with marked weight loss may need to increase their energy intake.

Dietary composition. Advice for diabetic patients has changed completely in recent years. Current recommendations are essentially those for the general population (Table 19.4). The traditional 'diabetic diet', low in all types of carbohydrate and with a relatively high fat content, may have predisposed to macrovascular disease.

Timing and size of meals. Meals must be coordinated with insulin injections and exercise. Twice-daily injection regimens fit best with a larger breakfast and evening meal, a small lunch, and snacks at mid-morning and bedtime. At present, judging insulin doses to cover meals is a matter of trial and error, rather than a science. Hyperlipidaemic patients should reduce their fat intake, and hypertensive patients their salt. A low-protein diet may slow the progression of diabetic nephropathy.

Diabetic education, lifestyle changes

The diabetic patient has to live with his/her disease every day and cope with treatment and self-monitoring procedures which many doctors and nurses do not understand fully. Careful education about diabetes, which may be best provided by the diabetes specialist nurse, can greatly improve diabetic control and quality of life.

Newly diagnosed patients need to learn a great deal, and every patient's understanding of diabetes should be checked and reinforced whenever possible. Some key points are:

- causes and effects of hyper- and hypoglycaemia
- treatment: doses of insulin or tablets; injection technique; diet
- monitoring: techniques; targets; how to respond to poor control
- 'sick-day rules': when and how to call for help.

Table 19.4 Current dietary recommendations for diabetic patients

Carbohydrate: >55% of total calories
Choose complex carbohydrates (starchy foods)
Avoid foods and drinks sweetened with sucrose or glucose

Fat: <30% of total calories
Choose poly- or monounsaturated fats (vegetable oils)
Avoid animal fats, dairy products and cholesterol-rich foods (eggs, fatty meats)
Avoid fried foods

Protein: 10–15% of total calories
Choose fish or vegetable protein (e.g. pulses)

Dietary fibre
Increase intake of vegetables, bran, pulses, etc.

Sweeteners
Avoid 'diabetic' foods (which contain sorbitol or fructose)
Aspartame is an acceptable calorie-free sweetener

This is not a 'diabetic' diet, but a guide to healthy eating suitable for the general population.

General suggestions for healthy living apply particularly to diabetic patients. Stopping smoking reduces the risks of macrovascular disease and probably of nephropathy and retinopathy. Alcohol, which is both a source of 'invisible' calories and a cause of hypoglycaemia, should be limited to 21 units/week in men and 14 units/week in women, and less in hypertensive patients. Regular exercise should be taken.

There are no employment restrictions on patients not receiving insulin and without complications but, because of the risk of hypoglycaemia, insulin treatment is a bar to joining the armed, police or fire-fighting forces and driving public-service or heavy-goods vehicles. Insulin-treated patients must inform the driving licence authorities and their insurance companies, and may need medical confirmation of fitness to drive. Special life insurance policies are available.

Novel and experimental treatments of IDDM

Immunosuppression can prevent insulitis and diabetes in animal models of IDDM and preliminary trials of prednisolone and cyclosporin given during the pre-diabetic phase of human IDDM suggests that the need for insulin treatment can be delayed or its dosage reduced. However, these drugs have serious side-effects and less toxic alternatives are being sought.

Pancreatic and islet transplantation. Segments of whole pancreas can be transplanted, with the exocrine ducts either occluded or drained into the bladder to prevent release of harmful enzymes into the peritoneal cavity. Islets isolated by partial enzymatic digestion of the pancreas can survive and secrete insulin in various anatomical sites including the liver, where they can be placed by injection into the portal vein. At present, however, both pancreas and islet transplants require immunosuppression and so are generally performed in patients undergoing renal transplantation, who will receive long-term immunosuppressive therapy. The best results with both techniques indicate that insulin dosage can be reduced, and in some cases withdrawn, for many months and even years.

NON-INSULIN-DEPENDENT DIABETES MELLITUS (NIDDM)

Three-quarters of British diabetic patients have NIDDM. This is often described as 'mild' diabetes, but these patients are nevertheless susceptible to chronic diabetic complications and most die prematurely, mainly from myocardial infarction. NIDDM is a common disease in well-fed societies, affecting perhaps 10% of Britons and North Americans over 70 years of age. There is a striking geographical and racial variation, which is totally different from that in IDDM. NIDDM is several times commoner in Asian immigrants to the UK than in the indigenous British population, and the highest recorded prevalence is in the Pima Indians of Arizona, of whom 50% are affected. Except for MODY (maturity onset diabetes of the young), most patients are over 40 years of age at presentation, and males predominate.

Aetiology and pathogenesis

NIDDM appears to be due to two separate defects – insensitivity of the tissues to insulin and defective insulin secretion – both of which may be partly inherited (Fig. 19.12).

Genetic factors

The concordance rate for NIDDM in identical twins exceeds 95%. Inheritance appears to be polygenic, except in MODY and certain other families, where NIDDM is transmitted as an autosomal dominant. No predictive HLA types or other genetic markers have yet been identified.

Insulin resistance

This signifies the inability of insulin at physiological concentrations to exert its normal metabolic actions. Investigation shows that insulin's action is reduced by about 40% in NIDDM. Liver, skeletal muscle and fat are all insensitive, so that increased hepatic glucose output and reduced peripheral uptake both contribute to hyper-

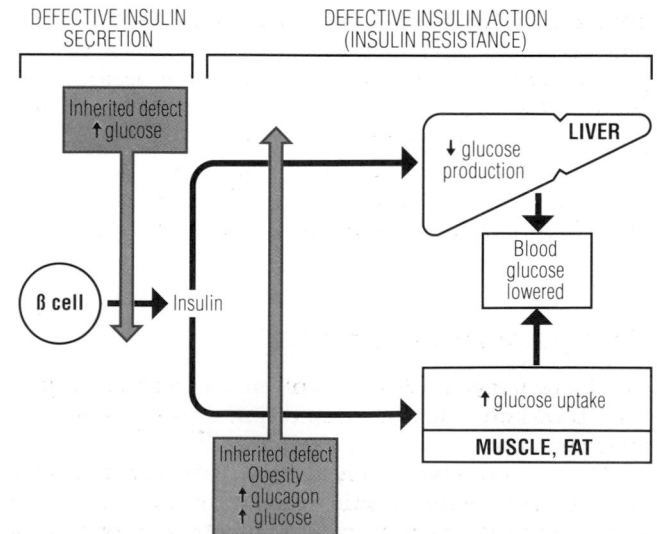

Fig. 19.12 Metabolic defects in NIDDM. Insulin secretion and insulin action (at the level of the liver and the peripheral tissues) are both impaired. The blood sugar rises as a result.

glycaemia (Fig. 19.12). The defect(s) causing insensitivity to insulin are unknown and apparently lie beyond its receptor. Possible contributory factors include obesity (which is strongly associated with NIDDM), an inherited predisposition and increased glucagon levels; hyperglycaemia itself also reduces insulin sensitivity.

Defective insulin secretion

Resting insulin levels as measured by conventional insulin radioimmunoassay may be normal, high or low in NIDDM patients. Much of this 'insulin' immunoreactivity is now known to represent biologically inert cleavage products of proinsulin which cross-react in the assay. True insulin levels (measured by a highly specific assay) are subnormal in most, if not all, NIDDM subjects. Furthermore, non-diabetic people exposed to hyperglycaemia would respond with far higher insulin levels than occur in NIDDM, and spontaneous pulses and the first phase of insulin secretion are absent in NIDDM.

The cause is unknown. β-cell numbers are reduced by 50% but there are no signs of autoimmune damage. The islets become infiltrated with amyloid deposits containing a peptide named amylin, or islet amyloid polypeptide. Amylin is synthesised by the β cells, but its possible aetiological role in NIDDM remains uncertain. Hyperglycaemia *per se* may also impair insulin secretion.

Biochemical abnormalities

There is hyperglycaemia, but enough insulin secretion remains to prevent lipolysis. Spontaneous ketosis and ketoacidosis therefore do not occur, even in extreme hyperglycaemia (hyperosmolar, non-ketotic coma).

Clinical features of NIDDM

Two-thirds of NIDDM patients in the UK are obese. At diagnosis, hyperglycaemic symptoms (polyuria, thirst, polydipsia) have usually been present for months or even years. An acute presentation and sudden marked weight loss are unusual but may occur, especially with intercurrent illness, introduction of diabetogenic drugs or carcinoma of the pancreas, which is associated with NIDDM in older people. Women often have troublesome pruritis vulvae due to candidiasis.

NIDDM often has a long subclinical course and many asymptomatic patients are diagnosed incidentally when screened routinely for glycosuria or hyperglycaemia. Others present with chronic diabetic complications such as myocardial infarction, retinopathy (especially maculopathy), or foot ulceration.

By definition, MODY presents in patients under 25 years of age, who do not need insulin for at least 5 years.

MODY is transmitted as an autosomal dominant trait. Some affected families appear to be relatively protected from chronic diabetic complications.

NIDDM is diagnosed and distinguished from IDDM as described on page 744 and in Table 19.2.

Management of NIDDM

NIDDM is often harder to treat effectively than IDDM. Diet is usually described as the 'cornerstone' of management, but unfortunately few patients are able to follow dietary advice continuously. Oral hypoglycaemic agents are ineffective in many patients, especially the obese majority, and insulin treatment introduces its own problems. A flow-chart for treating NIDDM is shown in Figure 19.13.

Diet and general lifestyle changes

All NIDDM patients should eat a 'healthy' diet (Table 19.4) and obese patients will also need to reduce their total intake of calories, especially of fat. This often causes

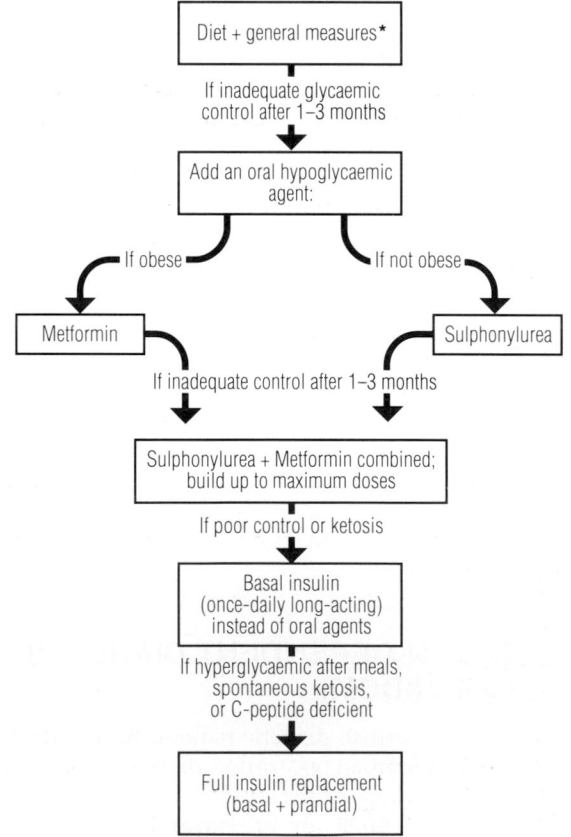

*Stop smoking; Reduce alcohol intake; Treat hyperlipidaemia; Treat hypertension; Regular exercise

Fig. 19.13 Flow-chart for treating NIDDM. Glycaemic targets are shown in Table 19.5.

an acute fall in blood glucose levels with symptomatic improvement; continued weight loss will produce a sustained reduction, and even normalization, of glycaemia. An acceptable rate of weight loss is about 0.5–1 kg per week, which corresponds to an energy deficit of at least 500 kcal/day. Weight loss, especially if combined with exercise, increases insulin sensitivity and also improves hyperlipidaemia and hypertension. Timing and distribution of meals is not critical in patients who are not taking insulin or sulphonylureas, as hypoglycaemia does not occur.

A sympathetic but firm dietitian, possibly reinforced by a slimming club, stands the best chance of success. Very low calorie diets (<700 kcal/day), which are very expensive, and weight-reducing drugs such as appetite suppressants (e.g. D-fenfluramine) and β_3-adrenergic agonists which increase energy expenditure, are being evaluated.

Weight-reducing diets must be given an adequate trial of 1–3 months but fewer than 20% of NIDDM patients will achieve either their target weight or acceptable glycaemic control (Table 19.5). The rest, given the gloomy label of 'dietary failures', need oral hypoglycaemic agents or insulin.

It is vital to tackle the risk factors for cardiovascular disease, which is the main cause of premature death in NIDDM. General measures include stopping smoking, moderating alcohol intake, taking regular exercise and controlling hyperlipidaemia and hypertension. Monitoring of NIDDM is generally assessed from once- or twice-weekly fasting glucose levels, although insulin-treated patients will need to test more frequently (p. 757).

Oral hypoglycaemic agents

The major oral hypoglycaemic agents (Table 19.6) are the sulphonylureas and metformin. Other drugs with

Table 19.5 Targets for diabetic control

	Ideal	Acceptable
Blood glucose (mmol/l)		
Fasting	4.4–6.7	<7.8
Postprandial	4.4–8.9	<10.0
Glycosylated haemoglobin (%)		
(with normal range of 5–8%)	6–8	8–10
Other targets		
Few hypoglycaemic episodes		
Body mass index <25*		
Normal plasma lipid concentrations		
Normal growth (in children)		
No diabetic complications	ultimate aims	
Normal lifespan		

*Body mass index = weight (kg)/height (m)².

Table 19.6 Oral hypoglycaemic agents

	Drug	Dosage schedule	Comments
First-generation sulphonylureas	Chlorpropamide	250–500 mg o.d.	Hypoglycaemia +++ (long half-life) Avoid in elderly and in renal failure Alcohol-induced flushing
	Tolbutamide	500 mg b.d., t.d.s.	Acceptable in mild renal impairment
Second-generation sulphonylureas	Glibenclamide	2.5–15 mg o.d.	Hypoglycaemia +++ (long biological action) Avoid in elderly or in renal failure
	Gliclazide	40–160 mg o.d., b.d	Acceptable in mild renal impairment
	Glipizide	2.5–15 mg o.d., b.d.	Acceptable in mild renal impairment
Biguanide	Metformin	500–850 mg b.d., t.d.s.	Contraindicated in renal, hepatic, cardiac or respiratory failures Does not cause hypoglycaemia

minor hypoglycaemic effects include soluble vegetable fibres such as guar, which interfere with intestinal glucose absorption, and the α-glucosidase inhibitors (e.g. acarbose and miglitol) which block the digestion of starch.

Sulphonylureas

These are derivatives of sulphonamides. 'First-generation' drugs include chlorpropamide and tolbutamide, and the newer 'second-generation' compounds include glibenclamide, gliclazide and glipizide (Table 19.6). Second-generation sulphonylureas are more potent, but seem to have few other specific advantages.

Mechanism of action and pharmacology. Sulphonylureas act primarily as insulin secretagogues. They restore the missing first phase of insulin release and enhance basal and prandial insulin secretion. As sulphonylureas depend on releasing endogenous insulin, they are ineffective in insulin-deficient IDDM patients. Sulphonylureas may exert an additional 'extrapancreatic' action, by slightly enhancing insulin sensitivity. Overall, sulphonylureas reduce fasting and postprandial glycaemia by about 25% in moderately hyperglycaemic patients, but usually have little effect if fasting glycaemia exceeds 14 mmol/l. They are ineffective at the outset in 5% of NIDDM patients, and subsequently fail in many of those who respond initially; poor compliance with treatment or progressive deterioration ('exhaustion') of β cells may be responsible.

Most sulphonylureas are cleared through the kidneys, although glipizide is metabolised in the liver. Chlorpropamide has a very long plasma half-life (36 hours) and glibenclamide has prolonged biological effects which outlast its survival in the circulation. These long-acting drugs are taken once daily. The others, especially the very short-acting tolbutamide and glipizide, are usually taken before breakfast and the evening meal.

Adverse effects of sulphonylureas. Hypoglycaemia is the main hazard, especially with the long-acting drugs in renal failure (when they accumulate) and in older people. Chlorpropamide and glibenclamide must therefore be avoided in patients over 60 years of age, and in renal failure. The short-acting agents are relatively safer in mild renal impairment but patients with nephropathy should be transferred to insulin when serum creatinine concentration rises above 250 μmol/l.

Weight gain further reduces insulin sensitivity and damages morale; it is probably due to the lipogenic effects of increased insulin levels, perhaps with relaxed dietary compliance in some cases.

Allergic skin rashes are fairly common. *Alcohol-induced facial flushing* is an idiosyncratic reaction in patients taking chlorpropamide. Rarer side-effects include water retention and hyponatraemia due to potentiation of ADH action and blood dyscrasias. Their hypoglycaemic effects are potentiated by drugs such as the sulphonamides, co-trimoxazole, fibrates, salicylates and probenecid, which compete for binding to plasma proteins and reduce the clearance of sulphonylureas.

Clinical use of sulphonylureas. They are indicated for dietary failure in NIDDM, especially in non-obese patients; obese subjects may benefit more from metformin which does not cause weight gain. Sulphonylureas are contraindicated in IDDM (C-peptide-negative) patients, or in NIDDM patients during intercurrent illness or surgery, because insulin is required.

Metformin

Metformin (Table 19.6) reduces hyperglycaemia by stimulating glucose uptake into peripheral tissues and by inhibiting gluconeogenesis from lactate in the liver. It does not stimulate insulin secretion and so does not cause hypoglycaemia in normoglycaemic subjects. Metformin reduces glycaemia by a similar degree to the sulphonylureas and is ineffective if fasting glycaemia exceeds 14 mmol/l.

Adverse effects of metformin. Lactic acidosis. Blocking lactate utilisation through gluconeogenesis inevitably causes lactate accumulation. Lactic acidosis occurs rarely with metformin, except in the 'organ failures' which either increase lactate production or prevent its utilization (p. 741).

Gastrointestinal problems, notably bloating, nausea, dyspepsia and diarrhoea are common; anorexia may help to prevent weight gain during metformin treatment. Metformin impairs vitamin B_{12} absorption and occasionally causes a megaloblastic anaemia.

Clinical use of metformin. Metformin is indicated in patients who fail to respond to diet, either alone or together with a sulphonylurea, especially if obese. It is contraindicated absolutely in renal, hepatic, cardiac and respiratory failures because the risks of lactic acidosis are greatly increased, and in insulin-deficient patients.

Insulin treatment in NIDDM

Diet with one or both types of oral agent will only achieve satisfactory long-term control (Table 19.5) in 50% of patients with fasting glycaemia of <10 mmol/l, and in few with higher glucose levels. Insulin is needed in patients with unacceptable hyperglycaemia or features of insulin deficiency (weight loss and spontaneous ketonuria).

Many NIDDM patients will be satisfactorily controlled by a single daily injection of ultralente or isophane insulin, as their remaining insulin secretion can cover mealtime requirements, but those with worsening insulin deficiency (low C-peptide levels) may ultimately need multiple injections, as for IDDM. Insulin treatment often causes weight gain, which further aggravates insulin insensitivity and increases insulin requirements, but the risks of hyperglycaemia probably outweigh those of obesity.

IMPAIRED GLUCOSE TOLERANCE (IGT)

This diagnostic category defines subjects whose blood glucose concentration lies between normality and diabetes, i.e. between 6.7 and 10.0 mmol/l 2 hours after a 75-g OGTT (p. 743 and Fig. 19.8). IGT is asymptomatic but must be distinguished from normal because long-term follow-up studies indicate that these subjects carry a considerably increased risk of cardiovascular disease (*not* microvascular disease, which only develops with truly diabetic glucose levels; see p. 764). Many are obese and display the hyperinsulinaemia, insulin insensitivity, hypertension and hyperlipidaemia which strongly predict cardiovascular disease (see p. 771).

After 10 years, most IGT subjects will remain in this category, but 25% will revert to normal while 25% progress to NIDDM. IGT has no specific management, but diabetogenic drugs (e.g. thiazides) should be withdrawn if possible and the patient strongly encouraged to lose weight (which tends to normalise glucose tolerance), stop smoking and reduce other cardiovascular risk factors.

Patients and their blood glucose levels should be reviewed annually, and the OGTT repeated if circumstances change.

SECONDARY DIABETES MELLITUS

Malnutrition-related diabetes mellitus (MRDM). Malnutrition can cause pancreatic damage and diabetes, through unknown mechanisms. MRDM is rare, and comprises two types:

- *Fibrocalculous pancreatic diabetes* is accompanied by chronic pancreatitis with recurrent abdominal pain, formation of large pancreatic calculi (easily visible on plain radiography or ultrasound scanning) and steatorrhoea.
- *Protein-deficient pancreatic diabetes* (PDPD) is less clearly defined.

Both types affect young adults who usually need insulin, sometimes in large doses in PDPD, but ketosis is rare.

Pancreatic disease. Diabetes may be caused by *chronic pancreatitis*, usually due to ethanol abuse. *Haemochromatosis* causes diabetes, cirrhosis and occasionally bronzing of the skin, due to iron deposition in the islets, hepatocytes and dermis. *Carcinoma of the pancreas* is associated with NIDDM in older people.

Endocrine diseases causing diabetes are *acromegaly* (60% of patients have IGT or diabetes), *Cushing's syndrome* (including iatrogenic causes), *phaeochromocytoma* and the very rare *glucagonoma*. These conditions produce excessive counter-regulatory hormones, whereas *Conn's syndrome* may cause IGT and sometimes diabetes through potassium depletion which impairs insulin secretion.

Gestational diabetes is described on page 760.

Diabetogenic drugs include the glucocorticoids, β_2-adrenergic agents (e.g. salbutamol or ritodrine) given intravenously, thiazide diuretics (which cause potassium depletion) and diazoxide (which blocks insulin release directly).

Other rare conditions associated with diabetes include the DIDMOAD syndrome (diabetes insipidus, diabetes mellitus, optic atrophy and deafness), lipoatrophic diabetes (with partial or total loss of subcutaneous fat) and 'leprechaunism', due to insulin receptor defects.

ASSESSING DIABETIC CONTROL

Diabetic treatment aims to keep glycaemia close to normal, to avoid the acute and long-term complications (p. 764). Various measures of immediate and medium-term glycaemic control are available (Table 19.5).

Blood glucose monitoring

The development of test-strips suitable for self-monitoring of blood glucose levels has revolutionised diabetes management. Most test-strips (e.g. BM sticks and Glucostix) contain glucose oxidase and a dye which reacts with the hydrogen peroxide generated by the oxidation of glucose in the blood sample. The colour developed can be read either visually against a colour-chart, or electronically by a reflectance meter. Newer 'sticks' measure glucose oxidation electrically.

Blood is usually obtained from the sides of the pulp of the finger and not the tip (which is a sensory organ), using various lancet devices. A generous drop is lowered carefully on to the reagent area, which must be covered completely, left in contact *exactly* for the reaction period stipulated, and then wiped off. The colour is allowed to develop for the correct time before reading. Inaccurate readings (sometimes dangerously misleading) are common in patients' own records and on ward charts. *All* doctors and nurses and all insulin-treated patients must be able to measure blood glucose with test-strips; the patient's technique and ability to interpret the results should be checked regularly.

For IDDM patients taking twice-daily insulin, the key time-points for testing are: before breakfast (when levels are determined by the previous evening's long-acting dose), before lunch and before the evening meal (determined by the morning's dose), and before bed (influenced by the evening's dose). Generally, readings can be made at different time-points on different days so that a pattern is built up. Patients should test whenever they feel unwell, and during the night if nocturnal hypoglycaemia is suspected (p. 751). Prandial doses of soluble insulin can be adjusted from the glucose level 90–120 minutes after eating. In NIDDM patients treated with oral agents and diet, occasional fasting values are a useful index of control.

Urinalysis for glucose and ketones

Urinalysis for glucose (using glucose oxidase test-strips) is inconvenient and usually unhelpful, as it reflects the average glycaemia above the renal threshold (which can lie anywhere between 7 and 13 mmol/l) since the bladder was last emptied. A crucial failing is that normo- and hypoglycaemia cannot be distinguished. Urinary glucose measurements are acceptable only in rare patients who cannot be persuaded to prick their fingers, and in NIDDM patients with a normal renal threshold who are not receiving insulin or who are not subject to hypoglycaemia.

Urinary ketone measurements provide useful warning of ketoacidosis and can be useful in children during intercurrent illness.

Glycosylated haemoglobin and fructosamine

Valine residues on the β-chain of the adult haemoglobin (HbA) molecule can react with glucose, and the resulting glycosylated haemoglobin (designated HbA$_1$) can be separated from native HbA and measured by electrophoresis. HbA$_1$ can be resolved further into subcomponents, of which HbA$_{1c}$ is the most stable and clinically useful. The proportion of HbA$_1$ which is glycosylated depends on its total exposure to glucose and is proportional to the average glycaemia during the half-life of the red blood cell, i.e. the preceding 6–8 weeks.

Non-diabetic HbA$_1$ values are about 5–8% of total HbA; well- and poorly-controlled diabetic values are about 8–10% and >12%, respectively. HbA$_1$ measurements are a useful index of medium-term glycaemic control but are invalidated if red-cell turnover is disturbed or if abnormally migrating Hb variants are present.

Serum albumin is also glycosylated and can be measured by the 'fructosamine' reaction. Albumin turns over faster than HbA$_1$ and indicates mean glycaemia during the previous 1–2 weeks. Current assays are cheaper, but less reliable and reproducible, than those for HbA$_1$.

ORGANISATION AND DELIVERY OF DIABETES CARE

Development of the diabetes care team, consisting primarily of doctors, specialist diabetes nurses, dietitian and chiropodist, has greatly improved efficiency by allowing effective division of labour. The diabetes specialist nurse is especially important, for educating patients about diabetes and starting and adjusting treatment. Other specialists, e.g. ophthalmologist, vascular surgeon and obstetrician, should be readily available for referral, and combined clinics, such as for diabetic foot problems, are particularly useful.

'Shared-care' schemes which involve both the general practice and the hospital team in looking after the patient are becoming popular, as are community 'miniclinics'.

However care is organised, all diabetic patients must be thoroughly reviewed annually, primarily to screen for complications (Table 19.7), and must have easy access to expert help.

INTERCURRENT EVENTS AND DIABETES

Infection

It is widely held that diabetic patients are generally more susceptible to infection than the non-diabetic population.

Diabetic patients are more likely to suffer infections with certain atypical or unusual organisms. These include tuberculosis; combined staphylococcal/streptococcal infections which result in a rapidly spreading cellulitis

Table 19.7 Annual review of the diabetic patient

Treatment and self-monitoring
Check and adjust as necessary
Coexistent risk factors and diseases
Strongly discourage smoking
Examination
Body weight and BMI*:   – determine target weight
Cardiovascular: – blood pressure, lying and standing; signs of heart failure; peripheral pulses (presence, strength, bruits)
Peripheral nerves: – examine limbs for neuropathy
Feet: – examine carefully
Eyes: – visual acuity (before mydriatics; ± glasses or pinhole); fundoscopy through dilated pupils; check for cataracts
Investigations
HbA$_1$
Plasma urea, creatinine and electrolytes
Fasting plasma lipid concentrations
Urinary albumin excretion
ECG if >40 years of age

*Body mass index; see Table 19.5.

('progressive synergistic gangrene'); mucormycosis (p. 281); and gas-forming organisms which infect the soft tissues of the feet or urinary tract.

Surgery

Surgery presents several potential hazards to diabetic patients. Firstly, the controlled trauma of surgery provokes a counter-regulatory stress response which causes catabolism and, especially in insulin-deficient patients, can rapidly cause hyperglycaemia and ketoacidosis. Secondly, insulin and the sulphonylureas can cause severe hypoglycaemia in fasted or anorexic patients and this is particularly dangerous during general anaesthesia. Finally, poorly controlled diabetes accelerates catabolism and delays wound healing postoperatively.

Diabetic control must therefore be meticulous. The risks of operating on diabetic subjects can be greatly reduced by agreeing a routine management policy between the diabetes care team, surgeons, anaesthetists and ward staff. Fitness for surgery should be carefully assessed in the light of cardiovascular or other complications. Patients should be admitted some days before surgery to stabilise their treatment if necessary, and blood glucose levels must be monitored regularly throughout the perioperative period. Basic treatment guidelines are as follows:

- *NIDDM patients who are well controlled by diet or oral agents and undergoing minor surgery only.* Change long-acting sulphonylureas (chlorpropamide, glibenclamide) to short-acting drugs (e.g. tolbutamide, gliclazide) some days before surgery to reduce the risk of hypoglycaemia; omit oral agents and breakfast on the morning of operation; monitor glycaemia carefully and treat persistent hyperglycaemia with the intravenous glucose–potassium–insulin regimen described below.

- *All other diabetic patients.* Stop regular insulin on morning of surgery, give a continuous intravenous infusion of balanced amounts of glucose, potassium and insulin ('GKI'), which will both maintain satisfactory glycaemic control (5–10 mmol/l) and prevent hypokalaemia (p. 851). This regimen (Table 19.8) should be started on the morning of surgery and continued until the patient is able to eat and drink normally, when the usual treatment can be resumed. Alternatively, insulin may be given as a variable rate infusion which provides greater flexibility.

Pregnancy

Pregnancy in diabetes poses problems for both mother and fetus. Two separate aspects need to be considered, namely pregnancy in women with established diabetes, and 'gestational' diabetes which is precipitated by pregnancy in a previously non-diabetic woman.

Pregnancy in established diabetes

Diabetes can cause difficulties at all stages of pregnancy; fortunately, most can be avoided by careful diabetic management.

Conception. Menstrual disturbance, anovulatory cycles and subfertility are common in poorly controlled diabetic women.

Risks to the mother during pregnancy. Pregnancy worsens hyperglycaemia, especially during the second and third trimesters, apparently because the hormones of pregnancy (e.g. placental lactogen) are diabetogenic. Pregnant diabetic women are at increased risk of hypertension and pre-eclampsia, and both retinopathy and nephropathy may deteriorate rapidly, possibly secondary to improved glycaemic control (p. 765). Delivery of overweight (macrosomic) babies also carries risks for the mother. Maternal mortality for diabetic women was previously high but is now comparable to that in the general population.

Risks to the fetus. Uncontrolled diabetes affects the fetus in several ways. *Congenital malformations*, especially cardiovascular and skeletal (e.g. agenesis of the sacrum), are three times commoner than in non-diabetic pregnancies and occur in up to 7% of cases. Diabetes is particularly teratogenic during the first 10 weeks of fetal life, when the major organs are being formed. The cause is not known. *Macrosomia* (increased body size and obesity) occurs because glucose crosses the placenta and high levels stimulate hyperplasia of the fetal β cells and insulin secretion; the resultant hyperinsulinaemia induces growth

Summary 6 Diabetes and pregnancy
Effects on the mother:
Insulin resistance and increased requirements
Microvascular complications may deteriorate
Risk of dystocia with macrosomic babies
Effects on the fetus:
Congenital malformations
Macrosomia
Effects on the neonate:
Birth trauma from macrosomia
Hypoglycaemia
Respiratory distress syndrome

and lipogenesis in the fetus. Gross macrosomia can cause dystocia and so threaten both mother and fetus.

Risks to the neonate. Babies of diabetic mothers are liable to hypoglycaemia in the neonatal period (because their hyperplastic β cells continue to secrete excessive insulin) and the respiratory distress syndrome (hyperglycaemia decreases surfactant synthesis and lung maturation). Perinatal mortality has fallen but remains higher than in non-diabetic pregnancies.

Diabetic women who intend to become pregnant require specific counselling and very tight diabetic control should be achieved before conception, to ensure near-normoglycaemia during the critical first few weeks of organogenesis. Patients must be encouraged to stop smoking and drinking alcohol, and other medical problems such as hypertension or retinopathy must be assessed and treated. Very tight glycaemic targets should be set (Table 19.5) and achieved if necessary by intensive insulin treatment with multiple daily injections or CSII. The few women taking oral agents should be transferred to insulin.

Fetal growth must be carefully monitored. Ultrasound scanning can identify macrosomia, manifested as an excessive increase in abdominal girth, and major malformations. Fetal lung maturation can be difficult to assess, because diabetes spuriously increases the commonly used lecithin:sphingomyelin ratio in amniotic fluid.

Macrosomia can be avoided by careful diabetic control, and full-term delivery (vaginal if possible) is preferred to reduce the hazards of prematurity, especially the respiratory distress syndrome. During labour, diabetes should be controlled by intravenous glucose–potassium–insulin infusion (see above and Table 19.8). Insulin requirements rise rapidly if dexamethasone is given to encourage fetal lung maturation or ritodrine to delay delivery, and dosages fall dramatically after the placenta is delivered. The neonate needs careful monitoring for hypoglycaemia (especially if macrosomic) and respiratory distress. The mother's usual diabetic treatment can be resumed soon after delivery, but oral agents must be avoided during breast-feeding as they enter the milk.

Table 19.8 Glucose–potassium–insulin ('GKI') regimen for surgery in diabetic patients

Indication
All diabetic patients *except* for NIDDM treated with oral agents or diet alone and undergoing minor surgery only

Infusion
15 U soluble insulin + 10 mmol KCl in 500 ml of 10% dextrose

Delivery
Infuse at 100 ml/hour
Check blood glucose level hourly:
– if glucose < 5 mmol/l: replace bag with one containing 10 U insulin + KCl
– if glucose > 10 mmol/l: replace bag with one containing 20 U insulin + KCl

Table 19.9 Causes of coma in a diabetic person

Diabetic ketoacidosis
Hyperosmolar, non-ketotic coma
Hypoglycaemia
Lactic acidosis
Others:
    Strokes (commoner in diabetes)
    Postictal (hypoglycaemia can cause fitting)
    Drug overdose (including insulin)
    Alcohol (can cause hypoglycaemia)

Gestational diabetes

This is diabetes occurring in 1–2% of pregnancies. The women were not diabetic before the pregnancy, although they may have been diabetic during previous pregnancies. Up to 70% subsequently develop NIDDM. The women are likely to be obese with a family history of NIDDM. The cause is the diabetogenic effects of the hormones of pregnancy, notably placental lactogen and perhaps oestrogens and cortisol. Gestational diabetes is virtually always an NIDDM-like syndrome, but most patients require insulin treatment to achieve adequate glycaemic control.

Hyperglycaemia is most pronounced during the second trimester and resolves after delivery. It is often asymptomatic and has little effect on the mother, but the fetus is at risk of macrosomia and the other hazards of diabetes described above. Early detection and treatment are therefore crucial.

Ideally, all pregnant women should be screened (by post-prandial blood glucose followed by OGTT if the value exceeds 7 mmol/l) early in pregnancy and during the second trimester. In practice, screening concentrates on the high-risk patients, namely those with gestational diabetes, hydramnios, malformed or macrosomic (>4.5 kg) babies in previous pregnancies; a family history of NIDDM; obesity; or glycosuria (which occurs in many normoglycaemic women during pregnancy because the renal threshold falls). Management targets are as above and insulin treatment, often intensive, is usually required.

DIABETIC METABOLIC EMERGENCIES

Coma in diabetic patients is commonly due to the disease's metabolic complications or its treatment, but other causes (Table 19.9) are very important and must be considered.

Diabetic ketoacidosis

Diabetic ketoacidosis (DKA) is severe uncontrolled diabetes with hyperglycaemia and metabolic acidosis due to high circulating ketone-body levels; acetoacetate and 3-hydroxybutyrate are organic acids. Ketone body overproduction is due to unrestrained lipolysis which only occurs with severe insulin deficiency. DKA therefore develops only in IDDM.

Before insulin, DKA killed most IDDM patients. It remains an important problem and the commonest cause of death in IDDM patients under 20 years of age. Overall mortality approaches 10% and exceeds 50% in older patients with severe intercurrent illness. Many deaths are due to avoidable delays and mistakes in diagnosis or treatment. The blood glucose level must always be checked in anyone who is ill.

Pathophysiology

DKA is due to insulin deficiency, compounded by excesses of glucagon and other counter-regulatory hormones. Insulin deficiency occurs in newly presenting, untreated IDDM patients and in established patients who omit or reduce their insulin, or fail to increase it during intercurrent illness (see p. 752). Counter-regulatory hormones are increased by the stress of intercurrent illness, such as infection (sometimes apparently trivial), trauma, surgery, burns or myocardial infarction. About 40% of episodes are unexplained, but patients often fail to take enough insulin during illness.

The result is runaway catabolism in all three branches of metabolism (see Figs 19.4–19.6). Unsuppressed lipolysis in fat yields FFA, which fuel ketogenesis, and glycerol, which together with alanine from proteolysis feeds hepatic gluconeogenesis. When hyperglycaemia exceeds the renal reabsorption threshold, glucose remains in the urine and, together with high ketone-body levels, causes an intense osmotic diuresis which takes sodium and potassium with it. This causes dehydration, hypovolaemia and renal underperfusion, which reduces the clearance of glucose through the kidneys (an important mechanism for limiting hyperglycaemia) and may lead to acute tubular necrosis (Fig. 19.14). Electrolyte and water depletion are exacerbated by vomiting, a direct central action of hyperketonaemia. DKA typically causes the loss of several litres of water and several hundred millimoles each (perhaps a week's normal intake) of sodium, potassium and chloride.

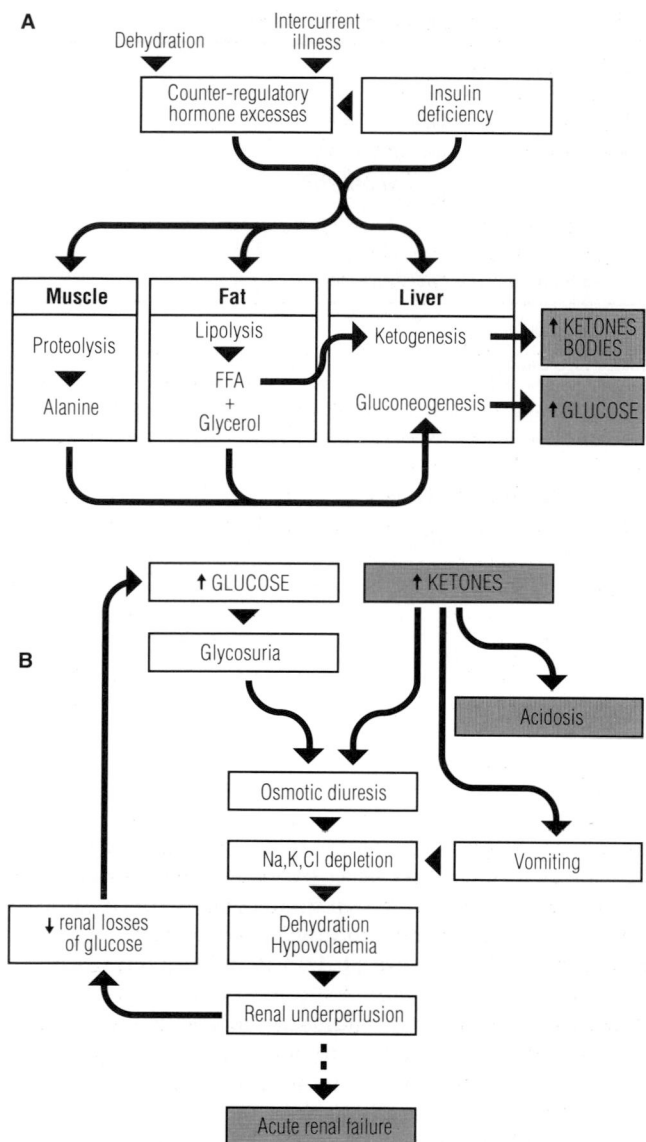

Fig. 19.14 Diabetic ketoacidosis. Biochemical basis (A) and pathophysiological disturbances (B).

Acidosis develops when acetoacetate and 3-hydroxybutyrate levels exceed the body's buffering capacity. Intracellular acidosis interferes with vital enzymes; death usually results from cardiac arrest.

Clinical features

The features of DKA are usually superimposed on those of untreated IDDM. Hyperventilation driven by acidosis may be mistaken for cardiac or respiratory dyspnoea. Acetone may be smelled on the breath. Nausea and vomiting are ominous, as dehydration can rapidly worsen.

Hypothermia, due to peripheral vasodilatation, may mask pyrexia of infection. Drowsiness and coma occur late.

Investigations and diagnosis

Once suspected, the diagnosis can be confirmed instantly by measuring blood glucose and urinary ketone levels with test-strips. Once diagnosed, treatment must begin immediately. Initial investigations aim to:

- *Assess the severity of DKA.* Venous blood is taken for glucose, urea and electrolytes; arterial blood for pH and gases; and urine is tested for ketones. Typical values are shown in Table 19.10. Blood ketone levels are measured by some laboratories and will exceed 5 mmol/l (normal range, <1 mmol/l). Plasma osmolality can be measured formally or calculated approximately (in mosmol/kg) as twice the sum of plasma sodium+potassium, plus the sum of urea+glucose (all in mmol/l). The 'anion gap' (plasma [Na+K] − [Cl+HCO$_3$]) will be increased above normal (>17 mmol/l) by the presence of acetoacetate and 3-hydroxybutyrate.
- *Identify the cause of DKA.* Tests should include a full blood count (note that DKA can cause a neutrophil leucocytosis, without infection), chest X-ray, ECG and cardiac enzymes in older patients, and blood and urine cultures.

Management of DKA

The first priority is to correct fluid and electrolyte depletion, as this is the immediate threat to life. Insulin replacement, to correct hyperglycaemia and restore glucose supply to the tissues, and treatment of any intercurrent illness are essential.

Fluid replacement

A large peripheral or central venous cannula is needed for intravenous fluids. Most patients recover rapidly with 2 litres of saline given in 2 hours, then 2 litres in 4 hours, then 4 litres in 24 hours. Fluid losses (in urine or vomit) should be added to these volumes. Replacement should be faster in shocked or oliguric patients (who may require plasma expanders), and slower in the elderly or those with cardiac disease or signs of fluid overload, cerebral oedema or respiratory distress. Fluid balance must be monitored continuously from urine output (catheterise if necessary), clinical signs, or measurement of central venous or pulmonary wedge pressures.

As sodium, chloride and potassium are depleted, the logical replacement fluid is saline with potassium chloride. Isotonic (0.9%) saline should be used until plasma glucose has fallen to 10–14 mmol/l, when 5% dextrose

Table 19.10 Investigations in diabetic ketoacidosis

Test	Normal range	Findings in ketoacidosis
Plasma glucose	4–8 mmol/l	>17 mmol/l (may be lower, especially in children)
Plasma Na	137–143 mmol/l	>155 mmol/l indicates hyperosmolality. May be depressed by very high glucose levels
Plasma K	3.5–5.0 mmol/l	Normal, high or low (total body K is always depleted)
Plasma urea	3.5–7.0 mmol/l	High in dehydration and renal failure
Venous HCO_3	18–28 mmol/l	Reduced (arterial blood pH and base excess are more useful)
Plasma osmolality	288–298 mosmol/kg	>350 mosmol/kg indicates severe hyperosmolality
Arterial blood pH	7.35–7.45	<7.0 indicates severe acidosis
Base deficit	−2 to +2 mmol/l	<−10 indicates severe acidosis
Urinary ketones	Negative	+ + or + + + (+ or + + may occur in starvation without ketoacidosis)

can be substituted; as this is given with insulin, the glucose is transported into cells and replenishes their stores. In severe hyperosmolality, half-isotonic (0.45%) saline may be given instead, as in hyperosmolar, non-ketotic coma (p. 763). Small amounts of sodium bicarbonate may be used in profound acidosis (see below).

Total body potassium is always depleted in DKA but acidosis causes potassium to leak out of cells, so that *plasma* levels can be low, normal or high. Plasma potassium often falls rapidly during treatment, as insulin carries it into cells together with glucose. Although potassium replacement is always needed, it must not be given during hyperkalaemia because it may precipitate cardiac arrhythmias.

Potassium chloride should be added to each litre of intravenous fluid as follows: 20 mmol if plasma potassium is normal (3.5–5.0 mmol/l), 40 mmol in hypokalaemia (<3.5 mmol/l), and none in hyperkalaemia (>5.0 mmol/l). Profound hypokalaemia may require additional potassium, which is best given by an infusion pump. Patients with severe potassium disturbances should be monitored electrocardiographically.

Insulin replacement

Soluble insulin given intravenously acts most rapidly and reliably in DKA; intramuscular and particularly subcutaneous absorption are too slow and erratic.

Insulin is best given by an infusion pump (50 U soluble insulin diluted in 50 ml saline, i.e. 1 U/ml), or as 50 U in a 500 ml bag of saline (0.1 U/ml). It should be infused initially at 10 U/hour, i.e. 10 ml/hour for the pump and 100 ml/hour for the drip, which should be regulated by a drip-counter or paediatric giving-set burette. Blood glucose must be measured hourly, and, when it starts to fall, the infusion rate should be titrated to achieve a glucose level of 10–15 mmol/l after 6–8 hours. Faster rates of fall are unnecessary and may cause hypoglycaemia. Most patients need 1–3 U/hour.

Other measures and problems

Frequent monitoring of glucose, electrolytes and clinical state is crucial. Any co-existent illness should be treated. Broad-spectrum antibiotics are usually given prospectively. Myocardial infarction with DKA has a very high mortality. Other problems include:

- *Shock*, which may cause acute prerenal and renal failure. This usually responds to adequate saline replacement, but plasma expanders and inotropes may be needed for severe hypotension (systolic BP<90 mm Hg).
- *Severe acidosis*. The use of bicarbonate in DKA is controversial, as it causes hypokalaemia and, although raising blood pH, may paradoxically worsen intracellular acidosis. Small volumes (250–500 ml) of *isotonic* sodium bicarbonate (1.4%) may be given if arterial pH is <7.0.
- *Cerebral oedema*. Subclinical brain swelling is probably common in DKA and may be exacerbated by water, ion or glucose shifts in the brain during rehydration. It particularly affects children, causing a decline in consciousness, sometimes with papilloedema. It carries a high mortality, but dexamethasone given intravenously before brain herniation occurs sometimes helps. Fluid overload should be avoided and corrected.
- *Adult respiratory distress syndrome (ARDS)*. Alveolar fluid accumulation, perhaps due to ion and water shifts, clinically resembles pulmonary oedema, but with a normal heart size on chest X-ray and low pulmonary wedge pressure. It is usually fatal. Treatment includes ventilation with high-concentration oxygen and correction of fluid overload.
- *Acute gastric dilatation*, with vomiting, a succussion splash and a ground-glass appearance on abdominal X-ray, requires nasogastric drainage to prevent aspiration, especially if consciousness is reduced.
- *Coma* requires standard nursing care, ideally in an intensive care unit.

Summary 7 Management of diabetic ketoacidosis

Fluid replacement
2 l in 2 hours, then 2 l in 4 hours, then 4 l in 24 hours (plus losses)
Isotonic saline initially
5% dextrose when blood glucose falls to 10–14 mmol/l

Potassium replacement
Replace according to plasma levels
Add 0, 20 or 40 mmol to each litre of i.v. fluid if plasma potassium is >5.0, normal or <3.5 mmol/l respectively

Insulin replacement
Continuous i.v. infusion of soluble insulin at 10 U/hour until blood glucose falls, then 1–3 U/hour according to blood glucose

Monitoring
Blood glucose (hourly)
Fluid balance and plasma electrolytes
Clinical condition

Identify and treat intercurrent precipitating illness
Broad-spectrum antibiotics

Identify and treat complications of ketoacidosis
Severe acidosis (pH < 7.0) – consider i.v. bicarbonate and ventilation
Shock – consider i.v. plasma expanders and inotropes
Cerebral oedema – i.v. dexamethasone, mannitol
Adult respiratory distress syndrome – ventilate

Afterwards
Stabilise insulin treatment
Education to prevent further episodes

- *Hypothermia* indicates a poor prognosis. It may respond to rewarming with a space blanket.

After the emergency is over

Intravenous fluids and insulin should be continued until the patient is able to eat and drink, and ketonuria has diminished. Standard subcutaneous insulin can then be resumed or started in newly-diagnosed patients using prolonged-acting insulin (p. 751). Patients who have had DKA require insulin for life. The cause of the episode must be identified if possible and discussed with the patient to prevent it from happening again.

Hyperosmolar, non-ketotic coma

This is distinguished from DKA by the absence of gross hyperketonaemia and metabolic acidosis. Hyperglycaemia is generally greater than in DKA and, together with a rise in urea due to dehydration and pre-renal failure, may elevate the plasma osmolality to >350 mosmol/kg.

Hyperketonaemia does not develop because these patients have enough insulin secretion to suppress lipolysis and ketogenesis, but not enough to prevent the liver from producing glucose. These patients are therefore C-peptide-positive patients with NIDDM, which is often previously undiagnosed. Precipitating factors include myocardial infarction, stroke, infection, and diabetogenic drugs such as glucocorticoids and thiazide diuretics.

Presentation is with severe hyperglycaemic symptoms (polyuria, intense thirst, weight loss, blurred vision), without the features of ketoacidosis. Confusion, drowsiness and coma are commoner than in DKA. Complications include stroke and thromboembolic disease (such as mesenteric artery thrombosis, deep venous thrombosis and pulmonary embolism) due to increased blood viscosity. Mortality exceeds 30% because these patients are old and often have a serious precipitating illness. The biochemical features are:

- *Hyperglycaemia*: often >50 mmol/l, sometimes >100 mmol/l
- *Hypernatraemia*: often >155 mmol/l (may be depressed by high glucose levels)
- *Uraemia*: due to dehydration, with or without renal failure
- *Hyperosmolality*: >350 mosmol/kg
- *Blood and urine ketone levels*: normal or slightly raised (in starvation)
- *Arterial pH, venous bicarbonate and anion gap*: normal.

Management is largely as for DKA. Saline replacement, using half-isotonic (0.45%) solution if plasma sodium exceeds 150 mmol/l or osmolality >350 mosmol/kg, must be cautious in older patients, in whom cardiac disease is common. Potassium levels must be carefully monitored and replaced as needed. Most patients respond rapidly to intravenous insulin infusion at low doses. Prophylactic low-dose heparin (5000 U s.c. 8-hourly) should be given, but full anticoagulation should be reserved for proven thromboembolism as the risks of fatal gastrointestinal bleeding are high.

Despite often impressive hyperglycaemia at presentation, these patients have NIDDM and many later do not need insulin. Drugs and other precipitating factors must be avoided subsequently if possible.

Lactic acidosis

Lactate is generated by glycolysis in muscle (Fig. 19.4). Lactate levels rise rapidly during tissue anoxia (e.g. shock, cardiac failure, pneumonia) and when the liver and kidney are prevented from utilising it (e.g. by hepatic impairment or biguanides). Lactic acidosis is rare with metformin as long as other predisposing factors (organ failures) are avoided.

It presents as coma with metabolic acidosis (reduced arterial pH and venous bicarbonate) and a wide anion gap (p. 854) due to lactate. Blood glucose levels are within the diabetic range. Treatment often fails to prevent death. Intravenous sodium bicarbonate may paradoxically aggravate intracellular acidosis (see above), which may be limited by vigorous ventilation to blow off carbon dioxide. Haemodialysis may both clear lactate hydrogen ions and remove sodium overload due to bicarbonate administration. Dichloroacetate, an experimental agent, decreases lactate synthesis.

CHRONIC COMPLICATIONS OF DIABETES

The chronic tissue complications of diabetes are the single greatest anxiety for most diabetic people. However, over 40% of IDDM patients survive for over 40 years, half of them without developing significant complications, and there is already encouraging evidence – notably the falling incidence of nephropathy during the last decade – that continuing advances in diabetic care will reduce the damage of diabetic complications.

Chronic diabetic complications are usually classified as:

- *Microvascular (microangiopathic) disease.* This is an essential component of retinopathy and nephropathy, and is characteristic of, and specific to, diabetes. The role in neuropathy is less certain. Common features are basement membrane thickening and abnormal leakiness in the microcirculation. The lesions affect particularly IDDM patients who developed the disease before puberty but can be devastating in NIDDM, even if 'mild'. Indeed, significant complications are often found in NIDDM patients at diagnosis, reflecting the long unsuspected presence of the disease.
- *Macrovascular (large-vessel) disease.* This is atherosclerosis, distinguished from that affecting non-diabetic people only by its rapid and extensive development.

Microvascular complications

Pathogenesis

Microvascular lesions in IDDM and NIDDM are identical, suggesting that hyperglycaemia or some other metabolic disturbance of diabetes is responsible. Epidemiological evidence indicates that microvascular complications are commoner in poorly-controlled and rarer in well-controlled diabetic patients.

The hypothesis that better control will diminish these complications has become testable with the advent of CSII and other intensified regimens able to maintain near-normoglycaemia for many months or years. Long-term, large-scale prospective studies are in progress, and

support the conclusions from previous shorter-term studies that tight control achieved by CSII can slow deterioration in the early stages of retinopathy (micro-aneurysm count), neuropathy (nerve conduction velocity) and nephropathy (albumin excretion rate and decline in glomerular filtration rate (GFR)). The long-term DCCT (Diabetic Chronic Complications Trial) in the USA has now confirmed that tight glycaemic control can halve the long-term incidence of retinopathy and nephropathy.

Suggested mechanisms of microvascular disease include:

- *Overactivity of the polyol pathway.* This alternative pathway converts glucose and other sugars to their respective polyols or sugar alcohols (e.g. glucose to sorbitol, galactose to dulcitol) through the action of aldose reductase. This enzyme is found in the retina, lens, glomerulus and Schwann cell of nerves, which are all damaged in long-standing diabetes. Glucose flux through the polyol pathway increases dramatically in hyperglycaemia, and this may cause accumulation of sorbitol in these tissues. How these changes might cause tissue damage is unknown.
- *Glycation of proteins.* Hyperglycaemia increases non-enzymatic glycation of many proteins which may impair their structural and metabolic functions.
- *Haemodynamic and coagulation disorders.* Resting blood flow is increased in the retinal, glomerular and other microcirculations and could cause microvascular damage. Smoking, hypertension and a tendency to enhanced coagulability of the blood may also contribute.
- *Other factors.* Since 60–70% of IDDM patients never develop nephropathy or proliferative retinopathy, an inherited susceptibility may be responsible.

Ocular complications

Diabetic eye disease, especially retinopathy, is the commonest cause of blindness in the British population of working age and, for most patients, is the most frightening complication of the disease. Fortunately, it is easily detected and now often treatable.

Diabetic retinopathy

Retinopathy is a readily visible sign of widespread microvascular damage. Background retinopathy (see below) affects 30% of patients with NIDDM at diagnosis and virtually all patients after 20 years of either IDDM or NIDDM; these changes therefore seem to result from hyperglycaemia or associated metabolic disturbances. By contrast, proliferative changes only ever develop in 30–50% of diabetic people, who may constitute a specific susceptible subset.

Early abnormalities include capillary dilatation with increased retinal blood flow, thickening of the capillary basement membrane, loss of the surrounding pericytes and increased leakiness of the capillaries. Focal occlusion of capillaries and later arterioles, possibly due to micro-thrombus formation, ultimately causes retinal ischaemia and infarction.

The progression of retinopathy is apparently accelerated by poor glycaemic control, smoking and possibly hypertension. Retinopathy may deteriorate acutely during pregnancy and after a sudden improvement in previously poor glycaemic control, probably because this reduces retinal blood flow and aggravates ischaemia in critically perfused areas of the retina.

Stages and lesions of retinopathy

The stages and lesions of retinopathy are detailed in Figure 19.15.

Background retinopathy. Capillary dilatation and leakage can only be demonstrated by fluorescein angiography (Fig. 19.16). The first lesions visible on fundoscopy are red dots, which are either *microaneurysms* (localised dilatations of weakened capillaries) or *haemorrhages* from ruptured capillaries. Haemorrhages deep in the retina appear as small dots or larger 'blots', whereas superficial ones fan out along nerve fibre bundles into a 'flame' shape. 'Hard' exudates are lipid-rich precipitates of

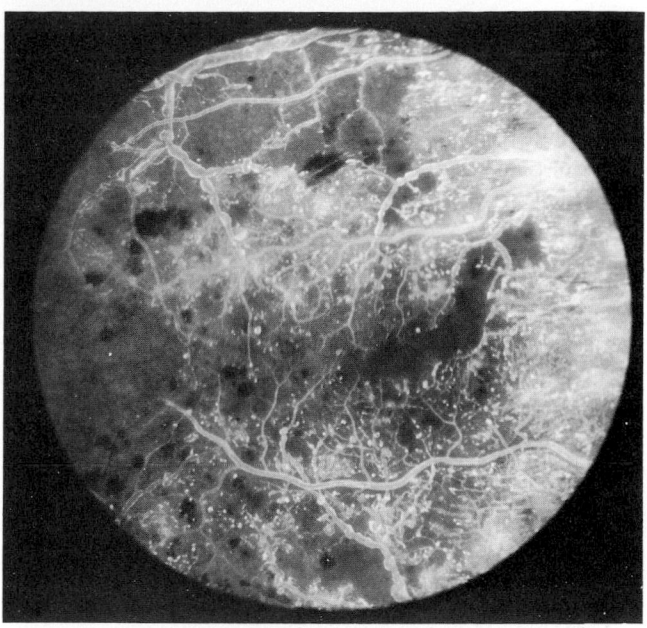

Fig. 19.16 Fluorescein angiogram. Severe background retinopathy showing microaneurysms, haemorrhages, and venous beading indicating early preproliferative changes. Diffuse fluorescence outside the vessels indicates extensive capillary leakage. (Photograph by courtesy of Mr H. Whitelocke.)

protein extravasated from leaky capillaries. These have a shiny, waxy appearance and are often clustered in arcs and rings around the macula. Background lesions alone do not impair vision, unless extensive exudates cause maculopathy, and in most cases do not progress to new vessel formation.

Preproliferative changes. These indicate worsening ischaemia, and 50% of cases develop new vessels within 12 months. *Multiple cotton-wool spots* ('soft' exudates) are fluffy, greyish-white patches of axoplasm released from retinal infarcts; they also occur in accelerated hypertension. *Venous abnormalities* include *beading* and *looping*. *Intraretinal microvascular abnormalities* (IRMA) are clusters of dilated capillaries (not new vessels). Vision is not affected by preproliferative changes alone.

Proliferative retinopathy. New vessels usually sprout from veins, especially where they bifurcate or enter the optic disc. They advance in leashes or arcades within the retina or into the vitreous, and may extend anteriorly to appear on the iris as *rubeosis iridis*. New vessels threaten vision because they are fragile and rupture easily, causing haemorrhages within the retina, in the vitreous, or in the potential preretinal (subhyaloid) space between the two. Vitreous haemorrhages appear as greyish opacities obscuring the fundus, whereas preretinal bleeds have a flat top if the red cells in the space are allowed to sediment. Extensive vitreous and preretinal haemorrhages

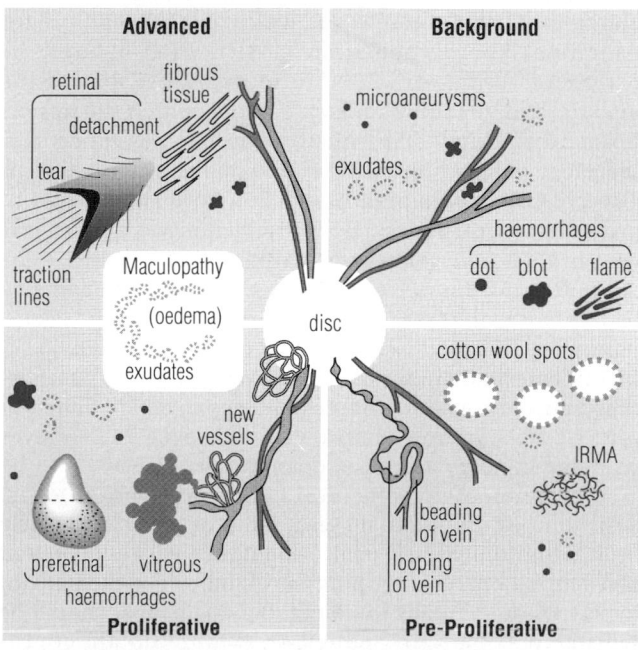

Fig. 19.15 Stages and lesions of diabetic retinopathy. Maculopathy, an important cause of blindness in NIDDM, can accompany any of these stages; macular oedema may be invisible on fundoscopy.

cause sudden loss of vision in the affected eye. Small haemorrhages may resorb almost entirely but bleeding usually recurs and ultimately impairs vision. Without treatment, 50% of patients with 'high-risk' new vessels (especially those involving the disc, which are particularly liable to bleed) will become blind within 5 years.

Advanced diabetic eye disease. Fibrous tissue proliferates with new vessels and following repeated haemorrhages, appearing as opaque, greyish membranes on fundoscopy. It tends to contract, so that strands attached to the retina exert traction, causing *retinal detachment* and *tears*. Detachment causes visual loss, which is permanent if the retina is not reattached within a few weeks. Warning symptoms include distortion of vision and a 'sparkling' sensation, and these therefore need urgent ophthalmological referral. Fibrosis also complicates rubeosis iridis, especially if the vessels bleed into the anterior chamber, and may block the filtration angle. This prevents reabsorption of aqueous and causes glaucoma, with a blind and extremely painful eye.

Maculopathy. The macula serves high-resolution central vision essential for daily activities such as reading. Unfortunately, it is particularly sensitive to damage by oedema and exudates from surrounding leaky capillaries and ischaemia. Maculopathy can complicate any stage of retinopathy and is the commonest cause of blindness in NIDDM. Significant maculopathy dramatically impairs vision and must be suspected if visual acuity is 6/12 or worse and cannot be explained by refraction errors, cataracts or vitreous opacities. *Fundoscopy may seem deceptively normal*; all patients with unexplained visual impairment must therefore be referred to an ophthalmologist. The diagnosis is confirmed by fluorescein angiography, which shows extensive capillary leakage, and slit-lamp examination which will reveal retinal thickening.

Screening and investigation of diabetic retinopathy

Visual acuity and fundoscopy should be checked routinely in every diabetic patient at diagnosis, annually thereafter, and 3- to 6-monthly if changes other than mild background are present. Acuity should be tested using the Snellen chart before mydriatics are given, and with any refractive errors corrected by the patient looking through his or her own distance glasses or a pinhole in a piece of card.

Fundoscopy must be performed through dilated pupils, as retinopathy, especially new vessel formation, often occurs far peripherally. Contraindications to mydriatics (e.g. 0.5% tropicamide) are glaucoma and previous eye surgery. The lens and vitreous, as well as the disc, major vessels and finally the sensitive macula ('look straight at my light'), must all be examined.

Table 19.11 shows guidelines for referring the patient to the ophthalmologist. Specialised investigations include

Table 19.11 When to refer diabetic patients to the ophthalmologist

Extensive or progressive haemorrhages or exudates
Preproliferative changes
Proliferative changes
Unexplained loss of visual acuity (6/12 or worse): possible maculopathy
Vitreous haemorrhage ⎫
Retinal detachment ⎬ urgent referral (within 24 hours)
Glaucoma ⎭

slit-lamp measurements of retinal thickness (which is increased in macular oedema), estimation of intraocular pressure, and fluorescein angiography. Fluorescein injected intravenously binds to albumin and so only leaves the circulation if the vessels are abnormally leaky. After a fluorescein bolus, rapid-sequence photographs using ultraviolet light demonstrate the retinal arteries, capillaries and veins. Fluorescence outside the vessels indicates leakage, notably in macular oedema and around new vessels (Fig. 19.16).

Management of diabetic retinopathy

With advances in laser photocoagulation and vitreoretinal surgery, many cases of severe diabetic retinopathy have become treatable.

Laser photocoagulation uses blue-green argon laser light which is absorbed by vascular structures. The laser can be used either to destroy localised targets such as clumps of new vessels or leaky capillaries, or for panretinal photocoagulation (PRP). PRP ablates the peripheral retina with 2000 or more burns, sparing the macula and maculopapillary bundle which carries its fibres to the disc. This destroys ischaemic retina and therefore removes the stimulus to neovascularisation; it also channels remaining blood flow into the macula to preserve central vision. With PRP the risks of patients with proliferative changes becoming blind within 5 years are reduced from 50 to 25%. Macular oedema can also be treated, using laser burns to seal surrounding leakage points.

Vitreoretinal surgery, by removing vitreous haemorrhage and fibrous membranes and repairing detached or torn retina, can now restore vision to over 50% of eyes rendered blind by advanced diabetic eye disease.

Prevention of diabetic retinopathy is a major priority. This hinges on regular screening of eyes and early ophthalmological referral, together with improved glycaemic control, stopping smoking and treatment of hypertension. Visually impaired diabetic people should be registered as partially sighted or blind to obtain appropriate State benefits. Sympathetic counselling and practical devices such as injection aids and speaking blood glucose meters may be very helpful.

Summary 8 Diabetic retinopathy

- The commonest cause of blindness in Britons of working age
- Background changes affect almost all cases after 20 years of diabetes
- Proliferative changes develop in only 30–50% of cases
- Maculopathy commonly causes blindness in NIDDM; it may be invisible on fundoscopy
- Laser photocoagulation prevents blindness in 50% of cases with new vessels
- Vitreoretinal surgery restores vision in 50% of cases with advanced eye disease

Other ocular complications of diabetes

Diabetes accelerates the formation of senile cataracts, and, rarely, 'snowflake' cataracts may develop rapidly during periods of very poor glycaemic control at any age. Cataracts must be distinguished from the blurred vision of hyperglycaemia, usually with hypermetropia, which may be due to osmotically-induced changes in lens shape. Normalisation of hyperglycaemia may also alter acuity for several weeks.

Diabetic nephropathy and other renal diseases

Diabetic nephropathy is a specific microvascular disease affecting mainly the glomerulus, although tubular lesions also occur. In the UK, diabetic nephropathy accounts for 25% of patients with end-stage renal failure. It is the commonest cause of premature death in IDDM, especially in patients who become diabetic before puberty, but is rarer when IDDM presents after 40 years of age. Only 30–40% of IDDM patients ever develop nephropathy and two-thirds of these ultimately enter end-stage renal failure. Nephropathy is rarer in NIDDM, but as this is commoner than IDDM, the numbers of renal failure patients with IDDM and NIDDM are comparable. Fortunately, the frequency of nephropathy is apparently falling.

Diabetes predisposes to urinary tract infections, especially in patients with incomplete bladder emptying due to autonomic neuropathy. Unusual organisms may be involved, including tuberculosis and gas-forming bacteria; a recognised complication is papillary necrosis, which may cause acute renal failure.

Pathophysiology of diabetic nephropathy

Nephropathy is one facet of generalised microvascular damage and is almost always associated with retinopathy, often proliferative. An extremely important association is with hypertension. This is present in virtually all patients with clinical nephropathy and, if untreated, accelerates the rate of decline of GFR. Susceptibility to nephropathy may relate to an inherited tendency to hypertension. Other predisposing factors include smoking and poor glycaemic control.

As in other capillary beds, the glomerular basement membrane is thickened. The mesangium is expanded by amorphous material and the glomerulus ultimately becomes sclerosed, forming the pathognomic Kimmelstiel–Wilson nodular lesions.

The first functional change is increased permeability of the glomerular capillaries to albumin. Urinary albumin excretion rate (AER) rises initially into the range of 30–300 mg/24 hours, known as 'microalbuminuria'. These albumin concentrations are below the detection limits of conventional dipsticks and are demonstrable only by radioimmunoassay or other sensitive methods. In two-thirds of these patients, AER continues to rise and at >300 mg/24 hours, the stage of clinical nephropathy ('macroalbuminuria') becomes detectable by dipsticks. In some patients, proteinuria ultimately exceeds 3.0–3.5 g/day, causing the nephrotic syndrome (Fig. 19.17).

GFR is initially normal, or even increased in some cases; this 'hyperfiltration' is associated with renal hypertrophy. Once AER reaches 100–300 mg/24 hours, GFR starts to decline linearly with an average loss of 10 ml/minute per year (Fig. 19.18). Rates of decline vary widely between individuals and may be slowed by controlling hypertension, reducing protein intake and possibly by stopping smoking. Serum creatinine levels begin to rise when GFR has fallen to 50 ml/minute and end-stage renal failure supervenes on average 5–7 years after macroalbuminuria appears.

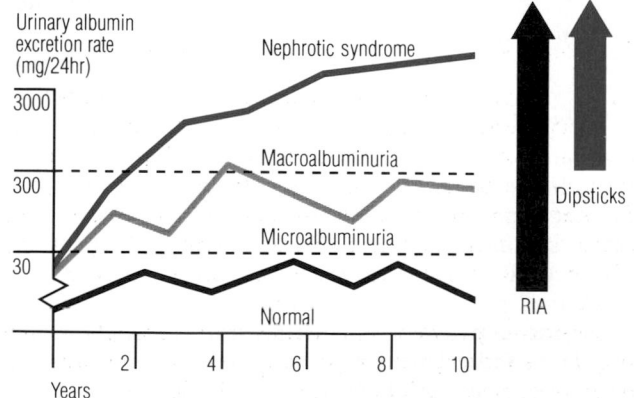

Fig. 19.17 Evolution of albuminuria in diabetic nephropathy.
'Microalbuminuria' represents an albumin excretion rate (AER) of 30–300 mg/24 hours, which is detectable by sensitive radioimmunoassay (RIA). In two-thirds of these patients, AER rises into the macroalbuminuric range (>300 mg/24 hours), detectable by routine dipstick testing. These patients are at risk of developing renal failure or the nephrotic syndrome.

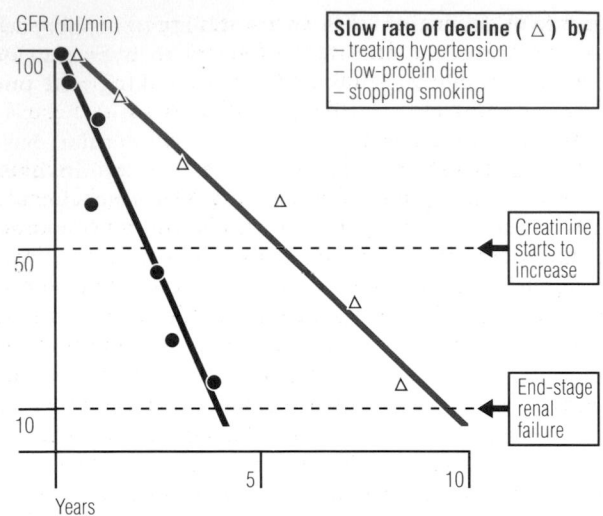

Fig. 19.18 Decline in GFR in established diabetic nephropathy. GFR falls linearly at an average rate of 10 ml/min per year; individual rates vary widely and may be slowed by treating hypertension, reducing protein intake and stopping smoking.

Investigations and diagnosis

Microalbuminuria can now be measured easily and cheaply, and tests suitable for screening spot urine samples are available. Screening should be performed annually. Blood urea and creatinine levels can be misleadingly normal until GFR has fallen by 50% (Fig. 19.18).

In about 10% of cases, renal failure or proteinuria in diabetic patients is not due to diabetic nephropathy. Atypical features, e.g. haematuria, rapid-onset renal failure, small kidney size, or the absence of retinopathy, should raise this possibility. The correct diagnosis is vital for therapeutic and prognostic reasons, and may have to be established by renal biopsy.

Management of diabetic nephropathy

Microalbuminuric stage. Much can be done at this stage to slow the pace of renal damage and delay progression to clinical nephropathy. Control of hypertension is crucial, as this significantly slows the rise in AER and fall in GFR. Many antihypertensive drugs are effective, and ACE inhibitors may confer additional benefits in reducing AER, possibly by specifically lowering intraglomerular pressure. Other measures are stopping smoking and improving glycaemic control.

Clinical nephropathy (macroalbuminuric stage). Effective treatment of hypertension (present in most patients) is again essential, and ACE inhibitors may markedly reduce proteinuria. Moderate restriction of dietary protein and stopping smoking may help to maintain GFR; optimising glycaemic control has little effect at this stage.

End-stage renal failure. Renal support therapy is needed when serum creatinine reaches 500 µmol/l. Prediction of this time from inverse creatinine (1000 ÷ creatinine in µmol/l) or GFR plots allows careful planning in advance (Fig. 19.18). The treatment options are the same as for non-diabetic people and are now nearly as successful. Patients must not be denied renal support simply because they have diabetes, although premature death (mainly from cardiovascular disease) is 10 times higher in diabetic than in non-diabetic patients receiving renal replacement therapy.

Renal transplantation is preferred for younger patients; live related donors are best, when 5-year survival exceeds 60%. Haemodialysis can be complicated by the difficulty of constructing arteriovenous fistulae in calcified arteries (which are common in nephropathy) and by postural hypotension due to fluid shifts. Chronic ambulatory peritoneal dialysis (CAPD) avoids these problems and is suitable for many patients, including the blind.

Other aspects of diabetic care can be difficult for renal failure patients. *Hypoglycaemia* is common, as insulin and most sulphonylureas are cleared partly through the kidneys and so accumulate in renal failure. Sulphonylureas are particularly dangerous and insulin should be substituted when creatinine levels begin to rise; metformin must never be given in renal failure, because of the very high risks of lactic acidosis. *Proliferative retinopathy* commonly coexists and may deteriorate during haemodialysis; early laser treatment is essential. *Neuropathy* causing foot ulceration is frequent, and autonomic neuropathy aggravates postural hypotension during haemodialysis. *Cardiovascular disease* ultimately kills most of these patients.

Diabetic neuropathy

Diabetic nerve damage involves both the somatosensory system, causing variable sensory and motor deficits, and the autonomic outflow to various organs. Pathological changes affect both the Schwann cells, with segmental peeling and loss of myelin, and the axons themselves. Axonal degeneration may be accompanied by regeneration and sprouting of nerve endings. Nerve conduction velocity is decreased and smaller fibres may fire spontaneously, a possible basis of the characteristic neurogenic pain. Causative factors in diabetic neuropathy are thought to include:

- *Hyperglycaemia.* Epidemiological studies have associated poor diabetic control with more severe nerve damage, and tightening glycaemic control with CSII has produced short-term neurophysiological and clinical benefits. Hyperglycaemia could damage nerves through glycation of proteins and/or polyol pathway overactivity.

Summary 9 Diabetic nephropathy

- The commonest cause of premature death in IDDM
- Microalbuminuria precedes macroalbuminuria (clinical nephropathy)
- In clinical nephropathy, GFR declines linearly
- Treating hypertension slows deterioration in renal function
- End-stage renal failure in diabetic patients should be treated as for non-diabetic people

- *Vascular damage.* Diffuse occlusion of the capillaries supplying the nerves (*vasa nervorum*) occurs in human diabetic nerves and may parallel functional impairment, presumably by causing hypoxia. The sudden focal palsies which affect single cranial and peripheral nerves may be due to occlusion of larger vessels, causing localised infarction and demyelination.

Somatosensory diabetic neuropathy

About 30% of diabetic clinic patients have evidence of neuropathy on formal testing, but this is mostly sub-clinical as only 10% have significant symptoms. Somatosensory nerve damage is of two types: a diffuse, symmetrical 'stocking and glove' pattern typical of metabolic or toxic neuropathies in which the longest nerves are most susceptible to damage; and focal or multifocal neuropathies in which individual nerves are picked off by discrete, presumably vascular, insults.

Diffuse, symmetrical neuropathies

These affect both sensory and motor function to a variable and overlapping extent, although the patient's symptoms often relate predominantly or exclusively to one or the other. Sensory symptoms are the commonest, typically consisting of unpleasant pins and needles, burning, shooting or electric shock-like sensations, often with 'allodynia', i.e. pain provoked by a normally innocuous stimulus such as contact with bedclothes. The feet and legs are usually affected and the hands only rarely. Pain is often worst at night, severely disrupting sleep and causing depression. Symptoms can either develop insidiously over many months or years, or acutely within a few days or weeks. The acute presentation often follows a period of severe hyperglycaemia, especially if accompanied by weight loss, and tends to resolve with time and improved glycaemic control. By contrast, the chronic form is less obviously associated with poor control and does not respond to intensified treatment.

Chronic sensory neuropathy also causes loss of sensation, sometimes profound. The most important loss is of pain perception, which is a major cause of damage to the neuropathic foot (see below). The patient may be unaware, for example, of full-thickness burns from hot-water bottles, scalds from bathwater, pressure damage from tight shoes, or having the foot impaled by stepping on a nail. Impaired touch and joint-position sense may give the impression of walking in thick socks, and cause a positive Romberg's sign.

Physical examination may reveal symmetrical 'stocking and glove' sensory loss affecting all modalities, but this is often patchy, usually spares the hands, and may be much less impressive than the symptoms would suggest; clinical testing may be normal in acute painful neuropathy. Tendon reflexes in the legs are often reduced or absent and there may be marked muscle wasting. Neuropathic foot problems – ulceration, increased skin blood flow and Charcot arthropathy – may develop through a combination of somatosensory and autonomic damage (see below).

Motor neuropathy with asymptomatic muscle wasting often accompanies primarily sensory syndromes, while a diffuse predominantly motor neuropathy may produce severe symmetrical wasting, which is typically worst in the hands and usually accompanied by intense pain. There is little sensory deficit and tendon reflexes are usually preserved. Older NIDDM patients, sometimes only mildly hyperglycaemic, are usually affected and recovery may be very poor.

Focal and multifocal neuropathies

These are palsies of one or more cranial or peripheral nerves. Cranial nerve palsies are common, especially affecting the third, sixth and fourth nerves. The third nerve palsy is characteristically painful and partial: diplopia and ptosis are present but the pupillary innervation is spared and pupil diameter and responses are unaffected. The palsy usually resolves spontaneously. Peripheral nerve palsies, particularly of the median, ulnar and lateral popliteal nerves, may be due to pressure damage and/or vascular insults and often recover slowly and incompletely. A phrenic nerve palsy may cause an elevated hemidiaphragm.

Diabetic amyotrophy may be due to vascular damage of a large nerve trunk or root (radiculopathy) supplying the leg. The femoral nerve is usually involved, causing acute pain, weakness and wasting in the quadriceps, with loss of the knee jerk. Muscles below the knee are less often affected. For an unknown reason, some patients have extensor plantar responses, a picture which must be differentiated from a spinal or cauda equina lesion. Amyotrophy often presents during a period of poor control and usually improves spontaneously within a few months, especially if diabetic control is tightened.

Diagnosis and management of diabetic somatosensory neuropathy

The history is usually diagnostic. Sensory modalities served by large fibres (vibration, joint position sense, light touch) and small fibres (pinprick, light touch) should be mapped, remembering that any deficit may not match the severity or extent of symptoms. Tendon reflexes and muscle bulk and power must be tested. Because of their different prognoses and treatments, diffuse and focal neuropathies must be distinguished. Sensory testing can be standardised by various bedside instruments. Electrophysiological testing will demonstrate slowed conduction velocities in affected nerves.

Diabetic neuropathy must be distinguished from other metabolic neuropathies, including vitamin B_{12} deficiency, uraemia and alcohol abuse, all of which can coexist with diabetes and require different treatments.

Treatment should begin by optimising glycaemic control, using intensified insulin regimens if necessary; this often helps acute painful syndromes but not those which develop slowly. Pain may respond to simple analgesics (aspirin, codeine), tricyclic antidepressants (imipramine, especially if combined with fluphenazine), membrane-stabilising drugs such as anticonvulsants (phenytoin, carbamazepine) or oral mexiletine or local anaesthetics (intravenous lignocaine). Some patients do not respond to any of these measures.

Autonomic neuropathy

Autonomic dysfunction commonly accompanies somatosensory neuropathy and presumably has a similar pathogenesis. About 40% of unselected diabetic patients have some features of autonomic neuropathy but most are not apparent clinically. Only a few suffer major symptoms, and these patients have a significantly reduced life expectancy.

Both sympathetic and parasympathetic divisions are involved. Clinically apparent features are commonest in patients with long-standing diabetes, and include:

- *Abnormal sweating*: this is usually reduced in the feet, but profuse 'gustatory' sweating of the face and trunk may be provoked by eating.
- *Postural hypotension*, with a systolic fall exceeding 20 mmHg on standing, is due to failure of the normal increase in cardiac output and vasoconstrictor tone, and causes dizziness and blackouts.
- *Gastrointestinal motility* is disturbed, causing gastric stasis with vomiting, diarrhoea (especially at night) which may be aggravated by bacterial overgrowth, and/or constipation.
- *Neuropathic bladder* problems include incomplete emptying, sometimes with a palpable bladder, which may cause overflow incontinence and predispose to ascending urinary tract infections.
- *Sexual difficulties* include failure of erection (a parasympathetic response mediated by the sacral nerves) and/or ejaculation (a sympathetic reflex trans-

mitted by the lumbosacral outflow). Erectile failure in diabetic men can also be due to depression (a common cause in non-diabetic men) or atheroma of the pudendal arteries which supply the corpora cavernosa.

- *Sudden unexplained death* is commoner in patients with severe autonomic symptoms; possible causes include cardiorespiratory arrest and hypoglycaemia, awareness of which is blunted in many patients with long-standing diabetes.

Investigation, diagnosis and management of autonomic neuropathy

Autonomic neuropathy is usually diagnosed clinically from non-invasive tests of cardiovascular reflexes, which demonstrate an excessive postural drop in systolic blood pressure (>20 mmHg), loss of the normal sinus arrythmia during deep breathing (<10 b.p.m. difference between inspiration and expiration), or loss of reflex bradycardia during the Valsalva manoeuvre. Special tests can demonstrate decreased pupillary responses, sweating and gastric and bladder emptying.

Symptomatic postural hypotension may be helped simply by raising the head of the bed at night, or by fludrocortisone which retains sodium and water and may aggravate coexistent supine hypertension. Vomiting often responds to metoclopramide or cisapride, and erythromycin often cures diarrhoea when bacterial overgrowth is present. Regular bladder training may improve emptying and incontinence. Impotence may be very difficult to treat. Artificial erections may be induced either by vacuum suction devices or by the injection of vasodilators such as papaverine into the corpus cavernosum.

Macrovascular (large-vessel) disease

Atherosclerosis is very common in both IDDM and NIDDM and the major cause of death in the latter.

Summary 10 Classification of diabetic neuropathy

Somatosensory	
Diffuse	– sensory and/or motor
	– acute or chronic
	– with or without pain
	– glove and stocking distribution
Focal	– peripheral nerves (ulnar, median especially)
	– cranial nerves (III especially; IV, VI)
	– amyotrophy
Multifocal	– more than one nerve involved
Autonomic	– Altered sweating, postural hypotension, fixed heart rate, gastric stasis, diarrhoea, bladder atonia, impotence, sudden death

Predisposing factors are those which operate in the non-diabetic population, amplified by hyperglycaemia.

Hyperglycaemia is an independent cardiovascular risk factor. Epidemiological studies indicate that the risk of macrovascular disease begins to increase when the 2-hour blood glucose value during an OGTT exceeds 7 mmol/l; this is the basis for defining the category of IGT (p. 744). The extent and severity of atheroma are related to the duration and degree of hyperglycaemia, suggesting that good glycaemic control may be preventative, but there is not yet evidence that it can reverse established disease.

Hypertension affects up to one-third of diabetic people and is two to three times commoner than in the general population. The association may be partly explained by sodium retention and altered vascular reactivity.

Hyperlipidaemia is common, with an atherogenic pattern of increased VLDL- and LDL-cholesterol and reduced HDL which is often more pronounced in NIDDM. Triglycerides are also increased in untreated diabetes (see p. 779).

Smoking is at least as common in diabetic as in non-diabetic people, and many diabetic people continue to smoke because they fear overeating and weight gain if they stop. The 10-year mortality in diabetic smokers is twice as high as in non-diabetic non-smokers and most premature deaths are from macrovascular disease.

Interestingly, *hyperinsulinaemia* has also been implicated as a risk factor for macrovascular disease, as epidemiological and experimental evidence has suggested that insulin and related molecules are atherogenic. The commonly associated features of hyperinsulinaemia, insulin insensitivity, obesity, hypertension and an atherogenic lipid profile may all stem from insulin insensitivity. This constellation of abnormalities has been termed 'Syndrome X' by Reaven and others.

Manifestations of macrovascular disease

Atheroma in diabetic patients is histologically identical to that in the general population but is often more extensive and multifocal and tends to involve more distal arteries. The main complications are as follows.

Coronary heart disease. Compared with the general population, this is at least twice as common in diabetic men and four times as common in diabetic women (especially before the menopause, when women are normally protected against atheroma). There is a very strong association with microalbuminuria, which identifies virtually all the patients at risk of premature cardiovascular death (p. 768). Myocardial infarction is the commonest cause of death in NIDDM. In diabetic people, it is commonly complicated by cardiac failure or cardiogenic shock and carries twice the general mortality. This may be due to a specific 'diabetic cardiomyopathy', independent of general ischaemic damage, as left ventricular function may be impaired in normotensive diabetic patients whose coronary arteries are devoid of atheroma. Cardiac failure, sometimes with normal findings on examination and chest X-ray, may cause dyspnoea. Angina and myocardial infarction may be painless in diabetic patients, especially those with autonomic neuropathy, presumably because of sensory denervation of the heart.

Stroke is two to five times commoner than in the non-diabetic population.

Peripheral vascular disease is common, with diffuse atheroma in the arteries below the knee as well as in the ilio-femoral vessels. Claudication, rest pain and gangrene may result; the latter is usually dry and may affect one or more digits or the whole foot. Diabetes accounts for one-half of all non-traumatic amputations. Other manifestations include *mesenteric artery occlusion* which causes anginal-type abdominal pain after eating and occasionally extensive infarction of the bowel.

Examination and investigations

All the peripheral pulses must be checked for their presence, strength and bruits. Signs of hypertension, cardiac failure and poor perfusion of the legs (slow capillary return after blanching the skin, thin skin and other 'trophic' changes) must also be sought. The arteries can be further investigated by non-invasive Doppler scanning or by arteriography.

Routine ECG and chest X-ray may reveal ischaemia, infarcts, cardiomegaly or pulmonary oedema but may be deceptively normal, and a stress ECG, echocardiography or isotopic cardiac scans may be needed to demonstrate dysfunction. Angiography of the coronary or peripheral arteries will localise stenoses and indicate the feasibility of surgery or angioplasty. Blood glucose and lipid levels should be monitored regularly.

Management of macrovascular disease

General measures to treat cardiovascular risk factors are crucial. The benefits of stopping smoking must always be stressed, especially as smoking may aggravate microvascular as well as macrovascular disease. Hypertension must be treated, preferably avoiding drugs which worsen blood glucose or lipid levels, such as high-dose thiazide diuretics and beta-blockers. Calcium-channel antagonists, ACE inhibitors and low-dose diuretics (e.g. 1.25–2.5 mg bendrofluazide) have no adverse metabolic effects. Hyperlipidaemia is treated as described on page 780, avoiding fish oils which aggravate hyperglycaemia in NIDDM. Glycaemic control should be optimised. Reducing obesity (to a BMI of <25) and taking regular exercise within the patient's capacity help to correct both hypertension and hyperlipidaemia.

Angina is treated conventionally (see Ch. 12, p. 395). The proportion of operable vessels and the outcome of bypass surgery are now comparable in diabetic and non-diabetic populations. Intermittent claudication often improves if the simple advice to 'stop smoking and keep walking' can be followed, but a rapidly shortening claudication distance or rest pain must be investigated by arteriography. The results of reconstructive surgery, including femoral-popliteal bypass and the use of the saphenous vein *in situ* for distal disease, are now very good, although the amputation rate remains high in diabetic people.

The diabetic foot

Diabetic foot problems are of great clinical and economic importance, as they are one of the commonest causes of hospital admission for diabetic patients; such admissions are often expensive, lasting several weeks. Fortunately, most problems are largely preventable by careful education, effective screening and prompt treatment of complications.

Causes of diabetic foot problems

There are four basic disorders – neuropathy, ischaemia, trauma and infection – which commonly coexist and reinforce each other.

Neuropathy involving sensory, motor and autonomic nerves commonly causes ulceration and other foot complications. Impaired sensation prevents tissue damage from being noticed. Distal motor neuropathy weakens the intrinsic muscles of the foot and the unopposed action of the long extensors lifts the arch, claws the foot and concentrates pressure damage on to the metatarsal heads and heel. Autonomic denervation reduces sweating, causing dry skin which cracks and encourages infection, and opens the arteriovenous anastomoses. This shunts blood past the capillary bed, reducing oxygen and nutrient supply to the tissues, and results in warm skin (sometimes approaching core temperature) and distended veins in the feet.

Ischaemia, due to peripheral vascular disease and possibly to impaired microcirculation, results in a cold, pulseless foot at risk of infarction.

The commonest form of *trauma* is pressure damage, especially to the metatarsal heads and heels in the clawed neuropathic foot and regions compressed by tight shoes or foreign bodies in the shoes. Pressure stimulates formation of callus, in which foci of liquefactive necrosis develop and break through to the skin surface to form an ulcer.

Infection enters the foot through ulcers or cracks in the skin, including self-inflicted damage from do-it-yourself chiropody. Mixed growths of pyogenic, anaerobic and occasionally gas-forming organisms are common and may cause extensive soft-tissue infection or spread to bone to cause osteomyelitis.

Clinical features

Ulceration is the commonest manifestation. This is often multifactorial, but the main contributory factors must be identified because their treatments differ. 'Purely' *neuropathic ulcers* occur at high-pressure sites and appear cleanly punched out of the surrounding callus. The ulcer is generally painless and sometimes goes unnoticed by the patient, who will complain of numbness with or without neuropathic pain in the feet. The foot is typically warm (unless peripheral vascular disease coexists), with distended veins, a clawed posture and sensory loss. *Ischaemic ulcers* are painful and tend to affect the edges of the foot, which are cold and pulseless. The history will be dominated by intermittent claudication, sometimes with rest pain. Infection may not cause obvious signs of acute inflammation, but osteomyelitis may cause deep tenderness.

Charcot arthropathy is disorganisation of the articular surfaces with resorption of bone, which can lead to total disruption of affected joints, sometimes accompanied by a large effusion. The metatarso–tarsal, mid-foot or ankle joints are usually affected. Sensory loss is usually profound and acute flare-ups of Charcot arthropathy, which can appear alarmingly like a septic arthritis, are often (but not always) relatively painless.

Investigation of the diabetic foot

Effective treatment depends on identifying the cause(s) of ulceration. Tests for neuropathy and ischaemia are

---

Summary 11 Features of diabetic foot ulcers

	Neuropathic	Ischaemic
Site	High-pressure zones (metatarsal heads, heel)	Margins of foot
Appearance	Cleanly punched out of surrounding callus	Ragged edges
Sensory function	Ulcer usually painless Foot numb	Ulcer usually painful Sensation preserved
Circulation	Foot pulses present Skin warm	Foot pulses absent Skin cold; trophic changes

N.B. *Neuropathy and ischaemia often coexist, and infection often complicates ulceration.*

described above. Swabs or curettings from deep in the ulcer should be cultured for both aerobic and anaerobic organisms. Plain radiography of the foot may show gas in the soft tissues or bony destruction due to osteomyelitis or Charcot arthropathy. Generalised loss of bone density (osteopenia) and tapering of the phalanges and metatarsals also occur in neuropathy. Osteomyelitis must be distinguished from Charcot arthropathy; ^{111}In labelled white cell scans are highly specific for infection (Ch. 11, p. 211). An acutely inflamed joint should be aspirated to exclude infection, even if Charcot arthropathy seems likely.

Management of diabetic foot problems

Predominantly neuropathic ulcers are treated with chiropody to remove callus and a lightweight plaster cast to unload pressure from the affected area, which accelerates healing while keeping the patient mobile. Extra-depth or custom-built shoes, or pressure-absorbing socks, will reduce pressure loading and help to prevent recurrence.

Ischaemia is treated as described above (p. 771) and if at all possible, aims to avoid or limit amputation. Rehabilitation after amputation is often difficult and the remaining limb is frequently threatened later by ischaemia.

Infection must be treated with appropriate antibiotics and repeated cultures may be needed to ensure that mixed infections, especially including delicate anaerobes, are completely covered. Soft-tissue infections may respond to oral broad-spectrum antibiotics such as co-trimoxazole, but extensive infections and osteomyelitis may require some weeks of intravenous treatment and surgical debridement. Amputation may be needed in refractory cases.

Acute Charcot arthropathy must not be treated surgically, as the joint often disintegrates further, and usually improves with immobilisation and non-steroidal inflammatory drugs. Even badly disrupted joints may remain functional, but chronically unstable joints require arthrodesis.

Diabetic foot problems are best managed in a combined specialist clinic. Prevention is extremely important. Many problems can be avoided by teaching the patients basic foot care, by regularly checking their feet and shoes, and by providing prophylactic chiropody and special footwear as appropriate.

Miscellaneous diabetic complications

Necrobiosis lipoidica diabeticorum is a striking lesion with a sunken, atrophic yellowish centre which usually affects the skin on the shins. Like *granuloma annulare*, a raised skin-coloured lesion with a depressed centre, necrobiosis

has been regarded as a cutaneous marker of diabetes, but both conditions also affect non-diabetic people. Connective tissue complications include thickening of the skin (sometimes resembling scleroderma) and *limited joint mobility* of the fingers.

HYPOGLYCAEMIA

Blood glucose concentrations are normally maintained between about 4 and 7 mmol/l. Lower concentrations are particularly hazardous to the brain, which depends critically on a steady supply of glucose, its sole metabolic fuel under normal circumstances. Hypoglycaemia is defined rigorously as an *arterial* blood glucose level of <2.2 mmol/l. In practice, the diagnosis is often made on the basis of venous blood glucose levels. The arterio–venous glucose difference may be particularly marked after meals because high prandial insulin levels promote glucose uptake and utilisation by skeletal muscle and fat.

Causes of hypoglycaemia

Hypoglycaemia occurs when glucose taken up into the tissues exceeds that entering the circulation from the liver and the gut. Factors predisposing to hypoglycaemia are therefore: high insulin levels; deficiencies of the counter-regulatory hormones, especially cortisol and growth hormone; hypothyroidism; damage to the liver, which depletes glycogen and impairs the liver's capacity to secrete glucose; intense exercise, which mobilises glycogen and stimulates glucose uptake into skeletal muscle; and prolonged starvation, which depletes liver glycogen. Specific causes of hypoglycaemia (Table 19.12) are discussed below.

Insulinoma and nesidioblastosis

Pancreatic β-cell tumours, or insulinomas, are the commonest cause of spontaneous hypoglycaemia. Insulinomas are often small (a few millimetres in diameter), sometimes multiple and may occur together with parathyroid and pituitary tumours in the multiple endocrine neoplasia syndrome type 1 (p. 706). About 15% of insulinomas are malignant and metastasise to the liver, when hypoglycaemia may be profound and intractable. Diffuse β-cell hyperplasia, rather than a discrete tumour, is termed *nesidioblastosis* and presents with hypoglycaemia usually in the neonate or infant.

Other tumours

Large *mesenchymal tumours* (e.g. retroperitoneal or pleural sarcomas) and *hepatomas* can cause severe hypogly-

Table 19.12 Causes of hypoglycaemia

Insulinoma (and nesidioblastosis in neonates)

Other tumours (producing insulin-like peptides)
Mesenchymal tumours
Hepatomas

Counter-regulatory hormone deficiencies
Addison's disease, congenital adrenal hyperplasia
Pituitary failure (ACTH, TSH, growth hormone deficiency)

Drugs and toxins
Insulin
Sulphonylureas
Pentamidine
Ethanol
Salicylate overdose (in children)

Hepatic disease
Acute hepatic necrosis, e.g. paracetamol overdose
Glycogen storage disease

Dumping syndrome (overdiagnosed)

Miscellaneous
Starvation ⎫ very rare in
Prolonged exercise ⎬ healthy subjects
Falciparum malaria
Neonatal (premature babies, or after diabetic pregnancy)
Autoimmune (antibodies activate insulin receptor)
Idiopathic (exceedingly rare)

caemia, by secreting insulin-like molecules (e.g. growth factors such as IGF-2) which structurally resemble insulin and so activate the insulin receptor.

Inadequate counter-regulatory hormone secretion

Hypoglycaemia may be a presenting feature of Addison's disease or hypopituitarism (in which growth hormone deficiency exacerbates hypoglycaemia), especially during vomiting. It also occurs in congenital adrenal hyperplasia (21-hydroxylase deficiency) and isolated ACTH deficiency.

Drugs and ethanol

Insulin and *sulphonylureas* commonly cause hypoglycaemia in treated diabetic patients (p. 749) and occasionally in non-diabetic subjects who take the drugs either inadvertently or deliberately. Self-induced 'factitious' hypoglycaemia, usually with insulin, is identified most commonly in medical or paramedical subjects or in those with a diabetic family member. *Pentamidine*, used to treat pneumocystis pneumonia in AIDS patients, can cause hypoglycaemia by inducing β-cell necrosis, which may then be followed by diabetes.

Ethanol directly inhibits hepatic gluconeogenesis and tends to cause hypoglycaemia, especially in treated diabetic patients who are unable to suppress their circulating insulin levels on demand, and in malnourished subjects or those with alcoholic and other liver diseases in which hepatic glycogen is depleted.

Hepatic diseases

Severe hepatocellular damage, such as alcoholic liver disease or acute hepatic necrosis in pregnancy or following paracetamol overdose, interferes with the mechanisms by which the liver normally secretes glucose. Certain glycogen storage diseases (p. 782) prevent mobilisation of hepatic glycogen and cause severe hypoglycaemia in infancy or childhood.

Gastrointestinal diseases

'Reactive' hypoglycaemia, i.e. that occurring after meals rather than during fasting, can occur following gastric and intestinal surgery and very rarely in normal subjects. The cause is inappropriately high insulin secretion, possibly stimulated by incretin hormones released from the gut by eating, which outlasts the absorption of glucose from the intestine (p. 740).

Miscellaneous causes

Starvation and *exercise* both have to be extreme for healthy subjects to become hypoglycaemic. *Neonatal hypoglycaemia* may occur in premature babies whose hepatic glycogen stores are limited, and in the babies of women who had poorly-controlled diabetes during pregnancy, because hypertrophied fetal islets continue to secrete excess insulin (see p. 759). *Falciparum malaria* causes hypoglycaemia, apparently by preventing hepatic glucose production, and this is exacerbated by quinine treatment which directly stimulates insulin secretion. *Autoimmune* hypoglycaemia is due to autoantibodies which bind to and activate the insulin receptor, analogous to the TSH-receptor antibodies which stimulate the thyroid in Graves' disease. This occurs rarely in autoimmune syndromes and following treatment with the antithyroid drug, methimazole.

Idiopathic spontaneous hypoglycaemia has long been a fashionable diagnosis, usually made for vague symptoms of hunger and shakiness which are relieved by eating. It is, in fact, very rare.

Effects and clinical features of hypoglycaemia

As described on page 750, hypoglycaemia causes 'autonomic' features due to sympathetic activation (tremor, sweating, tachycardia) and neuroglycopenic symptoms and signs including hunger, confusion, abnormal behaviour, specific neurological deficits which may suggest focal lesions, fitting and coma. Complaints may be nonspecific and hypoglycaemia may remain unrecognised for years: recurrent or chronic hypoglycaemia has caused people to be institutionalised for suspected psychiatric disease.

Most causes of hypoglycaemia will be exacerbated by lack of food and so present during fasting, the notable exception being the reactive hypoglycaemia which follows within a few hours of eating.

Investigation, diagnosis and management of hypoglycaemia

Confirmation of hypoglycaemia

It is crucial to document hypoglycaemia carefully, as many cases of suspected hypoglycaemia, especially those with 'reactive' symptoms, will not be confirmed; the high levels of psychosocial stress which many of these patients are under may contribute to their symptoms.

As a screening procedure, blood glucose levels may be measured before breakfast, but it is best to admit patients to hospital for a supervised 72-hour fast with regular exercise. This schedule will reveal over 99% of cases of spontaneous hypoglycaemia due to insulinomas (the commonest cause) and very few normal subjects will become hypoglycaemic during this time. Blood glucose levels should be checked regularly and, if symptoms develop, two blood samples should be taken for measurement of glucose (using a laboratory method, ideally in arterialised or capillary blood), insulin and C-peptide. Glucose should then be given to confirm that symptoms improve; this fulfils Whipple's triad, namely that symptoms are associated with fasting or exercise, that they are accompanied by demonstrable hypoglycaemia, and that they are relieved by glucose administration.

Investigation and treatment of causes of hypoglycaemia

A flow chart for investigating suspected hypoglycaemia is shown in Figure 19.19.

Hypoglycaemia not due to insulin excess normally suppresses insulin concentrations to <5 mU/l and C-peptide to undetectable levels (<0.1 pmol/l). Extrapancreatic tumours, endocrine diseases, gastrointestinal diseases and miscellaneous causes (Table 19.12) should be considered under these circumstances and appropriate tests performed to identify the cause.

High insulin levels are due either to endogenous hypersecretion, in which C-peptide levels will also be

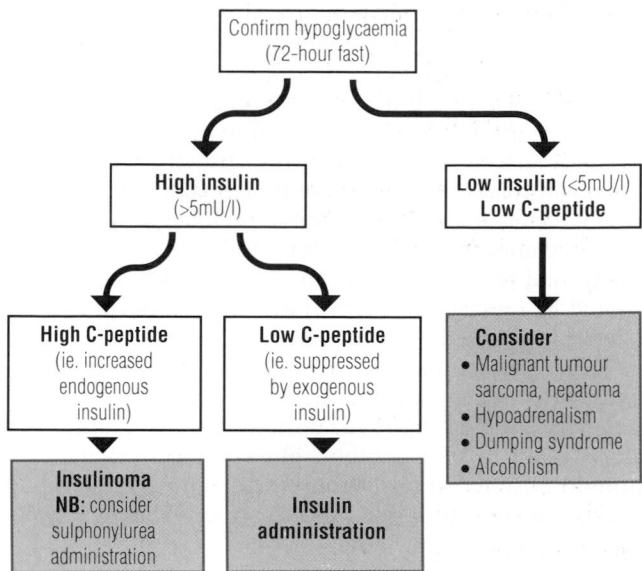

Fig. 19.19 Flow-chart for investigating suspected hypoglycaemia.

high, or to administration of exogenous insulin, which will suppress endogenous insulin and C-peptide secretion. Factitious hypoglycaemia induced by insulin injection can therefore be easily identified because C-peptide concentrations measured during hypoglycaemia are undetectable. Endogenous insulin hypersecretion with high C-peptide levels is almost always due to an insulinoma (or nesidioblastosis), when proinsulin levels may also be elevated because of defective processing of proinsulin in neoplastic β cells. The possibility of inadvertent or deliberate sulphonylurea administration, which stimulates insulin and C-peptide release, should be considered, especially if an insulinoma cannot be localised. Sulphonylureas can be detected by screening the urine.

Hypoglycaemia provocation tests, designed to demonstrate that endogenous insulin and C-peptide secretion from an insulinoma do not suppress normally during hypoglycaemia induced by exogenous insulin, are potentially dangerous and are now little used.

The flow-chart for diagnosing insulinoma is shown in Figure 19.19. The main problem is in localising the tumour; very small insulinomas may be missed by sophisticated imaging techniques including CT scanning and pancreatic arteriography, and even by palpation at operation. Ultrasound imaging may be helpful, either using a probe mounted on an endoscope which can visualise the head of the pancreas from the duodenum, or by scanning the pancreas exposed at operation. Selective venous sampling can also be used to determine which sector of the pancreas is secreting excess insulin. Treatment consists of surgical removal (which is curative for benign tumours) if the tumour can be localised. Nesidioblastosis is also treated by pancreatectomy. Medical treatment, for inoperable tumours or patients unsuitable for surgery, consists of suppressing insulin secretion, usually with diazoxide, a sulphonylurea derivative; its main side-effects are hypotension and hirsutism. Somatostatin analogues (e.g. octreotide) have been used to treat insulinoma and nesidioblastosis, but also suppress growth hormone and glucagon release so that hypoglycaemia, when it occurs, may be dangerously profound and prolonged.

Large mesenchymal tumours and hepatomas are easily diagnosed by CT scanning and biopsy. These tumours should be removed if possible; medical treatment consists of steroids and glucagon injections.

Idiopathic spontaneous hypoglycaemia is often investigated by the extended (5-hour) OGTT, which has a fairly high yield, as about 25% of normal, healthy subjects will show a fall in *venous* blood glucose levels to below 3 mmol/l during this test. When the diagnostic criteria for hypoglycaemia are applied strictly, true 'idiopathic' hypoglycaemia is extremely rare.

The management of acute hypoglycaemia is discussed on page 750 and individual causes of hypoglycaemia require the treatments described above.

PLASMA LIPOPROTEINS AND THEIR DISORDERS

Normal lipid metabolism

The two major lipids are *triglycerides*, a valuable energy source and store; and *cholesterol*, an essential component of cell membranes and a precursor in the synthesis of bile salts, steroid hormones and vitamin D. Both are absorbed from dietary fat (especially in meat, eggs and dairy products) and are also synthesised by the liver. Cholesterol is synthesised from acetyl-CoA, the rate-limiting enzyme being HMGCoA reductase (hydroxymethylglutaryl coenzyme A reductase). Cholesterol suppresses its own synthesis by inhibiting HMGCoA reductase, and bile-salt synthesis is inhibited by bile salts reabsorbed from the gut and returned to the liver through the enterohepatic circulation.

Triglycerides and cholesterol are insoluble and have to be complexed into soluble *lipoproteins* to allow their transport from the gut and liver to the tissues. The lipoproteins (Fig. 19.20) are spherical particles containing a hydrophobic core of triglyceride and esterified cholesterol surrounded by a hydrophilic coat of phospholipid, specific proteins termed *apoproteins*, and a little free cholesterol. Apoproteins are synthesised in the liver and gut and comprise six main classes (apos A to F). Lipoproteins can be classified by their density on ultracentrifugation, which decreases with increasing triglyceride content.

The lipoproteins are metabolised by two different pathways (Fig. 19.21). The *exogenous* pathway begins

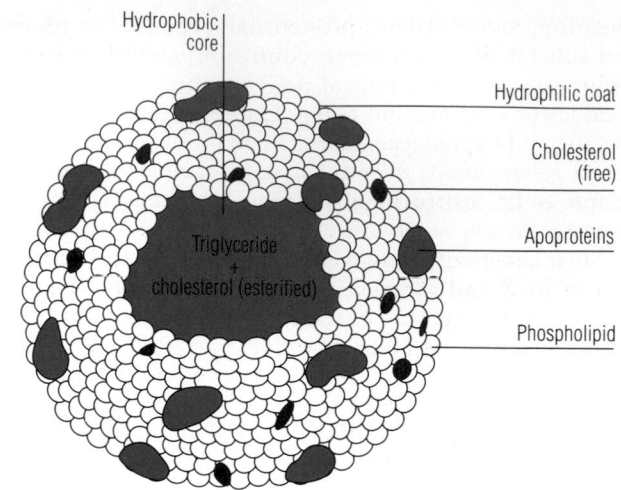

Fig. 19.20 Structure and composition of lipoproteins.

with dietary fat in the gut and employs triglyceride-rich chylomicrons to deliver FFA to the tissues and cholesterol to the liver. The *endogenous* pathway uses very low density

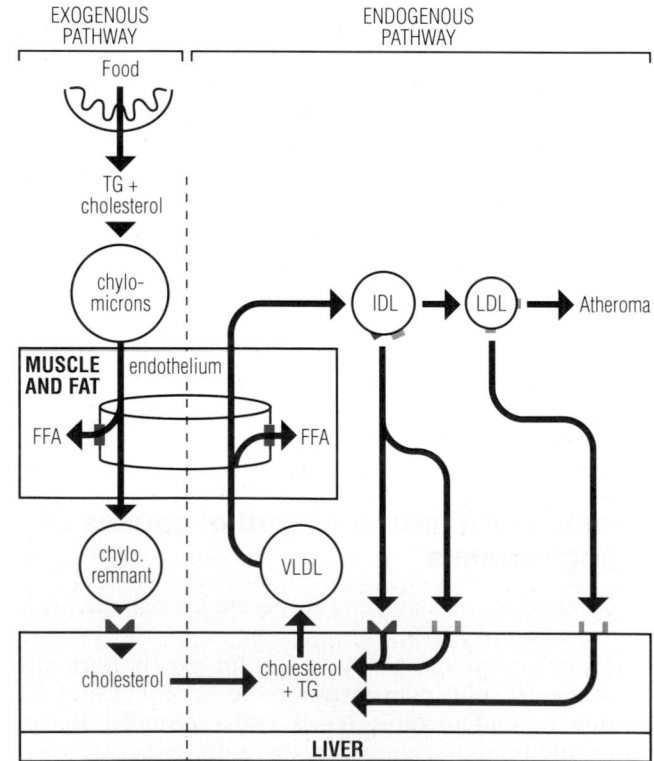

Fig. 19.21 The exogenous and endogenous pathways of lipid metabolism. FFA, free fatty acid; LPL, lipoprotein lipase (found in capillary endothelium); IDL, intermediate density lipoprotein; LDL, low density lipoprotein; VLDL, very low density lipoprotein. The chylomicron remnant binds to the hepatocyte via the apo-E receptor, as does the IDL. The LDL binds via the apo-B100 receptor (as does IDL also).

lipoprotein, containing triglyceride synthesised in the liver, to supply FFA and cholesterol to the peripheral tissues.

Exogenous pathway

- *Chylomicrons* are synthesised from dietary fat in the gut and have a very high triglyceride content, together with cholesterol and specific apoproteins (apos B48, C and E). Chylomicrons enter the circulation from the lymphatics and their triglyceride content is progressively depleted by lipoprotein lipase (LPL), an enzyme of the capillary endothelium in skeletal muscle and fat which is activated by apo CII in the chylomicrons. FFA liberated by triglyceride breakdown are used by the tissues as fuel or for storage as triglyceride.
- The residual *chylomicron remnants*, partly stripped of triglyceride and therefore denser, are taken up into hepatocytes by specific receptors which recognise apo E, so delivering cholesterol to the liver.

Endogenous pathway

- *Very low density lipoproteins* (VLDL) are synthesised in the liver and, like chylomicrons, have an initially high triglyceride content which is depleted by LPL in the periphery. VLDL also contain cholesterol and apos B100, C (including CII, which activates LPL) and E. Loss of triglyceride produces *intermediate density lipoprotein* (IDL).
- IDL is partly taken up by the liver (through receptors for apos B and E) to recycle cholesterol, and the rest is further stripped of triglyceride to yield *low density lipoprotein* (LDL).
- LDL is perhaps the most important lipoprotein in causing disease, as it is abundant (normally about three-quarters of total plasma cholesterol) and produces atheroma. It is taken up into the liver and other tissues by specific LDL receptors which recognise apo B100. LDL uptake has important effects on cholesterol metabolism and atherogenesis. LDL entering the liver 'down-regulates' (inactivates) LDL receptors and so reduces the liver's capacity to assimilate more LDL, and also inhibits HMGCoA reductase and therefore cholesterol synthesis. LDL is the only lipoprotein to deliver cholesterol to peripheral tissues, including the arterial intima, where its deposition causes atheroma formation (see p. 392).

Another atherogenic lipoprotein is *lipoprotein (a)*, or Lp(a), a quantitatively minor species synthesised in the liver, which contains apo B100 and apo(a). The latter structurally resembles plasminogen and may bind to fibrin, preventing fibrinolysis and promoting thrombosis, and inducing atherogenesis where fibrin is deposited at sites of vascular damage.

The final lipoprotein is *high density lipoprotein* (HDL), which is synthesised in the liver and gut and has a relatively high content of apoproteins, notably apo AI. HDL comprises about one-quarter of total plasma cholesterol and opposes the effect of LDL in that it protects against atheroma formation.

Measurement of plasma lipid levels

Plasma lipid concentrations, especially of cholesterol, vary widely between individuals and between different populations. For example, the mean plasma cholesterol is substantially lower in Africans and Asians than in Europeans, of whom about 50% have total cholesterol levels above the recommended limit of 5.2 mmol/l. Forty per cent of individual variability is genetically determined; environmental modifying factors include diet, exercise, body weight and alcohol intake. Both obesity and a diet rich in saturated fats cause the *atherogenic lipid profile* of increased LDL and reduced HDL levels, which can be reversed by a diet high in fibre and polyunsaturated fats and by regular exercise. Before the menopause, women have lower LDL and higher HDL cholesterol levels than men, which partly explains their relative protection against atherosclerosis.

For practical clinical purposes, total, LDL and HDL cholesterol, and triglyceride concentrations should be measured. A fasting sample is needed for accurate triglyceride measurements, as chylomicron levels rise considerably after meals. Lipid levels may be disturbed for several weeks after severe stress, such as myocardial infarction.

Large-scale, random population screening for hyperlipidaemia would be complicated, expensive and of doubtful benefit in the UK, where hypercholesterolaemia is so common. Plasma lipid estimations should therefore be confined to high-risk individuals with coronary heart or peripheral vascular disease (especially if present before 50 years of age), a strong family history of vascular disease, or other risk factors such as smoking, hypertension, diabetes or obesity.

Pathological significance of plasma lipid abnormalities

Epidemiological studies indicate that the incidence of atherosclerosis is strongly related to total plasma cholesterol and specifically to LDL cholesterol levels; as mentioned above, Lp(a) levels may also determine atherosclerosis in certain families or groups (e.g. diabetic patients with microalbuminuria). Conversely, HDL cholesterol concentrations are inversely related to coro-

Table 19.13 Lipoprotein levels and cardiovascular risks

| Lipoprotein | Concentrations (mmol/l) associated with: | | |
	Low risk	Borderline	Increased risk
Cholesterol			
Total	<5.2	5.2–6.5	>6.5
LDL	<4.0	4.0–5.0	>5.0
HDL	>1.0	0.9–1.0	<0.9
Triglycerides	<2.0	2.0–2.5	>2.5

These risk threshold values are more useful than 'normal' ranges, as about 50% of the British population have cholesterol concentrations which exceed the borderline risk threshold.

nary heart disease, especially in moderate hypercholesterolaemia. The current view is that there is a weak association with hypertriglyceridaemia, which becomes much stronger if LDL cholesterol is raised and HDL reduced. The risk thresholds for hyperlipidaemia (Table 19.13) are the basis for practical management.

Hyperlipidaemia

Increased concentrations of specific lipoproteins may be *primary*, i.e. due to hereditary defects in lipoprotein metabolism, or *secondary* to certain diseases. The lipoprotein class(es) involved may be identified precisely by lipoprotein electrophoresis, but this is superfluous to the routine clinical management of hyperlipidaemia, which can be guided satisfactorily by measuring the major cholesterol fractions and triglycerides.

Primary hyperlipidaemias

These conditions can be classified by the WHO/ Fredrickson system (Table 19.14). The molecular basis of several has been elucidated.

Familial hypercholesterolaemia (FH)

This is due to defects in the LDL receptor, which prevent uptake of LDL cholesterol into the liver and so increase plasma LDL levels. These are further raised by increased hepatic cholesterol synthesis, as feedback inhibition by cholesterol of HMGCoA reductase is reduced. Protective HDL cholesterol levels are reduced and triglyceride levels are either normal (type IIa) or increased due to VLDL (type IIb). These gene defects occur in about 1 in 500 in the UK. *Homozygotes* have grossly elevated LDL cholesterol (>15 mmol/l) and suffer greatly accelerated atherosclerosis, often dying of myocardial infarction in their teens or twenties. *Heterozygotes* (who have moderately reduced LDL receptor activity) have lower LDL cholesterol levels (>9 mmol/l) and present with coronary heart disease in their forties. Both often have tendon xanthomata, cholesterol deposits which thicken the Achilles tendon or cause nodules over the patellar or triceps tendons, as well as the corneal arcus and xanthelasmata which can occur in milder degrees of hypercholesterolaemia and also in people with normal cholesterol levels (see Table 19.15).

Polygenic hypercholesterolaemia

This is much commoner than FH and causes a similar but milder pattern of hypercholesterolaemia with normal (type IIa) or elevated (type IIb) triglyceride levels. Inheritance is polygenic; coronary heart disease develops in the forties and xanthomata do not develop.

Familial combined hyperlipidaemia

This is a variable combination of types IIa, IIb and IV, inherited as an autosomal dominant and which predisposes to atherosclerosis.

Table 19.14 Primary hyperlipidaemias (WHO modification of Fredrickson classification)

Type	Total plasma cholesterol	Total plasma triglyceride	Defect	Inheritance	Prevalence	Atherosclerosis risk increased
I	Normal	↑ (chylo)	Lipoprotein lipase deficiency or apo-CII deficiency	Recessive	Rare	No
IIa	↑ (LDL)	N	LDL receptor defect	Dominant (FH) or polygenic	Polygenic is common	Yes
IIb	↑ (LDL)	↑ (VLDL)	LDL receptor defect	Dominant	Common	Yes
III	↑	↑ (IDL)	Apo-E abnormality	–	Rare	Yes
IV	Normal or slight ↑	↑ (VLDL)	Overproduction of VLDL	Dominant	Common	No
V	Normal or slight ↑	↑ (chylo and VLDL)	Lipoprotein lipase deficiency or apo-CII deficiency	Recessive	Rare	No

Table 19.15 Features of hyperlipidaemia

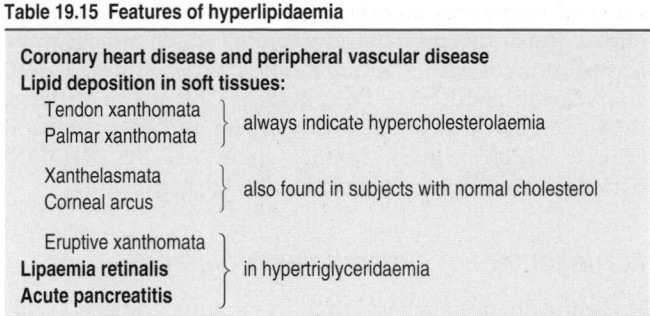

Coronary heart disease and peripheral vascular disease	
Lipid deposition in soft tissues:	
Tendon xanthomata Palmar xanthomata	always indicate hypercholesterolaemia
Xanthelasmata Corneal arcus	also found in subjects with normal cholesterol
Eruptive xanthomata **Lipaemia retinalis** **Acute pancreatitis**	in hypertriglyceridaemia

Familial hypertriglyceridaemia

This is due to either increased endogenous trigly-ceride synthesis (excess VLDL is produced by the liver, Fig. 19.21), or failure of exogenous triglyceride in chylo-microns to be cleared by LPL; defects in LPL itself or in apo CII, which normally activates it, can be responsible. Plasma triglycerides are grossly elevated (10–100 mmol/l); the fraction responsible can be identified simply by storing plasma for 18 hours at 4°C, when chylomicrons will form a creamy supernatant whereas VLDL or IDL cause uni-form turbidity. Severe hypertriglyceridaemia (>10 mmol/l) causes acute pancreatitis, eruptive xanthomata (itchy, reddish triglyceride deposits) and lipaemia retinalis (a milky appearance of the retinal vessels); coronary heart disease is not generally increased (see Table 19.15).

Secondary hyperlipidaemias

These may arise in hypothyroidism, untreated diabetes mellitus, oral oestrogen or thiazide diuretic therapy, alcohol abuse, the nephrotic syndrome and liver disease. Those causing an atherogenic lipid profile predispose to vascular disease. These conditions must be con-sidered and excluded in cases of lipid abnormality (Table 19.16).

Table 19.16 Secondary hyperlipidaemias

	Cholesterol				
Disorder	VLDL	LDL	HDL	Triglycerides	Complications
Diabetes	↑	↑	↓	↑ or ↑↑	CHD
Obesity	↑	↑	↓	↑	CHD
Hypothyroidism	↑	↑	—	—	CHD
Nephrotic syndrome	↑	↑	—	↑	CHD
Cholestasis (e.g. primary biliary cirrhosis)	—	↑	—	—	CHD
Alcohol abuse	↑	—	↑	↑ or ↑↑	Pancreatitis; not CHD

CHD, coronary heart disease.

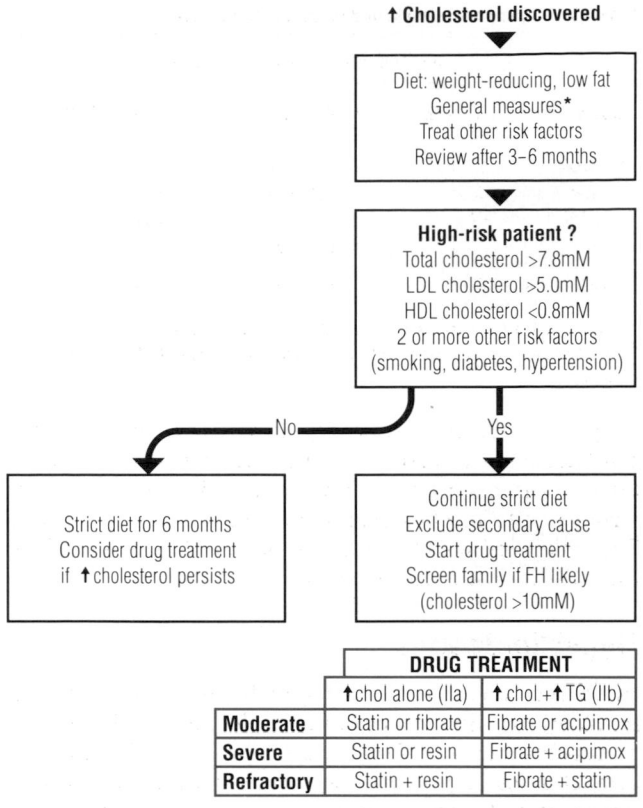

↑ Cholesterol discovered

Diet: weight-reducing, low fat
General measures *
Treat other risk factors
Review after 3–6 months

High-risk patient ?
Total cholesterol >7.8mM
LDL cholesterol >5.0mM
HDL cholesterol <0.8mM
2 or more other risk factors
(smoking, diabetes, hypertension)

No — Strict diet for 6 months
Consider drug treatment
if ↑ cholesterol persists

Yes — Continue strict diet
Exclude secondary cause
Start drug treatment
Screen family if FH likely
(cholesterol >10mM)

	DRUG TREATMENT	
	↑chol alone (IIa)	↑ chol +↑ TG (IIb)
Moderate	Statin or fibrate	Fibrate or acipimox
Severe	Statin or resin	Fibrate + acipimox
Refractory	Statin + resin	Fibrate + statin

* Stop smoking; Reduce alcohol intake; Take regular exercise; Treat hypertension

Fig. 19.22 Flow-chart for treating hypercholesterolaemia.

Management of hyperlipidaemias

Hyperlipidaemia must be managed as part of a general attack on cardiovascular risk factors. *Essential general measures* therefore include: stopping smoking (one of the most important independent risk factors); reducing exces-sive alcohol intake; controlling hypertension (avoiding drugs which raise blood lipid or glucose levels); reducing body weight towards a BMI of <25; and encouraging exercise (which raises HDL levels). A flow-chart for treating hypercholesterolaemia is shown in Figure 19.22.

Two recent studies have emphasised the value of both general and specific measures in reducing mortality from coronary heart disease in hyperlipidaemic people, namely diet and stopping smoking in the Oslo Trial, and gemfi-brozil treatment in the Helsinki Heart Study.

Lipid-modifying drugs

The principal classes of drugs are shown in Table 19.17. Those which primarily affect *cholesterol*, lowering total and LDL cholesterol and sometimes raising HDL, include the bile-salt sequestering resins and the HMGCoA reductase inhibitors (statins).

19 Diabetes Mellitus and Lipid Metabolism

Table 19.17 Lipid-modifying drugs

Drugs	LDL	HDL	TG	Side-effects	Indications
Resins Cholestyramine Colestipol	↓↓	—	↑	Flatulence, gut upset Block absorption of digoxin and warfarin	Hyperchol.
Statins (HMGCoA reductase inhibitors) Simvastatin Pravastatin	↓↓	↑	↓	Gut upset Myositis (rare) Long-term safety uncertain (as yet)	Hyperchol.
Fibrates Gemfibrozil Bezafibrate	↓	↑	↓	Gut upset Gallstones Myositis (rare) Potentiate anti- coagulants	Hypertrig. Combined
Nicotinic acid Acipimox (derivative)	↓	↑	↓	Gut upset, ulceration Flushing (less with acipimox) Glucose intolerance (less with acipimox)	Hypertrig. Combined
Fish oils Omega-3 marine oils	↑	—	↓	Gut upset Glucose intolerance (avoid in NIDDM)	Hypertrig.

Hyperchol., hypercholesterolaemia; hypertrig., hypertriglyceridaemia; combined, combined hyperlipidaemia; TG (triglycerides).

The *resins* (e.g. cholestyramine and colestipol) bind bile salts in the gut lumen, preventing them from returning to the liver in the enterohepatic circulation; this reduces negative feedback inhibition by the bile salts of their own synthesis and so increases cholesterol consumption by the liver. Resins are often effective in hypercholesterolaemia, including heterozygous FH, but have prominent gastrointestinal side-effects and must be introduced slowly. The resins have traditionally been first-line treatment for hypercholesterolaemia but are now being supplanted by the statins (e.g. simvastatin and pravastatin).

Statins block cholesterol synthesis and lower intracellular cholesterol levels, which up-regulates LDL receptors on the liver and stimulates LDL uptake from the blood. These powerful drugs are generally well tolerated and so far seem to have no long-term toxic side-effects.

Primarily *triglyceride-lowering* drugs are the fibrates, nicotinic acid and its derivatives, and fish oils; fibrates and nicotinic acid also improve the cholesterol profile, whereas fish oils may lower HDL levels. *Fibrates*, e.g. gemfibrozil and bezafibrate (which have generally replaced clofibrate), block VLDL and cholesterol synthesis, while *nicotinic acid* and its derivatives (e.g. acipimox) reduce VLDL synthesis by inhibiting lipolysis and therefore the supply of FFA from fat to the liver. Fibrates

are well tolerated; nicotinic acid has troublesome side-effects (flushing and hyperglycaemia) which appear to be less prominent with acipimox. The *fish oils* inhibit VLDL triglyceride synthesis. They have to be taken in large doses and cause gastrointestinal upset and glucose intolerance which argues against their use in NIDDM patients, who frequently have hypertriglyceridaemia.

Management of hypercholesterolaemia

Present evidence suggests that, in patients under 60 years of age, attempts should be made to lower elevated total and LDL cholesterol levels towards normal. Moderate (polygenic) hypercholesterolaemia should be treated initially for several months with a low-fat diet and general measures to reduce cardiovascular risk factors. A reduction in total fat intake and a relative increase in polyunsaturated fats (replacing fatty meats, dairy produce and fried foods with fish, chicken, vegetable oils and grilled or boiled foods) can reduce LDL cholesterol by up to 10% and be effective in mild hypercholesterolaemia. This healthy diet must be positively promoted.

Total cholesterol levels remaining above 7.8 mmol/l after this time, especially if HDL is <0.8 mmol/l, require a cholesterol-lowering drug. A statin or a resin are first-line agents for pure hypercholesterolaemia (type IIa), whereas a fibrate or acipimox are appropriate for combined hyperlipidaemia (type IIb). The treatment of FH is difficult. Heterozygotes usually respond to a combination of resin and statin, but homozygotes often do not and may require regular plasma exchange or ultracentrifugation of plasma to remove LDL.

Management of hypertriglyceridaemia

Dietary management of hypertriglyceridaemia should aim to achieve a BMI of <25 and a reduction in saturated fat intake. Severe hypertriglyceridaemia (>10 mmol/l) requires treatment to prevent attacks of acute pancreatitis. A fibrate or nicotinic acid are often effective, and bezafibrate is particularly useful in type III hyperlipidaemia. Hypertriglyceridaemia is frequently associated with glucose intolerance, and the latter may be exacerbated by either nicotinic acid (but not acipimox) or fish oils.

PORPHYRIA

The term porphyria refers to a heterogeneous group of inborn errors of metabolism causing enzyme defects in the biosynthetic pathway of haem, and the accumulation of its precursors, the porphyrinogens. These consist of four cyclised pyrrole rings and are classified into uro-, copro- and protoporphyrinogens by the distribution of side-groups around the porphyrin ring. Porphyrinogens are excreted in the urine if present in excess in blood. They are colourless compounds but are oxidised to yield highly coloured porphyrins which colour the urine dark in some cases of acute porphyria.

HAEM SYNTHESIS

Porphyrin biosynthesis occurs in a variety of cell types, but predominantly in liver and bone marrow (Fig. 19.23). The initial step is the condensation of glycine and succinyl CoA to form delta-amino-laevulinic acid (d-ALA) under the influence of mitochondrial ALA synthase. The single pyrrole ring, porphobilinogen (PBG) is then formed in the cytosol from two molecules of d-ALA. Four molecules of PBG are cyclised under the influence of PBG deaminase to form the porphyrin ring structure. There follows a series of decarboxylation and mitochondrial oxidation reactions, eventually yielding protoporphyrin IX. The addition of ferrous iron, catalysed by ferrochelatase, is the final step in haem biosynthesis. The pathway's activity is controlled by negative feedback of haem on d-ALA synthase.

CLASSIFICATION OF THE PORPHYRIAS

The porphyrias may be classified as hepatic or erythropoietic, according to the main site of the biosynthetic defect and excess precursor formation, but the clinical subdivision into acute or non-acute forms is more useful (Table 19.18).

All porphyrias are associated with increased d-ALA synthase activity because of decreased negative feedback, which is usually enhanced by an environmental factor. This is accompanied by increased PBG deaminase activity in the non-acute conditions, but normal or reduced activity in the acute varieties. The net result in the acute conditions is an accumulation of d-ALA and PBG which probably accounts for the neurological, psychiatric and acute gastrointestinal disturbances observed. In the non-acute conditions, specific uro- and coproporphyrins accumulate without PBG excess because increased activity of

Table 19.18 Classification of porphyrias

Acute	Non-acute
Acute intermittent porphyria	Porphyria cutanea tarda (cutaneous hepatic porphyria)
Variegate porphyria	
Hereditary coproporphyria	Erythropoietic – congenital porphyria – protoporphyria

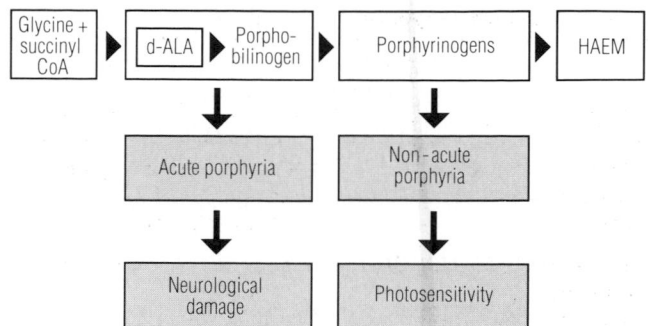

Fig. 19.23 Porphyrin metabolism. Increased d-ALA synthetase activity leads to increased porphyrin production (porphyria). In acute porphyria, porphobilinogen metabolism is normal or reduced, in contrast to non-acute porphyria in which it is increased.

the d-ALA synthase pathway is accompanied by increased PBG deaminase activity (Fig. 19.23).

Photosensitivity occurs in all porphyrias, except for the acute intermittent variety, and is due to accumulation of porphyrin within the epidermis as a result of photo-oxidation of porphyrinogens.

Acute porphyrias

Acute porphyrias are all inherited as Mendelian dominant traits. They are characterised by acute episodic neurological and gastrointestinal symptoms, usually followed by complete remission, although fatalities due to respiratory failure may occur. Episodes are rare before puberty, when a rise in the sex steroids enhances ALA synthase activity. Acute attacks are precipitated by alcohol, sex steroids (e.g. oral contraceptives) and many drugs, notably barbiturates, sulphonamides and other lipid-soluble enzyme-inducing drugs, which increase ALA synthase activity.

Acute intermittent porphyria

Acute intermittent porphyria is due to a defect in PBG deaminase. Most cases are clinically silent; women are more likely to manifest acute attacks, consisting in 95% of cases of abdominal pain and vomiting. Additional features include sinus tachycardia, hypertension and left ventricular failure (75%), sensorimotor peripheral neuropathy (50%), respiratory muscle paresis, fitting and coma. Psychiatric manifestations, which vary from depression to frank psychosis, may last throughout the acute episode. Renal impairment with proteinuria and inappropriate antidiuretic hormone (ADH) secretion (p. 847) may also occur.

The diagnosis may be suggested by a positive family history, or the passage of urine which turns red-brown on standing. Confirmation depends on testing urine for excess PBG using Ehrlich's aldehyde reagent, which produces a pink colour that is insoluble in chloroform.

Variegate porphyria

The defect is in protoporphyrinogen oxidase. Features are similar to those of acute intermittent porphyria, together with the cutaneous features of porphyria cutanea tarda (see below). The highest incidence is in South African whites.

Hereditary coproporphyria

Coproporphyrinogen oxidase is defective, causing features similar to variegate porphyria.

Management of acute porphyria

Prophylaxis in those at risk is of obvious importance. Suspected patients can be identified by urine testing (30% yield) and erythrocyte-enzyme assays. Those affected should avoid alcohol, barbiturates and oral contraceptives, and special observation during pregnancy is indicated.

Acute attacks may be curtailed by a high carbohydrate intake (e.g. 400 g/day of glucose intravenously) and perhaps intravenous haematin, both of which depress ALA synthase activity. Inappropriate ADH secretion may require fluid restriction. Tachycardia and hypertension should be treated with beta-blockade, psychiatric disturbances with phenothiazines, and fitting with benzodiazepines; barbiturates are absolutely contraindicated.

Non-acute porphyrias

Porphyria cutanea tarda

Porphyria cutanea tarda is due to a defect in hepatic uroporphyrinogen decarboxylase, which has a genetic element but is predominantly acquired; alcohol abuse is often important. It is characterised by bullae following sun exposure or minor trauma, usually affecting the face, back of the neck, and dorsum of the hands. The bullae heal with scarring and diffuse thickening of the skin, which can resemble scleroderma, and hypertrichosis also develops. Hepatomegaly (particularly with alcohol abuse) and hepatic siderosis and diabetes mellitus may occur. Urinary uroporphyrin excretion is increased but PBG is normal. Treatment includes avoidance of alcohol; venesection to achieve normal uroporphyrin levels in urine; and low-dose chloroquine, which increases urinary uroporphyrin excretion.

Congenital porphyria

Congenital porphyria is a rare autosomal recessively inherited condition which presents early in childhood. It is due to a defect in uroporphyrinogen cosynthetase and is characterised by photosensitivity with bulla formation and healing with scarring. Dystrophic nail changes and brown or pink tooth discolouration may also occur, and a normochromic anaemia with normoblastic marrow hyperplasia and splenomegaly are usual features. Low-dose chloroquine may be of value in treatment, and splenectomy may improve the anaemia.

Erythropoietic protoporphyria

Erythropoietic protoporphyria is an autosomal dominant condition due to a defect in ferrochelatase activity, which presents in childhood with photosensitivity (often with no rash), severe peripheral paraesthesia and hepatic dysfunction due to protoporphyrin deposition. The diagnosis is made by demonstrating characteristic erythrocyte fluorescence and elevated red cell protoporphyrin levels. Urinary and faecal protoporphyrin excretion may be increased. Treatment with oral beta-carotene may protect against the photosensitivity, and bile-salt sequestering agents (e.g. cholestyramine) may protect the liver by interrupting the enterohepatic circulation of protoporphyrin.

INHERITED DISORDERS OF CARBOHYDRATE METABOLISM

Glycogen storage diseases

Glycogen is synthesised from glucose by glycogen synthase and a branching enzyme which adds side-chains to the growing polymer. It is stored primarily in liver as a source of glucose for release into the circulation and in muscle as substrate for glycolysis (Fig. 19.4). Glycogen breakdown depends on several enzymes including phosphorylase (which removes glucose residues from the polymer), a debranching enzyme (amylo-1,6-glucosidase), and α-1,4-glucosidase which cleaves glucose from glycogen stored in lysosomes. In liver, glucose-6-phosphate is converted to glucose under the influence of glucose-6-phosphatase, whereas in muscle it undergoes glycolysis and is converted sequentially to fructose-6-phosphate, fructose-1,6-bisphosphate (catalysed by phosphofructokinase), pyruvate and lactate.

The glycogen storage diseases are due to defects in the above enzymes, which are all inherited as autosomal recessive traits. Twelve defects have been identified, and except for muscle phosphorylase deficiency (type V, McArdle), they present in early childhood. All are extremely rare. Glycogen synthase deficiency (very rare) causes severe depletion of liver glycogen. The other defects cause glycogen to accumulate in liver, muscle, myocardium, kidney or gut and cause features such as hepatomegaly, hypoglycaemia, muscle fatigue and cramps, and congestive cardiac failure. The commonest conditions are types I, II and V.

Type I (Von Gierke)

Hepatic glucose-6-phosphatase is defective, preventing hepatic glycogen mobilisation and presenting with hepatomegaly in infancy. The nervous system adapts to using ketone bodies as an energy source, but intercurrent illness precipitates severe hypoglycaemia and lactic acidosis. Affected infants are characteristically obese, grow poorly and exhibit hyperlipidaemia and hyperuricaemia. Blood glucose levels fail to increase after glucagon administration and the diagnosis is confirmed by liver biopsy. Untreated, the condition is usually fatal in early childhood. Successful therapy depends on frequent glucose feeds given day and night by nasogastric tube. This can restore normal growth, but impairs neurological ketoadaptation and so increases the hazards of acute hypoglycaemia.

Type II (Pompe)

α-glucosidase deficiency causes lysosomal glycogen to accumulate in cardiac and skeletal muscle and liver. Cardiomegaly and congestive cardiac failure usually present in infancy and prove fatal within months, but variants include childhood presentations with myopathy and an indolent onset in adult life. Hypoglycaemia does not occur.

Type V (McArdle)

Muscle phosphorylase deficiency is a rare condition which presents in adult life with muscle cramps and myoglobinuria after exercise. Victims are easily fatigued and develop proximal muscle wasting. Physical activity is restricted but lifespan is normal.

Galactosaemia

Galactosaemia is a rare autosomal recessive condition due to deficiency of the liver enzyme galactose-1-phosphate uridyl transferase, which catalyses conversion of galactose-1-phosphate to glucose-1-phosphate. Affected children are normal at birth, but develop symptoms soon after milk feeds are started: galactose in milk cannot be metabolised, causing accumulation of galactose-1-phosphate which is toxic to tissues. If undetected, the condition progresses from diarrhoea and vomiting to hepatomegaly and jaundice. Death within a few weeks is common, while survivors develop cataracts, cirrhosis and mental retardation. Fortunately, prompt detection in the neonate and avoidance of galactose in the diet allows relatively normal development, although some degree of mental retardation and ovarian failure may occur. Initial diagnosis is by detection

of reducing substances in the urine by a positive test with Clinitest but a negative result with enzyme-based sticks which are specific for glucose. Definitive diagnosis is based on assay of red-cell galactose-1-phosphate uridyl transferase levels. The effectiveness of therapy is assessed by red-cell galactose-1-phosphate concentration.

LYSOSOMAL STORAGE DISORDERS

Lysosomal storage disorders are a large group of inherited diseases in which there is an abnormal deposition of a substrate in vacuoles related to lysosomes as a result of an inborn error of metabolism. These disorders include lipid-storage diseases, mucolipidoses, mucopolysaccharidoses and glycoprotein storage diseases. These diseases are autosomal recessive, except for Hunter's disease (type II) and Fabry's disease, which are both X-linked. The disorders are generally characterised by excessive deposition of substrate in brain, spleen, liver and bone, causing neurological and skeletal problems with hepatosplenomegaly.

A few of the commoner disorders are briefly described below.

Sphingolipidoses

Gaucher's disease

Deficiency of β-glucocerebrosidase causes gangliosides to accumulate in nervous tissue (in the childhood form, causing mental retardation and spasticity) or in the liver, spleen and bone (in the adult form). The adult form is more common and presents with hepatosplenomegaly, bony symptoms including severe pain and deformity, and anaemia due to bone marrow infiltration. Typical Gaucher cells can be recognised on liver or marrow biopsy. Splenectomy may be helpful.

Niemann-Pick disease, Fabry's disease and Tay-Sachs disease

See Table 22.52, page 961.

Mucopolysaccharidoses

Mucopolysaccharidoses are a group of complex-carbohydrate storage disorders with abnormal accumulation in fibroblasts, chondrocytes and neural tissue. Common features include skeletal dysplasia, hepatosplenomegaly, coarse skin and corneal clouding. Gross mental retardation is present in the two best recognised variants, Hurler's syndrome and Hunter's syndrome, which overlap to some extent.

FURTHER READING

Bliss M 1987 The discovery of insulin. Macmillan Press, Basingstoke. *One of the best books of medical history ever written.*

Keen H, Jarrett J 1982 Complications of diabetes, 2nd edn. Edward Arnold, London. *A particularly good account of the morphological changes.*

Kritzinger E E, Taylor K G 1984 Diabetic eye disease. MTP Press, Lancaster. *A practical and well-illustrated handbook.*

Lehninger A L, Nelson D L. Cox M M 1993 Principles of biochemistry. Worth, New York. *The latest up-to-date edition of this unusually palatable and well-presented survey of biochemistry and metabolism.*

Marks V, Rose F C 1981 Hypoglycaemia, 2nd edn. Blackwell, Oxford. *A substantial but readable textbook.*

McLean T 1987 Metal jam. Coronet, London. *An entertaining but thought-provoking personal view of diabetes.*

Pickup J C, Williams G 1991 Textbook of diabetes. Blackwell, Oxford. *A large and up-to-date review of the subject.*

20
Renal and Urinary Disease

John Cunningham

Table 20.1 Functions of the kidney

Excretion of products of metabolism	Homeostasis
Urea	Body water
Creatinine	Body sodium
Urate	Body potassium
Oxalate	Acid–base status
Sulphate	Calcium
Phosphate	Phosphate
Hydrogen ion	
'Uraemic toxins'	
Water of metabolism	

Excretion of substances ingested in excess of requirement	Production of hormones
Water	Renin
Sodium	Angiotensin
Potassium	Erythropoietin
Calcium	1,25-dihydroxyvitamin D
Phosphate	

The function of the kidney in health falls into three main areas (Table 20.1). These are:

- excretion of waste products
- maintenance of the constancy of the internal environment
- biosynthesis of hormones.

The importance of these functions is vividly demonstrated in kidney disease, in which a wide variety of symptoms and signs are associated with disordered metabolism. The sophistication of the various functions of the kidney is evident from the striking contrast between the limited efficacy of the various forms of artificial dialysis treatment, and the virtual normalisation of body function that attends reversal of kidney dysfunction or successful transplantation.

EPIDEMIOLOGICAL CONSIDERATIONS

The annual incidence rate of end-stage renal disease (ESRD) in the UK is about 150 per million population. Of these, about 50% are suitable for renal replacement therapy (RRT), but in practice only about 70% of those suitable are given RRT. The remaining 30% die untreated.

In December 1990 the number of patients in the UK receiving treatment for ESRD by means of dialysis or transplantation was 18 300 (p. 810). Patients with the various forms of glomerulonephritis form the largest group receiving RRT, followed by those with tubulointerstitial diseases (including pyelonephritis) and diabetic nephropathy. The incidence of ESRD rises rapidly with age; its frequency is similar in males and females.

Urinary tract infection (UTI), though often not serious, is a considerable source of morbidity. It has been estimated that 1–2% of all general practice consultations are in relation to symptoms suggestive of UTI. Women are most frequently affected, and prevalence studies have shown symptoms of dysuria in as many as 21% of females aged between 20 and 65 years. Demonstrable infection has a prevalence of 4% amongst females between the ages of 16 and 45 years, rising to 10% between the ages of 55 and 64 years and 15% above 65 years of age.

For some renal diseases, there are marked racial and regional differences in incidence. For example, ESRD resulting solely from severe hypertension is much commoner in blacks than in whites. Renal amyloid is an uncommon cause of ESRD in Western Europe and the USA, but in Israel, with its large population of Sephardic Jews, familial Mediterranean fever leading to amyloidosis accounts for 7% of patients reaching ESRD. In some parts of the world, endemic parasitic infection may be associated with an unusually high incidence of certain types of renal or urinary disease. Examples are: East Africa, where immune complex glomerulonephritis with nephrotic syndrome due to chronic infection with *Plasmodium malariae* is common (accounting for up to 2%

of all hospital admissions); and Egypt and Sudan, where *Schistosoma haematobium* infection is associated with immune complex glomerulonephritis, obstructive uropathy and carcinoma of the bladder.

ANATOMY AND PHYSIOLOGY

THE KIDNEY AS AN ORGAN

In man, the kidneys are paired bean-shaped structures, measuring 10–12 cm in length, 5–6 cm in width and 3–4 cm in depth. The renal parenchyma consists of an outer cortex and inner medulla (Fig. 20.1A). The kidneys weigh about 150 g each, and are situated retroperitoneally on either side of the vertebral column, at the level of T12–L3, where they underlie the costovertebral angles posteriorly. The right kidney is about 1.5 cm lower than the left, and both move up and down about 3 cm during respiration. The functional unit of the kidney is the *nephron*. Each kidney contains about one million nephrons, each one made up of a glomerulus, a proximal

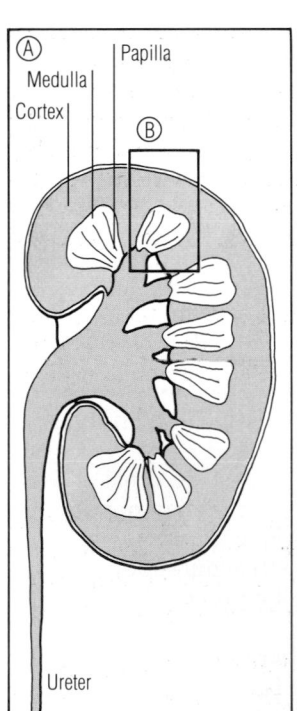
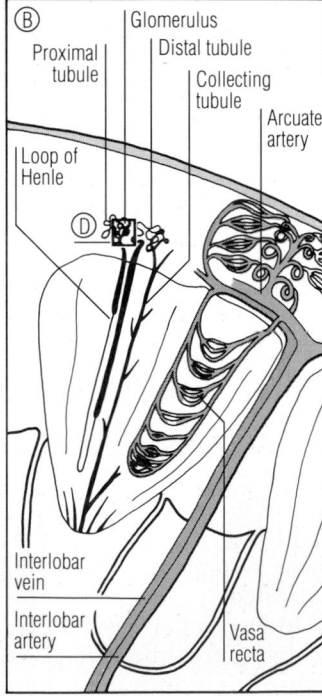
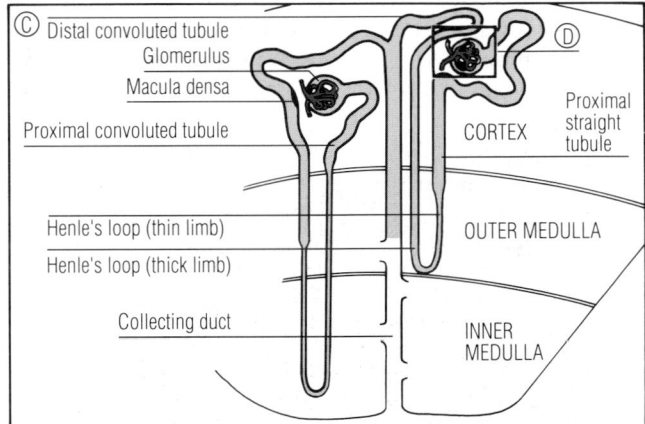
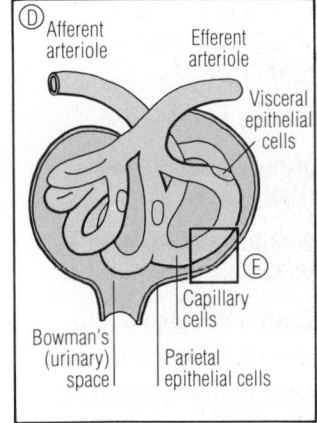
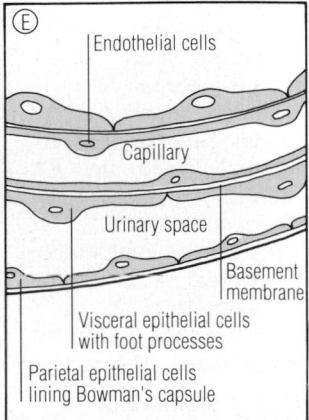

Fig. 20.1 Gross and microscopic anatomy of the kidney. A. Longitudinal section. **B.** Note that the loop of Henle dips deeply into the hypertonic medulla and, in the case of juxtamedullary nephrons (i.e. those with their glomeruli closest to the cortico-medullary junction area), the efferent arteriole is linked to the vasa recta, also dipping deeply into the medulla. **C.** A juxtamedullary nephron is shown on the left, and a cortical nephron on the right. **D.** and **E.** Microanatomy of the renal glomerulus.

tubule, a loop of Henle, a distal tubule and a collecting tubule (Fig. 20.1B).

Nerve supply. The renal capsule and ureters are innervated via the T10–T12 and L1 roots, and pain arising from the upper renal tract may be perceived over the corresponding dermatomes.

The blood supply is from the renal arteries, which may be single or multiple and which undergo a series of divisions within the kidney forming in succession *interlobar arteries* running radially as far as the corticomedullary junction, *arcuate arteries* running circumferentially along the corticomedullary junction and *interlobular arteries* running radially through the cortex towards the surface of the organ (Fig. 20.1B). *Afferent arterioles* arise from the interlobular arteries and supply the glomerular capillaries, which in turn drain into *efferent arterioles* (Fig. 20.2). The subsequent movement of blood depends on the location of the glomeruli within the kidney. Efferent arterioles from *outer cortical glomeruli* drain into a peritubular capillary network within the cortex, and thence into progressively larger and more proximal branches of the renal vein. In contrast, blood from *juxtamedullary glomeruli* passes into vasa recta in the medulla, where it maintains close proximity with the medullary portion of the tubules before turning back towards the area of cortex from which the vasa recta originated. The vasa recta have fenestrated walls which facilitate the movement of diffusable substances through the thin and thick limbs of Henle's loop.

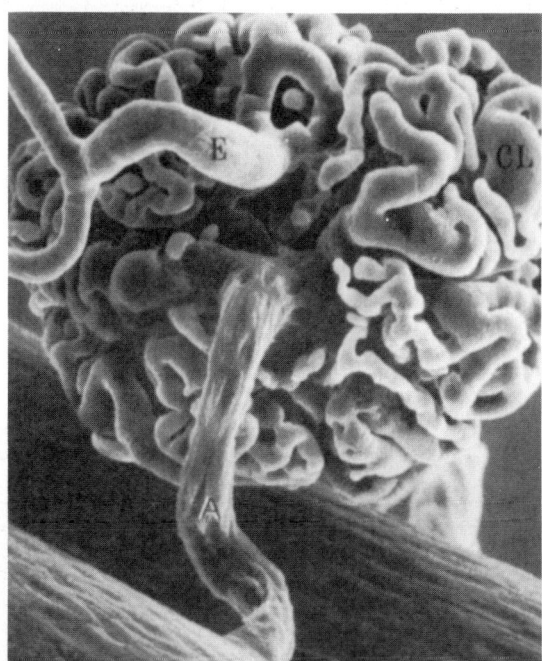

Fig. 20.2 Scanning electron micrograph of normal glomerulus. A, afferent arteriole; E, efferent arteriole; CL, capillary loop (one of many). (From: Brenner and Rector, The Liver, Vol 1, published by W B Saunders.)

Renal blood flow and glomerular filtration rate (GFR). Renal blood flow is high: about 25% of the resting cardiac output, or 1300 ml/min. This corresponds to a renal plasma flow of about 700 ml/min, of which 25% is ultrafiltered at the glomeruli, giving a GFR of 120 ml/min (180 l/day).

Collection of urine. The collecting tubules merge in the inner medulla to form the papillary ducts of Bellini, which in turn empty at the apices of the papillae into the calyces. The calyces are lined by a transitional cell epithelium which is continuous with that of the renal pelvis, ureters and bladder. Urine is passed to the bladder by active peristalsis in the ureters, pending intermittent discharge to the exterior by the process of micturition.

MICROANATOMY AND PHYSIOLOGY

The glomerulus

Each glomerulus consists of vascular and epithelial elements and is made up of three basic cell types:

- *Glomerular capillary endothelial cells.* These are unusual in that they are fenestrated with 500–1000 Å pores (Fig. 20.1E).
- *Epithelial cells.* These are designated parietal or visceral depending on their location (Fig. 20.1E).
- *Mesangial cells.* These specialised cells secrete the mesangial matrix of the glomeruli, and modify the filtration characteristics of the glomerulus, probably by the distribution of blood flow within the glomerulus. They are phagocytic, and are considered to be related to the macrophages of the reticuloendothelial system.

The basement membrane lies between the capillary endothelial and the visceral epithelial cells; this triad comprises the *glomerular sieve* across which glomerular filtration occurs.

The tubule

Throughout its length, the tubule is lined with epithelial cells which are cuboidal, except in the thin limb of Henle's loop where they are flat. A luminal brush border distinguishes the proximal tubular cells from those elsewhere in the tubule.

The anatomical arrangement of the different parts of the nephron and its blood supply is such that there is potential for events in a renal tubule to influence the behaviour of its own glomerulus. This phenomenon is called *tubuloglomerular feedback*. It is evident at the *macula densa*, where each distal tubule is in close proximity to the afferent arteriole of its own glomerulus, forming the *juxta-glomerular apparatus* (JGA) from which renin is released.

Although the nephrons differ in their anatomical location within the kidney and in their structure and function, each nephron is capable of undertaking most, if not all, of the functions of the complete organ. These functions are centred on the need for *selective* excretion in a *regulated* manner. Each nephron achieves this by producing a plasma ultrafiltrate and then modifying its composition to ensure reclamation of useful compounds and excretion of waste. These processes are conducted respectively in the glomerulus (formation of ultrafiltrate) and the tubules (modification of composition of the ultrafiltrate).

Formation of the glomerular filtrate

Hydrostatic, osmotic and electrostatic forces predominate in the formation of the glomerular filtrate (GF). The resistance to flow in the afferent and efferent arterioles is such that the hydrostatic pressure in the glomerular capillaries is much higher than in other capillary beds, approximating 40–60 mmHg. This favours the movement of water and other substances from the capillary lumen to the lower-pressure Bowman's space (Fig. 20.1D), and easily overcomes the opposing plasma osmotic pressure. Such movement requires passage across a functional 'sieve' which, as noted above, comprises the capillary endothelial cells, the visceral epithelial cells of Bowman's capsule and the basement membrane between them. The effective pore size in the sieve ensures that macromolecules are selectively retained within the capillaries, while water and other small and intermediate-sized molecules and ions pass through. Molecular charge is also important in determining movement across the sieve. The inner surface of the sieve is negatively charged and therefore repels anionic molecules such as albumin. The ease with which a substance will cross the glomerular sieve and so form a constituent of the GF thus depends on both its size and its charge. Plasma proteins are either too big (globulins) or both too big and unfavourably charged (albumin) to allow significant passage into the GF. However, immunoglobulin light chains (MW 22kD) normally appear in the urine.

Approximately 180 litres of GF are formed each day in an average man. As the composition of the GF is very close to that of plasma from which the macromolecules have been removed, the daily GF contains enormous amounts of low and middle molecular weight plasma constituents (in addition to water). Many, but not all, of these must be reclaimed from the GF if rapid depletion is to be avoided.

Modification of GF by tubular action

As the GF passes along the renal tubule, its composition is progressively altered by two simultaneous processes:

- *Tubular reabsorption,* i.e. the selective movement of substances from the tubular lumen prior to intrarenal catabolism or passage to the peritubular capillaries.
- *Tubular secretion,* i.e. the selective secretion of substances into the tubular lumen.

Both these processes may be passive or active and both change qualitatively and quantitatively along the length of the renal tubule. Important examples of tubular transport are given in Table 20.2 and an indication of their scale in quantitative terms in Table 20.3.

Selective filtration at the glomerulus, followed by tubular reabsorption and secretion, leads to the 'final urine'. Effective regulation of the processes of glomerular filtration, tubular reabsorption and tubular secretion ensures that the composition of the final urine is appropriate to the prevailing needs of the individual.

SPECIFIC HOMEOSTATIC FUNCTIONS

The specific homeostatic functions of the kidney are shown in Table 20.1.

Regulation of body water content

Body water, usually accounting for about 50% of adult body weight, is kept constant by a homeostatic system

Table 20.2 Tubular transport

Substance	Reabsorbed	Secreted
Water	Yes	No
Sodium	Yes	No
Potassium	Yes (proximally)	Yes (distally)
Calcium	Yes	No
Phosphate	Yes	No
Hydrogen ion	No	Yes
Bicarbonate	Yes	No
Glucose	Yes	No
Amino acids	Yes	No

Table 20.3 Quantitative aspects of tubular transport

Substance	Filtered load (per 24 hours)	Typical urinary excretion (per 24 hours)	% reabsorbed
Water	180 l	0.75–2.5 l	98.6–99.6
Sodium	25 000 mmol	100–250 mmol	99.0–99.6
Potassium	720 mmol	60–120 mmol	83.0–92.0
Calcium	234 mmol	5 mmol	98
Bicarbonate	4300 mmol	5 mmol	99.9
Glucose	810 mmol	1 mmol	99.9

(see also Ch. 21) in which both thirst and the renal handling of water are closely linked to the osmolality of the extracellular fluid (ECF). An increase in ECF osmolality is detected by osmoreceptors in the hypothalamus, stimulating both thirst and the release of ADH from the posterior pituitary. ADH activates an adenylate cyclase in the distal part of the nephron, increasing its permeability to water. Water then moves from the tubular lumen to the hyperosmolar medullary interstitium, the result being water conservation by the kidney (Fig. 20.3). In the absence of ADH, the distal nephron is relatively impermeable to water, and the reabsorption of Na^+ and Cl^- without water results in the formation of dilute urine.

In health, the kidney can adjust the rate of water excretion over an enormous range (0.5–25 l/day) in response to changing water intake and non-renal water losses. The lower limit is imposed by the need to excrete the daily load of 600–900 mosmol of solute (made up largely of urea and sodium chloride), and the inability of the kidney to increase urine concentration above 1200 mosmol/kg water. There is thus an obligatory water loss of 500–750 ml per day, the exact amount depending on dietary protein and sodium intake.

Abnormalities of body water content are described in Chapter 21.

Regulation of body sodium content

Body sodium content is governed by the balance between intake (from the diet) and output (mainly in the urine but also to a variable extent in sweat and faeces) (see Ch. 21). As with water, sodium ingestion varies widely, and the kidney is capable of modifying its handling of sodium in such a way as to maintain the constancy of body sodium (see Ch. 21, p. 843).

About 25 000 mmol of sodium is filtered at the glomeruli each day; to prevent overwhelming sodium depletion, the vast bulk of the filtered sodium must therefore be reabsorbed. To achieve a urinary sodium output of 100–250 mmol/day (the range typically seen in normal subjects eating a UK diet), 99% or more of the filtered sodium must be reabsorbed. When there is a need for extreme sodium conservation, as in subjects with a low sodium intake or who have become sodium-depleted as a result of non-renal sodium losses, tubular reabsorption can be increased further still, until a urinary sodium concentration as low as 1–2 mmol/l is reached.

Most (50–75%) of the filtered sodium is reabsorbed iso-osmotically with chloride and water in the proximal tubule, the remainder being reabsorbed in the ascending limb of Henle's loop and in the distal nephron (Fig. 20.3). The control of sodium reabsorption, and hence its excretion, is complex and incompletely understood, and is probably the result of a combination of hormonal (both systemic and local), neurogenic and vascular factors.

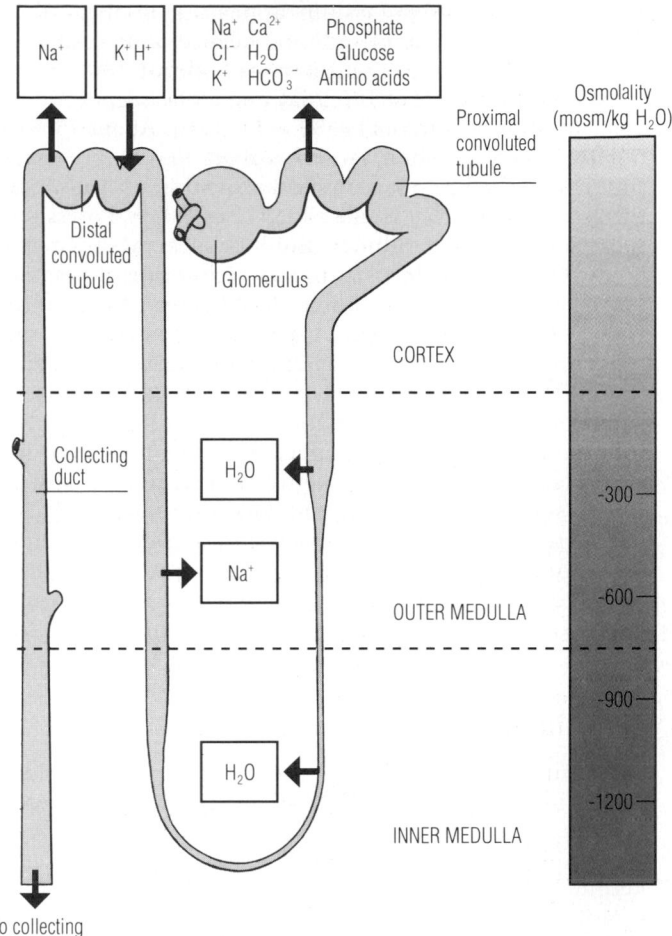

Fig. 20.3 Modification of the glomerular filtrate by tubular action.

Mineralocorticoids (predominantly aldosterone) are of great importance and act on the distal nephron to promote sodium reabsorption. These hormones are regulated in part by the activity of the renin-angiotensin system (itself influenced by the amount of sodium in the distal nephron in the vicinity of the macular densa) and in part by ACTH. Atrial natriuretic peptide (ANP) is stored in, and released from, the atria and promotes renal sodium excretion.

Regulation of body potassium content

As with sodium and water, the body content of potassium depends on the balance of intake (from the diet) and excretion, the latter being almost entirely renal. Potassium excretion by the kidney can also be varied over a wide range (approximately 10–700 mmol/day). Typical dietary intake (and thus urinary excretion rate) in the developed countries is about 60–120 mmol/day.

The amount of potassium appearing in the GF is much lower than that of sodium because of its relatively low concentration in blood plasma – about 720 mmol/day assuming a GFR of 180 l/day and a plasma potassium concentration of 4 mmol/l ($180 \times 4 = 720$). About 75% of the filtered potassium is reabsorbed in the proximal tubule and further potassium reabsorption occurs along the ascending limb of Henle's loop (Fig. 20.3). Potassium secretion into the tubular fluid occurs in the distal nephron, and it is here that the excretion rate of potassium is regulated by a combination of factors of which the action of mineralocorticoids, especially aldosterone, is the most important. Aldosterone increases potassium secretion in the distal nephron, but this effect is not entirely subjugated to the control of aldosterone by body sodium. Potassium itself also influences aldosterone secretion; high plasma potassium concentration stimulates aldosterone secretion by the adrenal cortex directly, and also indirectly by augmenting potassium-dependent renin secretion. By this mechanism, potassium excess thus tends to correct itself. Additional control of potassium excretion is exerted by the prevailing requirements for sodium excretion and acid–base status (Ch. 21).

Regulation of acid–base status

In quantitative terms, by far the most important acidic product of metabolism is CO_2, derived mainly from aerobic respiration, but also from the hepatic metabolism of lactic acid, and the oxidation of free fatty acids (FFA) and ketone bodies. An adult produces some 15 000–20 000 mmol of CO_2 per day, and virtually all of this is eliminated via the lungs. However, in addition to CO_2, the body produces a much smaller amount of non-volatile acid, some of which (amounting to 50–100 mmol/day or approximately 1 mmol/kg bodyweight per day) can only be excreted by the kidney. This is the result of the metabolism of cystine- and methionine-containing proteins and also of the incomplete oxidation of fat, carbohydrate and protein; all of these processes yield inorganic acids.

A helpful way to consider the role of the kidney in the maintenance of acid–base homeostasis (see Ch. 21) is in terms of balance. The kidney generates and releases into the circulation an amount of bicarbonate that precisely balances the net production of non-metabolisable, non-volatile acidic products of metabolism (i.e. 50–100 mmol of bicarbonate per day). To achieve this, a precisely equivalent amount of hydrogen ion (50–100 mmol/day) is excreted in the urine, the exact amount being regulated according to the prevailing production rate of non-volatile acids of metabolism.

The kidney achieves this balance in two ways (Fig. 20.4):

- proximal 'reclamation' of filtered bicarbonate
- urinary acidification in the distal nephron.

Proximal 'reclamation' of filtered bicarbonate. Bicarbonate ions in plasma are filtered at the glomerulus. The daily filtered load of bicarbonate is very large (about 4300 mmol/day) and, because its loss would rapidly lead to overwhelming bicarbonate depletion and acidosis, nearly all the filtered bicarbonate is reclaimed following titration in the tubular lumen by actively secreted H^+. The carbonic acid so formed is dehydrated to CO_2 and water (under the influence of brush border carbonic anhydrase). The CO_2 diffuses into the tubular cells and then combines with OH^- ions to form bicarbonate, before passing on to renal venous blood. Between 80% and 90% of the bicarbonate reclamation occurs in the proximal tubule.

Urinary acidification in the distal nephron. Reclamation of the 10–20% of the filtered bicarbonate load that reaches the distal tubule is also dependent on active secretion of H^+ ions. Additional H^+ secreted is trapped in the tubular lumen by two urinary buffers, ammonia (NH_3) and phosphate, although the role of ammonia as a urinary buffer is becoming controversial. It has been thought that ammonia (produced from the deamination of glutamine by the tubular cells), acts as a proton acceptor in the tubular lumen, being converted to ammonium (NH_4^+) and trapping secreted H^+ in the lumen. Monohydrogen phosphate (HPO_4^{2-}), derived from the GF, accepts H^+ forming dihydrogen phosphate ($H_2PO_4^-$). These mechanisms allow substantial amounts of acid to be excreted in the urine, while at the same time limiting the resulting decrease in urinary pH.

Certain features of this classical description of distal acidification mechanisms may soon require revision, however. It is now clear that most renal NH_4^+ production occurs in the proximal tubular cells, and that NH_4^+ is then transported to distal sites. The pK of ammonia is 9.4, indicating that, at physiological pH, nearly all the ammonia is present as NH_4^+. Thus, the ammonia produced from glutamine in the proximal tubular cells is immediately converted to NH_4^+. The tubular cell membranes are relatively impermeable to NH_4^+, but permeable to ammonia, and so NH_4^+ could only pass into the lumen by means of its equilibrium with ammonia (Fig. 20.4). Once in the tubular lumen, ammonia can accept H^+ and thereby act as a urinary buffer. However, the generation of ammonia in this way also leads to the production of an equivalent amount of H^+. Thus, although the mechanism allows the buffering of urinary H^+ by ammonia, it cannot directly influence overall acid–base status.

The regulation of acid secretion is extremely complex. From the foregoing account, it is apparent that changes in the filtered load of bicarbonate and/or its reabsorption, alteration of the distal secretion of hydrogen ion or of the availability of the urinary buffers, ammonia and HPO_4^{2-}, can singly or in combination affect the return of bicarbonate ions to the renal venous blood.

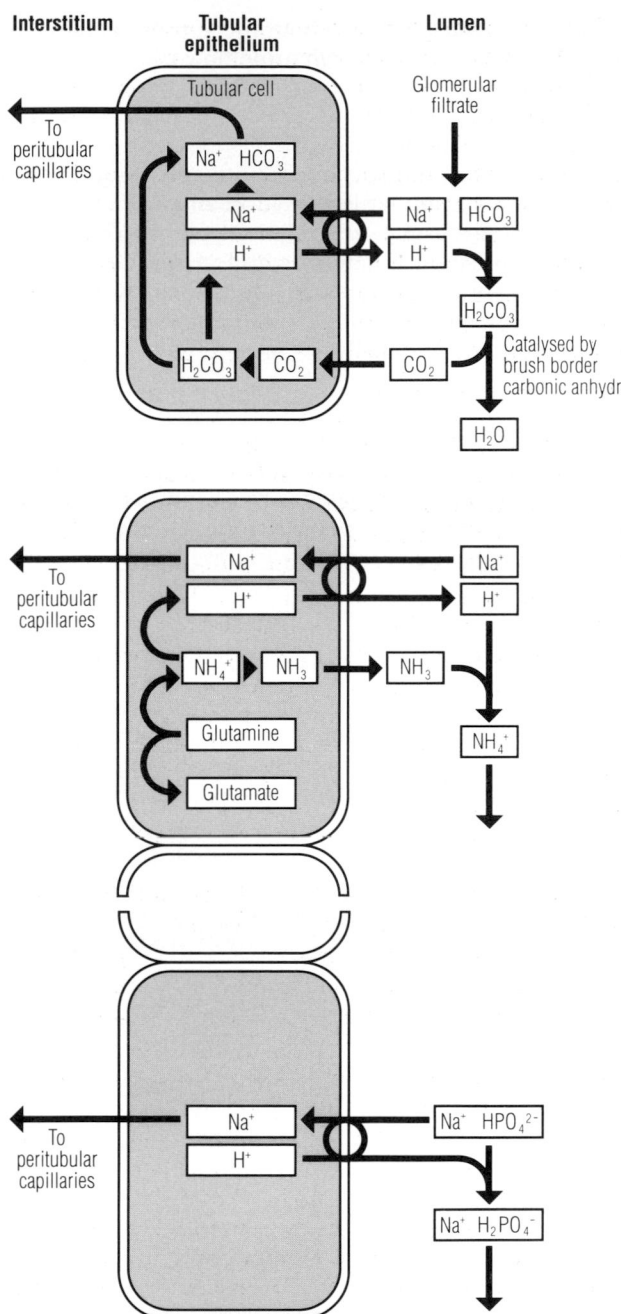

Interstitium **Tubular epithelium** **Lumen**

Tubular cell

To peritubular capillaries

Glomerular filtrate

Catalysed by brush border carbonic anhydrase

To peritubular capillaries

To peritubular capillaries

Fig. 20.4 Mechanisms of tubular action. Red = proximal tubular cell. Grey = distal tubular cells; the functions of the latter are separated for clarity.

Regulation of calcium and phosphorus metabolism

Calcium

Body calcium homeostasis (see Ch. 18) is dependent on:

- the movement of calcium between body fluids and the skeleton under the control of parathyroid hormone (PTH) and active metabolites of vitamin D
- the intestinal absorption of dietary calcium, also under the control of PTH (acting indirectly via the vitamin D endocrine system)
- the PTH-dependent regulation of the renal handling of calcium.

Ultrafiltrable calcium in blood plasma amounts to about 1.3 mmol/l of the 2.4 mmol/l of calcium normally present in plasma. This means about 230 mmol of calcium appears in the GF each day. Of this, 50–60% is reabsorbed in the proximal tubule and the remainder in the thick ascending limb of Henle's loop, the distal convoluted tubule and the collecting tubule. In health, the reabsorption is almost complete, only some 5 mmol of the initial 230 mmol of filtered calcium appearing in the urine per day. The most important controlling influence on urinary calcium excretion is PTH, which increases tubular calcium reabsorption. Additional effects are exerted by the level of sodium excretion and acid–base status (both natriuresis and acidosis increase calciuria). Increases in the filtered load of calcium, such as occur in hypercalcaemic states, also increase the urinary output of calcium.

Phosphate

Renal phosphate handling is the major determinant of ECF phosphate concentration. The 80% of plasma phosphate that is not protein bound is filtered at the glomerulus and 80–90% of this is then reabsorbed by tubular transport. The percentage of filtered phosphate that is reabsorbed can be varied over a wide range which, in health, is mainly in response to changes in dietary phosphate intake and PTH. The latter acts via cAMP to decrease tubular phosphate transport both in the proximal and distal nephron; PTH is thus a phosphaturic hormone.

THE ENDOCRINE FUNCTION OF THE KIDNEY

Hormone synthesis by the kidney. The hormones produced by the kidneys are listed in Table 20.4. They may act locally in the kidney or on remote target tissues. In the cases of 1,25-dihydroxyvitamin D, renin and erythropoietin, the kidney is the sole, or major site of production.

Hormone metabolism by the kidney. Polypeptide hormones (PTH, insulin), steroid and thyroid hormones are subject to varying degrees of renal catabolism, which may be altered in the presence of kidney disease.

Hormones with major renal actions. The kidney is a target organ for many hormones (Table 20.4), all acting

Table 20.4 Hormones and the kidney

Hormone	Synthesised in kidney	Action on kidney
1,25-dihydroxy-vitamin D	Yes	Increases tubular calcium reabsorption
Renin/angiotensin	Yes	Autoregulation and distribution of renal blood flow
Prostaglandins (PGE$_2$ and PGI$_2$)	Yes	Autoregulation and distribution of renal blood flow Increase renin release Influence water handling
Erythropoietin	Yes	None
Kallikrein	Yes	Autoregulation and distribution of renal blood flow Influences sodium and water handling
PTH	No	Increases phosphaturia Increases bicarbonaturia Increases tubular calcium reabsorption Increases synthesis of 1,25-dihydroxyvitamin D
Vasopressin	No	Increases antidiuresis
Aldosterone	No	Increases tubular Na$^+$ reabsorption Increases tubular K$^+$ and H$^+$ secretion
Catecholamines	No	Increase renin release
Atrial natriuretic peptide	No	Increases sodium/water excretion

to influence the kidney's performance of its various homeostatic functions.

ASSESSMENT OF RENAL STRUCTURE AND FUNCTION

Examination of the urine

Quantity

Most normal adults in temperate climates pass between 750 and 2500 ml of urine per day. *Anuria* is the complete absence of urine flow. *Oliguria* implies diminished urine flow and is present when the urine flow rate is less than the minimum required to allow excretion of the daily solute load (about 500 ml/day in an adult). *Polyuria* is a nebulous term, indicating passage of large volumes of urine, but implying nothing about the appropriateness (or otherwise) or cause of the high urine flow rate.

Specific gravity/osmolality

Measurements of the specific gravity and osmolality of the urine provide similar information and, in the absence of significant glycosuria, are functions of the urinary concentrations of sodium, chloride and urea. The range of specific gravity is 1.001–1.035 (equivalent to 50–1300 mosmol/kg water). Even heavy protein excretion alters these figures only minimally.

pH

Urinary pH varies from 4 to 8 and may be measured using paper strips impregnated with an indicator or, more accurately, by means of a pH electrode. Conditions associated with extremes of urinary pH are shown in Table 20.5.

Glucose

The use of glucose-oxidase-impregnated dipsticks provides a simple and specific semi-quantitative test for glucose in urine. The commonest cause of abnormal glycosuria is elevation of the plasma glucose concentration to above 8.3–10 mmol/l, at which point the tubular reabsorptive capacity for glucose is exceeded. In addition, a number of rare disorders of tubular function may be associated with glycosuria at normal plasma glucose concentrations; these disorders are collectively designated *renal glycosuria*.

Protein

Most people excrete less than 150 mg of protein per day in the urine and, with the exception of orthostatic proteinuria (see below), levels above this imply disease of the

Table 20.5 Conditions associated with extremes of urinary pH

Acid	Alkaline
High protein diet	Vegetarian diet
Acid ingestion (ascorbic acid, ammonium chloride)	Alkali ingestion (sodium bicarbonate, potassium citrate)
Metabolic acidosis	Infection with urea-splitting organisms
Respiratory acidosis (acute)	
Water deprivation	Metabolic alkalosis
Potassium depletion	Respiratory alkalosis (acute)
Hyperaldosteronism	Renal tubular acidosis (type I)
	Water diuresis

kidney or urinary tract. Semi-quantitative testing is done using dipsticks (sensitive to 200–300 mg protein per litre) or by the more cumbersome salicylsulphonic acid test (sensitive to 100–150 mg protein per litre). The latter has the advantage of detecting Bence-Jones protein (immunoglobulin light chains). Additional information may be obtained from quantitative measurement of the protein content of timed urine collections. Variation in the albumin excretion rate below the threshold for detection by dipsticks can now be followed using sensitive specific assays for urinary albumin. This is increasingly employed to detect very early glomerular damage. For example, in diabetics, urinary albumin excretion above the normal range (i.e. exceeding 30–40 mg/day) predicts the later development of clinical diabetic nephropathy.

The protein excretion rate is generally increased in the upright posture and, on occasion, this may lead to abnormally high protein measurements in timed collections or spot measurements in normal ambulant subjects. This is termed *orthostatic proteinuria* and the diagnostic difficulty may be resolved by demonstrating that an early morning urine specimen is normal while a specimen taken later in the day with the subject ambulant contains excess protein.

The diagnostic implications of abnormal protein excretion depend on both its *magnitude* (Table 20.6) and, to a lesser extent, its *selectivity*. Heavy proteinuria is always of glomerular origin, and albumin predominates over larger molecular weight protein such as globulins. In

highly selective proteinuria, only albumin is present in significant amounts, whereas, with non-selective proteinuria, the much larger globulins are present as well. Protein selectivity measurements are of little use in adults, but in children are helpful in predicting the nature and likely response to treatment of nephrotic syndrome (p. 811).

Blood

Blood in the urine may lead to a visible red or brown discolouration or smoky appearance when present in quantities exceeding 0.5 ml/l. Potentially confusing appearances may be seen in haemoglobinuria (as a consequence of haemoglobinaemia), porphyria, and dye or drug ingestion (e.g. beetroot, rifampicin). Smaller amounts of blood, insufficient to cause visible discolouration, may be detected by chemical tests for haemoglobin using dipsticks. A positive test for haemoglobin should always be followed by microscopic examination for red blood cells. This will distinguish haematuria from haemoglobinuria (in which no red cells will be seen). Careful assessment of red cell morphology using phase contrast microscopy may indicate whether they are derived from the renal parenchyma (dysmorphic red blood cells) or from the collecting system, ureters or bladder (normal red blood cells).

Culture

Although bladder urine should be sterile, voided urine is not and interpretation of bacteriological studies of the urine must take account of this. Contamination is minimised (though not eliminated) by use of the *midstream urine* (MSU) or *clean catch* technique, in which the initial part of the voided stream is discarded and the midportion of the stream collected in a sterile container. In the female, this should be preceded by cleaning of the external genitalia. The likelihood of significant infection is high if:

- a pure growth of a single organism is obtained (multiple organisms often indicate contamination)
- the number of bacteria exceeds 10^5/ml
- leucocytes are present in the spun deposit of fresh urine *(pyuria)*.

Deposit

The microscopic examination of a fresh unstained deposit of spun urine is an important part of the examination of any patient in whom disease of the urinary tract is suspected, especially if dipstick testing has shown blood or protein. A search is made for cells, casts and crystals (Table 20.7). Urinary casts consist of Tamm-Horsfall protein derived from the tubular epithelium, and are

Table 20.6 Diagnostic implications of proteinuria

Degree of proteinuria	Diagnostic implications
Mild (up to 500 mg/day)	Fever
	Benign hypertensive nephrosclerosis
	Renal tumour
	Obstructive nephropathy
	Prerenal uraemia
	Tubulointerstitial nephropathy
	Chronic pyelonephritis
	Orthostatic proteinuria
Moderate (up to 3 g/day)	Urinary tract infection
	Chronic pyelonephritis
	Acute tubular necrosis
	Acute glomerulonephritis
	Chronic glomerulonephritis
	Obstructive nephropathy
	Accelerated phase hypertension
	Orthostatic proteinuria
Heavy (more than 3 g/day)	Pre-eclampsia
	Myeloma
	Acute glomerulonephritis
	Chronic glomerulonephritis
	All causes of nephrotic syndrome

Table 20.7 The urinary sediment in various renal conditions

Condition	RBC	WBC	RBC casts	Granular casts	Hyaline casts
Acute glomerulonephritis	4	0–4	1–4	1–3	1–3
Chronic glomerulonephritis	1–3	0–1	0–2	1–3	1–3
'Minimal change' nephrotic syndrome	0–1	0	0	0–1	0–3
Acute tubular necrosis	1–3	1–3	0–2	1–3	1–3
Prerenal uraemia	0–1	0–1	0	0–1	0–2
Acute pyelonephritis	0–2	4	0	1–2	1–2
Chronic pyelonephritis	0–1	0	0	0–1	0–1
Benign hypertensive nephrosclerosis	0–1	0	0	0–1	0–1
Accelerated phase hypertension	1–4	0–1	0–2	0–2	0–2
Pre-eclampsia	0–1	0–1	0	0–1	0–3
Urinary tuberculosis	0–4	2–4	0	0–2	0–2
Tumour	0–4	0–1	0	0	0–1

The numbers 0–4 refer to the extent of the abnormality in each case. RBC, red blood cells; WBC, white blood cells.

Table 20.8 Characteristics of compounds used to measure GFR

Characteristic	Ideal marker	Inulin	Creatinine	Urea
Freely filtered at glomerulus	Yes	Yes	Yes	Yes
Tubular reabsorption	No	No	No	Yes (slight)
Tubular secretion	No	No	Yes (slight)	No
Ease of assay	Easy	Difficult	Easy	Easy
Endogenously produced	Yes	No	Yes	Yes*

* but variable rate

probably formed in the distal nephron. Hyaline casts contain no cellular elements or debris and may be seen in very small numbers in normal urine. Cellular casts, in which the Tamm-Horsfall matrix is studded with red or white blood cells are indicative of parenchymal renal disease. Granular casts are probably degenerate cellular casts and have a granular or grainy appearance. The number of cells and casts seen is usually expressed per high power field.

Measurement of GFR

The renal clearance of a substance is calculated from the formula:

$$\frac{UV}{P}$$

where U = urinary concentration, V = urine flow rate (usually expressed in ml/min) and P = plasma concentration. Calculation of GFR requires a test substance that is freely filtered at the glomerulus, but neither reabsorbed nor secreted by the tubules (Table 20.8). The polysaccharide, inulin, has ideal characteristics but the methodology is cumbersome, precluding its use in clinical practice. However, the renal handling of endogenously produced creatinine is similar to that of inulin and reliable estimates of GFR can generally be obtained from measurements of creatinine clearance. This requires only the measurement of plasma creatinine concentration in plasma and in a timed urine collection of known volume.

GFR can also be calculated simply from knowledge of the plasma creatinine concentrations and reference to 'normal values'. The formula for calculating creatinine clearance (UV/P) indicates that GFR is inversely related to plasma creatinine concentration (Fig. 20.5). Thus,

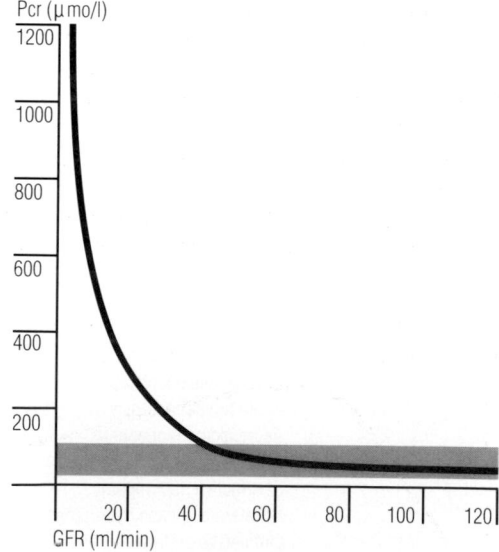

Fig. 20.5 Relationship between glomerular filtration rate (GFR) and plasma creatinine concentration (PCr). The normal range of PCr is shown hatched. At high levels of GFR, changes of GFR are associated with relatively small changes of PCr, which remains within the 'normal' range until GFR falls to about 45 ml/minute. At low levels of renal function, PCr becomes a much more sensitive indicator of GFR.

assuming a constant production rate of creatinine, a halving of GFR will lead to a doubling of plasma creatinine concentration, a fourfold decrease in GFR to a fourfold increase in plasma creatinine concentration, and so on. This method is very useful for monitoring *changes* in GFR in the same subject, but substantial individual variations in muscle bulk (and hence creatinine production rate) necessitate the inclusion of several correction factors before reasonably accurate GFR estimates can be made. Nevertheless, plasma creatinine measurement is one of the most frequently performed and useful tests of renal function.

Similar measurements can be made using urea instead of creatinine, but these are much less informative owing to wide fluctuations in urea production rate and substantial and variable tubular reabsorption of urea (Table 20.8).

Radionuclide methods

The GFR can be measured by injecting a radioactive substance that is handled by the kidney in the same way as inulin and then following its disappearance from plasma. ^{51}Cr-EDTA is a suitable radiopharmaceutical, and allows easy and reproducible calculation of GFR.

Range of GFR and effect of ageing

The GFR in a normal adult is about 120 ml/minute (Fig. 20.6). In children over 2 years of age, GFR is closely related to body surface area and should be expressed in relation to this. GFR peaks between the ages of 20 and 30 years, subsequently decreasing by 1 ml/minute per year, this decrease being paralleled by the slow decrease in muscle mass commensurate with ageing, such that plasma creatinine concentration changes little with advancing age. Appreciation of these age-related changes in GFR is important in clinical practice, particularly when considering dose modification of drugs prescribed to the elderly.

Measurement of renal plasma flow

The estimation of renal plasma flow requires a test substance that is both filtered at the glomerulus and rapidly secreted by the tubules such that none reaches renal venous blood. Para-aminohippuric acid has the required characteristics, but this measurement is almost never required in clinical practice; it remains important as a research tool, however.

Imaging of the kidney and urinary tract

Plain radiographs

In many people, one or both kidneys may be visible on plain abdominal radiographs or plain nephrotomograms, giving information about the presence, location, size and shape of the kidneys, as well as revealing certain types of renal stone or other calcifications.

Intravenous urography (IVU)

The injection of organic iodine compounds that are excreted by the kidneys opacifies first the renal parenchyma (nephrogram), and later the collecting system (pyelogram), ureters and bladder. As well as providing important structural information, the IVU also demonstrates the presence or absence of excretory function (Fig. 20.7). The quality of images may be poor if excretion is slow, as in severe renal disease, but can be enhanced by the administration of large doses of contrast medium and nephrotomography. Although the IVU is commonly employed and is often very useful, it carries a mortality of about 1 in 40 000 studies, with a substantial incidence of non-fatal adverse reactions to the injected contrast medium.

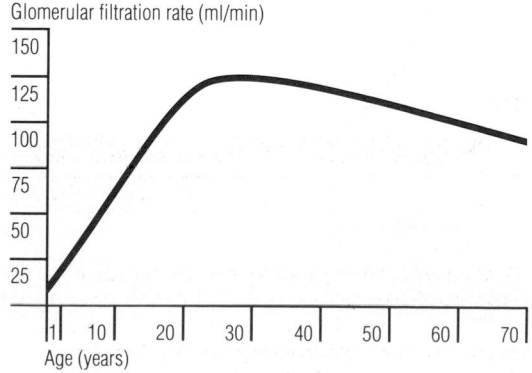

Fig. 20.6 Changes in glomerular filtration rate with age.

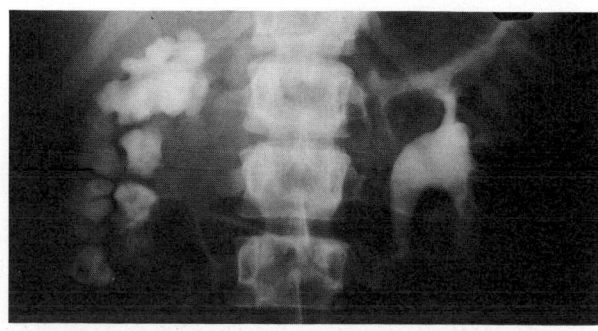

Fig. 20.7 Intravenous urogram showing obstructed right kidney. The IVU shows normal morphology on the left and dilation of the pelvicalyceal system on the right, due to pelviureteric junction obstruction.

Antegrade and retrograde urography

The morphology of the collecting system and ureters may not be demonstrated adequately by IVU if excretory function is poor. The direct introduction of contrast medium into the kidney (antegrade pyelography) or lower ureter during cystoscopy (retrograde pyelography) may yield further information if these invasive procedures are deemed appropriate (Fig. 20.8). Such investigations are most commonly used in the detailed assessment of patients with obstruction of the urinary tract.

Cystography

In cystography, the bladder is filled with contrast medium via the urethra and radiographs taken before, during and after micturition, usually to see whether urine refluxes up the ureters. The investigation is invasive, carrying the risk of introducing infection. It is usually performed in children with urinary infections in whom reflux nephropathy is suspected.

Ultrasonography

Ultrasonography allows totally non-invasive evaluation of gross renal morphology and visualisation of adjacent tissues (Fig. 20.9). It is useful in the diagnosis of cystic diseases of the kidney, renal tumours and renal obstruction. Unlike the IVU, renal ultrasound does not depend on the presence of excretory function, and so non-functioning

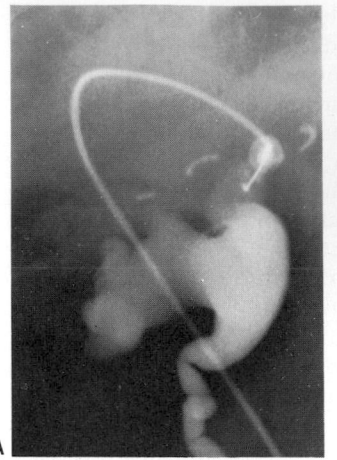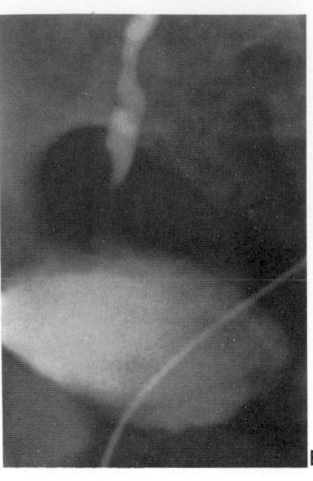

Fig. 20.8 Antegrade pyelograms showing obstruction of the right kidney due to a stricture in the lower part of the ureter. Contrast medium has been introduced directly into the dilated collecting system of the kidney via a percutaneously inserted catheter **(A)**. The obstruction is shown in the lower ureter in **B**.

kidneys can be seen just as well as functioning ones. On the other hand, ultrasonography yields no information on the relative function of the kidneys.

Computed tomography

Computed tomography (CT) gives detailed structural information about the kidneys and surrounding

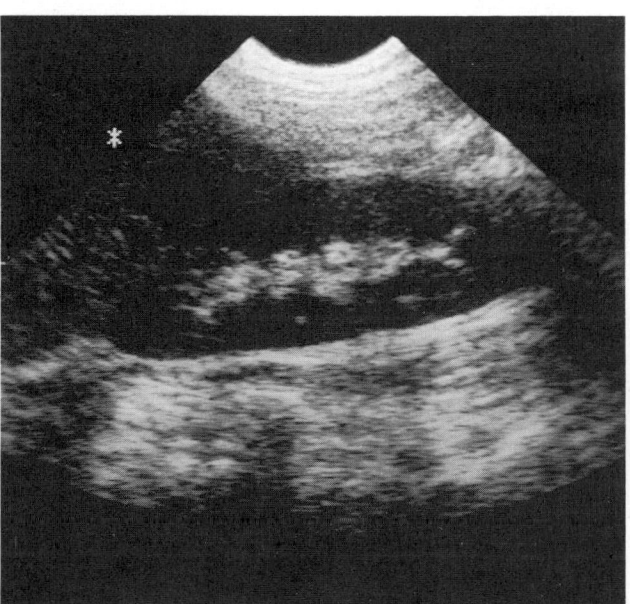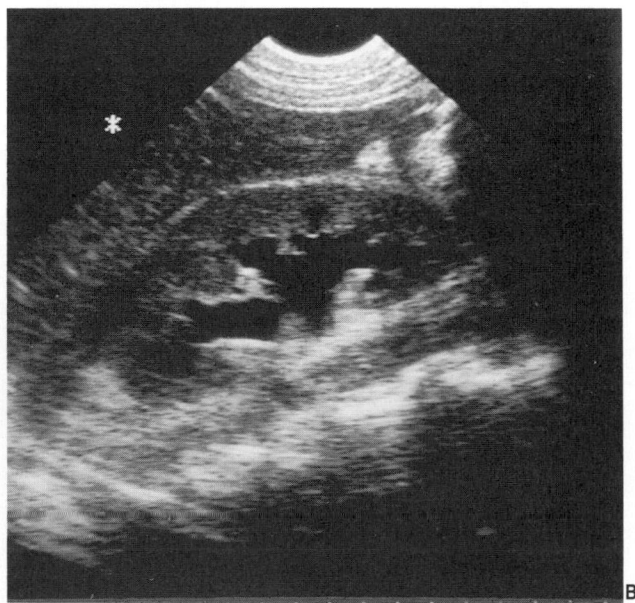

Fig. 20.9 Renal ultrasound examinations. A. Longitudinal scan of a normal kidney. The characteristic renal outline can be seen with the echogenic centre area representing the normal pelvicalyceal system and its associated fat. The surrounding elliptical renal parenchyma produces low level echoes and appears much darker. **B.** A dilated and obstructed collecting system. The large echo-free (i.e. black) renal pelvis and widened upper ureter can be seen in the centre of the picture.

tissues, the ureters and bladder. It is particularly useful in assessment of the retroperitoneum in cases of obstruction.

Arteriography and venography

The arterial and venous vasculature of the kidneys can be seen following direct injection of contrast medium into the renal artery or vein respectively (Fig. 20.10). These procedures are invasive and are used when compromise of the renal blood supply, leading to hypertension or impairment of renal function, is suspected. Pathological circulation to a renal tumour can be demonstrated in this way, although the advent of good quality ultrasonography and CT has made most arteriography redundant, except when the tumour is to be embolised. Venography is performed in cases where ultrasonography and/or CT have failed adequately to exclude renal vein thrombosis.

Radionuclide studies

Radionuclide studies allow both structure and functions to be evaluated and have the advantage of low associated radiation exposure compared with IVU. ^{99}Tc-DMSA (dimercaptosuccinic acid) is used to show gross renal morphology and either ^{99}Tc-DTPA (diethylenetriamine penta-acetic acid) or ^{131}I hippuran renograms to investigate function. In isotope renography, simultaneous counting over both kidneys is done and analysis of the resulting renograms (Fig. 20.11) may indicate the relative contribution of the two kidneys to total function (divided renal function), delay in perfusion (suggestive of renal vascular disease), or a progressive increase in activity with time (suggestive of obstruction).

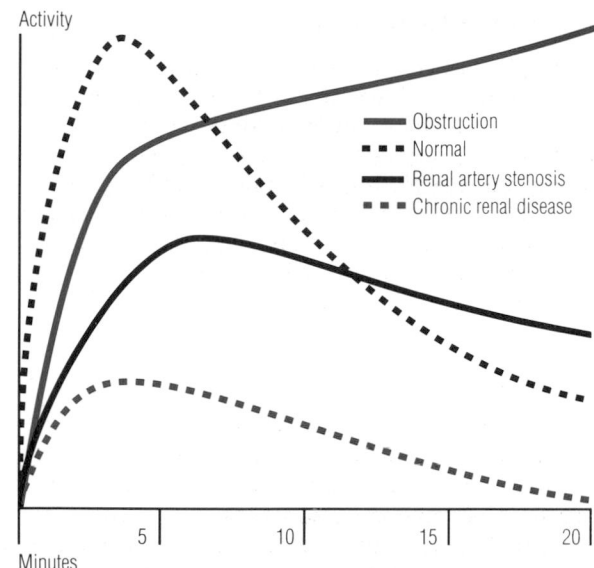

Fig. 20.11 **DTPA isotope renograms typical of various conditions.** In obstruction, the increase in activity up to 20 minutes results from the progressive accumulation of isotope within the obstructed collecting system. In renal artery stenosis, arrival of the bolus of isotope is delayed, leading to a delayed peak and subsequently slow clearance. In chronic renal parenchymal disease, arrival of the bolus is not delayed compared with normal, but is of much reduced intensity, reflecting low renal blood flow and low GFR.

Renal biopsy

The kidneys may be biopsied with relative safety using a cutting biopsy needle passed into the kidney through the renal angle under local anaesthetic. Preconditions that should be satisfied before biopsy is undertaken are:

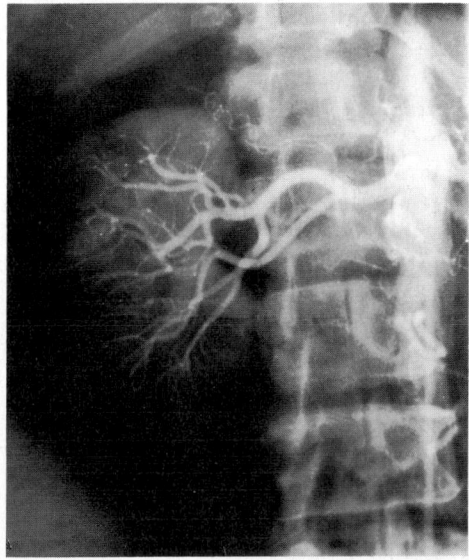

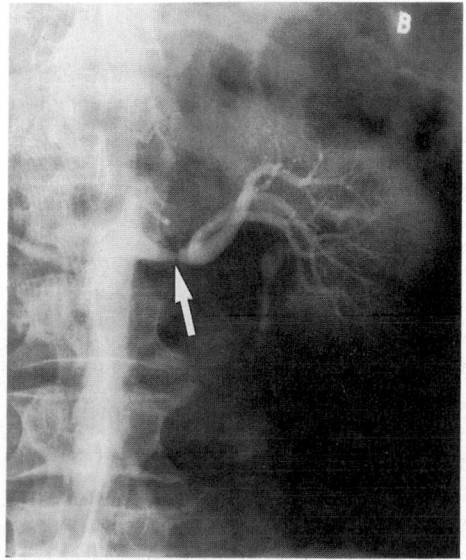

Fig. 20.10 **Renal arteriograms.**
A. Normal right kidney. **B.** Left renal artery stenosis.

Table 20.9 Usefulness of renal biopsy

Often helpful
Acute renal failure of uncertain cause
Rapidly progressive renal disease (especially if crescentic nephritis suspected)
Collagen disease, e.g. SLE, polyarteritis
Renal haematuria (cause unclear)
Proteinuria (cause unclear)
Nephrotic syndrome
Transplant assessment
Suspected amyloid

Sometimes helpful
Slowly progressive renal disease (with kidneys of normal size)
Diabetic nephropathy

Not indicated
Suspected renal infection
End-stage renal disease, especially if kidneys are small
Renal cystic disease

- an appropriate indication (Table 20.9)
- a cooperative patient
- absence of bleeding disorder
- prompt availability of blood for transfusion in the event of haemorrhage
- prior knowledge of the position, size and function of both kidneys. A solitary functioning kidney should rarely be biopsied.

The procedure is carried out with the patient lying prone and may be aided by simultaneous ultrasound localisation of kidney and biopsy needle. One or two small samples of renal cortex are taken, each containing 10–50 glomeruli, and used for light microscopy, electron microscopy and immunoperoxidase studies, allowing the presence and distribution of fibrin, complement, IgG, IgA and IgM to be defined.

The safety of renal biopsy is difficult to determine. Mortality appears to be well below 0.1% and serious morbidity, e.g. bleeding necessitating nephrectomy, occurs in about 0.1–0.2% of cases. Minor morbidity, such as significant pain or bleeding requiring transfusion, may arise in about 2% of cases.

MAJOR SYMPTOMS AND SIGNS OF RENAL AND URINARY DISEASE

The symptoms and signs associated with renal and urinary disease are diverse and often non-specific. In many patients, these features may remain subtle and nebulous, even when renal impairment is moderately severe, and this may lead to the patient seeking medical advice late in the course of the disease.

Haematuria

Haematuria may be macroscopic or microscopic, painful or painless, continuous or intermittent, persist throughout the act of micturition or be present only at the beginning or end of micturition. Haematuria due to renal parenchymal disease is usually continuous, painless and microscopic, although it may on occasion be macroscopic or intermittent. In contrast, haematuria arising from renal tumours is usually intermittent and painless and that from bladder tumours may be intermittent and sometimes painful.

Summary 1 Symptoms and signs of renal and urinary tract disease

- Uraemia
- Renal pain
- Oliguria/anuria

- Polyuria
- Frequency
- Nocturia
- Dysuria
- Incontinence

- Haematuria
  Macroscopic
  Microscopic
- Proteinuria
  Asymptomatic
  Symptomatic (nephrotic syndrome)
- Hypertension
- Oedema
  Peripheral
  Pulmonary

Proteinuria

Protein does not discolour the urine, and is therefore usually noticed as a result of routine urine examination, following the development of associated symptoms of renal disease or, in the case of heavy proteinuria, the development of the nephrotic syndrome (p. 811).

Hypertension

Hypertension is much commoner in people with renal disease than in those without. As many as 80% of patients with abnormal renal function, or who are receiving RRT by dialysis, will have experienced significant (and in many cases severe) hypertension at some stage during their illness. Conversely, there are occasions when severe hypertension may, by leading to vascular changes within the kidney, be the cause of renal disease (p. 828).

Oedema

Renal disease may give rise to oedema either as a consequence of inappropriate retention of sodium and water, leading to overexpansion of the ECF, or by reduction in

Table 20.10 Symptoms and signs of uraemic syndrome

Nervous system
Fatigue, malaise, depression, impaired thought, involuntary movements, nausea, fits, coma, pruritus, paraesthesiae, neuropathy

Cardiopulmonary
Pericarditis, pleurisy, Kussmaul breathing, dyspnoea

Dermatological
Pruritus, purpura, pallor, pigmentation, urea frost

Gastrointestinal
Anorexia, nausea, vomiting, GI bleeding, constipation, diarrhoea, peptic ulceration, angiodysplasia, colitis, foetor

Haematological
Anaemia (normochromic, normocytic), bleeding (disordered platelet function)

plasma oncotic pressure as a result of heavy urinary protein losses (nephrotic syndrome, see p. 811). In some cases, both these mechanisms are operative. Overexpansion of the ECF (in the absence of severe hypoalbuminaemia) may be accompanied by hypertension and expansion of the vascular compartment to the point where pulmonary oedema develops. This is particularly likely to occur in subjects with diminished cardiac reserve.

Uraemia

The *uraemic syndrome* is a group of symptoms and signs (Table 20.10), some or all of which are found in patients with serious reduction of excretory capacity (i.e. of GFR), from any cause. The uraemic syndrome rarely manifests itself clinically until the GFR has fallen to 20% of normal or less. The pathogenesis and management of the uraemic syndrome is discussed on pages 804–811.

Renal pain

Renal pain is usually felt in the loin or flank, although in the case of ureteric obstruction leading to renal pain, discomfort may be felt in the iliac fossa, testicle or labia, depending partly on the level of the obstruction. The commonest, and most spectacular, cause of renal pain is acute obstruction by a stone; this is of fairly rapid onset

Table 20.11 Causes of renal pain

Obstructive	Non-obstructive
Stone (kidney, ureter)	Renal swelling ± inflammation
Tumour	Acute pyelonephritis
Sloughed papilla	Renal vein thrombosis
Blood clot	Renal cysts
Pelviureteric obstruction	Renal tumour
	Acute nephritis (rare)
	Renal infarction
	Trauma

and great severity. Other causes of renal pain are listed in Table 20.11.

Oliguria/anuria

Oliguria is the passage of less than 500 ml of urine/day; anuria means cessation of urine flow. The causes may conveniently be divided into:

- *prerenal*, where primary decrease in renal blood flow leads to compromise of function in an otherwise normal kidney
- *renal*, i.e. intrinsic renal disease of any type
- *postrenal*, due to mechanical obstruction, which may be at any point from the collecting system in the kidney to the urethra. Acute obstruction to bladder outflow only results in impairment of renal function when the maximum bladder capacity is reached.

In general, the causes of anuria and oliguria are the same as those of acute renal failure (Table 20.15).

Polyuria

The causes of polyuria (increased urine flow) rate fall into three groups (Table 20.12). In some patients with diabetes insipidus, polyuria may be spectacular with daily urine output as great as 25 litres.

Frequency

Frequency of micturition results from polyuria or decreased functional bladder capacity (Table 20.13).

Nocturia

The absence of nocturia depends on the normal reduction in urine flow rate during the night and an adequate functional bladder capacity. Polyuria of any cause may thus result in nocturia, as may acute and chronic renal diseases, certain drugs such as corticosteroids and diuretics, and ingestion of large volumes of fluid late in the

Table 20.12 Causes of polyuria

Excessive water intake	Abnormal tubular water handling
Psychogenic polydipsia	Pituitary diabetes insipidus
Beer drinking	
Osmotic diuresis	Inherited nephrogenic diabetes insipidus (rare)
Diabetes mellitus (glucose)*	
Chronic renal failure (urea)*	Acquired nephrogenic diabetes insipidus
Diuretics (NaCl)*	Hypokalaemia
	Hypercalcaemia
	Obstructive uropathy
	Tubulointerstitial diseases

* The respective osmotic diuretics are given in parentheses.

Table 20.13 Causes of frequency and nocturia

Cause	Example
Infection*	Cystitis/urethritis/prostatitis Bacterial, including tuberculosis Fungal Parasitic (schistosomiasis)
Neoplasia*	Bladder tumour
Anatomical	Prostatic hypertrophy Urethral stricture
Neurological	Multiple sclerosis

* Often associated with dysuria also.

day; all of these, in one way or another, interfere with the normal diurnal variation in urine flow rate.

Reduction of functional bladder capacity due to local (e.g. infection, contracted bladder, outflow obstruction, tumour) or remote factors (e.g. neurological diseases) will also result in nocturia, in this case not associated with polyuria.

Dysuria

Dysuria is pain immediately before, during or immediately after micturition. The discomfort is often perceived as a 'burning' or 'scalding' sensation from the urine, and may be associated with frequency, decreased functional bladder capacity, urgency or hesitancy of micturition. Infection and neoplasia are the main causes; these and other causes of dysuria may also be associated with frequency.

Urgency of micturition, incontinence and enuresis

Urgency is the inability to postpone micturition significantly beyond the moment when the desire to micturate is first perceived. It may lead to *urge incontinence* if the patient cannot get to an appropriate place to void quickly enough.

Incontinence is the involuntary passage of urine and may result from disorders of the bladder, its nerve supply or within the CNS (see also p. 839). Incontinence occurring exclusively at night is termed *enuresis* and may be primary (failure to attain nocturnal bladder control in childhood) or secondary (development of enuresis following previous nocturnal continence). The above conditions are discussed further on page 838.

MAJOR RENAL SYNDROMES

Patients presenting with renal disease usually present with one of the renal syndromes discussed below (listed in Summary 2) and categorization by syndrome is an essential first step towards making a definitive diagnosis.

Summary 2 Major renal syndromes

- Acute renal failure (including acute tubular necrosis)
- Acute nephritic syndrome
- Rapidly progressive glomerulonephritis
- Chronic renal failure
- Nephrotic syndrome
- Recurrent gross haematuria
- Persistent, asymptomatic proteinuria and/or microscopic haematuria
- Renal tubular syndromes.

ACUTE RENAL FAILURE

Acute renal failure (ARF) is the rapid deterioration of renal function over a period of hours or days. Although oliguria and anuria are frequent accompaniments, this need not be the case; the cardinal index is a rapid decline in GFR, leading to nitrogen retention. This may arise de novo, or against a background of pre-existing stable chronic renal impairment (Table 20.14); distinguishing between these two possibilities is an important part of the diagnostic process.

The causes of ARF may be *prerenal, renal* and *postrenal*, and it is helpful to bear these categories in mind when assessing a patient with apparent ARF (Table 20.15).

Prerenal ARF

Prerenal ARF is associated with a low cardiac output (of any cause), intense renal vasoconstriction and reduced GFR with resulting oliguria, and avid salt and water retention. *The kidney is structurally normal but functionally compromised.* Removal of prerenal factors leads to rapid and complete recovery of renal function. The necessary measures may include correction of hypovolaemia with blood or saline, treatment of sepsis or improvement of cardiac function (if possible). If severe and/or prolonged, renal vasoconstriction may be severe enough to lead to ischaemic renal injury (*acute tubular necrosis*, ATN). Thus

Table 20.14 Diagnostic features distinguishing between acute and chronic renal failure

Favour acute	Favour chronic
Known recent onset	History of nocturia
Known precipitating factor(s)	Pigmentation
Near normal haematology	Small kidneys
Normal size kidneys (ultrasound, plain X-rays, IVU)	Bone disease (radiographic or biochemical)
	Normochromic anaemia

Table 20.15 Causes of acute renal failure

Prenal

Any cause of shock
Hypovolaemia:	haemorrhage, burns, salt and water depletion, perforated viscus, pancreatitis, postoperative (especially aortic, cardiac and biliary surgery)

Sepsis
Cardiogenic

Renal arterial or venous disease: renal artery stenosis, renal vein thrombosis

Inappropriate renal vasoconstriction, e.g. hepatorenal syndrome

Renal

Acute tubular necrosis following hypovolaemia or shock of any cause

Acute glomerulonephritis

Acute glomerulonephritis with multisystem disease, e.g. SLE, Henoch-Schönlein purpura, infective endocarditis

Disease of small/medium sized blood vessels, e.g. haemolytic uraemic syndrome, thrombocytopenic purpura, disseminated intravascular coagulation, polyarteritis vasculitis, systemic sclerosis, accelerated phase hypertension

Acute tubulointerstitial disease

Exogenous nephrotoxins, e.g. drugs, ethylene glycol, heavy metals, X-ray contrast media

Endogenous nephrotoxins, e.g. myoglobin, haemoglobin, bilirubin, uric acid, Bence-Jones protein

Postrenal

Any cause of obstruction
  Stone (bilateral or affecting solitary kidney)
  Ureteric obstruction by pelvic malignancy (cervix, bladder, prostate, rectum)
  Bladder outflow obstruction
  Retroperitoneal disease (lymphoma, aortic dissection, retroperitoneal fibrosis)

the identification and rapid correction of prerenal factors is of paramount importance in the management of these patients. An intractable type of prerenal ARF – the *hepatorenal syndrome* – is sometimes seen in patients with severe liver disease. The nature of the interaction between the liver and kidney is obscure. Renal recovery is unusual in the absence of hepatic recovery.

Renal ARF

In renal ARF, there are established structural abnormalities in the kidney. In some cases (e.g. postinfectious glomerulonephritis, acute tubulointerstitial nephropathy), the disease process may primarily involve the kidney with little evidence of disease elsewhere. Alternatively, there may be evidence of multisystem disease such as systemic lupus erythematosus, infective endocarditis, polyarteritis nodosa, Henoch-Schönlein purpura, or of nephrotoxic exposure.

The coexistence of any of the prerenal factors (given in Table 20.15) raises the possibility of established ATN,

and these factors should always be corrected as far as possible in the hope that progression from prerenal ARF to ATN may be averted. The distinction between established ATN and prerenal ARF in an oliguric patient is an important one; fortunately, it is generally straightforward. It may be made on the basis of one or more of the features listed in Table 20.16. Renal hypoperfusion is the commonest cause of ATN, although in some cases the lesion appears to develop as a result of a combined insult due to hypoperfusion and exposure to a nephrotoxin (Table 20.15). The renal vasoconstriction may be very severe and in many cases seems out of proportion to accompanying increases in systemic vascular resistance. Prevention of this 'inappropriately' severe renal vasoconstriction is a frequent therapeutic goal, but is difficult to achieve other than by avoiding or rapidly correcting shock states. The renal lesion is tubular necrosis with subsequent regeneration. The glomeruli are relatively spared. The process of repair may last from a few days to several weeks and generally leads eventually to complete or near complete recovery of renal function. If the ischaemic damage is very severe, however, varying degrees of cortical necrosis may occur and recovery of function is then limited or negligible. For reasons not fully understood, cortical necrosis is particularly likely to occur in relation to shock occurring during pregnancy, such as may arise following ante-partum haemorrhage.

Postrenal ARF

Important causes of postrenal ARF are given in Table 20.15. ARF will only develop if the obstruction is bilateral, or if it affects a solitary functioning kidney. Thus,

Table 20.16 Distinction between prerenal and renal causes of acute renal failure in an oliguric patient

Feature	Favours prerenal cause	Favours renal cause
Identifiable prerenal factor, e.g. shock, hypovolaemia	Yes	No
Urine		
Protein	0–1	1–4
Red blood cells	0	1–3
White blood cells	0	1–3
Casts	0–1	1–3
Osmolality (mosmol/kg/H_2O)	>500	<400
Sodium (mmol/l)	<20	>35
Urine/plasma urea ratio	>8	<3
Urine/plasma creatinine ratio	>40	<20
Fractional excretion of sodium*	<1%	>1%

* Fractional excretion of sodium is the percentage of the total filtered load of sodium that appears in the final urine (Table 20.3). The numbers 0–4 indicate the degree of urinary abnormality.

obstruction of one ureter by a stone does not lead to ARF, whereas obstruction of both ureters by pelvic malignancy does. Early identification of postrenal factors in a patient with ARF is most important if therapy is to be appropriately directed and irreversible obstructive injury to the kidneys averted. Assessment may be aided by prior knowledge of the presence of one of the potentially obstructing lesions. Physical examination may reveal a pelvic mass or enlarged kidneys or bladder. Ultrasound examination of the kidneys is valuable, both to give a positive diagnosis of obstruction, and to exclude obstruction as a likely factor in patients with ARF. In some cases, IVU may be undertaken, but the pictures can be equivocal and delayed films (up to 24 hours following the injection) may be needed. Invasive imaging of the urinary tract by antegrade or retrograde ureterography is rarely needed to make the diagnosis, but may, along with cystoscopy, be of help in the detailed assessment of the obstructed patient.

Management

Prerenal ARF will, by definition, respond promptly to correction of the prerenal factor(s).

Renal ARF may be of a type in which resolution usually occurs within days or weeks (e.g. ATN, postinfectious glomerulonephritis (GN), some toxic nephropathies), or it may lead to irreversible renal failure (e.g. renal infarction, some types of acute GN and renal vasculitis). In some cases (e.g. renal vasculitis), resolution of the renal lesion may follow therapy with steroids, cytotoxic drugs or plasma exchange.

Postrenal ARF is treated by relief of the obstruction, usually by mechanical means (e.g. insertion of ureteric stent, percutaneous nephrostomy, removal of stone) pending further assessment of the feasibility of definitive relief of the obstructing lesion. In a few patients, nonmechanical measures, such as radiotherapy, antitumour chemotherapy or steroids, may obviate the need for mechanical relief of obstruction.

Regardless of the underlying cause, any patient with prolonged ARF will require energetic supportive measures. These may be conservative, or involve the use of dialysis.

Conservative

Fluid intake

Fluid intake must be adjusted to ensure that the patient is neither hypovolaemic nor overloaded. *Euvolaemia* is the objective, and careful clinical assessment of volume status is of the utmost importance (p. 843). The volume of fluid given will depend initially on the patient's state of hydration at presentation. If overloaded, the patient

must be fluid-restricted to the lowest attainable level; conversely, hypovolaemia must be corrected promptly by oral or intravenous fluids. Maintenance of euvolaemia requires repeated clinical assessment of volume status, monitoring of external fluid losses, both measured (urine, faeces, nasogastric tube, fistula, etc.) and unmeasured (sweat, respiration), daily weighing (aiming to keep body weight near constant), and appropriate replacement.

Sodium intake

The hypovolaemic patient will require volume replacement with normal saline until euvolaemia is reached; sodium intake must then be adjusted to balance sodium losses. These may be very small (<30 mmol/day) in an oliguric, afebrile patient, or very large (e.g. from the gastrointestinal tract). The external losses of sodium should be quantitated by measurement of the sodium concentration and volume of the fluid, although in many cases knowledge of the source of fluid allows a reasonable estimate of its likely sodium concentration (p. 847). Sodium intake is then adjusted to match the total sodium loss.

Potassium intake

Potassium intake usually has to be reduced in an oliguric patient, typically to 30–40 mmol/day or less. The adequacy of potassium restriction may be monitored by serial measurements of plasma potassium concentration. Frequently, potassium restriction alone is insufficient to prevent hyperkalaemia; this progresses as a result of loss of potassium from the ICF due to accelerated tissue catabolism, and also by movement of potassium from the ICF to the ECF under the influence of developing renal acidosis. Sodium bicarbonate may be useful in this setting and, provided that its use is not precluded by body sodium and water overload, is very effective. Cation exchange resins (e.g. Calcium Resonium) given orally or rectally may increase external potassium loss, and the combination of insulin and glucose can also be useful in the short term for management of hyperkalaemia (p. 853).

Protein and energy provision

Many patients with ARF have severe associated disease (such as shock, sepsis and trauma) so that the usual considerations regarding protein restriction in renal failure (p. 808) may not apply. The management of *isolated ARF in an otherwise well and stable patient* should include dietary protein restriction to about 0.6 g protein/kg bodyweight per day. This should be accompanied by generous energy provision from carbohydrate and fat, to a total of at least

30 kcal/kg bodyweight per day. This accelerated tissue catabolism required to make up any shortfall in energy provision. In contrast, the patient with *ARF and severe associated illness* is likely to be in a hypercatabolic state and require as much as 50 kcal/kg bodyweight per day or more. Protein restriction has no place here; indeed, intake should be high (1.5 g/kg bodyweight per day).

Dialysis

Dialysis may be needed for one or more of the following indications:

- uraemic syndrome (p. 804)
- adverse biochemistry (urea levels > 40–45 mmol/l)
- severe hypervolaemia with hypertension and/or pulmonary oedema
- hyperkalaemia (potassium levels > 6.5 mmol/l)
- severe symptomatic acidosis
- the need to remove fluid to allow intensive feeding with high energy/high nitrogen diets or total parenteral nutrition (TPN). Such feeding usually requires an intake of at least 2500 ml/day.

Dialysis may be peritoneal or by haemodialysis (p. 810). *Peritoneal dialysis* has the advantage of simplicity, but may be difficult or impossible if there has been very recent abdominal surgery. *Haemodialysis* offers higher clearance of 'uraemic toxins' (p. 810), but requires partial anticoagulation of the patient and is more often associated with circulatory instability. *Slow continuous haemodialysis* and *slow continuous haemofiltration* are developments that have greatly improved the management of patients with ARF. Circulatory instability is avoided and these techniques are now widely used, especially with multiple organ failure.

ACUTE NEPHRITIC SYNDROME

Acute nephritic syndrome is characterised by the abrupt appearance of blood and protein in the urine, in association with a decline in GFR, sodium and water retention and hypertension. The haematuria may be macroscopic or microscopic and the spun deposit of fresh urine contains red blood cells and casts which are cellular, granular or both. The syndrome is often mild and transient, but may also be severe enough to present as ARF. The renal lesion is usually acute GN, which may be primary or secondary (discussed on pp. 816 and 820), although a minority of patients will be found to have acute tubulointerstitial disease (p. 826). The causes of acute nephritic syndrome are listed in Table 20.17. The management of the diseases causing this syndrome is discussed on pages 817–827.

Table 20.17 Causes of acute nephritic syndrome

Primary postinfectious	Secondary with underlying multisystem disease
Bacterial	SLE
Streptococci	Polyarteritis
Bacterial endocarditis	Wegener's granulomatosis
Ventriculo-atrial shunt	Goodpasture's syndrome
('shunt nephritis')	Henoch-Schönlein purpura
Typhoid	Haemolytic-uraemic syndrome
Brucella	
Meningococci	**Other**
	Idiopathic RPGN
Viral	Acute tubulointerstitial nephropathy
Cytomegalovirus	
Hepatitis virus	
Epstein-Barr virus	
Parasitic	
Plasmodium falciparum	

RAPIDLY PROGRESSIVE GLOMERULONEPHRITIS

The pathological process of rapidly progressive glomerulonephritis (RPGN) often appears confined to the kidney (idiopathic RPGN) but may also be present on a background of a multisystem disease such as polyarteritis, Henoch-Schönlein purpura, systemic lupus erythematosus (SLE) or infective endocarditis. There is usually a distinctive epithelial crescent within the glomerulus, leading to the alternative designation 'crescentic nephritis'. Fibrin deposition may be prominent. In this syndrome, renal function deteriorates progressively over days, weeks or months, usually with urine containing many casts, red blood cells and protein. The course is relentlessly downhill, and although some patients appear to respond to aggressive therapy with steroids, cytotoxic drugs, plasma exchange and in some cases antiplatelet and anticoagulant drugs, many progress to ESRD and require dialysis. Diagnosis is based on renal biopsy. The individual diseases causing RPGN, and their management, are discussed on pages 817–824.

CHRONIC RENAL FAILURE

Aetiology

Chronic renal failure (CRF) can result from any cause of parenchymal renal disease, including unrelieved obstruction (Table 20.18).

Clinical features and investigation

Assessment of the patient with suspected CRF is shown in Table 20.19. In all cases, it is important to decide

Table 20.18 Causes of chronic renal failure

Vascular Renal artery stenosis (only when bilateral or affecting solitary functioning kidney) Hypertensive nephrosclerosis Systemic sclerosis Haemolytic uraemic syndrome/thrombotic thrombocytopenic purpura Vasculitis (polyarteritis, Wegener's)
Glomerulopathy All causes of primary glomerulopathy (except minimal change) All causes of secondary glomerulopathy (with associated multisystem disease, e.g. SLE, Henoch-Schönlein purpura) Toxic glomerulopathy (mercurial diuretics, gold, penicillamine)
Tubulointerstitial nephropathy (TIN) Idiopathic Associated with multisystem disease (Sjögren's, sarcoidosis) Associated with metabolic disorders (e.g. urate, nephrocalcinosis) Toxic TIN, e.g. analgesic abuse, Bence-Jones protein in myeloma
Infection and/or reflux Chronic pyelonephritis Renal tuberculosis
Cystic disease Adult polycystic disease **Obstructive nephropathy** **Diabetic nephropathy** **Amyloid** **Renal dysplasia, hypoplasia, agenesis**

Table 20.19 Assessment of the patient who appears to have chronic renal failure

Clinical Symptoms or signs of uraemia Length of history Family history of renal disease Pointers to underlying multisystem disease (diabetes, SLE, etc.) Symptoms and/or signs of obstruction Palpably enlarged kidneys Volume depletion or expansion Blood pressure/signs of accelerated hypertension
Laboratory Urine analysis — for blood/protein — microscopy of fresh spun deposit — culture Assessment of GFR (plasma creatinine/clearance) 24-hour protein excretion Full blood count, ESR Immunological studies (optional, depending on case), e.g. immunoglobulins, complement, immune complexes, autoantibodies, ANCA Infection – HBsAg and blood cultures (where appropriate)
Imaging Plain abdominal X-ray with/without nephrotomography (renal size) Ultrasound of kidneys (renal size, obstruction) Radionuclide studies (level of renal function, obstruction) IVU (renal size, gross morphology and function) Hand X-rays (secondary hyperparathyroidism)
Histology Renal biopsy – only if kidneys are not small and there is doubt over chronicity

whether the renal impairment is indeed chronic or whether it is acute (Table 20.16). CRF rarely has the potential to improve significantly (although appropriate treatment may slow or arrest progression), but many patients with ARF have potentially recoverable lesions. It follows that diagnosis of CRF does not usually require more than general information regarding the renal pathology. Thus, renal biopsies are seldom of value in patients with CRF. There are, however, certain factors that require careful consideration, and attention should be directed in particular to the following:

- Is a prerenal factor exacerbating the CRF? The most likely of these is salt and water depletion (which may itself be a consequence of a concomitant renal concentrating defect) and its correction may dramatically improve the level of renal function.
- Has coexisting hypertension been controlled adequately?
- Have postrenal factors been adequately excluded? The importance of this is clear – relief of an obstructing lesion is likely to halt progression of the CRF, and may lead to its partial reversal.

Advanced CRF is always associated with the development of the *uraemic syndrome.*

Uraemia

The uraemic state eludes precise definition. A working description would be 'the constellation of symptoms, signs and altered body physiology and chemistry that arises when renal function is substantially impaired'. These features are listed in Table 20.10 (p. 799). Uraemia results mainly from toxic accumulation of waste products, but depletion of essential compounds and failure of biosynthetic functions of the kidney also contribute. Most organ systems are affected in one way or another. The conservative management of CRF is outlined in Table 20.20 (p. 805).

Uraemic toxins

There are many potential uraemic toxins, although urea itself is probably not one of them, at least in clinical practice. Other candidates are peptide hormones (PTH, gastrin, glucagon and calcitonin), purine metabolites, aliphatic and aromatic amines, phenols and indoles, all of which are demonstrably toxic in vitro. The demonstration of increased quantities of compounds of molecular weight 500–5000 daltons (so-called 'middle molecules') in

Table 20.20 Conservative management of the uraemic syndrome

Item	Comments
Identify and treat prerenal factors	Many patients with CRF cannot conserve sodium/water
Identify and treat post-renal factors	Exclude obstruction in all cases
Restrict dietary protein	GFR usually less than 25 ml/min. Early restriction might protect remaining nephrons
Adjust dietary sodium/potassium	Severe restriction unnecessary except in oliguria. Sodium supplementation needed in some cases
Fluids	Aim for urine flow rate of 1500–2000 ml/day
Prophylaxis or treatment of osteodystrophy	Restrict dietary phosphate. Give phosphate binders (calcium carbonate and/or aluminium hydroxide). Give calcium supplements. Consider vitamin D analogues (calcitrol, alfacalcidol)
Control blood pressure	Adjustment of body sodium/water by diet and diuretics. Beta-blockers, converting enzyme inhibitors, calcium antagonists if necessary
Look out for deficiency of vitamins and minerals	Iron is the most likely to require supplementation
Acidosis	Treat with sodium bicarbonate if (a) severe and (b) no contraindication

uraemic patients has led to speculation that one or more of these may be involved. Both small molecules, such as urea, and middle molecules are removed by dialysis (p. 810), and this is associated with amelioration of the uraemic syndrome. However, evidence relating these compounds directly to clinical uraemia remains circumstantial.

Haematopoietic system in uraemia

Anaemia

The majority of patients with significant renal impairment have normochromic normocytic anaemia. The following contribute to the anaemia (see also Ch. 24, p. 1050):

- decreased production of erythropoietin by the diseased kidney
- direct marrow suppression by uraemic toxins
- shortened red cell survival
- increased blood loss.

Most patients approaching ESRD or being treated by haemodialysis have haemoglobin concentrations in the region of 6–10 g/dl, although in those who have been nephrectomised, the anaemia is usually more severe.

Patients with polycystic kidney disease often continue to make erythropoietin and may have completely normal haemoglobin concentrations, even when on dialysis.

Haematinic deficiency may exacerbate the anaemia of CRF; iron and folate supply is often marginal in patients on restricted diets and, in addition, renal patients malabsorb iron and have increased iron needs as a result of mucosal bleeding.

Bleeding

Bleeding in uraemia is mainly from capillaries and is due to abnormal platelet function (platelet numbers are usually normal in uraemia). Treatment of uraemia by dialysis improves, but does not normalise, the platelet defect. The bleeding tendency manifests itself clinically with cutaneous ecchymoses and mucosal oozing.

Cardiovascular system in uraemia

Pericardium

Haemorrhagic pericarditis is a frequent complication of terminal uraemia, but may also arise in the less uraemic patient approaching ESRD or receiving dialysis. Its occurrence is loosely related to the severity of uraemia, as judged by plasma urea concentration. The onset may be insidious or abrupt, the latter leading to severe pain or cardiac tamponade which may be fatal. Management is that of any pericardial effusion (p. 426) combined with intensive dialysis. Surgical relief of tamponade or chronic constrictive pericarditis is needed occasionally.

Heart

Many patients with CRF, particularly those maintained for long periods on dialysis, appear to develop impaired cardiac function. Although this usually occurs as a consequence of hypertension or coronary artery disease, this is not always so. Chronic anaemia, volume overload, nutritional deficiency, high circulating levels of angiotensin II, and uraemic toxins may all contribute to a 'uraemic cardiomyopathy'. Rigorous control of intravascular volume, blood pressure (by dialysis and/or drugs) and anaemia (using erythropoietin) offers the best hope of prevention or amelioration of the condition. If necessary, symptomatic ischaemic heart disease and valve disease can be managed surgically without any great excess in morbidity or mortality.

Arteries

Chronically uraemic patients, whether treated by dialysis or not, have a greatly increased incidence of arterial disease, and cardiovascular disease is by far the largest single cause of death amongst patients on dialysis programmes. Uraemia is often accompanied by hyperlipidaemia, in which plasma triglycerides and very low density lipoproteins are elevated and high density lipoproteins are reduced (p. 777). These abnormalities, in combination with hypertension, may account for the accelerated arterial disease that appears to be part of the uraemic state. It is not yet known whether biochemical improvements from lipid-lowering diets and drugs translate to a reduction in vascular disease.

Skeletal and mineral metabolism in uraemia: renal osteodystrophy

Skeletal abnormalities are an invariable accompaniment of uraemia and comprise *hyperparathyroid bone disease, osteomalacia* and *osteosclerosis*. The pathogenesis of these conditions is dominated by two distinct processes, phosphate retention and intestinal calcium malabsorption (Fig. 20.12), both leading to secondary hyperparathyroidism.

Phosphate retention

Phosphate retention is a consequence of the decreasing filtered load of phosphate as GFR falls (p. 791). This

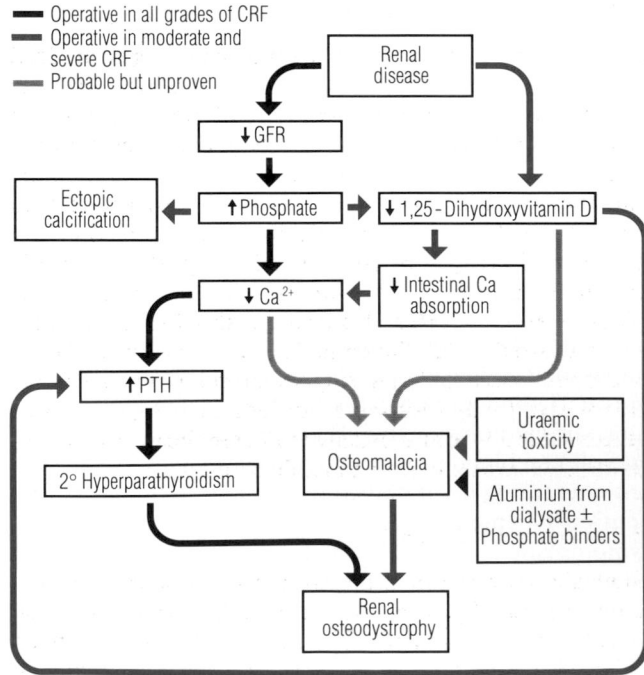

Fig. 20.12 Renal osteodystrophy. The process is dominated by a combination of phosphate retention (its consequences shown on the left side of the figure) and failure of the diseased kidney to synthesise 1,25-dihydroxyvitamin D (its consequences shown in the centre and right of the figure).

causes a reciprocal fall in plasma calcium which, in turn, provokes increased release of PTH. The result is normalisation of plasma calcium concentration and increased phosphaturia, such that plasma phosphate also returns to normal. Thus, with each decrement in GFR, a new steady state is reached with normal plasma concentrations of calcium and phosphate, but only at the expense of secondary hyperparathyroidism. The parathyroids compensate so well for the alterations in calcium and phosphorous homeostasis as renal function declines, that overt hyperphosphataemia develops only when GFR falls to 25 ml/minute or less. The price paid for this compensation is progressive PTH-mediated skeletal resorption.

Calcium malabsorption

Calcium malabsorption develops when renal damage has progressed to the point where the production of 1,25-dihydroxyvitamin D, the active hormonal form of vitamin D, from its precursor 25-hydroxyvitamin D (under the influence of 25-OHD-1α-hydroxylase) becomes significantly impaired (Fig. 20.13). Early in renal failure, plasma concentrations of 1,25-dihydroxyvitamin D are normal, probably because the accompanying hyperparathyroidism has the effect of stimulating the diseased kidney to maintain 1,25-dihydroxyvitamin D production (p. 728). In advanced renal failure (GFR <20 ml/minute), 1,25-dihydroxyvitamin D concentration falls to low or undetectable levels. This is partly as a result of decreased renal mass and loss of the cells that contain 25-hydroxyvitamin D 1α-hydroxylase (the proximal tubular cells), and partly as a result of the suppressive influence of hyperphosphataemia on the 1α-hydroxylase enzyme. The consequent intestinal calcium malabsorption further exacerbates the secondary hyperparathyroidism.

The dominant skeletal lesion is thus that of *hyperparathyroid bone disease*, with increased numbers and activity of osteoclasts, accelerated bone resorption, a coupled increase in osteoblastic activity, high bone turnover and variable degrees of peritrabecular fibrosis (osteitis fibrosa). These lesions can usually be reversed by therapy that alleviates the hyperparathyroidism (p. 809).

In addition, a proportion of patients show features of impaired mineralisation (*osteomalacia*), either in combination with hyperparathyroid bone disease, or in isolation. The pathogenesis of uraemic osteomalacia is less well understood than that of hyperparathyroidism, but it may be a direct consequence of 1,25-dihydroxyvitamin D lack, or a reflection of abnormal collagen synthesis or failure of transformation of calcium phosphate to hydroxyapatite in the presence of uraemia. Aluminium derived from dialysate or aluminium-containing phosphate binders may accumulate in the bone of some patients with uraemia and has been associated with severe and refractory osteomalacia (p. 809).

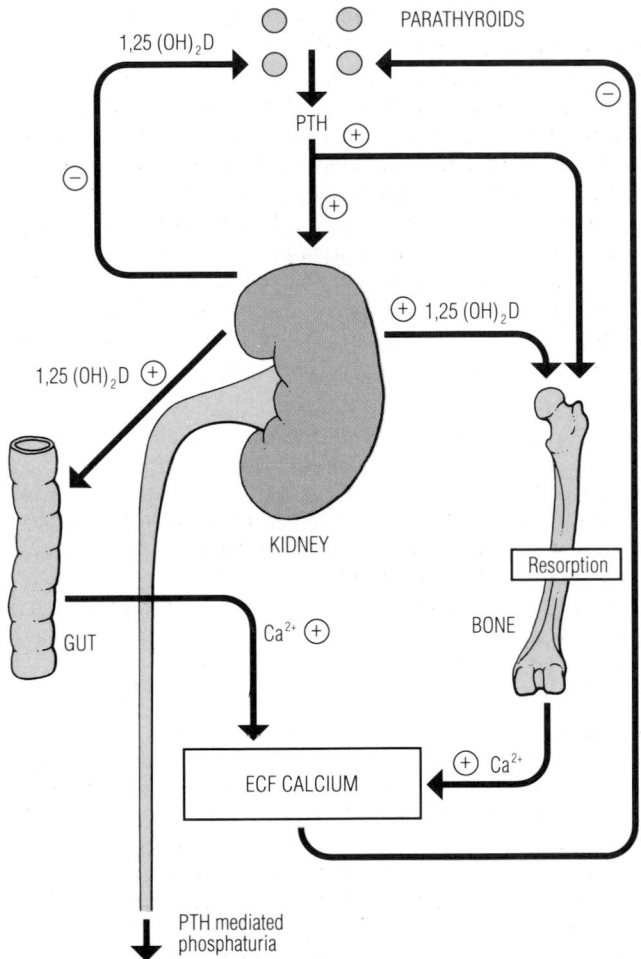

Fig. 20.13 Renal and hormonal control of calcium metabolism. PTF, secreted in response to decreasing ECF calcium, stimulates the production of 1,25 (OH₂)D in the kidney. 1,25(OH₂)D in turn stimulates bone resorption and intestinal calcium absorption, and feeds back negatively to inhibit PTH secretion.

Although hyperparathyroidism and osteomalacia both lead to osteopenia, some patients show *regional osteosclerosis*, particularly involving the trabecular bone of the spine. Its pathogenesis is poorly understood but it usually develops on a background of severe hyperparathyroidism. *Soft tissue calcification*, generally vascular, subcutaneous or corneal, may occur, especially in patients with chronic elevation of plasma phosphate concentration. *Metabolic acidosis* – from which all uraemic patients suffer to some extent and which is buffered by skeletal alkali – contributes little to the development of renal osteodystrophy except when the acidosis is severe and prolonged.

Clinical features are usually subtle when hyperparathyroidism dominates the condition, but, in the presence of significant osteomalacia, bone pain, deformity and pathological fractures may occur. Radiological evidence of hyperparathyroidism (subperiosteal erosions affecting particularly the phalanges and spinal osteosclerosis – *the rugger jersey spine*) or osteomalacia (osteopenia, Looser zones, non-healing fractures) may be present. Plasma biochemistry shows normal or low calcium concentration, raised inorganic phosphate and, often, raised alkaline phosphatase reflecting increased osteoblastic activity. If measured, PTH is high, 25-hydroxyvitamin D normal and 1,25-dihydroxyvitamin D low, indicating failure of renal bioactivation of vitamin D.

Gastrointestinal system and uraemia

Peptic ulcer disease is possibly more common in uraemic patients. Serum gastrin is elevated in uraemia, but basal and stimulated gastric acid secretion is often normal. Haemorrhagic complications of peptic ulcer disease are more likely in uraemia because of the associated haemostatic defects (p. 805) and, in the case of haemodialysis patients, exposure to anticoagulants. Treatment is along conventional lines with antacids and H₂-receptor antagonists. Small and large bowel changes are usually mild and of little functional significance, except in near terminal uraemia when bleeding may be severe. Angiodysplasia (Ch. 15, p. 567) is relatively common in uraemia and accounts for bleeding in a number of cases.

Nervous system in uraemia

Uraemic encephalopathy is a syndrome of global CNS dysfunction, probably resulting from retained uraemic toxins, although it is not clear which of these underlie the clinical manifestations. Its onset depends in part on the severity of uraemia (judged biochemically), but also on the rate of onset of uraemia, rapid onset being associated with earlier CNS decompensation. Higher mental functions are the first affected; poor concentration, apathy, insomnia and irritability occur frequently. Motor disturbances become evident later, leading to slurring of speech, tremors, asterixis (the 'uraemic flap'), myoclonus and even seizures. Nausea and vomiting are prominent in advanced uraemia and may respond to antiemetic drugs. 'Dialysis dementia' is a rare and usually fatal complication of severe aluminium intoxication in uraemic patients.

Peripheral nervous system

Uraemic neuropathy is a frequent complication of terminal uraemia. Symptomatic neuropathy may also develop in patients in whom the initiation of dialysis has been deferred for too long or who are underdialysed; clinical and electrophysiological evidence of asymptomatic neuropathy is very common. The neuropathy is mixed sensory and motor and is an axonal degeneration. A variable degree of improvement follows treatment of the uraemia.

Metabolic and nutritional considerations in uraemia

Protein. A mixed picture with elements of both deficiency and toxicity develops. Protein restricted diets predispose to protein malnutrition, while accumulation of nitrogenous compounds, some of which may be 'uraemic toxins', results from impaired renal catabolism and excretion of waste. Additional problems may be present in specific diseases (e.g. massive protein losses in nephrotic syndrome).

Carbohydrate. As a group, uraemic patients are slightly hyperglycaemic compared with normals, both when fasted and following glucose challenge. Peripheral insulin resistance appears to be the major cause, and this may be further exacerbated by a tendency of uraemia per se to inhibit insulin secretion. Conversely, the renal catabolism of insulin is normally considerable and decreases as renal disease progresses. As a result, although uraemic patients have mild carbohydrate intolerance, overtly diabetic patients with nephropathy require less insulin as nephropathy progresses.

Lipids. Plasma triglycerides and very low density lipoproteins are increased and high density lipoproteins decreased in uraemia. All these changes potentially contribute to the observed increase in atherogenesis amongst uraemic patients.

Conservative management of chronic renal failure

This section deals with the clinical management of the patient who has severe impairment of renal function but who has not yet reached ESRD and the need for renal replacement therapy (RRT). Because of the serious limitations of adaptive capacity in the diseased kidney, the central principles of conservative management are:

- to minimise the functional stresses and strains imposed on the kidney, by attempting to define the appropriate intake of food, minerals and water in such a way as not to exceed the kidney's limits of adaptation
- to identify and treat any coexisting factors that may further compromise renal function, e.g. hypertension, prerenal factors, postrenal factors
- to anticipate and, if possible, avoid future complications of uraemia, such as malnutrition, osteodystrophy, soft tissue calcification
- to anticipate and prepare for the initiation of RRT if needed.

Specific aspects of clinical management are as follows (and are summarised in Table 20.20).

Diet

Protein

Protein restriction is begun only when symptoms and/or signs of the uraemic syndrome become evident; this does not usually happen until GFR falls to 25 ml/minute or less. Protein restriction decreases the rate of production of uraemic toxins and the acid products of metabolism, and is very effective in alleviating the uraemic syndrome (though it has no immediate effect on underlying renal function). In the UK, normal dietary protein intake is 70–140 g/day. This can be reduced in a stepwise fashion (as GFR decreases) to a lower limit of 25–30 g/day (0.5 g/kg bodyweight per day) without serious risk of nutritional deficiency, provided that it is accompanied by adequate energy intake in the form of carbohydrate and fat. At these very low protein intakes, it is important that the protein is of animal origin, in order to avoid selective deficiency of essential amino acids; these may only be present in small amounts in vegetable protein. The essential amino acids in animal protein are present in proportions that approximate to their minimum daily requirement in man.

Although it is conventional practice to restrict protein only for symptomatic treatment of the uraemic syndrome, there is convincing laboratory and some clinical evidence that much earlier protein restriction will retard, and in some cases halt, the progression of renal deterioration (p. 809). If this proves correct, protein restriction is likely to be employed earlier in the course of renal failure in the future.

Sodium

In many patients, urinary sodium excretion is reasonably well maintained even at very low levels of GFR. However, in the salt-consuming developed countries, sodium restriction often becomes necessary; the indications are hypertension or evidence of expansion of body sodium and water. The dietary intake may be set at about 60 mmol/day (moderate salt restriction), compared with the 100–250 mmol/day in a normal diet. More severe sodium restriction may be used, but renders the diet increasingly unpalatable. Fortunately, potent loop diuretics often obviate the need for unpleasantly low sodium diets. Conversely, there are cases where inappropriate salt losses through the diseased kidney may dictate a high dietary sodium intake in order to avoid sodium and water depletion and prerenal exacerbation of the uraemic state.

Potassium

Even in advanced renal failure, the kidney is usually able to maintain adequate potassium excretion, provided that urine flow rate remains generous. Modest reduction of dietary potassium is required; 60–80 mmol/day is usually appropriate, compared with a typical 'normal' intake of 80–120 mmol/day. Severe hyperkalaemia may develop if there is oliguria, gross dietary indiscretion, acidosis (with shift of body potassium from ICF to ECF), or severe intercurrent illness with accelerated catabolism. Potassium-sparing diuretics (e.g. spironolactone, amiloride, triampterene) impair potassium excretion severely in uraemia and should be avoided. The treatment of hyperkalaemia is described on page 853, but, in patients with severely impaired renal function, a sudden rise in serum potassium may necessitate emergency dialysis.

Fluids

Fluid restriction is rarely necessary in a patient with CRF, unless oliguria or anuria supervene. On the contrary, it is important to ensure that the fluid intake is set at a level adequate to keep up with the relatively high obligatory urine flow rate in CRF, and thus prevent water depletion and prerenal exacerbation of the renal disease. In practice, the fluid intake should be such as to maintain urine flow at around 1500–2000 ml/day, i.e. minimum daily fluid intake should be 2000–2500 ml/day. A minority of patients with more severe urinary concentrating defects will require larger amounts of fluid to maintain water balance.

Calcium, phosphorus and vitamin D

CRF is associated with a tendency towards hyperphosphataemia, hypocalcaemia, hyperparathyroidism and impaired production of 1,25-dihydroxyvitamin D and consequent intestinal calcium malabsorption (p. 806).
    A number of therapeutic measures are employed.

● Moderate dietary phosphate restriction.
● Administration of oral 'phosphate-binders' with food. Aluminium hydroxide was routine, but fears of aluminium toxicity are leading to increased use of calcium carbonate and magnesium carbonate as phosphate binders.
● Maintenance of a high oral calcium intake. Calcium carbonate is convenient here. Doses of 25–150 mmol/day (2.5–15 g/day) given with food will often control plasma inorganic phosphate adequately, and also increase vitamin-D-independent intestinal calcium absorption, thereby lessening hyperparathyroidism.
● Use of potent analogues of vitamin D. The requirement is that they should bypass the vitamin D resistance of CRF, by not requiring renal 1-hydroxylation to achieve activity (Fig. 20.13). 1,25-dihydroxyvitamin D (calcitriol), 1α-hydroxyvitamin D (alfacal-

cidiol) and dihydrotachysterol are all effective. However, because they also augment intestinal absorption of phosphate, they should not be given until plasma phosphate has been controlled as described above.

Other vitamins and minerals

Clinical deficiency is rare in the well-managed patient with CRF, although subtle deficiency states may be more common. Iron status in particular may be marginal, reflecting intestinal iron malabsorption and increased requirements due to blood tests and occult bleeding. Overzealous and prolonged dietary protein restriction may lead to difficulties, but this usually reflects inappropriate persistence with conservative measures in a patient in whom dialysis should have been started earlier.

Acidosis

In some patients, uraemic acidosis is sufficiently severe, even after appropriate dietary protein restriction, to warrant attempts to relieve it. This may be done with sodium bicarbonate, although the need for concomitant sodium restriction may preclude or limit its use. Potassium bicarbonate is never used in this setting for fear of causing hyperkalaemia.

Control of blood pressure

The control of blood pressure is discussed on page 828. Its importance cannot be overemphasised.

Anaemia

Evidence of iron and folate deficiency should be sought and treated if appropriate. Replacement of the deficient hormone can now be delivered by regular injections of *synthetic human erythropoietin*; this approach is extremely effective and is being applied widely. Occasional, or even regular, blood transfusion is used in some patients. Symptoms (e.g. weakness, lethargy) and complications (angina, cardiac failure) of anaemia dictate the need for treatment; the absolute level of haemoglobulin is not, in isolation, a good indicator. Successful transplantation leads to rapid return of normal haematopoietic activity.

Measures to halt or retard the progression of chronic renal failure

Progressive renal disease usually causes a decrease in the number of functioning nephrons; therefore it follows that each of the remaining nephrons must process an unusually large amount of water and solute. Adaptive changes in the residual nephrons are many, but there is good evidence that single-nephron GFR (i.e. GFR per nephron) is increased in chronic renal disease and that this is associated with a raised hydrostatic pressure in the glomerular capillaries (glomerular hypertension). If sustained, this leads to glomerular sclerosis, loss of nephrons and progressive renal deterioration. In animals, this sequence of events can be prevented completely by dietary protein restriction or angiotensin-converting-enzyme (ACE) inhibition and it is likely, though not yet proven, that the same holds for some types of chronic renal disease in man. Experimentally, glomerular hypertension can be reduced by ACE inhibitors acting on the renal production of angiotensin II. At present, the clinical utility of these measures is not fully established. It is therefore not yet appropriate to implement them in all patients, although modest protein restriction (0.6–0.8 g/kg bodyweight per day) and early use of ACE inhibitors is reasonable.

Renal replacement therapy for chronic renal failure

Renal replacement therapy (RRT) for CRF can be achieved by haemodialysis, peritoneal dialysis or renal transplantation. Most centres offering RRT integrate all three treatment modalities, with the aim of providing each patient with the most appropriate management.

The requirement for RRT

It is estimated that 70–100 patients per million population (below the age of 70) reach ESRD in the UK each year and will die if RRT is not provided. The UK currently treats only about 50 patients per million population, a figure substantially lower than in most developed countries. Consequently, many people in the UK die from renal failure without receiving the benefits of RRT.

Dialysis treatment

Dialysis involves placing a large volume of artificial fluid (dialysate) in very close proximity to a large volume of the patient's blood, separating the two with a semi-permeable membrane.

Haemodialysis

In haemodialysis, the membrane is synthetic and semi-permeable, and is arranged to form an 'artificial kidney' through which blood passes at about 250 ml/minute before being returned to the patient (Fig. 20.14). The chemical composition of the dialysate is similar to that of ECF. Urea and other waste products, which are present

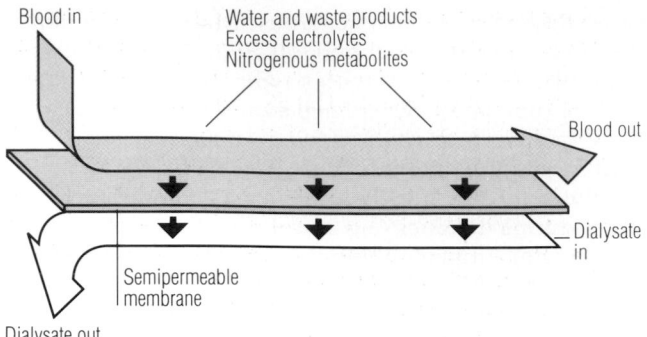

Fig. 20.14 Physical principles of haemodialysis.

only in plasma, diffuse down a concentration gradient across the membrane and into the dialysate. Changes in the composition of the dialysate and in the hydrostatic pressure gradient across the membrane allow 'tailoring' of the rate of removal of a variety of substances according to the patient's needs. Adequate access to the circulation is a prerequisite. This is obtained by percutaneous placement of large-bore central venous catheters (short-term treatment only), or by creation of an arteriovenous fistula at the wrist, thus increasing forearm blood flow and allowing large-bore needles to be placed in forearm veins (long-term treatment). Treatment is intermittent, typically three sessions of 4 hours each per week. In the UK, many patients undergoing this form of treatment conduct their own treatment at home.

Peritoneal dialysis

In peritoneal dialysis, the dialysate is fed into the peritoneal cavity via a flexible tube, and the peritoneum itself acts as a semi-permeable membrane. The dialysate is replaced with fresh fluid when chemical equilibrium is reached. Peritoneal dialysis takes the form of continuous ambulatory peritoneal dialysis (CAPD) in which 2-litre exchanges are performed three or four times per day. The technique is simple to learn and the vast majority of patients can carry out and supervise their own treatment at home.

Limitations of dialysis

Although dialysis can remove waste products, sodium, potassium and water reasonably well and thus control some aspects of the uraemic syndrome, it is, for the following reasons, inferior to normal functioning kidneys:

- The *average* clearance of urea or creatinine achieved by intermittent haemodialysis (approximately 12 hours treatment per week) is only 6 ml/minute and by CAPD about 7 ml/minute, compared with 100–120 ml/minute by normal kidneys.

- The permeability characteristics of the artificial membrane in haemodialysis and, to a lesser extent, the peritoneum in peritoneal dialysis (CAPD) are inferior to those of the physiological glomerular sieve.
- Dialysis has no equivalent of 'tubular action'; the dialysis membrane must therefore strike a compromise between being permeable enough to allow waste products to cross and not so permeable that excess loss of physiologically important compounds occurs. In practice, the membrane fails on both counts.
- Dialysis has essentially no adaptive capability.
- Endocrine functions of the kidney are not provided by dialysis. The anaemia (erythropoietin) and osteodystrophy (1,25-dihydroxyvitamin D) continue.

For these reasons most of the management considerations that apply to the non-dialysed patient with CRF also apply to the dialysed patient (Table 20.20).

Initiation of dialysis treatment

Because dialysis is inherently unnatural and invasive, its initiation should not be undertaken lightly. The optimum time to convert a patient with CRF from conservative management to dialysis is a finely judged clinical decision and is reached *just before* the development of uraemic complications (Table 20.21).

Renal transplantation

Successful renal transplantation is, compared with maintenance dialysis, a vastly superior form of treatment.

There is little that normal native kidneys can do in the way of excretory, homeostatic or endocrine function that cannot be done equally well by a good transplanted kidney. This is reflected in the clinical outcome; it is apparent that many transplanted patients are returned to a state of virtual normality. However, two problems continue to bedevil renal transplantation. These are inadequate supply of kidneys and graft rejection.

Kidneys are obtained from cadavers (usually with irreversible CNS injury due to trauma or stroke) or from fit, first degree relatives. ABO compatibility is essential and outcome is improved by good HLA matching. The transplanted kidney is placed in the left or right iliac fossa and anastamosed to the iliac vessels; the donor ureter is implanted into the recipient bladder. Immunosuppressive treatment is given routinely and comprises cyclosporin, often with steroids and/or azathioprine. These drugs are toxic; this is particularly unfortunate with cyclosporin which, as well as being an excellent immunosuppressive agent, also has marked acute and chronic nephrotoxicity. About 80% of cadaveric grafts function for 2 years or more and, because most graft loss occurs early, the majority of this 80% will continue to do well thereafter (Fig. 20.15). Living related-donor transplants do even better. Most patients receiving kidney transplants are already being dialysed and can return to dialysis treatment if the transplant fails.

NEPHROTIC SYNDROME

Nephrotic syndrome is best defined as the presence of heavy proteinuria (usually greater than 3 g/day), hypoalbuminaemia, hyperlipidaemia and oedema. It is not helpful to pursue the definition beyond this semi-quantitative statement, because there is much inter-patient variation in the clinical response to a given level of proteinuria.

Table 20.21 Indications for initiation of dialysis treatment

Suitability for long-term treatment and/or reversible cause of renal failure
Uraemic syndrome
Neurological
Coma, stupor, fatigue, abnormal mentation, fits, myoclonus, asterixis, peripheral neuropathy
Cardiovascular/pulmonary
Pericarditis, pleurisy, volume overload unresponsive to conservative measures
Skin
Pruritus
Gastrointestinal
Anorexia, nausea, vomiting, unremitting diarrhoea
Metabolic
Unremitting acidosis
Chemistry
Plasma urea more than 40 mmol/l on protein restricted diet
Plasma creatinine more than 1200 µmol/l
Creatinine clearance less than 5 ml/minute
Hyperkalaemia unresponsive to conservative measures

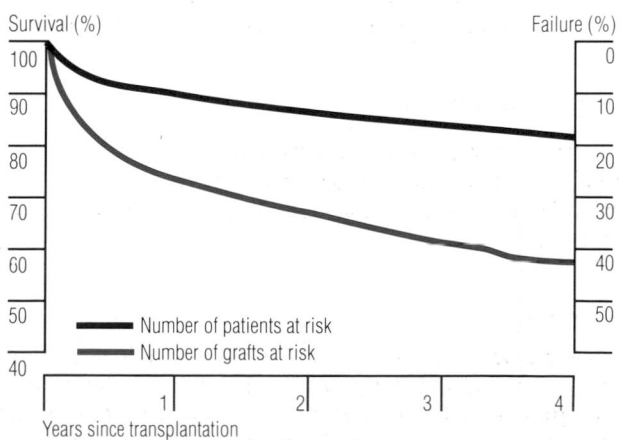

Fig. 20.15 Patient and graft survival following renal transplantation. (Data from UK Transplant Service).

Aetiology

Nephrotic range proteinuria, leading to the nephrotic syndrome, may result from a variety of different types of insult to the functional glomerular sieve (Table 20.22). The glomerular changes that result in nephrotic syndrome may reflect disturbances to the size selectivity or the charge selectivity (or both) of the glomerular sieve, such that substantial amounts of plasma proteins, particularly albumin, appear in the GF.

Pathophysiology

The amount of oedema is variable, but correlates better with the severity of hypoalbuminaemia than with the magnitude of proteinuria. The oedema is generalised and may be associated with pleural effusion and/or ascites, especially in children. The pathophysiological processes leading to oedema in the nephrotic syndrome are illustrated in Figure 20.16. This sequence predicts that the nephrotic patient has an expanded ECF, contracted vascular compartment, high plasma renin activity and aldosterone concentration, with avid renal sodium and water retention. This is indeed the case in many, though not all, nephrotic patients.

Investigation

In children, minimal change GN is the usual lesion. In such cases, the diagnosis can usually be made without

Table 20.22 Causes of nephrotic syndrome

Primary glomerular disease	Secondary glomerular disease
Minimal change GN	Infection (infective endocarditis,
Membranous GN	visceral sepsis, quartan malaria,
Focal segmental glomerulosclerosis	hepatitis B)
Mesangiocapillary GN	
Drug/toxin-induced	Neoplasia (carcinoma, lymphoma, leukaemia, myeloma)
Gold	
Other heavy metals	Multisystem diseases (SLE, Henoch-Schönlein purpura, rheumatoid arthritis, amyloid, diabetes mellitus)
Penicillamine	
Intravenous drug abuse	

recourse to renal biopsy. In a typical case, there is a normal GFR, an absence of significant numbers of red cells or casts in the urine and a highly selective urine protein excretion (p. 792). The abolition of proteinuria by steroid therapy is confirmatory. In children with steroid-resistant disease, or who have impaired GFR and/or red blood cells and casts in the urine, and in the majority of adults, identification of the renal lesion (Table 20.22) and appropriate management will usually necessitate renal biopsy.

Complications and management

The complications of the nephrotic syndrome may be serious, and an important therapeutic objective is therefore the amelioration or elimination of the proteinuria. (The specific glomerulopathies causing nephrotic syndrome are discussed on pp. 817–824.) Often this is not possible, but certain general measures remain appropriate regardless of the underlying renal lesion (Table 20.23). Diuretics should be used judiciously and in conjunction with dietary sodium restriction. Although, in some cases, very large doses of a potent loop diuretic will be needed to effect a diuresis, these drugs carry the risk of inducing severe contraction of the vascular compartment (hypovolaemia) and may lead to prerenal uraemia, shock and even ARF in some cases. Severe hypovolaemia can be corrected temporarily by administration of colloid in the form of plasma proteins, a manoeuvre that is also employed occasionally to initiate a diuresis. The use of the aldosterone antagonist, spironolactone, in these patients is both logical and useful.

Table 20.23 General measures in the treatment of nephrotic syndrome

- High protein diet
- Dietary sodium restriction
- Water restriction (rarely necessary)
- Diuretic therapy
- Intravenous proteins

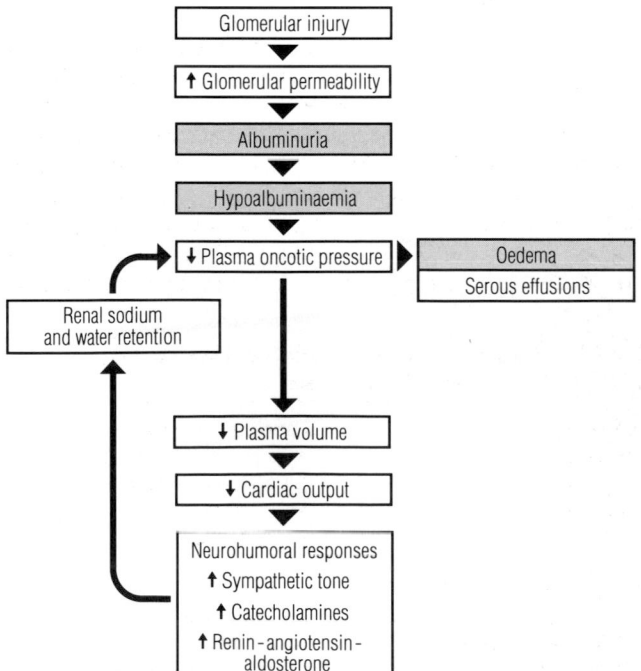

Fig. 20.16 Pathogenesis of oedema in nephrotic syndrome.

Summary 3 Complications of nephrotic syndrome

- Massive oedema

- Effusions/ascites

- Hypovolaemia (reduced blood volume)

- Protein malnutrition – growth retardation
  – poor wound healing
  – osteoporosis

- Hyperlipidaemia – probable increased atherogenesis

- Hypercoagulability – renal vein thrombosis
  – stroke

- Susceptibility to infection (especially in children)

Protein malnutrition is a major hazard in patients with nephrotic syndrome; the patients should maintain the highest possible protein intake, while ensuring adequate energy provision to prevent further acceleration of protein catabolism. Despite these measures, growth retardation, poor wound healing and reduced immune competence are frequent. The hyperlipidaemia is refractory to dietary measures, but responds to HMG CoA reductase inhibitors (pravastatin, simvastatin). Thrombotic problems resulting from the hypercoagulable state that attends the nephrotic syndrome are common. The hypercoagulability may be the result of urinary losses of antithrombin III. Thrombosis is particularly likely to involve the renal veins, leading to an abrupt decline in GFR that must be distinguished from progression of the underlying nephropathy. Diagnosis of renal vein thrombosis in a nephrotic is important, because anticoagulation almost certainly reduces the risk of subsequent pulmonary embolism and may allow eventual recanalisation of the occluded vessel and improvement in GFR. Careful ultrasound or CT examination of the renal veins may reveal the clot, but in some cases renal venography is required.

RECURRENT HAEMATURIA

Recurrent haematuria most frequently affects boys and young males. The syndrome is dominated by recurrent episodes of macroscopic haematuria, sometimes associated with loin pain and with a tendency to exacerbations following intercurrent viral upper respiratory infections or strenuous exercise. Microscopic haematuria usually persists between attacks and proteinuria is absent or modest (less than 1.5 g/24 hours).

In most cases, the renal pathology is characteristic, with florid mesangial deposition of IgA (or IgM) in the glomeruli; the nephropathy is then termed *IgA* (or *IgM*) *nephropathy* or *Berger's disease* (p. 821).

Investigation and management

Investigations should include measurement of GFR, examination of the urine and quantitation of protein output. An IVU should be performed in all cases. Children and young adults with a typical presentation can usually be spared cytoscopy, but middle-aged and elderly patients (in whom urological cancer becomes increasingly common) should undergo full urological assessment. Renal biopsy is needed to establish the diagnosis with certainty, especially if there is depression of the GFR, heavy proteinuria, hypertension, a low C3 complement, or a family history suggestive of hereditary nephritis (p. 822).

The course is often benign, although a proportion of patients go on to develop progressive renal disease. There is no specific treatment and management is therefore directed towards identifying and treating secondary hypertension and monitoring renal function.

PERSISTENT ASYMPTOMATIC PROTEINURIA AND/OR HAEMATURIA

The finding of abnormal proteinuria or microscopic haematuria in an apparently healthy person usually results from a routine medical examination for employment or insurance purposes, or is picked up incidentally during an unrelated illness. Table 20.24 lists the large number of conditions that may be associated with this syndrome.

Investigation

Inevitably, the question arises as to how far investigation should proceed in these otherwise healthy individuals. Assessment of renal structure and function by plasma biochemistry, creatinine clearance, 24-hour protein output, urine microscopy and culture, and either renal ultrasound or IVU should be undertaken in all cases. *Dysmorphic* red cells in the urine increase the probability of renal parenchymal disease rather than urological disease. Provided radiological investigation and GFR are normal, protein-

Table 20.24 Causes of asymptomatic persisting proteinuria and/or haematuria in an apparently healthy person

Primary glomerular disease	Miscellaneous renal
Mesangial proliferative GN	Tubulointerstitial nephropathy
Mesangiocapillary GN	Cystic diseases of the kidney
Membranous GN	Renal tumours
Focal segmental glomerulosclerosis	Renal tuberculosis
IgA nephropathy (often causes intermittent gross haematuria)	
	Non-renal
	Urothelial tumours
Multisystem disease	Prostatic disease
Henoch-Schönlein purpura	
SLE	

uria is modest and the urinary sediment does not show granular or cellular casts, it may be appropriate to adopt a 'wait-and-see' policy, only proceeding to invasive investigation, such as renal biopsy, if there is evidence of disease progression. However, early recourse to renal biopsy is usually justified in order to define prognosis or if there is suspicion that an active and progressive process may be present, particularly if this might be amenable to therapy.

RENAL TUBULAR SYNDROMES

Although most patients with renal disease will have evidence of disordered tubular function if a sufficiently diligent search is carried out, other manifestations of renal disease usually dominate the clinical picture. In a minority of patients, however, clinical disorders result directly from tubular dysfunction. In these cases, the disorder may be *inherited* with presentation generally in childhood, or *acquired*.

Renal glycosuria

Inheritance of renal glycosuria is autosomal recessive. The syndrome results from diminished proximal tubular glucose reabsorption, allowing glycosuria with normal blood glucose concentration. No clinical sequelae occur.

Aminoaciduria

The defects involved in aminoaciduria may be single or multiple. The most important is *cystinuria*, leading to recurrent cystine stone formation. Cystine solubility increases at alkaline pH and the disease is treated by a combination of high fluid intake and alkali ingestion. Penicillamine is also effective, although potentially toxic. Inheritance is autosomal recessive.

Phosphate transport defects

There are several types of phosphate transport defects, which result in inappropriate phosphaturia, hypophosphataemia and rickets. Inheritance is usually X-linked (the disorder is known as *vitamin-D-resistant rickets* (VDDR) or *X-linked hypophosphataemic rickets*) but sporadic inherited cases also occur. Treatment usually takes the form of oral phosphate supplementation with pharmacological doses of vitamin D, or smaller doses of 1,25-dihydroxyvitamin D (calcitriol). The latter combination is particularly effective in ameliorating the hypophosphataemia and healing rickets. A rare acquired form also exists, and is associated with certain mesenchymal tumours such as cavernous haemangioma, giant cell tumours of bone, and neurofibromata. In such cases of *oncogenous rickets*, the disordered phosphate metabolism is corrected by removal of the tumour.

Multiple tubular defects (Fanconi's syndrome)

Patients with Fanconi's syndrome have abnormal urinary excretion of amino acids, phosphate, bicarbonate, glucose and small proteins. The classification of this disorder is complex, reflecting its many inherited and acquired causes. All are relatively uncommon; some of the more important acquired ones are shown in Table 20.25. The defects of phosphate reabsorption and proximal bicarbonate reclamation often lead to clinical disease – hypophosphataemic rickets and proximal 'type II' RTA respectively. They require treatment with phosphate, 1,25-dihydroxyvitamin D, or alkali, as appropriate (pp. 814–816).

Renal tubular acidosis

Renal tubular acidosis (RTA) is metabolic acidosis of renal origin and is unrelated to the acidosis associated with severe impairment of GFR (uraemic acidosis). It is generally divided into three categories depending on the nature and site of the acidification disturbance (Table 20.26). Although the pathogenesis of the different types of renal tubular acidosis differs, all cause *hyperchloraemic metabolic acidosis* (low plasma bicarbonate, raised plasma chloride with normal anion gap) in contrast with the acidosis of uraemia (low bicarbonate, normal chloride and increased anion gap).

Distal RTA (type I RTA)

The causes of distal RTA are listed in Table 20.27. There is selective impairment of the distal tubules' ability to secrete H^+, such that urinary pH cannot be lowered below 5.5. Other distal tubular functions are unimpaired. The resulting inability of the distal tubule to reclaim all of the

Table 20.25 Causes of acquired Fanconi's syndrome

- Myeloma kidney
- Sjögren's syndrome
- Nephrotic syndrome
- Heavy metal poisoning
  Lead
  Mercury (organic and inorganic)
  Copper (Wilson's disease)
- Drugs
  Outdated tetracycline
  Salicylates
  Cisplatin

Table 20.26 Classification of renal acidosis

	Renal tubular acidosis (RTA)*			
	Proximal RTA (type II)	Distal RTA with hypokalaemia (type I)	Distal RTA with hyperkalaemia (type IV)	Uraemic acidosis
Defect	Decreased H$^+$ secretion	Decreased H$^+$ secretion	Decreased H$^+$ and K$^+$ secretion	Decreased nephron mass and decreased ammonia synthesis (controversial)
Acidosis				
Type	Hyperchloraemic	Hyperchloraemic	Hyperchloraemic	Normal plasma chloride
Anion gap	Normal	Normal	Normal	Increased
Severity	Moderate	Moderate or severe	Moderate	Usually moderate
Plasma K$^+$	Decreased	Decreased	Increased	Normal or increased
GFR	Usually normal	Normal or decreased	Usually decreased	Decreased
Treatment	Diuretics and alkali	Alkali	Mineralocorticoids K$^+$ restriction	Protein restriction, sometimes alkali, dialysis

* Type III RTA (not shown) is a rare condition where a patient has manifestations of both type I and type II RTA.

5–20% of filtered bicarbonate that normally escapes proximal reclamation leads to continuing bicarbonaturia, even in the presence of severe acidosis. It also limits the utility of urinary buffers such as HPO_4^{2-}, which require a low

Table 20.27 Causes and classification of distal renal tubular acidosis

With hypokalaemia (type I)	
Inherited	**Associated with nephrocalcinosis**
Sickle cell anaemia	Primary hyperparathyroidism
Medullary cystic disease	Vitamin D toxicity
Autoimmune disease	**Tubulointerstitial**
Cryoglobulinaemia	**nephropathy secondary to:**
Sjögren's syndrome	Obstruction
Systemic lupus erythematosus	Chronic pyelonephritis
Chronic active liver disease	Renal transplantation
	Drugs
	Amphotericin B
	Analgesics (in analgesic nephropathy)

With hyperkalaemia (type IV)	
Primary deficiency of mineralocorticoid	**Secondary deficiency of mineralocorticoid**
Isolated familial hypoaldosteronism (rare)	Hyporeninaemic hypoaldosteronism with underlying:
Generalised adrenocorticoid deficiency	Hypertensive nephrosclerosis
Addison's disease	Diabetic nephropathy
Adrenalectomy	Obstructive nephropathy
	Renal transplantation
Tubular resistance to mineralocorticoid	
Some cases of chronic renal impairment	
Spironolactone therapy	

urinary pH if they are to act as efficient proton acceptors. Distal potassium ion secretion is unimpaired and is often enhanced by mild ECF volume contraction and secondary aldosteronism, leading to hyperchloraemia and hypokalaemia.

Diagnosis depends on demonstrating an inappropriately high urinary pH (>5.5) during spontaneous or ammonium chloride-induced acidosis. Other diagnostic manoeuvres are available, but are rarely needed in clinical practice.

Treatment takes the form of alkali given in amounts sufficient to restore plasma bicarbonate and chloride concentrations to normal. Severe hypokalaemia is often present and should be treated *before* administration of alkali, to avoid the further drop in plasma potassium that would follow correction of the acidosis. The amount of alkali required is small (1–3 mmol/kg bodyweight per day) because bicarbonaturia is not severe and does not increase as plasma bicarbonate concentration rises on treatment.

Proximal RTA (type II RTA)

Proximal RTA may occur in several rare inherited diseases but is more commonly acquired in association with myeloma, Sjögren's syndrome or toxic nephropathy (especially lead or mercury). There is a diminished capacity of the proximal tubule to reclaim filtered bicarbonate ions. The resulting bicarbonaturia leads to progressive metabolic acidosis and decreased plasma bicarbonate concentration, in turn lessening the filtered load of bicarbonate. This chain of events progresses until the filtered load of bicarbonate has fallen to the point where the abnormal proximal tubule can again reclaim a normal percentage of the filtered bicarbonate load. This creates a new steady state in which bicarbonate losses cease, but only at the expense of stable metabolic acidosis. Administration of sufficient bicarbonate to these patients will reverse the sequence of events described above.

Treatment comprises long-term administration of bicarbonate. Large amounts (10–30 mmol/kg per day) are needed because, as plasma bicarbonate rises, so the magnitude of the bicarbonaturia also increases. The bicarbonate requirement can often be reduced by concomitant therapy with a thiazide diuretic. Hypokalaemia is often worsened by therapy, but can be countered by giving some of the bicarbonate as potassium bicarbonate or by the use of potassium-sparing diuretics.

Distal RTA with hyperkalaemia (type IV RTA)

In type IV RTA, there is generalised impairment of distal tubular function, usually on a background of a mild or moderate reduction in GFR. Both H^+ and K^+ secretion in the distal tubule are impaired (Tables 20.26 and 20.27), resulting in hyperchloraemic metabolic acidosis accompanied by disproportionately severe hyperkalaemia. This is the commonest form of RTA and, although the acidosis is mild, the accompanying hyperkalaemia may be severe or even life-threatening.

Type IV RTA may result from the following:

- *Primary lack of mineralocorticoid* due to adrenal disease in the presence of potentially normal distal tubular function (isolated hypoaldosteronism and Addison's disease).
- *Disease of the juxtaglomerular apparatus* (JGA) leading to impaired production of renin and secondary hypoaldosteronism (hyporeninaemic hypoaldosteronism). This is associated particularly with hypertensive nephrosclerosis or diabetic nephropathy.
- *Resistance of the distal tubule to mineralocorticoid action.* This is usually partial rather than complete, and may arise in some patients with chronic renal impairment. It is also, of course, a direct (and deliberate) consequence of spironolactone therapy.

Treatment depends on the underlying abnormality. Deficiency of mineralocorticoid – whether isolated, part of Addison's disease, or secondary to hyporeninaemia – requires replacement with mineralocorticoid in the form of 9α-fludrocortisone. When there is renal resistance to mineralocorticoid, control may often be achieved with pharmacological doses of 9α-fludrocortisone.

Salt-losing nephropathy and nephrogenic diabetes insipidus

In adults, salt-losing nephropathy and nephrogenic diabetes insipidus (failure to conserve sodium and/or water) are nearly always acquired. They can result from almost any cause of renal disease, particularly those predominantly affecting the renal medulla, such as urinary obstruction, papillary necrosis, chronic pyelonephritis and tubulointerstitial diseases. *Hypercalcaemia and hypokalaemia* cause a functional nephrogenic diabetes insipidus, initially reversible on correction of the metabolic abnormality. The severity of the polyuria in these acquired tubular syndromes rarely approaches that of pituitary diabetes insipidus, but, in contrast, accompanying salt losses may be massive. The importance of inappropriate renal salt and water loss is their tendency to cause severe volume contraction and prerenal uraemia; one should not be misled by the continuing production of large amounts of urine.

Treatment is usually straightforward. Underlying hypercalcaemia or hypokalaemia should be investigated and treated. In chronic renal disease, it is essential to ensure adequate intake of dietary salt and water, if necessary using salt tablets. This is especially important at times of intercurrent illness, when oral intake may fall. Some of these patients also have disordered renal acidification mechanisms (renal tubular acidosis) and it is then convenient to give the sodium supplementation as sodium bicarbonate.

PRIMARY GLOMERULAR DISEASE

IMMUNOLOGICAL AND OTHER MECHANISMS OF GLOMERULAR INJURY

Many glomerular diseases, whether occurring in isolation (primary) or as part of a multisystem disease (secondary) are associated with demonstrable immunological abnormalities. Although it is not always clear whether these are involved directly in the pathogenesis of the glomerular disease, much attention has been directed towards identification of the immunological disturbances and their manipulation as part of treatment. The final common path of immunologically mediated glomerular injury is the activation of various inflammatory mediators, both cellular and soluble, which then inflict damage on the glomerulus, or less frequently on other tissue elements in the kidney (Fig. 20.17). It is likely that the production and activation of the mediators (Table 20.28) requires the presence of antigen–antibody complexes in the kidney and also of specific cell types. Clearly, both the source of these immune complexes, the identification of their antigen component(s), and the factors that control the behaviour of the involved cells are of great importance in the understanding of the diseases, and in the development of rational treatment.

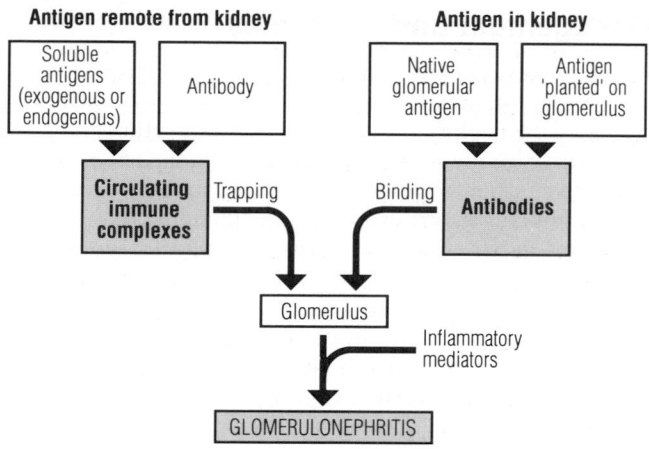

Fig. 20.17 Mechanisms of immunological glomerular injury.

Table 20.28 Initiators and mediators of glomerular injury

Cellular	Non-cellular
● Polymorphs	● Antibody
● Macrophages/monocytes	● Complement
● Lymphocytes (esp. T helper cells)	● Fibrinogen
● Platelets	● Histamine
	● Kinins
	● Prostaglandins
	● Some interleukins (esp. IL-1 and IL-2)
	● Tumour necrosis factor (TNF-α)
	● Free radicals

Two general mechanisms of immunological injury to the glomerulus are proposed.

In situ complex formation. The antigens may be an intrinsic part of the glomerulus, or may be derived from other parts of the body and be deposited or 'planted' in the glomerulus. In either case, formation of an antigen–antibody complex may occur in situ if an appropriate antibody is generated (Fig. 20.17).

Circulating complexes. The second mechanism of injury involves the generation of antibody directed against an antigen derived from sources other than the kidney. In this case, the antigen might be endogenous or exogenous. When the resulting antigen–antibody complex gains access to, or is produced in, the circulation, it can be deposited in the kidneys and there activate mediators of inflammation. Antigens suspected of mediating human glomerular disease through this mechanism are listed in Table 20.29.

The production of glomerular injury is complex and probably depends on linked cellular and non-cellular mechanisms. Immunohistopathological study or renal tissue obtained from renal biopsies or at postmortem

Table 20.29 Non-renal antigens linked with immune complex nephritis

Exogenous	Endogenous
● Bacterial	● DNA
Streptococcus	● Tumour specific
Staphylococcus	● Rbc membrane
Meningococcus	● Thyroglobulin
Treponema pallidum	● IgG
● Viral	
Hepatitis B	
Cytomegalovirus (CMV)	
● Parasitic	
Plasmodium malariae	
Schistosoma haematobium	
● Drugs	
Penicillin	
● Exogenous proteins	
Serum sickness	

sometimes reveals antibody (IgG, IgM or IgA) and complement components, the precise location and pattern of which can yield valuable diagnostic information. Furthermore, the common finding of monocytes/macrophages (producers of TNF and interleukin-1) and T helper lymphocytes (producers of interleukin-2) suggests, but does not prove, a role for these cells and cytokines in pathogenesis. Similarly, in only a minority of cases has it been possible to identify the antigenic component of the immune complexes, and even in cases where this has been achieved with certainty, it is still not clear what triggers the sequence of events that leads ultimately to glomerular injury; many patients with circulating immune complexes do not develop nephritis. Examples of human nephritis in which immune complexes are thought to play a role are given in Table 20.30.

CLINICAL PRESENTATION AND MANAGEMENT OF GLOMERULAR DISEASE

The specific glomerular diseases described below may present as one of the following:

● acute nephritic syndrome, with or without acute renal failure (p. 803)
● rapidly progressive glomerulonephritis (p. 803)
● chronic glomerulonephritis (p. 803)
● nephrotic syndrome (p. 811)
● hypertension (p. 828)
● asymptomatic haematuria and/or proteinuria (p. 813)
● recurrent macroscopic haematuria (p. 813)

Because some of these glomerular diseases may be part of a multisystem disease (e.g. SLE), problems unrelated to the kidney may dominate the clinical picture.

Table 20.30 Involvement of immune complexes in pathogenesis of nephritis

Probable	Possible
• Postinfectious GN	• Henoch-Schönlein purpura
• Infective endocarditis	• IgA nephropathy (Berger's disease)
• Shunt nephritis	• Mesangiocapillary GN
• Quartan malaria	• Idiopathic rapidly progressive GN
• Syphilis	• Membranous GN
• Hepatitis B infection	• Focal segmental glomerulosclerosis
• Systemic lupus erythematosus	

ACUTE POSTSTREPTOCOCCAL GLOMERULONEPHRITIS

Acute poststreptococcal GN is most common in children of school age, though it arises in adults and, rarely, also the very young. Males are more often affected. The preceding infection is usually in the upper respiratory tract, but can be in the skin or at other sites. There is usually a latency of 1–3 weeks. Group A, type 12, β-haemolytic streptococci are those most likely to cause acute GN.

Pathogenesis and pathology

Much circumstantial evidence points to a role for immune complexes, either circulating or formed in situ within the kidney. Immune complexes are demonstrable in serum in most cases, and activation of serum complement is frequent. A diffuse generalised proliferative glomerulonephritis is present, often with an infiltrate of polymorphs. The tubules and interstitium are relatively spared. Immunofluorescence studies show granular deposits of C3 complement and IgG in the glomeruli.

Clinical features and diagnosis

The illness typically presents as an acute nephritic syndrome with oliguria, fluid retention, hypertension, proteinuria and haematuria. The degree of renal impairment is variable.

The diagnosis is usually easy on clinical grounds alone. The urine is 'active' with red blood cells, cellular casts and protein. Evidence for preceding streptococcal infection is sought by means of swabs of throat or any suspicious skin lesion, and serological tests for streptococcal infection such as the ASO titre and anti-D-Nase B antibody. Hypocomplementaemia (low haemolytic complement and C3 with variable reduction of C2, C4 and C1q), due to alternative pathway activation (p. 84) and the presence of circulating immune complexes support the diagnosis. Renal biopsy is seldom required in children, although it may be in adults.

Management and prognosis

Antistreptococcal antibiotics (penicillin or erythromycin) are generally given although there is no evidence that they influence the nephritis. In most cases, observation and general supportive measures are sufficient. In oliguric patients, fluid retention is controlled by appropriate restriction of dietary salt and water; protein and potassium are restricted if uraemia or hyperkalaemia threaten. Hypertension is best managed by avoiding or correcting overexpansion of the ECF, with the aid of loop diuretics if necessary. Careful control of blood pressure is particularly important in children, in whom hypertensive encephalopathy may develop when the blood pressure is only moderately elevated. Rarely, severe renal failure may require temporary dialysis treatment (p. 803) pending recovery of renal function. Long-term antistreptococcal prophylaxis is not required.

Children have a better prognosis than adults. The early mortality is about 1% or less in children, but the minority in whom severe oliguria or proteinuria persist has a less favourable outcome. Long-term prognosis is uncertain, but a significant minority (up to 30%) may ultimately develop progressive renal disease, often 10 or more years later. Adults are more likely to show incomplete resolution after the initial attack and to progress thereafter to CRF.

GLOMERULONEPHRITIS IN ASSOCIATION WITH OTHER INFECTIONS

Pathology

The bacterial, viral or protozoan infections which may be complicated by GN are listed below in Table 20.31.

Bacterial

The most important bacterial-associated GN is that seen in patients with infective endocarditis. These patients usually have only mild impairment of GFR, with microscopic haematuria, proteinuria and urinary casts, in association with clinical and laboratory manifestations of endocarditis. Rarely, the renal disturbance may dominate

Table 20.31 Infections which may cause glomerulonephritis

Bacterial	Viral
Group A, β-haemolytic streptococci	Hepatitis B
Other streptococci	HIV
Staphylococci	Cytomegalovirus
Salmonella typhi	Epstein-Barr
Treponema pallidum	
Protozoan	
Plasmodium malariae	
Plasmodium falciparum	
Schistosoma haematobium	

the clinical picture with the syndrome of RPGN and renal failure. Circulating immune complexes are present and complement (C3 and C4) is reduced (classical pathway activation). Renal biopsy is only needed if the underlying diagnosis is in doubt or if renal impairment is severe and unremitting. A variety of renal lesions may be seen, but a focal proliferative GN is the commonest. Deposits of C3, IgG and IgM are conspicuous.

Other important chronic bacterial infections that may lead to GN include those arising on implanted devices (e.g. ventriculo-atrial shunts and synthetic vascular grafts) and in association with visceral abscesses.

Viral

The most important are HIV and chronic hepatitis B.

HIV. This may cause:

- HIV glomerulopathy
- acute renal failure
- electrolyte disturbances.

About 10% of HIV-infected subjects have proteinuria, in most cases with an underlying glomerulopathy (usually focal segmental glomerulosclerosis, FSGS). In most, this progresses to renal failure. The likelihood of HIV-associated glomerulopathy is greatest in full-blown AIDS, less so in AIDS-related complex, and infrequent in asymptomatic HIV infection.

ARF (with ATN) is seen in critically ill patients with sepsis and shock. Nephrotoxic drugs (pentamidine, aminoglycosides, amphotericin B) are important contributors. Hyponatraemia is the most common electrolyte disturbance, usually resulting from gastrointestinal sodium losses, or the syndrome of inappropriate ADH secretion in cases of pulmonary or CNS involvement.

Treatment. Progressive nephropathy is inevitable – no effective therapy has yet been found and survival on dialysis or after transplantation is poor.

Hepatitis B. This may lead to a variety of glomerular lesions, either in isolation or in association with hepatic involvement, or a more generalised process such as systemic vasculitis or cryoglobulinaemia.

Parasitic

Plasmodium malariae and *Schistosoma haematobium* infection are important causes of nephrotic syndrome in endemic areas. This is particularly so in children, where they must be distinguished from idiopathic nephrotic syndrome due to minimal change disease.

Management

Removal of the offending antigen, if possible, usually leads to resolution, although this may be incomplete in some cases. Renal failure is managed along conventional lines. There is no evidence that other manoeuvres, such as immunosuppressive drugs or plasma exchange, are of benefit.

MEMBRANOUS NEPHROPATHY

The majority of cases of membranous nephropathy are idiopathic, but this lesion may also arise in a variety of underlying diseases (Table 20.32).

Pathogenesis and pathology

The pathogenesis is unknown. Renal biopsies show thickening of the glomerular basement membrane, with a spike and dome pattern visible using special stains. Diffuse deposits of IgG, IgM and C3 complement are present in glomerular capillary walls. The presence of immune complexes in serum is variable and their role in the pathogenesis unsubstantiated.

Clinical features and diagnosis

Most patients present with asymptomatic proteinuria or nephrotic syndrome. In adults, membranous glomerulopathy is the commonest single cause of the nephrotic syn-

Summary 4 HIV and the kidney	
Glomerulopathy:	Present in 10% most likely in AIDS lesion is focal segmental glomerulosclerosis
Acute renal failure:	ATN sepsis, shock drug induced
Electrolyte disturbance:	hyponatraemia due to – sodium losses – inappropriate ADH

Table 20.32 Causes of membranous nephropathy

Idiopathic	Drugs/toxins
Infections	Mercury
Malaria	Organic gold (in treatment
Syphilis	of rheumatoid arthritis)
Hepatitis B	Penicillamine
	Captopril
Neoplasia	
Lymphoma } rarely	**Multisystem disease**
Leukaemia	Systemic lupus
Various carcinomas,	erythematosus
especially of the colon	Rheumatoid arthritis

drome, and a significant minority of adults will have an underlying neoplasm, colonic carcinoma being the most common. Renal function is usually normal, or nearly so, at the time of presentation, but progression to CRF is frequent, though difficult to predict. A proportion of patients, particularly those with underlying neoplasia, die of the non-renal cause of the disorder. Other complications, such as renal vein thrombosis and pulmonary emboli, are also a cause of morbidity and mortality. Hypertension becomes increasingly prevalent as the disease progresses.

The diagnosis rests on renal biopsy which should be carried out in adults and in those children whose nephrotic syndrome is resistant to corticosteroid drugs (see below).

Management

The nephrotic syndrome is managed conventionally (p. 812) and a watchful eye kept for renal vein thrombosis or pulmonary embolism, both of which are indications for anticoagulation. Treatment of the nephropathy is controversial. There is evidence that intensive immunosuppression (using corticosteroids and chlorambucil or cyclophosphamide) given for 6 months improves the long-term outlook.

MINIMAL CHANGE NEPHROPATHY

Minimal change nephropathy (known in the past as 'lipoid nephrosis') is by far the commonest cause of childhood nephrotic syndrome. It is also an important cause of nephrotic syndrome in adults.

Pathogenesis and pathology

The pathogenesis and aetiology of the condition are unknown. There is evidence of disordered T lymphocyte function, but the relevance of this to the pathogenesis is unproven. Of note, however, is the response of the lesion to steroids, alkylating agents and cyclosporin, all of which interfere with T cell function. The glomeruli are normal by light microscopy; immunofluorescence is negative. Electron microscopy shows fusion of the epithelial cell foot processes, but this is also seen in many other glomerular diseases; it is of significance only when the glomeruli appear normal under light microscopy. These features in the presence of nephrotic syndrome favour a diagnosis of minimal change nephropathy.

Clinical features and diagnosis

Children and adults usually present with oedema and are found to have nephrotic syndrome. Hypertension is rare, and renal function is usually normal. Males predominate amongst young children, but the sex incidence in adults is approximately equal. Progression to CRF is exceedingly rare, although ARF may supervene, particularly following excessive use of diuretics.

In adults, the diagnosis usually depends on renal biopsy. In children, however, the relative infrequency of other causes of nephrotic syndrome justifies a more empirical approach, especially if the proteinuria is highly selective (p. 793). In all age groups, urinary cells and cellular casts are infrequent or absent.

Management and prognosis

In 80–90% of cases, the lesion responds to steroids given at moderate to high dose for 8 weeks, most patients showing a response in less than 4 weeks. Subsequent withdrawal of steroids may be followed by prolonged remission, or lead to relapse of the nephrotic syndrome necessitating a further course of steroid treatment. In steroid-resistant patients, or in those in whom remission can only be maintained by the use of unacceptably heavy exposure to steroids (steroid dependence), cyclophosphamide or chlorambucil given for 8–10 weeks has led to prolonged remission or improved steroid responsiveness. The immunosuppressive agent, cyclosporin, is also capable of inducing remissions in previously refractory patients.

The renal lesion virtually never progresses to CRF, and since the introduction of steroids and cytotoxic therapy, the prognosis has been very good (Fig. 20.18), esp-

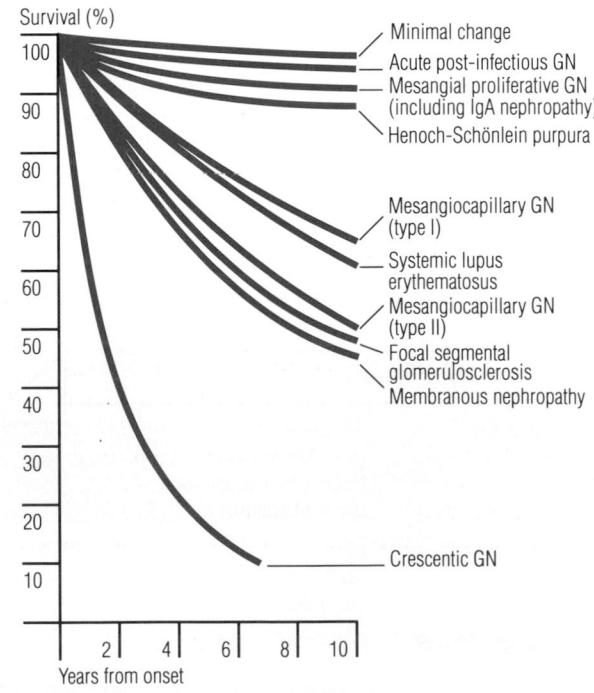

Fig. 20.18 Prognosis in various types of glomerulopathy.

cially in children. Initial failure to respond to steroids heralds a less favourable outcome. Despite the benefits of these therapies, a small number of deaths are the result of complications of treatment, particularly infection.

FOCAL SEGMENTAL GLOMERULO-SCLEROSIS

Focal segmental glomerulosclerosis (FSGS) is the second most common cause of nephrotic syndrome in children and, in contrast to minimal change GN, tends to progress to renal failure especially in children. Most cases are idiopathic, but some arise in association with underlying collagen vascular diseases.

Pathogenesis and pathology

The cause of FSGS is unknown. Although immune complexes may be found in as many as 70% of cases, there is no direct evidence of their involvement in the pathogenesis. The abnormal glomeruli are segmentally sclerosed, i.e. only a part of each glomerular tufts is affected. Early in the disease, only deep juxtamedullary glomeruli may be involved. IgM deposits are usually present, often with C3 complement.

Clinical features, diagnosis and treatment

Children present with nephrotic syndrome and adults with asymptomatic proteinuria and hypertension.

The diagnosis invariably depends on renal biopsy. In early cases, there may be confusion with minimal change nephropathy unless the biopsy contains juxtamedullary glomeruli; these may be the only ones affected early in the course of FSGS. Proteinuria is usually non-selective and urine often contains red blood cells and casts, helping to distinguish it from minimal change nephropathy.

Some cases respond to steroids, but this is unpredictable. Cytotoxic drugs have been tried without established benefit.

MESANGIOCAPILLARY GLOMERULO-NEPHRITIS

Mesangiocapillary glomerulonephritis (MCGN) comprises at least two, and possibly three, distinct diseases, each with its own characteristic glomerular pathology. The diseases best characterised are designated types I and II MCGN.

Pathogenesis and pathology

The pathogenesis is unknown and may well be different in the two types of MCGN. The glomerular pathology is characteristic. In *type I disease*, mesangial cell proliferation is marked and the glomerular basement membrane is intact, with subendothelial deposits easily visible on electron microscopy. *Type II disease* usually shows a lesser degree of mesangial cell proliferation and the electron-dense deposits appear to be intramembranous. IgG and complement are present, more consistently so, and in greater amounts, in type I MCGN. Persistent depression of plasma C3 complement is often found, particularly in patients with type II disease, and indicates complement activation by the alternative pathway. Circulating immune complexes are detectable in some patients.

Clinical features

Both types of MCGN may present with nephrotic syndrome, nephritic syndrome, hypertension or asymptomatic proteinuria/haematuria, and the majority of the presentations are in children or young adults. Slow progression to CRF is usual, though unpredictable. A minority of patients, usually with the type II variant, progress more rapidly and in a few patients there is a fulminant course to ESRD. It appears that those patients presenting with full-blown nephrotic syndrome do worse than those with asymptomatic urinary abnormalities.

Diagnosis and management

The diagnosis depends on renal biopsy. The glomerular morphology of type I MCGN may be seen in patients with underlying SLE, hepatitis B infection and chronic bacterial infection (such as infective endocarditis) and steps should be taken to identify or exclude these conditions.

Steroids, with or without cytotoxic drugs, are probably not useful and may be harmful. Antiplatelet drugs and anticoagulants have also been tried and may be of benefit, but this remains to be confirmed.

IGA NEPHROPATHY (BERGER'S DISEASE)

Pathogenesis and pathology

In IgA nephropathy (Berger's disease), the glomeruli show extensive mesangial deposits of IgA, often accompanied by C3 complement. This pattern is also seen in patients with Henoch-Schönlein purpura. Diffuse mesangial proliferation with superimposed segmental lesions are seen on light microscopy. A closely related variant, differing only by the presence of IgM in place of IgA, also exists, and has the same clinical features and management as IgA nephropathy.

Clinical features

This is predominantly a disease of young adult men, many of whom present with recurrent macroscopic haematuria sometimes accompanied by loin pain (p. 813). Proteinuria is variable, and cellular casts in the urine confirm the glomerular origin of the red blood cells. Relapses may show a temporal relation with upper respiratory infections. The condition has had a benign reputation, but undoubtedly may progress to CRF, particularly if hypertension or proteinuria is present early in the course. Occasionally, the disease may manifest itself with an acute nephritic syndrome.

Diagnosis and management

Although the clinical picture is often highly characteristic, renal biopsy is nearly always performed to establish the diagnosis with certainty. The IgA deposits that characterise the renal lesion are also evident in skin capillaries and this finding supports the diagnosis, even in the absence of renal biopsy. These patients should be spared fruitless and inappropriate urological investigation; a careful history and examination of the urinary deposit will usually indicate whether or not the haematuria is glomerular.

In many cases, the lesion is benign and observation only is required. No therapeutic intervention has been shown to alter the course of the progressive or relapsing disease.

IDIOPATHIC RAPIDLY PROGRESSIVE GLOMERULONEPHRITIS

Idiopathic RPGN is a serious condition which, as its name suggests, frequently progresses to renal failure.

Pathogenesis and pathology

There is little to suggest involvement of the immune system in this disease; neither circulating immune complexes nor glomerular deposits of immunoglobulin and C3 are evident in most cases. The hallmark is the presence of glomerular crescents containing large amounts of fibrin. Similar crescentic lesions are found in some patients with other types of GN, including those associated with polyarteritis, SLE and infective endocarditis.

Clinical features and diagnosis

The usual presentation is a sub-acute nephritic syndrome with malaise, hypertension, haematuria and proteinuria. Middle-aged and older adults predominate. Without treatment, the outlook is very poor.

RPGN should be suspected in any patient with apparent acute or sub-acute onset of renal impairment, particularly if the urine is 'active' with red blood cells and cellular casts. Assessment of renal size will identify those patients with normal-sized kidneys in whom CRF is unlikely. Renal biopsy is then required to establish the diagnosis.

Management

Empirical treatment with high doses of steroid drugs appears to be of some benefit, but these agents should not be given for more than 4 weeks unless there is clear evidence of a response. Cytotoxic drugs and plasma exchange have been tried and there are many anecdotal reports of success. Limited controlled studies suggest that standard therapy should comprise high-dose steroids, a cytotoxic drug such as cyclophosphamide or azathioprine (the latter possibly less effective) and intensive plasma exchange.

HEREDITARY NEPHRITIS (ALPORT'S SYNDROME)

Alport's syndrome is an inherited disorder that is characterised by progressive renal impairment and nerve deafness. Presentation is usually with microscopic or gross haematuria. Males tend to be more severely affected than females, particularly with regard to the nephropathy; and associated deafness is variable or even absent in some patients. The mode of inheritance is inconsistent, with some families showing a dominant, and others an X-linked pattern. The renal lesion is predominantly glomerular; although there are no specific features on light microscopy, electron microscopy reveals a thin, fragmented and sometimes split glomerular basement membrane. There is no known treatment.

RENAL INVOLVEMENT IN NON-RENAL AND MULTISYSTEM DISEASE

Involvement of the kidney occurs in many diseases. In most of these, the glomerulus is the site of damage, with a GN that may give rise to any of the syndromes of glomerular disease. The renal manifestations are of variable severity but, in some cases, dominate the clinical picture.

SYSTEMIC LUPUS ERYTHEMATOSUS

Renal involvement in SLE may manifest itself with haematuria/proteinuria, acute nephritic syndrome, nephrotic syndrome or chronic renal impairment. At least four glomerular lesions are described, all associated with deposition of complement and immunoglobulins within the glomeruli and with activation of complement and the presence of circulating immune complexes. The most benign lesion comprises deposition of Ig's and complement in an otherwise normal, or slightly abnormal, glomerulus. Focal and segmental proliferative GN and membranous GN both have an unpredictable prognosis, while diffuse proliferative GN with SLE progresses to renal failure in the majority of cases. In a few patients, tubulo-interstitial involvement dominates, with demonstrable Ig and C3 deposition on the tubular basement membrane.

Treatment. The need to treat is dictated by evidence of progressive renal disease and/or the presence of a renal lesion that is likely to progress. Steroids, often in combination with cytotoxic drugs such as cyclophosphamide or azathioprine, are used, sometimes with plasma exchange. Regimens that include a cytotoxic drug, especially cyclophosphamide given intravenously, are more effective at preventing progression of nephropathy than are steroids alone.

POLYARTERITIS

Polyarteritis usually affects the middle-aged and elderly, with males predominating. Renal involvement is frequent and in some cases the disease may appear to be limited to the kidneys at the time of presentation. Patients with involvement of medium-sized vessels, so-called *polyarteritis nodosa* or *classical polyarteritis*, suffer the consequences of renal ischaemia with hypertension, renal infarction and renal failure. Diagnosis can be made by skin biopsy, by visceral arteriography which may show multiple small aneurysms in the kidney or other viscera, or by renal biopsy in which arteritic lesions may be seen.

Microscopic polyarteritis on the other hand usually presents with an acute or subacute nephritic syndrome, often with purpura, arthropathy and myopathy. Clinically it may resemble Henoch-Schönlein purpura. Renal biopsies show a florid necrotising GN. Antineutrophil cytoplasmic antibodies (ANCA) are often present in serum.

Treatment. Both types usually respond to treatment with high-dose steroids and cyclophosphamide. (Polyarteritis is discussed further in Ch. 23, p. 1031).

WEGENER'S GRANULOMATOSIS

Wegener's granulomatosis (see also Ch. 23, p. 1031) has features in common with microscopic polyarteritis, including the presence of ANCA, but may be distinguished by its propensity for involvement of the upper airways and lungs and by the granulomatous nature of the arteritic lesions. Renal biopsies show necrotising glomerulitis, which usually manifests itself clinically with an

acute nephritic syndrome. The prognosis has improved greatly with the use of cyclophosphamide and steroids which control the disease in the majority of cases.

HENOCH-SCHÖNLEIN PURPURA

Henoch-Schönlein purpura is a condition of children and young adults who present with some or all of the following: GN, skin purpura, arthralgia/arthritis, abdominal pain. The renal lesion is a mesangial-proliferative GN with prominent IgA deposits. IgA is also deposited in skin and other tissues, in this respect resembling IgA nephropathy (Berger's disease). Disease activity is intermittent and tends to involve several organs at once. The GN is usually benign, especially in children, but may progress rapidly or slowly following a series of acute episodes with incomplete resolution. An immune complex aetiology is probable and no treatment has proven efficacy; immunosuppression with steroids, cytotoxic drugs and plasma exchange is often tried in severe cases.

SYSTEMIC SCLEROSIS

Visceral involvement in systemic sclerosis frequently includes the kidneys, in which marked thickening of the walls of the medium-sized arteries occurs (see also p. 1029). The glomerular lesions are those of ischaemia and severe accelerated-phase hypertension is a frequent complication. The aetiology is unknown and there is no effective treatment for the underlying condition. ACE inhibitors allow effective blood pressure control in most of these patients, and this results in a greatly improved renal prognosis, although other manifestations of the disease, particularly cardiac, remain potentially lethal.

RHEUMATOID ARTHRITIS

Renal disease in patients with rheumatoid arthritis is usually the result of secondary amyloid (AA type) or of adverse reaction to antirheumatic drugs such as gold, penicillamine or non-steroidal anti-inflammatory agents.

However, a few patients, particularly those with widespread vasculitis, may develop GN or renal vasculitis. Steroids and cytotoxic drugs have been effective in some cases.

GOODPASTURE'S SYNDROME

The term Goodpasture's syndrome refers to a disease in which the following features are present: lung haemorrhage, GN and formation of antibody to glomerular basement membrane (anti-GBM antibody). A *pulmonary-renal syndrome* can also arise in several other diseases, such as Wegener's granulomatosis, SLE and Legionnaire's disease, and often has clinical features indistinguishable from Goodpasture's syndrome. Anti-GBM antibody is absent in these conditions.

The reason for the formation of anti-GBM antibody is unknown; it probably plays a central part in the pathogenesis of the disease, and renal biopsies show linear deposits of IgG and C3 complement along the glomerular capillary walls, accompanied by a proliferative GN, often with crescent formation. The anti-GBM antibody is also demonstrable in lung, and deposits there probably mediate the lung haemorrhage.

The disease predominates in young male adults and there is considerable case-to-case variation. Either the pulmonary or the renal lesions may dominate the clinical picture.

Treatment centres around attempts to remove the offending antibody by means of plasma exchange, and to prevent its reappearance by the use of cytotoxic drugs. This approach, with dialysis support when needed, has greatly improved the outlook.

OTHER ACQUIRED COLLAGEN VASCULAR DISEASES

Mixed connective tissue disease (p. 505), essential mixed cryoglobulinaemia (p. 1101), sarcoidosis (p. 500) and Sjögren's syndrome (p. 999) may all be associated with GN, in addition to the more frequent association between Sjögren's syndrome and interstitial nephropathy (p. 826).

Table 20.33 Mechanisms of renal disturbance in malignant disease

Mechanism	Example
Obstruction	Carcinoma of prostate, bladder, cervix, rectum Para-aortic lymphadenopathy Intrarenal, e.g. urate, Bence-Jones proteinuria
Direct invasion of kidney	Leukaemia Hodgkin's disease and other lymphomas Myeloma
Secondary glomerulopathy Membranous nephropathy Minimal change glomerulopathy	Associated with carcinoma of lung, stomach, colon, breast, ovary Associated with Hodgkin's disease, lymphoma or leukaemia
Tumour-induced metabolic disturbance	Hypercalcaemia Urate nephropathy Syndrome of inappropriate ADH secretion (SIADHS)

NEOPLASTIC DISEASE

Malignancy may disturb kidney function in a number of ways (Table 20.33). Both isolated solid tumours or diffuse neoplasms of lymphoid tissue may be involved. *Tumour lysis syndrome* results from the very rapid release of urate and phosphate from a tumour undergoing necrosis, and may lead to acute renal failure from acute uric acid nephropathy. The specific instance of multiple myeloma and the dysproteinaemias is discussed below.

DYSPROTEINAEMIA, MULTIPLE MYELOMA AND RENAL AMYLOID

Multiple myeloma and the other dysproteinaemias may all involve the kidneys and at least 50% of patients with multiple myeloma will ultimately die of renal failure. The most important renal manifestations are *amyloid* (p. 1101) and *myeloma kidney* (Table 20.34).

Amyloid in patients with myeloma is of the AL type and its presence in the kidney (and an associated nephrotic syndrome) may antedate other clinical manifestations of myeloma. The nature of the renal lesion is similar, whether the amyloid is associated with underlying multiple myeloma, unassociated with malignant disease, or secondary to a chronic inflammatory process, such as sepsis or rheumatoid arthritis (amyloid of AA type). There is no specific treatment for the renal lesion, which usually progresses inexorably, although it is possible that chemotherapy of the myeloma at an early stage of the disease may slow or halt the progression of the amyloid as well.

Myeloma kidney is a tubulointerstitial nephropathy caused by nephrotoxic immunoglobulin light chains (Bence-Jones protein) in the glomerular filtrate. Recovery is unpredictable, and depends on successful treatment of the myeloma and reduction of the urinary Bence-Jones protein load. Even so, this lesion is often irreversible.

Table 20.34 Renal damage in multiple myeloma

- Bence-Jones proteinuria
- Myeloma kidney
- Hypercalcaemia
- Hyperuricaemia (especially at initiation of chemotherapy)
- Renal amyloid
- Dehydration ± X-ray contrast media (combination prone to induce ARF)
- Plasma cell infiltration
- Glomerulonephritis (immunologically mediated)
- Hyperviscosity syndrome (e.g. in macroglobulinaemia) may cause papillary necrosis
- Obstruction (by stone or sloughed papillae)

DIABETES MELLITUS

Diabetic glomerulopathy

Renal involvement in diabetes becomes progressively more common with increasing duration of disease, such that after 20 years, some 30% of diabetics will have proteinuria or other evidence of nephropathy. Surprisingly, the emergence of nephropathy more than 30 years after the initial diagnosis of diabetes is unusual, i.e. most diabetics who are destined for nephropathy will get it within 20–30 years. Type 1 and Type 2 diabetics are affected usually, though not always, with associated malignant vasculopathy and with other vascular complications of diabetes mellitus.

Glomerular changes predominate and are of two types:

- *diffuse glomerulosclerosis,* in which there is thickening of the glomerular basement membrane, capillary wall and mesangium. This lesion is common, but is not specific for diabetes mellitus
- *nodular glomerulosclerosis (Kimmelstiel-Wilson lesion),* which is specific for diabetes mellitus but is present in only a minority of patients.

The pathogenesis of diabetic nephropathy is unknown but attention has focused on two main possibilities:

- *Genetic.* The renal lesion is a manifestation of a genetic defect that also leads to carbohydrate intolerance. Various observations make this unlikely, in particular the finding of diabetic nephropathy in some 'non-genetic' cases, e.g. following pancreatectomy, and the appearance of diabetic lesions in 'normal' kidneys transplanted into diabetic recipients.
- *Acquired.* The renal lesion is acquired and is secondary to either lack of insulin, hyperglycaemia or both. This is now the favoured explanation, although the mechanism is unclear.

The disease generally passes through four recognisable phases:

- hyperfiltration with supranormal GFR
- microalbuminuria (but still dipstick-negative)
- proteinuria (dipstick-positive)
- heavy proteinuria (with nephrotic syndrome or renal failure).

Hypertension develops in virtually all these patients. Deterioration is inevitable, though its rate is unpredictable.

There is now, however, great interest in the possibility that reduction of the glomerular hypertension that is known to coexist with hyperfiltration early in diabetes may slow the development of nephropathy. In the short term, this can be achieved by means of very tight glycaemic control, protein restriction or use of ACE inhibitors (p. 810). Coexistent arterial hypertension accelerates progression; conversely, intensive antihypertensive therapy to the point of absolute normotension retards progression. There is no convincing evidence that good control of blood sugar prevents the development of nephropathy in clinical practice, although it is not yet clear whether this pessimistic view applies to the very tight control that is now available using insulin pumps. Certainly, some of the early functional abnormalities (hyperfiltration and microalbuminuria) can be reversed in this way, but this question is unlikely to be resolved for 10–20 years, because of the long latent period between the onset of diabetes and the appearance of complications.

Other renal complications of diabetes

Urinary tract infection (UTI) is more common in diabetics and is also more likely to be complicated by acute pyelonephritis, papillary necrosis and pyonephrosis. Autonomic neuropathy may impair bladder function, increasing the risk of ascending UTI.

Renal replacement therapy in diabetics

Haemodialysis, CAPD and renal transplantation are all used in diabetes, but coexisting retinopathy, cardiac and arterial disease (all frequently present) greatly reduce the success of those treatments and the survival prospects of diabetics with renal failure are poor.

SICKLE CELL DISORDERS

The most important renal complications seen in sickle cell disorders (discussed in Ch. 24, p. 1063) are recurrent gross haematuria, papillary necrosis and glomerulonephritis.

INTRAVASCULAR COAGULATION

Several conditions may lead to intravascular coagulation (Ch. 24, p. 1108) and renal impairment, but these two features are especially characteristic in *haemolytic uraemic syndrome* (HUS) and *thrombotic thrombocytopenic purpura.* In both these conditions, there is evidence of microangiopathic haemolytic anaemia (MAHA) and thrombocytopenia. Although laboratory features are similar, HUS is mainly a disease of children with prominent renal involvement, whereas thrombotic thrombocytopenic purpura usually affects adults and renal disease is more variable. The aetiology is uncertain, although HUS appears to follow viral or bacterial infections in children and also has shown case clustering in schools or families. Recent evidence has implicated verucytotoxin producing *E. coli* infection: patients with HUS produce antibody to verucytotoxin and the toxin itself can produce similar angiopathic lesions in rabbits. A rare disease indistinguishable from haemolytic uraemic syndrome has been recognised following apparently normal pregnancy and also in women taking the contraceptive pill. Treatment of these conditions is difficult, and the best prospects are offered by a combination of anti-platelet drugs and infusions of fresh plasma.

GOUTY NEPHROPATHY

Man excretes urate/uric acid in amounts that are very high considering the low solubility of uric acid at acid pH. Three types of clinical problem may arise:

Uric acid stone formation (p. 833).

Acute uric acid nephropathy. This is due to massive deposition of uric acid crystals in the tubules, renal pelvis and ureters and arises as a complication of accelerated uric acid production during treatment of widespread malignancy, such as lymphoma or leukaemia (Ch. 24, p. 1081). The xanthine oxidase inhibitor, allopurinol, usually provides adequate prophylaxis.

Chronic urate (gouty) nephropathy. This is a common accompaniment of prolonged hyperuricaemia, itself strongly associated with clinical gout. The renal damage is mainly interstitial, although glomerular changes also occur. Sodium urate crystals may be demonstrable in renal tissue in some cases. Management is prophylactic using allopurinol to decrease plasma and urine urate levels. Established chronic urate nephropathy is irreversible, although progression may be halted or slowed by allopurinol therapy.

DISEASES OF THE RENAL INTERSTITIUM

Diseases of the renal interstitium are sometimes collectively termed 'tubulointerstitial disease' or 'interstitial nephropathy'.

Aetiology and pathology

The tubulointerstitial nephropathies are distinguished from the glomerulopathies by relative sparing of the glomeruli and prominent changes affecting the nonglomerular components of the renal parenchyma, i.e. the interstitium and tubules. The causes of tubulointerstitial disease are given in Table 20.35.

Acute tubulointerstitial nephropathy is characterised by prominent interstitial oedema with a heavy infiltrate of inflammatory cells, amongst which neutrophils, eosinophils or mononuclear cells may predominate.

Table 20.35 Causes of tubulointerstitial disease

Cause	Acute	Chronic
Idiopathic	+	+
Drug hypersensitivity		
Penicillin	+	
Cephalosporins	+	
Sulphonamides	+	
Diuretics	+	
NSAIDs	+	
Toxin-induced		
Aminoglycoside antibiotics	+	
Cisplatin	+	+
Pentamidine	+	+
Analgesic abuse		+
Lithium		+
X-ray contrast media	+	
Heavy metals	+	+
Immunological disorders		
Sjögren's syndrome		+
SLE		+
Neoplasia		
Myeloma kidney	+	+
Leukaemic infiltration		+
Metabolic		
Hypercalcaemia	+	+
Hypokalaemia	+	+
Uric acid	+	+
Other		
Acute pyelonephritis	+	
Chronic pyelonephritis		+
Reflux		+
Obstruction	+	+
Sickle cell disorder		+

In contrast, *chronic tubulointerstitial nephropathy* is associated with marked tubular atrophy, interstitial fibrosis and an infiltrate of mononuclear cells.

Patients may present with ARF (p. 800), CRF (p. 803) or a tubular syndrome (p. 814). Heavy proteinaemia (>3 g/day) is exceedingly uncommon. In general, although by no means always, tubulointerstitial diseases are less likely to be associated with oliguria or anuria and are more likely to give rise to one or more of the renal tubular syndromes than are the glomerulopathies.

Many nephrotoxins act primarily on the interstitial tissues. In some cases, toxicity may be confined to the kidney, while others may involve several organs. Drugs are an important cause of toxicity, antibiotic and antirheumatic agents being particularly important (see p. 833). *Analgesic nephropathy* is a tubulointerstitial disease that results from prolonged exposure to certain mild analgesics. Phenacetin (now withdrawn) was implicated, but there is also evidence that aspirin, and NSAIDs may be involved in some cases. The disease eventually leads to ischaemic necrosis of the renal papillae and CRF; in the past, analgesic nephropathy was one of the major causes of ESRD in a number of developed countries.

Conditions such as renal obstruction (p. 835), reflux nephropathy and infection (p. 832) and multisystem diseases of the kidney (p. 822) may lead to severe interstitial damage. Obstruction (p. 835), reflux and infection (p. 830) are discussed in detail elsewhere, but nevertheless fall into the broad category of tubulointerstitial nephropathy.

Diagnosis and management

The frequency of drug-induced acute or chronic tubulointerstitial nephropathy indicates that the diagnosis should be carefully considered in any patient presenting with an unexplained acute or chronic renal disturbance. A history of relevant drug exposure should be sought, and in many cases a renal biopsy will be needed to define the renal lesion and the potential for recovery. In most cases, the treatment is expectant, with removal or avoidance of any relevant nephrotoxin if possible, and treatment of any underlying immunological disorder. Acute idiopathic cases and those associated with hypersensitivity reactions to drugs, such as penicillin, may benefit from a short course of steroids and generally have a good prognosis. Chronicity and the presence of marked tubular atrophy or

interstitial fibrosis on biopsy are adverse features, although progression may be very slow.

CYSTIC DISEASES OF THE KIDNEY

Renal cysts are relatively common and vary greatly in significance. Table 20.36 gives a classification of the important types, of which the most important are:

- adult polycystic kidney disease
- simple cysts (single or multiple)
- neoplastic cysts.

Less common are medullary cystic disease (MCD) and juvenile nephronopthisis.

ADULT POLYCYSTIC KIDNEY DISEASE

Adult polycystic kidney disease is an important cause of renal failure, accounting for 5–10% of all cases of ESRD. It is inherited as an autosomal dominant and the penetrance is 100%. Genetic counselling is therefore important. The gene has been localised to chromosome 16 close to the α-globin locus, enabling presymptomatic and prenatal diagnosis by DNA markers in some families.

Clinical features

Presentation may be with microscopic or macroscopic haematuria, hypertension, renal pain (associated with haemorrhage into a cyst or infection), CRF or identification of enlarged kidneys. Progressive enlargement of the cysts leading to impairment of renal function is the rule, about 10–20 years elapsing between presentation and ESRD in most cases. About 30% of patients also have hepatic cysts; these are not associated with hepatic dysfunction. There appears to be an increased incidence of subarachnoid haemorrhage in patients with adult polycystic kidney disease, and 10–22% of patients may have intracranial aneurysms.

Diagnosis and management

Diagnosis is easy in advanced cases, where the enlarged kidneys may be palpated and their gross morphology assessed by renal ultrasound. However, in early cases, particularly in children and young adult relatives of affected patients presenting for screening, diagnosis may be extremely difficult. Good quality renal ultrasound offers the best combination of accuracy, sensitivity and acceptability to the patient, although the sensitivity of CT scanning may be slightly better than that of ultrasound. Renal biopsy is not appropriate in these patients.

Table 20.36 Cystic diseases of the kidney

Cystic disease	Clinical and pathological features
Polycystic kidney disease	
Adult polycystic kidney disease	Common. Dominant inheritance. Renal failure. Associated with hepatic cysts but no hepatic disease
Juvenile polycystic kidney disease	Rare. Recessive inheritance. Hepatic cysts, renal and hepatic failure
Simple cysts	
Single / Multiple	Common. Often asymptomatic
Neoplastic cysts	Renal cell tumour (hypernephroma)
Medullary cysts	
Medullary cystic disease	Usually dominant inheritance; presents in adolescence. Renal failure
Juvenile nephronophthisis	Recessive; presents in childhood. Renal failure
Medullary sponge kidney	Tubular ectasia. Nephrocalcinosis. Recurrent urinary infections

Complications include hypertension, urinary infections and stone formation, and bleeding into cysts or the urine. Energetic treatment of these problems probably retards progression but, at present, there are no means of slowing or preventing the underlying process of cyst enlargement and renal damage.

SIMPLE CYSTS

Simple cysts may be single or multiple. If large enough, they may present with loin pain or a loin mass, but they are more frequently detected incidentally during the course of renal imaging for other reasons.

NEOPLASTIC CYSTS

Some renal tumours may exhibit cyst formation and it is therefore most important to distinguish accurately between benign simple cysts and neoplastic cysts. This can often be achieved with acceptable certainty by careful imaging, ultrasound or CT. However, it may be necessary to aspirate the cysts percutaneously and perform cytological examination of the fluid or renal arteriography in doubtful cases.

JUVENILE POLYCYSTIC KIDNEY DISEASE

Juvenile polycystic kidney disease is an uncommon recessively inherited disorder also associated with hepatic fibrosis and cysts. Renal and/or hepatic failure develop early.

MEDULLARY CYSTIC DISEASE AND JUVENILE NEPHRONOPTHISIS

Medullary cystic disease (autosomal dominant) and juvenile nephronopthisis (autosomal recessive) are causes of renal failure in early adulthood and childhood respectively. The prominent tubulointerstitial involvement leads to urinary concentrating defects and other tubular syndromes. There is no specific treatment.

RENAL DISEASE AND HYPERTENSION

The kidney and blood pressure interact in a number of ways and the final common paths of these interactions are such that:

● the kidney may cause hypertension
● the kidney may be damaged by hypertension.

Raised blood pressure as a consequence of renal or renal vascular disease

Hypertension is much commoner in patients with renal diseases than in the population at large, and the incidence of hypertension in such patients increases as renal function declines. By the time that CRF occurs, at least 80% of patients will be, or will have been, hypertensive.

It appears that two major processes, acting either in isolation or (probably more frequently) in concert, underlie the raised blood pressure in these patients. These are:

● increases in body sodium and water content
● inappropriately increased activity of the renin–angiotensin–aldosterone system.

Increased body sodium and water content. The most clear-cut example is the anephric patient receiving regular dialysis treatment. Here, the renin–angiotensin system is essentially non-functioning, and blood pressure is found to be closely related to the level of ECF expansion, rising as body sodium/water are allowed to increase and falling when sodium/water are removed by dialysis. Inhibition of the renin–angiotensin system by converting-enzyme inhibitors has only minor effects on blood pressure.

Increased activity of the renin–angiotensin–aldosterone system. In some patients in whom there is no evidence of excess body sodium and water, ACE inhibition dramatically reduces blood pressure, implying dependence of the elevated blood pressure on the renin–angiotensin–aldosterone system.

In practice, hypertension in most renal patients is probably a result of both mechanisms outlined above. Impaired ability to excrete sodium/water favours ECF expansion and a rise in blood pressure. In a normal individual, this would trigger a pressure-induced natriuresis and neurohumoral responses (including decreased renin release and increased release of atrial natriuretic peptide (ANP), both of which favour natriuresis (Fig. 20.19). The abnormal kidney, however, may show a blunted natriuretic response and may also fail to demonstrate appropriate suppression of renin release under these circumstances. Thus, volume expansion develops, the renin–angiotensin–aldosterone system is unsuppressed and hypertension ensues.

Renal damage as a consequence of raised blood pressure

The effect of raised blood pressure on the kidney depends on its severity, chronicity and whether or not the hypertension is in the *benign phase* or the *accelerated phase* (p. 431). It is doubtful whether hypertension in the benign phase poses a serious threat to renal function in the short or medium term, although there is evidence that black races

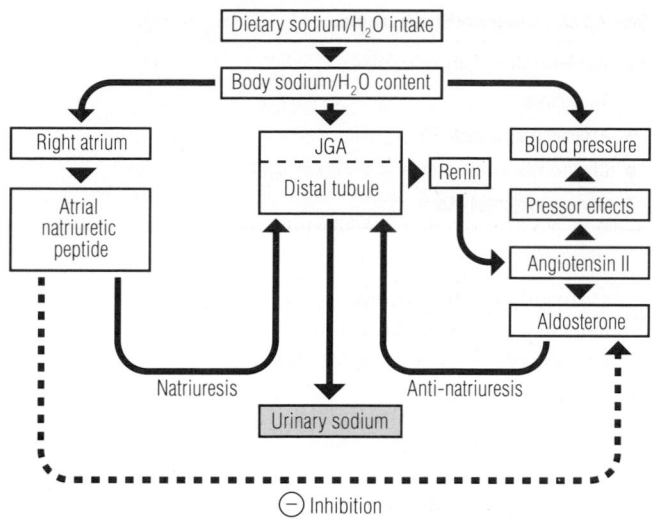

Fig. 20.19 Renal hypertension.

may be more susceptible to renal damage in this setting. In contrast, the accelerated phase of hypertension is associated with florid changes in the renal circulation, with fibrinoid necrosis and very marked endothelial cell proliferation giving rise to the so-called 'onion peel' appearance of the small blood vessels. These lesions are remarkably similar to those seen in patients with systemic sclerosis (p. 823). Rapid progression to renal failure is the rule, unless the spiral of increasing blood pressure and increasingly severe glomerular ischaemia is interrupted by means of effective hypotensive treatment.

Management

Hypertension with underlying renal parenchymal disease

The aim of treatment is the normalisation of blood pressure, achieved in most cases by a combination of dietary manipulation and drugs. The following possibilities must be considered:

- Is the patient fluid-overloaded? (Physical signs include raised JVP, peripheral oedema, pulmonary oedema.)
- Is the patient in the benign or the accelerated phase of hypertension? (The signs are mainly in the optic fundi; grade III or grade IV changes indicate accelerated phase and the need for immediate treatment.)

Those patients in whom volume expansion is a major factor will respond well to a combination of dietary sodium restriction and a loop diuretic such as frusemide (thiazides do not work well in patients with significant impairment of renal function). It is important not to cause excessive reduction in body sodium/water; to do so

would introduce a 'prerenal factor' which could further compromise renal function.

Patients in whom there is no evidence of volume overload, or who have not responded adequately to therapeutic reduction of body sodium/water, will usually respond well to inhibition of the renin–angiotensin system (ACE inhibitors), reflecting the overactivity of this system in the genesis of their hypertension.

Hypertension with underlying renal vascular disease

Regardless of the site of the arterial lesion (renal artery, branches of the renal artery, arcuate or interlobular vessels), the result is reduced renal blood flow, reduced pulse pressure at the baroreceptor in the JGA, and consequently increased release of renin by the JGA. In these patients, overactivity of the renin–angiotensin system is usually the dominant factor. Body sodium/water status is variable and successful inhibition of the renin–angiotensin system with a beta-blocker or ACE inhibitor is likely to control blood pressure, if necessary with the help of a diuretic or additional hypotensive agents. ACE inhibitors may cause a profound reduction in GFR in patients with critical renal artery stenosis, and are contraindicated if the stenosis is bilateral, or affects a solitary functioning kidney.

Disease of the renal artery

Disease of the renal artery poses a particular therapeutic problem because, in some cases, correction of the stenotic lesion will cure or ameliorate the hypertension and, if the stenotic lesion is severe, improve renal function. Stenosis of the renal artery is most often atheromatous and is therefore likely to be seen in middle-aged and elderly people with risk factors for arterial disease. A smaller number arise in young women in whom the pathology is fibromuscular hyperplasia of the renal artery. In both instances, the disease may be unilateral or bilateral.

Treatment, when indicated (see below), may be by open operation or balloon dilatation (angioplasty). Two considerations may lead to a decision to undertake angioplasty or surgery for renal artery stenosis:

- *The belief that correction of the lesion will cure or ameliorate the hypertension.* This is often very difficult to predict, but is more likely when the patient is young, when the hypertension is of very recent onset, when the disease is unilateral and confined to the renal artery, and when renal venous blood sampling shows plasma renin activity much higher on the affected side than elsewhere in the circulation.
- *The hope that renal function can be improved by correction of the stenotic lesion.* This usually involves

patients with bilateral atheromatous lesions in whom progression of the atheroma may lead to total occlusion, with catastrophic loss of renal function.

Unilateral renal disease and hypertension

Unilateral renal disease of any kind can cause hypertension. Nephrectomy may be considered in such cases, when the following indications apply:

- the kidney is dangerous, such as with renal tumour
- the kidney is useless and there is a good chance of 'surgical cure' of hypertension.

URINARY TRACT INFECTION, PYELONEPHRITIS AND TUBERCULOSIS

URINARY TRACT INFECTION

Infection of the urinary tract is exceedingly common, but in the vast majority of cases it is mild and easily treated. Table 20.37 lists the most common infecting organisms. A working definition of urinary tract infection (UTI) is the presence, in an appropriately collected mid-stream specimen of urine (MSU), of more than 10^{-5} colony forming units per ml of urine. However, this is merely an arbitrary limit above which significant infection is likely and below which infection is less likely. Exceptions are frequent. The diagnosis is made more likely if there is accompanying pyuria (evident on microscopic examination of the urine) and much less likely if more than one organism is isolated. *Sterile pyuria* is defined as white cells in the urine in the absence of significant bacterial growth. The causes of sterile pyuria are shown in Table 20.38. As UTI most frequently arises by means of ascending infection, faecal organisms predominate (Table 20.37). *M. tuberculosis* usually reaches the kidney by the haematogenous route.

Predisposing factors

Several factors predispose to development of UTI:

- *Female sex.* The male urethra is longer than the female one, which, together with the antibacterial action of prostatic secretions, probably accounts for the sub-

Table 20.37 Urinary pathogens

E. coli	Staphylococci
Enterococci	Klebsiella
Proteus	Candida (usually catheter associated)
Enterobacter	Mycobacterium tuberculosis
Pseudomonas	

Table 20.38 Causes of sterile pyuria

- Recently treated urinary infection
- Tuberculosis
- Acute interstitial nephritis
- Chronic interstitial nephritis (including analgesic nephropathy)
- Chronic pyelonephritis

stantially higher incidence of UTI in females of all ages as compared with males.
- *Failure of complete bladder emptying.* The most important causes are outflow obstruction due to prostatic hypertrophy in males and neurological diseases leading to functional disturbances of micturition in either sex.
- *Anatomical disorders of the bladder.* These may be congenital or acquired (e.g. bladder diverticulum, cystocoele).
- *Vesicoureteric reflux.* Reflux of urine into the ureters or kidney during micturition is abnormal, and, as well as predisposing to UTI, also renders ascent of the infection to the kidney much more likely. It is commonest in children and its importance lies in its likely role in the aetiology of chronic pyelonephritis (p. 832).
- *Pregnancy.* The ureters and renal pelves dilate during normal pregnancy and it is probable that this contributes to the substantially increased incidence of UTI and pyelonephritis seen in pregnant women.
- *Diabetes mellitus.* Diabetics as a whole suffer more UTIs than non-diabetics. This increase is confined largely to those patients with long-standing disease and neuropathic bladder dysfunction. Young diabetics are not at risk of UTI.
- *Tumours.* UTI may be the first sign of an underlying bladder tumour.
- *Stones.* The presence of stones anywhere in the urinary tract makes infection more likely and also renders it much harder to eliminate.
- *Foreign body.* Indwelling bladder catheters, nephrostomy tubes and ureteric stents all favour infection.

Clinical features

The presentation of UTI depends on the location and type of infection, though the relationship between apparent location of infection based on symptoms (i.e. bladder or kidney) does not always correlate with definitively demonstrated site of infection.

Urethral syndrome. Urethral syndrome is the combination of dysuria, frequency, urgency and strangury without demonstrable UTI as defined above. Women are affected exclusively and the disorder is probably heterogeneous, resulting from mechanical factors (sexual intercourse), chemical irritation (toiletries) or atypical infection (chlamydia, viruses or bacteria in small numbers).

Cystitis. Symptoms are those of the urethral syndrome and range from trivial to severe. They are accompanied by pyuria and significant bacteriuria. The urine is usually cloudy and may be foul smelling. A variable degree of constitutional disturbance is usually present and, in a minority of cases, the infection may ascend leading to acute pyelonephritis (see below).

Asymptomatic bacteriuria. In adults, the incidental finding of significant bacteriuria is generally of little consequence, although pregnant women show a propensity for the asymptomatic bacteriuria to progress to cystitis and acute pyelonephritis. However, in children the position is less clear, in that a significant minority will prove to have associated abnormalities of the urinary tract. In both children and adults, spontaneous resolution is quite common and, with the exception of pregnant women and children with vesicoureteric reflux, antibiotic therapy is not of value.

Acute pyelonephritis. This usually results from ascending infection and may be preceded by a clinical episode of cystitis. Rarely, it may be acquired haematogenously. There is usually a substantial constitutional disturbance, with fever, rigors and malaise. Renal pain and tenderness is usual, and the infection may occasionally be very severe with bacteraemia, shock and even death. Two types of patient are at particular risk of overwhelming acute pyelonephritis. These are: *diabetics*, who may suffer papillary necrosis during the course of such an infection; and subjects with *obstruction* of the urinary tract and acute pyelonephritis above the obstruction (most commonly arising in association with renal or ureteric stones). The latter may develop severe and permanent renal damage (pyonephrosis) over a very short period of time (hours or days), as well as being at high risk of bacteraemia.

Investigation

Investigation should focus on the isolation, identification and antibiotic sensitivity of the infecting organism. Fresh urine should be examined under the microscope for leucocytes and other formed elements. Patients with clinical evidence of acute pyelonephritis should have blood cultures. Additional investigations to be considered during or after treatment are ultrasound, IVU and cystourethroscopy.

Ultrasound. Often helpful during an acute episode of pyelonephritis to exclude obstruction.

IVU. This should be undertaken after the first infection in adult males and after the second or third in females, particularly if there was clinical evidence of pyelonephritis. Its purpose is to exclude the possibility of a functional or structural abnormality of the kidneys or urinary tract.

Cystourethroscopy. In men, this will often be needed after even a single infection because of the rarity of UTI in the absence of significant prostatic or bladder disease.

Management

General measures. Fluid intake should be generous and achieve a urine flow rate of at least 100 ml/hour. Analgesics may be required.

Antibiotic therapy. This is often begun before the results of bacteriological investigations are available, though it may be modified subsequently if the bacteriological results so dictate. Conventionally, a course of 5 days is given for *clinical cystitis* but effective treatment may also comprise a large single dose of an appropriate antibiotic. The most frequently used agents are:

● amoxycillin (250 mg t.d.s. for 5 days, or 3 g as a single dose by mouth)
● trimethoprim (300 mg once daily for 5 days)
● co-trimoxazole (960 mg or 2 tablets b.d.; or 2.88 g, 6 tablets as a single dose).

In complicated or severe infection, and where there is presumptive evidence of *acute pyelonephritis*, at least 7 days of high-dose chemotherapy should be given.

TUBERCULOSIS OF THE URINARY TRACT

Tuberculosis of the urinary tract almost always results from haematogenous spread, usually from a pulmonary focus, and involves one or both kidneys. A progressive interstitial nephropathy develops with extensive fibrosis and distortion of the gross anatomy of the kidney. Renal calcification is frequent, though not invariable. The disease spreads down the urinary tract, involving the renal pelves and ureters, and ureteric strictures frequently result. The bladder may be involved, leading to *tuberculous cystitis* and a contracted bladder, as may the epididymis, leading to tuberculous epididymitis. Renal damage is common, and may result from progressive destruction of parenchyma by the infection or from stricture formation leading to obstruction.

Clinical features and diagnosis

Unfortunately, some of these patients present with irreversible CRF. Others come to attention following painless haematuria, frequency or nocturia due to tuberculous cystitis, or with constitutional symptoms such as fever, malaise and weight loss. The urine shows a sterile pyuria. The epididymis may be hardened and calcified and renal imaging often shows intrarenal calcifications with irregular loss of renal parenchyma and, in some cases, obstruction. Ultimately, the diagnosis depends on successful isolation of acid-fast bacilli from the urine. Early morning urine specimens are used, and at least three should be obtained and examined by microscopy and culture for 6 weeks before excluding active infection.

Management

Treatment is with antituberculous chemotherapy (p. 473). Careful assessment of the anatomy of the renal tract is essential to exclude obstruction, and follow-up IVUs should be performed during the first year to identify late stricture formation. Surgical reimplantation of the ureters may be needed in some cases, and severe contraction of the bladder may require an enlargement procedure (caecocystoplasty) or urinary diversion to alleviate frequency and protect against further renal damage.

CHRONIC PYELONEPHRITIS AND VESICOURETERIC REFLUX

Chronic pyelonephritis (CPN) is a diagnosis based on abnormalities of gross morphology of the kidney (either at postmortem or by IVU or other forms of imaging). The cardinal features of the condition are:

- unilateral or bilateral parenchymal scars which give the kidney an irregular outline
- flattening of the renal papillae, giving a 'clubbed' appearance to the calyces. The parenchymal scars overlie the clubbed calyces.

Microscopically, there is severe interstitial fibrosis and scarring with tubular atrophy. The calyces and collecting system show mucosal thickening and inflammation. Glomerular lesions are variable.

Aetiology and pathogenesis

The aetiology of CPN is controversial. In the past, it was assumed that the scarring was the result of intermittent acute or chronic infection of the kidney. The main problem with this explanation is the absence of infection in many cases, and also the clear evidence that the disease may progress in the absence of persistent infection in the urine or in the kidney. It is now thought that a number of different factors, probably in association with transient infection in early life, may initiate and perpetuate the lesion that results in CPN. Of these, *vesicoureteric reflux* and *obstruction* are the two with the most clear-cut involvement, and it is therefore helpful to categorise CPN as follows.

CPN with vesicoureteric reflux. This association is far too frequent to be coincidental. It is likely that the repeated, and individually trivial, insults to the kidney following each episode of reflux (particularly in infancy, when the kidney is highly susceptible to damage) cause cumulative

damage. It appears that reflux of *infected* urine is particularly harmful, but whether the injury is mechanical, chemical or immunological is unclear.

CPN with obstruction. Evidence of obstruction is found in a proportion of patients who satisfy the diagnostic criteria for CPN; some of these have functional and structural disorders of the bladder.

CPN in isolation. In a sizeable proportion of cases, reflux is absent, and there is no evidence of back pressure or obstruction. In these idiopathic cases of CPN, an explanation that is increasingly accepted is that reflux in early childhood (probably associated with UTI) and with resolution in adolescence, may be the underlying cause.

Clinical features, investigation and treatment

Many patients present for the first time with symptoms and signs of CRF or hypertension. In addition, severe reflux may give rise to renal pain or predispose to clinically evident attacks of acute pyelonephritis.

In addition to the general assessment of renal function, a search should be made for factors that might accelerate the progression of the disease, in particular obstruction, presence of stone and active urinary infection. Reflux may be documented by micturating cystography, but surgical correction is rarely warranted and does not appear to retard progression of the disease even though it may make control of infection easier.

As in all patients with renal disease, close attention to maintenance of appropriate fluid and electrolyte balance and control of blood pressure are essential.

NEPHROPATHY DUE TO PHYSICAL OR CHEMICAL AGENTS

Radiation nephritis

Radiation nephritis most often arises in the context of radiotherapy for tumours in or adjacent to the kidneys, such as ovarian or testicular cancer, lymphoma, neuroblastoma or Wilm's tumour. Pathological changes are widespread, and involve glomeruli, tubules, interstitium and vascular elements. There is no treatment other than general supportive measures and control of blood pressure. Dialysis and/or transplantation may be appropriate in some cases.

Nephropathy due to chemical toxins

The importance of chemical toxins as a cause of nephropathy is illustrated by studies showing that nephrotoxins are implicated in 20–25% of cases of ARF. It is salutary to note that the vast majority of these cases are iatrogenic, with prescribed drugs identified as the offending agents. Chemical insult to the kidney may lead to any of the major renal syndromes.

The nephrotoxicity of many of the agents discussed below is enhanced by concomitant volume contraction; identification and correction of this and other 'prerenal factors' (Table 20.15) is thus of great importance when known nephrotoxins are being administered therapeutically.

Drug-induced nephrotoxicity (therapeutic)

Antibiotics are the major contributors, with those of the aminoglycoside group (gentamicin, tobramycin) prominent. Other frequently prescribed agents with nephrotoxic potential are NSAIDs, penicillamine, gold and lithium. Withdrawal of the offending agent will often allow renal function to return to normal but, in some cases, renal damage is permanent (Table 20.39).

Nephrotoxicity resulting from drug abuse

In epidemiological terms, by far the most important example is analgesic nephropathy (p. 826) following habitual consumption of large amounts of certain proprietary analgesic mixtures. Phenacetin (now withdrawn), paracetamol, aspirin, and ibuprofen can be obtained over-the-counter without prescription. Of these, paracetamol is the least toxic.

Heroin abuse may lead to immune complex GN or acute myoglobinuric renal failure due to rhabdomyolysis.

Other environmental nephrotoxins

X-ray contrast media are associated with a small risk of ARF, especially in patients with established renal disease, diabetes, jaundice and multiple myeloma. In these groups, an important predisposing factor is volume contraction, which should be corrected prior to injection of X-ray contrast media.

Other toxins include mercury, lead, organic solvents, ethylene glycol (antifreeze), paraquat and paracetamol (in large overdose).

URINARY STONE

Urinary stone, or urolithiasis, and the dramatic symptoms that may be associated with it have been recorded for at least two millennia. The true incidence is difficult to assess, but it is likely that clinical stone events afflict about 1% of the population at some time during their lives. Men are affected with about four times the frequency of women and, in both sexes, stone formation tends to be recurrent and unpredictable, putting a substantial onus on doctors to devise effective means of prophylaxis.

Types of stone

Details of the major stone types are given in Table 20.40, from which it can be seen that the large majority of stones are made up of calcium oxalate or a mixture of calcium oxalate with hydroxyapatite. Struvite stones (magnesium ammonium phosphate) usually contain calcium phosphate also and are invariably associated with infection. Uric acid stones and cystine stones are associated with elevated urinary excretion rates of these compounds.

Table 20.39 Iatrogenic toxic nephropathy

Drug	Renal disturbance
Aminoglycosides (gentamicin, tobramycin, amikacin)	ARF with or without oliguria
Penicillins (methicillin, benzylpenicillin, ampicillin)	Acute interstitial nephropathy
Sulphonamides	Precipitation in tubules
Cephalosporins (especially cephaloridine)	ARF
Demeclocycline	Nephrogenic diabetes insipidus
Amphotericin B	Decreased renal blood flow; tubular toxicity
Pentamidine	ARF
NSAIDs	Acute or chronic interstitial nephropathy
Penicillamine	Nephrotic syndrome
Organic gold	Nephrotic syndrome
Diuretics (thiazides, frusemide)	Interstitial nephropathy
Lithium carbonate	Tubular syndromes, chronic interstitial nephropathy
Cisplatin	Interstitial nephropathy
X-ray contrast media	ARF with or without oliguria

Table 20.40 Types of urinary stone

Composition	Radio-opaque	Frequency (%)
Calcium oxalate	++	35
Calcium oxalate + hydroxyapatite	++	45
Calcium phosphate	++	1–3
Magnesium ammonium phosphate + calcium phosphate (struvite)	++	10
Uric acid	0	5
Cystine	+	1–2

Pathogenesis

Stone formation is frequent because of the precariously high urinary concentration of compounds of relatively low solubility. Certain protective mechanisms are built in, such that immediate precipitation is not an inevitable result of supersaturation. Inhibitors of crystal formation in urine are inorganic (magnesium, pyrophosphate, citrate) and organic (glycoseaminoglycans, nephrocalcin) and it is possible that the action of these is at least as important a determinant of stone formation as the absolute concentrations of, for example, calcium, phosphate and oxalate in the urine. Uric acid is of particular importance, in that it is not only itself capable of precipitating and forming stones, but also appears to interfere with the action of the organic inhibitors, thus predisposing also to non-uric acid stone formation.

Calcium

About 30% of patients with calcium-containing stones will have hypercalciuria (arbitrarily defined as more than 7.5 mmol/day in men and more than 6.5 mmol/day in women). A minority of these will also be hypercalcaemic because of underlying hyperparathyroidism, sarcoidosis, vitamin D intoxication, milk alkali syndrome, malignant disease or hyperthyroidism. In these cases, the objective is to treat the underlying metabolic abnormality, thereby resolving the hypercalciuria.

However, the vast majority of hypercalciuric stone formers will be found to be normocalcaemic and, provided that there is no identifiable cause for hyperabsorption of calcium by the intestine (e.g. mild vitamin D intoxication), or of renal tubular disorder leading to hypercalciuria (e.g. renal tubular acidosis, high salt intake, chronic frusemide therapy), they are designated as suffering from *idiopathic hypercalciuria*. Detailed investigation of these patients suggests that they fall into three main groups:

- *absorptive hypercalciuria*, i.e. primary intestinal hyperabsorption of calcium with compensatory 'spillover' into the urine leading to hypercalciuria
- *renal hypercalciuria*, i.e. primary renal calcium leak with compensatory intestinal hyperabsorption of calcium (rare)
- *resorptive hypercalciuria*, i.e. primary acceleration of skeletal resorption with compensatory 'spillover' of calcium into the urine leading to hypercalciuria.

Oxalate

There is a positive relationship between urinary oxalate excretion and the likelihood of calcium oxalate stone formation.

Uric acid

Hyperuricosuric individuals have a greatly increased incidence of uric acid stone formation and a moderately increased incidence of calcium oxalate stone formation. This association probably reflects interference by uric acid with the action of urinary inhibitors of crystal formation.

Cystine

Cystinuria is inherited as an autosomal recessive and is associated with elevated excretion of other dibasic amino acids. Cystine stone formation is the only important clinical sequela.

Clinical features

Presentation is usually with renal or ureteric colic, resulting from partial or complete obstruction to the flow of urine. The pain is usually intense and is nearly always accompanied by haematuria, which may be macroscopic. If the stone has obstructed a single functioning kidney, ARF of postrenal type is inevitable.

However, less dramatic presentations are also common, with passage of tiny stones or gravel, usually with some associated discomfort. Symptoms may even be absent, or comprise merely dull backache which may lead to the erroneous diagnosis of a mechanical back lesion.

Fortunately, severe permanent renal damage is rare, and arises only when acute infection is present above an obstructing stone (leading to pyonephrosis) or following neglect of an obstructing stone.

Diagnosis and management

The diagnosis and treatment of urinary stone falls into an early phase of assessment and management of the immediate problems posed by the stone, and a late phase, concerned with the aetiology of the offending stone and strategy to prevent future episodes.

Early

Diagnosis is usually easy and is often made on clinical grounds alone. Plain X-ray of the abdomen will reveal the majority of calcium-containing stones, but their location in relation to the kidney and ureter requires an IVU. The IVU will also allow identification of non-radio-opaque uric acid stones, and usually demonstrates the position of the stone and the consequent dilatation of the upper urinary tract above the level of obstruction. Ultrasound examination of the kidney may be helpful in identifying stones within the kidney. Urine should be examined for blood and cultured, and all urine passed should be strained in the hope of catching the stone which can then be analysed. Renal or ureteric colic requires strong analgesia – opiates should be given promptly and in adequate dosage. The role of 'antispasmodics' such as anticholinergic drugs is not clear, but inhibitors of prostaglandin synthesis (e.g. indomethacin) may be highly effective. A generous fluid intake is maintained and the patient mobilised as quickly as possible. These measures alone will allow spontaneous passage of the stone in many cases. Factors favouring spontaneous passage are small size (<5 mm), and location in the lower third of the ureter.

Active intervention is required for unremitting obstruction and pain, associated infection, a large stone that is unlikely to pass, and ARF of postrenal type. Intervention may take the form of open surgery (nephrolithotomy or ureterolithotomy), endoscopic snaring from below during cystoscopy, or percutaneous removal from above via a nephrostomy. An important new development revolutionising the management of stone disease is external shock wave lithotripsy (ESWL). Here, appropriately directed ultrasound is used to shatter renal or ureteric stones in vivo, allowing spontaneous passage of the fragments.

Late

Analysis of the stone is desirable but not always possible. Routine metabolic tests to be undertaken in all cases are:

- plasma calcium, phosphate, alkaline phosphatase, urea, urate, creatinine, electrolytes
- 24-hour urine collection for simultaneous measurement of calcium, uric acid, oxalate, citrate and creatinine
- nitroprusside test for cystine.

Abnormalities in the initial screen may dictate measurement of serum PTH, fasting urinary calcium-excretion, tests of urinary acidification and plasma 25-hydroxyvitamin D concentrations to exclude vitamin D intoxication.

Depending on the results of the above assessment, the following specific measures should be taken (in addition to general advice to achieve fluid intake sufficient to maintain a urine output of at least 2 litres per day).

- *Hypercalciuria with hypercalcaemia.* Treat underlying cause of hypercalcaemia.
- *Idiopathic hypercalciuria.* Treat with thiazide diuretics to reduce urinary calcium excretion. In selected cases this may be combined with cellulose phosphate given orally (to decrease intestinal calcium absorption), with allopurinol (to reduce urinary uric acid excretion), or with potassium citrate.

- *Calcium stones with no metabolic abnormality.* The patient should avoid excessive oxalate-rich foods (tea, coffee, nuts, spinach, rhubarb). Treatment is with oral potassium citrate.
- *Uric acid stones.* Allopurinol.
- *Cystine stones.* Alkalinise urine with sodium or potassium citrate. Maintain urine flow at 3 l/day minimum. Consider penicillamine if the above measures are ineffective.
- *Struvite stones.* Surgical removal is the only effective treatment.
- *Hyperoxaluria and hypocitraturia.* When documented, hyperoxaluria should be countered by a low-oxalate diet and hypocitraturia should be treated with potassium citrate.

Dietary calcium restriction is sometimes recommended in patients with calcium-containing stones. However, this therapeutic dogma is of unproven benefit and may in some cases be harmful. A sensible compromise is to limit calcium intake only when excessive, and not to attempt to reduce it below 25 mmol/day (1 g of elemental calcium per day) except in those subjects shown to have absorptive hypercalciuria.

URINARY TRACT OBSTRUCTION

Aetiology

Some of the main causes of urinary tract obstruction are given in Table 20.41. The clinical presentation is varied and depends on age at onset and the site, severity and rate of onset of obstruction.

Table 20.41 Causes of urinary tract obstruction

Level of obstruction	Pathophysiology
Any	Stone, sloughed papilla, blood clot, trauma
Renal parenchyma	Uric acid, Bence-Jones protein, cysts
Collecting system	Urothelial tumour, TB, pelviureteric obstruction (stricture, aberrant vessel, fibrous band)
Ureter	Retroperitoneal or pelvic malignancy (carcinoma of bladder, prostate, cervix, rectum, lymphoma, carcinoma of ureter), aortic aneurysm, idiopathic retroperitoneal fibrosis, TB, schistosomiasis, obstetric trauma
Bladder	Benign prostatic hypertrophy, carcinoma of prostate or bladder, neurogenic bladder, TB, foreign body, trauma
Urethra	Urethral valves, phimosis, stricture, meatal stenosis, trauma, foreign body

Clinical features

The following clinical features are of importance in the management of patients suspected of having an obstructing lesion.

- *Pain.* Acute obstruction is usually associated with pain, regardless of the site of the lesion. In contrast, slowly progressive obstructions are likely to be pain-free and hence more likely to cause obstructive renal injury which may be severe and irreversible by the time the patient seeks help.
- *Renal failure* resulting from obstruction implies that both kidneys are obstructed, or that a solitary functioning kidney is obstructed.
- *Volume of urine.* The fact that a patient is passing normal volumes of urine does not exclude obstruction. While complete obstruction of the urinary tract of necessity causes anuria, the patient with partial obstruction will usually continue to pass normal, or even increased, volumes of urine at the expense of damaging back pressure on the kidney.
- *Renal impairment.* Because the early recognition and relief of obstruction is so important if unnecessary renal damage is to be avoided, the diagnosis must be considered in all patients presenting with acute or chronic renal impairment.
- eradicate should raise the suspicion of an anatomical and possibly obstructing lesion.

Effects of obstruction on the kidney

The earliest functions to be compromised by progressive obstruction are urinary concentration and acidification, followed by a decrease in GFR. Relief of obstruction may sometimes be followed by temporary concentrating defects leading to inappropriate salt and water losses.

Diagnosis and management

Clinical assessment may reveal symptoms and signs that point to obstruction and may also indicate its likely site and aetiology. This is particularly so in patients with urethral disease or bladder outflow obstruction. Alternatively, the clinical picture may suggest a disorder known to be associated with urinary obstruction, e.g. carcinoma of the cervix or lymphoma in a patient with unexplained renal failure. Although the existence of obstruction is usually clear-cut, major problems arise in some cases. These fall into three groups.

Is the 'obstruction' significant? The finding of a dilated collecting system does not necessarily imply current obstruction, but may be an anatomical hangover from previous obstruction.

Extent of renal damage. Is renal function likely to improve following relief of the obstruction? This problem arises when, in the presence of clear-cut obstruction, it remains uncertain whether renal damage has progressed beyond the point where useful recovery of function is likely. A variety of non-invasive and invasive tests can be helpful, but in some cases, the answer is only obtained following a trial of palliative drainage by means of a nephrostomy tube or bladder catheter.

Advanced malignancy. Should obstruction be relieved when it is the result of advanced malignancy? Malignant disease is an important cause of obstructive nephropathy (Table 20.41) and in these patients thought should be given to the likely prognosis of the tumour. If this is exceedingly poor, it may be kinder to allow the patient to die in uraemic coma, rather than as a result of uncontrolled pelvic malignancy.

Techniques used in the relief of obstruction include surgical bypass or urinary diversion through the skin, direct drainage from above via a nephrostomy tube, or internal stenting of an obstructing lesion.

NEOPLASIA IN THE KIDNEY AND URINARY TRACT

Cancers of the urogenital tract are common. The age-specific incidence rates for the UK are shown in Figure 20.20. In the kidney, renal cell carcinoma is the commonest tumour (75% of cases) with transitional cell carcinoma accounting for 15% of cases. Carcinoma of the prostate is the third largest cause of death from cancer in males.

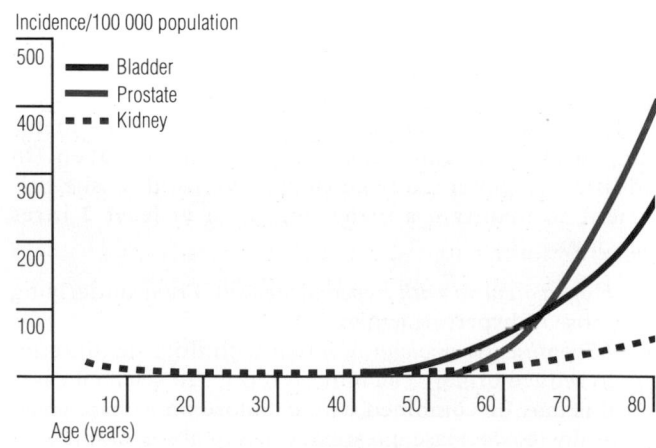

Fig. 20.20 Age-adjusted incidence of urinary tract cancer in the UK in 1983.

RENAL TUMOURS

Renal adenocarcinoma

Renal adenocarcinoma is three times commoner in men and may be related in part to cigarette smoking. It is also commoner in patients with von Hippel-Lindau syndrome (p. 913).

The tumour arises from the renal tubule cells. Lymphatic and haematogenous spread, and local spread through capsule mean that 30–40% of patients are inoperable when first seen.

Clinical features

Half of the patients have haematuria. Loin pain and an abdominal mass are frequently present. Presentation may also be with bone pain or cough and dyspnoea from metastases. Renal adenocarcinoma may also present with a variety of paraneoplastic symptoms including fever and night sweats, humoral hypercalcaemia, and polycythaemia due to excess erythropoietin production.

Investigation

Diagnosis can be difficult if the tumour is small. An IVU may show a space-occupying mass, but a negative X-ray does not exclude a small tumour. Ultrasound is more sensitive and a CT scan is helpful in difficult cases. These techniques have reduced the need for renal angiography.

Management and prognosis

Surgical resection offers the only hope of cure but over 30% of renal tumours are inoperable. Opinion is divided as to the extent of the operation. Lymph node dissection is usually carried out. Radiotherapy has a limited role, but is often used if extrarenal extension of the tumour is found at operation.

Chemotherapy is of little value. Alpha-interferon, interleukin-2 and vinblastine may cause regressions, and the tumour may spontaneously fluctuate in size. Although regression of metastases has been seen following removal of the primary, this is a rare event.

Of patients with small localised disease, 50% are alive at 10 years. Only 20% of patients with stage II disease (large tumours but no local or node spread) will be alive, and 5% of stage III cases (extracapsular spread). Cancer staging is discussed in Chapter 8, pages 131–132.

Nephroblastoma (Wilm's tumour)

Wilm's tumour is an embryonic renal tumour usually found in children, in whom it presents as an abdominal mass. Hypertension is common. Treatment is surgical

with adjuvant chemotherapy and radiotherapy in many cases. The combined approach has led to major improvements in the prognosis of the neoplasm.

Transitional cell carcinoma of kidney

The main symptoms of transitional cell carcinoma of the kidney are haematuria and renal pain, often with unilateral obstruction. The IVU shows a filling defect in the collecting system and the kidney may be obstructed. Cytological examination of the urine reveals malignant cells in 50% of cases.

Treatment is by nephro-ureterectomy where possible. Because the whole urothelium is unstable, stump recurrences are quite common. Radiotherapy may slow local progression but is not curative.

Transitional cell carcinoma of the bladder

Transitional cell carcinoma of the bladder was shown to be more common in workers in the aniline dye industry. The carcinogen was identified as β-naphthylamine. The tumour is also more common in the rubber industry, and in cigarette smokers. Worldwide, the major predisposing cause is bladder schistosomiasis (p. 312).

Staging

The staging notation (Fig. 20.21) is based on the mode of spread through the bladder wall.

Clinical features and investigation

The major symptom is haematuria which is usually painless. Urinary frequency, nocturia and back pain may all occur. Diagnosis is by cystoscopy. An IVU is essential to show renal anatomy, and simple renal function tests should be performed. Lymphography and CT scanning are increasingly used in staging.

Management

Small superficial lesions are treated transurethrally by cystodiathermy, and intravesical chemotherapy is being used increasingly. Up to 15% of such patients will develop more generalised intravesical recurrence requiring surgery.

For more advanced (T2–T3) tumours, treatment is with surgery or radical radiotherapy or a combination of the two approaches. Partial cystectomy may be possible in some cases, but in others, total cystectomy (with an ileal conduit for the ureters) may be needed. Recently, several studies have shown that radical radiotherapy produces results as good as radical cystectomy. Chemotherapy is

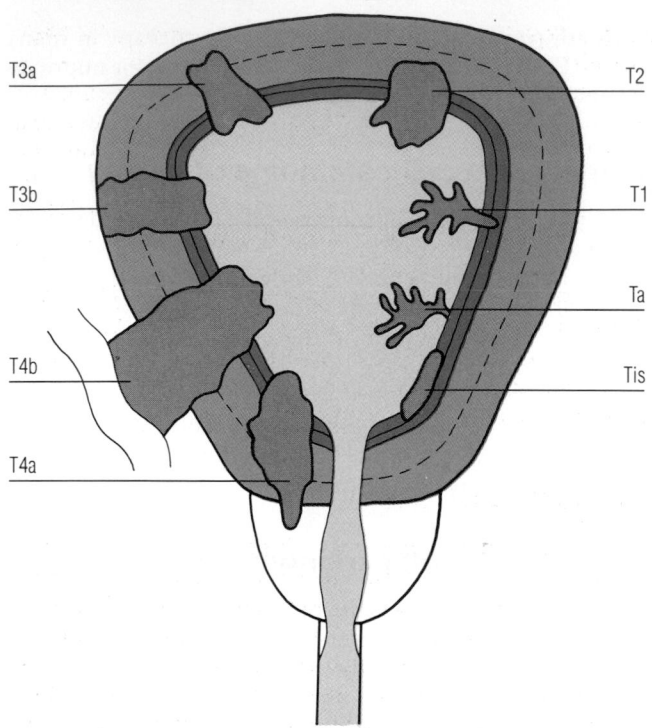

Fig. 20.21 Staging of bladder cancer. (After: Blandy JP 1986 Operative urology. Blackwell Scientific, Oxford). T1 tumours involve the bladder mucosa. T2 tumours involve the superficial muscle (dashed line), T3a extend into deeper muscle, and T3b involve the whole wall. T4a tumours invade the prostate (or vagina), and T4b the rectum and pelvic wall.

increasingly used in advanced and metastatic disease, with long survival in a minority of patients.

Carcinoma of the prostate

The age-specific incidence of this very common cancer is shown in Figure 20.20. In the last 50 years, mortality from this disease has increased in the UK. Little is known of its aetiology. The tumour is nearly always an adenocarcinoma. The majority are well-differentiated cancers, anaplastic tumours being only 15% of the total. The tumour grows in the gland (T1/T2) and then invades the capsule (T3) and, finally, adjacent structures (T4). Spread is to regional lymph nodes and then to bone and lung.

Clinical features and diagnosis

The tumour is often asymptomatic and may be diagnosed on rectal examination for some other reason. The commonest local symptoms are related to bladder outflow obstruction or infection, but presentation with backache from metastases is also frequent.

Measurements of serum acid phosphatase and/or prostate-specific antigen are useful for diagnosis and treatment monitoring. Histological confirmation may be obtained by biopsy, usually taken transrectally, or from curettings taken at transurethral prostatectomy. Further staging will include chest X-ray and bone scan. An IVU may show back pressure effects on the bladder and kidneys.

Management

For localised small tumours, both radical prostatectomy and radical radiotherapy have been used. With radical treatment, 30–40% of patients will be alive at 10 years, the proportion falling if there is extra-capsular extension of the tumour.

The mainstay of treatment is hormone manipulation, using orchidectomy, stilboestrol or the inhibitor of LH release, buserelin. For more advanced disease, radiotherapy may palliate both local symptoms and symptoms from bone metastases.

CONTINENCE AND INCONTINENCE

NORMAL MICTURITION

Functionally, micturition occurs in three phases:

- bladder filling
- postponement, comprising: perception of the need to void; movement to a suitable place to void; adoption of voiding posture
- voiding of urine.

Thus, micturition may be disturbed by intrinsic diseases of the bladder or its outlet, disordered afferent or efferent nerve supply of the bladder, spinal cord lesions, intracranial disease, psychological disturbance or locomotor disturbance.

Neuropathic bladder is a widely used (and abused) term denoting no more than bladder dysfunction resulting from any type of neurological disturbance; it implies nothing about the nature of that neurological disturbance.

The detrusor muscle of the bladder (parasympathetic innervation) and the bladder outlet (sympathetic innervation) act in a co-ordinated fashion, such that outflow resistance is high and detrusor tone low during filling. When the bladder is full and voiding is appropriate, micturition is accompanied by simultaneous contraction of the detrusor (mediated by increased parasympathetic activity) and relaxation of the bladder outlet (mediated by decreased sympathetic and pelvic floor activity) (Fig. 20.22). This is co-ordinated by a micturition centre in the brainstem, which is itself subject to a degree of cortical control (Fig. 20.23).

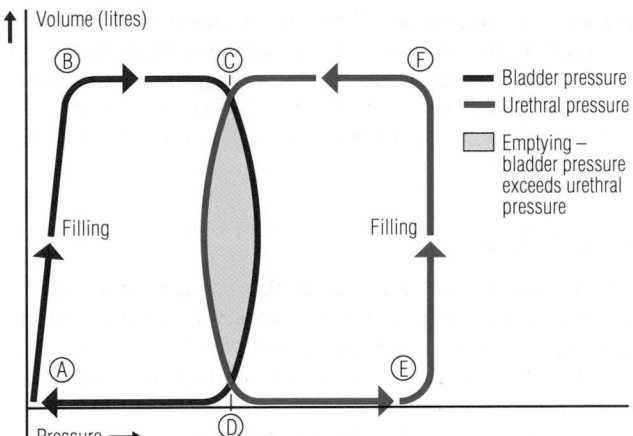

Fig. 20.22 The micturition cycle. Bladder emptying occurs at any time when bladder pressure is greater than urethral pressure (shaded area). During filling – (A) to (B) – bladder pressure rises little. Initiation of micturition at points (B) and (F) leads to a synchronous increase in bladder pressure and decrease in urethral pressure until, at (C), emptying begins. When emptying is complete (D), bladder and urethral pressures revert – points (A) and (E) – and filling resumes. (After Yeates WK in Hinman F (ed) 1983 Benign prostatic hypertrophy. Springer-Verlag, New York.)

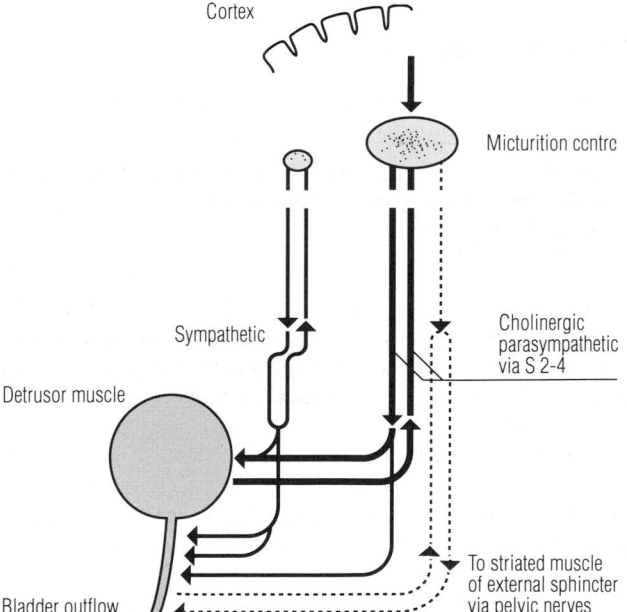

Fig. 20.23 Neurological control of micturition. The sympathetic efferent relaxes the detrusor muscle of the bladder and constricts the bladder outflow. The cholinergic efferent promotes contraction of the detrusor muscle. The pelvic nerve supply to the external sphincter stimulates further constriction of the bladder outflow. (After Yeates WK in Hinman F (ed) 1983 Benign prostatic hypertrophy. Springer-Verlag, New York.)

INCONTINENCE

Many of the causes of incontinence also result in a reduced functional bladder capacity which, of necessity, leads to frequency of micturition and/or nocturia (p. 798). The history and examination often yield a diagnosis but in some cases further investigations are needed to define the potential for pharmacological, urological or neurological treatment. Measurement of urine flow rate during the voiding phase is valuable in the assessment of bladder outflow obstruction. An IVU or ultrasound is often needed to determine the effects of the disordered bladder function on the upper urinary tract and kidneys. Residual urine after micturition can be demonstrated by IVU and/or ultrasound. Cine cystography shows the relevant anatomy during bladder filling and emptying, and may be combined with simultaneous pressure measurements to give a filling and voiding cystometrogram.

Stress incontinence

Stress incontinence is the involuntary passage of urine when intra-abdominal pressure is raised as in coughing, lifting, standing up, etc. In the main, it is a disease of women, in whom pelvic floor laxity, often the result of pregnancy and/or childbirth, compromises the closure of the bladder outlet. There is no neurological defect. The dysfunction should be confirmed by performing a cine voiding cystometrogram.

Treatment with pelvic floor exercises may be effective, and some patients are improved by α-agonist drugs, such as phenylpropanolamine. However, surgical intervention is often needed and is usually effective.

Urge incontinence

In urge incontinence, the perception of the desire to void is followed within seconds or minutes by voiding, even though the patient attempts to delay it. Voiding is usually complete. This problem may reflect:

- *increased afferent stimulation* from local disease, e.g. infective cystitis, bladder tumour, bladder hypertrophy
- *failure of central inhibition,* e.g. multiple sclerosis, cerebrovascular disease, cerebral tumour, spinal cord lesion
- *cortical stimulation,* e.g. incontinence provoked by the sound of running water.

In many female cases there is no detectable organic cause of incontinence (idiopathic 'bladder instability'). Sacral reflexes are preserved, and so usually is sacral sensation and voluntary control of the anal sphincter. Instability of the detrusor muscle is usually demonstrable in the neuropathic group.

Treatment should be directed at the underlying pathology when feasible. Pharmacological attempts to decrease detrusor hyperexcitability using anticholinergic drugs (e.g. probantheline), tricyclic antidepressants or calcium channel blockers (e.g. nifedipine) are sometimes successful. In severe cases of neurological origin in women (particularly multiple sclerosis), the bladder activity may be greatly reduced by the injection of phenol into the pelvic autonomic nerves through the bladder base.

Reflex incontinence

Reflex incontinence is where voiding occurs periodically without advance warning. The most important causes are spinal lesions above the level of the sacral outflow. Depending on the severity of the spinal lesion, neurological examination may show exaggerated sacral reflexes, a perianal sensory deficit and/or impairment of voluntary sphincter control. The interruption, not only of central inhibition but also of co-ordination, leads to detrusor hyperexcitability coupled with failure to relax the bladder outlet, a potentially dangerous combination that results in a high pressure bladder and risk of renal damage. Adequate decompression, by reduction of the resistance of the bladder outlet, is essential in these cases. Sometimes this can be achieved pharmacologically by α-adrenergic blocking drugs, such as phenoxybenzamine, or by endoscopic resection of the bladder neck and/or the external sphincter. The absence of bladder sensation, however, precludes the restoration of bladder control. In these circumstances, male patients nearly always require incontinence appliances. Female patients require continuous or intermittent catheterisation, and it is sometimes necessary to divert the urine by means of an ileal conduit.

Overflow incontinence

Overflow incontinence usually manifests itself with leakage of small amounts of urine, initially often at night only. The symptom is often quite subtle but it is important to recognise it because of the severe obstructive renal damage that usually ensues if the condition is neglected. The incontinence is always associated with a residual urine volume approaching that of the bladder capacity, usually resulting in a manifestly distended bladder. It is most often seen in a man with prostatic hypertrophy causing outflow obstruction. Other cases result from neurological lesions, either as an acute condition in spinal shock, or in sub-acute or chronic bladder dysfunction from prolapsed intervertebral disc, sacral plexus lesions or autonomic neuropathy (diabetes mellitus, tabes dorsalis) that decreases normal detrusor excitability. The urinary stream is slow.

Treatment is directed at correction of the mechanical outlet obstruction, e.g. by prostatectomy. In some neuropathic cases, α-blocking drugs (phenoxybenzamine, prazosin), or endoscopic resection or incision of the bladder neck or external sphincter, may improve matters by reducing outlet resistance. The outlook in those patients with local mechanical causes that increase bladder outlet resistance (e.g. prostatic hypertrophy) is usually excellent, whereas the prognosis in the long-standing neuropathic group is usually poor.

Enuresis

Enuresis denotes bed-wetting in, or beginning in, childhood, though strictly it means merely the voiding of urine. Bed-wetting is universal in infancy, affects about 50% of children at age 3 and about 15% at age 10. It is commoner in children with psychological problems and in those with organic diseases of the kidney and/or urinary tract. Primary nocturnal enuresis (i.e. present from birth) does not usually require detailed investigation, provided that daytime micturition is normal, and there is no evidence of present or past infection or of urinary tract obstruction.

Treatment, in the absence of associated abnormalities of the urinary tract, may involve bladder training, with voluntary postponement of voiding by day, or alteration of sleep pattern by means of a bell set to sound when the child wets a sensor pad in bed. The tricyclic antidepressants (e.g. imipramine) are effective in many cases, probably by multiple actions on the depth of sleep and on the detrusor muscle. An alternative approach is to give the vasopressin analogue, desmopressin, intranasally last thing at night. This decreases urine output during the night and is successful in selected patients.

Incontinence in the elderly

The overall problem of incontinence in the elderly is considerable. It has been estimated to afflict 5–15% of the elderly in the general population and many more in institutions. The mechanism is often multifactorial, particularly neuropathic; however, in depressed or demented patients, it may include loss of the will to be continent and loss of appreciation of what is a socially acceptable micturition site.

Treatment is similar to that in younger patients, but therapeutic options may be constrained by drug side-effects or unacceptable risks of surgery. As a result, relatively more of the elderly will require palliation in the form of incontinence appliances, pads or indwelling catheters. The latter, though an easy option for the doctor and nursing staff, should be avoidable in most cases. More detailed discussion is given in Chapter 9.

PRESCRIBING IN PATIENTS WITH RENAL DISEASE

The extensive renal excretion of therapeutic agents and their metabolites means that the prescription of drugs to

Table 20.42 Therapeutic considerations in renal disease

Pharmacological consideration	Example
Decreased therapeutic efficacy	
Target organ resistance	Diuretics less effective in patients with renal disease
Failure of diseased kidney to bioactivate agent	Vitamin D not bioactivated to 1,25(OH)$_2$D in severe renal disease
Increased nephrotoxicity	X-ray contrast media, aminoglycoside antibiotics more nephrotoxic to previously damaged kidneys
Decreased excretion of drug or metabolite	Digoxin, many antibiotics

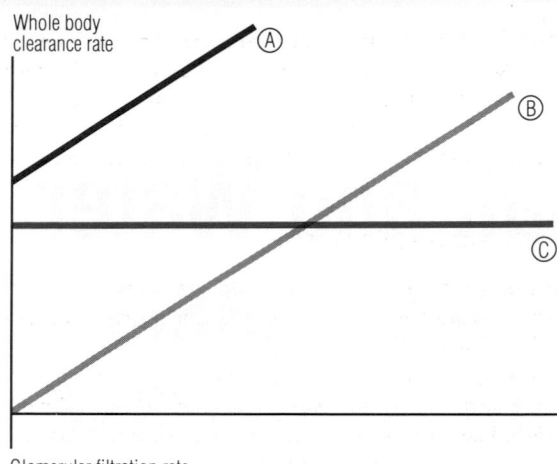

Fig. 20.24 Effect of changes of GFR on the elimination of different drugs. Drug (A) is cleared by both the kidney and the liver, and Drug (B) by the kidney alone. Drug (C) is cleared by the liver alone; its clearance rate is unaffected by changes in the GFR.

patients with renal disease must often be modified with regard to both the choice of drug and its schedule of administration. The main considerations (Table 20.42) are:

- decreased therapeutic efficacy
- increased nephrotoxicity
- decreased excretion of drug or metabolite.

Thus, some agents may have to be given in unusually large doses to patients with renal disease (e.g. diuretics) while others require dose reduction (e.g. digoxin) or should not be given at all if the risk of toxicity is too high.

Body clearance

As applied to a particular drug, body clearance is the sum of the clearances (i.e. hepatic, renal, skeletal, muscle, etc.) of that agent in all organs contributing to its removal. When the kidney is the sole route of exit, the renal clearance approximates the body clearance, while in the case of the drug that is removed exclusively by hepatic metabolism, the hepatic clearance approximates the body clearance and the renal clearance is zero. The effect of decreasing GFR on body clearance of different types of drug is illustrated in Figure 20.24.

Principles of dose modification

The decision to decrease the dose of a drug is based on both its potential to accumulate in renal failure and the potential for toxicity if accumulation occurs. Drugs with a very high therapeutic index (e.g. penicillin) require dose modification only if very large doses are being given or if

renal function is near zero. Conversely, drugs with a low therapeutic index (e.g. digoxin or aminoglycoside antibiotics) require dose modification even in the presence of slight impairment of renal function.

Depending on the pharmacokinetics of the drug, dose reduction may take the form of normal dose/increased dose interval, reduced dose/normal dose interval or a combination of the two. Appropriate modification can be aided by tables, nomograms and monitoring. In practice, tables and nomograms, used with an understanding of the relevant pharmacology, allow an educated guess of the correct dosage to be made; and subsequent monitoring of plasma concentrations of the drug helps to guide further dose adjustments.

FURTHER READING

Brenner B M, Coe F L, Rector F C 1987 Clinical nephrology. W B Saunders Company, Philadelphia. *Medium length text, with predominantly clinical emphasis. Well laid out and well referenced*

Brenner B M, Rector F C 1991 The kidney, 4th edn. W B Saunders Company, Philadelphia. *Comprehensive and detailed text with extensive coverage of renal physiology and pathophysiology as well as of clinical nephrology. Extensively referenced*

Raine A E G (ed) 1992 Advances in renal medicine. Oxford University Press, Oxford. *Excellent reviews covering clinical practice and scientific basis of nephrology*

Sweny P, Farrington K, Moorhead J F 1989 The kidney and its disorders. Blackwell Scientific Publications, Oxford. *Up-to-date, medium length textbook of nephrology*

21
Salt and Water Homeostasis and Acid–base Balance

John P Monson

WATER AND SODIUM HOMEOSTASIS

Total body water and sodium are maintained within narrow limits by neural and hormonal homeostatic mechanisms which ensure that water and salt intake and excretion are equal. Disease states may perturb salt and water balance either by exerting direct effects on one or more of these homeostatic mechanisms or by altering water or sodium loss or intake. The distribution of water between intracellular fluid and extracellular fluid depends on the

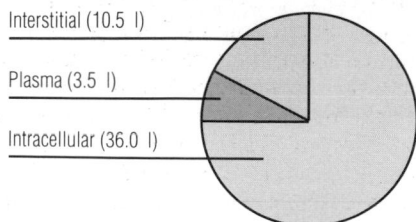

Fig. 21.1 **The distribution of total body water.** Osmolality is equal in all compartments.

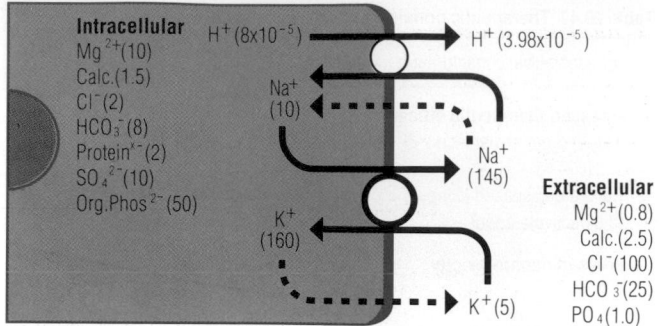

Fig. 21.2 **The intra/extracellular ion distribution.** Concentrations in mmol/l are shown in parentheses and those for calcium indicate the total of ionised and unionised. The solid arrows represent active transport mechanisms and the broken arrows passive diffusion, which depends on the electrochemical gradient.

osmolality of the two compartments (Fig. 21.1). Sodium is quantitatively the most important extracellular cation and, as 80% of total sodium is present in the extracellular space due to active sodium–potassium exchange across cellular plasma membranes (Fig. 21.2), the extracellular osmolality approximates to the molar concentrations of sodium and its anion equivalents, chloride and bicarbonate. It follows that extracellular fluid volume is largely dependent on the total body sodium. This applies to both intravascular and interstitial spaces, although the water distribution between these two components of extracellular space is further dependent on the osmotic effects of plasma proteins (oncotic pressure) and on hydrostatic pressure. Net *sodium loss* will result in shrinkage of both interstitial and intravascular volumes but, since such losses are frequently accompanied by loss of water, the osmolar changes will be slight and marked changes in intracellular volume will not occur. Net *water loss* will, however, result in an increase in extracellular osmolality, consequent free diffusion of water from the intracellular space, and therefore loss of water from all compartments.

Water homeostasis

Total body water is maintained primarily through the mechanism of action of *antidiuretic hormone* (ADH), also called *arginine vasopressin* (AVP), and by the sensation of thirst (Fig. 21.3).

Antidiuretic hormone

The net change in osmolality which follows any tendency to total body water deficit constitutes the most important stimulus to the secretion of ADH by neurosecretory cells in the supraoptic and paraventricular nuclei of the hypothalamus. Sensitive receptors which mediate this phenomenon are localised primarily in the hypothalamus. These osmoreceptors are particularly sensitive to increased

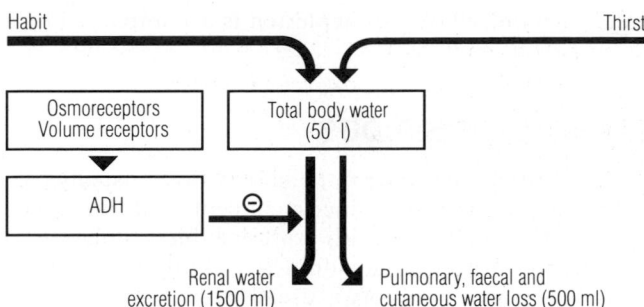

Fig. 21.3 Determinants of total body water balance. Water intake is initiated by habit and thirst. Total body water is maintained at a constant level by the thirst mechanism and by ADH modulation of renal water excretion; ⊙ denotes inhibition.

sodium concentrations, but less so to glucose or urea. Additional receptors, present in capacitance vessels near the heart and in the left atrium, mediate ADH release in response to vascular volume changes independently of changes in osmolality. This mechanism is less sensitive than that mediated by osmolar changes. Release of ADH may also be influenced by circulating angiotensin II, catecholamines and endogenous opiates.

ADH formed in the hypothalamus is transferred, as secretory granules, along the axons of the neurosecretory cells to the posterior pituitary, where it is released into the circulation in response to stimulation of osmo- or volume receptors. The major sites of action of ADH are the distal tubules and collecting ducts of the kidney. Permeability to water is increased by a cyclic-AMP-mediated phosphorylation mechanism, and water reabsorption occurs by virtue of medullary hypertonicity achieved by means of the counter-current system.

In addition to its effect on the kidney, ADH has recently been shown to influence glucose and urea production in the liver. The latter is of particular interest in view of the importance of urea in maintaining renal medullary hypertonicity.

The sensation of thirst

The sensation of thirst is predominantly mediated by hypothalamic osmoreceptors distinct from, but in close proximity to, those subserving ADH secretion. Vascular volume receptors may also contribute. However, except when water supplies are limited, much of everyday fluid intake occurs out of habit or on a social basis. For this reason, urine flow rates are generally far in excess of, and urine osmolality lower than, the values found when a significant degree of renal concentration occurs due to the action of ADH.

Sodium homeostasis

Sodium is lost to the body in cutaneous sweat and, via the kidney, in the urine. The former loss cannot be regulated

and is determined solely by environmental conditions. Maintenance of a constant total body sodium in the face of wide variations in sodium intake is therefore entirely dependent on appropriate variations in the rate of renal sodium excretion. This can achieve a constant total body sodium when daily intake ranges from 20 to several hundred millimoles. However, this mechanism is incompletely understood. Changes in adrenal aldosterone production, dependent on the renin–angiotensin system (p. 828), are undoubtedly important in the regulation of active sodium reabsorption in exchange for potassium and hydrogen ions in the distal tubule.

This mechanism alone cannot explain the observed capacity for variation of renal sodium excretion, however. It is probable that vascular receptors can sense changes in circulating volume, and mediate secretion of a circulating peptide, atrial natriuretic peptide (ANP), produced in the atrium which promotes renal sodium excretion. It would appear that secretion is stimulated by atrial stretch receptors activated by increases in blood volume due, for example, to increased sodium intake, congestive cardiac failure or renal failure. The precise mechanism of action of ANP is not known, but probably involves an increase in both renal blood flow and glomerular filtration rate together with inhibition of the renin–angiotensin–aldosterone system.

Clinical assessment of water and sodium balance

Derangements of sodium and water homeostasis are often obvious from the clinical history which may, for example, indicate abnormal losses of fluid and electrolytes from the gastrointestinal tract. Alternatively, symptoms of orthopnoea and oedema may suggest circulatory overload or heart failure.

Primary derangements in sodium balance alter the extracellular fluid volume and thus give rise to early alterations in circulating volume and consequent physical signs. Mild to moderate changes in water balance, on the other hand, are borne by intra- and extracellular compartments and are less obvious clinically. As a general principle, expansion or contraction of the circulating volume may be determined by examination of the jugular venous pressure (low in sodium depletion, raised in sodium excess) and of the lying and standing blood pressure (postural drop in sodium depletion). Peripheral oedema may also indicate a sodium retaining state (p. 849).

Estimating the state of hydration by clinical assessment of skin turgor or intraocular pressure is unreliable. Daily weighing, on the other hand, provides a sensitive index of changes and is often used to monitor intensive diuretic therapy. Further investigation of the patient's circulating volume and cardiac status may include measurement of central venous pressure and chest radiography, which will demonstrate cardiac enlargement and pulmonary venous congestion in heart failure.

Summary 1 Indicators of disturbed water and sodium homeostasis

- Raised venous pressure
- Weight gain
- Oedema
- Chest radiography (information on cardiac status)
- Postural hypotension
- Weight loss
- Skin turgor and intraocular pressure (unreliable)
- Reduction in urine output (if profound salt and water depletion)

Profound sodium and water depletion results in a reduction in urine output. The distinction between this prerenal oliguria and renal failure is discussed on page 859.

DISORDERS OF WATER HOMEOSTASIS

In some pathological conditions, dramatic changes in total body water may occur with little or no alteration in total body sodium or potassium; in others, water loss may be accompanied by significant losses of electrolytes. Even in the latter circumstance, however, the water deficit will usually be relatively greater than the sodium deficit, which has important implications for the interpretation of plasma sodium estimations (p. 850).

WATER DEPLETION

Water depletion may occur:

- as a result of failure of renal concentrating capacity
- by obligatory insensible water loss (through the skin, lungs and as concentrated urine) in situations when oral fluid intake is inadequate
- via the kidney when osmotically active solutes are present in tubular fluid in increased quantity
- via the gut
- by increased pulmonary loss in acute respiratory disease.

Because water depletion is borne by both intra- and extracellular compartments, the physical signs of fluid depletion may not be marked and, in particular, signs of reduced circulating volume occur late. With a severe reduction in total body water, a decreased level of consciousness is common and may persist for a considerable time after the deficit has been corrected. Severe water depletion results in both extra- and intracellular hyperosmolality (the rise in intracellular osmolality being highest in the central nervous system) and a tendency to intravas-

cular thrombosis. Water depletion is accompanied by a rise in plasma sodium.

DIABETES INSIPIDUS

This condition arises when the kidneys lose, usually partially, the capacity to produce a concentrated urine. The classical presentation is with excessive thirst (polydipsia) and the passage of large volumes of dilute urine (polyuria). The length of history is usually short, although mild failure of concentrating capacity may be present for a considerable time prior to diagnosis.

Causes

Diabetes insipidus occurs as a result of either deficiency of ADH secretion or failure of ADH action at renal tubular level. Important causes of the deficit, usually referred to as *cranial* or *neurogenic diabetes insipidus*, are listed in Table 21.1; postsurgical and so-called idiopathic causes are by far the most common. There is now considerable evidence that a proportion of apparently idiopathic examples are in fact due to autoimmunity and fit into the spec-

Table 21.1 Causes of diabetes insipidus

Cause	Example/comment
Cranial (neurogenic) diabetes insipidus	
Idiopathic	(Some autoimmune)
Familial	Autosomal dominant
	Autosomal recessive and including one or more of diabetes mellitus, optic atrophy, high tone deafness (DIDMOAD syndrome)
Postsurgical Traumatic	May be temporary
Tumours	Pituitary adenoma (rare)
	Craniopharyngioma
	Dysgerminoma } rare hypothalamic
	Teratoma } tumours
	Secondary carcinomas esp. lung, breast
Granulomata	Sarcoid
	TB
	Histiocytosis X
Infections	Meningitis/encephalitis
Vascular	e.g. Sheehan's syndrome – postpartum pituitary infarction (now rare)
Nephrogenic diabetes insipidus	
Familial	X-linked recessive
Hypercalcaemia	Malignancy, hyperparathyroidism
Hypokalaemia	Diuresis
Drug-induced	Lithium salts
	Demethylchlortetracycline

trum of organ-specific autoimmune diseases, which include autoimmune thyroiditis, adrenalitis, pernicious anaemia and some cases of diabetes mellitus. Pituitary adenomas rarely present with diabetes insipidus and, as a result of improvements in obstetric care, postpartum pituitary infarction is now rare. Diabetes insipidus secondary to pathological processes affecting the neurohypophysis, but sparing the pituitary stalk and neurosecretory cells, is frequently transient.

As adequate glucocorticoid is essential for water excretion, adrenocorticotrophic hormone (ACTH) deficiency may mask associated diabetes insipidus. The latter condition only becomes clinically evident when steroid replacement therapy is begun.

Failure of ADH action on renal tubules *(nephrogenic diabetes insipidus)* may occur as a primary inherited disorder, as a consequence of certain drugs, or secondary to hypercalcaemia or hypokalaemia (see Table 21.1). *Familial* nephrogenic diabetes insipidus is a rare X-linked recessive condition presenting in infancy. The underlying mechanism appears to be a defect either in the action of ADH on the renal tubule receptor, or in postreceptor activity. The disease is fully expressed in males inheriting the affected X chromosome, but subclinical defects in renal concentrating capacity may be found in female carriers.

Common *drug-induced* causes of failure of renal concentrating ability include lithium salts (used to treat manic-depressive disorders) and the long-acting tetracycline, demethylchlortetracycline. This action of demethylchlortetracycline is used to treat the syndrome of inappropriate secretion of antidiuretic hormone (SIADH) typically found in small-cell lung cancer. These agents probably produce their effects by impairing ADH-induced cyclic-AMP formation in renal tubular cells.

Hypercalcaemia reduces renal concentrating capacity by inhibiting chloride transport in the loop of Henle, with a consequent reduction in medullary hypertonicity, and by inhibiting the action of ADH on renal tubular cells. These effects may be marked in severe hypercalcaemia, and contribute to the vicious circle of dehydration and accelerating hypercalcaemia which may develop. Chronic *hypokalaemia* may produce the same effect, although usually to a lesser extent than with hypercalcaemia.

Investigation of polyuria and polydipsia

The approach to this combination of symptoms is outlined in Figure 21.4. Prolonged water deprivation is usually unnecessary, it being sufficient to continue only until 2-hourly measurements of osmolality have reached a maximum (normally achieved within 8 hours). It is important that the patient is weighed at hourly intervals and that the test is discontinued if weight loss exceeds 3% of total body weight. The latter outcome is virtually diag-

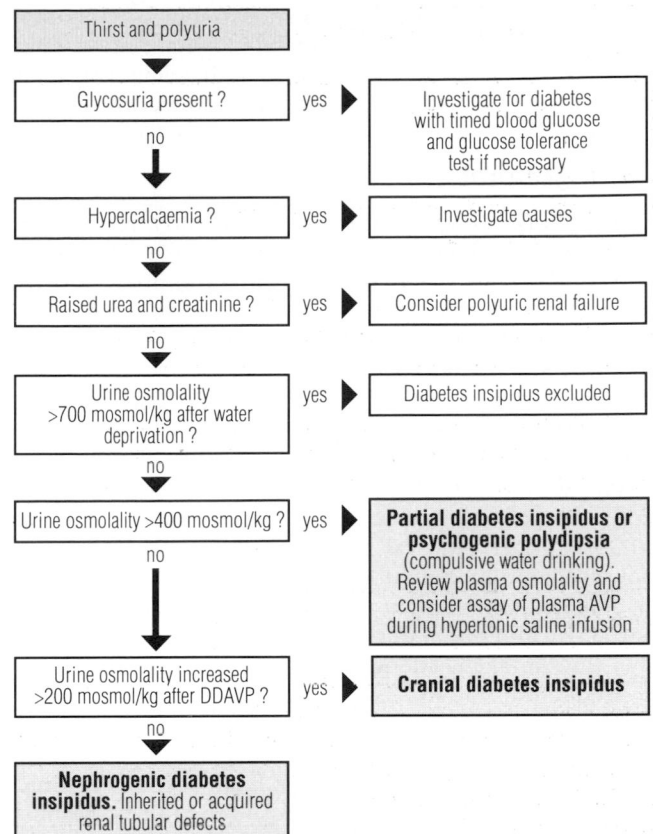

Fig. 21.4 The investigation of polyuria and polydipsia.

nostic of diabetes insipidus. Renal responsiveness to ADH is tested with an intranasal test dose (20–40 μg) of the synthetic ADH analogue, desmopressin (1-desamino-8-D-arginine vasopressin, DDAVP). Urine osmolality is measured in all specimens passed in the ensuing 9 hours.

The most difficult distinction to make is that between partial degrees of diabetes insipidus and compulsive water drinking. The latter condition, which represents an extreme of habit-mediated fluid consumption, results in renal medullary hypotonicity and a consequent secondary renal-concentrating defect. Some assistance in diagnosis may be provided by the plasma osmolality (or plasma sodium), which is characteristically less than 290 mosm/kg at commencement of water deprivation in compulsive water drinkers (because of some degree of overhydration), but is frequently higher than normal in partial diabetes insipidus because of water depletion. When the history and preliminary investigations still fail to distinguish between these possibilities, there is a place for measurement of plasma ADH (by radioimmunoassay) in response to a continuous intravenous infusion of hypertonic saline. In this test, patients with compulsive water drinking show a normal rise in plasma ADH as plasma osmolality increases; whereas any rise in patients with partial degrees of cranial diabetes insipidus is demonstrably less. It is vital that fluid intake should be controlled when test doses of DDAVP are administered, because of the danger of water intoxication in patients with compulsive water drinking.

Management

Cranial diabetes insipidus is most conveniently treated with the synthetic ADH analogue, desmopressin (DDAVP). This has a greater weight-for-weight antidiuretic activity than ADH and lacks the potentially hazardous vasopressor effects of ADH. It also has a prolonged half-life so that single doses act for up to 18 hours. For maintenance therapy, desmopressin is administered intranasally in doses of 2.5–20 μg once or twice daily. In partial disease, a single nocturnal dose may be sufficient. When intranasal administration is contraindicated, desmopressin may be given intramuscularly once or twice daily (0.25–2.0 μg). An oral preparation of desmopressin is now available but high doses are required.

The aim of treatment is to replace antidiuretic activity partially with normal thirst mechanisms, thereby ensuring that fluid intake is adequate and that overhydration and consequent intra- and extracellular dilution are avoided. Difficulties may arise with hypothalamic disorders which interfere with normal thirst mechanisms as well as ADH production. In these situations a fixed regimen of fluid intake and a carefully titrated dose schedule of desmopressin must be provided for the patient.

Nephrogenic diabetes insipidus, by definition unresponsive to desmopressin, is treated with thiazide diuretics and some limitation of sodium intake. The rationale is that the induced mild sodium depletion results in enhanced proximal renal tubular sodium and water reabsorption.

OTHER CONDITIONS IN WHICH WATER DEPLETION PREDOMINATES

Because of the effectiveness of the renal mechanism of sodium conservation, water depletion may predominate in a number of conditions simultaneously threatening to deplete both body salt and body water.

- It is most common in patients unable to maintain an adequate oral intake due to either upper gastrointestinal obstruction or a reduced level of consciousness. In this situation, continued obligatory insensible and renal loss of water results in slow, progressive intra- and extracellular dehydration. Urinary sodium loss is reduced to a minimum.
- Obligatory gastrointestinal loss of water also occurs in response to a large solute load. This may be produced by the administration of hyperosmolar solutions via a nasogastric tube to a partially conscious or paralysed patient.

- Virtually pure water loss may also occur as exaggerated insensible loss, via the lungs, in acute respiratory disorders such as asthma.
- Water depletion may be a feature of untreated diabetes mellitus, and is most likely to occur in the previously undiagnosed non-insulin-dependent diabetic who maintains a high intake of refined sugar (Ch. 19). A vicious circle of osmotic diuresis and rising extra- and intracellular osmolality may occur, especially if an intercurrent illness is present. Some increased renal loss of sodium occurs but this is relatively less than the water deficit. In the absence of ketosis, vomiting and consequent marked salt depletion is uncommon.
- High protein nasogastric feeds with subsequent protein catabolism may induce a solute diuresis.

Management

When oral fluid replacement is impractical, mild water depletion is treated by intravenous infusion of an iso-osmolar electrolyte-free solution (5% dextrose is the standard choice). However, this is unsatisfactory if some degree of salt depletion has also occurred, and in this situation infusions of isotonic saline (0.9%) are usually employed. Provided cardiac and renal function are adequate, any excess sodium replacement will be excreted via the kidneys. Alternatively, combinations of dextrose and saline solutions may be used. Maintenance daily intravenous fluid replacement for an adult patient taking nothing by mouth would aim to provide approximately 2.0–2.5 litres of water with 70 mmol of sodium and 60–80 mmol of potassium. This could be given as 2 litres of 5% dextrose and 0.5 litres of isotonic saline, with potassium chloride added in even distribution.

When water depletion has been sufficiently severe to elevate plasma osmolality markedly, there is a theoretical risk of cerebral oedema if water is rapidly replaced as 5% dextrose alone or in the form of hypotonic saline (e.g. half normal, 0.45%). For this reason, isotonic saline (0.9%) is often used to avoid an excessively rapid change in plasma osmolality. This policy may need to be modified, however, if the plasma sodium concentration continues to increase during isotonic saline administration. This may arise as a result of persistent water losses and of continuing aldosterone-mediated renal sodium reabsorption (stimulated by hypovolaemia). Nonetheless, profound water depletion should be corrected slowly, although the rate of fluid administration must keep pace with continuing renal loss of water in conditions of osmotic diuresis.

WATER EXCESS

An excess of total body water arises when water intake exceeds renal and cutaneous losses. Water excess is unlikely in the presence of normal renal function, except in

Table 21.2 Causes of reduced water excretion

Cause	Mechanism
Renal impairment	
Liver cirrhosis (hypoalbuminaemia)	
Cardiac failure	Reduced glomerular filtration rate leads to reduced solute delivery to distal tubule
Nephrotic syndrome (hypoalbuminaemia)	
Glucocorticoid deficiency	
Inappropriate ADH secretion (SIADH)	Increased renal tubular reabsorption of water

situations of increased water intake determined by psychological disturbance or, rarely, by hypothalamic disease. When water excretion is impaired, however, a rise in total body water is relatively common (Table 21.2), and is accompanied by a fall in plasma sodium (*dilutional hyponatraemia*).

The tendency to water excess in cardiac failure is usually compounded by diuretic therapy. This further impairs urinary dilution, and may result in stimulation of thirst as a result of increased activation of the renin–angiotensin system.

In SIADH, ADH secretion occurs despite hypotonicity of extracellular fluid and in the absence of depletion of circulating volume. The common causes are listed in Table 21.3. In many of these situations, the severity of the relative water excess and its clinical consequences may be aggravated by inappropriate administration of intravenous fluids.

Clinical features and diagnosis

Mild degrees of water excess cause few symptoms and the clinical features of the underlying disease predominate. However, with severe water excess, as may occur in some

Table 21.3 Causes of inappropriate ADH secretion (SIADH)

Source	Cause
Ectopic	Malignancies such as small-cell bronchial carcinoma
Hypothalamic	Inflammatory lung diseases
	CNS infections
	Drugs
	Carbamazepine
	Chlorpropamide
	Tricyclics
	Phenothiazines
	Syntocinon
	Cytotoxic drugs
	Cyclophosphamide
	Vincristine
	Wasting diseases

cases of SIADH, the reduction in intracellular osmolality in the central nervous system may produce symptoms ranging in severity from general lassitude to decreased levels of consciousness, coma and generalised convulsions.

The diagnosis of water excess is usually suggested at routine investigation by finding *hyponatraemia* in the absence of clinical or other evidence of volume depletion. Although sodium-depleting states may also result in hyponatraemia, this is only the case if the losses are marked. However, hyponatraemia may occur without water excess when the contribution of glucose to plasma osmolality is increased in untreated diabetes mellitus. The potential rise in plasma osmolality results in a movement of water from the intracellular to extracellular spaces, and a consequent fall in plasma sodium. Furthermore, an apparent hyponatraemia (*pseudohyponatraemia*) may be evident if marked hyperlipidaemia contributes significantly to plasma volume, thus reducing the water content per unit volume.

The assessment of the hyponatraemic patient is outlined in Figure 21.5. It will be noted that SIADH is characterised by hypotonicity of plasma (osmolality <280 mosm/kg) with inappropriate urinary concentration (>300 mosm/kg). This condition is associated with a normal or slightly increased circulating volume, so that

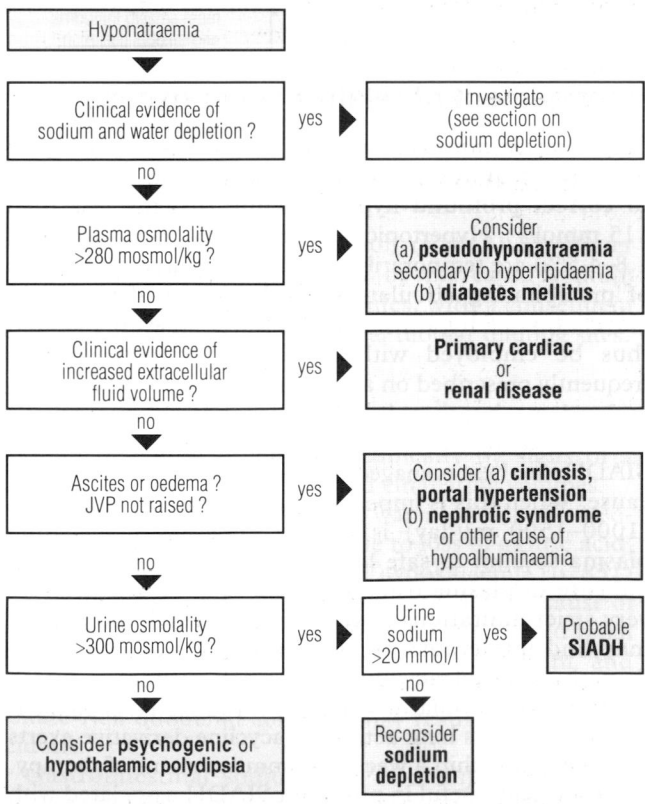

Fig. 21.5 The clinical and biochemical evaluation of hyponatraemia.

Table 21.6 Causes of net renal sodium loss

Intrinsic renal disease
Recovery phase of acute tubular necrosis
Relief of long-standing urinary obstruction
Some forms of chronic nephropathy, particularly tubulo-interstitial disease

Mineralocorticoid deficiency
Adrenal failure
Isolated aldosterone deficiency

Diuretic therapy

gastrointestinal cause. The causes of renal salt loss are given in Table 21.6. Sodium balance is particularly vulnerable in those forms of chronic renal disease which affect the medulla. Such patients lose the capacity to vary sodium excretion and are susceptible to dramatic salt depletion in the event of intercurrent gastrointestinal disturbance, with a resultant further and rapid reduction in glomerular filtration rate. In different circumstances, however, these patients are in potential danger of sodium retention (p. 848).

As a consequence of the reduction in circulating volume which accompanies marked sodium depletion, there is a fall in glomerular filtration rate and thus a rise in plasma urea and creatinine concentrations (Fig. 21.7). This is termed *pre-renal uraemia* (Ch. 20), and may, in some cases, prove difficult to distinguish from acute renal failure. In general, pre-renal states are associated with a disproportionate rise in the concentration of plasma urea compared with that of creatinine, and the haematocrit may also be raised consistent with haemoconcentration. However, other factors which affect plasma urea concentration, e.g. quantity of dietary protein or rate of body protein catabolism, may limit the usefulness of this comparison.

A low urinary sodium concentration distinguishes non-renal sodium depletion from acute renal failure (in which

urine sodium concentration is normal or increased). In the diuretic phase of acute tubular necrosis, or after relief of urinary obstruction, the aetiology of the sodium loss is usually obvious. The possibility of adrenal insufficiency should be borne in mind in any patient who presents with evidence of unexplained salt depletion.

Isolated aldosterone deficiency may occur in the absence of glucocorticoid deficiency and is a rare but well recognised complication of long-standing diabetes, particularly when complicated by autonomic neuropathy.

Management

Clinically obvious salt and water deficit almost always requires intravenous replacement with isotonic saline (sodium chloride, 0.9%). Potassium supplements are required for gastrointestinal losses. When it is impossible to distinguish definitely between salt depletion and established acute renal failure as the cause of the presenting oliguria and uraemia, it may be of benefit to administer 500 ml 0.9% saline rapidly and monitor urine output in response to this.

Salt-depleting chronic renal disease may necessitate regular oral sodium supplements (Ch. 20).

Interpretation of plasma sodium concentrations

The plasma sodium concentration reflects the degree of dilution of extracellular sodium. It thus tells us a great deal about total body water but relatively little about total body sodium. We learn more about the latter from clinical examination, from indirect indicators of glomerular filtration rate (dependent on circulating volume) such as plasma urea and creatinine, and from urine sodium excretion rates (Table 21.7).

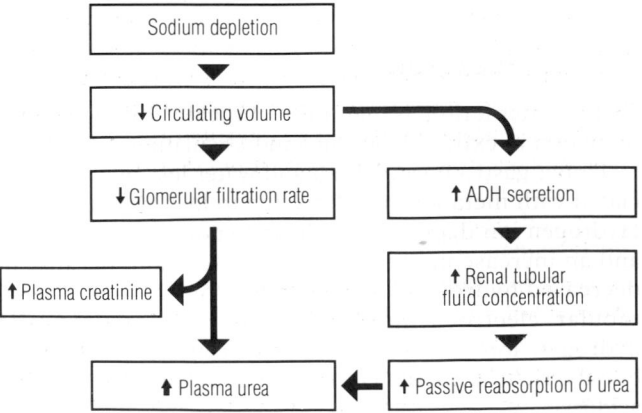

Fig. 21.7 The renal consequences of sodium depletion. The percentage increase in plasma urea exceeds that of creatinine by the mechanism shown, provided intrinsic renal function remains normal.

Table 21.7 Interpretation of the plasma sodium concentration

Diagnosis	Plasma Na$^+$	Plasma creatinine	Urine sodium (mmol/l)	Urine osmolality (mosm/kg)
SIADH	Low	↓	>20	>300
Adrenal failure	Low	↑	>20	>300
Renal failure	Low/normal	↑↑	>20	<300
Non-renal sodium loss	Low/normal	↑	<20	>300
Primary water deficit	High	N or ↑	>20	>300
Diabetes insipidus	High	N or ↑	<20	<300
Hyperosmolar diabetes mellitus	High	↑	Variable	>300

POTASSIUM HOMEOSTASIS

Potassium ions are predominantly intracellular, the concentration gradient depending on active Na^+/K^+ exchange across the plasma membrane (Fig. 21.2). The other major determinant of the distribution is pH. Alkalosis, associated with a fall in intracellular hydrogen ion concentration, results in a net flux of potassium into cells with a consequent fall in plasma potassium; acidosis has the reverse effect (Fig. 21.8). The mechanism of these changes is unknown but may be related to intracellular changes in hydrogen ion binding of negatively charged proteins. Cellular uptake of potassium is probably also partially insulin-dependent.

Maintenance of total body potassium depends on dietary intake (approximately 100 mmol per day in Western diets) and on control of renal potassium excretion. Potassium is actively reabsorbed in the proximal renal tubule. In the distal tubule, potassium excretion occurs by diffusion down its electrochemical gradient (Fig. 21.9). In the collecting ducts, passage of potassium into tubular fluid appears to be an active process shared with hydrogen ions, apparently in exchange for sodium ions in tubular fluid. This exchange is enhanced by increased concentrations of sodium in the tubular lumen and by aldosterone. Changes in intra- and extracellular pH alter concentrations of potassium in renal tubular cells and thus indirectly affect renal potassium excretion both by diffusion and in exchange for sodium. Under conditions of high potassium intake, renal tubular potassium secretion is increased.

HYPOKALAEMIA

A significant reduction in plasma potassium usually indicates profound depletion of total body potassium but may occasionally be due to temporary shifts of potassium ions from the extra- to intracellular spaces. The important causes of hypokalaemia and the proposed underlying mechanisms are outlined in Table 21.8.

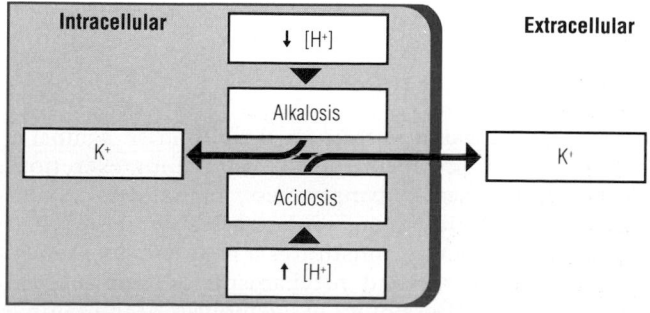

Fig. 21.8 The effect of acid–base changes on the distribution of potassium across cell membranes. The steady state distribution is altered by either acidosis or alkalosis in the directions shown.

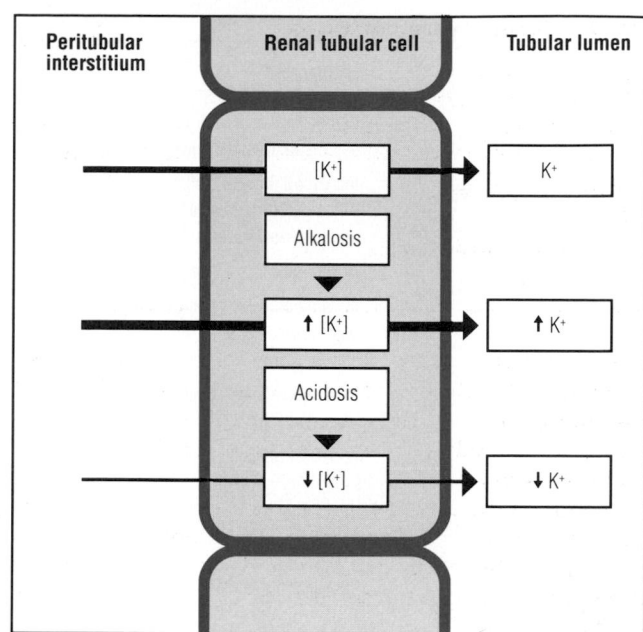

Fig. 21.9 The influence of acid–base changes on intracellular potassium concentration and renal excretion in the distal renal tubule. Diffusion of potassium into the tubular lumen is increased by alkalosis and decreased by acidosis as a consequence of changes in potassium concentration in renal tubular cells.

Clinical features

Non-specific symptoms of lethargy and weakness may accompany mild to moderate hypokalaemia (c. 2.8–3.5 mmol/l). Lower levels may give rise to marked muscular weakness, gut hypomotility, increased myocardial excitability and arrhythmias, and nephrogenic diabetes insipidus. A shift of hydrogen ions from extra- to intracellular spaces is thought to be responsible for the *metabolic alkalosis* which accompanies most cases of hypokalaemia. This apparent hydrogen ion shift may be due to a relative failure of cell membrane proton pumps (H^+ extrusion). In addition, chronic hypokalaemia may reduce renal chloride conservation, with a consequent increased delivery of sodium to distal tubular sites. This promotes sodium exchange for hydrogen ions with accentuation of the alkalosis.

Investigation

In many instances, the mechanism of hypokalaemia is obvious from the history and clinical observations. When this is not the case, investigation is directed initially at distinguishing gastrointestinal from renal loss of potassium by means of total 24-hour urine potassium estimations. These are very low in all non-renal mechanisms of potassium loss, with the exception of repeated vomiting which is complicated by alkalosis. It may prove very diffi-

Table 21.8 Causes of hypokalaemia

Cause	Mechanism
Alkalosis	Intracellular shift of K^+ in exchange for H^+; increased renal excretion
Diuretics Diabetes mellitus	Increased renal excretion secondary to enhanced distal tubular sodium delivery and increased tubular flow
*Conn's syndrome	Increased aldosterone effect
*Cushing's syndrome (esp. ectopic ACTH from malignant source)	Mineralocorticoid effect of increased glucocorticoids
*Steroid therapy (esp. high dose hydrocortisone)	Mineralocorticoid effect of increased glucocorticoids
*Carbenoxolone therapy for peptic ulcer	Mineralocorticoid effect
*Congenital adrenal hyperplasia (11-hydroxylase deficiency)	Mineralocorticoid effect of deoxycorticosterone
11β-hydroxysteroid dehydrogenase deficiency	Reduced peripheral metabolism of cortisol
Renal tubular acidosis (distal type)	Decreased Na^+/H^+ exchange in distal tubule (see Ch. 20)
Bartter's syndrome	Defective chloride absorption in loop of Henle with consequent solute loss and secondary hyperaldosteronism
Vomiting (esp. pyloric stenosis and bulimia nervosa)	Loss of gastric contents and effects of alkalosis
Secretory diarrhoea	Direct loss of potassium
Laxative abuse	Direct loss of potassium
Villous adenoma of rectum	Enhanced potassium loss from tumour cells
Hypokalaemic periodic paralysis	Intermittent shift of potassium into cells

*See Ch. 17

cult to diagnose surreptitious vomiting, or diuretic or laxative abuse. A finding of hypokalaemia with a *low* plasma bicarbonate always suggests the possibility of renal tubular acidosis and should prompt measurement of urinary pH (which will be inappropriately high in this condition). The rare combination of acidosis and hypokalaemia is also seen in the most severe examples of diabetic ketoacidosis, when potassium depletion is particularly marked.

Management

Hypokalaemia is usually corrected by oral potassium chloride in wax base (e.g. Slow K); if potassium depletion is profound and life-threatening, potassium chloride is given intravenously. The rate of administration depends on any continuing losses, but it should rarely be necessary to exceed 30 mmol/hour even at the initiation of therapy. Plasma potassium concentrations should be monitored regularly.

Rare causes of hypokalaemia

Bartter's syndrome

This rare syndrome, which may present in childhood, comprises a combination of hypokalaemic alkalosis, hyperreninaemia and secondary hyperaldosteronism. The precise pathogenesis is obscure but much evidence points towards defective chloride absorption in the ascending limb of the loop of Henle. Increased urinary prostaglandin excretion has been noted but is probably a secondary phenomenon. It is important to exclude diuretic abuse and surreptitious vomiting which may also present with unexplained hypokalaemic alkalosis and activation of the renin–angiotensin system.

Potassium supplementation and prostaglandin synthetase inhibition with indomethacin are effective in partially reversing the hypokalaemia. Inhibition of renin secretion with propranolol may be a useful addition.

Hypokalaemic periodic paralysis

In this condition paroxysmal episodes of profound muscular weakness may occur accompanied by hypokalaemia. The underlying mechanism is unknown but precipitating factors include high carbohydrate meals, sepsis, exercise and stress, all of which may promote shift of potassium into cells. The condition may be dominantly inherited. Certain susceptible patients with thyrotoxicosis may develop hypokalaemic periodic paralysis; this is rare in Caucasians but occurs in approximately 10% of oriental patients with Graves' thyrotoxicosis. Treatment of the thyroid disorder is curative.

11β-hydroxysteroid dehydrogenase deficiency

In this condition, which may present in childhood, peripheral metabolism of cortisol is impaired, with consequent increased renal mineralocorticoid effect of cortisol leading to hypertension and suppression of the renin–angiotensin system. Treatment with spironolactone or amiloride is effective.

HYPERKALAEMIA

Increases in plasma potassium usually arise against a background of decreased renal potassium excretion. Moderate increases are symptomless, but at levels exceeding 6.5 mmol/l, the risk of cardiac arrest increases, and severe hyperkalaemia constitutes a medical emergency. Aetiological factors and mechanisms are outlined in Table 21.9. The possibility of haemolysis of the sample causing artefactual hyperkalaemia should be considered in instances of isolated hyperkalaemia in the presence of normal renal function. Occasionally increased potassium

Table 21.9 Causes of hyperkalaemia

Cause	Mechanism
Acute renal failure	Decreased excretion which may be compounded by acidosis, cell necrosis (esp. when infection present), transfusions of stored blood and potassium retaining diuretics
Acidosis	Shift of potassium from intra- to extracellular spaces
Cell necrosis (e.g. after cancer chemotherapy)	Release of cellular potassium
Type 4 renal tubular acidosis (see Ch. 20)	Impairment of K^+ secretion in the distal nephron caused by: (a) Decreased mineralocorticoid activity due to adrenal failure (b) Reduced activity of renin–angiotensin system ('hyporeninaemic hypoaldosteronism') e.g. in diabetic neuropathy (c) Angiotensin converting enzyme inhibitors (d) Potassium retaining diuretics, i.e. direct inhibition of aldosterone action (spironolactone) or of Na^+/K^+ distal tubular exchange (amiloride, triamterene) (e) Tubular resistance to mineralocorticoid action

leakage from red cells may occur in blood stored at room temperature; this is a dominantly inherited phenomenon (familial pseudohyperkalaemia) of no clinical significance and is diagnosed by maintaining the sample at 37°C prior to potassium measurement.

Management

Marked hyperkalaemia (>7 mmol/1) should be reduced as a matter of urgency because of the risk of cardiac arrest. Simultaneous intravenous administration of glucose (50 g) and insulin (15 units) is temporarily effective; and intravenous bicarbonate (50 mmol) will cause some shift of potassium from the extracellular to the intracellular compartment. (The associated sodium load may be poorly tolerated, however, and dialysis may be necessary.) Renal potassium losses may be increased by loop diuretics such as frusemide. Intravenous calcium salts afford some protection against the cardiac consequences of hyperkalaemia. ECG monitoring is useful for acute assessment. Moderate hyperkalaemia is associated with peaking of T waves; more sinister changes include increasing width of QRS complexes. Longer-term control may be achieved by means of cation exchange resins (e.g. Resonium A-sodium, Calcium Resonium) which are given either orally or by retention enema.

The management of adrenal failure and hypoaldosteronism are considered in Chapter 17.

ACID–BASE HOMEOSTASIS

A large number of metabolic events are pH sensitive and maintenance of a stable acid–base status is therefore of critical importance. In the healthy individual, extracellular pH is held within narrow limits (pH 7.38–7.42). Intracellular pH is generally lower than extracellular pH and varies both from one tissue to another and according to nutritional status and exercise state (mean range pH 6.7–7.3). Under normal circumstances, homeostatic mechanisms are generally concerned with the buffering and disposal of hydrogen ions generated by intracellular metabolic events, particularly aerobic respiration (CO_2 production), glycolysis (lactic acid production) and lipolysis (fatty acid and eventual ketoacid production, see Table 21.10).

The acceptance of hydrogen ions by intra- or extracellular buffer base constitutes the first line of defence against deviations from normal pH. Important buffer systems include bicarbonate/carbonic acid, red cell haemoglobin, phosphate and intracellular proteins. Exhaustion of buffer capacity is prevented by short- or long-term elimination of hydrogen ions or by regeneration of bicarbonate. This occurs through respiration (acid eliminated in the form of CO_2); metabolism (hepatic metabolism of lactic acid, tissue metabolism of ketone bodies and free fatty acid); and renal excretion (buffered by ammonia and phosphate).

Lactic acid metabolism provides an interesting example of immediate buffering with subsequent hydrogen ion consumption and bicarbonate regeneration. Lactic acid (pK 4.6) is fully dissociated in plasma, and protons are consumed by normal buffering mechanisms (e.g. bicarbonate). The subsequent hepatic metabolism of lactate ions to produce glucose requires the stoichiometric consumption of hydrogen ions with consequent formation of bicarbonate from carbon dioxide and hydroxyl ions.

Table 21.10 Acid generation and elimination

Source	Acid	Elimination
Aerobic respiration	CO_2	Pulmonary
Glycolysis	Lactic acid	Hepatic metabolism to glucose or CO_2 (pulmonary elimination)
Lipolysis	Free fatty acids	Oxidation to CO_2 (pulmonary elimination)
Hepatic metabolism	Ketone bodies	Oxidation to CO_2 (pulmonary elimination)
Dietary protein catabolism	Inorganic acids	Renal

Henderson-Hasselbalch equation

The equilibrium relationship between the protonated and anionic forms of a buffer pair such as bicarbonate/carbonic acid may be indicated as follows:

$$[H_2CO_3] \underset{K_2}{\overset{K_1}{\rightleftharpoons}} [H^+] + [HCO_3^-]$$

$$\frac{K_1}{K_2} = \frac{[H^+][HCO_3^-]}{H_2CO_3} = K \text{ (equilibrium constant)}$$

$$[H^+] = \frac{K[H_2CO_3]}{[HCO_3^-]}$$

$$pH = pK + \log \frac{[HCO_3^-]}{[H_2CO_3]} \text{ (proportional to } P\text{CO}_2)$$

This is the classical Henderson-Hasselbalch equation which can be applied to all physiological buffer systems. Reference to the above equation indicates the change in concentration of a given buffer component which is required for pH to remain constant following a primary alteration in acid–base status. Thus, metabolic production of acid which leads to an immediate fall in HCO_3^- will lead to a fall in pH unless $P\text{CO}_2$ also decreases by increased respiration. Increases in $P\text{CO}_2$ consequent upon respiratory failure necessitate a rise in HCO_3^- concentration (by increased renal conservation of bicarbonate) if pH changes are to be minimised. Similar arguments can be applied to situations in which primary increases in HCO_3^-, or decreases in $P\text{CO}_2$, occur. Primary alterations in CO_2 are denoted as *respiratory acidosis or alkalosis* and primary changes in buffer base as *metabolic acidosis or alkalosis*. These terms apply regardless of whether or not appropriate compensatory mechanisms have been sufficient to maintain pH within the normal range (compensated metabolic or respiratory acidosis or alkalosis). Respiratory compensation is discussed in Chapter 13, page 449; see also Figure 13.7.

INVESTIGATION OF ACID–BASE STATUS

Blood gas analysis

Blood gas analysers measure pH and $P\text{CO}_2$ directly by means of specific electrodes, and bicarbonate concentrations are automatically calculated using the Henderson-Hasselbalch equation. Values are usually also given for the so-called 'standard bicarbonate' which represents the theoretical bicarbonate concentrations at a $P\text{CO}_2$ of 5.3 kPa (40 mmHg), and thus purports to show the extent

Table 21.11 Changes in $P\text{CO}_2$ and HCO_3 in acid–base disorders

	pH	$P\text{CO}_2$	HCO_3^-
Metabolic acidosis	N or ↓	↓	↓↓
Metabolic alkalosis	N or ↑	Slight ↑	↑↑
Respiratory acidosis	N or ↓	↑↑	↑
Respiratory alkalosis	N or ↑	↓↓	slight ↓

The primary derangements are denoted by double arrows.

of a given acid-base disturbance attributable to metabolic causes alone. In practice, however, clinical assessment and measurements of pH, $P\text{CO}_2$, $P\text{O}_2$ and bicarbonate are sufficient for the accurate classification of pure or mixed (e.g. acute metabolic acidosis and chronic respiratory acidosis) acid–base disturbances (Table 21.11).

Metabolic acidosis results in rapid respiratory compensation due to stimulation of carotid body, aortic and medullary chemoreceptors. *Metabolic alkalosis*, on the other hand, is less well compensated by respiratory mechanisms, probably because any decrease in ventilation is limited by hypoxic respiratory drive.

Chronic respiratory acidosis is partially compensated by a rise in plasma bicarbonate. This compensation occurs via increased hydrogen ion excretion and renal conservation of bicarbonate, a long-term effect occurring over 2–3 days.

Difficulties in interpretation may arise with *mixed acid–base disturbances*. This is most commonly seen with the superimposition of metabolic acidosis on chronic respiratory acidosis. This combination results in a low pH (by definition), an elevated $P\text{CO}_2$ (inability to respond to acidotic respiratory drive), and a fall in previously elevated bicarbonate level. The clinical presentation, history and critical evaluation of pH, $P\text{CO}_2$ and bicarbonate will usually indicate the dual diagnosis, and a decreased $P\text{O}_2$ will provide additional evidence of the respiratory component.

The anion gap

Subtraction of the total plasma concentrations of chloride and bicarbonate anions from sodium and potassium cations normally yields a 'gap value' of 10–20 mmol/l, made up of negatively charged proteins, phosphate, sulphate, lactate and small quantities of ketoacids. Calculation of this *anion gap* in metabolic acidosis is useful for distinguishing cases due to bicarbonate loss (e.g. pancreatic fistulae, renal tubular acidosis), in which the anion gap is normal, from those due to increases in endogenously produced acid (e.g. ketoacidosis, lactic acidosis and the acidosis of renal failure) in which the gap is increased. In the former cases, plasma chloride is increased (hyperchloraemic acidosis) to maintain electroneutrality.

Table 21.12 Causes of metabolic acidosis

Normal anion gap	Increased anion gap
Gut bicarbonate loss (e.g. pancreatic fistula)	Diabetic ketoacidosis
	Starvation ketoacidosis
Renal tubular acidosis (urine pH inappropriately high)	Lactic acidosis
Distal type (failure of proton secretion). Primary and secondary	Type A secondary to increased peripheral glycolysis in circulatory failure or hypoxia
Treatment with carbon anhydrase inhibitors	Type B secondary to failure of lactate metabolism or to net lactate production in liver, e.g. biguanide drugs, ethanol, methanol, ethylene glycol, fructose, liver disease
Proximal type (bicarbonate wastage). Primary and secondary	
	Acidosis of renal failure
	Salicylate poisoning

ACID–BASE DISORDERS

Metabolic acidosis

The common causes of metabolic acidosis are listed in Table 21.12.

The increased respiratory drive resulting from severe metabolic acidosis is clinically recognisable as deep, sighing respiration (*Kussmaul respiration*). Respiratory compensation for metabolic acidosis is dependent on adequate respiratory reserve. In many of the conditions listed in Table 21.12, accumulation of more than one acid may occur. If acidosis, from whatever cause, is severe, reduction in cardiac output may result in a superimposed lactic acidosis (Type A). This is due to increased peripheral glycolysis which occurs with tissue anoxia. Similarly, diabetic ketoacidosis is associated with salt and water depletion, and the resulting fall in circulating volume leads to

increased peripheral glycolysis and lactic acid accumulation. The situation is further complicated because acidosis itself partially inhibits the glycolytic pathway in peripheral tissues (Fig. 21.10), which tends to offset the increase in lactic acid production. However, acidosis directly inhibits hepatic gluconeogenic enzymes and, because lactate is an important gluconeogenic substrate, this may result in progressive lactic acid accumulation. Loss of the slight intracellular alkalinising effect of hepatic lactate metabolism further accentuates the effects of acidosis on hepatic lactate removal (Fig. 21.10).

The acidosis of renal failure has traditionally been attributed to decreased ammonia formation (from glutamine) in the diseased kidney, with consequent decreased buffering capacity in the urine. Decreased urinary buffer results in the minimum urinary pH being reached at a lower total hydrogen ion content, and thus leads to systemic acidosis. However, it has recently been pointed out that, because the metabolism of glutamine in renal tubular cells yields NH_4^+ rather than NH_3, this mechanism cannot be responsible for net hydrogen ion excretion by the kidney. The other route of glutamine metabolism is via urea formation in the liver. This mechanism results in net bicarbonate consumption and, since glutamine is diverted to hepatic metabolism when renal metabolism is impaired, it follows that the acidosis of renal failure may be primarily related to the acid-generating (i.e. bicarbonate-consuming) effect of hepatic ureagenesis (Fig. 21.11).

Details of renal tubular acidosis and salicylate poisoning are given in Chapters 21 and 4 respectively.

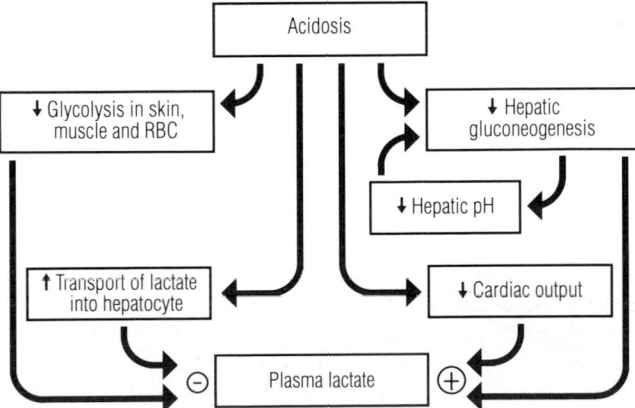

Fig. 21.10 The metabolic consequences of metabolic acidosis. Acidosis tends to decrease hepatic metabolism with resultant lactate and hydrogen ion accumulation. These effects are partially offset by a direct partial inhibition of glycolysis by acidosis and an increase in lactate transport into hepatocytes. (–) and (+) denote the potential changes in plasma lactate.

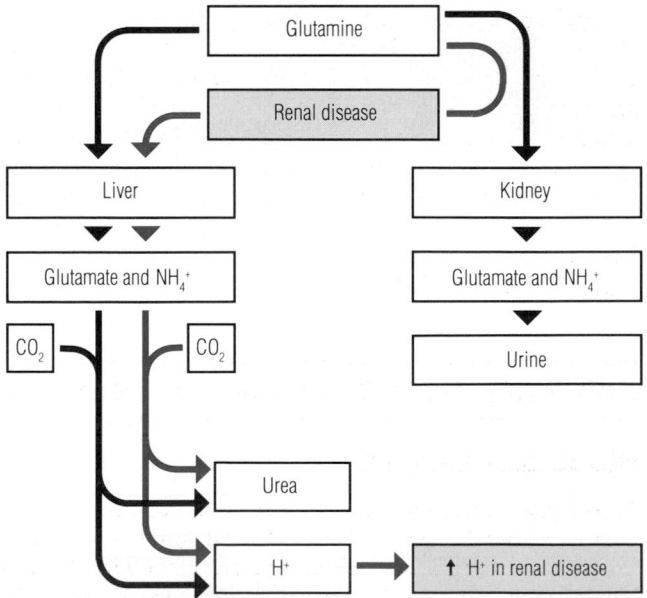

Fig. 21.11 Routes of glutamine metabolism in liver and kidney. Renal disease results in diversion of glutamine metabolism to the liver, with urea and hydrogen ion production.

Table 21.13 Causes of metabolic alkalosis

Gastric acid loss (esp. pyloric stenosis)
Potassium deficit / Hyperaldosteronism } leading to renal H⁺ loss
Ingestion of alkali or inappropriate intravenous administration

Metabolic alkalosis

Metabolic alkalosis results from direct loss of hydrogen ions or ingestion of bicarbonate (Table 21.13). Respiratory compensation is poor because hypoxia would be its direct consequence and possibly also because intracellular pH may increase relatively less than extracellular pH in some instances, leading to a lesser respiratory drive to compensate.

Respiratory acidosis

Carbon dioxide accumulation may occur as a result of many respiratory disorders (see p. 493, Table 13.31). The condition may be chronic (e.g. chronic obstructive airways disease) or acute (e.g. neuromuscular problems such as myasthenia). There are marked differences in compensatory responses in the two situations because several days are required for significant renal conservation of bicarbonate to occur. Thus, a new steady state of raised $P\mathrm{CO_2}$ and bicarbonate with maintenance of normal pH is frequently seen in chronic lung disease.

Respiratory alkalosis

An increase in ventilation and consequent fall in $P\mathrm{CO_2}$ usually arises as a primary event, as in hyperventilation due to anxiety or in hypoxic states (Table 21.14). When chronic hypoxia is the precipitating cause, some compensation may occur by means of increased renal bicarbonate excretion. In most instances, however, the fall in $P\mathrm{CO_2}$ is acute and pH rises rapidly.

Clinical consequences of acidosis

The clinical consequences of acidosis are outlined in Figure 21.12.

Acidosis is associated with a shift to the right of the oxygen dissociation curve (Fig. 21.13), thus tending to

Table 21.14 Causes of respiratory alkalosis

Stress hyperventilation	
Hypoxic stimulus to ventilation	**Drug-induced stimulus to ventilation**
Alveolar disease	
Right to left shunt	Salicylate poisoning
Altitude	

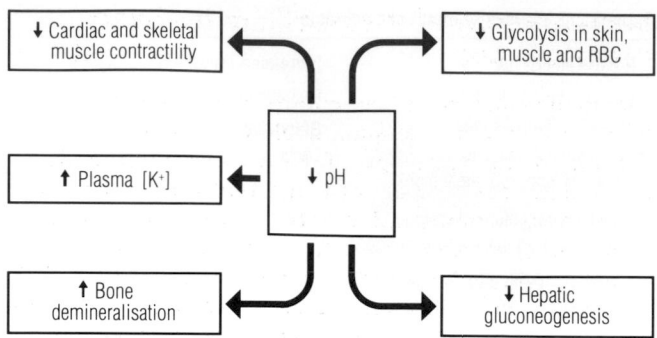

Fig. 21.12 The multiple effects of acidosis on heart, skin, red blood cells, liver and bone, and on plasma K⁺ concentration.

improve oxygen delivery to the periphery (provided pulmonary function is adequate). This effect is reduced to some extent by the fall in 2,3 diphosphoglycerate (2,3 DPG) concentration in erythrocytes, which occurs over a period of days. This has important implications for the management of metabolic acidosis.

Clinical consequences of alkalosis

In clinical terms, the most dramatic result of a rise in pH is a fall in ionised calcium resulting in tetany (carpopedal spasm). Milder symptoms, also suggesting a decreased ionised calcium, include peripheral and circumoral paraesthesia and are frequently found in patients with hyperventilation associated with stress.

Alkalosis has a hypokalaemic effect (p. 851) and also tends to increase peripheral glycolysis. In practice, however, raised lactic acid levels are not a feature of alkalotic conditions, with the possible exception of respiratory alkalosis accompanying liver failure, in which lactic acid metabolism is impaired.

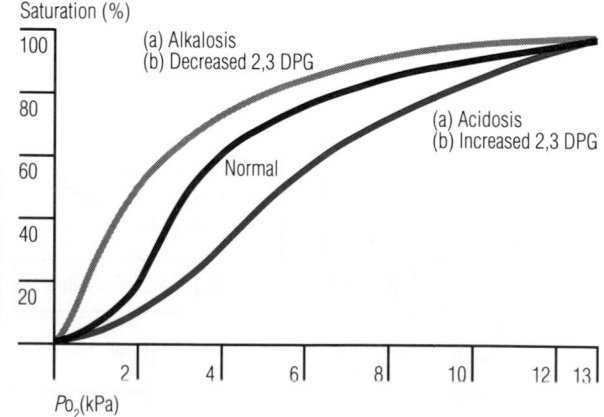

Fig. 21.13 The effects of (a) acid–base changes and (b) 2,3 DPG concentration on haemoglobin-oxygen dissociation. A shift to the right indicates increased oxygen delivery per unit fall in $P\mathrm{O_2}$. A shift to the left indicates decreased oxygen delivery per unit fall in $P\mathrm{O_2}$.

Management of metabolic acid–base disturbances

Metabolic alkalosis rarely requires more than correction of salt, water and potassium depletion, and treatment of the underlying pathology. However, metabolic acidosis, particularly some forms of lactic acidosis, may require intravenous administration of large quantities of sodium bicarbonate to counteract the negative inotropic effect and inhibition of hepatic lactate metabolism. The sodium load, which inevitably accompanies bicarbonate administration, may necessitate dialysis, particularly if there is co-existing renal impairment. Much controversy surrounds the use of bicarbonate in lesser degrees of acidosis. It has been suggested that rapid diffusion of CO_2 (formed by titration of hydrogen ions by administered bicarbonate) into cells may exacerbate intracellular acidosis. However, these arguments do not take account of the rapid pulmonary elimination of CO_2 in this situation and are probably not clinically relevant in most circumstances.

Mild to moderate diabetic ketoacidosis (pH >7.1) does not require alkali administration. In fact, such treatment may be potentially hazardous because of the risk of a leftward shift of the oxygen dissociation curve (Fig. 21.13) before peripheral perfusion has been improved by salt and water administration. This would exaggerate the adverse effects of lowered erythrocyte 2,3 DPG concentration on oxygen delivery. Restoration of circulating volume, lowering of blood sugar, and inhibition of lipolysis by insulin is followed by renal excretion and tissue metabolism of ketoacids (with net hydrogen ion consumption).

When administration of intravenous bicarbonate is necessary, it should be given in isotonic form (1.4%) if possible. The use of hypertonic solutions of bicarbonate (e.g. 8.4%, containing 1 mmol sodium/ml) is limited to the rapid administration of 50–100 mmol boluses in the management of cardiac arrest.

Renal tubular acidoses are treated by oral bicarbonate and/or potassium supplements (Ch. 20).

FURTHER READING

Arieff A I, De Fronzo R A (eds) 1985 Fluid, electrolyte and acid–base disorders, Vol I and II. Churchill Livingstone, Edinburgh. *A detailed treatment of this topic.*

Cohen R D 1990 The metabolic background to acid–base homeostasis and some of its disorders. In Metabolic and molecular basis of acquired disease (eds Cohen R D, Lewis B, Alberti KGMM, Denman A M) pp. 962–1001. Baillière Tindall, London. *An up-to-date appraisal of acid–base regulation with detailed consideration of the relative roles of liver and kidney in acid–base homeostasis.*

Häussinger D (ed) 1988 pH homeostasis – mechanisms and control. Academic Press, London. *A collection of definitive accounts on pH regulation and the relationship between pH homeostasis and metabolic processes.*

22

Neurological Disease

John W Scadding and Jeremy Gibbs

Table 22.1 Symptom review in neurological diagnosis

- Loss of consciousness
- Higher mental functions
- Headaches
- Vision
- Hearing
- Dizziness
- Unsteadiness
- Speech
- Swallowing
- Limb weakness
- Limb numbness and paraesthesiae
- Bladder and bowel control

or headache, for example, there are usually no physical signs. Anatomical localisation of lesions can also often be correctly identified from the history, and the timing and sequence of development of the symptoms will usually give some idea as to the nature of the underlying pathology. Supplementary history from relatives or witnesses is essential in patients with episodes of impaired consciousness or impairment of higher mental function. The major neurological symptoms which should be covered by the

Table 22.2 Neurological examination

1. Mental state	4. Motor system
Level of consciousness	Posture, involuntary movements
Orientation	Muscle bulk, fasciculation
Speech	Tone
General knowledge	Power
Memory	Coordination
Retention and recall	Reflexes
Reasoning and judgement	
Reading, writing, calculation	5. Sensory system
Object recognition	Light touch, pinprick, temperature, vibration and position sense
Praxis	Two-point discrimination
Perception	Stereognosis
Mood and affect	Tactile localisation
	Inattention
2. Gait and station	
Normal gait	6. General
Heel–toe walking	Bruits
Romberg's test	Skull size and shape
	Spinal deformity
3. Cranial nerves	Pes cavus
I: Olfaction	Neck rigidity
II: Acuity, fields, colour vision, fundi	Skin changes
III, IV, VI: Eye movements, nystagmus, pupils	
V: Facial and oral sensation. Masticatory muscles	
VII: Facial muscles, taste	
VIII: Hearing, Rinne and Weber tests	
IX: Pharyngeal sensation, gag reflex	
X: Speech, phonation, palatal movement, swallowing	
XI: Sternomastoids, trapezii	
XII: Tongue	

NEUROLOGICAL DIAGNOSIS

HISTORY-TAKING

Diagnosis in many patients with neurological disease depends entirely on the history; in patients with blackouts history are listed in Table 22.1; and in each section of this chapter, the typical features of the history are discussed.

PRINCIPLES OF EXAMINATION

Neurological examination can be performed quickly and efficiently if a routine is adhered to (Table 22.2).

Level of consciousness

The neurological examination starts with an assessment of the level of consciousness. When this is impaired to any significant degree, the patient's consciousness level is best described by the Glasgow Coma Scale (Table 22.3). This system has the advantage that it is simple, objective and easily applied by both medical and nursing staff without the use of imprecise terms such as 'drowsy', 'stuporose' or 'comatose'. It is particularly useful in sequentially monitoring the consciousness level.

Examination of the comatose patient

Detailed neurological examination in many patients permits an assessment of the site of the lesion. It is important to differentiate coma due to diffuse cerebral disease (either metabolic or inflammatory), from focal causes, either discrete brainstem lesions or focal cerebral hemisphere lesions associated with raised intracranial pressure and secondary brainstem compression (Table 22.4).

The first step in examining a patient in coma is to assess cardiorespiratory function. When vital functions and the level of coma have been assessed, general examination may provide important clues. A rash may indicate

Table 22.4 Causes of coma

Brainstem lesions	
Infarction	
Brainstem haemorrhage	particularly when complicated
Cerebellar haemorrhage	by hydrocephalus
Tumour	
Abscess	
Thiamine deficiency (Wernicke-Korsakoff syndrome)	
Brainstem encephalitis	

Cerebral hemisphere lesions with secondary brainstem compression	**Metabolic disturbances***
Extradural haemorrhage	Drug overdose
Subdural haemorrhage	Diabetes – hypoglycaemia
Intracerebral haemorrhage	ketoacidosis
Abscess	hyperosmolar coma
Tumour	Hyponatraemia
Large infarct	Hypernatraemia
Cerebral venous sinus thrombosis	Hypercalcaemia
	Uraemia
Diffuse neurological disease affecting cerebral hemispheres and brainstem	Hepatic failure
	Hypothyroidism
	Hypoadrenalism
	Hypopituitarism
Epilepsy	Respiratory failure (CO_2 narcosis)
Head injury	Severe heart failure
Subarachnoid haemorrhage	Hyperpyrexia
Meningitis	Hypothermia
Encephalitis	Porphyria
Hypertensive encephalopathy	
Encephalopathy in SLE	**Psychogenic coma**

*Also commonly cause an acute or subacute confusional state (p. 863).

Table 22.3 Glasgow coma scale

Category	Score
Eye opening	
Spontaneous	4
To speech	3
To pain	2
None	1
Best verbal response	
Orientated	5
Confused	4
Inappropriate	3
Incomprehensible	2
None	1
Best motor response	
Obeying commands	5
Localising	4
Flexing	3
Extending	2
None	1

The scores applied to each category of the grading system are summed to give an overall value, ranging from 3 to 14.

meningococcal septicaemia with meningitis, purpura may indicate a bleeding disorder associated with a cerebral haemorrhage, and signs of portal hypertension raise the possibility of hepatic encephalopathy. The skull and scalp should be examined for head injury.

Neurological examination should include:

- *Examination for neck stiffness*, indicating meningitis or subarachnoid haemorrhage. However, in deeply unconscious patients this nociceptive reflex may be absent.
- *Examination of the fundi*, primarily to look for evidence of raised intracranial pressure. Comatose patients frequently have small pupils which should not be dilated with mydriatics. Normal pupillary responses and reflex eye movements indicate that coma is likely to be due to diffuse disease, rather than focal brainstem pathology.
- *The pupils* are examined for equality of size and reaction to light. Cerebral hemisphere space-occupying lesions may cause herniation of the temporal lobe through the tentorium (coning); this frequently compresses the IIIrd cranial nerve, producing a large

unreactive pupil, with downward, outward gaze of one eye and limitation of all reflex movement of the affected eye, except abduction. Pupillary constriction (pinpoint pupils) are often seen in acute pontine lesions and opiate overdose. Metabolic causes of coma tend to cause loss of reflex eye movements, but preservation of pupillary reflexes.

- *Reflex eye movements* are examined by the doll's head manoeuvre or by caloric testing (p. 871). An acute cerebral hemisphere lesion may produce conjugate deviation of the eyes towards the side of the lesion. Lesions within the brainstem may produce a variety of partial or complete gaze palsies and pupillary abnormalities. Lesions in the pons tend to produce conjugate gaze away from the side of the lesion. Pressure from above, arising from cerebral hemisphere disease, causes progressive loss of brainstem function, with gradual loss of pupil reflexes, reflex eye movements and other brainstem reflexes.

- *Other brainstem reflexes* examined in comatose patients include the corneal reflexes (V), facial grimacing induced by pressure over the supraorbital nerve (V and VII), gag and coughing reflexes (IX and X), and the rate, depth and pattern of breathing. Most irregular patterns of breathing suggest brainstem pathology. The exception is Cheyne-Stokes breathing, which is now recognised to occur with both brainstem lesions and diffuse bilateral cerebral hemisphere disease.

- *Examination of the limbs* in the comatose patient should include observation of any spontaneous movements and, in particular, any asymmetry, indicating a unilateral hemisphere or brainstem lesion. Muscle tone is usually not diagnostically helpful, although in patients with drug overdose or in metabolic causes of coma, the tone is usually flaccid. Tendon reflexes and plantar responses are often of localising value, but may be abnormal, and sometimes asymmetrical, with diffuse cerebral insults such as metabolic causes of coma (Table 22.4).

An attempt can thus be made to differentiate the three main types of lesion causing coma.

With *intrinsic brainstem lesions*, there are focal abnormalities in the brainstem reflexes, often with cranial nerve abnormalities, which are present from the time of the first examination and often persist unchanged. In addition, there will be bilateral pyramidal tract signs in the limbs and there is likely to be an irregular breathing pattern.

In *brainstem compression* by lesions above the tentorium, brainstem signs appear in a progressive way. Early on, there is likely to be either a hemiparesis or asymmetrical bilateral pyramidal signs in the limbs. A unilateral IIIrd cranial nerve palsy may be an isolated early focal sign, due to compression of the nerve by herniation of the temporal lobe through the tentorium. Because pressure above the tentorium is raised, there may be papilloedema.

In *metabolic causes* of coma, pupillary and eye movement reflexes tend to be normal, although in deep metabolic coma, pupillary responses are preserved and reflex eye movements are lost. Pyramidal signs in the limbs are symmetrical. In overdose, particularly of opiates, breathing tends to be regular, but shallow.

Mental state examination

When it has been established that the conscious level is normal, examination of the mental state may proceed. Full testing is a lengthy process, which includes tests of cognitive function and sometimes a formal psychiatric assessment (Ch. 10). The broad outlines of the functions forming the mental state are described here, followed by a suggested scheme of testing of cognitive function, the 'mini-mental state' examination, which takes only 5–10 minutes to perform.

Some cognitive functions are clearly localised in the brain, e.g. language and calculation in the dominant hemisphere, and impairment provides information of localising value. Other functions, such as memory, are less clearly lateralised, and others, such as reasoning ability, are so complex as to be of little localising value. However, it is usually possible to decide whether there is a focal or a global impairment of cognitive function, this being the diagnostically important conclusion.

Speech

Speech will already have been assessed to some extent during the history. There are three major abnormalities.

Dysphasia is a difficulty with comprehension or expression of language, which results from a lesion of the dominant cerebral hemisphere. (Strictly, aphasia means a complete inability to comprehend speech or to communicate in speech, but the terms may be used interchangeably). In all right-handed people and 90% of left-handed people this is the left hemisphere. In *motor* or *expressive dysphasia*, there is no defect of comprehension of the spoken or written word and, through gesture or writing, the patient can demonstrate that he or she understands what is being said to him/her. In expressive dysphasia, the patient cannot find the right words and has grammatical difficulty. In mild forms, the speech will be hesitant, with pauses due to difficulty in finding particular words (nominal dysphasia). In severe cases, the patient may be speechless. Patients with expressive dysphasia usually appear frustrated by the defect.

By contrast, in *receptive* or *sensory dysphasia*, the patient does not fully comprehend spoken or written language. This results in an inability to understand what the examiner is saying and a failure to monitor his or her own speech. The speech is usually fluent and there is a tendency to talk in jargon.

Expressive dysphasia is produced by lesions of Broca's area in the frontal lobe, and receptive dysphasia is produced by lesions more posteriorly, in Wernicke's area in the temporal lobe. In many patients, the lesion produces a *mixed dysphasia*.

Dysarthria refers to a difficulty in articulation of speech. Any neuromuscular disorder affecting the control of the muscles involved in articulation may give rise to dysarthria.

Dysphonia refers to a defect in voice production. Neurological causes include Parkinson's disease, myasthenia gravis and recurrent laryngeal nerve palsy. Dysphonia may also result from disorders directly affecting the vocal cords or ventilatory function.

Attention, orientation and alertness

The patient should be orientated in time, place and person. He or she should be able to give the day, date, the name of the hospital and his or her home address. Alertness and attention may be simply tested by asking the patient to count backwards from 30; a time to do this exceeding 30 seconds is abnormal.

Both attention and immediate recall (registration) can also be tested by asking the patient to repeat back a series of digits, first forwards and then (with another sequence) in reverse order. If these tests show evidence of disorientation or marked inattention, more detailed testing of intellectual function is likely to be unreliable.

Memory

It is important to test both recent and remote memory. Recent memory is particularly affected in disease of the temporal lobes and certain nuclei in the thalamus. Short-term memory can be tested by asking the patient to remember a name and address, and some unrelated material such as the name of a flower and a colour. These should be repeated back immediately and then after an interval of 5 or 10 minutes. The patient's account of very recent personal events will also reflect the integrity of short-term memory. Remote memory is tested by asking questions about the patient's childhood, where he or she used to live, education, and previous employment. Impairment of remote memory occurs in more severe lesions of the temporal lobes.

Reasoning

The patient should have some *insight* into his or her condition and the ways in which it affects him/her. *Judgement* refers to the patient's ability to form an acceptable opinion given a particular set of circumstances. For example, if the patient is asked what he or she would do on seeing a set of keys lying in the road, and answers, 'Throw them in the dustbin', this would reasonably be considered to show poor judgement. *Abstraction* is tested by asking the patient the meaning of some proverbs. However, this is closely linked to academic achievement and, in some patients, a better test is to ask about similarities and differences between objects.

Impairment of insight, judgement and abstraction tend to occur together, and indicate disturbance of frontal lobe function.

Calculation

The ability to calculate depends on the integrity of the angular gyrus of the parietal lobe in the dominant hemisphere and is thus frequently disturbed in lesions producing dysphasia. *Dyscalculia* – the inability to perform simple calculations – is assessed by asking the patient to make serial deductions of 7 from 100, noting the time taken and the number of mistakes, and by other simple tests of mathematical ability.

Reading

Comprehension of the written word is also a function of the dominant hemisphere and impairment is often associated with dysphasia for spoken language. The patient is asked to read aloud. The patient is *dyslexic* if unable to read the words correctly or fails to understand what was read.

Writing

As with calculation and reading, writing is also a function of the dominant hemisphere, particularly the region of the angular gyrus. *Dysgraphia* – the inability to write – is usually associated with dysphasia.

Object recognition and agnosia

The inability to recognise objects in the absence of any defect of primary sensation is termed *agnosia*. To test for *visual agnosia*, the patient is presented with simple objects and asked to name them; failure indicates a lesion of the visual association cortex in the posterior parietal region. With extensive lesions in this area, the patient may be unable to recognise familiar faces (*prosopagnosia*) or familiar places, and be unable to find the way about his or her own home (*topographagnosia*). Visual agnosia can be tested in the presence of expressive dysphasia by asking the patient to match an object against a picture of a similar object.

Astereognosis, or tactile agnosia, is an inability to identify a simple object placed in the hand, with the eyes closed; this indicates a contralateral parietal lobe lesion.

With severe parietal lobe lesions, the patient may completely ignore and fail to identify a limb or the whole of the contralateral side of the body (*autotophagnosia*).

Agnosia is more easily recognised with lesions of the non-dominant hemisphere; with lesions in the dominant hemisphere, there is frequently associated dysphasia which makes it difficult to detect agnosia.

Praxis

Praxis is the ability to perform a planned motor task and *dyspraxia* (*apraxia*) is the inability to do this in the absence of paralysis. Motor dyspraxia may be due to a lesion of the dominant premotor frontal cortex, or the anterior corpus callosum, or to diffuse cortical disease. It is tested by asking the patient to mime simple tasks such as combing the hair or brushing the teeth, or to copy unusual hand postures demonstrated by the examiner. Constructional dyspraxia, which is more common with lesions of the non-dominant hemisphere, is the inability to construct shapes – by drawing or other means – either on request, or when asked to copy a particular design. It is usually tested by asking the patient to copy a drawing of a three-dimensional cube, or to draw a clock face or bicycle.

Perception

Disorders of perception are common in psychiatric disorders (p. 168), but also occur in organic brain disease. Visual, olfactory and gustatory hallucinations are relatively common in temporal lobe epilepsy. It is important to use the terms delusion, illusion and hallucination correctly. A *delusion* is a firmly held false belief. Delusions are common in normal people but tend to be more firmly held and more bizarre in patients with major psychotic illness. An *illusion* is a false interpretation of a sensory perception. Again, illusions may occur in normal people, but also occur with acute organic brain syndromes. *Hallucinations* are false sensory perceptions which have no external stimulus. Hallucinations occur with temporoparietal lesions, most commonly in temporal lobe epilepsy and with acute organic brain syndromes. Prolonged hallucinations, usually auditory, occurring without impairment of consciousness, are suggestive of a psychotic disorder.

Mood

Abnormalities of mood are often obvious from the way in which the patient presents his or her history. Depression, elation, lability, irritability and anxiety are the main disorders. Many patients will attempt to conceal abnormalities and will need to be questioned directly, sometimes with additional history from relatives. Abnormalities of mood usually indicate a psychiatric disorder but may also be an early feature of dementia or encephalopathy.

Excessive lability of mood, however, suggests bilateral frontal disease.

Affect

Affect is the emotional response to a particular situation. A patient with hemiplegia who is euphoric can be said to have an inappropriate affect, suggesting a frontal lesion. It can be difficult to decide whether affect is appropriate or not, particularly in patients with long-standing disease who have come to terms with their disability.

Mini-mental state examination

The mini-mental state examination (MMSE) provides a rapid means of testing cognitive function (Table 22.5).

Table 22.5 Mini-mental state examination

Test	Max. score	Patient's score
Orientation		
What is the (year) (season) (date) (day) (month)?	5	( )
Where are you (country) (county) (town) (hospital) (ward)?	5	( )
Retention		
Name 3 objects, then ask patient to repeat these.	3	( )
Give 1 point for each correct answer.		
Then repeat them until patient learns all 3.		
Count the number of trials and record		
Calculation and attention		
Serial 7's. 1 point for each correct answer.	5	( )
Stop after 5 answers. If patient cannot, or will not, do this, ask the patient to spell 'world' backwards.		
Score 0–5 points		
Recall		
Ask patient to name the 3 objects learned earlier.	3	( )
Give 1 point for each correct answer		
'Language'		
Name a pencil and a watch (2 points).	9	( )
Repetition: ask patient to repeat a short sentence (0 or 1 point).		
3-stage command: 'Take a piece of paper in your right hand, fold it in half and put it on the floor' (3 points).		
Read and obey the following:		
'Close your eyes' (0 or 1 point).		
Ask patient to write a sentence of his/her own choice.		
It must contain a subject and verb and make sense (0 or 1 point).		
Copying: ask patient to copy 2 intersecting pentagons (0 or 1 point)		
Total score	30	( )

Any abnormality detected using MMSE should prompt a more detailed psychological assessment. The MMSE can be applied to patients who are drowsy or stuporose but, if so, this must be recorded.

Acute confusional states

Acutely confused patients are, to a variable extent, disorientated; their ability to concentrate and their memory are impaired, they have difficulty following even simple instructions, their attention is poor, and they are often drowsy. Acute confusional states are often associated with delirium, a state characterised by restlessness, agitation, irritability and, sometimes, frightening hallucinations.

Acute confusional states can occur with focal cerebral hemisphere lesions, but are more common with metabolic disturbances, which may eventually result in stupor and coma (Table 22.4, p. 859), and with abrupt withdrawal of drugs, including barbiturates, alcohol and, occasionally, benzodiazepines.

Confusion is a feature of dementia and some psychiatric diseases, particularly the psychoses. However, in contrast to other causes of acute confusional states, psychiatric disease and dementia do not cause drowsiness.

GAIT AND STATION

The ability to stand and walk depends on the integrity of many different neurological functions, both motor and sensory. These include:

- position sense from muscles and joints in the limbs and also in the trunk and neck
- sensory input from vision and from the labyrinths in the inner ear
- motor functions, which include upper and lower motor neurones, the basal ganglia and cerebellum and, of course, the muscles and joints themselves.

Much can be learned from observing the gait carefully; certain types of gait disorder are easily recognised and provide immediate information about the causative lesion.

Station refers to the ability of the patient to stand and the posture of the stance. Examples of abnormalities include the stooped stance of a patient with Parkinson's disease, and the wide-based stance of a patient with cerebellar disease. It is relevant to observe how easily the patient is able to stand up, and whether assistance is required and, if so, how much. The ability to walk is then assessed. In patients whose gait appears normal, or only mildly abnormal, two further tests are useful.

Tandem gait. The patient is asked to walk heel-to-toe along a straight line (tandem gait). This is a fairly severe test of balance and coordination and, in the presence of normal power, failure usually indicates an impairment of cerebellar function, of vestibular function, or of postural sensation (sensory ataxia).

Romberg's test. If the tandem gait test is normal, the patient is asked to stand with the feet together and then to close the eyes (Romberg's test). An inability to maintain balance indicates either an impairment of postural sensation, or of vestibular function.

Some abnormalities of gait are easily recognised. For example, in a *spastic gait* the patient walks slowly, with obvious stiffness in the legs and, sometimes, with scissoring due to thigh adductor spasm. A hemiplegic gait is recognised by dragging, weakness and spasticity of one leg.

The patient with a *Parkinsonian gait* has a stooped posture and, when asked to walk, may have difficulty in initiating movement (start hesitation) and tends to take small shuffling steps, which quicken (the festinant gait).

With an *ataxic gait*, the patient is unsteady when standing and usually adopts a broad base; walking appears unsteady, with lurching from side to side, and the gait resembles that of a drunkard. There may be associated nystagmus.

In a *steppage gait*, resulting from bilateral footdrop (as found for example in a peripheral neuropathy), the patient has to flex the leg at the hip more than usual in order to prevent catching the toes. The gait has the appearance of someone trying to step up and there is usually an associated stamping as each foot hits the ground, particularly when weakness is combined with severe proprioceptive loss.

A *waddling gait* is produced by proximal weakness at the hip girdle. There is an inability to tilt the pelvis normally when swinging each leg through to take the next step, and this is compensated for by exaggerated lateral movements of the trunk, producing a waddling movement.

In an *apraxic* gait, the patient is able to stand but is unable to perform the planned motor function involved in walking. If the patient can walk, the gait is usually small-paced and shuffling.

A *limping gait* is very common, the usual cause being some painful musculoskeletal, rather than neurological, condition affecting the leg.

CRANIAL NERVES

Olfactory nerve

Testing of olfactory function is not essential in every patient but it is paticularly important in certain situations. In patients with frontal lobe tumours, e.g. olfactory groove meningiomas, there may be unilateral anosmia due to direct compression of the nerve. Bilateral anosmia or hyposmia is common following colds and with sinusitis. Impairment of smell is common in heavy smokers. Bilateral anosmia may also be produced by head injuries which damage the nerves as they pass through the cribriform plate; this is usually permanent. Smell is tested in each nostril separately. Test substances include camphor, peppermint, cloves, lavender and other distinctive strong-smelling substances, but not chemical irritants, such as ammonia, which stimulate trigeminal afferents.

Optic nerve

The assessment of optic nerve function includes measurement of visual acuity, colour vision, the visual fields, and examination of the fundi. The efferent pupillary responses are mediated by the IIIrd nerve (p. 867); the optic nerve provides the afferent limb of the light reflex.

Visual acuity

Distant and near vision are examined. Distance vision is assessed using a Snellen chart. The patient is positioned 6 metres from the chart, and each eye is tested separately. If the patient has glasses, these should be worn. The patient is asked to read the smallest line that can be seen, and the acuity is recorded as 6 (which is the numerator and is the maximum distance at which a subject with normal vision can clearly read the type) over the number of the smallest size of print which the patient can see. Normal vision is 6/6. Since refractive error is common, acuity should be retested, using a pinhole, if abnormal. Near vision is tested using standard test types and, again, it is important to state whether glasses have been used.

Colour vision is particularly dependent on macular and optic nerve function. Colour desaturation, particularly to red, is the earliest and most sensitive indicator of impaired optic nerve function. Standard charts (Ishihara) for testing colour vision are available and should be used in patients suspected of having any lesion of the retina, optic nerve or optic chiasm, as long as acuity is not severely impaired.

Visual fields

A working knowledge of the neuroanatomy of the visual pathway is essential when examining the visual fields (Fig. 22.1). Light from the temporal half of the visual field is focused on the nasal half of the retina, and light from the nasal half of the visual field on the temporal half of the retina, with inversion of the images. There are no rods or cones over the optic nerve head, producing a blind spot in the visual field situated a few degrees lateral to central vision.

The optic nerve exits from the orbit through the optic foramen and, with the optic nerve from the other side, forms the optic chiasm. The fibres from the temporal halves of each retina pass through the chiasm, without decussating, into the optic tract on the same side. The nasal fibres decussate, the optic tract on each side therefore consisting of fibres from the nasal half of the contralateral retina and the temporal half of the ipsilateral retina. The fibres pass to the lateral geniculate body and thence, via the optic radiation, to the occipital cortex. The fibres concerned with pupillary reflexes pass from the lateral geniculate body to the pretectal nucleus in the mid-brain. The upper and lower fibres of the visual radiation pass through the parietal and temporal lobe respectively before reaching the occipital cortex. Lesions at different points in the optic pathway produce characteristic visual field defects (Fig. 22.1).

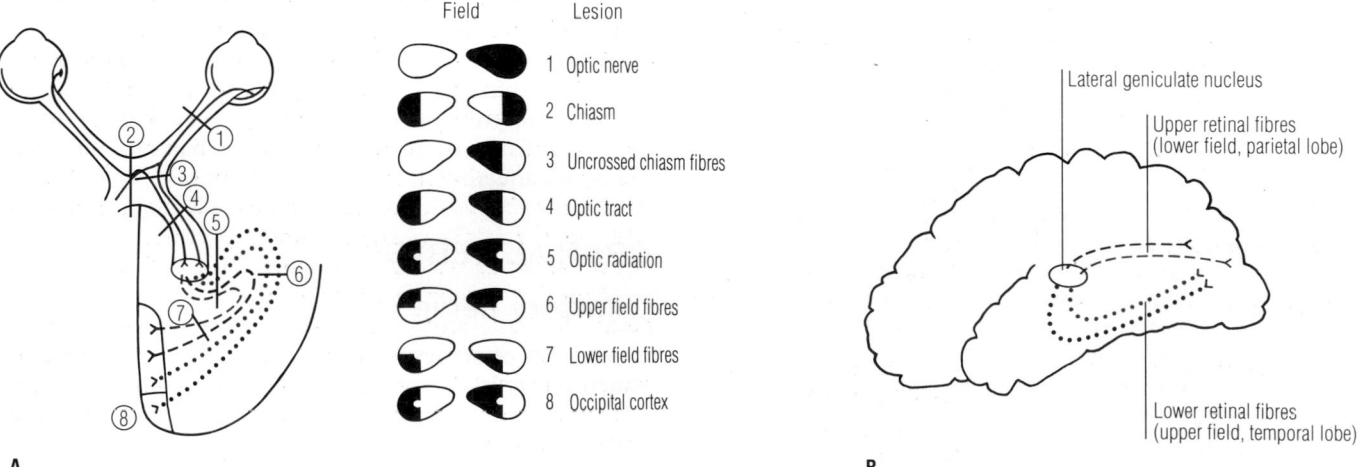

A

B

Fig. 22.1 Anatomy of the visual pathway. A. Lesions at points 1–8 produce the visual field defects shown. **B.** The arrangement of the visual radiation is shown in a lateral view. Lesions of the upper and medially situated part of the radiation in the parietal lobe produce a lower quadrantanopia, and lesions of the lower and laterally placed part of the radiation in the temporal lobe produce an upper quadrantanopia. Note that macular sparing occurs with lesions of the radiation or cortex.

1. Complete destruction of one optic nerve results in blindness in that eye and loss of the direct pupillary light reflex.
2. A midline lesion of the optic chiasm produces a bitemporal hemianopia.
3. Lesions involving the optic chiasm and the optic tracts often produce incongruent field defects, with more marked involvement of one monocular field. Lesions involving the optic radiation or the occipital cortex are usually congruent and symmetrical.
4. An expanding pituitary tumour from below will produce an upper bitemporal quadrantanopia, due to the inversion of the image in the retina.
5. Pressure on the optic chiasm from above, usually due to a suprasellar meningioma, produces a lower bitemporal quadrantanopia.
6. A lesion involving the optic tract will produce a homonymous hemianopia.
7. A lesion in the parietal lobe involving the medial part of the optic radiation will result in a lower homonymous quadrantanopia.
8. A lesion in the temporal lobe involving the lateral fibres of the optic radiation will produce an upper homonymous quadrantanopia.
9. A lesion involving the whole of the optic radiation or the occipital cortex will produce a homonymous hemianopia.
10. A complete lesion of both occipital lobes will produce cortical blindness, but pupillary reflexes will be preserved.

The visual fields are tested by comparing the patient's visual field with that of the examiner. Each eye is tested separately. The peripheral field is usually screened briefly using movements of the examiner's fingers in the four quadrants, but when suspicion of a defect is high, more detailed assessment is necessary using a small white target, or comparing the quality of the colour of a red-headed pin in different quadrants. Any visual field loss can be mapped out by placing the pin within the area of

Table 22.6 Common visual field defects

Defect	Causes
Homonymous hemianopia	Stroke Tumour
Quadrantanopia	Stroke Tumour
Bitemporal hemianopia	Pituitary tumour Craniopharyngioma
Monocular field loss	Vascular occlusion Retinal disease Optic neuritis Optic nerve compression
Enlarged blind spot	Papilloedema

loss and moving it from this position into the areas of normal vision. In this way, it is possible to detect all quadrantic and hemianopic defects and discrete areas of visual field loss (scotomas). The patient's blind spot, which represents a discrete scotoma, can be mapped out. A red pin is more sensitive for detecting central scotomas in which the only defect may be impairment of colour vision, e.g. as may be the case in optic neuritis.

Visual field defects can be documented more fully by using a perimeter for the peripheral fields and a Bjerrum screen for testing the central fields. The common causes of visual field defects are given in Table 22.6.

Optic fundi

Examination of the optic fundi should include scrutiny of the blood vessels, retina and choroid and the optic discs. The anterior part of the eye can be examined using the 10 + lens on the ophthalmoscope.

Abnormalities of blood vessels

Hypertensive and sclerotic changes are the most commonly seen blood vessel abnormalities. Hypertensive changes are graded thus:

- *Grade 1.* Arteriolar narrowing.
- *Grade 2.* Narrowing with arteriovenous nipping where arteries cross veins.
- *Grade 3.* Changes as for grade 2, together with haemorrhages and/or exudates.
- *Grade 4.* Changes as for grade 3 with papilloedema.

Sclerotic changes in retinal arterioles are commonly associated with hypertension, but also occur in normotensive people and are increased in diabetes and hyperlipidaemias. The changes are narrowing, tortuosity and an increase in the light reflex (silver wiring).

Arterial emboli. Emboli, usually arising from atheromatous plaques in the carotid artery in the neck at the level of the bifurcation, are occasionally seen. They may be cholesterol emboli, which are highly refractile and often multiple, or platelet emboli which appear white. Small emboli may be asymptomatic, and usually move peripherally fairly rapidly. Larger emboli produce amaurotic attacks affecting part or the whole of vision of that eye.

Central retinal artery occlusion causes complete monocular blindness and is associated with a pale retina with very narrow pale vessels. The blood supply of the macular region is from the choroidal circulation, so this part of the retina has a pinker appearance, sometimes described as a cherry-red spot.

Venous occlusion. Thrombosis of the central retinal vein occurs in polycythaemia rubra vera but may occur spontaneously. Vision may be relatively well preserved; the ophthalmoscopic appearances are venous engorgement and multiple haemorrhages, together with swelling of the optic disc.

Other causes of retinal haemorrhage. Any cause of raised intracranial pressure will produce venous engorgement, which may produce retinal haemorrhages and papilloedema. In subarachnoid haemorrhage, subhyaloid haemorrhages may occur, which are large and well-defined and have a horizontal level in the upright posture. Bleeding disorders may produce retinal haemorrhages.

Abnormalities of the retina and choroid

Pigmentary degeneration of the retina. Retinitis pigmentosa is the most common type of pigmentary degeneration affecting the retina. It is hereditary in the great majority of cases, usually as an autosomal recessive trait although sometimes as an autosomal dominant or sex-linked recessive trait. Ophthalmoscopy shows a lace-like network of thin pigmented lines, sometimes with larger areas of confluent pigmentary change. Similar pigmentary changes may be seen in other conditions, including spinocerebellar degenerations (p. 929), Refsum's disease (p. 949), and mitochondrial cytopathy (p. 956).

Chorioretinitis. Inflammatory disease of the retina and underlying choroid may produce scarring, with pale areas where the retina has been destroyed, together with pigmentary change. Chorioretinitis may be caused by intra-uterine infection with toxoplasmosis or cytomegalovirus; syphilis may produce similar changes.

Optic discs

The normal optic disc has clearly defined margins and a central depression (optic cup) where the arteries and veins enter and leave the eye. In most people, venous pulsations can be seen in the large veins on the optic disc, but, when intracranial pressure rises, these pulsations disappear. The two main abnormalities of the optic disc are papilloedema and optic atrophy.

Papilloedema means oedema of the optic disc, caused either by local haemodynamic changes, raised intracranial pressure or inflammation of the optic disc (Table 22.7). Early changes include hyperaemia of the disc, and venous dilatation with absent venous pulsation. Swelling of the optic disc produces elevation and blurring of the disc margins. Small haemorrhages may appear at the disc margin. With more severe papilloedema, haemorrhages become larger, and the disc becomes further elevated and enlarged, giving rise to an enlarged blind spot in the visual field, usually detectable by confrontation. Folds may appear in the retina, together with white exudates with indistinct margins ('soft' exudates).

Indistinct optic disc margins are often present in hypermetropic people, but should not be confused with papilloedema. Occasionally, hyaline bodies are present on the optic nerve head; these may mimic papilloedema and are known as drusen. The other condition which is sometimes confused with papilloedema is the presence of myelinated nerve fibres spreading from the optic disc onto the surrounding retina.

Optic atrophy may result when papilloedema has been present for a prolonged period, whatever the cause, and it may also develop gradually in a number of other disease processes (Table 22.8). The appearance is a pale white optic disc, which is flat and has sharp margins.

Table 22.7 Causes of papilloedema

Raised intracranial pressure	**Central retinal artery occlusion**
Tumour	Occlusive
Abscess	Embolic
Hypertension	
Hydrocephalus	**Optic nerve tumours**
Venous sinus thrombosis	Glioma
Meningitis	Meningioma
Encephalitis	
Subarachnoid haemorrhage	**Blood disease**
Intracerebral haemorrhage	Severe anaemia
CO_2 retention	Polycythaemia rubra vera
Cerebral oedema due to	DIC
trauma	Thrombocytopenic purpura
	Leukaemia
Venous obstruction	Sickle cell disease
Central retinal vein thrombosis	
Cavernous sinus thrombosis	**Toxic and deficiency**
Carotico-cavernous fistula	Methyl alcohol
(carotid aneurysm)	Uraemia
Thrombosis or obstruction of SVC	Arsenic
Orbital lesions, e.g. cellulitis,	
tumour, thyroid eye disease	**Raised CSF protein**
	Guillain-Barré syndrome
Anterior optic neuritis (papillitis)	Spinal cord tumour
Isolated lesion	
Multiple sclerosis	
Meningitis, tuberculosis, syphilis	
Sarcoidosis	

Table 22.8 Causes of optic atrophy

Optic nerve compression	Tobacco
Pituitary tumour	Quinine
Carotid aneurysm	Ethambutol
Glaucoma	Lead and arsenic
Optic nerve tumour	Anaemia
Sphenoid meningioma	
Olfactory groove meningioma	**Secondary to retinal disease**
	Senile macular degeneration
Optic neuritis	Retinitis pigmentosa
	Severe chorioretinitis
Following long-standing	
papilloedema	**Secondary to trauma**
	Orbital fracture
Central retinal artery occlusion	
	Hereditary
Toxic/metabolic	Leber's optic atrophy
Diabetes	Hereditary ataxias
Methyl alcohol	Spinocerebellar degenerations

IIIrd, IVth and VIth cranial nerves

Clinical anatomy

The *IIIrd nerve* contains motor fibres to the extraocular muscles (excluding lateral rectus and superior oblique), afferent proprioceptive fibres from these muscles, and motor parasympathetic fibres to the pupil which produce constriction.

The motor fibres arise from the IIIrd nerve nucleus in the mid-brain, ventral to the aqueduct. The important relations of the nerve between the brainstem and the eye are its proximity to the posterior communicating artery (site of aneurysm), its course over the tentorial edge close to the uncus of the temporal lobe (compression during 'coning'), and its passage through the lateral wall of the cavernous sinus, before entry into the orbit through the superior orbital fissure.

The motor parasympathetic fibres to the pupil arise in the upper part of the oculomotor nucleus (Edinger-Westphal nucleus), pass through the mid-brain and reach the orbit together with the oculomotor motor fibres. Within the orbit, the parasympathetic fibres enter the ciliary ganglion; from here, the postganglionic fibres pass to the ciliary and sphincter pupillae muscles as the short ciliary nerves.

The *IVth nerve*, supplying superior oblique, has its nucleus in the mid-brain ventral to the aqueduct at the level of the inferior colliculus. The nerve follows a similar course to the IIIrd nerve and runs along the lateral wall of the cavernous sinus, entering the orbit through the superior orbital fissure.

The *VIth nerve*, supplying the lateral rectus muscle, arises from the nucleus in the upper pons, ventral to the floor of the fourth ventricle. The fibres pass forwards and downwards to emerge near the midline, in the sulcus between the pons and medulla. The nerve lies on the ventral surface of the pons, and enters the cavernous

sinus below the posterior clinoid process. It passes through the sinus and enters the orbit through the superior orbital fissure.

The directions of gaze for testing individual extraocular muscles are summarised in Figure 22.2. The oblique muscles are attached to the eye behind the equator of the globe. Thus, superior oblique depresses the eye and inferior oblique elevates the eye during adduction. Elevation of the eyelid involves two muscles, the levator muscles supplied by the IIIrd nerve, and Muller's muscle supplied by the cervical sympathetic. Thus, any lesion affecting the superior division of the oculomotor nerve is likely to be associated with ptosis.

Pupillary reflexes

The anatomy of the light and near vision pupillary reflexes is shown in Figure 22.3.

Size. The pupils should be round and regular and equal in size. Mild degrees of inequality (anisocoria) can be normal, but a major difference in the size of the pupils is pathological.

Light reflex. The pupils are first tested to light, with observations of the direct response in the ipsilateral eye

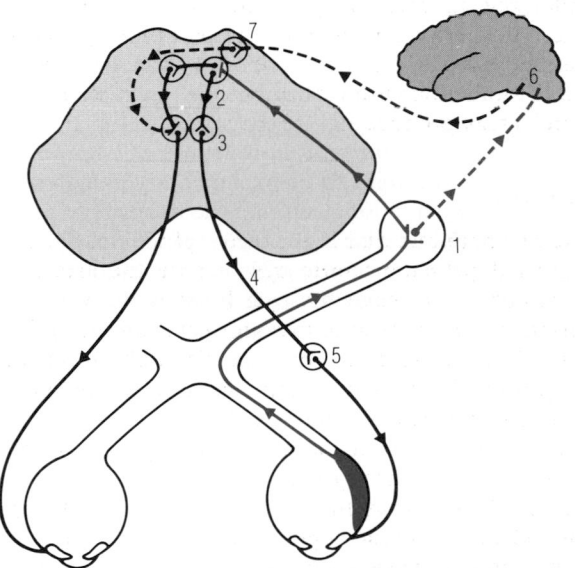

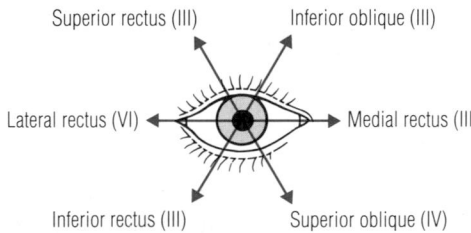

Superior rectus (III) Inferior oblique (III)

Lateral rectus (VI) ← → Medial rectus (III)

Inferior rectus (III) Superior oblique (IV)

Direction of weakness	Nerve palsy
up and out	III
up and in	III
medially	III
down and out	III
down and in	IV
laterally	VI

Fig. 22.2 Actions and innervation of the extraocular muscles (right eye).

Fig. 22.3 Light and near vision pupillary reflexes. The afferent pathways to the brainstem for the light reflex are shown as a continuous red line and that to the occipital cortex for the near vision reflex is shown as a dashed red line. For the light reflex, fibres from the lateral geniculate nucleus (1) pass to the pretectal nucleus (2) in the mid-brain. After synapsing, fibres pass to the ipsilateral and contralateral Edinger-Westphal nucleus (3), which is part of the oculomotor nuclear complex. From here, fibres travel in the IIIrd nerve (4) to the ciliary ganglion (5) and postganglionic fibres pass from here to innervate the iris and ciliary muscles. Afferent fibres for the near vision reflex pass to the occipital cortex (6); impulses are then relayed to the nucleus of the superior colliculus (7). From here, there are bilateral connections to the Edinger-Westphal nucleus (3). For clarity, only the contralateral connection is shown on the diagram.

and the consensual response in the contralateral eye. Both should respond equally and briskly. Cataracts or corneal opacities will reduce the light stimulus. Degenerative disease of the retina results in a reduced afferent input, as may lesions of the optic nerve, chiasm or optic tracts. Local disease of the eye, such as iridocyclitis, may cause adhesions preventing pupillary constriction. A lesion of the IIIrd nerve nucleus or IIIrd nerve, or of the ciliary ganglion or short ciliary nerves will also result in an impaired or absent pupillary reflex. By examining the direct and consensual light reflexes in the two eyes, it is possible to determine whether a pupillary abnormality is due to a lesion of the afferent or efferent limb of the reflex.

Near vision reflex. The near vision or convergence reflex is tested by asking the patient to fix his/her gaze on an object held at a comfortable distance from the patient's eyes, and then to follow the object as it is brought nearer. The reflex depends on an intact visual pathway to the visual cortex, and from there to the pretectal area and on to the Edinger-Westphal nucleus. From here, the efferent limb of the reflex is the same as for the light reflex.

The *tonic pupil* (Holmes-Adie syndrome) is a large pupil which has a poor or absent response to light, but does show constriction on convergence. The response to near vision is usually slow, and the pupil then gradually reverts to its previous size. The tonic pupil usually affects one eye initially but may then become bilateral. It may be an isolated abnormality or occur in association with diminished or absent tendon reflexes. The lesion of the tonic pupil is thought to be in the ciliary ganglion, with defective reinnervation such that the majority of regenerated fibres are involved in the convergence reflex only.

The *Argyll-Robertson pupil* is usually associated with neurosyphilis. In contrast to a tonic pupil, the Argyll-Robertson pupil is often small and irregular. The response to light is reduced or absent and the pupil fails to dilate in the dark. The response to near vision is better than the response to light. The lesion producing the Argyll-Robertson pupil is probably immediately rostral to the Edinger-Westphal nucleus, affecting the light reflex but not the fibres serving the near vision reflex (which are located in a more ventral position).

Horner's syndrome is produced by a lesion of the cervical sympathetic fibres. It comprises miosis (whereby the pupil is smaller than the normal contralateral pupil), ptosis, apparent enophthalmos due to the ptosis, and loss of sweating on the ipsilateral side of the face.

The sympathetic pathway which supplies the head originates in the hypothalamus, passes down through the lateral brainstem and cervical spinal cord and then exits in the T1 and, to a lesser extent, C8 anterior spinal roots. The fibres leave these roots via the white rami communicans and enter the cervical sympathetic ganglia. From the cervical ganglia, branches travel with the carotid artery into the head. A lesion affecting any part of this pathway will produce Horner's syndrome.

Examination of eye movements

The range of movement in each eye is assessed and the patient is asked to report any diplopia. In disturbances of conjugate gaze there will be no diplopia, but movement of both eyes will be incomplete in certain directions. Diplopia may be caused by lesions at the level of the nuclei in the brainstem supplying the extraocular muscles or their internuclear connections, or lesions affecting the peripheral nerves or the extraocular muscles themselves. The eye movements are routinely tested by asking the patient to look up, down, and to each side and then to follow the examiner's finger moving laterally and medially, upwards and downwards. The eyes are also observed for nystagmus – an involuntary rhythmic movement of the eyes which may be present at rest or in certain directions of gaze, and which persists when the eyes are still.

Conjugate eye movements

Conjugate movements are both voluntary and reflex in nature. A disturbance of voluntary conjugate movement refers to an inability to gaze in a particular direction on command. A disturbance of reflex conjugate eye movement refers to an inability to follow a moving object presented to a conscious patient who understands the command. Reflex conjugate eye movements may also be tested in unconscious patients, by observing the eyes and moving the head in a horizontal or vertical plane. If the reflex eye movements are intact, this induces movements of the eyes known as *doll's eye movements*.

Destructive or irritative lesions involving supranuclear pathways to the eye movements may produce conjugate deviation of the eyes at rest. An acute destructive lesion in one frontal lobe causes conjugate deviation of the eyes towards the side of the lesion, whereas an irritative lesion leads to conjugate deviation of the eyes away from the side of the lesion. A destructive lesion involving supranuclear fibres below the decussation of the fibres in the upper part of the brainstem leads to conjugate deviation of the eyes away from the side of the lesion. An extensive lesion in the upper mid-brain may involve the supranuclear fibres bilaterally. This leads to severe impairment of involuntary eye movements, but the eyes remain conjugate and there is no diplopia. Reflex eye movements produced by head turning (doll's eye movements) or by vestibular (caloric) stimulation are normal.

Physiology of eye movements

Conjugate gaze is coordinated in the pons. There are inputs from a number of centres in the visual and frontal cortex, the vestibular system, and the cerebellum. Fibres from the pons pass to the nuclei controlling the extraocular muscles, the medial longitudinal fasciculus being one of the pathways. Reflex conjugate eye movements when following an object depend on visual perception; thus, visual acuity and all the structures on which this depends must be normal. From the primary visual area, fibres pass anteriorly to the associated visual cortical areas in the occipital lobe. From here, corticotectal fibres concerned with upward gaze pass to the tectum in the mid-brain, and corticotegmental fibres concerned with horizontal gaze pass to the pons. Impairment of upward gaze may occur with lesions involving the corticotectal pathway; the causes include cerebral infarction, multiple sclerosis and, occasionally, a pineal tumour.

Doll's eye movements. The centres controlling eye movements receive a vestibular input which is responsible for the reflex conjugate doll's eye movements. In an unconscious patient, doll's eye movements depend on the vestibular apparatus and its brainstem connections with the centres for conjugate eye movements. The head is turned from side to side and, if intact, the reflex will induce lateral conjugate deviation of the eyes in the direction opposite to the direction of the head movement. Similar eye movements will be induced by flexion and extension of the neck. The absence of doll's eye movements indicates bilateral lesions of the brainstem connections and is usually associated with a very poor prognosis.

Eye movement disorders due to pontine lesions

Lesions in the pons are commonly associated with disorders of eye movements. The common abnormalities include involvement of the VIth nerve or its nucleus. This leads to paralysis of the lateral rectus and, if the lesion is at nuclear level, there may be conjugate gaze paralysis to the ipsilateral side. It is often associated with a facial nerve palsy, due to the proximity of the VIIth nerve nucleus. Lesions of the medial longitudinal fasciculus lead to paralysis of the ipsilateral medial rectus, producing defective adduction of the ipsilateral eye. On gaze to the contralateral side, there may be nystagmus, greater in the abducting eye (ataxic nystagmus). This combination of signs is known as an internuclear ophthalmoplegia, which, particularly in younger adults, is likely to be due to demyelinating disease (multiple sclerosis, p. 957). Pontine lesions affecting the medial longitudinal fasciculus may also produce skew deviation, in which one eye is elevated relative to the other eye. This usually leads to tilting of the head to compensate for the dysconjugate position of the eyes.

Paralysis of extraocular muscles

IIIrd nerve palsy leads to outward and, usually, slightly downward deviation of the eye on the affected side. If the pupillary constrictor fibres are also involved in the lesion, there will be dilatation of the pupil (internal ophthalmoplegia). Ptosis is also present.

VIth nerve palsy. A lesion of the VIth nerve produces paralysis of the lateral rectus muscle, leading to inward deviation of the affected eye at rest and an inability to abduct this eye.

IVth nerve palsy is difficult to detect and the changes induced by a complete IVth nerve palsy may be very mild. There is limitation of depression of the affected eye when adducted; this leads to diplopia, with the false image being below and lateral to the true image and also oblique to it. On covering the normal eye, the eye with the IVth nerve palsy deviates downwards and inwards. The head tends to be tilted towards the normal side to compensate for the oblique separation of images.

Nystagmus may be congenital or may occur as a result of disturbances of visual acuity, vestibular function or cerebellar function; it may be drug-induced. Nystagmus is discussed in more detail on page 871.

Trigeminal nerve

Clinical anatomy

The anatomy of the trigeminal nerve is shown in Figure 22.4. Figure 22.6 (p. 882) shows the cutaneous territories of the divisions of the trigeminal nerve, and

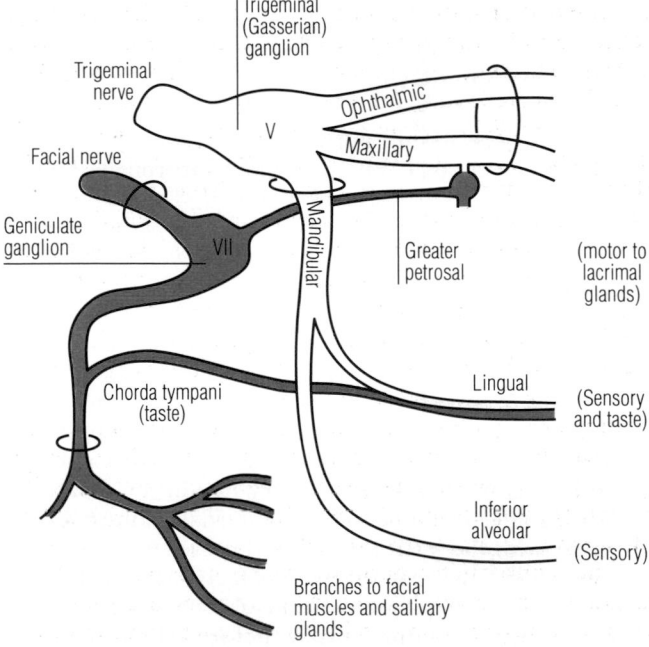

Fig. 22.4 Anatomy of the trigeminal and facial nerves. The motor branches of the fifth nerve are not shown; these come off the mandibular division at various points along its course to supply the muscles of mastication. See text for details of the central connections and intracranial course of the two nerves.

Table 22.15 (p. 882) lists the non-cutaneous innervation. The sensory root of the trigeminal nerve passes from the Gasserian ganglion to enter the pons at the junction of the pons and the middle cerebellar peduncle. The main sensory nucleus subserves tactile sensation; fibres subserving pain and temperature sensation enter the spinal tract and nucleus, which extends downwards into the upper segments of the cervical spinal cord as low as C4. The fibres entering the spinal nucleus are arranged so that those from around the mouth enter the spinal nucleus in the medulla, and fibres from further out on the face enter the nucleus at progressively lower levels.

Examination

The routine examination of the trigeminal nerve consists of assessment of both motor and sensory functions. The masseter and temporalis muscles are palpated with the jaw tightly clenched, and the pterygoids are tested by asking the patient to move the jaw laterally and resist pressure to maintain this posture. Sensation is tested to light touch and pinprick in all three divisions of the nerve, and the corneal reflex should also be tested. The afferent limb of this reflex is the ophthalmic division of the trigeminal nerve, and the efferent limb producing a blink response is the facial nerve. A small wisp of cotton-wool is gently stroked on the cornea. It is important that the patient is asked to look to one side, so that the approaching cotton-wool is not seen, since the visual threat will produce a blink response. The reflex produces bilateral blinking; thus, if there is an ipsilateral VIIth nerve palsy, a blink will still occur on the contralateral side.

The jaw jerk should normally be present, but a brisk jaw jerk indicates bilateral upper motor neurone lesions.

VIIth cranial nerve

Clinical anatomy

The complex anatomy of the VIIth cranial nerve is shown in Figure 22.4. The functions of the facial nerve tested routinely are the power of the facial muscles and taste. The VIIth nerve has its nucleus in the lower part of the pons, the nerve emerging between the pons and the medulla just medial to the VIIIth nerve in the cerebello-pontine angle. It then enters the internal auditory canal, together with the VIIIth nerve, and passes to the geniculate ganglion. The main part of the facial nerve enters the facial canal, where it gives off the chorda tympani and a branch to the stapedius muscle, before leaving the skull through the stylomastoid foramen. The taste fibres from the anterior two-thirds of the tongue pass through the lingual nerve and then join the facial nerve via the chorda tympani. The cell bodies of these fibres are in the genicu-late ganglion and, after joining the facial nerve, they enter the tractus solitarius and synapse with cells of the dorsal visceral grey nucleus. From here, there are projections to the thalamus and hypothalamus.

Examination

Severe facial weakness may be obvious at rest, with loss of the nasolabial fold, sagging of the lower eyelid and drooping of the side of the mouth. Partial weakness may not be obvious at rest. To test the facial muscles, the patient should be asked to close the eyes tightly and resist attempts to open the eyelids; and to grimace, hold the lips together tightly, and blow out the cheeks.

With an upper motor neurone lesion, the lower facial muscles are much weaker than the upper facial muscles. This is because there are bilateral corticobulbar projections to the neurons of the VIIth nerve nucleus supplying the upper facial muscles, while that to the neurones supplying the lower facial muscles is unilateral. In lower motor neurone lesions, all the muscles are usually equally affected. If the nerve is affected distal to the stylomastoid foramen, there is paralysis of the facial muscles but preservation of taste. A lesion of the nerve proximal to the point where the chorda tympani joins it will involve taste on the same side of the anterior two-thirds of the tongue. An injury of the facial nerve in the facial canal proximal to the origin of the nerve to the stapedius muscle will also produce an abnormal loudness of sound in the ear on the same side (hyperacusis). A lesion of the facial nerve proximal to the geniculate ganglion will additionally produce absence of lachrymation on the same side, due to involvement of the greater superficial petrosal nerve.

Finally, damage to the facial nerve in the pons is often associated with a VIth nerve palsy producing weakness of abduction of the eye.

To test taste, four solutions – sweet, salt, sour and bitter – are applied carefully on each side of the tongue.

VIIIth cranial nerve

Clinical anatomy

The VIIIth cranial nerve comprises the cochlear and vestibular nerves. The cochlear nerve passes from the inner ear through the internal auditory canal and enters the upper medulla at the level of the inferior cerebellar peduncle. Within the medulla, the auditory fibres reach the dorsal and ventral cochlear nuclei, where they synapse; fibres from these nuclei cross the midline as the trapezoid body, and enter the lateral lemniscus on the opposite side. They terminate in the inferior colliculus and the further projection is thence to the medial geniculate body and the auditory radiation to the temporal cortex. There are bilateral connections in the cochlear nuclei and at sites above this level, so that unilateral lesions of the temporal cortex and the brainstem do not produce deafness. Unilateral lesions of the cochlear nucleus or the VIIIth nerve will produce unilateral deafness.

Examination of hearing

The ability to hear a watch ticking a few inches from the ear indicates normal hearing; alternatively, the examiner whispers numbers at a slight distance from the ear, with the contralateral ear occluded, and asks the patient to repeat what was said. In most instances, this assessment of hearing is adequate, but audiometry may be required in some patients.

In *Rinne's test*, air and bone conduction are tested using a 128 cycles per second tuning fork. Air conduction should be better than bone conduction, and this is tested firstly by placing the tuning fork in front of the ear and secondly, by placing the base of the tuning fork on the mastoid process. If the latter is heard more loudly than the former, it indicates a conductive deafness due to disease of the middle ear. In nerve deafness, both air and bone conduction are diminished compared with the other side, but air conduction should still be better than bone conduction.

In *Weber's test*, the tuning fork is placed on the middle of the forehead and the patient is asked whether the sound is heard in the middle or off to one side. In conductive deafness, the sound is lateralised towards the affected side, whereas, in disease of the cochlea or nerve deafness, the sound is lateralised towards the unaffected side.

Vestibular division

The vestibular division of the nerve carries fibres from the vestibular apparatus, comprising the saccule, utricle and three semicircular canals. The cell bodies of these fibres lie within the internal auditory meatus, and the centrally directed axons of the cell bodies pass to the upper medulla, together with the auditory division of the VIIIth nerve, and then pass to the flocculo-nodular lobe of the cerebellum and the four vestibular nuclei. All four vestibular nuclei have connections with the cerebellum and with the medial longitudinal fasciculus, by which they are connected with the IIIrd, IVth and VIth cranial nerves. The cortical projections from the vestibular nuclei are diffuse and poorly understood.

Vertigo

The major symptom of vestibular disease is vertigo. This can be defined as an hallucination of movement, either of the patient himself, or the world surrounding him. It is often associated with sympathetic overactivity, producing nausea, vomiting, tachycardia and, rarely, diarrhoea. When it is severe, balance will be impaired and the patient will be unable to walk or even stand. Vertigo is discussed more fully on page 884.

Nystagmus

Nystagmus is a rhythmical involuntary movement of the eyes, usually evident during maintenance of horizontal or vertical gaze but occasionally in the primary position as well. It may result from any disorder of the mechanisms maintaining conjugate gaze (p. 868), most often from lesions involving the vestibular system or cerebellar pathways. Vestibular lesions may be peripheral (labyrinthine) or central (in the brainstem). Nystagmus may also be a drug-induced phenomenon, typically caused by anticonvulsants or benzodiazepines and probably as a result of their effects on the brainstem and cerebellum. Rarely, nystagmus may occur as a congenital disorder, either in isolation or as a secondary consequence of lifelong visual impairment.

The typical clinical appearance of nystagmus is of failure to sustain gaze with a slow drift back towards the primary position, which is rhythmically interrupted by rapid corrective jerks in the direction of attempted gaze ('sawtooth', or 'jerk' nystagmus). In severe unilateral vestibular lesions or during provocative tests, the jerks may persist in the mid position (second degree nystagmus) or even when looking in the direction of the slow component (third degree nystagmus). Congenital ocular nystagmus is also present in all positions of gaze but the movements are usually pendular, having equal velocity and amplitude in each direction. Non-ocular congenital nystagmus may be pendular or 'sawtooth' in type, sometimes variable in amplitude and often very marked with little accompanying visual disturbance. Acquired nystagmus of similar severity is usually accompanied by vertigo, or at least oscillopsia, an unpleasant awareness of movement of the visual environment, which may impair acuity.

A systematic approach to nystagmus is summarised in Table 22.9.

Tests of vestibular function

Vertigo is often accompanied by nystagmus, due to an abnormal stimulus arising in one labyrinth or to acute loss of function in one labyrinth. The slow phase of the nystagmus is induced by vestibular stimulation; it is in the direction of the movement of the endolymph and has a fast phase of recovery. Vestibular nystagmus is increased on turning the head or the eyes in the direction of the fast phase. Vestibular nystagmus can be induced either by sudden head movements (of which the most reliable technique is the use of a rotating chair), or by *caloric testing*, which is simpler to perform. The labyrinth is stimulated

Table 22.9 Analysis of nystagmus

	Site of lesion	Pathophysiology	Clinical features
Vestibular system	Labyrinth	Idiopathic Inflammatory Trauma Ménière's disease Vascular Toxic (alcohol, aminoglycosides)	Horizontal or rotatory. Beats *away* from side of labyrinthine lesion
	Eighth nerve (rare)	Acoustic neuroma	
Cerebellar system	Brainstem (Vestibular nuclei and cerebellar connections)	MS Vascular lesions Wernicke's encephalopathy Trauma	Horizontal, rotatory or vertical. May be complex and dysconjugate, as in internuclear ophthalmoplegia (p. 969)
	Cerebellum	Drugs Degenerative disorders Brainstem encephalitis Tumours	Usually horizontal, beating *towards* side of cerebellar lesion. Downbeating with flocculo-nodular lesions (rare)
Congenital nystagmus	Ocular disease	Albinism, cataracts, retinal lesions	Usually rapid and pendular, present in all directions of gaze
	Normal vision, site unknown	Pathology unknown	May be pendular in mid-position Often very marked on lateral gaze

by irrigating each external auditory meatus with water, first at 30°C and then at 44°C. For most purposes, only the cold water test is necessary. The test is performed with the patient lying on his/her back with the head held flexed to about 30° above the horizontal. Nystagmus is induced by the cold water and normally persists for about 2 minutes. The response is absent if there is total destruction of the vestibular apparatus or vestibular division of the VIIIth nerve; less severe degrees of damage produce impairment, rather than absence, of the response. If the vestibular lesion is irritative and nystagmus is already present, it will increase with caloric testing.

IXth cranial nerve

Of the many functions of the glossopharyngeal nerve, sensation of the posterior third of the tongue and the pharyngeal wall is the only one tested routinely. As well as supplying sensation to this area, the nerve also supplies motor fibres to the stylopharyngeus muscle, secretor-motor fibres to the parotid gland, and taste to the posterior third of the tongue. The nerve passes between the internal jugular vein and the internal carotid artery, enters the skull through the jugular foramen and joins the medulla between the inferior olive and the inferior cerebellar peduncle.

Light touch of the posterior third of the tongue and the pharyngeal wall can be tested using an orange stick. All but the lightest stimuli in this area will produce a gag reflex. This consists of elevation of the palate, retraction of the tongue and contraction of the pharyngeal muscles. The afferent limb of this reflex is the glossopharyngeal nerve, and the efferent limb is the vagus nerve. The gag reflex is more likely to be absent with lesions of the glossopharyngeal nerve than of the vagus.

Xth cranial nerve

As well as supplying general visceral efferent preganglionic fibres to the thoracic and abdominal viscera and visceral afferents, the vagus nerve supplies motor fibres to the intrinsic muscles of the larynx, the cricothyroid muscle and the pharyngeal musculature; it also supplies sensation to the pharyngeal wall, the epiglottis, the base of the tongue and the larynx, and a small sensory branch to the external auditory meatus.

The nerve rises from the dorsal nucleus and the nucleus ambiguus in the medulla. It exits from the medulla, passes through the jugular foramen, and then enters the carotid sheath and passes down through the neck and into the thorax. The recurrent laryngeal nerve winds around the subclavian artery on the right side, before ascending between the oesophagus and the trachea to enter the larynx. On the left, the recurrent laryngeal nerve winds around the arch of the aorta and ascends to the larynx.

Examination

Articulation of speech, the ability to phonate, palatal movement and swallowing are the principal clinical tests of vagal function.

Dysarthria may occur with impairment of vagal function, but may also occur in edentulous people or those with poorly fitted dentures. Other causes include facial weakness, weakness of the tongue, or impaired coordination of movement due to a pyramidal, extrapyramidal or cerebellar defect. Some causes of dysarthria produce characteristic speech abnormalities:

- Edentulous people have difficulty in pronouncing the consonants 's', 'th' and 't'.
- Patients with a VIIth nerve palsy have particular difficulty with lip movements and, thus, most difficulty in pronouncing the consonants 'b' and 'p'.
- Weakness of the tongue leads to difficulty in the pronunciation of the consonants 'd' and 't'.
- Palatal paralysis causes a nasal quality to the voice, and difficulty in pronouncing the consonants 'k', 'q' and 'ch'. This is more marked if the paralysis is bilateral.
- Cerebellar lesions produce so-called scanning speech, which has an interrupted quality.
- Bilateral upper motor neurone lesions induce speech which is slow, spastic and sometimes grunting.
- Extrapyramidal disease causes dysarthria which is slurring and is often associated with dysphonia. The speech may peter out in mid-sentence and there may be difficulty in initiating speech.

Soft palate. Movement of the soft palate is tested by asking the patient to say 'ah'. This produces palatal elevation and the uvula should remain in the midline as the palate rises. A palatal paralysis on one side will produce deviation of the uvula towards the normal side.

Laryngeal function is tested by listening to the voice. This may be hoarse or husky and of low volume. The ability to sing is lost in either unilateral or bilateral vocal cord paralysis.

Swallowing is tested by asking the patient to drink some water. Regurgitation of liquid through the nose indicates palatal weakness and the patient with dysphagia may cough as fluid spills into the trachea.

XIth cranial nerve

The XIth cranial nerve supplies the sternomastoid and trapezius muscles. The motor cells lie in the upper five cervical segments, the nerve passing upwards through the foramen magnum and into the posterior fossa, where it joins the bulbar accessory nerve which is part of the vagus nerve. Together, they leave the skull through the jugular foramen with the glossopharyngeal and vagus nerves. The spinal accessory fibres then descend in the neck to supply the sternomastoid and trapezius muscles. The sternomastoid muscles contract together to flex the neck, and each one acts to turn the head towards the opposite side. The patient's ability to turn the head against resistance is tested and the sternomastoid can be both seen and palpated. The trapezius is tested by asking the patient to shrug his or her shoulders against resistance.

XIIth cranial nerve

The hypoglossal nucleus lies in the dorsal part of the medulla. The nerve leaves the medulla and passes out of the posterior fossa through the anterior condylar foramen. It then passes anteriorly through the neck and reaches the tongue.

To test the tongue, the patient is first asked to open his or her mouth and the tongue is examined lying at rest in the floor of the mouth. The bulk of the tongue is assessed. Wasting and fasciculation indicate a lower motor neurone lesion. Tremor in the tongue can be difficult to distinguish from fasciculation. Protrusion of the tongue should be in the midline. A weakness on one side will lead to the tongue being protruded towards the weak side. Lower motor neurone lesions produce ipsilateral wasting of the tongue with weakness. Only occasionally, with an acute severe upper motor neurone lesion, is there deviation to the opposite side.

THE MOTOR SYSTEM

The motor unit – consisting of an anterior horn cell or motor neurone of a cranial nucleus, the peripheral axon and the muscle it supplies – is influenced by activity in the cortex, via the corticospinal tracts, the cerebellum, the basal ganglia, the vestibular system and afferent information, largely postural sensation. Routine examination of the motor system allows the identification of dysfunction of one or more of these centres influencing movement.

Motor system lesions

Cortex and corticospinal (pyramidal) tract lesions

Lesions of the cortex or corticospinal tract lead to an increase in tone without muscle wasting, except after long periods, as a result of disuse. There is no fasciculation. The distribution of weakness with pyramidal lesions is characteristic. In the upper limbs, the flexor muscles remain stronger than the extensors and, in the leg, the extensors remain stronger than the flexors. The tendon reflexes are brisk and the plantar response is extensor.

Basal ganglia

The term *extrapyramidal disease* is loosely used to refer to disease of the basal ganglia; this causes a number of motor abnormalities, including a rest tremor (which often disappears or is reduced with purposeful movement), and other involuntary movements including chorea, athetosis, dystonia and ballismus. Basal ganglia lesions may also lead to akinesia or hypokinesia (poverty of movement), difficulty in initiating movements, slowness of movement (bradykinesia) and rigidity in the muscles, with a characteristic irregular increase in tone, producing 'cogwheeling' (p. 919). The tendon reflexes in extrapyramidal disease are usually normal.

Cerebellum

Cerebellar disease produces incoordination. There is often a tremor which develops on action, and this may involve the trunk as well as the limbs. Head tremor is called *titubation*. Speech may be involved, typically producing a scanning dysarthria. Muscle tone is normal, or sometimes reduced, and reflexes may be sluggish. Cerebellar lesions do not lead to weakness, though incoordination may cause disabling loss of function (p. 929).

Lower motor neurone lesions

Lesions of the anterior horn cell or the lower motor neurone at any point will lead to denervation of the muscle supplied. This produces muscle wasting, fasciculation, a reduction in muscle tone and depressed or absent tendon reflexes.

Muscle disease

Disease of the muscles themselves produces weakness. In many acquired muscle diseases, weakness is mainly in the large proximal hip and shoulder girdle muscles, and is often accompanied by wasting. Tendon reflexes are preserved and plantar responses are flexor. Muscle tone is reduced, in proportion to the degree of muscular wasting and weakness.

Examination of the motor system

The motor system is examined in the following order.

1. Posture and involuntary movements

Inspection of the patient may reveal a number of abnormalities of posture which are helpful in diagnosis, e.g. the patient with a hemiplegia whose affected arm is held flexed, or the patient with Parkinson's disease with mask-like facies and a flexed posture of the trunk. The patient is also observed for involuntary movements at rest. These are common in extrapyramidal disease.

2. Muscle bulk

The bulk of the muscles in the limbs and on the trunk is assessed. Wasted muscles should be carefully examined for fasciculation.

3. Muscle tone

With complete relaxation, there should be little resistance to passive movement of limbs. With pyramidal tract lesions, there is a spastic increase in tone, which is usually a constant resistance to movement. However, with rapid passive movement the clasp-knife phenomenon may be elicited, in which there is an increase in tone followed by a sudden decrease. Sudden passive movement about a joint may elicit clonus, which reflects a disinhibited stretch reflex. This is most easily obtained at the ankle in the calf muscles, though it may be present in any spastic muscle group. In extrapyramidal disease, the increase in tone is intermittent and feels like a ratchet (cogwheel rigidity). Tone may be reduced in a severe neuropathy or myopathy leading to marked muscle wasting, and also, occasionally, in cerebellar disease.

4. Power

Power should be tested with attention to the segmental innervation of the muscles being tested. It is usual to do this in the order set out in Table 22.10. Power of trunk flexion and extension should be tested as well as muscles in the limbs.

It is useful to grade power in each muscle group. A number of scales have been suggested. In the UK, the most widely used scale is that of the Medical Research Council:

Grade 0 – no movement at all
Grade 1 – flicker of movement
Grade 2 – movement with gravity eliminated
Grade 3 – movement against gravity
Grade 4 – movement against resistance. This covers a wide range of power and is usually subdivided in grades 4−, 4 and 4+.
Grade 5 – normal power.

5. Coordination

Tests of coordination are of little value if marked weakness is present. In the upper limbs, the finger–nose test assesses the presence of an action tremor, and coordination is further tested by rapid repetitive movements, such as tapping the back of one hand with the other, and fine finger movements, such as touching each finger in turn

Table 22.10 Innervation of muscle groups*

Muscle/muscle group	Segmental/nerve innervation	
Diaphragm	C3, 4, 5	
Rhomboid	C4, 5	
Serratus anterior	C4, 5, 6	
Supraspinatus	C4, 5, 6	
Infraspinatus	C4, 5, 6	
Pectoralis major	C5, 6, 7, 8, T1	
Deltoid	C5, 6	
Biceps/brachialis	C5, 6	
Triceps	C6, 7, 8	Radial
Brachioradialis	C5, 6	Radial
Wrist extensors	C5, 6, 7, 8	Radial
Wrist flexors – carpi radialis	C6, 7	Median
carpi ulnaris	C7, 8, T1	Ulnar
Finger extensors	C6, 7, 8	Radial
Finger flexors	C7, 8, T1	Median
Abductor pollicis brevis	C8, T1	Median
Abductor pollicis longus	C7, 8	Radial
Interossei	C8, T1	Ulnar
Upper abdominal	T6–9	
Lower abdominal	T10–L1	
Iliopsoas	L1, 2, 3	
Adductors of hip	L2, 3, 4	
Abductors of hip	L4, 5, S1	
Extensors of hip	L5, S1, 2	
Knee flexion	L4, 5, S1, 2	
Knee extension	L2, 3, 4	
Dorsiflexion of foot	L4, 5	
Plantarflexion of foot	S1, 2	
Toe extension	L5, S1	
Extensor hallucis longus	L5	
Extensor digitorum brevis	S1	
Toe flexion	S1, 2	
Inversion of foot	L4, 5	
Eversion of foot	L5, S1	

*Those shown in bold type are those routinely tested

Table 22.11 Segmental reflex levels

Reflex	Level
Glabellar	Corticopontine
Snout	Corticopontine
Sucking	Frontal
Palmomental	Frontal
Grasp	Frontal
Jaw	Pons
Biceps	C5, 6
Supinator	C5, 6
Triceps	C7, 8
Finger	C7, 8, T1
Abdominal – upper	T9, 10
lower	T11, 12
Knee	L2, 3, 4
Ankle	S1
Plantar	Corticospinal tract (afferent L5, S1)
Cremasteric	L1, 2
Anal	S3, 4, 5

with the thumb of the same hand. Physiological tremor is a fine tremor of the outstretched hands and fingers which does not impair coordination to any significant degree. Incoordination due to an action tremor on finger–nose testing is termed *past-pointing* or *dysmetria*, and is seen in cerebellar disease. Impairment of rapid repetitive movements is *dysdiadochokinesis*. Further tests of coordination in the upper limbs are writing and use of a knife and fork. In the legs, the heel–shin test is the equivalent of the finger–nose test, and foot-tapping on the examiner's hand is a test of rapid repetitive movement.

6. Reflexes

The main reflexes tested are listed in Table 22.11. In routine practice, it is usually necessary only to test the jaw jerk, the tendon reflexes, the plantar reflexes and the abdominal reflexes. The reflexes may be absent in peripheral neuropathy. They may be reduced in cerebellar disease or, in the case of a corticospinal tract lesion, be increased and accompanied by an extensor plantar response.

The *abdominal reflexes* may be absent with a corticospinal tract lesion. They are otherwise usually present in the young, but may disappear with age and obesity.

The *glabellar reflex* is performed by tapping the forehead between the eyebrows with a finger, from behind the patient so that the finger cannot be seen. This is positive if there is persistent closing of the eyes, the reflex indicating damage of the frontopontine pathways to the facial nerve nucleus. It is an early sign in Parkinson's disease and it is also seen in dementia, with cerebral atrophy and with frontal lobe tumours.

The *snout reflex* is elicited by tapping the nose and is positive if this induces excessive grimacing of the face. Like the glabellar reflex, it indicates frontal lobe disease.

The *sucking reflex* is also a frontal lobe sign. It is positive when stroking of the lip produces pouting and sucking movements of the lips. It is a normal reflex in young babies but usually disappears within the first 18 months of life. It is seen with diffuse lesions affecting the frontal lobes. The *chewing reflex* also indicates diffuse frontal disease. A tongue depressor is placed in the mouth, and this provokes reflex chewing movements. The *grasp reflex* also indicates frontal lobe disease. The patient's palm is stroked and this elicits reflex grasping which becomes stronger if attempts are made to remove the fingers from the grasp. Sometimes stroking of the dorsum of the patient's fingers of the same hand will inhibit the reflex and allow release of the examiner's fingers from the grasp. These reflexes, indicating frontal lobe damage, are collectively known as the *primitive reflexes*.

Table 22.12 summarises the main findings on examination of the motor system with various types of neurological deficit.

SENSORY SYSTEM

Primary sensations

The primary sensations tested are light touch, pinprick, temperature, vibration and joint position sense. A working knowledge of peripheral nerve and dermatomal anatomy is essential (Fig. 22.5). Light touch is tested with a wisp of cotton-wool; pinprick with a disposable pin, not a hypodermic needle. Temperature sensation is tested with tubes filled with hot or cold water, vibration with a 128 cycles per second tuning fork and joint position should be tested initially in the distal interphalangeal joints of the fingers and toes. Body charts are useful to record the sensory abnormalities.

Sensory system lesions

Sensory tract lesions

Lesions of the spinal cord and lesions rostral to this may affect the sensory tracts in a differential way. For example, in cervical spinal cord compression from a prolapsed disc, it is common to find that loss of postural and vibration sense (dorsal columns) is more marked than pinprick and temperature sensation, whereas, with an intramedullary lesion of the spinal cord involving decussating spinothalamic tract fibres, there will be a dissociated impairment of pain and temperature at the level of the lesion.

Cortical sensation

More complex types of sensory disturbance occur with lesions affecting the parietal lobe.

Two-point discrimination, the ability to detect two separate stimuli closely applied on the finger, is normally 3–5 mm on the finger pulps. Parietal lesions impair discrimination. Sensory extinction of one of a pair of simultaneously applied stimuli on each side of the body is also a feature of parietal lobe lesions. The patient is asked to close the eyes, and the examiner then touches one side of the body with a pin and asks the patient to report on which side the stimulus was felt. The patient with a parietal lobe lesion will be able to identify correctly a single right-sided or left-sided stimulus, but, with paired stimuli, will only report feeling the pin on the side contralateral to the normal parietal lobe.

Graphaesthesia is the ability to identify figures or letters drawn on the palm of the hand with an orange stick, with the eyes closed. This ability may be lost in the hand contralateral to a parietal lobe lesion.

Stereognosis is the ability to manipulate objects within the hand and correctly identify them. Coins are usually used for this purpose. A contralateral parietal lobe lesion may lead to astereognosis.

Tactile localisation is the ability to identify the part of the body touched briefly by the examiner. The patient is asked to localise the point touched by the examiner by placing his or her own finger on the same spot. Again, this is impaired with a contralateral parietal lobe lesion.

Identification of body parts is also impaired with a parietal lobe lesion. Such a patient is unable to identify correctly his or her different fingers and show them to the examiner. With severe lesions, this agnosia of parts of the body may lead to denial of the existence of part of the body or even the whole of one side of the body. Some patterns of sensory deficit are included in Table 22.13.

Table 22.12 Motor system examination

Deficit	Muscle bulk	Fasciculation	Tremor	Tone	Power	Coordination	Reflexes	Plantars	Gait
Lower motor neurone (including anterior horn cell)	Reduced	Usually	–	Reduced	Reduced	Impaired with severe weakness	Reduced or absent	Flexor	Steppage
Upper motor	Normal	–	–	Increased (spastic)	Usually reduced	Sometimes impaired	Increased	Extensor	Spastic or hemiplegic
Extrapyramidal	Normal	–	+ (At rest)	Increased (cogwheel)	Normal	Impaired (slow)	Normal	Flexor	Stooped hypokinetic
Cerebellar	Normal	–	+ (On action)	Normal or reduced	Normal	Impaired	Normal or reduced	Flexor	Ataxic
Myopathy	Wasting proximally	–	–	Reduced	Proximal weakness	Impaired in proportion to weakness	Normal or reduced	Flexor	Waddling

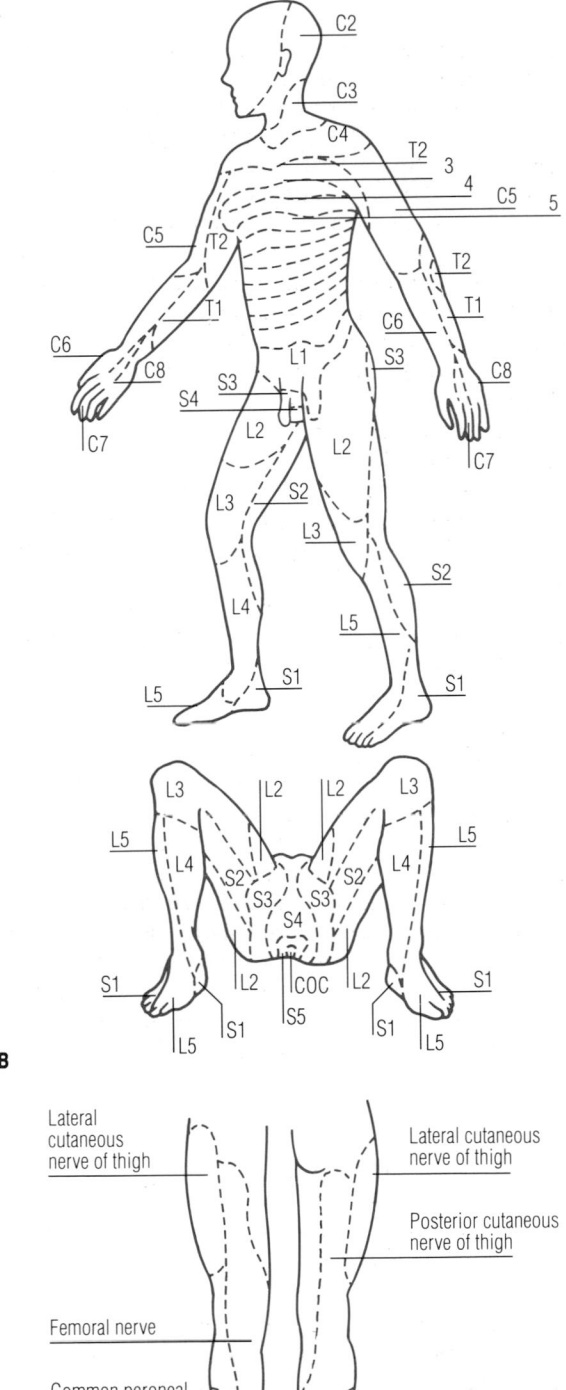

Fig. 22.5 Peripheral nerve and dermatomal anatomy. A. Dermatomal fields. **B.** Sensory territories of selected peripheral nerves of clinical importance.

LESIONS OF THE LOBES OF THE BRAIN

Localised lesions of the different lobes of the brain produce readily recognisable clinical syndromes. The lesions most often producing focal deficits are tumours and areas of infarction.

Frontal lobe

Lesions of the frontal lobe commonly produce a contralateral hemiparesis due to involvement of the motor area and upper part of the corticospinal tract. However, a hemiparesis is not invariable with frontal lobe lesions. Involvement of Broca's area will produce an expressive aphasia. Mental changes are common with frontal lobe lesions. There is often some degree of intellectual impairment, consisting of poor attention span, some loss of retention and recall, impairment of judgement and loss of insight. Mood changes are prominent, with periods of euphoria or depression. The affect is typically fatuous or frivolous, and behaviour may become disinhibited; these effects together may lead to considerable social disruption. Bladder and bowel control may be lost, leading to incontinence, sometimes with an inappropriate lack of concern. Fits are common with frontal lobe lesions.

Parietal lobe

Abnormalities of cortical sensation are prominent (see above). Impairment of tasks involving visuospatial skills and apraxia is common. Topographagnosia is the difficulty experienced by patients, particularly those with non-dominant parietal lobe lesions, in finding their way in familiar places. Prosopagnosia is the inability to recognise familiar faces. Apraxia leads to serious practical problems, such as an inability to dress and perform other simple tasks, e.g. eating and shaving. Involvement of the visual radiation produces a lower homonymous quadrantanopia.

Temporal lobe

A lesion involving Wernicke's area, which lies in the anterior part of the temporal lobe, produces a receptive aphasia. In addition, temporal lobe lesions produce memory impairment. Involvement of the visual radiation leads to an upper homonymous quadrantanopia.

Occipital lobe

A lesion involving the visual cortex will produce a hemianopic visual field defect. Lesions more anterior in the occipital lobe, in the visual association areas, may lead to visual agnosia and agnosia for colours. Fits are commonest with frontal and temporal lobe lesions, less common with parietal lesions, and least common with occipital lesions.

Table 22.13 Common patterns of neurological deficit

- **Diffuse cerebral**
  Dementia, with or without physical signs, depending on cause
  Fits
  Gait dyspraxia

- **Cerebral hemisphere**
  Hemiparesis, dysphasia, sensory loss, visual loss (hemi- or quadrantanopia) and other specific features, depending on lobe affected
  May be raised intracranial pressure, sometimes with false localising signs (e.g. IIIrd nerve palsy)
  Fits, focal or generalised

- **Extrapyramidal**
  Akinesia, bradykinesia
  Abnormal posture
  Rest tremor
  Cogwheel rigidity
  Chorea, dystonia, ballismus

- **Cerebellum**
  Ataxia of trunk with midline lesions
  Ipsilateral ataxia of limbs and nystagmus with cerebellar hemisphere lesions
  Dysarthria

- **Expanding pituitary lesions**
  Bitemporal visual field loss, usually asymmetrical
  Hypopituitarism – usually partial
  Sometimes optic atrophy
  Sometimes ocular movement palsies

- **Brainstem**
  Cranial nerve lesions at the level of the brainstem lesion
  UMN signs in brainstem below level of lesion, and in limbs
  Limb signs often bilateral
  Sensory impairment variable – often contralateral spinothalamic (ST) loss
  Bulbar (medulla) involvement common – dysarthria, dysphagia, impaired breathing
  Variable bladder and bowel involvement
  Cerebellar signs very common
  Impairment of consciousness common with acute lesions, unless ventrally placed
  Mass lesions may be associated with hydrocephalus due to aqueduct obstruction

- **Spinal cord**
  May be root signs at level of lesion
  UMN (pyramidal tract) weakness below level of lesion
  Extensor plantars and brisk reflexes below lesion
  Abdominal reflexes reduced or absent
  May be sensory level on trunk – this may be at or below the level of the lesion
  Sensory loss in limbs may be of dorsal column (DC) or spinothalamic (ST) type, or affect all modalities
  Intrinsic cord lesions more likely to cause ST loss
  Compressive cord lesions more likely to cause DC loss
  Bladder and bowel involvement very common and may be the major early symptom.

- **Anterior horn cell**
  Wasting, fasciculation, weakness. In motor neurone disease, a combination of LMN and UMN signs.

- **Cauda equina**
  Multiple lumbosacral root lesions. Often asymmetrical
  Bladder and bowel involvement common
  Absent reflexes at affected root levels

- **Roots**
  Motor (LMN) and/or sensory loss in a root distribution
  Tendon reflex absent if it affects appropriate root

- **Peripheral nerve**
  Mononeuritis: motor (LMN) and/or sensory loss in distribution of a single peripheral nerve

  Mononeuritis multiplex: asymmetrical, patchy motor and/or sensory deficit attributable to multiple peripheral nerve lesions

  Polyneuropathy: symmetrical motor (LMN) and/or sensory deficit most marked distally. Usually legs more affected than arms. Reflexes variably absent, depending on type and extent of neuropathy

- **Neuromuscular junction**
  Fatigable weakness affecting any voluntary muscle

- **Muscle disease**
  Usually proximal wasting and weakness
  Reduced or absent reflexes if wasting severe
  Plantars flexor. No sensory deficit
  No bladder or bowel involvement

HEADACHE

Headache is one of the commonest symptoms in medicine (Table 22.14). It usually does not indicate serious intracranial disease and often accompanies systemic illnesses as a non-specific symptom. In most patients presenting with headache, there are no abnormal physical signs, so that the diagnosis depends entirely upon an accurate history.

Aetiology

A number of intracranial and extracranial structures may give rise to headache. It may be due to referred pain from the muscles and joints of the cervical spine; disease of the sinuses, temporomandibular joints, teeth, ears and eyes may all produce headache, rather than local pain. Raised and reduced intracranial pressure can both cause headache. Intracerebral arteries innervated by the trigeminal nerve are sensitive to stretch and pressure, and the

Table 22.14 Causes of headache

Migraine	Postictal headache
Tension headache	**Postconcussional headache**
Without any demonstrable underlying structural abnormality	**Diseases of the skull and sinuses**
Headache associated with cervical spine disease	Sinusitis
	Fractures
	Mastoiditis
	Paget's disease
	Tumours of bone
Diseases affecting blood vessels	
Intracranial	**Ear disease**
Intracerebral haemorrhage	Acute otitis media
Cerebral thrombosis	Chronic suppurative otitis
Cerebral embolism	media
Berry aneurysm	
Arteriovenous malformation	**Diseases of the eyes and orbits**
Cortical thrombophlebitis	Glaucoma
Hypertensive encephalopathy	Iritis
Cerebral arteritis	Orbital tumour
Extracranial	
Giant cell arteritis	**Toxic and metabolic causes**
	Infections with fever
Raised intracranial pressure	Hypercapnia
Tumours	Hypoxia
Abscess	Hypoglycaemia
Encephalitis	Alcoholic hangover
Hydrocephalus	
Benign intracranial hypertension	**Haematological disease**
Pituitary tumours	Anaemia
Acute trauma with oedema	Polycythaemia
Subdural haematoma	
	Coital cephalgia
Meningeal irritation	
Meningitis	**Psychogenic headache**
Subarachnoid haemorrhage	

leptomeninges are also very sensitive to distortion and inflammation. Subarachnoid haemorrhage and meningitis usually produce severe headache. Spasm, dilatation or inflammation of branches of the external carotid artery may lead to headache. A number of metabolic disturbances such as hypoglycaemia and hypercapnia are associated with headache; in these, the mechanisms of pain are largely unknown.

Taking a history

When taking a history of headache, a structured approach along the following lines is suggested:

1. When did the headaches start?
2. How often do the headaches occur? Are they continuous or episodic?
3. How long does each headache last?
4. How severe is the headache and how does it affect daily activities including work and sleep?
5. Where is the headache felt? Is it localised or generalised?
6. Are there associated symptoms, particularly any visual or gastrointestinal symptoms?
7. What has been the effect of treatment already tried?

TENSION HEADACHES AND HEADACHES ASSOCIATED WITH CERVICAL ARTHRITIS

Tension headaches

Tension headaches are by far the commonest type of headache. Pain is usually described as continuous, occurring every day with a tendency to worsen during the day. They rarely disturb sleep, and patients are usually able to continue their activities. There are no specific associated symptoms and analgesics have limited or no effect. Periods of relaxation, such as holidays, often have a beneficial effect. The headaches are generalised, occipital or frontal, are often described as a dull ache, a band around the head or a pressure feeling, and may be associated with pain and stiffness in the neck. There may be a history of domestic or work stress or anxiety. Neurological examination is normal, but there may be tenderness of the neck muscles.

The basis for the pain of tension headache is uncertain. The frequent occurrence of muscular tenderness suggests that undue sustained contraction plays a part. Treatment with analgesics is not usually successful. Explanation, reassurance and instruction in techniques of relaxation by a physiotherapist is often all that is required, though some tension headaches prove extremely refractory to treatment.

Cervical osteoarthritis

Headaches associated with cervical osteoarthritis are very similar, although neck symptoms are more prominent and neck movements are limited and painful. Disease of the joints of the cervical spine probably causes referred headache, and there is often associated muscle spasm. Physical measures are usually more helpful than analgesics, although NSAIDs may be useful in some patients.

MIGRAINE

Migraine affects up to 5% of the population and is more common in women. It may start in childhood, adolescence or early adult life, but rarely after the age of 35.

Clinical features

In children the development of obvious migraine attacks may be preceded by episodic vomiting associated with abdominal pain (bilious attacks), headache often being a relatively minor symptom at this stage. Migraine is defined as episodic headache usually lasting 6–24 hours, and which is associated with transient visual and/or gastrointestinal disturbances. Headache is often preceded by a visual aura of teichopsia (flashing moving dots) or fortification spectra (zig-zag scintillating lines partly obscuring vision), scotomas (discrete areas of loss of vision), blurring of vision or hemianopic obscurations. Photophobia and phonophobia are common. Additional prodromal symptoms include hemiparaesthesia, occasionally mild unilateral weakness and dysphasia, but these are present in only a small minority of patients. The prodromal disturbances last for 5–30 minutes and are followed by the headache. This is unilateral or generalised, some patients always experiencing pain on the same side. It is often severe, leading to prostration, and is described as throbbing or continuous in nature. In some instances, it is relieved by sleeping, in others by vomiting. Nausea and vomiting are experienced by the majority of patients in some attacks at least.

Provoking factors include fatigue, alcohol, menstruation and hunger. In some patients, there is a history suggesting food allergy and migraine appears to be induced by dietary factors; the common provoking foods are chocolate, cheese, shellfish and red wine.

Rare forms of migraine

Hemiplegic migraine. This is a rare form of migraine, in which a profound hemiplegia, sometimes with dysphasia and hemianopia, precedes the development of headache by 30–60 minutes. The weakness and other focal deficits usually resolve quickly; occasionally, however, they may improve only gradually and, very occasionally, a permanent deficit may result. Hemiplegic migraine sometimes occurs as a familial condition, in which case only this type of migraine occurs.

Basilar migraine. This is an unusual form of migraine, in which brainstem disturbances are common, including impairment of consciousness, vertigo, dysarthria, diplopia and limb weakness.

Ophthalmoplegic migraine. In this very rare condition headache is followed by transient unilateral ophthalmoplegia with ptosis, which may last for several days.

Pathophysiology

The pathophysiology of migraine remains controversial. Migraine was traditionally considered to have a vascular basis, the prodromal visual and other symptoms of neurological deficit being attributed to vasospasm affecting intracerebral and meningeal vessels, and the subsequent headache to dilatation of extracranial arteries. However, this theory does not account satisfactorily for the gradual progression of focal symptoms across the territories of different cerebral arteries, or for the profound systemic symptoms, heightened sensitivity to various stimuli, and autonomic disturbance that often accompanies a migraine attack. These features, and the results of research studies of cerebral activity and blood flow during migraine, suggest that there is also a disturbance of neuronal function during attacks, the vascular changes being possibly a secondary phenomenon. Several neurotransmitters may be important in migraine and much attention has been focused on 5-hydroxytryptamine (5-HT): the complexity of its role in the disorder is illustrated by the fact that a 5-HT antagonist such as pizotifen is effective in migraine prophylaxis, whereas treatment of the established acute attack is based on 5-HT agonists such as ergotamine and sumatriptan.

Management

Acute attacks

Most patients will experience attacks less frequently than once a month. In these patients, vigorous early treatment of the acute attack with an adequate dose of an analgesic, such as aspirin, paracetamol or dihydrocodeine, together with an antiemetic, such as metaclopramide, domperidone or prochlorperazine, is often all that is necessary. Emphasis should be placed on early treatment. Often, patients will have up to 30 minutes of prodromal symptoms before the onset of headache. Many patients are helped by lying in a darkened room, others by sleeping.

Identification and avoidance of provoking factors is an important and often neglected aspect of treatment.

Ergotamine is an effective drug in migraine, but is frequently associated with side-effects of nausea and vomiting. Usually, the drug is not necessary; however, in a few patients, relief of headache can only be achieved with ergotamine, which can be taken either orally or by suppository. Regular frequent use of ergotamine can actually induce headaches and, rarely, cause peripheral ischaemia and gangrene. A promising new acute treatment is the 5-HT agonist sumatriptan, which is apparently free of most of the side-effects of ergotamine and is at least as effective.

Frequent attacks

Patients with frequent attacks should be considered for prophylactic therapy. The two drugs most frequently used are propranolol and pizotifen, although many patients do not respond to either. Other agents used in prophylaxis include amitriptyline, calcium antagonists, cyproheptadine and the potent 5-HT antagonist methysergide. The latter should only be prescribed when all other treatment has failed and when migraine is disabling, because the drug has serious unwanted effects, including retroperitoneal fibrosis.

MIXED HEADACHE

Patients who have migraine seem more prone than average to develop tension headaches, the result being a confusing presentation of the two different kinds of headache. Often, it is found that all the headaches are being inappropriately treated as if they were migraine, when the majority of the headache is tension headache.

Some persistent, benign headaches defy diagnosis and treatment, and some of these undoubtedly have a psychological basis. Such patients are often extensively investigated without a cause becoming apparent. Their headaches are often of several years' duration and are resistant to all treatment.

INTRACEREBRAL BLOOD VESSELS AND HEADACHE

A number of diseases affecting the cerebral circulation may cause headache. The most dramatic is subarachnoid haemorrhage, most commonly caused by rupture of a berry aneurysm (p. 906). Headache is abrupt in onset, usually very severe and often associated with vomiting and impairment of consciousness. Any headache of instantaneous onset should raise the possibility of an aneurysm. Small leaks from aneurysms, causing headache alone, are common in the weeks or months before a larger, more severe bleed. In some instances, enlargement of an aneurysm, rather than rupture, may cause headache, and this type of headache is usually not so severe. Haemorrhage within the brain substance itself may occur in arteriovenous malformations or with hypertension, but many occur as apparently spontaneous events without any underlying hypertension or demonstrable vascular pathology. Bleeding causes an acute rise in intracranial pressure which usually causes severe headache. Cerebral thrombosis or embolism is usually painless, but a small number of patients with thrombotic stroke will complain of headache, which can be transiently severe.

Hypertensive encephalopathy (p. 903) may cause headache, but this is usually overshadowed by fits and impairment of consciousness.

Giant cell (temporal) arteritis is a cause of severe headache in the elderly (p. 1032), and headache is often a prominent symptom in the much rarer intracranial arteritides.

OTHER INTRACRANIAL CAUSES OF HEADACHE

With the exception of those due to diseases of the cerebral circulation, most intracranial causes of headache do so by irritation, traction or displacement of the dural lining of the brain, or distortion of blood vessels. It is likely that this is also the mechanism of headache due to raised intracranial pressure. Expanding pituitary tumours cause pain by local pressure in the pituitary fossa. Headache immediately following cranial trauma is very common (p. 924) and a minority of patients will continue to complain of postconcussional headaches for months, or even years, after head injury. The mechanism of such headaches is unknown. Suggestions of a relationship with impending litigation in some patients may hold some truth, but for most this is not the case.

Meningeal irritation

Headache with meningeal irritation is usually associated with neck stiffness. Meningitis and subarachnoid haemorrhage are the main causes. Localised disease involving the meninges, such as meningioma, focal metastatic tumour deposits and subdural haematoma, may each cause headache which may be felt as localised or generalised pain.

Postictal headache

Epileptic convulsions are often followed by headache. This usually lasts for less than 24 hours, but may be severe. There is often postictal drowsiness, confusion and fever; in addition, the cerebrospinal fluid (CSF) cell count and protein level may both be slightly elevated. This means that unless a clear history of a fit is obtained from a relative or friend, the situation can be diagnostically difficult and, in particular, meningitis should be considered.

Other causes of headache

Table 22.14 lists several other focal conditions which may present with headache, rather than pain localised to the region of pathology. Coital cephalgia is a rare condition, seen mainly in men, in which headache, often of abrupt onset, occurs during or just after intercourse. It may be severe, and the clinical picture may resemble that of subarachnoid haemorrhage (which, of course, may also be provoked by intercourse). Patients require careful assessment, and it is better in doubtful cases to examine a normal CSF than to miss a subarachnoid haemorrhage. Headache as a symptom of psychiatric disease is extremely common.

FACIAL PAIN

Most patients with facial pain have no signs. The presence of trigeminal sensory loss or other abnormal physical

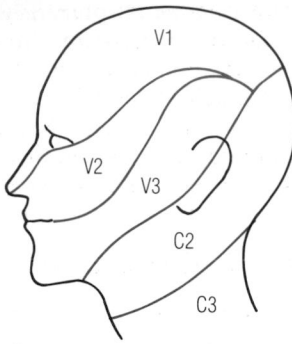

Fig. 22.6 Cutaneous fields of the three trigeminal divisions (V1, V2, V3) and two upper cervical dermatomes (C2, C3).

signs suggests a structural cause. A working knowledge of the cutaneous and non-cutaneous innervation of the trigeminal nerve is necessary (Fig. 22.6 and Table 22.15), and a recognition that pain may be referred onto the face from diseases affecting deeper structures.

It is clinically useful to classify the causes of facial pain according to the site of the lesion, these being local causes (Table 22.16), lesions between the cavernous sinus and

Table 22.15 Non-cutaneous trigeminal innervation

Division	Structures innervated
Ophthalmic	Eye, including cornea
	Mucosa of frontal sinus and upper part of nose
Maxillary	Lateral wall and floor of nasal cavity
	Upper jaw and teeth
	Roof of mouth
	Mucosa of maxillary sinus
Mandibular	Anterior wall of external auditory meatus
	Temporo-mandibular joint
	Lower jaw and teeth
	Floor of mouth
	Anterior two-thirds of tongue

Table 22.16 Disease of local structures causing facial pain

Teeth	Salivary glands
Impacted wisdom teeth	Infection, e.g. mumps
Dental abscess	Inflammation due to duct obstruction
	Granuloma, e.g. sarcoidosis
Sinusitis	Tumour, e.g. lymphoma,
	primary tumour
Giant cell arteritis	
	Eye
Temporo-mandibular joint	Glaucoma
disease	Iritis
	Optic neuritis
Nasopharynx	
Tumour	

Table 22.17 Lesions causing facial pain between cavernous sinus and pons

Root	Basal meninges
Trigeminal neuralgia	Granuloma, e.g. TB, sarcoid, syphilis
Cerebellopontine angle tumour	Tumour, e.g. lymphoma, carcinoma
Acoustic neuroma	
Meningioma	**Ganglion**
	Herpes zoster
	Middle fossa fracture

Table 22.18 Central lesions causing facial pain

- Thalamic infarcts
- Brainstem glioma
- Posterior inferior cerebellar artery thrombosis (Wallenberg syndrome)
- Syringomyelia/syringobulbia
- Tabes dorsalis

Table 22.19 The facial neuralgias

- Trigeminal neuralgia
- Postherpetic neuralgia
- Migrainous neuralgia (cluster headache)
- Atypical facial pain

the pons (Table 22.17) and central lesions (Table 22.18). The facial neuralgias (Table 22.19) cause the greatest diagnostic difficulty. Most lesions which involve the trigeminal nerve produce sensory impairment and, sometimes, paraesthesia rather than pain.

TRIGEMINAL NEURALGIA

Trigeminal neuralgia (tic douloureux) is a severe paroxysmal pain with a lancinating shock-like quality. It occurs in women more than men with a ratio of 3:1, with onset usually over the age of 50, though it may occur much earlier than this. It is sometimes seen in association with multiple sclerosis, but it may occur in young people without any associated disease.

Pathology

The cause of the condition is uncertain. The fact that there is no detectable trigeminal sensory impairment on routine testing indicates that the lesion must be minimal. In patients with intractable trigeminal neuralgia coming to operation, it has been observed that, in the posterior fossa, the superior cerebellar artery may be unusually tortuous, producing compression of the trigeminal root. Histologically, minor degenerative changes are seen both in the trigeminal ganglion and in trigeminal root fibres.

Clinical features

Trigeminal neuralgia nearly always occurs in a maxillary or mandibular distribution, and ophthalmic division pain is rare. It is always unilateral at any time, though later development on the contralateral side is described. The commonest sites are shown in Figure 22.7. Pain either originates in the region of the upper lip and radiates upwards over the cheek towards the eye, or originates from the angle of the mouth and radiates backwards and upwards towards the ear. Occasionally, pain is migratory, occurring in different sites in different bouts of pain. Between the paroxysms of pain, which last from 10 to 60 seconds, there is usually no pain, although patients with long-standing trigeminal neuralgia may describe a dull background ache. There is always triggering of the pain in trigeminal neuralgia. Innocuous cutaneous stimuli in the upper lip or at the angle of the mouth, any movement of the face or jaw, eating or drinking, may all provoke the pain. This usually occurs in bouts of weeks or months with long periods of freedom from pain of up to several years. In long-standing trigeminal neuralgia, there may be no remission. Neurological examination reveals no abnormal physical signs, although the pain can often be provoked by cutaneous stimulation or by asking the patient to open the mouth. Many patients will be loath to speak, eat or drink during a bout of severe pain.

Management

Carbamazepine

Most patients respond initially to carbamazepine, which may be effective for many years. In some patients, however, although the pain is controlled, side-effects from the drug are intolerable; these include drowsiness, unsteadiness of gait, nausea and vomiting. If pain becomes unresponsive to carbamazepine, it is worthwhile trying phenytoin, but surgical treatment will often need to be considered. Of the treatments currently available, the least invasive is thermocoagulation gangliolysis. This involves making a controlled radiofrequency heat lesion to the peripheral branch of the trigeminal nerve in the territory of which the pain is felt. More than 90% of patients with trigeminal neuralgia respond to this treatment and there is a low incidence of complications.

POSTHERPETIC NEURALGIA

Shingles affecting the trigeminal nerve nearly always involves only the ophthalmic division (Fig. 22.6, p. 882). Herpes zoster ophthalmicus is a disease of middle and old age, and is rare in people under 55. There is usually acute shingles and obvious scarring within the ophthalmic nerve territory. The acute zoster infection produces damage in the nerve, causing numbness and hyperalgesia. The pain is usually continuous, and has a burning or stinging quality. There may be superimposed lancinating pains which, in contrast to the pain in trigeminal neuralgia, often disturbs patients during the night.

Management

Postherpetic neuralgia is extremely difficult to treat. Local measures, such as cold, sometimes heat, vibration, ultrasound and acupuncture may all have a limited symptomatic effect. Simple analgesics have little effect. Amitriptyline and, occasionally, anticonvulsants have a beneficial effect. Opiate analgesics should not be used.

There is no convincing evidence that local or systemic corticosteroid treatment decreases the incidence of postherpetic neuralgia, although acute neuralgia may be lessened. Idoxuridine applied locally to the rash may hasten recovery, but has no effect on the incidence of postherpetic neuralgia. Systemic acyclovir does not lessen the incidence of postherpetic neuralgia.

MIGRAINOUS NEURALGIA (CLUSTER HEADACHE)

Migrainous neuralgia (cluster headache) is usually considered as a migraine variant. The cause and underlying pathology of the condition are unknown. The condition occurs much more frequently in men than women, with a ratio of around 7:1.

Clinical features

Migrainous neuralgia is characterised by bouts of daily pain occurring for a few weeks or months at a time, with long periods of complete freedom from pain between these bouts. This pattern of the pain has given rise to the alternative name of cluster headache.

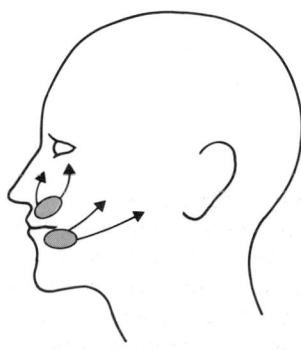

Fig. 22.7 Trigeminal neuralgia. The two most common sites of origin and radiation of pain are shown; mouth–ear and nose–orbit. The pain usually starts in the region of the encircled area and radiates in the directions shown.

The pain is always unilateral and it is centred on the eye and the upper part of the cheek. It may be very severe and, characteristically, occurs once a day, waking the patient from sleep in the early hours.

Each episode of pain lasts from 20 to 60 minutes and there may be associated unilateral facial flushing, nasal secretion on the affected side and profuse watering of the eye with conjunctival hyperaemia. Occasionally, an ipsilateral Horner's syndrome will develop. This is usually transient, but may persist and become permanent. Alcohol provokes attacks during a cluster.

Examination between the bouts of pain is usually normal though there may be a Horner's syndrome.

Management

Treatment for migraine is usually ineffective for this type of pain. Drugs are useless once the pain has started, since, by the time the drug is absorbed from the gut, the pain will have come to an end. Prophylactic treatment is thus necessary and, in most cases, is successfully achieved with ergotamine. This drug may be taken orally, sublingually, by inhalation, by suppository, or by subcutaneous injection. It is usual to advise oral or sublingual treatment in the first instance, and the patient is instructed to take 2 mg a few hours before the pain is due. In some patients, parenteral ergotamine is more effective. The drug should be stopped periodically to see whether a spontaneous remission has occurred. Most clusters of this type of headache last for less than 3 months. Occasionally, the pain will not respond to ergotamine by any route. A number of other treatments have been advocated, and may be successful in occasional patients. These include oxygen inhalation at the time of the pain, lithium and corticosteroids.

ATYPICAL FACIAL PAIN

Pain in the face is a surprisingly common symptom of psychological disturbance, usually depression. It is much more common in women, and the onset is usually in middle-age. Differentiation of this type of facial pain from organic causes can be extremely difficult. The pain is usually unilateral and is often confined to a trigeminal distribution. In patients in whom the pain is bilateral and clearly extends outside trigeminal territory, the diagnosis is made more easily. The pain is usually described as being continuous and severe, and may have lasted months or even years. Many patients will attribute the pain to minor dental surgery and some will have had repeated dental procedures. The pain often has a burning quality and may involve the tongue and other intraoral structures. There is, in some patients, an obvious associated depression and the response to a tricyclic antidepressant drug is usually good.

Summary 1 Facial pain

- Disease of deep structures innervated by the trigeminal nerve may produce pain referred onto the face.

- Trigeminal neuralgia is a paroxysmal, lancinating pain, lasting less than a minute, in maxillary or mandibular division territory, which is triggered by cutaneous or oral stimuli.

- Postherpetic neuralgia nearly always affects the ophthalmic division. It is usually a continuous pain, with cutaneous hyperaesthesia.

- Migrainous neuralgia (cluster headache) is much more common in men. The pain is in the eye and on the cheek, lasts 20–30 minutes, often occurs at night and is very severe.

- Atypical facial pain may be bilateral and often extends outside trigeminal territory. It is continuous, and is often associated with depression. Treatment of the depression usually relieves the pain.

Despite careful clinical assessment and sometimes extensive investigation, the cause of facial pain in a few patients cannot be detemined. A trial of a tricyclic antidepressant in such patients is always worthwhile.

DIZZINESS AND VERTIGO

'Dizziness' is an extremely common presenting complaint and the word may be used by different patients to describe not only vertigo but light-headedness, faintness, visual disturbance, confusion, loss of balance due to ataxia, and even feelings of weakness or loss of sensation in the legs. There are often no physical signs in patients with dizziness, and, as with headache, the diagnosis depends largely on a careful history.

A normal feeling of equilibrium depends on being fully conscious and receiving appropriate afferent information from the eyes, the vestibular system, and sensory pathways from the neck, trunk and limbs. The coordinating nuclei in the brainstem also receive modulating inputs from the cerebral cortex, basal ganglia, cerebellum and reticular formation. The *vestibular system* refers to the end organs in each inner ear (semicircular canals, ampullae, utricle and saccule), the VIIIth nerve, the vestibular nuclei in the pons and upper medulla, and more central projections. There is continuous tonic input from each labyrinth. Changes of head posture increase the input from one side and decrease it from the contralateral side, causing corrective eye movements via pathways subserving the vestibulo-ocular reflex (VOR) and preventing a disconcerting awareness of the movement that has occurred.

Any pathological process that disturbs the balance of vestibular inputs may lead to a feeling of disequilibrium which is characterised by a false perception of movement. It is this specific feature that distinguishes *vertigo* from other sensations of dizziness and faintness. The apparent motion of vertigo may be clearly rotatory, particularly when severe, but in many patients the sensation has a side-to-side, up-and-down, leaning or falling quality that is difficult to describe. Vertigo may arise from lesions in the labyrinth (most common), the brainstem, or rarely in the VIIIth nerve itself; it may also occur briefly at the onset of a complex partial seizure, probably due to disturbance of central vestibular projections in the temporal lobe. Vertigo is often elicited or exacerbated by movement, and when severe, it may be accompanied by nausea, vomiting, pallor and sweating. Some patients find it difficult to describe in detail their sensation of dizziness, so that the division into vertiginous and non-vertiginous dizziness may not always be certain from the history.

Clinical features and diagnosis

An acute brief episode of vertigo is usually due to a peripheral labyrinthine disturbance, although central lesions, such as temporal lobe epilepsy and, very occasionally, vertebrobasilar insufficiency, can produce this isolated symptom. Ménière's disease may, in the early stages, cause episodes of vertigo lasting less than a minute, but episodes lasting 1 or 2 days are more usual in later attacks. Vertigo from vestibular neuronitis may be severe for several days. Central lesions causing vestibular disturbances as the only symptom usually lead to vertigo of gradual onset, which is less severe than that caused by peripheral lesions. Acute severe vertigo may occur with central vascular lesions, most commonly lateral medullary infarction due to occlusion of the vertebral or posterior inferior cerebellar artery, but there are always associated neurological symptoms and signs.

Non-vertiginous dizziness is a common symptom in anxious patients, sometimes associated with overbreathing, and in patients with depression.

Central vs. peripheral lesions

Flow charts are useful in the diagnosis of vertigo (Fig. 22.8). Having established that the patient's complaint is a symptom of a vestibular disturbance, the next important clinical distinction to make is whether the symptom is due to a central or peripheral lesion.

Peripheral

Associated deafness, tinnitus or pain in the ear, particularly when unilateral, suggests a peripheral disturbance. A very gradually progressive unilateral deafness associated with vertigo raises the possibility of an acoustic neuroma. If, in addition to a sensory neural deafness, there is a cerebellopontine angle syndrome – comprising an ipsilateral lower motor neurone facial weakness, trigeminal

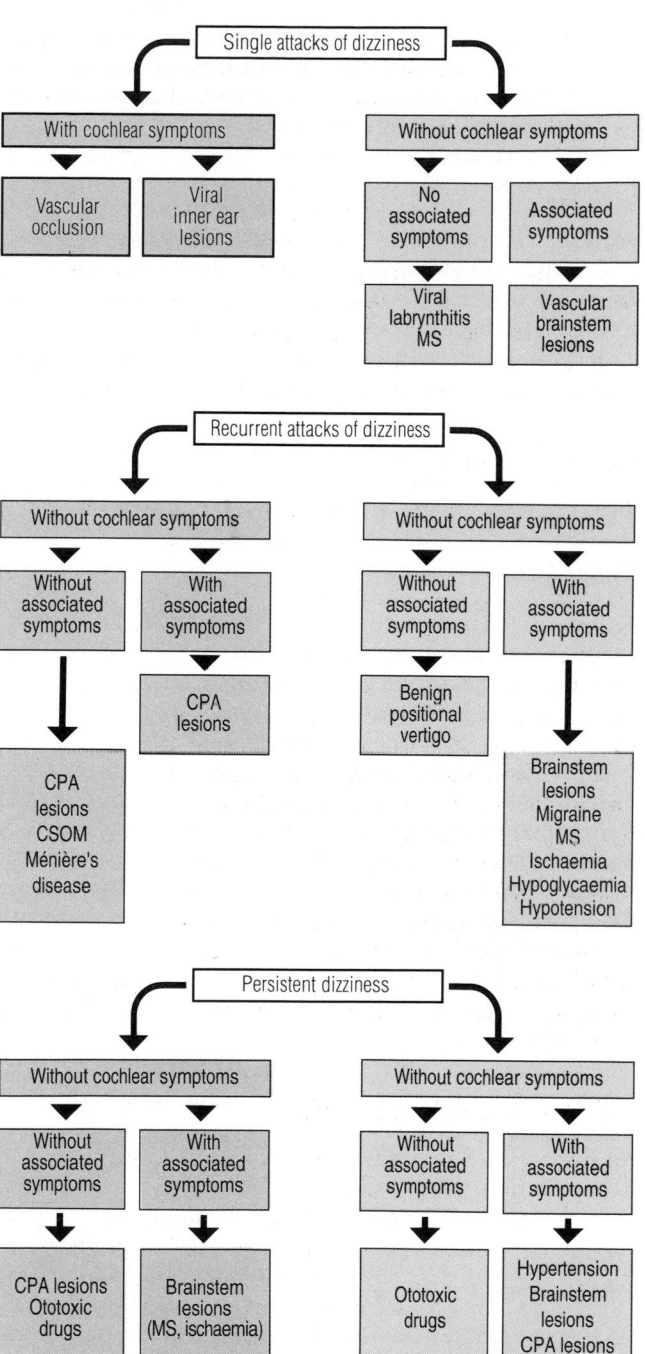

Fig. 22.8 Diagnostic flow diagrams for dizziness and associated symptoms.
CPA = cerebello-pontine angle; CSOM = chronic suppurative otitis media; MS = multiple sclerosis.

hypoaesthesia and ipsilateral limb ataxia – an acoustic neuroma is by far the likeliest diagnosis, although other tumours such as meningiomas may also produce this syndrome. An abrupt mild deafness or tinnitus with acute severe vertigo suggests a viral labyrinthitis or an acute vascular occlusion affecting the inner ear. Intermittent episodes of tinnitus, deafness, vertigo and pain in the ear are characteristic of Ménière's disease (p. 887).

Central

With the exception of acoustic neuromas, the presence of associated neurological symptoms usually indicates that the cause of vertigo is a central lesion. Many brainstem lesions may affect the vestibular nuclei and pathways, and these pathologies will tend to produce symptoms and signs in other systems, including the cranial nerve nuclei, pyramidal and sensory tracts together with cerebellar deficits.

The aura of temporal lobe epilepsy may include vertigo, but there will be other symptoms (p. 891), the most important being impairment of consciousness.

Other causes of dizziness

Any cardiac disease leading to a low cardiac output, whether chronically, exacerbated by exertion (as in aortic stenosis) or as a result of dysrhythmia, may cause dizziness. Dizziness is a common first symptom in a vasovagal fainting attack, but, again, is not the only symptom.

Other important causes of dizziness include ototoxic drugs, such as the aminoglycosides or treatment with tranquillisers, antidepressants, or neuroleptic drugs. A previous history of ear disease may also be relevant. Impaired visual acuity or eye movement disorders causing diplopia or oscillopsia may all cause patients to complain of dizziness rather than a visual symptom.

Examination

The examination is often normal, particularly in younger patients. General examination, including lying and standing blood pressure, are as important as the neurological examination. Some patients have mild disturbances of gait and nystagmus. Clinical testing of hearing is an important part of the neurological examination.

Romberg's test

In Romberg's test, a patient with an acute peripheral vestibular lesion will tend to fall towards the affected side. Patients with non-organic illnesses tend to fall backwards, without immediate appropriate attempts to correct their posture; however, they will usually avoid injury by acrobatic manoeuvres to maintain balance at the last moment.

Vestibulo-ocular testing

Examination of the eye movements (vestibulo-ocular testing) should first establish that there is a full range of movement in each eye and that gaze remains conjugate. Slow following eye movements (pursuit) and rapid eye movements (saccadic) should be normal.

Nystagmus (p. 871). A unilateral vestibular disturbance upsets the balance of impulses from each labyrinth tending to cause deviation of the eyes towards the side of the lesion. This is balanced by a rapid saccadic movement of the eyes towards the opposite side. Nystagmus, described in the direction of the fast component, therefore beats away from the side of the lesion. Mild nystagmus of this sort may be seen only with caloric or rotational stimulation.

Routine testing for nystagmus is relatively crude and is greatly helped by *electronystagmography*. In a peripheral vestibular lesion, spontaneous nystagmus at 30° of lateral gaze occurs only in one direction, the eyes always remain conjugate and the nystagmus is increased by removing fixation using Frenzel's glasses. The nystagmus is most marked with acute lesions, and the central nervous system (CNS) compensates over a period of weeks so that nystagmus (and dizziness) tends to improve. In central vestibular lesions, compensation tends not to occur, the nystagmus may occur in more than one direction of gaze, the eye movements are sometimes dysconjugate, and removal of fixation has little effect.

Caloric testing (p. 871) is an easily performed and reliable measure of vestibulo-ocular reflexes. If the response to caloric testing is reduced on one side, there is said to be *canal paresis*, which indicates a peripheral lesion (labyrinth, nerve or vestibular nucleus). A *directional preponderance* refers to an increase in the nystagmus in one direction. This occurs when there is an imbalance of the peripheral vestibular inputs or a central imbalance. In some patients, there will be a mixture of these abnormalities.

Optokinetic nystagmus is the normal reflex oscillation of the eyes induced by movements of the subject's surroundings. It is disturbed in central vestibular lesions, but not with peripheral lesions.

Testing for positionally induced nystagmus is particularly helpful when there is a history of dizziness provoked by certain positions of the head, usually lying down or extending the neck to look upwards. Placing the patient's head in the position which induces dizziness may also induce nystagmus. A better test is the *Hallpike manoeuvre*, in which the patient's head is rapidly lowered from a sitting position backwards and over the end of the bed with head turned either to the right or the left. In benign positional vertigo (see below) of peripheral origin, nystagmus is provoked with a latent period of 2–20 seconds, disappears (adapts) within 1 minute, is associated with vertigo and fatigues with repeated testing; the fast phase of the nystagmus is towards the lower ear with the head in this posture. Positional nystagmus may sometimes be a feature of central vestibular lesions, but the

Hallpike manoeuvre in these patients characteristically provokes nystagmus without vertigo. There is no latent period, nor any fatigability, on repeated testing. The direction of the saccadic phase of nystagmus is variable.

Hearing

Cochlear function is routinely tested as described on page 871, supplemented by audiometry.

Aetiology

There are a number of common causes of vertigo (Table 22.20).

Acute labyrinthine failure

Although this condition is often referred to as 'labyrinthitis' or 'vestibular neuronitis', an inflammatory basis is seldom evident or proven. Typically the onset of vertigo is abrupt on waking in the morning. It may be severe for 1–3 days, is minimised by keeping the head still and is provoked by any head movement. It is often associated with nausea and vomiting. There is gradual resolution of the symptoms over a few weeks, although mild symptoms may be provoked by sudden head movement for up to several months later. Examination during the acute stage

Table 22.20 Causes of dizziness

Vertiginous	Non-vertiginous
Labyrinthine	**Cardiovascular**
'Labyrinthitis'	Vasovagal syncope
Post-traumatic vestibular damage	Postural hypotension
Benign positional vertigo	Cardiac arrhythmias
Vascular occlusion affecting labyrinth	Aortic stenosis
Ménière's disease	HOCM
Secondary to middle ear disease	Low-output cardiac failure
Alcohol	
	Haematological
Eighth nerve	Anaemia
Ototoxic drugs	Polycythaemia
Acoustic neuroma	
Herpes zoster (Ramsay Hunt	**Metabolic**
syndrome with VIIth nerve	Hypoglycaemia
involvement)	Hyperventilation
Brainstem	**Ocular**
Multiple sclerosis	Poor acuity
Vertebrobasilar TIA or stroke	Diplopia
Migraine	Oscillopsia
Encephalitis	
Tumours	**Drugs**
	e.g. Benzodiazepines
Cerebral	Tricyclics
Temporal lobe seizures	Anticonvulsants

Summary 2 Dizziness

- In the majority of patients presenting with dizziness, the cause is a peripheral labyrinthine disturbance or syncope.

- Acute episodes of vertigo with nausea and vomiting, but without other neurological symptoms, are nearly always due to a peripheral labyrinthine disturbance.

- Episodes of vertebrobasilar ischaemia may produce vertigo, but almost always with other neurological symptoms.

- Peripheral labyrinthine disturbances are much more likely to be associated with tinnitus and/or deafness than central lesions.

- When there is doubt whether vertigo is due to a peripheral or central lesion, caloric testing is useful; a canal paresis indicates a peripheral lesion.

- Long-term use of vestibular sedative drugs, such as prochlorperazine or cinnarizine, is rarely necessary.

- When dizziness occurs in association with other neurological symptoms and signs, the patient should be referred for a neurological opinion.

may reveal nystagmus, either spontaneously present on forward gaze or only on lateral gaze. Later, nystagmus will be absent, but caloric testing shows a unilateral canal paresis. The audiogram is normal. Complete resolution of symptoms eventually occurs in most patients, although mild symptoms may persist for months.

Up to 50% of patients with acute labyrinthine failure will have had a cold or other viral infection shortly before the onset of the symptoms; it is thus often regarded as a viral or postviral syndrome. Treatment for a few days is often necessary during the acute stage. The vestibular sedatives, cinnarizine or prochlorperazine, are effective.

Benign positional vertigo

Benign positional vertigo is produced by certain head postures, most commonly lying down with the head turned on one side or extending the neck. Vertebrobasilar ischaemia is often invoked as the cause of such vertigo, but this is probably very unusual (see below). Vertigo, often positional, is a common symptom following head injury.

The labyrinth is the likely site of the lesion. The Hallpike manoeuvre is particularly helpful in eliciting nystagmus in this condition, which has the features of a peripheral lesion. A vestibular sedative, such as cinnarizine, is occasionally necessary when symptoms are severe or persistent.

Ménière's disease

Ménière's disease results from endolymphatic hydrops (increased pressure in the membranous labyrinth) and is of unknown cause. It is characterised clinically by attacks of severe vertigo occurring several times in a few weeks, followed by long periods of remission of months or years. The onset of Ménière's disease is usually between 40 and 60 years of age and the condition is more common in men. It is always initially unilateral, although in about 25% of patients the other ear is later affected.

Each attack is usually preceded by a sensation of pressure in the ear. The subsequent onset of vertigo may be severe and is associated with nausea, vomiting, deafness and tinnitus. Between attacks, the tinnitus and deafness persist and gradually worsen. Recurrent attacks lead to increasing deafness; when hearing is completely lost, the attacks of vertigo cease.

Audiometry shows a sensorineural deafness, and caloric testing an ipsilateral canal paresis. During a bout of attacks, a vestibular sedative, such as cinnarizine, may be helpful. In very severe cases, surgical measures to destroy the labyrinth can be considered, but should not be contemplated if there is deafness in the other ear. Surgical procedures which ablate the labyrinth, but preserve residual cochlear function, are now increasingly used.

Vertebrobasilar ischaemia

Vertigo is a common symptom of vertebrobasilar ischaemia, but the diagnosis must rest on a description of attacks, which also include one or more of the following symptoms: diplopia, bilateral visual obscurations, bilateral facial numbness or paraesthesiae (commonly circumoral), bilateral facial weakness, dysarthria, dysphagia, dysphonia, weakness or sensory loss in the limbs, and impairment of consciousness (p. 898).

Ototoxic drugs

Many drugs are potentially ototoxic, and some cause permanent vestibular damage, particularly streptomycin and gentamicin.

Multiple sclerosis

Plaques of demyelination in the brainstem quite frequently cause vertigo (p. 958).

Acoustic neuroma

Acoustic neuromas do not usually cause major vestibular involvement; when it does occur, vertigo is usually mild (p. 911).

Geniculate herpes zoster (Ramsay Hunt syndrome)

Geniculate herpes zoster is a rare condition, but important to recognise. It is due to involvement of the genicu-late ganglion by *Herpes zoster* and there is often involvement of neighbouring nerves. Severe earache is the first symptom, and a discrete vesicular rash develops within 1–3 days of the onset of pain. The rash is present on the tympanic membrane and external auditory meatus, and spreads onto the concha. It is occasionally also present on the palate and pharynx. The rash is often discrete, with only a few visible vesicles spreading onto the concha. There is a lower motor neurone facial palsy, which may be the only neurological abnormality; however, vertigo is common, together with some impairment of hearing, and, very occasionally, there is involvement of the glossopharyngeal and vagus nerves. Like other forms of shingles, it tends to affect an older age group, and, occasionally, can produce a very severe illness, with meningitis and an acute confusional state.

SYNCOPE AND EPILEPSY

The term 'blackout' means different things to different people and it is important to establish in what sense the patient is using the word. When describing disturbed consciousness, a patient's recollection of events is bound to be incomplete, and a detailed independent account of the episode is invaluable.

The great majority of patients presenting to their doctors with blackouts will have no physical signs. The diagnosis rests entirely on a meticulous history.

Differential diagnosis of epilepsy and syncope

Syncope is defined as loss of consciousness due to transient impairment of cerebral blood flow.

Epilepsy is a paroxysmal, abnormal cerebral electrical discharge associated with a clinical change; this may take a wide variety of different forms, but usually includes some impairment of consciousness.

Features which help in distinguishing epilepsy from syncope, the commonest clinical differential diagnostic problem, include the following:

The time of day and circumstances of the attack

Attacks during the night, while the patient is recumbent in bed, are not likely to be syncopal. Nocturnal attacks which the patient cannot remember, but which wake other members of the family, are likely to be fits. Syncopal attacks may occur during the night on getting up, often during micturition.

Events causing squeamishness, or bad news, may provoke syncope. Patients with photosensitive epilepsy may have a history of attacks provoked by watching television (usually when sitting too close), or flickering lights.

Posture

Standing for long periods, particularly in hot surroundings, often provokes syncope.

Warning of the attack

Loss of consciousness in syncope is nearly always preceded by a period of malaise with dizziness, nausea, visual blurring and dimming, and a feeling of impending loss of consciousness. Many patients will have discovered that lying down promptly during this prodromal phase will prevent loss of consciousness.

Period of unconsciousness and postictal state

Syncope usually causes brief loss of consciousness of less than a minute. Exceptions are usually due to attempts by onlookers to sit the patient up. This merely intensifies the period of unconsciousness and may, on occasions, provoke a secondary hypoxic convulsion. Such attacks are then often mislabelled as being epileptic. Minor fits may cause a period of absence which may be momentary (see below) and which may appear to witnesses as absent-mindedness, rather than impairment of consciousness. Convulsions are associated with loss of consciousness of more than 1 minute (and sometimes up to 10 or 15 minutes), followed by a period of postictal drowsiness and confusion; this is often accompanied by irritability and, sometimes, aggressive, irrational behaviour if the patient is disturbed. Patients recovering from syncope are orientated and rational.

Appearance during the period of unconsciousness

A history from witnesses of convulsive tonic or tonic-clonic movements of the limbs, with facial grimacing, jaw clenching, tongue biting and grunting noises, and irregular breathing, clearly indicate a fit. A patient who lies limp while unconscious, appears pale and sweaty, whose pulse is difficult to feel and who rapidly regains consciousness, is likely to have had a syncopal attack. Nevertheless, patients with fits may also appear pale and sweaty and tonic-clonic movements may be discrete or absent. The differential diagnosis can sometimes be impossible from the accounts given by some patients and witnesses of their attacks.

Incontinence

Incontinence of urine, and, sometimes, faeces is relatively common in epilepsy, and urinary incontinence occasionally occurs in syncope.

SYNCOPE

Syncope is very common. In a healthy young adult, a blood pressure of less than 50 mmHg will reduce cerebral blood flow sufficient to cause loss of consciousness. The conditions most commonly leading to syncope are:

- Vasovagal attacks
- Cardiogenic syncope
- Cough, sneeze and micturition syncope
- Breath-holding attacks
- Orthostatic hypotension
- Carotid sinus sensitivity.

Vasovagal syncope

Vagal overactivity produces a bradycardia and a fall in blood pressure, which is associated with peripheral vasodilatation. Such attacks are often reflex in nature and provoked by emotional or painful circumstances. Vasovagal faints often occur in adolescents and young adults who are otherwise entirely healthy and, occasionally, children of less than 10 years are prone to fainting. Faints are more common soon after getting up. They are always postural, the symptoms starting while standing or sitting. They are more frequent in women than men, may be associated with menstruation or intercurrent febrile illness, and are more frequent after sleep deprivation and prolonged fasting.

Cardiogenic syncope

Heart disease may cause syncope in three main ways:

- by acute dysrhythmias, as in supraventricular tachycardia or heart block
- by obstruction to flow, as in aortic stenosis
- in low output states, as with a pericardial effusion.

Cardiac causes of syncope are particularly important in the older population. Syncope on exertion suggests the possibility of cardiac disease.

Cough, micturition and sneeze syncope

Prolonged bouts of coughing raise intrathoracic pressure, impair venous return to the heart, and cause syncope. Sneezing occasionally induces syncope, probably by a vagal reflex mechanism. Coughing or sneezing in patients with cerebellar tonsillar herniation through the foramen magnum (Arnold-Chiari malformation) may provoke syncope, the mechanism of which is uncertain. Fainting may occur during micturition in men, particularly during the night, due to a postural fall in the blood pressure, reflex vagal activity stimulated by a full bladder, and reduced venous return caused by straining.

Breath-holding attacks

These usually occur in very young children as a reaction to emotional stress. They are sometimes seen with prolonged crying. There is prolonged breath-holding, leading to cyanosis and, eventually, loss of consciousness. Attacks usually start before the age of 18 months and stop by the age of 5 years. In severe prolonged attacks, secondary hypoxic convulsions may be induced and the child is frequently mislabelled as epileptic.

Orthostatic hypotension

Orthostatic hypotension refers to a fall in blood pressure on standing, which may be sufficiently profound to cause a loss of consciousness. There are numerous causes (Table 22.21).

Postural hypotension may be a result of impaired sympathetic activity, as occurs in some neuropathies (diabetes being the commonest), and in central autonomic failure; the latter may occur as an isolated phenomenon, as part of the Shy-Drager syndrome associated with Parkinsonism or as part of a multiple systems atrophy (p. 921).

Many drugs, in addition to hypotensive agents, can lower blood pressure sufficiently for loss of consciousness to occur. Corticosteroid deficiency, which may be due to Addison's disease, abrupt withdrawal of administered steroid or hypopituitarism, leads to hypotension exacerbated by standing.

Chronic idiopathic orthostatic hypotension is a rare condition, in which there is no cardiovascular sympathetic response to a fall in blood pressure induced by standing. Tachycardia, vasoconstriction and sweating (the normal responses to hypotension) are all absent.

Table 22.21 Causes of orthostatic hypotension

Venous pooling	**Reduced muscle and vascular tone**
Prolonged standing	Prolonged bed rest
Severe varicose veins	
	Fluid depletion
Impaired vasomotor activity	
Peripheral neuropathy	**Drugs**
Diabetes	Hypotensive therapy
Guillain-Barré syndrome	Tranquillisers
Surgical sympathectomy	Phenothiazines
Spinal cord lesions	Levodopa
Syringomyelia	
Tabes dorsalis	**Steroid deficiency**
Familial dysautonomia	Hypopituitarism
Shy-Drager syndrome	Addison's disease
	Chronic idiopathic orthostatic hypotension

> **Summary 3 Differential diagnosis of syncope and epilepsy**
>
> - Always try to obtain an eye-witness account of an episode of loss of consciousness; do not diagnose epilepsy on insufficient grounds.
> - Syncope is usually postural, with prodromal symptoms before loss of consciousness. Fits often occur without any warning.
> - Loss of consciousness in syncope usually lasts less than a minute, in contrast to most fits.
> - Confusion, headache and drowsiness are common after fits, but not after syncope.
> - Excessive alcohol – either binge drinking or chronic alcoholism – is a common cause of isolated fits.
> - The interictal EEG may be normal in epilepsy. The diagnosis of epilepsy is essentially clinical and does not depend on the EEG.

Carotid sinus sensitivity

Carotid sinus sensitivity is the result of atherosclerotic disease affecting the carotid artery at its bifurcation in the neck. It is usually seen in middle-aged or elderly people in the setting of widespread vascular disease. Mild pressure over the sinus, such as that which might be caused by a tight shirt-collar, combined with head turning, causes an excessive bradycardia, hypotension and, occasionally, transient asystole which may last 10–15 seconds (Ch. 12).

EPILEPSY

A number of terms are used to describe the clinical and associated electrical abnormalities of epilepsy. Epileptic attacks, fits, seizures and convulsions all refer to the same phenomenon – a paroxysmal electrical discharge affecting a group of neurones, starting in one part of the brain, but often spreading to become a generalised abnormality.

Classification

Fits are clinically and electrically heterogeneous. Aetiological classifications are useful reminders of the many causes of fits but must be supplemented with a classification of the type of fit (Table 22.22). Fits are disturbing events, but there is a great difference to the patient in the impact of, for example, an absence attack of petit mal and a generalised tonic-clonic convulsion. It is thus helpful to qualify a diagnosis of epilepsy with a statement about the type of attack or attacks suffered by a particular patient.

Pathophysiology

Partial seizures

In focal epilepsy (partial seizures), paroxysmal discharges develop in one part of the cerebral hemispheres, the temporal lobe being the most common site. If it remains

Table 22.22 Types of fit – WHO classification

Generalised seizures
Absence attacks
    Petit mal – 3 Hz spike and wave
    Atypical absences
Myoclonic seizures
    Myoclonic jerks, single or multiple
    Clonic seizures
Tonic-clonic seizures
    Grand mal, major fits
Tonic seizures
Atonic or akinetic seizures

Partial seizures
Simple, without impairment of consciousness
    Motor, sensory, aphasic, cognitive, affective, amnesic, illusional, olfactory,
    psychic. Includes Jacksonian, temporal lobe, psychomotor epilepsy
Complex partial seizures with impairment of consciousness
    Simple partial onset, followed by impairment of consciousness
    Impairment of consciousness from the onset
Partial seizures, either simple or complex, evolving into generalised tonic-clonic
seizures
Generalised tonic-clonic seizures, with EEG but not clinical evidence of focal onset

Table 22.23 Causes of fits

Idiopathic/constitutional

Hereditary and familial
Petit mal
Some patients with temporal lobe
epilepsy
Aminoacidurias
Trisomy 21
Lipidoses

Developmental defects
Phakomatoses
Intrauterine rubella, CMV,
toxoplasma
Irradiation

Birth trauma
Perinatal anoxia
Cerebral contusion
Cerebral haemorrhage and
thrombosis

Anoxia in infancy and childhood

Tumours
Primary and secondary

Vascular
Mature infarcts/arteriovenous
malformation

Infection
Febrile convulsions
Viral encephalitis
Bacterial meningitis
Tuberculous meningitis
Cerebral abscess
Cysticercosis
Neurosyphilis
Echinococcus
Toxocariasis
Toxoplasmosis

Inflammatory
SLE/PAN/multiple sclerosis

Metabolic
Uraemia/water intoxication/
hyponatraemia/hypo-
glycaemia/hypocalcaemia/
hypomagnesaemia

Toxic
Alcohol/drugs, e.g.
barbiturates, amphetamines,
lignocaine, tricyclic antidepressants,
phenothiazines, lead

Degenerative
Alzheimer's disease/
Creutzfeldt-Jakob
disease/Huntington's disease

focal, such activity will produce a minor fit in which the type of symptom experienced depends on the region of the brain involved; there may or may not be impairment of consciousness. In many minor temporal lobe attacks, the impairment of consciousness takes the form of brief lapses of awareness without obvious loss of consciousness observable by witnesses of the attack. In focal motor fits that remain focal, there may be no impairment of awareness or consciousness, so that the patient will be in a position to provide a complete account of events. However, focal epileptic activity may become generalised, in which case there is loss of consciousness and, usually, clinical evidence of a convulsion. Many patients will have both focal attacks and fits which are preceded by symptoms of the focal electrical disturbance.

Generalised seizures

Paroxysmal discharges are generated in deep sites at the hypothalamic, thalamic or upper brainstem level, and rapidly spread to both hemispheres simultaneously to produce generalised epileptic discharges. This type of abnormality is present in many patients with so-called idiopathic or constitutional epilepsy, and is also responsible for petit mal attacks.

Aetiology

Particular causes of fits (Table 22.23) may produce fits of different kinds. Perinatal anoxia, for example, may cause either generalised or partial seizures.

Idiopathic or constitutional epilepsy is a term used to refer to patients with recurrent fits in whom no cause can be identified. This is by far the largest group of epileptic patients, and probably includes those who have had intra-uterine, birth and neonatal insults. In some patients, there is a strong family history; this is often the case with petit mal and in some patients with temporal lobe epilepsy. In most idiopathic epileptics, however, there is no family history.

Apart from the rare degenerative disorders which may cause epilepsy (see below and Table 22.25), genetic factors are also important in febrile convulsions and petit mal. In the latter, the typical EEG abnormality has been found in nearly 50% of siblings whether or not they have clinical fits.

Factors provoking fits

Some agents may cause fits in people not normally prone to having fits, e.g. alcohol (both bingeing and abrupt withdrawal, p. 979) and drug abuse (particularly with barbiturates and amphetamines). In epileptics, sleep deprivation is a common provocative factor. In some patients, there is a clear relationship between fits and stressful life events. Some patients have fits only, or mainly, at night, the epileptic threshold being reduced during sleep. In some women with epilepsy, their fits tend to occur just before or during menstruation (catamenial epilepsy).

Photosensitivity is important in a relatively small proportion of epileptics, particularly those with petit mal and myoclonic epilepsy. Rarely, fits can be induced by music, looking at certain patterns, and reading.

Types of fit

Generalised seizures

Petit mal

Petit mal refers to brief (10–15 second) absence attacks associated with a generalised 3-second spike-and-wave discharge on the EEG. The fits always start in childhood, and consist of a brief cessation of activity associated with a blank staring look and, occasionally, nodding of the head, fluttering of the eyelids and (very occasionally) small convulsive movements of the limbs. Objects may be dropped, but postural control is maintained if the child is sitting or standing. It is common for petit mal to continue into adolescence, but only occasionally into adult life. About 50% of children with petit mal will later develop grand mal fits.

Tonic-clonic fits (grand mal epilepsy, major fits)

In tonic-clonic fits (grand mal epilepsy, major fits), there is abrupt loss of consciousness associated initially with a *tonic phase*, in which there is sustained muscular contraction affecting all muscles, including respiratory, facial and jaw muscles. Breathing may cease and the patient becomes cyanosed. It is during this phase that the tongue may be bitten and incontinence occurs. After a short period (usually less than 30 seconds) a *clonic phase* supervenes, in which there are repeated violent jerking movements of the trunk and limbs. Self-inflicted injury is common during this phase, which may last for several minutes. On cessation of the fit, consciousness is slowly regained, passing through a stuporose phase. There is often postictal confusion, irritability and headache; irrational behaviour may occur during this stage, of which the patient is later amnesic.

Many patients will have a few seconds' warning of a fit. The symptoms are often non-specific, and include malaise, dizziness and a feeling of detachment. Patients who come to recognise these symptoms may have time to sit or lie down before losing consciousness. However, others will have no such prodrome.

Management. A patient having a fit should be turned onto his/her side to prevent the tongue obstructing the airway, and self-injury should be prevented as far as possible. It is a mistake to attempt to force open the mouth. Most fits are single, self-limiting events. It is unnecessary to admit known epileptics to hospital after a single fit.

Partial seizures

Focal epileptic discharges may arise in any part of the cerebral hemispheres, causing partial seizures. *Focal motor* fits characteristically cause convulsive twitching of one side of the body, starting in the face, arm or leg and gradually spreading (Jacksonian epilepsy). *Focal sensory* fits arising in the postcentral gyrus cause a similar march of sensory symptoms. *Versive fits*, in which the eyes and head are turned to one side, are produced by contralateral posterior frontal epileptic activity.

Temporal lobe epilepsy

Temporal lobe epileptic attacks are by far the commonest type of partial seizure. These may occur as a *simple* type of partial attack without loss of consciousness (psychomotor fits) with aphasia or cognitive, affective, amnesic, olfactory, illusional or psychic symptoms; or they may be *complex* partial seizures, in which the symptoms are followed by a period of impaired consciousness. The term 'temporal lobe epilepsy' is often used to refer to all complex partial seizures, but such attacks can arise from other parts of the brain, particularly the frontal lobes.

In temporal lobe attacks, the patient appears vacant and this may be associated with inability to talk, though simple commands may be obeyed. Olfactory, epigastric and psychic phenomena, such as déjà-vu and jamais-vu, are very common. During an attack, repetitive motor behaviours may occur; lip-smacking, chewing and grimacing movements are the commonest. In simple attacks, at least partial awareness is preserved, while, in complex partial seizures, the patient will be amnesic for part of the attack and may not afterwards realise that anything has happened. Like other partial seizures, minor temporal lobe fits may progress to a generalised convulsion.

Febrile convulsions

In young children, sudden rises in body temperature may provoke convulsions. Such fits are usually generalised and brief; they occur between the ages of 6 months and 5 years, and only occur with fever. There is a small increased risk of later development of epilepsy in children who have had febrile fits.

Rarer types of fit

Other, rarer types of fit are described in Table 22.24.

Pseudo seizures

It can be difficult to determine clinically whether or not attacks are organic or 'hysterical' in nature. Many patients who have simulated or hysterical attacks also suffer

Table 22.24 Rarer types of epilepsy

Atypical absences
Clinically the same as petit mal; slower EEG, other abnormalities and often associated mental retardation and atrophy (Lennox-Gastaut syndrome); seizures hard to control

Tonic seizures
Tonic posturing only of limbs (sometimes trunk)

Infantile spasms
Brief sudden head flexion – 'salaam' attacks often with failure of development and regression. Onset at 3–9 months. May be refractory to treatment

Myoclonic epilepsy
Single (or repetitive) sudden convulsive movements of limbs and trunk

Mostly children with idiopathic epilepsy; attacks early in the morning

Photosensitive myoclonus and epilepsy

Hereditary myoclonic epilepsies – generalised seizures and myoclonus with degenerative disease, e.g. Lafora body disease: children/adolescents with myoclonus, major seizures and dementia. Death occurs within a few years. Intracellular inclusion bodies present

Gangliosidoses

organic seizures. EEG monitoring during an attack may be helpful, but, in some instances, continuous 24-hour recording with simultaneous video recording is necessary to establish whether the attacks are epileptic or not.

Investigation

A diagnosis of epilepsy cannot be made from an EEG, but an abnormal EEG showing clear epileptic activity supports the clinical diagnosis. An EEG should be done in any patient presenting with an unprovoked first fit. Where alcohol or drug abuse is suspected as the underlying cause, the EEG is likely to be normal. The investigation is of most value when there is a history of focal onset and the presence of abnormal physical signs suggests a structural abnormality. Further investigation with a CT scan is then essential.

Meningovascular syphilis is now uncommon and a Wasserman test is rarely of value. Lumbar puncture is of very limited value. In children in whom a metabolic disturbance is suspected, special investigation is necessary, as is the case with the phakomatoses and lipidoses.

Management

Principles of medical treatment

A single fit is rarely an indication to start anticonvulsant treatment. Exceptions are patients with a clear history of focal seizures, in whom an underlying structural cause is likely, and patients who have abnormal physical signs following a fit, indicating a hemisphere lesion. Otherwise,

most neurologists would wait until two or three fits have occurred within a period of 2 years or less before starting treatment.

Patients with fits clearly related to alcohol withdrawal (p. 979) should not be given anticonvulsants.

Having decided that treatment is necessary, the choice of drug will depend on the type of seizure, the age of the patient, the possibility of pregnancy, interaction with other medication and the likelihood of producing unacceptable side-effects. It is best to use a single drug, starting at a dose which will avoid excessive side-effects and increasing to a therapeutic level. Monitoring of blood levels of anticonvulsants is sometimes indicated, either to ensure therapeutic levels in patients who continue to have fits on treatment or if symptoms and signs of toxicity develop. Blood levels of the shorter-acting anticonvulsants, such as valproate and clonazepam, are of little value.

Follow-up is important to monitor the efficacy of treatment and the occurrence of drug side-effects. Patients must understand the details of their treatment. A card carried by the patient with drug information can be invaluable in an acute situation. Periodic review of the continuing need for treatment is necessary. In patients with adult onset of relatively infrequent fits, it is reasonable to consider gradual withdrawal of treatment when they have been free from fits for 2 years.

Choice of drug

For petit mal, ethosuximide is the drug of choice, though alternatives in resistant cases are valproate and clonazepam (Table 22.25). For tonic-clonic seizures, or for partial seizures alone, several drugs are appropriate. Carbamazepine is now probably the drug of choice, mainly due to its low incidence of long-term side-effects, both in children and adults. Phenytoin and phenobarbitone are alternatives. For tonic-clonic seizures associated with petit mal, valproate is better than carbamazepine, phenytoin or phenobarbitone, but, as with other forms of epilepsy, there is considerable individual variation. Vigabatrin is a new anticonvulsant agent which is used most often as a supplementary drug in patients with seizures that are not responding to front-line drugs. Infantile spasms are usually refractory to all treatment, but ACTH and nitrazepam have been effective in some cases.

All major anticonvulsant drugs (apart from valproate) induce liver enzymes, and this is important with concurrent drug therapy including the oral contraceptive pill.

Anticonvulsant drugs in pregnancy

Establishing definite evidence of teratogenicity with a particular drug is difficult, but all are thought to have some teratogenic effects, except perhaps for phenobarbi-

Table 22.25 Anticonvulsant drugs in adults

Drug	Average dose	Unwanted effects	Comment
Phenytoin	250–400 mg o.d.	Sedation, ataxia, dizziness, intellectual impairment, hirsutism, seborrhoeic skin thickening, gum hypertrophy	Avoid in pregnancy
Carbamazepine	300–800 mg per day, as b.d. dosage	Sedation, ataxia, nausea and vomiting. Rarely, bone marrow suppression and hepatotoxicity. Skin rash	Screen for neural tube defects in pregnancy
Phenobarbitone	30–90 mg per day, as b.d. dosage	Sedation, intellectual impairment	Safe in pregnancy
Clonazepam	1.5–6.0 mg per day, as t.d.s. dosage	Sedation with initial treatment	? Safe in pregnancy
Primidone	250–750 mg per day, as b.d. dosage	Sedation. As for phenobarbitone. May be better tolerated than phenobarbitone	Avoid in pregnancy
Valproate	600–1500 mg per day, as t.d.s. dosage	Occasional sedation, nausea and vomiting	Least sedating A/C drug. No liver enzyme induction. Screen for neural tube defects in pregnancy
Ethosuximide	250–750 mg per day, as t.d.s. dosage	Occasional sedation	Of greatest value in children and adolescents, with little effect in adults

tone. Phenytoin causes harelip and cleft palate, and cardiac malformations. Valproate and carbamazepine both lead to an increased incidence of neural tube defects (spina bifida, p. 937). This can be screened for early in pregnancy, at a stage when the fetus can be aborted if necessary.

Blood levels of anticonvulsant drugs tend to fall during pregnancy. Monitoring of levels is advisable, particularly in women whose epilepsy is normally difficult to control.

Newer anticonvulsant drugs

In patients with severe epilepsy, not adequately controlled by one of the first-line drugs or a combination of these drugs, the new anticonvulsants vigabatrin, lamotrigine or gabapentin may be added. The place of these three drugs in the treatment of epilepsy is still under evaluation.

Serial epilepsy and status epilepticus

A succession of convulsions in a single day constitutes *serial epilepsy*. When fits follow each other without consciousness being regained, this is known as *status epilepticus*. Urgent treatment is necessary to stop the fits, since continuing epileptic activity leads eventually to exhaustion and cerebral damage. Initial treatment with a slow bolus of intravenous diazepam (10–30 mg) may terminate status, but its anticonvulsant action is short-lived. Further doses are likely to produce increasing sedation and the need for ventilation. A continuous infusion of diazepam may occasionally be successful. A slow bolus of clonazepam (0.5–1.5 mg) is often more effective than diazepam, due to its longer duration of action.

Chlormethiazole, given as a ready-made 8.4% solution at a rate of 20–60 ml per hour, is the treatment of choice in status, having a good therapeutic ratio. The drug has a short half-life, so that if an excessive dose is given, causing respiratory depression, the effect is short-lived. If this is ineffective, an alternative is an infusion of thiopentone which is very long-lasting and which may take several days to clear from the body after stopping the drug, particularly in obese patients. When all else fails, paraldehyde (10 ml) by intramuscular injection of 5 ml into each buttock, followed at 4-hourly intervals by single 5 ml doses up to a total of 30 ml, is sometimes effective.

It is unwise to paralyse patients in status epilepticus who require ventilation unless continuous EEG monitoring is available; removal of the observable manifestations of convulsive cerebral activity by paralysing the patient leaves no indication of whether the anticonvulsant treatment is being effective or not.

Partial seizures may also occur continuously (*epilepsy partialis continua*). In focal motor epilepsy, this takes the form of continuous jerking of one side, or part of one side, of the body. In psychomotor (temporal lobe) status, the patient is confused and disorientated, will appear detached and may not respond to questions, but will be conscious. An EEG is invaluable in identifying the cause of the confusion.

Surgical treatment

Since epilepsy may be a symptom of a progressive cerebral lesion, surgical treatment may become part of overall therapy, but may not abolish fits. In a selected group of patients with intractable temporal lobe epilepsy, in whom it can be shown that epileptic discharges arise entirely unilaterally, a temporal lobectomy may produce marked improvement. Histological examination of the resected temporal lobe often reveals no abnormality, but mesial temporal sclerosis and, occasionally, small benign tumours have been found.

Prognosis

With the exception of patients with progressive structural or metabolic cerebral disease, in childhood or adult life, the overall prognosis is relatively good. In one large series, 20 years after initial diagnosis about 50% of patients were free from fits and off anticonvulsant treatment; a further 20% continued to take anticonvulsants and were fit-free; and fits continued in about 30% of patients who remained on treatment. Fits are less likely to remit in patients with mental retardation, abnormal neurological signs, clustering of fits, and complex partial and grand mal seizures.

Psychiatric and social factors

In most patients, the timing of fits is unpredictable and there is no, or only the briefest, warning of an impending attack. This alone may lead to social withdrawal and avoidance of public places. Patients are limited in their choice of work and may feel victimised by employers unwilling to continue their employment. There is still considerable social stigma attached to epilepsy, which may cause difficulties in personal relationships. Psychotic disorders may develop in a few patients with complex partial seizures.

Few restrictions need to be imposed on most patients. However, the law concerning epilepsy and driving is understandably cautious. A distinction is made between nocturnal and daytime fits. Patients who have had only nocturnal fits for a period of at least 3 years may hold a licence; patients who have had a single daytime fit may not drive for 1 year; in all other cases, where there have been two or more fits, the licence will be withdrawn and will not be reinstated until a period of at least 2 years fit-free has elapsed. Holders of HGV licences who have fits will have their licence permanently removed. Discussion of the law and driving is an issue that often threatens the relationship between doctor and patient. It is the doctor's duty to inform the patient not to drive after a fit and to seek the advice of the licensing authorities.

NARCOLEPSY

In narcolepsy, episodes of sleep occur during the day with a prodrome of an irresistible desire to sleep. The attacks occur in inappropriate circumstances and can usually be distinguished from normal daytime postprandial drowsiness. Narcolepsy is associated with an abnormal EEG pattern of rapid eye movement (REM) sleep, REM sleep occurring quickly during the daytime sleeping episodes. There are three associated clinical phenomena in narcolepsy.

- *Cataplexy* is an abrupt reduction in muscle tone leading to collapse to the ground, induced by emotion, often laughter and loud noises. Consciousness is preserved and recovery usually occurs within a few minutes.
- *Sleep paralysis* describes episodes of complete paralysis (without respiratory involvement) which occurs transiently on waking. It is usually short-lived, a few minutes at most.
- *Hypnagogic hallucinations* are a feature in some patients. These are vivid, sometimes frightening hallucinations which occur as the patient is falling asleep.

Narcolepsy and the related symptoms are thought to be due to abnormalities of monoaminergic pathways in the brainstem reticular-activating formation, and there is a very strong association with HLA-DR2. There is often a family history of the condition. Combination treatment with a tricyclic antidepressant and amphetamine is usually effective.

OTHER SLEEP DISORDERS

Narcolepsy is a rare disorder which accounts for only a proportion of patients complaining of daytime drowsiness. In many cases the primary problem is a disturbance of nighttime sleep; this may result from depressive illness, drugs (including alcohol), or sometimes intermittent nocturnal respiratory failure – sleep apnoea (p. 491). The interruption of respiration may be mechanical (obstructive sleep apnoea) or, less commonly, due to failure of neurogenic respiratory drive during sleep (central sleep apnoea). Many patients have persistent daytime drowsiness for no identifiable reason.

CEREBROVASCULAR DISEASE

The term cerebrovascular disease embraces all the pathological and clinical manifestations of the following:

- disease of the cerebral arteries (atheroma being by far the commonest cause) and of the major neck vessels supplying the brain
- disease of the heart, which may cause embolism to the brain or, rarely, ischaemia due to a critical fall in cardiac output

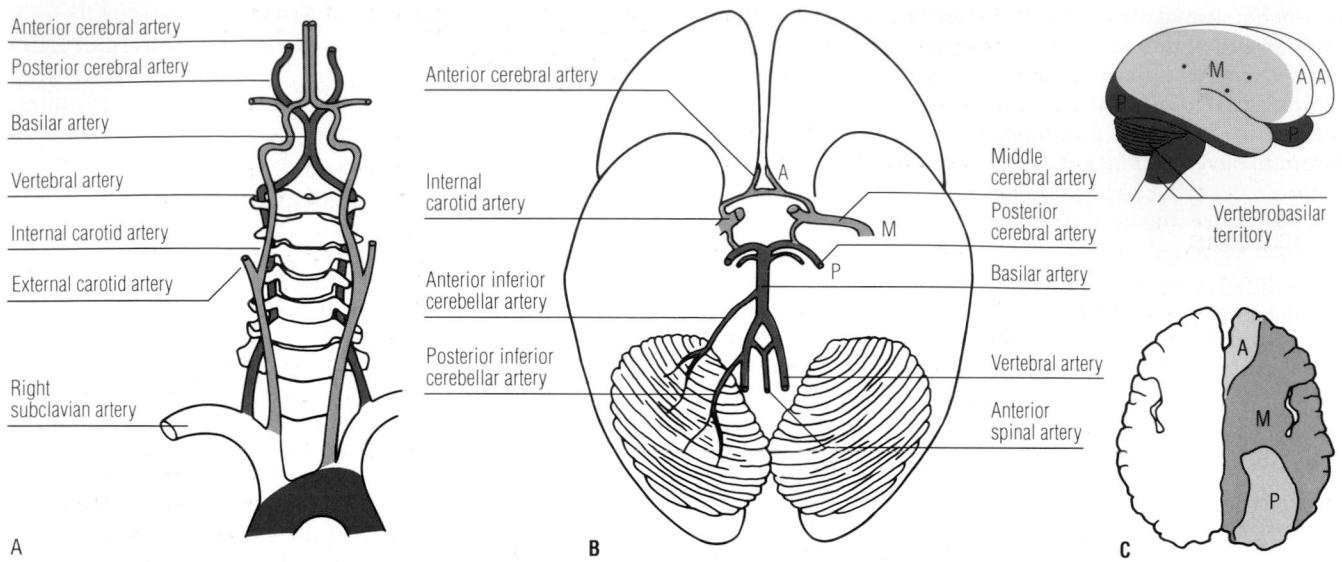

Fig. 22.9 The cerebral arterial supply. A. The origins of carotid (pale red) and vertebral (dark red) arteries are shown, as is their relationship to the cervical spine. **B.** The major branches of the circle of Willis at the base of the brain are shown. **C.** The distribution of the anterior (A), middle (M) and posterior (P) cerebral arteries are shown. The middle (M) and anterior (A) areas comprise carotid territory. Note in the upper diagram that vertebrobasilar territory includes the branches supplying the brainstem and cerebellum as well as the distribution of the posterior cerebral arteries (P). The lower section is at the level of the internal capsule.

- disorders of the blood, which may lead to impaired clotting, causing haemorrhage, hyperviscosity or hypercoagulable states, which increase the tendency to cerebral thrombosis.

Thus, in a patient presenting with a stroke, particularly younger patients, the diagnostic net must be cast wide.

Definitions

Stroke and transient ischaemic attack

A stroke is an acute or subacute event in which a neurological deficit develops over minutes or hours, sometimes in a stepwise fashion, persists for at least 24 hours, and is caused by a vascular disturbance in the brain. Recovery is variable in its speed and extent, but it can eventually be complete. Vascular events lasting less than 24 hours are defined by convention as transient ischaemic attacks (TIAs), although the distinction is not absolute. Some apparent TIAs may be associated with infarction on a CT scan, whereas more prolonged symptoms are not always accompanied by a visible structural lesion in the brain. In practice, most TIAs are very brief, lasting only minutes or 1–2 hours at most.

Most strokes are due to arterial occlusion and consequent ischaemic focal infarction of the brain, primary intracerebral haemorrhage being comparatively much less common. Subarachnoid haemorrhage, although clearly an acute intracranial vascular event, is primarily extracerebral in its origin and the underlying pathophysiology, clinical presentation and management are all quite distinct from a typical 'stroke' as defined above.

The term 'cerebrovascular accident' has found widespread usage, but 'stroke' is preferable, not least because it is a term understood and used by both doctors and patients.

Epidemiology

Stroke is the third commonest cause of death in the UK, after heart disease and cancer. It has an incidence of 1–2 per 1000 population per year, but is much higher than this in older age groups. The incidence in men is slightly higher than in women at all ages. Stroke has a prevalence of around 5 per 1000 population. It has been estimated that about 80% of intracranial vascular events are due to cerebral infarction, 10% to spontaneous intracerebral haemorrhage and 10% to subarachnoid haemorrhage.

While TIAs are probably mainly due to emboli, the proportion of strokes which are embolic rather than thrombotic in situ remains uncertain.

Anatomy and physiology

Cerebral circulation

Figure 22.9 shows the origins of the great vessels from the aortic arch, the circle of Willis and its branches, and the areas of the brain supplied by the major intracerebral arteries. There are four branches from the terminal part of the internal carotid artery: the anterior and middle cerebrals, the anterior choroidal and the posterior communicating artery. A number of small branches are given off within the cavernous sinus. The most important of these is the ophthalmic artery, which passes anteriorly into the orbit where it divides, the central retinal artery being one of the branches. The other branches form anastamotic connections with branches of the external carotid artery. These anastamoses are a source of an important collateral circulation, which may develop after occlusion of the internal carotid artery in the neck.

The vertebral arteries arise from the subclavian artery. The arteries join to form the basilar artery at the level of the lower pons. In addition to the terminal branches shown in Figure 22.9, the vertebral arteries give off the anterior and posterior spinal arteries.

Autoregulation

Cerebral blood flow (CBF) is maintained in the normal subject despite a wide range of blood pressures. A fall in blood pressure causes compensatory cerebral vasodilation, and a rise produces vasoconstriction. Above a certain level, however, this autoregulation fails and, with high enough pressures, cerebral oedema develops, eventually resulting in hypertensive encephalopathy (p. 903). Conversely, a fall of systemic blood pressure below the range of autoregulation will reduce cerebral perfusion and lead to haemodynamic cerebral ischaemia.

Causes of cerebrovascular disease

Atheroma

Of all the causes of cerebrovascular disease listed in Table 22.26, atheroma is by far the most important, and patients presenting with a stroke often have evidence of peripheral or coronary vascular disease. The coexistence of cerebral and peripheral vascular disease is emphasised by the fact that a patient presenting with a first stroke is as likely to have a myocardial infarction in future as a further stroke. Atheroma tends to be most marked at branch points in the major vessels and in the carotid syphon. In relation to the cerebral circulation, the origins of the arteries from the aorta, brachiocephalic trunk and subclavian artery, the carotid bifurcation, the basilar artery and the origins of the anterior, middle and posterior cerebral arteries are all sites for atheroma formation.

Atheroma may cause stenosis or complete obstruction, but thrombus commonly forms on atheromatous plaques in the absence of any haemodynamically significant stenosis. Fragments of thrombus may then break off and become lodged in a smaller artery distally. Partial obstruction or rapid lysis may lead to prompt restoration of the circulation producing the clinical picture of a TIA, but infarction results if the circulation is interrupted for

Table 22.26 Causes of cerebrovascular disease

ARTERIAL DISEASE	
Atheroma	In situ thrombosis
	Artery-to-artery embolism
	Rupture and haemorrhage
Hypertension	Exacerbates all the above
	Small vessel disease (lipohyalinosis)
Congenital	Aneurysms
	Arteriovenous malformations
	Fibromuscular dysplasia
	Pseudoxanthoma elasticum
	Cystic medial necrosis
Inflammatory	Arteritis: PAN, giant cell, Wegener's, SLE, intracerebral, Behçet's, sarcoid
	Radiation angiopathy
	Infection: basal meningitis (TB, fungi, pyogenic), syphilis, local infection in the neck
	Cortical thrombophlebitis secondary to infection
Trauma	Whiplash injury, direct trauma to the neck, angiography, producing vascular dissection or occlusion
CARDIOVASCULAR	
Cardiac embolism	Numerous causes (see Table 22.27)
Cardiac arrest	Patchy infarction in watershed areas
Prolonged hypotension	Diffuse hypoxic-ischaemic damage
HAEMATOLOGICAL DISORDERS	
Prothrombotic	Polycythaemia, thrombocythaemia
	Sickle cell disease
	Antiphospholipid antibody syndrome
Hyperviscosity	Myeloma, Waldenström's macroglobulinaemia
	Leukaemias
Haemorrhagic disorders	Thrombocytopenias
	Factor deficiencies
	Iatrogenic: heparin and warfarin

more than a few minutes. Alternatively, thrombus forming on an atheromatous plaque causing stenosis may lead to complete obstruction in situ. The presence of bruits in the neck and supraclavicular fossa indicates arterial stenosis, but partial stenosis may occur without thromboembolism or any significant haemodynamic effects. The natural history of asymptomatic carotid bruits is still controversial, but recent studies suggest that it is more benign than previously thought.

Other causes of cerebral embolism

There are numerous other causes of cerebral embolism apart from atheroma in the great vessels (Table 22.27). Emboli or local occlusion of the intracerebral vessels may each present with either a TIA or a stroke; it is often impossible to distinguish between local thrombosis and embolism.

Table 22.27 Causes of cerebral embolism

● Carotid or vertebral artery disease	– Atheroma
	– Dissection
● Cardiac	
Aortic or mitral valve disease	– Endocarditis
	– Rheumatic
	– Prosthetic valve thrombosis
Left atrium	– Mural thrombosis with AF
	– Myxoma
Left ventricle	– Mural thrombus after myocardial infarction or with aneurysm or cardiomyopathy
● Air embolism	– Cardiac surgery
	– Trauma
● **Paradoxical embolism** (from venous circulation)	– Latent foramen ovale
	– ASD

Risk factors

The most important risk factor for stroke (Table 22.28) is hypertension. Recent studies have clearly shown that both smoking and alcohol are risk factors.

TRANSIENT ISCHAEMIC ATTACKS

TIAs are generally considered to be due to embolism, which seems the most likely explanation, particularly when repeated stereotyped episodes occur. The proportion of TIAs caused by emboli arising from the heart has probably been overestimated in the past; a recent estimate is 5–10%.

Clinical features

Carotid territory TIA

Transient ischaemia in the carotid territory usually produces a contralateral hemiparesis (with or without hemisensory or hemianopic disturbance), and dysphasia if the dominant hemisphere is affected. Attacks last from a few minutes to several hours; by definition, all symptoms and signs have resolved within 24 hours. Amaurosis fugax is the term used to describe transient monocular blind-

Table 22.28 Risk factors for TIA and stroke

● Hypertension	● Previous TIA
● Cardiac disease	● Cervical bruit
Ischaemic heart disease	● Hyperlipidaemia
Causes of embolism (Table 22.27)	● Raised haematocrit
● Peripheral vascular disease	● Alcohol
● Diabetes	● Oral contraceptive pill, particularly in smokers
● Smoking	

ness. It is most often caused by embolism of the retinal circulation, but similar transient loss of vision may occasionally occur in glaucoma, or with papilloedema, retrobulbar neuritis, orbital tumours, retinal haemorrhage and retinal detachment.

Vertebrobasilar TIA

In the vertebrobasilar territory, TIA may cause vertigo, diplopia, visual blurring or loss (due to occipital cortical ischaemia), facial paraesthesiae and numbness (often circumoral and bilateral), facial weakness, dysarthria, dysphagia and dysphonia, nausea and vomiting, ataxia, hemiparesis or tetraparesis, and hemisensory or four-limb sensory impairment. There is frequently impairment or loss of consciousness. It is an error to make a diagnosis of vertebrobasilar TIA on the basis of dizziness or loss of consciousness alone, in the absence of other symptoms suggesting a brainstem lesion. Isolated dizziness on head movement is much more likely to be due to a peripheral vestibular lesion. On rare occasions, with vertebral artery stenosis, neck movement (particularly extension) may further impair blood flow by cervical compression, leading to a vertebrobasilar TIA.

Subclavian steal syndrome

Subclavian steal syndrome is rare and is due to subclavian stenosis proximal to the origin of the vertebral artery. During exercise of the arm, there is peripheral vasodilatation and blood flows retrogradely from the vertebral artery into the subclavian artery, causing vertebrobasilar ischaemia. There is usually a substantial reduction in blood pressure on the side of the subclavian stenosis, and a palpable difference between the pulses in the two arms.

Examination

It is rare to witness a TIA, and patients seen between attacks will have no neurological signs, apart from, occasionally, a cervical bruit. General examination is directed towards identifying associated factors such as hypertension, peripheral vascular disease and cardiac abnormalities. During an attack of amaurosis fugax, emboli can occasionally be seen in the retinal arterioles; platelet emboli are white, cholesterol emboli are yellowish.

Investigation of TIA and stroke

Investigation and management after TIA (or a minor stroke) are directed towards minimising the risk of a disabling cerebral infarct in the future. A scheme of investigation is shown in Table 22.29, the more specialised tests on the right being applied selectively in appropriate cases. CT scanning is usually of little value but it may

Table 22.29 Investigation of TIA and stroke

All patients	Selected cases
● Full blood count, ESR	● Fasting lipids
● Urea and electrolytes, MSU	● Clotting screen
● Blood glucose	● Autoantibodies
● Chest X-ray	● Blood cultures
● ECG	● Treponemal serology
	● Lumbar puncture
	● Echocardiography
	● CT scan
	● Doppler studies
	● Angiography

show unsuspected cerebral infarcts, and if these are bilateral, there is a greater likelihood of recurrent embolism from the heart. Doppler ultrasonography may show evidence of ulcerative or occlusive carotid disease in the neck, but if surgery is seriously contemplated, angiography is usually necessary as well. Other indications for angiography are considered below.

Management and prognosis

The risk of stroke in patients with TIAs varies between 5 and 15% per annum, depending on the type and frequency of attacks and their cause. Numerous episodes associated with a 90% stenosis of one carotid artery carry a much worse prognosis than a single attack in a patient with mild hypertension. Nevertheless, high blood pressure remains the most important treatable risk factor for all types of stroke. Diabetes should be controlled, smoking stopped, alcohol consumption reduced if high, and weight loss encouraged if appropriate (although obesity is not a clear independent risk factor for stroke). There is no firm evidence that reduction of hyperlipidaemia reduces stroke risk, but this should be treated in younger patients with high levels. Attention should also be directed to the high risk of myocardial infarction in patients presenting with TIA or stroke.

There has been much uncertainty about the value of antiplatelet agents, anticoagulants and reconstructive arterial surgery in the prevention of stroke.

Antiplatelet therapy

Drugs in this category include aspirin, dipyridamole, ticlopidine and sulphinpyrazone. Only aspirin has been conclusively shown by adequate trials to reduce stroke risk after TIAs. The lowest dose of proven value is 300 mg daily, although studies are in progress to evaluate much smaller doses. Review of all the methodologically sound trials for both stroke and cardiac disease indicates that aspirin reduces the incidence of non-fatal stroke or myocardial infarction by about 30%, and all vascular

deaths by 15%. It is therefore reasonable to prescribe regular aspirin for all patients who have had TIAs or an ischaemic stroke, providing there is no contraindication on other grounds. Caution should be exercised in patients with uncontrolled hypertension and whenever there is suspicion of a haemorrhagic or potentially haemorrhagic lesion in the brain.

Anticoagulants

The use of heparin and warfarin following TIA and stroke has not been adequately studied. There is no evidence supporting the use of anticoagulants in patients with TIAs due to carotid artery disease. However, warfarin is indicated for patients with a demonstrable source of embolism in the heart. Those with prosthetic valves or rheumatic valvular disease with atrial fibrillation are at greatest risk, but anticoagulation is also justifiable in patients with left ventricular thrombus associated with myocardial infarction, cardiomyopathy or ventricular aneurysm, and when embolism from the left atrium is suspected in patients with non-valvular atrial fibrillation. The use of heparin infusion for a slowly progressing ischaemic stroke is often suggested but not supported by any objective evidence of its efficacy. Anticoagulation in the acute phase after an embolic cerebral infarct carries some risk of inducing haemorrhage into the lesion, but this must be balanced against the threat of further emboli (p. 905).

Reconstructive arterial surgery

In patients with TIAs or minor stroke due to platelet embolism from ulcerative plaques or stenotic lesions in the internal carotid artery, carotid endarterectomy has the theoretical value of removing the source of embolism and preventing a subsequent and more disabling stroke. The indications for this procedure have remained controversial since its invention in 1954, but preliminary results of recent trials in Europe and the USA have clarified the issue to some extent: in patients with recent or continuing ischaemic symptoms attributable to severe carotid stenosis (i.e. between 70 and 99% reduction of luminal diameter), there is a high risk of an ipsilateral stroke, which is significantly reduced by carotid endarterectomy by an expert in the field. The major complication of this procedure is the very catastrophe it is designed to prevent. In certain circumstances, endarterectomy may also be justifiable to reverse a state of critically low perfusion pressure beyond a tight stenosis, but prevention of embolism is the major indication, in highly selected cases.

The innovative procedure of extracranial to intracranial arterial bypass surgery was practised actively for many years, particularly in North America, until a definitive controlled clinical trial showed clearly that the operative morbidity far outweighed any potential benefits.

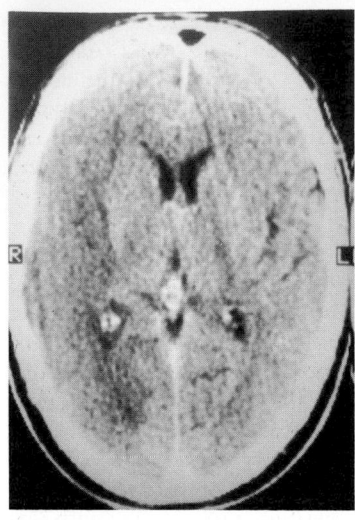
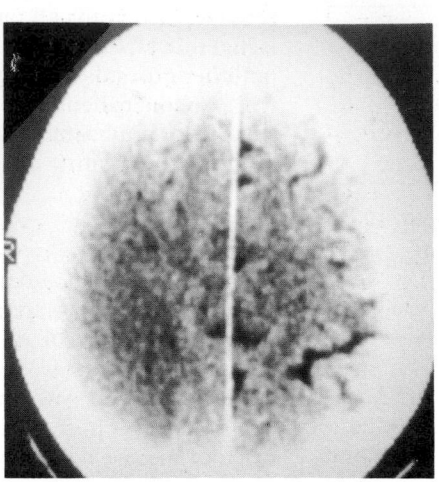

Fig. 22.10 Acute cerebral infarction. There is an extensive right cerebral hemisphere infarct in this patient, scanned 24 hours after the onset of a complete left hemiparesis with left hemisensory loss and a left homonymous hemianopia. An ill-defined area of low attenuation, occupying most of the right hemisphere, is not causing midline shift, but there is obliteration of the overlying sulci, indicating mass effect.

STROKES DUE TO CEREBRAL INFARCTION

The causes of cerebral infarction are the same as for TIAs, but it is generally considered that fewer strokes than TIAs have an embolic basis. Most cerebral infarcts swell during the first few days after the acute event with surrounding oedema (Fig. 22.10). Large infarcts may exert considerable mass effect, sometimes causing life-threatening herniation at the tentorium. Cerebral oedema is usually at its most severe 4–7 days after infarction and then gradually resolves over 2–4 weeks (Fig. 22.11).

There is always a possibility that an ischaemic infarct may become haemorrhagic. This is most likely if the infarct is due to an embolus which is then cleared at an early stage, allowing blood under arterial pressure to enter the fresh infarct. An infarct may also become haemorrhagic due to the collateral blood supply at the boundaries of the infarct.

Clinical features

The cardinal clinical feature of a stroke is its abrupt onset. Occasionally, there is a slow worsening over hours, or a stepwise deterioration in function over a day or two (stroke in evolution). Strokes vary enormously in both their severity and the combination of symptoms and signs. When occlusion of a major cerebral artery occurs, the extent of infarction will depend on the degree of collateral blood supply. For example, occlusion of the internal carotid artery, either at the carotid bifurcation or in the syphon (the two common sites for atheroma formation in the carotid), may cause no deficit at all if the circle of Willis is complete and flow through the other carotid and vertebrals is sufficient.

Major cerebral vessel occlusion syndromes

Carotid territory

Middle cerebral artery occlusion

Middle cerebral artery and internal carotid artery occlusion may be indistinguishable clinically, and the extent of infarction after either is very variable. Preceding amau-

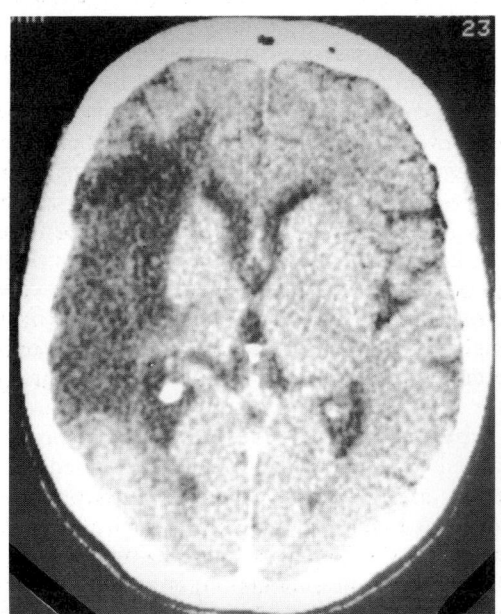

Fig. 22.11 A mature cerebral infarct, in the distribution of the right middle cerebral artery. The infarct has a lower attenuation than adjacent normal brain, there is no mass effect, and there is a clear line of demarcation between infarct and normal brain.

rosis fugax may indicate either internal carotid artery occlusion or embolic occlusion of the middle cerebral artery. The middle cerebral artery is also the most frequent vessel occluded by emboli from the heart. However, some middle cerebral artery territory strokes are probably due to in situ thrombosis of the main trunk of the middle cerebral artery or its branches.

The usual deficit after middle cerebral artery occlusion is a contralateral hemiparesis, affecting the arm and face more than the leg. When the dominant hemisphere is affected, dysphasia is usually expressive more than receptive. Contralateral homonymous hemianopia and a mild contralateral hemisensory loss may also be present.

Anterior cerebral artery occlusion

Unilateral occlusion of the anterior cerebral artery results in contralateral hemiparesis and hemisensory loss, in which the leg is often more severely affected than the arm. After anterior cerebral artery occlusion in the dominant hemisphere, there may be an expressive dysphasia; in either hemisphere, there may be marked motor dyspraxia, causing particular difficulty in walking.

Vertebrobasilar territory

Ischaemic lesions in the posterior circulation, due to vertebral, basilar or branch artery occlusions, are very variable in extent. There are many described discrete syndromes but, in clinical practice, the deficit in a particular patient usually does not correspond exactly to one of these. It is usually sufficient to recognise the major area of infarction within the brainstem.

Infarction of the medulla

Hemiparesis, tetraparesis or triparesis with lower cranial nerve palsies may occur after vertebral artery occlusion, together with disturbances of breathing and cardiovascular control due to involvement of the medullary reticular formation. Respiratory irregularities, apnoea, hypotension or hypertension, and a number of cardiac arrhythmias may result.

Posterior inferior cerebellar artery occlusion (Wallenberg syndrome, lateral medullary infarction)

The posterior inferior cerebellar artery (PICA) occlusion syndrome is as often due to vertebral occlusion as to occlusion of the PICA. The clinical syndrome is striking, and occurs sufficiently frequently to be recognisable as a separate entity. Symptoms usually consist of ipsilateral facial paraesthesiae or pain due to involvement of the spinal nucleus and tract of the trigeminal nerve, severe vertigo and vomiting due to involvement of

the vestibular nucleus and its medullary connections, dysphagia, dysphonia, ataxia and contralateral limb sensory impairment.

Examination reveals an ipsilateral Horner's syndrome from involvement of descending sympathetic fibres in the medullary reticular formation, horizontal nystagmus towards the side of the cerebellar lesion, ipsilateral trigeminal pain and temperature sensory impairment. There is also, occasionally, an ipsilateral lower motor neurone facial palsy, ipsilateral palatal, vocal cord, pharyngeal and lingual palsies (which may cause severe dysphagia), ipsilateral limb ataxia, and, sometimes, ataxia of gait. In addition, there is a contralateral spinothalamic limb and trunk sensory impairment. Rarely, there is a contralateral hemiparesis, but this only occurs with extensive infarcts.

Pontine infarction

Pontine infarction, due to basilar artery thrombosis, is often fatal. The signs are coma, quadriplegia, multiple cranial nerve signs (usually involving gaze palsies), nystagmus, facial paralysis and cardiorespiratory abnormalities. Bilateral infarction of the basis pontis, with relative sparing of the more dorsal parts of the pons, results in quadriplegia and, often, anarthria, and jaw, facial, palatal and tongue paralysis with preservation of consciousness. This is the so-called 'locked-in' syndrome, in which patients are only able to communicate with movement of the eyes.

Paramedian infarction of the pons causes patchy damage, involving the pyramidal tracts, pontine cranial nerve nuclei and fibres passing to the middle cerebellar peduncle.

In lateral infarction of the pons, the trigeminal nucleus, medial lemniscus and the middle cerebellar peduncle are mainly affected, with some involvement of the pyramidal tract to the legs more than to the arms.

In tegmental infarction of the pons, the trigeminal, abducens and facial nuclei, together with the medial longitudinal fasciculus and superior cerebellar peduncle, are affected; this causes a variety of conjugate gaze palsies, ipsilateral trigeminal, abducens and facial lower motor neurone lesions, and ipsilateral cerebellar signs.

Mid-brain infarction

Mid-brain infarction occurring alone is unusual. Syndromes of ipsilateral third nerve palsy with contralateral hemiparesis (Weber's syndrome) and ipsilateral third nerve palsy with contralateral cerebellar signs (syndrome of Benedikt) are described, but are rare. Superior cerebellar artery thrombosis causing infarction of the midbrain–pontine junction leads to an ipsilateral Horner's syndrome, ipsilateral nystagmus and cerebellar signs, ipsilateral lower motor neurone facial weakness, contralateral spinothalamic sensory loss in the limbs, and, sometimes, Parkinsonian signs from involvement of connections to the substantia nigra.

Cerebellar infarction

Pure cerebellar infarction probably occurs only rarely; most infarcts also involve the brainstem, although cerebellar signs predominate.

Posterior cerebral artery occlusion

The posterior cerebral arteries supply the upper part of the mid-brain, the cerebral peduncles, parts of the thalamus and the subthalamic nuclei, as well as the occipital lobes. Thus, although homonymous visual field defects predominate in posterior cerebral artery occlusion, hemiparesis, sensory disturbances and, occasionally, hemiballismus (p. 923) may also occur. In addition to the primary visual cortex, the more anteriorly placed association cortex may also be damaged. Patients with extensive lesions here may deny being blind (Anton's syndrome); they will describe objects incorrectly and may wrongly be thought to be confused.

Thalamic pain is a rare consequence of stroke. It arises from infarction of the lateral part of the thalamus. Thalamic stroke causes contralateral sensory loss, often with only a mild hemiparesis. The pain may come on weeks or months later and is usually continuous, severe and chronic; it has a burning quality, often with associated cutaneous hyperaesthesiae. Treatment with antidepressants, benzodiazepines or anticonvulsants is occasionally successful. Thalamic electrical stimulation may give partial relief.

Lacunar infarcts

Lacunar infarction refers to small deep infarcts in the region of the internal capsule, basal ganglia, thalamus and brainstem, particularly the pons (Fig. 22.12). These are often multiple. The deficit from such strokes is usually mild. Lacunar infarction is most common in hypertension but also occurs in normotensive subjects. Lacunae are thought to be caused by occlusion of small branch arteries, or by microaneurysm formation (Charcot-Bouchard aneurysms) followed by rupture, producing a small haematoma which resolves leaving an area of infarction. The common lacunar syndromes are listed in Table 22.30.

Diffuse small vessel disease

The third, least common pattern of ischaemic cerebrovascular disease is diffuse small vessel disease. It is more common in hypertensive patients. The typical presenta-

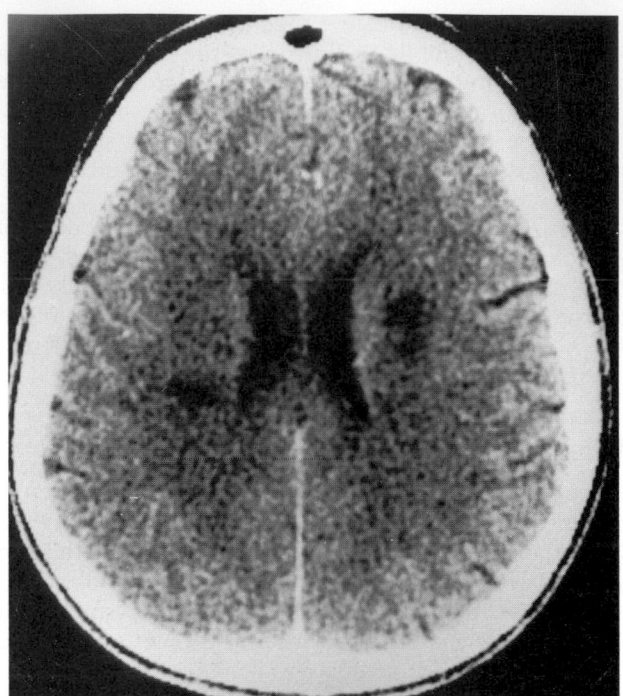

Fig. 22.12 CT scan showing bilateral small lacunar infarcts in the internal capsule.

Table 22.30 Common lacunar syndromes

Type	Clinical features	Lesion
Pure motor stroke	Partial hemiparesis	Internal capsule
Pure sensory stroke	Partial hemisensory impairment	Internal capsule
Hemiparesis with ataxia	Partial hemiparesis Ataxia of cerebellar type Dysarthria	Internal capsule or pons

tion is difficulty in walking and dementia, which is usually progressive. There is sometimes urinary incontinence. Examination reveals intellectual impairment, often with prominent primitive reflexes, and bilateral pyramidal tract signs which affect the cranial nerve nuclei as well as the limbs. There may be a brisk jaw jerk, dysarthria (of spastic type), and dysphagia (the lower cranial nerve signs constituting a pseudobulbar palsy). The signs in the limbs are often asymmetrical, with little or no sensory impairment. The gait is characteristically small-paced, unsteady and slow, the so-called 'marche à petits pas'. It resembles a Parkinsonian gait in some respects, but the patient walks more upright and with a wider base.

CT scanning (Fig. 22.13) shows a variable degree of cortical atrophy and a characteristic diffuse periventricular low attenuation indicating deep white matter loss (sometimes known as Binswanger's disease).

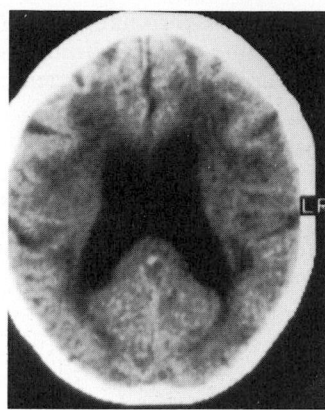

Fig. 22.13 Diffuse small vessel disease. The scan shows cerebral atrophy, with well-marked low attenuation diffusely in the subcortical white matter surrounding the ventricles. (Reproduced by permission of Dr J Stevens and Dr A Valentine.)

Multi-infarct dementia

Patients presenting with a history of progressive dementia are sometimes found to have multiple cerebral infarcts of differing size. They usually have physical signs corresponding to some, if not all, of the lesions (Fig. 22.14). Vascular dementia is discussed more fully on page 909.

Other patterns of cerebrovascular disease

Migrainous infarction. Extremely rarely, a persistent deficit may follow a focal migraine attack, usually in the form of a hemianopia. It is likely that cerebral infarction is due to in situ thrombosis within a vessel critically narrowed by either spasm or oedema within its walls, or to this process of narrowing alone. Women with complicated migraine who take the contraceptive pill may be at slightly greater risk of having this type of stroke.

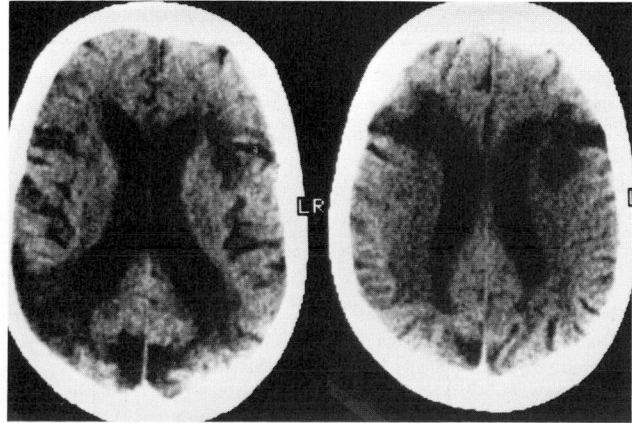

Fig. 22.14 Multiple bilateral cerebral infarcts in a middle-aged man with a history of coronary artery and peripheral vascular disease.

Hypotensive cerebral infarction. Prolonged severe hypotension (e.g. after cardiac arrest) may lead to focal cerebral infarction even with normal cerebral vessels, although diffuse cortical damage is more common. Patients with pre-existing cerebral arterial narrowing are particularly at risk.

Watershed infarction most commonly affects the boundary parieto-occipital area between anterior, middle and posterior cerebral artery territories.

Hypertensive encephalopathy. The encephalopathy resulting from severe hypertension is characterised by coma, fits and a very high blood pressure, in excess of 220/130 mmHg. Papilloedema is invariably present. There is cerebral oedema and multiple small cerebral haemorrhages.

Reduction of the blood pressure is essential (Ch. 12) and recovery is often surprisingly rapid and complete. Gradual reduction of the blood pressure over a few hours is preferable to an abrupt lowering, which is more likely to lead to ischaemia and infarction.

STROKES DUE TO PRIMARY INTRACEREBRAL HAEMORRHAGE

Aetiology

The causes of spontaneous intracerebral haemorrhage are listed in Table 22.31. Haemorrhage is most commonly due to hypertension or intracerebral extension of bleeding from a ruptured berry aneurysm. Subarachnoid haemor-

Table 22.31 Causes of spontaneous intracerebral haemorrhage

- **Hypertension**
- **Cerebrovascular disease without hypertension**
- **Subarachnoid haemorrhage, with intracerebral extension**
- **Arteriovenous malformations** (alone, or as part of Sturge-Weber syndrome*)
- Other cerebrovascular disease: Mycotic aneurysms
    Cortical thrombophlebitis
    Capillary haemangiomas
    Haemorrhagic telangiectasia**
    Cavernous haemangiomas
    Haemangioblastomas***
    Congophilic (amyloid) angiopathy
- Bleeding into cerebral tumours (rare)
- Haematological disease: Thrombocytopenia from any cause
    Haemophilia
    Sickle cell disease
    Iatrogenic – anticoagulants
            – cytotoxic drugs

Common causes are shown in bold type.
*Sturge-Weber syndrome – AVM with ipsilateral trigeminal cutaneous capillary angioma ('port-wine' stain).
**Osler-Rendu-Weber syndrome – haemorrhagic telangiectasia in brain and retina
***Von Hippel-Lindau disease — CNS haemangioblastomas, particularly in cerebellum, brainstem and spinal cord, with retinal haemangioblastomas, renal or pancreatic cysts, hypernephroma and adrenal tumours.

rhage is considered on page 906. Cerebral infarction is about eight times as common as primary cerebral haemorrhage as the cause of stroke. Although haemorrhage without hypertension occurs, haemorrhage is much more common in hypertensive subjects. Many cerebral haemorrhages are thought to arise from Charcot-Bouchard microaneurysms, situated deep in the cerebral hemispheres, cerebellar hemispheres and pons. Lesions situated superficially in the cerebral hemispheres are more likely to be due to one of the less common causes of haemorrhage.

Surrounding oedema develops within a few hours of cerebral haemorrhage; this exacerbates the space-occupying effect, which is much greater with haemorrhage than with infarction. Extension of a cerebral haemorrhage into the lateral ventricle carries a worse prognosis.

Clinical features

The clinical presentation of cerebral hemisphere haemorrhage is often indistinguishable from cerebral infarction. However, because intracranial pressure is more likely to be raised with haemorrhage, severe headache, vomiting and impairment of consciousness are more common with haemorrhage. The presence of meningism indicates blood in the subarachnoid space, and therefore haemorrhage extending either from an intracerebral haemorrhage or from a primary subarachnoid source.

Haemorrhage in the cerebellum produces a typical presentation of ataxia, headache and vomiting, often with vertigo. This is followed by progressive impairment of the conscious level, resulting both from brainstem compression directly due to the haematoma, and from hydrocephalus due to obstruction of CSF flow through the aqueduct of Sylvius (Fig. 22.26). Pontine haemorrhage usually causes rapid loss of consciousness, a quadriplegia, multiple brainstem signs, and is usually fatal.

The diagnosis is usually confirmed by CT scanning, which, in more severe cases, may also show focal ischaemic lesions or early hydrocephalus. When there is doubt and the patient is conscious without focal hemisphere signs, examination of the CSF may also be necessary.

Differential diagnosis of stroke

The abrupt onset of a neurological deficit, often with a distribution corresponding to a single vessel territory, and with a tendency to improve slowly, usually leaves little doubt about the diagnosis of a stroke. Other diagnoses should be considered when the history is atypical, inadequate or unreliable. These include:

- chronic subdural haematoma, sometimes bilateral
- cerebral abscess
- encephalitis (particularly due to Herpes simplex)
- cerebral tumour.

Other conditions may occasionally produce stroke-like presentations, including demyelinating disease, cerebral venous thrombosis and acute hypoglycaemia.

Complications of stroke

The complications of a disabling cerebral infarct or haemorrhage are listed in Table 22.32. Death from the stroke itself usually occurs within the first 2 weeks. Pneumonia is an early and sometimes fatal complication. Incontinence, a poor prognostic feature, is associated with recurrent urinary tract infections.

Investigation of acute stroke

Since 80–90% of strokes are ischaemic rather than haemorrhagic, the basic approach to investigation is the same as for patients with TIAs (Table 22.29, p. 899). Screening for the more obscure causes of stroke is performed selectively, depending on the age of the patient and the type of lesion.

CT scanning

Not all patients require a CT scan, but when performed, it usually provides more precise diagnostic and prognostic information, and it is an essential investigation in the following circumstances:

- *Uncertainty about the diagnosis.* Particularly when the history is inadequate or the patient is deteriorating, a scan is required to exclude a subdural haematoma, expanding intracranial haematoma, tumour or focal intracranial infection.
- *Distinction between infarction and haemorrhage.* When there is doubt on clinical grounds and active intervention is planned with anticoagulants or even aspirin, it is important to exclude a haemorrhagic lesion.

Table 22.32 Complications of stroke

Neurological	Renal and metabolic
Cerebral oedema (early)	Urinary infection
Epilepsy	Renal failure
Spasticity	Dehydration
Contractures, frozen shoulder, shoulder	Electrolyte abnormalities
subluxation	SIADH (early)
Depression	Hyperglycaemia/diabetes (early)
Incontinence	
	Skin
Respiratory and cardiovascular	Pressure sores
Neurogenic pulmonary oedema (early)	
Cardiac arrhythmias (early)	**General**
Pneumonia	Weight loss
DVT	Weight gain
Pulmonary embolism	Malnutrition
	Dependent oedema

- *Young patients.* Those with vascular events at an unexpectedly early age require full investigation to exclude unusual causes of stroke, including unsuspected multiple lesions or a vascular malformation.
- *Cerebellar stroke.* Expanding cerebellar haematomas or acute hydrocephalus due to swelling of a cerebellar infarct are rare but life-threatening vascular events that may require immediate surgical intervention.

Lumbar puncture

This is rarely indicated in the acute phase, but CSF examination may necessary if there is suspicion of an underlying inflammatory disorder causing the stroke, e.g. low-grade meningitis (especially TB and fungi), neurosyphilis, cerebral arteritis, SLE and HIV infection.

Angiography

Development of tomographic imaging (both CT and MRI) has left relatively few indications for cerebral angiography in stroke patients. The following are fairly clear-cut, however:

- In patients with continuing carotid ischaemic events (despite aspirin) being considered for endarterectomy, cervical angiography is necessary unless Doppler studies are (a) available and (b) have shown that there is definitely no potentially operable lesion. Digital subtraction angiography with venous contrast injection is usually adequate for visualisation of the carotid and other neck vessels.
- To identify a suspected intracerebral arteriovenous malformation or aneurysm in patients with intracerebral haemorrhage for whom active surgical management is contemplated.
- To identify features of macroscopic cerebral arteritis or other rare arteriopathies such as dissection or fibromuscular dysplasia (Table 22.23).
- Diagnosis of cerebral vein or venous sinus thrombosis (MRI can also do this).
- Investigation of primary subarachnoid haemorrhage (see p. 907).

Management of stroke

Acute phase

Cerebral infarction

Many medical treatments, including anticoagulants, putative cerebral vasodilators, haemodilution, dextran, hyperbaric oxygen, hypercapnia and hypocapnia, have been advocated as measures which may improve the prognosis of acute cerebral infarction. However, none has been proven to be of benefit in adequate clinical trials.

Dexamethasone. There is some evidence that reducing cerebral oedema with dexamethasone may enable some patients to survive. However, life-threatening cerebral oedema is associated with large infarcts, so that the quality of survival in the few patients who may be saved in this way is poor.

Anticoagulation. There is no place for routine anticoagulation in stroke, except in patients in whom a cardiac source for emboli is certain, or strongly suspected.

For patients with a cerebral infarct who have a cardiac lesion likely to be the source of an embolus, the timing of anticoagulation is problematical. Immediate anticoagulation carries a risk of turning a soft cerebral infarct into a haemorrhagic one, but, against this, is the possibility of further cerebral embolism. This issue has not yet been the subject of a proper clinical trial. A reasonable course is to wait 10 days after the onset of the stroke before starting oral anticoagulation. The duration of anticoagulant therapy will vary, from a few weeks after an embolus from a mural thrombus, to lifelong treatment for an embolus due to rheumatic mitral or aortic valve disease.

Cerebral emboli occurring during the course of acute bacterial endocarditis or subacute endocarditis are usually considered to be a contraindication to anticoagulants; this is because of the high risk of haemorrhage from mycotic aneurysms, which are formed from spread of infection from the embolus into the vessel wall.

Hypotensive treatment. Many patients presenting with stroke have transient high blood pressures on admission. However, a sustained diastolic pressure of 110 mmHg or more is an indication for hypotensive treatment.

Surgery. All the available evidence indicates that surgical revascularisation procedures have no place in the management of acute stroke, mainly because of the high incidence of reperfusion haemorrhage and oedema within the infarcted tissue treated in this way.

Summary 4 Stroke

- Cerebral infarction causes about eight times as many strokes as cerebral haemorrhage.
- Probably only a minority of cerebral infarcts are caused by emboli from the heart. Overall, few patients require anticoagulants to prevent further strokes.
- Primary intracerebral haemorrhage may cause strokes which are clinically indistinguishable from cerebral infarction, but impairment of conscious level, vomiting and signs of raised intracranial pressure are more common with large haemorrhages.
- Secondary prevention of cerebral infarction includes treatment of hypertension, diabetes and severe hyperlipidaemia if present, weight loss, cessation of smoking and low-dose aspirin.
- Carotid surgery should be considered in patients with continuing symptoms due to a severe internal carotid stenosis.
- Unusual causes of stroke are more common in younger patients.

Intracerebral haemorrhage

As with large infarcts, dexamethasone may improve the number of patients surviving but not the quality of survival. Expanding haematomas in the cerebellum constitute an acute neurosurgical emergency, and immediate evacuation may return a moribund patient to a good quality of life. Surgical evacuation of large supratentorial haematomas is of doubtful value, however, as surviving patients are usually left profoundly disabled.

The early management of most patients with acute stroke, irrespective of the pathology, therefore consists mainly of the provision of good supportive medical and nursing care, directed towards the prevention and early treatment of secondary complications (Table 22.32, p. 904).

Rehabilitation

The mainstay of treatment after strokes from all causes is rehabilitation. This involves nursing and medical staff, physiotherapists, occupational therapists and speech therapists. Even in patients with considerable residual deficit, return home is often possible with sufficient support.

Secondary prevention

As for TIAs, secondary prevention after stroke involves minimising exposure to risk factors, by following the procedures outlined on page 899.

Prognosis

Most patients show some recovery after cerebral infarction, but this is very variable and difficult to predict. In general, the more severe the initial deficit, the less complete will be the eventual recovery. Certain features are of poor prognostic significance; these include impaired consciousness, incontinence and sustained lateral deviation of gaze. About 20% of all patients with strokes due to cerebral infarction die within the first month, and the long-term death rate is about 5–10% per annum. These late deaths are as likely to be due to myocardial infarction as to further stroke.

The recovery from spontaneous intracerebral haemorrhage (excluding subarachnoid haemorrhage) is not as good as from infarction. Mortality during the first few weeks is considerably greater than for infarction.

SUBARACHNOID HAEMORRHAGE

The majority of spontaneous subarachnoid haemorrhages are caused by berry aneurysms which develop at proximal branch points in the major cerebral vessels at the base of the brain. The common sites are the bifurcation of the middle cerebral artery, the terminal carotid, the anterior cerebral artery and the posterior communicating artery. Basilar artery aneurysms are uncommon. Aneurysms are sometimes multiple. Although mainly congenital, aneurysms may develop as a result of degenerative and hypertensive changes. Subarachnoid haemorrhage can occur at any age, but is a particularly important cause of death and disability in the 20–40 year age group. In a minority of cases, the predisposing causes listed for intracerebral haemorrhage (Table 22.32) may be responsible. In about 10% of patients, no cause for the haemorrhage is found.

Clinical features

The typical history of subarachnoid haemorrhage is severe headache of abrupt onset accompanied by neck pain and stiffness, and vomiting. Drowsiness is common, and there is often confusion and impairment of consciousness. Some patients will be deeply unconscious at presentation. In such patients, neck stiffness may be absent.

Focal hemisphere signs may be present, due to either intracerebral bleeding or vasospasm, which may affect the aneurysm-bearing vessel or other vessels. A third cranial nerve palsy (due to direct compression) often occurs with posterior communicating artery aneurysms and, less commonly, with carotid and middle cerebral artery aneurysms.

There may be papilloedema and subhyaloid haemorrhages, seen only in subarachnoid haemorrhage.

Investigation

If done within 8 hours of the haemorrhage, the CSF may not contain blood, though the pressure is usually raised. Xanthochromia – the yellowish discolouration of the supernatant CSF in a spun sample, due to haemoglobin breakdown products – does not develop for at least 24 hours. The CSF in subarachnoid haemorrhage is often obviously uniformly bloodstained. Cell counts of CSF in three separate bottles distinguishes a traumatic tap from true subarachnoid haemorrhage.

It is potentially hazardous to perform a lumbar puncture in an unconscious patient or one with focal hemisphere signs. In each case, it is likely that there is an intracerebral haematoma, with an increased supratentorial intracranial pressure. CT scanning demonstrates even quite small quantities of subarachnoid blood (Fig. 22.15), and also intracerebral blood if present.

Angiography is contraindicated in stuporose or comatose patients, but should be done at an early stage if the patient is fit enough, because of risk of re-bleeding (maximal between 7 and 14 days). Many of those not fit enough initially will improve over a few days, and angiography can then be undertaken with reasonable safety.

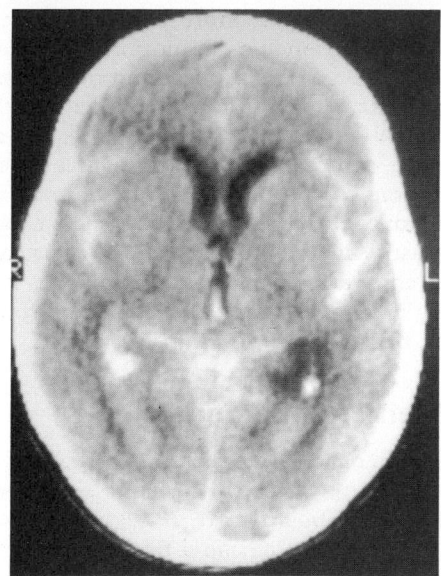

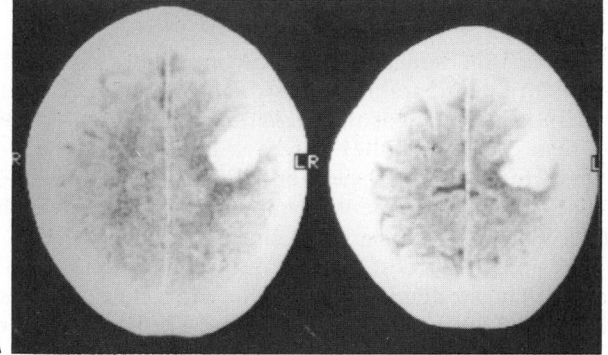

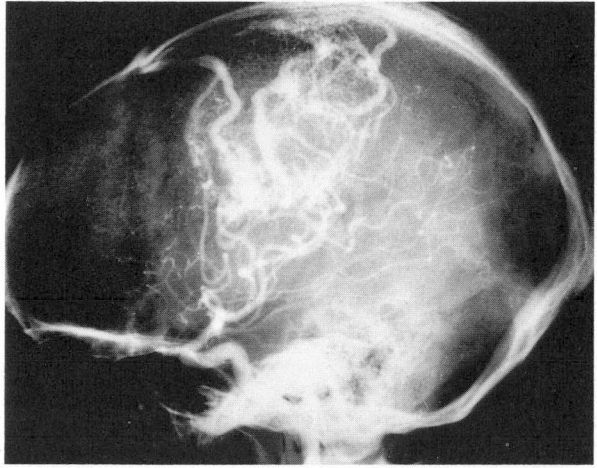

Fig. 22.15 Extensive subarachnoid haemorrhage from an anterior communicating artery aneurysm. In the unenhanced scan, blood (showing as a dense white image) is present in the interhemispheric fissure anteriorly, the Sylvian fissures, the IIIrd ventricle and the posterior parts of the right lateral ventricle.

Patients may deteriorate after subarachnoid haemorrhage, due to re-bleeding, vasospasm or hydrocephalus. CT scanning will often identify the cause.

Management and prognosis

Many aneurysms are accessible to surgical treatment by clipping. However, many, perhaps 30–40% of all patients with subarachnoid haemorrhage from aneurysms, do not survive for more than a few hours, and some will never reach hospital alive. A further 30% of patients die within the first month; the remainder survive with a re-bleed risk of about 2% per annum, unless the aneurysm can be successfully clipped.

Arteriovenous malformations

Arteriovenous malformations (AVM) tend to bleed from the venous side. Haemorrhage terminates at an earlier stage, probably because the pressure is lower, and the clinical effects are often less severe than bleeding from aneurysms. There can be episodes of bleeding over a period of many years, causing a relatively mild neurological deficit. Epilepsy is common with AVM. The diagnosis can be made on an enhanced CT scan, but the definitive test is an angiogram (Fig. 22.16). Many AVM, due to their deep situation and extent, are best left alone. Others are amenable to partial, or sometimes total, excision. Embolisation of feeding vessels offers an alternative method of treatment but, as with surgery,

Fig. 22.16 Arteriovenous malformation. A. CT scan showing an acute left frontal cerebral haemorrhage, with surrounding oedema. **B.** Left carotid angiogram in the same patient, showing an extensive arteriovenous malformation.

this often carries an unacceptable risk of producing a major deficit due to infarction of surrounding normal brain.

DEMENTIA

Dementia can be broadly defined as a persistent, and usually progressive, deterioration of intellect, behaviour and personality. The process is not necessarily irreversible. Progression of dementia usually leads to global cognitive impairment, but some dementing disorders are more focal in the early stages. Distinction must be made from acute or subacute confusional states (delirium) which are usually associated with impairment of consciousness and more rapidly reversible with appropriate treatment. Deterioration of intellect and performance may also be a major presenting feature of psychiatric disorders, particularly depression; the impairment of function is no less real but the term 'pseudodementia' is generally used in this setting.

Causes of dementia

A diagnosis of dementia should always lead to a search for a potentially treatable cause (Table 22.33). A useful general clinical rule is that patients have an organic basis for their dementia if they also have abnormal neurological signs. However, in Alzheimer's disease (the commonest cause of dementia), mental symptoms and signs invariably precede the physical signs, usually by months or years.

It is probably best to consider dementia as a whole, rather than subdivide the condition into senile and presenile on the basis of age. The younger the patient, the less likely it is that Alzheimer's disease is the cause.

Clinical diagnosis

Assessment of intellectual function is discussed on pages 860 and 861. Amnesia or dysphasia in isolation do not constitute a state of dementia, although they may be presenting features of a more global disorder. Severe language dysfunction makes more general assessment very difficult. The mode of onset and rate of progression of symptoms may give some indication about the underlying cause of dementia. Alzheimer's disease and other degenerative disorders typically progress slowly over years; more rapid deterioration should raise the possibility of spongiform encephalopathy (Creutzfeldt-Jakob disease), paraneoplastic encephalitis, communicating hydrocephalus or cerebral arteritis. Vascular dementia may have a fluctuating or stepwise course, punctuated by acute focal symptoms, but this is by no means invariable.

Investigation of dementia

All younger demented patients should have a CT scan. Table 22.34 lists the investigations which should be undertaken in a demented patient without physical signs. Pointers to an underlying cause from history or examination will permit a more selective approach to investigation in some patients.

ALZHEIMER'S DISEASE

The great majority of patients over the age of 60 with progressive dementia have Alzheimer's disease. It has been estimated that approximately 7–8% of all people over the age of 65 have this disease.

Aetiology

Alois Alzheimer described the histological abnormalities in the atrophied brains of patients dying with dementia, and these changes remain the defining characteristics of the condition; however, none of the histological changes is, in itself, unique to Alzheimer's disease. In addition to atrophy and reduced numbers of cortical neurones in all areas, many surviving neurones contain neurofibrillary tangles. Senile plaques (amyloid plaques) – structures of about 50 µm diameter – are invariably present. Both changes are found to some extent in the brains of elderly non-demented patients, so may be considered normal ageing changes. With the growth of our understanding of

Table 22.33 Causes of dementia

Cause	Examples
Degenerative	Alzheimer's disease Pick's disease Huntington's chorea Multisystem atrophy Steele-Richardson syndrome Friedreich's ataxia and other spinocerebellar degenerations Some patients with Parkinson's disease
Vascular	Multiple cerebral infarcts Diffuse small vessel disease Cerebral arteritis
Toxic	Alcohol/lead/carbon monoxide poisoning/solvent abuse
Drugs	Hypnotics, tranquillisers, barbiturates, neuroleptics
Trauma	Head injury, including subdural haematoma
Neoplastic	Frontal tumours, multiple metastases Posterior fossa tumour with hydrocephalus Paraneoplastic dementia
Hydrocephalus	Tumour Normal pressure hydrocephalus
Infection	TB meningitis, syphilis, encephalitis, toxoplasmosis, SSPE, PML, AIDS-related dementia, Kuru, CJD
Inflammatory	MS, SLE, sarcoidosis
Metabolic	Hypothyroidism, uraemia, hepatic failure, B_{12} deficiency, prolonged hypoglycaemia, prolonged hypoxia, respiratory failure, low output cardiac failure, Wilson's disease
'Pseudodementia'	Depression

SSPE = subacute sclerosing panencephalitis; PML = progressive multifocal leucoencephalopathy; CJD = Creutzfeldt-Jakob disease

Table 22.34 Investigation of dementia

● Full blood count, ESR	● Glucose
● Renal function	● Vitamin B_{12}
● Liver function	● HIV (selected patients)
● Thyroid function	● Chest X-ray, ECG
● Calcium	● CT scan
● Toxicology (selected patients)	● EEG (selected patients)
● Treponemal serology	● CSF (selected patients)

brain histochemistry, a number of theories based on altered chemistry have been proposed. Much attention has focused recently on the degenerative changes in the wide cortical cholinergic projection from the nucleus basalis of Meynert, deep in the frontal lobe.

Occasional families are found in which Alzheimer's disease is clearly inherited as an autosomal dominant trait, and in these families the onset of symptoms tends to occur at a younger age.

Clinical features

Loss of recent memory with a complaint of forgetfulness is the most common presenting symptom. Loss of interest in life and personality change, sometimes with antisocial and disinhibited behaviour, are also common early symptoms. Dysphasia, dyslexia, dysgraphia and dyscalculia are sometimes particularly marked. Dyspraxic symptoms, such as topographagnosia (inability to find one's way about in familiar surroundings) and dressing apraxia, are frequent. Loss of bladder and bowel sphincter control may be an early or late feature. Sleep disturbance is common. Wandering may become a serious problem. Increasing confusion and complete social disintegration eventually occur. The most common physical complaint in Alzheimer's disease is unsteadiness of gait. The gait may appear ataxic or Parkinsonian, and a combination of cerebellar, extrapyramidal and pyramidal signs may be found later in the disease. Myoclonus is common in the advanced stages.

The course of Alzheimer's disease is very variable, average survival being between 5 and 10 years.

Investigation and management

There is no single diagnostic test for Alzheimer's disease. The finding of diffuse cerebral atrophy on CT scanning (Fig. 22.27) and exclusion of other treatable causes of dementia usually leaves little doubt about the diagnosis.

Management is largely supportive, though there is much current interest in a possible therapeutic effect of cholinergic drugs. The disease imposes huge strains on

---

Summary 5 Dementia

- Alzheimer's disease (AD) is the commonest cause of dementia in people over 60 years of age.

- In the elderly, depression may closely mimic dementia.

- AD nearly always presents at over 55 years of age.

- Dementia in younger patients must always be thoroughly investigated, including CT scanning.

- Dementia with abnormal neurological signs as an early feature is unlikely to be AD.

---

the spouse and family of the patient. Inevitably, many patients eventually require institutional care.

PICK'S DISEASE

Pick's disease is rare. It consists of dementia with selective impairment of speech function associated with focal atrophy of frontal and temporal lobes. It is frequently inherited as an autosomal dominant condition.

HUNTINGTON'S CHOREA

Huntington's chorea is a dominantly inherited condition consisting of chorea and progressive dementia of unknown cause. It is not common, with an estimated prevalence of 1 in 20 000.

Clinical features

The onset of symptoms is gradual, usually between 30 and 50 years, beginning with either chorea or early symptoms of dementia, often taking the form of a change in personality. Chorea gradually becomes more marked, and eventually interferes with all voluntary movements. A feature of the early stages of the dementia is some retention of insight which, associated with a knowledge of the family history, can lead to severe depression, and sometimes suicide. The average duration of the disease from onset of symptoms to death is about 15 years. In the advanced stages, there is increasing dementia, akinesia and rigidity.

Management

Treatment is purely symptomatic. Neuroleptic drugs such as sulpiride, pimozide or haloperidol may help the chorea to some extent. Genetic counselling is vital. The children of a parent with Huntington's chorea have a 1 in 2 risk of developing the disease, and their children have a 1 in 4 risk. A recent advance has been the identification of a gene marker for Huntington's chorea, which should permit identification of those carrying the abnormal gene.

NORMAL PRESSURE HYDROCEPHALUS

This disorder is relatively rare but important because of its potential reversibility by surgical treatment with a vertriculo-peritoneal shunt. Patients classically present with dementia, bladder disturbance and a disorder of gait (p. 918).

DEMENTIA DUE TO VASCULAR DISEASE

This condition is probably overdiagnosed, since autopsy studies show many suspected cases to have degenerative pathology of Alzheimer type as well as the vascular lesions recognised during life. However, dementia can result from various patterns of cerebral vascular disease (see pp. 902–903):

- multiple large cortical infarcts, typically embolic from the heart
- multiple subcortical lacunar infarcts, typically due to hypertensive small vessel disease, but possibly embolic in some cases
- diffuse subcortical small vessel disease ('Binswanger encephalopathy'), also seen most often in hypertensive subjects
- diffuse patchy ischaemic damage following cardiac arrest or profound hypotension
- Cerebral arteritis (very rare).

The diagnosis of vascular dementia is likely to be made on the basis of the CT scan appearances and other evidence of vascular disease. Investigation and management involves attention to all vascular risk factors (Table 22.28, p. 898), particularly hypertension and potential sources of cardiac embolism.

CEREBRAL TUMOURS

Primary cerebral tumours account for about 10% of all tumours, and about a quarter of all intracranial tumours are metastatic. Some are much more common than others (Table 22.35 and Fig. 22.17).

There are considerable differences between tumours in children and adults. In children, most tumours arise in the posterior fossa, whereas in adults, most are supratentorial. Gliomas and meningiomas are rare in children.

Clinical features

Cerebral tumours present in four main ways:

- with symptoms and signs of focal neurological deficit
- with epilepsy, either focal or generalised (when supratentorial)
- with symptoms and signs of raised intracranial pressure
- with endocrinological effects (pituitary tumours).

Table 22.35 Classification of cerebral tumours

Tumour	Origin	Site	Age
Astrocytoma grades I–IV	Astrocytes	Mainly cerebral hemisphere. Also cerebellum and optic nerves	20 years or more, occasionally in children
Oligodendroglioma	Oligodendrocytes	Cerebral hemisphere	20 years or more
Ependymoma	Ependyma	Ventricles	Mainly children
Medulloblastoma	Neurones	IVth ventricle and cerebellum	Children
Ganglioneuroma	Neurones	IVth ventricle	Mainly children
Primary lymphoma/microglioma	Lymphoid	Hemisphere or cerebellum	Mainly adults, particularly in HIV infection
Pinealoma	Pineal	Pineal gland	Mainly children
Haemangioblastoma	Uncertain	Cerebellum	Children and young adults
Pituitary adenomas	Adenohypophyseal cells	Pituitary gland	Mainly adults
Craniopharyngioma	Epithelial cell rests in Rathke's pouch	Hypothalamus	Children and adults
Chordoma	Notochord remnants	Clivus and pituitary fossa	Young adults
Meningioma	Arachnoid	Any site of meninges	Adults (40–50 years)
Schwannoma	Schwann cells	VIIIth nerve	Mainly adults
Glomus tumour	Nodose ganglion of vagus	Jugular foramen	Adults
Cholesteatoma	Uncertain	Cerebello-pontine angle/petrous temporal bone	Adults
Skull tumours Osteoma Osteosarcoma Myeloma Metastatic carcinoma		Any part of skull	Mainly adults
Metastases	Lung, breast, kidney, colon, thyroid, etc.	Hemisphere or cerebellum	Mainly adults

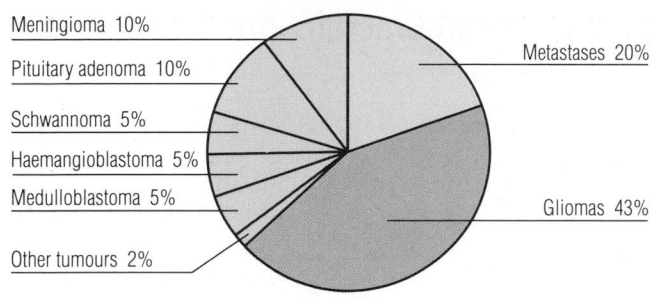

Meningioma 10%
Pituitary adenoma 10%
Schwannoma 5%
Haemangioblastoma 5%
Medulloblastoma 5%
Other tumours 2%
Metastases 20%
Gliomas 43%

Fig. 22.17 Relative frequencies of cerebral tumours.

Cerebral hemisphere tumours

A tumour arising in one cerebral hemisphere will eventually cause symptoms and signs of focal neurological deficit. Surrounding cerebral oedema often leads to focal deficit, which is greater than that caused by the tumour itself. Epilepsy is a common manifestation, whereas headache is a very variable symptom. Local invasion of the meninges by tumour may cause localised headache. A large hemisphere tumour may cause hydrocephalus, which may occasionally be accompanied by an abrupt clinical deterioration. In general, the deficit produced by tumours is contralateral to the lesion, but a swollen hemisphere may compress the contralateral cerebral peduncle against the free edge of the tentorium, causing a hemiparesis ipsilateral to the tumour. The ipsilateral IIIrd nerve may be compressed. These signs of tentorial coning occur as a late feature of a cerebral hemisphere tumour.

Papilloedema may, or may not, accompany raised intracranial pressure and, when present, is often more marked on the ipsilateral side.

Posterior fossa tumours

Tumours arising in the cerebellum cause gait ataxia if situated medially in the vermis, or of the ipsilateral limbs if situated in one cerebellar hemisphere. Later, compression of the brainstem produces local effects and involvement of the long tracts. Tumours within the brainstem itself (usually gliomas) are rare. Mid-brain and pontine tumours lead to ocular gaze palsies, internuclear and upper cranial nerve palsies, and long tract signs. Lower cranial nerve palsies occur with intrinsic medullary tumours, but are commoner with extrinsic tumours, such as glomus tumour or meningeal infiltration by carcinoma or lymphoma.

Enlarging posterior fossa tumours of any type may obstruct the aqueduct of Sylvius and cause hydrocephalus, with abrupt clinical deterioration. Coning at the foramen magnum may occur with large posterior fossa tumours. The cerebellar tonsils are pushed downwards through the foramen magnum, with accompanying compression of the medulla.

Pituitary tumours

Pituitary tumours rarely increase intracranial pressure, but may cause headache due to expansion within the pituitary fossa. Pituitary adenomas may be secretory, presenting with endocrine effects (Ch. 17). Pituitary tumours which expand out of the pituitary fossa impinge on the optic chiasm (Fig. 22.18). The characteristic visual field defect is a bitemporal hemianopia, but temporal field loss in one eye only may occur. Occasionally, pituitary tumours expand laterally into the cavernous sinus, involving the oculomotor and trigeminal nerves. Craniopharyngiomas may impinge on the optic chiasm, producing visual field loss identical to that of a pituitary tumour.

Cerebellopontine angle tumours

The commonest cerebellopontine angle (CPA) tumour is the acoustic neuroma (Fig. 22.19), but meningiomas and, less frequently, other tumours (e.g. epidermoids) also occur at this site. An enlarging extrinsic CPA mass produces progressive deafness (VIIIth nerve), facial sensory loss (trigeminal nerve), facial weakness (facial nerve) and then ipsilateral cerebellar signs. Eventually, brainstem compression leads to brainstem and long tract symptoms and signs, and hydrocephalus develops.

Investigation

Clinical suspicion of cerebral tumour comes from a history of insidious onset and gradual progression. The

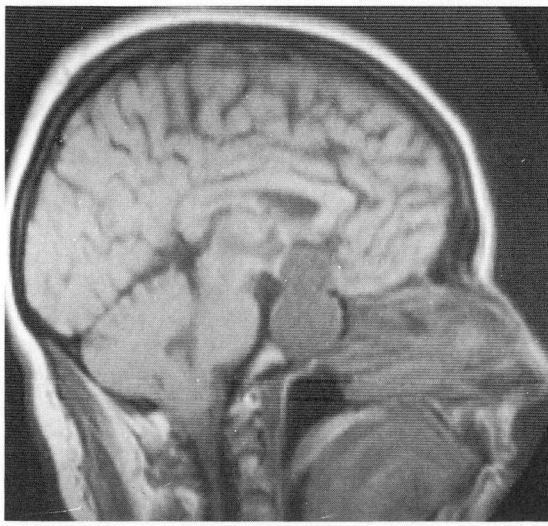

Fig. 22.18 Magnetic resonance scan, showing a large pituitary tumour in sagittal section. The tumour, an adenoma, has extended upwards, out of the pituitary fossa, and is compressing the optic chiasm. (Reproduced by permission of Dr J Stevens and Dr A Valentine.)

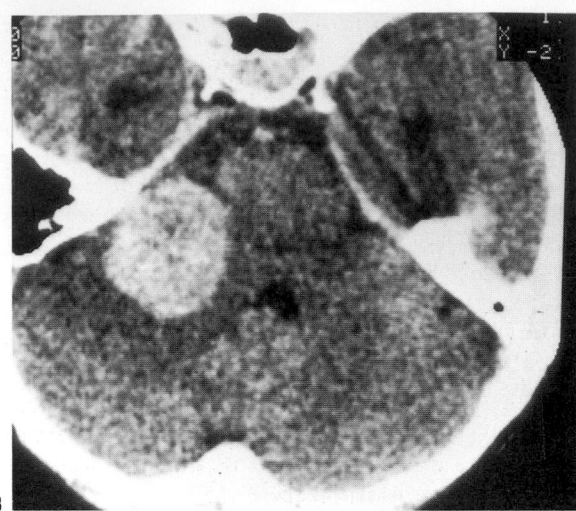

Fig. 22.19 Acoustic neuroma. After contrast enhancement, the tumour is easily seen as a mass in the cerebellopontine angle compressing the brainstem. These appearances are typical of an acoustic neuroma. Tumours of this size frequently produce cerebellar and long tract signs, and an obstructive hydrocephalus.

absence of neurological signs does not exclude a cerebral tumour. Raised intracranial pressure may give rise to subtle intellectual impairments, and careful assessment of the mental state is an important part of the examination.

Skull X-ray. The skull X-ray is of limited value but may be diagnostic in pituitary tumours, in which the pituitary fossa is often enlarged, or in CPA tumours, in which views of the internal auditory meati may demonstrate unilateral enlargement due to bony erosion from an acoustic neuroma. In meningiomas, the skull vault overlying the tumour may become thickened (hyperostosis) and the impression of large draining veins may be apparent. Chronically raised intracranial pressure causes erosion of the skull vault giving rise to a 'copper beaten' appearance, and there may also be erosion of the posterior clinoid processes. In adults, in whom the pineal may become calcified, shift from the midline by an expanding hemisphere tumour may be seen. Certain tumours, particularly oligodendrogliomas and slowly growing astrocytomas, may become calcified, and this is sometimes visible as speckled calcification on a plain skull X-ray.

CT scanning, with and without intravenous contrast enhancement, is the definitive investigation in patients suspected of having a cerebral tumour (Figs 22.19–22.22). Early gliomas and small tumours, particularly in the posterior fossa, may be missed on CT scans. MR scanning may demonstrate these lesions.

Angiography. Although vascular tumours such as meningiomas can usually be confidently identified on CT scans, neurosurgeons often require detailed information about blood supply only obtainable from angiography.

Individual cerebral tumours

Astrocytomas

Astrocytomas are the commonest primary malignant cerebral tumours. They are of variable malignancy, grade I being the least and grade IV being the most malignant. Grade IV astrocytomas are known as *glioblastoma multiforme* (Fig. 22.20). Survival times of 20–30 years are possible with a grade I astrocytoma, while only about one patient in five will survive longer than 1 year with a glioblastoma multiforme.

In adults, the great majority of astrocytomas arise in the cerebral hemispheres, brainstem astrocytomas being rare. A relatively benign form of astrocytoma occasionally occurs in the cerebellum in adults.

In children, cerebellar gliomas are often cystic, and long survivals have been reported after resection of these tumours. The optic nerve and hypothalamus are other preferential sites of astrocytoma formation in children.

Most astrocytomas remain unilateral in the cerebral hemisphere, but some grow through the corpus callosum to the contralateral hemisphere. These tend to be the histologically more malignant tumours.

Slowly growing tumours are associated with less surrounding oedema than rapidly growing tumours. Partial relief of oedema with dexamethasone may produce considerable clinical improvement, but the effect is usually short-lived.

Oligodendrogliomas

Oligodendrogliomas are slowly growing tumours, often partly calcified, arising in the cerebral hemispheres in adults. They carry a relatively good prognosis.

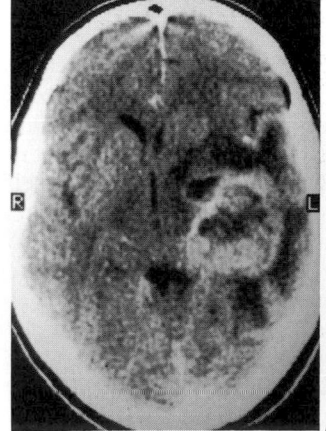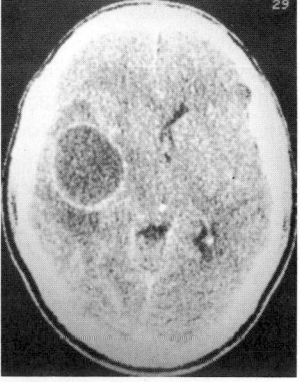

Fig. 22.20 Astrocytoma. A. A highly malignant astrocytoma, grade IV (glioblastoma multiforme), showing marked mass effect and irregular contrast enhancement. **B.** A grade II astrocytoma in the anterior part of the right temporal lobe. This tumour is cystic; there is some associated oedema and ring enhancement around the cystic part of the tumour.

Ependymomas

Ependymomas arise from the ependymal cells lining the IVth and lateral ventricles. They usually present in childhood or adolescence, and tend to run a fairly malignant course. Spread of these tumours may occur via the CSF; thus, wide dissemination sometimes results.

Medulloblastoma

Medulloblastoma is the commonest CNS tumour in children. The tumour arises in the roof of the IVth ventricle, causing ataxia, local brainstem signs, long tract signs and, eventually, hydrocephalus. They are of variable malignancy, but almost always fatal within 3 years.

Primary cerebral lymphoma/microglioma

These are rare tumours which only arise in the cerebral hemispheres in adults. They are diffusely spreading, highly malignant tumours, resistant to treatment. There is an increased incidence in AIDS.

Meningioma

Meningiomas arise from the arachnoid and are benign tumours. The most common sites are the parasagittal region arising from the falx, the meninges of the convexity over the hemispheres, the olfactory groove, and the wing of the sphenoid (Fig. 22.21). They are more common in women, and tend to present over the age of 40 years. Involvement of bone is common in meningioma, with erosion and hyperostosis. These slowly growing tumours are extremely vascular and often calcify. Surgical resection may be technically difficult and the tumours tend to regrow if incompletely removed. Occasionally, malignant change to meningosarcoma occurs.

Pituitary tumours

The endocrinological aspects of pituitary tumours are discussed in Chapter 17. Prolactinomas are associated with weight gain, amenorrhoea and galactorrhoea. Growth-hormone-secreting tumours produce gigantism in childhood and acromegaly in adults. ACTH-secreting tumours cause Cushing's syndrome. Symptoms and signs of hypopituitarism are frequent.

Schwannoma

Schwannomas arise from the Schwann cells of the peripheral nerves and nerve roots. Within the cranium, acoustic neuromas are by far the commonest (p. 911), but Schwannomas may occasionally arise on other cranial nerves.

Less common primary cerebral tumours

Pinealomas are rare tumours seen mainly in children. They affect the dorsal mid-brain, causing a characteristic failure of upward gaze, pupillary abnormalities and, sometimes, other ocular palsies.

Ganglioneuromas are uncommon tumours of relatively low malignancy. They occur in children and arise from the floor of the IIIrd ventricle.

Haemangioblastomas arise in the cerebellum in children or young adults. They may be either solitary tumours, or occur as part of the rare Von Hippel-Lindau syndrome (haemangioblastoma in CNS and retina, with renal or pancreatic cysts, hypernephroma and adrenal tumours). Haemangioblastomas are often cystic, with a vascular enhancing area of solid tissue seen on CT scanning. They present with ataxia and then symptoms of brainstem compression and hydrocephalus. Occasionally, they secrete erythropoietin, causing polycythaemia. Many are amenable to surgery.

Chordomas arise from the primitive notochord structures, the sella and clivus. They cause multiple lower cranial nerve palsies and sometimes invade the brainstem.

Craniopharyngiomas arise from epithelial cells in the pituitary stalk. They are slowly growing and often calcify. They cause optic chiasmal compression and compression of the IIIrd ventricle, leading to hydrocephalus.

Glomus jugulare tumours are highly vascular tumours, the precise cellular origin of which is uncertain. They may

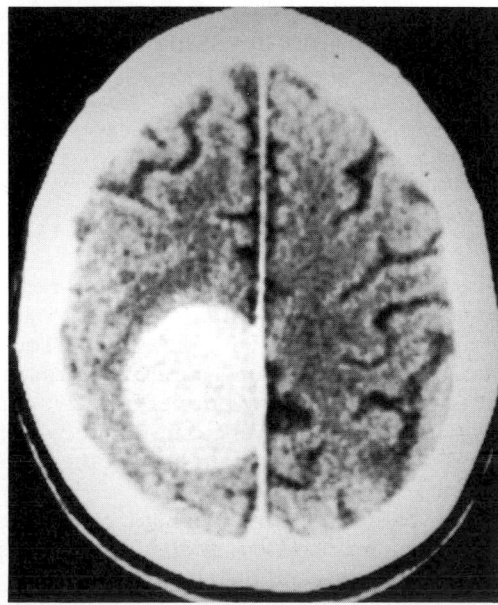

Fig. 22.21 An enhanced scan showing a right-sided parasagittal meningioma, arising from the falx. This tumour had produced a slowly progressive left hemiparesis developing over 5 years.

arise from the nodose ganglion of the vagus nerve. They give rise to the characteristic jugular foramen syndrome, which includes IXth, Xth, XIth and XIIth cranial nerve palsies on one side, accompanied by an ipsilateral Horner's syndrome, due to involvement of the cervical sympathetic fibres travelling with the carotid artery. Extension into the petrous temporal bone and middle ear causes conductive deafness, and the tumour is often visible through the tympanic membrane. With intracranial extension, brainstem and cerebellar compression may occur. Occasionally, these tumours extend into the upper part of the neck, where they may form a visible mass. Bruits over these vascular tumours are common.

Cholesteatomas within the petrous temporal bone probably arise from epithelial elements. Their relationship to middle ear disease remains uncertain. They usually present as a CPA syndrome and may involve the middle ear, producing conductive deafness.

Cerebral and cerebellar metastases

Although metastases commonly cause symptoms, many clinically silent metastases are found at post-mortem.

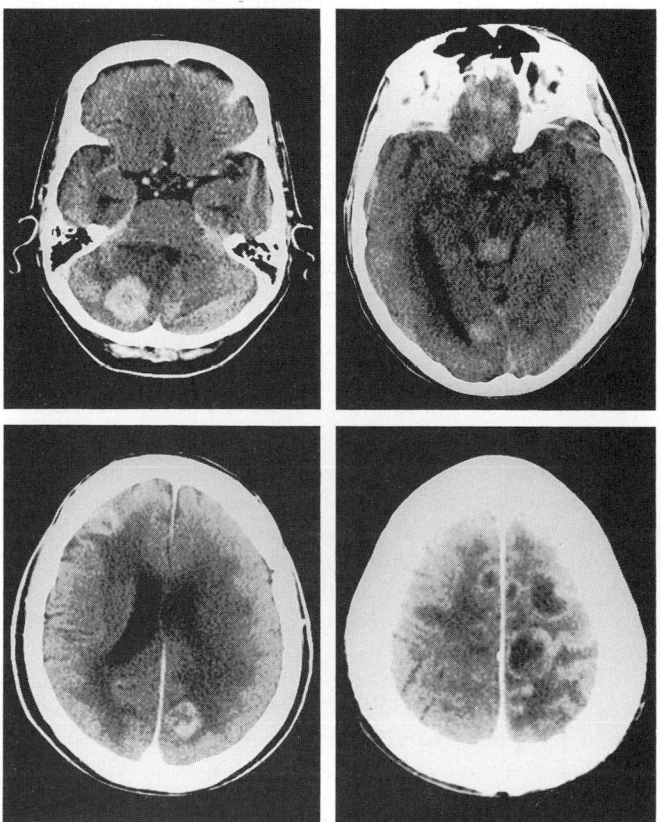

Fig. 22.22 Multiple cerebral metastases. These four contrast-enhanced scans show a cerebellar metastasis and multiple hemisphere metastases, in a patient with primary bronchogenic carcinoma.

Many are multiple (Fig. 22.22) and the cerebellum seems to be a preferential site. The commonest primary tumours are bronchus, breast, kidney, colon and thyroid; leukaemia and lymphoma are also common tumours, leading to intracranial metastases. Secondary spread may also occur to other intracranial structures, particularly the meninges, producing a malignant meningitis.

The neurological non-metastatic effects of systemic malignancy are considered on page 978.

Differential diagnosis

The differential diagnosis of cerebral hemisphere tumours is wide, and includes cerebral abscess, tuberculoma, chronic subdural haematoma, vascular disease and, occasionally, encephalitis. In the posterior fossa, demyelinating disease needs to be considered, together with structural abnormalities such as an Arnold-Chiari malformation (p. 938).

Management

The urgency of treatment of cerebral tumours depends on whether there is raised intracranial pressure, due either to the mass effect of the tumour itself, or to associated hydrocephalus.

Fits require anticonvulsants but sometimes prove resistant to therapy. Raised intracranial pressure leading to impairment of consciousness is an indication for urgent treatment to reduce cerebral oedema. Dexamethasone (10 mg immediately, followed by 4 mg 4-hourly) is usually effective, an alternative being mannitol (200 mg of a 20% solution given intravenously over 15–30 minutes). Dexamethasone is used pre- and postoperatively to protect against the development of excessive cerebral oedema induced by surgery.

Surgery

Whenever possible, the aim of treatment for benign cerebral tumours is complete surgical resection. However, inaccessibility and potential damage to normal tissue often dictates a less ambitious surgical approach. Some benign tumours may recur, but very slowly, and many patients with residual meningioma tissue will have no further problems after the main bulk of the tumour has been resected.

The role of surgery for malignant primary cerebral tumours remains uncertain. Biopsy of the tumour to establish the diagnosis and plan further treatment is often advisable. Hydrocephalus should be relieved as soon as possible by ventriculoperitoneal shunting.

While malignant primary cerebral tumours are not curable by surgery, removal of a large part of a tumour

Summary 6 Presentation and investigation of cerebral tumours

- Cerebral hemisphere tumours may present with epilepsy, progressive focal neurological deficit, or signs of raised intracranial pressure (ICP).

- Posterior fossa tumours often present with ataxia, with or without focal brainstem and long tract signs. Raised ICP is common with larger lesions, due to hydrocephalus.

- Raised ICP may not be associated with either symptoms or papilloedema.

- Pituitary tumours present with a variety of endocrine effects and, characteristically, a bitemporal hemianopia.

- Cerebellopontine angle tumours present with unilateral deafness (VIII), facial sensory loss or pain (V), facial weakness (VII), and later, ataxia and long tract signs due to brainstem and cerebellar compression; eventually, hydrocephalus occurs.

- If a cerebral tumour is suspected, a CT scan is the investigation of choice

- Lumbar puncture should never be done if a focal cerebral lesion or raised ICP is suspected.

- Cerebral metastases are single or multiple and may be indistinguishable on CT from primary tumours.

- Stroke, cerebral abscess, tuberculoma or chronic subdural haematoma may mimic cerebral tumour.

may produce improvement and relieve the effects of raised intracranial pressure. Surgery is not without risk of damaging normal cerebral tissue. The usual practice with probable malignant primary cerebral tumours presenting with epilepsy and/or a mild neurological deficit, is to delay craniotomy and biopsy until a significant neurological deficit develops. In most cases, a definite early diagnosis is unlikely to lead to any change in management.

Metastases, both cerebral hemisphere and cerebellar, are often separable from surrounding brain tissue and can, occasionally, be completely surgically removed.

Radiotherapy

The role of radiotherapy in the management of malignant gliomas remains controversial. Recent studies have shown very limited benefit in any type of adult glioma, and the morbidity of the treatment has to be weighed against the marginal benefits. Radiotherapy is particularly upsetting in older patients, producing headache, nausea, vomiting, malaise and, sometimes, exacerbation of the neurological deficit. At the start of treatment, there is often an increase in cerebral oedema, necessitating the use of large doses of dexamethasone.

Radiotherapy is usually advised for the more malignant histological types of astrocytoma but not for astrocytomas grade I. The effect in glioblastoma multiforme (grade IV)

is, however, disappointing, and the prognosis is probably not significantly altered (20% survival at 1 year). For grade II astrocytoma, the prognosis is marginally improved by radiotherapy.

The overall prognosis for astrocytomas grades I–III is about 50% survival at 5 years (Fig. 22.23). However, some low-grade tumours remain clinically static for many years. Survival for 20–30 years is possible with such tumours.

Whole neuraxis radiotherapy for childhood medulloblastoma improves the prognosis, though overall survival rates are poor (between 1 and 3 years).

Ependymomas are variably radiosensitive. Radiotherapy is usually recommended after surgery for pituitary adenomas and craniopharyngiomas.

Multiple metastases are often palliated with a combination of radiotherapy and dexamethasone.

Chemotherapy

The role of chemotherapy for primary cerebral tumours remains uncertain. Cis-platinum is the most frequently used agent. Intracerebral and meningeal leukaemia and lymphoma are often treated with a combination of radiotherapy and intrathecal methotrexate (p. 978).

BENIGN INTRACRANIAL HYPERTENSION

Benign intracranial hypertension (BIH) is also known as pseudotumour cerebri, since it may mimic a cerebral tumour. There is raised intracranial pressure without a demonstrable mass or hydrocephalus.

Aetiology and pathology

The cause of BIH is unknown. There is a strong association with obesity and an empty sella. Occasionally, there is a history of a preceding episode of dural sinus thrombosis. Hypervitaminosis A in children may cause BIH,

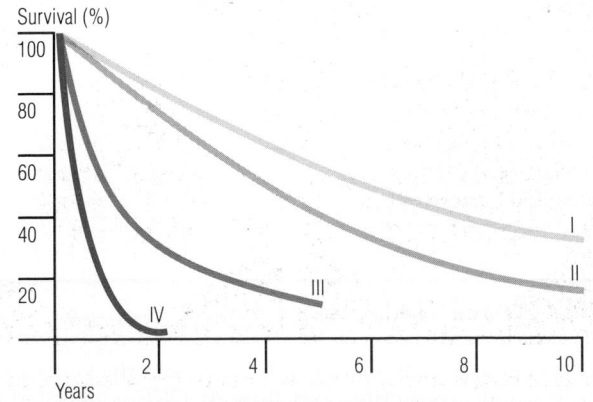

Fig. 22.23 Survival curves for astrocytoma grades I to IV.

and the prescription of certain antibiotics (including tetra-cycline and nitrofurantoin) and, occasionally, cortico-steroids may precede the development of the condition.

Cerebral blood volume is increased in BIH and a disorder of autoregulation has been proposed. There is no evidence that vasogenic oedema occurs in BIH, and the syndrome is probably not due to overproduction of CSF. Reduced absorption of CSF has been demonstrated, but it is not clear why hydrocephalus does not develop if this is the major abnormality.

Clinical features and investigation

BIH is a rare condition most commonly affecting young women. There is headache, with associated malaise and nausea. Visual obscurations are frequent, resulting from papilloedema. Visual acuity may be impaired when papilloedema is severe, with enlarged blind spots and, some-times, constriction of the visual fields. Reduced colour vision is common. About a third of patients develop diplopia, due to an associated VIth nerve palsy. Many patients are grossly obese.

Patients require a CT scan to investigate a possible mass lesion. The CT scan is either normal or shows small ventricles. When CT scan has excluded a mass lesion, lumbar puncture is safe and the diagnosis is confirmed if an opening pressure of more than 200–250 mmHg is recorded. The CSF is normal. Angiography is often needed to exclude venous sinus thrombosis.

Management and prognosis

The most important complication of BIH is permanent loss of vision. To prevent this, treatment is directed at reducing intracranial pressure. This can be achieved by repeated lumbar puncture, with removal of 20–30 ml of CSF several times a week, which may induce a remission. Some patients respond to a few weeks of high doses of prednisolone. Diuretics and carbonic anhydrase inhibitors (acetazolamide) may reduce the pressure in some patients. In obese patients, there is usually a reduction in pressure with weight loss. In a few patients resistant to all other treatment, lumboperitoneal shunting may be necessary, or optic nerve sheath decompression to protect vision.

Spontaneous remission usually occurs after a few months or years, but a small proportion of patients develop recurrent symptoms.

HYDROCEPHALUS

Hydrocephalus is an excess of CSF within the ventricles. The normal production and flow of CSF is detailed in Figure 22.24. Most CSF is absorbed through the arach-

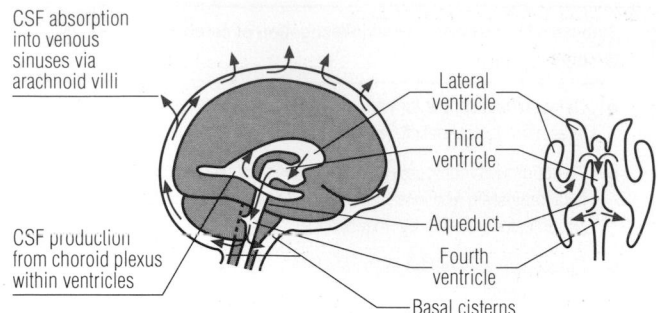

Fig. 22.24 The normal production and flow of CSF. The fluid is secreted by the choroid plexus within the lateral, third and fourth ventricles. The direction of flow is from the lateral ventricles into the third ventricle, then via the cerebral aqueduct into the fourth ventricle; from there it passes down the central canal of the spinal cord and (via the foramina of Magendie and Lushka) into the subarachnoid spaces of the basal cisterns; CSF flows within the subarachnoid space downwards around the spinal cord and upwards over the whole surface of the brain before being absorbed into the dural venous sinuses via the arachnoid granulations.

noid villi into the dural sinuses, although some is absorbed through the veins of the arachnoid. When there is obstruction to the flow of CSF, and CSF pressure rises, fluid may be forced through the ependymal lining of the ventricles directly into the brain substance. This oedema, most evident in the periventricular white matter of the lateral ventricles on CT scanning (Fig. 22.25), is charac-teristic of acute obstructive hydrocephalus.

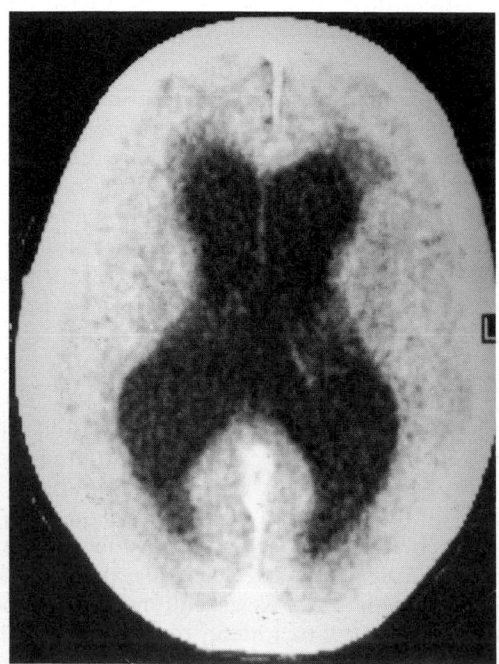

Fig. 22.25 Acute hydrocephalus, showing grossly dilated lateral ventricles, with periventricular lucency, particularly anteriorly, indicating periventricular white matter oedema. From a patient with obstruction at the level of the IIIrd ventricle.

Table 22.36 Causes of hydrocephalus

Cerebral dysgenesis	**Impaired CSF absorption** Subarachnoid haemorrhage Meningitis

Obstruction to flow of CSF
At level of third ventricle
  Hemisphere tumour
  Tumour involving third ventricle
At level of aqueduct
  Aqueduct stenosis
  Posterior fossa tumour
At level of fourth ventricle
  Atresia of exit foraminae
  Dandy-Walker syndrome
  Arnold-Chiari malformation
	Excess production of CSF
	Choroid plexus papilloma
	
	Secondary to cerebral atrophy
	
	Unknown cause
	Includes normal pressure hydrocephalus

Causes of hydrocephalus

The causes of hydrocephalus are listed in Table 22.36.

Cerebral dysgenesis

Maldevelopment or absence of any part of the brain will lead to a compensatory excess of CSF.

Obstruction to flow of CSF

This may occur within the ventricular system (non-communicating hydroccphalus) or within the subarachnoid space as a result of failure of absorption or flow through the subarachnoid space (communicating hydrocephalus). A large cerebral hemisphere lesion may compress the IIIrd ventricle and obstruct the flow of CSF, producing hydrocephalus in one, or both, lateral ventricles. Very often, a mass lesion in one hemisphere will produce compression of the ipsilateral lateral ventricle and an obstructive hydrocephalus of the contralateral lateral ventricle. Any mass lesion in the posterior fossa may obstruct the flow through the cerebral aqueduct, causing enlargement of the lateral and IIIrd ventricles (Fig. 22.26).

Impaired CSF absorption

Dilatation of the lateral IIIrd and IVth ventricles indicates a communicating hydrocephalus and may result from impairment of reabsorption of CSF. However, in many cases of communicating hydrocephalus, the CSF pressure is found to be normal (normal pressure hydrocephalus, see p. 918). Communicating hydrocephalus may occur in acute meningitis, and is seen particularly with tuberculous meningitis. It may also occur after subarachnoid haemorrhage, and in diseases in which the CSF protein remains greatly elevated over long periods of time.

Excess production of CSF

This occurs very rarely and usually indicates a papilloma of the choroid plexus.

Atrophic

Any acquired disease leading to loss of brain volume will result in a compensatory increase of CSF volume and often ventricular size. However, this is pathophysiologically distinct from hydrocephalus as discussed above. By far the commonest cause is the atrophy associated with Alzheimer's disease (pre-senile dementia). In this disease, there is both ventricular dilatation and cortical atrophy, giving characteristic CT scan appearances in most cases

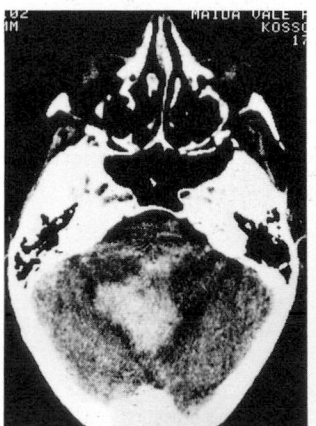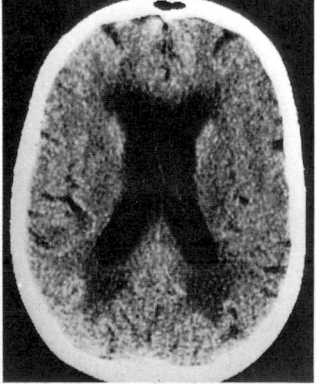

Fig. 22.26 CT scans trom a patient with an acute cerebellar haemorrhage.
Blood has a high attenuation and appears as a white mass in the cerebellum. The haemorrhage and surrounding oedema are obstructing the cerebral aqueduct, causing acute hydrocephalus with well-marked periventricular lucencies.

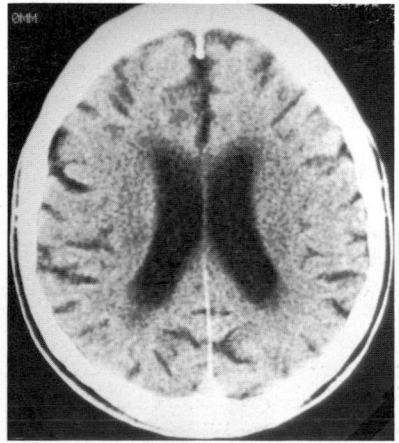

Fig. 22.27 Generalised cerebral atrophy, from a patient with Alzheimer's disease. Note the cortical atrophy, with widened sulci, and the ventricular dilatation.

(Fig. 22.27). Diagnostic difficulties arise when the degree of ventricular enlargement is out of proportion to the extent of cortical atrophy, raising the possibility of an obstructive hydrocephalus.

INFANTILE HYDROCEPHALUS

Most infants with hydrocephalus appear normal at birth.

Aetiology

Occasionally, hydrocephalus leading to enlargement of the head may be present in utero and cause birth difficulties. About half of those affected have associated malformations of the brain. Congenital cerebral aqueduct stenosis, atresia of the exit foramina of the IVth ventricle and the Dandy-Walker syndrome are the commonest abnormalities. In the *Dandy-Walker syndrome* there is atresia of the foramen of Magendie, with a failure of development of the vermis of the cerebellum, and a grossly enlarged IVth ventricle, which occupies most of the posterior fossa. In the *Arnold-Chiari malformation*, there is elongation of the medulla with herniation of the cerebellar tonsils through the foramen magnum, associated with obstruction of the outflow of CSF from the IVth ventricle (see also p. 936). Very occasionally, a posterior fossa tumour in infancy may be the cause of hydrocephalus.

Trauma leading to subarachnoid haemorrhage and subsequent hydrocephalus is probably a fairly common cause of infantile hydrocephalus, as is meningitis. In many children, however, the cause of the hydrocephalus cannot be identified with certainty.

Clinical features, investigation and management

Progressive enlargement of the head is the earliest clinical feature, with delayed development, mental retardation, fits, spastic limb weakness (particularly in the legs), optic atrophy and limitation of upward gaze. The condition is often fatal if untreated, but, occasionally, children may survive with a state of arrested hydrocephalus into adult life. They are almost invariably physically and mentally retarded.

Investigation of infantile hydrocephalus includes the sequential measurement of head circumference. In suspected cases, investigations include skull X-rays (which show cranial enlargement and separation of the sutures), CT scanning and, in selected cases, contrast radiology.

Treatment is with a shunt, which usually arrests further hydrocephalus and neurological deficit.

NORMAL PRESSURE HYDROCEPHALUS

The term normal pressure hydrocephalus refers to the presence of ventricular enlargement affecting all the ventricles without cortical atrophy (Fig. 22.28), and with normal CSF pressure (as measured at lumbar puncture).

Clinical features, investigation and management

Patients present in adult life with dementia, and, usually, an associated physical neurological deficit, comprising ataxia of gait, pyramidal signs in the limbs and incontinence of urine. In patients with pre-senile dementia, but without physical abnormalities, diagnostic difficulties may arise in distinguishing normal pressure hydrocephalus from Alzheimer's disease (p. 908). There may be similar difficulties distinguishing normal pressure hydrocephalus from diffuse small vessel cerebrovascular disease (p. 902).

The pathogenesis of normal pressure hydrocephalus is unknown in most patients. A single measurement of CSF pressure at lumbar puncture is likely to be normal, but monitoring of intracranial pressure over 24–48 hours reveals intermittent periods of raised pressure.

In patients shown to have periods of sustained increased intracranial pressure, the results of ventriculoperitoneal shunting are fair; about half of the patients show some improvement both in intellectual and physical deficits. Occasionally, this improvement is dramatic and occurs within days of shunting.

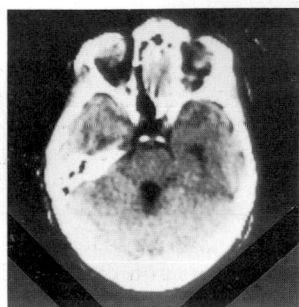
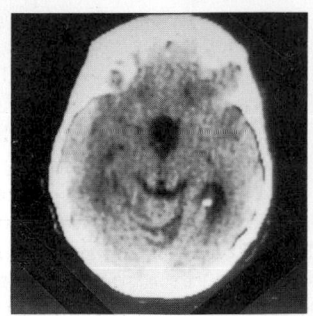
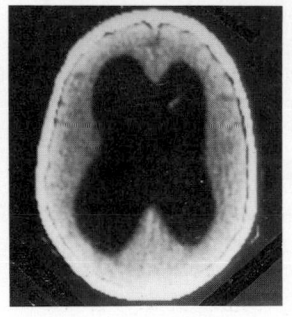

Fig. 22.28 Normal pressure hydrocephalus. There is gross enlargement of the entire ventricular system This patient has been treated with a ventriculoperitoneal shunt; the shunt tube can be seen in the right lateral ventricle.

EXTRAPYRAMIDAL DISEASE

The term extrapyramidal disease is used to refer to disorders produced by lesions affecting the basal ganglia. Diseases of the extrapyramidal system may be divided into:

- the *akinetic-rigid syndromes*, such as Parkinson's disease, which lead to a poverty of movement associated with an increase in tone
- the *dyskinesias*, in which occur involuntary movements.

Major symptoms of extrapyramidal disease

Akinesia means a loss or poverty of movement and is usually the most striking and disabling feature of Parkinson's disease. The terms hypokinesia and akinesia are used interchangeably. Bradykinesia refers to the slowness of movement seen in patients with Parkinsonism.

Rigidity refers to the increase in tone in the limbs and trunk which frequently accompanies akinesia. It is typically of a cogwheeling type, and may be increased in a limb by asking the patient to perform a repetitive movement, such as turning the head from side to side (reinforcement, or synkinesis).

Dyskinesia includes a number of different types of involuntary movement. *Tremor* is a rhythmical movement of variable amplitude and frequency. The main causes are noted in Table 22.38 (p. 922). *Chorea* refers to irregular jerky movements of variable amplitude usually involving all limbs, the trunk and sometimes the facial muscles, though not simultaneously. In its mild forms, chorea may be a discrete physical sign mimicking fidgeting movements. In its severe form, e.g. as in Huntington's chorea (p. 909), it is readily recognisable. The causes of chorea are listed in Table 22.39.

Dystonia refers to the adoption of an abnormal posture of any part of the body of variable duration. Dystonia is often not static, but associated with slow writhing movements of the affected part (athetosis). The term dystonia is now preferred to describe such dynamic abnormal movements in the setting of an abnormal posture. The causes of dystonia are listed in Table 22.40.

Myoclonus is a rapid jerking movement, usually of large amplitude, affecting one or several limbs and the trunk. It may occur as a single involuntary movement, or may be repetitive. The causes of myoclonus are listed in Table 22.41.

Tics are rapid repetitive, sometimes semi-purposeful movements, which may look like myoclonic jerks. Unlike other involuntary movements, it is usually possible for patients to voluntarily control tics, but this leads to increasing anxiety and, eventually, resumption of the tic.

Table 22.37 Akinetic-rigid syndromes

Parkinson's disease	Parkinsonism with other neurological features
Pure Parkinsonism	Wilson's disease
Postencephalitic Parkinsonism	Huntington's chorea
Neuroleptic drugs	Cerebral palsy
MPTP toxicity	Progressive supranuclear palsy
Cerebral anoxia	Multiple system atrophy

PARKINSON'S DISEASE

Parkinson's disease is an akinetic-rigid syndrome affecting about 1 in 1000 adults and about 1 in 200 over the age of 65. First described as the 'shaking palsy' by James Parkinson in 1817, this is a slowly progressive condition in which there is akinesia, a rest tremor, cogwheel rigidity and postural abnormalities. Several other disease processes may produce an identical akinetic-rigid clinical presentation; Parkinsonism is the term used to refer to such patients. The causes of Parkinsonism are listed in Table 22.37.

Aetiology

The cause of Parkinson's disease is unknown. Pathology shows degeneration of the substantia nigra and other brainstem pigmented nuclei. It is currently thought that about 85% of substantia nigra neurones must be lost, with a corresponding decrease in dopamine, before symptoms and signs of Parkinson's disease develop. The search for possible environmental factors has increased following the recent discovery that a synthetic opiate analogue, MPTP, mistakenly synthesised by opiate addicts a few years ago, can cause an illness identical to Parkinson's disease.

Clinical features

The mean age of onset of Parkinson's disease is 55 years. Tremor is the most common early symptom. Akinesia is often not noticed by the patient in the early stages, but may be commented on by relatives.

Tremor is initially only present at rest, disappearing transiently on voluntary action. It is a slow (4–6 Hz) tremor, and usually affects the hands first, producing a typical pill-rolling tremor. It may involve the whole limb, the legs and sometimes the trunk. It is exacerbated by stress and anxiety and is worse in company. The tremor is often also present on maintained posture, and may thus cause increasing difficulty with everyday tasks, such as eating and drinking. The increase in tone causing rigidity is usually of cogwheeling type.

Akinesia is frequently the most disabling feature of Parkinson's disease. There is slowness and difficulty in initiating movement which affects all voluntary activity.

Postural abnormalities are common in Parkinson's disease, a stooped flexed posture being typical. There is loss of postural control leading to falls, both standing and while walking.

The abnormalities of motor control outlined above combine to produce all the clinical features of Parkinson's disease. These include the abnormal posture, with facial masking, dribbling of saliva due to reduced swallowing, dysphonia, dysphagia and dysarthria. The combination of dysphonia and dysarthria produces the typical quiet monotonous speech with a tendency to peter out with continued effort. Difficulty initiating movement leads to pausing before walking (start hesitation), and sudden freezing when attempting to change direction. Difficulty in stopping walking, once started, may lead to festination.

There is an increased incidence of dementia in patients with Parkinson's disease.

Natural history

The course of Parkinson's disease is very variable. Quality of survival has undoubtedly been improved by levodopa treatment, but the drug has probably not greatly altered average survival, which is in the region of 10 years from the onset of symptoms.

With initial treatment at the time of diagnosis, about one-third of patients with Parkinson's disease improve markedly, one-third show some improvement and one-third show no significant improvement in terms of regaining function. When there are no signs of improvement at all, the diagnosis should be reassessed and one of the causes of Parkinsonism should be considered (Table 22.38). As a rule, Parkinsonism which is not Parkinson's disease does not respond to drug treatment.

Management

The pharmacological approach recognises both that there is a deficiency of dopamine in the corpus striatum and that a balance exists between dopaminergic and cholinergic activity. Side-effects of the anticholinergic drugs used include blurred vision due to impairment of accommodation (these drugs should not be used in glaucoma), a dry mouth, constipation and urinary hesitancy. Injudicious use in men with prostatic enlargement may precipitate urinary retention. The cerebral side-effects of these drugs include mental agitation, a toxic confusional state, psychosis and occasionally fits.

Levodopa. The introduction of levodopa revolutionised the treatment of Parkinson's disease. The drug exerts its greatest effect on akinesia. It is now given in combination with an extracerebral decarboxylase inhibitor, either as Sinemet (levodopa plus carbidopa) or Madopar (levodopa plus benserazide), which prevents systemic metabolism of levodopa, thereby promoting higher CNS levels. Much smaller doses of levodopa can thus be given, leading to a reduction in the systemic side-effects of the drug which include nausea and vomiting, postural hypotension and cardiac arrhythmias. Nausea and vomiting can be further reduced by taking levodopa after food. The drug may produce agitation, poor concentration, hallucinations and a frank psychosis. These effects frequently limit or prevent the use of the drug and are more common in elderly patients, and in those with long-standing Parkinson's disease or coexistent dementia. Excessive levodopa treatment often leads to dyskinetic movements.

Anticholinergic drugs have most effect on tremor and relatively little on the akinesia in Parkinson's disease. Anticholinergics are useful, but are now usually given in conjunction with levodopa therapy.

Amantadine, which increases synthesis and release of dopamine, has a weak anti-Parkinsonian effect and is occasionally helpful when there is intolerance to anticholinergic or levodopa therapy.

In the early stages, Parkinson's disease does not merit drug treatment. If tremor is the major disability, without symptomatic akinesia, either benzhexol (2 mg t.d.s.) or orphenadrine (50 mg t.d.s.) are recommended. Amantadine (100 mg b.d.) is an alternative.

When akinesia is severe enough to lead to disability, Sinemet or Madopar (62.5 mg of either three times a day after meals) should be started. The dose can be gradually increased. Common dose-limiting side-effects are nausea or mental changes. In patients intolerant of therapeutic doses of levodopa, bromocriptine (a dopamine receptor agonist) can be tried. It is not superior to levodopa in its therapeutic effects and causes the same side-effects.

Summary 7 Management of Parkinson's disease

- When symptoms and disability are mild, in the early stages, drug treatment may not be required.

- If tremor is the main problem, start with an anticholinergic drug, unless contraindicated (glaucoma, prostatic hypertrophy).

- If akinesia is the main problem, start dopamine with a decarboxylase inhibitor.

- Aim to alleviate, rather than abolish, the symptoms and signs.

- Be aware of the major side-effects of the drugs, which become much more common in the later stages of the disease.

- Intolerance to the drugs, particularly dopamine, is common later in the disease, and often necessitates reduction of dose and sometimes withdrawal.

- Dose-related motor oscillations may be reduced in some patients by giving divided doses more frequently.

- In later stages, motor oscillations are frequently not related to dosage.

- Selegiline is useful in some patients with the on-off phenomenon, and may slow progression of the disease in the early stages.

Levels of dopamine may be increased by the selective monoamine oxidase B inhibitor, selegiline. This drug has an effect in some patients with long-standing Parkinson's disease who develop the *on-off phenomenon*, in which, unrelated to timing of dosage of levodopa, there is an abrupt onset of severe akinesia which lasts for up to 2 hours, followed by an equally abrupt restoration of mobility.

It has been shown recently that patients with mild, early Parkinson's disease may be helped by selegiline, which slows progression of the disease, prolonging the period before treatment with levodopa is needed. Whether selegiline has any such influence in the later stages of the disease is the subject of current research.

In long-standing Parkinson's disease there is often decreasing responsiveness and increasing intolerance to treatment. However, many patients do relatively well and eventually die of causes unrelated to Parkinson's disease.

OTHER AKINETIC-RIGID SYNDROMES

Encephalitis lethargica (postencephalitic Parkinsonism)

Encephalitis lethargica is now a rare illness. It is a Parkinsonian syndrome which may occasionally follow encephalitis. The great flu epidemics of the 1920s resulted in many cases of encephalitis lethargica. All the features of Parkinson's disease may be present, but there is a limited response to drug treatment.

Multiple system atrophy

The term multiple system atrophy (MSA) is now used to refer to three overlapping degenerative conditions in which Parkinsonism is an important feature.

Progressive autonomic failure

In progressive autonomic failure (*Shy-Drager syndrome*), there are degenerative changes in the basal ganglia, cerebellum, brainstem and the intermediolateral column of the spinal cord (producing sympathetic dysfunction). Patients often present initially with a syndrome indistinguishable from Parkinson's disease, although tremor is uncommon. Incontinence and impotence are early symptoms and, later, an obvious widespread autonomic disturbance develops, with postural hypotension, failure of sweating and respiratory problems, including sleep apnoea.

Olivopontocerebellar degeneration

In olivopontocerebellar degeneration, there are severe degenerative changes in the cerebellum, pons and medulla. Clinically, a progressive cerebellar, limb and gait ataxia, with dysarthria and nystagmus, overshadows Parkinsonism. Pyramidal signs are also present.

Striatonigral degeneration

In striatonigral degeneration, there are extensive degenerative changes in the basal ganglia. This is the akinetic syndrome most likely to be confused with Parkinson's disease.

All three syndromes comprising MSA are essentially untreatable, there being little or no response to levodopa therapy. Syndromes are relentlessly progressive and death usually occurs within 5 years of onset.

Steele-Richardson-Olszewski syndrome (Progressive supranuclear palsy)

Steele-Richardson-Olszewski syndrome is characterised by Parkinsonism without tremor, and a progressive supranuclear ocular (gaze) palsy, widespread pyramidal signs and, sometimes, dementia. Patients present with difficulty in walking or visual symptoms, particularly with reading or looking downwards. The syndrome is rarely helped by levodopa or other drug treatment.

Cerebral anoxia

Diffuse cerebral anoxia (usually resulting from cardiorespiratory arrest) occasionally leads to Parkinsonism, due to bilateral basal ganglia infarction with relative preservation of other parts of the CNS. In younger people, carbon monoxide poisoning and severe hypotension with hypoxia in opiate overdosage are the usual causes of this syndrome. The Parkinsonism is unresponsive to drug treatment and is sometimes progressive.

Wilson's disease (hepatolenticular degeneration)

Behavioural changes and dyskinesias are the common neurological manifestations of Wilson's disease in childhood, but Parkinsonism, often with dyskinesias, is the more common adolescent and early adult presentation (p. 643). Presentation of Wilson's disease in adult life is almost invariably with the neurological manifestations, and patients may present as late as the fifth decade. Although the basal ganglia bear the brunt of neurological damage in Wilson's disease, copper deposition in the CNS is widespread, with dementia developing in untreated patients. Wilson's disease must be considered in any child or young adult presenting with an extrapyramidal syndrome. Copper deposition in Descemet's membrane at the margin of the cornea may produce a Kayser-Fleischer ring. Copper deposition in the lens may cause a cataract, and deposits in the nail beds a bluish discolouration.

DYSKINESIAS: ABNORMAL MOVEMENTS

The dyskinesias include tremor, chorea, hemiballismus, dystonia and myoclonus.

Tremor

Tremor (see also p. 919) may be classified as:

- *postural* tremor when it is maximal with maintained posture
- *rest tremor*, characteristic of extrapyramidal diseases
- *action tremor*, due to diseases affecting the cerebellum directly or its connections in the brainstem (Table 22.38).

Normal physiological tremor may be exaggerated by anxiety and is also enhanced in thyrotoxicosis, by sympathomimetic drugs and by alcohol.

Essential tremor

Essential tremor (also known as benign essential tremor, familial tremor and senile tremor) is the commonest of the dyskinesias. It is usually mild. The cause remains uncertain. It is a postural tremor which is also present on, but not exacerbated by, action. This differentiates it from cerebellar or Parkinsonian tremor. There are no other neurological abnormalities.

Emotional circumstances increase the tremor, and unlike other forms of tremor, small amounts of alcohol

Table 22.38 Causes of tremor

Tremor	Cause
Postural tremor	
Exaggerated physiological tremor	Anxiety
	Alcohol
	Thyrotoxicosis
	Drugs – some tricyclic antidepressants
	Lithium
	Sympathomimetics, e.g. bronchodilators
Benign essential tremor	Uncertain
Severe cerebellar disease (rubral tremor)	
Rest tremor	Parkinson's disease
	Causes of Parkinsonism (Table 22.38)
Action tremor	
Cerebellar and brainstem disease	
	MS
	Infarction or haemorrhage
	Tumours
	Hereditary ataxias and spinocerebellar degenerations
Benign essential tremor	Uncertain

have a therapeutic effect. There is a positive family history in at least 50% of cases, and the condition is thought to be dominantly inherited with variable penetrance.

Beta-receptor-blockers, such as propranolol, help about one-third of patients. Judicious use of alcohol can be recommended in certain patients, and benzodiazepines are occasionally helpful.

Asterixis

The term asterixis is used to refer to the flapping tremor seen in the severe metabolic disturbances of respiratory, renal and hepatic failure. It is a postural tremor, and is best seen in the outstretched hands.

Chorea

Chorea (see also p. 919) has a number of causes, listed in Table 22.39.

Huntington's chorea

Huntington's chorea is discussed on page 909.

Sydenham's chorea

Sydenham's chorea, a complication of rheumatic fever, is now rare. The onset is usually gradual, most cases occurring between 7 and 12 years of age. In only 30% of cases is there a clear preceding history of a streptococcal infection with rheumatic fever.

More widespread cerebral disturbance occurs in some patients, who may develop a confusional state or behavioural changes. The pathogenesis of these neurological complications of streptococcal infection is uncertain, but immune complex deposition is likely.

Chorea is of variable severity. All the neurological manifestations resolve gradually over 1–6 months. Symptomatic treatment with neuroleptics, such as chlorpromazine or tetrabenazine, may be necessary. A history

Table 22.39 Causes of chorea

Sydenham's chorea	**With systemic disease**
	Thyrotoxicosis
Chorea gravidarum	Polycythaemia rubra vera
	Encephalitis lethargica
Chorea with oral contraceptive pill	SLE
	Hypocalcaemia
Huntington's disease	Hypernatraemia
Drug-induced	**Hemiballismus or hemichorea**
Neuroleptic drugs	Infarction
Phenytoin	Tumour
Alcohol	
Levodopa	

of Sydenham's chorea predisposes to the later development of chorea gravidarum, or chorea with the oral contraceptive pill or other drugs, such as phenytoin.

Hemiballismus

Hemiballismus, or hemichorea, is a dramatic type of involuntary movement in which there are large amplitude throwing movements of the limbs on one side. It usually occurs acutely in elderly patients, and is the result of infarction involving the contralateral subthalamic nucleus. It very occasionally occurs with a tumour or after head injury. Hemiballismus is usually an isolated abnormality, but may be accompanied by a hemiparesis or hemisensory impairment. It usually resolves spontaneously within a few months, but symptomatic treatment with neuroleptic drugs is necessary when the movements are severe.

Dystonia

The causes of dystonia are listed in Table 22.40. Acute drug-induced dystonia is the most common type; it is usually mild and reversible on stopping the offending drug.

Spasmodic torticollis

Spasmodic torticollis may occur as an isolated phenomenon or as part of a generalised dystonia. There is involuntary turning of the head to one side, which may be a maintained posture or a rhythmical movement, and

Table 22.40 Causes of dystonia

Focal dystonia
Writer's cramp
Spasmodic torticollis
Cranial dystonia
Hemiplegic dystonia due to, e.g., strokes, tumours, encephalitis, trauma

Generalised dystonia	
Drug-induced acute and tardive dystonias	
Anti-emetics; prochlorperazine, metaclopromide	
Neuroleptics	
Levodopa and dopamine agonists	
Torsion dystonia	
Dystonia with other cerebral diseases	
Hereditary –	Gangliosidoses
	Metachromatic leucodystrophy
	Wilson's disease
	Huntington's disease
	Homocystinuria
Acquired –	Cerebral palsy
	Encephalitis lethargica
	Mitochondrial cytopathy

there is frequently associated extension of the neck (retrocollis). Onset is usually in adult life without obvious provocation, although occasionally there is a history of trauma to the neck. It may last a few weeks or months, remit and not recur. However, recurrent episodes are common, and in some patients there is no remission.

Treatment is difficult. Neuroleptic drugs may help, but may eventually induce extrapyramidal disease. A combination of diazepam and benzhexol can be effective and is safe if long-term treatment becomes necessary. Surgical denervation of the neck muscles is rarely successful. Intramuscular injection of botulinum toxin is helpful in selected cases.

Torsion dystonia (dystonia musculorum deformans)

Torsion dystonia is a rare and disabling generalised dystonia of unknown cause. When it presents in childhood, there is often a family history, or examination of other family members may reveal milder forms of the condition. Inheritance as an autosomal dominant or recessive trait has been reported. The disease tends to be more severe in children than in the adult-onset group. Typically, dystonic posturing of the trunk and limbs is provoked or exacerbated by voluntary actions.

Large doses of benzhexol (up to 120 mg a day), sometimes combined with diazepam, offer the best chance of improvement. Attempts at stereotaxic surgery may have to be considered, but bilateral thalamotomy necessarily carries substantial risks.

Cranial dystonia

Cranial dystonia includes: *blepharospasm*, an involuntary closure of the eyelids due to spasm of the orbicularis oculi muscles; and *oromandibular dystonia*, which refers to involuntary dystonic movements of the tongue, jaw and face which may seriously interfere with speech and eating. The cause of these dystonias is unknown. Cranial dystonia usually starts in middle-age and does not remit.

Treatment, as in other dystonias, is unsatisfactory. Neuroleptic drugs are sometimes helpful and the best combination is high-dose benzhexol and diazepam. Injection of botulinum toxin into the orbicularis oculi muscles may relieve blepharospasm for up to 3 months.

Writer's cramp

Some cases of writer's cramp are probably psychogenic, but the condition is widely regarded as being a focal dystonia with an organic basis, albeit of unknown nature. It almost always occurs as an isolated abnormality. Observation of the patient writing demonstrates the problem.

The pen is usually gripped awkwardly and/or too tightly with an abnormal posture of the hand and arm and sometimes of the trunk and head. Writing is slow and laborious, and becomes increasingly illegible with continued effort. The condition may also affect other repetitive, fine manipulative tasks, e.g. musicians often present with a similar difficulty in playing their instruments.

Myoclonus

The causes of myoclonus are listed in Table 22.41. Myoclonus may be divided into two major categories, generalised and focal or segmental myoclonus.

Generalised myoclonus may be divided into three subgroups:

- *Essential myoclonus* refers to myoclonus which is not associated with any other neurological abnormality. It is often familial and runs a benign course.
- *Myoclonic encephalopathies* are generalised progressive or static encephalopathies in which myoclonus is a frequent or recognised feature.
- *Myoclonus associated with epilepsy* (see page 893).

Focal myoclonus is rare. Lesions of the cortex or cerebral hemisphere may occasionally be the cause. Hemifacial spasm sometimes takes the form of myoclonic jerking, but a more continuous, less myoclonic type of involuntary muscular contraction is more usual. The pathophysiology in hemifacial spasm remains unknown. In some cases, a peripheral nerve basis is suggested by the occasional occurrence of hemifacial spasm with posterior fossa compressive tumours, and following Bell's palsy.

Table 22.41 Causes of myoclonus

Type of myoclonus	Cause
Generalised myoclonus	
Essential familial myoclonus	
Myoclonic encephalopathies	Degenerative cerebral diseases, e.g. gangliosidoses, Lafora body disease, hereditary ataxia
	Encephalitis lethargica
	Subacute sclerosing panencephalitis
	Creutzfeldt-Jacob disease
	Metabolic – uraemia, hypocalcaemia, hepatic failure, hyponatraemia, respiratory failure (CO_2 narcosis), alcohol withdrawal
	Post-traumatic myoclonus
	Post-anoxic myoclonus
Myoclonus with epilepsy	
Focal myoclonus	Cortical or cerebral hemisphere lesions
	Brainstem degeneration or infarction
	Spinal myoclonus

Palatal myoclonus is indicative of a brainstem lesion involving olivodentatorubral pathways. Myoclonus occurs very rarely with spinal cord lesions.

Drug-induced extrapyramidal disease

Chlorpromazine and related drugs (the neuroleptics) may produce a number of extrapyramidal side-effects including Parkinsonism, acute dyskinesias, tremor and tardive dyskinesia. The anti-emetics, metaclopramide and prochlorperazine, also have neuroleptic properties, and may produce acute and chronic extrapyramidal syndromes. Most tremors and dystonias resolve on withdrawing the offending drug, and involuntary movements can often be acutely stopped by intravenous anticholinergic drugs, such as benztropine. Tardive dyskinesias are the exception. Excessive levodopa therapy is a common cause of dyskinesia and dystonia in patients with Parkinson's disease.

Tardive dyskinesia

Tardive dyskinesia is the most serious side-effect of neuroleptic treatment; it requires at least 6 months of continuous neuroleptic administration. The usual manifestations are orofacial dyskinesias with a variety of chewing, pouting and lip-smacking movements, combined with a discrete dystonia, or choreiform limb movements and, sometimes, rocking trunk movements. Occasionally, the dyskinesias may be incapacitating. Withdrawing the drug responsible leads to gradual improvement in about half the patients, with resolution over a period of up to 3 years. However, in other patients there is no improvement and in a small minority the dyskinesia is progressive and resistant to all treatment, despite stopping the neuroleptic drug.

The frequent prescription of drugs with neuroleptic properties, such as prochlorperazine and metaclopramide, emphasises the need to take a careful and detailed drug history in all patients presenting with symptoms and signs of extrapyramidal disease.

HEAD INJURY

In the UK, approximately 5000 people die each year as a result of head injury and many others survive, but with some disability. Road traffic accidents are the commonest single cause, and alcohol can be implicated both in many of these and in other causes of severe head injuries. Fracture of the skull occurs in only a small proportion of head injuries. Its absence does not imply a mild head injury, but the presence of a skull fracture is associated with a greatly increased incidence of intracranial haemorrhage.

Effects of head injury

Immediate

Severe blows to the head cause shearing forces within the brain, causing both diffuse axonal injury, particularly to the white matter, and also focal areas of damage in the cortex and deeper parts of the brain. Haematomas may develop deep within the hemispheres, often distant from the site of impact. The inferior surfaces of the frontal and temporal lobes are particularly common sites of haematoma formation, because of their rough bony surfaces. Lacerations of the cortex may be produced by depressed skull fractures.

Secondary

Haematoma formation

Haematomas may form at the time of the head injury, but often develop during the first 24 hours after injury and sometimes over longer periods. Their maximum effect on cerebral function may occur at much longer intervals, the most extreme example being chronic subdural haematomas.

Intracerebral haematomas may be multiple and are of very variable size (Fig. 22.29). Oedema developing around haematomas will further contribute to a rise in intracranial pressure. Extradural haematomas (Fig. 22.30) develop within hours of head injury in which the skull vault is fractured. They are due to bleeding from torn meningeal arteries, commonly the middle meningeal artery. On arrival at hospital, the patient may be alert and orientated, but the conscious level then rapidly deteriorates. Extradural haematomas may be fatal, or lead to perma-

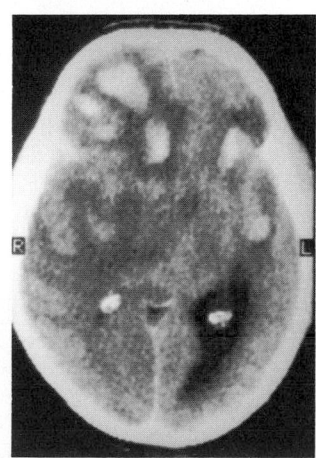

Fig. 22.29 Multiple, bilateral intracerebral haematomas in a young man with a severe closed head injury. In the right hemisphere, there is massive oedema, causing midline shift and obstruction of CSF flow, leading to hydrocephalus of the left lateral ventricle.

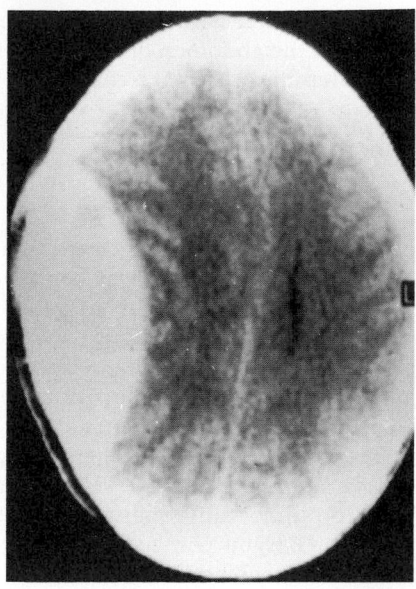

Fig. 22.30 Right-sided extradural haematoma, associated with a skull fracture. There is acute severe cerebral compression. (Reproduced by permission of Dr J Stevens and Dr A Valentine.)

nent brain damage, unless promptly treated. Large acute subdural haematomas may produce similar effects, but are less likely than extradural haematomas to lead to a rapid early deterioration of cerebral function. Acute subdural haematomas are relatively uncommon, probably because bleeding is due to rupture of cortical veins crossing the subdural space, which occurs more slowly than arterial bleeding. Bleeding into the subdural space usually presents later as a chronic subdural haematoma (p. 926).

Cerebral oedema and raised intracranial pressure

Cerebral oedema may result from diffuse cerebral injury without haematoma formation; it also develops around haematomas. The effect is a rise in intracranial pressure which may be life-threatening.

Infection

There is a risk of meningitis or cerebral abscess with any penetrating injury of the skull. Leakage of CSF through the nose (rhinorrhoea) or the ear (otorrhoea) indicates a basal skull fracture and the potential for development of meningitis. Fractures involving the nasal sinuses may also lead to infection.

Extracranial factors complicating the effects of head injury

A compromised airway, chest injury or infection and, rarely, the adult respiratory distress syndrome may all lead to hypoxia. Together with hypotension, usually the result of bleeding in the abdomen or associated with other injury, hypoxia intensifies cerebral ischaemia.

Management

Early management

The first consideration in the management of head injury is resuscitation (Ch. 14). The airway must be cleared. Intubation and artificial ventilation may be necessary. Shock in head-injured patients is almost always the result of other major injury, and requires immediate correction.

Having resuscitated the patient, an initial neurological examination is undertaken. This includes a thorough examination of the skull and scalp, determining any CSF leaks, and assessing the conscious level; it is particularly important to monitor subsequent improvement or deterioration. The Glasgow coma scale (p. 859) provides a simple means of assessment.

Neck injuries are a common accompaniment of head injury. The neck must therefore be handled with care until cervical spine X-rays have excluded major bony injury.

Controversy surrounds the necessity for skull X-rays in mild head injury. Definite indications are a history of loss of consciousness at any time, the presence of scalp bruising or swelling, any neurological signs, a CSF leak or evidence of a penetrating injury. The absence of a skull fracture does not exclude serious intracranial problems in an individual patient, but for patients with a fracture whose conscious level is impaired, there is a 1 in 4 risk of intracranial haemorrhage. This compares with a 1 in 30 risk of haemorrhage in patients with a fracture but with a normal conscious level; a 1 in 120 chance in patients without a skull fracture, but with impairment of conscious level; and a 1 in 6000 chance in patients without skull fracture or impairment of conscious level.

It is important to know what the conscious level was immediately after the head injury; a history of a lucid interval of consciousness suggests the possibility of an extradural haemorrhage, for which urgent CT scanning and treatment is necessary.

Neurosurgical referral

Many patients with minor head injury can be rapidly discharged if there is no history of loss of consciousness, no evidence of skull fracture and no abnormal neurological signs. Any patient in whom there has been loss of consciousness for any period must be admitted and observed for 24 hours. Neurosurgical referral in obvious severe head injury is clearly essential. Neurosurgical advice should also be sought for any patient who has suffered a period of unconsciousness lasting for more than an hour, who has abnormal neurological signs persisting for more than a few hours, or who has a skull fracture. Referral is particularly important if there is a basal skull fracture, a compound depressed fracture, or evidence of a penetrating injury.

Treatment of intracranial haematomas

Extradural haematomas often increase in size during the first few hours after head injury, and prompt evacuation is crucial. Acute subdural haemorrhage is less common, and deterioration in the hours following head injury is not characteristic of this type of bleeding. Large subdural collections need to be evacuated.

Large intracerebral haematomas are evacuated, particularly if associated with neurological deterioration or a very poor initial neurological state. Multiple small haematomas are best managed conservatively.

CSF leaks usually resolve within a few days and surgical treatment is not necessary. Prophylactic antibiotics should be given.

Depressed skull fractures alone do not necessarily require treatment, but if there is cortical damage, reduction is necessary, and open fractures require surgical closure of the dura and skin.

Cerebral oedema frequently develops after major brain injury, compounding the neurological deficit. Mannitol and frusemide are effective in reducing this, but the use of dexamethasone in the treatment of cerebral oedema resulting from head injury is controversial. Artificial ventilation is often necessary in severe head injury, and ventilation is sometimes used electively to reduce arterial CO_2 levels in order to reduce intracranial pressure (see Ch. 14). Whether or not this alters the outcome of brain damage due to head injury is uncertain.

Late complications of head injury

Persistent physical neurological deficit is the rule after severe head injury. In addition to hemiparesis or quadraparesis, dysphasia and visual field defects are common. Cranial nerves are commonly affected (e.g. diplopia is a common and troublesome post-head-injury symptom). Cerebellar deficits are fairly common. Brain injury may eventually lead to focal or generalised cerebral atrophy, as well as hydrocephalus. Epilepsy usually develops later, sometimes years after the injury.

Chronic subdural haematoma

Chronic subdural haematoma is more common in older patients. In at least 50% of cases there is no history of any preceding head injury, and in others, the injury recalled is usually trivial and not associated with loss of consciousness or other immediate neurological sequelae. Degradation of the subdural blood produces smaller molecules with greater osmotic effect, and the subdural haematoma increases in size over weeks or months, changing into a straw-coloured fluid. This may present with hemisphere symptoms and signs, together with symptoms and signs of raised intracranial pressure. A mild hemiparesis with intellectual deterioration and a fluctuating level of consciousness is the classical, but by no means the only, presentation of chronic subdural haematoma. Papill-oedema is often present. Chronic subdural haematomas are bilateral in a proportion of cases (Fig. 22.31).

The differential diagnosis includes cerebral tumour or abscess, and chronic subdural haematoma is often mis-diagnosed as cerebrovascular disease. Treatment by drain-age of the haematoma through burr holes often produces a marked improvement, regardless of the age of the patient.

Boxing encephalopathy

A combination of progressive cognitive impairment, dys-arthria, ataxia, extrapyramidal and pyramidal signs may develop in some boxers. This 'punch drunk' syndrome is the result of repeated blows to the head, and a similar syndrome may result from repeated minor head injury in other sports, e.g. rugby football or diving. The cerebral damage is irreversible. CT scans usually show diffuse atrophy.

Psychological effects of head injury

Amnesia for events after the injury (post-traumatic amnesia) is always longer than that before the event (pre-traumatic or retrograde amnesia). The period of post-

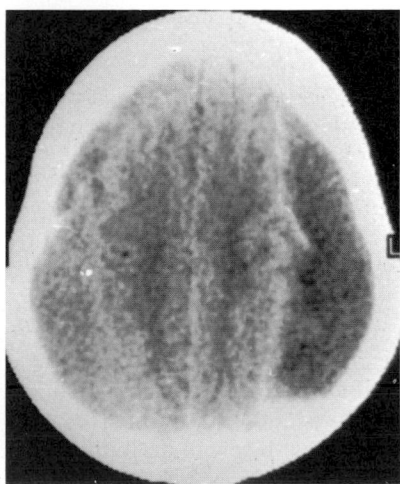

Fig. 22.31 Chronic bilateral subdural haematomas. On the left hemisphere, there is a clear line of demarcation between compressed brain and the subdural collection. The attenuation of the subdural is mainly low, indicating that it is chronic, but there is fresh blood, producing a fluid level in the posterior part of the subdural. There is a smaller right chronic subdural haematoma.

traumatic amnesia is related to the severity of the head injury. Some intellectual impairment after severe head injury is inevitable. Most improvement occurs within the first few months, but can occur for up to 2 years. Increasingly, multidisciplinary rehabilitation units are adapting to the needs of increasing numbers of head-injured patients, many of whom are young.

Some patients develop a variety of persistent and disabling symptoms after apparently minor head injuries. Their symptoms usually include headache, positional vertigo, irritability, poor memory and concentration, and a general failure to cope with their usual activities. There are often associated depressive symptoms, and there has been much unproductive debate as to whether such symptoms are due to 'organic' brain damage or psychological factors. In practice the distinction is not possible or helpful. Certainly there are demonstrable neuropsychological deficits in many such patients, and these may result from microscopic shearing lesions affecting axonal fibres in the subcortical white matter and brainstem, attributable to the distortion of brain substance by linear and torsional forces during sudden acceleration and deceleration. This view is supported by the occurrence of very similar symptoms in many patients with whiplash injuries, in whom there has been no direct trauma to the head at all. In some patients with prolonged post-traumatic symptoms, there seems little doubt that the degree and duration of disability is determined to some extent by the patient's personality and the circumstances under which the injury occurred. Legal proceedings may complicate the issue further, but more often by perpetuating anxiety and uncertainty than by inducing a state of frank malingering. In helping the patient to return to a more normal life, explanation and reassurance about residual symptoms is generally more effective than a dismissive approach.

CEREBRAL PALSY

The term cerebral palsy refers to a variety of neurological deficits, mainly affecting motor function, which arise as a result of prenatal insult, birth injury or some illness in early infancy. Implicit in the diagnosis is the assumption that the deficit is static, but it is usually impossible in early life to establish the extent of the cerebral injury, which only becomes fully manifest in late childhood. In addition to motor deficits, intellectual impairment and behavioural problems are common. The majority of children with cerebral palsy survive into adult life.

Incidence and aetiology

The incidence of cerebral palsy varies from country to country, but is of the order of 2–5 per 1000 live-born children surviving to school age.

Table 22.42 summarises the many factors known to be important in the development of cerebral palsy.

Major types of cerebral palsy

The classification of the cerebral palsies is descriptive, and is based on the major motor deficit (Table 23.43).

Spastic hemiplegia is the commonest type of cerebral palsy. In addition to the hemiplegia, there may be a hemisensory and hemianopic visual field defect, and sometimes dysphasia. There are often bilateral lesions, and up to half of these children have learning difficulties. Some have associated choreoathetosis and many develop epilepsy.

Spastic paraplegia causes difficulty in walking; the legs often do not develop properly and are short. The upper limbs are relatively spared, although the reflexes are brisk, and there is sometimes clumsiness of the hands. Learning difficulties, fits and squints are all common.

Tetraplegia is the result of extensive bilateral cortical damage, which leads to mental retardation and, often,

Table 22.42 Factors important in causation of cerebral palsy

Antenatal
Developmental abnormalities
Infections, e.g. CMV, rubella, toxoplasma, syphilis
Hypoxia, e.g. placenta praevia, placental haemorrhage, maternal hypotension
Pre-eclamptic toxaemia
Irradiation
Maternal age <20 or >35 years
Twins

Natal	
Trauma	Intracerebral haemorrhage
Breech delivery	Subdural haemorrhage
Prolonged or precipitous delivery	Intraventricular haemorrhage
	Subarachnoid haemorrhage
Prematurity	
Postmaturity	

Postnatal in preterm infants
Cerebral ischaemia
Cerebral haemorrhage
Hypoxia secondary to respiratory distress syndrome
Acidosis
Hypothermia
Hypoglycaemia

Postnatal in children with normal CNS at birth
Encephalitis
Meningitis
Hypoxia, e.g. during cardiac surgery
Kernicterus
Trauma, including non-accidental injury

Table 22.43 Classification of cerebral palsy

Spasticity	Cerebellar ataxia
Hemiplegia	
Paraplegia (diplegia)	Mixed syndromes
Tetraplegia	
Involuntary movements	
Choreoathetosis	
Dystonia	

visual and sensory deficits, in addition to a spastic tetraplegia. The visual defect may be cortical in origin, or due to optic nerve atrophy. Squints are common, as is epilepsy. The bilateral upper motor neurone deficit leads to a pseudobulbar palsy. Many children do not survive for more than a few years.

In *choreoathetosis and dystonia*, choreoathetoid movements may not develop for some months postnatally. The early brief choreiform movements may be subtle, and athetosis may not develop until the child is about 2 years old. The involuntary movements often lead to dysarthria, but these children are usually of normal intelligence. In the past, kernicterus was a common cause of this type of palsy.

Ataxia, a form of pure cerebellar ataxia thought to be usually due to maldevelopment of the cerebellum, is occasionally seen; it is often associated with mental retardation.

Mixed syndromes are common, the most frequent being a combination of a spastic paraplegia and ataxia. There is often associated hydrocephalus, possibly the result of intraventricular haemorrhage prenatally, or birth trauma.

Management

The full extent of disability in children with cerebral palsy may not be evident for some years, and it is important from an early stage to recognise potentially treatable additional deficits such as squints, epilepsy and deafness. Physiotherapy has a large role to play, but contractures and other deformities inevitably develop in some children and may require surgical treatment. Dislocation of the hip is common in spastic legs. The combined efforts of therapists from various disciplines are necessary, together with family counselling and social support. Many children require special education. Specially adapted equipment, such as typewriters and communicators, may be needed to enable the child with severe disability but normal intelligence to communicate. Lack of mobility is a major problem, threatening to deprive children of many educational and recreational opportunities, and special wheelchairs may be needed. Many less severely affected patients with cerebral palsy are able to lead reasonably independent lives.

CEREBELLAR ATAXIAS

Impairment of cerebellar function is common in neurological disease. The cerebellum is responsible for monitoring afferent activity and influencing the cerebral cortical control of movement. Afferents to the cerebellum arise from muscle and joint receptors via fibres travelling in the spinocerebellar tracts; there is also some input from cutaneous afferents, the vestibular system and some visual afferents. For clinical purposes, the cerebellum may be divided into the two hemispheres and the midline vermis. Lesions of one hemisphere produce ipsilateral limb incoordination (ataxia), hypotonia and, sometimes, nystagmus. Vermis lesions cause disturbance of control of truncal movement, leading to the characteristic wide-based unsteady gait. It is also important to recognise that cerebellar signs may be caused either by lesions of the cerebellum itself, or its connections within the brainstem. Thus, lesions confined to the brainstem often produce cerebellar signs.

Limb or gait ataxia may also be caused by weakness or sensory impairment, particularly proprioceptive loss.

Hereditary ataxias, spinocerebellar degenerations and hereditary spastic paraparesis

The neurological deficit in cerebellar ataxias ranges from a pure cerebellar ataxia (as in autosomal dominant inherited, late-onset cerebellar ataxia), through mixed syndromes, involving spinal as well as cerebellar features (*spinocerebellar degenerations*), to a pure spastic paraplegia. There are often other neurological and non-neurological associated features.

The hereditary ataxias

Most hereditary ataxias are rare; many are of concern principally to the paediatric neurologist, as those affected usually fail to survive into adult life.

Early-onset hereditary ataxias

Friedreich's ataxia, an autosomal recessive condition, is much the most common type of hereditary ataxia. Progressive ataxia of gait and limbs usually develops in childhood and always before the age of 25 years, and is associated with dysarthria, nystagmus, a spastic paraparesis and extensor plantars, but with areflexia due to an axonal sensory neuropathy. A cardiomyopathy is present in about two-thirds of patients, and diabetes in about 10%; some patients are of low intelligence. The ataxia is relentlessly progressive and death usually occurs during

the fourth decade from cardiac failure. A similar, but more benign, autosomal recessive condition (also arising in childhood) occurs, in which there is no evidence of neuropathy.

Ataxia telangiectasia – an autosomal recessive syndrome of progressive cerebellar ataxia with onset in childhood – is associated with conjunctival and cutaneous telangiectasia.

Two important and treatable disorders which include ataxia amongst other presenting neurological symptoms are Wilson's disease (p. 921) and Refsum's disease (p. 949).

Late-onset hereditary ataxias

A number of hereditary ataxias do not develop until the patient is more than 20 years of age. It is clinically useful to consider these cases as a single group. A pure cerebellar ataxia of onset at over 50 years is occasionally seen. In all patients with dominantly-inherited, late-onset ataxias, the major feature is a slowly progressive gait and limb ataxia, with dysarthria and nystagmus.

Cerebellar ataxia also occurs as a minor feature of many other inherited metabolic defects, most of which produce widespread neurological deficits, e.g. mitochondrial cytopathy.

Acquired ataxias

Mild unsteadiness of gait is extremely common in elderly patients and is often multifactorial in origin. A degree of cerebellar degeneration is common in old age. Iatrogenic, drug-induced ataxia is also common, particularly in the elderly, the offending drugs including phenytoin, carbamazepine and benzodiazepines. An acute reversible ataxia is produced by alcohol, but chronic alcohol abuse may lead to a predominantly midline vermis degeneration which is largely irreversible (p. 981). Cerebellar involvement is common in multiple sclerosis (MS). Mild ataxia is quite common in hypothyroidism and may occasionally be the presenting factor. Cerebellar tumours and some

Table 22.44 Causes of cerebellar ataxia in children

Congenital malformations	Infectious
Cerebellar agenesis/hypoplasia	Secondary to bacterial meningitis
Dandy-Walker syndrome*	Secondary to encephalitis
Arnold-Chiari malformation**	
	Hydrocephalus*
Hereditary ataxias	
Friedreich's ataxia	Tumours
	Medulloblastoma
Trauma	Astrocytoma
Birth trauma*	Haemangioblastoma
Head injury in childhood*	

* May persist into adult life. ** May present in adult life

paraneoplastic syndromes can cause ataxia. Pyogenic abscesses and tuberculomas occasionally develop in the cerebellum. Encephalitis may produce a cerebellar ataxia, particularly in children, in whom a pure syndrome of cerebellar ataxia is now recognised. Other causes of ataxia in childhood are listed in Table 22.44.

Ataxia arising as a result of foramen magnum and posterior fossa congenital malformations, particularly Arnold-Chiari type I malformations (p. 938), may present in adult life, without any neurological deficit in early life.

DISEASES OF THE SPINAL CORD

Anatomy and physiology

The spinal cord extends from the foramen magnum to the level of the lower border of the first lumbar vertebra. The essential features of spinal cord lesions are bilateral symptoms and/or signs, together with impairment of bladder and bowel control, impairment of sexual function in men and, sometimes, a sensory level on the trunk. Partial spinal cord lesions do not produce all these effects; when the signs are unilateral, they may be difficult to distinguish from lesions at higher levels in the nervous system.

The major motor pathways in the spinal cord are the *corticospinal tracts*. These decussate at the level of the lower medulla and descend in the anterolateral columns of the spinal cord, ending on anterior horn cells.

The two major sensory pathways are the dorsal columns and the spinothalamic tracts. *Dorsal column* fibres convey joint position and vibration sensation and some touch. *Spinothalamic tract* fibres convey information about pain, temperature and some touch. Some spinal cord lesions produce selective sensory tract damage, giving rise to dissociated sensory loss on the trunk and in the limbs. A sensory level on the trunk is a hallmark of spinal cord disturbances, but is present only in a minority of lesions. The sensory level is often several segments below the actual level of the lesion in the spinal cord.

The abdominal reflexes are occasionally helpful in determining the level of a thoracic cord lesion. However, the abdominal reflexes are lost with increasing age and are absent in obese patients. The segmental level of the upper abdominal reflexes is T9, and of the lower T11.

It is often not possible to localise the precise level of a spinal cord disturbance on clinical grounds; in most cases, special investigation is necessary. Compressive spinal cord lesions may be complicated by disturbances of blood supply which cause additional damage to the cord.

Any acute spinal cord lesion may give rise to a flaccid paraplegia with areflexia and non-reactive plantar responses, rather than a spastic paraparesis. It can be difficult to distinguish a spinal cord lesion from a peripheral lesion causing widespread weakness, e.g. an acute Guillain-Barré syndrome. However, involvement of the bladder and the presence of a sensory level will clearly indicate that the lesion is within the spinal cord in most cases.

Clinical differentiation of extradural, intradural, extramedullary and intramedullary lesions is often not possible. Some intramedullary lesions, e.g. syringomyelia, give rise to a highly characteristic evolution of symptoms and signs.

Patterns of spinal cord deficit

Cervical lesions

The two commonest causes of cervical cord lesions are demyelinating disease and cervical spondylosis. Degenerative change is usually most pronounced in the midcervical region at C5–6, and the myelopathy which may be associated with cervical spondylosis is often maximal at this level. Any cervical cord lesion may produce a combination of root signs (leading to lower motor neurone signs in the upper limbs), radicular sensory impairment and a spastic paraparesis.

A lesion at C5 or 6 results in sluggish or absent biceps and supinator reflexes with brisk reflexes below this, including the triceps jerk and lower limb reflexes. The occurrence of a finger jerk when eliciting the biceps or supinator reflexes is referred to as an *inverted supinator reflex*.

Cervical cord compression may give rise to dorsal column sensory impairment in the legs, while intrinsic lesions tend to produce spinothalamic disturbances more often than compressive lesions.

Bladder symptoms usually consist of urgency and frequency, eventually with incontinence. Acute cervical cord lesions may result in retention with overflow. Impotence in males is common in cervical cord disturbances.

Lesions at C3 or above affect the phrenic nerve outflow and cause respiratory paralysis.

Many cervical lesions produce minor symptoms in the upper limbs, such as reflex asymmetry, but the major problem is a spastic paraparesis. Careful examination of the upper limbs is essential in all patients presenting with a paraparesis, since there may be signs helpful in localising the lesion to the cervical region.

Thoracic cord lesions

Thoracic cord lesions cause a spastic paraparesis, with bladder, bowel and sexual impairment, and sensory loss as with cervical lesions. A sensory level on the trunk is particularly helpful in establishing the level of the lesion but, as mentioned above, a level on the trunk may be caused by a lesion in the cervical region.

Brown-Séquard syndrome

The clinical features of hemisection of the spinal cord were first described by Brown-Séquard (Fig. 22.32). This syndrome may be produced by compression or inflammatory disease of the spinal cord and, occasionally, with vascular lesions. There is ipsilateral sensory loss over one or several segments at the level of the lesion, and also ipsilateral dorsal column sensory impairment. Ipsilateral pyramidal signs occur and, sometimes, bilateral pyramidal signs, but these are always worse on the ipsilateral side; there is also contralateral spinothalamic sensory impairment. Bladder and bowel involvement is variable.

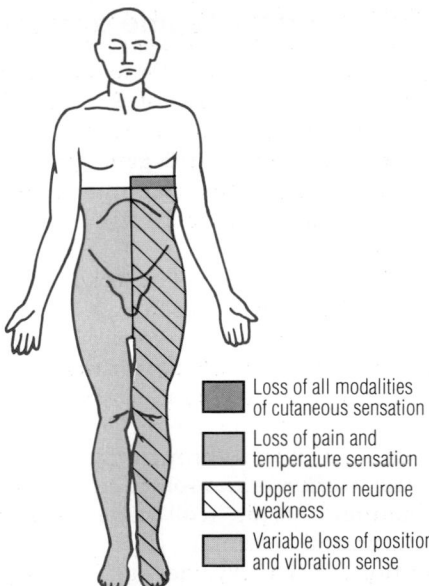

Loss of all modalities of cutaneous sensation

Loss of pain and temperature sensation

Upper motor neurone weakness

Variable loss of position and vibration sense

Fig. 23.32 The features of hemisection of the spinal cord, the Brown-Séquard syndrome. In addition to the signs shown, there is sometimes border zone hyperaesthesia, either at the upper limit of the contralateral spinothalamic sensory loss, or the ipsilateral root sensory loss, or both.

Conus medullaris

Lesions at the conus produce a mixture of upper and lower motor neurone lumbosacral root signs, and are usually caused by a tumour, such as an ependymoma or Schwannoma. The bladder disturbance is usually retention and overflow in a large atonic bladder.

Investigation and management of paraplegia

It is essential in any patient presenting with a spinal cord syndrome – particularly when of acute or subacute onset – to exclude spinal cord compression, as this is potentially surgically remediable. Complete loss of bladder function for more than 24 hours cannot be reversed, even if a compressive lesion is relieved, though there may be partial recovery of complete motor and sensory deficits after this time. Table 22.45 lists the many causes of acute and subacute spinal cord lesions and Table 22.46 lists the causes of chronic progressive paraplegia.

Initial investigations include a chest X-ray, which may demonstrate a primary carcinoma or metastases. Plain X-rays of the cervical and thoracic spines may show spondylotic change, lytic change or collapse of a vertebra. Plain CT scans of the spine may be helpful, but most patients

Table 22.45 Causes of acute or subacute paraplegia

Trauma to a previously normal spine	
Vertebral disease	**Infection**
Metastatic carcinoma	Epidural abscess
Cervical spondylosis*	TB abscess
Dorsal disc prolapse*	Syphilitic myelitis*
Paget's disease	HIV infection
Rheumatoid arthritis*	Vascular myelopathy
Pott's disease of spine*	
	Vascular
Tumours	Anterior spinal artery occlusion
Extradural or intradural	Infarction secondary to hypotension
carcinoma, lymphoma, myeloma,	Embolic infarction
leukaemia	Infarction secondary to
Dorsal meningioma*	aortic dissection
Neurofibroma*	Arteriovenous malformation:
	infarction or haemorrhage
Haematological disease	Primary intramedullary haemorrhage
Any cause of	Vasculitis – PAN
thrombocytopenia	
Other clotting	**Inflammatory**
disorders	Epidural or	Myelitis of unknown cause
Leukaemia	intra-	Multiple sclerosis
Anticoagulant	medullary	SLE
treatment	haemorrhage	Sarcoidosis*
	Metabolic
	Subacute degeneration of the cord*

* May also cause chronic progressive paraplegia

Summary 9 Spinal cord compression

- Progressive weakness of the legs and bladder symptoms should be considered to be due to spinal cord compression until proved otherwise.

- Total loss of bladder control for more than 24 hours, due to spinal cord compression, is likely to be permanent, even if the compression is subsequently relieved.

- Urgency of investigation of cord compression will depend on the speed of progression of symptoms, but is always urgent when bladder function is threatened.

- Minimum investigation includes chest X-ray, plain X-rays of the spine, full blood count and ESR and then a myelogram.

- Investigation of suspected cord compression should always be performed in close consultation with a neurosurgeon.

presenting with an acute or subacute paraplegia will require a myelogram. If there is spinal block, a lumbar puncture may occasionally lead to an abrupt deterioration and myelography should be performed in consultation with a neurosurgeon.

Myelography is the definitive test in establishing spinal cord compression, and is sometimes combined with CT scanning. MRI now offers an alternative to CT myelography. In patients in whom no structural lesion is demonstrated, examination of the CSF is particularly important. A raised lymphocyte count and protein content suggest an inflammatory cord lesion.

Management. Where there is substantial loss of cord function, and in particular when there is bladder or bowel disturbance, surgical decompression is usually necessary. In the case of destructive malignant disease, decompression may have to be combined with procedures to stabilise the spine. With a less severe deficit, a combination of radiotherapy and dexamethasone may produce improvement. However, operation is often required in order to establish a histological diagnosis.

Table 22.46 Causes of chronic progressive paraplegia

- **Causes marked ***
  from Table 22.45

- Tumours
  Meningioma
  Neurofibroma
  Glioma
  Ependymoma
  Chordoma
  Lipoma

- Syringomyelia
  With Arnold-Chiari
  malformation
  With tumour

- Subacute combined degeneration of the cord

- Hereditary spastic paraplegia

- Radiation myelopathy

- Arachnoiditis

- Ankylosing spondylitis

- Tropical spastic paraparesis (HTLVI infection)

- Motor neurone disease

CAUSES OF SPINAL CORD LESIONS

Spinal cord injury

Many spinal cord injuries are the result of road traffic accidents and sports injuries. Initially, a spinal cord injury may not be suspected, particularly when there is associated head injury. All patients with severe head injury require cervical spine X-rays to investigate an associated spinal injury. If cervical spine X-rays show no bony displacement or fracture, the patient can be managed conservatively. If X-rays demonstrate a fracture or displacement indicating instability, great care is necessary with movement of the patient. Surgical reduction of fractures may be necessary, but many patients are treated with traction in the hope that some neurological recovery will occur.

In the elderly with associated cervical spondylosis, spinal cord injury is likely to occur with relatively minor trauma. Hyperextension injuries lead to contusion of the cord in a canal narrowed by spondylotic change. When examining a patient suspected of having a cervical spine injury, it is important not to move the neck excessively. Neck X-rays must be obtained urgently and neurosurgical advice taken. The management of severe paraplegia due to spinal cord injury is best undertaken in spinal injury units. The condition often results in permanent paralysis.

Spinal cord injury in the dorsal region is less common than in the cervical region.

Degenerative cervical spine disease

Degenerative cervical spine disease may present with local neck pain, symptoms and signs of a radiculopathy, or evidence of a myelopathy.

Neck pain due to a cervical degenerative arthritis is extremely common in middle-aged and elderly people, but in most cases there is no associated neurological deficit.

Cervical radiculopathy is caused by narrowing of the exit foraminae by osteophyte encroachment combined with disc degeneration and loss of disc space height. The most common level for cervical radiculopathy in degenerative cervical spine disease is at C5 and C6. This causes pain which radiates over the shoulder and into the upper arm and, sometimes, diffusely throughout the arm. Signs include wasting, weakness and sometimes fasciculation in deltoid, spinati and biceps, with loss of the biceps and supinator reflexes and sometimes sensory impairment in a root distribution. If there are no signs of an associated myelopathy, it is best to treat initially with a firm cervical collar by day, and a soft cervical collar at night. Root pain often settles within a few weeks with this treatment and motor signs may also improve. In a few patients with evidence of a persistent or progressive radiculopathy, investigation with myelography may be necessary, followed by surgical treatment to decompress the root.

Myelopathy. In patients with a myelopathy, with progressive paraparesis, myelography is necessary. With a disc prolapse, surgery is by an anterior approach in which the degenerative disc material is removed and a bone graft inserted (Cloward procedure). For diffuse cervical canal stenosis, which usually occurs in old people, it is often not possible to perform the Cloward procedure at multiple levels and, when indicated, a posterior decompression is preferred.

Thoracic disc

Prolapse of a thoracic disc is relatively rare. It may present as a progressive paraparesis. Following myelography, decompression is necessary, usually via an anterior approach.

Paget's disease

Paget's disease occasionally produces localised vertebral involvement in one or several adjacent vertebrae in the thoracic region, which can cause compression. Surgical decompression is followed by treatment with calcitonin.

Pott's disease of the spine

Tuberculosis affecting the spine usually occurs in the thoracic region of children or young adults. A single vertebra, or several adjacent vertebrae, may be affected and the onset is insidious. The first symptom is usually back pain and this is sometimes severe. With gradual destruction of one or more vertebrae, a kyphosis may develop. Infection by tuberculosis starts in an adjacent disc and then involves the vertebral body. This leads to collapse of the vertebra, with eventual wedge collapse of one or several adjacent vertebrae and the development of a paravertebral cold abscess. A slowly progressive paraparesis is the usual neurological presentation. X-rays demonstrate rarefaction of the bones and loss of disc space height. The differential diagnosis includes pyogenic infection (which may produce similar X-ray changes) and malignancy.

When Pott's disease of the spine is not associated with neurological involvement, antituberculous drugs are usually all that is required. When there is neurological involvement, decompression may be necessary, followed by antituberculous chemotherapy.

Rheumatoid arthritis

Rheumatoid arthritis (Ch. 23) may produce diffuse cervical arthritis, but the characteristic lesion is atlanto-axial subluxation. Narrowing of the upper cervical canal is produced by subluxation of the odontoid process. This may present as a chronic progressive tetraparesis. Occi-

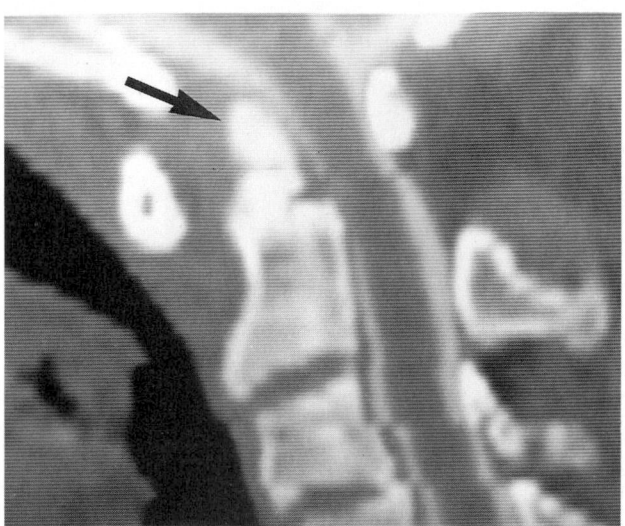

Fig. 22.33 CT myelogram of upper cervical region in a patient with rheumatoid arthritis. There is atlanto-axial subluxation, with upward and posterior displacement of the odontoid (arrowed), which is causing compression at the cervico-medullary junction.

pital neuralgia, due to compression of the upper cervical sensory roots (C2), is a common early symptom. Occasionally, the onset of symptoms is abrupt and provoked by minor head trauma. There may also be symptoms of brainstem dysfunction – dysarthria and dysphagia being the commonest – due to compression of the anterior spinal artery or vertebral arteries by upward displacement of the odontoid process.

The upper cervical region is sometimes difficult to visualise by myelography, and CT myelography is usually the most helpful investigation (Fig. 22.33). Elderly, very disabled patients with atlanto-axial subluxation can be managed conservatively with a firm cervical collar, but if there is evidence of a progressive myelopathy, surgery is usually recommended. This involves removal of the odontoid process and posterior stabilisation of the upper cervical spine.

Metastases

Metastatic deposits of cancer or lymphoma are common causes of acute or subacute paraplegia. Cord compression usually results from extradural deposits, and there is often associated vertebral collapse (Fig. 22.34). Surgery followed by radiotherapy is usually required. In some cases of relatively mild cord compression, urgent radiotherapy is performed with careful neurological observation.

Primary spinal cord tumours

Meningiomas occasionally occur in the thoracic region, usually in middle-aged or elderly women (Fig. 22.35).

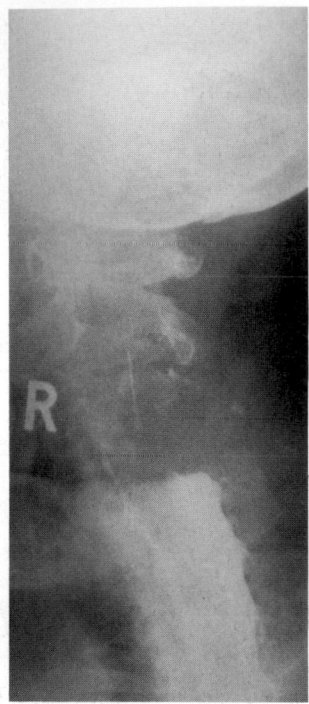

Fig. 22.34 Cervical myelogram, showing complete block to flow of contrast at C4/5, associated with extensive vertebral bony destruction at this level. The spinal cord is compressed by a large extradural mass. This was metastatic carcinoma of the lung.

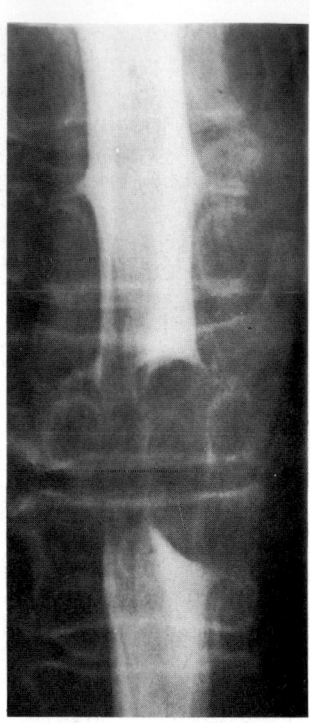

Fig. 22.35 Myelogram showing the mid-thoracic region, in an elderly woman presenting with a slowly progressive spastic paraparesis and a sensory level on the trunk at T10. A large rounded mass is compressing the spinal cord. At operation a meningioma was removed.

They present with a gradually progressive paraparesis. The results of surgical removal are usually good.

Neurofibromas may develop on spinal roots at any level (Fig. 22.36). These gradually enlarge, producing bony erosion of the exit foraminae and then spread into the spinal canal, compressing the theca and spinal cord. The history is usually of a gradually progressive paraparesis or tetraparesis. Plain X-rays of the spine will often suggest the diagnosis of neurofibromatosis, showing extensive bony erosion (Fig. 22.36A).

Intramedullary tumours are rare. They include gliomas, which usually occur in the cervical region in young adults. Some are amenable to partial surgical resection. When an intrinsic tumour causes enlargement of the cord, bony decompression of the spinal canal by laminectomy may be helpful. Some spinal cord gliomas are radiosensitive, so that prolonged survival, with slow progression, can occur; other tumours, however, run a much more aggressive course.

Ependymomas may arise at any level of the spinal cord and are often associated with cysts. Although these tumours are histologically benign, they are often difficult to remove surgically.

A *lipoma* may occur anywhere in the cervical or thoracic spinal cord, as well as the cauda equina where they are associated with spina bifida and spinal dysraphism. When

they cause neurological deficit, partial surgical resection is usually necessary.

Chordomas are rare tumours, derived from remnants of the embryonic notochord. In the head, they arise in the region of the clivus, and in the spinal canal, usually in the sacrococcygeal area.

Myelitis

Acute inflammation of the spinal cord may occur at any level and is usually of unknown cause. In some patients, there is a history of preceding viral infection, and myelitis commonly occurs as part of MS. There is usually a history of weakness and sensory loss in the legs progressing over a few days, sometimes leading to a severe paraparesis with a clear sensory level on the trunk. A Brown-Séquard syndrome may result from myelitis. Bladder and bowel involvement are common, and back pain at the level of the lesion is also a common feature.

Investigation and management

Many patients will require myelography to exclude spinal cord compression. The CSF shows a raised lymphocyte count and protein level. Treatment is with steroids or ACTH. In myelitis due to MS, there is usually partial

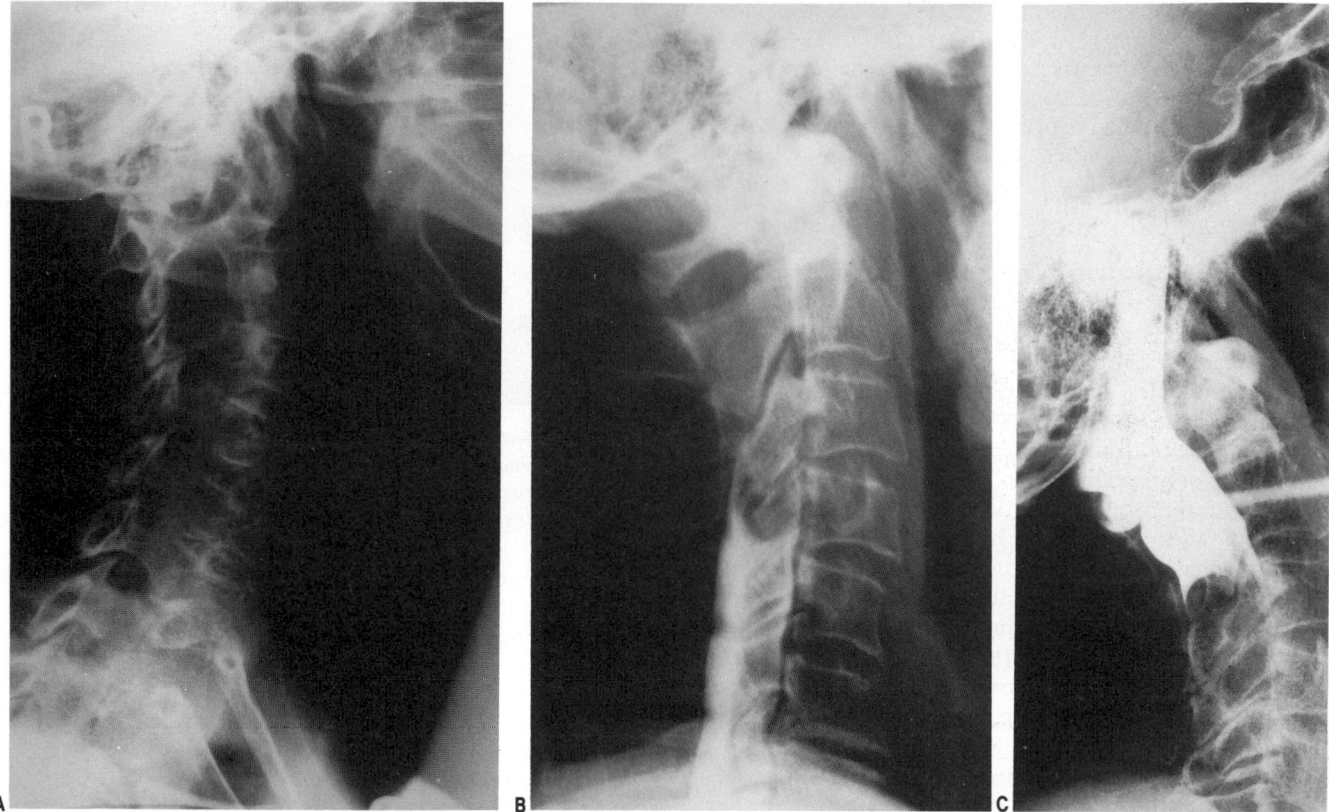

Fig. 22.36 Cervical neurofibroma. A. Plain oblique view of the cervical spine in a woman of 63 years with a spastic tetraparesis. A grossly enlarged exit foramen is present at C3/4. **B.** and **C.** Cervical myelograms in the same patient. In (B), with contrast injected in the lumbar region, there is a block to flow at C4. In (C), with contrast injected above the lesion at C2, the upper border of the rounded neurofibroma is shown.

recovery of function. In idiopathic myelitis, when severe paralysis occurs, many patients are left with a severe residual deficit.

Epidural abscess

Epidural abscesses are usually pyogenic and most often due to staphylococcal infection, usually blood-borne from another site of infection. The history is of a rapidly progressive paraparesis with local back pain and tenderness, and there is often fever. Urgent surgical decompression and antibiotic treatment are necessary.

Vascular disease

Vascular disease affecting the spinal cord is relatively uncommon, although some of the neurological deficit seen with compressive lesions may be due in part to interruption of the blood supply to the cord. Anterior spinal artery occlusion produces an acute paraparesis, often with predominantly spinothalamic sensory impairment. Recovery is variable. Generalised hypotension, embolism

and dissection of the aorta can all impair spinal cord blood supply.

Arteriovenous malformations are the commonest cause of vascular lesions of the spinal cord. These usually present acutely due to infarction or haemorrhage, but there is sometimes a stepwise or gradually progressive paraparesis. The diagnosis may be apparent at myelography and is then confirmed by spinal angiography. Some are amenable to surgical treatment.

Vasculitis occasionally leads to acute spinal cord lesions; this occurs most commonly in polyarteritis nodosa.

Syringomyelia

In syringomyelia, a large fluid-filled cavity develops within the spinal cord; it is in communication with the central canal and contains CSF. Syrinxes may be long cysts extending over the whole length of the spinal cord, but are often more localised. They are most common in the cervical region, where they are often associated with Arnold–Chiari malformations (p. 938). Syrinxes may also be associated with spinal cord tumours and can occur as a late sequel of trauma. The pathogenesis of most syrinxes remains uncertain. However, the fact that there is a frequent association with Arnold-Chiari malformations suggests that partial obstruction to the flow of CFS from the foramina in the roof of the IVth ventricle may play some part.

Clinical features

The clinical presentation of a syrinx is characteristic of an intrinsic cord lesion. The developing cyst impinges on anterior horn cells, and produces unilateral or bilateral (often asymmetrical) wasting, affecting particularly the small hand muscles, but eventually also other muscles in the upper limbs. Interruption of the decussating spinothalamic fibres centrally in the spinal cord leads to a dissociated sensory impairment in the upper limbs involving pain and temperature sensation, with preservation of other modalities. Since the spinothalamic fibres from the lower limbs have decussated lower down in the cord and their fibres lie laterally in the spinothalamic tracts, there is no impairment of spinothalamic sensation in the lower limbs. Eventually, the corticospinal tracts become involved, producing a spastic paraparesis; a late feature is involvement of dorsal column sensation (joint position and vibration sensation).

The dissociated sensory impairment in the hands leads to painless traumatic lesions of the fingers. The upper limb reflexes are usually absent. In the legs, a mild paraparesis develops. Syringomyelia is usually slowly progressive and the chronic loss of pain sensation may lead to the development of Charcot joints in the hand, elbow or, occasionally, shoulder joints.

Occasionally, cervical syrinxes may extend into the brainstem (syringobulbia), affecting the lower cranial nerve nuclei producing dysphagia and dysarthria. There may be sensory loss on the face of spinothalamic type, due to the involvement of the spinal nucleus and tract of the trigeminal nerve.

Investigation

Myelography usually shows an expanded cord in the region of the syrinx (Fig. 22.37) and delayed CT scanning after myelography may demonstrate contrast medium within the syrinx itself. MRI also demonstrates syrinxes clearly.

Management and prognosis

When there is an associated Arnold-Chiari malformation, foramen magnum decompression may arrest the further progression of the syrinx in some but not all patients. The more recent operation of syringoperitoneal shunting is now preferred by some neurosurgeons.

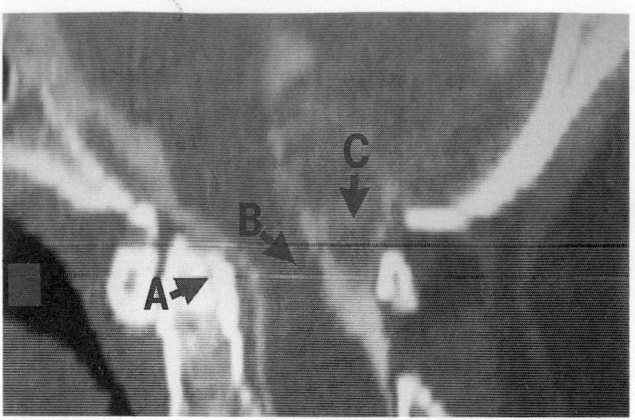

Fig. 22.37 CT myelogram showing syringomyelia associated with an Arnold-Chiari malformation. Odontoid peg (A), spinal cord (B). The cerebellar tonsils (C) are in an abnormally low position and the upper cervical spinal cord is grossly expanded due to the syrinx.

The prognosis is variable. In some patients the neurological deficit arrests after a time, while in others there is relentless progression.

Subacute combined degeneration of the cord

Long-standing B_{12} deficiency in pernicious anaemia may lead to degeneration of the lateral and posterior columns of the spinal cord, together with a peripheral neuropathy. This produces the clinical syndrome known as subacute combined degeneration of the cord. There may be an associated mild dementia and optic atrophy. Patients with subacute combined degeneration are usually middle-aged or elderly. Paraesthesiae or pain in the hands and feet are frequent presenting complaints; there are often few signs in the early stages, but a progressive paraparesis soon develops.

Only some patients are anaemic; a normal haemoglobin does not exclude this diagnosis, but a macrocytosis is invariably present (Ch. 24). Treatment with parenteral B_{12} is usually beneficial, but an established severe paraparesis and peripheral neuropathy may not respond well.

Motor neurone disease

Motor neurone disease (MND) may present as a slowly progressive spastic paraparesis. MND is considered further on page 940.

Radiation myelopathy

Occasionally, damage of the cervical spinal cord occurs following radiotherapy to the neck for conditions such as

Hodgkin's disease. Symptoms of a progressive myelopathy usually develop between 6 months and 5 years after radiotherapy. The myelopathy may be mild, but in some cases it is steadily progressive and leads to a severe deficit.

Sarcoidosis

Sarcoidosis has many neurological manifestations (p. 974) and is an occasional cause of myelopathy.

Hereditary spastic paraplegia

Hereditary spastic paraplegia – of dominant inheritance often with variable penetrance – takes the form of a slowly progressive paraplegia without sensory deficit. Bladder and bowel involvement is often a late feature and may be absent. Onset is usually in the second or third decade. Paraparesis associated with the spinocerebellar degenerations is considered on page 929.

Tropical spastic paraparesis

A slowly progressive paraparesis is seen in the tropics and migrants from these countries. There is sometimes an associated mild peripheral neuropathy. The condition was previously known as Jamaican neuropathy, but the spinal cord disturbance tends to dominate the clinical picture. Occasionally other lesions such as optic atrophy and ataxia are present. The paraparesis is usually slowly progressive and may remain mild. There is now strong evidence that HTLVI infection is the cause of tropical spastic paraparesis.

DEVELOPMENTAL ANOMALIES AFFECTING THE SPINAL CORD

Spina bifida

Spina bifida refers to defective fusion of the vertebral arches.

Aetiology

The cause of spina bifida in most patients is unknown, but there is an association with trisomy 13 or 18 in a few infants. The condition is commoner in girls. There has been a decrease in incidence of spina bifida in recent years, the reason for which is uncertain. There is now evidence that folic acid deficiency early in pregnancy causes spina bifida. The anticonvulsant drugs sodium valproate and carbamazepine are also associated with a slightly increased incidence of spina bifida.

Clinical features

Defective fusion of the vertebral arches is most common in the lumbar region. It is extremely common in a single lumbar vertebra and is an incidental radiological finding of no significance in many normal people. However, when the defect of the vertebral arches extends over several segments, there may be associated abnormalities. These include:

- a tuft of hair overlying the defect
- a low, tethered spinal cord extending below the lower border of L1
- a dermal sinus extending towards the spinal canal
- intraspinal lipoma
- sometimes, diastematomyelia (splitting of the spinal cord).

Neurological problems associated with this type of bony abnormality are collectively known as *spina bifida occulta*. However, an extensive bony abnormality may be present without any neurological deficit.

Spina bifida cystica

Spina bifida cystica refers to a more severe defect, in which the meninges prolapse through the bony defect of the vertebral arches. The meninges may prolapse without including neural tissue (a *meningocele*), or may include neural elements (a *meningomyelocele*). In its most severe form, spina bifida leads to a wide-open defect without covering of the cauda equina; this is known as *rhachischisis*. With meningocele and meningomyelocele, there is nearly always an associated Arnold-Chiari type II malformation (see below), with hydrocephalus and a kyphosis.

Management. Meningoceles require closure, but following this, some infants develop hydrocephalus and will require shunting. Spina bifida cystica is associated with obvious cauda equina problems at birth with paralysis of the legs. The decision whether to treat some of these infants or not remains controversial. If nothing is done, death from meningitis is almost inevitable. Treatment consists of closure of the defect and shunting for hydrocephalus. With these measures many of these children will survive. However, most will be severely handicapped and will require further operations later for contractures and other problems resulting from their severe neurological deficit.

Spina bifida occulta

Spina bifida occulta may present in childhood, adolescence or in adult life. Many of these patients have a partial cauda equina syndrome. There is often a longstanding history of bladder difficulties with enuresis, frequency and, sometimes, incontinence during the day. The signs of cauda equina deficit in the legs may be relatively mild or be fairly obvious, with underdeveloped, short legs and muscle wasting.

Investigation and management. Patients whose symptoms (particularly bladder symptoms) are progressing, warrant investigation with myelography. This may demonstrate a low tethered cord, some degree of spinal dysraphism and, occasionally, a lipoma or haemangioma. Surgical intervention seldom produces improvement; the aim is to prevent further progression. This may be achieved when a lipoma or haemangioma is present, and in some cases of spinal dysraphism, but release of a tethered cord alone does not usually produce any benefit.

Arnold-Chiari malformations

Arnold-Chiari malformations are of two types.

In *type I malformations*, there is cerebellar tonsilar herniation through the foramen magnum, often associated with syringomyelia (Fig. 22.37). Most patients present in adult life, either with symptoms and signs attributable to the syringomyelia, or with ataxia, lower cranial nerve palsies, nystagmus and a mild spastic tetraparesis. Treatment is initially by foramen magnum decompression, and sometimes later shunting of the syrinx.

In *type II malformations*, there is herniation of the cerebellar vermis and tonsils, and of the lower part of the brainstem through the foramen magnum. There is associated hydrocephalus, and, as mentioned above, there is a strong association of the type II malformation with meningomyeloceles. The type II malformation usually presents in infancy with dysphagia causing feeding difficulties. There may be associated platybasia, an upward displacement of the skull base. The treatment is to shunt the hydrocephalus and perform a foramen magnum decompression.

Dandy-Walker syndrome

Dandy-Walker syndrome is a severe congenital abnormality in which there is hypoplasia of the vermis of the cerebellum, with massive cystic dilatation of the IVth ventricle and expansion of the posterior fossa; there is secondary hydrocephalus. This malformation is often associated with other major brain and spinal cord malformations. The abnormality is usually obvious at birth, though it occasionally presents later in childhood, with ataxia. Shunting of the hydrocephalus is necessary, sometimes together with posterior fossa surgery.

Klippel-Feil deformity

The Klippel-Feil deformity consists of fusion of two or more cervical vertebrae, sometimes involving most of the cervical spine. There may be abnormal and unstable joints in the cervical spine. The neck is short and the posterior hairline is low. There is often associated platybasia and other abnormalities of the petrous temporal bone, which lead to conductive deafness in some patients. There is also an association with syringomyelia. The presence of incomplete decussation of the pyramidal tracts often produces the curious physical sign of mirror movements. Patients with the Klippel-Feil deformity may present with a gradually progressive tetraparesis or a cervical radiculopathy but, occasionally, with a sudden onset of tetraplegia following minor neck trauma, as a result of instability in the cervical spine. They may also present with symptoms and signs of syringomyelia.

DISEASES AFFECTING SPINAL ROOTS

Anatomy and physiology

Dorsal and ventral spinal roots are given off by every segment of the spinal cord; thus, there are 8 cervical, 12 thoracic, 5 lumbar, 5 sacral and 1 coccygeal pair(s). The dorsal and ventral roots join in the intervertebral foramina. The lumbar and sacral roots pass downwards, below the lower end of the spinal cord, which terminates at the lower border of the L1 vertebral body (conus medullaris); the lower lumbosacral roots form the cauda equina below this level. The sympathetic outflow from the spinal cord travels in the T1 to L1 roots; the caudal parasympathetic outflow is localised to the S2-S4 roots.

An important part of the blood supply to two watershed regions of the spinal cord enters via roots, one in the lower cervical region, one at the thoraco-lumbar junction, the artery of Adamkiewicz. Interruption of the arteries travelling on these roots may critically impair the blood supply of the cord, causing infarction.

Effects of root lesions

The clinical effects of root lesions may be both negative and positive. Negative effects include segmental wasting and weakness, sometimes with reflex loss if an appropriate root is affected, and a dermatomal sensory impairment. Positive effects are sensory – root pain which may or may not be clearly localised, paraesthesiae and hyperaesthesiae. Root pain due to structural lesions which tether the root and inhibit movement may be exacerbated by spinal movement and by manoeuvres which increase intraspinal pressure, such as coughing, sneezing and straining.

The commonest cause of root lesions is degenerative spine disease affecting the lower cervical and lumbar regions.

Cervical spondylosis

Spondylosis is the term used loosely to describe the degenerative changes which often occur in the cervical and lumbar regions (Ch. 23). The spinal canal is narrowed by these degenerative changes which, in the cervical spine, are usually most marked at C4–5, C5–6 and C6–7.

Clinical features

Cervical spondylosis presents in three ways:

- with local pain related to the degenerative changes, but without neurological involvement
- with root compression, either motor, sensory or both
- with spinal cord compression.

Root or cord compression may develop gradually over long periods of time, or may present acutely, usually as the result of a disc prolapse.

If a root is compressed by the disc protrusion, pain and paraesthesiae in a radicular distribution are usually the first symptoms, sometimes followed by motor symptoms and signs appropriate to the root involved. Acute disc protrusions may also cause symptoms and signs of cord compression.

Diagnosis

In many patients, the signs indicating a root (rather than a peripheral nerve or brachial plexus) basis for the symptoms are not clear-cut. EMG and nerve conduction studies are often helpful. Other investigations include cervical spine X-rays with oblique views to show the intervertebral foramina.

Although root pain is usually due to a disc protrusion, there are a number of other causes including compression in malignant vertebral body collapse, and other spinal tumours. Malignant invasion of the brachial plexus must also be considered (p. 949).

Management

In patients with minor symptoms of cervical root compression, a period of rest in a firm cervical collar, together with analgesia, will often help the pain and aid the spontaneous resolution of the signs over several weeks. Continuing severe pain, the failure of signs (particularly motor) to improve or progression of signs are indications to investigate further with myelography. Myelography is also indicated if there are signs of cord compression (p. 931). A disc causing continuing pain and neurological deficit may be surgically removed via facetectomy or foraminotomy from a posterior approach, or anteriorly through the disc with vertebral body fusion, using a bone graft (Cloward's procedure).

Lumbar spondylosis

Low back pain is experienced by virtually all adults at some time (Ch. 23). The cause of pain in most patients with back pain cannot be identified with confidence. Pain radiating down one leg is not always due to root compression; musculoskeletal pain may radiate in a similar way. The two roots most commonly compressed by prolapsed lumbar discs are the L5 root (by a prolapsed L4–5 disc) and the S1 root (by an L5–S1 prolapse). L5 root pain is felt on the lateral aspect of the leg and dorsum of the foot, while S1 pain tends to radiate down the back of the leg to the sole of the foot. However, many patients are unable to clearly localise their pain. With L5 root compression, there is partial weakness of dorsiflexion and eversion of the foot. As extensor hallucis longus is supplied by L5 alone, it is relatively weaker, and this is of help in distinguishing a root lesion from a peroneal nerve lesion. Sensory loss will be within an L5 distribution. With S1 lesions, it is difficult to detect minor degrees of weakness of gastrocnemius soleus because of its strength. However, there may be reduction or loss of the ankle jerk and, on sensory testing, impairment of sensation on the lateral border of the foot, and on the sole. In either L5 or S1 lesions due to compression by a disc, the tethering of the root by the disc may cause a positive root stretch test; straight leg raising is the standard test for this.

Back and/or leg pain with focal neurological signs may settle with a period of bed rest, and traction is sometimes helpful. However, the continuing presence of focal signs is an indication for investigation with myelography, with a view to decompressive surgery.

Lumbar canal stenosis

The combination of a congenitally narrow lumbar canal with subsequent degenerative change leads to canal stenosis. This may cause low back pain, together with focal signs, sometimes indicating a lesion of more than one root. The syndrome of cauda equina claudication is almost always associated with lumbar canal stenosis; its symptoms are thought to be due to impairment of the blood supply of the roots of the cauda equina, secondary to the canal stenosis.

The history is pain, numbness, paraesthesiae or weakness in the legs or buttocks, provoked by exertion and relieved by resting; symptoms often resolve more rapidly when the lumbar spine is flexed, i.e. in a sitting posture. The symptoms may mimic vascular claudication in the legs, but numbness and paraesthesiae (when present) are a helpful clue to the diagnosis. There may be no abnormal neurological signs at rest, but sometimes, immediately after exertion, focal signs may develop. Foot pulses are normal. Myelography confirms the stenosis, which is often most pronounced at several disc levels, presenting a formidable surgical challenge.

Cauda equina lesions

Cauda equina lesions usually cause bilateral leg symptoms and signs, together with bladder and rectal involvement. The bladder symptoms comprise reduced sensation, both of bladder filling and of urethral sensation, with difficulty voiding, a poor stream, and incomplete emptying. Eventually, painless retention with overflow incontinence develops. Constipation and faecal soiling may occur.

It is essential to examine sensation on the buttocks and perineum in any patient with unexplained loss of bladder or rectal sphincter control. The development of bladder symptoms is an indication for urgent myelography.

Other lesions occasionally affecting the cauda equina include neurofibromas, Schwannomas, lipomas, meningiomas and ependymomas. Spina bifida is considered on page 937.

Thoracic disc prolapse

Thoracic disc prolapse is relatively rare. It usually causes cord compression rather than root symptoms. The diagnosis is confirmed by myelography. Surgical treatment is hazardous, and a lateral or anterior approach is necessary.

ANTERIOR HORN CELL DISEASES

The acquired condition, motor neurone disease (MND), is the commonest of these disorders. Spinal muscular atrophy comprises a rare group of hereditary diseases in which there is slow degeneration of anterior horn cells. The polio virus shows a selective tropism for anterior horn cells. Poliomyelitis is discussed on page 969.

Summary 10 Diagnosis of motor neurone disease (MND)

- Never make a diagnosis of MND in the presence of sensory loss or bladder symptoms.

- Upper motor neurone (UMN) and lower motor neurone (LMN) signs in the upper and lower limbs may be produced by a combination of cervical and lumbar spondylosis.

- Do not make a definite diagnosis of MND until there are UMN and LMN signs in the same muscle groups in the limbs, and similar signs affecting cranial nerve-innervated muscles.

- If there is any doubt that a spinal cord lesion is present, myelography is essential.

MOTOR NEURONE DISEASE

MND is a progressive degenerative disease of unknown cause which affects upper and lower motor neurones in the brain and spinal cord. It is rare, with a prevalence of about 4–5 per 100 000, and usually affects middle-aged or elderly people. The disease is usually rapidly progressive, with death within 3–4 years of onset of symptoms.

Pathology

The pathology of MND is degeneration of anterior horn cells in the spinal cord, and lower motor neurones in the cranial nerves; the upper cranial nerves controlling eye movements, and the motor neurones to the bladder and bowel sphincters are spared. Cortical upper motor neurones supplying both cranial nerves and spinal motor neurones also degenerate, leading to the characteristic combination of widespread upper and lower motor neurone signs. In most patients, there is no intellectual impairment. Sensory tracts and nuclei remain normal.

Aetiology

In a very small number of cases, there is a family history. HLA typing shows no consistent trends. The pathology is not inflammatory, and there is no evidence of an immune mechanism. Searches for toxic factors have been fruitless.

Clinical features

MND may present with almost any combination of upper and lower motor neurone symptoms and signs, and is often asymmetrical in the early stages. As the disease progresses, however, a common pattern emerges.

Patients present with bulbar problems or limb symptoms or a combination of both. Early bulbar symptoms are dysarthria and dysphonia, dysphagia and difficulty in chewing, with nasal regurgitation of fluids. There may be recurrent chest infections, and respiratory muscle weakness may cause dyspnoea. In the limbs, the common presentations are weakness of a hand or whole arm, often with wasting which the patient has noticed, or, in the leg, progressive foot drop. Cramps are common.

Examination often reveals wasting, fasciculation and weakness in the muscles innervated by the cranial nerve nuclei. A particularly important sign is fasciculation in a wasted tongue. In the limbs, a combination of fasciculation and weakness, with brisk reflexes in wasted muscles, in the absence of any sensory abnormality, is strongly suggestive of MND.

Differential diagnosis

In many patients, a confident diagnosis can be made at the initial presentation, but in some, particularly those without cranial nerve signs, diagnostic difficulties may arise. A progressive bulbar palsy without limb signs may resemble myasthenia gravis. Multiple bilateral cerebral hemisphere infarcts or diffuse subcortical small vessel disease can produce bulbar problems similar to those of MND. When there are no cranial nerve signs, a cervical lesion producing a combination of motor root signs in the upper limbs with myelopathic upper motor neurone signs in both upper and lower limbs must be considered. This is the presentation of the *amyotrophic lateral sclerosis* variant of MND. Any sensory deficit or the presence of bladder symptoms suggests that the diagnosis is not MND. When limb signs are entirely lower motor neurone, a pure motor neuropathy is a possibility. In cases with predominantly proximal weakness and wasting, diabetic amyotrophy may be considered, and in occasional patients with signs confined to the legs, a cauda equina lesion may require exclusion.

Investigation

The diagnosis of MND is essentially a clinical one. Needle EMG shows denervation but not its cause. Surface EMG of all the limbs is often the more helpful test, in that it may demonstrate widespread denervation even in the absence of physical signs. Muscle biopsy is seldom necessary.

Prognosis and management

There is relentless progression. In older patients, and particularly those presenting with limb, rather than bulbar problems, the disease may last for 5–10 years from onset of symptoms to death. In others, death may result in less than a year. A few patients become demented. There may be emotional lability.

There is no cure for MND, which is invariably fatal. Only supportive measures can be provided. For patients with dysarthria and dysphonia, a range of communicators is now available. In the earlier stages, these symptoms, together with dysphagia, may be considerably ameliorated by speech therapy. Dysphagia requires careful attention to consistency of the food. Thin liquids and solids often lead to choking, while a blended diet may cause fewer problems. Nonetheless, eating usually imposes increasingly severe problems. A nasogastric tube or gastrostomy may be helpful in many patients. Dribbling of saliva may be helped by oral atropine or a tricyclic antidepressant, the latter also sometimes having a beneficial effect on mood. Progressive respiratory paralysis with aspiration pneumonia is the usual cause of death. Some patients with troublesome nocturnal dyspnoea and sleep disturbance are helped by non-invasive ventilation, but artificial ventilation via an endotracheal tube merely prolongs suffering.

Most patients become immobile and eventually require full nursing care. Patients remain alert to the end, and drug treatment to alleviate distress is often indicated.

HEREDITARY SPINAL MUSCULAR ATROPHY

Several rare disorders are described, but the two commonest are:

Werdnig-Hoffman disease

Werdnig-Hoffman disease is an autosomal recessive condition presenting either neonatally as a floppy baby, or with progressive weakness and wasting within the first year of life, due to widespread lower motor neurone degeneration. Death occurs within the first 4 years of life.

Kugelberg-Welander syndrome

Kugelberg-Welander syndrome is a progressive spinal muscular atrophy of either autosomal dominant or recessive inheritance. The disease sometimes affects children over the age of 2, but onset is usually in adolescence or early adult life, when there is degeneration of lower motor neurones, with relative sparing of cranial nerve nuclei. Kugelberg-Welander syndrome often presents with a predominantly proximal weakness, which may give a similar picture to a limb girdle dystrophy. This form of spinal muscular atrophy is relatively benign, but most patients eventually become disabled.

DISEASES OF PERIPHERAL NERVES AND PLEXUSES

PERIPHERAL NEUROPATHY

Peripheral nerves contain motor, sensory and autonomic fibres, with their cell bodies in the anterior horn, dorsal root ganglia, and autonomic ganglia, respectively. Nerve fascicles are surrounded by connective tissue, the perineurium, which forms a blood–nerve barrier maintaining a special environment in the endoneurium, the intrafascicular compartment in which the fibres lie. Myelinated nerve fibres are of varying size, the largest in diameter conducting at velocities of up to 70 m/second, the smallest at about 5 m/second. Unmyelinated axons conduct at less than 1 m/second. The Schwann cells provide axons with a certain amount of physical support, form the myelin of myelinated fibres and probably act in a nutritional capacity to axons. Most of the synthesis in nerve fibres occurs in the cell bodies, with subsequent transport down axons.

Pathophysiology

The principal pathology in diseases affecting peripheral nerves is either axonal degeneration or demyelination. *Axonal degeneration* may take the form of a neuronopathy, in which the cell body and whole axon are affected, or an axonopathy, in which the part of the axon furthest from the cell body is first affected. In *demyelinating neuropathies*, the primary pathological process is demyelination. This may lead to conduction block with consequent loss of function. Severe demyelination may lead to secondary axonal degeneration.

Regeneration in axonal neuropathies may occur after a period of Wallerian degeneration. Regeneration proceeds at only 1–2 mm per day. Remyelination in demyelinating neuropathies initially leads to short internodes and thin myelin sheaths, causing greatly reduced conduction velocities. A severely reduced nerve conduction velocity on electrophysiological testing indicates a demyelinating neuropathy; this may be generalised, e.g. as in Guillain-Barré syndrome (acute inflammatory polyneuropathy), or focal, as in an entrapment neuropathy such as the carpal tunnel syndrome.

The fibres in peripheral nerves are occasionally damaged by diseases which primarily affect the connective tissue, particularly the blood vessels of the nerve. Examples are the neuropathies due to vasculitis seen in polyarteritis nodosa, or SLE.

Clinical classification

Neuropathies may be divided into:

- *Mononeuropathy*, when a single nerve is involved
- *Multiple mononeuropathy* (mononeuritis multiplex or multifocal neuropathy), in which more than one, and sometimes many, individual nerves are affected in a patchy distribution. Multifocal neuropathy is typical of some diseases (Table 22.47).

Table 22.47 Causes of mononeuritis multiplex (multifocal neuropathy)

- Diabetes
- Connective tissue disease, e.g. SLE, RA, PAN
- Inflammatory, e.g. sarcoid
- Infective, e.g. leprosy, Herpes zoster (usually a mononeuritis)
- Familial disposition to entrapment neuropathy (tomaculous neuropathy)
- Other physical injury, e.g. radiotherapy, electrical injury, thermal injury, ischaemia
- Neoplastic, e.g. carcinomatous or lymphomatous infiltration, neurofibromatosis, malignant nerve tumours, related to paraproteinaemia

- *Polyneuropathy*, in which there is a diffuse symmetrical involvement of the peripheral nerves. Some diseases, notably diabetes, may also produce a multifocal neuropathy. Some polyneuropathies (e.g. Guillain-Barré syndrome) also affect the spinal roots, and in such cases the terms *polyradiculoneuropathy* or *polyradiculopathy* are more accurate.

Clinical features

Neuropathies may affect motor and sensory fibres or each differentially. Autonomic involvement is prominent in certain neuropathies, the commonest being diabetes.

Motor nerve involvement

The major symptom of motor nerve involvement is weakness. Examination reveals wasting and weakness, which, in the case of mononeuropathies, is appropriate to the distribution of a particular nerve; in the case of polyneuropathy, it is usually most marked distally in the limbs. Most peripheral neuropathies involve the lower limbs before the upper limbs. Occasionally, a predominantly proximal weakness may result from peripheral neuropathy, e.g. as in Guillain-Barré syndrome. Fasciculation is sometimes seen in peripheral neuropathy, usually in patients with rapidly progressive denervation. Tendon reflexes are often absent, usually as a result of sensory loss rather than motor impairment. Loss of the ankle jerks is common in normal elderly people.

Sensory nerve involvement

Sensory involvement includes the negative symptom of numbness and the positive symptoms of paraesthesiae and pain. Some neuropathies differentially affect large and small fibres. Those selectively affecting large fibres (e.g. uraemic neuropathy) impair touch, pressure, two-point discrimination and joint position sense; pain and temperature sensation are unaffected. Neuropathies selectively affecting small fibres (e.g. small fibre diabetic neuropathy or amyloid neuropathy) produce loss of pain and temperature sensation with relative preservation of other modalities. All the tendon reflexes may be present, since these depend on large fibre function. Substantial loss of pain and temperature sensation may lead to neuropathic feet ulcers.

In mononeuropathy, sensory impairment is within the distribution of a single nerve. In polyneuropathy, a stocking and glove, distal sensory impairment is typical.

Autonomic involvement

A severe type of burning pain (*causalgia*) occurs after injury to major limb peripheral nerves, e.g. the median, ulnar and sciatic nerves, and occasionally with injury to smaller nerves. Causalgia is often associated with evidence of local or regional reflex sympathetic disturbance, including vascular and sweating changes, and trophic changes in the skin and nails. Causalgia may be partly or completely relieved by sympathetic blockade, indicating the role of sympathetic activity in maintaining such pain. Similar burning pain, together with sympathetic changes, is sometimes a feature of polyneuropathy, most notably alcoholic neuropathy.

In a minority of patients, autonomic involvement is sufficiently severe to cause symptoms. Loss of blood pressure control leads to syncope. There may be impairment of sweating, sometimes severe enough to cause hyperpyrexia in hot weather; impairment of bladder and bowel sphincter function may lead to incontinence.

Diagnosis and investigation

In cases where the history and examination leave doubt about the presence of a neuropathy, motor and sensory nerve conduction studies are valuable.

Small fibre neuropathies pose particular diagnostic difficulties in that, with large fibre preservation, tendon reflexes are not lost and sensory loss is selective and often discrete. Recording of thermal thresholds for warming and cooling offers a simple way of assessing small fibre sensory function.

Nerve biopsy is only occasionally helpful in establishing the cause of a neuropathy. It is most often useful in patients with multifocal neuropathy, in those suspected of having amyloid, and in a number of the rare inherited metabolic disorders which lead to abnormal depositions in peripheral nerves, such as metachromatic leucodystrophy.

Mononeuropathy

The more common entrapment neuropathies are described below and Table 22.48 lists the main features of a number of less common traumatic mononeuropathies.

Summary 11 Peripheral neuropathy

- Peripheral neuropathy is classified clinically into mononeuropathy (mononeuritis), mononeuritis multiplex (multifocal neuropathy) and polyneuropathy.
- Polyneuropathies may be motor or sensory, but are usually mixed (sensorimotor).
- The clinical type of the neuropathy may be helpful in identifying the cause.
- In polyneuropathies, legs are affected before the arms.
- Tendon reflexes may be partly preserved in a polyneuropathy in the early stages, or when the neuropathy predominantly affects the legs, or is predominantly motor rather than sensory.
- Autonomic involvement characteristically occurs with some neuropathies.
- Some neuropathies (e.g. Guillain-Barré) may affect respiratory function.

Brief periods of nerve compression cause focal demyelination, leading to conduction block, but without loss of axonal continuity (*neurapraxia*). Remyelination will restore both conduction and function over days or weeks. With more severe compression, which often occurs over a longer period, axonal interruption may result; this leads to Wallerian degeneration of the axons distal to the site of compression, but with continuity of the connective tissue elements of the nerve. Axonal regeneration and remyelination with relief of compression occur over a much longer period after such injury, but good restoration of function is possible. With severe, penetrating injuries causing division of the nerve, connective tissue continuity is also lost, and regeneration is always incomplete, even with the most careful surgical apposition of nerve ends.

Median nerve

Carpal tunnel syndrome

Compression of the median nerve at the wrist beneath the flexor retinaculum gives rise to the carpal tunnel syndrome. This is most common in middle-aged women, and more likely to occur after wrist fracture, in pregnancy, in rheumatoid arthritis with involvement of the wrist joint, in myxoedema and in acromegaly. The median nerve may also be damaged by penetrating trauma at the wrist. Symptoms may be provoked by occupational use of the hands.

The symptoms of carpal tunnel syndrome are pain, numbness and paraesthesiae in the hand. The symptoms are often diffuse, affecting the whole hand. Pain may radiate through the forearm and, occasionally, may involve the whole arm. Typically, pain is most troublesome at night or first thing in the morning. Sensory symptoms are more common than motor symptoms, but some patients notice weakness of the thumb. On examination, there is weakness of abductor pollicis brevis (APB), with or without wasting, and also weakness of opponens. There is sensory impairment in a median distribution (Fig. 22.38). The Tinel sign is positive when gentle tapping over the

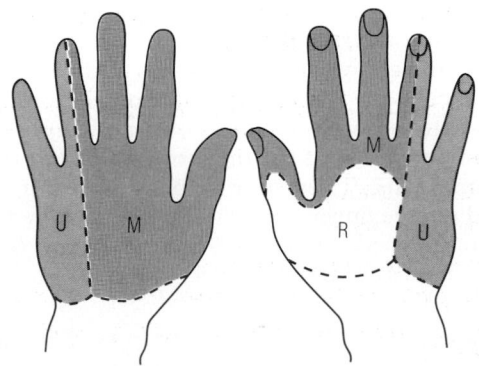

Fig. 22.38 The cutaneous sensory territories of the median (M), ulnar (U) and radial (R) nerves.

Table 22.48 Causes and features of individual nerve lesions (See also Figure 23.5)

Nerve (root)	Site and cause of lesion	Clinical features
(Median, ulnar and radial nerves: see text*)		
Axillary (C5, 6)	Brachial plexus. Crutches. Sleeping partner's head – 'honeymoon palsy'	Paralysis of shoulder abduction, deltoid
Musculocutaneous (C5, 6)	Humeral fracture with brachial plexus injury	Paralysis of biceps, brachialis. Sensory loss on lateral aspect of forearm
Femoral (L2–4)*	Fracture of pelvis or femur Dislocation of hip Hip operations Psoas abscess or psoas haematoma in haemophilia	Paralysis of iliacus, quadriceps, sartorius. Sensory loss over anterolateral thigh and saphenous distribution. Absent knee jerk
Lateral cutaneous nerve of thigh (L2, 3)*	Pressure of inguinal ligament Obesity. 'Meralgia paraesthetica'	Sensory loss over anterolateral thigh. Often with burning pain and paraesthesiae
Obturator (L2, 4)	Neoplastic or radiotherapy damage in pelvis. Fetal head pressure, or forceps injury	Weakness of hip adductors. Sensory loss over lower medial thigh
Sciatic (L4, 5, S1–3)*	Pelvic mass. Fracture/dislocation of femur. Penetrating trauma Baker's cyst in popliteal fossa Pressure palsy in drug addicts and alcoholics	Paralysis of all lower leg and foot muscles. Absent ankle jerk. Sensory loss of whole foot, extending up lateral aspect of lower leg. Often painful
Common peroneal/lateral popliteal (L4, 5, S1, 2)*	Compression at neck of fibula: squatting, sitting cross-legged, pressure under anaesthesia Fibular fracture	Foot-drop and weakness of eversion. Sensory loss over lateral aspect of lower leg and dorsum of foot
Tibial (L4, 5, S1–3)	Trauma in thigh and popliteal fossa Distal injury in tarsal tunnel	Paralysis of plantar flexion and inversion. Sensory loss on sole. Pain common. In tarsal tunnel syndrome, paralysis of medial foot muscles and sensory loss on sole
Sural (L5, S1–2)	Pressure in lower calf and at ankle, e.g. from tight boots	Sensory loss over lateral border of foot

The most important lesions are marked*

carpal tunnel causes paraesthesiae in part of the cutaneous distribution of the nerve.

In mild cases, a wrist splint to reduce movement at the wrist may help, and an injection of hydrocortisone into the carpal tunnel may give temporary relief. In cases where there is sensory loss or weakness, surgical decompression of the carpal tunnel is required. Mild carpal tunnel syndrome symptoms often resolve spontaneously.

Proximal lesions

More proximal injuries of the median nerve are unusual. A lesion at the elbow causes weakness of the long finger flexors (except the ulnar half of flexor digitorum profundus), together with weakness of flexor carpi radialis, pronator teres, most of the thenar muscles and the two radial lumbricals. There is weakness of flexion of the index and middle fingers and distal phalanx of the thumb, in addition to weakness of APB and opponens. Sensory loss is the same as in carpal tunnel syndrome.

Ulnar nerve

Ulnar nerve lesions usually follow entrapment at the elbow. Above the elbow, the nerve gives rise to branches supplying the medial part of the deep finger flexors and flexor carpi ulnaris. In the forearm, the nerve gives off the dorsal branch which supplies the skin over the medial part of the dorsal aspect of the hand, the medial one-and-a-half digits, and the medial part of the palm over the hypothenar eminence (Fig. 22.38). The deep branch of the nerve supplies the hypothenar muscles, the interossei, adductor pollicis, the third and fourth lumbricals and part of flexor pollicis brevis.

Sensory symptoms from ulnar nerve lesions include pain, paraesthesiae and numbness in the hand; as with carpal tunnel syndrome, these symptoms may not be confined to the anatomical distribution of the nerve. Weakness is often asymptomatic.

A lesion of the nerve in the region of the elbow may lead to palpable thickening of the nerve in the ulnar groove. The muscles in the forearm are spared. In the hand, there is wasting of the first dorsal interosseus and abductor digiti minimi, and wasting of the other interossei, causing guttering between the metacarpals with weakness of finger abduction. In severe lesions, a claw-hand posture develops. This is due to paralysis of the interossei and medial two lumbricals, which normally flex the fingers at the metacarpophalangeal joints, and extend the fingers at the interphalangeal joints. In claw-hand, there is extension at the metacarpophalangeal joints due to the unopposed action of the long extensors of the fingers, and flexion at the interphalangeal joints due to the action of the flexor digitorum superficialis. The posture mainly affects the little and ring fingers, since, although all the interossei are weak, the radial lumbricals supplied by the median nerve prevent extension of the lateral metacarpophalangeal joints.

Lesions of the ulnar nerve above the elbow produce weakness of finger flexion and flexor carpi ulnaris. Lesions at the wrist and in the hand spare the dorsal branch, so that sensation on the dorsum of the hand and fingers is preserved. Lesions at the wrist involve the superficial branch, so that sensory loss occurs on the medial palm and palmar aspects of the ring and little fingers; lesions within the hand usually spare this branch.

Radial nerve

The radial nerve lies on the posterior surface of the humerus in the radial groove, and supplies triceps in the upper arm and the skin on the back of the upper arm. In the forearm, the nerve gives branches to brachioradialis, and extensor carpi radialis longus and brevis. The deep branch supplies supinator, extensor digitorum, extensor carpi ulnaris and extensor digiti minimi. The extension of the deep branch is the posterior interosseous nerve, which supplies abductor pollicis longus, extensor pollicis longus and brevis, and extensor indicis. The terminal superficial radial nerve innervates the skin over the lateral part of the dorsum of the hand and thumb, index and middle fingers.

When the radial nerve is injured in the axilla or in fractures of the humerus, there is paralysis of all these muscles, including triceps. 'Saturday night palsy' is a neurapraxia in which the nerve is damaged in the upper arm when compressed over the arm of a chair, the result of going to sleep in this position when drunk. Triceps is spared, but there is weakness of all other muscles supplied by the nerve, producing a wrist-drop, together with sensory loss over the dorsum of the hand (Fig. 22.38). Recovery takes place over several weeks; function in the hand is improved by a splint to correct the wrist-drop.

Mononeuritis multiplex (multifocal neuropathy)

By comparison with polyneuropathy, mononeuritis multiplex has relatively few causes (Table 22.47). Biopsy of an affected sensory nerve may reveal specific pathological changes much more often than in polyneuropathy.

Polyneuropathy

The many possible causes of polyneuropathy are shown in Table 22.49. Despite extensive investigation, the

Table 22.49 Causes of polyneuropathy

Inflammatory	
Acute inflammatory polyneuropathy: Guillain-Barré syndrome	Chronic progressive inflammatory polyneuropathy (CPIP)
Chronic relapsing inflammatory polyneuropathy (CRIP)	Serum sickness
	Sarcoidosis
	SLE
	PAN
Metabolic	
Diabetes	Myxoedema
Uraemia	Amyloid
	Ischaemia
Nutritional	
Beri-beri (thiamine deficiency)	Burning feet syndrome
Pellagra (niacin deficiency)	Sprue
Vitamin B_{12} deficiency	Malabsorption
Neoplastic	
Non-metastatic	Paraproteinaemia
Myeloma	Macroglobulinaemia
Infections	
Leprosy	Mumps
Diphtheria	Infectious mononucleosis
Measles	Brucellosis
	HIV
Toxic	
Alcohol	Thallium
Lead	Triorthocresyl phosphate (TOCP)
Arsenic	Insecticides
Gold	Acrylamide
Mercury	N-hexane
Drugs	
Isoniazid	Sulphonamide
Nitrofurantoin	Emetine
Vincristine	Phenytoin
Metronidazole	Pyridoxine
Disulphiram	Griseofulvin
Clioquinol	Cisplatinum
Dapsone	Amiodarone
	Tricyclic antidepressants
Hereditary	
HMSN type I	Porphyria
HMSN type II	Dystrophy
HMSN type III	Metachromatic leucodystrophy
Hereditary sensory neuropathy	Fabry's disease – angiokeratoma
Friedreich's ataxia	corporis diffusum
Familial dysautonomia (Riley-Day)	

cause of some neuropathies is never established. In such cases, it is particularly important to examine family members, both clinically and electrophysiologically, as this may establish the diagnosis of an hereditary neuropathy.

COMMON CAUSES OF NEUROPATHY

Endocrine and metabolic neuropathies

Diabetic neuropathy

In many countries, diabetes is the commonest cause of neuropathy.

Mononeuropathy and multifocal neuropathy

Entrapment neuropathies, e.g. carpal tunnel syndrome, are much more likely to develop in diabetes. In addition, peripheral nerves may be affected by the small vessel disease of diabetes. This microangiopathic pathology underlies the IIIrd cranial nerve palsy, which typically produces an ophthalmoplegia but spares the pupil. This is because the fibres to the pupil are distributed in the outer part of the nerve, and the ischaemia produced by small vessel occlusion affects predominantly central parts of the nerve. Other cranial nerves may be affected. A multifocal neuropathy in the limbs is occasionally seen, and is presumed to have a microangiopathic basis.

Diabetic amyotrophy

Diabetic amyotrophy is a proximal multifocal neuropathy which affects the femoral nerve and, to a lesser extent, other nerves supplying proximal muscles in the leg. It occurs in middle-aged or elderly diabetics, commonly in those with poor diabetic control. The condition is usually unilateral. The first symptom is pain in the thigh lasting for weeks or months. Weakness rapidly develops; this is most marked for hip flexion and knee extension, but usually also involves other muscles at the hip and the hamstrings. Distal power is normal. The knee jerk is absent. Recovery begins within weeks or months and is usually good.

Polyneuropathy

Polyneuropathy is the commonest type of diabetic neuropathy. It is a sensory motor neuropathy, but in many patients it remains predominantly sensory. Numbness and paraesthesiae are the main symptoms, occasionally with hyperaesthesiae on the soles of the feet. Pain, either a continuous aching or burning, or of a shock-like stabbing nature, may occur. The onset is usually insidious over weeks or months.

A much rarer type of painful polyneuropathy affects predominantly the small myelinated and unmyelinated fibres, leading to impaired pain and temperature sensation. Tendon reflexes, which depend on large fibre afferents, are preserved. Patients with this type of neuropathy complain of severe pain in the feet, often associated with hyperaesthesia. Another type of acute peripheral polyneuropathy in diabetes affects all fibre types. The onset is preceded by rapid weight loss. This neuropathy, which is very painful, resolves after 9 months to a year in most patients.

Autonomic neuropathy

An autonomic neuropathy is common in diabetes and is nearly always seen in association with a sensory motor polyneuropathy. The pupils may be affected, with reduced response to light. There may be dysphagia if the oesophagus is involved. Gastric atony causes vomiting, and denervation of the lower bowel leads to diarrhoea. Postural hypotension with syncope is the commonest early symptom. Diagnostically, postural hypotension and the absence of the normal cardiac beat-to-beat interval variation are useful observations. Erectile impotence, retrograde ejaculation, retention of urine and incontinence may all be troublesome features.

Management

The mainstay of treatment of diabetic neuropathy is good control of the diabetes (Ch. 19). This particularly helps the mononeuritis and multifocal neuropathies. Symptomatic treatment for neuropathic pain is often unsatisfactory. Simple analgesics, anticonvulsants and benzodiazepines may all occasionally help.

Treatment of autonomic neuropathy is always difficult. Usually, the most troublesome symptom is postural hypotension. Tight stockings to prevent venous pooling in the legs rarely have a major effect. The blood pressure tends to be at its lowest in the morning and rises gradually during the day. Patients with autonomic failure tend to lose excess sodium and water during the night. This can be counteracted to some extent by sleeping with the head of the bed raised. This lowers the recumbent blood pressure, leading to renin release and a reduction in the nocturnal sodium and water loss.

Fludrocortisone, which causes sodium and water retention, is also effective. A dose of 0.1–0.2 mg daily is usually sufficient, but excessive sodium and water retention, particularly in elderly patients, may lead to heart failure. Pressor drugs are seldom useful.

Other endocrine and metabolic neuropathies

Uraemic neuropathy is described on page 976. Myxoedema causes an axonal, predominantly sensory polyneuropathy, but this is a much less common manifestation than either the proximal myopathy (p. 956) or cerebellar ataxia (p. 929) that occur in hypothyroidism. Amyloid, of either the hereditary or acquired type, may cause a peripheral sensory motor neuropathy, which particularly affects small fibres and is characteristically painful. A helpful diagnostic sign in this type of neuropathy is palpable thickening of the peripheral nerves. Long-standing lower limb ischaemia may lead to peripheral nerve damage, giving rise to signs of a peripheral polyneuropathy in the legs.

Inflammatory polyneuropathies

Guillain-Barré syndrome

Guillain-Barré syndrome (acute inflammatory polyneuropathy) is an acute, demyelinating, predominantly motor polyradiculoneuropathy which affects people of all ages.

Aetiology

In some (but not all) patients there is a preceding history of a viral illness, often an upper respiratory infection. A number of specific preceding infections have been identified, including enterovirus and mycoplasma infections. It is thought that preceding infection or some other immune stimulus may trigger a mainly cell-mediated process causing demyelination of spinal roots and peripheral nerves. There is little evidence that circulating antibodies are involved in this process.

Clinical features

Maximum weakness usually occurs between 10 and 14 days after the onset of the neuropathy. Occasionally, profound paralysis may develop within 24 hours. The first symptoms are usually sensory, with distal paraesthesiae, numbness and sometimes pain. Cranial nerve involvement occurs in 30–40% of patients, with bilateral facial weakness being the common manifestation. Bulbar weakness predisposes to aspiration pneumonia. The autonomic nervous system is sometimes involved, causing lability of blood pressure and arrythmias. Bladder dysfunction is rare. The CSF protein is sometimes raised to very high levels, causing impaired reabsorption in the arachnoid granulations, leading to papilloedema.

Examination reveals weakness, with variable cranial nerve involvement. There is no wasting, as the neuropathy is acute in onset. Reflexes are nearly always all absent. Despite prominent sensory symptoms, objective signs of sensory loss are slight. Occasionally, there is an ascending dense sensory loss affecting first the limbs and then the trunk.

Investigation

The CSF is under normal pressure and shows a normal cell count, or slight pleocytosis of lymphocytes, and a markedly elevated protein of between 1 and 10 g/l. Demyelination quickly spreads distally and, by the time electrodiagnostic tests are done, there is usually some slowing of conduction, which later may become severe. The vital capacity must be measured regularly.

Differential diagnosis

The diagnosis is obvious in the majority of cases. Acute cervical spinal cord lesions, acute myaesthenia gravis and poliomyelitis all require consideration. In acute poliomyelitis, weakness is often asymmetrical and, in contrast to Guillain-Barré syndrome, the CSF always shows a raised cell count of 10–200 cells/mm^3.

Management and prognosis

With supportive treatment alone, 85–90% of all patients with Guillain-Barré syndrome recover completely over several months. Others are left with some residual deficit, usually mild. A few patients show a slowly progressive course (chronic progressive inflammatory polyneuropathy) but may respond to corticosteroid and other anti-inflammatory treatments and, occasionally, to plasma exchange. A variant of this chronic demyelinating neuropathy is one showing a relapsing course (chronic relapsing inflammatory polyneuropathy), which may respond to similar treatment.

There is no evidence that corticosteroids or other anti-inflammatory drugs improve the outcome in acute inflammatory polyneuropathy. However, plasma exchange improves the prognosis if used early in patients who are rapidly deteriorating and severely affected.

Even those patients who require ventilatory support may make a complete recovery. The best prognostic guide is the compound motor action potential which, if reduced to 20% or less of normal, indicates a poor prognosis.

Miller Fisher syndrome

Miller Fisher syndrome is a variant of acute inflammatory polyneuropathy, in which there is an ophthalmoplegia, probably of peripheral origin, due to demyelination of any or all of the IIIrd, IVth and VIth cranial nerves, together with ataxia and areflexia, with little or no weakness in the limbs. The prognosis is good; no treatment has been found to have an effect.

Nutritional neuropathies

The neurological consequences of vitamin B$_{12}$ deficiency are discussed on page 936. In addition, a number of other nutritional deficiencies may cause polyneuropathies which are characteristically painful. The burning feet syndrome, described in Japanese prisoners of war, was probably the result of multiple nutritional deficits. Peripheral neuropathy – one of the neurological manifestations of pellagra due to niacin deficiency – is a sensory motor polyneuropathy in which severe burning of the feet with tenderness and hyperaesthesia of the lower legs and feet is prominent. A painful neuropathy also occurs in beriberi due to thiamine deficiency.

Neoplastic neuropathies

The neoplastic neuropathies are described on page 977.

Paraproteinaemic neuropathy

Myeloma and other malignancies, such as some types of lymphoma and Waldenström's macroglobulinaemia, which produce a monoclonal gammopathy may be associated with a demyelinating neuropathy. In addition, a benign IgM gammopathy associated with a chronic, slowly progressive demyelinating neuropathy is now recognised; there is evidence that the neuropathy is caused by the abnormal IgM. Some patients respond to immunosuppression or plasma exchange.

Infective neuropathies

Worldwide, leprosy (p. 270) is the most frequent infective cause of peripheral neuropathy. It produces a multifocal neuropathy and there is marked nerve thickening.

Both brucellosis and infectious mononucleosis are rarely associated with an acute, predominantly motor, polyneuropathy, similar to acute inflammatory polyneuropathy. The neuropathy occurring with infectious mononucleosis may respond to steroid treatment. A mononeuritis or multifocal neuropathy may also develop with either of these infections. Mumps and measles are very rarely complicated by a transient polyneuropathy.

Diphtheria (p. 259) may cause a profound demyelinating peripheral neuropathy, due to the action of the exotoxin. The first symptom is palatal weakness, usually occurring about 2 weeks after pharyngeal infection. Weakness of the external ocular muscles may develop after about 4 weeks, and a generalised polyneuropathy after about 7 or 8 weeks. This may include respiratory weakness, for which ventilation is necessary. Remyelination with gradual recovery occurs over several months, but the commonly associated myocarditis may prove fatal.

Neuropathies occurring with HIV infection are considered on page 973.

Toxic neuropathies

Alcoholic neuropathy, described on page 981, is easily the most important of the toxic neuropathies.

Other toxic causes of neuropathy are listed in Table 22.50. These produce axonal neuropathies and many cause widespread CNS damage in addition.

Table 22.50 Classification of the muscular dystrophies

X-linked	Autosomal dominant
Duchenne	Facioscapulohumeral
Becker	Scapuloperoneal
	Oculopharyngeal
Autosomal recessive	Ocular
Limb-girdle	
Childhood dystrophy	

Drug-induced neuropathy

Certain drugs almost inevitably cause a neuropathy if given in sufficiently large dosages for long enough. Examples include vincristine and metronidazole. Other drugs show a strong tendency to produce neuropathy but depend on host susceptibility. For example, isoniazid neuropathy (preventable with small doses of pyridoxine) is much more likely to develop in patients whose liver is only capable of slow acetylation of the drug.

Hereditary neuropathies

HMSN types I and II (peroneal muscular atrophy, Charcot-Marie-Tooth disease)

Peroneal muscular atrophy (Charcot-Marie-Tooth disease) is the commonest of the hereditary neuropathies, subdivided into hereditary motor and sensory neuropathy (HMSN) types I and II, on the basis of motor nerve conduction velocity.

Type I HMSN tends to present in the first decade of life, with difficulty walking and pes cavus or equinovarus foot deformity. Associated kyphoscoliosis is common. There is severe distal wasting in the legs and, later, in the upper limbs. The wasting in the legs sometimes spares the upper part of the thighs, producing the so-called 'inverted champagne bottle legs'; however, a diffuse pattern of wasting in the legs is as common. In the upper limbs, in addition to wasting, weakness and generalised areflexia, there is frequently tremor and a cerebellar type of ataxia. Respiratory muscle weakness can occur. Peripheral nerves are sometimes thickened. Nerve conduction velocity is reduced to less than 38 m/second, and is often severely slowed, indicating a severe demyelinating type of neuropathy.

Type II HMSN is of later onset, with a peak onset in the second decade but with many cases presenting much later than this. It is primarily an axonal neuropathy. Weakness and wasting are less marked than in type I, and tend to be confined to the lower limbs. Foot and spinal deformity are less common than in type I and there is no palpable nerve thickening. The tendon reflexes are absent in the legs, but are often preserved in the arms. Motor conduction velocities are reduced, but not below 38 m/second.

In both types of HMSN, the inheritance is usually autosomal dominant, although sporadic cases occur of both types and a few cases probably have an autosomal recessive mode of inheritance. In both types, men tend to be more severely affected than women.

Porphyria

An axonal neuropathy may develop in attacks of acute intermittent porphyria (p. 781). The neuropathy is unusual in distribution, in that a predominantly proximal weakness may develop together with a proximally distributed sensory impairment.

Refsum's disease

Refsum's disease is a condition with autosomal inheritance which results from defective metabolism of the long-chain aliphatic alcohol, phytol. Metabolism cannot proceed past the stage of phytanic acid due to deficiency of the enzyme, phytanic acid alpha hydroxylase. Phytanic acid thus collects throughout the body and affects the nervous system, producing a demyelinating sensory motor polyneuropathy, cerebellar ataxia, sensory neural deafness, retinal pigmentary degeneration and anosmia. A cardiomyopathy is also common. Presentation is usually in the second decade but, occasionally, patients may present much later.

Phytol is derived from chlorophyll in the diet and the condition may be alleviated by a chlorophyll-free diet.

DISEASES AFFECTING BRACHIAL AND LUMBOSACRAL PLEXUSES

Brachial plexus lesions

The brachial plexus is a relatively infrequent site of peripheral nerve damage.

Trauma

Lesions involving the upper part of the brachial plexus (C5 and C6, upper trunk) result from downward traction of the arm or forceful downward trauma on the shoulder. Severe trauma may avulse the C5 and C6 roots completely, causing extensive proximal weakness at the shoulder and sensory loss involving the outer aspect of the arm and the thumb, index and middle fingers. Trauma causing damage to the lower part of the plexus (C8 and T1) usually occurs with upward traction on the arm. There is paralysis of the small hand muscles and weakness of wrist and finger flexors, with sensory loss on the medial aspect of the arm and the little and ring fingers. Horner's syndrome is often present.

Birth injuries exemplify these two types of damage. In Erb's palsy, due to excessive traction on the head or a breech delivery, there is an upper brachial plexus lesion in which paralysis of abduction occurs with the arm internally rotated at the shoulder, the elbow extended, and the forearm pronated in the 'waiter's tip' posture. In Klumpke's paralysis, due to traction with the arm abducted and extended, a lower brachial plexus lesion occurs.

In adult life, trauma to the brachial plexus most commonly occurs as a result of motor-cycle accidents.

Cervical rib

Cervical rib is either a bony rib or fibrous band arising from the seventh cervical vertebra and attached anteriorly to the first rib. The C8 and T1 roots and the subclavian artery may be distorted as they pass over the cervical rib. Symptoms arise in adult life and may be either vascular or neurological, but rarely both together. Neurological symptoms are pain in the arm along the medial border and on the ulnar aspect of the hand, with weakness of grip. Very often symptoms are provoked by carrying heavy objects. Examination shows wasting and weakness of the small hand muscles and the medial finger and wrist flexors, with sensory loss affecting the little and ring fingers extending along the ulnar border of the forearm. Vascular symptoms comprise ischaemia in the hand, sometimes embolic symptoms and Raynaud's phenomenon. Treatment is surgical resection of the rib or band.

Neuralgic amyotrophy

Neuralgic amyotrophy, also called cryptogenic brachial plexus neuropathy, is an acute patchy lesion of the brachial plexus, usually involving mainly C5 and C6 innervated muscles. Occasionally, the condition may follow immunisations or be associated with a connective tissue disorder. The first symptom is severe pain around one shoulder. Weakness develops within a few days of onset of the pain, and most often affects the deltoid, spinati and serratus anterior, less commonly biceps and triceps, and rarely forearm and hand muscles. There is sometimes sensory loss, but this is usually mild. Demyelination is the likely underlying pathology. The prognosis is good.

Occasionally phrenic nerve involvement causes diaphragm weakness and breathlessness. Phrenic nerve damage may not recover.

Malignant invasion of the brachial plexus

The commonest tumours invading the brachial plexus are carcinomas of the lung and breast. Lymphoma, spreading from cervical glands, is occasionally responsible. Virtually complete brachial plexus lesions may be seen with malignant invasion, and pain is a common and usually very troublesome symptom.

Benign nerve tumours, such as neurofibromas, occasionally arise in the brachial plexus; very occasionally, primary malignant tumours involve the plexus.

Radiation brachial plexus lesions

Radiation may cause delayed damage to the brachial plexus, and considerable diagnostic difficulties arise when it is difficult to distinguish malignant invasion from radiation damage. MRI may be particularly helpful in some patients. Radiation lesions usually develop several years after treatment.

Lumbosacral plexus lesions

A wide variety of lesions may affect the lumbosacral plexus. The main diagnostic problem is confirming that the lesion is of the lumbosacral plexus, rather than an intraspinal lesion causing a lumbosacral radiculopathy. The two commonest lumbar root lesions due to discs are at L5 and S1 (p. 939). Lumbosacral plexus lesions will often affect root levels higher than L5 and the presentation of an atypical lumbar radiculopathy syndrome should always raise the possibility of a plexus lesion. The commonest cause is malignant invasion from carcinoma of the cervix, rectum, uterus, bladder, prostate and, occasionally, lymphoma. As with malignant invasion of the brachial plexus, pain is a prominent symptom, with progressive wasting and weakness, and sensory impairment. The lumbosacral plexus may be involved in pelvic fractures. The fetal head is occasionally responsible for damage during parturition.

Neurophysiological investigation is often helpful in demonstrating that the extent of denervation is greater than would be found with a single root. CT scanning and MRI are used to visualise the posterior pelvic region if a lumbosacral plexus lesion is suspected.

DISEASES AFFECTING THE NEUROMUSCULAR JUNCTION

These are rare disorders, in which there is defective transmission at the neuromuscular junction. The commonest is myasthenia gravis, with a prevalence of approximately 1 in 30 000.

MYASTHENIA GRAVIS

Myasthenia gravis (MG) is a disease characterised by fatigable weakness of striated muscle. This may be localised or generalised and is due to a defect of transmission at the neuromuscular junction. Women are affected twice as often as men, with the onset usually in early adult life. However, it may appear at any age. Neonatal MG, which occurs in 1 in 8 babies born to mothers with MG, resolves over a few weeks.

There is an association of MG with the presence of a thymoma in older patients. Such tumours may be benign or malignant. MG also shows a strong association with thyrotoxicosis and associations also exist with diabetes mellitus, rheumatoid arthritis and SLE, suggesting an autoimmune basis. There are antibodies to the acetylcholine receptor and, while the antibody titre does not correlate well with disease severity, the presence of a raised titre of acetylcholine receptor antibody is a useful diagnostic test.

Apart from thymoma, thymic histology is often abnormal in MG, showing hyperplasia. This does not usually cause gross thymic enlargement.

Clinical features

The commonest initial presentation is weakness, often affecting only the external ocular muscles, and usually with ptosis (ocular myasthenia). However, any muscle may be involved, including bulbar and neck muscles, respiratory, shoulder girdle and pelvic girdle muscles. MG may be very localised at the onset but usually becomes generalised with time. There is a tendency for the condition to relapse and remit, and intercurrent illness, particularly infection, may provoke severe exacerbations.

Initially, diplopia may only be noticeable at the end of the day. Bulbar weakness causes difficulty in chewing, weakness of the facial muscles, dysarthria, palatal weakness leading to regurgitation of fluids, and dysphagia and dysphonia. Neck weakness is common when there is bulbar weakness. In the limbs, symptomatic weakness is usually proximal and affects shoulder girdle more than pelvic girdle muscles.

The hallmark of myasthenic weakness is fatigability, and this must therefore be tested in the physical examination. Ptosis tends to appear more rapidly on sustained upward gaze. Eye movements should be tested with maintained gaze in different directions, and the patient questioned for the appearance of diplopia. Repetitive counting may reveal bulbar weakness. In the limbs, power is tested before and after repetitive proximal limb movements.

In early MG, muscle bulk is normal. However, in advanced MG, permanent, often non-fatigable, weakness with wasting sometimes develops. Even in wasted, weak muscles reflexes are present and may be brisk.

Diagnosis

The diagnosis can usually be made with confidence on clinical grounds, but can be confirmed or established in cases of doubt by the intravenous edrophonium (Tensilon) test. This anticholinesterase drug has a duration of action of only a few minutes. A test dose of 1–2 mg is given to ensure no major adverse effects, followed by 5–10 mg as an intravenous bolus. Myasthenic weakness is usually improved with this drug, but the success of the tests depends on timing and a certain degree of clinical expertise. Eye movements in ocular MG may appear not to be improved even when this is the correct diagnosis, since the improvement may be limited.

EMG can be helpful, showing a decremental response to supramaximal repetitive stimulation of a muscle nerve. Acetylcholine receptor antibody titres are raised in about 90% of patients with MG. A chest X-ray and thoracic CT should be done to investigate the possibility of thymic enlargement. There is a strong association of thymoma with striated muscle antibody.

Management

Initial treatment is with the long-acting anticholinesterase, pyridostigmine, a usual starting dose being 60 mg three or four times a day. Atropine is given if muscarinic side-effects are troublesome. Larger doses of pyridostigmine are given if there is deterioration. Large doses of pyridostigmine (more than 12–15 doses of 60 mg daily) are capable of producing a cholinergic block at the neuromuscular junction; this leads to weakness which may be indistinguishable from myasthenic weakness. When there is uncertainty as to whether weakness is due to a cholinergic or myasthenic crisis, a test dose of Tensilon should be given, with an anaesthetist and full resuscitation equipment on hand.

Thymectomy in MG is likely to benefit most patients if it is undertaken relatively early in the course of the disease. It is nearly always done in patients suspected of having a thymoma, the exceptions being old age and other associated illness. Thymectomy may produce a long period of remission, particularly in younger patients.

Immunosuppression with prednisolone and azathioprine is beneficial in patients with a limited response to pyridostigmine. The use of these drugs at an early stage of the disease remains controversial. Many patients are maintained in reasonable health for long periods with a combination of these drugs.

Plasma exchange improves weakness in MG, probably by removing circulating acetylcholine receptor antibody. It is extremely helpful as an immediate life-saving measure in severe MG with respiratory involvement.

A number of drugs with membrane stabilising properties may profoundly worsen the weakness of MG. These drugs include suxamethonium (the initial diagnosis of MG may be made after prolonged paralysis with this anaesthetic drug), beta-blockers, the aminoglycoside antibiotics and anticonvulsant drugs.

Prognosis

The prognosis is variable. Some patients, young or old, run a progressive downhill course despite all treatments, and die within a few years. Others remit for variable periods. The prognosis is much worse for patients with a thymoma (usually patients in the older age group).

LAMBERT-EATON MYASTHENIC SYNDROME

In the rare Lambert-Eaton myasthenic syndrome (LEMS), the defect at the neuromuscular junction is prejunctional, due to failure of release of acetylcholine. Typical fatigable weakness develops proximally in the limbs and trunk, and there is occasionally ptosis. Bulbar muscles are unaffected. In some patients, there is no clear history of fatigable weakness. In contrast to MG, tendon reflexes are usually absent, but can be reinforced by a brief maintained isometric contraction. This is the so-called *post-tetanic potentiation*, a useful sign in diagnosis.

Autonomic symptoms, due to failure of acetylcholine release in the parasympathetic nervous system, are common, and include a dry mouth, sphincter dysfunction and erectile impotence.

About half the cases of LEMS arise in patients with small cell cancer of the lung, while half are not associated with any disease. Both types appear to have an autoimmune basis and may be helped by prednisolone and azathioprine. Guanidine and 3,4-aminopyridine have both been used to increase release of acetylcholine at the neuromuscular junction.

BOTULISM

The exotoxin of *Clostridium botulinum* binds irreversibly to the presynaptic terminals of nerves whose impulse transmission is mediated by acetylcholine. Those include neuromuscular junctions, autonomic ganglia and parasympathetic nerve terminals. The toxin acts by preventing release of acetylcholine. Antitoxin has no effect once the toxin has become bound, but recovery of transmission is achieved by terminal axonal sprouting and formation of new synaptic contacts. Botulism results from eating food contaminated with *Cl. botulinum*, which produces the toxin under anaerobic conditions. The toxin is neutralised within 60 seconds by heating to above 85° and botulism thus usually results from eating home-made food preserves, small outbreaks being the rule. It is a rare disease in the UK, but is more frequent in other parts of the world where preparation of uncooked food preserves is common.

Clinical features

The first symptoms, which occur 12–72 hours after ingestion, are a dry mouth, abdominal distension with constipation, hesitancy of micturition, blurred vision (due to failure of accommodation), nausea and vomiting. Weakness of cranial nerve innervated muscles occurs early, so that diplopia is often the first symptom of weakness. Widespread weakness, including respiratory paralysis, then develops.

Diagnosis and management

The symptoms and signs of autonomic cholinergic dysfunction distinguish botulism from Guillain-Barré syndrome, MG and diphtheria. EMG may also be helpful. Sensory action potentials and conduction velocities are normal, and there is a reduced compound motor action potential to stimulation of motor nerves. However, as with LEMS, in which a similar prejunctional defect occurs, tetanic stimulation of the nerve gives rise to an increase in the amplitude of the muscle action potential (post-tetanic potentiation). Injection of the patient's serum into mice will reproduce the weakness.

Treatment involves intensive supportive measures with ventilation in many patients. Botulinum antitoxin is given to neutralise any remaining circulating unbound toxin, and benzyl penicillin to destroy any *Cl. botulinum* in the gut. With these measures, the mortality is low.

MUSCLE DISEASE

The term *myopathy* refers to any condition which primarily affects muscle physiology, structure or biochemistry. The functional unit of muscle is the motor unit, which comprises a variable number of muscle fibres all innervated by a single anterior horn cell via a motor axon. Muscle fibres are of three types, subdivided on the basis of histology and enzyme content (Fig. 22.39).

- *Type I* fibres are smaller than type II and contain larger numbers of mitochondria and oxidative enzymes, and a larger amount of fat. They are relatively slow contracting and relaxing, and are important in postural control.
- *Type II* fibres have a higher content of glycogen and certain enzymes, including phosphorylase, necessary for anaerobic metabolism. These fibres are rapidly contracting, so-called *fast twitch* muscle fibres. Type II fibres are further subdivided into *types IIa* and *IIb* on the basis of oxidative enzyme content.

Histochemical and biochemical techniques are increasingly used in the recognition and diagnosis of metabolic defects which affect muscle function.

Dystrophy is the term used to describe inherited degenerative muscle diseases.

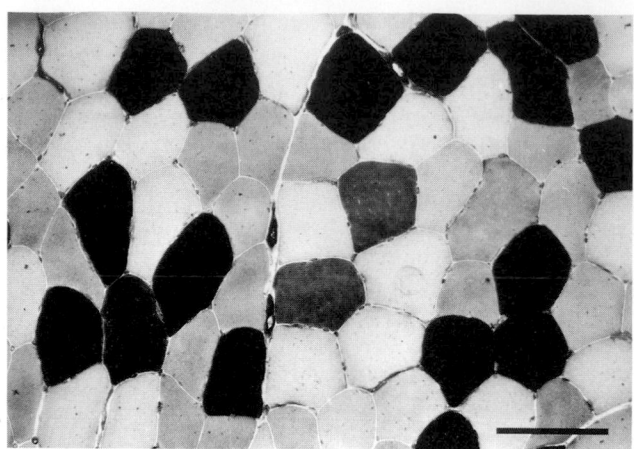

Fig. 22.39 Transverse frozen section through a biopsy sample of human vastus lateralis, stained for myosin ATPase. The black fibres are type I, the intermediate staining fibres type IIb, and the remainder of varying paler shades type IIa. Scale bar = 100 μm. (Photomicrograph by courtesy of Prof D N Landon.)

Clinical features

The major categories of muscle disease are:

- the dystrophies (hereditary)
- the myotonic disorders (hereditary)
- inflammatory muscle disease
- a number of endocrine and metabolic disorders (some hereditary).

Symptoms

The main symptoms of muscle disease are weakness, wasting (often a symptom as well as a sign), pain and fatigability. Less common symptoms are cramps and muscle twitching.

Weakness. The distribution of wasting and weakness is characteristic for many myopathies, particularly the dystrophies. The time course of development of weakness is also diagnostically helpful.

Muscle pain. Pain is particularly a symptom of inflammatory muscle disease and may be present at rest as well as on exertion. Metabolic disorders often lead to exertional pain. Other muscle diseases are less likely to cause pain.

Fatigability. Fatigability is a leading symptom of the myasthenic syndromes (p. 950).

Cramps. Cramps usually occur at night and are only rarely a symptom of myopathy. They may be relieved by a small dose of quinine sulphate.

Other important points in the history are details of any current or past systemic illnesses which may be associated with myopathy, and – in view of the many inherited disorders of muscle – a family history.

Wasting and weakness are the major signs of muscle disease. The distribution is characteristic for the various dystrophies. Most acquired myopathies have a proximal limb girdle type of distribution. Muscle hypertrophy is an occasional feature of muscle disease. Muscle tone is usually reduced in wasted muscles, though this is not specific for muscle disease. Myotonia is a delayed muscular relaxation following voluntary contraction seen in dystrophia myotonica and myotonia congenita. Tenderness of the muscles is usually seen only in inflammatory disorders.

Tendon reflexes are preserved in myopathies until wasting is severe. In some dystrophies, reflexes in affected muscle groups are absent from an early stage.

Investigation

Nerve conduction tests and EMG will distinguish neurogenic and myopathic electrical changes, and are the most reliable quick methods of identifying the underlying cause of wasting and weakness when there is clinical doubt.

Diseased muscle fibres tend to release the enzyme, creatine kinase (CK). In Duchenne dystrophy and polymyositis, very high serum levels may be found; in other myopathies, the CK may be raised to a lesser degree. However, it is important to recognise that any generalised denervating process may cause a modest rise in CK; MND is the commonest cause of this. Other enzymes, including aminotransferases and aldolase, are also released from diseased muscles, but are not specific for muscle.

Tests of thyroid and adrenal function are appropriate in some patients, while in those with the periodic paralyses, investigation of potassium levels and balance may be necessary. The complex mitochondrial myopathies and the glycogen storage diseases require special investigation.

Muscle biopsy is only occasionally needed to settle diagnostic doubt as to whether a myopathy is present. A combination of histology and histochemistry in muscle biopsy now permits characterisation of the disease process in many patients with muscle disease.

THE MUSCULAR DYSTROPHIES

The muscular dystrophies are classified according to the mode of inheritance (Table 22.50). The Duchenne type is the commonest of all the dystrophies; the rest are much rarer. The symptoms, signs and rate of progression are extremely variable in the different dystrophies. Skeletal deformities and contractures are common in some types.

Duchenne muscular dystrophy

Duchenne muscular dystrophy (DMD) has an incidence of 13–33 per 100 000 live births.

Clinical features

DMD usually presents in the third year of life with weakness of the pelvic girdle muscles, leading to delay and difficulty in walking, falls, difficulty in rising from the floor and climbing stairs. Hypertrophy of the calf muscles and, sometimes, the deltoids occurs. This is probably a true hypertrophy resulting from relative sparing of these muscles. Exaggeration of the normal lumbar lordosis develops, together with an equinovarus deformity due to weakness of the tibialis anterior and peroneal muscles, with relative sparing of the calf muscles; this leads to a tendency to walk on tiptoe. When rising from the floor, a characteristic method of climbing up the legs is adopted (Gowers' sign). Contractures at the knees and elbows are common. The condition is relentlessly progressive, so that most boys are in a wheelchair by 10 years of age, and have died before the age of 20. Cardiac failure, due to cardiac muscle involvement, and respiratory failure are the commonest causes of death. Some boys with DMD are of low intelligence. Diagnosis of DMD over the age of 3 is usually not difficult on clinical grounds, though diagnosis in the early stages can be difficult. The condition must always be suspected in boys with delayed walking past the age of 18 months. The CK is raised from birth.

Genetics of DMD

Much recent research has been devoted to the genetics of DMD and the gene has been localised on the short arm of the X chromosome, in a region designated Xp21. With a number of DNA probes (p. 68), it is now possible to identify the gene in carriers and affected fetuses. However, accuracy of identification depends on the availability of DNA samples from many members of a particular family because, in DMD, different mutations may occur over a long stretch of the gene. A number of cases of DMD result from spontaneous mutations in maternal ovarian cells, the exact proportion of all cases of DMD being uncertain. Thus, the risk of the sister of a DMD boy being a carrier of the abnormal gene is less than the 50:50 expected if half the mother's X chromosomes carry the DMD gene inherited from her mother. The identification of carriers does enable the incidence of DMD to be reduced in families with a known history of the condition, but not when DMD occurs as a result of spontaneous mutation. Affected boys can be identified in utero and aborted, but this tends to lead to an increased number of female children, many of whom will be carriers of the DMD gene.

Other dystrophies

Becker dystrophy

Becker dystrophy is an X-linked dystrophy similar in its distribution of weakness to DMD, but more benign. Onset of symptoms occurs between 5 and 25 years, with inability to walk occurring about 20 years after the onset of symptoms. Muscle hypertrophy is a common prelude to development of weakness. Cardiac muscle is not involved in this type of dystrophy. As Becker patients survive into adult life, they may pass on the abnormal gene to their daughters, who may then have affected sons.

Limb girdle dystrophy

Limb girdle dystrophy – an autosomal recessively inherited condition – begins in the second or third decade of life and affects the sexes equally. Initially, the onset of weakness may be in either the shoulder girdle or pelvic girdle muscles. Severe disability usually results within 20 years of onset, though benign forms do occur. Wasting and weakness may become widespread in the limbs, and the condition can be confused with spinal muscular atrophy (p. 941). It is now recognised that many patients with the clinical syndrome of limb girdle dystrophy have an underlying defect of mitochondrial metabolism (p. 956).

Childhood dystrophy

The term childhood dystrophy refers to dystrophy in children of autosomal recessive inheritance. Occasionally, a Duchenne-like dystrophy is seen in girls, often when the parents are consanguinous. The disease is more benign than DMD in boys.

Congenital muscular dystrophy is a rare condition presenting at birth with severe generalised hypotonia, and then progressive wasting and weakness. The condition mimics the infantile form of anterior horn cell degeneration, Werdnig-Hoffman disease. The prognosis is very poor.

Facioscapulohumeral dystrophy

Facioscapulohumeral dystrophy is an autosomal dominant condition affecting boys and girls with onset during childhood or early adult life. Facial muscle weakness leads to a typical drooping appearance around the mouth, with difficulty closing the eyes. Weakness around the scapula causes winging and riding up of the scapulae on the chest wall on abducting the arms. There is associated wasting of pectoralis major and other shoulder girdle muscles. Later, weakness of the anterolateral muscles in the lower legs develops, causing foot drop and weakness of eversion. Other muscles in the legs are sometimes affected. There is no cardiac muscle involvement and many patients have a normal lifespan.

MYOTONIC DISEASES

Myotonia – the continuing contraction of a muscle after voluntary contraction ceases – is usually seen as a feature of dystrophia myotonica but also occurs in the rarer myotonia congenita.

Dystrophia myotonica

Dystrophia myotonica is an autosomal dominant condition, and the gene locus is now known to be on chromosome 19. The features are initially a distal muscle dystrophy with myotonia, with later involvement of proximal muscles, causing respiratory failure, facial muscle weakness and ptosis. Other features of the condition are low intelligence or progressive dementia, cataracts, frontal balding in males, cardiomyopathy, diabetes and gonadal atrophy. Dysphagia is common due to dystrophic change and incoordination of contraction caused by the myotonia. Occasionally, external ophthalmoplegia occurs. Somnolence is common.

The condition usually presents in the third and fourth decades. The degree of myotonia is variable. Most men are infertile. Survival is usually not beyond middle-age.

Myotonia may be helped by procainamide (250–500 mg t.d.s) or phenytoin (300 mg daily), but these drugs should only be given when myotonia impairs functional ability.

Myotonia congenita (Thomsen's disease)

Myotonia congenita is a dominantly inherited condition in which myotonia is present from birth, when it may cause feeding difficulties. There is no dystrophy; indeed, in some children there is muscular hypertrophy. Myotonia tends to improve with age. It is usually worst at rest and in the cold, and is relieved to some extent by exercise.

INFLAMMATORY MUSCLE DISEASE

Inflammatory diseases of muscle can be divided into those in which a causative infective organism can be identified, and those in which the cause is unknown (Table 22.51). In the UK, all types of infective myositis are uncommon.

Infective causes

Bacterial myositis

In the UK, clostridial myositis develops in dirty wounds with anaerobic conditions. *Clostridium welchii* produces a toxin and enzymes which cause necrosis of muscle with

Table 22.51 Inflammatory myopathies

Infective	
Bacterial	– Clostridial myositis (gas gangrene)
	Staphylococcal myositis
Viral	– Postviral myalgia
	Influenza myositis
	Coxsackie A & B
	Echo
Parasitic	– Cysticercosis
	Trichinosis
	Toxoplasmosis
	Trypanosomiasis
Unknown cause	– Polymyositis
	Dermatomyositis
	Polymyositis with connective tissue disease
	Sarcoidosis
	Other granulomatous myositis
	Eosinophilic polymyositis

inflammation and haemorrhage. Urgent treatment with surgical debridement and penicillin is necessary.

In tropical countries, acute suppurative tropical myositis is relatively common (it is rarely seen in temperate zones). The initiating lesion may be a penetrating or crush injury, or it may be secondary to a staphylococcal arthritis. *Staphylococcus* is the usual infecting organism. Proximal lower limb muscles are usually most affected.

Viral myositis

A number of viruses regularly produce myositis. Myalgia with a bad cold (adenovirus or rhinovirus) is a non-specific effect. A more severe polymyalgia may arise after influenza infections. It affects the thigh or calf muscles, which may swell, and the CK is raised.

Two of the Coxsackie viruses occasionally cause myositis. Bornholm disease and epidemic myositis affecting muscles in the trunk, particularly the chest, is now known to be caused by Coxsackie B5. Polymyositis with myoglobinuria may be caused by Coxsackie B6. Other viruses, notably the echoviruses, have occasionally been associated with myositis.

Parasitic myositis

Myositis may occur as part of a number of parasitic infections, none of them common in the UK.

In *cysticercosis*, ingested larvae spread from the gut to all parts of the body. Their presence in muscles and the nervous system may be asymptomatic at the time of infestation. In the muscles, an acute painful myositis may result or, as the encysted larvae gradually enlarge, a diffuse hypertrophic myopathy may occur. In the brain, epilepsy may result.

In *trichinosis*, larvae of the nematode *Trichinella spiralis*, eaten in inadequately cooked pork, spread widely via the blood, including to muscles. There, they cause an acute, painful myositis, together with conjunctivitis, periorbital oedema and, often, a generalised rash.

Toxoplasma gondii occasionally causes a myositis. Collections of parasites (pseudocysts) are found in the muscles.

Trypanosomiasis causes an acute polymyositis, often with encephalomyelitis and myocarditis. The treatment of all these diseases is considered in Chapter 11.

Myositis of unknown cause

Polymyositis refers to a group of conditions the cardinal feature of which is a myopathy, usually proximal in distribution, and of acute, subacute or chronic presentation, in which the CK is variably raised, myopathic changes are present on EMG, and muscle biopsy shows an inflammatory infiltrate with varying degrees of muscle necrosis. Polymyositis and dermatomyositis are discussed in Chapter 23, page 1029.

Sarcoidosis may cause a proximal myopathy, usually subacute in onset, in which typical non-caseating granulomas are found on muscle biopsy. Other conditions which occasionally produce an inflammatory proximal myopathy are polyarteritis nodosa and Wegener's granulomatosis. In eosinophilic polymyositis, muscle involvement is only one part of a multisystem disease associated with eosinophilia, which includes heart and lung involvement, peripheral neuropathy, encephalopathy, skin changes and hypergammaglobulinaemia.

Prognosis of polymyositis and related disorders

The prognosis for polymyositis not associated with other disease at presentation is good. Childhood, adolescent and early adult dermatomyositis similarly has a good prognosis. However, in later-onset dermatomyositis, particularly in men, the prognosis is poor, due to the 50% incidence of underlying cancer. The outlook is also worse for polymyositis associated with collagen disease. The prognosis for polymyositis with sarcoidosis is variable.

ENDOCRINE MYOPATHIES

Thyroid disease

In some patients with uncontrolled thyrotoxicosis, a symptomatic proximal myopathy develops, and mild degrees of asymptomatic proximal weakness can be demonstrated in many thyrotoxic patients. This resolves with treatment of the thyrotoxicosis. About 5% of all patients with MG also have thyrotoxicosis. A normokalaemic periodic paralysis is occasionally seen in thyrotoxicosis (see below).

Hypothyroidism is occasionally associated with a proximal myopathy, typically leading to pain in the muscles after exertion.

Myopathy with adrenal and pituitary disease

In Cushing's syndrome, there is usually some evidence of a proximal myopathy with wasting and weakness. Steroids given therapeutically for any reason may lead to a similar proximal myopathy. The rate at which this appears in different people is extremely variable.

Patients who have had adrenalectomy for Cushing's disease may develop a proximal myopathy, thought to be caused by raised levels of circulating corticotrophin. In acromegaly and pituitary gigantism, generalised weakness, particularly proximally, is common. In Addison's disease and hypopituitarism, weakness is a leading symptom, usually secondary to salt and water abnormalities.

Parathyroid disease

In hyperparathyroidism, a painful proximal myopathy may develop. A particularly painful myopathy characteristically occurs in osteomalacia, often without much wasting or weakness.

TOXIC MYOPATHIES

Various drugs may cause a myopathy, of which the most important are the corticosteroids. Steroid myopathy is usually reversible if the drug is withdrawn. Other drugs which occasionally cause myopathy include vincristine, chloroquine and amiodarone, all of which also cause a neuropathy. Emetine and epsilon aminocaproic acid also cause a myopathy. Penicillamine leads to the development of a myasthenic syndrome indistinguishable from MG. This is sometimes reversible on withdrawal of the drug, but in many patients it is permanent.

Alcohol may produce an acute myopathy with myoglobinuria, usually following an alcoholic binge. Many cases of reported chronic alcoholic myopathy probably have a neuropathic rather than a myopathic basis (p. 982).

An acute reaction to halothane anaesthesia, malignant hyperpyrexia, is now known to have a muscular basis, though the mechanism remains unclear. The condition is familial and is rare. Dantrolene has been used to prevent the reaction but, if suspected from a family history, it is best to use alternative anaesthetic agents.

METABOLIC MYOPATHIES

Glycogen storage diseases of muscle

The most important of the glycogen storage diseases of muscle is *McArdle's disease*, due to deficiency of myo-phosphorylase in muscle leading to impaired utilisation of muscle glucose. The disease presents with muscle pain and stiffness which is made worse by exertion. The condition usually comes on in early adult life and, although usually non-progressive, some patients develop increasing wasting and weakness.

Many other biochemical abnormalities affecting muscle glucose utilisation have been described, most leading to multiple system disorders and disability and death in children. Acid maltase deficiency is one important exception, which may present with a limb girdle dystrophic picture. The specific underlying metabolic defect is suspected when biopsy shows characteristic glycogen-containing vacuoles. None of the glycogen storage diseases affecting muscle is yet treatable.

The periodic paralyses

These are dominantly inherited conditions in which episodic weakness is associated with a change in plasma and muscle potassium concentrations. There are two major types: the commoner hypokalaemic periodic paralysis and the less severe hyperkalaemic variety.

In the *hypokalaemic type*, episodes of weakness are provoked by exertion, but usually occur on the following day during a period of rest. In some patients, attacks are provoked by large carbohydrate meals. Each attack may last several hours. During the episodes of weakness, plasma potassium is below 3.0 mmol/l, with some accumulation of potassium within muscle cells. Acetazolamide or a thiazide diuretic usually prevents attacks, and some patients respond to oral potassium. The disease usually starts in the second or third decade, and attacks tend to gradually improve during adult life.

In the *hyperkalaemic type*, attacks of generalised weakness of about 30 minutes are also provoked by exertion, but the weakness immediately follows the exercise. During the attack, the plasma potassium concentration increases. Acetazolamide helps this type of attack.

Mitochondrial myopathies (cytopathies)

The mitochondrial myopathies are rare, and their numerous clinical manifestations have only recently been recognised. Since tissues and organs other than muscle, notably the CNS, may also be affected, producing multi-system diseases, the broader term *mitochondrial cytopathy* is now used. Some of the disorders are confined to muscle, but clinical syndromes also include dementia, fits, ataxia, pigmentary retinopathy, stroke-like episodes, extrapyramidal syndromes, deafness and peripheral neuropathy without clinically obvious myopathy. A number of underlying mitochondrial defects are responsible for these disorders. In muscle biopsies, the common feature is the so-called *ragged red fibre*, in which there are accumulations of abnormal mitochondria at the periphery of the muscle fibres. Ultrastructurally, mitochondria are abnormal in size and shape, and often contain paracrystalline inclusions. These mitochondrial abnormalities, however, are not always present.

At least 25 different biochemical abnormalities have now been described.

CHRONIC FATIGUE SYNDROME

Pathological fatigue is a well recognised feature of certain neurological disorders, notably myasthenia, certain myopathies and MS, and is also encountered in some types of peripheral neuropathy. However, some patients with a primary complaint of chronic fatigue do not have any identifiable neurological disease. Their condition is sometimes referred to as 'myalgic encephalomyelitis' (ME) or 'postviral fatigue', but there is no rational basis for the use of either of these diagnostic labels. The available evidence suggests that as many as 70% of such patients have a treatable depressive disorder, although this explanation may be resisted. A few may eventually be found to have MS or other specific disorders; in others there may indeed have been an unidentified viral myositis, in which case the prognosis is good. Some patients, however, remain persistently and severely incapacitated by their symptoms. As in the case of the post-traumatic disorder following head injury (p. 927), it seems likely that the degree of long-term disability reflects the complex interaction between a relatively minor illness and the patient's personality and individual circumstances at the time.

DEMYELINATING DISEASES

Demyelinating disease refers to a group of CNS disorders in which the primary pathological process is demyelination without axonal degeneration. By far the most important of these is multiple sclerosis (MS). Demyelination is also the result of a number of rare inherited disorders of sphingolipid metabolism; these include the leucodystrophies and some lipid storage diseases.

MULTIPLE SCLEROSIS

MS is a disease of unknown cause, in which discrete areas of demyelination develop at many sites in the brain and spinal cord. Lesions develop in different sites at different times, usually with some capacity for regeneration and restoration of function. This leads to a characteristic relapsing and remitting history in many patients; in others, a slowly progressive deficit occurs. Although demyelination is the primary pathology in MS, extensive areas of demyelination are associated with axonal loss and, in most patients, there is a slowly cumulative neurological deficit.

Epidemiology

The prevalence of MS shows a strong geographical variation, being essentially a disease of temperate climates. Even within the UK there are considerable variations in prevalence, e.g. around 30 per 10 000 in Shetland and Orkney, compared with 6 per 10 000 in England.

MS is very rare in childhood and uncommon in early adolescence. There is an increasing incidence with age, peaking at about 30 years. It is uncommon over the age of 50. In late presentations it is often possible to obtain a history of a previous minor neurological episode in earlier life which was likely to have been due to MS. This emphasises the relatively benign course of the disease in some patients. Slightly more women than men are affected by MS.

Aetiology

There have been many hypotheses about the cause of MS. Acute demyelination is an inflammatory process and the most favoured explanation, at present, is that acute demyelination is the result of an abnormal immune response to an antigen, perhaps of viral origin. Genetic factors may be important in some instances, as there is an association of MS with HLA-A3 and DR2 antigens. Studies of migrants show that if migration occurs before the age of 15, the risk of developing MS becomes that of the country to which the patient has migrated. This evidence emphasises the importance of an environmental factor or factors.

Pathology

Acute demyelination occurs in discrete areas known as plaques, which may be single or multiple. The lesions may occur anywhere in central white matter, but common sites are the optic nerve, the brainstem and cerebellum, the periventricular regions and the cervical spinal cord. Later, glial scarring results in the whitish appearance of the chronic plaque. Some remyelination may be possible, but this is limited. Resolution of oedema in and around plaques reverses conduction block and improves function. Even without symptoms or signs, slowing of conduction can often be demonstrated in visual, auditory and somatosensory pathways by electrophysiological testing.

Clinical features

Since plaques may occur at any site in central white matter, the clinical manifestations of MS are extremely variable. However, early in the disease a number of presentations are characteristic.

Optic neuritis

Inflammation of the optic nerve may be symptomatic or asymptomatic. When it affects the optic nerve head, it is sometimes termed *papillitis*; when inflammation occurs in the optic nerve further away from the eye, it may be called *retrobulbar neuritis*.

Symptoms. In acute optic neuritis (which is nearly always unilateral), there is dimming of vision, blurring, loss of acuity and reduced colour vision. These symptoms usually progress over hours or a few days. Rarely, vision may be lost altogether. Patients may be aware of the central or paracentral scotoma characteristic of this condition. Pain in and around the eye, particularly with movement of the eye, is common. The symptoms may be mild and transient, lasting only a few days, and may not cause patients to present to their doctors.

Signs. Examination during acute symptomatic optic neuritis will usually show impaired visual acuity, but formal visual field mapping may be necessary to detect small scotomas. The pupillary reaction to light shone in the affected eye will be sluggish in both the affected and unaffected eyes; a brisker response is obtained in both eyes when the same light is shone into the unaffected eye, indicating an afferent pupillary defect. On fundoscopy, there may be no abnormality if inflammation is located proximally in the optic nerve, but with inflammation near to the optic nerve head, there may be papilloedema.

Optic neuritis usually resolves within a few weeks, often without residual symptoms. However, a degree of optic atrophy is often detectable as pallor of the optic disc, a useful diagnostic sign in MS. Some patients will be aware of continuing impairment of visual acuity and colour vision and, rarely, there is severe visual impairment after a single episode.

Repeated acute episodes of optic neuritis during the course of MS are common. Sometimes, a slowly progressive visual impairment results from indolent optic neuritis. Other rare causes of optic neuritis include sarcoidosis, syphilis, Herpes zoster and SLE. About 30% of patients presenting with optic neuritis have no other evidence of MS, and do not develop the disease.

Cervical cord

Involvement of the cervical spinal cord is very common early in the course of MS, presenting with motor, sensory or bladder, bowel and sexual disturbances. Symptoms may be unilateral, but pyramidal signs are usually bilateral. Although there are usually no symptoms in the upper limbs in the early stages, brisk reflexes are often found.

Sensory symptoms include tingling paraesthesiae and numbness. Examination reveals disturbance of dorsal column function (impaired joint position and vibration sensation) and, less often, of spinothalamic sensation. A common early manifestation of MS is the L'Hermitte symptom, in which the patient notices tingling paraesthesiae in the legs and sometimes trunk and upper limbs on flexing the neck. This is probably due to mechanical sensitivity of dorsal column fibres in an area in, or surrounding, a plaque of demyelination. It may occasionally occur after cervical cord trauma, with cervical tumours and in subacute combined degeneration due to vitamin B_{12} deficiency.

Bladder disturbances are common in MS and are occasionally the presenting complaint. Urgency and frequency of micturition, then incontinence, are characteristic. Constipation is the main bowel disturbance early in MS, but urgency of defaecation with soiling may occur. Erectile impotence and ejaculatory failure are common symptoms.

Brainstem and cerebellum

Visual disturbances other than optic neuritis are frequent, and include diplopia due to either VIth nerve palsy or an internuclear ophthalmoplegia (INO). In INO, due to a lesion of the medial longitudinal fasciculus, eye movements are dysconjugate on lateral gaze; thus, on right lateral gaze there is incomplete adduction of the left eye, and there may be associated nystagmus, which is of greater amplitude in the abducting right eye, so-called ataxic nystagmus. Nystagmus without any ocular palsy is a common manifestation of brainstem demyelination, and may be horizontal, vertical or rotatory.

Vertigo is a fairly common early symptom of MS, due to plaque formation involving the vestibular nuclear complex. Ataxia involving limbs and/or trunk is also frequent early in the disease, and is due to plaque formation within the cerebellum or affecting its connections in the brainstem. Long motor and sensory tracts may also be involved in the brainstem; this produces symptoms and signs similar to those of cervical cord demyelination.

Later features

Depression in long-standing MS is common, and requires vigorous treatment. Widespread cerebral hemisphere demyelination leads to intellectual impairment. Often, there is a predominantly frontal impairment, producing disinhibition and other frontal features (p. 877).

Brainstem demyelination leads to complex ocular palsies, ataxia and long tract signs. Trigeminal neuralgia shows an assocation with MS, and there is also an increased incidence of atypical neuralgic pains in a trigeminal distribution. Rubral tremor is a particularly disabling type of cerebellar tremor; it is postural and of large amplitude, preventing purposeful actions in the arms. Myokymia refers to a continuous rippling twitching of the facial muscles on one side. It is probably due to irritation of the facial nucleus. Progressive bulbar involvement producing dysarthria, dysphagia and dysphonia indicates a particularly poor prognosis. Lower motor neurones are rarely affected in MS.

Other factors

Patients with MS frequently remark that their symptoms are worse in hot weather, after a hot bath, during fever or after exertion, all of which raise body temperature. Conduction in demyelinated axons is blocked by small rises in body temperature.

There is probably no increased risk of relapse during pregnancy but there is in the puerperium.

Course and prognosis

MS can be a remarkably benign disease with long periods of remission and relatively little neurological deficit. However, in most patients an increasing neurological deficit accumulates. The end stage of MS is characterised by dementia, quadriplegia, incontinence, blindness, pressure sores and recurrent respiratory and urinary tract infections.

In about three-quarters of patients, the disease has a relapsing and remitting course, and in the remainder, a chronic progressive course. In about 20% of patients there is no significant disability after 5 years, and the average life expectancy overall from the onset of symptoms is 20–30 years. In about 5% of patients, the disease is rapidly progressive and fatal within 5 years. Poor prognostic factors are an older age at onset, the development of dementia and the early development of ataxia.

Diagnosis

In many patients the diagnosis is straightforward and established on clinical evidence of more than one lesion in the nervous system, together with a characteristic relapsing and remitting history. The finding of optic atrophy in a patient presenting with a brainstem or cervical cord lesion is particularly helpful diagnostically.

Evoked potentials, either visual, auditory or somatosensory from the limbs, are sensitive measures of damage in these sensory pathways. Visual evoked potentials are recorded from the scalp over the occipital cortex. A flash or regular pattern reversal stimulus produces a small visual evoked potential, which can be averaged. The latency is prolonged if there has been significant demyelination at any time in the past. Similar information can be obtained concerning brainstem auditory pathways and large fibre, dorsal column somatosensory pathways from

the limbs. The evoked potentials are often delayed in the absence of any present or past symptoms.

CSF protein content may be raised. The IgG fraction of this may be greater than 10%, and CSF electrophoresis may show discrete bands in the gamma 4 and gamma 5 regions (*oligoclonal bands*). These immunoglobulins are synthesised locally within the CNS. Oligoclonal bands are not unique to MS, and occur occasionally in other conditions, including neurosyphilis and neurosarcoidosis. However, the finding of oligoclonal bands in the clinical setting of suspected MS lends support to this diagnosis.

CT scans are usually normal in the early stages. Large areas of acute demyelination may be seen, and chronic plaques, particularly in the periventricular regions, give rise to discrete abnormalities. *MRI* is a much more sensitive means of imaging the white matter (Fig. 22.40).

Management

There is no specific treatment for MS. Corticosteroids may accelerate remission in relapse, probably by reducing inflammation and oedema in acute plaques. Steroids have no effect on the outcome of a particular relapse and do not protect against further relapse. Long-term immunosuppression with cytotoxic agents is of no proven benefit.

Dietary restrictions or supplements are frequently recommended, but there is no evidence of their efficacy. Hyperbaric oxygen has also had a vogue in recent years. Carefully controlled clinical trials have not shown any benefit.

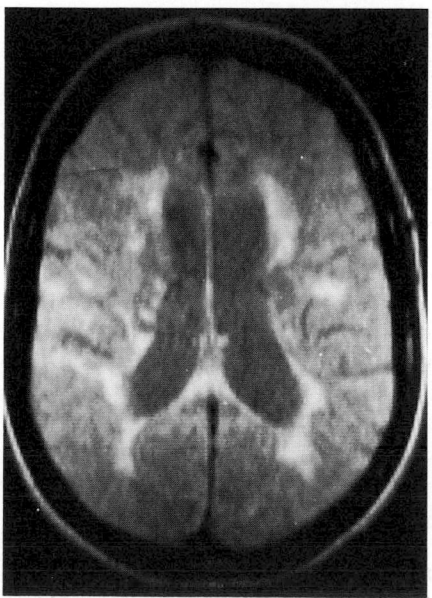

Fig. 22.40 Magnetic resonance scan in multiple sclerosis. Multiple areas of abnormal signal, here shown in white, are visible in the cerebral hemisphere white matter, particularly adjacent to the lateral ventricles.

Summary 12 Multiple sclerosis (MS)

- MS is the commonest progressive disabling neurological disease affecting young adults in the UK.

- Common sites of symptomatic demyelination are the optic nerves, cervical cord, brainstem, cerebellum and, usually later in the course of the disease, the cerebral hemispheres.

- MS may run a relapsing–remitting or chronic progressive course. The former is more likely to occur with younger age of onset.

- Prognosis is better with young onset and a relapsing–remitting course, but is very variable.

- Corticosteroids may shorten relapse, but immunosuppressive treatment has no effect on the long-term course of the disease.

- There is no clear-cut evidence that dietary restrictions or supplements, or hyperbaric oxygen, alter the course of the disease.

The treatment of MS remains symptomatic and supportive. Physiotherapy and occupational therapy have a large role to play. Spasticity may be relieved by anti-spastic drugs, such as baclofen and dantrolene, but these may exacerbate weakness.

Urinary urgency and frequency are often partly relieved by anticholinergics. Other patients will require urinary devices, such as sheaths and pads, and some patients eventually need permanent catheterisation. An alternative, increasingly used and suitable for many patients, is intermittent self-catheterisation.

Counselling in MS

MS is a common neurological disorder, and patients with a wide variety of symptoms think – often incorrectly – they have MS. The lay view of MS and its prognosis is often more gloomy than the reality. In patients with a single neurological episode possibly due to MS, it is usually ill-advised to discuss the possibility of MS unless directly asked by the patient. When the diagnosis is definite, however, it is nearly always best to inform the patient. Time must be set aside to discuss the disease, its effects and its prognosis with the patient and relatives. Open discussion and allaying fears, which are often misguided or ill-founded, is usually helpful.

OTHER ACQUIRED DEMYELINATING DISEASE

Postviral and postvaccinial encephalomyelitis

In postviral and postvaccinial encephalomyelitis, widespread acute inflammation with demyelination in the brain and spinal cord follows a viral illness – either one of the exanthemata or an intercurrent viral infection. Occasionally, a similar disease follows smallpox vaccination and other inoculations, particularly rabies. Because of the frequency of the exanthemata in childhood, children are affected by this type of encephalomyelitis more often than adults. Occasionally, there is no preceding history of infection or inoculation.

The illness is characterised by subacute onset of malaise, headache, vomiting, drowsiness, convulsions and fever, together with focal symptoms and signs. A hemiparesis, brainstem and cerebellar signs, and evidence of a myelitis are the principal focal features. Occasionally, optic neuritis occurs. Coma and death may ensue, but the majority of patients recover, some with residual intellectual and physical deficit, including epilepsy. Occasionally, there are recurrent episodes. Rarely, an initial severe episode of MS presents in this way. The acute illness resembles an encephalitis due to direct viral infection and, clinically, it can be impossible to distinguish the two (p. 969).

Acute haemorrhagic leucoencephalopathy, in which there are accompanying multiple areas of haemorrhage, probably represents a particularly severe form of encephalomyelitis.

The demyelinating condition of central pontine myelinolyis is discussed on page 982.

Disorders of sphingolipid metabolism

Many rare disorders of myelin metabolism exist. These fall into two broad groups, the leucodystrophies and the lipid storage diseases (Table 22.52). Demyelination is common to both groups. They are primarily of relevance to paediatric practice. Most lead to progressive mental deterioration and a multiplicity of neurological signs, often including spasticity in the limbs, fits, ataxia and optic atrophy. Death within months or 1–2 years occurs in many of these disorders; metachromatic leucodystrophy, adrenoleucodystrophy and Fabry's disease are exceptions. There is no specific therapy for these conditions.

Metachromatic leucodystrophy

Metachromatic leucodystrophy is an autosomal recessive condition, due to deficiency of aryl sulphatase A, in which there is tissue accumulation of metachromatic lipids in the white matter of the CNS and in peripheral nerves. The effects are widespread, with onset of symptoms usually in early childhood, but sometimes as late as adolescence. There is weakness, ataxia, dementia and fits. Examination shows signs of peripheral neuropathy, in addition to pyramidal weakness, ataxia and dementia, and there is often optic atrophy. The diagnosis is made by assay of the enzyme in leucocytes, and metachromatic material can be seen on rectal or peripheral nerve biopsy.

Table 22.52 Disorders of sphingolipid metabolism

Disease	Biochemical defect	Clinical features
The leucodystrophies		
Metachromatic leucodystrophy	Aryl sulphatase A deficiency	See text
Adrenoleucodystrophy	Unknown	X-linked dementia, spasticity, neuropathy, hypoadrenalism
Globoid cell leucodystrophy	Galactocerebroside β-galactosidase deficiency	Onset in infancy Irritability, motor regression, nystagmus, spasticity or hypotonia, optic atrophy, fits. Death within 1 year
Lipid storage diseases		
Gangliosidoses, e.g. Tay-Sachs disease	β-acetyl hexosaminidase deficiency causing accumulation of GM2 ganglioside	Motor regression in infancy. Optic atrophy. Death within 2 years
Gaucher's disease	Glucocerebrosidase deficiency	Progressive neurological deterioration after birth. Death within 1 year
Niemann-Pick disease	Sphingomyelinase deficiency	Onset at 6 months. Progressive mental and neurological deterioration. May survive many years
Fabry's disease	Ceramide trihexosidase deficiency	Cardiac, renal and nervous system involvement

BACTERIAL INFECTIONS OF THE NERVOUS SYSTEM

ACUTE BACTERIAL MENINGITIS

Bacterial meningitis is infection of the leptomeninges and the CSF which diffusely affects the whole meninges and subarachnoid space and, sometimes, the ventricles (ventriculitis). The three bacteria most commonly causing meningitis, *Neisseria meningitidis*, *Haemophilus influenzae* and *Streptococcus pneumoniae*, gain access to the meninges and subarachnoid space via the bloodstream from the nasopharynx, through the walls of the intracranial venous sinuses. Once in the CSF, bacteria rapidly multiply. Other bacteria may also cause meningitis (Table 22.53; see also Ch. 11); any bacterium causing septicaemia may enter the CSF and cause meningitis. Haematogenous spread may also occur from infective endocarditis, osteomyelitis and pyelonephritis.

Mechanisms of infection

Direct infection occurs from penetrating trauma, including compound skull fractures, and gunshot wounds. Fractures of the skull with CSF leaks are common causes of meningitis. Septic foci closely adjacent to the meninges (and thus potential causes of meningitis) include sinusitis, middle ear and mastoid infection, and osteomyelitis of the skull bones. Lymphatic spread of infection to the spinal cord occurs from retropharyngeal, retroperitoneal and psoas abscesses. Congenital abnormalities, particularly meningomyeloceles, provide a further route of infection.

Despite the most careful aseptic precautions, meningitis still remains a serious complication of neurosurgical procedures. Shunts are particularly likely to lead to infection. Meningitis is a much more common illness in immunocompromised patients; these include patients undergoing organ transplantation and patients with HIV infection.

Complications of meningitis

Meningitis may be complicated by *ventriculitis* or *intracerebral abscess*. There may be obstruction of CSF flow through the foramina between the ventricles and cerebral

Table 22.53 Treatment of bacterial meningitis in adults

Organism	Treatment
Neisseria meningitidis	Benzyl penicillin (4 megaunits, 4-hourly) or chloramphenicol (20 mg/kg, 6-hourly) in hypersensitivity to pencillin
Streptococcus pneumoniae	Benzyl penicillin or chloramphenicol, doses as for *N. meningitidis*
Haemophilus influenzae	Cefuroxime (3 g, 8-hourly) or chloramphenicol (20 mg/kg, 6-hourly) or ampicillin (2 g, 6-hourly for 2 days, then 1 g, 6-hourly) or co-trimoxazole (160 mg trimethoprim and 800 mg sulphamethoxazole, 12-hourly)
Staphylococcus aureus *Staphylococcus epidermidis*	Flucloxacillin (3 g, 6-hourly) or vancomycin (500 mg, 6-hourly) or gentamicin (5 mg/kg/day*) in penicillin hypersensitivity
Pseudomonas aeruginosa	Piperacillin (4 g, 6-hourly) with tobramycin (3–5 mg/kg/day) or ticarcillin (5 g, 6-hourly) with gentamicin (5 mg/kg per day*)

*Gentamicin blood levels necessary

aqueduct, causing *hydrocephalus*. Purulent exudate may cause reduced reabsorption of CSF in the arachnoid granulations, also leading to hydrocephalus; and septic thrombosis of the venous sinuses can occur, leading to an increase in intracranial pressure with a communicating hydrocephalus. The purulent exudate in the basal meninges may affect the cranial nerves and arteries which cross the subarachnoid space; *cranial nerve palsies* are thus common complications of bacterial meningitis. The IIIrd and VIth cranial nerves may also be affected by direct pressure from downward displacement of an oedematous brain with raised intracranial pressure. The major arteries at the base of the brain may, occasionally, become occluded by the purulent arteritis, leading to major *strokes*, affecting either the cerebral hemispheres or brainstem. Cortical veins may also become occluded, which may lead to areas of infarction.

Infection may also spread into the subdural space, causing a *subdural empyema*. Localised *epidural abscesses* may occur over the cerebral hemispheres and epidural abscesses may develop secondary to meningitis in the spinal cord, leading to spinal cord compression.

Late sequelae of acute bacterial meningitis include persistent cranial nerve palsies, though the acute palsies usually improve to some extent. *Deafness*, due to VIIIth nerve damage, is often bilateral, severe and permanent. This has been estimated to occur in 5–40% of all patients. In young children, diffuse cerebral damage with *mental retardation* often results from acute meningitis, particularly with *H. influenzae* infection.

Clinical features

In adults, the main symptoms of meningitis are headache, vomiting, irritability, photophobia and drowsiness. Fits are usually a later symptom. In meningococcal meningitis, the progression of symptoms may be extremely rapid, the patient presenting in coma within hours of the onset of symptoms.

The signs are fever, neck stiffness, drowsiness, stupor or coma; sometimes, there is neurological deficit – cranial nerve palsies, hemiparesis or other focal signs – which result from occlusion of the basal cerebral arteries. Focal deficit is more common in advanced, untreated cases of meningitis. Neck stiffness may be mild or absent in deeply comatose patients. Meningeal irritation may cause a positive Kernig's sign, and Brudzinski's sign, in which neck flexion causes flexion of the legs. Later, there may be a posture of extension of the neck and spine. The typical rash of meningococcal septicaemia may be present (p. 221 and Plate 11, p. 247).

In neonates and young children, the symptoms and signs of meningitis may be minimal. Fits are a much more common presenting feature in the young, and irritability, fever and drowsiness may be the only signs. Likewise, in the elderly, there may be few signs and, in some cases, a much more insidious onset.

Differential diagnosis

The commonest alternative cause of severe headache, neck stiffness and vomiting, with or without focal signs, is subarachnoid haemorrhage. This is usually, but not always, of abrupt onset. CT scanning is helpful in demonstrating subarachnoid blood in such cases. Aseptic viral meningitis is the other main differential diagnosis. Other types of meningitis may cause an identical presentation to acute bacterial meningitis. The onset of tuberculous meningitis can be acute, but is more often subacute and may be insidious. In immunocompromised patients, fungal (cryptococcal or candida) or amoebic meningitis must be considered and an India ink stain of the CSF performed. The opisthotonos of tetanus may mimic meningeal irritation. In children, acute fever is fairly often associated with neck stiffness as a non-specific sign.

Investigation

Examination of the CSF is diagnostic but lumbar puncture can be a dangerous procedure in certain instances, e.g. in the presence of a developing cerebral abscess complicating the meningitis. Intracranial pressure is nearly always raised in meningitis, but in the presence of papilloedema, focal signs or coma, it is safest to perform a CT scan to exclude hydrocephalus or a focal mass lesion prior to performing lumbar puncture. When scanning is not available, clearly a risk must be taken and the CSF examined.

At lumbar puncture, the opening pressure should be measured before samples are taken for a Gram stain, culture, cell count, protein and glucose estimation. Typical findings in acute bacterial meningitis are a neutrophil count of more than $1000/mm^3$, a glucose which is less than 40% of the blood glucose or below 1.7 mmol/l, and a considerably raised protein concentration. Blood cultures, and any other relevant cultures, from suspected foci of infection should be taken. However, it cannot be overemphasised that prompt treatment of acute meningitis is essential for survival and prevention of complications. Meningococcal meningitis may be fatal within 24 hours. In immunocompromised patients, unusual pathogens must be looked for, such as *Listeria monocytogenes*, tuberculosis, amoeba and fungal infections, particularly *Cryptococcus*.

Findings similar to those of acute bacterial meningitis may be found in viral meningitis. The pleocytosis in the CSF usually comprises lymphocytes but can be due to neutrophils, and the CSF glucose is occasionally low. CSF glucose may also be low in malignant meningitis, subarachnoid haemorrhage, tuberculous meningitis and malignant hypertension.

Summary 13 Lumbar puncture in meningitis

- Lumbar puncture (LP) is safe in patients with meningitis without focal signs and whose conscious level is no worse than drowsy.

- If there are focal signs or the patient is in coma, a complication of meningitis (e.g. cerebral abscess, hydrocephalus) may have supervened. There is a risk of coning with LP. Get a CT scan.

- If in doubt, ask for neurological advice before doing an LP.

- Minimum examination of the CSF in suspected meningitis includes cell count, protein, glucose, Gram stain, and Z-N stain.

- In any patient who may be immunocompromised, ask for special microbiological CSF tests for fungal, Listerial, amoebic and other rare organisms.

- Tuberculous meningitis rarely causes a white cell count of more than 1000/mm³, and a Z-N stain may be negative. If there is strong clinical evidence, treat for TB.

- Never give intrathecal antibiotics.

Failure of the patient's clinical state to improve within 24–36 hours of starting antibiotic treatment is an indication for further CSF examination. This is particularly important when there is microbiological doubt about the causative organism. A rise in cell count in the second CSF, with a persistently low glucose, implies an inadequate antibiotic treatment which must therefore be changed. With correct treatment, the cell count rapidly falls.

If signs indicate a spinal cord lesion in a patient with meningitis, a spinal epidural abscess should be suspected and, in consultation with a neurosurgeon, myelography should be urgently performed.

Management

Antibiotics

Antibiotic treatment must be started immediately the CSF has been taken. In rare instances where there is likely to be delay in performing a lumbar puncture, treatment must be started blind. Table 22.54 sets out the antibiotics used for different organisms; these are usually given intravenously. Chloramphenicol should not be used in neonates, due to bone marrow and renal toxicity occurring as a result of inadequate metabolism by the liver. Chloramphenicol is effective against the rarer *Listeria monocytogenes*.

For patients suspected of being immunosuppressed and who may thus be infected with one of the less common bacteria, an initial broad-spectrum antibiotic combination is given, such as gentamicin and cefuroxime.

Bacterial culture is usually available within 24 hours, by which time some clinical improvement should have occurred. If not, the CSF must be re-examined.

High-dose intravenous antibiotics should always be continued for at least a week. As meningeal inflammation decreases, the blood–brain barrier is gradually restored, allowing less of the drug to gain access to the infected meninges. An identified focus of infection, e.g. sinusitis or suppurative otitis media, is an indication for a longer period of treatment, during which time the focus must be treated on its own merits. Immunosuppressed patients also require longer periods of treatment.

Intrathecal penicillin makes no difference to outcome and is potentially dangerous. Large doses cause an encephalopathy with fits, which is usually fatal.

Fits

Fits are common, particularly in children with meningitis. Treatment of status epilepticus or serial epilepsy is as described on page 894. Regular oral anticonvulsant treatment should be started in all patients having fits. It can be given via a nasogastric tube, but phenytoin may also be given by slow intravenous injection, and phenobarbitone by intramuscular injection. Loading doses are necessary, followed by regular maintenance doses. Phenytoin competes with chloramphenicol for glucuronation in the liver and so increases levels of this antibiotic.

Raised intracranial pressure and hydrocephalus

Generalised cerebral oedema may produce life-threatening rises in intracranial pressure. This is treated urgently with mannitol and then dexamethasone. Hydrocephalus may develop after several days; in such cases, there is typically clinical improvement after initiation of treatment, followed by a deterioration. The diagnosis is established by a CT scan. Some patients with progressive hydrocephalus will require treatment with a ventricular drain.

Cerebral abscess

Despite adequate treatment, some patients will develop cerebral abscesses. The development of fits and focal signs also raises the possibility of venous sinus thrombosis (p. 965). Clinical deterioration, with or without focal signs or fits, is an indication for an urgent CT scan. If the CT scan is normal, the CSF must be re-examined.

Prevention

Treatment of close contacts (family, medical and nursing staff) of patients with *Strep. pneumoniae* meningitis is not necessary, but it is recommended with *H. influenzae* or *N. meningitidis*. Rifampicin (600 mg b.d. for adults or 20 mg/kg per day for children for 2 days) is effective prophylaxis for both bacteria.

Vaccines for *N. meningitidis* may be used in family members when the meningococcus occurs in small epidemics, and for contacts at particular risk, such as the immunocompromised, the very young and the elderly.

Prognosis

Overall mortality for the three common pathogens ranges from as low as 3% for *H. influenzae* to as high as 60% for *Strep. pneumoniae*. In the very young and the elderly, mortality is highest.

INTRACRANIAL ABSCESS

Intracranial abscesses are most commonly intracerebral, but pus may collect in the subdural space (subdural empyema) or in the extradural space. Subdural empyema or intracerebral abscesses may extend to the meninges and cause meningitis, or, conversely, infection may spread from the meninges. Intracerebral abscesses may rupture into the ventricles, causing a ventriculitis.

An intracerebral abscess starts as an area of cerebritis which then develops into a pus-filled cavity surrounded by a wall of variable thickness, and, outside this, cerebral oedema. The oedema is often extensive and, together with the abscess itself, leads to increased intracranial pressure and mass effect on surrounding structures. Some abscesses are single, others multilocular or multiple (Fig. 22.41).

Aetiology

Cerebral abscesses. Excluding cerebral abscesses occurring in AIDS (which are usually multiple and are most often

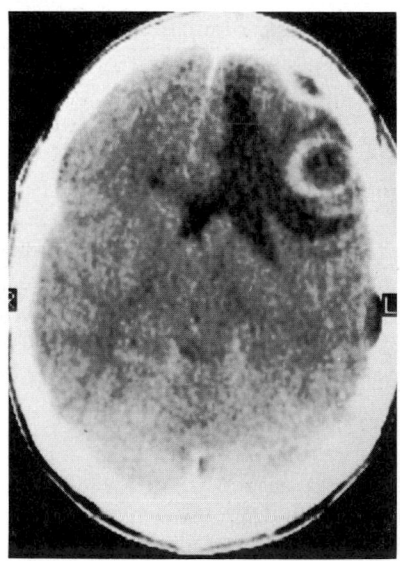

Fig. 22.41 Cerebral abscess. Enhanced CT scan of a patient with a left frontal acute pyogenic abscess. Note the typical ring enhancing lesion with massive surrounding cerebral oedema, causing midline shift. There is also a small subdural collection of pus (subdural empyema). The intracranial abscess in this 21-year-old man was secondary to frontal sinusitis.

caused by *Toxoplasma gondii*, p. 973), about 60% of intracerebral abscesses are caused by middle ear infection and are situated in the temporal lobe or cerebellum. About 20% are secondary to frontal sinusitis, which results in frontal lobe abscess; approximately 10% are due to bacteraemia or septicaemia from the lung (abscess, empyema or bronchiectasis), the heart (infective endocarditis), dental sepsis, or some other peripheral site, with penetrating skull trauma accounting for a small proportion of cases; and, in about 10% of cerebral abscess, no source for the infection is found. Cerebral abscess is more likely to occur in patients with debilitating illness and in the immunocompromised.

Subdural empyema usually results from frontal sinusitis or penetrating injury, and sometimes middle ear infection. In infants, it is often secondary to meningitis. In adults it is occasionally secondary to septicaemia. Extradural abscess has similar causes and may also be secondary to osteomyelitis of the skull, now a rare condition.

Bacteriology

In contrast to meningitis, intracranial abscesses are often due to mixed infection. The organisms most frequently causing abscesses are *Strep. viridans*, *Staph. aureus*, *Klebsiella*, and, occasionally, other Gram-negative bacteria. Infection with one of these is frequently associated with an anaerobe, either anaerobic streptococcus or bacterioides. In immunocompromised patients, a wide range of bacteria may be responsible, together with occasional amoebic or fungal abscesses.

Clinical features

Intracerebral abscess. An acute pyogenic abscess is likely to cause symptoms which progress quickly over days rather than weeks. Multiple abscesses may cause a plethora of symptoms and signs. A combination of headache, rapidly progressive neurological deficit, symptoms of raised intracranial pressure, with or without fever, and a deteriorating conscious level suggests the possibility of an intracerebral abscess. Fits are also very common.

Fever is very variable in cerebral abscess. Meningism is quite common. A careful search for a systemic source of infection must be made in every case of suspected abscess.

Subdural empyema. Patients with subdural empyema are usually very ill. The pus spreads rapidly over the surface of the hemisphere, producing hemiparesis, raised intracranial pressure, fits and meningism.

Extradural abscess. Extradural abscesses are often well localised and may present less acutely. They usually cause localised, severe headache and are associated with sinusitis, mastoiditis or penetrating trauma.

Investigation

The most important immediate investigation is a CT scan. Most acute pyogenic abscesses are rounded lesions of low attenuation with ring enhancement and much surrounding oedema, producing mass effect (Fig. 22.41). However, these appearances are not specific to abscess and may occur with tumours. In the earlier stage of spreading cerebritis, there is no ring enhancement.

Plain radiology should include skull X-rays, to look particularly for evidence of sinusitis or mastoiditis and middle ear infection, and a chest X-ray. Culture of any possible source of infection, together with blood cultures, should be done. Lumbar puncture is contraindicated.

Management

Rapidly rising intracranial pressure is usually the life-threatening factor in pyogenic intracerebral abscess, and urgent drainage of the pus is necessary. Although Gram stain of the aspirated pus may give some guide to antibiotic treatment, initial treatment must be guaranteed to be effective against a wide range of organisms. A combination of benzyl penicillin, cefuroxime, gentamicin and metronidazole is reasonable, until bacterial results are available.

All patients with supratentorial abscess, with or without fits at presentation, should be given an anticonvulsant, because of the high incidence of fits. Cerebral oedema may require treatment either with mannitol or dexamethasone, and ventilation is sometimes necessary.

Some abscesses only need to be drained on one occasion, but others may need several evacuations. Serial CT scanning permits frequent monitoring of abscess size. Surgical treatment for supratentorial abscesses is usually limited to regular aspiration. Eventual healing with antibiotic treatment is often good, with little or no neurological deficit. In cerebellar abscess, many surgeons will attempt complete excision, both because of the dangers of hydrocephalus and because it is possible to excise sizeable lesions with relatively little risk of producing neurological deficit. Subdural empyema and extradural abscesses require surgical drainage and high doses of intravenous antibiotics.

Prognosis

The prognosis is related to the clinical state at the time of presentation. The overall mortality of intracerebral abscess is in the region of 10%. In survivors, lasting neurological deficit is often not severe. Persistent fits are a problem in 30–50% of patients with supratentorial abscess.

CORTICAL VENOUS THROMBO-PHLEBITIS AND VENOUS SINUS THROMBOSIS

Thrombosis of cortical veins and thrombosis of the dural venous sinuses are relatively rare. Thrombosis of the dural sinuses is nearly always preceded by cortical vein thrombosis. The exception to this is cavernous sinus thrombosis.

Aetiology

The causes of cortical thrombophlebitis and dural venous thrombosis are listed in Table 22.54. The commonest causes are infection and the hypercoagulable state which occurs postpartum.

Clinical features

There is an acute or subacute onset of severe headache, fits, hemiparesis, drowsiness and then a progressive impairment of conscious level due to cerebral oedema, together with an increase in intracranial pressure. Focal signs, such as aphasia or hemianopia, sometimes occur. A low-grade fever is often present, even in patients without a primary infective cause.

Investigation

Skull X-ray may reveal evidence of sinus or middle ear infection. CT scans may show patchy or confluent areas of cerebral cortical oedema, sometimes with haemorrhage. In cases of doubt, cerebral angiography may reveal reduced or absent filling of one of the dural sinuses. Lumbar puncture should not be done in the presence of severe cerebral oedema, as judged from the CT scan. The CSF is under raised pressure and may be normal or, frequently, lightly bloodstained.

Table 22.54 Causes of cortical vein and dural sinus thrombosis

- Infection of scalp, skull, sinuses, face, middle ear, mastoiditis. Also secondary to meningitis and septicaemia
- Postpartum (days or weeks following delivery)
- Dehydration, e.g. dysentery, cholera
- Diabetes mellitus
- Trauma (open or closed head injury)
- Catheterisation of jugular veins
- Blood dyscrasias, particularly leukaemia
- Postoperative hypercoagulability
- Severe heart failure
- Tumour invasion of sinuses
- Rare non-metastatic effect of malignant disease
- Contraceptive pill, particularly in smokers

Management

Fits must be urgently controlled, and raised intracranial pressure is treated with dexamethasone. In patients with an infective cause, appropriate antibiotics should be given. The use of anticoagulants remains controversial. There is evidence for a beneficial effect in some patients, but also a risk of causing or exacerbating cerebral haemorrhage. The prognosis is good, with resolution of all symptoms and signs in most cases.

CAVERNOUS SINUS THROMBOSIS

Cavernous sinus thrombosis is usually secondary to infective lesions originating on the face or to sinusitis of the frontal sphenoidal or ethmoidal sinuses. Untreated unilateral thrombosis often spreads to become bilateral within a few days.

Clinical features

The onset of the illness is with fever, then headache, severe malaise, pain in the eye and diplopia, and, eventually, loss of visual acuity in the affected eye. There is sometimes also nausea and vomiting. Examination reveals orbital oedema, sometimes with proptosis, normal or impaired visual acuity, and there may be papilloedema. There is a partial or complete ophthalmoplegia with ptosis. The pupil is not spared. The trigeminal nerve is sometimes involved, leading to sensory impairment on the face and cornea.

Differential diagnosis

Caroticocavernous fistula, either due to rupture of an intra-cavernous carotid aneurysm or occurring secondary to head injury, may produce a similar clinical picture. However, the degree of proptosis is often greater with a caroticocavernous fistula and the proptosis is pulsatile. There is usually a loud bruit in the region of the eye which may be altered by ipsilateral carotid artery compression.

Investigation and management

Venography by injection of contrast medium into the frontal vein demonstrates non-filling of the thrombosed cavernous sinus.

Treatment is with high-dose intravenous antibiotics and fluids, and sometimes by surgical treatment of associated sinusitis.

TUBERCULOUS MENINGITIS

Tuberculous meningitis (TBM) is now uncommon in the UK but is still a major problem in developing countries. In the past, the peak incidence was in children, but nowadays a larger proportion of patients with TBM are adults.

Pathology

TBM is nearly always due to infection with *Mycobacterium tuberculosis* and only rarely with the atypical mycobacteria. Infection reaches the meninges via haematogenous spread during miliary infection. A granulomatous inflammation develops, particularly affecting the basal meninges, where it involves the large arteries and the cranial nerves. The optic chiasm may also be affected, leading to a variety of visual field defects. Reabsorption of CSF may be impaired by granulomatous inflammation, leading to hydrocephalus, which may also be caused by obstruction of CSF outflow from the fourth ventricle.

Granulomatous inflammation over the cerebral hemispheres may lead to cortical infarction. Fits are common in TBM. Tuberculomas may develop deep within the brain, behaving as tumours. Generalised cerebral oedema with raised intracranial pressure is common.

TBM frequently leads to spinal arachnoiditis, which may cause root or cord lesions. These are often transient, but severe cord lesions with complete spinal block (as demonstrated at myelography) may develop.

Clinical features

TBM usually presents subacutely. There is often a prodrome of general malaise, without specific symptoms, of up to 6 weeks, followed by headache, lethargy and vomiting. Examination may reveal no focal abnormal neurological signs, and even meningism may be mild or absent in the early stages. A low-grade fever is usual, but may be intermittent.

Focal signs include cranial nerve palsies in about 25% of patients. These may occur as single or multiple palsies, those most commonly affected being the IIIrd, IVth, VIth, IInd, VIIth and VIIIth nerves. Fits, either focal or generalised, occur in about 25% of patients. Raised intracranial pressure, due to generalised cerebral oedema or hydrocephalus, produces papilloedema. Hemiparesis, dysphasia or hemianopia may be caused by cortical infarction, major vessel occlusion at the base of the brain, or the development of a tuberculoma (Fig. 22.42). Many patients are drowsy or stuporose at the time of presentation, but coma during the course of TBM indicates a poor prognosis; only about 50% of patients survive from this state. Finally, inappropriate ADH secretion may develop.

Investigation

The most important investigation is examination of the CSF. This is safe in patients without signs of raised intra-

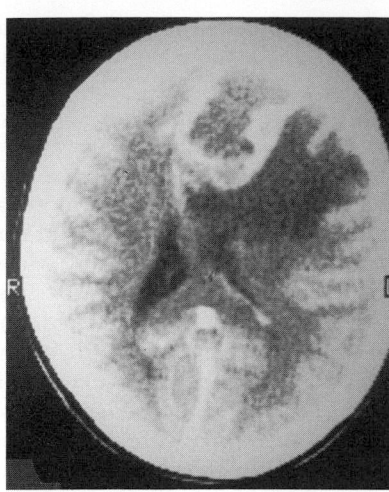

Fig. 22.42 Large left frontal tuberculoma. Contrast enhanced scan shows appearances indistinguishable from an acute pyogenic cerebral abscess with mass effect, substantial cerebral oedema and ring enhancement. Although the tuberculoma in this patient was solitary, they are frequently smaller and multiple.

cranial pressure or focal signs (excluding cranial nerve palsies). In any patient suspected of having TBM with papilloedema or focal hemisphere signs, a CT scan should be done prior to lumbar puncture to exclude hydrocephalus or tuberculoma. Obtaining CSF for diagnostic purposes in these patients should be done after consultation with a neurosurgeon. Likewise, in patients with signs of a myelopathy, spinal block and the possibility of exacerbating the cord lesion by lumbar puncture must be considered. Again, close collaboration with a neurosurgeon is necessary.

The CSF in TBM usually contains 50–500 cells/mm³ and only rarely more than 1000 mm³. In the early stages, these are mainly neutrophils; later, lymphocytes predominate. The protein is raised, sometimes to very high levels. The glucose is nearly always low. This is helpful in differentiating aseptic meningitis due to tuberculosis, from viral meningitis. Ziehl-Neelsen staining of the CSF is not infrequently negative, even when tubercle bacilli are later cultured. A lengthy and careful search of a stained centrifuged deposit of CSF is necessary.

Immunological tests for the presence of mycobacterial antigen in the CSF are becoming available, but at present the incidence of both false positive and false negative results is still too high to make this a reliable diagnostic screening procedure.

Differential diagnosis

Viral meningitis is excluded if the CSF glucose is low; however, malignant meningitis, whether carcinoma-

tous, leukaemic or lymphomatous, may cause a similar picture.

Fungal meningitis may also cause a similar clinical presentation and CSF findings. India ink staining is useful. Meningovascular syphilis and sarcoidosis are two rare causes of aseptic meningitis.

Management

It is important in TBM to start treatment as soon as possible. Even with prompt chemotherapy, complications such as hydrocephalus, cerebral infarction, tuberculomas and cranial nerve palsies are common. Drugs normally given are isoniazid, rifampicin, pyrazinamide and, sometimes, ethambutol (see Ch. 13, p. 473).

Streptomycin is not commonly used; if it is used, there is no advantage in giving the drug intrathecally. Penetration of cycloserine, ethionamide and pyrazinamide is better than that of the other antituberculous drugs, but this is not an important factor when the meninges are inflamed. Second-line drugs are used only when sensitivities from culture indicate their use.

Clinical improvement in TBM is slow. Clinical deterioration suggests the possibility of hydrocephalus, and the diagnosis is confirmed by CT scanning. Persistence of fever after 3 weeks is cause for concern, and the CSF should be re-examined after obtaining a CT scan, if possible. A minimum of 18 months of treatment is necessary and 2 years is recommended by most authorities.

Anticonvulsants are often needed but should not be given unless fits occur.

Tuberculomas (Fig. 22.42) may arise during the course of treatment even when the organism is sensitive to the drugs being given. They may be solitary or multiple. Most resolve with continued medical treatment, but larger lesions may have to be surgically drained.

The place of corticosteroids in treatment remains controversial. Claims have been made for lessening of the basal and spinal arachnoiditis with prevention of hydrocephalus, cranial nerve palsies, strokes and spinal cord syndromes, but none of these claims has been substantiated by careful clinical trial. Steroids are often given when one of these complications arises, or in very sick patients, but there is as yet no clear indication for such treatment.

Prognosis

The mortality of TBM in the UK is still high (15–30%) and, in developing countries, is higher. Adverse factors affecting prognosis are coma at presentation, pregnancy and an age of less than 2 years or more than 65 years. Persistent problems in survivors include major cranial nerve palsies causing blindness, squints and deafness;

strokes causing hemiparesis, dysphasia, and other focal hemisphere signs; and a paraparesis from spinal arachnoiditis. In a small proportion of patients, hydrocephalus develops as a late complication, sometimes years after successful treatment.

VIRAL INFECTIONS OF THE NERVOUS SYSTEM

Viral infection of the nervous system produces illness by two mechanisms: either direct invasion, or as a post-infectious illness, in which initial infection leads to an immunological reaction which itself causes damage soon after infection. This damage is usually predominantly demyelination, and it is likely that viruses cause some type of sensitisation to CNS myelin. The clinical spectrum of viral diseases comprises meningitis, encephalitis and myelitis, occurring either alone or, quite frequently, in combination. In addition, it has recently been recognised that some progressive fatal encephalitides may be the result of persistent viral infection. These include subacute sclerosing panencephalitis, progressive multifocal leucoencephalopathy and Creutzfeldt-Jakob disease.

Viruses

Some viruses are very selective in the regions and cell types within the nervous system which they affect. For example, the polio virus affects predominantly anterior horn cells, while others may produce a wide variety of illnesses; Coxsackie, for example, may cause either meningitis or a diffuse encephalitis.

Viral meningitis is most often caused by Coxsackie, Echo, measles, mumps, Herpes simplex, Herpes zoster, adenoviruses and EB virus. Direct HIV infection must now be added to this list, and is of increasing importance.

The viruses causing encephalitis vary in different parts of the world. In the UK, mumps, Echo, Coxsackie, measles, Herpes simplex, Herpes zoster, EB virus and adenoviruses are the commonest causes, in this order of frequency. HIV is now also recognised to produce encephalitis. In Asia, Japanese B virus is the commonest cause of encephalitis, while in North America, Herpes simplex is the leading pathogen.

Myelitis is caused by Coxsackie, Echo, Herpes zoster, EB virus and, occasionally, polio and rabies viruses. Immediate identification of the virus causing many presumed viral meningitides and encephalitides is often difficult, retrospective diagnosis often resting on the result of antibody titres in paired sera. In postinfectious encephalomyelitis, diagnosis often depends entirely on serological testing, except when the cause is one of the exanthemata. The common causes of postinfectious en-

cephalomyelitis are measles, varicella, vaccinia, mumps, rubella, influenza and, occasionally, rabies vaccine.

Pathology of viral infection

Most viruses reach the nervous system via blood spread from the initial site of infection, often the respiratory or gastrointestinal tracts. Some viruses spread centripetally via the nerves, e.g. the Herpes viruses, which may lie dormant in sensory ganglia for many years. It is not clear why some viruses remain confined to the meninges and others invade the brain or spinal cord, nor why some viruses show such a predilection for certain sites in the nervous system.

Within the brain and spinal cord, viruses lead to destruction of neurones, followed by phagocytosis, demyelination, vascular inflammatory change with perivascular lymphocytic cuffing, diffuse inflammatory change with a predominantly lymphocytic infiltrate, and a variable amount of oedema. Oedema may cause life-threatening rises in intracranial pressure. These pathological changes occur both in direct viral invasion and in postinfectious encephalomyelitis, but in the latter, demyelination in association with oedema is the predominant pathological change.

VIRAL MENINGITIS
Clinical features and investigation

In a minority of cases of viral meningitis there is a history suggesting viral infection. The meningitis may be of acute or subacute onset, with headache, fever, neck stiffness, nausea and vomiting, and diagnosis is not usually difficult. It is indistinguishable clinically from bacterial meningitis.

The crucial investigation is examination and subsequent culture of the CSF. The pressure is usually raised, with a pleocytosis up to several 1000/mm^3; this is usually of lymphocytes but sometimes predominantly polymorphs. The protein is increased but, in contrast to bacterial meningitis, the glucose is only very occasionally low. No organisms are seen on Gram staining. These changes may be seen in other causes of aseptic meningitis, including partly-treated bacterial meningitis.

The blood count may show a lymphocytosis, and antibody titres on acute and convalescent sera may enable a retrospective aetiological diagnosis to be made.

Management and prognosis

Treatment is symptomatic in the majority of cases. Herpes simplex or Herpes zoster meningitis is treated with a 5-day course of intravenous acyclovir. A history of steroid or other immunosuppressive treatment, or of systemic disease likely to produce an immunocompromised host, should lead to a search for unusual pathogens.

The prognosis of viral meningitis is excellent. However, HIV infection is an exception to this (p. 973) and Herpes simplex meningitis is sometimes recurrent.

VIRAL ENCEPHALITIS

Clinical features

As with meningitis, there is usually no prodromal illness in viral encephalitis. The symptoms and signs are drowsiness, headaches, nausea and vomiting, confusion, fits and, sometimes, focal signs. Occasionally, a predominantly brainstem encephalitis occurs. In severe cases, stupor and coma develop. A low-grade fever is usual. Raised intracranial pressure due to oedema is common. An associated meningitis may cause neck stiffness. The onset can be rapid, with coma developing within 12–24 hours, but the onset usually occurs over 24–72 hours.

In Herpes simplex encephalitis, focal temporal lobe lesions are common, in the setting of a diffuse encephalitis. This may be apparent both clinically with dysphasia, a visual field defect or temporal lobe epilepsy, and on investigation with EEG or CT scan. However, other viruses may cause a similar clinical picture.

The *differential diagnosis* of viral encephalitis includes other infections, particularly cerebral abscess, cerebral malaria (p. 292), metabolic encephalopathies (p. 975), cerebral tumours, and occasionally the presentation may mimic subdural haematoma or stroke.

Investigation

It is wise to do a CT scan before examining the CSF if there is an impaired consciousness level, signs of raised intracranial pressure or focal signs. Scanning may demonstrate an abscess. Focal low density in one or both temporal lobes suggests Herpes simplex infection. Often, there is no abnormality on the CT scan, or else diffuse cerebral oedema. MRI is more sensitive than CT in detecting early changes.

The CSF usually shows a modest rise in the cell count, usually lymphocytes; the protein is raised with a normal glucose, and the pressure is increased. Detection of viral antigen in CSF in Herpes simplex encephalitis at an early stage of infection is now available in some centres.

The EEG in encephalitis usually shows diffuse changes of encephalopathy, sometimes with focal features.

Management and prognosis

Treatment is largely supportive. Acyclovir is beneficial in Herpes simplex and Herpes zoster encephalitis, and it is reasonable practice to give a course of intravenous acyclovir to all patients with encephalitis in whom Herpes simplex may be the cause.

Commonly, it is not clinically possible to differentiate direct viral infection from postinfectious encephalomyelitis, unless there is a clear preceding history of an identifiable viral illness, or a preceding vaccination or immunisation.

The position of steroid treatment in postinfectious viral encephalitis is uncertain. A reasonable approach is to reserve steroids for very sick patients with encephalitis, and to give steroid with acyclovir.

The prognosis of known causes of encephalitis is very variable. Rabies encephalitis is always fatal. Mortality rates for other viruses include 40–75% for Herpes simplex, 10–20% for measles, and less than 1% for mumps. There may be permanent deficit after severe encephalitis due to any virus, whether direct viral or postinfectious. Physical deficits such as hemiparesis are less common than intellectual impairment and behavioural disturbances.

POLIOMYELITIS

Poliomyelitis remains a major health problem in developing countries and sporadic cases of polio are still seen in the UK. Following a viraemia, the virus spreads to the meninges and gains access to the CNS, where it shows an extraordinary tropism for anterior horn cells in the spinal cord and brainstem, with inflammation and cell destruction.

Clinical features

Only in 1% of those infected with the virus does a paralytic illness occur. The onset of this is 3–4 days after the initial febrile illness has resolved. However, the minor illness may be very mild in adults and may pass unnoticed. Predisposing factors to the development of the paralytic form of the illness are a history of recent tonsillectomy, recent inoculation and pregnancy. The site and severity of the paralysis is probably partly determined by physical exertion during the period between the minor illness and the onset of the paralysis (major illness).

The major illness is heralded by fever and neck stiffness, and then paralysis with myalgia develops. In the spinal form there is involvement of spinal anterior horn cells only, and there is often temporary bladder paralysis.

In the bulbar form, there is paralysis of the muscles supplied by the IXth, Xth and XIIth cranial nerves, causing pharyngeal, laryngeal and lingual paralysis. Vasomotor centres in the brainstem are also involved, causing tachycardia and lability of the blood pressure. In the bulbospinal form, there is a mixture of bulbar and spinal paralysis.

Respiratory paralysis may result either from the spinal form, with paralysis of the diaphragm, intercostal and abdominal muscles, or from bulbar paralysis, which is usually complicated by a pharyngeal paralysis leading to severe dysphagia. Paralysis is generally worse in adults than in children, with less capacity for recovery.

Differential diagnosis

Diagnosis of polio in epidemics is not difficult, but the diagnosis in isolated cases is often not suspected until paralysis develops. Occasionally, other viruses may lead to temporary paralysis, including Coxsackie, Echo and arboviruses. Differential diagnosis from Guillain-Barré syndrome is occasionally a problem, but the CSF in Guillain-Barré shows no increase in cell count, and the presence of sensory symptoms and signs in this syndrome usually leaves no doubt about the diagnosis.

Investigation and management

The CSF in poliomyelitis shows normal or slightly increased pressure, a pleocytosis of 10–200 cells/mm^3 (initially polymorphs changing to lymphocytes within 24–36 hours), a moderate increase in protein and a normal glucose. Virus may be isolated from a throat swab for a few days only, but is present in the stool for many months.

Treatment may be prophylactic if the minor illness can be recognised (in epidemics), by advising strict rest in order to reduce the risk of severe paralysis. Analgesia is often needed for the severe myalgia, and ventilation for respiratory paralysis. Regular measurement of vital capacity is essential. Pneumonia is a common complication. Many patients are left with severe paralysis and require the full resources of rehabilitation. Patients with severe respiratory paralysis require long-term respiratory support.

UNUSUAL VIRAL INFECTIONS OF THE CNS

Subacute sclerosing panencephalitis

Subacute sclerosing panencephalitis (SSPE) is subacute encephalitis occurring in children, due to persistent infection with measles virus. It is more common when there is a history of infection at an early age, often less than 2 years. After a latent period of months or, in some cases, several years, there is an insidious onset of intellectual decline, behavioural change (particularly apathy), then ataxia, myoclonic jerking and, often, a hemiparesis or tetraparesis. Other features include a retinitis and choroiditis, papilloedema, optic atrophy and cortical

blindness. The disease is relentlessly progressive and death usually occurs within 2 years of onset.

CT scans in SSPE show patchy, low-density lesions in the cerebral hemisphere white matter, and progressive cerebral and cerebellar atrophy.

There is no effective treatment.

Progressive multifocal leucoencephalopathy

Progressive multifocal leucoencephalopathy (PML) is an illness occurring only in immunocompromised patients, particularly those with lymphoma. It is now also being increasingly seen in AIDS. The causative viruses are the JC and SV40 papovaviruses. Oligodendrocytes are preferentially affected, producing widespread demyelination, spreading from many different foci in the white matter. Patients present with progressive dementia, and focal signs including hemiparesis, hemianopia, dysphasia and ataxia. The disease is progressive and death usually occurs within a few months.

CT scans in PML show multiple low-density lesions, with atrophy in the later stages. The CSF is normal. Treatment with cytosine arabinoside may slow the progress of the disease in some patients, but a fatal outcome is inevitable.

Creutzfeldt-Jakob disease

Creutzfeldt-Jakob disease (CJD) is a very rare disease which has been shown to be transmissible and which is thought to be due either to a viral infection or infection with a virus subparticle (prion). There is a family history in about 6% of cases. The pathology is a progressive neuronal loss without inflammation. In man, CJD has been transmitted to children in growth hormone made from pituitary extracts and in corneal grafts. The transmissible agent is apparently resistant to both heat and formalin.

The clinical features of CJD include myoclonus, ataxia, extrapyramidal rigidity, dementia, hemiparesis, aphasia and fits. The onset may be gradual or subacute. In the early stages, the differential diagnosis includes PML or cerebral tumour. CT scans eventually show atrophy but may be surprisingly normal early in the disease. There is no treatment.

NEUROSYPHILIS AND OTHER RARE INFECTIONS

SYPHILIS

The major features of syphilis infection are described in Chapter 11. *Treponema pallidum* may invade the CNS weeks or months after the initial infection, but only causes a meningitic illness in about a quarter of these cases. Occasionally, the meningitis is severe, with transient cranial nerve palsies and convulsions; usually, however, it is mild or even asymptomatic.

All the clinical manifestations of late or tertiary syphilis have a chronic meningitis as the underlying pathological process. This process leads to arterial involvement (syphilitic arteritis), affecting meningeal and parenchymal vessels. Tertiary syphilis may present as:

- chronic meningovascular syphilis
- parenchymatous involvement as general paralysis of the insane (GPI) or tabes dorsalis. Syphilitic amyotrophy is a rare form of parenchymatous involvement.

Diagnostic tests

Details of the serological tests for syphilis are discussed in Chapter 11. In active neurosyphilis of any type, the CSF is always abnormal, showing a raised cell count with positive antibody tests (VDRL, TPHA, FTA and TPI). The protein content is also usually raised, and there is evidence of local synthesis of IgG, with oligoclonal bands on electrophoresis. Difficulty arises when positive antibody tests are found, without a rise in the cell count, in a patient with a neurological presentation not typical for one of the syndromes of neurosyphilis. Under these circumstances, it is important to give a full course of antibiotic treatment and to re-examine the CSF 6 months later.

Meningovascular syphilis

In meningovascular syphilis, there is a combination of chronic basal granulomatous meningitis and syphilitic arteritis.

The condition presents within 10–12 years of primary infection, either with a generalised illness, including headache, neck stiffness, convulsions, and confusion or psychosis, usually without fever, or with focal neurological symptoms, often cranial nerve palsies and, sometimes, strokes affecting either the hemispheres or brainstem. Optic atrophy is a common feature. Although meningovascular syphilis is relatively uncommon, it is important to recognise since it usually responds well to treatment in the earlier stages.

Syphilitic gumma

Gummas are large granulomatous lesions arising in the meninges with central necrosis. They usually remain superficial over the hemisphere, and present with fits, hemiparesis, dysphasia and other focal deficits. Gummas occasionally occur in the spinal meninges and cause cord compression.

Parenchymatous syphilis

In all three forms of parenchymatous syphilis – GPI, tabes dorsalis and syphilitic amyotrophy – the pathology is a meningoencephalomyelitis. The meninges show changes of chronic granulomatous inflammation and thickening, and there are both degenerative changes within the brain with neuronal loss, and glial changes, together with endarteritis obliterans. In about 50% of cases, *Treponema pallidum* can be demonstrated. There is generalised cerebral atrophy. In tabes dorsalis and amyotrophy, there are usually diffuse pathological changes but the spinal cord bears the brunt of the disease.

General paralysis of the insane

GPI is characterised by progressive mental deterioration (dementia), which is usually insidious in onset but may be abrupt, together with a variety of physical deficits. The condition develops 15–20 years after initial infection. Younger patients presenting with dementia should have serological tests for syphilis. Dysarthria and tremor – either cerebellar or extrapyramidal in type, affecting limbs, trunk and tongue – are common, as are fits, brisk reflexes and extensor plantars. The tremor is frequently the most disabling of the physical manifestations. Occasional focal features, such as dysphasia or hemiparesis, occur.

The Argyll-Robertson (AR) pupil may occur with all forms of tertiary syphilis but is most often seen in GPI and tabes dorsalis. The AR pupil is usually, but not always, small. It fails to react to light, but does react normally to convergence. It is nearly always bilateral. The pupils are often irregular and unequal in size (anisocoria).

Differential diagnosis. The differential diagnosis of GPI includes Alzheimer's disease, diffuse cerebrovascular disease, or multi-infarct dementia, metabolic encephalopathy, chronic alcoholic cerebral degeneration, traumatic encephalopathy and subdural haematoma.

Treatment. Prompt treatment in the early stages will arrest progression and, in some patients, there is reversal of the deficits. Without treatment, death occurs within a few years.

Tabes dorsalis

Tabes dorsalis develops 10–25 years after initial infection and may be accompanied by GPI in some cases. There is degeneration, initially in the dorsal roots, and then in the posterior columns of the spinal cord.

Lightning pains are virtually pathognomic of tabes, and often occur for years before other manifestations of the condition. They are usually in the legs, but may also occur in a girdle distribution around the trunk and, very occasionally, in the face. They last only seconds, are lancinating and severe.

Tabetic crises are sudden attacks of epigastric pain and vomiting, lasting hours to days. This may mimic an acute abdomen but there is cutaneous hyperaesthesia without any peritonism. Similar crises may rarely affect the bladder, uterus, rectum and genitalia.

Ataxia with a slapping, steppage gait is characteristic, and is sensory in type due to the dorsal column degenerative change. Examination shows loss of joint position and vibration sensation in the legs. Distal cutaneous numbness and paraesthesiae are common, and there is sometimes hyperaesthesia of the feet. Loss of deep pain sensation leads to the development of neuropathic (Charcot) joints, and severe loss of cutaneous sensation causes penetrating ulcers on the feet. There is often a breastplate area of sensory impairment on the thorax, with a butterfly distribution of sensory loss on the face. There is areflexia in the legs, and the plantars may be flexor or extensor. A neurogenic bladder is common.

Syphilitic amyotrophy

Syphilitic amyotrophy is an uncommon manifestation of spinal cord involvement in neurosyphilis. There is a progressive neuronal loss in the anterior horns of the spinal cord. The condition mimics amyotrophic lateral sclerosis (one form of motor neurone disease, see p. 941).

Congenital syphilis

The features of congenital syphilis are those of combined GPI and tabes dorsalis, so-called *taboparesis*. In addition, there are other stigmata, including interstitial keratitis, sensory neural deafness, Hutchinson's teeth (wide spaced, notched teeth), a saddle nose deformity and evidence of periostitis and osteochondritis on X-rays. Congenital syphilis is discussed in more detail in Chapter 11.

Management

The management of syphilis is considered in detail in Chapter 11. The CSF must be re-examined 6–8 weeks after therapy and, if the cell count is still raised, a further course of penicillin is given. The CSF must then be re-examined at annual intervals for several years, to ensure eradication of infection.

MYCOPLASMA

Mycoplasma infection may be associated with neurological complications, including meningo-encephalitis, cranial nerve palsies, myelopathy or peripheral neuropathy (see also p. 466).

LYME DISEASE

This disorder, caused by the tick-borne spirochaete *Borrelia burgdorferi*, is characterised by skin lesions (erythema chronicum migrans), a systemic illness and various neurological features: these may include cranial nerve lesions (esp. VII), painful radiculopathies, myelopathy or meningo-encephalitis.

LISTERIA

Listeria is a rare cause of meningitis or meningo-encephalitis, encountered most often in immunocompromised subjects (see below).

RICKETTSIA

Rickettsial infections often produce pronounced headache and a non-specific encephalopathic state, but some are characterised by a frank encephalitis or immune-complex cerebral vasculitis.

FUNGAL INFECTION

Fungal infections of the nervous system may take the form of low-grade meningitis (often with secondary communicating hydrocephalus), multiple abscesses, or localised sinus invasion with tissue destruction. Possible organisms include cryptococcus, nocardia, aspergillus, mucormycosis, actinomycosis and coccidiomycosis. These infections usually arise in the context of AIDS, other immune deficiency states, steroid treatment or diabetes (see below).

NEUROLOGICAL MANIFESTATIONS OF AIDS

The human immune deficiency virus (HIV) is a highly neurotropic virus and has widespread effects on the central and peripheral nervous system. Nervous system involvement is common both in established AIDS and as a result of acute infection at the pre-conversion stage, before antibodies to the virus are detectable. The full extent of nervous system involvement in HIV infection is still uncertain, with new syndromes currently being recognised. It has been estimated that about 75% of AIDS patients have evidence of nervous system involvement, as determined at necropsy. In about 10% of patients, one of the neurological manifestations is the presenting illness of

AIDS; the problems include encephalitis, meningitis, cerebral abscesses, cerebral tumours, myelopathy, peripheral neuropathy and retinitis. There is an increased incidence of syphilis in patients with AIDS.

Encephalitis

Subacute. The subacute form of encephalitis is a major problem in about 30% of AIDS patients, but probably affects all patients, to some extent, who survive long enough. In the majority, the subacute encephalitis is thought to be caused by direct HIV infection, but other pathogens may produce a similar clinical picture, including CMV, Herpes zoster, Herpes simplex, atypical mycobacteria and diffuse lymphoma. It nearly always arises in patients who have already had other manifestations of AIDS, but there have been recent reports of subacute encephalitis being the presenting illness. It usually develops as an insidious onset of intellectual failure, but sometimes more acutely, with a confusional state provoked by another illness. Depression, itself common in AIDS, may initially be thought to be the explanation of the symptoms. There is progression to a severe dementia in many cases. The leading physical manifestation is ataxia, and pyramidal signs are also common.

The CT scan may be normal in the early stages but later shows progressive atrophy. CSF usually shows a lymphocytic pleocytosis and a raised protein content.

Acute. An acute, recoverable encephalitis is now recognised within 3 months of HIV infection, occurring at about the time antibodies are first detectable. This illness lasts about a week and is characterised by headache, fits, confusion and decreased level of consciousness.

Meningitis

AIDS patients may develop a preconversion acute aseptic meningitis with typical or atypical features of meningitis, presenting with headache, neck stiffness, fever and, sometimes, cranial nerve lesions (the Vth, VIIth and VIIIth being the commonest), together with long tract signs. This type of meningitis may be recurrent or become chronic.

Many pathogens may cause meningitis in established AIDS. These include all the common bacteria producing meningitis, as well as many less common organisms. *Cryptococcus neoformans* is particularly important (p. 279). Here, the CSF shows a modest increase in cells, an increase in protein and a reduced glucose, and the organism can be demonstrated with an India ink stain. The detection of cryptococcal antigen in the CSF (and blood) is diagnostically useful. The possibility of other types of fungal infection, and of amoebae and *Listeria monocytogenes*, has also to be considered when examining the CSF.

Cerebral abscess

Cerebral abscess is common in AIDS. Multiple abscesses are more usual than single lesions, and are most often caused by *Toxoplasma gondii* (about 70%). Multiple tuberculomas, primary cerebral lymphoma and *Candida albicans* may all cause a similar clinical picture. Patients present with headache, focal deficits and fits. Because of the predominance of toxoplasma (and unless there is a life-threatening increase in intracranial pressure), a reasonable approach is to give a 1–2-week trial of treatment for toxoplasma (p. 288) in the first instance. If there is no clinical improvement, biopsy of an easily accessible lesion is undertaken.

Tumour

Primary cerebral lymphoma is not infrequent in AIDS, and may present either as a progressive dementia or with focal deficits, headache and fits. The CT appearances may be indistinguishable from multiple abscesses.

Myelopathy

A myelopathy alone is uncommon in AIDS but may occur in association with subacute encephalitis. It is thought to be due to direct HIV infection. An acute preconversion myelopathy has also been described.

Peripheral neuropathy

Acute preconversion neuropathies include: a cranial neuropathy, most often involving the facial nerve, which usually recovers over several months; and a mononeuritis multiplex (multifocal neuropathy) affecting the limbs. Commoner than either of these is a symmetrical painful sensory motor polyneuropathy. It is thought to be due to direct HIV infection, and is usually progressive.

Retinitis

A retinitis caused by CMV occurs in AIDS patients. Blurred vision, loss of acuity, and scotomas are early features. It may progress in some cases to complete blindness. Fundoscopy shows retinal vessel irregularity and narrowing, with perivascular exudates and haemorrhages, and later, arteriolar occlusion causing retinal infarction. Many patients respond to treatment with gancyclovir.

Myopathy

A myopathy has been described in a few patients. In some, this is related to treatment with zidovudine.

NEUROLOGICAL ASPECTS OF SYSTEMIC DISEASE, INCLUDING MALIGNANCY

SYSTEMIC DISEASES WHICH AFFECT THE NERVOUS SYSTEM

Connective tissue disorders

Systemic lupus erythematosus

The vasculitis of systemic lupus erythematosus (SLE, see Ch. 23) affects the CNS of at least 30% of patients at some stage during the illness. Mental changes, most commonly depression, but also psychosis and mania, occur. These can also be the result of high-dose steroid treatment. Fits and cerebral microinfarcts due to vasculitis are further manifestations. The CSF is often abnormal in CNS involvement, which helps to distinguish this from steroid-induced changes. In the spinal cord, vasculitis can cause infarction leading to paraplegia. The peripheral nervous system may be affected by a mononeuritis multiplex, again thought to be due to vasculitis. Occasionally, a diffuse sensory motor neuropathy may arise, and very uncommonly a Guillain-Barré syndrome. Neurological illness may be the presenting manifestation of lupus.

Systemic sclerosis

Neurological involvement in systemic sclerosis (Ch. 23) is fairly common. It usually takes the form of a slowly progressive proximal myopathy, in which there is atrophy without inflammatory change. Occasionally, a more rapidly progressive myopathy occurs, with increased creatine phosphokinase levels and inflammatory change on muscle biopsy, indistinguishable from isolated polymyositis. This latter form responds to anti-inflammatory and immunosuppressive treatment (p. 1030). Despite the often extensive skin and subcutaneous thickening, entrapment neuropathies are relatively infrequent. A cranial neuropathy may develop, most commonly affecting the trigeminal nerve and, occasionally, the facial nerve. Sensory loss on the face may be bilateral and severe. It is not certain whether the peripheral nerve lesions have a vasculitic basis or are simply due to sclerosis. Very occasionally, sclerotic change can affect the major neck vessels, causing strokes.

Rheumatoid arthritis

Peripheral nerve involvement. Entrapment neuropathies, particularly carpal tunnel syndrome and ulnar neuropathy at the elbow, are common in rheumatoid arthritis (Ch. 23) and are simply related to the disorganisation of the joints. A digital entrapment neuropathy also occurs. A mononeuritis multiplex with a vasculitic basis is frequent; occasionally a symmetrical polyneuropathy develops. Both patterns of neuropathy are often associated with a cutaneous vasculitis.

Muscle. Muscle wasting and weakness due to atrophy are universal in advanced rheumatoid arthritis. Rarely, an inflammatory polymyositis occurs.

Cervical myelopathy (p. 933) is the most serious neurological complication of rheumatoid arthritis.

Polyarteritis nodosa

In polyarteritis nodosa (p. 1031), which affects many more men than women, medium- and small-sized arteries are patchily involved in an inflammatory process of unknown cause throughout the body. Peripheral nerve involvement is common, CNS involvement is less usual. The inflammatory change in arteries leads to occlusion and infarction, and occasional aneurysm formation with subsequent haemorrhage. A mononeuritis multiplex is the commonest manifestation. Muscle pain and focal areas of necrosis are common.

The many CNS manifestations are often transitory. They include an aseptic meningitis, fits, mental disturbances (particularly psychosis) and, sometimes, small strokes.

Diseases of unknown cause

Sarcoidosis

Peripheral nerve involvement, including cranial neuropathy, is relatively common in sarcoidosis (p. 500), while CNS manifestations are rare. Nervous system involvement is much more common in blacks than Caucasians. The hypercalcaemia of sarcoidosis may lead to neurological symptoms.

The commonest neurological manifestation of sarcoidosis is a lower motor neurone facial palsy indistinguishable from a Bell's palsy. The weakness improves over weeks or months. Optic neuritis may also occur in sarcoid, but other cranial nerves are affected relatively infrequently. A mononeuritis multiplex may arise, and patchy muscle involvement, sometimes with palpable lumps of sarcoid tissue, can occur.

Sarcoid granulomas can arise in any part of the CNS and can achieve a large size. The hypothalamic area is particularly favoured. Here, the disease causes diabetes insipidus, appetite disturbances and, commonly, hypersomnolence. The spinal cord may be affected, producing a paraparesis. Since the CSF is often abnormal, with an increased cell count and oligoclonal bands, diagnostic confusion with MS occasionally arises.

Diagnosis of neurosarcoidosis can be difficult in the absence of obvious systemic disease (p. 503).

Treatment of the neurological lesions in sarcoidosis with steroids is often unrewarding, although some patients with peripheral neuropathy or spinal cord lesions do improve. CNS supratentorial involvement may occasionally be amenable to surgery.

Wegener's granulomatosis

Wegener's granulomatosis is a necrotising midline granulomatous vasculitic condition, in which a cranial or peripheral mononeuritis multiplex occurs in about a third of patients.

Behçet's disease

Behçet's disease is characterised by a relapsing and remitting clinical picture over many years, with oral and genital ulceration, uveitis and, often, arthritis and rash. The cause of this disease is unknown. Nervous system involvement occurs in at least a quarter of patients at some time during the illness, and its relapsing and remitting nature may cause diagnostic confusion with MS. The pathology is a vasculitis causing small areas of infarction and demyelination. This often affects the brainstem, producing disorders of ocular movement, and cerebellar and long tract signs. With cerebral hemisphere involvement, a hemiparesis may result. There are no diagnostic tests for Behçet's disease; diagnosis rests on the clinical combination of oral and genital ulceration and sometimes other systemic features, with a typical neurological presentation.

GENERAL METABOLIC DISTURBANCES

Anoxia

The causes of diffuse cerebral anoxia are shown in Table 22.55. The brain can only withstand 3 minutes of anoxia. Diffuse anoxia for shorter periods may cause focal areas of infarction in older patients in whom there is a pre-existing partial vessel occlusion, causing critical hypoperfusion.

Table 22.55 Causes of diffuse cerebral anoxia

● Cardiac arrest	● Fat embolism
● Severe hypotension, e.g. due to drug overdose, bleeding	● Cerebral malaria
	● Anaesthetic catastrophe
● DIC	● Cardiopulmonary bypass surgery

The immediate effects of prolonged anoxia are loss of consciousness and of brainstem reflexes. The pupils are widely dilated and fixed, reflex eye movements are absent, there is no respiratory effort, and the limbs are flaccid with absent reflexes. If resuscitation is to prove successful, some clinical improvement should be evident within a short period. Pupillary reactions and spontaneous breathing are the earliest signs of improvement. If pupils remain fixed and there is still no ventilatory effort within an hour or so, the outlook is almost always very poor. Recovery to a state in which brainstem reflexes return to a variable extent, but the patient remains unconscious, is common, and recovery may become arrested at this stage. Further gradual recovery over weeks and months can occur from this state, but if consciousness is lost for 24 hours or longer after diffuse cerebral anoxia, some permanent physical and intellectual deficit is the rule.

Rarely, satisfactory recovery is followed weeks later by a delayed deterioration in neurological function.

Hypoglycaemia

Hypoglycaemia (Ch. 19) produces life-threatening coma, and the more profound and prolonged it is, the more likely it is that recovery will occur with neurological deficit. Hypoglycaemia may present as unexplained coma, confusion, with fits which may be partial or generalised, or with focal deficit of abrupt onset mimicking a stroke. Very rarely, a picture resembling MND is seen in patients with chronic hypoglycaemia due to insulinoma.

In all cases of unexplained coma, intravenous glucose should be given. In the Wernicke-Korsakoff syndrome (p. 979) glucose given without thiamine may cause further deterioration, since glucose cannot be metabolised easily without thiamine. Given the increased incidence of Wernicke-Korsakoff syndrome in the UK, glucose and thiamine should now be given to all patients with unexplained coma.

Respiratory failure

Carbon dioxide retention (Ch. 13) causes headache, drowsiness, stupor and eventually coma. A metabolic tremor (asterixis) is common, and myoclonic jerking and fits are occasional features. Papilloedema secondary to venous distension is present in a few patients.

Uraemic encephalopathy

Untreated acute and chronic renal failure (Ch. 20) lead to a progressive decrease in the consciousness level, associated with hyperventilation, asterixis, myoclonic jerking, tetany and convulsions. Rapid dialysis may lead to the so-called *disequilibrium syndrome*, in which plasma urea, electrolytes and osmolality are rapidly corrected while brain concentrations remain high. Water enters the hyperosmolar brain, producing a form of water intoxication.

A predominantly sensory axonal peripheral neuropathy is a common complication of uraemia, and may be partially reversible with dialysis.

Hepatic encephalopathy

Hepatic encephalopathy is discussed on page 980 and in Chapter 16.

Hyponatraemia

Neurological effects of hyponatraemia (p. 847) are much more likely to appear if the latter develops rapidly; they comprise agitation, confusion, fits, myoclonus, asterixis, and then coma when the plasma sodium concentration falls below 110–115 mmol/l. Central pontine myelinolysis (p. 982) can rarely occur.

Hypernatraemia

Hypernatraemia (p. 848) occurs in hyperosmolar diabetic coma and in untreated diabetes insipidus, particularly when the hypothalamus is affected by the lesion producing the diabetes insipidus, abolishing thirst. Such lesions include large pituitary tumours, craniopharyngiomas, eosinophilic granulomas and sarcoidosis, together with hypothalamic tumours. A falling level of consciousness and convulsions develop when the plasma sodium concentration reaches 155–160 mmol/l.

Hypokalaemia

Hypokalaemia (p. 340) produces muscle weakness and fatigue, followed by a decreasing level of consciousness with confusion and delirium. Death may occur from ventricular tachycardia.

Hypomagnesaemia

Hypomagnesaemia usually occurs with severe vomiting or diarrhoea, particularly if fluid replacement is given without adequate magnesium. It is commonly associated with hypocalcaemia. Symptoms of hypomagnesaemia include irritability, confusion, muscle twitching, hallucinations, myoclonus, chorea, coma and fits.

Hypermagnesaemia

Hypermagnesaemia is rare, but may occur in renal failure due to administration of magnesium salts, usually inadvertently in the form of antacids. Magnesium is important

in acetylcholine release at the neuromuscular junction, and hypermagnesaemia results in generalised weakness, lethargy, coma and death from respiratory paralysis.

Hypercalcaemia

The neurological symptoms of hypercalcaemia (p. 729) are agitation, confusion, hallucinations and, sometimes, delirium and fits. Papilloedema is occasionally a feature.

Hypocalcaemia

In chronic hypocalcaemia (p. 733), mental blunting is the rule and patients are often thought to be demented or retarded. Other features are fits and raised intracranial pressure. Tetany, which may be symptomatic, can be demonstrated as a positive Chvostek sign. Cataracts and basal ganglia calcification occur in long-standing hypocalcaemia.

Porphyria

Of the two types of porphyria (p. 780), erythropoietic and hepatic, only the latter (acute intermittent porphyria) is associated with neurological consequences. Aminolaevulinic acid (ALA) binds to GABA receptor sites in the CNS and the neurological complications are thought to be due in part to facilitation by ALA of transmission at GABA receptors.

In acute intermittent porphyria, mental changes are prominent, with agitation, mania, tremor, delirium, hallucination, fits and eventually coma. Strokes and retinal ischaemia may occur, and are thought to be due to cerebral arterial spasm. A polyneuropathy in the limbs may also occur, as may multiple cranial neuropathies, together with brainstem signs, in particular ocular movement abnormalities. These neurological manifestations are usually preceded and accompanied by abdominal symptoms.

NEUROLOGICAL MANIFESTATIONS OF ENDOCRINE DISEASE

Diabetes

Peripheral neuropathy (p. 946) and hypoglycaemia are common problems. Uncontrolled hyperglycaemia (Ch. 19) also causes coma. Diabetes is a major predisposing cause of atheromatous vascular disease and therefore of cerebral infarction.

Hyperthyroidism

The general neurological effects of hyperthyroidism (p. 688) include anxiety and tremor. Proximal myopathy is common in untreated thyrotoxicosis (p. 690). Chorea is a rare sign of hyperthyroidism. Dysthyroid eye disease may occur while the hyperthyroid patient is thyrotoxic or euthyroid. In some cases, the symptoms arise only after a euthyroid state has been achieved with treatment; in other patients, the eye disease arises in the absence of any preceding toxicity. In dysthyroid eye disease, there is an enlargement of the external ocular muscles due to a lymphocytic infiltration, with oedema. The eye muscles can become enormously swollen (Fig. 22.43), causing impaired venous drainage from the orbit; this leads to papilloedema and reduced visual acuity. The pathogenesis of these changes remains uncertain (p. 690).

The first symptom of the exophthalmic ophthalmoplegia is diplopia. The changes may be asymmetrical in the early stages. Examination reveals unilateral or bilateral proptosis, an ophthalmoplegia which usually affects all movements with sparing of downward gaze and lid retraction; corneal ulceration may also occur.

Treatment is urgent in patients with reduced visual acuity or papilloedema. Oral steroids usually relieve orbital pressure, with rapid recession of the exophthalmos. Failure to respond to steroids requires surgical decompression. Tarsorrhaphy may be necessary to protect the cornea.

Dysthyroid eye disease usually runs a course of 1–2 years. Surgical measures to correct residual squint should be reserved until this stage.

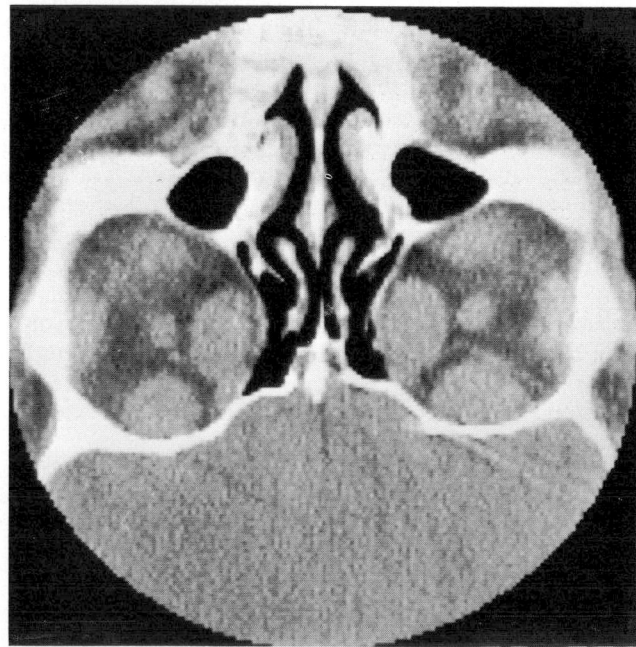

Fig. 22.43 Coronal CT scan in a patient with dysthyroid eye disease. There was marked proptosis, bilateral papilloedema and severe ophthalmoplegia. The scan shows gross enlargement ot the extraocular muscles.

Hypothyroidism

The neurological manifestations of myxoedema include mental slowing and, sometimes, dementia. Alternatively, behavioural disturbances, psychosis and even mania may result ('myxoedema madness'). A predominantly sensory polyneuropathy is associated with hypothyroidism. Occasionally, patients with myxoedema present with ataxia of gait without other obvious abnormal signs. A proximal myopathy can be a feature.

Apart from the mental slowing, a common neurological complication of hypothyroidism is unilateral or bilateral carpal tunnel syndrome, due to compression of the median nerve by myxoedematous tissue.

Cushing's syndrome

Mental changes in Cushing's syndrome can take the form of a mild euphoria associated with an increase in appetite or, occasionally, psychotic illnesses. A proximal myopathy is inevitable with large doses of steroids taken over a period of months but the tendency to develop this complication is extremely variable.

Hypoadrenalism

In Addison's disease, hypoadrenalism causes hyponatraemia, hyperkalaemia and, often, hypotension; together, these factors cause lethargy and weakness. In severe Addisonian crises, coma develops and fits may occur.

NEUROLOGICAL MANIFESTATIONS OF MALIGNANCY

About 20% of all malignancies are associated with some type of neurological involvement. Metastatic spread may occur to the brain, spinal cord substance, epidural space or vertebral body. Direct invasion of the brachial or lumbosacral plexus is common with breast and pelvic tumours. Occasionally, individual peripheral nerves may be directly infiltrated.

A number of tumours are also capable of producing remote neurological effects without direct invasion of the nervous system – the so-called non-metastatic or paraneoplastic effects of malignancy. Neurological problems may also result directly from treatment, e.g. the peripheral neuropathy due to vincristine. Opportunistic infection of the nervous system is an important problem following immunosuppressive therapy.

Cancer

Metastatic spread of cancer to the brain or spinal cord is particularly common with primaries in breast, lung, bowel, skin, kidney and testes. Direct invasion of the meninges (malignant meningitis) is relatively unusual.

The two commonest non-metastatic effects of cancer are a predominantly sensory polyneuropathy and a cerebellar ataxia. Cancer of the lung is by far the commonest primary associated with these non-metastatic effects. A proximal myopathy has been described, sometimes associated with an elevated CPK. There is an increased incidence of inflammatory polymyositis associated with cancer, but it still remains relatively uncommon. The incidence of underlying cancer in patients presenting with polymyositis (p. 955) has been greatly overestimated in the past, except in the case of adult-onset dermatomyositis. A rapidly progressive encephalomyelitis has been described as a non-metastatic complication of carcinoma, but is very rare. Finally, the Lambert-Eaton myasthenic syndrome (p. 951) is occasionally seen with small cell carcinoma of the lung. This condition, due to a failure of acetylcholine release at the neuromuscular junction, is characterised by a progressive proximal myopathy, sometimes with fatigability mimicking myasthenia gravis.

Lymphoma

Lymphomas rarely metastasise to cause intracerebral mass lesions, but malignant meningitis is not uncommon. Localised masses of lymphoma tissue present occasionally in the nasopharynx, and invade either upwards to involve the lower cranial nerves, or within the orbit, causing a progressive ophthalmoplegia, proptosis and, eventually, visual loss. The spinal cord may be compressed by epidural collections of lymphomatous tissue.

Non-metastatic neurological complications are more common with lymphoma than with cancer, except perhaps cancer of the lung. A degenerative cerebellar ataxia occurs, together with a variety of different types of polyneuropathy. An encephalitic illness is also described with lymphoma. Opportunistic nervous system infection is particularly likely to occur with this malignancy.

Although not exclusive to lymphomas, the condition of progressive multifocal leucoencephalopathy occurs most frequently with this type of tumour. It is thought to be caused by a papovavirus, which leads to progressive massive areas of demyelination (p. 970).

Leukaemia

By far the most common form of neurological involvement in leukaemia (Ch. 24) is a malignant meningitis; this often occurs at a time of systemic remission. It is thought that small numbers of leukaemic cells which are relatively immune to the effects of systemic chemotherapy cross the blood–brain barrier during periods of systemic relapse. These cells are then able to proliferate later, causing a malignant meningitis. The frequent development of CNS relapse in leukaemia led to the early adoption of prophylactic therapy. This is standard in younger patients to avoid CNS relapse. Malignant meningitis is occasionally complicated by hydrocephalus, due to a reduced capacity for reabsorption of CSF.

As in lymphoma, opportunistic infection is very common in leukaemia; progressive multifocal leucoencephalopathy is an occasional development.

Myeloma

Spinal cord compression resulting from vertebral collapse is particularly common in myeloma. Surgical decompression is complicated by the special difficulties of spinal stabilisation when several adjacent vertebral bodies are involved. A painful neuropathy may be a non-metastatic complication and, in contrast to other non-metastatic neuropathies, may show some improvement with tumour treatment. Occasionally, myeloma neuropathy is complicated by the development of amyloid, which is an independent cause of peripheral neuropathy (p. 948).

Large quantities of paraprotein occasionally lead to a hyperviscosity syndrome with the development of multiple cerebral infarcts, a situation not unlike that seen with polycythaemia rubra vera. Finally, severe hypercalcaemia is common with myeloma, and may cause neurological symptoms (p. 976).

Radiation damage to the nervous system

Radiotherapy can cause neurological damage. Treatment of malignant invasion of the brachial or lumbosacral plexuses seems particularly likely to cause damage, with symptoms of progressive, often painful, plexopathy starting 1–5 years after radiotherapy. Radiation to the spinal cord may rarely produce an acute myelopathy, which usually resolves slowly after radiotherapy is stopped. A delayed, slowly progressive, radiation myelopathy with onset 1–5 years after radiotherapy is more common.

In children with acute leukaemia treated prophylactically, the somnolence syndrome, consisting of drowsiness, lethargy, irritability and anorexia, is common. It resolves after radiotherapy is stopped. The question of whether radiotherapy produces permanent intellectual damage in children remains controversial. There is some evidence that this may occur in adults.

ALCOHOL AND THE NERVOUS SYSTEM

Alcohol causes a wide range of neurological effects.

Acute intoxication and coma

Alcohol is absorbed rapidly from the gut and easily crosses the blood–brain barrier. The cerebral effect of alcohol taken acutely is due to a direct inhibitory effect on membranes, which leads to a reduction in neurone excitability. In non-alcoholics, blood ethanol concentrations of 30–70 mg/100 ml will affect coordination, sensory perception and intellectual functions. Drunkenness is associated with levels of between 50 and 150 mg/100 ml. The effects of acute intoxication are well known. A feeling of well-being and relaxation is associated with loss of inhibition, loss of judgement and an inability to sustain or follow critical argument. Mood changes depend to a large extent on personality and pre-existing mood. There may be excitement, depression or paranoia. Memory for events during the period of intoxication is usually impaired and, with very high levels of alcohol, there may be amnesic periods of several hours or longer. These are sometimes known as alcoholic blackouts, though there is no loss of consciousness. The effects of acute intoxication are associated with dysarthria, ataxia and increased sympathetic activity, producing flushing, pupillary dilatation and tachycardia; the respiratory rate is often increased. With increasing levels of alcohol, disorientation is followed by stupor and then coma, with a reduced respiratory rate. Death may occur due to the direct toxic effects of very large amounts of alcohol; more commonly, vomiting leading to aspiration pneumonia is the cause of death. In certain susceptible people, hypoglycaemia occurs, particularly when alcohol has been taken without food.

In chronic alcoholism, tolerance to ethanol develops, so that at levels well in excess of 100 mg/100 ml there may be no apparent impairment of intellectual or motor function.

Alcoholic coma is rare; disorientation and stupor are more common. Patients should be allowed to rest, and many will sleep. On the day following acute alcohol excess, there is dehydration, sometimes tremulousness, headache, malaise and nausea.

Many patients in coma also abuse other drugs; the combination of alcohol and barbiturate is particularly dangerous. The association of alcoholism and cranial trauma leads to an excess of subdural haematomas in this group.

Delirium tremens

Delirium tremens is an acute psychosis seen in chronic alcoholics during alcohol withdrawal. The effects are probably due to withdrawal of sedation, and release of autonomic activity and neuronal irritability.

There is a change in personality, the patient becoming withdrawn, restless, irritable, anorexic and sleepless; there are often frightening hallucinations, which tend to be visual more than auditory. Disorientation, dysarthria and progressive clouding of consciousness also occur. Fits occur 12–48 hours after alcohol withdrawal and, when present, always precede the period of delirium. Death

occasionally occurs from ventricular tachycardia secondary to hypokalaemia.

The mainstay of treatment is sedation, and the drug of choice is chlormethiazole, given either orally or as a continuous intravenous infusion. In severe refractory cases, it may be necessary to use paraldehyde. It is necessary to correct fluid and electrolyte imbalance, ensure adequate nutrition at an early stage, and to give thiamine to prevent the development of a Wernicke-Korsakoff syndrome (see below).

Alcoholic fits

Alcoholic fits, sometimes known as 'rum fits', are a common complication of alcoholism, and they may also be seen in non-alcoholics after a single acute excess of alcohol. Fits occur 12–48 hours after alcohol withdrawal, and nearly always take the form of generalised convulsions. Fits rarely occur during a period of drinking; if they do, it is usually related to a rapidly falling blood alcohol level. The majority of patients with alcohol withdrawal fits have not had previous fits, and the subsequent EEG is normal.

Alcoholic dementia and cerebral degeneration

Chronic alcoholism may cause a slowly progressive dementia associated with generalised cerebral atrophy. There is often associated depression. Dementia in alcoholics may also be due to repeated head injuries, undetected subdural haematoma, insidious hepatic encephalopathy and chronic fits.

In the early stages, some degree of dementia may be reversible if the patient abstains completely from alcohol. Depressed patients should respond to antidepressant drugs. Many patients, however, continue to drink.

In some alcoholics, without any clinical evidence of dementia or other brain damage but with cerebral atrophy on CT scanning, the CT scan appearances improve with abstinence from alcohol. This improvement occurs slowly over a period of 6 months to 3 years. Similar, partly reversible cerebral atrophy has also been observed in anorexia nervosa, kwashiorkor and in patients treated with corticosteroids.

Wernicke-Korsakoff syndrome

In 1881, Karl Wernicke described three patients with confusion, ataxia and ophthalmoplegia with nystagmus. All were dead within 2 weeks of the onset of the illness. Independently, Sergei Sergeyevich Korsakoff described 20 chronic alcoholics with severe impairment of short-term memory associated with disinhibition, leading to a confabulatory dementia. Most patients also had a peripheral neuropathy, and this led Korsakoff to describe the syndrome as psychosis polyneuritica. It was not until some years later that the close association of the two conditions was recognised, and it is now clinically useful to consider them together as the Wernicke-Korsakoff syndrome.

Aetiology

The syndrome does not only occur in alcoholics. It is due to thiamine deficiency, and may therefore be seen in severe starvation, malnutrition, intravenous feeding without vitamin supplementation, occasionally in hyperemasis gravidarum and in vomiting due to high gastrointestinal obstruction.

Clinical features

The clinical features of the syndrome initially include a triad of ophthalmoplegia, ataxia and confusion. The ophthalmoplegia and ataxia may precede the mental symptoms by several days. In the early stages, the mental changes are dominated by confusion and restlessness, followed by drowsiness, disorientation and then coma. The Korsakoff confabulatory dementia often only becomes evident after treatment. The eye signs consist of nystagmus, VIth and IIIrd nerve palsies, gaze palsies and, occasionally, ptosis.

Hypothermia due to hypothalamic involvement may occur, and sudden death is a feature of the syndrome.

The confabulatory dementia is selective, in that the ability for retention and recall and short-term memory are severely impaired, while other intellectual functions are relatively well preserved. A peripheral neuropathy is present in up to 80% of patients.

The pathology of the syndrome includes punctate haemorrhages and non-haemorrhagic areas of necrosis in periventricular sites around the third and fourth ventricles.

Diagnosis and treatment

The diagnosis of Wernicke-Korsakoff syndrome is essentially clinical. A high index of suspicion is needed. There may be associated alcohol withdrawal and acute delirium tremens in the early stages, and making a definite diagnosis of the Wernicke-Korsakoff syndrome can be difficult. Thiamine should be given to all alcoholics who present acutely with problems associated with alcohol withdrawal.

Biochemical abnormalities in Wernicke-Korsakoff syndrome include a raised blood pyruvate level and a reduced red cell transketolase, and these may be of retrospective diagnostic value.

The response to thiamine of the ocular signs in Wernicke-Korsakoff syndrome is often dramatic, occurring within 24–48 hours. The ataxia shows some recovery, and the confusion and restlessness also improve fairly rapidly. In contrast, the Korsakoff confabulatory dementia shows a limited response to treatment.

Despite early recognition and prompt treatment, about 20% of patients die during the first few days.

Hepatic encephalopathy

From a neurological point of view, three types of hepatic encephalopathy (Ch. 16) are recognised:

- acute coma associated with fulminating hepatic failure
- reversible hepatic encephalopathy in cirrhotics with a recognisable precipitating cause
- hepatocerebral degeneration syndrome, which is a consequence of the portosystemic shunting of long-standing liver disease. This is a slowly progressive condition and responds poorly to treatment.

The neurohistopathological abnormalities are minimal in acute fulminant hepatic failure. However, in chronic hepatic encephalopathy, there is neuronal loss, diffuse gliosis and many astrocytes containing enlarged irregular nuclei, with astrocytic proliferation.

Clinical features

Acute fulminant hepatic failure is accompanied by confusion, delirium, stupor and then coma. Eye movements become disconjugate and tone is increased in the limbs with brisk reflexes; eventually, with deepening coma, decerebrate posturing, loss of tendon reflexes, fits and then death occur.

In *reversible chronic hepatic encephalopathy* a hallmark of the condition is a fluctuating level of consciousness with confusion. Euphoria may be present and, characteristically, there is marked intellectual impairment in a patient who is alert and may have no other abnormal neurological signs. Constructional apraxia, which can be measured serially from day to day, is a useful index of improvement or deterioration. With worsening encephalopathy, drowsiness, dysarthria, asterixis, myoclonic jerks, fits, choreoathetosis and extrapyramidal rigidity, together with pyramidal signs, appear. Recovery from a deeply comatose state is unusual, since this reflects severe hepatic dysfunction.

In the *hepato-cerebral degeneration syndrome*, there is a progressive dementia, extrapyramidal rigidity, asterixis and pyramidal signs in the limbs. The neurological deficit may remain stable for many months before deteriorating.

Investigation and treatment

The most helpful neurological investigation in hepatic encephalopathy is the EEG. This shows progressive slowing of activity, loss of the normal alpha rhythm, paroxysmal slow waves, and, in many patients, triphasic waves. The value of the EEG is that the sequence of changes in a particular patient is a reliable index of the severity of the encephalopathy, and that the EEG changes may precede any obvious change in the clinical state.

The treatment of hepatic encephalopathy is that of hepatic failure (Ch. 16). There are suggestions that large doses of L-dopa or bromocriptine may partially reverse the encephalopathy, associated with an improvement in the EEG.

Cerebellar degeneration

Cerebellar degeneration is a fairly common consequence of chronic alcoholism, and is probably due to a combination of nutritional deficiency and alcohol toxicity. There is marked atrophy of the upper part of the vermis, but the cerebellar hemispheres are relatively spared. This leads to ataxia which is most marked for the trunk, leading to gait ataxia. Nystagmus is uncommon. A fairly acute form of cerebellar syndrome may respond well to abstinence, but recovery from chronic cerebellar degeneration is limited.

Peripheral neuropathy

Signs of a peripheral neuropathy may be present in up to 10% of all chronic alcoholics; in most cases it is mild and asymptomatic. The neuropathy is usually, but not exclusively, seen in malnourished patients. In well-nourished alcoholics, the neuropathy tends to be less painful than in malnourished patients. In the early stages, the neuropathy is predominantly sensory and, characteristically, there is severe burning pain with paraesthesiae and hyperaesthesia of the feet and lower legs. The hands are usually affected later, and distal wasting and weakness develops. Some patients may be unable to walk because of pain and hyperaesthesia. Treatment is abstinence from alcohol and an adequate diet. Pain responds poorly to analgesics, and symptoms improve slowly over several months. Patients find they can relieve their severe symptoms with alcohol and many therefore return to excessive drinking.

Alcoholic amblyopia

Impairment of vision in one or both eyes due to an optic neuropathy may occasionally occur in chronic alcoholics. Fundoscopy shows optic atrophy. The pathology of the condition is a loss of ganglion cells in the retina and necrosis of central parts of the optic nerve and chiasm.

Table 22.56 Disorders caused by drugs and toxins

Dementia	
Alcohol	Manganese
Mercury	Aluminium
Lead	Solvent abuse
Acute or subacute encephalopathy	
Lead (esp. children)	Thallium
Mercury	Solvent abuse
Manganese	(many others)
Drug-induced confusional state of psychosis	
Antiparkinsonian drugs	Lithium
Steroids	Amphetamines
Isoniazid	Cannabis
Tricyclics	LSD
Alcohol withdrawal	(many others)
Lowered threshold for seizures	
Alcohol	Tricyclics
Amphetamines	Other antidepressants
Neuroleptics	
Parkinsonism	
Neuroleptics	Amiodarone
Flupenthixol	Manganese
Antiemetics	MPTP
Reserpine	
Chorea and/or dystonia	
L-DOPA	Phenytoin
Bromocriptine	Benzhexol
Antiemetics	Manganese
Neuroleptics (often 'tardive')	
Tremor	
Beta$_2$-agonists (salbutamol, etc.)	Alcohol (esp. withdrawal)
Lithium	Thyroxine
Sodium valproate	Mercury
Amiodarone	Manganese
Amphetamines	
Cerebellar syndrome	
Alcohol	Solvent abuse
Phenytoin	Mercury
Ototoxicity	
Aminoglycoside antibiotics	Frusemide
Quinine	Aspirin (in overdose)
Ethacrynic acid	
Optic neuropathy	
Ethambutol	Clioquinol
Chloroquine	Chloramphenicol
Methyl alcohol	?Pipe tobacco
Lens opacities	
Steroids	
Chloroquine	
Amiodarone	*(continued over)*

Table 22.56 (cont'd)

Myelopathy
Nitrous oxide abuse
Lathyrism (plant toxins)

Peripheral neuropathy

Gold	Industrial solvents
Lead	Solvent abuse
Arsenic	Numerous drugs (Table 22.49,
Thallium	p. 945)
Mercury	

Neuromuscular blockade

Botulinum toxin	Penicillamine
Organophosphorous compounds	Aminoglycosides (and other antibiotics)
'Nerve gases'	may exacerbate myasthenia

Myopathy

Steroids	Amiodarone
Chloroquine	Zidovudine (AZT)
Clofibrate	Alcohol

Alcoholic myopathy

Rarely, an acute destructive alcoholic myopathy occurs, and the consequent myoglobinuria can cause acute renal failure. A chronic, predominantly proximal, alcoholic myopathy has also been described.

Central pontine myelinolysis

Central pontine myelinolysis (CPM) is a rare condition. It is usually seen in chronic alcoholics, but there is also an association with hyponatraemia, particularly in children, liver disease being the major cause. The development of CPM often coincides with over-rapid correction of the hyponatraemia. The pathology is a massive, progressive demyelination affecting the basis pontis and involving pontocerebellar fibres, long tracts and myelinated fibres in the pontine nuclei. The clinical features are confusion and cranial nerve palsies, particularly affecting the IVth, Vth and VIth nerves, with gaze palsies and bulbar signs; there are pyramidal signs in the limbs, occasionally cerebellar signs and, often, disturbances of vasomotor control with hypotension.

The differential diagnosis includes vascular lesions affecting the pons, multiple sclerosis and brainstem encephalitis.

In 75% of cases, death occurs within 1 month, but occasionally it runs a chronic course over several months, sometimes with a partial recovery. There is no specific treatment.

TOXIC AND DRUG-INDUCED DISORDERS

Table 22.56 includes the more commonly encountered drugs and other toxic agents responsible for the various neurological syndromes listed, but it is not totally comprehensive. For example, a 'toxic confusional state' may sometimes result from almost any drug, particularly in the elderly.

FURTHER READING

Aminoff M J 1989 Neurology and general medicine. Churchill Livingstone Inc, New York. *A multi-author book, written from the perspective of the general physician needing to know more about neurological involvement in systemic disease. It provides information about a wide range of common and rare neurological problems associated with systemic disease.*

Bradley W G, Daroff R B, Fenichel G M, Marsden C D Neurology in clinical practice 1991, Vols 1 & 2 Butterworth-Heinemann, London. *An outstanding and comprehensive neurological textbook. Volume 1 starts with an approach to the evaluation of common presenting complaints and clinical states, then deals with investigations of principles of management. Volume 2 provides systematic coverage of neurological diseases and includes a section on neurology in other parts of the world. A very useful reference work for the inquisitive student.*

Harrison M J G 1987 Neurological skills. Butterworths, London. *About half of this short book deals with a very practical approach to history-taking and examination; the remainder is concerned with common neurological symptoms and brief descriptions of selected common diseases affecting the nervous system.*

Lindsay K W, Bone I, Callander R 1991 Neurology and neurosurgery illustrated. 2nd edn. Churchill Livingstone, Edinburgh. *The richly illustrated text covers all the common neurological and neurosurgical disorders.*

Aids to the examination of the peripheral nervous system, 1986, Ballière Tindall, London. *An invaluable slim volume showing the details of the peripheral motor and sensory systems, with photographs demonstrating the correct technique for examining individual muscles and muscle groups.*

Patten J 1989 Neurological differential diagnosis. 2nd edn. Harold Stacke Ltd, London and Springer-Verlag, New York. *Another very well-illustrated volume, which deals particularly well with applied anatomy and physiology and the neurological deficits caused by lesions at different sites in the nervous system.*

23

Musculoskeletal and Connective Tissue Disease

Brian Hazleman

In the UK each year, an estimated 20 million people experience some form of rheumatic complaint and eight million seek help from their general practitioner. At least half a million people have rheumatoid arthritis (RA) and around five million are affected by osteoarthritis (OA). There are 500 000 patients with gout and about the same number with ankylosing spondylitis; while low back pain and soft tissue rheumatic disorders together account for over 50% of the rheumatic causes of working days lost annually in the UK (in total about 88 million days). These are consequently important causes of morbidity. By recognising arthritis early, much can be done to help these patients.

STRUCTURE AND FUNCTION OF JOINTS

Synovial joints have a capsule (Fig. 23.1) which is continuous with the periosteum covering the bone. The non-articular surfaces within the joint are covered by synovial tissue. Articular cartilage lies on subchondral bone. Additional 'spacers' may be present in the form of fibrocartilage (e.g. knee menisci) or fat pads covered by synovium. Muscles acting across joints have an important function in maintaining joint stability.

Joint capsule

In most joints, the capsule is composed of bundles of collagenous fibres arranged somewhat irregularly, in con-

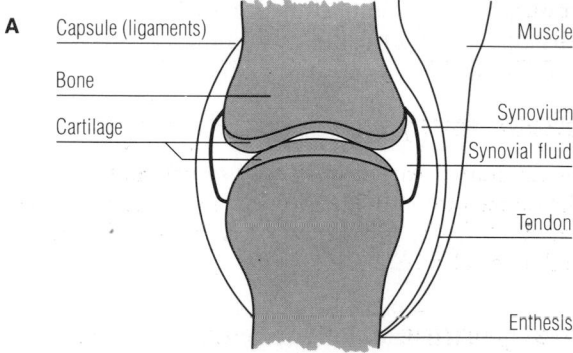

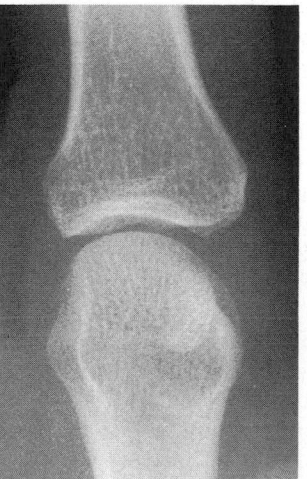

Fig. 23.1 Schematic cross-section (A) and X-ray of normal synovial joint (B).

trast to their more regular arrangement in tendons and many ligaments. These bundles tend to spiral, thus making them sensitive to tension in most positions that the joint adopts. Change in tension stimulates proprioceptive nerve endings in the capsule and ligaments. Most ligaments have both mechanical and proprioceptive functions.

The joint is covered by the 'soft tissues', including tendons, bursae and ligaments. The junction of tendon and bone is called an enthesis; this can become inflamed.

Synovial tissue

The synovial membrane is a specialised connective tissue lining the capsule of diarthrodial joints, bursae and tendon sheaths. Its main function is to produce synovial fluid.

The normal synovium – glistening, slightly pebbly and with multiple redundant folds in its gross appearance – has only three or four cell layers lining its surface. It is customary to divide the synovial lining cells into:

- *Type A*, which are macrophage-like and have a primarily phagocytic function
- *Type B*, which are secretory and similar to fibroblasts, with a large amount of endoplasmic reticulum.

Neither the structure of the synovium nor the composition of the synovial fluid suggests that there is a major barrier to fluid movement between the synovial capillaries and the synovial cavity. Furthermore, fenestrated capillaries have been described in the superficial part of synovium, and this type of capillary is usually found in tissues where there is a relatively high fluid and plasma protein flux between blood and tissues.

Synovial fluid

The normal joint contains only a small volume of synovial fluid, essentially a dialysate of blood plasma with the addition of hyaluronic acid, which is secreted by synovial lining cells and imparts to the fluid its stickiness and high viscosity. Both the concentration of hyaluronic acid (normally about 3.5 g/l of fluid) and its molecular weight are reduced in conditions of inflammatory synovitis, particularly rheumatoid arthritis, with a resulting decrease in fluid viscosity. Most of the protein (60–75%) in synovial fluid is albumin; the larger globulin molecules are present in relatively lower concentrations. Plasma proteins of high molecular weight are present in small amounts in normal synovial fluid. When the synovium becomes inflamed, the protein content of the synovial fluid increases and the quantity of large molecular weight proteins is greater than in normal fluid.

The functions of synovial fluid are lubrication (in association with articular cartilage) and nutrition of cartilage cells.

Articular (hyaline) cartilage

Like other connective tissues, hyaline cartilage consists of three components:

- *Cells*. The cells are chondrocytes, and they synthesise the other components.
- *The matrix*, which consists of proteoglycans linked to hyaluronate to form large aggregates.
- *The fibres*, consisting of collagen which binds the cartilage to bone and entraps the proteoglycan aggregates. Because proteoglycans absorb water, they swell to distend the collagen network and give cartilage elastic properties.

Joint sensation

Synovial membrane is relatively insensitive to pain but, in contrast, capsule, ligaments and periosteum have a rich sensory supply and these tissues are probably the main source of pain in arthritis, haemarthrosis and septic joints. With advanced joint damage, sensory fibres from bone are also stimulated, due to the release of chemical mediators.

Arthritis tends to produce a 'flexion deformity' because there is an increase in synovial fluid and the joint is held in the position in which the capacity of the synovial cavity is greatest.

CLINICAL ASSESSMENT

In arriving at a specific diagnosis, the information obtained from a detailed history and careful clinical examination must be collated with the radiological and laboratory findings. In addition, it should be remembered that often no single physical sign, laboratory test or radiological appearance is unique for a particular disease.

Table 23.1 summarises the terms commonly used in rheumatology.

Table 23.1 Rheumatological terminology

Term	Meaning
Arthralgia	Pain arising in the joints
Arthritis	Objective joint abnormality
Bursitis	Inflammation of a bursa
Enthesopathy	Inflammation or abnormality of an enthesis
Monoarthritis	Affects one joint
Oligoarthritis/pauciarticular	Affects two, three or four joints
Polyarthritis	Affects more than four joints
Synovitis	Inflammation of synovial joint
Tendinitis	Inflammation of tendon
Tenosynovitis	Inflammation of tendon sheath
Seropositive arthritis	Rheumatoid factor present in serum
Seronegative arthritis	Rheumatoid factor absent in serum

HISTORY

General

Age, sex and race

Age and sex are of some diagnostic value. Systemic lupus erythematosus (SLE), RA and Reiter's syndrome predominately affect the young and middle-aged, while polymyalgia rheumatica and giant cell arteritis tend to affect the elderly. RA and SLE are more common in females, whilst ankylosing spondylitis, Reiter's syndrome and polyarteritis nodosa are more common in males. Gout is more common in men, the sex ratio being 20:1 and the mean age at onset 40 years; in women, the onset of gout is postmenopausal.

There is a higher incidence of SLE in female American blacks than in black males and whites of either sex, and familial Mediterranean fever is common in Sephardic Jews.

Occupation

Repeated minor trauma resulting from occupational factors, unaccustomed exercise, leisure activities or changes in lifestyle may lead to arthropathy or soft tissue inflammation involving tendons, bursae or ligaments. OA may be caused by minor trauma, as in the proximal interphalangeal joints in wicket-keepers' hands. Arthritis may be due to a specific toxic agent, e.g. saturnine gout (lead), acrosteolysis (polyvinyl chloride) or avascular necrosis of the femoral head (nitrogen in deep sea divers). In RA and OA, the dominant hand may be preferentially, or more severely, affected.

Family history

A genetic factor is present in some rheumatic diseases, e.g. ankylosing spondylitis, gout, psoriasis and haemophilia. First-degree relatives of RA patients have an increased incidence of RA, as well as other autoimmune diseases, e.g. myxoedema and pernicious anaemia. There is an association between RA and histocompatibility antigens DR1 and DR4. Most patients with ankylosing spondylitis have the histocompatibility antigen B27.

Social history

A detailed assessment of the patient's functional capacity, both at home and at work, is important. Practical details of the patient's occupation, mode of transport to work, and leisure pursuits are also important, as is the involvement of friends, family, community and social services. In addition, the patient's cooperation, motivation and goals must be assessed.

Drug history

The introduction or withdrawal of many drugs may exacerbate or precipitate existing rheumatic conditions. Attention must be paid to the dosage and duration of steroid therapy, as this can cause vertebral crush fractures and, less commonly, avascular necrosis of bone. Exacerbation of symptoms is common if steroids are withdrawn too quickly. Details of previous drug therapy, the response to these agents and any adverse effects should be noted.

Gout and SLE may be precipitated by drugs in susceptible individuals (Table 23.2).

Previous medical history

Inquiry should be made about similar illnesses in the past and their response to treatment (e.g. salicylates in rheumatic fever, colchicine in gout), as well as results of investigations. Previous aches and pains, rashes, venereal diseases or other recent infections may have a bearing on the present illness.

Prodromal illness

A recent history of streptococcal sore throat is usual in rheumatic fever, and non-specific rashes or upper respiratory tract infection commonly precede viral arthritis. Previous episodes of diarrhoea, iritis or urethritis may indicate Reiter's syndrome or arthropathy complicating inflammatory bowel disease.

Constitutional symptoms

Constitutional symptoms are usually non-specific. Low-grade fever, fatigability, lethargy and night sweats are common in the connective tissue diseases and inflammatory joint disease, but are absent in OA. These symptoms may be present in acute RA, as well as in patients with an underlying malignancy. A swinging fever characteristically occurs in Still's disease, and in connective tissue diseases such as polyarteritis. A persistent low-grade fever may accompany tuberculous arthritis.

Table 23.2 Drugs precipitating gout and lupus syndrome

Gout	Lupus syndrome
Thiazide diuretics	Hydralazine
Aspirin (low dosage)	Procainamide
Allopurinol/uricosuric agents	Phenytoin
(initial therapy)	Isoniazid
Cytotoxic therapy for malignancy	Oral contraceptives (may
or polycythaemia	exacerbate pre-existing SLE)
	Penicillamine

History of presenting complaint

It should be clearly established which joints are the most troublesome and whether the patient is affected by pain, stiffness, impaired function or immobility.

Pain is the chief symptom and major cause of disability in most rheumatic diseases. Its site, nature, duration, aggravating and relieving factors, radiation and relation to any specific incident must be determined. Some causes of pain have characteristic features: the pain of malignancy is constant, persists at night and is usually unrelieved by rest; that due to ankylosing spondylitis may be relieved by exercise; pain from the hip may often radiate to the knee.

Stiffness may be particularly marked in the mornings, or after immobility. The former is typical of RA and is a useful guide to disease activity.

The nature of onset of joint symptoms must be noted: e.g. whether this is acute and abrupt (as in infection or crystal synovitis) or chronic and insidious (as in RA and OA). RA may be of acute onset in the elderly. It should also be determined whether the progression of symptoms is episodic (as in gout) or migratory (as in rheumatic fever); and the number and order in which joints are involved. Many rheumatic diseases have characteristic patterns of joint involvement, for example:

- *monoarticular* as in infective and crystal arthritis
- *oligo-* or *pauciarticular* as in juvenile arthritis
- *polyarticular* as in RA and SLE.

Problem identification

It is necessary at the beginning to identify the major clinical problems. Once the doctor has established the reason for the consultation, then the site and principal symptoms can be clearly identified. In particular, symptoms arising from the joints should be differentiated from those due to bursitis, tendinitis, myalgia, vascular insufficiency, peripheral neuropathy or radicular or spinal compression. In peripheral arthritis, pain is usually maximal over the joint; in soft tissue rheumatism (including low back pain), it is less easy to localise.

PHYSICAL EXAMINATION

Many rheumatic complaints are part of a multisystem disorder, and a complete physical examination is necessary. Special attention must be paid to those organs which are most frequently involved in rheumatic conditions, such as the skin and mucous membranes, the eyes, and the gastrointestinal and genitourinary systems.

The patient's posture in bed may indicate 'protection' of affected joints from movement or undue pressure. Mouth ulcers may be a manifestation of disease, e.g. Behçet's (painful) or Reiter's syndrome (painless). These conditions are often associated with genital ulcers or circinate balanitis and, in Reiter's syndrome, plaque-like lesions on the glans penis. Ulcers in the mouth and throat may also be caused by infection secondary to the neutropenia of Felty's syndrome or drug therapy, particularly the use of gold and immunosuppressive agents. Leg ulcers are a feature of Felty's syndrome (p. 999). Dryness of the conjunctiva and mucous membranes, as a result of reduced lacrimal and salivary gland secretions, occurs in the sicca syndrome (p. 999). Splenomegaly and hepatomegaly are found in Still's disease, Felty's syndrome and SLE.

Abnormalities of the skin and its appendages may be associated with joint disease (Table 23.3). The eyes are commonly involved in connective tissue disorders, and symptoms may antedate those due to joint disease (Table 23.4).

Table 23.3 Dermatological signs in joint disease

Rash
Localised
    Butterfly rash and light-sensitive rash in SLE
    Psoriatic plaques
Generalised
    Macular rash in Still's disease
    Drug rash
    Erythema marginatum in rheumatic fever

Ulcers
Leg ulcers in Felty's syndrome and rheumatoid vasculitis
Ischaemic ulcers of fingertips in systemic sclerosis

Infarction
Nail fold infarcts in RA, SLE and vasculitis

Nodules
Sited over pressure areas and tendons in RA
Tophi in gout

Nails
Pitting and onycholysis in psoriasis

Hair
Alopecia or loss of frontal hair in SLE

Table 23.4 Ophthalmic complications of joint disease

Disease	Structure(s) affected
Gonococcal arthritis	Conjunctiva
Sicca syndromes (e.g. Sjögren's syndrome)	Lacrimal gland and conjunctiva
Rheumatoid arthritis	Sclera and episclera
Ankylosing spondylitis, Reiter's	Iris, uveal tract
Behçet's syndrome	Iris
Vasculitis in SLE	Retina
Drug treatment of joint disease	Cataract (e.g. due to steroids in children) Retinopathy (e.g. due to chloroquine)

Table 23.5 Patterns of polyarticular disease

Peripheral (small joints of hands, feet and wrists)

Symmetrical
  Rheumatoid arthritis

Asymmetrical
  Psoriatic arthritis
  Osteoarthritis
  Gout

Central (sacroiliac joints, spine, lower limb joints)

Ankylosing spondylitis, enteropathic arthritis, Reiter's syndrome, etc.

Table 23.6 Factors contributing to joint deformity

- Synovial hypertrophy
- Bony or cartilaginous overgrowth
- Urate deposits
- Joint subluxation/dislocation
- Bone absorption/misalignment
- Muscle contracture
- Tendon rupture

Musculoskeletal system

Clinical assessment involves inspection, palpation and assessment of function based on the range of joint movement. Most joints and muscle groups are paired and can therefore be compared. Inflamed joints are painful and must be examined gently. The nature of the joint swelling, together with the temperature and tenderness of the joint, can be ascertained by palpation;

- if joint swelling is soft, warm and tender, it is usually due to synovitis
- if hard, it is usually due to bony overgrowth
- if fluctuant, it is usually due to an effusion.

Type and distribution of joint involvement. Many rheumatic diseases have characteristic patterns of joint involvement (Table 23.5). However, clinical variants are not uncommon and the pattern may be atypical in the early stages of disease.

In the hand (Fig. 23.2), RA usually affects the metacarpal phalangeal (MCP) and proximal interphalangeal (PIP) joints, while sparing the distal interphalangeal (DIP) joints. In contrast, primary OA involves the PIP and DIP

joints as well as the first carpometacarpal joints and tends to spare the MCP joints.

Joint swelling may be caused by fluid, subcutaneous tissue, synovial or bony overgrowth (e.g. Heberden's nodes in OA). Fluid may result from effusion within either a joint or bursa. It is often tense but, when present in small amounts, may be squeezed from one side of the joint to the other. Subcutaneous tissue is often warm and tender indicating acute disease, commonly septic arthritis, gout or tendinitis. Pitting oedema of tissues overlying a joint is also a sign of acute inflammation and may occur in early RA.

Synovial or *capsular thickening* is confined to the anatomical boundaries of the joint. It feels doughy and can best be felt by pinching the soft tissues gently and rolling the synovium over the joint.

Deformity is usually a feature of established disease and has many causes (Table 23.6). It may limit both function and movement and should be accurately described. Many conditions are associated with characteristic deformities (e.g. at the knee)(Fig. 23.3) but no deformity is pathognomonic of one disease.

Tenderness may be localised when caused by meniscal tears, inflamed Heberden's nodes and bony spurs. Synovial inflammation, however, is diffusely tender over the joint surface and its severity is a useful parameter in the assessment of disease activity.

Range of movement of an individual joint is determined by its anatomical configuration. Active movement may be limited by damage to the articular surfaces, muscle weakness and tendon involvement. Passive move-

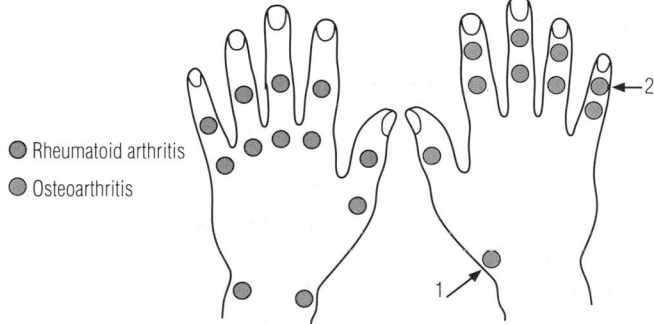

○ Rheumatoid arthritis
○ Osteoarthritis

Fig. 23.2 Joints of the hands involved in rheumatoid arthritis and osteoarthritis. Note how OA affects the carpometacarpal joint of the thumb, and RA affects the wrist. ① OA of the first carpometacarpal joint gives an appearance of a 'square hand' due to enlargement of the joint and adductive deformity of the metacarpal joint. ② Osteophytes of the terminal interphalangeal joints are called 'Heberden's nodes'.

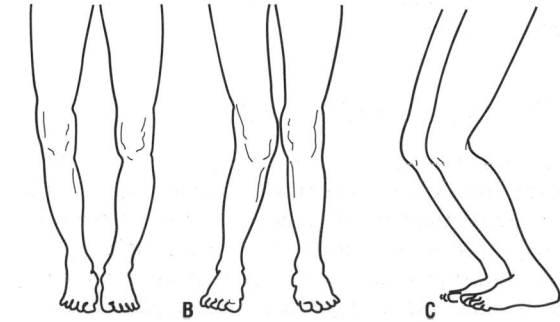

Fig. 23.3 Types of knee deformities. A. Varus – due to medial compartment damage; typical of OA. **B.** Valgus – seen when both compartments are damaged; typical of inflammatory arthritis. **C.** Flexion deformity – common in many arthritides.

ment may produce pain or discomfort, resulting in reflex spasm or voluntary contraction of muscles which reduces the actual range of movement. When the active and passive ranges are not equal, the passive is usually the greater and is a more reliable indicator of the actual range of movement. Reproducible measurements may be made with a goniometer. This is useful for the knee and elbow and for assessing the results of surgery, but is of limited value in reflecting moderate changes in synovial activity in peripheral joints, with the exception of finger joint motion.

The range of movement may be increased in hypermobility syndromes, such as Ehler's-Danlos and Marfan's (p. 78). Approximately 10% of people also fall into the hypermobile spectrum. Although normal, such hypermobility may contribute to locomotor problems, e.g. dislocation, enthesopathy. Generalised hypermobility can be assessed using a modified Beighton score (Table 23.7).

During movement, crepitus may be felt. This is a sensation of creaking or grinding which is a sign of damage to the bearing surfaces. Characteristically, this is coarse in OA and fine in RA. Crepitus may also arise from tendon sheaths.

Instability is usually caused by a combination of ligament laxity, rupture or joint displacement. The knee and ankle joints should be tested with the patient bearing weight, as well as on the examination couch.

Gait should be observed with the patient wearing shoes. The patient's ability to rise from a chair, bend and undress will provide valuable clues in diagnosis.

Muscle power. The muscles should be evaluated for both atrophy and weakness. In patients with joint disease, these usually involve muscles adjacent to the affected joints. Muscle tenderness is uncommon, except in patients with inflammatory muscle disease.

INVESTIGATION

There are few specific and reliable tests in rheumatology, so results should not unduly influence clinical judgement.

Table 23.7 Modified Beighton scoring system

Manoeuvre	Score
1. Extend little finger >90°	1 point for each finger
2. Bring thumb back parallel to or touching forearm	1 point for each thumb
3. Extend elbow >10°	1 point for each elbow
4. Extend knee >10°	1 point for each knee
5. Touch floor with palms of hand, keeping the legs straight	1 point

A score of 6 or more indicates hypermobility

Haematological and immunological investigations

Haemoglobin

A moderate anaemia is the commonest systemic manifestation of inflammatory joint disease, and its severity reflects disease activity (Table 23.8). Though the anaemia is often hypochromic and sometimes microcytic, it generally reflects the inability of the reticuloendothelial cells to release sequestered iron, and only occasionally a genuine iron deficiency.

The avid retention of iron by the reticuloendothelial system and synovial membrane is reflected by a rise in both serum ferritin concentration and normal iron stores within the bone marrow. In this situation, measurement of serum iron and transferrin is often unreliable: the serum iron level may fall, as it is no longer released, and transferrin synthesis by the liver may be depressed, causing a slow fall in the total iron-binding capacity (the anaemia of chronic disease, see p. 1070).

Serum ferritin concentrations fluctuate during episodes of inflammation, the percentage change within the individual (rather than the absolute concentration) reflecting the degree of inflammation. Consequently, serial measurements of serum ferritin concentration can be used to monitor inflammatory activity. An initial high concentration in patients presenting with early RA has been suggested as being an indicator of severe disease.

Macrocytic anaemia is five times more common in rheumatoid patients than in the general population. There is reduced folate release from red blood cells (the body's main store of folate), and an increased uptake by proliferating synovial tissue. Megaloblastic marrow appearances are unusual.

Table 23.8 Anaemia in rheumatoid arthritis

Measurement	Typical value in RA	
Haemoglobin	Males	12.5 g/dl
	Females	11.0 g/dl
Mean corpuscular haemoglobin concentration	28–32.0 g/dl (normal 32–36 g/dl)	
Serum iron	Low	
Transferrin	Normal or low	
Ferritin	Lower limit of normal (without iron deficiency); low with iron deficiency	
Serum folate	Low	
Red blood cell folate	Occasionally low	
Bone marrow	Normoblastic; very occasionally megaloblastic	

White cell count

A raised white cell count, of 12 000–20 000/mm³ with a neutrophilia, occurs in infective arthritis, acute gout, juvenile chronic polyarthritis and in rheumatoid patients receiving corticosteroids. Higher counts of 30 000/mm³ or more, with or without eosinophilia, may be a feature of polyarteritis nodosa (PAN). Eosinophilia also occurs in rheumatoid patients as a result of gold sensitivity and, rarely, in association with nodular, vasculitic, erosive and strongly seropositive disease. RA with splenomegaly and neutropenia is referred to as *Felty's syndrome*; anaemia and a slight thrombocytopenia are also common. Drug sensitivity, e.g. to gold or penicillamine, may cause a pure agranulocytosis, whereas cytotoxic drugs tend to cause a more general depression of the white cell count. Leucopenia is a feature of SLE, although counts of under 2×10^{-9}/l are infrequent, and the response to infection is usually preserved.

Platelets

Thrombocytosis is found in approximately one-third of patients with RA, and has been observed to correlate directly with disease activity.

Thrombocytopenia occurs in SLE and may be sufficiently low to cause purpura. More commonly, thrombocytopenia is related to therapy with antirheumatoid drugs, such as penicillamine, gold and cytotoxic agents. Regular platelet counts are necessary when these agents are used.

Erythrocyte sedimentation rate

The erythrocyte sedimentation rate (ESR) is a non-specific indicator of inflammation and is rarely of diagnostic value. In *RA* the ESR is measured to follow the course of disease. However, patients with long-standing disease and hyperglobulinaemia may have persistently raised values. Conversely, patients with progressive erosive disease may have only a mildly elevated ESR. Similarly, in other inflammatory arthritides, normal values do not exclude active disease. In *polymyalgia rheumatica* (PMR) an ESR of over 50 mm in the first hour is usual and alerts the clinician to the possibility of this disease in patients with rheumatic symptoms but minimal joint signs. A normal ESR can occur even in active PMR.

Viscosity

Plasma viscosity has replaced the ESR in some laboratories, as the test can be automated and the results are not influenced by age, sex or haematocrit. Both measurements are mainly dependent upon changes in fibrinogen and other globulins.

Acute-phase proteins

The acute-phase proteins, which include C-reactive proteins (CRP), fibrinogen, haptoglobin, caeruloplasmin and α_1-antitrypsin, are raised in 'active' inflammatory joint disease. In RA patients, measurement of both CRP and ESR may be more helpful than either alone in assessing disease activity. As acute-phase proteins are single proteins, measurement is less influenced by anaemia, changes in size and shape of red cells, serum immunoglobulins and cholesterol concentrations. In some centres, all are measured to give a corporate picture of disease activity in RA. All fall sooner than the ESR in response to treatment, and are particularly useful in penicillamine or gold therapy.

Rheumatoid factors

Rheumatoid factors (RFs) are autoantibodies directed against antigenic determinants on the Fc fragment of immunoglobulin G (IgG). RF is locally produced in the rheumatoid synovium. While RF may also belong to immunoglobulin classes IgG and IgA, the standard tests measure IgM RF. The commonly used tests are those in which indicator cells (sheep red cells) or particles (latex), coated with IgG, are agglutinated (Fig. 23.4). The latex test is more widely used and is cheaper than the more specific but time-consuming sheep cell agglutination test (SCAT). Patients whose sera cause agglutination at levels selected to exclude most non-rheumatoid subjects (usually 1:20 in the latex test or 1:32 in the SCAT), are termed seropositive.

Although RF is found in up to 80% of patients with RA, its presence is by no means diagnostic: it is also present in other connective tissue diseases (Table 23.9),

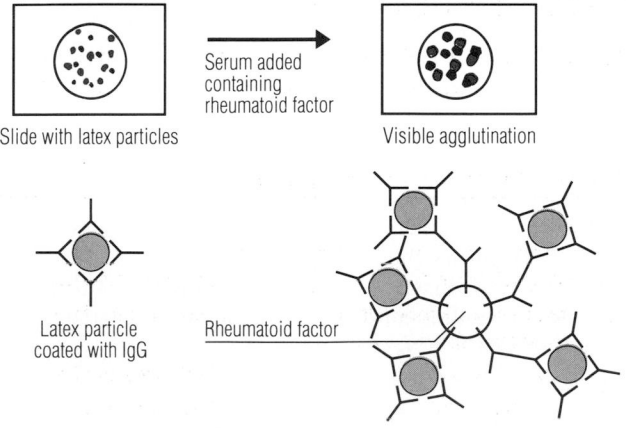

Fig. 23.4 The RA latex test. Latex beads passively coated with human IgG are cross-linked by rheumatoid factor to produce visible flocculation.

Slide with latex particles

Serum added containing rheumatoid factor

Visible agglutination

Latex particle coated with IgG

Rheumatoid factor

Table 23.9 Seropositivity and antinuclear antibodies in connective tissue disease

Disease	IgM rheumatoid factor (%)	Antinuclear antibodies (%)
Rheumatoid arthritis	70	20–30
Sjøgren's syndrome	90	60–80
Systemic lupus erythematosus		90–100
Systemic sclerosis	30	70
Dermatomyositis		30
Polyarteritis nodosa		10–20
Juvenile chronic arthritis	10	30
Other diseases		
Chronic hepatitis		65
Fibrosing alveolitis	15	30
Sarcoidosis		–

chronic infections, other immunological disorders, and in 4% of the general population. The incidence in the general population increases with age (25% over the age of 75 years) and is higher in relatives of people with positive tests, whether or not they have RA. Recent work suggests that a common factor may be a defect in glycosylation of the IgG molecule, leading to a reduction of terminal galactose and an increase of N-acetyl glucosamine. This has revived interest in the idea that mycobacteria or streptococci (which also express this sugar) may be involved in the aetiology of RA. This defect in galactosylation appears to be related to disease activity, becoming less marked with disease remission.

RF may be absent in early RA. Indeed, it commonly takes up to six months from the onset of symptoms before RF is detectable. The role of IgM RF is not entirely clear, but evidence suggests that it is capable of fixing complement and it may facilitate the phagocytosis of immune complexes by neutrophils in the synovial fluid.

Lupus erythematosus cells and antinuclear antibodies

The basis of the tests for lupus erythematosus (LE) cells and antinuclear antibodies is described on page 1024. Table 23.9 shows the incidence of antinuclear antibodies in connective tissue disease. Antinuclear antibodies include antibodies binding to a wide range of structures, including DNA, RNA, histones, etc.

Serum complement

The serum complement level (total haemolytic complement, C3 or C4) is a useful investigation in SLE. Low complement levels in the presence of a high DNA-binding titre are diagnostic of active SLE. Serial measurements of complement are useful in following the clinical course of lupus, as the level drops by about 50% before, and remains low during, an exacerbation. Particularly low levels of complement components, especially C3 and C4, are strongly indicative of active lupus nephritis, as a result of complement being continuously consumed by the immune complexes deposited in the glomeruli.

Individuals with a genetic deficiency of C2 appear to have an excessive incidence of SLE.

Biochemical investigations

Biochemical screening results are frequently abnormal in connective tissue diseases but, apart from a markedly raised serum urate in gout, have little diagnostic value. Tests of renal function are essential, since the kidney is frequently affected by glomerulonephritis in SLE and may be affected by amyloid in RA and ankylosing spondylitis.

Synovial fluid examination

Synovial fluid examination is critically important if septic arthritis is a possibility. The appearance, cell count, Gram stain and culture all contribute to the diagnosis. For other rheumatic conditions, results must be interpreted in the light of biochemical and other laboratory features because considerable overlapping of diagnostic groups can occur.

Skill in joint aspiration is easily acquired and it is a virtually painless procedure; indeed, removal of fluid often relieves pain. Fluid for a differential cell count should be placed in anticoagulant, and is best examined within a few hours; fluid for culture and for crystal examination should be placed in a sterile container without anticoagulant or preservative and, if necessary, can be kept overnight in a refrigerator.

Examination of the synovial fluid identifies urate and calcium pyrophosphate crystals by using the effect of polarising light to demonstrate the differences in crystal lattice structure of the compounds. When viewed under the compensated polarised light microscope, urate crystals show strong negative birefringence and calcium pyrophosphate shows weak positive birefringence (Fig. 23.5).

Synovial biopsy

Tissue may be obtained by open surgery, arthroscopy or needle biopsy. Needle biopsy has the disadvantage of possible sampling error. Synovial biopsy is indicated in monoarthritis, when the diagnosis is in doubt.

Specific histological features are found in tuberculosis, amyloid and Whipple's disease.

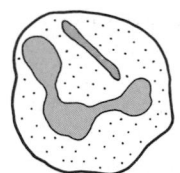 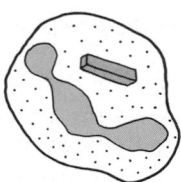

Urate
Size: 2-10 µm
Birefringence: strongly negative, needle shaped

Pyrophosphate
Size: 1-10 µm
Birefringence: weakly positive, cuboidal in shape.

Fig. 23.5 Identification of joint crystals by polarised light microscopy.

Radiological investigations

X-rays of clinically involved joints are often helpful in the investigation of rheumatic disease. X-rays of the hands and feet are the most valuable films, as the bones and joints of the hands and wrist are involved in many types of arthritis, the connective tissue diseases and some metabolic disorders. X-rays may demonstrate diagnostic features despite the absence of symptoms and signs in these joints; this is particularly so in RA, juvenile arthritis and psoriatic arthropathy.

Radiological changes in rheumatoid arthritis

The radiological changes seen in RA (Fig. 23.6) are:

* *Soft tissue changes.* An increase in soft tissue shadows due to an effusion.
* *Juxta-articular osteoporosis.* Rarefaction of bone due to decreased use caused by pain.
* *Uniform narrowing of joint spaces.* This implies loss of cartilage.
* *Erosions at margins of joints* (near origin of synovium and capsule). This is the most definitive radiological change and implies removal of bone substance.

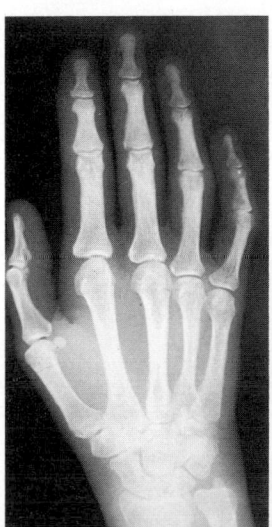 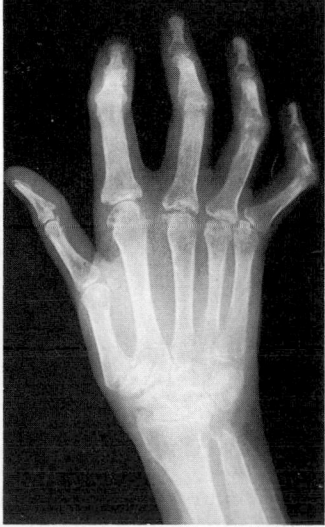

Fig. 23.6 Rheumatoid arthritis of the wrist and hands: progressive radiological changes over a five-year period.

In most patients, it takes at least three months for bone changes to appear (e.g. cartilage thinning or bone erosion).

Radiology is helpful in the diagnosis of conditions mimicking RA. In the case of gout, tophi may erode bone outside the joint capsule (unusual in RA) and frequently tophi have greater density than surrounding soft tissue. In degenerative arthritis, reactive bone formation is prominent and distal interphalangeal joint involvement is common, whereas osteopenia around joints and metacarpophalangeal joint damage is rare. It should be remembered that degenerative changes in joints are a feature of ageing and should not be used indiscriminately to explain musculoskeletal symptoms in the elderly.

Chondrocalcinosis (Fig. 23.7) is a radiological finding characteristic of 'pseudogout' or calcium pyrophosphate arthropathy (p. 1023).

Other investigations

An arthrogram, produced by injection of radio-opaque dye into the joint, may show the meniscus or a ruptured joint capsule.

A

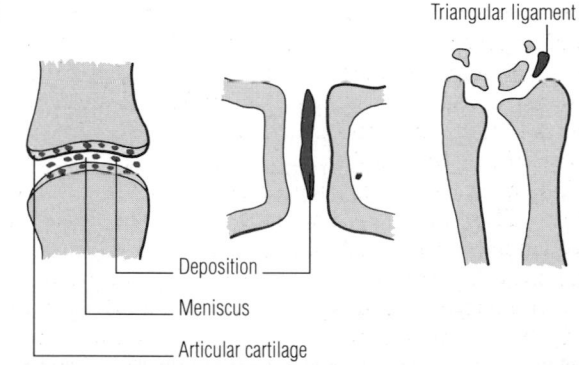

Triangular ligament

Deposition

Meniscus

Articular cartilage

B

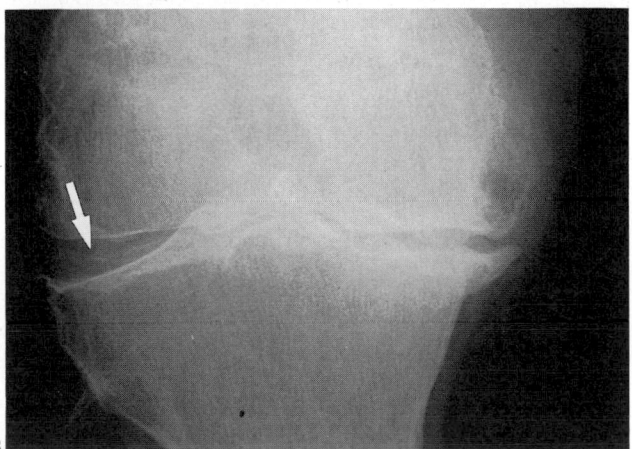

Fig. 23.7 Chondrocalcinosis. A. Common radiological sites for pyrophosphate deposition (knee, symphysis pubis and wrist). **B.** Chondrocalcinosis in the knee joint. Calcification is present in the menisci and the joint shows degenerative changes, with loss of joint space, osteophyte formation and cysts.

A bone scan shows increased uptake in inflammatory arthritis and is useful in demonstrating malignancy.

Arthroscopy is useful for demonstration of mechanical lesions, particularly in the knee, where a torn meniscus can be demonstrated and partially removed.

DIFFERENTIAL DIAGNOSIS OF POLYARTHRITIS

Chronic rheumatic disorders, with their characteristic deformities and clinical, radiological and serological abnormalities, do not usually pose problems in differential diagnosis. However, an acute polyarthritis may be the presenting feature of many rheumatic diseases (Table 23.10) and, at this early stage, diagnosis may be difficult: there is wide variation in the severity of acute attacks and the number of joints involved, and the pattern may change with recurrent attacks of the same illness.

It must be stressed that an acute polyarticular presentation is not the only mode of onset in the diseases listed in Table 23.10, and the list itself is by no means exhaustive.

A practical approach to differentiate diagnosis is to separate RA from the rest. General points that may help in the differential diagnosis of polyarthritis are given in Table 23.11.

Certain types of arthritis tend to be commoner in particular sexes and age groups (Table 23.12). Determining the balance of joint and systemic symptoms may also be helpful in diagnosis (Table 23.13).

The combination of symptoms in well-recognised clinical syndromes can help in the diagnosis, e.g. Reiter's syndrome presents as a classic triad of acute polyarthritis, urethritis and conjunctivitis. The major clinical features

Table 23.10 Diseases that may present as acute polyarthritis

- Rheumatoid arthritis and palindromic rheumatism
- Adult and childhood Still's disease (juvenile chronic arthritis)
- Rheumatic fever
- Systemic lupus erythematosus
- Infections – viral (rubella), rarely pyogenic and tuberculous
- Reiter's disease
- Seronegative arthritides, e.g. psoriatic arthritis
- Gonococcal arthritis
- Gout and pyrophosphate arthropathy
- Serum sickness
- Acute sarcoidosis with erythema nodosum
- Familial Mediterranean fever
- Henoch-Schönlein purpura
- Type II hyperlipoproteinaemia
- Leukaemia

Table 23.11 Clinical clues in the differential diagnosis of polyarthritis

- Family history – of gout and familial Mediterranean fever
- Similar episodes in the past, and response to treatment, e.g. salicylates in rheumatic fever and colchicine in gout
- Genitourinary symptoms suggest Reiter's syndrome; in homosexual males, suspect gonococcal arthritis
- Symptoms of inflammatory bowel disease suggest enteropathic arthritis
- Immunosuppressive therapy, e.g. corticosteroids may predispose to septic arthritis
- A history of photosensitivity, Raynaud's phenomenon or recurrent abortions suggest SLE

Table 23.12 Types of arthritis according to age and sex

Age/sex	Type of arthritis
Child	Juvenile arthritis, viral infection, rheumatic fever
Adolescent	Traumatic synovitis, ankylosing spondylitis, infectious mononucleosis
Adult	Reiter's syndrome, rheumatoid arthritis
Elderly	Degenerative joint disease, pyrophosphate arthropathy (pseudogout)
Female	Rheumatoid arthritis, systemic lupus erythematosus
Male	Gout, Reiter's syndrome

Table 23.13 The balance between joint and systemic symptoms* in acute polyarthritis

Conditions in which joint disease predominates
Acute onset RA
Rheumatic fever
Reiter's syndrome
Gonococcal arthritis
Gout and pseudogout (pyrophosphate arthritis)

Conditions in which systemic disease predominates
SLE
Still's disease – adult and juvenile systemic type
Acute sarcoidosis with erythema nodosum
Polyarteritis nodosa

* Systemic features include fever, rash, lymphadenopathy and hepatosplenomegaly

of rheumatic fever are carditis, chorea, arthritis, subcutaneous nodules and erythema marginatum.

Patterns of arthritis and progression

In addition to the anatomical distribution (Table 23.5) of joint involvement, the temporal pattern and progression of polyarthritis is helpful in arriving at a probable diagnosis.

Temporal patterns

Migratory pattern. Joints that were initially inflamed remit, while other joints simultaneously become acutely inflamed. Although occasionally seen in RA and SLE, this pattern is more common in acute rheumatic fever, postviral arthritis, gonococcal arthritis and meningococcal septicaemia.

Additive pattern. Here, features tend to accumulate during the disease while the original features persist. This pattern is non-specific and is seen in RA, SLE and postrubella arthritis.

Palindromic or intermittent pattern describes conditions associated with recurrent attacks of synovitis which remit completely without sequelae. Short episodes (two to three days) are seen in RA and gout, and may occur in sarcoidosis and familial Mediterranean fever (FMF). Longer episodes (seven to ten days) occur in the peripheral synovitis of spondylitis, the arthropathy of inflammatory bowel disease, Behçet's syndrome and also in FMF.

Concerning progression, polyarthritis may be transient, e.g. in viral infections; recurrent, as in palindromic rheumatism; or may develop into a chronic disorder, e.g. in RA.

Palindromic rheumatism is a descriptive term for acute episodes of joint pain, swelling, redness, tenderness and stiffness recurring at irregular intervals, developing spontaneously and lasting a few hours. Up to one-third of cases subsequently develop RA.

RHEUMATOID ARTHRITIS

Introduction

Rheumatoid arthritis is the most common chronic inflammatory disease of joints. Although the brunt of the disease falls on the joints, this is a systemic condition and may affect other organs.

Epidemiology

RA is a condition of unknown aetiology whose distinctive features include a persistent and symmetrical peripheral inflammatory arthritis. RA remains the major disease against which other forms of arthritis are compared, because it is the most common (2–3% of the population) and the most disabling of the inflammatory arthritides. There is a female preponderance of 3:1 and 70% of cases begin between the ages of 25 and 59, although it can begin at any age (Fig. 23.8). The contraceptive pill may protect against development of the disease. There is some evidence for a declining trend in the incidence. Differences in prevalence rates have been reported for various ethnic populations. In black rural Africans a low prevalence rate of 0.1% for definite RA was reported, whereas the prevalence rate in an urban black population was

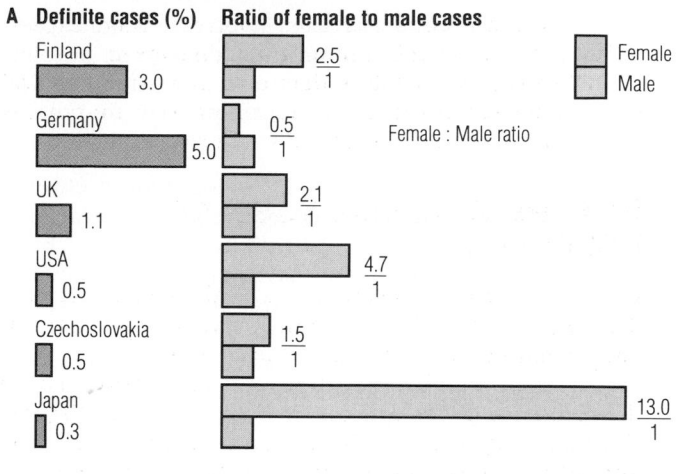

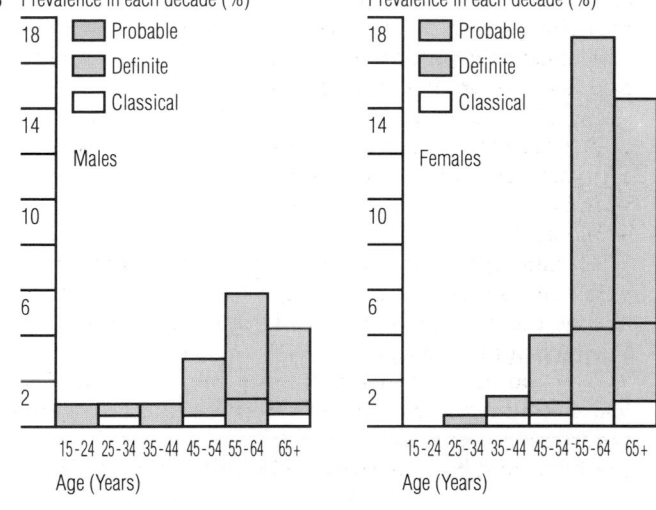

Fig. 23.8 Epidemiology of rheumatoid arthritis. A. Estimates of prevalence of RA (probable and definite) in different countries derived from surveys conducted at similar times. **B.** Prevalences of RA in the UK 1954–62 using American Rheumatism Association criteria. (After Lawrence JS, 1977.)

more similar to rates in the Western World. The onset appears more common in winter.

Aetiology

The aetiology of RA remains unknown. Of interest is its relatively recent development as a major disease (the first description only appeared in the middle of the 19th century), the high risk conferred by HLA D4, and its high prevalence in women.

From experimental models in animals, two main hypotheses have been proposed which may not be mutually exclusive.

- *Infection.* It is proposed that RA is caused by infectious agents such as bacteria, mycoplasma or viruses.

● *Autoimmune*. It may be that the disease is the expression of disordered immunity leading to an autoimmune attack on the body's own constituents. The current suggestions are autoimmunity to type II collagen or to IgG.

In addition, it is clear that the development of chronic arthritis in animals is partly dependent on genetic factors.

Although mycoplasma and diphtheroids have been demonstrated in synovium, as have antibodies to peptidoglycans (a constituent of bacterial cell walls), it seems unlikely that these are causative agents. Attempts to demonstrate viruses in tissues have generally been unsuccessful. Recent interest in the Epstein-Barr virus has been stimulated by the finding of an antibody in rheumatoid sera which cross-reacts with a nuclear antigen extracted from Epstein-Barr virus infected lymphocytes.

Genetic factors

Genetic studies of the distribution of RA in families and in mono- and dizygotic twins show that there is a small but definite contribution of genetic factors to the disease. In twin studies, there is around 30% concordance of the disease in identical twins and around 5% in non-identical twins. Recent studies have shown an association between HLA-DR1, HLA-DR4 and seropositive disease.

Pathology

In the rheumatoid synovial membrane there is a marked increase of macrophage-like cells (type A cells, see p. 984) and the synovium becomes oedematous, thickened and vascular, with surface deposition of fibrin. The synovium is also infiltrated by lymphocytes, predominately helper T cells. Lymphoid follicles can form and plasma cells are present. Active inflammation of the synovium is also associated with inflammatory changes in the synovial fluid, which contains large numbers of granulocytes (these are not present in the synovium).

The inflamed synovium produces a chronic inflammatory *pannus* which grows from the joint margins to cover the articular cartilage and leads to cartilage and bone destruction. This bone damage usually first appears as a marginal erosion at the site of synovial proliferation, where bone is unprotected by hyaline cartilage. Subsequent bone destruction leads to subluxation and deformity.

Pathological effects of RA are also found in the lymph nodes (which may show reactive hyperplasia), blood vessels (which may show vasculitis) and in nodules. Only the nodules are pathognomonic of RA. They are seen at sites of pressure, such as the extensor surface of the forearm. Palisaded tissue macrophages (histiocytes) surround a central area of hyaline necrosis. Around the histiocytes are scattered lymphocytes and the occasional plasma cell.

Pathogenesis

Much evidence supports the view that the immune system plays a central role in the pathogenesis. Of particular relevance are the observations that removal of circulating lymphocytes by thoracic duct drainage brings about a temporary remission of joint symptoms, and that immunosuppressive regimens are effective therapies.

The major events in the pathogenesis of RA are shown in Figure 23.9. The inflamed synovial membrane produces large quantities of immunoglobulin, mainly as rheumatoid factors (RFs). The cellular basis for production of RFs is well established, although the factors which initiate this process are unknown. RFs, like other immunoglobulins, are products of plasma cells.

Lymphokines. The inflamed synovium also contains activated T lymphocytes; these produce lymphokines which can be found in synovial fluid. Lymphokines have a number of properties; they can activate additional T lymphocytes, act as helper factors for B cell proliferation, stimulate fibroblasts to produce collagen and stimulate macrophages. Activated macrophages produce prostaglandins and other inflammatory mediators and enzymes, in particular collagenase, interleukin 1 (IL-1) and tumour necrosis factor (TNF), which may play a part in destruction of bone and cartilage.

IL-1 and TNF have potent effects on synovial fibroblast and chondrocyte functions that may involve stimulation of prostaglandin and collagenase production as well as modulation of the synthesis of proteoglycans, collagen and fibronectin. In organ culture, both IL-1 and TNF cause cartilage cells to resorb matrix. In addition, macrophage-derived IL-1 can act on osteoblasts to generate osteoclast activation. It also induces the acute-

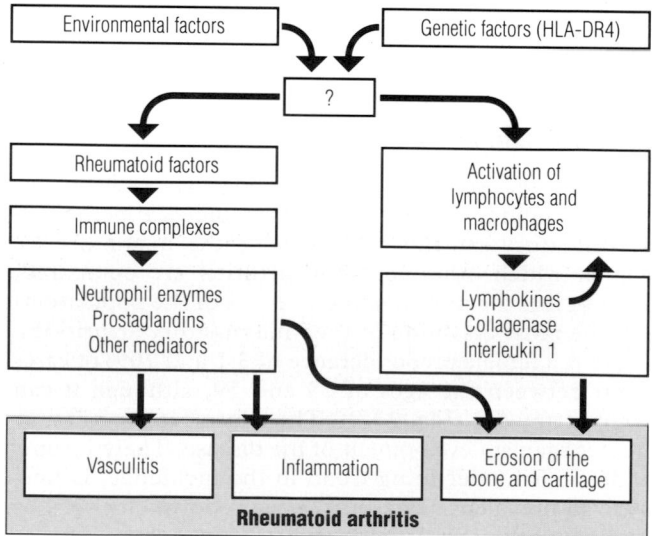

Fig. 23.9 A schematic representation of the major events thought to be involved in the immunopathogenesis of rheumatoid arthritis.

phase response and fever and may potentiate chronic inflammation by induction of lymphocyte growth factors such as IL-2 and its receptor.

Rheumatoid factors. Immunological abnormalities in the serum of patients include hypergammaglobulinaemia and the presence of RFs. IgG RF, in particular, readily undergoes self-association through its binding affinity for its own Fc determinants, forming immune complexes. These complexes have been detected in the synovial membrane, synovial fluid, serum and surrounding blood vessels; they are phagocytosed by neutrophils, monocytes and macrophages, with the release of a number of inflammatory mediators and enzymes. In addition, immune complexes containing RF can activate the complement cascade, which generates inflammatory and chemotactic factors with further accumulation of inflammatory cells. High titres of RFs, both IgG and IgM, correlate closely with the presence of severe erosive joint disease, nodules, vasculitis and extra-articular complications of RA.

Inflammatory mediators. Local release of inflammatory mediators leads to increasing exudation of high molecular weight proteins such as fibrinogen. This results in local fibrin deposition, with activation of the fibrinolytic system and release of further inflammatory and destructive enzymes. Local fibrin deposition may be a further immunological stimulus to the cellular phase of the inflammatory response.

Enzymes. Local destruction of bone and cartilage is brought about by local enzyme release. These include neutral proteinases such as collagenase, elastase and cathepsins secreted by macrophages, and lysosomal enzymes secreted by leucocytes.

Diagnosis

Diagnostic criteria (Table 23.14) are useful in standardising groups of patients in comparative studies.

Clinical features

Disease onset

In most cases, RA begins insidiously or subacutely, which may be associated with a worse prognosis. In 10–20% of

Table 23.14 Diagnostic criteria for rheumatoid arthritis

Arthritis of three or more joints (soft tissue swelling or fluid)
Arthritis of hand joints (wrist, metacarpal; metacarpal or wrist; metacarpal and wrist)
Symmetrical swelling of same joint areas
Serum rheumatoid factor
Radiographic features of RA

Revised by American Rheumatism Association

patients, the onset is very sudden and may be associated with systemic symptoms, including fever. Many patients describe prodromal symptoms such as aches and pains in a variety of joints. The classical presentation is of a woman in her mid-thirties with pain, stiffness and swelling of several weeks' duration in the small joints of her hands, wrists and feet. There may be associated lethargy, weight loss and depression. Gradually more joints are affected, accompanied by morning stiffness. Carpal tunnel syndrome or episodic arthritis (palindromic rheumatism) may antedate acute symptoms by months or years.

Articular features

The characteristic pattern of joint involvement at onset – occurring in 65% of cases – is symmetrical and peripheral. Large joints are involved in 30% of cases, and both large and small joints in 5%. In a few patients, involvement of a single joint may occur, the disease remaining localised to that joint and then spreading slowly. Joint pain and swelling, and stiffness on waking in the morning and after periods of rest, are the main symptoms. Stiffness may be related to fluid retention in the peri-articular tissues; it is a valuable semi-quantitative measure of the activity of the inflammatory process.

In the early stages of RA, the inflammatory changes may not be localised to the joints. Tender swelling of the entire hands or forearms, or swollen feet and ankles may be the earliest findings. As joint destruction progresses, the anatomical changes themselves produce increasing functional disability. The distinctive features of RA are the symmetry, the prominent signs of inflammation and, to a lesser degree, the location. The most commonly affected joints (in order of decreasing frequency) seem to be proximal interphalangeal, metacarpophalangeal, metatarsophalangeal, wrists, knees and ankles. Any joint can be affected. Persistent inflammation leads to destruction of cartilage and bone, stretching and rupture of tendons and, eventually, to subluxation and dislocation of the joints themselves; this results in the characteristic rheumatoid deformities of the peripheral joints (Fig. 23.10).

Hands and wrists

The typical patient shows fusiform inflammatory swellings, often with a dusky cyanosis over the inflamed joints. Later, there may be marked synovial hypertrophy on the dorsum of the wrist with involvement of the extensor tendon sheath, which may cause rupture of the tendons. In the palmar aspect of the wrist, synovial hypertrophy may lead to the carpal tunnel syndrome. The ulnar head may be prominent and extremely tender. Early synovial swelling of the wrist is highly characteristic and is a valuable sign in distinguishing inflammatory from degenera-

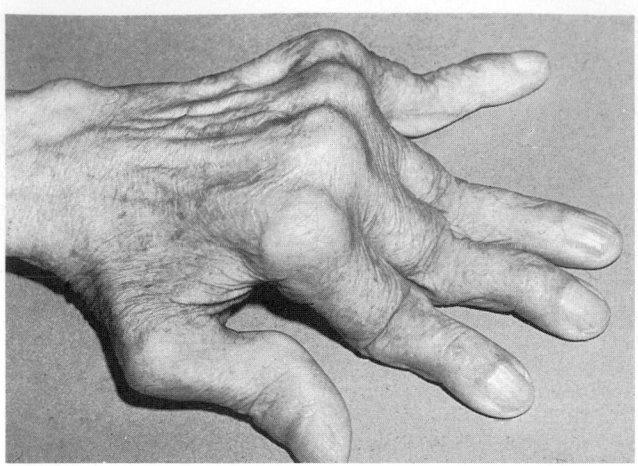

Fig. 23.10 Rheumatoid arthritis in the hands, illustrating ulnar deviation, metacarpal phalangeal swelling and swan-neck deformity.

tive disease. Wasting of the dorsal interosseous muscles is often marked, and RA is the commonest cause of wasting of the small muscles of the hand.

Synovial infiltration of flexor tendon sheaths often causes a trigger finger. Palmar erythema is common. Other mild vasomotor disturbances are frequent in RA. Typical Raynaud's phenomenon may occur, but if it is severe in the presence of only mild arthritis, then one should consider the diagnosis of scleroderma.

Deformity of the hands takes the form of ulnar deviation of the fingers, the button-hole or boutonniere deformity and the swan-neck deformity (Fig. 23.10). Involvement of the distal interphalangeal joint is rare. Anterior subluxation of the wrist may occur.

Knee joint

Involvement of the knee joint accounts for a great deal of disability. Synovial hypertrophy and effusion are often marked, and the bursae in the popliteal fossa may be swollen and may communicate with the joint cavity. These enlarged bursae are called Baker's cysts and may sometimes rupture. Quadriceps wasting is often marked, even in the early stages of the disease. Flexion contractures may develop, and these are especially important because of the disability that they produce. Both the cruciate and lateral ligaments may be destroyed, resulting in gross joint instability and valgus or varus deformity.

Rupture of the joint or a Baker's cyst, as a consequence of the high intra-articular pressure developed during exercise, causes acute pain in the knee radiating into the calf, which becomes swollen and tender on pressure. This may lead to a misdiagnosis of deep vein thrombosis, but an arthrogram or ultrasound scan will demonstrate the lesion.

Cervical spine

The upper cervical discs are frequently involved in RA, in contrast to lower cervical involvement in OA (p. 1011). The cervical vertebrae may become subluxed and this may cause serious neurological involvement.

The atlantoaxial articulations and their associated ligaments are frequently involved. This is detected by taking lateral radiographs in both flexion and extension, where separation between the odontoid process and the first cervical vertebra exceeds the normal 2–3 mm. Patients with this involvement often complain of pain radiating along the distribution of the first and second cervical nerves. Pain commences in the cervical spine and radiates upwards over the occiput and vertex to the forehead. Symptomatic relief may be found with a well-fitting cervical collar.

Atlantoaxial dislocation may cause vertebrobasilar insufficiency or may produce neurological signs by direct pressure on the cord. However, neurological sequelae are less common than might be expected. The abnormality is present in 25% of patients requiring joint reconstructive surgery, and it is important that anaesthetists are aware of the potential dangers of neck manipulation.

Involvement of other joints

Pain in the forefoot is commonly due to downward metatarsal head subluxation. The patient complains of a feeling of 'walking on pebbles', and the metatarsal heads are readily palpable on the sole of the foot. The most common deformities are subluxation of the metatarsophalangeal joints with the toes displaced upwards, together with fixed flexion deformities of the interphalangeal joints.

The hip joint is less commonly involved than the knee or metatarsophalangeal joints, but when it occurs, it causes serious disability. The femoral head may penetrate the acetabulum (protrusio acetabuli) and the femoral head may collapse. This is often referred to as *aseptic necrosis* and is more common in corticosteroid-treated patients.

Extra-articular manifestations

RA is a systemic disease; some 75% of patients have two or more extra-articular features at some stage. Systemic involvement occurs in patients with more active disease, and warrants a more aggressive therapeutic approach. Systemic features also increase the likelihood that there will be premature death from RA.

Active RA is associated with a number of systemic features including low-grade fever, anorexia, weight loss and malaise.

Anaemia

Anaemia is the commonest extra-articular manifestation of RA and is present in about two-thirds of patients with active disease. Usually, it resembles the anaemia of chronic disease (Table 26.4).

Osteoporosis

Spontaneous fractures of the long bones, neck of femur and the pelvis are well recognised in patients with RA (whether or not they are receiving corticosteroid therapy). Osteoporosis occurs early in active RA, and rarefaction of the bones in the neighbourhood of an affected joint is one of the first radiological signs of the disease.

Lymph node enlargement

Generalised lymphadenopathy is a common feature of Still's disease, but is rare in adult arthritis. Some patients, particularly those with seropositive RA, develop marked enlargement of nodes proximal to the inflamed joint. Biopsy shows large germinal centres and, occasionally, hyperplasia is so marked as to resemble giant follicular lymphoma.

Infection

Infections are common in patients with RA. Patients with severe chronic seropositive RA, or with Felty's syndrome, are particularly susceptible.

Summary 1 Extra-articular manifestations of rheumatoid arthritis

Common	Uncommon
● Fever, weight loss, malaise	● Hearing impairment
● Anaemia	● Myositis
● Osteoporosis	● Episcleritis
● Lymphadenopathy	● Systemic vasculitis
● Infection	● Pericarditis
● Depression	● Pulmonary fibrosis
● Muscle wasting	● Pulmonary nodules
● Peripheral oedema	● Splenomegaly
● Nodules	● Amyloidosis
● Tendinitis and bursitis	
● Scleritis	
● Keratoconjunctivitis sicca	
● Carpal tunnel syndrome	
● Nail fold vasculitis	
● Peripheral neuropathy	
● Pleural effusion	

Periarticular manifestations

Subcutaneous rheumatoid nodules

Rheumatoid nodules occur in approximately 25% of patients at some time in the course of their disease. Nodules are found in patients with high titres of RF and indicate severe, potentially more destructive, disease. The nodules are a few centimetres in diameter and are not tender on palpation. Normally, they are subcutaneous, but can be intracutaneous or attached to periosteum. They vary in size and number with the activity of the disease. They are found along the extensor surfaces of the forearms, but also occur over pressure areas or may be related to tendons. The nodules can ulcerate and can be painful over the ischial tuberosities and on the feet. Excision is rarely helpful since they reform.

Tendons and bursae

Rheumatoid synovitis can extend to the synovial sheaths of tendons and bursae, particularly in the hands, where pressure from the granulation tissue may contribute to extensor tendon rupture. In addition, nodules can form in the tendons and can impact in the flexor tendon sheaths of the fingers to produce triggering. Local steroid injection will often relieve this condition.

When the ulnar styloids become unduly prominent, because of erosions and/or dorsal subluxation at the inferior radio-ulnar joint, there may be progressive rupture of the extensor tendons, starting from the ulnar side.

Some bursae become inflamed in almost all cases of RA and, since there are more than 150 bursae, there are numerous ways bursitis can present. The following are common:

● *Olecranon bursitis* is a common problem; rarely it becomes infected.
● *Prepatella bursitis* (housemaid's knee); this is uncommon in RA.
● *Subacromial bursitis*, which is a common cause of shoulder pain.
● *Trochanteric bursitis*; this may cause pain down the antero-lateral aspect of the thigh.

Myositis

Muscle wasting is very common in RA, mainly due to disuse associated with painful joints. In addition, ischaemic atrophy can result from vasculitis and, very rarely, true polymyositis can occur (p. 1029).

Corticosteroid therapy can cause proximal myopathy. Chloroquine can also cause a myopathy associated with characteristic vacuolation of muscle fibres. Rarely, penicillamine therapy may lead to polymyositis.

Oedema

Recurrent oedema of the lower limbs is commonly found in association with RA. In some cases it develops around an acutely inflamed ankle joint. In many instances there is no clearly defined cause.

Organ involvement

Heart

Cardiac involvement takes the form of pericarditis and effusion, rheumatoid granulomata, myocarditis and coronary arteritis.

In patients with RA, clinical evidence of pericarditis is not common, but at post-mortem it is found to be present in about 40%. Clinical evidence of pericarditis is found in 10% of patients admitted to hospital and, using echocardiography, subclinical pericardial effusions can be detected in one-third. Effusions are usually small and posterior. The pericardial fluid is an exudate characterised by very low levels of glucose and complement. Gammaglobulin and lactate dehydrogenase levels are increased.

Rheumatoid granulomata can occur in any layer of the heart or in the valves. They are found in 1–3% of post-mortem studies. The valve lesions are usually mild and of no haemodynamic significance.

Non-specific interstitial myocarditis and endocarditis occasionally occur, presumably secondary to vasculitis; they can be associated with patchy valvular fibrosis. Coronary arteritis is rare, and is usually part of a generalised vasculitis.

Lungs

The main syndromes are shown in Table 23.15.

Pleural effusion. Typically, pleural effusion is unilateral and occurs in seropositive males over 45 years of age. It may precede the arthritis and, unlike most other extra-articular lesions, can occur early in the disease. The effusion can be chronic and be associated with considerable pleural thickening.

Table 23.15 Pulmonary complications of rheumatoid arthritis

- Infection
- Pleural effusion
- Rheumatoid nodules or granulomata
- Fibrosing alveolitis
- Rheumatoid pneumoconiosis (Caplan's syndrome)
- Pulmonary hypertension
- Empyema
- Obliterative bronchiolitis

Rheumatoid nodules. These are usually symptomless and solitary, and are found, by chance, on a routine chest X-ray. Like pleural effusions and pericarditis, with which they can be associated, they are commoner in males with seropositive nodular disease. Rarely, they can precede the arthritis, but even at that stage the patient is usually seropositive. The nodules are often subpleural and may be multiple and recurrent. The histology resembles subcutaneous nodules. They may disappear, remain unchanged for years or, rarely, cavitate, become infected or even rupture. Biopsy is sometimes necessary to exclude tuberculosis, fungal infection or malignancy.

Fibrosing alveolitis. This condition may occur in isolation (Ch. 13, p. 509) or be associated with a variety of disorders, including RA.

Obliterative bronchiolitis. Recently, an association has been suggested between this condition and rheumatoid disease. The illness is characterised by a rapid onset of breathlessness, progressing over a few months to complete incapacity or death. Lung function tests show gross reduction in vital capacity, with severe hyperinflation. The chest radiograph is virtually normal. The condition may also be associated with penicillamine therapy.

Nervous system

Both the peripheral and central nervous system (CNS) can be involved in RA. CNS involvement may occur due to cervical cord and vertebral artery compression (p. 933), while peripheral neuropathy may be:

- due to entrapment
- symmetrical – either sensory or sensory and motor
- due to mononeuritis multiplex.

Entrapment neuropathies develop where the nerve is enclosed by a tight soft tissue band, or where a nerve passes over a bony area close to the skin. The usual presentation is an insidious onset of pain and paraesthesiae in the distribution of a peripheral nerve; weakness is sometimes the main problem. The median nerve at the wrist, the ulnar nerve at the elbow, the tibial nerve at the ankle and the lateral popliteal nerve at the head of the fibula are the most common sites.

Sensory or *mixed motor and sensory peripheral neuropathies* present with a glove and stocking distribution. The cause is probably a vasculitis of the vasa nervorum. A sensory neuropathy is most common and is benign; a mixed neuropathy occurs with systemic vasculitis.

Mononeuritis multiplex is caused by vascular lesions in several different peripheral nerve trunks. The sites of involvement are similar to the entrapment neuropathies.

The neurological consequences of cervical subluxation are unpredictable, but survival tables suggest that they do not, in themselves, significantly shorten life expectancy in rheumatoid disease.

Splenomegaly

Splenomegaly occurs in about 5% of patients with RA, but only 1% develop leucopenia as well. Felty's syndrome is the association of RA, lymphadenopathy, splenomegaly, anaemia, thrombocytopenia and neutropenia. Patients have severe RA. Leg ulcers are also common.

[handwritten: FELTY'S (S) = RA, L, S, A, T, N]

Skin

Skin complications are common. The elderly rheumatoid patient has thin fragile skin often made worse by corticosteroid therapy. Ulceration frequently occurs, particularly on the legs where it may be due to trauma (often minimal), stasis and poor venous return due to inactivity, Felty's syndrome or vasculitis.

Rheumatoid nodules can also ulcerate, particularly over pressure points.

Sjøgren's syndrome

Sjøgren's syndrome is the association of keratoconjunctivitis sicca and/or xerostomia with RA or another connective tissue disorder. The lacrimal glands are infiltrated by chronic inflammatory cells, producing acinary atrophy and fibrosis, and a reduction of tear and saliva secretion. The same pathological process may affect other exocrine glands, such as bronchial, pancreatic and vaginal glands. Patients may have a high incidence of adverse drug reactions, particularly to antibiotics and gold therapy, and have an increased risk of developing lymphomas.

Gastrointestinal tract

Most of the gastrointestinal symptoms in RA are related to drug therapy. However, vasculitis can cause ischaemic colitis and infarction, and amyloidosis can result in malabsorption. Apart from amyloidosis, no histological abnormality is found on jejunal biopsy, although malabsorption can be demonstrated in up to one-quarter of patients with active arthritis.

Gastrointestinal ulceration and haemorrhage frequently occur from the ingestion of aspirin and other nonsteroidal anti-inflammatory drugs (NSAIDs).

Kidney

Although infections are common in patients with RA, the urinary tract is seldom affected. However, structural changes are commonly found in the kidney at autopsy. It is difficult to assess the role of drug therapy in these changes (see Ch. 20, p. 826). Paracetamol alone is probably not nephrotoxic. NSAIDs can cause an acute or chronic tubulo-interstitial nephropathy. All patients receiving drug treatment for RA should have their renal function intermittently assessed. With gold, proteinuria

may present at any time or with any dose, and a clear association has been described between the presence of HLA-DR3 and/or HLA-B8 and the development of proteinuria.

Drug-induced proteinuria may persist or initially increase after stopping therapy, before decreasing gradually and resolving completely in more than 80% of cases by two years. In those with persistent proteinuria, moderate impairment of renal function may occur, but this has not been shown to progress to chronic renal failure. Proteinuria in RA may also be caused by amyloidosis.

Amyloidosis

RA is the commonest cause of amyloidosis in the Western world. It is found in 20–60% of cases at post-mortem, but is rarely evident during life, when it is usually manifested by proteinuria (see Ch. 20, p. 824). Renal amyloidosis is rarely associated with hypertension. Involvement of the gastrointestinal tract can result in malabsorption or intractable bloody diarrhoea. The liver, spleen, or kidney can be infiltrated but are seldom greatly enlarged.

Arteritis

Approximately 25% of patients with RA have been found to have vasculitis at post-mortem examination. Arteritis may conveniently be considered in three categories:

- *Obliterative endarteritis* of small end-arteries, such as the anterior ciliary arteries and those in the nail folds, obstruction of which produces minute ischaemic areas. These changes are of great significance in the eye (see below).
- *Necrotising arteritis* of large arteries, e.g. mesenteric or major limb vessels, leads to peripheral gangrene, mesenteric occlusion or cerebrovascular accident.
- *Subacute inflammatory arteritis* of small and medium-sized arteries, such as those of the vasa nervorum and muscle. The larger the vessel affected, the more severe is the histological abnormality. Thus, the nail-fold lesions result from intimal hyperplasia, but when the medium-sized arteries are involved, there is a much more active process with fragmentation of the elastic lamina and cellular infiltration. These destructive changes, which may lead to gross necrosis of the arterial wall, can be indistinguishable from PAN; unlike the latter, however, they tend to spare the kidneys and only rarely lead to hypertension. In peripheral nerves, a mononeuritis multiplex can result.

The eye

RA and other rheumatic diseases frequently involve the eye. Keratoconjunctivitis sicca, scleritis and uveitis are the commonest manifestations. In RA, 11% of patients have keratoconjunctivitis sicca, and 0.5% develop scleritis with a marked predilection for severe cases with a bad prognosis. Uveitis is a complication of juvenile chronic arthritis.

A large number of drugs used for the treatment of the rheumatic diseases can themselves cause eye lesions, including chloroquine, mepacrine, allopurinol, indomethacin and ibuprofen.

In summary, although RA is chiefly a disease of joints, there are often major systemic manifestations. Indeed, these features may impose a prognosis far more serious than that of the patient's joint disability. The presence of extra-articular features indicates that aggressive therapy should be started at an early stage. In the vast majority of patients, complete or adequate control of the disease can be achieved.

Principles of management

The progressive destructive inflammatory process in RA may cause not only crippling deformity, but systemic illness and changes outside the joints that may prove fatal. In its early stages, before joint destruction and deformity have occurred, it can be a reversible disease.

It is important to remember that drug treatment is just one component in the total management of arthritic patients. Management must also include advice about rest and exercises, splintage, the provision of appliances designed to reduce dependence upon others, and advice about employment.

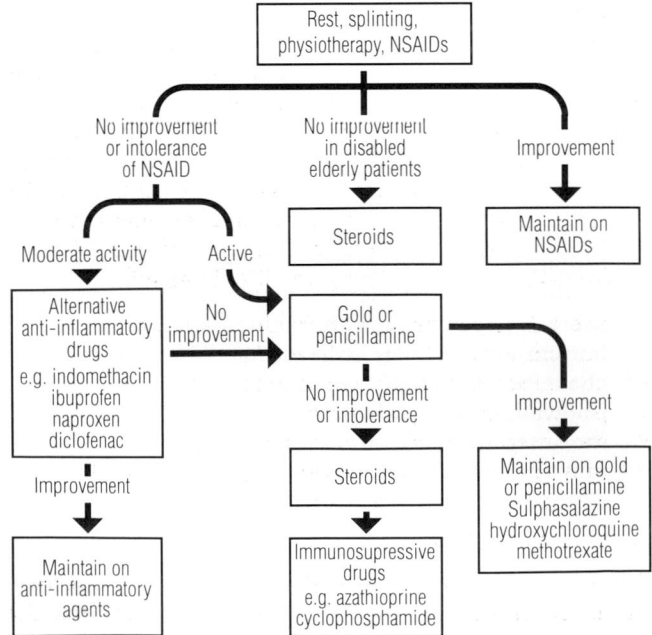

Fig. 23.11 A flow chart of the treatment regimens for rheumatoid arthritis.

The general principle of drug therapy is to use the least number of agents in the lowest effective dosage. Drug regimens must be tailored to the needs of the individual patients (see Fig. 23.11).

RA is often badly treated; patients are kept on anti-inflammatory drugs alone for long periods, in the face of obvious deterioration, or corticosteroids are given early with considerable immediate effect but at the cost of complications later on. There is an understandable tendency to gradually increase the dose of drugs to alleviate the patient's symptoms. This is dangerous, however, and often unnecessary.

The inflammatory process can usually be suppressed, with symptomatic improvement, better function, less stiffness and considerable pain relief, but the disease cannot be cured. Hence, adequate patient education is required from the outset, stressing the importance of controlling the disease, to help give the patient realistic expectations.

The aims of treatment are to reduce inflammation, maintain function and prevent deformities. Adequate suppression of chronic inflammation allows secondary manifestations, such as anaemia, to revert to normal.

Physiotherapy and occupational therapy

The physiotherapist can help in relieving musculoskeletal symptoms of pain and stiffness, improve joint movement and muscle power and re-educate function of the joints. Heat, ice, wax baths and other local external applications may relieve symptoms and aid relaxation. Patients are also instructed to exercise at home to maintain joint movement and muscle power in order to prevent deformities. Hydrotherapy has an important role, allowing muscles to relax and joints to move freely in a warm environment. It is particularly useful for painful hips and backs.

The value of rest cannot be overemphasised. Patients with acute lesions should have complete bed rest; patients with chronic lesions should alter their domestic and work patterns so that they are less stressful. The dangers of short-term rest have been exaggerated; joints do not stiffen in days, and muscles cannot be strengthened if a joint is inflamed. However, as soon as pain and inflammation are controlled, mobility and strength can be restored.

Splints may be used to rest joints, to prevent deformity or to aid power and functions of a limb. Splints are useful in active disease as rest is important, but daily exercises to maintain joint motion and muscle bulk are necessary. In chronic disease, wrist splints may aid power when finger movement is impaired by pain and deformity, or inflammation at the wrist; back splints for the knee may prevent flexion contractures. Orthoses are more permanent appliances used to prevent instability and move-

---

Summary 2 Principles of management of RA	
Pain control	**Preservation of**
Rest	**function**
Splints, collar	Ice and exercise
Joint aspiration and steroid	Splints
injection	Hydrotherapy
Analgesics	Joint protection advice
NSAIDS	
Joint replacement	
Prevention of disability	
Aids, appliances	
Domestic adaptation	
Job retraining	
Financial support	

ment, and require fitting to each patient. They include spinal supports and braces, and T-straps to control ankle instability.

A variety of simple aids and appliances may transform the lives of disabled patients, as joint deformity may prevent normal function. Occupational therapists assess the difficulty encountered in daily tasks and advise about aids to daily living such as toilet seat raises, long-handled combs and handles for taps. These and similar appliances can often allow independent living. A home visit is often helpful.

Drug therapy

The drugs used can be classified into seven groups (Table 23.16). Alteration in disease activity in response to a drug treatment can be assessed by a number of subjective and objective parameters (Table 23.17). Pain remains the parameter which correlates best with the overall assessment of a change in disease activity.

Table 23.16 Drugs used in rheumatoid arthritis

Type of drug	Example
Simple analgesics	Paracetamol
Analgesics with minor anti-inflammatory properties	Propionic acid derivatives
Analgesics with major anti-inflammatory properties	Indomethacin Aspirin
Pure anti-inflammatory drugs	Corticosteroids
Compounds with more specific action in rheumatoid arthritis	Gold and salazopyrin Penicillamine
Anti-inflammatory immuno-suppressives	Azathioprine
Intra-articular radioactive colloids	

Table 23.17 Assessment of disease activity

- Assessment of pain
- Measurement of joint tenderness
- Measurement of grip strength
- Measurement of joint size
- Assessment of joint stiffness
- Functional evaluation
- Aspirin or paracetamol consumption
- Patient's drug preference
- Radioactive technetium bone scans
- Laboratory correlates (ESR, acute phase proteins)

Simple and opioid analgesics

Simple analgesics such as paracetamol and weak opioid analgesics such as dihydrocodeine have no anti-inflammatory activity and should not normally be used alone in an inflammatory arthropathy.

Non-steroidal anti-inflammatory drugs

The class of NSAIDs encompasses both aspirin and its derivative, indomethacin, the more recently introduced propionic acid derivatives, oxicams and phenylacetic acids. These drugs must be given in full dosage to achieve a continuing anti-inflammatory effect, lower dosage merely producing analgesia.

There is little to choose between the non-steroidal anti-inflammatory analgesics in terms of pain relief, nor is it likely that using them in combination will provide any more relief than using them singly. Because of the increasing evidence of pharmacokinetic interaction between these drugs, pain should, whenever possible, be controlled with a single drug.

There is a large variation in an individual's response to NSAIDs. It is often necessary to try a number of drugs for a particular patient before finding one that provides adequate relief of symptoms. Each drug should be given for two weeks to assess its efficacy. Aspirin has now been replaced by newer NSAIDs as first-line treatment as the newer NSAIDs can be given in a convenient dosage schedule and they have a lower incidence of side-effects.

Guidelines for prescribing an NSAID include:

- use a drug you are familiar with
- prescribe cheaper, established drugs
- prescribe only one drug at a time
- prescribe an adequate dose
- encourage compliance by flexible dosing
- prescribe for two weeks and review.

Aspirin (acetylsalicylic acid)

Aspirin has analgesic and anti-inflammatory properties, but it requires blood levels of 250–300 mg/l for adequate anti-inflammatory effect; this requires a daily dose of 3–6 g. As the therapeutic level is near toxic levels, salicylism (tinnitus, deafness, nausea and vomiting) may occur.

The content of standard aspirin BP tablets is 300 mg. These are seldom used, however, because they consistently cause gastric mucosal injury. Soluble aspirin is better tolerated, as are enteric-coated preparations. Aspirin has been combined with other substances, such as aluminium oxide and glycine; these have the advantage of containing 500 mg and 600 mg of aspirin respectively, which reduces the number of tablets required. The paracetamol ester of aspirin, benorylate, causes less gastrointestinal bleeding. It is given as a suspension, and can be added to drinks such as tea or coffee. Because of its long duration of action, it only has to be given twice a day.

Indomethacin

Indomethacin is a potent anti-inflammatory agent. It is particularly useful in reducing morning stiffness when given at a dosage of 50–100 mg at night. The daily dose is up to 150 mg and the main restrictions on the drug are its side-effects, which occur in 10–20% of patients. The two common problems are gastric irritation and ulceration (even when given as a suppository), and cerebral symptoms. These include headaches, muzziness and dizziness and seem to be dose-related. Other infrequent side-effects include leucopenia, thrombocytopenia, skin rashes, oedema and hypertension.

Other non-steroidal drugs

The major advantage of these compounds is a reduction in adverse effects rather than an improvement in efficacy. They also have advantages over aspirin in the smaller number of tablets required and often, using drugs such as benorylate and naproxen, less frequent administration is needed. When NSAIDs have been compared in controlled studies, no significant differences have been found in terms of pain relief or the patient's assessment of efficacy.

NSAIDs can be divided broadly into those with a short half-life (ibuprofen) or those with a long half-life (piroxicam). Many of the short half-life NSAIDs can be effective in a twice-daily dosing regimen. Long half-life NSAIDs remain in the body for longer once administration has ceased; adverse effects may persist for many days. Also a steady state level is not reached for two weeks and the onset of action is slow.

All anti-inflammatory drugs can cause gastrointestinal bleeding, partly by a local action on the stomach and partly by a systemic effect.

About 20% of all cases of ulcer haemorrhage and perforation are directly attributable to the use of NSAIDs. The risk is increased in elderly females. If patients develop severe indigestion or peptic ulceration it is best to discontinue the NSAID. If this is not possible, an H_2-

Table 23.18 Main side-effects of NSAIDs

Gastric	Skin
Indigestion	Erythema multiforme
Ulceration	Photosensitivity
Haemorrhage	Urticaria
Small bowel perforation	
	Pulmonary
Renal	Bronchospasm
Hypertension	
Renal impairment	**CNS**
Fluid retention	Dizziness
	Confusion
Hepatic	Headache
Hepatocellular damage	
Reye's syndrome	**Haematological**
	Thrombocytopenia
	Neutropenia

antagonist may allow healing to occur; this is less likely with a gastric ulcer. There is increasing evidence that prophylactic use of prostaglandin analogues (e.g. misoprostol) may reduce the incidence of peptic ulceration.

There are many other side-effects of NSAIDs, and these are listed in Table 23.18.

More specific antirheumatic drugs

If an adequate trial of treatment with a combination of physical therapy and anti-inflammatory drugs fails to reduce inflammation after two to three months, then treatment with gold salts, chloroquine, sulphasalazine or penicillamine should be considered. The aim is to initiate disease-suppressing treatment before irreversible joint destruction has occurred. Of the three, gold salts are particularly popular and effective, although their adverse effects have led to periods when their use has fallen into disfavour. None of these drugs has a short-term effect in relieving symptoms; however, they suppress the underlying disease process in a proportion of patients when given over a period of months (Table 23.19). Major side-effects include renal and haematological toxicity.

Sulphasalazine

Sulphasalazine, an acid azo compound of sulphapyridine and 5-aminosalicylic acid, is an effective antirheumatoid

Table 23.19 Characteristics of antirheumatic drugs

- Slow action. Begin working after four to six weeks and may take six months to produce full benefit
- Improvement in joint symptoms accompanied by fall in ESR and RF
- May retard progression of erosive change seen on X-ray
- Patients feel much improved in general health

agent. Its mode of action is unknown, but sulphapyridine appears to be the active moiety. It is as well tolerated as gold or penicillamine over two- to five-year periods, and has fewer serious adverse effects; its principal problem is the symptom complex of nausea, dyspepsia and depression encountered early in treatment. The usual dosage is 2 g/day.

Gold salts

Gold salts have been used in the treatment of RA for over 50 years. In the UK, the gold preparation sodium auro-thiomalate has been used for longer than any other. It is given by weekly intramuscular injections of 50 mg, after a 10 mg test dose, either until a total dose of 1 g has been given or disease remission has occurred. It does not produce a disease-suppressing effect before two to three months of treatment. After remission, gold is continued indefinitely with a monthly maintenance regime. About one in three patients develop toxic adverse effects, which include rashes, stomatitis, thrombocytopenia, leucopenia and, occasionally, bone marrow aplasia, glomerulone-phritis and pneumonitis. Regular monitoring of platelet and white cell counts, and of urine for proteinuria, is essential.

Auranofin is an orally active gold preparation; it has a lower incidence of adverse effects compared with intra-muscular gold. The most common reaction is diarrhoea or loose stools. Dosage is 6–9 mg/day.

D-penicillamine

D-penicillamine is a sulphur-containing amino acid related to cysteine. It has similar indications and incidence of adverse effects to gold therapy. Loss of taste is an early adverse effect, but this usually disappears if the drug is continued. Myasthenia gravis and a drug-induced lupus syndrome rarely occur as complications. Dosage is 375–750 mg/day.

Chloroquine and hydroxychloroquine

These antimalarial drugs also have antirheumatic properties. The main factor limiting their use is ophthalmic complications; progressive accumulation of the drug in the retina can lead to blindness. The risk of retinal toxicity is minimised if the daily drug dosage is kept at or below 250 mg of chloroquine phosphate or 400 mg of hydroxychloroquine. Vision should be assessed at six-monthly intervals.

Corticosteroids

Corticosteroids are the most powerful agents in suppressing the inflammation of arthritis, but there is little evidence that they affect the ultimate course of rheumatoid disease, including joint destruction. Because of their many adverse effects, it is important that they be given only after NSAIDs have had an adequate trial. Most patients with early RA are as well-controlled symptomatically and objectively on aspirin, but steroids are useful in the presence of systemic disease, e.g. vasculitis, and are valuable in a patient severely incapacitated by acute disease when there is an urgent need for symptomatic relief. Incapacitating morning stiffness is also relieved, and the elderly rheumatoid may be kept independent on a small dose of prednisolone. Corticosteroids are also used in intractable iritis, common in juvenile arthritics or in Reiter's syndrome. It should be remembered that most patients who begin steroid treatment remain on it more or less permanently, although repeated attempts should be made to wean patients from the drug.

Joint aspiration and steroid injection

Corticosteroids can also be given as an intra-articular injection, usually after the aspiration of fluid; 2–30 mg of triamcinolone hexacetonide is commonly used, depending on the size of the joint. Its local effect in preventing recurrent effusion and pain may be dramatic. Repeated injections may result in joint destruction resembling a neuropathic joint, and for this reason it is often recommended that weight-bearing should be reduced immediately after an injection. Stringent aseptic precautions are required. Therapy should only be considered when one or possibly two joints are actively inflamed, while others are under good control from general treatment. The major contraindication to intrasynovial steroid administration is the presence of infection; this procedure should, therefore, never be performed without a definite diagnosis and previous synovial fluid examination. An injection of corticosteroid can relieve the symptoms of carpal tunnel compression and localised areas of tenosyn-ovitis, although injections directly into a tendon can lead to rupture.

Immunosuppressive drugs

Immunosuppressive drugs are reserved for the treatment of severe RA and its complications and for use in patients who have not responded to gold and pencillamine. Azathioprine and cyclophosphamide are the drugs most commonly used.

Methotrexate is widely used in N. America and increasingly in the UK; it is given once a week. A drug-induced pneumonitis is an occasional severe complication. There may also be an interaction with trimethoprim which must be avoided. Long-term experience with the drug in RA is being evaluated and it is not thought or considered that there is a significant increase in hepatic disease or late malignancy. Although this drug is being increasingly used in the treatment of RA, its use should still be carefully monitored.

Patient support

RA is not a disease the patient should contend with alone. Patients with any chronic disease must know something of their disability, how to control it, and how to live with and adapt to it.

Surgery

Combined clinics with physicians and orthopaedic surgeons are now common in most rheumatology centres, surgical treatment being an important stage in a patient's continuing therapy and management. This team approach allows surgery to be carried out at the optimum time, rather than only when patients become seriously disabled from joint damage and wasted muscles.

Surgery has two main objectives, depending on the stage of the disease: prophylactic, designed to prevent joint damage and deformity; and reconstructive, aimed at restoration of function and stability and the correction of deformity (Table 23.20). Excision of inflamed synovium will often relieve pain and swelling although, contrary to earlier expectations, it does not halt the progress of the disease. Persistent synovitis of the wrist and extensor-tendon sheath of the hand commonly leads to rupture of the tendons, which can be prevented by synovectomy and excision of the ulnar head. If the tendons rupture, suture or transfer of a slip of adjacent tendon corrects 'dropped fingers'.

The reconstructive surgical procedures used include arthroplasty (provision of a new joint), arthrodesis, osteotomy, tendon repair and transplantation. Joint replacements are most successful in the hip, and usually both acetabular and femoral components are replaced.

Prognosis

The course of RA is variable and it is often not possible to predict at onset those patients who will develop severe disease. In general, 25% remain fit for all normal activities, 40% have moderate impairment of function, 25% are quite badly disabled and 10% become wheelchair patients.

A poor prognosis is indicated by high titres of rheumatoid factor, early appearance of erosions, rheumatoid nodules, systemic manifestations and the presence of HLA DR4. Patients who have remissions generally do better than those with continuous disease, and explosive onset is often associated with a good outcome.

SERONEGATIVE SPONDARTHRITIDES

The seronegative spondarthritides (spondyl: joint of the backbone) are a group of disorders characterised by a consistent absence of RFs in the serum, by involvement of the sacro-iliac joints and by peripheral inflammatory arthritis. These conditions are, as a group, clinically distinguishable from RA (Table 23.21). Clinical evidence of overlap exists between the various seronegative spondarthritides. Thus a patient with psoriatic arthropathy may develop uveitis or sacro-iliitis, and a patient with inflammatory bowel disease may develop ankylosing spondylitis or mouth ulcers. Pathological changes are concentrated at

Table 23.20 Indications for surgery in rheumatoid arthritis

Stage of disease	Surgical procedure
Proliferation of synovium	Synovectomy and debridement
Destruction of tendon	Tendon reconstruction
Moderate to advanced destruction and deformity	Interposition arthroplasty Total joint replacement or excision arthroplasty

Table 23.21 Comparison of seronegative spondarthritis and seropositive rheumatoid arthritis

Feature	Seronegative	Seropositive
Peripheral arthritis	Asymmetrical	Symmetrical
Spinal involvement	Ankylosis	Cervical subluxation
Cartilaginous joints	Commonly affected (especially SI joints)	Rarely affected
Tissue typing	HLA-B27	(HLA-DR4)
Eye involvement	Anterior uveitis, conjunctivitis	Scleritis, keratoconjunctivitis sicca
Skin involvement	Epidermal dysmaturation (psoriasis keratoderma blenorrhagica), mucosal ulceration, erythema nodosum	Cutaneous nodules, vasculitis
Heart involvement	Fibrosis of aortic root, aortic regurgitation, conduction defects	Pericarditis
Pulmonary involvement	Chest wall ankylosis	Alveolitis, nodules, effusions
Gastrointestinal involvement	Ulceration of small or large intestine	Drug-induced symptoms
Genitourinary involvement	Urethritis/prostatitis, genital ulceration	

sites of insertion of ligaments or tendons (enthesopathy) rather than the synovium, and changes may also be seen in the eye, aortic valve and skin. There is a tendency to familial aggregation and the disorders are linked as a group by association with histocompatability antigen HLA-B27. This association ranges from 50% for psoriatic and enteropathic spondylitis to over 95% for ankylosing spondylitis.

The concept of seronegative spondarthritis is useful in a clinical context for a number of reasons:

- the prognosis is better than for RA
- a knowledge of the clinical associations can allow an earlier diagnosis to be made
- physical management differs from that of RA
- awareness of sacro-iliitis in this group can avoid the error of labelling back pain as lumbar disc disease
- awareness of the frequency of familial associations may help the patient or undiagnosed relative.

In the differential diagnosis of arthritis, seronegativity is of wider importance than these spondarthritic conditions and includes all forms of inflammatory polyarthritis in which the RF is absent. For this reason, the term seronegative *spond*arthritis should only be applied when there is spinal involvement.

Radiological examination of the affected joints aids diagnosis because bony ankylosis, marginal periostitis and asymmetrical involvement are found more often in the seronegative group. These differences suggest separate underlying pathological processes between the two groups.

Pathogenesis

The pathogenesis of these disorders is poorly understood, even in those conditions where the infective agent (e.g.

Yersinia, *Shigella* or *Salmonella* infection) is known. The term 'reactive' refers to an inflammatory arthropathy that is distant in time and place from the original infective trigger. However, *Chlamydia* and *Yersinia* antigens may be found in the synovial tissue.

Hereditary factors play an important role. Individuals with HLA-B27 have a 1–2% chance of developing disease, whereas the risk for HLA-B27-positive relatives of HLA-B27-positive patients with ankylosing spondylitis is about 10%. Approximately 10–20% of HLA-B27-positive individuals develop Reiter's syndrome after exposure to *Shigella* or other infectious agents. The explanation for the link between HLA-B27 and the spondarthropathies remains unknown. Three hypotheses have been put forward:

- HLA-B27 acts as a receptor site for an infective agent
- HLA-B27 is a marker for an immune response gene that determines susceptibility to an environmental cause
- HLA-B27 may induce tolerance to foreign antigens with which it cross-reacts.

ANKYLOSING SPONDYLITIS

Epidemiology

Ankylosing spondylitis occurs in both sexes but is usually milder, and therefore less frequently diagnosed, in women. Recent estimates suggest that it is three times more common in men. Clinical features of ankylosing spondylitis are seen in 0.5% of males. The prevalence in different ethnic groups is related to the frequency of HLA-B27 in these populations (Fig. 23.12A). Ankylosing spondylitis is uncommon in African blacks and in the Japanese, who have a low frequency of B27, while the North American Haida Indians have a high frequency of both HLA-B27 and ankylosing spondylitis. An abnormal response to bacteria, such as *Klebsiella*, which carry an antigen that mimics B27, has been suggested as the underlying cause of ankylosing spondylitis. Identical twins homozygous for HLA-B27 may be discordant for ankylosing spondylitis.

Pathology

The early histological changes in the synovial joints resemble RA; however, the most important effects are in the cartilaginous joints. Bony ankylosis is more frequent and the sacro-iliac joints often become fused. The apophyseal joints are involved and the discs show replacement of the nucleus pulposus, the annulus fibrosus and parts of the vertebral body by vascular fibrous tissue without any evidence of marked inflammatory changes. In the spine, the lesion is in the ligamentous attachment to

---

Summary 3 Conditions that overlap to form the seronegative spondarthritides, and their common features

The seronegative spondarthritides

- Ankylosing spondylitis
- Psoriatic arthritis
- Enteropathic arthritis (associated with ulcerative colitis, Crohn's disease and Whipple's disease)
- Reiter's syndrome/reactive arthropathy
- Behçet's syndrome

Common features

- Negative tests for rheumatoid factor
- Absence of rheumatoid nodules
- Inflammatory peripheral arthritis
- Radiological sacro-iliitis
- Evidence of clinical overlap between members of the group
- Tendency to familial aggregation

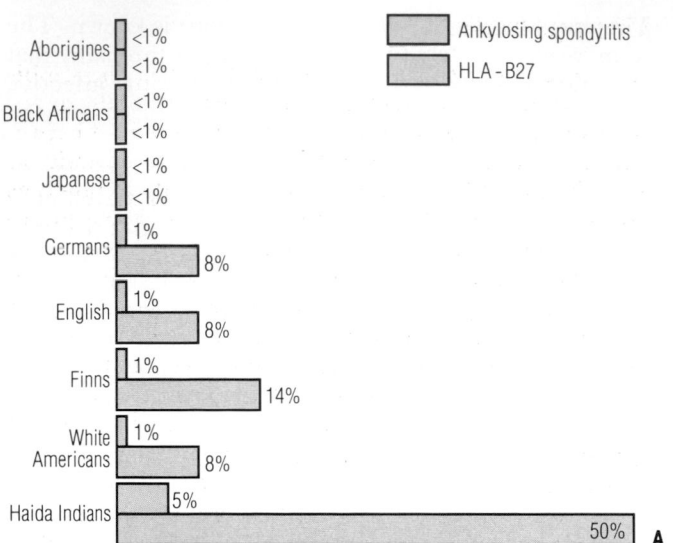

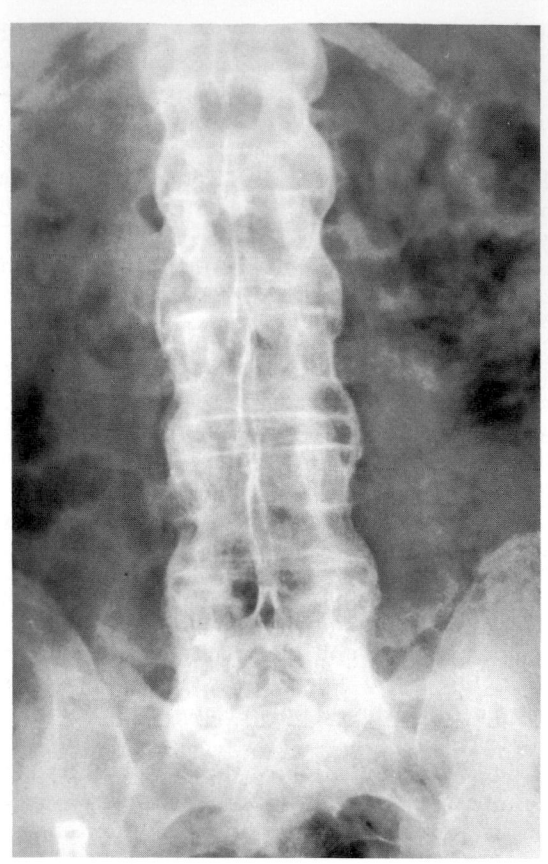

Fig. 23.12 Ankylosing spondylitis. A. Prevalence of ankylosing spondylitis and HLA-B27 in different parts of the world. (After Lawrence JS, 1977.) **B.** X-ray of the spine in severe ankylosing spondylitis; there are extensive syndesmophytes ('bamboo spine') and the sacro-iliac joints are fused.

bone (the enthesis) and this is characteristic of the disorder.

The disease is characterised by bilateral sacro-iliitis. The sacro-iliac joint is a composition joint with the lower half to two-thirds a synovial joint, and the upper part ligamentous. Early inflammatory changes occur in the synovial joint.

As the disease extends up to the intervertebral joints, there is 'squaring' of the vertebral bodies radiologically, seen on the lateral view (Fig. 23.12B) and calcification of the annulus fibrosus giving the characteristic syndesmophytes which fuse to form the classic 'bamboo spine'. This is caused by inflammation of the anterior corners of the vertebrae which extends into the outer layers of the annulus fibrosus.

Calcification of the intervertebral ligaments occurs. At this stage, there is osteoporosis of the vertebra, and fractures of the spine after minor trauma can occur. Other cartilaginous joints, such as the sternomanubrial joint and symphysis pubis, can be affected with erosions and bony ankylosis.

Clinical features

The disease most commonly begins between 16 and 40 years of age.

Articular features

Back pain is the usual presenting symptom. Its onset is gradual and is often accompanied by constitutional disturbances. The pain usually disturbs sleep and is associated with morning stiffness and stiffness after immobility. In the late stages of the disease, there may be reduction in spinal pain as the axial skeleton becomes ankylosed. Involvement of the costovertebral joints may result in chest pain and, later, decreased chest expansion. Symptoms improve with exercise.

Diagnosis is often delayed, symptoms being ascribed to lumbar disc disease. In spondylitis, spinal mobility is limited in all directions in contrast to disc prolapse, when lateral flexion is usually normal. The lumbar spine becomes flattened and the normal lordosis is lost. Sacro-iliac tenderness may be present. In an advanced case, the diagnosis is easy, as posture, gait and limitation of back movements are typical. However, only a few patients exhibit marked kyphosis and spinal rigidity.

Peripheral joints are involved in about a quarter of patients, and involvement of the hip is important because of the functional implications. Sometimes, pain and tenderness at the site of tendinous insertions can be a prominent feature, with the back, pelvic brim and ischial tuberosities being characteristic sites. Several joints are involved, usually the large joints of the lower limb.

Extra-articular features

Although primarily an articular disease of the axial and peripheral skeleton, other organs may be involved.

Iritis may be a presenting feature; it occurs in 25% of cases and can cause blindness. Aortitis and myocarditis are causes of death, as is uraemia from amyloidosis. Spinal cord or cauda equina compression may occur because of atlanto-axial subluxation or fracture of a rigid spine. Patients with severe ankylosing spondylitis may exhibit chronic fibrotic changes in the upper lung that resemble tuberculosis.

Features suggestive of inflammatory spinal disease are:

- insidious onset of discomfort
- age at onset of less than 40 years
- persistence for more than three months
- association with morning stiffness
- improvement with exercise.

Investigation

The ESR is often elevated in active phases of the disease. There is little correlation with disease severity. Tissue typing for HLA-B27 is both expensive and unnecessary, as diagnosis can be made on the clinical findings and X-rays. Raised IgA levels are associated with activity.

Anterio-posterior views of the sacro-iliac joints and lateral X-rays of the lumbar spine should be obtained. Both may be normal in early disease. The earliest changes are of sclerosis and erosions in the sacro-iliac joints, usually bilateral. Later, complete fusion may occur.

Early changes in the lumbar spine are erosions of the edges of the vertebral bodies with squaring of the vertebrae and syndesmophyte formation (Fig. 23.12B). In the most severe cases, ossification of the anterior longitudinal ligaments and apophyseal joints occur with production of a 'bamboo spine'.

Management

A long-term programme of active mobilisation in combination with anti-inflammatory drug therapy are the mainstays of management. Indomethacin is usually effective. The aim is to ease pain and stiffness, to keep deformity to a minimum and to maintain spinal mobility as much as possible. In contrast to the patient with RA, who is put to bed during an exacerbation, the patient with ankylosing spondylitis stiffens with bed rest and should be encouraged to remain active. Lumbar supports should not be prescribed. The patient must understand that the purpose of anti-inflammatory drugs is to reduce pain and stiffness so that an active exercise programme can be followed. Phenylbutazone can still be prescribed for ankylosing spondylitis and sulphasalazine can help the peripheral synovitis.

Advice should be given about posture. A firm bed with one pillow is appropriate at night. The patient should be taught exercises which can be performed daily at home and these should include spine extension and breathing exercises. Support groups and group physiotherapy sessions may help in providing advice and support in carrying out exercises.

Surgical intervention is most often carried out for hip involvement. Rarely, spinal osteotomy is used for severe spinal curvature.

Genetic counselling

Most patients with ankylosing spondylitis are HLA-B27-positive, and 50% of their offspring will carry this antigen. If HLA-B27-positive, a son or daughter has a 33% chance of developing ankylosing spondylitis. Parents should be advised that if the child develops symptoms such as swollen joints or painful eyes, they should seek medical advice.

Prognosis

With suitable treatment, the prognosis is excellent and 85% of patients never lose a day's work. After the early, painful phase, the back may be stiff but disability is minimal unless hip involvement is present. About 5% of patients have an unfavourable course from the outset.

PSORIATIC ARTHRITIS

Psoriasis occurs in about 2% of the population. Arthritis occurs in about 10% of patients with psoriasis, particularly in those with nail involvement. It affects the sexes equally. The skin and nail changes involved in psoriatic arthritis are described on page 1135.

Clinical features

The onset of arthritis usually follows a long history of psoriasis and can be acute, insidious, monoarticular or polyarticular. Occasionally it precedes the skin lesions. There does not appear to be a correlation between the severity of the skin lesions and the development of the arthropathy, although the joint lesions are usually associated with involvement of the nails.

The severity and ultimate deformity caused by the disease is usually less than that due to RA, and remissions are more frequent. There may be some synchrony of activity of joint and skin manifestations. Different types of psoriatic arthropathy are recognised:

- *Asymmetric oligoarthritis*, which involves one or two joints of fingers or toes, but can affect large joints.
- *Symmetrical polyarthritis*, which resembles RA.
- *Arthritis mutilans*, the most severe form of destructive arthritis.
- *Psoriatic spondylitis* in which radiological sacro-iliitis occurs in 20% of cases.
- *Psoriatic nail disease* and *distal interphalangeal joint involvement*.

The histological synovial changes resemble RA, but the joints involved and the pattern of destruction are different. While any joint can be affected, the most characteristic are the distal interphalangeal joints of the hands and feet.

Investigation

Radiological features of psoriatic arthritis are erosions in the distal interphalangeal joints with ankylosis, reabsorption of the terminal phalanges, and marginal bone overgrowths at the tendon insertions. When this last feature is

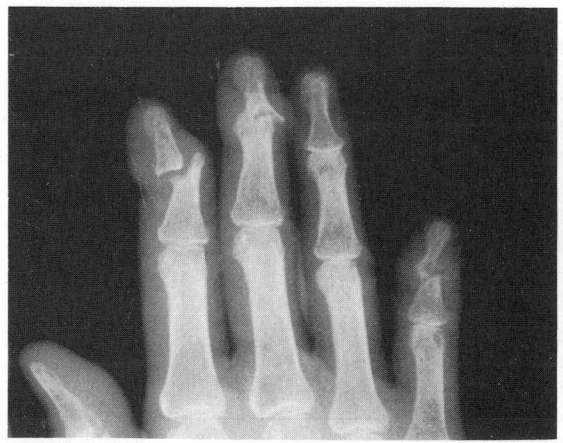

Fig. 23.13 Psoriatic arthropathy, with extensive involvement of the distal interphalangeal joints.

associated with osteolysis of the middle phalanx the radiological 'pencil in cup' deformity appears. If osteolysis progresses to 'telescoping' of the phalanges, the condition is known as *arthritis mutilans* (Fig. 23.13).

Sacro-iliitis is found in up to 30% of cases in which erosions, sclerosis and ankylosis may occur. Unlike ankylosing spondylitis, the involvement is usually asymmetrical. It is particularly common in patients with the severe arthritis mutilans form of disease. Paravertebral calcification and occasional large syndesmophytes may be seen. However, the incidence of typical ankylosing spondylitis is also higher in psoriatics and relatives than might be expected in the general population. Hyperuricaemia can occur in up to 20% of all psoriatics and the arthropathy should not therefore be confused with gout.

Management and prognosis

The treatment of the peripheral arthritis is similar to that of RA. Methotrexate therapy may be required for the more severe cases. Spinal disease is treated in the same way as ankylosing spondylitis.

In most cases, the prognosis is good and joint function is barely impaired, but deformity and disability occur in some patients.

REITER'S SYNDROME

Reiter's syndrome was described several times before 1916, when Hans Reiter described the case of a Prussian cavalry officer serving on the Balkan Front who developed an acute febrile illness characterised by arthritis, urethritis and conjunctivitis. The attack followed an episode of bloody diarrhoea. Although the venereal form of the disease is commoner in the UK, the postdysenteric form predominates in Europe. The incidence in patients with dysentery is approximately 0.2% and 0.8% of patients with non-specific urethritis develop Reiter's disease.

Aetiology

The disease follows an infection of either the bowel or lower genital tract. In the dysenteric form, several organisms have been implicated, chiefly *Shigella flexneri*, *Salmonella typhimurium* and *Yersinia enterolitica* but, in many cases, no causal agent has been found. *Salmonella* and *Yersinia* are also associated with 'reactive arthritis' without concomitant urethritis and conjunctivitis.

In the urogenital form, there is evidence that *Chlamydia* may be responsible for at least some of the cases. There is a genetic predisposition to the disease, since 60–90% of patients have the tissue antigen HLA-B27.

Clinical features

The diagnostic triad in Reiter's syndrome is urethritis, conjunctivitis and arthritis. One of this triad may be absent, and it should be noted that urethritis can occur even in the postdysenteric form of the disease. Most cases of Reiter's syndrome occur in the age range 16–35 years, and the male to female ratio is 20:1. However, urethritis is often not clinically apparent in females, and women presenting with an inflammatory arthritis in association with the HLA-B27 antigen may have Reiter's syndrome. Postdysenteric Reiter's syndrome has an equal sex distribution.

Urethritis is usually the first feature to appear, and occurs up to one month after sexual exposure. It is often mild but, rarely, there is a bloodstained discharge. The complaint of dysuria is almost invariable and there is frequency and suprapubic discomfort due to bladder involvement and prostatitis.

Mucocutaneous lesions in the glans penis are characteristic. Superficial ulcers often coalesce to form circinate patches. Involvement of the mucous membranes of the mouth is found in 10% of patients. The lesions are often painless and subside spontaneously.

The typical cutaneous lesion of Reiter's disease is *keratoderma blenorrhagica*. Initially a red macular eruption, it becomes hyperkeratotic and histologically identical to pustular psoriasis. This can occur anywhere on the body, but is most characteristically seen on the palms of the hands and soles of the feet. The crust is eventually shed leaving no scar.

Sterile conjunctivitis is the most common form of eye involvement and is usually mild. Occasionally, ocular involvement may be very severe, with almost all parts of the eye being involved, although the disease has a predilection for the conjunctiva and anterior uveal tract. Frequently, there are transient abnormalities of cardiac conduction which may progress to complete heart block. Pericarditis and aortic valve lesions also occur. Transient pulmonary shadowing has been described.

The *arthritis* varies in severity from a mild, transient synovitis to a chronic destructive arthritis. It tends to involve large weight-bearing joints and although it may on occasion be monoarticular, this is uncommon; it is usually asymmetrical, involving fingers and toes. In a typical case, arthritis may last for weeks or months, although in a few cases permanent joint damage may result. A feature of the condition is its liability to recurrences. Over 60% of cases have two attacks or more. Symptom-free intervals of 10 years or more are not uncommon, but in a small number, no clear-cut remission occurs.

Investigation

The ESR is elevated, sometimes markedly in the acute phase. Radiological examination in the early weeks may

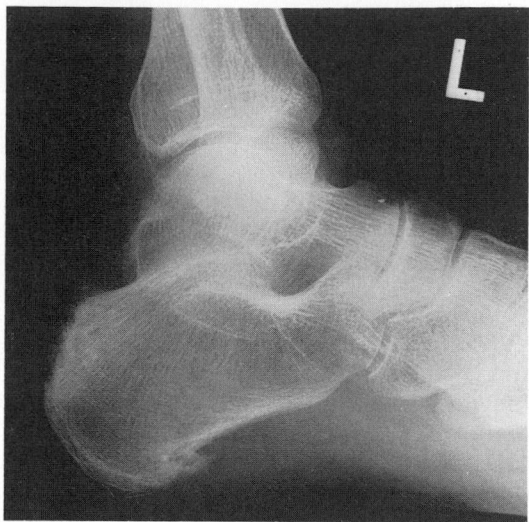

Fig. 23.14 Reiter's disease; X-ray showing plantar spur.

reveal no abnormality or only juxta-articular osteoporosis. Periostitis is a characteristic finding, especially in the metatarsals and in the phalanges of the feet. The new bone formation has an exuberant, fluffy appearance. Plantar spurs occur in 20–45% of cases (Fig. 23.14). Unilateral or bilateral changes are seen in the sacro-iliac joints, the frequency increasing to 50% after five years, and changes of ankylosing spondylitis may be seen in the spine.

The skin lesions and the arthropathy may resemble psoriasis. There have been cases when apparently typical Reiter's disease has progressed to typical psoriatic arthropathy. The link is emphasised by family studies where, among the male relatives of patients with Reiter's disease, the prevalence of psoriasis is 13%.

Management and prognosis

For most patients, an NSAID is useful. Methotrexate or azathioprine should be considered for severe intractable disease. Uveitis should be evaluated by an ophthalmologist if it does not respond rapidly to steroid eye-drops.

Spouses are often concerned that they may catch the disease from the patient. This does not occur. Most patients with Reiter's syndrome do not seem to have sexually acquired disease.

Tetracycline is effective in the treatment of non-specific urethritis, but has no effect on the other manifestations of the disease.

Reiter's syndrome was, at one time, considered to be a self-limiting condition. It is now known to be persistent in many patients; about 80% of patients have evidence of disease activity when they are examined after five years.

ENTEROPATHIC ARTHROPATHIES

The term enteropathic arthropathy means arthropathy associated with bowel disease (usually ulcerative colitis and Crohn's disease). There are two main clinical patterns:

- an episodic synovitis mainly involving weight-bearing joints
- sacro-iliitis.

About 50% of individuals with both inflammatory bowel disease and ankylosing spondylitis are HLA-B27-positive.

Synovitis occurs in 12% of patients with ulcerative colitis and 21% of those with Crohn's disease. The synovitis correlates with exacerbations of ulcerative colitis and is more likely when the bowel disease is extensive or when complications such as perianal suppuration occur. A total proctocolectomy abolishes the synovitis. In Crohn's disease, surgery seldom offers a radical cure, but synovitis tends to correlate with bowel activity. In both cases, the synovium shows non-specific inflammatory changes and, irrespective of the number of recurrences of the condition, progression to radiological joint destruction does not occur.

Radiologically typical ankylosing spondylitis or sacro-iliitis occurs in 17% of cases of inflammatory bowel disease. This frequently antedates the bowel symptoms and the progress of the two manifestations are not synchronous. In ulcerative colitis, radical excision of the colon does not provide a cure for the spondylitis. Involvement of the peripheral joints may lead to confusion with enteropathic synovitis; however, the presence of sacro-iliac and spinal disease, the lack of association of joint and bowel symptoms, and the presence of radiological changes in the involved joints all help in differentiation.

Family studies show an increased evidence of sacro-iliitis and ankylosing spondylitis in relatives. This supports the view that the spondylitis is an hereditary accompaniment, rather than a complication, of the disease.

WHIPPLE'S DISEASE

Whipple's disease is a rare condition. The finding of bacilliform bodies on electron microscopy and the good response to long-term antibiotic therapy suggest that it has an infectious aetiology.

An episodic arthritis is a common presentation, and may precede the gut symptoms by several years. The pattern of joint disease is similar to that seen in intestinal inflammatory disease, but the absence of overt gut symptoms should alert one to the possibility of Whipple's disease.

Prolonged antibiotic therapy leads to improvement. It is usual to give tetracycline 1 g daily for 12 months, following an initial 10 days' treatment with parenteral penicillin and streptomycin.

BEHÇET'S SYNDROME

Behçet's syndrome was first described in Turkey and is common in Eastern Mediterranean countries and Japan, though rare in England. It is of unknown aetiology and is characterised by the triad of aphthous-type oral and genital ulceration and iritis. Other features that commonly occur include thrombophlebitis, erythema nodosum, pustules and folliculitis. Some patients show the phenomenon of pustule formation where the skin is subjected to trivial injury, e.g. venepuncture. Large vessel thrombosis and bowel disease resembling ulcerative colitis can occur. The CNS can be involved, with meningo-encephalitis, cranial nerve palsies, hemiparesis and transient episodes resembling strokes. Vascular involvement of the eye is one of the most serious aspects of Behçet's syndrome, with blindness being a frequent outcome.

Arthritis occurs in 60% of cases, affecting mainly the weight-bearing joints, and the course tends to be chronic. The inclusion of Behçet's syndrome in the seronegative group is somewhat speculative. There is association with HLA-B5 but not HLA-B27, and eye disease is particularly associated with HLA-B51.

Acute episodes, especially those involving the eye, usually require high-dose corticosteroid therapy. Colchicine is useful for some aspects of the disease, especially the orogenital ulceration. Cyclosporin A has shown promise, particularly for controlling the eye disease.

OSTEOARTHRITIS

Osteoarthritis (OA) is defined pathologically and radiologically by reduced joint space secondary to loss of cartilage, by sclerosis of subchondral bone and by osteophyte formation. The term primary OA is used to distinguish cases with no apparent cause from secondary OA, when a number of localised or generalised pre-existing disorders are present (Table 23.22).

Table 23.22 Secondary causes of osteoarthritis

• Previous inflammatory arthritis	• Congenital dislocation of hip
• Previous joint infections	• Perthe's disease
• Avascular necrosis	• Acromegaly
• Intra-articular fracture	• Ochronosis
• Joint dysplasias	• Haemochromatosis

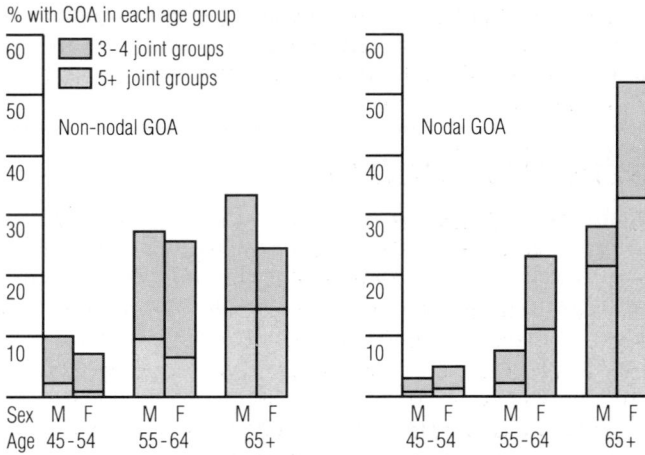

Fig. 23.15 Age and sex distribution of generalised osteoarthritis (GOA) in the UK in patients with and without Heberden's nodes. (After Lawrence JS, 1977.)

Epidemiology

Radiographic evidence of OA is found in 35% of people under 30 years of age, and in 85% of 80-year-olds (Fig. 23.15). OA of the hip is more common in men under 35 years of age, but in later years it is more common and more severe in women. Although radiographic evidence of OA appears to have an equal sex ratio, symptoms are three times more common in women. There is a marked familial tendency, particularly in association with Heberden's nodes, and the geographical distribution of joint involvement varies. Certain occupations have a high frequency of OA, e.g. coal miners develop OA of the spine and knees. OA is seen in all cultural groups, though the pattern of involvement varies. Hip disease is uncommon in Mongoloids and hand disease is seldom seen in Afro-Caribbeans.

Aetiology

A number of processes are involved in the development of OA:

- failure of bone and cartilage remodelling
- inflammation
- ageing
- abnormal joint loading
- deposits of apatite and calcium pyrophosphate are common, but how they affect the joint remains unknown
- alterations of the complex reflex neurological and muscle function around a joint, resulting in an impaired shock-absorbing capacity
- enzymic destruction of cartilage.

The development of OA appears to be a 'final common pathway' in joint malfunction, but age and loading patterns appear to be the most important predisposing factors. Once the natural history of the disease has been established, the course varies from rapid progression, through relapsing phasic activity to apparent stabilisation.

Pathology

The early stages of OA include an increase in proteoglycan turnover, a change in proteoglycan composition and an increase of type II collagen production. The relationship of these changes to ageing is uncertain.

Cartilage shows thinning, erosions, fibrillation, clefts and loss of joint surface congruity with areas of chondrocyte loss. Subchondral bone becomes sclerotic with increased vascularity and bone distant from the joint undergoes remodelling. Proliferation of the cartilage produces osteophytes, which is usually a late phenomenon. In the later stages, cysts are formed in the underlying subchondral bone, and the articular surface may collapse.

A mild synovitis may be seen, and the synovial fluid may contain apatite and pyrophosphate crystals.

Clinical features

The main initial symptom of OA is pain made worse by movement and eased by rest. Stiffness may be present after inactivity, but morning stiffness is not a feature. As the joint deteriorates with loss of joint movement and joint instability, the pain becomes more pronounced, and is present at rest and in the night. Only about a third of patients with radiological OA have symptoms, and the cause of pain is not understood, as there are no pain receptors in cartilage. Pain may also arise from the ligaments or bursae around the joint.

Examination shows deformity and bony enlargement of the joint, with occasional synovial thickening and effusion. There is coarse crepitus on joint movement. The pattern of joint involvement varies, but those most commonly affected include the first metacarpophalangeal joint, the first metatarsophalangeal joint and the distal interphalangeal joint of the hands (Fig. 23.2). The hip and knee are affected less frequently and the shoulder and ankle are seldom involved. In the spine, the apophyseal joints around C5–C7 and L3–L5 are commonly involved.

OA is not a single static condition but a family of conditions, with widely different pathogenetic factors. Generalised OA affects several joints and there are usually Heberden's nodes present. 'Inflammatory' OA affects particularly the interphalangeal joints, and is associated with cartilage erosion. Hip arthritis can be confined to one area of the hip, particularly the superior pole or the medial pole, or may involve the entire joint. Similarly, there are different patterns of knee involvement. Lateral compartment changes seldom occur without medial compartment changes. Predominate patello-femoral disease is a feature of pyrophosphate arthropathy (p. 1023).

Investigations

OA can only be diagnosed by X-ray, showing bone sclerosis and osteophyte formation. All blood tests are normal in uncomplicated OA.

Management

The natural history of OA is poorly documented. There is evidence that the process may stop, or even improve, in some patients, and in those that have progressive disease, severe joint failure tends to occur in a weight-bearing joint in a minority of patients.

Generalised OA tends to progress slowly, and prognosis with respect to preservation of joint function is excellent. Patients should be reassured that they do not have a relentlessly progressive disease such as RA. Pain relief can be achieved with analgesics such as paracetamol. NSAIDs have more side-effects, but may be necessary when pain is severe. Intra-articular steroid injections and aspiration of joints may help in restoration of function if there are effusions and inflammatory changes.

Physical therapy

OA in a weight-bearing joint may be helped by physiotherapy. This may restore the function of wasted muscles, improve mobility and compensate for some instability. Heat may provide pain relief. Hydrotherapy helps to reduce the load on the joint allowing mobilisation. Fixed flexion deformity of the knee can be helped by serial splinting. A walking stick is useful for hip or knee involvement. Splints may support unstable joints, and walking aids may be helpful.

Surgery

Surgery is indicated if pain and loss of function have failed to respond to conservative measures. Surgical procedures include removal of loose bodies, osteotomy to relieve pain and arthrodesis and arthroplasty (joint replacement) (Table 23.23). Proper assessment is the key to a successful outcome and surgery should only be carried out when there is a clear indication that function will be improved. Joint replacement will continue to develop. There is still

Table 23.23 Some surgical procedures in arthritis

• Synovectomy/debridement	• Arthrodesis
• Arthroplasty	• Tendon repairs
• Osteotomy	• Nerve decompression

much basic research to be done into biomechanics of joints under normal conditions and after prosthetic replacement, and on the problems of lubrication.

INFECTIVE ARTHRITIS

Arthritis may arise from direct infection of joints by micro-organisms, or as a reaction to a preceding infection. Infection must be considered in all cases of acute arthritis, particularly when only one joint is affected. Delay in treatment may lead to permanent joint damage or septicaemia.

BACTERIAL INFECTIONS

Most cases of bacterial arthritis result from haematogenous spread; much less frequently, infection results from joint aspiration or injection, or spread from osteomyelitis. The most frequent organisms are *Staphylococcus aureus*, *Streptococcus pyogenes*, *Diplococcus pneumoniae* and *Neisseria gonorrhoeae*. Certain organisms appear to exhibit a tropism for joints: for instance, septic arthritis complicates about 1% of pneumococcal and salmonella infections when treatment is delayed, whereas about 80% of patients with gonococcal septicaemia develop arthritis. The frequency with which different organisms are associated with septic arthritis is partly age-dependent. The organisms which cause septic arthritis in young children are usually not the same as those causing it in adults.

Septic arthritis may occur at any age, but is particularly common under the age of 15 years and in the elderly. Other predisposing factors include debilitating disease, hypogammaglobulinaemia, corticosteroid and immunosuppressive therapy, and RA.

Clinical features

Usually, a single joint is involved and there is marked inflammation with severe pain, tenderness, erythema and swelling. There may be minimal signs of inflammation in patients receiving corticosteroids or with a debilitating illness. In an infant, there may also be little systemic illness and the child may present with sudden refusal to move a limb.

An infected joint is commonly associated with a fever, often accompanied by rigors, and the patient looks ill. When the organism is the gonococcus, a migratory polyarthritis may precede localisation in a single joint. Ten to 20% of staphylococcal infections and 75–85% of gonococcal infections involve two or more joints. More than one joint may also be involved in immunosuppressed and debilitated patients. The identification of a septic joint in RA can prove difficult, but must be considered whenever there is increase in pain, swelling or other evidence of inflammation in one or a limited number of joints. The development of low-grade infection in prosthetic joints is an increasing problem, and recognition may take several months. Organisms of low virulence, especially *Staphylococcus albus*, predominate.

Diagnosis

Diagnosis of septic arthritis depends on demonstrating the organism in joint fluid or tissue, and synovial fluid and blood should be sent for culture. In addition to routine aerobic and anaerobic cultures, special media are needed for the isolation of *N. gonorrhoeae*, and additional culture of sputum, urine and cervical mucus may prove helpful in special circumstances.

Osteomyelitis should be considered if the site of maximal tenderness extends beyond the joint. If there is any doubt about the bone adjacent to an infected joint, an isotope scan will demonstrate bone involvement.

The condition known as *transient synovitis of the hip* can prove a difficult differential diagnosis. No definite cause has been established for this disorder and it may represent a number of conditions. It affects children between the ages of two and 12 years, who present with pain, a low-grade fever and slight elevation of the ESR. It is safest to treat this as an infection until the diagnosis of septic arthritis has been excluded.

Management

Antibiotics should be started as soon as specimens have been sent to the laboratory. Changes in therapy can be made once the sensitivities of the infecting organism are known. Therapy should be administered intravenously for up to two weeks and then oral therapy given for at least six weeks. Intra-articular therapy is not required. The joint should be splinted in a suitable position to relieve pain until the inflammation has subsided.

Synovial fluid should be aspirated when it reaccumulates, since the presence of purulent material may inhibit the action of antibiotics. Gross joint destruction and the presence of contiguous osteomyelitis are indications for surgical drainage, as is failure of response to drug therapy within 72 hours. Once the acute inflammation has subsided, passive, then active exercises can be given. Weight-bearing can be resumed when signs of inflammation have subsided.

Specific bacterial arthritides

Gonococcal arthritis

Gonococcal arthritis is most common in females and homosexual males, in whom the primary infection is often asymptomatic.

Clinical features. The most common pattern of joint involvement is a migratory polyarthritis associated with tenosynovitis, with the synovitis localising in one or two joints. Joint symptoms occur within three weeks of infection and are accompanied by fever and rigors. There is a tendency for the small joints of the upper limbs to be involved, rather than larger joints; however, the knee is also frequently affected. A sparse erythematous skin rash, which may be macular, vesicular or pustular, occurs in one-third of cases and is found adjacent to involved joints. It appears before, or within a few days of, the arthritis and may be painful at the outset.

Diagnosis. The gonococcus is difficult to grow, and repeated blood and synovial fluid cultures may be required to confirm the diagnosis. The organism is identified in joint fluid in only 25% of patients.

There should be little difficulty in distinguishing between Reiter's disease and gonococcal arthritis. There is an 80% female preponderance of gonococcal arthritis, compared with a high proportion of males with Reiter's disease. In gonococcal arthritis, pyrexia is more common, the upper limb joints are involved more frequently, and the arthritis is less symmetrical than in Reiter's disease. Reiter's disease is associated with the tissue antigen B27; gonococcal arthritis is not.

Treatment. Benzylpenicillin is given intravenously until there is a clinical response. Penicillinase-producing strains of gonococci are resistant to penicillin and cephaloridine. For such patients spectinomycin or cephoxitin is the treatment of choice.

Meningococcal arthritis

Meningococcal infection is complicated by arthritis in 5–10% of patients. Characteristically, it affects large joints, and sometimes flits from one to another. The onset is a few days after the beginning of the illness. Once on therapy, resolution occurs in one to four weeks.

Infective endocarditis

Joint manifestations are present in about half the patients with infective endocarditis. Large joint involvement is usual, and symptoms vary from mild arthralgia to an acute, red, swollen, painful joint. The combination of fever, arthritis and cardiac murmur may initially suggest rheumatic fever.

Lyme arthritis

This was first described in Old Lyme, Connecticut (USA) in 1972. Symptoms include a recurrent asymmetrical arthritis involving a few large joints. The arthritis follows one to 24 weeks after an erythematous rash, erythema chronicum migrans. The causative agent is a tick-borne spirochaete, *Borrelia burgdorferi*, which is transmitted by *Ixodes dammini* or related ixodid ticks. Penicillin or tetracycline therapy given at the time of the rash may shorten the early illness and prevent arthritis. Later stages respond to high dose intravenous penicillin.

Lyme disease usually begins in summer with erythema chronicum migrans; this is the unique clinical marker, which begins as a red macule or papule that expands to form a large annular lesion. Skin involvement is often accompanied by fever, headache and regional lymphadenopathy, and migratory musculoskeletal pain and arthritis. Meningeal irritation and cardiac involvement may follow.

Tuberculous arthritis

Tuberculosis should be considered in the differential diagnosis of chronic joint disease. It is most common in immigrant children and in the middle-aged or elderly. Only about 1% of all patients with tuberculosis have skeletal involvement; of these, approximately 50% have spinal disease, 30% infection of hips or knees, and 20% arthritis of other joints, particularly the sacro-iliac joints. Involvement of the knee is more common in adults, and the spine and hips in children. About half the patients do not have pulmonary disease. It is assumed that haematogenous dissemination infects subchondral bone adjacent to a joint or to a spinal intervertebral disc. The resulting osteomyelitis may remain dormant for years before there is reactivation. Alcoholism and chronic debilitating disease may predispose to reactivation.

When the vertebral column is involved, dissection along fascial planes may cause a psoas abscess. Spread of infection to involve adjacent vertebrae may lead to wedging and kyphosis. The anterior portions of the vertebrae between the sixth thoracic and fifth lumbar level are usually involved. Bone biopsy may be necessary to confirm the diagnosis.

Peripheral joint involvement is usually monoarticular and destruction of cartilage occurs later than in pyogenic arthritis. The usual organism is *Mycobacterium tuberculosis* but atypical organisms (e.g. *M. kansasii*, *M. trivale*) have been isolated from infected joints, and the bovine strain has been implicated in carpal tunnel infection.

Diagnosis and treatment. The diagnosis is made by biopsy and culture of the synovium, since the bacilli are rarely grown from synovial fluid. Treatment is with antituberculous therapy (p. 473).

Syphilitic arthritis

Direct invasion of the synovium by *Treponum pallidum* is uncommon. A migratory polyarthritis occurs infrequently during the secondary stage of acquired syphilis and may resemble rheumatic fever.

Congenital syphilis may cause:

- acute epiphysitis or osteochondritis, most commonly of the humerus and usually in the first weeks of life
- 'Clutton's joints', painless bilateral swelling of the knees between the ages of eight and 16 years
- rarely, a neuropathic arthropathy secondary to tabes dorsalis (Charcot's joint).

FUNGAL INFECTIONS

Fungal infections of joints are rare. Culture of pus, synovial fluid or biopsy material permits diagnosis. Surgical drainage and excision of necrotic tissue may facilitate recovery.

Actinomycosis commonly affects the mandible, but involvement of vertebrae occasionally occurs from local spread. Bone abscesses develop. Blastomycosis, coccidiomycosis, histoplasmosis and sporotrichosis can all affect the joints.

ARTHRITIS IN VIRAL DISEASE

Several viral infections may be accompanied or followed by an arthropathy. Joint symptoms may coincide with, follow, or even precede the onset of other signs and symptoms; they are usually mild and tend to resolve spontaneously in a few weeks. In contrast to bacterial infections, viral arthropathies are usually polyarticular. It is thought that the synovitis results from immune complex deposition. Only in rubella arthritis has the virus been isolated from an affected joint. A viral arthritis should be suspected if the patient has a low white count with a relative lymphocytosis.

Rubella

In rubella (see p. 239) the arthritis involves the metacarpophalangeal or proximal interphalangeal joints (85%), elbows, wrists and knees, in a symmetrical fashion. Morning stiffness, painful tenosynovitis, the occasional occurrence of carpal tunnel syndrome and a positive latex test for RF may make the resemblance to RA even more striking, and differentiation between the two conditions in the early stages is not always possible on clinical grounds alone. The ESR is usually normal or slightly elevated. Rubella antibodies may be demonstrable in high titre.

Complete resolution of the arthritis occurs within a few weeks to a few months. Only in rare cases are symptoms so severe that a short course of corticosteroids is required. Arthralgia may persist for several months.

Rubella vaccination produces musculoskeletal symptoms in up to 20% of cases. An arthritis similar to that associated with the natural infection occurs two to four weeks after vaccination and lasts for a few days, although it can persist for several weeks. Occasionally, synovitis continues for months. Joint pain affecting the arms or legs two to 10 weeks after rubella vaccination is caused by radiculoneuritis, and may be associated with paraesthesia.

Infectious hepatitis

During the early incubation period of viral hepatitis, some patients may experience joint symptoms; these may be mild and transient (usually type A infections) or acute and prolonged (usually type B). It is rare before adolescence.

There is bilateral and symmetrical involvement of the proximal interphalangeal joints and the spine is occasionally involved. Other symptoms are a rapid onset of morning stiffness, and warm, red and tender joints with slight effusions, associated with fever, anorexia, malaise and an occasional urticarial rash. The arthritis usually resolves with the appearance of jaundice. Joint disturbances can also be prominent in anicteric cases.

Mumps

Arthritis caused by mumps is most common in male teenagers. Overall, less than 1% of those affected by mumps develop arthritis, usually one to four weeks after the start of the illness. It is usually migratory and asymmetrical, involving large joints. When the pattern of joint movement is accompanied by pericarditis, it can resemble rheumatic fever. During an epidemic, children may have an arthritis but no parotitis.

Chickenpox

Chickenpox may be complicated by bacterial arthritis with spread from infectious scabs. A transient, acute arthritis may occur at the time of the rash.

Adenoviral arthritis

The arthritis associated with adenovirus infections usually occurs in children. It begins with fever, coryza and pharyngitis, followed by a macular erythematous rash and symmetrical arthritis.

Infectious mononucleosis

In infectious mononucleosis, widespread lymphadenopathy, splenomegaly, rash, fever and transient arthritis or arthralgia may mimic both rheumatic fever and systemic juvenile chronic arthritis. However, the skin lesions tend to be larger and raised and do not recur as often as those of juvenile arthritis. This is a disorder of adolescents. In children, cytomegalovirus can cause a similar picture.

Arboviruses

Viral infections endemic to certain parts of the world can give rise to illnesses with prominent musculoarticular symptoms. The Ross River virus, a group A arbovirus found in Australia, causes a macular rash and fever, and a polyarthritis usually involving the small joints of the hands. Dengue fever, of South and South-East Asia, can cause a haemorrhagic rash, fever and severe joint and muscle pains. Both these illnesses are self-limiting. Arboviruses are discussed further in Chapter 11, page 240.

Parvoviruses

In adults, joint involvement (transient arthralgia and arthritis) is common (80–90%) but is less common in children (<10%) (see Ch. 11, p. 234).

Rheumatic manifestations of HIV infections

Increasingly, HIV-infected individuals are presenting to rheumatologists, and, in some, rheumatic symptoms are the first manifestation of infection. Patients may present with Reiter's syndrome, or an acute oligoarthritis, which predominantly affects lower limb joints, in the absence of clinical features of Reiter's syndrome.

Other rheumatic syndromes which have been associated with HIV infection include myositis, vasculitis and lupus-like illness with low-titre antinuclear antibodies. It is difficult to attribute these clinical features exclusively to HIV infection, as many patients are likely to be exposed to other infections.

Summary 5 Viral causes of arthritis

- Rubella and rubella vaccination
- Infectious hepatitis
- Mumps
- Infectious mononucleosis
- Adenovirus infections
- Arbovirus infections
- Chickenpox
- Parvovirus infections
- HIV

CHILDHOOD ARTHRITIS

There are a number of causes of arthritis in children (Table 23.24) and the diagnosis can be difficult. The commonest cause used to be rheumatic fever but there has been a marked reduction in its incidence in the past 40 years. Children seem to suffer less discomfort from arthritis than adults. Arthritis may be first suggested by joint swelling, or by a limp or guarding of the joints.

JUVENILE CHRONIC ARTHRITIS

Juvenile chronic arthritis (JCA) is a generic term covering several overlapping patterns of disease (Table 23.24).

Systemic JCA (Still's disease)

The most common age of onset of systemic JCA is under five years, when boys are affected as frequently as girls; but the disease can present later in childhood, and even in adult life (see below). With later presentation, girls are affected more commonly than boys.

Clinical features

Fever and rash are the main clinical features. The fever is characteristic. It differs from that of rheumatic fever in that the temperature may be normal or subnormal in the morning, and the child may then appear to be reasonably well. By the late afternoon, however, a temperature of up to 40°C may be recorded and the child looks ill. Salicylates or paracetamol usually control the fever. When high fever precedes arthritis, diagnosis can prove difficult and is often aided by the appearance of the rash.

About 40% of children develop a rash, which is evanescent, often appearing when the temperature is high. It is usually pink, macular, discrete and non-pruritic, and affects the trunk and limbs, although it can be widespread and involve face, palms and soles.

Table 23.24 Differential diagnosis of arthritis in children

- Joint infections (bacterial, tuberculous)
- Virus infections (rubella and mumps in particular)
- Juvenile chronic arthritis (JCA)
  - Still's disease (systemic JCA)
  - Pauciarticular JCA
  - Polyarticular-onset JCA
- Still's disease in young adults
- Rheumatic fever
- Henoch-Schönlein purpura
- Leukaemia and haemorrhagic disease
- Trauma and synovitis

Generalised lymph node enlargement may be marked, so that the clinician may suspect leukaemia or lymphoma, but histology shows reactive hyperplasia and the nodes regress as the disease subsides. Enlargement of the mesenteric glands may cause abdominal pain. Splenomegaly is moderate. If it persists, the complication of amyloidosis should be considered.

Initially, there may be no joint symptoms, minor arthralgia or definite arthritis. Ultimately, however, most patients develop arthritis affecting the knees, wrists and ankles. Flexor tendon involvement of the hands is common. Involvement of the cervical spine occurs and leads to pain and limitation of movement.

Pericarditis is detected in 7% of patients, but is found in approximately 45% of necropsies. Myocarditis may also occur.

Subcutaneous nodules are less common in children than in adults. Interestingly, their histology resembles that of the nodules of rheumatic fever.

Differential diagnosis

The diagnosis is a clinical one. Infective causes of fever and arthritis must be excluded. In the first few days, it can be difficult to distinguish systemic JCA from a viral infection, but the persistent spiking fever and recurrent maculopapular eruptions, together with a rising white blood count, are helpful. In the past, the most difficult differential diagnosis was rheumatic fever, but this is now unusual.

Pauciarticular JCA

In pauciarticular JCA, four or less joints are involved in the first three months, and this is by far the commonest mode of presentation. The knee, ankle and elbow are most commonly affected, although involvement of a single finger or toe is also common. There are probably several different patterns of illness, the most common being that seen in younger children. Here, the most serious complication is chronic iridocyclitis, which is either present at the onset or develops within the next year. The iridocyclitis affects both sexes and is associated with antinuclear antibody in the serum. The danger to these children is therefore not from joint involvement, which is usually mild, but from serious eye involvement. Slit lamp examination is therefore important in all children diagnosed as having JCA. Children that present in their teens often have the early features of ankylosing spondylitis.

The diagnosis of monoarticular arthritis can be difficult. Infection, trauma and foreign bodies in the joints are possible causes which may not be readily apparent at onset.

Polyarticular-onset JCA

Polyarthritis (defined as involvement of five or more joints) can develop at any time in childhood. Females and older children are predominantly affected. Patients are usually seronegative; however, 10% have persistent IgM RF, tend to be older (over 10 years) and have a slightly different prognosis and distribution of joint involvement. They often progress to severe RA.

Clinical features

The disease may begin acutely or insidiously. The most commonly involved joints are the knees, the wrists and the ankles, with relative sparing of the metatarsophalangeal joints. There is flexor tenosynovitis of the hands, neck involvement is seen early and lymphadenopathy may be present. Although there may be an occasional spike of fever, the marked spiking of systemic illness is absent. When IgM RF is present, joint involvement has a clinical appearance and course indistinguishable from adult RA, i.e. polyarticular, peripheral and symmetrical. Large joints may be involved, but usually in association with small joint involvement. Systemic features are similar to those of the adult disease: nodules occur and the prognosis is poor.

Management of JCA

Around 80% of patients with JCA are able to lead useful independent lives, although one-third may require anti-inflammatory drugs to control pain, and up to 10% die from infection or chronic renal disease secondary to amyloidosis.

The aim of treatment is to achieve a state in which the child lives at home with minimal residual joint deformity. A successful outcome depends on two main factors: support from the child's family who must understand the aims of treatment; and liaison between the general practitioner and hospital, social and educational services. Drugs form only part of the treatment.

Daily exercises are important. Bed rest is indicated only in children with severe systemic features because it can result in muscle wasting and joint ankylosis. Weight-bearing is restricted only if there is severe pain or a flexion deformity which requires serial splinting. Hip and knee flexion is discouraged by daily periods of lying prone. Night splints are used during the acute phase, to rest the joints in a good position.

In view of the association with aspirin therapy and Reye's syndrome, an NSAID such as naprosyn is often used. If the disease progresses, gold or penicillamine can be given; methotrexate is being increasingly prescribed. There are few indications for using corticosteroids; they do not influence the ultimate prognosis or prevent complications, and can cause alarming iatrogenic effects which cannot be justified in a disease with a good prognosis. They are, however, indicated in severe systemic disease, chronic iridocyclitis that does not respond to local steroids, and progressive disease that is resistant to other drugs. Alternate day dosage is preferred; this allows for some skeletal growth and does not suppress growth spurts, sexual maturation or reaction to stress. Surgery is restricted to synovectomy in children old enough to cooperate with postoperative physiotherapy. Correction of joint deformities, or joint replacement, is carried out in adolescence or adult life after growth has ceased.

ADULT STILL'S DISEASE

Adult Still's disease is a distinct entity, almost exclusively affecting young adult females. Characteristically, it is a flitting polyarthritis with a similar distribution to that encountered in the childhood variety. Systemic features are also similar. The fever, which usually responds to salicylates, may sometimes be prolonged, requiring treatment with corticosteroids. A meticulous search for sources of sepsis must be made before embarking on steroid therapy. Recurrences are frequent.

RHEUMATIC FEVER

Rheumatic fever was at one time the commonest cause of acute polyarthritis in childhood, but has been declining in incidence for many years. It is seldom seen before four years of age; the peak age for first attacks is around six years and they are rare after 15 years. The sexes are equally affected. Rheumatic fever starts one to five weeks after a throat infection with a group A β-haemolytic streptococcus.

Clinical features

Articular symptoms

Arthritis is the most common major manifestation and is usually the presenting symptom. Joint involvement may vary from arthralgia, where patients have acutely painful and tender joints with little objective signs of inflammation, to an acute arthritis with effusion and involvement of pericapsular structures. The overlying skin is hot and red. Carditis is frequent and severe in the younger child, while arthritis is frequent and severe in the adolescent and adult.

The onset of arthritis is typically acute and polyarticular, affecting mainly the knees (75%) and ankles (50%), and occasionally the wrists and elbows. In contrast to RA, involvement of the small joints of the hands (8%) and feet (15%) is uncommon. Historically, the arthritis of rheumatic fever was described as 'migratory' or 'flitting', conveying the erroneous impression that, as the inflammation flits from one joint to another, the joint involved earlier may revert to normal. In practice, particularly if untreated, many joints may remain actively involved at the same time, and give the appearance of a symmetrical polyarthritis.

Symptoms of a throat infection may be so mild as to have passed unnoticed. A preceding streptococcal infection can be demonstrated by a rising antistreptolysin 0 titre (greater than 250 units for adults; greater than 333 for children), and lack of evidence of recent streptococcal infection makes the diagnosis less likely. A leucocytosis is common, and a raised ESR is invariable unless cardiac failure is present.

Systemic symptoms

Systemic symptoms are prominent but non-specific. Fever usually starts at the onset of joint involvement, is usually high (up to 40°C) and sustained. It is accompanied by sweating, anorexia, malaise and vomiting, all of which could also result from salicylate therapy. When abdominal pain occurs with nausea and vomiting, it is usually caused by mesenteric adenitis and may simulate an acute abdomen. The subcutaneous nodules of rheumatic fever, like those of RA, occur at pressure points – elbows, knees and the soles of the feet – but (unlike RA) they occur early in the course of the disease, are smaller and more numerous, and tend to last for a shorter period. Histologically, they are distinguishable from those of seropositive RA by the lack of necrosis and palisade layer.

Erythema marginatum

Erythema marginatum is strongly suggestive of, but not entirely specific for, rheumatic fever and occurs in only a small proportion of patients. It is a fleeting, non-pruritic, pink or red, macular or papular rash which extends centrifugally (in contrast to fixed drug eruptions) to become circinate or leaf-like while fading at the centre. It occurs most frequently in children, in association with carditis and subcutaneous nodules, and is most apparent at the height of the fever. It mainly affects the trunk, and less frequently the proximal parts of the limbs, but never the face. (Note that in SLE and adult Still's disease, the face is involved.)

The appearance of signs and symptoms and ECG evidence suggestive of carditis (p. 420) in the presence of a rash and fever are strongly suggestive of rheumatic fever. The difficulty in establishing a diagnosis has led to the development of diagnostic criteria (Table 23.25).

Management

Complete bed rest is important to minimise cardiac work and rest painful joints. Penicillin should be given to eradi-

Table 23.25 Criteria for diagnosis of rheumatic fever*

Major manifestations	Minor manifestations
● Carditis	● Fever
● Polyarthritis	● Arthralgia
● Chorea	● Previous rheumatic fever or rheumatic heart disease
● Erythema marginatum	● Elevated ESR or CRP
● Subcutaneous nodules	● Prolonged PR interval

* These criteria are a revised version of the Jones criteria. Diagnosis is based on one major and two minor criteria plus supporting evidence of preceding streptococcal infection.

cate any streptococci. Fever and joint pain can be controlled with salicylates. Although the initial response to salicylates (in adequate dosage) and corticosteroids can be equally dramatic in RA and Still's disease, the response to salicylate in rheumatic fever seems to be more complete and longer lasting. With clinical improvement, all but penicillin should be withdrawn slowly and activities gradually increased. In severe carditis, steroids will often prevent or resolve cardiac failure. Neither steroids nor salicylates have any other effect on the disease, on the likelihood of recurrences, or on the final cardiac state.

ANAPHYLACTOID (HENOCH-SCHÖNLEIN) PURPURA

Anaphylactoid purpura is due to a widespread vasculitis involving arterioles and small capillaries. It can occur at any age, but primarily in children, especially boys. The disease occurs most often in the spring, and usually follows an upper respiratory tract infection. The onset is acute, with fever, headache and rash. Initially, macules or urticarial papules occur on the buttocks and the extensor aspects of the limbs. These become flat, purpuric, and may coalesce or even ulcerate. Localised oedema of the face, scalp, hands and feet occurs; in young children, it can mimic arthritis. Haemorrhage into the gut wall can cause colic, melaena or haematemesis.

Usually the joint involvement is mild, consisting of transient, non-migratory synovitis typically affecting more than one joint. The ankles, knees, hips, wrists and elbows are usually affected, with a tendency to lower limb involvement. The synovial fluid is inflammatory in character. Joint destruction does not occur.

A mild focal glomerulonephritis (p. 823), producing proteinuria and microscopic haematuria, occurs in 50% of cases. Occasionally, it progresses to the nephrotic syndrome and, very rarely, to renal failure. The disease usually settles in four to six weeks without sequelae, but may recur.

CRYSTAL SYNOVITIS

GOUT

Gout is the principal clinical manifestation of sustained hyperuricaemia. Clinical features include acute arthritis (tenosynovitis, bursitis), tophaceous deposits, renal disease and urolithiasis.

Epidemiology

Gout occurs mainly in developed countries, with a prevalence in the UK and USA of 0.3%. The prevalence of hyperuricaemia is about 5%. Men are 10 times more likely to have gout than women. At puberty, male blood uric acid levels rise and remain higher than those of females until the menopause, when female uric acid levels also rise. Gout is very uncommon before puberty, when it usually suggests an enzyme defect.

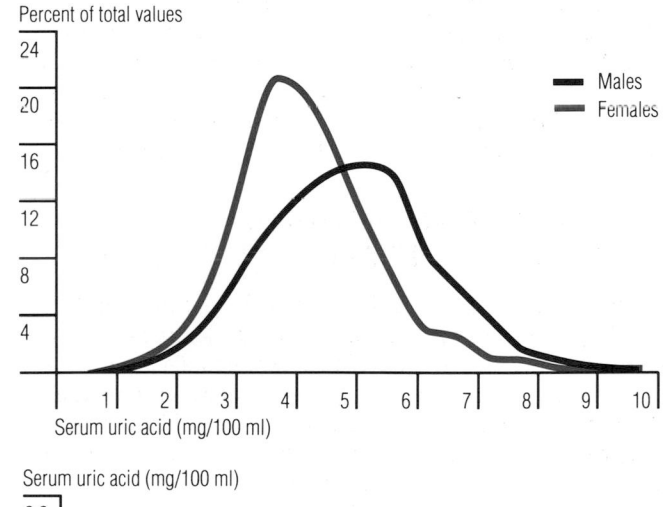

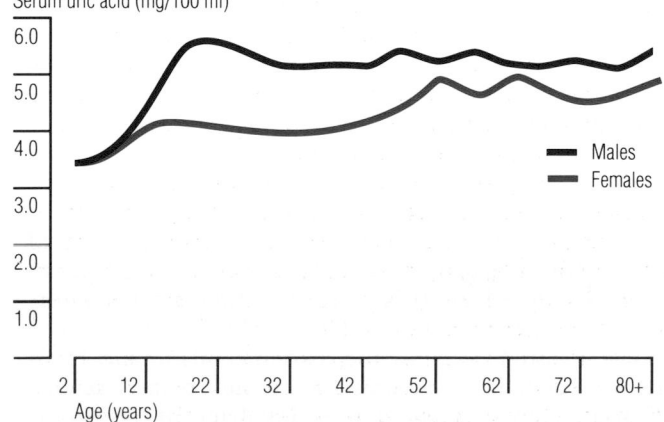

Fig. 23.16 **Age and sex distribution of serum uric acid levels. A.** Distribution of serum uric acid levels by age in males and females after the age of six. **B.** The mean serum acid levels in males and females for different age groups.

Serum uric acid concentrations are related to several demographic factors, the most important being age, sex, body bulk and genetic constitution (Fig. 23.16). Values are higher in urban than in rural communities and correlate positively with social class, weight and a high protein diet. Values are distributed in a population as a continuous variable, with a skew towards the higher values. Hyperuricaemia can be defined as the mean plus two standard deviations, which gives values of above 0.42 mmol/l in adult males and above 0.36 mmol/l in adult females.

Uric acid production and disposal

Uric acid is derived from the breakdown of purine bases (Fig. 23.17). These are the products of essential nucleotides which are synthesised in the liver. Adenine and guanine are re-utilised. About 60% of uric acid is replaced daily; the quantity produced is directly proportional to body size. Less than 10% comes from preformed dietary nucleotides.

Seventy-five per cent of uric acid is excreted in the kidneys and the remainder is lost in the gut. The uric acid is freely filtered at the glomerulus and 90% is then resorbed. Renal handling of uric acid involves glomerular filtration, proximal tubular reabsorption, tubular secretion, and postsecretory reabsorption. The paradoxical effects of high and low dose aspirin on uric acid excretion can be explained by differential effects on active secretion and reabsorption.

Uric acid circulates as monosodium urate, but is found mainly as the free acid in the urine. In hyperuricaemia,

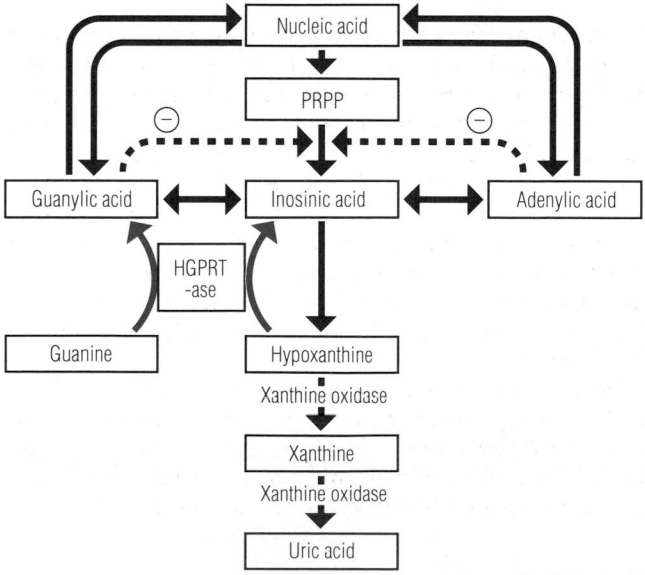

Fig. 23.17 **A simplified diagram of some of the metabolic pathways involved in the formation of uric acid.** PRPP = phosphoribosyl pyrophosphate. HGPRTase = hypoxanthine-guanine-phosphoribosyl-transferase.

urate is usually present in the blood as a supersaturated solution. Lowering of the pH lessens the solubility and increases the likelihood of crystal formation.

Causes of hyperuricaemia

Diuretic drugs are the main cause of hyperuricaemia, accounting for some 60% of cases, but clinical gout is an uncommon association. Hyperuricaemia occurs with renal failure, but here too gout is surprisingly rare. Other genetic and environmental factors lead to hyperuricaemia by decreasing the excretion, or increasing the production, of uric acid (Table 23.26). In most patients, although there is often a family history, no definite cause can be found.

Dietary purines have only a modest effect on plasma urate levels and avoidance will lead to a fall of uric acid of some 1 mg/100 ml.

In only 10–15% of patients is gout due to overproduction of uric acid. These patients can be detected by measuring the excretion of uric acid on a 70 g protein, purine-free diet. Overproducers excrete more than 3.6 mmol/24 hours (600 mg/24 hours).

Gout and hyperuricaemia are often associated with obesity, type IV hyperlipoproteinaemia, impaired glucose tolerance, hypertension and ischaemic heart disease.

Hyperuricaemia may occur when large quantities of nucleoprotein are broken down during treatment of leukaemia or lymphoma, and prophylactic therapy is sometimes given to avoid the risk of urate nephropathy (Ch. 20, p. 826).

Enzyme defects may, rarely, cause overproduction of uric acid. Hypoxanthine-guanine phosphoribosyl transferase deficiency is associated with accelerated purine synthesis, childhood gout and renal stones. Complete deficiency is a rare, X-linked, inborn error of metabolism in which gout is associated with spasticity, a variable degree of mental deficiency and a compulsive self-mutilation (the Lesch-Nyhan syndrome).

Phosphoribosyl pyrophosphate synthetase overactivity is another X-linked inborn error of metabolism associated with gout and increased purine synthesis.

Many drugs affect renal elimination of uric acid. For example, aspirin reduces clearance at low doses but is uricosuric at high doses. Other drugs reducing clearance include diuretics (except amiloride and spironolactone), pyrazinamide and ethambutol. Lead also reduces clearance (saturnine gout).

Pathology

Prolonged hyperuricaemia leads to the formation of small crystal aggregates. These accumulate in the synovium and at external sites, such as the ear, cartilage and olecranon, and may eventually become visible tophi. Crystal deposition may proceed over several years without symptoms. Uric acid and urate deposition in the kidney can lead to a variety of pathological effects, including interstitial nephritis, renal stones and acute tubular damage (Ch. 20, p. 826).

Joint inflammation is the result of uptake of crystals by polymorphonuclear leucocytes. When crystals are phagocytosed they enter an endocyte vacuole (phagosome). Fusion with lysosomes occurs and these contain hydrolytic digestive enzymes. There is interaction between the crystals and the phospholipid of the lysosomal membrane, possibly due to the weak acidic groups on the surface of the crystal forming hydrogen bonds. Disruption of the membrane follows, with release of lysosomal enzymes and the crystal. Phagocytosis of urates leads to increased production of lactic acid which causes further precipitation of crystals.

Crystal ingestion stimulates the production of a chemotactic factor producing further recruitment of leucocytes. Hageman factor is activated and this leads to a series of further reactions releasing chemical mediators of inflammation, including kinins. Colchicine has been shown in vitro to stabilise the lysosomal membrane, block the release of chemotactic factor and hinder the assembly of intracellular microtubules involved in lysosomal release. These factors are less pronounced in pyrophosphate arthropathy; this is consistent with the relative ineffectiveness of colchicine in this condition.

Table 23.26 Causes of hyperuricaemia

Increased production of uric acid
Increased purine synthesis
Hypoxanthine guanine phosphoribosyl transferase deficiency
Phosphoribosyl pyrophosphate synthetase overactivity
Increased turnover of preformed purines
Lymphoproliferative and myeloproliferative disorders
Secondary polycythaemia
Chronic haemolytic anaemia
Severe psoriasis
Carcinomatosis
Decreased renal excretion of uric acid
Chronic renal disease
Drug administration
Diuretics
Salicylates (low dosage)
Pyrazinamide
Reduction in fractional urate clearance
Increased levels of organic acids (exercise, starvation, alcohol, ketoacidosis)
Hypertension
Hyperparathyroidism
Hypothyroidism

Table 23.27 Factors provoking an acute attack of gout

- Joint trauma
- Unusual physical exercise
- Alcohol
- High protein diet or starvation
- Surgery
- Drugs
  Diuretics
  Initiation of uricosuric or allopurinol therapy
- Severe incidental illness

Clinical features

Classical gout is easily diagnosed. The typical patient is young or middle-aged, male, and wakes in the early hours of the morning with severe pain, usually in the big toe. On average, three out of four attacks affect the big toe and one attack in 10 affects more than one joint. Several factors may provoke an attack (Table 23.27).

The affected joint is usually red, swollen and warm. The overlying skin is often shiny, with periarticular oedema, and there is often fever. The joint is extremely painful and tender. Untreated, the attack lasts days or weeks before subsiding spontaneously. Patients may have just one attack, or may have recurrences at monthly or yearly intervals. Recurrent attacks may merge into each other, leading to destruction of cartilage, bony erosion

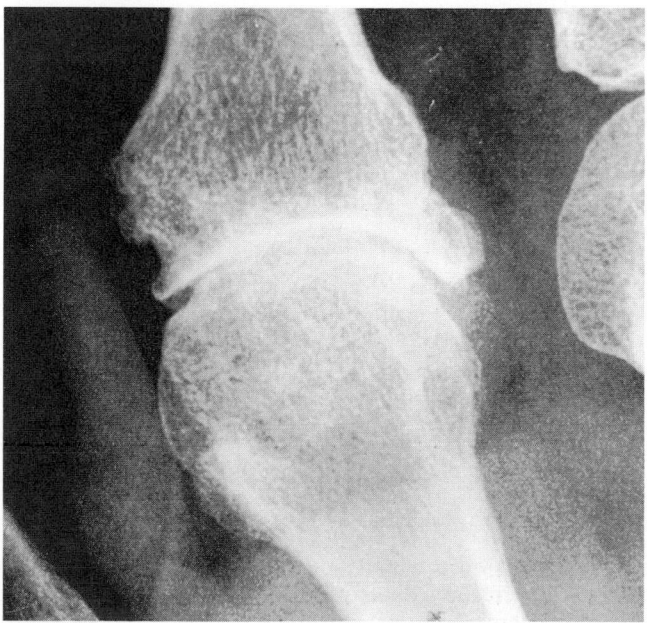

Fig. 23.18 Gout; X-ray proximal interphalangeal joint showing erosion with no surrounding osteoporosis.

(Fig. 23.18) and disability. No synovial joint is immune from gout, but feet, ankles, knees, wrists and fingers are the most susceptible. Bursitis, especially of the elbow, may occur.

Polyarthritis as an initial manifestation of gout is unusual, but when it occurs, it can mimic RA. Similarly, about 5% of patients with pyrophosphate arthropathy have multiple joint involvement with subacute attacks lasting from four weeks to several months. The diagnosis of crystal synovitis should be considered in patients whose joints are inflamed sequentially (rather than together as in RA), and when osteophytes are present; diagnosis is proven by the demonstration of crystals in the joint fluid.

Tophi. Recurrent acute attacks of gout lead to asymmetrical, hard swellings, and tophaceous deposits may also occur in periarticular tissues, the cartilage of the ear (Fig. 23.19), bursae and tendon sheaths. Tophi may occur at atypical sites (e.g. fingertips), especially in elderly patients receiving diuretics.

Renal calculi. A history suggestive of renal calculi is present in up to 10% of gout patients; this is higher in hot climates. Uric acid calculi may be radiolucent (composed of uric acid alone) or radio-opaque (combined with calcium salts). They are produced by dehydration and excessive purine ingestion, or may be associated with defects in tubular reabsorption of uric acid, or the use of uricosuric drugs. All patients should be instructed in the necessity for a high fluid intake.

Diagnosis and investigation

A number of conditions should be considered in the differential diagnosis of acute and chronic gouty arthritis (Table 23.28).

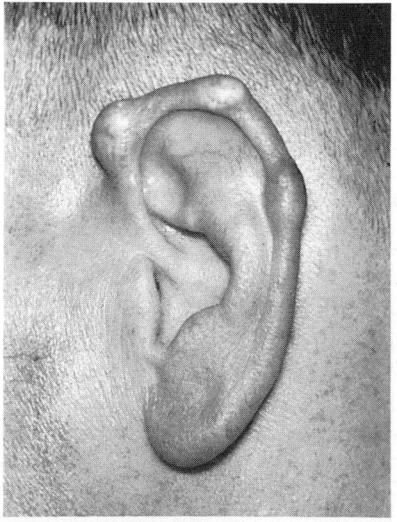

Fig. 23.19 Gouty tophi in the ear.

Table 23.28 Differential diagnosis of gout

Acute arthritis

Infective arthritis
Another crystal arthritis, e.g. pseudogout due to pyrophosphate crystals, or apatite arthritis
Traumatic arthritis
Rheumatoid arthritis
Seronegative arthritis

Chronic arthritis

Nodular rheumatoid arthritis
Osteoarthritis with Heberden's and Bouchard's nodes
Xanthomatosis

In all cases of suspected gout, details of previous rheumatic symptoms and those of urinary tract calculi should be elicited. The patient's family history should be recorded and serum uric acid measurements made. Synovial fluid should be examined under polarising light for monosodium urate crystals, and possible causes of secondary hyperuricaemia should be investigated.

Serum uric acid measurements. A high serum level of uric acid with a typical history is almost diagnostic of gout. However, a raised serum uric acid alone does not justify the diagnosis of gout, because of the many factors which raise the serum level.

Polarised light microscopy. Diagnosis can only be made with certainty by demonstrating crystals in joint fluid taken during an attack. In gout, the synovial fluid is turbid, and although other inflammatory joint conditions and sepsis can have similar appearances, the diagnosis is made by the presence of monosodium urate crystals. Urate crystals show strong negative birefringence and calcium pyrophosphate weak positive birefringence, when viewed under the compensated polarised light microscope (Fig. 23.5).

Management

There are three main aims: to reduce acute synovitis, prevent further crystal formation, and identify associated disease.

Reduction of acute synovitis

The first line of treatment of acute synovitis is with an NSAID. Indomethacin is the drug of choice, at a dose of 50 mg four-hourly until the attack subsides. Other anti-inflammatory drugs can be used; azapropazone (standard dose 600 mg twice daily) is both uricosuric and anti-inflammatory.

Colchicine is effective, but has to be taken every two hours until control is achieved. Main side-effects include nausea, vomiting, intestinal colic and diarrhoea. These develop at the time of clinical improvement. Intravenous colchicine is effective, but is not generally used because of the small risk of serious toxicity. If long-term management is to be instituted, then allopurinol or uricosuric drugs should not be started for several weeks, as they may prolong the acute attack or trigger further episodes. Salicylates and diuretics should also be avoided.

Prevention of crystal formation

A single attack of gout does not justify preventive drug treatment. Obese patients should lose weight, alcohol should be reduced and the need for diuretics causing hyperuricaemia should be reconsidered. Indications for long-term therapy include recurrent attacks, tophaceous gout and renal disease. During the reduction of plasma urate, there is a risk of provoking acute gouty arthritis and therefore prophylactic anti-inflammatory drugs or colchicine should be prescribed concomitantly for the first three months. Successful lowering of plasma urate abolishes the risk of gout and tophi will eventually disappear. If the underlying cause of hyperuricaemia cannot be modified, indefinite hypouricaemic therapy is required. Treatment is aimed at keeping the serum uric acid level below the solubility level (0.45 mmol/l).

Uricosuric drugs (probenecid and sulphinpyrazone) act by blocking the renal tubular transport of uric acid which allows the filtered load to be excreted. Side-effects are uncommon, but include nephrotic syndrome and skin rashes. These drugs are less effective than allopurinol in severe disease, and often ineffective in patients with renal failure. They are best avoided in patients with urolithiasis or purine overproduction, because they do not reduce the risk of nephropathy or stone, and are best reserved for underexcretors of uric acid.

Allopurinol, a xanthine oxidase inhibitor, reduces the oxidation of hypoxanthine to xanthine, and of xanthine to uric acid (Fig. 23.17). The more soluble xanthine is excreted. Indications for this drug include extensive tophaceous gout, renal impairment, hyperuricaemia due to antimitotic drug therapy and intolerance or failure of response to uricosuric therapy. Side-effects are few, and include dyspepsia and skin rash. Therapy is usually for life.

Asymptomatic hyperuricaemia

Provided blood pressure, weight and renal function remain normal no therapy is required for asymptomatic hyperuricaemia. Some authorities recommend treatment if the serum uric acid is consistently above 9 mg/100 ml.

PYROPHOSPHATE ARTHROPATHY (CALCIUM PYROPHOSPHATE DIHYDRATE DEPOSITION DISEASE)

Pyrophosphate arthropathy is the term used to describe the clinical presentation of acute and chronic arthritis, whereas *chondrocalcinosis* refers to the radiological appearance due to the deposition of calcium pyrophosphate crystals in cartilage. Fibrocartilage is most commonly involved, especially the menisci of the knee, but articular hyaline cartilage also calcifies as do other articular structures, including ligaments and joint capsules. This leads to a degenerative arthropathy which usually affects old people, but can occur earlier in life if there is a strong family history.

Aetiology

The pathogenesis of both the chronic crystal deposition and acute arthritis (*pseudogout*) are poorly understood. Acute attacks of arthritis are precipitated by shedding of crystals from preformed deposits in cartilage into the joint cavity. The mechanism leading to the formation of these deposits is unknown. Present evidence suggests a local articular, rather than a systemic metabolic, disturbance of pyrophosphate metabolism.

A large number of other conditions have been associated with calcium pyrophosphate deposition, including diabetes mellitus, hypertension and hypothyroidism. Not all are necessarily of aetiological significance, because patients are often elderly and multiple diseases might be expected to be present. However, 7% of patients prove to have hyperparathyroidism, and pyrophosphate deposition also occurs in haemochromatosis and Wilson's disease.

Clinical features and diagnosis

Pyrophosphate arthropathy may present as an acute arthritis affecting particularly the knees and wrists, which resolves within one to four weeks. Trauma, surgery or medical illnesses may precipitate an attack. Less frequently, RA may be mimicked as there may be multiple joint involvement and associated joint inflammation.

Pyrophosphate deposition may present as asymptomatic chondrocalcinosis and is a common finding in the elderly. Common sites of chondrocalcinosis include pubic symphysis, triangular ligament of the wrist and knee menisci. Deposition may also be seen with severe generalised OA. There may, or may not, be inflammatory exacerbations. The knees are most frequently affected, and hips, shoulders, elbows, ankles and wrists may also be involved.

The diagnosis is made on the basis of clinical features, chondrocalcinosis on X-ray and demonstration of crystals by polarising microscopy of synovial fluid from an involved joint (Fig. 23.5).

Management

Primary metabolic disorders should be identified and treated appropriately. Treatment of an acute attack of pyrophosphate arthropathy is similar to that for acute gout, although drugs are less effective; joint aspiration together with the injection of corticosteroid gives relief.

Unfortunately, there is no effective means of preventing further attacks of pyrophosphate arthropathy, although colchicine may sometimes prove helpful. Management is that of OA, with analgesics, physiotherapy and local measures when appropriate.

SYSTEMIC LUPUS ERYTHEMATOSUS

Systemic lupus erythematosus (SLE) is a disease of unknown aetiology; it affects predominantly young women and has a marked tendency to exacerbation and remission. The diverse clinical features reflect the multisystem involvement that is characteristic of the disease.

Currently, there is much interest in the possibility that the disease may arise from an interaction of genetic factors and viral infection. The high prevalence of SLE in women of reproductive age suggests that female hormones may modify the immune response. There are a number of haematological and serological abnormalities, of which the key one is the formation of antinuclear antibodies (ANAs). The use of DNA-antibody and complement estimations has improved the clinical management of SLE patients and led to a greater understanding of their role in immune-complex-mediated tissue damage.

Epidemiology

The prevalence of SLE appears to vary from country to country; in the UK, it is about 1 per 10 000 of the population. Females are affected six to nine times more frequently than males, and the disease is especially common during the childbearing years. Blacks and Chinese are particularly susceptible; in the USA 1 in 250 female blacks of childbearing age may be affected.

There is an increased prevalence of SLE in the families of patients with the disease, and the incidence of ANAs, hypergammaglobulinaemia and false positive serological tests for syphilis are also increased in healthy members of these families. There may therefore be a genetically determined susceptibility to the development of SLE in appropriate environmental circumstances in some individuals. A null or absent allele for C4 on the sixth chromosome has been noted in family studies, and twin studies show a greater than 60% concordance of SLE in monozygotic twins.

Pathology

Many of the histological changes are non-specific. Two findings suggestive of SLE are the periarteriolar or onion-skin fibrosis in the spleen, and the haematoxylin body – the tissue counterpart of the LE cell. There is usually widespread small and medium vessel vasculitis, portions of the walls of which may become necrotic and be found to contain fibrinoid deposits. These deposits contain immune complexes consisting chiefly of DNA, anti-DNA antibody and complement components.

Immunological features of SLE

Antinuclear antibodies

ANAs are a constant feature of SLE and are directed at different antigenic components. The demonstration of ANAs, by immunofluorescence, provides the most widely used screening test for SLE. The test is very sensitive but is negative in about 5% of patients (uraemia may render an ANA result negative). However, positive tests are found in many other conditions. A frozen tissue section is incubated with the test serum to allow antibodies to fix, washed thoroughly to remove any unfixed antibodies and then stained with a fluorescent antibody to human globulin. This will bind to any fixed antibody. The tissue is then examined using an ultraviolet microscope. The value of the ANA test has been enhanced with the use of human cell lines such as the HEp^{-2} cell line. Sometimes, the pattern of nuclear staining gives a clue to the antigen involved (e.g. chromatin pattern staining is associated with antibody to nucleoprotein) and carry some diagnostic significance; for example the rim (or ring) staining patterns represent antibodies to double-stranded DNA and are thus more specific for SLE.

In 1957, a number of groups reported findings of antibodies against native (double-stranded) DNA in the serum of patients with SLE. It later became apparent that the antibodies were a heterogeneous group, binding to a variety of sites on the DNA molecule. Antibodies against native DNA were found to be almost always specific for SLE. The measurement of DNA antibodies by immuno-assay has proved a major advance in the management of SLE. Problems remain in standardisation of the DNA and in the exclusion of denatured DNA fragments or strands. In most patients with SLE, fluctuations in DNA-binding parallel clinical activity. It may rise before a clinical exacerbation becomes apparent. In diseases such as Sjøgren's syndrome, RA and scleroderma, where positive ANA tests are common, DNA antibodies are usually absent or in low titre. The methods used to detect these antibodies include:

- *Farr technique (DNA-binding test)*. The serum containing antibodies is mixed with a preparation of radiolabelled DNA, and the immune complexes so formed precipitated with 50% ammonium sulphate. The radioactivity in supernate and precipitate is then measured, and a formula used to calculate the DNA-binding value (expressed as a percentage).
- *Counter-immune electrophoresis*. This is a sensitive and rapid test for precipitating antibodies to DNA. It is not quantitative.
- *Crithidia-immunofluorescence test*. Trypanosomes have nuclei which do not contain nucleohistone and also have a large kinetoplast containing a high concentration of ds-DNA. This has been found useful in the diagnosis of SLE. Species of *Crithidia* which are not pathogenic for man are grown easily in rats. A film of these, treated with a serum containing DNA antibodies and then stained with fluoresceinated anti-human gammaglobulin, gives a strong staining of the kinetoplasts. This is a reliable screening test for antibodies to ds-DNA.
- *ELISA*. ELISA anti-DNA antibody assays are now widely available and distinguish IgG, IgM and IgA isotypes.

RNA antibodies

Antibodies to both single-stranded and double-stranded RNA can be detected in SLE by a variety of techniques. The occurrence of antibodies to double-stranded RNA is interesting, as human RNA is single-stranded with the exception of small helical regions on transfer RNA. Some viral RNA, on the other hand, is double-stranded and this finding has stimulated speculation on the possibility of a viral aetiology in this disorder.

Serological tests for syphilis

False positive tests for syphilis are found in up to one-third of SLE patients. Rarely, a positive TPHA test occurs; this is probably caused by antibody reacting against the DNA in the treponeme.

Other autoantibodies in SLE

Table 23.29 demonstrates the wide variety of antibodies that occur, the pattern varying from patient to patient. They appear to reflect a general immunological disturbance, which results in an exaggerated production of humoral antibodies. Sometimes, the antibodies precede the clinical manifestations of SLE by years. They only rarely give rise to clinical abnormalities, although antibodies to platelets, red cells, leucocytes and clotting factors may

Table 23.29 Autoantibodies in SLE

Antinuclear antibodies

Anti-DNA histone (LE cell)
Anti-DNA (double-stranded)
Anti-DNA (single-stranded)
Anti-RNA
Antinucleoprotein (soluble or particulate)
Antinuclear glycoprotein (Sm antigen)
Antiextractable nuclear antigen (ENA) – Ro(SSA), La(SSB)

Other antibodies

Anticytoplasmic antibodies (mitochondrial and microsomal)
Rheumatoid factors (IgG and IgM – 33% of cases)
Cryoglobulins
Lymphocytotoxic antibodies
Antiphospholipid (cardiolipin, lupus anticoagulant)
Organ-specific autoantibodies
Elevated titres of antiviral antibodies (e.g. measles)
Antibodies against: red cells
 lymphocytes
 leucocytes
 platelets

cause haematological disorders. Patients may also have scrum antibodies which are apparently lymphocytotoxic.

Clinical subsets of SLE have been defined by antibody typing, as certain antibodies appear to be associated with specific clinical features. Anti-Ro antibodies are associated with the development of congenital heart block in the offspring of SLE patients. Anti-phospholipid (cardiolipin) antibodies are responsible for the false positive VDRL and the circulating lupus anticoagulant, and are associated with an increased thrombotic tendency and a high incidence of recurrent abortion. Patients with raised serum anticardiolipin may also have thrombocytopenia, livedo reticularis, neurological disorders other than stroke, and aortic and mitral valve disease. Although the antiphospholipid syndrome may be related to SLE and other autoimmune diseases, it may also exist as a distinct entity.

Serum complement

The serum complement level (either total haemolytic complement, or C3 or C4) is a useful investigation in SLE. Low complement levels in the presence of a high DNA binding titre is diagnostic of active SLE. Serial measurements of complement are useful in following the clinical course, as the level drops about 50% before, and remains low during, an exacerbation. Particularly low levels of complement components, especially C3 and C4, are strongly indicative of active lupus nephritis, during which complement is continuously consumed by the immune complexes deposited in the glomeruli.

Individuals with a genetic deficiency of C2 appear to have an increased incidence of SLE. SLE is not associ-ated with any particular HLA antigen, but associations have been described with HLA-B8, DR2 and DR3.

Aetiology

The cause of SLE is unknown. There is some evidence for a viral aetiology.

A strain of mice known as New Zealand Black/New Zealand White Fl hybrid develop a lupus-like disease. Immune complexes in the kidney can be shown to contain DNA and various oncorna virus antigens. These findings suggest a viral aetiology, but no oncorna virus has been isolated in human SLE. The disease is more severe in females, and can be partially reversed by testosterone. Immunosuppression selective for T cells (such as with cyclosporin A) also reduces severity.

Pathogenesis

There is considerable evidence that the lesions of SLE are due to immune complexes causing local damage. Immune complexes can be detected free in the serum, and precipitated in the kidneys on the mesangium and glomerular basement membrane. These would be expected to fix complement, and complement breakdown products (e.g. C3d) are present in the serum. Patients possessing anti-DNA antibodies and entering a relapse will have free circulating DNA, and must therefore go through a stage where immune complexes form. At this stage, the serum complement levels fall. DNA itself will bind to glomerular basement membrane, and this membrane-bound DNA can react with antibody and complement to give a nephrotoxic type of damage.

Clinical features

The clinical features of SLE are extremely variable both in nature and severity (Table 23.30). An exacerbation may be precipitated by exposure to sunlight, an infection, drugs or pregnancy. Common initial features are general

Table 23.30 Relative incidence of the major clinical manifestations of SLE*

Manifestations	Incidence (%)
Musculoarticular	95
Cutaneous	81
Fever	77
Neuropsychiatric	59
Renal	53
Pulmonary	48
Cardiac	38

*After Estes D and Christian CL 1971 Medicine 50; 85.

malaise, with fever, fatigue and loss of weight. SLE presents in the majority of patients with articular or cutaneous features.

Musculoskeletal features

The commonest musculoskeletal complaint is of joint or muscle pains, occasionally presenting years before other features become obvious; the pain often appears out of proportion to the degree of synovitis. The small joints are most commonly involved and the arthritis is symmetrical. Erosions are rare. Occasionally, a patient develops a deforming arthritis, as a result of capsular and ligamentous laxity. Tendon involvement may be prominent, leading in some cases to flexion contractures at the forearm and wrist. A proximal myopathy occurs in 5% of patients; this differs from steroid myopathy in that the shoulder girdle is more commonly involved and the serum muscle enzymes are usually elevated. Aseptic necrosis affecting the weight-bearing joints occurs in patients who have been receiving high doses of corticosteroids for long-standing SLE.

Skin manifestations

The skin lesions appear most often on sun-exposed areas. The classical eruption is the 'butterfly' rash, an erythematous eruption over the nose, spreading to the cheeks. It occurs in less than half of all patients. The scalp is frequently involved in patients with cutaneous LE, producing patches of permanent alopecia. Photosensitivity is particularly common in patients with anti-Ro. Livedo reticularis, a reticular blotchy pattern especially common on the lower extremities, is often associated with anticardiolipin antibodies. Diffuse alopecia occurs in about 60% of patients and is an important sign of active systemic disease. The hair tends to regrow when the disease enters a remission. Erythema, telangiectasia and capillary infarcts in the proximal nail folds are often seen. Chilblain-like purplish-red swellings on the digits, and vasculitic lesions which can ulcerate, also reflect involvement of the cutaneous vasculature.

Skin biopsy can be helpful in diagnosis; immunoglobulin and complement are demonstrated at the dermal epidermal junction both in discoid lesions and generally in SLE, including unaffected skin.

Purpura may occur, usually associated with thrombocytopenia. Mucosal ulcers, affecting mouth and genitalia, occur in active SLE but settle in remission, unlike skin lesions which may persist.

Cardiovascular features

Pericarditis frequently occurs during acute exacerbations of the disease. Myocardial disease is common in SLE, and may lead to arrhythmias and, uncommonly, to cardiac failure. Hypertension occurs following severe renal involvement. A non-infective endocarditis occurs (Libman-Sacks endocarditis); this most commonly affects the mitral valve and is usually clinically insignificant. Murmurs are frequently heard in SLE, often in the absence of any anatomical proof of endocarditis, and are an unreliable guide to its diagnosis.

A vasculitis may produce scleritis, myocardial infarction, Raynaud's phenomenon, digital ulceration and atrophic skin changes, bowel perforation and chronic leg ulceration. Thrombophlebitis also occurs, and may be recurrent or migratory.

Respiratory system

Pleurisy is common and usually bilateral, and pleuritic pain may remain a problem long after all other evidence of disease activity has regressed. LE cells may be present in pleural fluid and complement levels decreased. Recurrent pneumonitis may occur, with patchy, plate-like atelectasis or diffuse basal infiltration. Loss of lung volume from vascular damage leads to gradual elevation of both hemidiaphragms and restrictive lung defects. The diaphragm may also be affected by a myopathy. Acute pulmonary lesions are responsive to steroid therapy. Bacterial pneumonia is common.

Renal system

Sixty per cent of patients have renal involvement, and its extent and severity significantly affect the patient's prognosis. According to current concepts of immune complex disease, renal involvement probably occurs transiently in the majority of cases. Mesangial deposition of immunoglobulin may be a reversible change. Diffuse proliferative glomerulonephritis often leads to nephrotic syndrome, hypertension and uraemia and the mortality is greater than 60% at three years. Patients with the membranous form of nephritis almost all develop the nephrotic syndrome, but hypertension and uraemia are less frequent.

Nervous system

The importance of neuropsychiatric involvement in SLE has recently become apparent, because of both its prevalence and its association with a poorer prognosis than renal disease. The commonest abnormalities are disorders of mental function and seizures; other manifestations include cranial nerve palsies, chorea, tremor, headache.

CNS involvement is most frequent in well-established cases of lupus, and 50% of patients with renal involvement also have some CNS abnormality. The CNS symptoms are likely to be the result of small vessel vasculitis in the CNS. Peripheral neuropathy may occur and is probably due to vasculitis.

Haematological features

Neutropenia and/or absolute lymphocytopenia is a frequent finding. An autoimmune haemolytic anaemia may antedate the other manifestations of the disease by many years. This responds well to corticosteroids but not to splenectomy. The normochromic anaemia of chronic disease, and the hypochromic anaemia that may accompany drug therapy or bleeding from vasculitis lesions, are more frequent causes of anaemia in SLE than are immune mechanisms.

A low platelet count, with or without demonstrable platelet antibodies, is common and may be sufficiently low to cause all the signs and symptoms of idiopathic thrombocytopenic purpura. Response to splenectomy is good. Lymphadenopathy is common; the pathological changes are those of reactive hyperplasia. Splenomegaly is rarely gross.

Bacterial infection occurs frequently in SLE, and infections with opportunistic organisms are more common in patients on suppressive therapy.

Syndromes related to SLE

Discoid lupus erythematosus

Discoid lupus erythematosus is a chronic skin disease characterised by erythema, scaling, plugging of the sebaceous glands and scarring, often on the cheeks and bridge of the nose. There may be marked alopecia. It is generally benign, but a small proportion of patients do develop systemic disease. A variety of serological abnormalities may be found in otherwise healthy discoid patients, e.g. ANA may be positive.

Mixed connective tissue disease

In a small group of patients, the features of SLE, myositis and systemic sclerosis occur in sequence or concurrently. The original description was of a good prognosis and a low incidence of renal disease. The term 'mixed connective tissue disease' has been proposed for this group. The sera of these patients do not have anti-DNA antibodies, but show both a strongly positive 'speckled' pattern of ANA tests, and antibodies to extractable nuclear antigen, an RNA protein. Whether or not it is clinically useful to so define a group of patients remains a subject of debate.

Antiphospholipid syndrome

High titres of IgG antiphospholipid antibodies identify a population at risk of recurrent arterial and venous thromboses and recurrent abortions. Antiphospholipid syndromes may be primary (not associated with a known underlying disease) or secondary (associated with SLE or another connective tissue disease). The syndrome has a wide spectrum of clinical manifestations; apart from thromboses they include recurrent fetal loss, thrombocytopenia, haemolytic anaemia and transient ischaemic attacks and strokes. Coagulopathy rather than vasculitis appears to be the pathogenetic mechanism.

Drug-induced lupus

A large number of drugs may, in certain individuals, give rise to a syndrome closely resembling SLE, with rashes, fever arthritis, polyserositis and pulmonary manifestations (see Table 23.2, page 985). Steroids are occasionally required to suppress symptoms, even after discontinuing the drug. Circulating ANAs develop in the majority. In drug-induced lupus, anti-DNA antibodies are usually present in low titre, and renal disease is absent in most cases. Furthermore, the disease is usually reversible on stopping the drugs, though up to 70% of patients with hydralazine-induced lupus have a more prolonged course.

Management

The high incidence of emotional and neuropsychiatric problems, together with the unpredictability of the disease, call for particularly sympathetic care of patients with SLE. There is no evidence that treatment during periods of remission alters the long-term prognosis, and it is usual policy not to treat patients in remission with normal complement levels.

Chloroquine salts should be considered before corticosteroids in patients where the skin and joint manifestations predominate, although many of the joint symptoms respond to salicylates alone. The possibility of retinal damage by chloroquine must be borne in mind. Local application of steroids can be helpful for rashes. Effective sun screens should be used routinely on light-exposed skin.

Measures designed to help prevent a relapse include the avoidance of sunlight and all non-essential drugs, and prompt treatment of infections. Regular measurement of anti-DNA antibodies will often show a rise preceding clinical relapse.

In the management of active SLE, prednisone dosage should be the lowest sufficient to control symptoms and signs. Some features, such as pericarditis or haemolytic anaemia, respond well to corticosteroids. Others, particularly CNS manifestations, are difficult to manage. It is now realised that the steroid dose may be fairly rapidly reduced once the acute episode is over, and most patients are maintained on dosages of 10 mg daily or less. There is evidence that immunosuppressive drugs, e.g. azathioprine or cyclophosphamide, are of value. Most controlled studies have been of patients with renal lupus, where it appears that the combination of prednisone with an immunosuppressive drug is superior to the use of either drug alone.

Prognosis

Unless there is severe renal or CNS involvement, the outlook in SLE is now much improved. The estimated five year survival is now over 90%. There is no contra-indication to pregnancy in a patient who is in reasonable remission and who has good renal function.

For those with renal disease, however, the prognosis is less good; the outlook for diffuse proliferative nephritis is poor, with a five year survival of around 50%. Causes of death in SLE include renal failure and sepsis. There is an increased mortality from the complications of atherosclerosis in later years; corticosteroids probably predispose to atheroma.

Pregnancy in SLE

Fertility is normal, except when there is severe renal involvement or when high-dose steroid therapy causes amenorrhoea. Recurrent abortion can occur before or during the clinical course of SLE; this may be due to the presence of anticardiolipin antibodies. Although remission of the disease occurs in 30% of patients, an exacerbation may occur at any time during pregnancy. A postpartum deterioration is common, and may occur very early after delivery. Patients with active renal disease have a much worse prognosis; they seldom become pregnant and the fetal mortality is around 30%. Increasing proteinuria and hypertension may mimic pre-eclamptic toxaemia.

Neonatal SLE is uncommon; it may be associated with a lupus rash, anaemia, thrombocytopenia, splenomegaly and cardiac conduction abnormalities. The complication occurs almost exclusively in the offspring of women with anti-Ro antibodies.

SYSTEMIC SCLEROSIS

Systemic sclerosis is an uncommon multisystem disorder caused by fibrosis of connective tissue throughout the body. It is three times more common in women than men, and its peak age of onset is between the third and fifth decades. *Scleroderma* is the name used for the fibrosis and hardening of the skin but, occasionally, patients have limited or absent skin involvement.

Aetiology and pathology

There are familial cases reported suggesting that genetic and environmental factors may be important in the aeti-

ology of systemic sclerosis. Chromosomal abnormalities have been reported, and there are weak associations with HLA antigens DR3 and DR5.

There is extensive deposition of collagen in the skin, internal organs and blood vessels. The sequential changes of inflammation, fibrosis and atrophy are most frequent in the skin, but occur to a lesser extent in the gut, heart, lungs and kidneys.

The widespread vascular changes involve both small and medium-sized arteries as well as arterioles and capillaries, and the relationship between the fibrosis and vascular abnormalities remains to be determined. The characteristic changes include concentric proliferation and thickening of the intima, with fibrosis of the adventitia. The capillary abnormalities can be seen at the nail fold. Raynaud's phenomenon occurs in up to 90% of patients.

Classification of scleroderma

Scleroderma-like changes occur in diseases other than systemic sclerosis, e.g. carcinoid syndrome, and systemic sclerosis varies from a mild, limited disease with a good prognosis to a severe disease with diffuse skin involvement and a high risk of renal disease.

The *CRST syndrome* is a benign variant associated with calcinosis (C), Raynaud's phenomenon (R), sclerodactyly of the fingers (S), telangiectasiae (T) and sometimes also oesophageal involvement.

Localised forms of scleroderma include *morphoea* where there are discrete cutaneous plaques of induration, sometimes yellowish in colour and often with violaceous borders; and linear scleroderma, where a band of fibrosis may involve subcutaneous tissue, muscle and even bone (Table 23.31). These localised forms are rarely associated with systemic disease and are usually self-limiting:

- *Sclerodema* is a painless self-limiting oedema of the face, neck and upper trunk which occurs in children.

Table 23.31 Classification of scleroderma

Classification	Example
Localised	Morphoea Linear scleroderma
Generalised	With diffuse visceral involvement CRST syndrome Overlap with other connective tissue disease
Chemical or drug-induced scleroderma	Polyvinylchloride Bleomycin
Diseases with skin changes mimicking scleroderma	Scleroderma
Eosinophilic fasciitis	

- *Eosinophilic fasciitis* is a rare disorder associated with acute swelling and thickening of forearms and legs, often following trauma or unaccustomed exercise. There is eosinophilia, a high ESR associated with a typical histological appearance. This condition responds to corticosteroids.

Clinical features

Skin involvement

There are three stages in evolution of the skin disease. Firstly, there is an oedematous phase associated with bilateral painless oedema of hands, legs and face. This is followed by thickening and tightening of the skin affecting the fingers, face and hands and spreading sometimes to involve the limbs and trunk. Finally, atrophy occurs and limb contractures can occur, often with areas of hyperpigmentation, vitiligo and alopecia. The face becomes pinched, microstomia develops, and telangiectasiae are seen on face, lips, mouth, palms and nail folds. There is intracutaneous and subcutaneous calcification which affects the fingertips and may also affect the forearm; this may ulcerate.

Raynaud's phenomenon may precede cutaneous changes by many years. It occurs in many connective tissue disorders, and the risk of patients with Raynaud's developing systemic sclerosis is less than 2% in females and about 6% in males. In severe disease, there may be ischaemic changes of the fingertips and gangrene may develop.

Musculoskeletal involvement

Tendon involvement leads to friction rubs and flexion contractures. Arthralgia and arthritis are often early features of systemic sclerosis; the arthritis can be erosive and progressive. Muscle weakness and wasting is common, and muscle biopsy shows deposition of collagen and myofibrillar degeneration; florid inflammation is uncommon.

Gastrointestinal involvement

After the skin, the gut is the most common organ to be involved. The oesophagus is frequently affected, and barium swallow shows decreased or absent peristalsis with oesophageal dilatation. The commonest clinical complaint is of dysphagia for solid foods and heartburn, but the patient can be asymptomatic. The small bowel is involved in about 50% of patients, causing symptoms from intestinal stasis or malabsorption. Large bowel involvement is fairly common but usually asymptomatic; wide-mouthed colonic diverticulae are characteristic in the condition.

Other clinical features

Cardiac abnormalities include conduction defects, pericarditis and cardiomyopathy; these are often asymptomatic. Renal involvement is the major cause of death in systemic sclerosis, the onset being acute or chronic. Chronic renal failure is associated with proteinuria and hypertension. Acute renal disease presents with malignant hypertension, rapid renal failure and microangiopathic haemolytic anaemia. Pulmonary complications, which occur in 50% of patients, include interstitial fibrosis, pleurisy and pulmonary hypertension.

Antinuclear antibodies are positive in about 70% of patients; a nucleolar or speckled pattern of fluorescence is characteristic. Anticentromere antibodies occur in patients with the CRST syndrome. Anti-Scl-70 antibodies are present in 20% of scleroderma patients. The antigen has recently been identified as a topoisomerase enzyme.

Management

No treatment has been shown to alter the long-term progression of systemic sclerosis. The natural tendency of the disease is towards skin softening, which complicates the assessment of new treatments. D-penicillamine may have some therapeutic effect, and is commonly used.

Oesophagitis due to oesophageal involvement responds to antacids and H_2-antagonists. Strictures of the gastro-oesophageal junction may require surgery or dilatation. In patients with hypertension, control of blood pressure improves survival. Raynaud's phenomenon may be particularly troublesome. Patients should be told to avoid both smoking and exposure to cold. Nifedipine can be helpful, as can thymoxamine. Prostaglandin infusions can improve peripheral blood supply in severe Raynaud's.

DERMATOMYOSITIS AND POLYMYOSITIS

Polymyositis is an inflammatory disease of muscle which may occur either alone or in association with another connective tissue disease. It is characterised by symmetrical proximal muscle weakness, and when associated with a rash, the term *dermatomyositis* is used. Polymyositis is less common than SLE, and of similar frequency to systemic sclerosis. Both dermatomyositis and polymyositis may occur in childhood and there is an association with underlying malignancy in a minority of cases. Peak ages of onset are in childhood and in the fifth and sixth decades.

Aetiology

The aetiology of polymyositis is unknown. Several viruses, including rubella, influenza and Coxsackie, can cause acute myositis, and cellular immunological mechanisms are also implicated. Cytotoxic lymphocytes from patients have been shown to kill muscle cells. There is a weak association with HLA-B8 and DR3. A number of autoantibodies have been detected including Jo-1; sera with anti-Jo-1 activity bind histidyl-t-RNA and block its aminoacylation. Jo-1 is associated with myositis and pulmonary involvement.

Clinical features

The hallmark of polymyositis is progressive proximal muscle weakness, often insidious in onset. In severe acute forms, there is muscle pain and tenderness, but there is usually little pain. Typical presenting features are difficulty in climbing stairs and weakness of the neck muscles. There may be dysphagia and weakness of the respiratory muscles and, with progressive disease, muscle wasting and muscle contractures. Arthralgia occurs in about 25% of patients but is usually mild. Fever may be present.

Cutaneous features include oedema and erythema and a characteristic rash causing a lilac (heliotrope) discolouration of the eyelids and periorbital oedema. A scaly erythematous rash involves the dorsum of the hands, knuckles and extensor surfaces of other joints. Long-standing disease is associated with skin deposits of calcium, which can present as nodules that may ulcerate. Calcinosis of subcutaneous tissue and fascial planes between muscles can occur, particularly in children. Vasculitis may involve the skin and internal organs, especially the gastrointestinal tract. Involvement of cardiac muscle can cause arrythmias and congestive cardiac failure. Pulmonary problems can be severe. Weakness of the respiratory muscles may result in breathlessness and ventilatory failure. Weakness of upper airway musculature combined with disordered swallowing predispose to aspiration, and impaired cough predisposes to pneumonia. Fibrosing alveolitis may also occur.

An underlying malignancy is present in up to 20% of adults, particularly with dermatomyositis, and treatment can lead to resolution of the skin and muscle changes. The commonest neoplasms are carcinoma of the bronchus, breast, stomach and ovary.

Investigation

The most important investigations are serum muscle enzyme measurements, electromyography (EMG) and muscle biopsy. Any one of these investigations may be normal, even during active disease. The creatine phosphokinase (CPK) is usually the most sensitive muscle enzyme to measure, and may be used in following the course of the disease. Serial measurement of muscle strength can also be useful in assessing progress.

EMG abnormalities are well described and are useful in establishing the diagnosis and in distinguishing between myositis and steroid myopathy. Muscle biopsy changes include necrosis, muscle fibre regeneration and lymphocytic infiltration.

A search for underlying cancer should be made in adults over the age of 50 with dermatomyositis. The skin and muscle disease may, however, appear one to two years before the cancer is apparent.

Management

Corticosteroids usually control the disease, and are given initially in dosages of 40–60 mg of prednisolone daily. Immunosuppressive therapy with azathioprine, methotrexate or cyclophosphamide is frequently used, particularly if the disease is difficult to control with steroids. Treatment may be required for years. Plasma exchange has been used but without clear evidence of benefit.

VASCULITIS

The vasculitides are characterised by inflammation of blood vessels. They are commonly classified on the basis of vessel size and histology (Table 23.32).

Giant cell arteritis is common in the elderly, but many of the other vasculitides are uncommon; the most frequent are those associated with the connective tissue diseases and drug hypersensitivity. Biopsy is central to the diagnosis, and the changes reflect a spectrum ranging from pure arteritis without granuloma formation to pure granulomatosis without vasculitis. Thus, PAN and the arteritis of RA are at one end of the spectrum, while

Table 23.32 Classification of vasculitis

Group 1
Systemic necrotising arteritis involving small and medium-sized arteries
Polyarteritis nodosa
Wegener's granulomatosis
Kawasaki's disease
Arteritis of connective tissue disease
Group 2
Small vessel vasculitis
Henoch-Schönlein purpura
Essential mixed cryoglobulinaemia
Vasculitis of connective tissue disease
Group 3
Giant cell or Large artery arteritis
Temporal arteritis
Takayasu's arteritis

rheumatoid nodules and midline granulomata are at the other.

POLYARTERITIS NODOSA

PAN is a systemic necrotising arteritis which may be associated with cutaneous as well as systemic features (p. 1144). The disease affects men more frequently than women.

Pathology

Muscular arteries throughout the body are affected, particularly in the kidneys, heart, gastrointestinal tract and peripheral nervous system. All layers of the vessel wall are affected, and acute vasculitis is associated with fibrinoid necrosis and an inflammatory infiltrate of predominantly polymorphonuclear leucocytes. Multiple aneurysm formation is common. Chronicity of the lesion leads to fibrosis and narrowing of the vessel lumen with thrombosis.

The vascular lesions may be due to local deposition of immune complexes, and a similar disorder can be produced in animals by intravenous immunisation. Some cases may be associated with hepatitis B infection.

Clinical features and diagnosis

Systemic features include fever, myalgia and weight loss (Table 23.33), and these may be the presenting complaint. Cutaneous features include peripheral gangrene, rashes and livedo reticularis. The commonest neurological manifestation is mononeuritis multiplex. Renal involvement is common; the clinical features include haematuria, loin pain, acute and chronic renal failure and hypertension. Abdominal pain is a common presenting symptom and may reflect severe arteritic involvement. Articular features are usually mild.

The diagnosis is made on the basis of typical multi-system disease features. There is frequently anaemia, leucocytosis and a raised ESR. Angiography may demonstrate microaneurysms, especially in renal arteries and the

Table 23.33 Relative incidence of features of polyarteritis

Clinical feature	Incidence (%)
Systemic symptoms (fever weight loss)	80
Renal	75
Arthritis/myalgia	60
Cutaneous	55
Neurological	50
Abdominal	45

coeliac axis. Arteritis can also be detected in about 50% of renal biopsies, and rectal or sural nerve biopsies may also be diagnostic.

Management

Untreated the prognosis is poor. Prompt treatment with corticosteroids and immunosuppressive drugs, initially given intravenously, is associated with an improved prognosis. The prognosis improves markedly after the first three months, and most patients do not have further attacks after the first year.

KAWASAKI'S DISEASE

Kawasaki's disease (mucocutaneous lymph node syndrome; see also p. 1127) is a rare acute systemic illness of infants and children, characterised by fever, exanthematous rash, mucous membrane involvement, conjunctival congestion and cervical lymphadenopathy. There is a necrotising arteritis, and coronary arteritis can be detected angiographically in up to 60% of cases. The disease is usually self-limiting, although sudden death may be caused by acute myocardial ischaemia resulting from coronary artery occlusion, myocarditis or aneurysm rupture.

CHURG-STRAUSS DISEASE

Churg and Strauss described a vasculitic syndrome that differed from PAN in that pulmonary vessels were frequently affected. Patients have a history of allergy, and asthma develops in adult life. The high frequency of pulmonary symptoms, peripheral eosinophilia and the absence or mildness of the renal disease help to distinguish the disease from PAN (p. 496).

WEGENER'S GRANULOMATOSIS

Wegener's granulomatosis is often classified separately from the other systemic arteritides, because of the severity of pulmonary, sinus and nasopharyngeal symptoms in this condition. However, vasculitis is a common feature and the range of the vessels involved is similar to that seen in Churg-Strauss syndrome. Wegener's granulomatosis is discussed in Chapter 13, page 505 and Chapter 20, page 823.

SMALL VESSEL VASCULITIS

Small vessel vasculitis is a feature of a number of different disorders including the connective tissue diseases. A number of distinct clinical syndromes are characterised by small vessel vasculitis including Henoch-Schönlein purpura and cryoglobulinaemic vasculitis.

A characteristic feature of small vessel vasculitis is a nonthrombocytopenic purpura which is caused by inflammation of small cutaneous capillaries, particularly in dependent parts of the body. Disease features include purpura, haematuria, polyarthritis, abdominal pain and peripheral neuropathy. The progress of this type of vasculitis is influenced by the underlying disease process, but these vasculitides are often self-limiting.

GIANT CELL ARTERITIS AND POLYMYALGIA RHEUMATICA

Giant cell arteritis predominantly affects elderly patients. It is often associated with polymyalgia rheumatica. Although almost any large artery may be involved, the majority of clinical signs and symptoms result from involvement of the carotid artery or its branches.

Both polymyalgia rheumatica and giant cell arteritis are more common in the elderly and in women. The incidence is probably about 1 in 10 000. Giant cell arteritis and polymyalgia are well-recognised in the UK and in Scandinavia. In the USA, most reports derive from Northern states, few cases are reported from Southern states or in blacks, but the diseases are recognisable worldwide.

Aetiology and pathology

The aetiology of polymyalgia and temporal arteritis is unknown. The constitutional features suggest a viral infection, and many patients notice a distinct prodromal illness resembling influenza. There is little evidence of primary muscle disease in polymyalgia. Muscle biopsy shows only mild atrophic changes and the EMG is normal. Muscle enzymes are not elevated.

Giant cell arteritis affects large and medium-sized arteries and involvement is patchy, 'skip lesions' often being found. The arteritis is a panarteritis with giant cell granuloma formation, often in close relationship to a disrupted internal elastic lamina. The gross features are not characteristic. The vessels are enlarged and nodular, having little or no lumen due to marked intimal proliferation.

There may be widespread vasculitis, with involvement of the aorta and its branches, the abdominal vessels and the heart. The pulmonary and renal vessels and the small arterioles are generally not involved, and this may be useful in differentiating between this condition and PAN.

Clinical features

Giant cell arteritis

Headache is common and may be either a non-specific tension type, or well localised, severe, continuous and with associated scalp tenderness. There can be pain in the face on chewing, due to claudication from facial artery involvement. Tingling in the tongue, and loss of taste and pain in the mouth and throat can also occur, presumably due to vascular insufficiency. Infarction of the skin can rarely occur.

The great danger, particularly but not exclusively in patients with symptoms of arteritis, is sudden irreversible blindness. This may be preceded by transient visual disturbances, e.g. field defects. Blindness results from ischaemic optic neuritis caused by arteritis of the posterior ciliary and branches of the ophthalmic arteries. The ocular complications usually occur within weeks or months of the onset of systemic manifestations of the disease. If temporal arteritis is suspected, steroid therapy, in adequate dosage, should be started immediately before further investigation of the patient in order to protect sight. The blindness is irreversible and often bilateral, and loss of sight in the second eye may follow within hours of the first.

Arteritis can involve the carotid, vertebral, meningeal and, rarely, the intracerebral vessels, leading to hemiplegia, epilepsy or focal vertebral or occipital lobe lesions. Aortic involvement can lead to an aortic arch syndrome; aortic aneurysm is rare.

The amount of constitutional upset is variable, but lassitude, arthralgia, anorexia, weight loss, a low-grade fever and depression are all common. A transient synovitis can occur, particularly in the knee and often with an effusion. The systemic features can be vague and easily overlooked; conversely, they can be striking.

Polymyalgia rheumatica

Approximately 50% of patients have features of polymyalgia rheumatica. The initial symptoms of polymyalgia rheumatica may be sudden, with pain and severe stiffness of proximal muscles and periarticular tissues. Stiffness is usually the predominant feature; this is particularly severe after rest, and may prevent the patient getting out of bed in the morning. The muscular pain is often diffuse, and worse after resting. The musculoskeletal symptoms are almost always bilateral and there is tenderness of muscle and periarticular structures.

There is often little to find on examination of patients with polymyalgia rheumatica, although anaemia and obvious weight loss are quite frequent. The muscles may be tender, but there is no muscle weakness. Classically, when the temporal artery is involved, the vessel is thickened and tender, with absent pulsation, but usually the signs are limited to diminished or absent pulsation, perhaps with tenderness of the scalp. Tenderness in areas distant from arteries may be present even when the vessels are clinically normal. Bruits are often present over large arteries and there may be tenderness, particularly over the subclavian; these are presumably due to arteritis as they disappear with treatment.

Investigation

Investigations in polymyalgia and giant cell arteritis are essentially normal apart from a high ESR and increases in the acute phase proteins. The ESR is usually at least 70 mm/hour and is often over 100 mm/hour, particularly if arteritis is present: this provides a useful means of monitoring treatment. A normal ESR does not exclude the diagnosis.

Anaemia, usually of a mild hypochromic type, is common and resolves without specific treatment, but a marked normocytic anaemia occasionally occurs and may be responsible for presenting symptoms.

Abnormalities of thyroid and liver function have been described. Hypothyroidism or hyperthyroidism can occur. Raised serum values for alkaline phosphatase are found in 20% of patients. Liver biopsy specimens may show portal and intralobular inflammation, with focal liver cell necrosis and small epithelioid cell granulomas.

Temporal artery biopsy is the most important diagnostic procedure, but, in view of the patchy nature of the arteritis, a negative biopsy does not exclude the disease. Steroids reduce the inflammatory infiltrate within days, so temporal artery biopsy should be carried out before treatment is started if possible, but if there is any delay, then steroids should be started immediately, in order to prevent visual complications.

Diagnosis

The diagnosis of polymyalgia rheumatica is initially one of exclusion. The differential diagnosis (Table 23.34) in elderly patients with muscle pain, stiffness and a raised ESR is wide because the prodromal phases of several serious conditions can mimic it. In practice, non-specific clinical features and the frequent absence of physical signs makes diagnosis difficult.

Management

Most of the symptoms of polymyalgia rheumatica are improved with salicylates or other anti-inflammatory agents. However, these drugs do not control the under-

Table 23.34 Differential diagnosis of polymyalgia rheumatica

• Neoplasm	• Lymphoma
• Connective tissue disease	• Polymyositis
• Multiple myeloma	• Dermatomyositis
• Leukaemia	• Myopathy

lying arteritis or stop the development of vascular complications. Corticosteroids dramatically relieve myalgic symptoms and suppress the arteritis, and are used in almost every case of polymyalgia.

It is rarely necessary to exceed 20 mg of prednisolone to control the myalgic symptoms, the ESR being used to titrate the dosage. In proven arteritis, doses of 40 mg of prednisolone usually suppress the disease. The dramatic response to steroid therapy supports the diagnosis. Patients must be reviewed regularly for exacerbations of the disease or for the development of arteritis and the steroid dosage adjusted accordingly. Once there is no clinical evidence of disease activity, the steroids can be gradually discontinued, but recurrences are common, sometimes many years later.

TAKAYASU'S ARTERITIS

Takayasu's arteritis is a large vessel arteritis in which giant cells are rarely detected. It is a rare disease, predominantly of young women. Features include systemic symptoms, with weight loss and fever. The arteritis involves the aortic arch and its branches, and the inflammation results in stenosis, which may be demonstrated angiographically. Features of arterial stenosis include dizziness, fainting, exertional dyspnoea and reduced or absent peripheral pulses. The acute symptoms may respond to steroid therapy, but vascular reconstruction may be helpful in later stages of the disease.

LOW BACK PAIN

Although back pain results in the loss of millions of working days each year, most individuals recover without medical attention. Of the small proportion of people who consult a general practitioner, only a very small proportion ultimately undergo surgery.

Anatomy and biomechanics

The spine is a weight-bearing structure. Movement occurs at the apophyseal joints, which are synovial, and at the intervertebral discs. These structures are closely related, and disease or deformity of one often affects the other. In the lumbar spine, the apophyseal joints resemble a mortise and tenon arrangement, which provides strength at the expense of mobility. There is very little rotation, and flexion is 45° (Fig. 23.20).

Lumbar disc lesions usually cause root syndromes, because the spinal cord ends at L2. The lumbar nerve root exits high in its foramen, and is usually above a prolapsing disc which compresses the nerve root passing to the interspace immediately below.

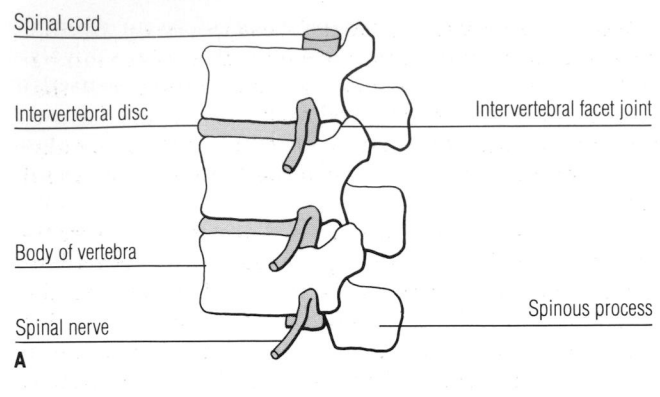

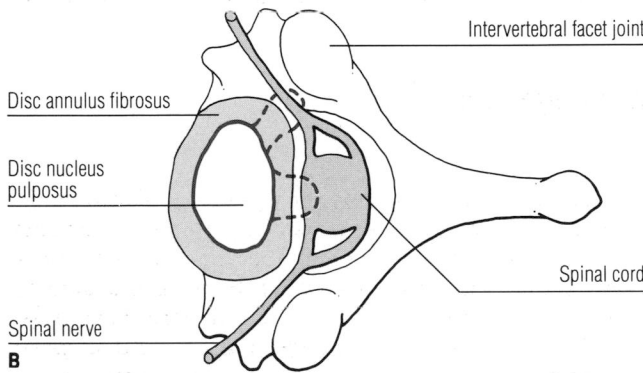

Fig. 23.20 Diagram showing the position of the nerve roots and spinal nerve in relation to skeletal structures. A. Lateral aspect of the lumbar spine. **B.** Superior aspect of a cervical vertebra. The precise position of the union of the ventral and dorsal nerve roots, to form the spinal nerve, in the intervertebral foramen is a little variable. Dotted lines indicate the usual sites of disc herniation.

Pain fibres are present within the spinal ligaments, in the apophyseal joint capsules, in the periosteum at the fascial and tendon attachments and in blood vessels, but only in the outer layers of the intervertebral discs. Pain is produced by pressure on these structures from disc protrusions, osteophytes or trauma. The healthy nucleus pulposus behaves like a gel, and distributes pressure equally in all directions. With age, this property declines, and localised points of high pressure develop. The pressures within the discs are increased most by lifting whilst bending forwards or sitting.

Pathology

Disc protrusions usually occur posterolaterally, because here the annulus fibrosus is no longer reinforced by the posterior longitudinal ligament. Occasionally, pain is produced when there is a tear in the annulus but no protrusion. Disc lesions heal by fibrosis but there is always a risk of recurrence. Degenerative changes are present in the intervertebral discs of all subjects by middle-age. These are more marked, and occur earlier,

after disc prolapse. There is a direct relationship between the degree of disc degeneration, osteophyte formation on the margins of vertebral bodies and apophyseal joint changes, suggesting that disc degeneration is the primary event leading to degenerative spondylosis.

Aetiology

The mechanical and non-mechanical causes of backache are listed in Table 23.35. A detailed history and examination, with the appropriate laboratory studies, usually identifies non-mechanical causes (Table 23.36). The age groups at particular risk are listed in Table 23.37. In general practice, it is people between the ages of 50 and 60 that attend most commonly with low back pain.

Clinical features

History

Mechanical and inflammatory back pain must be differentiated: the former is exacerbated by movement and improved by rest, while the latter is associated with stiffness after rest. These distinctions are not absolute, since inflammation involves some local swelling (i.e. mechanical change) and trauma generates some inflammation.

Table 23.35 Causes of backache

Cause	Example
Mechanical	Prolapsed intervertebral disc
	Apophyseal osteoarthritis
	Ankylosing hyperostosis
	Spinal stenosis
	Spondylolisthesis and other congenital abnormalities
	Scheuermann's osteochondritis
	Fractures
	Non-specific
Inflammatory	Ankylosing spondylitis and related seronegative spondylarthritides
	Rheumatoid arthritis
	Infection
Neoplastic	Bone – primary or secondary
	Spinal tumours
Metabolic	Osteoporosis
	Osteomalacia
	Ochronosis
	Chondrocalcinosis
Paget's disease	
Referred	Pelvic/abdominal disease
	Posture
Depression	

Table 23.36 Clinical features of low back pain

Feature	History	Examination
Mechanical	Precipitating strain Previous episodes Unilateral leg/buttock pain Worse on movement and coughing Eased by rest	Asymmetrical restriction of movement and of straight leg raise Uniradicular signs
Systemic disease	Constant or progressive Worse on rest or at night Morning stiffness Bilateral or alternating pain Systemic illness Diffuse pain and tenderness	Features of ill health Rigid lumbar spine Symmetrical restriction of movement and straight leg raise Multiradicular signs Other neurological signs Wasting of paraspinal muscles High ESR
Non-specific	Postural factors Depression Gynaecological symptoms Diffuse pain	Normal movement Local tenderness

Table 23.37 Causes of low back pain related to specific age groups

Age group (years)	Cause of pain
Children	Osteochondritis (Scheuermann's disease) Scoliosis – primary or secondary
15–30	Ankylosing spondylitis Prolapsed intervertebral disc and fractures Spondylolisthesis Postural pain from pregnancy
30–50	Degenerative joint disease Prolapsed intervertebral disc Malignancy
50 and over	Degenerative joint disease Osteoporosis Paget's disease Malignancy

Back pain also occurs when bone is affected by tumour, infection or metabolic disease. The patient experiences unremitting pain, which is worse at night and exacerbated by movement.

Examination

The way in which a patient moves should be noted. Painful conditions can cause scoliosis through a protective muscle spasm. Sometimes this is only present on forward flexion, whereas secondary scoliosis (e.g. that caused by unequal leg length) disappears on flexion. Inflammatory conditions cause flattening of the lumbar lordosis. Patients with degenerative disease and disc lesions typically have restricted back movements, but with limitation of lateral flexion to one side; whereas, in ankylosing spondylitis, there is bilateral limitation of lateral flexion.

Neurological examination identifies nerve root irritation. Straight-leg raising is performed with the patient supine. The sciatic nerve is stretched by raising the straight leg until this becomes painful; a restriction to 45° or less indicates significant root irritation. The femoral stretch test is often misinterpreted. Root irritation is present if pain is produced in the anterior thigh on flexing the knee, with the patient *prone*.

Investigation

Radiology

Plain radiographs of the lumbar spine are of little diagnostic help. Radiographs are normal in 25% of patients with disc prolapse confirmed at operation, in early ankylosing spondylitis and early metastases. Bone density appears unchanged until 50% of the mineral has disappeared. In contrast, marked degenerative and disc space changes can be present in the absence of any symptoms or can easily be falsely interpreted as the cause of symptoms. In localised bone disease, isotope scanning is often helpful.

CT scans and MRI scans are increasingly used as the investigations of choice. The accuracy that can be obtained with MRI and CT scans is such that radiculography is seldom necessary. Intravenous gadolinium can enhance the contrast, allowing differentiation between residual disc material and granulation tissue resulting from a previous surgical procedure.

Laboratory investigations

Only simple screening tests are usually required (Table 23.38). The ESR is the most useful.

Prolapsed intervertebral disc

Only a few patients with back pain have a disc prolapse and the condition is often diagnosed erroneously. The diagnosis is *unlikely* if there is:

- no evidence of nerve root compression
- more than one root involved
- bilateral and symmetrical nerve involvement
- diffuse pain and tenderness
- unremitting pain, worse on resting at night.

The leg symptoms and signs are the result of pressure on the dura mater and nerve roots. Straining or sneezing

Table 23.38 Radiological and laboratory findings in back pain

Cause of back pain	Radiological features	ESR	Calcium	Phosphate	Alk. Phos.
Mechanical	Normal or degenerative changes	N	N	N	N
Inflammatory	Sacro-iliitis Osteomyelitis Psoas abscess	↑	N	N	N
Neoplastic	Osteolytic or sclerotic deposits Vertebral collapse	↑	N or ↑	N	↑
Osteoporosis	Reduced bone density Vertebral collapse	N	N	N	N
Osteomalacia	Osteoid seams Reduced bone density	N	↓ or N	↓	↑
Paget's disease	Sclerosis and expansion of bone	N	N	N	↑↑

exacerbate disc pain by raising pressure within the spinal canal. A central protrusion may cause cauda equina compression, with saddle-shaped sacral anaesthesia, flaccid paralysis of the legs and sphincter involvement (usually urinary retention). This constitutes a surgical emergency. The presenting symptoms may be no more than impairment of urethral sensation. Early surgical exploration is indicated to preserve sphincter control (p. 939).

Back pain or sciatica is very occasionally caused by a cauda equina tumour. Diagnosis is difficult, but bladder or bowel symptoms, impotence, and wasting of the legs require urgent investigation.

Management

The causes of back pain are not well understood and treatment is largely empirical. Prophylactic exercises, advice on future activities and general back care should form the basis of management. However, for more severe back pain, treatment may include bed rest, traction, manipulation, the wearing of a surgical corset and surgery.

Mechanical back pain

Complete prolonged bed rest, usually no more than one week, and analgesics successfully treat most cases of mechanical back pain. The mattress should be firm (boards can be placed underneath), and muscle relaxants may help. After a period of immobilisation, exercises are started gradually. Isometric exercises (sometimes combined with traction) give better results than active mobilising exercises (which increase the load on the lumbar spine). A surgical corset may be useful if there is residual pain.

Traction. Although symptoms are often relieved during traction, there is no evidence that it improves the rate of recovery. Patients with root pain, who find that it is relieved by lying down, benefit most from traction. It is seldom effective in chronic back pain or severe sciatica with neurological signs.

Manipulation can help in both acute and chronic low back pain. Unfortunately, one cannot identify in advance those patients who will respond. Trials suggest that manipulation gives significant immediate benefit but, after one to two weeks, manipulated and non-manipulated groups of patients show equal improvement. Manipulation should be restricted to mechanical back pain without neurological involvement or any spinal instability.

Lumbar supports probably act not so much by immobilising the spine as by raising the intra-abdominal pressure, so that some body load is transmitted through the abdomen, rather than through the spine. They can be helpful if:

- the patient remains ambulant
- heat and intermittent traction are ineffective
- manipulation is contraindicated
- bed rest has not relieved pain
- back pain recurs in spite of prophylactic exercises and back care.

The spinal support should be worn continuously during the acute episode, and then during the day for several weeks. However, it is important to avoid dependence, and trunk muscle bulk must be maintained during immobilisation by static and then active exercises. Prophylactic use during hard physical work and long car journeys is recommended.

Epidural injections of local anaesthetic and steroid may reduce pain and allow a patient to return to work earlier. The main indications are chronic sciatica, and sciatica with root interruption. This presents as severe pain unrelieved by rest. It improves spontaneously after several days, but an epidural injection can give immediate relief. The benefit may result from the anti-inflammatory action of the steroid, or by the large volume of fluid freeing adhesions around nerve roots.

Chemonucleolysis. An injection of chymopapain into the nucleus pulposus leads to a reduction in disc size and results in improvement in 80% of selected patients.

Surgical treatment is seldom necessary, unless severe pain either persists in spite of adequate treatment or recurs often, or if neurological signs are progressing. Laminectomy is successful in 80% of selected patients.

General rehabilitation. Patients should be encouraged to resume normal activities, and advised on lifting and bending, exercises, weight control, posture, beds, chairs and the correct height for work surfaces. Prolonged sitting without lumbar support (e.g. by a small cushion or bedrest), stooping and carrying should be avoided. Patients with recurrent pain may have to accept some limitations on their previous activities.

Chronic low back pain. Despite treatment, less than 50% of patients with low back pain of over six months' duration ever return to full employment. A rehabilitation unit may be beneficial; confidence may be increased through a progressive exercise regimen and advice given on employment. Caution and restraint are required when contemplating back surgery.

Other causes of back pain

Degenerative disease of the lumbar spine is accompanied by central low back pain and buttock or thigh pain. Neurological signs are uncommon. Many patients respond to heat and mobilising exercises, while others benefit from gentle manipulation. Surgery is rarely required.

Paget's disease is a common radiographic finding, but not always the cause of symptoms (p. 735).

Metabolic bone disease (Ch. 18). In osteoporosis and osteomalacia, sudden pain may result from compression fractures of the vertebral bodies or from microfractures not visible on the radiograph. Nerve root and cord compression are uncommon, even when there is gross deformity of the spine. Chondrocalcinosis and ochronosis also cause premature disc degeneration and back pain. Patients with any of these conditions should be encouraged to be mobile, since immobility aggravates bone loss.

Short leg syndrome. Differences in leg length of greater than 12.5 mm may lead to the gradual onset of backache (usually in middle-age), which may be initiated by minor trauma. Provided there are no structural changes, correction of discrepancies of greater than 12.5 mm should relieve or prevent pain.

Infections of the spine are uncommon. Early diagnosis can be difficult, as backache may develop insidiously with few signs of systemic illness. Tuberculosis of the spine is an important cause. Both tuberculosis and brucellosis may produce unilateral sacro-iliitis.

Congenital abnormalities are usually identified radiologically. Common abnormalities include spondylolisthesis, spondylolysis, transitional vertebrae, spina bifida and abnormalities of the posterior articular facets. *Spondylolisthesis*, in which there is forward subluxation of the body of one vertebra onto the one below, usually occurs at L5–S1 in athletic adolescent boys. It is usually secondary to *spondylolysis* (a bony defect of the neural arch), which is symptomless by itself. Approximately 70% of patients with spondylolisthesis have back pain, but only 10% have sciatica. Pain usually responds to conservative treatment, including the use of a corset.

Sprung back. Tears in ligaments or paraspinal muscles cause acute localised pain and tenderness. Pain is often exacerbated by lifting or by a period of inactivity and may radiate to the buttocks. There are no articular or dural signs.

Neoplastic disease. Persistent pain, particularly at night, with associated tenderness should always be investigated. A bone scan may confirm the presence of metastases before there are any radiological changes. Vertebral collapse may precipitate root pain, and intraspinal tumours may mimic prolapsed disc. However, there are a number of distinguishing features: no response to treatment, progressing neurological signs, sphincter disturbance, multiple root involvement, nocturnal pain and pain unrelated to exercise, presence of an upper motor neurone lesion and signs of ill health. Bony metastases are much commoner than primary intraspinal tumours of the vertebral column, particularly from carcinomas of the breast, bronchus, kidney and thyroid (all osteolytic), or of the prostate (osteosclerotic). Primary bone tumours are rare.

Spinal stenosis. Variations in the size and shape of the spinal canal are common. Narrowing can result in pressure on the spinal cord or on nerve roots, or can leave less space to accommodate a prolapse or osteophytes.

Scheuermann's osteochondritis occurs in adolescent males and causes a dull ache in the lower thoracic region. Radiographs are diagnostic. They show fragmentation of the vertebral epiphysial end-plates and, later on, narrowing of the disc space and wedging of the vertebrae, producing a smooth kyphosis. The cause is unknown.

Ankylosing hyperostosis. In this syndrome, bony spurs usually form on the anterolateral aspect of several dorsolumbar vertebral bodies and fuse to form bridges. There is progressive stiffening of the spine but little pain or disability.

Psychological factors are important in chronic back pain. Such pain is common in patients who are unhappy at work or at home. In many of these patients, no overt psychiatric symptoms are present, and they may prove very difficult to treat.

Compensation neurosis. Some patients develop symptoms following an accident that are totally resistant to treatment, and which may remain even after the claim has been settled.

SOFT TISSUE RHEUMATISM

Lesions of tendons and their sheaths, fasciae, bursae, joint capsules and the tenoperiosteal junction (the enthesis) cause much morbidity and loss in productivity. They constitute a significant proportion of the workload of general practices and hospital accident, orthopaedic and rheumatology departments. As biopsy and surgery are rarely employed in their diagnosis and treatment, histological data are scanty and their pathologies are poorly understood. While there are adequate anatomical and clinical features to allow identification of individual conditions, diagnosis is often imprecise and management remains largely empirical.

Any or all of these lesions may occur in association with overt systemic disease, as, for example, in inflammatory arthritis or infection. A large proportion, however, occur in the absence of systemic disease. In these circumstances, local causes, such as chronic repetitive low-grade trauma, or excessive and unaccustomed use either at work or at play, may be responsible. These factors may also cause partial interruption of the blood supply, resulting in incomplete attempts at healing and degeneration; this renders these structures more vulnerable in the middle-aged and elderly, in whom these lesions predominate.

Classification

Conditions can be divided into generalised and localised.

Table 23.39 Generalised soft tissue lesions

With evidence of inflammation
Polymyalgia rheumatica and cranial arteritis
Prodrome of inflammatory arthropathies and connective tissue diseases
Viral and bacterial infections
Without inflammation
Fibromyalgia
Hypothyroidism
Drug-related painful states associated with steroid withdrawal, chronic barbiturate abuse and the contraceptive pill
Dyskinetic phase of Parkinson's disease
Chronic brucellosis, Bornholm's disease
Associated with malignancy, e.g. myeloma, carcinoma
Osteomalacia
Fibrositis
Associated with weakness
Prodrome of polymyositis or dermatomyositis
Carcinomatous neuromyopathy (some forms)
Hypokalaemic states
Psychogenic rheumatism

Generalised soft tissue lesions

Generalised soft tissue lesions (Table 23.39) may result from underlying disease, and most of the primary conditions can be diagnosed by careful clinical and laboratory assessment. Polymyalgia rheumatica is considered on page 1032.

The diagnosis of *psychogenic rheumatism* must be made with caution and after exclusion of other disease. Chronic pain may itself lead to psychological problems. Several features suggest a psychological illness, including written lists of symptoms, inconsistent or negative physical findings on repeated examinations and inappropriate concern with serious future disability.

Localised soft tissue lesions

The major structures involved in localised soft tissue lesions and the associated lesions are listed in Table 23.40. Examination should permit accurate localisation of the anatomical structure involved. Figure 23.21 shows common sites of soft tissue lesions.

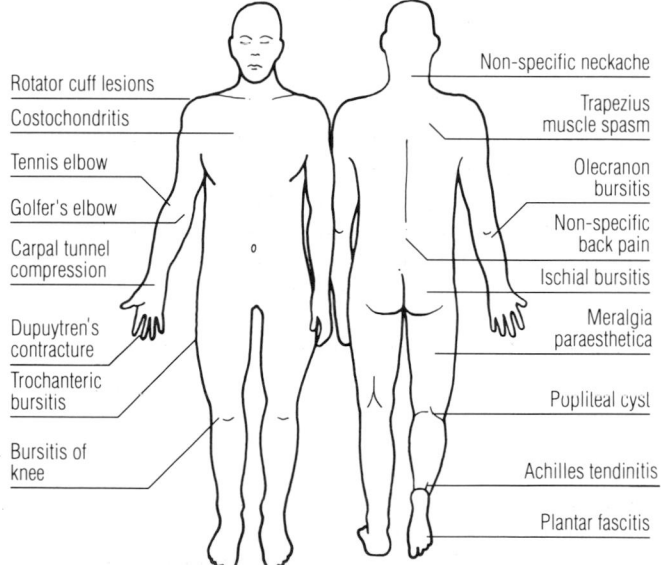

Rotator cuff lesions
Costochondritis
Tennis elbow
Golfer's elbow
Carpal tunnel compression
Dupuytren's contracture
Trochanteric bursitis
Bursitis of knee

Non-specific neckache
Trapezius muscle spasm
Olecranon bursitis
Non-specific back pain
Ischial bursitis
Meralgia paraesthetica
Popliteal cyst
Achilles tendinitis
Plantar fascitis

Fig. 23.21 Common sites of soft tissue lesions.

Table 23.40 Localised soft tissue lesions

Structure	Lesion
Tendons and tendon sheaths	Rupture, degenerative tendinitis, peritendinitis, tenosynovitis, ganglia
Bursae	Bursitis – acute or chronic
Tenoperiosteal junction	Enthesopathies, apophysitis
Fasciae	Fasciitis, Dupuytren's contracture
Ligaments	Sprain, strain, tear

The painful shoulder

More than 90% of lesions causing a painful shoulder result from extracapsular soft tissue lesions. Trauma is often slight or unnoticed. Night pain and inability to lie on the affected shoulder are common to all the lesions, but careful clinical assessment with particular attention to the presence of a painful arc, location of tenderness and manoeuvres that increase pain (Table 23.41) usually permit accurate diagnosis. Bony crepitus, when present, is of limited diagnostic value.

Rotator cuff tendinitis

While any of the tendons of the rotator cuff may be affected by tendinitis, it most commonly affects the supraspinatus portion of the cuff close to its insertion to the humeral head. Overuse, with resultant wear and tear and relative avascularity, may be important in inducing tendon degeneration. The lesion often remains asymptomatic, but can manifest itself as pain and limitation of active (and sometimes passive) movement, especially abduction. A painful arc on abduction and tenderness over the tendon insertion may be noted.

Calcific supraspinatus tendinitis

Some cases of supraspinatus tendinitis are associated with calcific deposits visible on X-ray (Fig. 23.22). The exact mechanism responsible for the deposition of the calcium hydroxyapatite crystals in the tendon is unclear. The deposits may remain asymptomatic, or produce chronic symptoms with nagging discomfort in the region of the

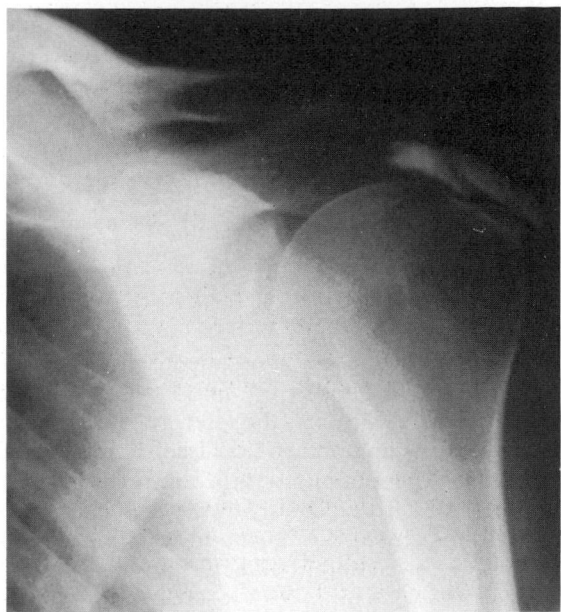

Fig. 23.22 X-ray of shoulder showing calcification of supraspinatus tendon.

affected tendon. The crystal may also be extravasated into the subacromial bursa, causing acute bursitis with intense shoulder pain, loss of movement, severe tenderness, swelling and muscle spasm. Fever, sweating and other systemic symptoms may be present, mimicking gout or septic arthritis.

Infraspinatus and subscapularis lesions

Infraspinatus and subscapularis lesions are less common and seldom calcify. While the symptoms are usually similar to those of supraspinatus tendinitis, pain induced by resisted external or internal rotation (Table 23.41) usually allows the correct diagnosis to be made.

Rupture of the rotator cuff

Rupture of the rotator cuff is most common in patients over the age of 50 years, and almost always begins in the supraspinatus tendon. It probably follows long-standing tendon degeneration. Partial tears are more usual and are a cause of the painful arc syndrome, although they may also be asymptomatic. Complete tears are associated with marked weakness and inability to initiate active abduction; passive movement is full. Pain can be severe and there may be a history of injury. Partial tears may be difficult to differentiate from tendinitis and local anaesthetic infiltration, and contrast arthrography may be necessary. Atrophy of supra- and infraspinatus muscles often follows.

Table 23.41 Clinical features of some extracapsular shoulder lesions

Lesion	Painful arc	Pain increased by
Supraspinatus tendinitis, calcific deposit or incomplete tear	Yes	Resisted abduction
Infraspinatus tendinitis	Yes	Resisted external rotation
Acromioclavicular joint disease	Yes. Pain begins later in abduction (not below 90°) and increases as full elevation is reached	Local palpation Resisted adduction
Subscapularis	No	Resisted internal rotation
Bicipital tendinitis	No	Resisted flexion and supination of the elbow Tender bicipital groove

Bicipital syndromes

Tendinitis of the long head of the biceps is less common than are rotator cuff lesions, but may lead to rupture of the tendon.

Subacromial bursitis

Subacromial bursitis is almost always secondary to tendinitis or another adjacent lesion.

Frozen shoulder (adhesive capsulitis)

Frozen shoulder may occur spontaneously but can follow other rotator cuff lesions or trauma. In addition, conditions that produce pain (e.g. the referred pain of myocardial infarction) or immobility (e.g. stroke or polymyalgia rheumatica) of the shoulder or arm can predispose to the development of a frozen shoulder. Severe night pain and pain on all movement develops and lasts for four to 12 weeks. Severe restriction of all active and passive movements is noted, lasting six to 18 months, before improving to near normal. Early arthrography may reveal a small, shrunken, thickened capsule.

Patients with even minor degrees of frozen shoulder may develop a secondary reflex sympathetic dystrophy syndrome – the shoulder-hand syndrome. The symptom complex is characterised by an immobile painful shoulder associated with a swollen, painful, cold and dystrophic-looking hand. The lesion may progress until the patient is left with a painful, tender and useless hand.

Fibromyalgia syndrome

This is a syndrome of widespread pain characterised by:

- poor sleep pattern
- multiple painful sites affecting right and left sides of the body and upper and lower segments

- fatigability and lethargy
- hypersensitivity of tender sites.

The role of sleep, psychological factors, repetitive trauma, physical and emotional stress and physical inactivity all seem important in the initiation and perpetuation of symptoms.

The painful elbow

Pain round the elbow is commonly caused by soft tissue lesions, but care must be taken to exclude referred pain from the cervical spine, brachial plexus, shoulder and wrist.

Humeral epicondylitis

In humeral epicondylitis, lateral involvement (tennis elbow) is much more common than medial involvement (golfer's elbow). In spite of their sporting connotations, both occur more frequently in those performing repetitive movements with their arms, such as operating machinery, using a screwdriver or doing housework.

In tennis elbow, there is pain over the lateral aspect of the elbow with localised tenderness near the lateral epicondyle. Resisted dorsiflexion of the wrist exacerbates the pain and there is a reduction in grip strength. Thermography usually shows a discrete 'hot spot' on the side of the elbow.

In golfer's elbow, there is a tender spot at the medial epicondyle and pain is induced by flexing the wrist against resistance, with the elbow fully extended. An enthesopathy has recently been suggested as a unifying pathological basis for lesions, including humeral epicondylitis and shoulder tendinitis, but many other histological changes have also been reported.

Olecranon bursitis (miner's elbow)

The superficial bursa over the olecranon process is commonly involved in RA (with nodule formation) or gout, but can also be affected by trauma or infection. In the acute stage, it distends with fluid, with prominent

---

Summary 6 The painful shoulder

Rotator cuff lesions

Tendinitis	– supraspinatus
	– acute calcific supraspinatus
	– infraspinatus and subscapularis
Rupture	– partial
	– complete

Bicipital syndromes

Tenosynovitis of long head
Rupture of long head

Subacromial bursitis

Usually secondary to adjacent pathology

Frozen shoulder (adhesive capsulitis)

Shoulder-hand syndrome and referred pain

Summary 7 The painful elbow

Humeral epicondylitis

Lateral – tennis elbow
Medial – golfer's elbow

Olecranon bursitis

Traumatic – student's elbow
Secondary to inflammatory joint disease

Friction neuritis of ulnar nerve

signs of acute inflammation. If it becomes chronic, the wall can be greatly thickened. As the posterior wall of the bursa is so close to the periosteum of the olecranon, pain can be felt down the border of the ulna.

The painful wrist and hand

Both seropositive and seronegative arthritides have a predilection for inflammatory involvement of the synovial structures of the tendons and joints in the wrist and hand. Tenosynovitis denotes an inflammation of the synovial lining of the tendon sheath usually accompanied by inflammation of the contained tendon. The clinical manifestations are pain, tenderness and swelling, with 'crepitus' that is palpable when the tendon moves within the inflamed sheath.

Stenosing tenosynovitis

Stenosing tenosynovitis is primarily a disorder of fibrosis of the tendon sheaths with intrathecal narrowing of the lumen, especially involving sites near bony prominences where tendons pass through fibrous rings. This more commonly affects the flexor than extensor tendons in the hand. If a fibrous nodule develops in the flexor tendons, a 'trigger finger' can result, which further limits function. The finger often locks in flexion. Extension can be forced with difficulty and is often painful. Palpation during muscle action may reveal a mobile nodule within a tendon sheath of a finger or palm.

De Quervain's tenosynovitis

De Quervain's tenosynovitis is a common lesion. It is caused by repeated minor trauma, and results from involvement of the tendon sheaths of the abductor pollicis longus and extensor pollicis brevis. The patient complains of pain on using the thumb or wrist. Tenderness is maximal in the 'snuffbox' area between the two tendons, and there is often a visible tender swelling about the radial styloid. Pain can be elicited by forced ulnar deviation after placing the patient's thumb in the palm (Finkelstein's sign).

Summary 8 The painful wrist and hand
● Stenosing digital tenosynovitis
● Tenosynovitis – De Quervain's and others
● Dupuytren's contracture
● Rupture of tendons
● Ganglion
● Median nerve compression – carpal tunnel syndrome

Acute frictional tenosynovitis

Acute frictional tenosynovitis occurs after unusually active use of the wrist over a period of days or weeks. Pain is felt at the back of the wrist and lower forearm, and affects the extensor tendons of the wrist and thumb. A characteristic fine crepitation, caused by the fibrin-covered tendon gliding within the inflamed paratendon, is felt if the examiner's hand is placed over the swollen wrist while the patient extends and flexes the affected wrist and digits.

Dupuytren's contracture

The condition of Dupuytren's contracture, of unknown aetiology, produces progressive thickening of the palmar fascia and causes flexion contracture predominantly affecting the ring and little fingers. It is commonly bilateral and can also involve the plantar fascia. The palm of the hand becomes indurated, and lines of fibrosis, with nodules and skin puckering, run along the tendons causing progressive fixed flexion of the metacarpophalangeal and proximal interphalangeal joints.

The rate of progression is variable. Surgical fasciectomy should be performed when disability is severe, and should be considered before amputation becomes the only alternative.

Repetitive strain injury

This can be defined as a chronic pain syndrome affecting usually the whole of one or both neck-arm regions and usually occurs in the context of activities requiring a controlled posture, usually of a repetitive nature. Psychological factors contribute to the syndrome. The condition affects predominantly female employees engaged in low-paying, monotonous, low-prestige occupations.

Symptoms include chronic pain in the neck, arm and hand and are associated with weakness of grip and tight proximal muscles. There may be dysaesthesiae and variable hand and forearm swelling. These symptoms lead to an inability to perform previous work tasks or leisure activities which relate to repetitive movement. There are accompanying mood changes associated with a poor sleep pattern.

Ganglia

Ganglia are tense uni- or multilocular cystic swellings that develop in relation to a joint capsule or tendon sheath, and contain a clear jelly-like substance. They vary in size and can be so tense that they may be mistaken for a bony swelling. They are sometimes provoked by injury or arthritis but often occur spontaneously.

Entrapment neuropathy (carpal tunnel syndrome)

Nerve compression can occur at any site where a peripheral nerve passes though an opening in fibrous tissue or an osseofibrous canal. If the clinical diagnosis is in doubt, it may be confirmed by EMG.

Entrapment of the median nerve in the carpal tunnel at the wrist is the commonest entrapment lesion. It is more common in females. Most cases are idiopathic or caused by unaccustomed repetitive use, but carpal tunnel compression may be associated with RA, myxoedema, acromegaly, pregnancy and the contraceptive pill. Fracture, deformity or dislocation of the carpal bones can cause similar problems. Early symptoms include painful tingling in the wrist and hands, mainly affecting the thumb, index and middle fingers, but often symptoms are poorly localised. The pain may occasionally extend up the arm well above the wrist and often interferes with sleep. Patients try to obtain relief by hanging the affected limb out of the bed. Later, weakness (first in the abductor pollicis brevis) develops. Diminution of sensation to touch and pinprick, usually over the palmar aspects of the distal phalanges of the index and middle fingers, may be found. Untreated, wasting of the muscles of the thenar eminence develops. EMG is helpful where the clinical diagnosis is in doubt. A delay in motor or sensory conduction velocity across the wrist confirms the diagnosis, although no electrical abnormality may be detected in early cases.

The painful knee

Tendons, ligaments and bursae are the soft tissue structures around the knee from which pain may originate. When assessing the knee, the clinical history is more valuable than the findings of clinical examination. The patient's account of the symptoms and their onset will usually make it possible to decide which structures in the knee have been damaged and how seriously.

Patellar tendinitis

The ligamentum patellae may become painful and tender at its attachment to the upper or lower pole of the patella or at its distal attachment to the tibia. Prolonged and heavy exercise, such as jogging, predisposes to this condition which usually occurs in adults. Steroid injections may be effective but should be used cautiously; surgical exploration is occasionally necessary.

Osgood-Schlatter disease

Apophysitis of the tibial tubercle at the insertion of the patellar tendon occurs predominantly in adolescent children and is another common cause of pain in front of the knee. The condition is more common in boys, and symptoms include localised tenderness and swelling at this site. Pain can be reproduced by resisted knee extension, and radiographs may be abnormal and show an isolated spicule of bone at the site of the swelling. Most patients improve spontaneously but, sometimes, the pain may persist for several years, and injection, plaster immobilisation or even excision of the bony spicule may then be required. A similar, but rare, condition can occur at the lower pole of the patella (*Sinding-Larsen disease*).

Bursitis

Some bursae are in direct contact with the knee joint while others are separate. Like bursae elsewhere, acute or chronic inflammation, infection and involvement in systemic diseases, such as gout and arthritis, can occur.

Acute bursitis is characterised by classical signs of acute inflammation with intense localised tenderness and marked restriction of movement. Chronic bursitis may follow acute episodes but is much more commonly associated with repeated trauma. The bursal lining becomes thickened and cells degenerate; adhesions, villi and calcaneous deposits eventually develop. The degree of inflammation, muscle weakness and wasting and limitation of movement can vary widely, making diagnosis difficult.

Prepatellar bursitis (housemaid's knee). Here, the bursa is subcutaneous, and inflammation usually results from repeated kneeling, but can follow a fall onto the patella. Infection of the prepatellar bursa gives a characteristic red, shiny appearance over the knee, and is often mistaken for an infected knee joint. When chronic, fibrous bodies and fibrous bands form in the thickened enlarged bursa.

Infrapatellar bursitis. This small, deep bursa occupies the space between the upper part of the tibial tuberosity and ligamentum patellae, separated from the synovium by a fat pad. When inflamed, the fluid obliterates the depression on each side of the ligament, the fluctuant swelling being most marked when the knee is actively extended.

Popliteal cysts (Baker's cysts). Synovial cysts in the popliteal fossa are usually referred to as Baker's cysts. They may arise from the semi-membranous bursa when they communicate with the knee joint, or from a posterior rupture of the knee joint capsule. Cysts are common in children and are of no serious significance although, in young adults, there may be quite severe pain after exercise. The most common course is gradual resolution. If the cyst does not resolve, it may extend into the calf or burst, with fluid tracking down the fascial planes of the calf, mimicking an acute deep venous thrombosis. Arthrography of the knee joint establishes the diagnosis but must be performed early after the onset of symptoms, as the leak may seal off after a few days.

Anserine bursitis. The tendons of sartorius, gracilis and semitendinosus all cross the lower medial side of the femur and attach by a common tendon. The anserine bursa lies beneath this tendon. Pain is felt diffusely on the medial aspect of the knee, but tenderness can usually be localised to the area of the bursa. Knee range is normal, but contracting the hamstrings induces pain. The bursa is often inflamed in elderly obese women with a valgus deformity, and is also a common source of pain in inexperienced joggers, often being mistaken for joint injury.

Ligament injuries

If a patient has injured the knee in such a way that the structures on the medial side have been stressed, damage to the medial ligament must be suspected. Clinical examination may reveal tenderness localised to the attachment of the ligament to the femur or tibia. The diagnosis can be confirmed by stressing the medial ligament; this will reproduce the pain or demonstrate ligament laxity.

Tendinitis

The popliteus tendon runs through the knee joint from the lateral femoral condyle, between the lateral meniscus and the capsule, to the back of the tibia. Inflammation may cause lateral knee pain.

The biceps tendon is attached to the head of the fibula, and inflammation will cause pain around the tendon insertion, felt particularly when the knee is flexed against resistance and the area pressed firmly.

Pain in the back of the knee may arise from a hamstring injury. The pain usually develops acutely after sudden activity without adequate warming-up.

Anterior tibial syndrome

The anterior tibial syndrome consists of severe pain in the anterior aspect of the leg, associated with foot drop,

---

Summary 9 The painful knee
• Patellar tendinitis
• Rupture of quadriceps apparatus
• Apophysitis of tibial tubercle – Osgood-Schlatter disease

• Bursitis
    Prepatellar
    Intrapatellar
    Popliteal cysts – semimembranous
                  – Baker's cyst
    Anserine

• Infrapatellar fat pad lesions
• Medial and lateral ligament injuries
• Tendon lesions
• Anterior tibial syndrome

---

occurring after exercise and relieved by rest. It is thought to be the result of a tight fascia compressing the muscles in the anterior tibial compartment of the leg. There are many predisposing factors, of which exercise is the commonest. Surgery gives relief.

The painful heel

Pain can arise from either the posterior or plantar aspects of the heel. Most lesions occur in people who walk or stand a great deal and are particularly common in athletes. Whatever the cause, the pain tends to be aggravated by walking and relieved by rest. Accurate localisation of tenderness is important in diagnosis.

Pain behind the heel

Tendon rupture

Complete or partial tendon rupture may occur after vigorous activity. In the young, the musculotendinous junction tends to be the site of rupture, while in the old, the tendon itself is at risk. Complete rupture is easily recognised by loss of anatomical continuity and function. Partial rupture is more difficult to diagnose. Initially, swelling and marked tenderness is noted just above the tendon insertion, with exquisite pain on movement. Later, a more irregular swelling due to fibrous tissue develops, with continuing pain on movement.

Central core degeneration of the Achilles tendon

Central core degeneration of the Achilles tendon must be differentiated from the more common peritendinous lesion, as tendon rupture is much more likely and local steroid injections are contraindicated. Onset is less dramatic than partial rupture, but other clinical findings can be similar.

Pain gradually increases as the day progresses. Careful examination also reveals a localised tender nodule or thickening, 3–6 cm above the insertion to the calcaneum.

Peritendinitis (Achilles tendinitis)

Peritendinitis is the common cause of chronic, persistent and often annoying pain at the back of the heel. It occurs most commonly, but by no means exclusively, in athletes, especially long-distance runners. In the acute stage, there is diffuse swelling and tenderness on both sides of the tendon, sometimes accompanied by crepitus. Later, signs become less obvious, but pain and tenderness recur with exercise. The symptoms usually develop gradually, distinguishing the condition from rupture of the tendon, and occasionally the tendon may calcify. Inflammation of the peroneal tendons behind the lateral malleolus causes pain when the muscle is contracted, as when walking over rough ground. If this tendinitis is chronic, RA should be considered.

Bursitis

Subachilles (retrocalcaneal) bursitis may also cause pain at the lower end of the Achilles tendon. Physical examination reveals the bulging tender bursa on either side of the Achilles tendon with normal ankle joint movement. Dorsiflexion of the foot aggravates the pain by compressing the bursa. Frequently, the patient can recall a traumatic incident.

Subcutaneous (postcalcaneal) bursitis

A more superficial bursitis can develop over the tendon attachment as a result of poorly fitting shoes; here, the swelling is lower down, large and fluctuant. Inflammatory changes in the overlying skin are common.

Retrocalcaneal apophysitis (Sever's disease)

The insertion of the Achilles tendon into the calcaneum can become inflamed, resulting in symptoms of pain and tenderness behind the heel. This usually occurs in boys aged between nine and 15 years.

Pain under the heel

Plantar fasciitis

In weight-bearing, stress is placed on the long plantar ligament and fascia which support the longitudinal arch of the foot. An enthesopathy can develop at the point of attachment of the ligament to the heel. Pain and tenderness may be confined to the point of attachment but can be much more widespread; it is always aggravated on walking. The presence of a calcaneal spur on the X-ray is not necessarily significant, as it is also commonly seen on films of asymptomatic heels. Plantar fasciitis may be associated with the seronegative arthritides, such as Reiter's syndrome and ankylosing spondylitis.

Tender heel pad

The condition of tender heel pad causes pain in the hind part of the heel on standing or walking. The tough fibro-fatty pad beneath the prominent weight-bearing part of the calcaneus is tender to finger palpation. The area of tenderness is well localised and may be a result of simple contusion; in most cases, there is no history of trauma and, in these patients, the tenderness may result from obesity combined with excessive walking in unsatisfactory footwear, or from mild inflammation of uncertain origin.

Summary 10 The painful heel

Pain behind the heel

Achilles tendon lesions
  Rupture – partial/total
  Central core degeneration
  Ossification
  Peritendinitis (Achilles tendinitis)

Bursitis
  Subachilles (retrocalcaneal)
  Subcutaneous (postcalcaneal)

Retrocalcaneal apophysitis
(Sever's disease)

Pain under the heel

Plantar fasciitis
Calcaneal apophysitis and spurs
Tender heel pad

The painful foot

'Flat feet'

'Flat feet' rarely cause symptoms in the young. In adolescents they may be part of a general postural defect. At this age, especially in boys, spasmodic flat foot is caused by peroneo-extensor spasm. The foot is rigid and painful and symptoms are worse on walking. Flat foot usually leads to osteoarthritis of the midtarsal joint in later life.

'Spring' ligament

The 'spring' or plantar calcaneonavicular ligament supports the talonavicular joint from below; it may be strained, leading to deep-seated pain on weight-bearing.

Metatarsalgia

Patients with anatomical abnormalities of the feet, such as claw-toes or equinus deformity, are liable to develop pain in the metatarsal heads on walking. Metatarsalgia, or pain around the metatarsal heads, is not itself a diagnosis. Between the metatarsal heads and the skin lie the flexor tendons and their sheaths and, in the case of the great toe, the sesamoids in the flexor hallucis brevis. Inflam-

---

Summary 11 The painful foot

- Anterior flat foot – dropped transverse arch
- Injuries to the spring ligament
- Plantar digital neuritis – Morton's metatarsalgia
- Tarsal tunnel syndrome
- Plantar warts and callosities
- Hallux valgus (bunion)
- Dorsal exostoses with bursae

matory joint disease can cause inflammation of the tendon sheaths and causes generalised pain.

Hallux valgus

Hallux valgus (bunion) is an example of an adventitious bursa resulting from prolonged pressure over a bony prominence as a result of valgus deformity of the hallux. It is frequently inflamed. Initially, treatment consists of padding to reduce pressure and advice on suitable footwear. If these measures prove unhelpful, surgical treatment may be necessary.

Tibialis anterior and posterior

Pain in the mid-foot may arise around the insertion of the tibialis anterior after strenuous walking. Pain on the medial side of the foot, at the point of insertion of the tibialis posterior tendon on the navicular, is more common; it is particularly severe if the patient has an accessory navicular bone.

Dorsal exostoses

Some patients develop a bony prominence on the dorsum of the foot at the joint between the navicular and the cuneiform bone. Excessive friction may lead to the formation of a bursa.

Entrapment syndromes in the foot

Tarsal tunnel syndrome. Compression of the posterior tibial nerve under the flexor retinaculum below the medial malleolus can lead to burning pain under the medial side of the longitudinal arch of the foot.

Morton's metatarsalgia (plantar digital neuritis). In this condition, patients complain of a sharp pain in the forefoot shooting through to the toes, usually the third and fourth. There may be tingling, or even numbness, in the adjacent sides of the third and fourth toes. The pain is localised between the metatarsal heads, and the transverse metatarsal compression may produce a palpable click. The condition is caused by interstitial fibrosis compressing the digital nerve just before it divides into its two terminal branches. In the early stages, well-fitting shoes, with or without a metatarsal bar, give relief. Excision of the thickened tissue effects a cure.

Other common entrapment syndromes in the lower limb

Lateral popliteal nerve lesions

The lateral popliteal branch of the sciatic nerve lies superficially against the head and neck of the fibula, where it is susceptible to compression, especially when sitting with legs crossed, kneeling or wearing knee pads. Anaesthesia and periods of unconsciousness present particular risks. The symptoms are pain and tingling in the lateral aspect of the leg and dorsum of the foot, associated with weakness of dorsiflexion and eversion of the foot. Wasting of tibialis anterior, peroneal and extensor digitorum brevis can occur. The high-stepping gait is typical. EMG can confirm the diagnosis.

Lateral femoral cutaneous nerve entrapment (meralgia paraesthetica)

The lateral cutaneous branch of the femoral nerve traverses a tunnel formed by the lateral attachment of the inguinal ligament as it runs towards the anterior superior iliac spine. Entrapment produces paraesthesia and burning pain over the lateral thigh with reduced sensation. Local trauma, obesity or pressure from tight garments are known predisposing factors.

Management of patients with soft tissue rheumatism

One feature common to all of the soft tissue rheumatism syndromes is a tendency to spontaneous remission. Many of the syndromes take weeks to improve, and few persist with significant symptoms beyond six months. A clear diagnosis therefore allows the physician to reassure the patient that arthritis is not present and that the prognosis is good. Failure to resolve is often due to further injury. Few of the conditions require complete rest; most respond to selective rest of the involved region.

Immobilisation

Tenosynovitis around the wrist may respond to immobilisation in a light forearm splint, maintaining the wrist in a position of optimum function (10–15° extension), and median nerve compression may respond to night-splinting alone. The acutely painful shoulder also benefits from rest, mobility being maintained by pendular exercises. Physiotherapy in the acute stages only exacerbates the condition. Rest is essential for the painful heel and foot. Raising the heel of the shoe reduces tension on the Achilles tendon, and Elastoplast strapping will help immobilise the ankle. If there is flattening of the medial arch of the foot, then physiotherapy and an arch support may be helpful.

Drug therapy

The short-term use of NSAIDs may be necessary. Their immediate use is beneficial in limiting the pain and swelling of soft tissue trauma. Many soft tissue lesions respond to a local injection with steroid and anaesthetic. Some experience in the various techniques is necessary before reasonable success can be obtained.

The choice of steroid and local anaesthetic varies between physicians but, for most purposes, the shorter-acting hydrocortisone acetate is suitable. After injection, there may be an increase in symptoms for up to 48 hours and patients should be warned of this possibility. About 80% of patients gain symptomatic benefit from these injections. It is important not to inject the tendoachilles itself, as this may predispose to rupture. In spite of decades of use of ultrasound in treating a wide spectrum of musculoskeletal disorders, its effectiveness remains unproven. Persistent lesions may require further injections, and if conservative measures fail, surgery may be required.

FURTHER READING

Anderson J 1987 Epidemiological, sociological and environmental aspects of rheumatology, Vol 1. No 3. Baillières. *Clinical rheumatology. An epidemiological account of the rheumatic diseases.*

Dixon A St J (ed) 1979 Soft tissue rheumatism. Clinics in rheumatic diseases, Vol 5. W B Saunders, London. *A good review of soft tissue rheumatism*

Doherty M, Hazleman B, Blake D, Maddison P, Perry D 1992 Rheumatology examination and injection techniques. W B Saunders, London/Philadelphia. *A clear review of examination techniques*

Ebringer A, Shipley M (ed) 1988 Pathogenesis of ankylosing spondylitis and rheumatoid arthritis. British Journal of Rheumatology (Suppl Issue 11). *A good review of the pathophysiology of these two diseases*

Hadler N 1984 Medical management of the regional musculoskeletal diseases. Grune and Stratton. *A good review of regional disorders.*

Hughes G R V 1987 Connective tissue diseases, 3rd edn. Blackwell Scientific Publications. *An excellent introduction to these disorders, including current ideas on pathogenesis and treatment*

Kelly W N, Harris E H, Ruddy S, Sledge C B 1989 Textbook of rheumatology, 3rd edn. W B Saunders, Philadelphia. *A good textbook of rheumatology*

Moll J M H, Bird H A, Rushton A (ed) 1986 Therapeutics in rheumatology. Chapman and Hall, London. *A good introduction to the drugs used in treatment and the management of rheumatic disorders*

Woo P, White P, Ansell B (eds) 1990 Paediatric rheumatology update. Oxford University Press, Oxford. *The most recent review of paediatric rheumatology*

24

Haematological Disorders

David C Linch

HAEMOPOIESIS

Haemopoiesis is the process by which blood cells are derived from multipotential stem cells.

Ontogeny of haemopoiesis

In the human embryo, nucleated erythrocytes develop in the extraembryonic membranes and synthesise specific embryonic haemoglobins. In the sixth week of gestation, erythropoiesis transfers to the fetal liver and the embryonic haemoglobins ($\alpha_2\varepsilon_2, \zeta_2\varepsilon_2$) are replaced by fetal haemoglobin ($\alpha_2\gamma_2$). Bone marrow haemopoiesis is established between the 11th and 22nd week of gestation. Hepatic haemopoiesis declines in the third trimester and ceases soon after birth. Finally, at about the time of birth, fetal haemoglobin is replaced by adult haemoglobin (HbA, $\alpha_2\beta_2$).

These sequential changes in haemoglobin synthesis during development represent the orderly activation of the globin genes from the 5' to 3' end of the globin gene clusters (Fig. 24.1). The δ gene is never fully expressed and HbA$_2$ ($\alpha_2\delta_2$) represents only 2% of adult haemoglobins. The molecular mechanism of Hb gene switching is incompletely understood.

At birth, most of the bone marrow cavity is haemopoietically active but, during the first decade, this active red marrow is replaced by inactive fatty yellow marrow. In adults, red marrow and hence haemopoiesis is restricted to the upper ends of the femora and humeri, the vertebrae, ribs, sternum, clavicles, scapulae, skull and pelvis.

There is very limited granulocyte and monocyte production until the end of gestation. Lymphoid cells first appear during the first trimester and, by the second trimester, leucocytes in the blood are phenotypically mature T and B lymphocytes. However, full functional integrity of the immune system is not achieved until after birth.

Haemopoietic differentiation

The mature elements of the blood probably all arise from a multipotent haemopoietic stem cell. Such cells may self-replicate (and so replenish the stem cell pool) or, alternatively, may proliferate and enter the differentiation

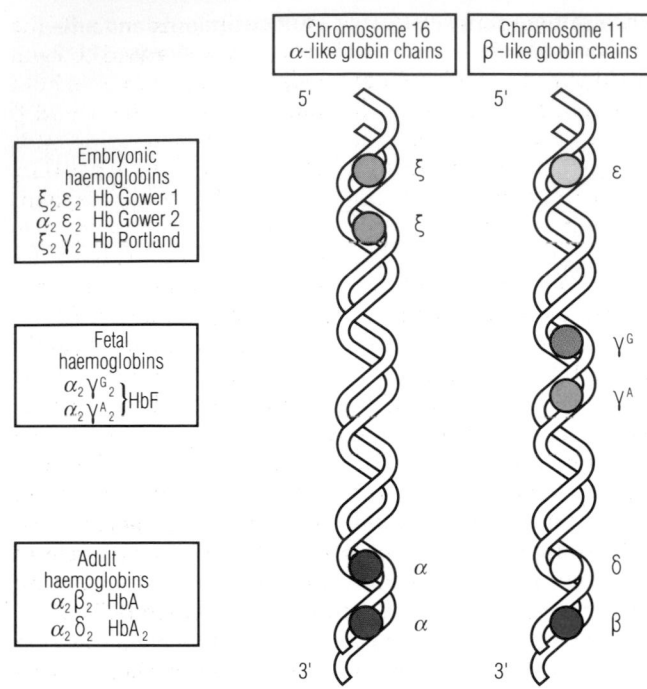

Fig. 24.1 Diagrammatic representation of the α-like globin gene cluster and β-like globin gene cluster on chromosomes 16 and 11 respectively. Hb switching during ontogeny represents the orderly expression of the globin genes from the 5' to 3' end of the globin gene clusters.

Progenitor cells appear as undifferentiated blast cells, but in the final five or six divisions of the differentiation pathway, the cells progressively acquire the morphological features and functional attributes of the mature cell. These recognisable precursor and end cells account for more than 95% of normal marrow cells.

Myeloid end cells have a limited life-span. The steady state is maintained by a continuous influx of stem cells and progenitor cells into the precursor cell pool. Mature lymphoid cells, on the other hand, are capable of clonal expansion or, alternatively, of transition to a resting 'memory cell' which is able to divide at a later date when appropriately stimulated.

Regulation of haemopoiesis

Haemopoiesis is regulated, at least in part, by a series of glycoproteins referred to as haemopoietic growth factors (HGFs). Erythropoietin, produced in response to hypoxia by the peritubular adventitial cells of the kidney, is a true hormone, whereas the other HGFs probably act in a paracrine manner.

From in vitro and in vivo studies, the HGFs can be grouped into three broad categories (Fig. 24.3). The *late-acting factors* are relatively lineage restricted and stimulate the terminal divisions of the maturation pathway with associated differentiation to mature cells. These include erythropoietin, granulocyte colony-stimulating factor (G-CSF), monocyte colony-stimulating factor (M-CSF) and eosinophil colony-stimulating factor, known as IL-5. Proliferation of rather more primitive cells in the pathway is regulated by the *multi-CSFs*, IL-3 and granulocyte–macrophage colony-stimulating factor (GM-CSF), which stimulate the early divisions of several cell lineages, including granulocytes, monocytes, eosinophils, mega-

pathway (Fig. 24.2). With each division there is increasing loss of multipotentiality and the stem cells thus become committed to one or more lineages. Monocyte and neutrophil (though not eosinophil) lineages appear to be closely related, as are red cells and megakaryocytes. Committed myeloid progenitor cells do not self-replicate, leading to the production of functional end cells.

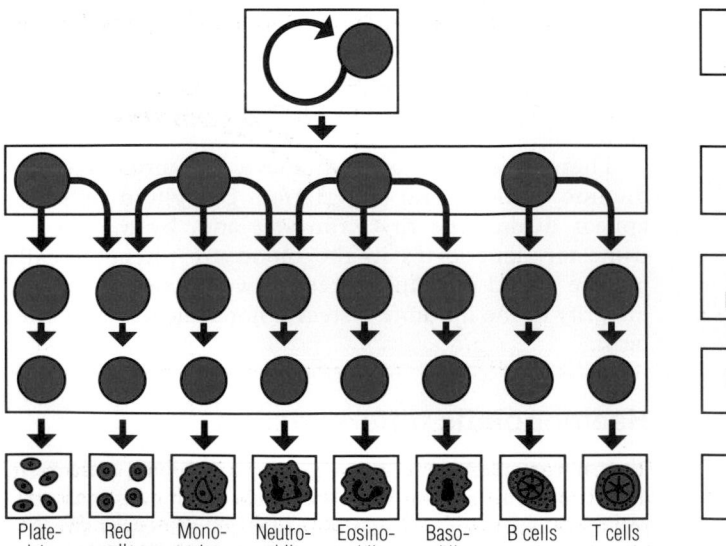

Fig. 24.2 Diagrammatic representation of the differentiation of haemopoietic stem cells.

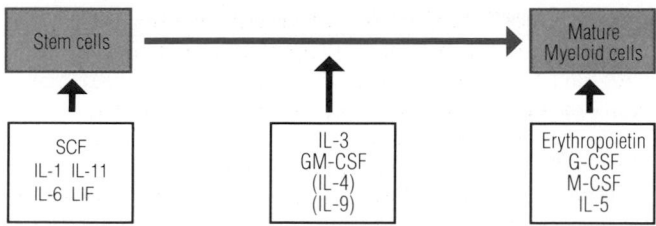

Fig. 24.3 Haemopoietic growth factors.

karyocytes and red cells. IL-3 also stimulates mast cell progenitors and some early lymphoid cells. Both IL-1 and IL-6 are extremely promiscuous in their target cell reactivity, but appear to act on the most primitive stem cells. *Stem cell factor* (SCF), also known as Steel Factor (SF), is produced by bone marrow stromal cell and has synergistic activity on primitive haemopoietic cells. The categorisation of the HGFs into three groups is undoubtedly an oversimplification and G-CSF and M-CSF may have some effects on primitive progenitor cells.

The specialised environment provided by bone marrow stromal tissue is essential for effective haemopoiesis, particularly for the survival, self-renewal and proliferation of stem cells.

The activity of the HGFs is not restricted to immature cells. G-CSF enhances many of the functional activities of mature neutrophils, GM-CSF enhances neutrophil, monocyte and eosinophil function, and M-CSF and IL-3 primes some monocyte functions, the latter also modulating eosinophil and mast cell function.

The HGFs are produced by a wide range of cell types, including activated T cells, monocytes, endothelial cells and fibroblasts. Many such cells are found in inflammatory sites and several of the HGFs probably serve as inflammatory mediators. GM-CSF produced at local inflammatory sites might increase phagocyte expression of cellular adhesion molecules, promote adhesion to the local vascular endothelium, induce migration into the inflammatory site, and increase phagocytic activity.

Several of the HGFs are now available for the treatment of neutropenia. Both G-CSF and GM-CSF accelerate neutrophil recovery following cytotoxic chemotherapy. Further developments in this field will include the use of synergistic combinations of HGFs.

FUNCTION OF HAEMOPOIETIC CELLS

RED CELLS AND HAEMOGLOBIN

Erythrocytes package haemoglobin for the delivery of oxygen from the lungs to the tissues; carbon dioxide is carried by red cells in the reverse direction. Haemoglobins have a molecular weight of approximately 65 000.

Each molecule consists of two α-like and two β-like polypeptide chains, with a haem group attached to each chain within a hydrophobic pocket. The tetramer is held together predominantly by bonds between the α and β chains. Because these bonds are not irreversible, the molecule exists in equilibrium between two configurations, one with a low, and one a high affinity for oxygen. Binding of oxygen to a haem group destabilises the low affinity form, thus increasing the oxygen affinity of the molecule. Due to this cooperative binding, a sigmoid oxygen dissociation curve is produced (Fig. 24.4). In the lungs, P_{O_2} is approximately 14 kPa and the haemoglobin is nearly fully saturated. In the tissues, where the P_{O_2} is about 5.4 kPa, haemoglobin saturation is about 70%. If tissue oxygen consumption rises, a small fall in tissue P_{O_2} will bring about a large further release of oxygen because these values of P_{O_2} correspond to the steep part of the oxygen dissociation curve. Various other factors also influence oxygen dissociation. A fall in pH or a rise in P_{CO_2} decreases the oxygen affinity (moves dissociation curve to right). This tends to increase oxygen delivery to tissues where the pH is lower and the P_{CO_2} higher than in the lungs. A rise in temperature, e.g. during heavy exercise, also decreases the oxygen affinity. Haemoglobin's affinity for oxygen is also modulated by 2,3-diphosphoglycerate (2,3-DPG). The mechanism is shown in Figure 24.5.

2,3-DPG is an intermediate on the glycolytic pathway (Fig. 24.6) and is present in relatively high concentrations within the red cell. Hypoxia within the red cell tends to increase 2,3-DPG levels in two ways. Firstly, the increased quantity of deoxygenated haemoglobin means that more 2,3-DPG is bound, thereby reducing product inhibition of DPG mutase. Secondly, deoxyhaemoglobin is a weaker acid than its oxygenated form, so red cell pH rises. This increases 2,3-DPG levels both by stimulating glycolysis in general and by inhibiting DPG phosphatase.

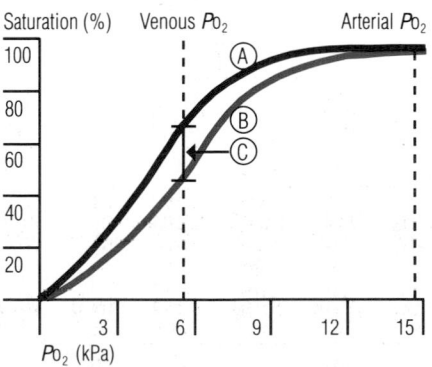

Fig. 24.4 **The sigmoid nature of the oxygen dissociation curve.** (A) represents the normal steady state. (B) represents the shift of the curve to the right seen with decreased pH, increased P_{CO_2} or increased 2,3-DPG. At a given venous P_{O_2}, this results in a larger amount of oxygen (marked C) being given to the tissues.

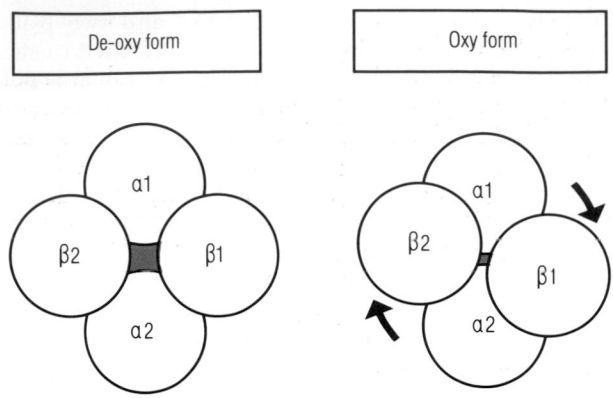

Fig. 24.5 Diagrammatic representation of the change in configuration of the haemoglobin molecule associated with oxygenation. Oxygenation is accompanied by a rotation of the α_1-β_1 dimer about the contact point between α_1 and β_2, thus closing up the pocket in which 2,3-DPG binds. Insertion of 2,3-DPG into this pocket prevents this rotation and stabilises the deoxy configuration, which reduces the oxygen affinity.

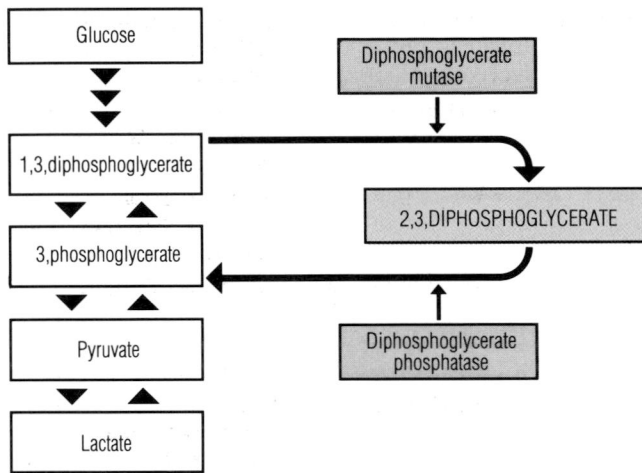

Fig. 24.6 The production of 2,3-diphosphoglycerate.

With an anaemia of 7.5 g/dl, the tissue hypoxia causes a rise in 2,3-DPG levels sufficient to increase oxygen delivery by about 25%. If, however, the hypoxia is sufficiently severe to cause acidosis within the red cell, 2,3-DPG levels will be depressed. Fortunately, this effect on oxygen affinity is balanced by the direct effect of H^+ on oxygen affinity (Bohr shift). This is of considerable importance in patients with a severe acidosis treated with bicarbonate. Sudden correction will immediately negate the Bohr shift and move the dissociation curve to the left; while the compensatory rise in 2,3-DPG will take many hours to occur. During this interim period, tissue oxygenation will be further impaired.

Some of the CO_2 released from the tissues diffuses into the red cells and is rapidly hydrated to carbonic acid

Table 24.1 Changes in haemoglobin concentration with age

Age	Haemoglobin concentration (g/dl)
First 3 days of life	13–21
First month thereafter	10–18
1–12 months	10–13.5
1–12 years	11.5–15.5
Adult males	13.0–18.0
Adult females	12.0–16.0

(H_2CO_3) because of the high levels of carbonic anhydrase. The H_2CO_3 dissociates to H^+ and HCO_3^- and the H^+ is buffered predominantly by deoxyhaemoglobin while the HCO_3^- re-enters the plasma. In the lungs, this process is reversed with the resultant CO_2 released into the alveoli.

The normal red cell mass is 25–35 ml/kg in men, and 20–30 ml/kg in women. The more readily measured haemoglobin concentration has a wide normal range which changes with age and sexual development (Table 24.1).

Leucocytes

Neutrophils

Neutrophils are mobile phagocytic cells able to recognise, phagocytose and then kill micro-organisms opsonised by IgG or C3b. They also migrate to non-infective sites of tissue damage, where they contribute to the inflammatory process. The neutrophil count is high in the first weeks of life but thereafter remains between 2.0 and 7.5×10^9/l.

Eosinophils

Eosinophils are phagocytes particularly effective in the elimination of parasites. They also participate in hypersensitivity reactions, especially in the skin, lungs and gut. The normal eosinophil count is less than 0.4×10^9/l.

Basophils

Basophils are involved in the pathogenesis of immediate hypersensitivity. When IgE is bound to their surface, they release histamine, which causes increased vascular permeability and smooth muscle contraction. The normal count is less than 0.1×10^9/l.

Monocytes

Monocytes are phagocytic cells which remove micro-organisms, damaged cells and cell fragments. They also have a central role in the generation of the immune response, through presentation of antigen to lymphocytes, regulation of many T and B cell functions, and cytotoxic activity towards antibody-coated cells. The monocyte count can be relatively high in the neonate (up to 4 x 10^9/l) but falls rapidly during early childhood. By four years of age, the normal adult values of 0.2–0.8 x 10^9/l are attained.

Lymphocytes

Neonates and young children have a high lymphocyte count, but this falls at puberty to the normal adult range of 1.5–4.0 × 10^9/l.

Thymus-dependent T cells are the major population of lymphocytes in the blood, accounting for approximately 70% of all lymphocytes. Two-thirds of T cells express the CD4 antigen on the cell surface and one-third the CD8 antigen. CD4+ cells are predominantly involved in interactions with other cells in association with class II HLA antigens, and serve to initiate and regulate the immune response (helper/inducer cells). The CD8+ population includes cells with cytotoxic activity which is usually specific for antigen recognised in association with class I HLA antigens, and also cells which suppress the immune response.

B cells account for 5–10% of peripheral blood lymphocytes. They have the potential to synthesise and secrete antibody and express surface immunoglobulin. Several heavy chain isotypes may be expressed, but only one light chain is expressed by a single cell.

The remaining 10–25% of peripheral blood lymphocytes are *non-T, non-B lymphocytes*. Some of these cells have a large granular appearance and non-MHC-restricted cytotoxic activity (natural killer cells).

CLASSIFICATION AND CAUSES OF ANAEMIA

Anaemia occurs when the haemoglobin concentration [Hb] falls below the normal range for the age and sex of the individual. [Hb] may be altered when living at high altitudes (which elevates the normal range), and in states such as pregnancy and splenomegaly, which lead to an increased plasma volume so that a normal red cell mass is maintained at lower haemoglobin concentrations.

True anaemia arises when there is an imbalance between red cell production and red cell destruction (Fig. 24.7). Increased red cell destruction can be compensated for in part by increased marrow production, so that chronic anaemia only occurs when red cell survival is less than half normal. Many causes of anaemia have multiple mechanisms. In thalassaemia, for example, both ineffective erythropoiesis and haemolysis occur.

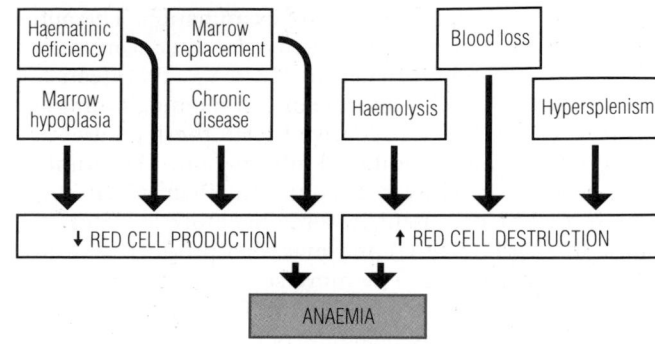

Fig. 24.7 The aetiology of anaemia.

From the practical standpoint, the classification of anaemia is based on routine haematological investigation – viz. automated cell counter analysis – considered in the

Table 24.2 Classification of anaemia according to the MCV

Type of anaemia	Cause	Features on blood film
Microcytic	Iron deficiency	Marked anisocytosis and poikilocytosis Pencil cells
	Thalassaemia	Target cells Nucleated red cells Reticulocytes
	Chronic disease	May be neutrophilia Target cells – liver disease Burr cells – renal failure
	Sideroblastic anaemia	Red cells often dimorphic
Normocytic	Acute haemorrhage	Reticulocytosis
	Haemolysis	Reticulocytosis
	Marrow hypoproduction	Pancytopenia May be abnormal cells, e.g. leukaemia
	Chronic disease	
	Combined iron and folate deficiency	Microcytes and oval macrocytes
Macrocytic	Megaloblastic change	Prominent oval macrocytes Pancytopenia Multisegmented polymorphs
	Reticulocytosis (haemorrhage, haemolysis)	Polychromasia and reticulocytosis
	Alcohol	
	Liver disease	Target cells
	Myxoedema (rare)	
	Aplastic anaemia (rare)	Pancytopenia
	Leukaemia and related disorders (rare)	Abnormal cells Normoblasts and myeloid precursor cells in blood

context of the clinical history and examination. The automated counters measure the haemoglobin concentration, red cell count and mean cell size (MCV). The mean cell haemoglobin (MCH) and mean cell haemoglobin concentration (MCHC) are derived from these parameters and provide limited additional information. The counters also produce a white cell count (nucleated red cells, which may be prevalent in some haemolytic states, are counted as white cells) and may also produce an automatic platelet count. The more sophisticated machines are able to perform a white cell differential count. The anaemias are initially characterised in terms of red cell size (Table 24.2). The precise cause of the anaemia can often be surmised from the combination of automated counter analysis and clinical situation, while examination of the blood film provides further clues as to aetiology. Further specific investigations are individually planned, depending on the results of these screening tests.

IRON DEFICIENCY ANAEMIA

PATHOPHYSIOLOGY

Iron deficiency is the commonest form of anaemia and is particularly prevalent in underprivileged communities. The daily intake of iron is closely related to the calorific value of the diet, so that individuals with poor diets (especially menstruating women) are particularly at risk. Even in Western societies, over 5% of such women have iron deficiency anaemia. Others at risk include: premature babies, as they have low iron stores and a milk diet which is relatively low in iron content; children during rapid growth periods; and women during pregnancy and lactation, when iron requirements are high.

The average Western diet contains 10–15 mg of iron per day and about 10% of this is absorbed. In iron deficiency, absorption is increased and may be as high as 30% of the total ingested. Iron enters the mucosal cells of the upper small intestine and is bound to apoferritin for transport across to the inner membrane of the mucosal cell, where it is given up to plasma transferrin. The level of transferrin saturation thus regulates absorption. Transferrin transports iron to the bone marrow where it is incorporated into haemoglobin. Iron is taken up by the reticulo-endothelial (RE) system and other tissues, where some is bound to enzymes and myoglobin but most is stored as ferritin and haemosiderin. Iron is lost from the body in sweat, urine, desquamated cells and in breast milk, but most of the iron released from effete red cells is recycled. Any bleeding is a major source of iron loss; menstruating women, for example, are only in marginal iron balance.

When iron loss exceeds iron absorption, the iron stores become depleted and the transferrin saturation in the blood then falls. When this drops to below around 10%, abnormal, iron deficient, erythropoiesis occurs. The MCV falls, with signs of abnormal erythropoiesis on the blood film such as variation in size (poikilocytosis) and shape (anisocytosis). As the iron deficiency progresses, microcytic anaemia develops, the anisocytosis and poikilocytosis becomes more marked and very narrow elliptocytes known as pencil cells may be seen. In more severe cases, target cells appear. The red cells are hypochromic in appearance, but this is more a reflection of their small size than poor haemoglobinisation, as the MCHC only falls below the normal range when the anaemia is severe.

Clinical features

There is a gradual onset of the symptoms of anaemia, with lethargy, weakness, dizziness and palpitations particularly on exertion. In addition, the hair and nails may become brittle and the nails spoon-shaped (koilonychia). Pruritus vulvae may occur and, in severe cases, cerebral irritability and even cerebral oedema may arise. Very rarely, a postcricoid web develops which initially causes dysphagia for solids but not liquids.

Aetiology and investigation

The aetiology of iron deficiency is illustrated in Fig. 24.8. Nearly one-half of patients who have had a partial gastrectomy develop iron deficiency if not given iron supplements, due primarily to rapid gastrojejunal transit. Achlorhydria may also cause iron deficiency as hydrochloric acid is important for the absorption of iron contained in foodstuffs. The cause of iron deficiency must always be established and particular attention paid to possible gastrointestinal bleeding. Malignancies of the gastrointestinal tract may present with iron deficiency anaemia in the absence of any other symptoms.

Diagnosis

This is suggested by microcytosis on the automated counter printout and associated changes on the blood

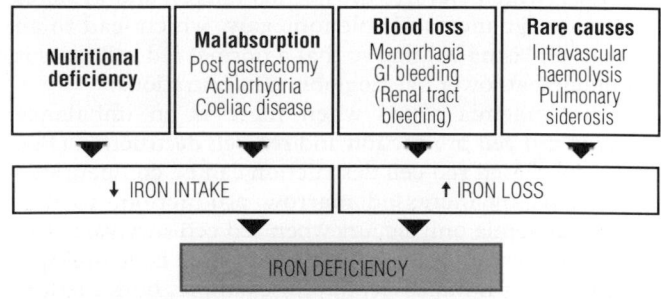

Fig. 24.8 The aetiology of iron deficiency.

film, and is confirmed by finding a low serum iron and high/normal total iron binding capacity (TIBC). The percentage TIBC saturation is less than 10%. In the anaemia of chronic disease (p. 1070), which may also be microcytic, the serum iron is also low, but the TIBC is reduced and the percentage saturation is thus usually above 10%. In thalassaemia, the percentage saturation is high due to ineffective erythropoiesis, haemolysis and transfusion. Where difficulties in interpretation occur, the serum ferritin may be useful. This is usually below 40 µg/l in iron deficiency (normal range 15–300 µg/l), but may be higher if there is coexistent inflammatory disease. A bone marrow examination gives definitive evidence of the status of the iron stores, as there is no Prussian Blue-stainable iron in marrow fragments in iron deficiency anaemia.

Management

The treatment of iron deficiency requires identification and correction of its cause where possible. The iron deficiency anaemia itself is usually correctable with oral iron supplements. Ferrous sulphate (200 mg t.d.s.) is cheap and usually well tolerated. If gastric intolerance occurs, reduction of the dosage to 200 mg once or twice per day will usually be acceptable and provide sufficient iron. Therapy should be continued until the anaemia has resolved, and then for a further three months to replete the iron stores. Parenteral iron is only necessary if oral preparations cannot be tolerated, or if inadequate iron is absorbed by that route. The response to parenteral iron is no faster than that to oral iron. Intramuscular iron is usually given as an iron–sorbitol–citric acid complex (Jectofer). Iron dextran can be given intravenously to correct the iron deficiency in a single infusion, but this therapy can be hazardous and is not generally advisable.

SIDEROBLASTIC ANAEMIA

Sideroblastic anaemia is characterised by anaemia in which ring sideroblasts are found in the bone marrow. Ring sideroblasts are normoblasts with an interrupted ring of iron around the nucleus revealed by a Perl's iron stain. There is a disorder of haem synthesis, with accumulation of iron within the mitochondria.

Aetiology

Sideroblastic anaemia may be inherited or acquired (Table 24.3). The inherited form is usually X-linked. Sideroblasts are a frequent finding in clonal disorders of the myeloid stem cell. The presence of anaemia and ring sideroblasts is classified as a form of myelodysplasia (see

Table 24.3 Causes of sideroblastic anaemia

Congenital
Acquired
Myeloid stem cell disorder
Myelodysplasia
Acute myeloid leukaemia
Myeloproliferative disorder
Drugs and toxins
Isoniazid
Alcohol
Lead
Miscellaneous
Connective tissue disorders
Widespread carcinoma

p. 1089) but if there are no other abnormalities, the prognosis is relatively good, with many patients surviving many years without transformation to acute leukaemia.

Haematological features

There is, typically, a dimorphic blood film with both normal and microcytic red cells apparent. The bone marrow shows ring sideroblasts and often other features of dyserythropoiesis. Other haematological findings depend on the cause of sideroblastosis: in myelodysplasia/leukaemia, disorders of the white cell lineage, including an increase in blast cells, may be apparent in blood and bone marrow; in lead poisoning, punctuate basophilia may be seen in the red cells.

Management

Any cause must be identified and, if possible, treated. Pyridoxine is always worth trying. It helps in occasional cases of both congenital and acquired disease. Blood transfusion may be necessary and consideration must be given to iron chelation therapy.

THE MEGALOBLASTIC ANAEMIAS

The megaloblastic anaemias are caused by impaired DNA synthesis and are almost always due to a deficiency of either B_{12} or folate. These anaemias are characterised by the abnormal morphology (megaloblastosis) of all cell lines within the bone marrow and blood. While the precise biochemical mechanism of megaloblastic change is unknown, it is clear that DNA replication is blocked whilst synthesis of cytoplasmic RNA and protein continues. The production of mature end cells is thus reduced and many precursor cells die within the marrow (ineffective haemopoiesis).

Clinical features

The onset of megaloblastic anaemia is usually insidious and the disease can be very advanced before presentation. The patients have symptoms and signs of anaemia and a slight yellow tinge due to the haemolytic component of the ineffective erythropoiesis. The tongue may be red and sore, and slight splenomegaly may be present. In severe cases, there may also be a low grade pyrexia together with infections and purpura secondary to pancytopenia. In the elderly, the gradual onset of anaemia may produce heart failure. In megaloblastic anaemia secondary to B_{12} deficiency, there may be neurological symptoms and other signs including optic atrophy, peripheral neuropathy, subacute combined degeneration of the cord and dementia. Due to considerable individual variation in the susceptibility of the nervous system to B_{12} deficiency, severe neurological sequelae can occur even with relatively minor anaemia.

Haematological features

There is a macrocytic anaemia with a subpopulation of very large, oval macrocytes usually visible on the film. Excessive alcohol intake and liver disease are also frequently associated with a macrocytic anaemia, as is a reticulocytosis; but the blood film will often resolve any diagnostic difficulties. In megaloblastic anaemia, the white cells and platelets are also affected and the counts may be low. This may also be the case in liver disease with hypersplenism but, in megaloblastic change, the neutrophils are typically multisegmented. In very severe anaemia, nucleated red cells may appear in the blood and have the appearance of megaloblasts.

The definitive diagnosis of megaloblastic anaemia is made by examination of the bone marrow. In the red cell series, the nucleus looks 'open' with delayed maturation relative to the haemoglobinising cytoplasm; the white cell series is also abnormal with giant metamyelocytes present. It is not essential to examine the bone marrow in all cases of macrocytic anaemia.

Aetiology and investigation

Megaloblastic change may be due to either B_{12} or folate deficiency and very rarely to other inherited and acquired anaemias. In patients with *macrocytic* anaemia, samples for serum B_{12} and red cell folate (which is less affected by recent diet than serum folate) should be taken immediately; liver function tests and plasma thyroxine should also be measured. If an examination and blood film suggest megaloblastic change, therapy with B_{12} and folate should be started immediately, as delay could result in the development of neurological problems. Bone marrow examination can usually be restricted to those patients where there

is considerable initial uncertainty about the diagnosis, or where a rapid response to therapy is not achieved. Further investigation will then depend on whether the cause of the megaloblastic anaemia is deficiency of B_{12} or folate.

B_{12} DEFICIENCY

Animal products are the main source of B_{12} in the diet. Ingested B_{12} binds to intrinsic factor (IF) secreted by the gastric parietal cells, and the B_{12}–IF complex is then absorbed in the terminal ileum. Large stores of B_{12} are contained in the liver so that B_{12} deficiency takes three or four years to develop in the face of normal requirements. The normal serum B_{12} level is 150–950 pg/ml and may be measured by bioassay or radioimmunoassay. The major function of B_{12} is as a cofactor to production of formate, which is used in purine synthesis, conversion of deoxyuridine to thymidine and in the formation of folate polyglutamate (the major red cell form of folate). In B_{12} deficiency, red cell folate levels are also low, although serum folate is normal or high.

Aetiology

The causes of B_{12} deficiency are shown in Fig. 24.9. Nutritional deficiency occurs predominantly in vegans and chronic alcoholics. IF deficiency occurs following gastric surgery and in pernicious anaemia – a relatively common condition (6000 cases/year in the UK) which occurs mainly in the elderly. In pernicious anaemia, there is an autoimmune-mediated atrophic gastritis resulting in achlorhydria and inability to produce IF. It may be associated with other autoimmune diseases such as myxoedema, diabetes mellitus and vitiligo. There may be a family history of other autoimmune disorders and sometimes a

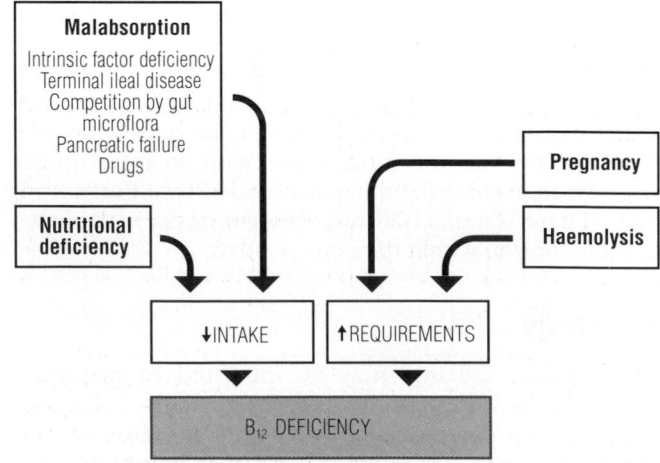

Fig. 24.9 The aetiology of vitamin B_{12} deficiency.

history of premature greying of the hair. The disease is more common in individuals with blood group A.

Malabsorption of B_{12} due to terminal ileal disease occurs most commonly in Crohn's disease, when there is often concomitant iron and folate deficiency. Pancreatic failure may also cause B_{12} malabsorption, probably by reducing the pH and Ca^{2+} concentration of the terminal ileal fluid to below the optimum for absorption. A variety of drugs have been reported as inhibiting B_{12} absorption, including the biguanides and high dose potassium supplements. Bacterial overgrowth, such as occurs with intestinal 'blind loops' (p. 579), may consume ingested B_{12}. The Scandinavian fish tapeworm is a more exotic cause of such intestinal competition.

Diagnosis

The diagnosis of the cause of B_{12} deficiency is made by the *Schilling test*, in which the fasting patient is given a loading dose of parenteral vitamin B_{12} to saturate both plasma and liver binding sites, and is then given oral radioactive B_{12}. The principles of the test are shown in Fig. 24.10. Parts I and II of the Schilling test can be done simultaneously if two different cobalamin isotopes are used – one to label free B_{12} and one to label B_{12} complexed to IF.

The diagnosis of pernicious anaemia is confirmed by the presence in the serum of autoantibodies to both parietal cells (in over 90% of patients with pernicious anaemia, but also in 15–20% of normal elderly people) and IF (in over 50% of patients). Histamine-fast achlorhydria and a raised serum gastrin are also present, but rarely need to be measured.

Management

B_{12} deficiency is treated with hydroxycobalamin supplements. These may be given orally in patients with a dietary deficiency (5–10 μg/day), but must be given intra-muscularly when malabsorption is present. It is usual to give five or six loading doses of 1000 μg over a period of one to two weeks, followed by 1000 μg every three months. A brisk reticulocyte response is usually seen after one week, although this may be delayed if the patient has other coexistent disease such as alcoholism. Hypokalaemia and gout may develop during treatment of severe megaloblastic anaemia. Therapy with B_{12} may also disclose and exacerbate incipient iron deficiency. Blood transfusion is rarely necessary and is best avoided.

FOLIC ACID DEFICIENCY

Folic acid is the parent compound of the folates, which facilitate the transfer of one-carbon units necessary in the synthesis of purine and pyrimidine bases. Folates are found in fresh fruit and vegetables, liver and kidney, and are destroyed by thorough cooking. Folate is absorbed in the upper small intestine and stored in a number of tissues, but particularly the liver. These stores provide about four months' supply of folate in the absence of further intake.

Aetiology

The aetiology of folate deficiency is illustrated in Figure 24.11. Dietary deficiency is seen particularly in milk-fed premature babies, the elderly (especially if living alone), and in chronic alcoholics. As coeliac disease and tropical

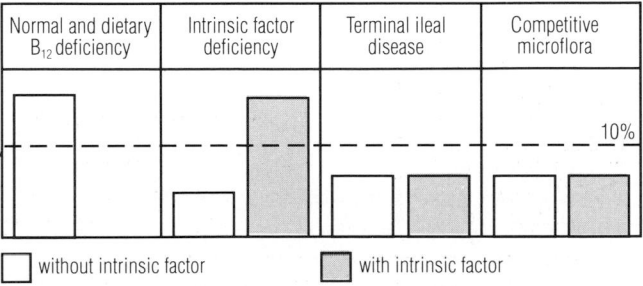

Fig. 24.10 **The Schilling test.** The urinary excretion of orally administered radioactively labelled vitamin B_{12} is measured. Low levels are excreted if there is malabsorption of B_{12} for any reason. If malabsorption is due to pernicious anaemia (IF deficiency), there is correction with simultaneous oral administration of IF. This correction does not occur when the cause of malabsorption is terminal ileal disease or competitive gut microflora.

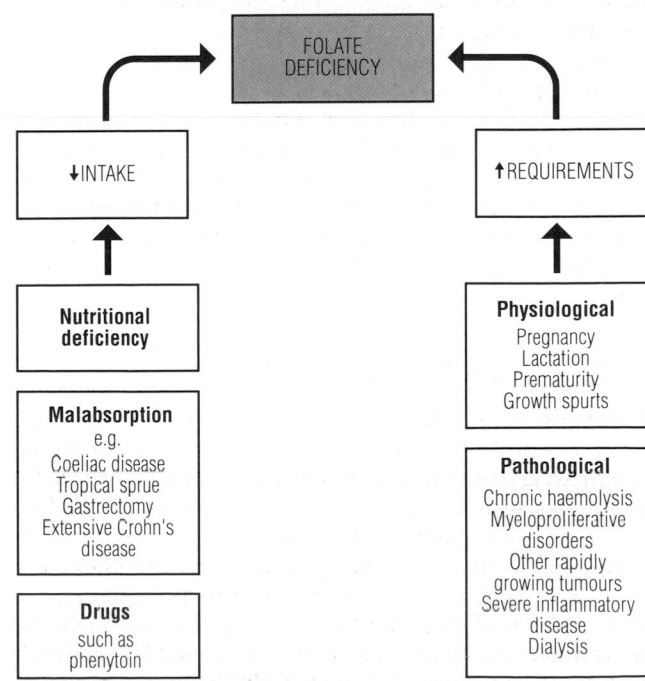

Fig. 24.11 **Aetiology of folate deficiency.**

sprue primarily affect the jejunum, folate deficiency is also very common in these diseases. They are also often associated with iron deficiency and the combined deficiency may result in normocytic indices on the automated printout. Examination of the blood film may reveal evidence of both iron deficiency and macrocytosis (dimorphic picture). Megaloblastic change is still apparent on bone marrow examination and pancytopenia and multisegmented polymorphs may be seen in the blood. Folate deficiency is also common (though less so than B$_{12}$ deficiency) after gastrectomy; both decreased dietary intake and rapid gastro-jejunal transit may contribute to its development. Drugs such as phenytoin may inhibit folate absorption, probably through a direct effect on the enterocyte brush border. Other drugs may interfere with folate utilisation, giving rise to megaloblastic anaemia in the presence of normal folate levels. These include the antifolate cytotoxic drugs (e.g. methotrexate), trimethoprim and anticonvulsants (e.g. phenytoin and phenobarbitone). Alcohol may also interfere with folate utilisation and this may account in part for the macrocytosis seen with excess consumption.

Management

The underlying cause of folate deficiency must be found and treated. The deficiency is treated with oral folic acid supplements (5–15 mg/day) which is usually adequate, even in malabsorption states. Folic acid is also given prophylactically to pregnant women, premature babies, patients receiving dialysis and in severe chronic haemolytic states. Folic acid should not be given alone in megaloblastic anaemia until B$_{12}$ deficiency has been excluded, since folate administration may precipitate neurological changes in B$_{12}$ deficiency.

THE HYPOPLASTIC ANAEMIAS

The hypoplastic or aplastic anaemias are a group of disorders in which there is anaemia due to a decrease in erythropoietic marrow. Although there is usually pancytopenia with reduction of all marrow elements, selective cytopenias do occur.

CONGENITAL/INHERITED HYPOPLASTIC ANAEMIAS

Congenital forms of hypoplastic anaemia occur in childhood. In *Fanconi's anaemia* (an autosomal recessive condition), pancytopenia usually develops between 5 and 10 years of age. Many of the children also suffer from other congenital abnormalities, including skeletal malformations (especially affecting the radii and thumbs), renal anomalies, microcephaly and congenital heart disease. This type of aplastic anaemia is characterised by a high red cell MCV, increased levels of HbF, a high ESR and a high incidence (5–10%) of transformation to acute leukaemia. Without successful bone marrow transplantation, the disease is invariably fatal.

Pure red cell aplasia (*Diamond-Blackfan syndrome*) may also be inherited, although the pattern of inheritance is not clear. Again, other congenital abnormalities may be present but are not as common as in Fanconi's anaemia. The anaemia usually appears in the first few weeks of life, although the diagnosis may be made considerably later. Steroids induce remissions in many patients but the majority become transfusion dependent.

Other familial and congenital hypoplastic states have also been described but are far less common.

ACQUIRED HYPOPLASTIC ANAEMIAS

Aetiology

The causes of the chronic acquired aplastic anaemias are shown in Table 24.4. Most cases are idiopathic in origin. It has been suggested that, in many such cases, there is an immunological suppression of haemopoiesis, but definite proof is lacking.

Transient episodes of marrow hypoplasia also occur, particularly following infections and idiosyncratic drug reactions. For example, very transient selective erythroid hypoplasia accompanies parvovirus infections. In normal individuals, this results in a transient reticulocytopenia, but in patients with haemolytic disease, there can be a dramatic fall in the haemoglobin level. Chronic pure red cell aplasia also occurs in adults, associated in nearly half the cases with a benign thymoma.

Clinical features

Patients with chronic aplastic anaemia present with insidious onset of the symptoms of anaemia, infections sec-

Table 24.4 Aetiology of chronic acquired aplastic anaemia

- Idiopathic
- Drugs
  Cytotoxic drugs
  Idiosyncratic reaction to drugs (including choramphenicol, phenylbutazone and thiouracils)
- Irradiation
- Chemicals, e.g. benzene
- Associated with infections, particularly viral hepatitis
- Associated with autoimmune disease
- Associated with pregnancy
- Paroxysmal nocturnal haemoglobinuria

ondary to the granulocytopenia, and bleeding due to thrombocytopenia. Examination may reveal signs of the above, but is otherwise usually normal. Splenomegaly, which occurs in less than 10% of cases, always suggests that the pancytopenia may be due to another cause.

The differential diagnosis of pancytopenia is shown in Table 24.5. In the marrow replacement states, the anaemia is often leucoerythroblastic, i.e. with nucleated red cells and granulocyte precursor cells in the blood.

Laboratory features

The anaemia of aplastic anaemia is usually normocytic but may be slightly macrocytic. There is an absolute reticulocytopenia. HbF levels may be modestly increased. Granulocytopenia and monocytopenia are present but the lymphocyte count may initially be near normal. The platelets are generally reduced. In a patient with a hypocellular marrow, severe aplastic anaemia is indicated by two of the following: reticulocytes $<1\%$, neutrophils $<0.5 \times 10^9/l$, platelets $<20 \times 10^9/l$. The diagnosis of aplastic anaemia is made by examination of a large bone marrow biopsy (preferably from two sites). Fat spaces predominate and there is markedly reduced haemopoiesis. Islands of haemopoiesis may be found and can be particularly confusing on a small biopsy specimen.

Management

Support

The successful management of aplastic anaemia is dependent on aggressive supportive care. Infections must be actively sought, recognised early and treated with intravenous antibiotics. In patients with a neutrophil count below $0.5 \times 10^9/l$, it is usual to give prophylactic oral antifungal agents such as nystatin or amphotericin. Some centres also give prophylactic oral cotrimoxazole or ciprofloxacin. Isolation facilities are advisable for severely neutropenic inpatients, but severe neutropenia alone is not an indication for hospitalisation. Therapy should be started empirically in patients with significant fever (above 38°C) sustained for two hours (less if clinical signs or symptoms are present). If there is a fever, the antibi-

otics must be broad-spectrum and cover Gram-negative organisms including the coliforms and pseudomonas. A third-generation cephalosporin or a combination of a ureidopenicillin and an aminoglycoside are usually used. Ciprofloxacin is also of value. Before initiating such therapy, a throat swab, sputum (if available), midstream specimen of urine, swabs from intravenous catheter sites, and blood taken from both a peripheral site and from any central intravenous lines, should be sent to microbiology for culture. The antibiotics can be rationalised later, if and when an organism is isolated and the sensitivities determined. A serum sample should be saved for possible viral antibody titres at a later date. A chest X-ray should be performed.

In patients who fail to respond to broad-spectrum antibiotics within three days, an opportunistic infection with fungus or pneumocystis should be suspected. If the chest X-ray shows pulmonary infiltration, bronchoscopy and alveolar lavage may help in diagnosis. Intravenous amphotericin therapy is used for suspected fungal infection, while pneumocystis infection may respond to high-dose cotrimoxazole therapy.

Red cell transfusions should be given as required and leucocyte-poor red cells used if sensitisation to white cell antigens occurs. Although repeated transfusions do increase the risks of graft rejection in patients who are later treated by bone marrow transplantation, it is more important to keep the patient in a good general condition.

Platelet transfusions are given to all patients with thrombocytopenia and evidence of bleeding. The use of platelets prophylactically in aplastic anaemia is limited by the chronic nature of the disease and the sensitisation that may occur to HLA and platelet-specific antigens. Granulocyte transfusions are not given prophylactically, and their use is limited to the treatment of life-threatening infections in severely neutropenic patients who are not responding to broad-spectrum antibiotic therapy. Even in this situation, their value is unproven.

Table 24.5 Differential diagnosis of pancytopenia

- Aplastic anaemia

- Bone marrow replacement
  Leukaemias, lymphomas and myeloma
  Non-haematological malignancies
  Fibrosis
  Osteopetrosis (rare)
  Gaucher's disease (rare)

- Hypersplenism

Summary 1 Management of hypoplastic anaemia

Supportive

Early treatment of infection with intravenous antibiotics (initially broad-spectrum, rationalised later)
Prophylactic oral anti-fungal agents
(Isolation facilities, if severely neutropenic)
Red cell transfusion
Platelet transfusion

Specific therapy

Androgen therapy (oxymethalone)
Haemopoietic growth factors
Intensive immunosuppression
Bone marrow transplantation

Specific therapy

The traditional therapy for aplastic anaemia has been *androgen therapy*, continued for at least three to six months. Oxymethalone is used, as it is less virilising than the testosterone derivatives. Proof of efficacy is lacking, however, and in severe cases androgens are not used alone. *Haemopoietic growth factors* (G-CSF, GM-CSF) may raise the neutrophil count in mild aplasia but are rarely effective in severe aplasia.

Intensive immunosuppression usually consists of high-dose methylprednisone and/or a course of anti-lympho-cyte serum. In some series, up to half the patients show a significant response, although there is considerable variation in the response to different batches of anti-lympho-cyte globulin. This type of therapy is intensive, and requires inpatient support similar to that required for transplantation. In the patients who do not respond, the response is usually only partial and completely normal haemopoiesis is not re-established.

Bone marrow transplantation is usually limited to those individuals under 40 years of age with an HLA identical sibling. Patients are usually prepared for transplantation with cyclophosphamide (50 mg/kg) on four successive days. In multiply transfused patients, some centres use total nodal irradiation to reduce the risk of graft rejection, but similar results can be achieved with cyclosporin A. The marrow inoculum required for transplantation in aplastic anaemia is probably higher than that for acute leukaemia, and at least 2×10^8 cells/kg should be given. The development of graft-versus-host disease (GVHD) can be minimised by administration of methotrexate or cyclosporin A. The removal of mature T cells from the marrow inoculum has been shown to be very effective in reducing GVHD, but there may be increased graft rejec-tion, particularly in multiply transfused aplastic patients.

Complications of bone marrow transplantation

GVHD is an ill-understood immunological reaction of mature donor lymphoid cells against host tissue. The acute form arises coincident with, or shortly after, haemo-poietic regeneration, and manifests as a maculopapular rash involving the hands and feet, hepatocellular liver toxi-city and diarrhoea. In its severest forms, there can be erythroderma (p. 1144), widespread bullae and then desquamation and torrential diarrhoea. Acute GVHD is treated with a course of high-dose methylprednisone. Severe cases may respond but the mortality is appreciable. Chronic GVHD develops several months after transplan-tation and is not necessarily preceded by the acute form. It takes the form of sclerodermatous skin changes and obstructive liver disease which can be debilitating and refractory to treatment. Immunosuppressive agents, such as azathioprine, are usually tried in this situation.

Immediately following preparative chemo/radiotherapy the patients with aplastic anaemia become even more pancytopenic. The risks of bacterial and fungal infection are thus very high in the 2–3 week period before graft regeneration occurs. Following engraftment the patient remains immunosuppressed for a variable time and opportunistic infections may still occur. *Pneumocystis* infection typically arises between four and 12 weeks and cytomegalovirus (CMV) infection between six weeks and six months. Some centres give prophylactic Septrin and ganciclovir for *Pneumocystis* and CMV, respectively.

However, over half the patients survive transplantation for aplastic anaemia and obtain haematological normality. In some centres, the success rate is in excess of 70%.

HAEMOLYTIC ANAEMIAS

The aetiology of haemolysis (excessive destruction of red cells) is given in Table 24.6.

Clinical and laboratory features

Patients with acute haemolysis develop profound symp-toms of anaemia. However, in the chronic haemolytic states quite severe anaemia can be tolerated with symp-toms only arising on exercise. The patient is jaundiced but this is often mild and easily missed. The urine is dark (especially after standing), due to the oxidisation of uro-bilinogen to urobilin. The spleen tends to be enlarged to a degree dependent on the underlying cause of the haemol-ysis. Leg ulcers, usually over the lateral malleolus, occur in the congenital haemolytic anaemias, particularly sickle cell disease.

The presence of haemolysis is usually established in the laboratory by a raised level of unconjugated bilirubin and reticulocytosis. Examination for urine haemoside-rinuria is particularly useful in low-grade chronic haemol-ysis. Red cell survival studies with ^{51}Cr-labelled red cells

Table 24.6 Aetiology of haemolysis

Congenital	Acquired (non-immune)
Defects of haemoglobin synthesis and structure	(see p. 1068, Table 24.9)
Thalassaemia	**Acquired (immune)**
Sickle cell disease	(see p. 1067, Summary 5)
Unstable haemoglobins (rare)	
Membrane defects	
Hereditary spherocytosis	
Hereditary elliptocytosis	
Red cell enzyme defects	
G6PD deficiency	
Pyruvate kinase deficiency (rare)	

are rarely required, but may be useful when combined with surface counting to estimate the role of the spleen in the haemolysis. The normal half-life of ^{51}Cr-labelled red cells is 25–35 days. The marrow can compensate for a half-life reduced to about 15 days, but below this anaemia occurs.

Investigation

The history will often indicate whether a haemolytic anaemia is familial or congenital. Particular attention must be paid to coexistent systemic disease and drug ingestion, both of which may be associated with haemolytic anaemia. Examination of the peripheral blood film may show red cell changes indicative of the underlying cause (Table 24.6). White cell abnormalities, such as the atypical mononuclear cells of infectious mononucleosis or the lymphocytosis of chronic lymphocytic leukaemia, may also indicate the cause of haemolysis. If an acquired haemolysis is suspected, the initial investigation is the direct antiglobulin test to determine whether this has an immune aetiology.

DEFECTS OF HAEMOGLOBIN SYNTHESIS AND STRUCTURE I: THE THALASSAEMIAS

Defects of haemoglobin synthesis and structure are one of the major congenital causes of haemolysis. The major examples are the thalassaemias and sickle cell disease.

The thalassaemias are inherited disorders in which there is a reduced synthesis of one or more globin chains. This results in unbalanced globin chain synthesis, globin precipitation, ineffective haemopoiesis and haemolysis. The α-thalassaemias are mainly found in the Far East, Middle East and Africa, while the β-thalassaemias are particularly prevalent in the Mediterranean. Thalassaemic genes are found in all racial groups.

The primary defect occurs either in the DNA sequences coding for the globin chains or in the intervening sequences between these coding regions. Chromosome 16 contains two genes coding for α chains, and there is a single gene coding for the β globin chain on chromosome 11 (Fig. 24.1, p. 1048). In the α-thalassaemias, the α genes are usually deleted, but such whole gene deletions are rare in the β-thalassaemias. In these cases, small aberrations in the gene may lead to decreased or absent transcription of the gene and intervening sequences, or they may prevent processing of the nuclear RNA to cytoplasmic RNA (during which the intervening sequences are removed). Rarely, cytoplasmic RNA is produced but cannot be translated into protein, e.g. where point mutations have introduced a stop sequence. A thalassaemic β gene may thus produce no β globin (β^0 gene) or low levels of β globin (β^+ gene).

β-THALASSAEMIAS

Clinical features

Clinically, the β-thalassaemias fall into three broad categories – thalassaemia minor (trait), intermedia and major. Individuals with *thalassaemia trait* are heterozygous for the thalassaemic gene and are usually fit and well; however, anaemia may develop during pregnancy, or in association with infections. In *thalassaemia major*, both β genes are abnormal so that the α : β chain synthesis imbalance is sufficient to cause a severe anaemia several months after birth. At birth, most of the haemoglobin is HbF ($\alpha_2\gamma_2$) and haemoglobin levels are normal. After birth α chain production continues, γ chain synthesis diminishes, but there is little or no β chain production (which would normally replace synthesis of γ). The result is a gradual onset of severe anaemia. Infants with thalassaemia major become listless, have a poor appetite and fail to thrive. Mental development is normal but walking is frequently delayed, and untreated children are grossly incapacitated and fail to develop. Expansion of the marrow cavities of the skull and facial bones results in a typical *mongoloid facies*, with frontal bossing of the skull and a 'hair on end' appearance on skull X-ray. Hepatomegaly and marked splenomegaly occur, and leg ulcers are frequent. Without transfusions, these children die in childhood or adolescence, usually from high output cardiac failure. Sexual maturity is not attained.

In *thalassaemia intermedia*, both β genes are affected but the clinical course is less severe, with haemoglobin levels typically in the range 6–9 g/dl. The molecular basis of β-thalassaemia intermedia is varied and includes:

- homozygosity for mild β^+ thalassaemic genes
- combinations of β^+ thalassaemia genes and δβ thalassaemia genes, in which there is decreased δ and β globin production but raised production of γ chains

---

Summary 2 Clinical features of thalassaemia major

Features of severe anaemia (if not transfused)

- Failure to thrive and growth retardation
- Thalassaemic facies
- Hepatosplenomegaly
- Leg ulcers
- High output cardiac failure

Features of iron overload (if transfused)

- Growth arrest
- Endocrine failure
- Liver damage
- Cardiac failure

- homozygotes with β-thalassaemia in whom there is a genetic predisposition to high HbF production.
- The combination of β-thalassaemia with α-thalassaemia trait, which also results in less chain imbalance and decreased severity of the disease.

Growth is not retarded and diagnosis is frequently delayed for several years until an intercurrent infection precipitates an acute fall in haemoglobin. These patients frequently survive into adulthood without transfusion and achieve normal sexual maturity, but pigment gallstones and leg ulceration are often a major problem.

Laboratory features

The thumbprint of thalassaemic genes is the appearance of microcytic red cells in the peripheral blood. In the β-thalassaemia traits, the haemoglobin concentration is normal or slightly reduced. The diagnosis is made by exclusion of iron deficiency and the anaemia of chronic disease, and the demonstration of a raised HbA_2 in a blood haemolysate. Levels of HbA_2 ($\alpha_2\delta_2$) are typically in the range 4–6% (normal 1.5–3%). In patients with homozygous β-thalassaemia, there is marked anaemia to a degree dependent on the nature of the underlying genetic defect. Poikilocytes and target cells are seen in the blood as well as polychromasia, and nucleated red blood cells are also present in the most severe cases. Haemoglobin electrophoresis usually shows HbF to be the major component. The level of HbA_2 is very variable. HbA is present in β^+ cases (Fig. 24.12).

In very difficult diagnostic cases – usually β-thalassaemia traits with microcytosis but a normal HbA_2 – the

thalassaemic defect can be demonstrated by showing imbalance of α and β globin synthesis in reticulocytes, following in vitro pulse labelling with radioactive leucine.

Management

Patients with thalassaemia minor require no specific therapy, but the nature of the genetic defect should be thoroughly explained. In thalassaemia major, blood transfusion is administered once every four to six weeks from the time of diagnosis, to maintain a normal [Hb]. This enables a young child to grow satisfactorily and live a relatively normal life. Unfortunately, repeated blood transfusions result in iron overload and iron accumulates in many tissues. Although much remains within the RE system, some enters and damages other tissues and multiple organ failure develops, most notably in the liver, the endocrine glands and the heart. The iron overload leads to slowing of growth and failure to attain sexual maturity. Death may occur in adolescence as a result of cardiomyopathy secondary to iron toxicity. Serum ferritin levels provide information about the kinetics of iron accumulation, but the absolute levels do not correlate closely with tissue toxicity.

Iron overload can be reduced by regular administration of an iron chelator – generally desferrioxamine given subcutaneously (approximately 60 mg/kg/day) by infusion pump over eight hours, five or six days a week. Ideally, the individual dose should be adjusted in accordance with iron balance studies. Oral vitamin C is also sometimes given to improve iron excretion. Children given desferrioxamine from the age of two to three years have grown well and developed sexually, but their ultimate life expectancy is not yet known. There is, moreover, the major problem with subcutaneous desferrioxamine of being attached to a pump for a quarter of one's life. Compliance is often poor and constant encouragement for the patients and family is required. Orally active iron chelators are being developed and offer hope for the future.

Hypersplenism frequently exacerbates the anaemia of thalassaemia, and splenectomy is therefore indicated if the transfusion requirements progressively increase or other cytopenias develop. Antipneumococcal vaccine may be of value if given before splenectomy, and oral penicillin V should be given as prophylaxis against pneumococcal infections. In recent years the results of allogeneic bone marrow transplantation from matched sibling donors have been encouraging.

Antenatal diagnosis

Antenatal diagnosis of thalassaemia with abortion of affected fetuses is acceptable in some communities, and appropriate facilities are available in specialist centres. Prenatal diagnosis begins with screening of all pregnant women attending their first antenatal clinic. In thalas-

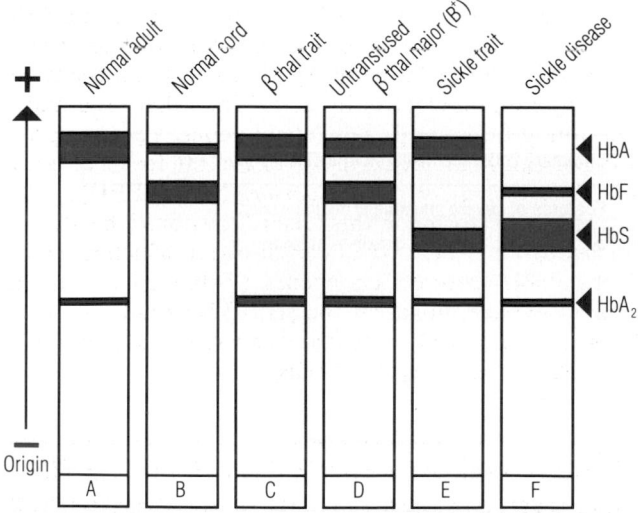

Fig. 24.12 Diagrammatic representation of haemoglobin electrophoresis at pH 8.9. HbD migrates in the same position as HbS, and HbC and HbE in the same position as HbA_2.

saemia trait, the MCV is low and the MCHC is normal; the MCH is a product of these measurements and is therefore a useful screening index. Patients with MCH values below 27 pg should have haemoglobin electrophoresis performed to look for a raised HbA$_2$. The iron status should also be determined, as patients with β-thalassaemia trait and iron deficiency may have a normal HbA$_2$. If the mother is found to have thalassaemia trait, the father should also be screened. Where both parents have the trait and the fetus is therefore at risk, prenatal diagnosis can be offered after both full discussion of the implications of the disease and consideration of the ethical issues involved. Prenatal diagnosis can be performed in the second trimester of pregnancy through globin chain synthesis studies on fetal blood obtained by fetoscopy. Diagnosis may also be made by DNA analysis of first-trimester chorionic biopsy specimens. This has the great advantage of being possible earlier in gestation, at a time when termination of pregnancy is less traumatic.

α-THALASSAEMIAS

The α-thalassaemias have a wide spectrum of clinical manifestations, partly because there are four genes coding for α globin. The commonest genetic abnormality is a complete deletion of one or more genes.

- Where only one gene is defective, the condition is often clinically silent, with a normal [Hb] and only a slight reduction in the MCV.
- In α-thalassaemia trait, there are usually two genes involved. Here, the [Hb] tends to be in the low/normal range, and microcytosis, poikilocytosis and some target cells are present in the blood. Supravital staining of the red cells may reveal inclusion bodies, which are precipitates of β chain tetramers known as HbH. HbA$_2$ levels are not raised. In newborn infants with α-thalassaemia trait, approximately 5% of the haemoglobin is in the form of γ chain tetramers known as Hb Barts.
- The more severe form of this disorder (haemoglobin H disease) is frequently due to the presence of three abnormal α genes. The patient usually has a mild anaemia, which may worsen rapidly with intercurrent infections or during pregnancy. The blood film shows the typical changes of thalassaemia and 5–20% of the total Hb is HbH. HbA$_2$ is not raised. Patients with HbH disease tend to become folate-deficient and should be given prophylactic supplements. Intercurrent infections should be treated vigorously.
- If all four α chains are deficient, there is no α chain synthesis and no production of HbF, HbA or HbA$_2$. The fetus dies in utero of hydrops fetalis and examination of the blood shows that about 80% of the haemoglobin is Hb Barts (γ_4), with small amounts of

Table 24.7 Causes of a raised [HbF]

- β-thalassaemia major
- Hereditary persistence of HbF
- Marrow expansion states
    Pregnancy
    Recovery from hypoplasia
- Abnormal erythroid clone
    Chronic myeloproliferative diseases, especially juvenile chronic myeloid leukaemia
    Acute leukaemia
    (Paroxysmal nocturnal haemoglobinuria)
- Other
    Some cases of acquired aplastic anaemia

HbH (β_4) and small amounts of the embryonic haemoglobin Hb Portland ($\varepsilon_2\gamma_2$).

OTHER FORMS OF THALASSAEMIA

Haemoglobin Constant Spring is a variant of the normal α globin, in which there is elongation of the α chain. Synthesis of this globin is reduced, resulting in an α-thalassaemic syndrome.

Alpha-thalassaemic genes may be associated with β-thalassaemic genes or abnormal chain variants. In general, this results in a reduction in severity of the underlying β-thalassaemic disease. Thus, a combination of β-thalassaemic genes that might otherwise be expected to cause thalassaemia major, may give rise to thalassaemia intermedia if there is concomitant α-thalassaemia.

The β-thalassaemic syndromes sometimes involve δ chain production, in which case no increase in HbA$_2$ occurs. In Hb Lepore there is low production of a hybrid formed from a part of the δ and part of the β chain, giving another form of thalassaemic syndrome with an abnormal haemoglobin on electrophoresis. When there is a major deletion in both the β and δ chain genes, γ gene expression remains high, giving rise to one of the forms of *hereditary persistence of fetal haemoglobin* (HPFH). The heterozygous form of this disorder should be distinguished from the variety of conditions in which reactivation of HbF production occurs (Table 24.7). In the marrow expansion states, the [HbF] is usually less than 3% and is often only detected as a rise in the number of red cells containing HbF (F-cells).

DEFECTS OF HAEMOGLOBIN SYNTHESIS AND STRUCTURE II: SICKLING DISORDERS

The sickle cell gene has a single base substitution which results in a change of valine for glutamine in the sixth

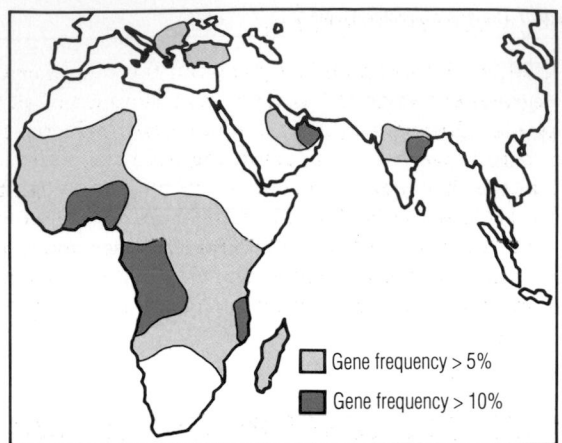

Fig. 24.13 Geographical incidence of the sickle cell gene.

Gene frequency > 5%

Gene frequency > 10%

amino acid position of the β chain. In the deoxygenated form, HbS forms non-hydrophobic bonds with adjacent HbS molecules, resulting in fibril formation and the appearance of distorted sickle-shaped cells. Initially, this process is reversible when the haemoglobin becomes oxygenated, but eventually the red cell membrane becomes damaged and leads to the formation of irreversibly sickled cells. The sickle gene originates primarily in areas where the malarial parasite (*Plasmodium falciparum*) is endemic, and owes its prevalence to the selective advantage conferred by the sickle cell trait on young children infected with this organism (Fig. 24.13).

SICKLE CELL TRAIT

In sickle cell trait (heterozygous state), at least 50% of the haemoglobin is HbA. The concentration of HbS is relatively low, so that sickling only occurs under anoxic conditions such as occur with non-pressurised air travel, poor anaesthetics, or (rarely) in conditions of marked acidosis and dehydration as may occur with severe infections. Individuals with sickle cell trait are not anaemic and are usually asymptomatic. However, the sickle cell screening test – in which an HbS haemolysate precipitates and becomes cloudy at pH 7.1 – is positive. Haemoglobin electrophoresis reveals 35–50% HbS, which runs as a slow band at alkaline pH (Fig. 24.12), with the remainder nearly all HbA. [HbA$_2$] and [HbF] are not raised.

SICKLE CELL DISEASE

Clinical features

Symptoms occur from the second half of the first year of life onwards, as the HbF levels fall. The major problems caused by sickling in young infants are haemolytic anaemias and dactylitis. Later, the main problem is the occurrence of painful vasocclusive crises caused by the sickled cells. These crises are frequently provoked by minor infections or dehydration.

The pain may be mild or so agonising as to require large doses of opiate analgesics. Fever and malaise are common, making it difficult to determine whether there is an underlying infection. Pain may arise in the limbs, back, abdomen or trunk. In childhood, splenic infarcts are frequent, leading to splenic atrophy and functional hyposplenism. Aseptic necrosis of the femoral head is a common and disabling complication.

Small vessel occlusions in the retinae lead to ischaemia and vascular proliferation, with visual impairment and a high risk of vitreous haemorrhage and retinal detachment. Retinopathy is particularly common in sickling disorders with a high [Hb], such as HbS/C disease. Haematuria occurs frequently due to papillary necrosis, but even in patients without such overt renal episodes, there is an acquired tubular reabsorption defect with inability to produce a concentrated urine. Priapism may occur due to sickling in the corpora cavernosa. This is extremely painful and, unless decompressed rapidly, results in impotence.

The anaemia of sickle cell disease may be exacerbated by episodes of erythroid hypoplasia (aplastic crises) precipitated by parvovirus infections, acute splenic and rarely hepatic sequestration of red cells, or folate deficiency. The chronic haemolytic anaemia frequently leads to ankle ulceration and the development of gallstones.

Patients with sickle cell disease also have an increased risk of infection, which is only partly explained by splenic atrophy. Fulminating pneumococcal infections may occur, and there is an unusually high incidence of *Salmonella* osteomyelitis which, initially, can be difficult to differentiate from a vasocclusive infarction.

Summary 3 Clinical features of sickle cell disease

- Painful 'crises'
- Sickle lung syndrome
- Symptoms of anaemia
- Aseptic necrosis of the femoral head
- Retinopathy
- Renal tubular damage
- Priapism
- Leg ulcers
- Gallstones
- Increased risk of pneumococcal and salmonella infections
- Dactylitis (infants)
- 'Hypoplastic' anaemic crises
- 'Sequestration' anaemic crises

Acute pulmonary episodes are the most common, and also potentially most dangerous, complications of sickle cell disease. The pulmonary lesions may be infective, ischaemic or a combination of the two. Minor lung changes can progress rapidly with development of widespread intra-alveolar consolidation and respiratory failure within hours.

Laboratory features

Haematological investigations reveal a mild to moderate normocytic anaemia. Anisocytosis, poikilocytosis and sickled cells can be seen on the blood film while, in older children and adults, target cells and Howell Jolly bodies are also seen as a result of the hyposplenic state. The sickle screening test is positive and haemoglobin electrophoresis shows most of the haemoglobin to be HbS. HbA$_2$ levels are normal. HbF levels are raised in a minority of patients (Fig. 24.12).

Management

Appropriate measures should be taken to prevent sickling crises. Patients should avoid severe cold and dehydration, and infections must be treated early and aggressively. Prophylactic penicillin V should be given to all children in view of the hyposplenism, with some centres recommending continued use throughout life. Hypoxia with anaesthesia or unpressurised air travel must be avoided. In patients with very frequent and severe sickling episodes, a hypertransfusion regime can be instituted to replace HbS with HbA. This is mainly of value as a relatively short term measure prior to surgery (particularly ophthalmic surgery), and in the management of major complications.

It is essential to keep the patient undergoing a sickle crisis warm, hydrated and well oxygenated. Large quantities of opiate analgesics are often required. Possible infections must be investigated and treated appropriately. It is common practice to give all patients with sickle crises a course of ampicillin after appropriate cultures have been taken, though proof of beneficial effect is lacking. Where a pulmonary infection is suspected, broad-spectrum cover should be given. If a sickle-lung syndrome develops, regular blood gases should be performed and the patient ventilated early if hypoxia develops.

Contraception

Double barrier techniques, such as the cap and spermicidal foam and pessaries, are safe and effective if used correctly. The intrauterine contraceptive device (IUCD) and low-dose contraceptive pill are used in some circumstances, but there is little firm data on their safety in sickle cell disease.

Management of pregnancy

Folate supplements should be given but there is otherwise little agreement as to the correct management of sickle cell disease during pregnancy. Many centres institute a three to four-weekly transfusion regime during the last trimester, with the aim of achieving normal haemoglobin levels with 70–80% HbA at the expected time of delivery. If there is a history of first or second trimester abortions, transfusion is started as soon as possible in the pregnancy. Other specialists feel that transfusion during pregnancy is unnecessary.

SICKLE CELL GENES IN ASSOCIATION WITH OTHER ABNORMAL Hb GENES

Sickle cell genes frequently interact with thalassaemic genes. In α-thalassaemia, the severity of sickle cell disease in β^s (sickle gene) homozygotes is often reduced, possibly a result of the slightly decreased concentration of HbS in the red cells.

If a heterozygote β^s interacts with a β-thalassaemia gene, the HbS level is higher than in a usual HbS trait leading to clinical symptoms. If the thalassaemia gene is a β^0 gene, a severe sickle cell syndrome may arise.

Interaction of β^s with an HPFH (Table 24.7) results in virtually no normal β chain production. However, although the level of HbS may be as high as 80%, the high levels of HbF present reduce the risks of sickling. Other forms of 'high F gene' exist and may also reduce the sickling tendency.

The sickle gene may also interact with other β gene haemoglobinopathies. Thus, HbS/C disease, for example, results in a moderate or reasonably mild anaemia. The blood film shows sickle cells and many target cells, and haemoglobin electrophoresis shows that approximately half is HbS and half HbC, the latter running behind HbS in the same position as HbA$_2$ (Fig. 24.12). The clinical picture is very varied, but ocular complications are particularly common. In contrast to adult sickle cell disease, splenomegaly is often present.

OTHER HAEMOGLOBINOPATHIES CAUSING HAEMOLYSIS

HbC

HbC is very common in West Africa, particularly Ghana. The heterozygous state is symptomless and the [Hb] normal. In the homozygous state, however, the [Hb] may be slightly reduced, the spleen is usually large, gallstones may develop and ocular lesions are frequent.

HbD

HbD is found in many ethnic groups. It migrates with HbS on standard agar gels at pH 8.6 but not at acid pH. The heterozygous state is asymptomatic, with a mild anaemia occurring in the homozygous state. An asymptomatic patient with apparent homozygosity for HbS may in fact be HbS/D.

HbE

HbE is found predominantly in South-East Asia. It migrates on standard agar gels with HbC and HbA$_2$. The trait (heterozygous state) is symptomless, with a mild microcytic haemolytic anaemia in the homozygous state.

Unstable haemoglobins and methaemoglobinaemia

A variety of unstable haemoglobins have been described which tend to precipitate and cause a haemolytic anaemia. Heinz bodies are seen within erythrocytes on a reticulocyte stain. Some forms of autosomal dominant congenital methaemoglobinaemia are due to amino acid substitutions in the region of the haem pocket of globin. The patient is cyanosed and may have a mild haemolytic state.

CONGENITAL RED CELL MEMBRANE DEFECTS

Haemolysis can be due to congenital red cell membrane defects, the commonest of which are hereditary spherocytosis and hereditary elliptocytosis.

Hereditary spherocytosis

The commonest membrane defect is hereditary spherocytosis, an autosomal condition affecting 1 in 5000 individuals. The abnormality usually resides in the spectrin molecule of the cytoskeleton. Clinically, the disease is very varied. Haemolysis may be well compensated with no anaemia, or anaemia may be severe. There may also be acute exacerbations of anaemia, such as haemolytic crises associated with intercurrent infections and aplastic crises associated with parvovirus infections or folate deficiency. The spleen is usually palpable and not tender, but may become so during haemolytic crises. There is usually mild jaundice but, in the neonate, it may be sufficiently severe to cause kernicterus. Gallstones may arise in late childhood and adult life.

There is usually a mild normocytic anaemia, but during crises the [Hb] may fall below 8 g/dl. The blood film reveals spherocytes and a reticulocytosis. The diagnosis is confirmed by demonstration of increased red cell osmotic fragility (Fig. 24.14), and by exclusion of other causes of spherocytosis such as autoimmune haemolysis. Family studies may also prove useful.

Children, non-splenectomised adults and pregnant women should receive folate supplements. Transfusion may be required for aplastic crises. Splenectomy reduces the haemolysis, prevents acute haemolytic crises and reduces the incidence of pigment gallstone formation; but this is usually delayed until adolescence because of the risks of postsplenectomy infections. If splenectomy is to be performed, gallstones should first be looked for using ultrasound and a simultaneous cholecystectomy considered. Following splenectomy, prophylactic penicillin should be given.

Hereditary elliptocytosis

Hereditary elliptocytosis is an autosomal dominant condition in which an abnormality of the cytoskeleton results in oval red blood cells. The osmotic fragility is normal. In some (usually mild) cases, the inheritance is linked to the rhesus genes. Most patients are asymptomatic, but a small proportion have the signs and symptoms of chronic haemolysis, which may necessitate splenectomy.

Other hereditary red cell membrane defects

These include: hereditary stomatocytosis, in which the red cells have a slit-like central pallor resembling a mouth; hereditary pyropoikilocytosis in which there is marked haemolysis and in vitro fragmentation of red cells

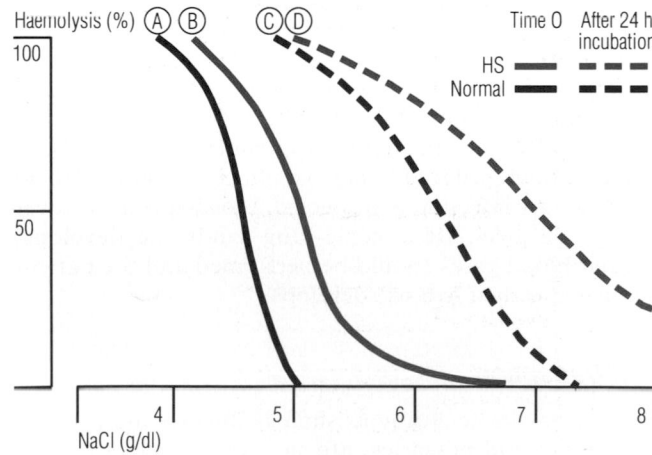

Fig. 24.14 Osmotic fragility curves showing lysis of red cells at low salt concentrations. (A) represents the normal curve and (C) represents normal cells pre-incubated for 24 hours at 37°C. (B) and (D) represent fresh and pre-incubated hereditary spherocytic cells respectively.

upon gentle heating; and hereditary acanthocytosis. This last condition is inherited in an autosomal recessive manner and is associated with abetalipoproteinaemia, malabsorption, retinitis pigmentosa and diffuse nervous system abnormalities.

CONGENITAL RED CELL ENZYME DEFECTS

The glycolytic enzymes in the erythrocyte generate two moles of ATP for each mole of glucose metabolised (Fig. 24.15). ATP is required for transmembrane iron transport and for the maintenance of the shape and flexibility of the red cell. NADH is also produced by the glycolytic pathway and is required for the maintenance of haem iron in the ferrous state. NADPH, produced by the hexose monophosphate shunt, is necessary for the reduction of glutathione which protects the red cell from oxidant stress. 2,3-DPG is derived as an offshoot of the glycolytic pathway and is important for its modulating effects on haemoglobin-oxygen affinity. The tricarboxylic cycle, protein synthesis, and nucleic acid synthesis do not occur in the erythrocyte.

Glucose-6-phosphate dehydrogenase deficiency

Glucose-6-phosphate dehydrogenase (G6PD) deficiency is the commonest inherited disease in the world. G6PD is the first enzyme in the hexose monophosphate shunt, so a deficiency leads to a fall in NADPH and increased sensitivity of the erythrocytes to oxidant stress. The G6PD enzyme is coded on the X chromosome, so that disease due to deficiency of this enzyme mainly affects males. Female heterozygotes (carriers) have about 50% of normal levels overall, but within individual red cells the G6PD levels are either completely normal or grossly deficient so that clinical disease may also occasionally occur in females. Many isoenzymes of G6PD have been described. The predominant isoenzyme – found in Caucasians and 60% of blacks – is designated B+. A normal African variant found in 25% is designated A+. Other isoenzymes, however, lead to G6PD deficiency. In the African A– variant, G6PD is produced in normal quantities and initially has full functional activity. However, the enzyme is unstable, so that the G6PD activity of an erythrocyte declines with time. In Mediterranean-Oriental type G6PD deficiency, the enzyme usually has low or absent functional activity from the beginning.

Clinical features

The clinical spectrum of G6PD deficiency is wide. The commonest presentation is that of an *acute haemolytic episode*, precipitated by infection, acute illness or drugs. Many drugs have been implicated in causing acute haemolysis in G6PD deficiency, but only a few commonly used drugs consistently have this effect (Table 24.8). In the African-type G6PD deficiency (A–), the haemolysis leads to a brisk reticulocytosis and, as the reticulocytes have adequate levels of G6PD, is thus self-limiting. However, in G6PD deficiency variants where reticulocyte G6PD levels are low, the intravascular haemolysis may be sufficiently severe to cause collapse and death. *Favism* is the condition when acute haemolysis is precipitated in G6PD deficiency following exposure to broad beans,

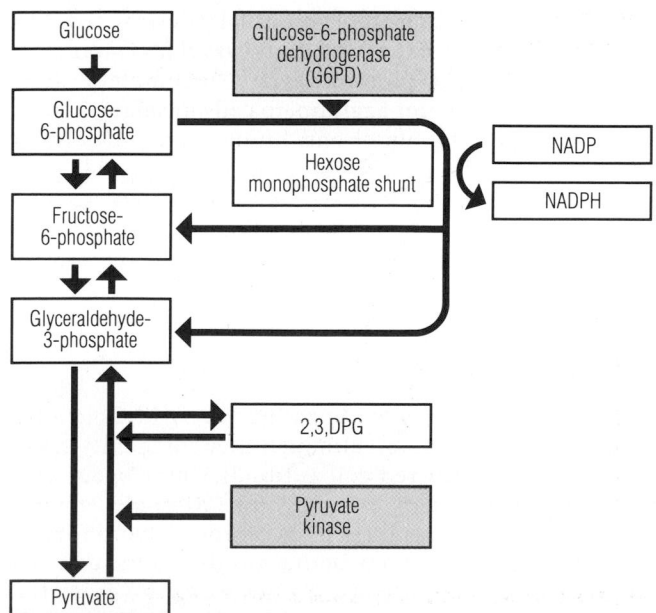

Fig. 24.15 Simplified scheme of glycolysis and the hexose monophosphate shunt.

Table 24.8 Drugs which may precipitate acute haemolysis in G6PD deficiency

Type of drug	Example
Analgesics	Aspirin
Antibiotics	Sulphonamides
	Nitrofurantoin
	Chloramphenicol
	Quinolones
	Para-aminosalicylic acid
Antimalarials	Quinine
	Chloroquine
	Primaquine
Antileprotics	Dapsone
Miscellaneous	Vitamin K
	Vitamin C

either as lightly cooked food or as pollen. It is mostly confined to the Mediterranean variants of G6PD deficiency and mainly affects young children. The *chronic haemolytic anaemia* of G6PD deficiency is rare but has been described with many different variants. The anaemia is usually mild. *Neonatal haemolysis* occurs mainly in Mediterranean and Oriental variants, and is an important differential diagnosis of immune haemolysis of the newborn in these areas. The administration of vitamin K may precipitate or exacerbate some cases.

Laboratory features

During haemolytic episodes there is a non-spherocytic anaemia with anisocytosis. Vital staining of the blood film reveals a reticulocytosis and many Heinz bodies (precipitated haemoglobin). Erythrocyte G6PD levels can be measured in a commercially available enzyme kit, but it must be borne in mind that in the African type of G6PD deficiency, the level may rise into the female heterozygote range during acute episodes with a reticulocytosis. In these circumstances, definitive assays should be delayed until the convalescent period.

Management

Patients with G6PD deficiency should receive prompt therapy of all infections and avoid drugs known to precipitate haemolysis. Blood transfusion is occasionally required for severe episodes of haemolysis, and exchange transfusion may be needed in cases of neonatal jaundice.

Pyruvate kinase deficiency

Pyruvate kinase (PK) deficiency is rare compared with G6PD deficiency. It is generally an autosomal recessive condition (although occasionally heterozygotes may have minor haemolysis), and is most common in Caucasians. PK deficiency results in the reduced generation of ATP and NADH and inability of the cells to maintain electrolyte balance. Haemolysis is extravascular, with removal of defective cells by the RE system.

Clinical and laboratory features

There is a congenital non-spherocytic anaemia of very variable severity. Severe anaemia is partially ameliorated by the high 2,3-DPG levels present (distal block) which help maintain tissue oxygenation (p. 1049, Fig. 24.6). The anaemia is often exacerbated by infections. Splenomegaly is common and severe cases may require regular transfusions.

Examination of the blood film reveals poikilocytosis and reticulocytosis. The diagnosis is confirmed by measurement of erythrocyte PK enzyme activity.

General approach to erythrocyte enzymopathies

When haemolysis due to an enzyme defect is suspected, the G6PD level should be measured first, as this is the commonest enzymopathy. If this is normal, PK activity should be measured. Many other enzyme deficiencies have been reported, but these are extremely rare. The family and clinical history may provide clues, and measurement of 2,3-DPG levels may help localise a defect in the Emden-Myerhof pathway.

AUTOIMMUNE HAEMOLYTIC ANAEMIAS

Autoimmune haemolytic anaemias (AIHA) are generally categorised according to whether the anti-red cell antibody is cold or warm. Warm antibodies react with red cells at 37°C, tend to be IgG and usually destroy red cells by means of opsonisation and extravascular clearance in the RE system. IgG antibodies are 'incomplete' antibodies and thus do not agglutinate cells in saline; hence, the addition of albumin or anti-human gamma globulin (direct antiglobulin test, DAT; see p. 1072, Fig. 24.19) is required. Cold antibodies are usually IgM complete antibodies which agglutinate cells in saline at room temperature. The thermal amplitude of such antibodies is very variable.

Aetiology

AIHA is most commonly idiopathic in origin. Cold antibodies are most common although they frequently cause little problem. Anti-red cell antibodies may occur secondary to malignancies, especially the low-grade lymphoproliferative disorders such as chronic lymphocytic leukaemia. The warm antibodies produced in such circumstances are polyclonal, do not originate from the malignant clone, and are indicative of the overall immune dysregulation that occurs in these conditions. However, when cold antibodies are produced in lymphoma they are frequently monoclonal. AIHA can occur in association with all the autoimmune diseases but is most common in systemic lupus erythematosus when it may occasionally be the presenting feature. Viral infections frequently predate warm antibody AIHA in children and young adults. Infectious mononucleosis may lead to production of cold antibodies with *i* blood group specificity and mycoplasma pneumoniae with *I* specificity.

Drugs may cause AIHA by several mechanisms.

- Certain drugs, such as methyldopa, L-dopa and mefanamic acid, induce the production of autoantibodies directed against red cell antigens through an unknown mechanism. With chronic methyldopa use, up to 20% of patients acquire a positive direct antiglobulin test, although haemolytic anaemia occurs in less than 1%. If haemolysis does occur, it usually ceases within two weeks of stopping the drug, although the DAT may remain positive for several years. In this case, the antibody is usually a warm IgG reactive with the rhesus antigen system.
- Some drugs cause haemolysis by acting as a hapten. This occurs most frequently with high-dose parenteral penicillin. It is absorbed onto the red cell and in that form stimulates antibody production. IgM antibodies are frequently produced without clinical effect, but if IgG antibodies are produced, haemolysis may be severe.
- Immune complex-mediated haemolysis is rare but has been reported with a wide range of drugs. In these cases, the patient has usually received the drug before and has become sensitised to it. On rechallenge, immune complexes containing the drug are formed, bind to the red cells and precipitate complement-mediated intravascular haemolysis.

Immune haemolysis may complicate blood transfusion, and this and haemolytic disease of the newborn are discussed on pages 1074–1077.

Summary 5 Aetiology of autoimmune haemolytic anaemia

- Idiopathic
- Secondary
  Neoplasms, especially lymphoproliferative disorders
  Autoimmune disorders
  Infections
  Drugs – Induction of 'true autoantibodies'
       – Drugs acting as haptens on red cell surface
       – Passive absorption of drug–antibody complex onto erythrocyte
- Complication of blood transfusion (transient)
- Immune haemolytic disease of the newborn

Clinical features

Warm antibodies do not generally cause complement activation and intravascular haemolysis. Instead, the red cells are opsonised and removed in the RE system, resulting in anaemia which may be either acute and severe or a mild chronic disorder. Occasionally, AIHA may be complicated by immune thrombocytopenia and, in these cases, bruising and petechial haemorrhages may occur.

Cold antibodies may be asymptomatic or, alternatively, give rise to cold haemagglutinin disease (CHAD). The idiopathic form occurs mainly in the elderly. On exposure to the cold, acute episodes of haemolysis may occur and peripheral cyanosis and Raynaud's phenomenon are also frequent. In between episodes, the haemoglobin may be normal or only slightly reduced. Rarely, there is a chronic severe anaemia which is refractory to treatment. Infection-induced cold haemolysis is usually characterised by acute onset of anaemia, jaundice and haemoglobinuria which subsides after several weeks.

Paroxysmal cold haemoglobinuria (PCH) is a very rare form of cold antibody haemolysis, in which the antibody is a cold IgG specific for the P blood group system. It may be idiopathic or postinfective, particularly following syphilis. The degree of cold exposure required to precipitate attacks is very variable.

Laboratory features

The anaemia is usually slightly macrocytic due to the reticulocytosis. If haemolysis is severe, nucleated red cells may be seen in the blood. Spherocytes are frequently seen and the osmotic fragility may be increased, although usually to a lesser extent than in hereditary spherocytosis. Red cell aggregates are commonly found on the blood film, particularly with cold antibodies. The ESR is usually markedly raised.

Hyperbilirubinaemia is present and reflects in part the severity of the haemolysis. Haemoglobinuria occurs with acute intravascular haemolysis, and haemosiderinuria with chronic intravascular haemolysis (p. 1069).

The diagnosis of AIHA is made by demonstrating the presence of a red cell autoantibody. With warm antibodies (active at 37°C in DAT), this is usually IgG and only occasionally IgA or IgM. Cold antibodies are usually IgM and agglutinate at room temperature (less so at 37°C). The DAT is usually positive with anti-C3d, and in some cases only C3d can be demonstrated on the cell surface.

Management

Warm antibody haemolysis

In primary (idiopathic) cases, remission induction is attempted with a course of high dose steroids (prednisone

1 mg/kg per day), which is then tailed off gradually according to the response. Blood transfusion may be necessary, and this causes considerable difficulties with the cross-match. Splenectomy is usually tried if steroids fail; and immunosuppression with azathioprine, chlorambucil or cyclophosphamide may prove effective in splenectomy resistant cases. In cases of chronic haemolysis, folic acid supplements should be given.

In secondary AIHA, appropriate treatment of the underlying disease will often terminate the haemolytic process. Drugs suspected of causing haemolysis should be withdrawn. Spontaneous remissions may occur, particularly in postinfective AIHA in children.

Cold antibody haemolysis

If the haemolysis is mild and well compensated, no specific therapy is required but the patient must avoid exposure to cold. During acute episodes (especially following infections), confinement to a very warm room may be necessary; and if transfusion is required, washed cells should be given (reduced complement) through a blood warmer. Steroids and splenectomy rarely help in cold haemagglutinin disease; if the haemolysis is chronic and severe, chlorambucil or cyclophosphamide should be tried.

ACQUIRED NON-IMMUNE HAEMOLYTIC ANAEMIAS

The aetiology of acquired non-immune haemolytic anaemias are shown in Table 24.9.

Hypersplenism

Hypersplenism is defined as a peripheral blood cytopenia which can be cured by splenectomy. The spleen is usually enlarged (splenomegaly), the causes of which are shown in Table 24.10.

The mechanism of hypersplenism is multifactorial and includes both pooling of cells within the spleen and rapid destruction of cells within the spleen. The plasma volume is usually increased in splenomegaly and a dilutional factor contributes to any anaemia. Assessment of hypersplenism can be difficult. The diagnosis is usually suggested by the finding of a peripheral blood cytopenia, an active cellular marrow and splenomegaly. However, if there is an underlying haematological disease such as a haemolytic anaemia, it can be difficult to separate out the effects of this from the hypersplenism. In some cases, radioactive isotope studies may be of value. Using ^{51}Cr-labelled red cells, a shortened red cell survival can be demonstrated, and surface counting can then be per-

Table 24.9 Aetiology of acquired non-immune haemolytic anaemias

Hypersplenism

Toxic states
Infections, e.g. malaria
Uraemia
Drugs
Chemicals, e.g. lead poisoning
Venoms, e.g. cobra bites

Microangiopathic haemolytic anaemias
Disseminated intravascular coagulation (DIC)
Haemolytic uraemic syndrome (HUS) and thrombotic thrombocytopenic purpura (TTP)
Malignant hypertension

Trauma to red cells
Cardiac prostheses
March haemoglobinuria
Burns

Acquired red cell membrane defects
Paroxysmal nocturnal haemoglobinura (PNH)
Liver disease
Vitamin E deficiency, especially in premature babies

Table 24.10 Causes of splenomegaly

Primary haematological disorders
Haemolytic anaemias, especially if severe and chronic
Lymphoproliferative disorders
Myeloproliferative disorders

Non-haematological disorders
Congestive splenomegaly
    Portal hypertension
    Hepatic or portal vein thrombosis
    Chronic congestive cardiac failure

Infections
    Bacterial, e.g. septicaemia, typhoid, tuberculosis
    Viral, e.g. hepatitis, infectious mononucleosis
    Tropical, e.g. malaria, kala-azar

Collagen vascular diseases

Metabolic 'storage disease'

Sarcoidosis

formed over the spleen. In extravascular haemolytic anaemias, the role of the spleen in red cell destruction can be partly assessed by comparison of the spleen and liver uptake of ^{51}Cr-labelled red cells over a period of 10 days. A ratio greater than 4 suggests that considerable splenic destruction is occurring, and that splenectomy may be beneficial.

Blood changes following splenectomy

If hypersplenism was present, the cytopenias should resolve following splenectomy. A number of other changes in the blood also occur (Table 24.11). It must be noted that these changes also occur in other hyposplenic states (Table 24.12).

Microangiopathic haemolytic anaemias

The microangiopathic haemolytic anaemias include disseminated intravascular coagulation, haemolytic uraemic syndrome and thrombotic thrombocytopenic purpura. These are discussed on pages 1108–1110.

Trauma to red cells

Trauma to red cells may occur in a number of situations, including cardiac prostheses, march haemoglobinuria and burns.

Cardiac prostheses. Trauma to red cells due to cardiac prostheses occurs predominantly with prostheses on the left side of the heart where systolic pressures are high. It is particularly common with faulty valves through which there is regurgitation. The anaemia is usually mild, and red cell fragments (schistocytes) are seen on the blood film. The platelet count may also be low.

March haemoglobinuria. In march haemoglobinuria, red cells are ruptured in the small vessels of the feet in some otherwise healthy individuals when they engage in long marches or runs. It may be sufficiently severe to cause frank haemoglobinuria, nausea and abdominal cramps.

Paroxysmal nocturnal haemoglobinuria

Paroxysmal nocturnal haemoglobinuria (PNH) is a rare disorder of multipotential stem cells in which an affected clone gives rise to abnormal red cells, leucocytes and platelets. It is caused by a mutation in an X-linked gene involved in the formation of membrane phosphatidyl inositol anchors. Why the PNH clone should obtain a selective advantage over normal haemopoietic clones is not known. The membranes of these cells are deficient in those proteins normally anchored to the cell membrane through a phosphatidyl inositol linkage. As these include complement deactivating factors, the cells are very sensitive to complement lysis activated by the alternative pathway. There is a high incidence of aplastic anaemia and acute leukaemia reflecting the aberrant nature of the stem cell.

Clinical features

This disorder usually presents in adults, and is more common in women. The clinical manifestations are wide. Paroxysmal haemolysis and haemoglobinuria during sleep is reported in only 25% of patients. Severe bouts may be associated with jaundice and low back pain.

Chronic low-grade intravascular haemolysis is more common than the severe form and usually leads to iron deficiency. Mild neutropenia and thrombocytopenia are also common, and occasionally severe aplastic anaemia may arise or be the presenting feature. The thromboses that occur are usually venous, though occasionally arterial. The sites of thromboses are often atypical and include the hepatic veins and cerebral sinuses.

Summary 6 Clinical features of PNH

- Paroxysmal nocturnal haemoglobinuria
- Chronic haemolysis
- Mild cytopenias
- Severe aplastic anaemia
- Thromboses
- Leukaemic transformation

Diagnosis and management

Non-immune intravascular haemolysis should always raise the suspicion of PNH, but haemosiderinuria may be the only evidence of haemolysis. Iron deficiency and cytopenias are frequent. The neutrophil alkaline phosphatase score is usually low in PNH (unless aplastic anaemia occurs) and is a useful diagnostic indicator. The standard diagnostic test has been the *Ham's test*, in which PNH (but not normal) red cells lyse during a one hour 37°C incubation with normal sera, but do not lyse if complement is first removed from the sera by inactivation at 56°C. Diagnosis can also be made by immunophenotype analysis for deficient antigen expression. (CD59 for red cells and platelets, CD67 for granulocytes, CD14 for monocytes and CD24 for B cells.)

There is no specific therapy for PNH and treatment is supportive. Initiation of iron therapy for haemolysis may cause a reticulocytosis and a temporary exacerbation of the haemolytic process.

Table 24.11 Blood changes postsplenectomy

Blood cell type	Change
Red cells	Howell-Jolly bodies (nuclear remnants)
	Siderocytes
	Target cells
	Normoblasts
Leucocytes	Neutrophil leucocytosis (usually transient)
	Myelocytes appear in the blood during infections
Platelets	Thrombocytosis (usually transient)

Table 24.12 Causes of hyposplenism

• Splenectomy	• Congenital absence (rare)
• Sickle cell disease	• Systemic lupus erythematosus (rare)
• Coeliac disease	• Senile atrophy (rare)

ANAEMIA OF CHRONIC DISEASE

The anaemia of chronic disease is multifactorial. Haematinic deficiency, poor iron utilisation, relative erythroid hypoplasia and a slightly decreased red cell survival may all contribute to the anaemia, while other factors may also contribute in specific diseases.

The anaemia is usually mild or moderate and may be microcytic or normocytic. The serum iron is usually low, but the total iron binding capacity is also reduced, giving a percentage saturation greater than 10%. Marrow iron is present and the serum ferritin is normal or raised. There may be a leucocytosis and the blood film may show features specific to the underlying disease process. Several chronic diseases merit special attention.

Renal failure

The anaemia may be severe in chronic renal failure. Retained toxic metabolites may directly suppress erythropoiesis, but the major cause of anaemia is decreased production of erythropoietin. This is largely due to destruction of erythropoietin-producing tissue, but is also a result of the acidosis and raised phosphate levels (including 2,3-DPG) that occur in renal failure. Red cell survival is often shortened and, in severe renal failure, there may be a microangiopathic haemolysis. Examination of the blood in renal failure reveals a normocytic anaemia with crenated cells and often also red cell fragments.

Despite the multifactorial nature of the anaemia of chronic renal failure, a normal haemoglobin can be obtained in most patients by the administration of erythropoietin.

Liver disease

In liver disease, there is a mild anaemia which may be normocytic but is frequently macrocytic. Target cells are usually seen on the blood film. There may be a slight reticulocytosis, as mild haemolysis occurs as well as decreased erythropoiesis. Excessive bouts of alcohol intake in patients with chronic liver disease can produce frank haemolysis associated with abdominal pain, jaundice and hyperlipidaemia (Zieve's syndrome). The anaemia may be exacerbated by the complications of cirrhosis, i.e. hypersplenism and blood loss.

Malignant disease

The anaemia of non-haematological malignancy is multifactorial, and that which may occur in carcinoma of the bronchus is shown as an example in Figure 24.16.

BLOOD TRANSFUSION

Donors

All blood products should ideally be obtained from volunteer donors to reduce both the expense and the risks of infection transmission. The risks to the donor are very small, consisting mainly of bruising at venepuncture (and rarely arterial puncture) sites. The commonly used criteria for the acceptability of donors are shown in Table 24.13.

Blood from all donors is screened for syphilis serology, HIV and hepatitis C antibodies, and hepatitis B surface antigen.

Red cell antigens and antibodies

All blood is classified according to its ABO and rhesus antigen phenotype.

ABO system

There are three alternative genes which act on the product of the H gene to produce the O (H), A and B

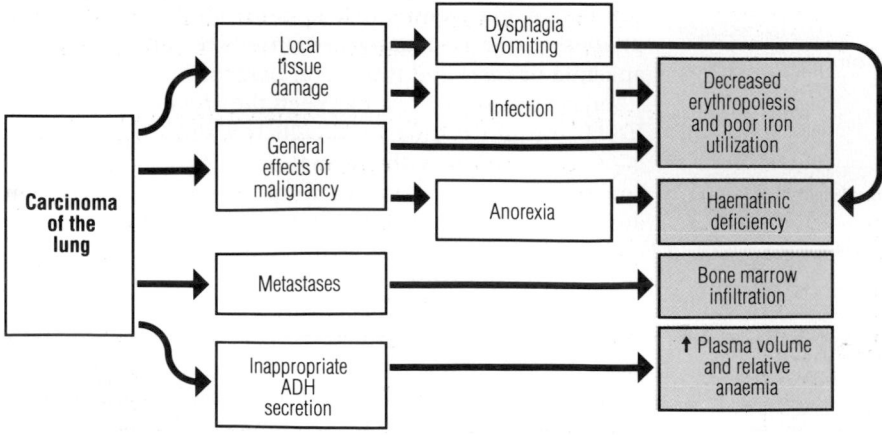

Fig. 24.16 Development of anaemia in carcinoma of the bronchus showing the multiple mechanisms involved.

Table 24.13 Criteria for the acceptability of blood donors in the UK

- Aged 18–65 years

- Good general health and 'feeling well'

- [Hb] greater than 13.1 g/dl (men)
  greater than 12.5 g/dl (women)

- Not pregnant at present or in the last year

- Never suffered from:
  Cancer
  Syphilis
  Brucellosis

- No recent:
  Malaria
  Infectious mononucleosis
  Hepatitis/jaundice

- Nor had (in last 6 months):
  Blood or blood products
  Surgery, tattoos, ears pierced
  Contact with hepatitis

- Nor in high-risk group for AIDS

- Nor in tropics for 3 months

Table 24.14 Incidence (%) of ABO blood groups in various racial groups

Blood group	Caucasians	Asians & Indians	African Blacks
A	36	24	21
B	14	24	29
AB	3	9	5
O	47	33	43

antigens (Fig. 24.17). The approximate incidence of the ABO antigens in various racial groups is shown in Table 24.14. At approximately six months of age, so-called *naturally occurring antibodies* arise to the ABO system as shown in Table 24.15. These antibodies probably arise as cross-reactions to antigens on gut flora. They are IgM antibodies which will agglutinate red cells in the cold in saline (*complete antibodies*). Subgroups of A are recognised. Approximately 80% of Caucasians are A1 and 20% are A2.

parent. The D antigen is clinically most important and approximately 85% of Caucasian individuals are D^+. In Chinese populations, nearly 100% are D^+ and in black people the incidence is approximately 95%. For general blood transfusion purposes, a recipient is called Rh-negative if he or she is d/d, but a Rh-negative donor is defined as cde/cde. Some patients have an abnormal D antigen (D^u) which may type very weakly, or even as d.

Naturally occurring antibodies to the rhesus system do not occur. However, antibody formation occurs following sensitisation during pregnancy or after mismatched transfusion. The antibodies formed are warm reacting IgG antibodies that do not agglutinate in saline (incomplete antibodies). They can be detected on addition of albumin or by using anti-immunoglobulin as a cross-linking reagent. Anti-Rh antibodies are most important in the context of immune haemolytic disease of the newborn (p. 1075).

Other antigen systems

Many other red cell antigen systems have been described but are not routinely typed. However, preformed antibodies to these antigens will be detected in a cross-match and can then be identified with panels of *typing cells*.

Blood grouping and cross-matching

ABO typing is performed by adding known anti-A and anti-B sera to a red cell suspension at room temperature, and then looking for agglutination (Fig. 24.18). The serum is also typed against known red cells as a back

Rhesus system

The rhesus system is composed of three closely linked allelic genes, one group of three being inherited from each

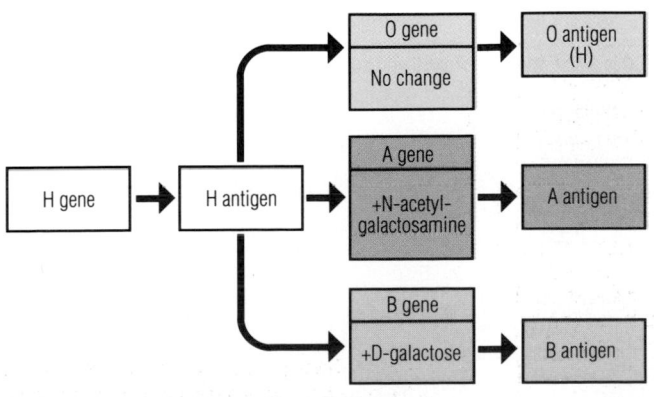

Fig. 24.17 The ABO antigen system.

Table 24.15 ABO genotype, phenotype and natural occurring antibodies

Genotype	Phenotype	Antibodies
AA	A	Anti-B
AO	A	Anti-B
BB	B	Anti-A
BO	B	Anti-A
OO	O	Anti-A+ Anti-B

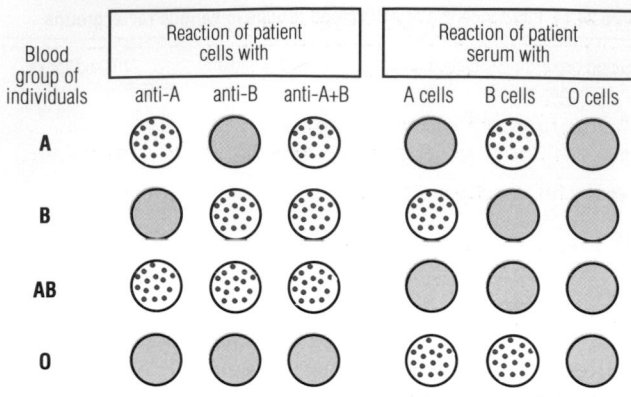

Blood group of individuals	Reaction of patient cells with			Reaction of patient serum with		
	anti-A	anti-B	anti-A+B	A cells	B cells	O cells
A						
B						
AB						
O						

Fig. 24.18 ABO tile grouping.

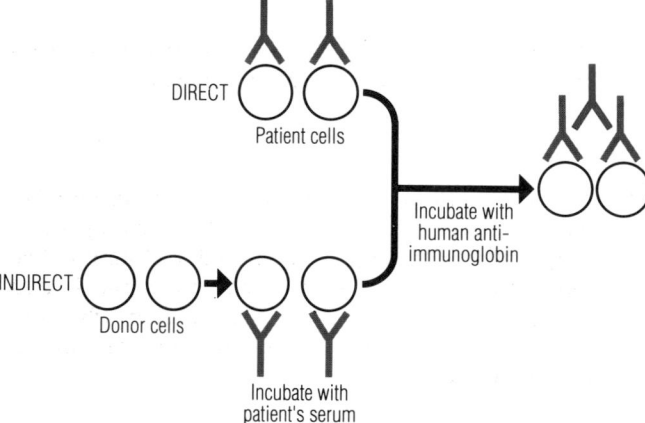

Fig. 24.19 Diagrammatic representation of the direct and indirect antiglobulin test. Human anti-immunoglobulin is shown in red.

check. Rhesus typing with anti-D cannot be performed in saline at room temperature, but must be carried out at 37°C in the presence of albumin or anti-human globulin in an *indirect antiglobulin test* (Fig. 24.19). At least two anti-D reagents should be used.

When the patient's ABO and rhesus group have been determined, a cross-match between the potential donor cells and the recipient serum is performed. A control is also performed using the recipient's own cells and serum to check for autoagglutinins. The cross-match should be performed both in saline at room temperature to detect cold complete antibodies, and in albumin at 37°C to detect warm incomplete antibodies. An indirect antiglobulin test at 37°C is also performed and is generally the most sensitive test available.

To speed up compatibility testing, an antibody screen on the serum of all potential recipients can be carried out using two batches of carefully selected target cells. If any antibodies are found, they must be identified, appropriate antigen-negative blood found and a full cross-match performed. If no antibodies are found, cross-matching is only

performed in surgical cases, such as cardiac surgery or a Wertheim's hysterectomy, in which there is a very high chance of blood being used. Blood is not cross-matched in surgical cases where blood is not usually required. If blood is then required urgently, group matched blood is issued after a 5–10 minute rapid (spun) cross-match.

Use of blood, blood products and substitutes

Whole blood

Whole blood should only be used in circumstances such as acute haemorrhage, where there is a need to restore the intravascular volume as well as the oxygen carrying capacity of the blood (Table 24.16). For exchange transfusions in neonates, the blood should be less than 48 hours old and CMV negative.

Red cell concentrates

It is essential that packed cells are used for patients with anaemia but without hypovolaemia. Otherwise the national blood transfusion service would be unable to obtain enough plasma to provide the required amounts of plasma products (Table 24.17). It should also be noted that the majority of patients with anaemia due to haematinic deficiency do not require transfusion, unless very ill, pregnant, or being prepared for surgery.

Table 24.16 Indications for the use of whole blood

- Acute blood loss
- Exchange transfusions
  Sickle cell disease
  Haemolytic disease of the newborn
- Priming extracorporeal circulations
  Heart–lung machines
  Some dialysis equipment

Table 24.17 Blood products and substitutes

Cellular products	Plasma products
Whole blood	Fresh frozen plasma
Packed red cells	Plasma protein fraction
Washed red cells	Freeze-dried, salt-poor albumin
Filtered blood	
Frozen red cells	Artificial plasma expanders
Red cell substitutes	Clotting factors
Platelet concentrates	Cryoprecipitate
Granulocyte concentrates	Factor VIII concentrates
	Factor IX concentrates
	Freeze-dried fibrinogen

Washed red cells

Red cells washed three times in saline contain few white cells and platelets, and reactions to platelet and leucocyte antigens in patients with preformed antibodies are thus reduced. In general, the use of washed cells for this purpose is now replaced by use of filtered blood. As the plasma is removed, reactions to plasma products, especially IgA, are avoided. Washed blood must be used within 12 hours of washing.

Filtered blood

Modern filters, which are expensive, effectively remove over 95% of leucocytes, and filtered blood is thus very useful in patients with antileucocyte antibodies causing febrile reactions.

Frozen red cells

Frozen red cells (after thawing and washing) are free of leucocytes. Filtered blood is now generally used for sensitised patients and red cell cryopreservation is mainly of value for the indefinite storage of blood with rare phenotypes.

Red cell substitutes

Emulsions of perfluorocarbons can be used to transport oxygen and carbon dioxide in the blood. However, they have a short half-life in the circulation and require the patient to inhale 50% oxygen to be effective. Their use is therefore limited to the management of individuals with religious objections to blood products, and perhaps also as a reserve for the treatment of large numbers of casualties after a major disaster.

Platelet concentrates

Platelet concentrates can be obtained from the donor units of blood by centrifugation, or in larger quantities using cell separators. As platelet concentrates are invariably contaminated with red cells, ABO and rhesus compatibility between donor and recipient should be maintained. Platelets are best stored at room temperature, preferably with constant agitation, and should be used as soon as possible (and not at all after three to four days from collection). Platelets stored at 4°C survive less well but have greater initial activity in the recipient.

Fresh frozen plasma

Fresh frozen plasma (FFP) contains the plasma proteins and labile clotting factors. The uses of FFP are confined to those in Table 24.18, as it is essential that fresh plasma

Table 24.18 Indications for use of fresh frozen plasma

Acquired coagulation disorders
Liver disease
Over anticoagulation with oral anticoagulants
Following massive transfusion with stored blood (if indicated by clotting screen)
Congenital coagulation disorders
Factor XI deficiency
Minor bleeds in von Willebrand's disease
Factor V deficiency
Factor VII deficiency
Factor X deficiency
Factor XIII deficiency
Thrombotic thrombocytopenic purpura
Angioneurotic oedema (FFP provides C1 esterase inhibitor)

is used primarily for the production of other plasma products. It should not be used as a plasma expander.

Plasma protein fraction

Plasma protein fraction is the solution remaining after removal from plasma of cryoprecipitate, fibrinogen and immunoglobulins. It is largely composed of albumin. The solution is heat-treated to destroy HIV, hepatitis and CMV viruses and is used as a volume expander when red cells are not required, and for replacement therapy in hypoalbuminic states.

Freeze-dried salt-poor albumin

Freeze-dried, salt-poor albumin is of limited use but may be of value in some patients with nephrotic syndrome or liver disease.

Artificial plasma expanders

Hydroxethyl starch is a very useful and safe plasma expander. High molecular weight dextrans are also used, but anaphylactic reactions occasionally occur and there may also be occasional interference with subsequent cross-matching (rouleaux formation). Gelatin solutions are also safe but only remain in the circulation for a relatively short period.

Cryoprecipitate

When FFP is just thawed to between 4°C and 8°C, a white gelatinous material remains as cryoprecipitate which can be removed and refrozen. This substance enters solution when thawed at 37°C. Cryoprecipitate contains approximately 50% of the original factor VIII present, including von Willebrand factor. It also contains high levels of fibrinogen but no factor IX. It is now rarely used except in some cases of disseminated intravascular coagulation (DIC) where fibrinogen is required as well as other clotting factors.

Factor VIII concentrates

Highly concentrated factor VIII preparations are available in freeze-dried forms. They are less bulky than cryoprecipitate, can be stored at 4°C, and contain less fibrinogen than cryoprecipitate, all of which properties make them suitable for major bleeds. Because they are produced from pooled plasma collections, they potentially contain viruses, including HIV. Heat treatment appears to eliminate HIV and hepatitis viruses. The process reduces the functional factor VIII content and is therefore very expensive.

Porcine and bovine factor VIII concentrates are occasionally useful in patients who have developed antifactor VIII antibodies. Genetically engineered factor VIII has now become available. This expensive product is not contaminated by viruses.

Factor IX concentrates

Factor IX concentrates are used in the treatment of congenital factor IX deficiency not responding to FFP, and occasionally in liver disease. These preparations also contain factors II, VII (depending on the method of preparation) and X. Activated clotting factors may also be present, which makes the concentrate potentially thrombogenic, but provides a way to bypass the factor VIII requirement in haemophiliacs with anti-factor VIII antibodies. Special 'activated' factor IX concentrates are available for this purpose, but must be used with great caution.

Freeze-dried fibrinogen

Freeze-dried fibrinogen is available for use in congenital fibrinogen deficiency and dysfibrinogenaemia.

Complications of blood transfusion

Serological reactions

If blood has been incorrectly cross-matched (or not cross-matched), or if (more commonly) there has been a clerical error and the patient has antibodies to donor red cell antigens, rapid complement-dependent lysis of the transfused cells may occur. Rarely, immediate haemolysis may also be due to high titre anti-A or anti-B IgG antibodies in the donor blood, when group O blood is given to A or B recipients. Symptoms may arise within minutes or up to several hours after the transfusion has started, and include fever and rigors, headache, lumbar back pain,

abdominal discomfort and vomiting, and chest pain. In severe cases, the patient becomes shocked and then suffers acute renal failure and DIC. When an immediate serological reaction is suspected, the transfusion must be stopped immediately and appropriate action taken (Table 24.19).

Serological reactions may also be delayed. This occurs when an antibody to donor red cells, which was not present in the patient's serum at the time of transfusion, develops rapidly afterwards. This is almost invariably a secondary antibody response in previously transfused individuals. Haemolysis usually occurs between one and two weeks after transfusion.

It should also be noted that a transfusion may produce sensitisation to donor red cells. Although this may not cause haemolysis, future transfusions may be compromised and there may be a risk in young women of haemolytic disease of the newborn.

Febrile reactions

In multiply transfused patients, febrile reactions frequently accompany transfusion due to the development of antibodies to leucocyte and platelet antigens. The fever usually develops several hours after starting the transfusion and may last for up to 12 hours. Filtered blood, slow rate of transfusion, and intravenous chlorpheniramine or hydrocortisone will reduce this problem.

Table 24.19 Plan of action for a suspected immediate haemolytic transfusion reaction

1. STOP TRANSFUSION

2. Maintain venous access (give saline initially)

3. Check names, groups and numbers on the blood pack and blood transfusion report forms

4. Return blood pack to laboratory with:
   Clotted blood sample
   – re-check group of patient and donor pack
   – perform a direct antiglobulin test
   – repeat cross-match and identify any antibodies
   Heparinised blood sample
   – check for free Hb in plasma
   Citrated sample
   – check clotting screen
   Sequestrene sample
   – check [Hb] and platelet count

5. Give intravenous hydrocortisone and chlorpheniramine

6. Maintain venous return if shock develops – give saline, plasma and whole blood if necessary

7. Maintain urine output by using intravenous diuretics *after* establishment of adequate venous return

8. Replenish clotting factors and platelets if DIC develops

Infections

Blood rarely becomes contaminated with bacteria, but organisms able to grow at 4°C (such as *Pseudomonas* and coliforms) produce bacteraemic shock and can be rapidly fatal. Many viruses can be transmitted by blood transfusion. Blood donations are screened for hepatitis B and C and transmission of these agents is rare. CMV transmission may occur as the virus can be dormant in leucocytes. In immunocompromised patients without anti-CMV antibodies, and in neonates, blood from CMV-negative donors should be given. The extremely small risk of HIV transmission from blood donated in the UK has been further reduced by screening the donated blood for anti-HIV antibodies. Infectious mononucleosis may occasionally be transmitted. Other contaminating organisms include brucella, plasmodia, trypanosomes, leishmania and filaria. Syphilis transmission is rare as all blood is pre-screened for antibodies to *Treponema pallidum* and positive units discarded.

Transfusion siderosis

Each unit of blood contains about 0.25 g of iron and so, with frequent transfusions, iron overload with parenchymal tissue damage may occur. Serious problems arise after about 30 g of iron accumulation. When repeated transfusion is anticipated, desferrioxamine therapy must therefore be considered.

Ion toxicity

Blood is stored in citrate which can chelate calcium and sometimes cause tetany. However, as citrate is rapidly metabolised in the liver, citrate toxicity only occurs in severe liver disease and during rapid and massive blood transfusion.

Stored blood leaks $[K^+]$ from red cells, which may cause problems in patients who already have a raised plasma $[K^+]$, or with massive transfusions, especially exchange transfusion in neonates. Stored blood also contains high levels of NH_4^+ and should therefore be avoided in liver disease.

Problems of massive transfusion

Large volume blood transfusions given over a short period of time may be associated with special problems. Where stored blood has been used, there is a theoretical risk of toxicity from citrate, hydrogen ions (acidosis) and potassium ions, but these problems are in fact rare. Dilution of platelets and clotting factors does occur, and must be corrected by replacement therapy.

IMMUNE HAEMOLYTIC DISEASE OF THE NEWBORN

Aetiology

In immune haemolytic disease of the newborn (HDN), IgG antibodies produced by the mother against fetal red cell antigens cross the placenta and produce haemolysis in the fetus (Fig. 24.20). In 90% of cases, the antibodies are directed to antigens of the rhesus group and severe disease is mainly caused by anti-D antibodies. Other antibodies causing occasional problems are shown in Table 24.20. In the UK, 85% of the population are Rh-positive (D+) and 13% of UK marriages are between a dd (D–) woman and a D+ man. Three in four of their children will

---

Summary 7 Complications of blood transfusion

- Haemolytic reactions
  Serological – immediate
  – delayed
  – sensitisation
  Thermal – faulty blood warmers
- Febrile reactions
- Infections
- Circulatory overload
- Thrombophlebitis at transfusion site
- Transfusion siderosis
- Air embolism (with use of central lines)
- Ion toxicity (e.g. citrate and potassium)
- Special problems associated with massive transfusion

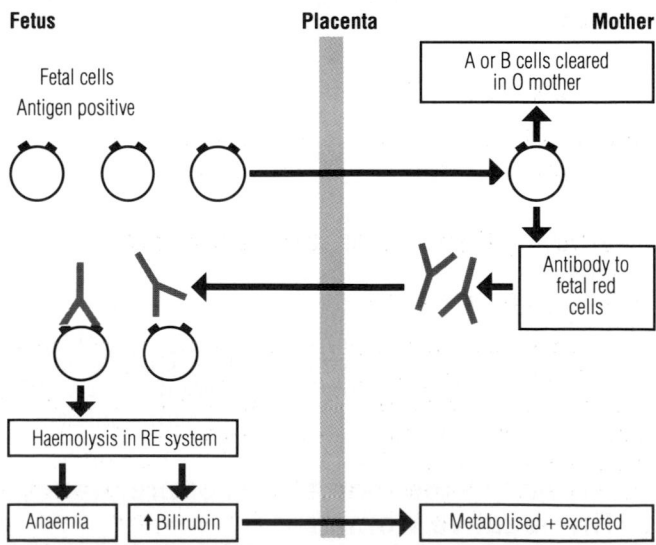

Fig. 24.20 Diagrammatic representation of the prenatal mechanism of haemolytic disease of the newborn (HDN).

24 Haematological Disorders

Table 24.20 Antibodies causing haemolytic disease of the newborn*

Anti-rhesus (in order of incidence)	Anti-Kell
Anti-D	
Anti-C + D	Anti-Duffy
Anti-E	
(Anti-C) (often severe)	Anti-Kidd
(Anti-D + E)	
(Anti-C + E)	Anti-A + Anti-B
(Anti-e)	

*Parentheses indicate rarity

be D+. Sensitisation of the mother requires passage of a considerable quantity (approximately 0.5 ml) of fetal cells into the maternal circulation and this usually happens at birth. Firstborn children are therefore rarely affected. However, the mother is now primed, and can produce a secondary antibody response to the small quantity of fetal red cells that enter the maternal circulation during a subsequent normal pregnancy. Group O mothers are less frequently sensitised if the fetus is Group A or, to a lesser extent, Group B – presumably because the fetal cells are rapidly cleared from the maternal circulation by naturally occurring anti-A and anti-B antibodies. It should also be noted that rhesus sensitisation can occur with antepartum haemorrhages, obstetric manipulations, Rh-positive blood transfusions and other blood products.

ABO incompatibility is a rare cause of HDN, as most individuals produce only IgM antibodies which do not cross the placenta. Only occasional Group O women will produce high titre IgG anti-A or anti-B when carrying an A+ or B+ fetus. It should be noted in these cases that, at birth, the cord cells often give a negative DAT (probably due to the low ABO antigen density on cord cells), and this may make the diagnosis very difficult.

Clinical features

The affected fetus becomes anaemic, and produces a reticulocytosis and many nucleated red cells in the peripheral blood (erythroblastosis fetalis). As the anaemia progresses, cardiac failure develops with scalp oedema, pericardial effusions and ascites (hydrops). Hyperbilirubinaemia is not a problem in utero because of placental clearance but, after birth, haemolysis continues until all the maternal antibody has been used up, and severe jaundice may develop quickly. High levels of unconjugated bilirubin can cause severe damage to the central nervous system, especially in premature infants.

Approach to the monitoring of pregnancy in Rh-negative women

All pregnant women should have a red cell group performed at the booking clinic at 12 weeks gestation. The serum should also be screened against a cell panel at this stage to look for antibodies which, if found, must then be identified. This should not be restricted to Rh-negative women (cde/cde) as anti-c antibodies, as well as other rarer antibodies, would then be missed. In the case of Rh-negative women, it is also usual to genotype the father to determine whether he is Rh-positive and DD or Dd. Antibody screening should ideally be repeated in Rh-negative women at 24 weeks, 34 weeks and at delivery if it is a first pregnancy, and even more frequently in later pregnancies. If an antibody screen is positive, it should be repeated at four-weekly intervals throughout the second trimester and at two-weekly intervals during the last trimester. Rising antibody levels indicate an affected fetus, and amniocentesis should be performed if the anti-D titre is greater than 1:16 (4 µg/ml). If high levels of antibody are present before amniocentesis is feasible, the fetus should be monitored by ultrasound for evidence of hydrops. It must be noted that the level of maternal antibody correlates poorly with the severity of HDN, and amniocentesis should therefore be performed whenever doubt arises. In these circumstances, the previous obstetric history must be taken into account. In first-affected fetuses, it is likely that the disease will be mild; whereas the disease is more likely to be severe in subsequent pregnancies, with a five-fold greater mortality. If a mother has had a previous severely affected fetus, she should be monitored by ultrasound from 16 weeks gestation and by amniocentesis from 25 weeks gestation, even if the antibody titres are low.

The purpose of amniocentesis is to measure the bile pigment levels in the fetal blood. This is measured spectrophotometrically by absorption at 450 nm. The value obtained must be plotted on a graph of optical density of the amniotic fluid versus gestation, and interpretation is made using well standardised criteria (Fig. 24.21). If a value is obtained in zone A, the fetus is severely affected and at high risk of death. Therapeutic intervention is therefore necessary. If in zone B, great vigilance is

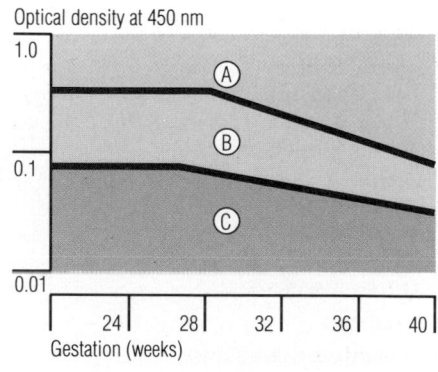

Fig. 24.21 Chart of optical density of the amniotic fluid versus gestation, showing ranges of risk. (A) Fetus at high risk. (B) Fetus at risk. (C) Fetus at low risk.

required and amniocentesis should be repeated after two weeks.

Management of HDN

Antenatal

Intrauterine transfusions can be given to severely affected fetuses, either by the intraperitoneal route from 24 weeks of gestation onwards, or by injection (fetoscopic or ultrasound-guided) into an umbilical blood vessel from 16 weeks onwards. The blood given is washed O Rh-negative (cde/cde) and is cross-matched with the mother's serum. It should also be from an anti-CMV negative individual.

Maternal plasmapheresis is sometimes used in cases with high antibody titres early in pregnancy, in an attempt to reduce the severity of the haemolysis. To be effective, very large exchanges are required three or four days a week from about 10 weeks gestation onwards. The plasma replacement should be from Rh-negative donors to prevent contamination with Rh-positive red cell stroma.

The mainstay of management remains the induction of premature labour. In most severely affected fetuses, this is done at 32 weeks, and at later dates in less severely affected fetuses. Measurement of lecithin:sphingomyelin ratios in the amniotic fluid at the time of amniocentesis provide some indication of lung maturity, and may assist in the decision of when to induce labour.

Postnatal

Exchange transfusion should be performed immediately after birth in severely anaemic or hydropic infants. The best indicator of severity at birth is the cord blood haemoglobin concentration: values below 12.5 g/dl are indicative of the need for exchange. The bilirubin level is less useful but a value above 70 µmol/l probably indicates the need for exchange. At a later stage, bilirubin estimations are paramount and exchanges must be performed to keep this well below an accepted value, i.e. below 240 µmol/l for infants delivered between 30 and 31 weeks; below 290 µmol/l for infants delivered between 31 and 34 weeks; and below 350 µmol/l for 'older' infants. These values should be lowered if the infant is clinically unwell. In exchange transfusion, fresh blood collected into citrate phosphate dextrose is used. The blood should be O-negative, compatible with both the mother's and infant's serum, and CMV-negative. Usually a two-volume exchange (1 vol = wt (kg) × 90 ml) is performed; this removes antibody-coated red cells which would eventually be destroyed, removes unbound antibody and reduces the bilirubin level.

In mildly affected infants, phototherapy may augment bilirubin breakdown and avoid the necessity for exchange transfusion.

Prevention of HDN

Rh-negative women should not be given Rh-positive blood or blood products.

At childbirth, Rh-negative women should be given intramuscular anti-D within 72 hours of delivery of an Rh-positive child, in order to neutralise any fetal cells in the circulation and prevent sensitisation. The dose of 100 µg usually given should be sufficient to neutralise approximately 4 ml of fetal blood. A Kleihauer test should be performed on the mother's blood (fetal cells stain darkly, adult cells very weakly) and, if fetal cells are detected at a frequency of more than 1 in 600, further anti-D should be given. Anti-D should also be given to Rh-negative women for threatened abortions, abortions, haemorrhages and obstetric manoeuvres. Fifty micrograms is given before the twentieth week of pregnancy, and after this, 100 µg. The antibody only crosses the placenta slowly and the fetus is not harmed.

Despite such measures, nearly 1% of women still become sensitised during their first pregnancy. It has therefore recently been recommended that all Rh-negative women with a potential Rh-positive child should receive 100 µg of anti-D at 28 weeks and 34 weeks gestation, to minimise sensitisation from silent fetal to maternal blood transfer in utero.

NON-MALIGNANT LEUCOCYTE ABNORMALITIES

Leucocyte abnormalities can be considered as qualitative or quantitative.

Infection is the commonest cause and the response usually varies with different organisms and at different phases of the disease. Thus, acute pyogenic infections cause an initial neutrophilia, but may give rise to monocytosis in the recovery period. Parasitic infections typically give rise to eosinophilia, and viral infections to lymphocytosis, although considerable variation to this general rule may occur. The reactive lymphocytes may appear atypical, and this is particularly prominent in infectious mononucleosis. Neutrophilia also occurs in response to all forms of tissue injury or inflammation, whereas eosinophilia is usually associated with inflammation which has an allergic basis. Basophilia is only rarely a reactive condition, and always suggests an underlying myeloproliferative disorder.

The causes of a decreased neutrophil or lymphocyte count are shown in Table 24.21. Minor components of the leucocyte population may also decrease, but this is not usually detected on a routine differential count. Although the cytopenias must be due to either decreased production or increased loss/destruction, it is difficult to classify the causes in this way as some are multifactorial

Table 24.21 Causes of low leucocyte count in the peripheral blood

Neutrophils	Lymphocytes
Marrow aplasia	Severe marrow aplasia
Marrow infiltration	Severe marrow infiltration
Megaloblastic anaemia	Severe megaloblastic anaemia
Cyclical neutropenia	
Congenital agranulocytosis (Kostman's syndrome)	
	Congenital immunodeficiency disorders
Some acute infections	Rarely in acute infections
Typhoid, brucella, miliary TB	
Protozoa	
Fungi	
Rickettsia	
Viral	
HIV infection	**HIV infection**
Collagen disorders	**Collagen disorders**
	Lymphomas
Exposure to high-dose irradiation	**Exposure to irradiation**
Immune destruction	Immune destruction
Idiopathic	
Associated with drugs	
Hypersplenism	Hypersplenism
	Intestinal loss due to lymphatic obstruction

Bold type indicates that the relevant cytopenia is common in that condition; it does *not* mean that the particular condition is a common cause of the cytopenia.

(e.g. neutropenia in acute infections) and the mechanism is not always well understood (e.g. lymphopenia in advanced Hodgkin's disease). Qualitative lymphocyte abnormalities are discussed in Chapter 6.

Functional abnormalities of phagocytes also occur and may be primary or secondary (Table 24.22). The primary abnormalities include:

Table 24.22 Aetiology of phagocytic functional abnormalities

Abnormal phagocytic function	Disorder	
	Primary	Secondary
Movement	Lazy leucocyte syndrome	Renal failure Diabetes Malnutrition
Recognition		Immunoglobulin and complement (opsonins) deficiency
Phagocytosis	Chediak-Higashi syndrome	Severe malnutrition Vitamin E deficiency
Killing	Chronic granulomatous disease	Severe iron deficiency Postirradiation

- *Chediak–Higashi syndrome*, a rare autosomal recessive disorder in which there is oculocutaneous albinism, neurological deficit, a bleeding tendency and frequent pyogenic infections. Inclusion bodies are visible in the leucocytes.
- *Chronic granulomatous disease*, which is usually X-linked but may be autosomal recessive. There is an absence of cytochrome b or some other component of the oxidase system, such that phagocytosis does not lead to a respiratory burst with ultimate free radical production and bacterial killing. It presents with chronic and recurrent infections during infancy, with abscess and granuloma formation.

The secondary causes of abnormal neutrophil function are extensive, but their true significance in vivo is not clear.

HAEMATOLOGICAL MALIGNANCY

The nature and aetiology of haematological malignancies has been more extensively studied than in other tumours, largely because of the ease with which single cell suspensions can be obtained from blood, marrow and lymph nodes. However, the insights gained from these studies can probably be applied to many other types of neoplasia.

Pathogenesis

Nearly all haematological malignancies examined have been shown to be clonal in origin. The B cell malignancies express light-chain-restricted surface immunoglobulin (if the cells are sufficiently mature to express surface immunoglobulin), and nearly all cases show a clonal rearrangement of the immunoglobulin genes. Similarly, T cell malignancies have been shown to have clonal rearrangements of the T cell antigen-receptor genes. Some of these malignancies (and also the myeloid leukaemias) may have clonal chromosomal abnormalities, such as alterations in chromosome number or chromosome translocations. Other myeloid leukaemias have been shown to be clonal by studies in women heterozygous for G6PD isoenzymes or other X-linked polymorphic gene markers. (G6PD is coded on the X-chromosome and, as one X-chromosome is inactivated in each cell early in embryogenesis, a clonal population expresses only one G6PD isoenzyme.)

The phenotype of malignant cells is almost always similar to that of their normal counterparts. The phenotype of blast cells in acute myeloid leukaemia (AML) is thus usually identical to that of a rare population of normal primitive cells, although the Auer rods sometimes seen in AML cells are not seen in normal adult cells. No leukaemia-specific surface antigens have been defined (but see p. 1080). The common-ALL antigen (p. 1089) is a normal early lymphoid differentiation antigen. Leukaemic cells may, however, express an unusual combination of antigens not seen in normal cells.

Blast cells in acute leukaemia are not completely homogeneous. Some cells have a more primitive phenotype than the main cell population. In chronic myeloid leukaemia (CML), G6PD isoenzyme studies have shown that, although most malignant cells are late granulocytic cells, the clonal disorder also affects red cells, platelets and some B lymphocytes. The 'leukaemic hit' must therefore have occurred at the multipotential stem cell level. Similar findings have been reported in cases of adult AML. The oncogenic event occurs at a multipotential stem cell level but the malignant cells are still able to differentiate in part down all the myeloid pathways. A 'differentiation block' is, however, present at the myeloblast stage and these cells therefore accumulate. This level of differentiation block may change over time and the blastic transformation that occurs in CML probably represents such a process.

In vitro studies have demonstrated that leukaemic cell growth is often not autonomous. In polycythaemia rubra vera (PRV), the erythroid progenitors will (like their normal counterparts) only grow in the presence of erythropoietin, although their sensitivity to erythropoietin is considerably greater.

The growth rate of leukaemic cells is also thought to be about the same as (or even slower than) that of normal cells, so that expansion of the leukaemic mass is not due to markedly accelerated growth. In the chronic leukaemias, it is likely that there is instead an alteration in the balance between stem cell self-renewal and commitment/differentiation. Initially, a malignant clone with a slightly higher self-renewal rate will produce fewer end cells, but eventually it will produce an exponentially increasing population of end cells. A similar process may occur in the acute leukaemias, but, here, cell population growth is also affected by the differentiation block, which reduces the cell death rate associated with terminal differentiation.

Summary 8 Features of haematological malignancies

- Clonal
- Malignant cells have normal counterparts
- Malignant populations have stem cells more primitive than the majority of the malignant population
- The level of 'differentiation block' may change
- Growth is not autonomous
- The growth rate is not necessarily higher than in normal cellular counterparts
- Growth rates are not always constant

It should be noted that the growth rate in the haematological malignances is not necessarily constant over time. In multiple myeloma, for example, treatment will often induce a plateau phase during which the tumour is kinetically quiescent and resistant to further chemotherapy. If chemotherapy is stopped at this stage the plateau phase is often maintained for many months.

Aetiology

The aetiological factors associated with haematological malignancies have been widely studied.

Hereditary/congenital factors

Familial tendencies to acquire haematological malignancies are relatively weak, with the exception of identical twins. Here, if one twin develops acute leukaemia, the risk of the remaining twin is reported to be 25%, although most of this high risk is accounted for by twins presenting with leukaemia in the first 18 months of life where there has been prenatal transmission of the leukaemia via the linked circulation. There are in addition a variety of congenital disorders, such as Down's syndrome, Bloom's syndrome and Fanconi's anaemia, in which the incidence of leukaemia is markedly increased.

Ionising radiation and drugs

Exposure to excessive ionising radiation increases the risk of all haematological malignancies except chronic lymphocytic leukaemia. Many drugs have also been proposed as carcinogens, but the data are only firm for benzene. Both ionising radiation and benzene directly damage DNA.

Gross chromosomal abnormalities

Gross chromosomal abnormalities, such as additional chromosomes, deletions or major translocations, can be detected in many cases of leukaemia or lymphoma and certain of these have prognostic significance. Thus, acute lymphoblastic leukaemia patients with a 4:11 translocation have a very poor prognosis, whereas patients with hyperdiploid (more than 50 chromosomes) blast cells respond very well to treatment.

Proto-oncogenes

At a finer level, great interest has recently been focused on proto-oncogene expression in malignant cells. In any one case of leukaemia or lymphoma, there may be high levels of multiple proto-oncogene mRNA, which may be indicative of a multistep oncogenic process in which more than one oncogene is involved. This finding must be viewed with some caution, however, because the normal levels of gene expression in cells of the same lineage at the same stage of differentiation have not always been determined. The cellular myc gene is highly expressed in many haematological malignancies, but is also high in normal primitive myeloid cells and in mitogen-activated lymphoblasts. It thus appears that c-myc expression can be a feature of the proliferating cells rather than a primary oncogenic process. Of particular interest is the anatomical siting of certain proto-oncogenes in relation to common translocations in the haematological malignancies. In Burkitt's lymphoma, for example, most patients have a translocation of the long arm of chromosome 8 to the long arm of chromosome 14, close to the region coding for immunoglobulin heavy chains. The break point on chromosome 8 is close to the 8q 24 band, which is the site of the c-myc oncogene. It is probable that the high c-myc expression found in this tumour is due to the ectopic siting of the c-myc oncogene either in proximity to a different promoter, or beyond the influence of a local suppressing sequence.

In other situations, the aberrant location of a proto-oncogene can lead to production of an abnormal mRNA species and protein product. Thus, in the Philadelphia (Ph') chromosome, which is present in most cases of CML, there is a translocation between chromosome 9 and chromosome 22. The translocation site on chromosome 9 is within the c-abl sequence, at a splicing site between the 5' and 3' end of this gene. In the Ph' chromosome, a region of chromosome 22 known as the *break-point cluster region (bcr)* becomes joined to the 3' end of c-abl, leading to the production of a unique fusion gene product (Fig. 24.22).

The precise functions of most oncogene products are still unknown, but many of the proto-oncogenes studied to date have been found to code for tyrosine kinases or growth factor receptors, and are therefore likely to be important metabolic regulatory proteins.

In addition to the possible role of structural abnormalities in, or ectopic siting of, proto-oncogenes in malignant transformation, there may be further gene sequences which normally suppress proto-oncogene expression. Such genes have been called *anti-oncogenes*, and mutations in these genes might also give rise to malignant change. Mutations of the p53 gene have been implicated in some cases of blastic transformation in CML, and absence of the retinoblastoma gene product has been found in some ANLs.

Viruses

Although many malignancies in the animal kingdom can be transmitted by retroviruses containing sequences similar to cellular proto-oncogenes, this has not been described in man. *Human T cell lymphotrophic virus I*

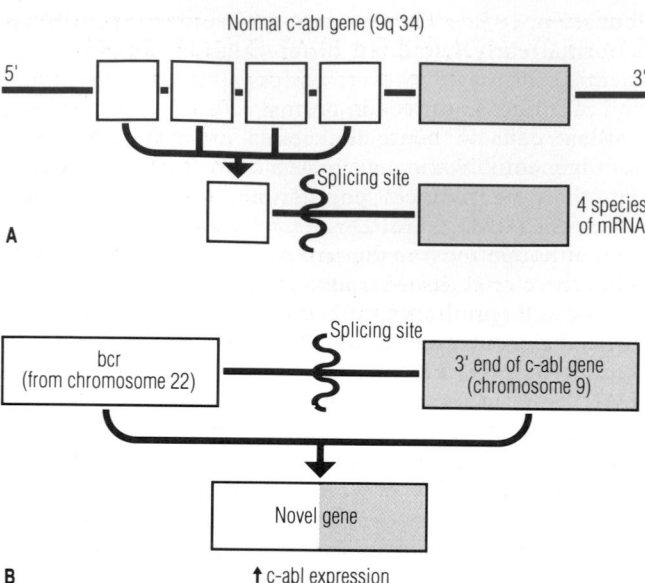

Fig. 24.22 Diagrammatic representation of c-abl gene. A. In the normal gene there is variable spacing to give four species of mRNA. **B**. In the Philadelphia (Ph') chromosome the bcr from chromosome 22 joins the 3' end of the c-abl gene to give a novel hybrid gene.

(HTLV I) is a retrovirus and is undoubtedly associated with certain T cell leukaemia/lymphomas, but it does not contain a gene sequence with a normal cellular counterpart. The precise mechanism of oncogenesis is not known, but may involve an indirect increase in growth factor (interleukin-2) receptor expression. The vast majority of patients infected with HTLV I do not develop lymphoproliferative diseases. HTLV I neoplasms nonetheless comprise a large proportion of the haematological malignancies in South-West Japan and the Caribbean basin, but only a small proportion elsewhere.

The *Epstein Barr virus* is associated with Burkitt's lymphoma. The mechanism of transformation, which occurs in small numbers of individuals (mainly in areas of Africa), is again obscure. The virus may also be implicated in the pathogenesis of some cases of Hodgkin's disease.

Summary 9 Aetiological factors in haemotological malignancies

- Familial and congenital associations
- Ionising irradiation
- Chemical carcinogens
- Chromosome abnormalities including over-expression of proto-oncogenes
- Viruses: HTLVI, EBV

MYELOPROLIFERATIVE DISORDERS

The myeloproliferative disorders are defined as neoplastic proliferations of the myeloid stem cell and its progeny. This is a simplification in that the multipotential stem cell may also be involved in the malignant process, with additional involvement of the lymphocyte series. Although the level of leukaemic transformation is at the most primitive stem cell level, the individual disease entities are recognised by the predominant cell type accumulating in the blood and marrow (Fig. 24.23). Intermediate states and transitions between one entity and another may occur. AML is clearly a myeloproliferative disorder although it is common to consider only the chronic proliferations under this heading. Fibrosis frequently occurs as a reaction to the malignant proliferation, especially if there is a prominent megakaryocytic element. Occasionally, marked fibrosis is the presenting feature and is then known as primary myelofibrosis; it is, nonetheless, a secondary process.

CHRONIC MYELOID LEUKAEMIA

Chronic myeloid leukaemia (CML) is a disorder of the multipotent stem cell in which the myeloid progenitor cell compartment, and subsequently the maturing granulocytic cell compartment, becomes grossly expanded. The erythroid, megakaryocytic and B lymphoid cells are also part of the malignant clone; their accumulation is not

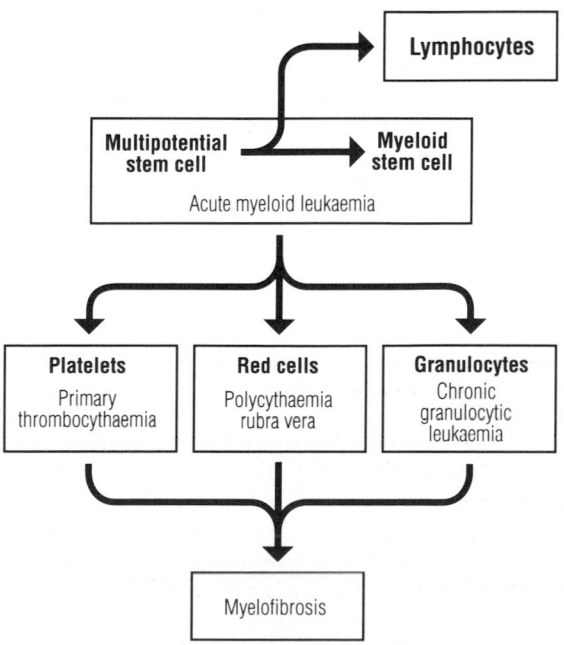

Fig. 24.23 The myeloproliferative disorders.

usually prominent, although polycythaemia and thrombocytosis may occur. Over 90% of cases have the Philadelphia chromosome, in which there is a translocation from the long arm of chromosome 22 to the long arm of chromosome 9 with the resultant production of an abnormal c-abl gene product (p. 1080). Even in cases of apparent Philadelphia-negative CML, detailed molecular analysis has often shown a translocation involving the c-bcr-abl gene regions. The mechanism by which the c-abl product is associated with malignant transformation is not known.

Clinical features of chronic phase CML

CML occurs predominantly in those over 30 years of age, although childhood variants do occur (p. 1082). Males and females are equally affected and the annual incidence in the UK is approximately 1 in 100 000. CML is initially an indolent disease that can, in the chronic phase, be readily controlled by chemotherapy, but transformation to an *accelerated phase* is almost invariable. Typically, there is slow onset of symptoms of anaemia, often accompanied by weight loss. Infections and bleeding are rare at presentation. The spleen is almost always palpable and may become enormous. Splenic pain due to infarction may arise. Lymphadenopathy does not generally occur.

Haematological features of the chronic phase

The most striking peripheral blood abnormality is the rise in white cell count; there is an increase in neutrophils, basophils and eosinophils. Many precursor cells, particularly myelocytes, are present and up to 5% of the circulating leucocytes may be blast cells. The haemoglobin tends to fall as the white cell count rises, although, occasionally, it may be high at presentation. The platelet count is variable. The bone marrow shows myeloid hyperplasia and sometimes an increase in reticulin.

Differential diagnosis

The main differential diagnosis of CML is that of reactive leucocytosis due to infection or inflammation. A *leukaemoid reaction* (a non-neoplastic leucocytosis of marked degree) can usually be distinguished from CML, as splenomegaly is not common in the former, and eosinophilia and basophilia are not usually a component of the leucocytosis. The neutrophil alkaline phosphatase (NAP) level (detected by cytochemical staining) is typically very low in CML and high in reactive leucocytoses. The final arbiter in difficult cases is the demonstration of the Philadelphia chromosome or bcr-abl rearrangement in CML.

Chronic myelomonocytic leukaemia with a high count may also cause confusion but, in this condition, monocytes are plentiful and eosinophils and basophils are not usually increased (p. 1090). Primary myelofibrosis may also be associated with an initial leucocytosis but, in this disease, there are also usually red cell changes attributable to marrow fibrosis, the NAP score is raised, and the Philadelphia chromosome is absent.

Management of chronic phase CML

Therapy is essentially palliative for most patients. Blood transfusions should be given as necessary and any infections treated vigorously. Allopurinol is often given to prevent secondary gout, especially if there is hyperuricaemia. Chemotherapy is given in an attempt to normalise the blood count and shrink the spleen. This undoubtedly improves the quality of life but does not delay acute transformation. Alkylating agents (e.g. busulphan) may be given as a small daily dose (2–6 mg/day) or in larger doses at less frequent intervals. Hydroxyurea is an alternative to busulphan, and has the advantage that its effects are readily reversible. Alpha interferon will normalise the white count and may prolong chronic phase. Occasionally, a very high leucocyte count at presentation can lead to hyperviscosity and thrombotic events such as confusion and priapism. Should this occur, or if the leucocyte count is over 200×10^9/l, leucopheresis is advisable until chemotherapy has decreased the rate of white cell production.

Attempts have been made to eliminate the Philadelphia-positive clone during the chronic phase by using intensive acute leukaemia regimens, but these have almost invariably proved ineffective. For younger patients who have an HLA identical sibling, massive chemo/radiotherapy and allogeneic bone marrow transplantation during the chronic phase is the treatment of choice. The immediate mortality is less than 25% and many patients will have prolonged disease-free survival.

Clinical features of acute transformation

Acute transformation of CML may take the form of increasing myelofibrosis or transition to an acute leukaemia. On average it occurs within three years of onset, although there is considerable individual variation. Many clinical events may herald transformation, including increasing anaemia, fever, increasing spleen size and bone pain. A patient is considered to have entered an accelerated phase when the therapy (which was previously effective) can no longer control the symptoms, signs and haematological features of the disease. In a myelofibrotic transformation, there is progressive anaemia, thrombocytopenia and possibly even neutropenia. The spleen enlarges markedly and may cause severe discomfort. In blastic transformation, the features are those of marrow failure, as they are with other types of acute leukaemia (p. 1056).

Haematological features of acute transformation

Acute transformation may be heralded by a fall in the haemoglobin or platelet count, or by a rise in the white cell count while still on therapy. There may be a rise in the basophil and blast cell count and in the NAP score. In a myelofibrotic transformation, the blood picture is similar to that seen in any case of marrow fibrosis, with leucoerythroblastic anaemia (primitive red and white cell precursors in the blood) and marked poikilocytosis with tear-drop forms.

In a blastic crisis, blast cells predominate in the blood and marrow. In about 80% of cases, these are myeloblasts; but in the remaining 20% of cases they are pre-B lymphoblasts, which express the common acute lymphoblastic leukaemia antigen (CD10). This illustrates the fact that CML involves a multipotent stem cell with both myeloid and lymphoid potential.

At the time of accelerated phase or blast crisis, cytogenetic analysis frequently reveals clonal abnormalities additional to the Philadelphia chromosome.

Management of the acute phase

In a myelofibrotic transformation, transfusion should be given for symptomatic anaemia. Splenectomy should be considered for spleen pain, or if splenic pooling in a big spleen is considered to contribute to the anaemia or other cytopenia. Local irradiation may ease splenic pain, but it rarely causes a long-lasting reduction of spleen size.

In blastic transformation, acute leukaemia therapy of appropriate type is given (p. 1087). Remissions, in which there is return of chronic phase CML, may be achieved, but they are usually of brief duration.

Allogeneic transplantation in *acute* phase CML has not been very successful.

Chronic myeloproliferative disorders in childhood

Diseases resembling CML may occur (rarely) in infancy and childhood. So-called *juvenile* CML presents in infancy with anaemia, infection, facial rashes, lymphadenopathy and hepatosplenomegaly. The white cell count is elevated with a prominent monocytosis. The HbF is markedly raised in most cases. The disease is rapidly progressive, with death usually due to marrow failure rather than transformation to acute leukaemia. Therapy is currently unsatisfactory.

A variant form of juvenile CML which occurs in infancy is the myeloproliferative disease associated with monosomy 7 in the malignant clone. The HbF level is not markedly raised in this condition. The prognosis is again very poor.

Adult-type CML with a Philadelphia chromosome occasionally occurs in older children and has a natural history similar to that seen in adults.

POLYCYTHAEMIA RUBRA VERA

Polycythaemia refers to an increase in the red cell mass. If due to a malignant myeloproliferative disorder, it is known as *polycythaemia rubra vera* (PRV); if due to a raised level of erythropoietin, it is known as *secondary polycythaemia*. A raised haemoglobin concentration may also occur due to a decreased plasma volume without an increase in the red cell mass; this is known as *pseudopolycythaemia* or *stress polycythaemia* (Fig. 24.24).

PRV is a malignant disorder of the multipotential haemopoietic stem cell, with predominant expansion of the mature erythroid cell population. The erythroid progenitors have increased sensitivity to erythropoietin, although the mechanism is not known. There is often also an increase in granulocytic cells and platelets, in keeping with the stem cell nature of this disease.

Clinical features

PRV is largely a disease of the middle-aged and elderly. It has been reported slightly more often in males than females.

The symptoms and signs of the disease are shown in Table 24.23, but it should be noted that symptoms may be minimal. Splenomegaly is present in 75% of cases, but diagnostic difficulties mainly arise in patients without

Table 24.23 Clinical features of polycythaemia rubra vera

Cause	Effect
Haemopoietic proliferation	Gout Hepatosplenomegaly Splenomegaly
Increased haematocrit	Hypertension Cerebral ischaemia Myocardial ischaemia Other thrombotic events
Multifactorial	Pruritus Peptic ulceration Bleeding

splenomegaly. The major symptoms and causes of death are due to the hyperviscosity associated with a raised haematocrit (Fig. 24.25A). Despite the elevated [Hb], blood flow and oxygen delivery is actually reduced to critical organs, particularly the brain (Fig. 24.25B). Pruritus is common and may in part be related to basophil production; iron deficiency may exacerbate this complaint. Peptic ulceration is very common. This is mainly due to hyperviscosity but may be exacerbated by excessive histamine release from basophils. Gastrointestinal bleeding from gastric erosions is not infrequent.

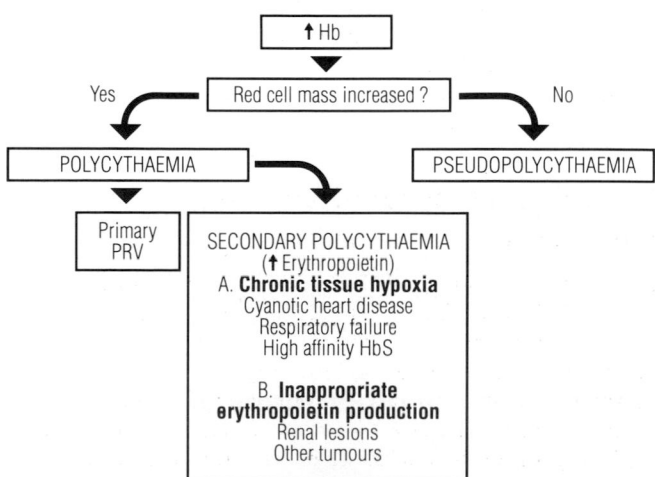

Fig. 24.24 Approach to the diagnosis of a raised haemoglobin (Hb) level.

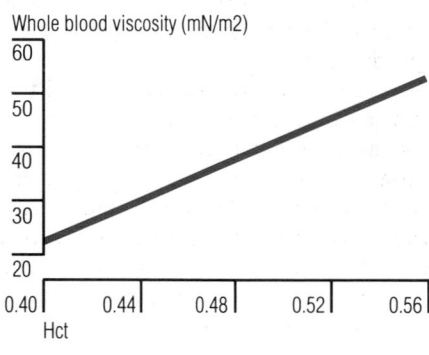

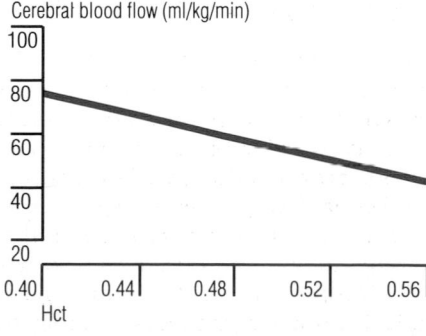

Fig. 24.25 Relationship of (A) blood viscosity and (B) cerebral blood flow to the haematocrit (Hct). As the haematocrit rises, there is a marked rise in viscosity and fall in blood flow.

Haematological features

Haematological investigations show that the [Hb] and red cell count are usually raised, but if iron deficiency occurs the [Hb] may fall to within the normal range. The red cells are then microcytic and the red cell count remains high. The neutrophil count is modestly raised in three-quarters of patients and the platelet count in about one-half. The increased neutrophil production gives rise to a raised B_{12} level, secondary to an increased B_{12} binding protein release. The NAP score is usually raised (unlike the situation in CML). The bone marrow shows gross erythroid hyperplasia. Some fibrosis may be apparent. Chromosome analysis is usually normal at presentation.

Diagnosis

The first step in diagnosis is to demonstrate a raised red cell mass. The patient's red cells are labelled with ^{51}Cr, the total radioactivity bound to the red cells measured, and the red cells reinjected. Samples are taken after equilibration and the red cell mass calculated from:

$$\text{Red cell mass} = \frac{\text{Total counts/min injected}}{\text{Counts/min per ml of sample}} \times \text{haematocrit}$$

The result is expressed in ml/kg body weight.

The next stage is to exclude secondary polycythaemia. The Pa_{O2} should be measured and renal ultrasound performed. Polycystic kidneys and even hydronephrosis can cause a rise in erythropoietin, although polycythaemia of renal origin usually indicates a renal tumour. Other investigations to exclude an underlying cause of polycythaemia should be performed if the clinical situation merits it. If there is no splenomegaly and no raised white cell or platelet count, particular care must be taken to exclude a secondary cause. An Hb–oxygen dissociation curve is essential (especially in younger patients) to exclude the possibility of a high affinity haemoglobin. This is an inherited abnormality which gives rise to tissue hypoxia in the presence of a normal Pa_{O2}.

It might be thought that measurement of erythropoietin levels would readily differentiate between primary

Table 24.24 National (USA) PRV Study Group criteria for the diagnosis of polycythaemia rubra vera

A	↑Red cell mass Normal O_2 saturation
B	Splenomegaly
C	↑Platelets ↑Leucocytes (more than 12×10^9/l) ↑AP score ↑B_{12} (more than 900 pg/ml)

PRV is diagnosed if both A and B group symptoms are present; or if group A symptoms are present with any two symptoms from group C.

and secondary polycythaemia, but the results of erythropoietin assays are not always discriminatory. The criteria adopted for the diagnosis of PRV are shown in Table 24.24.

Patients with a raised red cell mass and normal Pa_{O2} who do not have splenomegaly or two category C features should be referred to as having *idiopathic erythrocytosis*. Although most patients will develop a myeloproliferative disorder, this is not invariable, and they should not therefore receive cytoreductive therapy at this stage.

Management

Supportive measures should include allopurinol for the prevention of secondary gout, especially if the uric acid level is high or if cytoreductive therapy is to be commenced. Antihistamines may help pruritus, and the symptom often improves with control of the disorder.

Once PRV has been diagnosed, venesection should be commenced. Approximately one unit of blood should be removed every second day until a normal haematocrit is obtained. Younger patients may tolerate more intensive initial venesection, while the converse applies in the elderly. Regular venesection alone can also be used to maintain the haematocrit below 0.46–0.48. Venesection may cause a thrombocytosis, and cytoreductive therapy should be instituted if platelet levels rise above 600×10^9/l, as this may exacerbate the thrombotic tendency of PRV.

Cytoreductive therapy is usually with hydroxyurea or an alkylating agent such as busulphan. ^{32}P (3–8 mCi) may also be used. It is given as a single i.v. bolus, and results in suppression of haemopoiesis with minimal systemic disturbance. The injection of ^{32}P can be repeated if necessary, but only after an interval of several months as the full effects of ^{32}P may take this long to be seen. It is usual to discontinue ^{32}P when a total dose of 30 mCi has been given.

Prognosis

Untreated, the median survival is only two years, most deaths being due to strokes and myocardial infarctions. With adequate therapy, however, the median survival is over 13 years. About 10% of cases transform to a myelofibrotic state and a similar number transform to an acute leukaemia (usually myeloid). Leukaemic transformation is higher in patients receiving cytoreductive therapy, particularly with ^{32}P, which is avoided in younger patients.

Management of other forms of polycythaemia

The problems of hyperviscosity in other forms of polycythaemia are similar to PRV. Patients with idiopathic erythrocytosis and pseudopolycythaemia should be venesected to achieve a haematocrit below 0.48. In secondary polycythaemia, the situation is more complex as erythrocytosis is secondary to hypoxia. Nonetheless, the increased oxygen-carrying capacity of the erythrocytosis is often more than offset by the decreased blood flow to critical organs; a trial of venesection is worthwhile in patients with neurological symptoms. It can be very difficult to maintain a lowered haematocrit.

ESSENTIAL THROMBOCYTHAEMIA

Essential thrombocythaemia (ET) is a myeloproliferative disorder in which there is a predominant proliferation of the megakaryocyte series. It occurs predominantly in the middle-aged and elderly.

The clinical features are shown in Table 24.25. Splenomegaly may be present but is frequently absent due to repeated infarction. The [Hb] is often reduced, especially if there is iron deficiency. The red cells frequently display the features of hyposplenism. The white cell count is often modestly raised and the NAP score increased. The platelet count is usually in excess of 1000×10^9/l. The bone marrow is hypercellular, with a marked proliferation of megakaryocytes; myelofibrosis is often present.

Diagnosis

The diagnosis of ET can be difficult, especially when the thrombocytosis is modest and there is no splenomegaly. Causes of secondary thrombocytosis must be excluded (p. 1110) and platelet function tests may be helpful, as there is often an aggregation defect in ET.

Management

Patients with a raised platelet count and a thrombotic history should be treated with anti-platelet aggregating agents, such as aspirin and dipyridimole. Cytoreductive therapy with hydroxyurea, busulphan or ^{32}P should be given to reduce the platelet count to below 500×10^9/l; α interferon is a useful alternative. Many patients survive for more than 10 years with appropriate therapy, but transformation to acute leukaemia or, more commonly, myelofibrosis may occur.

Table 24.25 Clinical features of essential thrombocythaemia

Cause	Effect
Myeloproliferation	Anaemia
	Splenomegaly (frequently absent)
High/abnormal platelets	Arterial and venous thromboses
	Haemorrhage
Multifactorial	Peptic ulceration

PRIMARY MYELOFIBROSIS

Primary myelofibrosis is a misnomer, in that it is a reaction to an underlying myeloproliferative disorder (although this primary cause may be occult).

The disease mainly affects the middle-aged and elderly, and presents with anaemia due to marrow failure and massive splenomegaly. The blood film reveals a leucoerythroblastic anaemia. A bone marrow aspirate is usually dry and a trephine biopsy shows extensive fibrosis. The diagnosis is not usually difficult, but it should be remembered that infections (particularly tuberculosis) can cause extensive marrow fibrosis.

Treatment is largely supportive, with regular transfusions. Splenectomy may be indicated if the large spleen is causing local symptoms, if there is an excessive transfusion requirement, or if there is marked granulocytopenia or thrombocytopenia.

The median survival is approximately five years. Progression to acute leukaemia occurs in 5–10% of cases.

ACUTE LEUKAEMIA

In acute leukaemia, there is accumulation in the blood and marrow of primitive haemopoietic cells (blast cells). Untreated, the course is rapidly progressive in the large majority of patients. The disease is rare, with an annual incidence of 4.4 per 100 000, although in children, acute leukaemia – particularly acute lymphoblastic leukaemia – is the commonest form of malignancy.

Acute leukaemia is divided into:

- acute lymphoblastic leukaemia (ALL)
- acute non-lymphoblastic leukaemia (ANLL), which is also called acute myeloid leukaemia (AML).

Each broad category can be further divided using morphological, cytochemical, immunological and genetic criteria.

Clinical features

Acute leukaemia typically presents with the features of marrow failure – anaemia, infection and bleeding. The latter may be particularly severe in promyelocytic variants of AML, where disseminated intravascular coagulation is a common complication. Onset is nearly always rapid in ALL, but there may be a preceding myelodysplastic phase in AML, with variable cytopenias lasting months or even years. In ALL, there is no such preleukaemia phase, although occasional cases present with an *aplastic* picture; the malignant proliferation then becomes apparent during the ensuing three months.

Hepatosplenomegaly is common in acute leukaemia, and lymphadenopathy is often present in ALL. Bone and joint pain may occur, particularly in ALL. Infiltration of soft tissues such as skin, gums and perineum may occur, and usually indicates a monocytic type of AML. CNS disease is rare at presentation although it is a common site of relapse in ALL. A wide range of metabolic disturbances may also be present at diagnosis, including hyperuricaemia, hyponatraemia and hypokalaemia. These changes may all be exacerbated by treatment.

ACUTE MYELOID LEUKAEMIA

The annual incidence of AML is approximately 3.4 per 100 000. Although the disease does occur in children and young adults, it is more common in the middle-aged and elderly (Fig. 24.26).

Diagnosis

The blood count typically reveals a normocytic or macrocytic anaemia, often with marked anisocytosis and poikilocytosis on the blood film. The platelet count is usually reduced, and the white count is usually – although not invariably – raised, with myeloblasts the predominant cells. Neutrophils are usually reduced in number and may appear dysplastic. There are relatively few intermediate myelocytes in the blood (unlike the situation in CML).

The bone marrow is hypercellular but may produce a dry tap. The majority of cells are myeloblasts (over 30% required for diagnosis) and the remaining haemopoietic cells may show marked dysplastic changes. In some cases, pathognomonic 'Auer' rods are seen in the myeloid cells.

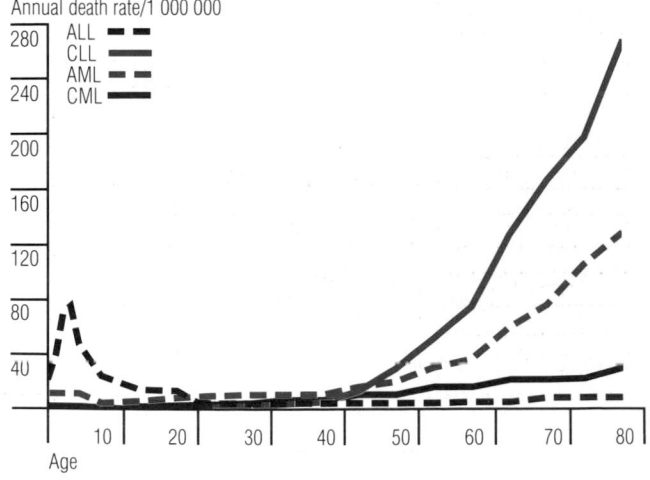

Annual death rate/1 000 000

Fig. 24.26 Annual death rate for different types of leukaemia at different ages.

Classification

Most cases of AML can be readily identified using morphological criteria, although some cases may be difficult to distinguish from ALL (especially the L2 subtype). The diagnosis of AML can be supported by cytochemical, immunological and genetic studies where appropriate (Table 24.26).

The subdivisions of AML are based on the nature of any differentiation that is present, using morphological and cytochemical criteria (Table 24.27).

Chromosome analysis

Chromosomal abnormalities are seen in about 50% of cases using Giemsa banding analysis, and more frequently with high resolution techniques. Trisomy 8, loss of the Y chromosome and monosomy 7 are the most common defects found. Specific translocations are also seen. A chromosome 8:21 translocation is associated with some M2 leukaemias and probably also with an improved pro-

Table 24.26 Differentiation between myeloblasts and lymphoblasts

	Myeloblasts	Lymphoblasts
Morphology		
Cell size	Moderate to large	Small to moderate
Cytoplasm	Moderate to abundant	Scanty to moderate
Granules in cytoplasm	Often in some cells	Rare
Auer rods	May be present	Absent
Nucleoli	Often more than two	One or two
Cytochemistry		
Peroxidase/ Sudan black	+	–
PAS	–	+
Immunology		
Nuclear terminal deoxynucleotidyl transferase (Tdt)	– (Occasionally +)	+
CD10 antigen (CALLA)	–	+
CD19 antigen (pan-B)	–	+ (common ALL and null ALL)
CD7 antigen (pan-T)	– (rarely +)	+ (T-ALL)
CD33	+	–
HLA-DR	+	+ (– in T-ALL)
Genetics		
Ig light chain gene rearrangement	–	+ (common ALL and null ALL)
T cell receptor gene rearrangement	–	+ (T-ALL)

Table 24.27 Subdivisions of acute myeloid leukaemia

M0   **AML without maturation**: Blasts are Sudan black and peroxidase negative but show CD13 or CD33.

M1   **AML without maturation:** More than 3% peroxidase or Sudan Black positive blasts; some blasts may have occasional granules or Auer rods.

M2   **AML with maturation:** Evidence of maturation at, or beyond, the promyelocyte stage.

M3   **Promyelocytic leukaemia:** Majority of cells promyelocytes. Note that leukaemic promyelocytes may be hyper- or hypogranular.

M4   **Myelomonocytic leukaemia:** Monocytic cells more than 20% of blood or marrow. Granulocytic cells more than 20% of marrow. Demonstration of fluoride-sensitive non-specific esterase staining aids the diagnosis of monocytic cells.

M5   **Monocytic leukaemia:**
     a)   Poorly differentiated monoblasts
     b)   Monoblasts, promonocytes and monocytes. Granulocytic cells less than 20% of marrow.

M6   **Erythroleukaemia:** Erythropoietic component exceeds 50% or 30% if associated with severe dyserythropoiesis. Myeloblasts must still constitute more than 30% of marrow cells.

M7   **Megakaryocytic leukaemia:** Identification of megakaryoblasts aided by electron microscopic demonstration of platelet-specific peroxidase or platelet-specific surface antigens. This disease often presents as acute myelofibrosis in which the blasts are few in number in the marrow.

gnosis; while a 15:17 translocation occurs in many cases of M3 leukaemia. The 8:21 and 15:17 translocations are associated with a relatively good chance of survival; –7 and +8 a relatively poor prognosis.

Management

The treatment strategy for AML is outlined in Figure 24.27. The *induction therapy* used in AML is very intensive as it is necessary to induce a hypoplastic marrow in order to achieve remission. The most effective drugs used are the anthracyclines and antimetabolites, and a typical induction regime is illustrated in Figure 24.28. Intensive blood product, antibiotic and psychological support is required during the hypoplastic period (p. 1056). In cases of M3 leukaemia, low-dose heparin therapy is probably advisable, to reduce the risks of disseminated intravascular haemolysis associated with tumour lysis. Retinoic acid may also induce maturation of the leukaemia alone and reduce cytotoxic drug induced DIC.

Remission is obtained in about 70% of younger patients, although this may take several induction courses. Once remission has been obtained, it is usual to give several further courses of induction type therapy; this is referred to as *consolidation*. Cycles of less intensive therapy (which exclude an anthracycline because it causes cumulative cardiotoxicity) are often given as *maintenance therapy* for one to two years, although evidence of the

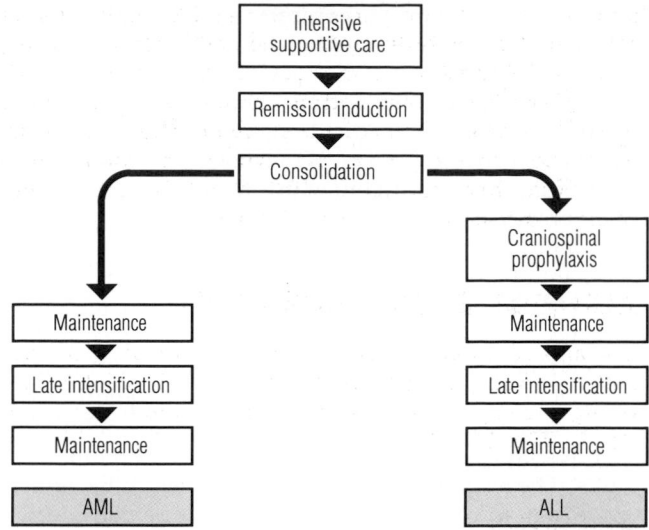

Fig. 24.27 Schematic representation of the treatment of acute leukaemia.

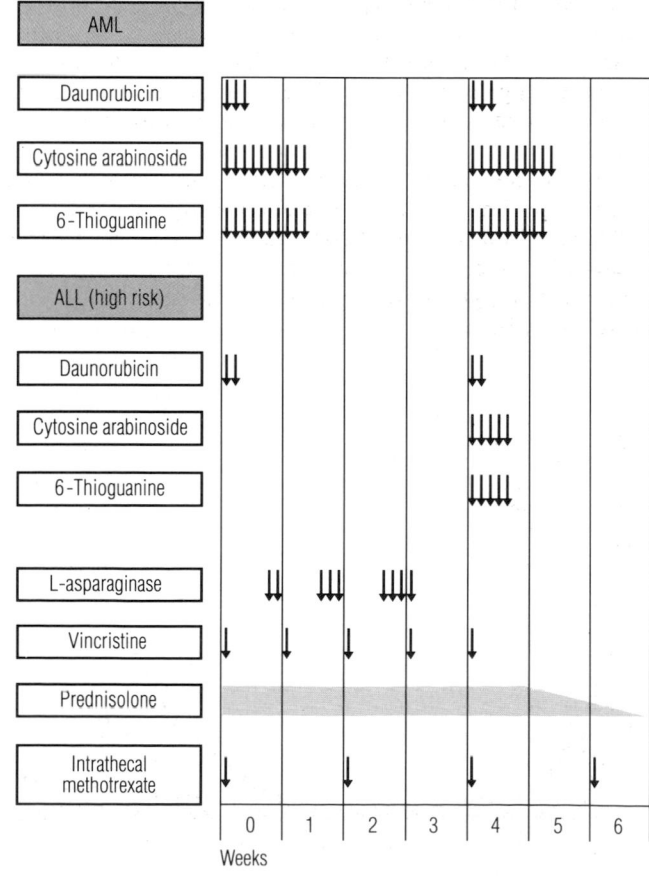

Fig. 24.28 Typical drug regimens used for induction therapy in acute myeloid leukaemia and high-risk acute lymphoblastic leukaemia.

benefits of maintenance therapy is slight. In some regimens, *late intensification* therapy similar to the induction regimen is given.

Allogeneic bone marrow transplantation is an alternative form of late intensification therapy, available for young patients who have an HLA matched sibling donor (only a minority of patients with AML). The cytoreductive therapy usually given is a combination of cyclophosphamide and total body irradiation. This is the treatment of choice in patients below 30 years of age, but in the 30–40-year-old age group the benefits are presently marginal. This situation might change if early deaths due to GVHD and infection fall without a rise in graft failure or leukaemia recurrence. High-dose chemo/radiotherapy with *autologous* marrow rescue has been used as a form of late intensification therapy, with promising preliminary results. The advantages are that every patient is his or her own donor and much older patients can be considered due to the absence of GVHD. The main disadvantages are the possibility of reinfusing untreated leukaemic cells with the marrow inoculum, and the absence of any graft-versus-leukaemia effect.

In patients who relapse, a second remission can sometimes be obtained. The chances are better in patients who relapse after ceasing chemotherapy. However, second remissions are almost invariably short-lived unless an allogeneic transplant can be performed. The results of transplantation at this stage are less good than in first remission.

Prognosis

The complete remission rate is close to 70% and, although most patients relapse on conventional therapy, approximately 30% of complete responders will still be alive after five years. Recipients of allogeneic grafts have an overall long-term (five year) survival of approximately 50%, this figure being somewhat higher in the under 25's. Half of the deaths are due to transplant-related complications, and half to leukaemic relapse.

Various factors influence response and survival on conventional therapy. On the more intensive regimens, children fare better than adults; and monocytic variants probably do less well than the non-monocytic variants. There is a higher early death rate in M3 leukaemia, due to haemorrhage; but in those achieving complete remission the survival may be longer than in other types of AML. The presence of nuclear terminal deoxynucleotidyl transferase (Tdt) and some chromosomal abnormalities are thought to be poor prognostic indicators (p. 1087).

ACUTE LYMPHOBLASTIC LEUKAEMIA

The annual incidence of ALL in the UK is approximately 1.0 per 100 000. The incidence peaks in mild-childhood (Fig. 24.26). There is a slight excess in males.

Diagnosis

The haematological findings are similar to those found in AML (p. 1087), except that the anaemia is nearly always normocytic; myelodysplastic features are not seen; and lymphoblasts predominate in the marrow and usually also the blood.

Classification

The morphological, cytochemical, immunological and genetic features of malignant lymphoblasts are shown in Table 24.27. ALL has been subdivided into three morphological variants (L1–L3) by the French–American–British (FAB) Co-operative Group, although this is of limited value in determining prognosis and therapy (Table 24.28). ALL may also be classified on immunological and genetic criteria (Table 24.29).

Chromosome analysis

Cytogenetic abnormalities are detected in about two-thirds of cases by routine banding techniques. Both

Table 24.28 Subdivisions of acute lymphoblastic leukaemia based on morphology

Feature	L1	L2	L3
Cell size	Small	Small to moderate Heterogeneous	Moderate Homogeneous
Amount of cytoplasm	Scanty	Scanty to moderate Heterogeneous	Moderate Homogeneous
Cytoplasmic basophilia	Minor	Minor to moderate	Marked
Cytoplasmic vacuolation	Minor	Minor	Marked
Nuclear irregularity	Unusual	Frequent	Unusual
Discernability of nucleoli	Often difficult (usually small)	Easy (often large)	Prominent
Nuclear chromatin pattern	Homogeneous	Heterogeneous	Homogeneous

Table 24.29 Subcategories of acute lymphoblastic leukaemia based on lineage and differentiation stage

Cell lineage	Differentiation stage	Alternative name	Incidence in children	Incidence in adults
B lineage	Very early	Null cell ALL	12%	38%
	Early	Common ALL	75%	50%
	Late	B cell ALL	<1%	2%
T lineage	Very early and early	T cell ALL	12%	10%

numerical and structural changes are seen. Unlike AML, hyperdiploidy (less than 50 chromosomes present) is not infrequent, and may be associated with a good prognosis. The Philadelphia chromosome (9:22 translocation) is present in 5% of childhood ALL and approximately 20% of adult cases. These patients have a poor prognosis. Other specific translocations also occur, for example an 8:14 translocation is found in most cases of L3 leukaemia (as well as in Burkitt's lymphoma).

Management

The treatment strategy in ALL is shown in Figure 24.27. In the early 1970s, remission was *induced* with vincristine and prednisone; both drugs have specificity for lymphoblasts and do not cause severe haematological suppression. Since then, regimens have become more intensive, and the differences from induction regimens used in AML are less marked (Fig. 24.28). With modern anthracycline-containing regimens, over 95% of children and over 85% of adults with ALL obtain remission although there is concern about the long-term cardiotoxic effects of anthracyclines particularly in young children. Most induction regimens also contain L-asparaginase (Fig. 24.28).

Once remission is obtained, it is now common practice to give a further intensive *consolidation* course before commencing *maintenance* therapy. Maintenance is less intensive than induction therapy, and cyclical combinations of 6-mercaptopurine, methotrexate, vincristine and prednisone are usually given. Unlike the situation in AML, there is reasonable evidence that maintenance should be given for at least two years in ALL. In many centres, a further ablative therapy course is given after about six months; this is known as *late intensification*, and appears to be particularly valuable in high risk cases.

Craniospinal prophylaxis must also be given during remission, to prevent relapse in this 'privileged site'. It is usual to give 18 Gy in 10 daily fractions to the cranium, and repeated injections of intrathecal methotrexate or cytosine arabinoside to treat the spinal compartment. Drugs which cross the blood–brain barrier are currently being investigated. Testicular irradiation has also been used as prophylaxis against relapse at this site (10% of relapses in boys); but this has made little impact on survival and causes hypogonadism and infertility.

The role of allogeneic bone marrow transplantation in ALL is still not fully defined. It is not justified in the large majority of children in first remission, because recent intensive regimens are so effective even in high-risk cases. It may have a role in first remission adults. Once a relapse has occurred, bone marrow transplantation in second remission is probably the treatment of choice if the patient is below 40 years of age and a matched donor is available.

Prognosis

Nearly all patients with ALL achieve remission, but relapse is still a major problem. The factors influencing survival are shown in Table 24.30. The immunological phenotype is clearly related to prognosis, with common ALL doing well and T- or B-ALL badly; but phenotyping probably provides little additional prognostic information, beyond that obtained from the age, sex and presenting white cell count. Many regimens identify the high-risk group at presentation and more intensive therapy is then given. With some regimens, this has removed the survival difference between the good and poor risk cases, both groups having a projected five year survival in excess of 60%. Death usually follows once relapse occurs, but second remissions may be protracted, especially if relapse occurs late after stopping therapy. Allogeneic bone marrow transplantation may cure some patients in second remission, but the relapse rate is high; long-term survival is probably less than 30%.

Table 24.30 Factors at presentation of acute lymphoblastic leukaemia indicative of a poor prognosis

- High peripheral white count
- Age less than two years or over 10 years
- Male sex
- Certain chromosomal abnormalities
- Morphological L3, and possibly L2, subtype
- Immunological
  Null ALL
  T cell ALL   ↑ Worsening prognosis
  B-cell ALL

MYELODYSPLASIA

Myelodysplasia refers to an acquired state of haemo-poietic dysfunction, in which there is cytopenia (involving one or more cell lines) without evidence of peripheral destruction and a cellular marrow. Haemopoiesis is ineffective, and morphological abnormalities are prominent in blood and marrow. Anaemia is common and there is frequently a mild to moderate macrocytosis, anisocytosis and poikilocytosis. The neutrophil count is often low, and the neutrophils exhibit abnormalities of granulation. The platelet count may also be reduced. A monocytosis may occur in some cases. The bone marrow shows dysplastic changes in one or more cell lines, the blast cell count may be raised, and an iron stain may reveal ringed sidero-blasts. Clonal chromosomal abnormalities are detected in 50–60% of cases, and many other cases also undoubtedly represent a clonal expansion. The myelodysplastic syndromes (MDS) have been subdivided by the French–American–British (FAB) Group and are shown in Table 24.31. It should be noted that while this terminology refers to 'refractory anaemia', it does in fact include 'refractory neutropenia or thrombocytopenia' due to ineffective production. Also, although chronic myelomonocytic leukaemia is included in the MDS, and although anaemia is almost invariable in this condition, the white cell count may be raised suggestive of a myeloproliferative disorder.

Clinical features

The MDS are a group of diseases that occur predominantly in the elderly, but can arise at any stage of adult life. Patients usually present with symptoms attributable to the cytopenia. Fever not related to infection, bone pain and splenomegaly occasionally occur.

The MDS clearly represent a spectrum of disorders, from mild marrow dysfunction to almost frank leukaemia. Many cases of refractory anaemia with ringed sideroblasts and normal white count and platelets remain stable for many years; whereas refractory anaemia with excess blasts can be difficult to differentiate from acute leukaemia at presentation, and usually progresses rapidly. The features suggestive of a poor prognosis are the involvement of more than one cell lineage and a high blast cell count; but, even in these cases, the term 'preleukaemia' is best avoided. This is because the term can only be used with certainty in retrospect, and because many of the deaths in severe MDS arise from worsening cytopenias, rather than transformation to acute leukaemia.

Management

The conventional approach to the management of the MDS is to provide supportive therapy, only instituting acute leukaemia therapy when leukaemic progression occurs. The response to treatment at this later stage is not good, and it may therefore be appropriate to institute more aggressive therapy earlier in young patients with MDS who exhibit poor prognostic features. Haemo-poietic growth factors may increase the white count but the clinical benefit is uncertain.

MALIGNANT LYMPHOPROLIFERATIVE DISORDERS

There is a spectrum of neoplastic proliferations of lymphoid and other cells (such as histiocytes) which comprise the normal lymphoreticular system. The lymphoid leukaemias – both acute and chronic – are usually considered as distinct from the lymphomas, which preferentially involve nodes and spleen. Overlap is frequent, however.

Lymphocyte proliferation is a normal response to antigenic challenge and diagnostic confusion between reactive and neoplastic nodes can arise. Features suggesting malignancy include: effacement of the normal node archi-

Table 24.31 FAB classification of the myelodysplastic syndromes

Syndrome	Blasts in marrow	Blasts in blood	Auer rods	Monocytes $>1 \times 10^9$/l in blood	Ringed sideroblasts >15% of nucleated bone marrow cells
Refractory anaemia (RA)	<5%	<1%	–	–	–
Acquired idiopathic sideroblastic anaemia (AISA)	<5%	<1%	–	–	+
Refractory anaemia with excess blasts (RAEB)	5–20%	<5%	–	–	±
Refractory anaemia with excess blasts in transformation (RAEBT)	21–30%	>5%	+	±	±
Chronic myelomonocytic leukaemia (CML)	<20%	<5%	–	+	±

tecture; extension beyond the usual confines of the node; and the presence of a uniform population of cells. The latter is often absent, however, partly because the malignant clone may be represented by cells at more than one stage of differentiation, and partly because a marked reactive proliferation may also occur in the same node.

It is possible on clinical, morphological and immunological criteria to define distinct entities within the spectrum of the lymphoproliferative disorders, but it is difficult in some cases to relate a malignant proliferation to the differentiation level of its normal cell counterpart. The cell lineage of some lymphomas (particularly Hodgkin's disease) is uncertain as, in contrast to the myeloid system, the morphology of the lymphoid cells reflects the proliferative status of the cell as much as its stage of differentiation. Figures 24.29 and 24.30 outline B and T cell differentiation pathways, and give an approximation of the corresponding malignancies.

HODGKIN'S DISEASE

Hodgkin's disease (HD) is a clinically and histologically distinct malignant lymphoma, although the cell of origin is uncertain. Some cases appear to be of B cell origin, although it is possible that the disease is in fact heterogeneous in origin.

Clinical features

The annual incidence of HD in the UK is approximately 2.4 per 100 000. It is uncommon in childhood, with peak incidence in early adulthood and again in the elderly. Patients most commonly present with lymphadenopathy, especially in the cervical region. When more than one region is involved, the areas are usually contiguous, consistent with the view that spread is predominantly through the lymphatics. The lymph nodes may or may not be

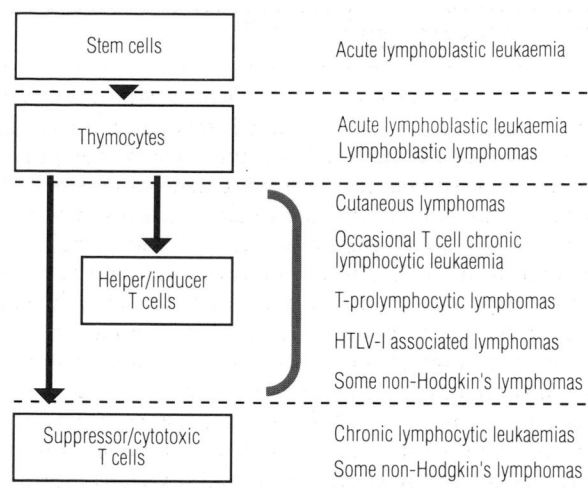

Fig. 24.30 T cell-lymphoproliferative diseases and their putative relationships to normal T lymphocytes. The HTLV I associated malignancies typically have a helper inducer phenotype (CD4+) but have suppressor function in vitro.

tender, and may initially fluctuate in size. Alcohol-related pain in the nodes may occur but is rare. Hepatosplenomegaly occurs with more advanced disease, and there can be infiltration of almost all organs. Systemic symptoms are frequent, especially in disseminated disease, although some patients with extensive tumour bulk feel well. Intense generalised itching (pruritis) is common. Anaemia occurs in about 35% of patients, and is correlated with advanced disease rather than marrow infiltration, which is found in less than 10% of cases. Neutrophilia is common and eosinophilia occurs in 15% of patients. Lymphopenia is frequent in disseminated disease but, even in patients with normal lymphocyte numbers, there is often a functional T cell deficit, the cause of which is not fully understood. Clinical depression of cell mediated immunity is most clearly manifest as *Herpes zoster* infection.

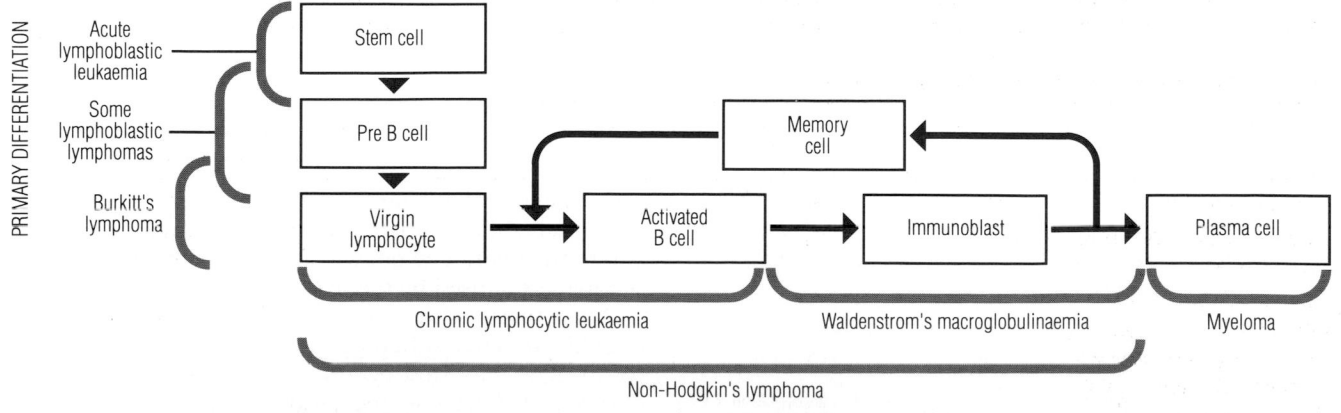

Fig. 24.29 B cell-lymphoproliferative diseases and their putative relationships to normal B lymphocytes.

Histological classification

The diagnosis of HD is made from histological diagnosis of affected tissue, usually lymph node. The malignant Reed Sternberg cells and their mononuclear counterparts are present in variable (often small) numbers in an appropriate reactive background of lymphocytes, eosinophils and fibrous tissue. The Reed Sternberg cell is classically a large binucleate cell with vesicular nuclei and prominent eosinophilic nucleoli. These cells may appear to be in lacunae, especially if fibrosis is present. The classification of HD is shown in Table 24.32 and is primarily dependent on the composition of the reactive elements. In the original classification by Lukes and Butler, nodular sclerosis (subdivision of node by fibrous tissue and presence of lacunar cells) was not subdivided, but this broad category accounts for over 70% of cases. Nowadays, subdivision of nodular sclerosis into high- and low-grade is often made, with reference to the reactive cellular elements. The presence of easily recognised areas of lymphocyte depletion or of numerous pleomorphic Hodgkin's cells is indicative of high-grade (grade II) nodular sclerosis. Lymphocyte-depleted HD is rare (less than 5% of cases) and has a very poor prognosis.

Staging

Accurate staging provides important prognostic information and dictates the appropriate treatment strategy. The Ann Arbor staging system is usually used (Table 24.33).

Table 24.32 Histological classification of Hodgkin's disease and relation to prognosis

Lymphocyte predominant Nodular sclerosis – low-grade	**Good prognosis**
Nodular sclerosis – high-grade Mixed cellularity Lymphocyte depleted	**Poor prognosis**

Table 24.33 The Ann Arbor staging system

Stage I	Single lymph node region involved, sometimes with local spread to extralymphatic tissue (IE).
Stage II	Involvement of two or more node regions on the same side of the diaphragm, sometimes with local spread to extralymphatic tissue (IIE).
Stage III	Involvement of nodes on both sides of the diaphragm. (The spleen is considered as a 'node'.)
Stage IV	Diffuse or disseminated involvement of one or more extralymphatic organs.

Each stage is also divided into A or B according to absence or presence of systemic symptoms; these include a sustained fever (>38°C), weight loss (more than 10% of body weight in six months) and night sweats, but not pruritus.

A thorough history and examination is required, involving chest X-ray, liver function tests and good quality imaging of the abdomen, such as ultrasound, computed tomography or nuclear magnetic resonance scanning. With the increasing availability of these techniques, lymphangiography is performed less often, although the latter will demonstrate abnormal node architecture in relatively small nodes. Laparotomy and splenectomy were introduced to improve tumour localisation, but these are now performed infrequently. This degree of detailed staging may now add little to overall survival because most patients with occult intra-abdominal disease, treated inappropriately with radiotherapy to the lymph nodes above the diaphragm, can later be rescued with chemotherapy when intra-abdominal relapse occurs.

Management

Localised disease (stages IA and IIA, Table 24.35) without symptoms is conventionally treated by radiotherapy alone. It is usual to irradiate all node areas above or below the diaphragm, according to the site of the disease. These extended fields are known as *mantle fields* and *inverted Y fields* (Fig. 24.31). It may be acceptable to irradiate only the involved nodal areas, but there is then a higher relapse rate in adjacent node regions. These nodes are, however, amenable to further radiotherapy, and the more localised therapy has fewer side-effects. The overall relapse rate following a mantle field for supradiaphragmatic disease is high (approximately 40%). Most relapses are outside the irradiated field. It is usual to give chemotherapy as well when there is a large mediastinal mass, since the risk of local relapse is higher. Some centres give adjuvant chemotherapy for many other cases of localised disease. This minimises relapse but does not necessarily improve survival, as chemotherapy salvage is highly effective.

Patients with stage IIB disease have a very high relapse rate following radiotherapy, and are therefore usually treated by chemotherapy. This is particularly appropriate in centres which do not perform a staging laparotomy, since the probability of intra-abdominal disease is high. Stage IIIA disease can be effectively treated by total nodal irradiation (mantle and inverted Y) but, again, most centres prefer to use chemotherapy rather than employ such extended radiation fields. If the patient relapses soon after total nodal irradiation has been given, it is very difficult to treat with chemotherapy because of lasting myelosuppression caused by the radiotherapy.

All patients with stage IIIB and IV disease must be treated with chemotherapy. The standard treatment was six to eight monthly cycles of 'MOPP' (mustine, vincristine, procarbazine, prednisone) combination therapy, or minor modifications of this. Chlorambucil can replace mustine with less toxicity. There is no value in protracted

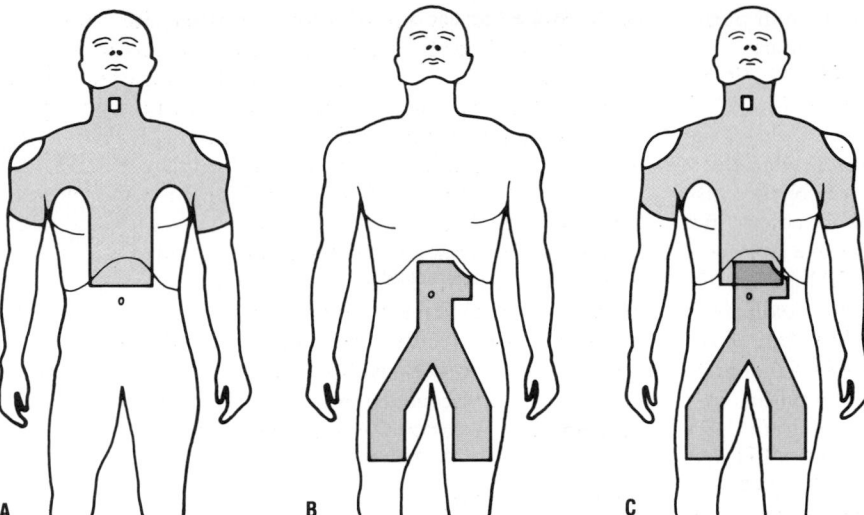

Fig. 24.31 Irradiation fields used in the treatment of Hodgkin's disease. (A) Mantle field. (B) Inverted Y field. (C) Total nodal irradiation.

maintenance therapy. Improved results have been obtained with the addition of other drugs (such as ABVD – adriamycin, bleomycin, vinblastine, dacarbazine), either alternating with MOPP or in combined 'hybrid' regimens. In some centres, radiotherapy to sites of previous bulk disease is also given following chemotherapy, but its value is unproven.

Relapse of local disease may be amenable to further radiotherapy if tissue limits have not been reached in that region. Alternatively, chemotherapy can be used. If relapse occurs many months after stopping therapy in those patients who received initial chemotherapy, it is often possible to induce a further remission with the same drugs. If the patient is resistant to primary therapy, or if relapse has occurred soon after stopping the initial drugs, then a so-called non-cross-resistant regimen such as ABVD should be tried. The clinical situation is very difficult in patients relapsing soon after alternating or hybrid regimens. High dose chemotherapy and autologous bone marrow transplantation may be indicated.

Prognosis

The overall 10 year survival in HD is approximately 60%, but both the complete remission (CR) rate and the long-term survival is influenced by the stage and histological grade of the disease (Table 24.34). Age is also very important, with patients over 50 years faring much worse. Most relapses occur in the first few years, although late relapses do occasionally occur.

NON-HODGKIN'S LYMPHOMAS

Non-Hodgkin's lymphomas (NHL) are more common than HD; the annual incidence in the UK is approx-

Summary 10 Treatment of Hodgkin's disease according to stage

IA	
IB	} Radiotherapy
IIA	

| IIB | |
| IIIA | } Chemotherapy (occasionally radiotherapy) |

IIIB	
IVA	} Chemotherapy
IVB	

Table 24.34 Prognosis in Hodgkin's disease

Stage	% total cases	Histological grade	5 year survival (%)
IA	20	I	92
		II	83
IB	0–1	–	–
IIA	21	I	94
		II	77
IIB	7	I	78
		II	70
IIIA	17	I	80
		II	71
IIIB	13	I	77
		II	55
IVA	6	I	74
		II	56
IVB	14	I	64
		II	46

imately 8.2 per 100 000. Although there is a small peri-adolescent peak, they are most common in the elderly.

Clinical features

Most patients have lymphadenopathy at presentation but, unlike the situation in HD, the spread is not contiguous and disseminated disease at presentation is common. Patients with histologically low-grade disease are frequently asymptomatic; whereas patients with high-grade disease tend to have symptoms of fever, anorexia and weight loss. A multiplicity of local symptoms can arise from nodal pressure or extranodal disease. These include: obstruction of the superior vena cava; abdominal distension and back pain due to enlarged para-aortic nodes; bone pain from erosion or metastases in bone; chylous ascites and chylothorax from rupture of lymphatic channels; and cutaneous, pulmonary and hepatic infiltration. NHL can also arise as primary tumours of the gastrointestinal tract, brain, thyroid, bone, orbit and testis and are discussed in these chapters. Anaemia may arise from marrow infiltration, hypersplenism or auto-immune haemolysis; this is particularly common in the low-grade lymphomas. Low levels of paraprotein are often present in the low-grade lymphomas, although hypergammaglobulinaemia in NHL is usually polyclonal.

Histological classification

There are many classifications of NHL, all of which have their advocates. The working formulation shown in Table 24.36 has the advantage of simplicity, being based largely on cell size and shape and the presence of malignant follicles. It is also particularly useful in translating from one classification to another. The working formulation considers lymphomas in three prognostic categories but, in practice, they are usually divided into two categories (low and high grade) as shown in Table 24.35.

Most NHL (70%) are tumours of the follicular centre cell, which appear either as small cells with a cleaved nucleus (centrocyte) or as larger cells with less marked nuclear cleavage (centroblasts). In these follicular centre cell lymphomas, the tumour may make large follicles (follicular appearance) or the node may be diffusely replaced by sheets of tumour cells (diffuse appearance).

There is not always a clear dividing line between the two, and different lymph nodes may show both diffuse and follicular change in the same patient. As the follicular lymphoma progresses, it may also change to a diffuse appearance.

The lymphomas may also be classified according to their cell of origin. The follicular centrocytic/centroblastic lymphomas are B cell tumours, as are many of the diffuse lymphomas. A significant proportion of the diffuse large cell and lymphoblastic lymphomas are of T cell origin, as

Table 24.35 Classification of non-Hodgkin's lymphomas

Grade	Working formulation	
Low grade	Small lymphocytic cell Follicular small cleaved cell (centrocytic) Follicular mixed small cleaved and large cells (centrocytic/centro blastic)	commonly referred to as **low grade** or indolent
Intermediate grade	Follicular large cleaved cell (centroblastic)* Diffuse small cleaved cell (centrocytic)	

High grade	Diffuse mixed small and large cell (centrocytic/centroblastic)
	Diffuse large cell (centroblastic)
	Diffuse large cell (immunoblastic)
	Lymphoblastic
	  – convoluted
	  – non-convoluted
	Small non-cleaved cell
		commonly referred to as **high grade** or aggressive

Miscellaneous	Including mycosis fungoides and composite lymphomas	

* Many consider this to be a high grade tumour.

are the cutaneous T cell lymphomas such as mycosis fungoides. T cell lymphoblastic lymphomas and some mature T cell lymphomas have a very poor prognosis, but it is not yet clear that all patients with T cell lymphomas fare badly. A very small proportion of diffuse large cell lymphomas may be of true histiocytic origin.

Staging

The Ann Arbor staging system is used in NHL, but is less useful than in HD as most cases of low-grade disease are already stage IV at presentation. Marrow infiltration is particularly common in these cases. Accurate staging is important if patients are involved in clinical trials, since stage may affect prognosis; but invasive investigations, particularly laparotomy, are rarely justified.

Management

There has been a paucity of controlled clinical trials in NHL and, in many circumstances, the optimal therapy has not been defined. In general terms, the *low-grade lymphomas* only require treatment if they are symptomatic or have a critical organ dysfunction. If the disease appears localised to one or two node regions, then local radiotherapy is probably the treatment of choice. If the disease is generalised, systemic chemotherapy is usually given,

Table 24.36 Prognosis in the non-Hodgkin's lymphomas

Histological grade	Stage	CR rate (%)	Five year survival (%)
Low grade	I & II	85	80
	III & IV	60	65
High grade	I	95	75 (90% in large cell lymphomas)
	IIA	70	60
	IIB	50	40
	IIIA	70	60
	IIIB	45	40
	IVA	50	35
	IVB	30	25

Figures given are approximate values obtained from the British National Lymphomas Investigation data bank.

Summary 11 Therapeutic strategies in non-Hodgkin's lymphomas

Low grade

Stages I & II (excluding gut)	Local radiotherapy if symptomatic
Stages III & IV	Single agent chemotherapy with/without radiotherapy if symptomatic

High grade

Stage I	Local radiotherapy/combination chemotherapy
Stage II	Combination chemotherapy
Stage III	Combination chemotherapy
Stage IV	Combination chemotherapy

---

with or without radiotherapy to any particularly troublesome node region. Single agent therapy such as chlorambucil (5–10 mg/day) is usually sufficient to induce a response. Most patients obtain a good response (Table 24.36) but relapse frequently occurs. Once a good response has been achieved, therapy can be discontinued and the patient carefully followed up.

In the high-grade lymphomas, intensive therapy should be instituted immediately. The patients are already symptomatic or will soon become so. Uncommonly, a high-grade lymphoma is truly stage I and, in these cases, full dose local radiotherapy is often curative. Chemotherapy is given for all other disease stages and many centres also use chemotherapy in stage I disease. The CHOP regimen (cyclophosphamide, doxorubicin, vincristine, prednisone) has been standard therapy for high grade NHL but, in recent years, attempts have been made to improve results by adding further drugs to this regimen, e.g. bleomycin and methotrexate; by using alternating regimens of CHOP and other potentially non-cross-resistant regimens; or by using hybrid regimens in which two different drug combinations are combined into a single drug cycle. Preliminary results with these more intensive regimens were encouraging, but none have yet been proved to be superior to CHOP. Most treatments are continued for about three months after complete remission is obtained, and there is no benefit from protracted maintenance therapy. In patients with lymphoblastic lymphomas or small non-cleaved cell lymphomas, the risk of relapse in the CNS is high and CNS prophylaxis is therefore essential.

It should be noted that some low-grade lymphomas do behave in a very aggressive manner either at presentation or during the course of the disease. These patients can be recognised clinically and should receive combination chemotherapy. Progression to a more aggressive course may not indicate a change in histology, but about 25% of low-grade lymphomas do transform to high-grade histology.

Prognosis

The complete remission and five year survival rates are dependent on the histological grade and stage (Table 24.37). In the low-grade lymphomas, relapse and a continuing death rate are the rule; whereas in the high-grade lymphomas, about two-thirds of patients who obtain a complete remission are probably cured. By 10 years, therefore, the overall survival of the low-grade and high-grade lymphomas cross-over (Fig. 24.32).

Cutaneous T cell lymphomas

Many mature T cell tumours involve the skin; the major example is mycosis fungoides and its leukaemic counterpart, the Sézary syndrome, both of which occur most commonly in middle-aged males. In both cases, the malignant cell is a CD4+ mature T cell the nucleus of which frequently has a highly convoluted and bizarre morphological appearance. These *Sézary cells* may also occur in the blood in light-sensitive eczemas. As mycosis

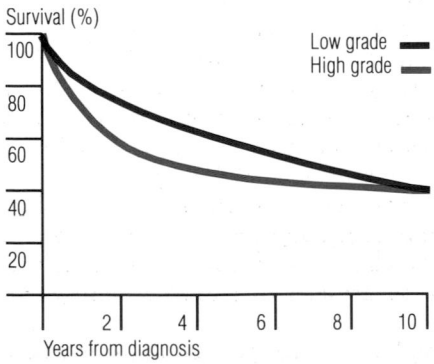

Fig. 24.32 Comparison of survival with low- and high-grade non-Hodgkin's lymphoma. The initial death rate is high with high-grade tumours, but the curve then flattens with 40% of patients cured. A steady, slower, death rate occurs with low-grade tumours, with no evidence of cure.

fungoides often begins as an eczematous reaction, precise definition of when the disorder should be considered malignant is difficult; however, demonstration of clonality by T cell receptor gene rearrangement may be of value. In the later stages of mycosis fungoides, the skin lesions form plaques, tumours and fungating ulcers. Erythroderma (p. 1144) may occur, which is often highly pruritic. In the Sézary syndrome, there is leukaemia, generalised lymphadenopathy and hepatosplenomegaly in addition to skin infiltration (usually erythroderma).

Lesions of mycosis fungoides can be treated with topical steroids, topical cytotoxic agents, PUVA (p. 1135) or radiotherapy. When visceral involvement is present, systemic cytotoxic therapy is required, although the responses are often of brief duration. The median survival of mycosis fungoides is five years but is much less if there is a leukaemic element.

Adult T cell leukaemia/lymphoma

This entity is rare in the UK but is common in South-West Japan and the Caribbean basin. It is of particular interest because it is caused by the human T cell lymphotropic virus (HTLV 1). The infectivity of this virus is low, and only a small proportion of patients who have been infected with HTLV 1 develop T cell lymphomas. These lymphomas involve phenotypic CD4+ cells and often behave in a very aggressive manner. Widespread visceral involvement with a leukaemic element is usual, and cranial involvement and hypercalcaemia are common. The response to chemotherapy is usually poor.

Angio-immunoblastic lymphadenopathy

Angio-immunoblastic lymphadenopathy is a spectrum of disorders characterised clinically by lymphadenopathy, hepatosplenomegaly and hypergammaglobulinaemia. The patient is often febrile and autoimmune haemolytic anaemia is common. Histologically, the node is infiltrated by a mixed proliferation of immunoblasts, plasma cells, lymphocytes, eosinophils and small blood vessels. In some cases, this is a self-limiting condition often responsive to steroids. In other cases, a lymphoma develops, most of which are T cell lymphomas.

Histiocytic medullary reticulosis

This is a rare malignant proliferation of monocytic/histiocytic cells that usually presents with fever and pancytopenia. The histiocytes in the marrow exhibit haemophagocytosis. The disease responds poorly to chemotherapy and is rapidly fatal. This condition may be difficult to differentiate from virus-induced histiocytosis which is a potentially self-limiting disorder.

Histiocytosis X (Langerhans cell histiocytosis)

Histiocytosis X refers to a spectrum of disorders (Table 24.37). They are proliferations of Langerhans cells (histiocytes found in the dermis) and are of uncertain malignancy. The lesions are characterised by variable proliferation of histiocytes, with formation of giant cells and granuloma, and infiltration by eosinophils, foam cells and fibrosis. The Langerhans cells have characteristic EM inclusions.

The lesions are responsive to intralesional steroids, local radiation and systemic chemotherapy. Since remissions occur spontaneously, especially in childhood, a conservative approach is adopted whenever possible.

Childhood lymphomas

The malignant cells in childhood lymphomas usually have an immature phenotype, with T cell-lymphoblastic lymphomas and small non-cleaved cell lymphomas predominating. The small non-cleaved lymphomas may be associated with Epstein Barr virus (EBV) infection (Burkitt's lymphoma). With recent intensive therapy, it appears that many of the Burkitt's lymphomas are curable, but reports of high cure rates in the T lymphoblastic lymphomas have not been universally upheld. Hodgkin's disease may also occur in childhood. The principles of treatment are similar to in adults but wide field irradiation is avoided whenever possible because of skeletal deformity in later life.

CHRONIC LYMPHOCYTIC LEUKAEMIA

The annual incidence of chronic lymphocytic leukaemia (CLL) in the UK is approximately 6 per 100 000. It does

Table 24.37 Classification and treatment of histiocytosis X

Classification	Symptoms	Treatment and prognosis
Unifocal eosinophilic granuloma	Usually single destructive bone lesions	Curable by curettage and radiotherapy
Multifocal eosinophilic granuloma (Hand-Schuller-Christian disease)	Multiple osseous and extraosseous lesions Triad of bone lesions, exophthalmos, diabetes insipidus occurs in 25%	Local lesions treated by curettage and radiotherapy Permanent remissions rare
Letterer-Siwe syndrome	Bone lesions, skin infiltration, lymphadenopathy and hepatosplenomegaly	Partial response to cytotoxic drugs Usually fatal

not occur in children and is rare in young adults, but the incidence rises steeply with advanced age. It is nearly twice as common in males as females (p. 1086).

Clinical and laboratory features

CLL usually presents with lymphadenopathy with or without splenomegaly. Some early cases are discovered on an incidental blood count. As the disease progresses, there is insidious development of anaemia. Occasionally, the onset of anaemia may be rapid and of severe degree. This usually indicates the development of autoimmune haemolytic anaemia. There is also an increased incidence of bacterial and, to a lesser extent, viral infections.

Laboratory investigations show that the lymphocyte count is very variable, from just above normal up to $300 \times 10^9/l$. Most are small, mature lymphocytes and a variable number are larger cells with a nucleolus but still a mature nuclear chromatin pattern (prolymphocytes). Smudge cells are also numerous on the blood film.

In over 95% of cases, the lymphocytes are B cells which express low levels of light-chain-restricted surface immunoglobulin. They also express pan-B antigens detectable by monoclonal antibodies and the CD5 antigen – a pan-T antigen expressed on cells transiently during B cell differentiation. CLL cells also express receptors that cause them to form rosettes with mouse red cells. Surface marker analysis with demonstration of light chain restriction may be particularly helpful in making the diagnosis of CLL when the lymphocyte count is only marginally raised.

Biopsy of affected nodes (which is seldom necessary to make the diagnosis), shows a low-grade diffuse lymphocytic lymphoma, with cells identical to those in the blood.

Hypogammaglobulinaemia due to suppression of normal immunoglobulin production occurs at some stage of the disease in about one-third of cases; paraproteins (usually IgM) occur in about 5% of cases.

Management

As with the low-grade lymphomas, treatment is only indicated if the patient is symptomatic or has critical organ dysfunction. Initial treatment is usually with chlorambucil (2–10 mg/day). In good responders, it is often possible to stop therapy as it is not necessary or feasible to strive for a complete remission. Steroids are of value if the patient has thrombocytopenia or an autoimmune haemolytic anaemia. As the disease progresses, resistance to chemotherapy occurs with an increasing lymphocyte count, lymphadenopathy, hepatosplenomegaly and bone marrow failure. In such patients, combination chemotherapy will frequently bring the disease under control,

but this is usually only temporary. In some patients, progression is associated with increasing numbers of prolymphocytes in the blood; rarely, there is transformation to a histologically aggressive lymphoma (Richter's syndrome).

Prognosis

The median survival exceeds five years, but patients presenting with advanced disease have a much shorter survival. Poor prognostic features at presentation include large numbers of prolymphocytes on the blood film, massive splenomegaly and marrow failure.

Prolymphocytic leukaemia

Prolymphocytic leukaemia (PLL) is a variant of CLL in which the majority of peripheral blood cells are prolymphocytes. In most cases, these are B cells but a significant proportion of cases are of mature T cell origin. In PLL, the leucocyte count tends to be high and massive splenomegaly is common, often with little lymphadenopathy. The prognosis is poor compared to typical CLL.

Hairy cell leukaemia

This is a chronic B cell lymphoproliferative disorder in which the malignant cells have a typical 'hairy appearance' with multiple fine cytoplasmic projections. Pancytopenia and splenomegaly are usual, and lymphadenopathy is uncommon. There is often fibrosis of the marrow with a dry tap. Therapy is not usually required unless there is marked neutropenia. Splenectomy may be of value, and good responses may be obtained with α-interferon deoxycoformycin, or 2 chlorodeoxyadenosine therapy. The median survival is in the order of five years.

T cell chronic lymphocytic leukaemia

T cell chronic lymphocytic leukaemia encompasses several rare entities with distinct natural histories. CD4+ proliferations generally have an aggressive natural history, whereas the CD8+ proliferations are comparatively benign. The cells in CD8+ T cell CLL are usually large granular lymphocytes, the lymphocyte count is only moderately raised and, although the marrow infiltration is usually not total, very severe red cell aplasia or neutropenia may occur. The precise pathogenesis of these cytopenias is not clear. The disease may remain stable for many years and a complete remission is often obtained with single agent cytotoxic therapy. T cell CLL has been associated with rheumatoid arthritis.

TUMOURS OF IMMUNOGLOBULIN-PRODUCING CELLS

This term refers to monoclonal proliferations of B cells at a relatively late stage of differentiation. The cells are usually secreting immunoglobulin, in which case the abnormal proliferation is accompanied by an abnormal band on serum protein electrophoresis. The monoclonal immunoglobulin is called a paraprotein.

Multiple myeloma

Multiple myeloma is a malignant B cell proliferation in the bone marrow, in which the predominant cell type is the plasma cell. This disease occurs predominantly in the elderly, and the annual incidence is approximately 5.9 per 100 000.

Clinical and laboratory features

The development of the symptoms and signs of multiple myeloma is shown in Figure 24.33.

Direct effects of plasma cell proliferation

The proliferation of plasma cells within the marrow leads to *skeletal destruction*. The bone destruction may be due to the release of an osteoclast activating factor (OAF) by the plasma cells, rather than to a direct expansion of the plasma cells within the bones. Widespread osteoporosis and lytic lesions without osteoblastic reaction (no sclerosis and normal alkaline phosphatase) occur in most cases. Multiple lytic lesions of the skull and crush fractures of the spine are particularly common. Hypercalcaemia in association with bone resorption occurs in 30% of cases at some stage of the disease, not infrequently at presentation. This gives rise to thirst, polyuria, and dehydration, constipation and abdominal pains, lethargy, confusion and coma.

The plasma cell proliferation frequently causes *a mild to moderate anaemia*. This is in part due to replacement of the marrow space by tumour, but the proliferation may also suppress haemopoiesis. Neutropenia and thrombocytopenia are rarely severe at presentation, but may become so following chemotherapy or with very advanced disease. The cytopenias may also be exaggerated by the increase in plasma volume that may accompany paraproteinaemia.

Plasma protein abnormalities

Paraproteins do not usually cause symptoms, but when in sufficient quantity they may cause *hyperviscosity* with lethargy, confusion, loss of vision and coma. This is particularly likely to occur with IgA paraproteins, since the IgA molecules have a tendency to polymerise, thus greatly increasing their intrinsic viscosity. Paraproteins may cause a haemorrhagic tendency mainly through non-specific coating and interference with platelet function. Some paraproteins are also cryoglobulins (p. 1101) and may give rise to Raynaud's phenomena.

More importantly, myeloma is accompanied by suppression of normal immunoglobulin production (*hypogammaglobulinaemia*) and infection is thus a major cause of morbidity and mortality. The mechanism of suppression of normal antibody production is obscure, but it is severe and usually persists even in patients whose paraprotein disappears on treatment.

Multifactorial

Renal dysfunction commonly occurs at presentation or with advancing disease. There are multiple causes, including light chain precipitation in the renal tubules and amyloid deposition in the glomeruli. Hypercalcaemia causes impaired glomerular function and a failure of renal tubular function, resulting in an inability to concentrate the urine. As a result, many patients are dehydrated at presentation; the prerenal element in the renal failure must be recognised and treated by salt and water replacement. Other causes of renal damage include hyperuricaemia with tubular deposition of urate, and myeloma infiltration of the kidney.

Myeloma deposits extruding from bone (particularly collapsed vertebrae) may cause cord compression or root

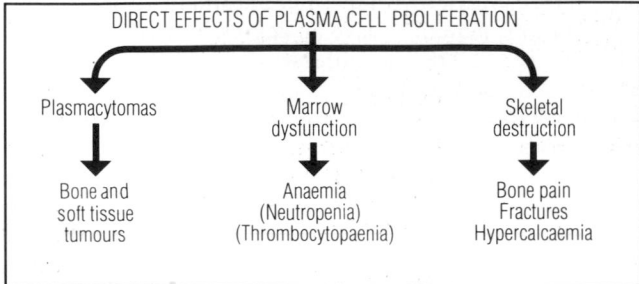
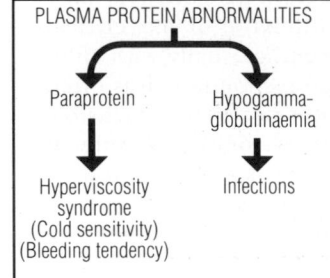
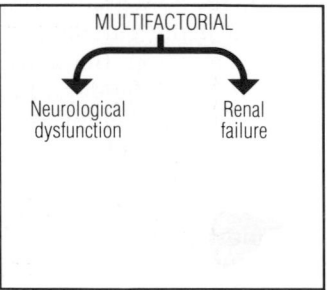

Fig. 24.33 Development of symptoms and signs in multiple myeloma.

lesions. Cranial nerve lesions due to compression occur rarely. Peripheral neuropathies may also arise as a non-metastatic manifestation of malignancy.

Investigation

Mild anaemia is common, leucopenia and thrombocytopenia less so unless as a result of treatment. Plasma cells are only rarely seen in the peripheral blood. If a paraprotein is present, rouleaux formation and a high ESR are usually found. Bone marrow examination usually shows a plasmacytosis (more than 10%), but the disease can be 'patchy' and the sample not fully representative. The plasma cells often have an abnormal appearance with a centrally placed nucleus, which is often binucleate or trinucleate. The total serum gammaglobulin level is usually increased due to the paraprotein, and the serum albumin often reduced. Plasma protein electrophoresis reveals a narrow monoclonal band in over 75% of cases (Fig. 24.34). The incidence of the different types of immunoglobulin production in myeloma is shown in Table 24.38). Light chains are rapidly metabolised and often do not give rise to a serum paraprotein. They can nearly always be detected by immunoelectrophoresis of the urine; free light chains can also be detected in the urine of many patients who have a paraprotein composed of intact immunoglobulin – so-called Bence-Jones proteinuria.

Serum β_2 microglobulin (a protein associated with class I HLA antigens) levels are usually raised and give an indication of the myeloma mass.

The investigation of the patient with suspected myeloma should also include a skeletal survey, and esti-

mation of urea, creatinine and electrolytes, calcium, phosphate and uric acid.

Diagnostic criteria

The three major diagnostic criteria for myeloma are:

- Bone marrow plasmacytosis (greater than 20%, but lower level acceptable if proven to be monoclonal).
- Lytic lesions on X-ray (severe osteoporosis is acceptable if marrow plasmacytosis is greater than 30%).
- Paraprotein in blood or urine.

At least two of these criteria should be present for a definitive diagnosis, as each feature alone can be due to other diseases (Table 24.39). Where there is doubt, it is often advisable to wait and reassess later.

Table 24.38 Approximate incidence of different types of immunoglobulin production in myeloma

Immunoglobulin	Incidence (%)
IgG	55 (IgG + urinary light chain in 35%)
IgA	20 (IgA + urinary light chain in 15%)
Light chain only	20
IgD	2
IgE	
IgM	very rare
Non-secretory	

Table 24.39 Differential diagnosis of myeloma

Symptom	Differential diagnosis

Paraproteinaemia	Benign monoclonal gammopathies
	Malignant lymphoproliferative disorders
	Reactive – Infections
	      Autoimmune disease
	      Liver disease
	      Non-lymphoid tumours

Bone marrow plasmacytosis	Chronic infections Chronic inflammatory disorders Liver disease Other tumours
Lytic lesions	Multiple metastases 'Spotty osteoporosis' Multiple eosinophilic granulomas Hyperparathyroidism Primary amyloid Hydatid disease Fibrous dysplasia

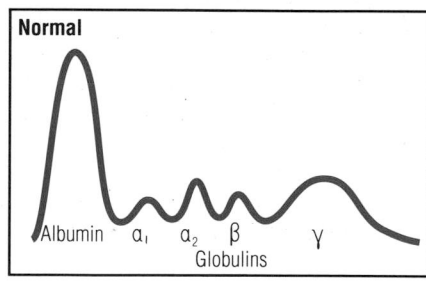
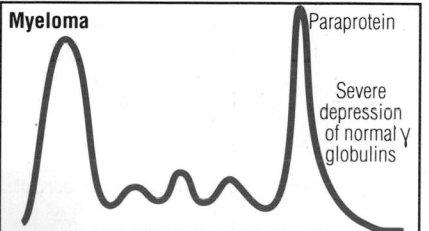

Fig. 24.34 Densitometry traces of serum protein electrophoresis from a normal individual and a patient with multiple myeloma.

Management

Most patients are symptomatic at presentation and merit immediate therapy. Occasionally, patients are asymptomatic and do not have advanced bone disease, a high level of paraprotein or organ dysfunction. Treatment can be delayed in these patients.

Supportive therapy

Immediate therapy is supportive. Pain must be controlled and, if there are fractures, this may require continuous infusion of opiates. Local radiotherapy is often strikingly effective in the relief of bone pain. Vertebral collapse and spinal pain must be treated promptly, as there is a risk of cord compression resulting in paraplegia. Radiotherapy is the treatment of choice. Careful attention must be paid to the fluid status; in patients with renal dysfunction or hypercalcaemia, a high fluid intake is essential. Prompt rehydration will often prevent permanent renal damage. In some patients with renal tubular damage, there is a chronic inability to conserve fluid, and the weight and standing and lying blood pressures must be carefully followed in these patients. Hypercalcaemia is treated in the usual way with fluids, loop diuretics and steroids (p. 734). Infections are common and must be treated vigorously. The hyperviscosity syndrome will respond temporarily to plasma exchange.

Specific therapy

Standard specific therapy for myeloma is with the alkylating agent melphalan, approximately 7 mg/m^2 daily for four days every three weeks, providing renal function is normal. Intermediate dose prednisone (60 mg/m^2 per day) is usually given in addition over the treatment days, but is of limited value in the absence of bone pain or hypercalcaemia. Approximately 50% of patients have a good initial response, with a decrease in myeloma mass and fall of paraprotein to a stable plateau level. Improved responses may be obtained with combination regimens containing doxorubicin (adriamycin) but these are more toxic. Disappearance of paraprotein with normalisation of the marrow is rare (5% of cases). In the plateau phase, therapy can be discontinued until progression occurs. Continuous α interferon may prolong the plateau phase. In patients who become resistant to melphalan, second line therapies are available; these include drugs such as anthracyclines, nitrosoureas, vinca alkaloids and very high-dose steroids. These regimens are less effective if these drugs have been used initially. The duration of response is usually short.

Very high-dose melphalan is sometimes used as initial therapy in younger patients, while cyclophosphamide, total body irradiation and allogeneic transplantation has been used in some patients under 45 years of age. Preliminary results with such approaches are encouraging, although very few patients are young enough to be considered for an allogeneic transplant.

Prognosis

The overall survival is poor, with a median survival of approximately two years (marginally better in younger patients), although occasional long-term survivors do occur. It is possible to categorise patients at diagnosis into good, intermediate and poor prognostic groups on the basis of the [Hb], urea (posthydration) and the performance status (Table 24.40). The β$_2$ microglobulin level is also a valuable prognostic indicator. Good prognosis patients have a two year survival of about 75%, and poor prognosis patients about 10%.

Plasmacytomas

Plasmacytomas are collections of plasma cells at a single site. They are usually part of a more generalised myeloma, but isolated tumours do occur without evidence of widespread disease. Many of the latter patients will go on to develop myeloma. Full dose radiotherapy should be given to solitary plasmacytomas, followed by chemotherapy if there is persistence of paraproteinaemia (usually only at low levels). Careful long-term follow-up is required.

Waldenstrom's macroglobulinaemia

This is a rare, low-grade, B cell malignancy presenting in the elderly as a lymphoma or chronic leukaemia. Biopsy of affected tissue shows a diffuse lymphocytic lymphoma with plasmacytoid differentiation. Similar cells are seen in the marrow and in the blood. The hallmark of this disease is the production of large quantities of IgM paraprotein leading to symptoms of hyperviscosity, haemorrhagic tendencies and cold sensitivity (cryoglobulins in 30%). Weight loss, lymphadenopathy and hepatosplenomegaly are all common, but lytic bone lesions and renal failure are rare (unlike the situation in myeloma).

Table 24.40 Prognostic categories in myeloma

Prognosis	Criteria
Good	Posthydration urea less than 8 mmol/l [Hb] greater than 10 g/dl No or few symptoms
Intermediate	Patient in neither good nor poor prognostic categories
Poor	Posthydration urea greater than 10 mmol/l and restricted activity; or [Hb] less than 7.5 g/dl and restricted activity

No therapy is necessary in asymptomatic patients, although they must be followed up carefully. When symptoms arise, therapy with alkylating agents such as chlorambucil will often produce a satisfactory response, though not a complete remission. Hyperviscosity syndrome may respond to plasmapheresis while the disease is being brought under control with chemotherapy. The median survival is about five years.

Cryoglobulinaemia

Cryoglobulins are immunoglobulins which precipitate when cooled. They may be monoclonal, polyclonal or mixed. The monoclonal cryoglobulins are usually indicative of a lymphoproliferative disease and the polyclonal varieties are often reactive and transient. A mixed monoclonal and polyclonal cryoglobulin is not infrequently associated with autoimmune disease. Clinically, their presence may give rise to Raynaud's phenomena, acrocyanosis, vascular purpura, arthralgia and – in the most severe cases – renal failure, hepatic failure and isolated neurological lesions.

The blood film typically shows marked agglutination of red cells, and the ESR may be spuriously low at room temperature although normal if performed at 37°C.

The mainstay of treatment is avoidance of cold and treatment of any underlying conditions such as a lymphoma. Plasmapheresis may have a role if there are severe symptoms.

Heavy chain disease

Heavy chain disease (HCD) refers to rare B cell proliferations in which there is secretion of heavy chains uncoupled to light chains. Serum electrophoresis usually shows hypogammaglobulinaemia without a clear monoclonal band. Immunoelectrophoresis is therefore required to demonstrate the abnormal heavy chain unassociated with light chain. Immunoelectrophoresis of the urine is often helpful.

Alpha-HCD occurs mainly in the Mediterranean countries, Asia and South America. It typically presents with abdominal pain, malabsorption and clubbing. Lymphadenopathy and hepatosplenomegaly are not usually present and (because of the malabsorption) coeliac disease is often suspected. In the early phases, the mucosa is infiltrated with polyclonal plasma cells and lymphocytes, and the disease is called immune proliferative disease of the small intestine. Later, a frankly invasive lymphoma develops. The production of α chains diminishes as the lymphoma progresses. The disease may respond to tetracycline in its early stages, but the established lymphoma is not very responsive to treatment.

Gamma-HCD mainly occurs in the elderly, and presents with weakness, fever, palatal oedema, lymph-adenopathy and hepatosplenomegaly. The marrow is usually infiltrated with lymphocytic cells, and pancytopenia is common. The course is variable but death occurs in most cases.

Mu-HCD is rare and is usually associated with typical chronic lymphocytic leukaemia in which the plasma contains μ heavy chains.

AMYLOIDOSIS

Amyloidosis is a generic term for a group of conditions in which there is waxy infiltration of the tissues, the amyloid infiltrate staining pink with haematoxylin and eosin stain, and green with Congo red. The amyloid material is birefringent and is composed of fibrils formed into β-pleated sheets. These infiltrates ultimately damage normal tissue by means of pressure, atrophy and hypoxia.

Classification

The amyloidoses are best classified on an aetiological basis. The amyloid associated with immunoglobulin-producing tumours includes what was formerly known as *primary amyloid*, as well as that associated with myeloma. The primary amyloid is best thought of as early myeloma without lytic bone lesions. A monoclonal band on serum electrophoresis is present at diagnosis or appears during the course of the disease in nearly all cases. The amyloid deposits in this type of amyloidosis are made up of intact immunoglobulin light chains or parts of the variable domains; it is clear that certain myeloma proteins are more amyloidogenic than others. In reactive systemic amyloidoses – which typically occur in association with chronic infections (e.g. bronchiectasis), chronic inflammatory disorders (e.g. rheumatoid arthritis) or neoplastic disorders – it is thought that the amyloid is primarily composed of an acute phase protein called amyloid A protein.

The heredofamilial amyloidoses include familial Mediterranean fever and Portuguese nephropathy. The amyloid seen around some endocrine tumours is thought to be composed of hormone precursors. Finally, amyloid occurs in many tissues in the elderly, especially brain and heart. It is usually asymptomatic.

Summary 12 Aetiological classification of amyloidosis

- Amyloid associated with immunoglobulin-producing tumours
- Reactive systemic amyloidosis
- Heredofamilial amyloidosis
- Local amyloid associated with endocrine tumours
- Amyloid of ageing

Table 24.41 Clinical features suggestive of amyloidosis

- Nephrotic syndrome and renal failure
- Peripheral neuropathy with or without a carpal tunnel syndrome
- Restrictive cardiomyopathy
- Malabsorption and protein losing enteropathy
- Polyarthropathy
- Skin nodules, infiltrates and periorbital purpura
- Macroglossia

Clinical features

Amyloid can cause diverse organ dysfunction but the features shown in Table 24.41 should always raise the possibility of amyloidosis. It appears that renal amyloid is more prominent in the reactive amyloidoses, with cardiac and gut amyloid predominating in those associated with immunoglobulin-producing tumours; but the overlap is wide.

Diagnosis

The diagnosis is made by histological inspection of infiltrated tissues. Where tissue is not readily accessible, a renal or rectal biopsy often gives the diagnosis. Appropriate tests should also be performed to exclude myeloma, even when the patient has another chronic disorder.

Management and prognosis

This is primarily supportive, with specific treatment of any underlying disease. Care should be taken with the administration of diuretics or digitalis, as these can precipitate severe hypotension or dysrhythmias respectively.

The median survival of patients with myeloma and amyloid is probably less than two years, but is nearly 10 years with the reactive systemic amyloidoses.

NORMAL HAEMOSTASIS

The haemostatic processes involve a complex sequence of interacting events which serve both to protect the integrity of the vascular system and to re-establish patency of small segments which become occluded (Fig. 24.35). There is initial vasoconstriction at the site of injury, but this is transient and not a major component of the haemostatic mechanism. The major component of haemostasis is the formation of a platelet plug followed by the laying down and cross-binding of fibrin.

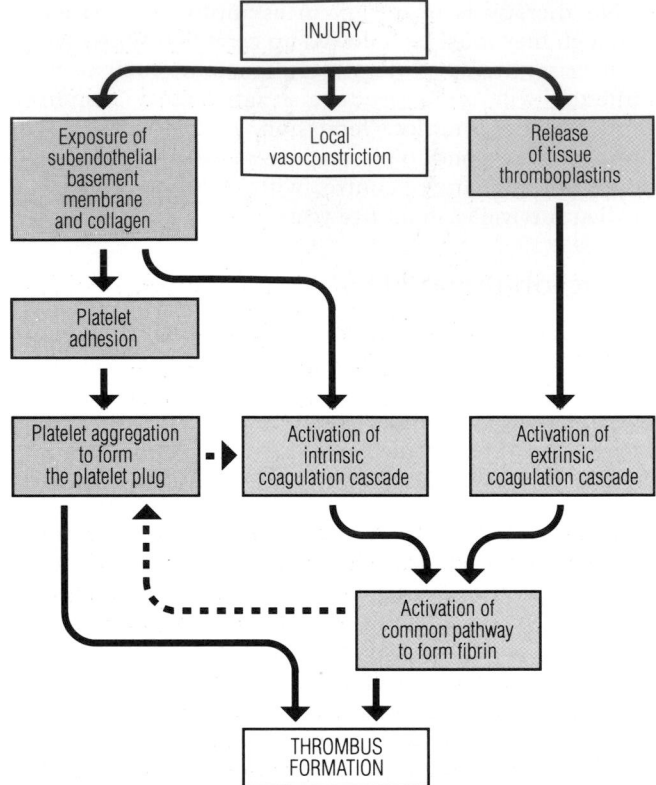

Fig. 24.35 The mechanisms of haemostasis. The process of platelet aggregation and activation is shown in grey; and the formation of fibrin in red.

Platelets

Injury exposes collagen and the subendothelial basement membranes. Circulating platelets adhere to these structures, aided by fibronectin and high molecular weight multimers of factor VIII complex (factor VIII/von Willebrand factor = fVIIIvWF, p. 1104) which coat the surface of the platelets. Following the adhesion of a single layer of platelets to the damaged vascular endothelium, further platelets stick to one another, aggregate, become activated, and ultimately form a platelet plug. The aggregation is mediated via a large range of factors which are produced at the site of injury and react with receptors on the platelet surface. Many of these factors – such as ADP, serotonin and thromboxane A_2 – are themselves released by activated platelets (Fig. 24.36), producing a positive feedback loop. ADP is also released from damaged red cells at the site of injury. Thrombin is a potent aggregatory agent, so the activation of the common pathway in the coagulation cascade (p. 1104) further stimulates the formation of a platelet plug.

The process of platelet aggregation and activation is mediated by at least two separate biochemical pathways.

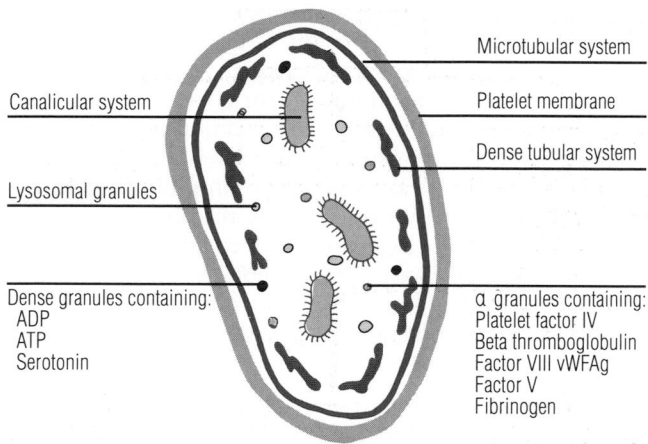

Fig. 24.36 Diagrammatic cross-sectional view of a platelet.

- Ligands such as ADP, or collagen in low doses, bind to specific receptors. This leads to activation of membrane phospholipases with the release of arachidonic acid from the platelet membrane phospholipids. A proportion of arachidonic acid is then converted to the cyclic endoperoxides, and then to thromboxane A_2 (TXA_2). TXA_2 is biologically highly active, and mediates a rise in intracellular $[Ca^{2+}]$ and platelet granule release (Fig. 24.37) which promotes further platelet aggregation.
- Thrombin and high doses of collagen bring about a rise in intracellular $[Ca^{2+}]$ and degranulation by a mechanism distinct from that of arachidonic acid metabolism and TXA_2 generation.

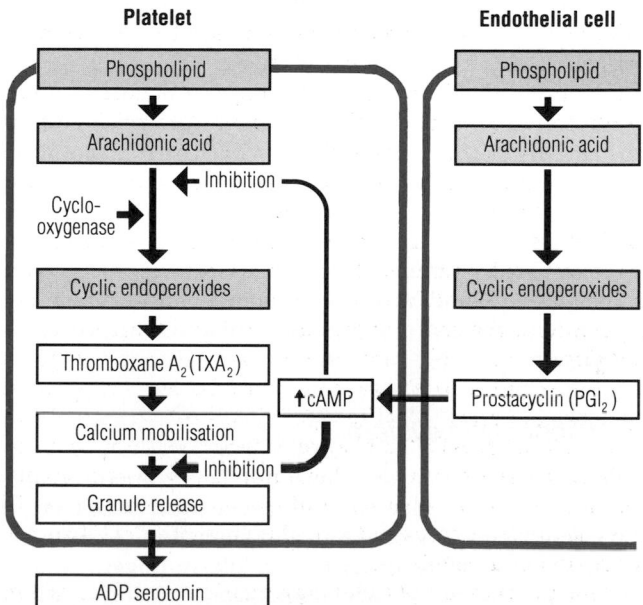

Fig. 24.37 Arachidonic acid metabolism in platelets and endothelial cells.

Platelet activation and aggregation also has a role in the coagulation cascade that becomes activated at the site of injury. Factors VIIIvWF, V and fibrinogen are stored in granules and are released on activation; but more importantly, the platelet undergoes a configurational change during the activation process, such that phospholipid micelles on the platelet surface become available to facilitate the action of factors VIII and V. Activated platelets may also actually trigger the coagulation cascade by directly activating factors IX and X.

The coagulation cascade

This is conventionally divided into intrinsic and extrinsic pathways, converging on a common pathway, but this is an oversimplification although useful in practice.

Intrinsic coagulation cascade

Exposure of negatively charged endothelial surfaces following injury or damage leads to the adsorption of both factor XII and high molecular weight kininogen (Fig. 24.38). Prekallikrein and factor XI then bind to the

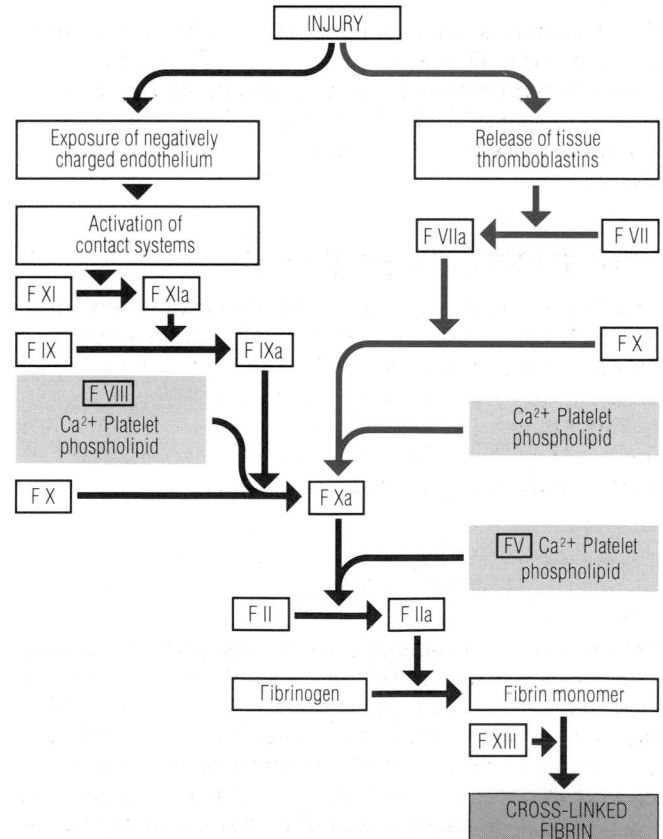

Fig. 24.38 The coagulation cascade. The extrinsic pathway is shown in red.

high molecular weight kininogen, with activation of factor XI by factor XII. There follows a series of amplification reactions, during which an inert precursor is converted to an active serine protease with ultimate formation of fibrin. Factor XI activates factor IX which in turn activates factor X at the site of tissue injury. This reaction requires calcium ions, a platelet or phospholipid surface and factor VIII as a cofactor.

The factor VIII molecule is a complex structure. The component with procoagulant activity is referred to as factor VIIIC (antibodies to this moiety detect factor VIIICAg). Factor VIIIC has a molecular weight of approximately 220 000 and is synthesised in the spleen, other parts of the RE system, and the kidney. The factor VIIIC moiety then binds to factor VIIIvWF (Fig. 24.39). This is synthesised in vascular endothelial cells and (to a much lesser extent) in megakaryocytes. The VIIIvWF protein consists of subunits with a molecular weight of 200 000–240 000 (detected immunologically as factor VIIIvWFAg, previously called factor VIII related antigen (factor VIIIRag)). The subunits polymerise to form multimers of varying size. These are required for functional activity, both to prolong the half-life of factor VIIIC and to participate in platelet adhesion to the damaged vessel wall. Ristocetin-induced platelet aggregation is dependent on the high molecular weight factor VIII multimers, and this test is therefore used to measure factor VIIIvWF (also known as ristocetin cofactor VIII-RiCoF).

Extrinsic coagulation cascade

Trauma produces release of tissue thromboplastins. These bind to and activate factor VII, which then cleaves factor X to produce factor Xa. As with the intrinsic system, this reaction requires calcium ions and phospholipid.

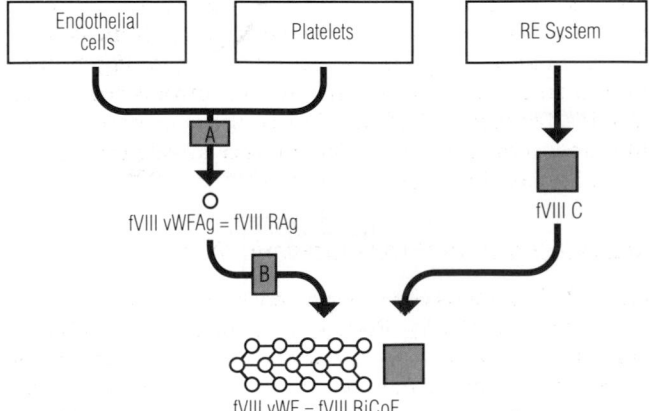

Fig. 24.39 Schematic representation of the production and structure of factor VIII. A and B refer to blocks in formation of fVIIIvWFAg which give rise to different types of von Willebrand's disease (see p. 1112).

The common pathway

Factor Xa, generated via the extrinsic and intrinsic cascades, converts prothrombin (factor II) to the serine protease thrombin (factor IIa). The reaction again requires calcium ions and phospholipid, and is accelerated by factor V which serves as a cofactor. Thrombin then digests fibrinogen to form fibrin, which is readily converted to fibrin polymers. The digestion of fibrin (and fibrinogen) is associated with release of fibrinopeptides (fibrin degradation products). The loose fibrin polymer is stabilised by a cross-linking reaction employing factor XIII as a catalyst.

Haemostatic inhibitory systems

A complex system of physiological inhibitors and feedback control mechanisms exists to control and limit excessive or inappropriate activation of the haemostatic system and thus help maintain vascular patency.

Endothelial cell inhibitors

Vascular endothelial cells synthesise prostacyclin from arachidonic acid (Fig. 24.37). Prostacyclin causes vasodilation and potent inhibition of platelet adhesion and aggregation. It is released in increased quantities when the vessel wall is stressed or injured, and binds locally to specific platelet membrane receptors which mediate activation of adenylate cyclase and a consequent rise in cyclic-AMP. This blocks aggregation through inhibition of platelet arachidonic acid metabolism and calcium flux. Endothelial cells also synthesise plasminogen activator, and a heparin-like anticoagulant.

Coagulation inhibitors

A natural system of coagulation inhibitors exists to limit the activity of the coagulation cascade. Antithrombin III is the major inhibitor of thrombin (factor IIa) and also inhibits factors IXa, Xa and XIa. Other plasma thrombin inhibitors include α_2-macroglobulin and α_2-antitrypsin. Protein C is a vitamin K dependent protein which inactivates factors V and VIII; and protein S – also a vitamin K dependent protein – serves as a cofactor for protein C activity.

The fibrinolytic system

The fibrinolytic system is activated simultaneously with the intrinsic coagulation system via the contact factor system of factor XII kallikrein and kinin (Fig. 24.40). The inactive circulating pro-enzyme, plasminogen, is converted to the active serine protease plasmin, which hydrolyses fibrin into soluble fibrin degradation products and also inactivates factors V and VIII.

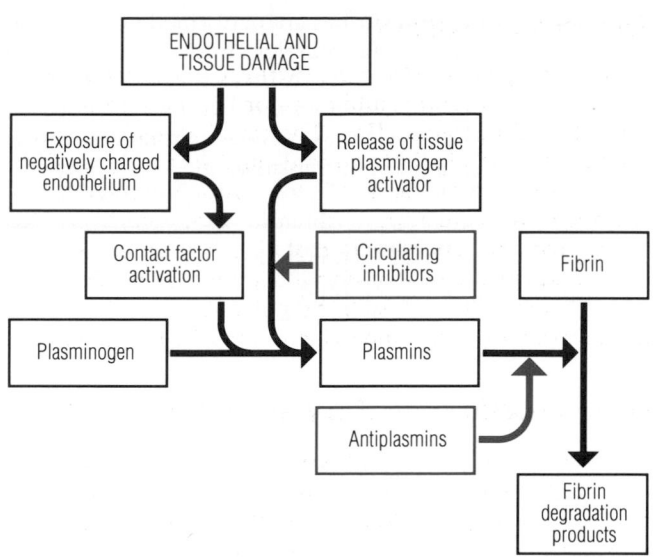

Fig. 24.40 The fibrinolytic system.

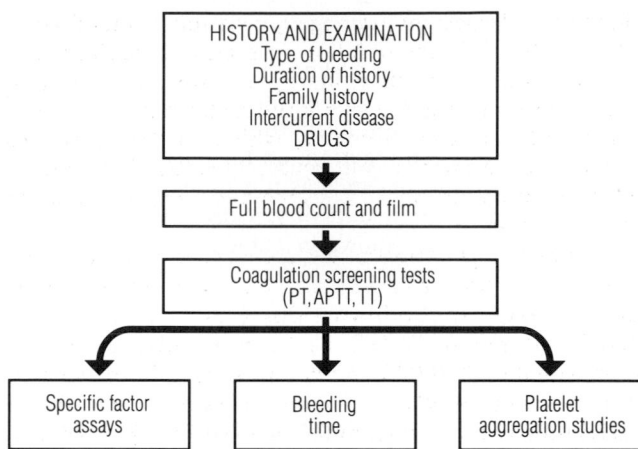

Fig. 24.41 Approach to investigation of a patient with a bleeding disorder.

Plasminogen can also be activated by tissue plasminogen activator (tPA) released from endothelial cells and from traumatised tissues. Several factors ensure that plasminogen conversion to plasmin is largely restricted to the site of trauma and thrombus formation.

- Tissue plasminogen activators are inactivated by circulating inhibitors and are also degraded in the liver.
- The affinity of tPA for plasminogen is greatly increased when the tPA is bound to a fibrin complex.
- Any circulating plasmin is rapidly bound to α_2-antiplasmin, which has far less affinity for plasmin bound to fibrin.

DIAGNOSIS OF DISORDERED HAEMOSTASIS

History and examination

A detailed history and examination is of paramount importance and will often indicate the cause of bleeding (Fig. 24.41). Firstly, it must be determined whether bleeding is a localised problem, such as a gastric ulcer, or a generalised bleeding tendency (although it must be remembered that minor defects in haemostasis may only be brought to light by specific injuries). Secondly, the type of bleeding should be ascertained: purpura and mucosal bleeding usually suggest a platelet disorder, whilst confluent skin bruises and haemarthroses are more indicative of coagulation disorders. The length of the bleeding history and the age at onset must be noted and a family history taken. It is often informative to ask specific

questions, e.g. 'has any member of the family had excessive bleeding after dental extractions?'. Attention must be paid to any previous medical history of the current illness. A detailed drug history is essential.

Screening tests

A full blood count and blood film will detect anaemia and thrombocytopenia (the commonest platelet defect), and platelet morphology should be noted. Occasionally, the blood film also reveals the cause of bleeding, such as DIC or acute leukaemia. The coagulation screening tests – the prothrombin time (PT), activated partial thromboplastin time (APTT) and the thrombin time (TT) are then performed.

Prothrombin time

The PT examines the extrinsic and common pathways. Citrated plasma is recalcified, excess tissue thromboplastin is added, and time to clot formation measured. The normal range is 10–14 seconds and prolongation of more than two seconds compared to control is suggestive of defective factors VII, X, V or II or the presence of an inhibitor to these factors. The PT is relatively insensitive to the level of fibrinogen.

Activated partial thromboplastin time

The APTT screens the intrinsic coagulation cascade and the common pathway. Platelet-poor plasma is incubated with kaolin to provide *contact activation* in the presence of added phospholipid, and the clotting time after recalcification is noted. The normal range is approximately 38–45 seconds but this varies between laboratories. An abnormal result indicates deficiencies or inhibitors to one or more of factors XII, XI, IX, VIII, X, V, II or I (i.e. not factor VII).

Thrombin time

The TT is performed by adding thrombin to plasma, thus bypassing the extrinsic and intrinsic systems, and measuring the time to clot formation. It is a measure of thrombin-fibrinogen reaction, and is particularly useful for detecting inhibitors such as fibrin degradation products or heparin. The results of screening tests in several clinical conditions are shown in Table 24.42.

Further tests

Where an abnormality is detected in the intrinsic or extrinsic coagulation cascade, the test is repeated using a 50/50 mixture of the patient's plasma and normal plasma. If this corrects the test, there is a deficiency in one or more of the factors assayed by the test. If full correction does not occur, then this implies the presence of a coagulation inhibitor.

Specific factors can be measured functionally by the use of mixtures of the patient's serum with serum known to be deficient in a single factor. Thus, if a prolonged APTT is obtained which is corrected by normal plasma but not by plasma from a patient with factor IX deficiency, then this implies that the patient is also deficient in factor IX. Some factors can also be measured immunologically, and the measurement of factor VIIIvWFAg is often of value in differentiating between haemophilia and von Willebrand's disease. The functional activity of factor VIIIvWF is determined by ristocetin platelet aggregation studies.

When a bleeding disorder is strongly suspected and the platelet count and clotting screen are normal, a template bleeding time should be done; if prolonged (normal bleeding time is less than 10 minutes), this is indicative of a vessel wall or platelet defect. The latter includes von Willebrand's disease in which the platelet/vessel wall interaction is defective; the bleeding time may be abnormal in mild von Willebrand's disease when the APTT is within the normal range.

Platelet aggregation studies are performed both to help detect the rare congenital platelet abnormalities and to determine the level of fVIIIvWF (ristocetin cofactor). Platelet aggregation is based on the fact that platelet-rich plasma is turbid but clears as platelets aggregate; this is measured by increased light transmission.

PLATELET DISORDERS I: THROMBOCYTOPENIA

Thrombocytopenia is the commonest disorder of platelets and may be due to either decreased production or increased destruction (Table 24.43). The two mechanisms can usually be differentiated by bone marrow examination: megakaryocyte numbers are decreased in production thrombocytopenias, and increased where there is excessive platelet destruction. In some circumstances (e.g. severe infection), both mechanisms may be operative.

PRODUCTION THROMBOCYTOPENIAS

Production thrombocytopenias may be congenital or acquired. There are a number of rare congenital disorders in which thrombocytopenia occurs, or where there are normal numbers of qualitatively defective platelets. Several of these rare disorders have a storage pool defect such that there are defective platelet nucleotide stores

Table 24.42 Results of coagulation screening tests in different clinical conditions (N = normal)

Clinical condition	Platelet count	PT	APPT	TT
Haemophilia A	N	N	↑	N
Von Willebrand's disease	N	N	↑	N
Factor VII deficiency	N	↑	N	N
Liver disease	N or ↓	↑	↑	N or ↑
Disseminated intravascular coagulation	↓	↑	↑	↑↑
Warfarin	N	↑	↑	N
Heparin	N	↑	↑	↑

Table 24.43 Causes of thrombocytopenia

Decreased production of platelets

Congenital

Acquired
   Marrow hypoplasia
   Marrow replacement
   Megaloblastic anaemia
   Specific platelet suppression by drugs
   Occasional viral infections

Increased destruction of platelets

Immune thrombocytopenia
   Idiopathic
   Viral infections (including HIV)
   Associated with drugs
   Isoimmune neonatal thrombocytopenia
   Post-transfusion purpura

Microangiopathic platelet destruction
   Disseminated intravascular coagulation
   Haemolytic uraemic syndrome
   Thrombotic thrombocytopenic purpura

Severe sepsis

Massive transfusions

resulting in defective aggregation at sites of vascular injury. In vitro, this is manifest as loss of the secondary aggregation wave to ADP.

The acquired production thrombocytopenias may be due to:

- generalised marrow hypoproduction as in aplastic anaemia
- megaloblastic anaemia
- less commonly, a megakaryocyte-specific suppression. This may occur with chronic alcohol ingestion and (rarely) with some drugs such as the thiazide diuretics.

INCREASED PLATELET DESTRUCTION I: IMMUNE THROMBOCYTOPENIC PURPURA

The commonest cause of thrombocytopenia is immune destruction. In many children, immune thrombocytopenic purpura (ITP) follows a recent viral infection, while in some adults there is an underlying predisposing cause, such as a collagen vascular disease or a lymphoproliferative disorder. In many cases, however, they are idiopathic. Whatever the aetiology, the mechanism of platelet destruction is similar, namely opsonisation of platelets by platelet-specific autoantibodies, leading to phagocytosis of the platelets by the RE system. It should be noted that it is not possible to identify platelet-associated antibodies in every case. This may reflect lack of sensitivity of the test used, but should always alert one to alternative diagnoses.

Clinical and laboratory features

The peak incidence in childhood is between the ages of two and five years, at a time when children are most at risk for the common exanthemata. In both children and adults there is sudden onset of purpura, easy bruising and frequently also epistaxis. Gastrointestinal bleeding occurs occasionally, but clinically significant intracerebral bleeding is rare. Fatalities in children are extremely unusual even with very low platelet counts. The exception is babies born to mothers with ITP, who become affected owing to transplacental passage of antibody. If severely affected, such babies are at risk, during delivery and in the early neonatal period, of cerebral haemorrhage and even death.

The haemoglobin and white cell count are usually normal, although atypical lymphocytes may be seen on the blood film if there has been a recent viral infection. Very occasionally, the haemoglobin is reduced either due to blood loss or concomitant immune haemolysis. The platelet count is variably reduced, but in the presence of purpura is usually less than 50×10^9/l. Some of the platelets may appear large.

Management

Childhood

ITP in childhood is usually self-limiting, and treatment is rarely necessary even with a very low platelet count. Occasionally, bleeding may be troublesome and prednisone should be given (approximately 1 mg/kg and reduced as quickly as possible). Rarely, the disease becomes chronic and splenectomy may be considered; this is seldom justifiable, however, as the benefits must be balanced against the operative risks and problems of post-splenectomy infection. It must be remembered that late spontaneous remissions in children do occur.

Adults

In adults, it is usual to give a trial of oral corticosteroids if the platelet count is very low. High dose i.v. methylprednisolone may produce a more rapid response. The response is often suboptimal or the dose of steroids necessary is high with unacceptable side-effects. Splenectomy is then beneficial in 50–75% of cases. This may reduce antibody levels and, more importantly, removes a major site of RE platelet destruction. In splenectomy-resistant patients, immunosuppression with azathioprine, cyclophosphamide or chlorambucil may be of value. Vinca alkaloids may also be effective. Temporary respite can often be achieved by intravenous infusion of large doses of immunoglobulin preparations, which result in RE blockade. This is extremely expensive, but may be warranted in a life-threatening situation. In Rh-positive individuals, an injection of anti-D immunoglobulin will often produce similar RE blockade; unfortunately, anti-D is in short supply.

At birth

The neonate born to a mother with ITP merits further consideration. The neonate is usually only severely affected if the mother has severe ITP but this is not invariable. Particular attention must be paid to women with ITP who have had a successful splenectomy; their platelet count may be normal but their babies severely affected. If the mother has a low platelet count, a course of steroids or intravenous immunoglobulin should probably be given several days before delivery (if this can be anticipated). The birth should be as atraumatic as possible, and protracted labours must be avoided. At birth, the baby's platelet count must be checked and monitored daily for several days, as late falls are not infrequent. If the thrombocytopenia is very severe in the neonate, it is probably wise to give a short course of steroids and to minimise bouts of crying (which increase intracerebral pressure). Some centres would consider exchange transfusion to reduce the antibody titre.

Drug-induced immune thrombocytopenia

Drugs may induce immune thrombocytopenia by serving as haptens, with subsequent absorption of immune complexes onto the platelets. Quinidine may produce thrombocytopenia by this mechanism. Alternatively, the drug may interact with a platelet protein, with the production of specific drug-platelet protein antibody. When drug-induced thrombocytopenia occurs, it is usually reversible within several days of stopping the offending drug.

Isoimmune neonatal thrombocytopenia

The mechanism of isoimmune neonatal thrombocytopenia is similar to that of isoimmune neonatal haemolysis and usually occurs when the mother (but not the baby) lacks the platelet A1 antigen present in 98% of the population. Treatment of the infant is usually not necessary, but in extreme situations maternal (PLA-1 negative) platelets should be given. Intrauterine transfusion should be considered where a previously affected fetus died in utero.

Post-transfusion purpura

This is an unusual cause of thrombocytopenia which occurs in PLA-1-negative individuals about one week after a transfusion of blood containing PLA-1 positive platelets. The antibodies formed to the PLA-1 antigen bind to autologous platelets, probably as preformed immune complexes, and cause thrombocytopenia.

INCREASED PLATELET DESTRUCTION II: MICROANGIOPATHIC DESTRUCTION

Microangiopathic platelet destruction occurs in the presence of extensive small vessel disease. As blood passes through the damaged vessels, the platelets are removed and the red cells subjected to extreme shearing stresses, resulting in a concomitant haemolytic anaemia. Thus, the blood film typically shows red cell fragmentation and polychromasia (reticulocytosis), as well as thrombocytopenia.

Haemolytic uraemic syndrome/ thrombotic thrombocytopenic purpura

Haemolytic uraemic syndrome (HUS) and thrombotic thrombocytopenic purpura (TTP) are related syndromes whose aetiology is poorly understood. In many cases, there appears to be breakdown in the normal platelet/ vessel wall interaction, with excessive adhesion of platelets to intact endothelium.

Clinical features

HUS usually presents in young children with the triad of haemolytic anaemia, purpura and acute renal failure. TTP occurs predominantly in young adults (18–40 years). There is haemolytic anaemia, purpura, hepatic damage and neurological impairment which, in the acute form, may cause clouding of consciousness and coma. Digital ischaemia and small vessel infarcts may occur. Renal function is initially well preserved. TTP may also become chronic or undergo multiple relapses.

The mortality in HUS with good supportive care is below 10%, and in TTP about 10–25%.

Laboratory features

In the appropriate clinical setting, the finding of a microangiopathic blood film is highly suggestive of the diagnosis. At least in the early stages, the clotting screen is virtually normal, thus differentiating this cause of thrombocytopenia from disseminated intravascular coagulation (DIC). The hydroxybutyrate dehydrogenase level (HBD) is raised as a component of the haemolysis and this parameter is often valuable in assessing daily progress.

Management

Vigorous medical support for organ failure is paramount. Early dialysis in HUS is indicated. Large quantities of fresh frozen plasma appear to be beneficial in many cases and this usually requires daily plasma exchange. The mechanism of action is unclear. A short course of steroids is recommended in TTP.

Disseminated intravascular coagulation

In DIC there is widespread deposition of fibrin and platelets within the microcirculation with consumption of coagulation factors and platelets (Fig. 24.42). The presence of fibrin degradation products exacerbates the

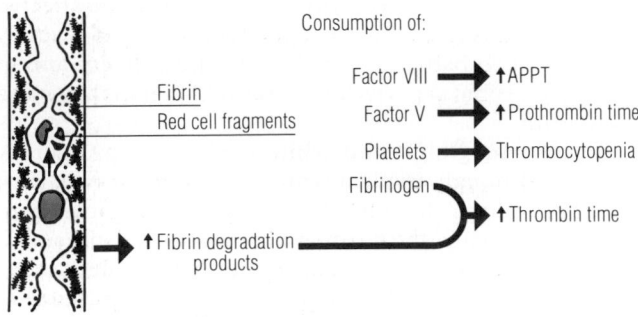

Fig. 24.42 The pathogenesis of disseminated intravascular coagulation.

bleeding tendency, by inhibiting the polymerisation of fibrin.

Clinical features

The causes of DIC are varied (Table 24.44) but sepsis is the most common cause. Precipitating factors include the release of procoagulant materials from damaged leukocytes and endothelial cells, and widespread activation of the contact factor system. In severe cases, there is widespread bruising and oozing from mucous membranes and venepuncture sites; but DIC is more often subclinical and merely a laboratory finding. Although small vessel occlusions do occur, clinically apparent thromboses are not commonly detected.

Laboratory features

Thrombocytopenia and a normocytic anaemia with red cell fragmentation are seen, although the latter may not be noticed in mild cases. There is prolongation of the PT, APPT and TT, the last being most affected, especially in mild cases. Fibrin degradation products (FDPs), produced by the proteolytic action of plasma on fibrin and fibrinogen, are found in raised amounts in the serum, although it must be remembered that serum FDPs are also raised after major trauma or surgery and in renal failure without DIC. The measurement of FDPs is therefore not the primary screening test for DIC and is only indicated if the TT is significantly prolonged.

Table 24.44 Causes of disseminated intravascular coagulation

Sepsis

Gram-negative septicaemia
Meningococcal septicaemia

Shock

Hypovolaemia
Anaphylactic

Obstetric complications

Amniotic fluid embolism
Intrauterine death
Abruptio placentae

Tissue factor release

Severe trauma
Burns
Promyelocytic leukaemia
Haemolytic transfusion reactions
Acute pancreatitis

Management

The underlying cause of DIC should be treated vigorously, and full supportive measures given. Hypoxia and hypovolaemia must be corrected, and platelets and clotting factors replaced as necessary; this usually requires both fresh frozen plasma and factor VIII concentrates. Although there was a vogue at one time for the use of heparin in DIC, to try and break the vicious cycle of thrombosis and haemorrhage, such treatment is dangerous and now has few advocates. Low-dose heparin

Table 24.45 Congenital primary platelet disorders

Syndrome	Inheritance	Platelet count	Platelet aggregation	Other features
Fanconi's anaemia	Autosomal recessive	↓	Normal	Multiple skeletal/organ abnormalities (p. 1056)
Amegakaryocytic thrombocytopenia	Variable	↓	Normal	Absent radii and skeletal abnormalities in some cases
Wiskott-Aldrich syndrome	X-linked	↓	Reduction in secondary aggregation wave (storage pool defect)	Eczema Immunodeficiency
May-Hegglin syndrome	Autosomal dominant	↓ (variable) Giant size	Normal	Inclusion bodies in leucocytes
Bernard-Soulier syndrome	Autosomal recessive	Normal or ↓ Giant size	↓ aggregation to ristocetin	
Glanzmann's thrombasthenia	Autosomal recessive	Normal	↓ aggregation to ADP, adrenaline and collagen. Normal aggregation to ristocetin	
Grey platelet syndrome		Slightly ↓		Myelofibrosis may occur
Chediak-Higashi syndrome	Autosomal recessive	Normal	Reduction in secondary aggregation wave to ADP (storage pool defect)	Oculocutaneous albinism, phagocytic defect Neurological impairment
Hermansky-Pudlak syndrome	Autosomal recessive	Normal	Reduction in secondary aggregation wave to ADP (storage pool defect)	Albinism

may have a role, however, in the prevention of DIC during induction therapy for acute promyelocytic leukaemia.

Other causes of microangiopathic thrombocytopenia

Microangiopathic haemolytic anaemia and/or thrombocytopenia may also occur in malignant hypertension, pre-eclampsia and in association with giant haemangiomas.

QUALITATIVE PLATELET ABNORMALITIES

There are several rare congenital disorders in which platelet function is abnormal (Table 24.45) as well as the more common von Willebrand's disease.

Qualitative platelet abnormalities may also be acquired in a variety of systemic disorders (particularly uraemia and liver disease), and the platelet defect may contribute to any bleeding diathesis in these conditions. Platelet function may also be abnormal in the myeloproliferative diseases due to both the production of abnormal platelets from a malignant stem cell, and to a poorly understood failure to produce normal high molecular weight multimers of factor VIII. Platelets may also function poorly in the presence of paraproteinaemia due to non-specific protein coating of the platelets.

The commonest acquired platelet abnormality, however, is due to the ingestion of aspirin and other antiplatelet drugs (p. 1115).

PLATELET DISORDERS II: THROMBOCYTOSIS

The myeloproliferative disorders may give rise to very elevated platelet counts, especially in essential thrombocythaemia. If the platelet count is only moderately raised, it may be difficult to differentiate primary from secondary causes (p. 1086). The platelet count rarely exceeds $1500 \times 10^9/l$ in secondary thrombocytosis, but may do so following splenectomy. Here, the platelet count rises within hours or days and usually falls to the high normal range in the ensuing weeks, although the thrombocytosis is occasionally persistent. The thrombocytosis postsplenectomy is accompanied by a modest leukocytosis (usually transient) and the permanent appearance of abnormal shaped red cells, spherocytes, target cells and Howell-Jolly bodies. Probably the commonest cause of secondary thrombocytosis is in response to the stress of major surgery. Other forms of stress such as exercise may also cause the platelet count to rise. Both bleeding and haemolysis may stimulate a thrombocytosis, and this may be more marked if there is concomitant iron deficiency.

Summary 13 Aetiology of thrombocytosis

Primary

Myeloproliferative disorders

Secondary

Postsplenectomy
Bleeding or haemolysis
Postoperative period
Following extreme exercise
Inflammatory states
Collagen vascular diseases
Malignant neoplasms
Vinca alkaloid drugs

This may imply that the physiological stimuli for increased red cell production cross-react with megakaryopoiesis, but the detailed mechanisms are not understood. All forms of inflammation can cause a rise in the platelet count, but it appears to be particularly common in the inflammatory bowel disorders and in sarcoidosis. The neoplasms most often associated with thrombocytosis are lymphomas and gut carcinoma.

Clinical features

Patients with primary thrombocytosis may present with bleeding or thrombotic problems (p. 1085). Thrombotic phenomena attributable to a secondary thrombocytosis are unusual, and rarely require treatment. In patients with thrombocytosis in whom thrombotic events have occurred, treatment with antiplatelet agents is advisable.

HEREDITARY COAGULATION DISORDERS

HAEMOPHILIA A

Haemophilia A (classical haemophilia) is an X-linked recessive disorder which affects males and is transmitted by female carriers. The incidence in the UK is approximately 12 per 100 000. There is low or absent factor VIIIC but factor VIIIvWFAg and factor VIIIvWF activity are normal (p. 1104).

Clinical features

The clinical severity of haemophilia A is very variable and is dependent on the level of factor VIIIC (Table 24.46). In the absence of trauma or surgery in the first few months of life, the disease does not usually present until the child starts to crawl or walk. In mild cases the diagnosis may be further delayed. There is easy bruising, soft

Table 24.46 Severity of haemophilia A

Clinical manifestations	Factor VIIIC levels (% of normal)
Severe	less than 1%
Moderate	1–5%
Mild	over 5%

tissue muscle bleeding and haemarthrosis often appearing spontaneously and not related to obvious trauma. The repeated joint bleeds may lead ultimately to restriction of movement and deformity. Less commonly, there is retroperitoneal haemorrhage, spontaneous haematuria and pseudotumour formation in the long bones or pelvis, secondary to recurrent subperiosteal haemorrhage and new bone formation. Severe psychological and family problems may also arise as a result of the chronic disease and its treatment.

Diagnosis

The diagnosis is suspected from the history and the finding of a prolonged APTT, and proven by demonstration of a low factor VIIIC level in a specific assay.

Assessment of the ratio of factor VIIIC:VIIIvWFAg can be used in about 80% of cases to identify female carriers. Daughters of haemophiliacs are of course obligate carriers (p. 72). Prenatal diagnosis is available for male fetuses of known carriers by analysis of factor VIIIC levels in the fetal blood or by analysis of DNA from chorionic villus samples.

Management

Bleeding episodes require prompt treatment by factor VIII replacement. Approximately 0.5 units are required per kg body weight to raise the factor VIII level by 1%. Thus, if a level of 100% is required in a severe 70 kg haemophiliac, then a dose of approximately 3500 units should be given. The injections are repeated to maintain a trough level above 20% for minor bleeds, and above 60% for major trauma or surgery. The half-life of injected factor VIII is approximately 12 hours and so it is usual to give twice-daily factor VIII during an acute episode. The dose and frequency of administration can be modified according to pre- and postinjection factor VIIIC levels. Some patients keep a stock of factor VIII at home and will inject themselves at the first sign of a bleed, thereby often averting a severe problem. In very severe cases, prophylactic factor VIII injected by the patient at home twice a week may markedly reduce the frequency of haemorrhagic incidents.

Bleeding episodes (especially into joints) are very painful and adequate analgesia must be given, often with opiates. During acute bleeds, rest is required followed by

Summary 14 Management of haemophilia A

Treatment
Factor VIII replacement
Pain relief
Rest
Oral antifibrinolytics (e.g. tranexamic acid)
DDAVP

Complications
Development of inhibitory antibodies
Transmission of viral infection, e.g. HIV
Psychological trauma

gradual mobilisation. The optimal management of haemophilia requires a team approach, with interested haematologists, physiotherapists and orthopaedic surgeons working together to minimise permanent joint damage.

Oral antifibrinolytics (e.g. tranexamic acid) may aid haemostasis, and are particularly useful in mild haemophiliacs after dental procedures. For minor procedures in very mild haemophiliacs, DDAVP (1-deamino-8-D-arginine vasopressin) may circumvent the need for factor VIII, as it may lead to a temporary rise in autologous factor VIII production.

Complications of therapy

Inhibitory antibodies develop in some severe haemophiliacs after factor VIII administration, which make treatment extremely difficult. Should this occur, massive doses of factor VIII may temporarily swamp an inhibitor, or factor IX concentrate containing some factor IXa may be used to circumvent the need for factor VIII. Although the latter approach carries some risk of precipitating thrombosis, it is probably small with modern material. In life-threatening situations, purified porcine factor VIII can be given as the antibodies do not usually cross-react with the pig protein. However, antiporcine antibodies tend to form rapidly, and limit recurrent use. In desperate situations, immunosuppression and even plasmapheresis may have a role in reducing the inhibitor level.

Transmission of viral infections, especially HIV, was a serious complication of factor VIII concentrate administration, and many severe haemophiliacs are now HIV antibody positive. There are some differences in the natural history of HIV infection in haemophiliacs compared with other patient groups, with Kaposi's sarcoma rarely occurring. Current sterilisation of factor VIII concentrates has virtually eliminated this problem. The risk of transmission of hepatitis C is now also very small.

The treatment of haemophilia may contribute to psychological trauma, with 'needle phobias' in children and narcotic analgesic abuse in adults being uncommon, but severe, problems.

VON WILLEBRAND'S DISEASE

Von Willebrand's disease is a syndrome, rather than a single disease entity, which is usually transmitted as an autosomal dominant condition. The incidence is greater than that for haemophilia A. Different types are recognised. In the commonest variety (type I) there is deficiency of factor VIIIvWFAg (shown as **A** in Fig. 24.39), with consequent low factor VIIIvWF activity as measured by ristocetin aggregation. Factor VIIIC levels are also low, as the half-life of factor VIIIC is reduced when not bound to the vWFAg. In type II, factor VIIIvWFAg is quantitatively normal, but unable to form high molecular weight multimers, so that factor VIIIvWF activity is reduced (shown as **B** in Fig. 24.39). In the rare type III, fVIIIvWFAg is completely absent and fVIIIc barely detectable. In almost all forms of von Willebrand's disease, the bleeding time is prolonged.

Clinical features

Bleeding is generally less severe than in haemophilia A, with skin and mucous membrane bleeding predominating. Many cases only become apparent after dental extractions.

Diagnosis

The bleeding time is usually prolonged and is the best indicator of clinical severity. Factor VIIIvWF is usually reduced, as is factor VIIIvWFAg in most cases. The factor VIIIC level is more variable, but is usually low and thus causes a prolonged APTT with a normal PT. However, it must be noted that factor VIII levels rise as acute phase reactants, and one set of normal factor VIII parameters does not exclude von Willebrand's disease.

Management

Minor bleeding or surgical episodes can often be contained by use of DDAVP and tranexamic acid, although DDAVP is likely to be less effective in variants where factor VIIIvWFAg is qualitatively abnormal and unable to form high molecular weight multimers, or is totally absent. In more serious circumstances, factor VIIIvWFAg replacement should be given in the form of fresh frozen plasma or factor VIII concentrate.

OTHER CONGENITAL COAGULATION FACTOR ABNORMALITIES

Other congenital coagulation factor abnormalities are summarised in Table 24.47.

Table 24.47 Less common congenital coagulation factor deficiencies

Abnormal factor	Inheritance	Bleeding disorder
Factor IX (haemophilia B or Christmas disease)	X-linked	Severe
Factor XI	Autosomal recessive	Mild
Factor VII	Autosomal recessive	Severe
Factor XII	Autosomal recessive	Very mild
Factor V	Autosomal recessive	Mild
Factor XIII	Variable	Mild
Fibrinogen		
Afibrinogenaemia	Autosomal recessive	Surprisingly mild
Dysfibrinogenaemia	Autosomal recessive	Mild

ACQUIRED COAGULATION DISORDERS

The causes of acquired coagulation disorders are outlined in Figure 24.43.

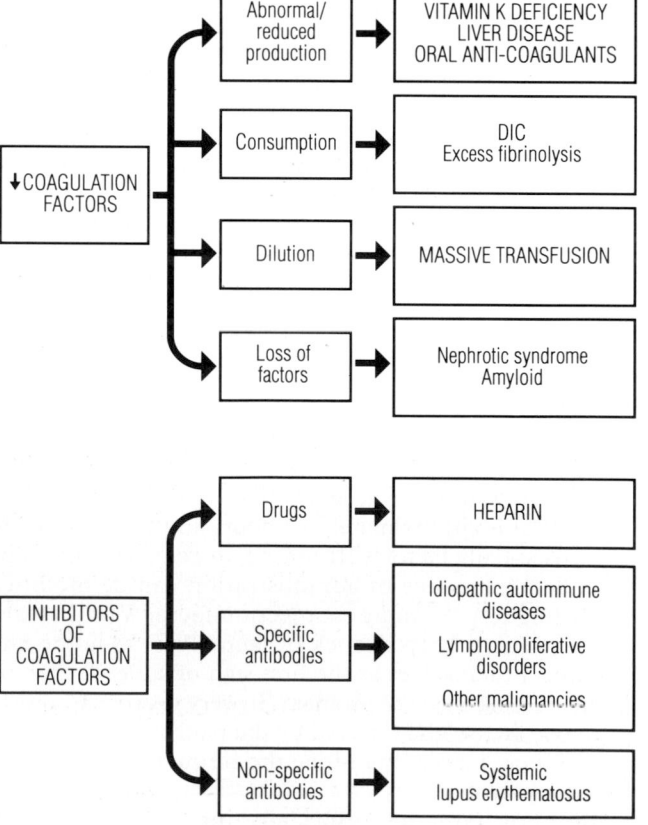

Fig. 24.43 Acquired coagulation disorders and their causes. Capital letters indicate the commoner causes.

Vitamin K deficiency

Vitamin K is a fat-soluble vitamin which carboxylates the glutamic acid residues on factors II, VII, IX and X. This enables them to bind to phospholipid in the presence of calcium and thus rapidly activate the next part of the cascade. Vitamin K deficiency may arise readily in newborn infants, in malabsorption states and also in patients with marginal stores who are severely ill and receive protracted broad-spectrum antibiotic therapy. In addition, oral anticoagulants of the warfarin and phenindione family lead to increased accumulation of phylloquinone epoxide (an inactive product of vitamin K_1), with a consequent net reduction in carboxylation of factors II, VII, IX and X.

Vitamin K deficiency leads to a bruising tendency, with a prolonged PT and APTT but a normal TT. It is reversible following vitamin K administration, although its effects take several hours to appear.

Liver disease

The aetiology of the bleeding tendency in liver disease is multifactorial (p. 620). There is decreased production of the vitamin K dependent factors, followed by decreased factor V production and (in some cases) the production of decreased or abnormal fibrinogen (dysfibrinogenaemia). If there is biliary disease, the clotting factor deficiencies may be exacerbated by malabsorption of vitamin K. This, together with the presence of ill-defined inhibitors, accounts for the difficulty in correcting the coagulation defects with fresh frozen plasma. The liver is the major site of degradation of activated factors, and hepatic insufficiency may therefore lead to DIC and excessive fibrinolysis. There may also be hypersplenism and thrombocytopenia associated with the liver disease, and qualitative platelet defects have been reported. Excessive alcohol may also directly suppress platelet production.

In liver disease the PT and APTT are frequently prolonged. Prolongation of the TT – indicating hypo/ dysfibrinogenaemia or DIC – is less common. A five-day course of vitamin K should be given if there are bleeding problems, although the benefit is marginal. Fresh frozen plasma can be given if clinically required, although the clinical and laboratory response is often poor. Platelets should be given to bleeding thrombocytopenic patients.

Disseminated intravascular coagulation and fibrinolysis

DIC is discussed on page 1108. Very rarely, excess fibrinolysis occurs without DIC, due to high levels of plasminogen activator. This may follow major trauma, extensive surgery and carcinoma (especially prostate) in which there is excessive release of tPA; some snake venoms; and in severe liver disease in which there is failure to inactivate tPA. Generalised fibrinolysis is also produced by streptokinase therapy.

Acquired inhibitors

Specific anti-factor VIIIC antibodies may arise in severe haemophiliacs following factor VIII therapy. They may also arise in other individuals, often in association with autoimmune disease (such as rheumatoid arthritis, lymphoproliferative disease and other malignancies); but they are also frequently idiopathic in origin. Less commonly, antibodies to other clotting factors may also develop.

Anti-factor VIII antibodies may be produced in systemic lupus erythematosus, but more commonly there is a non-specific *lupus anticoagulant*, which inhibits the coagulation reactions that occur on phospholipid surfaces. There is prolongation of the APTT, which becomes disproportionately longer upon dilution of the thromboplastin. Patients with lupus anticoagulants do not bleed, but may have thromboses and spontaneous abortions. Many are asymptomatic.

ANTICOAGULANTS AND ANTI-THROMBOTIC DRUGS

This group of drugs includes both inhibitors of platelets and the coagulation cascade, and activators of fibrinolysis.

HEPARIN

Mechanism of action

The heparins are a group of negatively charged polysaccharide sulphates which combine with antithrombin III, thereby increasing its activity against the activated serine proteases: thrombin and factors XI, IX, X and XIII. The effect is almost immediate. Heparin may also have some effects on platelets but these are of lesser importance.

Indications

The indications for the use of heparin are outlined in Table 24.48. Intravenous heparin helps prevent pulmonary embolism in patients with popliteal femoral and iliac vein thromboses. Its value in more superficial, or calf vein, thromboses is less certain, but it is usually given if the patient has significant symptoms. Heparin is also frequently used to prevent the development of thromboembolism in high-risk situations, e.g. following major gynaecological or abdominothoracic surgery. The low-

Table 24.48 Indications for the use of heparin

- Treatment of deep vein thrombosis
- Treatment of pulmonary embolism
- Treatment of acute arterial occlusions
- During cardiac bypass surgery
- Thromboembolic prophylaxis

Table 24.49 Indication for use of oral anticoagulants

- Pulmonary embolism (following heparin therapy)
- Deep vein thrombosis (following heparin therapy)
- Prosthetic heart valves
- Rheumatic heart disease
- Following myocardial infarction

dose subcutaneous heparin given in these circumstances has some antithrombotic effect, but does not in general cause postoperative haemorrhage.

Administration

Full-dose heparin is given as a loading dose of 5000–10 000 units, followed by a continuous infusion of 25 000–40 000 units/day depending on patient size and laboratory tests. Heparin affects all the routine coagulation tests, but none are entirely satisfactory for control of heparin therapy. The APTT is usually used and should be 1.5–2.5 times the normal control. Measurement of factor Xa is a better test but is expensive. Following a thromboembolic episode, heparin should be given for five to seven days. Low molecular weight heparins have a longer half-life and only need daily administration, which is valuable for long-term use. They can only be monitored by factor Xa assay.

Low-dose subcutaneous heparin is usually given into the abdominal wall or thigh in a dose of 5000 units b.d. Laboratory control is not necessary.

Complications

If bleeding occurs, the heparin should be reversed with protamine sulphate and the response monitored by laboratory tests such as the APTT or TT. Heparin may cause hypersensitivity reactions and acute thrombocytopenia, but this is rare before seven days of therapy. In patients receiving long-term heparin, alopecia and osteoporosis may occur. Low molecular weight heparins produce less thrombocytopenia and possibly osteoporosis.

The most common complication is haemorrhage, and full anticoagulation should therefore be undertaken with great caution in patients with an active, or potentially active, bleeding site, severe hypertension, liver disease, haemorrhagic tendency of any form, or immediately following surgery (especially to the eye or CNS).

ORAL ANTICOAGULANTS

Mechanism of action

Bishydroxycoumarin (warfarin) and phenindione (dindevan) interfere with vitamin K metabolism by aug-

menting the formation of the inactive phylloquinone epoxide. This leads to the formation of factors II, VII, IX and X in which the glutamic residues have not been carboxylated. These *acarboxy factors* cannot interact with calcium and phospholipids and cannot therefore participate in the rapid clotting cascade.

Indications

The indications for use of oral anticoagulants (Table 24.49) are still controversial in many circumstances due to conflicting trial results. This particularly applies to their use following myocardial infarction. An isolated deep vein thrombosis or pulmonary embolus merits four weeks' therapy, although a second episode should be treated for three months. Recurrent pulmonary embolism is an indication for lifelong therapy.

Administration

Anticoagulation is usually started with intravenous heparin, commonly given for five days. Oral anticoagulants are also started at the same time, their maximum effect taking five days to develop. A loading dose of warfarin (10 mg/day for three days, or similar regimen) is given, and the dose adjusted thereafter according to the results of a PT. The therapeutic range is an *international normalised ratio* (INR = ratio of patient's PT to control PT) of 2–4, depending on the indication for anticoagulation. If the patient is also receiving heparin, the heparin in the sample must first be neutralised with protamine sulphate if the APTT is greater than 2.5 times control. The half-life of warfarin is 30–60 hours, so daily administration gives rise to fairly stable steady state levels. Once good control has been achieved, monthly checks on the PT are usually acceptable. Drugs which inhibit liver enzyme degradation of oral anticoagulants, such as cimetidine and sulphonamides (including co-trimoxazole), will potentiate the anticoagulant effect. By contrast, barbiturates and rifampicin (which induce liver enzymes) will decrease the activity of oral anticoagulants. Broad-spectrum antibiotics, which interfere with vitamin K biosynthesis by intestinal flora, will augment the action of oral anticoagulants; cholestyramine reduces their effect by preventing anticoagulant absorption. The list of possible drug interactions is enormous; some of the more common

Table 24.50 Drugs modulating warfarin activity

Type of drug	Drugs potentiating warfarin activity	Drugs diminishing warfarin activity
Gut	Cimetidine (moderate) Liquid paraffin (minor)	Cholestyramine (minor)
Circulation	Sulphinpyrazone (marked) Clofibrate (moderate) Amiodarone (moderate) Dipyridamole (minor)	
CNS		Carbamazepine (minor) Primidone (minor) Barbiturates (minor)
Endocrine	Thyroxine (moderate) Anabolic steroids (moderate) Steroids (minor)	Oral contraceptives (minor)
Anti-inflammatory	Salicylates (moderate) Phenylbutazone (moderate) Mefenamic acid (moderate) Azapropazone (moderate)	
Antibiotics	Cotrimoxazole (moderate) Metronidazole (moderate) Erythromycin (minor)	Rifampicin (minor)

are shown in Table 24.50. It is essential to use a reference source of drug interactions when changing concurrent drug therapy, and the PT must be monitored frequently in these circumstances.

Complications

The major complication of anticoagulation is bleeding. As with heparin, some patients are at particular risk (p. 1114), but haemorrhagic disaster can occur in any patient and diligent control is therefore essential at all times. Most importantly, patients should not receive long-term therapy unless it is absolutely necessary. If the PT is found to be between 4.5 and 7 (INR), warfarin should be withheld for one or two days, and then restarted at a lower dose. If the PT is greater than 7, either vitamin K (1 mg i.v.) should be given or fresh frozen plasma (FFP) infused. FFP should be given immediately if there is any sign of bleeding. Additional (but rare) side-effects of warfarin include skin rashes, diarrhoea, jaundice and alopecia.

ANTICOAGULATION IN PREGNANCY

Pregnancy is itself a prothrombotic state, due to both local pressure on the venous system from an enlarged uterus, and also an increase in coagulability and decrease in fibrinolysis. Thromboembolic disease occurs in approximately two per 1000 pregnancies. Other pregnant women require prophylactic anticoagulation because of previous thromboses, or high risk situations such as prosthetic heart valves.

Warfarin crosses the placenta and may cause chondrodysplasia punctata and abnormal development of the brain and face. The risk is greatest in the first three months, but is still present in the second trimester. Heparin should therefore be used instead as it does not cross the placenta. For an acute thromboembolism in the first trimester, full intravenous heparinisation should be given, followed by subcutaneous heparin (10 000 units b.d.). Some clinicians change to warfarin for the second trimester, but this still carries some risk of fetal malformation. In the third trimester, subcutaneous heparin should again be used, as warfarinisation may cause serious bleeding in both mother and baby at the time of delivery. Warfarin can be started 10 days after delivery, even in mothers who are breast-feeding.

Unfortunately, subcutaneous heparin is not as effective as full-dose intravenous heparin or oral warfarin, and is probably not therefore acceptable for the safety of mothers with the most high-risk prosthetic heart valves. A difficult compromise must be achieved after detailed discussion with the parents, if the pregnancy is to continue.

Some women become pregnant whilst taking warfarin and may not report it to their doctor until the pregnancy is well advanced into the first trimester. Clearly, all fertile women should be warned about the problems of pregnancy when warfarinisation is commenced.

ANTIPLATELET AGENTS

Mechanism of action

The mechanisms of action of the more commonly used antiplatelet agents are shown in Table 24.51. The inhibition of platelet cyclo-oxygenase by aspirin is irreversible, and the effects of a single dose will last several days until new platelets are produced. Aspirin also inhibits endothelial cyclo-oxygenase which blocks prostacyclin production, a potent natural antiplatelet agent. Endothelial cells (unlike platelets) are nucleated, and continue to synthesise cyclo-oxygenase; as a result, the aspirin effect is short-lived. Thus, in theory, the maximal antiplatelet effect of aspirin may be achieved simply by a twice-weekly

Table 24.51 Drugs interfering with platelet function

Drug	Mechanism of action
Aspirin	Irreversible acetylation of platelet cyclo-oxygenase with blockade of platelet prostaglandin production
Sulphinpyrazone (Anturan)	Competitive inhibitor of cyclo-oxygenase
Dipyridamole (Persantin)	Reversible inhibition of platelet phosphodiesterase

regimen, although most trial evidence is based on daily doses. Sulphinpyrazone similarly blocks cyclo-oxygenase, but its effect is reversible. Dipyridamole reversibly suppresses platelet cyclic AMP levels with consequent inhibition of agonist-mediated rises in intracellular calcium ions.

Indications

Some of the possible indications for antiplatelet agents are shown in Table 24.52, although it must be noted that the data from clinical trials are not conclusive in all circumstances, particularly in the last three indications listed.

Administration and complications

There is no universally accepted optimum regimen. Aspirin (300 mg daily) with or without dipyridamole (50–200 mg q.d.s. – higher doses may not be tolerated) is widely used. Antiplatelet agents do increase the bleeding time, but this alone causes a few problems. Aspirin may, however, lead to gastric erosions and major bleeding from this site. Dipyridamole causes migrainous type headaches in many patients at the start of therapy, although these usually subside within a few weeks.

INTRAVASCULAR FIBRINOLYTIC THERAPY

Mechanisms of action

Streptokinase (which is derived from β haemolytic streptococci) combines with plasminogen and leads to the formation of the fibrinolytic compound plasmin. *Urokinase* (which is isolated from human urine) has a similar mechanism of action. It is a less toxic, naturally occurring compound, but is very expensive to purify. More recently, the naturally occurring *tissue plasminogen activators* (tPAs) have been produced by recombinant DNA technology; tPA is used in a patient who has had streptokinase in the previous year.

Table 24.52 Possible indications for the use of antiplatelet agents

- Cerebrovascular transient ischaemic attacks
- Prethrombotic states in which there is thrombocytosis or increased platelet aggregation
- Acute myocardial infarction
- Maintenance of A-V shunts
- Valvular disease of the heart
- Prevention of deep vein thromboses after surgery

Indications

The major indication is in acute myocardial infarction (Ch. 12, p. 403). Other uses are shown in Table 24.53.

Administration

Streptokinase is antigenic and most patients have circulating antibodies due to previous streptococcal infections. These must first be neutralised by a loading dose, which is then followed by continuous infusion for three to seven days. There is no consensus as to the optimum dosage schedule, although after myocardial infarction a single infusion dose has been shown to be effective. Fibrinolytic therapy reduces the fibrinogen level, markedly prolongs the TT, and causes a rise in serum fibrin degradation products; these data are of little help, however, in monitoring the dosage. Ideally, streptokinase is infused locally, i.e. using a pulmonary artery catheter for pulmonary embolism.

Complications

Streptokinase therapy is potentially hazardous. Bleeding, especially from drip sites, is very common and can be fatal. All patients receiving streptokinase should therefore have blood cross-matched and available. Fevers and other allergic phenomena are not infrequent, and it is common practice to give prophylactic steroids. Hopes that tPA would have fewer side-effects have not been realized.

Oral fibrinolytic agents

A variety of oral drugs such as the biguanides (e.g. metformin) and anabolic steroids (e.g. stanozolol) increase fibrinolytic activity, and may have occasional value in patients with recurrent venous and arterial thromboses who are on oral anticoagulants. These agents do, however, have major potential side-effects, e.g. hypoglycaemia and masculinisation, unrelated to their fibrinolytic function.

Table 24.53 Indications for the use of intravascular fibrinolytic agents

- Pulmonary embolism (acute massive)
- Major deep vein thrombosis
- Acute arterial thrombo-embolism
- Acute myocardial infarction (within 6–12 hours)
- Unblocking indwelling central venous catheters and arteriovenous shunts

PRETHROMBOTIC STATES

A *prethrombotic state* is any situation in which there is an increased risk of thromboembolism. Possible causes with examples are shown in Table 24.54.

The full investigation of a potential prethrombotic state is both extremely time-consuming and expensive. All patients presenting with a thromboembolic episode should be thoroughly examined to exclude local causes of circulatory stasis, and systemic diseases associated with hypercoagulability. A full blood count should be performed to exclude polycythaemia or thrombocytosis. Further studies (Table 24.55) are only cost-effective in selected cases. The criteria for selection of patients (Table 24.56) are designed primarily to allow detection of the hereditary prethrombotic states.

Interpretation of the laboratory investigations for a prethrombotic state is not always easy. Firstly, raised clotting factors or increased levels of activated factors may be secondary to a recent (possibly subclinical) thrombosis, rather than the cause of a prethrombotic state. Similarly, increased levels of platelet release products, such as platelet factor 4 (PF4) or β-thromboglobulin (β-TG), within the serum may reflect ongoing thrombosis rather than a primary platelet/vessel wall abnormality. Secondly, many patients requiring investigation will already be

Table 24.54 Possible causes of a prethrombotic state

Mechanism	Example
Circulatory stasis	
Immobilisation	Prolonged bed rest
Mechanical obstruction	Pelvic tumours
Increased Hct	Polycythaemia
Greatly increased WBC	Chronic myeloid leukaemia
Increased plasma viscosity	Myeloma
Abnormalities of platelet/vessel wall interaction	
Thrombocytosis	Essential thrombocythaemia
Increased platelet aggregability	Diabetes
Decreased vessel wall prostacylin production?	Thrombotic thrombocytopenic purpura
Coagulation abnormalities	
Clotting factors	Increased levels of VIIIC and VIIC associated with risk of coronary death
	Antithrombin III deficiency
	Lupus anticoagulant
Coagulation inhibitors	Protein C deficiency
	Protein S deficiency
Fibrinolytic abnormalities	
Plasminogen activators	Found in some patients with
Inhibitors of plasminogen	thrombotic episodes
Increased antiplasmin	(significance uncertain)

Table 24.55 Investigation of a prethrombotic state

- Full blood count
- Liver function tests
- Analysis of plasma lipids
- Protein electrophoresis to exclude hypergammaglobulinaemia
- Coagulation screen with particular attention to abnormalities due to dysfibrinogenaemia, or a lupus anticoagulant
- Euglobin clot lysis time as an index of the fibrinolytic pathway
- Antithrombin III levels
- Protein C levels (also protein S levels if available)
- Platelet aggregometry to detect hyperaggregable platelets
  or
- Measurement of platelet release products (PF4, β-TG) within the plasma

Table 24.56 Possible criteria for the selection of patients for detailed investigation of a prethrombotic state

- Patient with DVT in whom there is a positive family history
- Thrombosis in unusual site, e.g. mesenteric vein
- DVT or pulmonary embolism in early pregnancy
- Recurrence of DVT while on oral anticoagulants
- Recurrent DVT in a patient under 35 years of age

taking oral anticoagulants; determining deficiencies of vitamin K dependent proteins such as antithrombin III and protein C is then very difficult.

Antithrombin III deficiency

Antithrombin III (AT-III) deficiency may be either congenital or acquired.

Congenital

This is an autosomal dominant condition in which there is decreased synthesis of AT-III or synthesis of a dysfunctional molecule. The incidence is estimated to be 20–50 per 100 000. Affected individuals have functional AT-III levels of 40–70% (normal range 70–130%).

The disease typically presents with venous thromboses in early adulthood. Thromboses are particularly common after starting the contraceptive pill, during pregnancy or following surgery. Heparin is usually given in the short term, but is less effective here than in other situations, as AT-III is required as a cofactor for heparin. The administration of heparin also actually causes the AT-III level to fall further. For these reasons, fresh frozen plasma (or AT-III concentrates if available) should also be given in the acute stages. Long-term oral anticoagulants do reduce the incidence of recurrent thromboses and increase the circulatory levels of AT-III.

Acquired

As noted above, AT-III levels fall with the contraceptive pill, during surgery and after major surgery or trauma, and this may contribute to the prethrombotic state in these situations. AT-III levels may also fall with severe proteinuria, thereby contributing to the documented thrombotic tendency in the nephrotic syndrome. AT-III synthesis is reduced in liver disease, but bleeding (rather than thrombosis) is usually the problem in this situation.

Protein C and protein S deficiency

Protein C deficiency is an autosomal dominant condition, with an incidence probably similar to that of AT-III deficiency. The clinical course is also similar. Extensive skin necrosis has been noted in some patients following the initiation of anticoagulants.

Protein S deficiency (autosomal dominant) is probably less common, but may still account for up to 10% of thromboses in the high risk categories shown in Table 24.56.

Lupus anticoagulant

The lupus anticoagulant is associated with an increased incidence of thrombosis, although it is detected by the prolongation of the APTT. It is discussed on page 1116.

FURTHER READING

Colman R W, Hirsh J, Marder V J, Salzman E W (eds) 1987 Haemostasis and thrombosis, 2nd edn. J B Lippincott, Philadelphia. *An authorative, multi-author textbook.*
Dacie J V, Lewis S M 1991 Practical haematology, 7th edn. Churchill Livingstone, Edinburgh. *The classical reference work for laboratory technology.*
Hoffbrand A V, Petit J E (eds) 1988 Clinical haematology. Gower Medical, London. *An illustrated guide to haematology with excellent photomicrography.*
Hoffman A V, Benz E J, Shattil S J, Furie F, Cohen H J 1991 Haematology: Basic principles and practice. Churchill Livingstone, Edinburgh. *A comprehensive, up-to-date textbook of haematology.*
Leukaemia and lymphoma 1990. Published by the Leukaemia Research Fund, London. *The epidemiology of haematological malignancies in the UK.*
Linch D C, Yates A 1986 Colour aids: Haematology. Churchill Livingstone, Edinburgh. *An inexpensive atlas of haematology.*
Mollison P L 1990 Blood transfusion in clinical medicine. Blackwell Scientific, Oxford. *The standard UK textbook on blood transfusion.*

APPENDIX: NORMAL HAEMATOLOGICAL VALUES

The following are guidelines only – ranges may vary with the methods of assay used.

Measurement	Range	Units	Measurement	Range	Units
Red cell count	M 4.5–6.5	10^{12}/l	Monocytes	0.2–0.8	10^9/l
	F 3.8–5.8	10^{12}/l	Eosinophils	<0.4	10^9/l
Haemoglobin	M 13.0–18.0	g/dl	Basophils	<0.1	19^9/l
	F 11.5–16.5	g/dl	Platelet count	150–400	10^9/l
PVC	M 0.4–0.5	ratio	Serum iron	12–32	mmol/l
	F 0.35–0.47	ratio	TIBC	45–72	mmol/l
MCV	78–96	fl.	B_{12}	150–900	ng/l
MCH	27–32	pg.	Serum folate	3–15	ng/l
MCHC	30–34	g/dl	Rbc folate	160–640	ng/l
Reticulocytes					
Percentage	0.2–2.0	%	ESR <50 years	<20	mm/h
Absolute count	10–100	10^9/l	ESR >50 years	<30	mm/h
Total wbc	3.5–11.0	10^9/l	Prothrombin time	<3 s over control	
Differential wbc count:					
Neutrophils	2.0–7.5	10^9/l	Activated partial thromboplastin time	<7 s over control	
Lymphocytes	1.5–4.0	10^9/l	Thrombin time	<3 s over control	

25

Skin Disease

Cameron T C Kennedy and
Robin A C Graham-Brown

Table 25.1 Incidence of skin diseases*

Rates of consultation (general practice) per 1000/year	
All skin diseases	120.0
Dermatitis and eczema	45.6
Virus warts	14.3
Rash	13.3
Acne	9.6
Urticaria	8.6
Psoriasis	4.6
Chronic ulcer	2.4
Malignant neoplasms	0.8
Some comparisons	
Back pain	32.8
Osteoarthritis	23.5
Diseases of stomach	19.7
Irritable bowel	18.4
Rheumatoid arthritis	5.6

*Data from Office of Population Censuses and Surveys, Third National Study. HMSO, 1986.

Skin disorders are a common reason for seeking medical advice (Table 25.1). Apart from diseases which primarily affect the skin, many systemic diseases may produce dermatological manifestations.

When a skin disease is widespread and interfering with skin functions, systemic consequences follow – sometimes, as in untreated pemphigus vulgaris, with fatal results. More limited skin diseases can cause distress or hardship. The psychological impact of readily visible skin lesions, even if biologically trivial, should not be underestimated. Another common problem associated with skin disorders is fear (often not expressed) that a skin disease is contagious, or a manifestation of cancer.

In this chapter there is a brief account of the biology of the skin, the principles of diagnosis and therapy, and then a description of those skin diseases which are either common or important. Diseases presenting as changes in the skin, but whose major impact is on other systems, are discussed in other chapters. Because of the great importance of the visual aspects of dermatology, a colour atlas, or whenever possible, patients, should be viewed in conjunction with the text. Therapy is considered in terms of general principles.

BIOLOGY OF THE SKIN

The skin is a protective barrier between a hostile environment and internal tissues. Its principal functions are to reduce the loss of water, electrolytes and other solutes, and the entry of unwanted molecules, microbes and radiation. It has a complex and specialised sensory innervation and contains a network of antigen-processing cells. The cutaneous vasculature and sweat glands are vital to heat regulation. Vitamin D is synthesised in the skin. By virtue of its smell, colour and texture, the skin has psychological and sexual roles.

The skin is composed of three layers: epidermis, dermis and fat (Fig. 25.1).

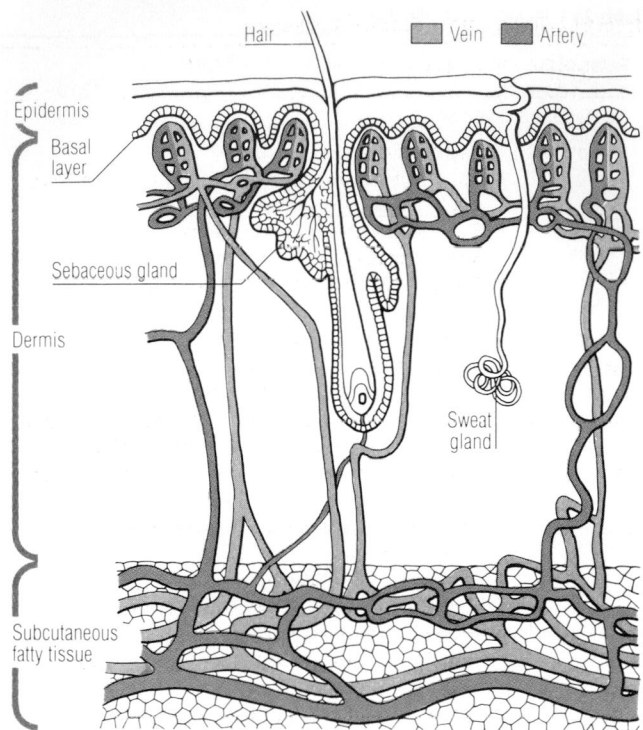

Fig. 25.1 Cross-section of the skin.

Labels in figure: Hair, Vein, Artery, Epidermis, Basal layer, Sebaceous gland, Dermis, Sweat gland, Subcutaneous fatty tissue

Epidermis

The epidermis is a stratified epithelium, comprised mainly of keratinocytes, which are of ectodermal origin. They divide in the basal layer, where they are separated by the basal lamina from the dermis, progressively produce the sulphur-rich fibrous protein keratin, and become flattened and dead by the time they reach the surface. These cells have a lipid-rich envelope. Keratinocytes are linked to one another by specialised cell junctions, notably the desmosomes, and in health the horny layer is tough, flexible and relatively impermeable. At the surface they are constantly shed as squames. Removal of the horny layer virtually destroys the barrier function of the skin with respect to water and solutes. The effectiveness of the horny layer is reduced if its production is faulty (e.g. in psoriasis), if the water content drops below a critical level (e.g. chapping), or if it is damaged (e.g. by detergents and lipid solvents).

Resident in the epidermis are the melanocytes, Langerhans cells and Merkel cells:

- *Melanocytes* migrate early in fetal life from the neural crest and become established along the basal layer so that there is approximately one melanocyte per 10 basal keratinocytes. Via their dendritic processes, the yellow or brown pigmented protein melanin is passed in membrane-bound particles, called melanosomes, into the keratinocytes; here most of it is distributed over the surface of the nucleus which faces the sun. Melanin absorbs ultraviolet radiation and thus helps protect against DNA damage. In its absence, in albinism, skin cancer on exposed sites is common at an early age.
- *Langerhans cells*, also dendritic, are of bone marrow origin. They are located in the mid-epidermis, function as antigen-trapping and antigen-presenting cells and can migrate to regional lymph nodes. Together with lymphocytes, they constitute a vital outpost of the immune system.
- *Merkel cells*, best recognised on electron microscopy by their dense-cored granules, are closely associated with sensory nerve endings, and may represent a mechanoreceptor system. They are most numerous on the lips, digital pads and in hair follicles.

The epidermis is separated from, and attached to, the dermis by a basal lamina, across which all nutrients must pass. A component of the basal lamina is the target of immunological attack in the blistering disease bullous pemphigoid (p. 1145).

Dermis

The dermis is a three-dimensional, fibrous tissue network of collagen and elastin associated with water-rich glycosaminoglycans, in which are embedded the blood and lymphatic vessels, neural elements and epidermal appendages – sweat glands, sebaceous glands and hair follicles (Fig. 25.1). The dermis is manufactured by fibroblasts, and other cells seen in normal tissue include dermal phagocytes and mast cells. The dermis has visco-elastic properties, allowing body movements without permanent distortion, yet considerable mechanical strength. It is essential to the well-being and repair of the epidermis. The superficial part of the dermis, containing capillaries and nerve endings, is more loosely woven than deeper layers, and projects into the undersurface of the epidermis as papillae.

Blood flow through the skin can be greatly in excess of nutritional demands, and skin vasculature contributes to thermoregulation and maintenance of blood pressure. There are networks of blood vessels at the levels of the deep fascia, the fat–dermis junction and in the papillary dermis, where capillary loops follow the contour of the dermo-epidermal junction. There are also numerous arterio-venous shunts which allow blood to bypass capillaries, conserving heat. Vascular control is by autonomic nerves and chemical mediators. The skin is also provided with an extensive plexus of lymphatics which act both as a drainage system for lymph and in the recirculation of lymphocytes.

There are afferent sensory nerves subserving touch, pain, temperature and itch, and also the specialised Meissner and Pacinian corpuscles, which are probably mechanoreceptors. The autonomic supply is sympathetic, with adrenergic, cholinergic and purinergic terminals.

Collagen and elastin disorders are described on page 78.

Epidermal appendages

Eccrine sweat glands consist of secretory coils connected by straight ducts to the surface. There is a rich blood supply and a predominantly cholinergic sympathetic innervation. Because of the sodium resorptive properties of the ducts, sweat is hypotonic. The basal level of fluid loss through the skin of about 600 ml/day can be greatly increased in response to the need for heat loss.

Apocrine sweat glands are found in the axillae, anogenital regions, on the breast and on the scalp. They open into hair follicles and on to the skin surface. Their secretion is low in volume and after bacterial alteration it has a characteristic odour. Very similar glands produce wax in the ears and occur on the eyelids.

The *pilosebaceous follicles* produce both hairs and sebaceous glands. In man, hair is largely of cultural and sexual significance. There are three types of hair: lanugo, which covers the fetus; vellus hair, which is fine and short; and terminal hair, which is coarse and occurs on the scalp, eyebrows, axillae and pubic regions. A residual protective value of hair is seen when its absence in bald males is accompanied in later life by sun-induced neoplasms. An important characteristic of hair follicles is their cyclical activity: for each follicle a period of active growth (anagen) is followed by a transition period (catagen) and then a resting phase (telogen), when the hair is shed and a new hair begins. Individual follicles are normally asynchronous, hence humans do not moult.

Nails are hard plates of keratin which protect the ends of the digits and facilitate many of the functions of the hands.

EXAMINATION OF THE SKIN

It is essential to examine all the skin, together with the mouth, genitalia, hair and nails, in a good light. The skin should be palpated as well as inspected, to appreciate the thickness of lesions and of the whole skin. Skin lesions should be described in terms of:

- the individual characteristics (shape, colour, etc.)
- their arrangement in relation to each other (if any)
- their distribution.

The terms used have precise meanings (Table 25.2).

Table 25.2 Terms used to describe skin lesions

Skin lesion	Definition
Appearance	
Erythema	Redness due to vasodilatation
Macule	Flat, circumscribed, impalpable area of colour change. There may be scaling, as in pityriasis versicolor
Papule	Small (less than 0.5 cm), solid, elevated lesion, most of which is above the plane of the skin
Plaque	Elevated lesion with relatively large surface area in relation to height
Nodule	Large (greater than 0.5 cm diameter) solid lesion
Vesicle	Blister less than 0.5 cm diameter
Bulla	Blister greater than 0.5 cm diameter
Pustule	Elevation of the skin containing fluid and leucocytes, usually yellow or green in colour, but not necessarily infective
Weal	Elevation due to dermal oedema, lasting minutes to several hours
Angio-oedema	Massive oedematous reaction in loose dermis or subcutaneous tissue
Purpura	Extravasated red cells (see Diascopy, p. 1122). Small purpuric lesions are called petechiae, large ones ecchymoses. They are not obliterated by pressure. The colour varies from red, through purple and brown, to yellow, depending on the age of the lesion
Telangiectasia	Permanent dilatation of capillaries
Atrophy	Thinning, often with loss of normal skin markings, and increased transparency
Sclerosis	Hardening due to changes in the dermis
Ulcer	Loss of (at least) the epidermis
Excoriation	Scratch mark
Crust	Dried exudate
Scaling	Desquamating horny layer
Burrow	Irregular linear elevation of horny layer, characteristic of scabies
Shape and arrangement	
Linear	In a line
Annular	Ring-shaped
Target	Erythematous ring or rings separated by relative pallor with a purplish centre
Herpetiform	Clustered, like herpes simplex
Zosteriform	Clustered and following a dermatome
Reticular	Net-like

Distribution

The following points should be noted:

- Is the rash localised, regional or generalised?
- Is there symmetry? Endogenous disorders are often symmetrical.
- Is there localization by exposure to light, cold or some other environmental factor?
- Has non-specific trauma, e.g. scratching, caused new lesions (Koebner phenomenon), as in psoriasis and lichen planus?
- Is there an underlying anatomical basis, e.g. the vascular or nerve supply, the flexures or hair follicles?

Many conditions have characteristic patterns of distribution, the basis for which is obscure, e.g. dermatitis herpetiformis on elbows and knees, scalp, shoulders and buttocks.

DERMATOLOGICAL DIAGNOSIS

There is a great variety of dermatological diagnoses. However, the practised observer can describe changes that suggest a diagnosis or differential diagnostic group. The history is important, narrowing the possibilities (Table 25.3). Diagnostic procedures and investigations may be useful.

Diascopy

Having pressed the skin with a microscope slide or Perspex spatula, purpura (which does not blanch) can be distinguished from erythema (which does).

Nikolsky sign

The Nikolsky sign involves the production or extension of a blistering process by the combination of pressure with a sliding action. It is characteristic of pemphigus and some other blistering diseases.

Wood's light

Wood's light is produced by a long-wave UV lamp, which shows red fluorescence with erythrasma, green fluorescence with some common scalp fungal infections, and pale yellow fluorescence with pityriasis versicolor. It enhances the pallor of vitiligo and is helpful in screening for the ash leaf macules of tuberous sclerosis.

Biopsy

Biopsies are carried out for histopathology and, when relevant, immunological studies, microbiological culture and electron microscopy.

Mycological techniques

Mycological techniques are described on page 1127.

Patch testing

Patch testing is described under 'Contact dermatitis' (p. 1138).

Scabies mite scraping

Scabies mite scraping is described on page 1133.

DERMATOLOGICAL THERAPY

Dermatological treatment includes *topical and systemic pharmacy*, *physical modalities* such as liquid nitrogen cryotherapy, ultraviolet radiation, radiotherapy, laser and surgical procedures, and *dietary measures*. Topical therapy is the traditional province of the dermatologist.

Vehicles

Active ingredients are applied to the skin in a vehicle (Table 25.4). A vehicle may be used therapeutically: a lotion to cool and dry, a cream to soothe, an ointment to moisturise dry skin, and a paste to protect.

When an active ingredient is included, the vehicle must deliver it appropriately and maintain its integrity against oxidation and bacterial contamination. Therefore vehicles, especially creams, often contain preservatives and stabilisers. Some preparations contain substances to enhance drug penetration, e.g. urea. When adverse reactions to topical agents occur, it should be remembered that not only the active ingredient but also the components of the vehicle should be considered as possible causes.

For most active ingredients the major barrier to penetration is the horny layer. Penetration is greater through facial and genital skin, flexures (e.g. axillae, crural folds) and is increased by occlusion (e.g. by rubber gloves), diseases altering the horny layer (e.g. eczema and psoriasis), and pharmaceutical penetration enhancers, such as urea. In contrast, when the horny layer is very thick, as on the palms and soles, there is reduced penetration.

Table 25.3 Taking a history

History of the skin eruption
When and where did the problem start?
Has it spread, and how?
Has it changed in character? What was it like if different before?
Does it itch?
Does it come and go?
What has been used or taken for it (prescribed and self-medication)?
Have any other medications – oral, injected or topical – been used?
Is there any relation to sunlight?
Any past history of skin disease?
Does anyone the patient knows have anything similar?
What does the patient think is the cause?
Background
Age, sex, race. Pregnant? Pubertal?
General medical, past and family history
Personal and family history of eczema, asthma or hay fever
Social history: occupation, hobbies, travel
Any known allergies?

Table 25.4 Composition and properties of vehicles for topical treatment

Vehicle	Composition	Properties
Lotion	Liquid (water or alcohol)	Cools inflamed skin. Useful in hairy areas. Miscible with exudate
Shake lotion	Water + powder	Powder increases area for evaporation, so has cooling properties
Cream	Water + grease + emulsifier	Aqueous phase gives some cooling effect and miscibility with exudate. Grease increases hydration. Properties will vary depending on whether the emulsion is oil-in-water or water-in-oil
Ointment	Grease	Moisturises dry skin by trapping water passing through the epidermis. Hydrophobic (e.g. vaseline) or hydrophilic (e.g. lanolin)
Paste	Grease + powder	Moisturising and protective
Dusting powder	Powder	Reduces friction. Absorbs water

Topical corticosteroids

Topical corticosteroids have anti-inflammatory and other actions, with useful suppressive effects in a number of skin disorders, but they do not cure disease. They can worsen skin infection and modify physical signs, and the more potent preparations easily produce side-effects.

In general, the efficacy of topical steroids goes hand in hand with the ability to cause side-effects, and a preparation of the lowest potency that is effective should be used (Table 25.5). Applications are usually once or twice daily, with bland creams or ointments at other times if necessary. Efficacy is determined by the steroid molecule, its concentration, the vehicle, and also by factors favouring increased absorption. Adverse effects (Table 25.6) are very unlikely with topical 1% hydrocortisone.

Table 25.5 Potency of topical corticosteroids

Group	Potency	Examples
1	Very high	Clobetasol propionate
2	High	Betamethasone valerate Hydrocortisone butyrate
3	Moderate	Clobetasone butyrate
4	Low	Hydrocortisone

Table 25.6 Adverse effects of topical steroids

Adverse effects	Factors increasing risk
Pituitary–adrenal axis suppression; growth suppression in children	Potency group 1 Potency groups 1 and 2 with occlusion Widespread skin inflammation Infancy Hepatic failure
Spread of skin infection	Overt infection Body folds
Atrophy (thin, red, fragile skin)	High risk sites, e.g. face, body folds Occlusion Prolonged use
Striae (stretch marks)	Potency groups 1 and 2 Body folds
Increased hair growth (hypertrichosis)	Potency groups 1 and 2 Prolonged use
Peri-oral dermatitis	Face
Exacerbation of skin disease on withdrawal	Psoriasis Facial dermatoses

Other topically used drugs

A selection of drugs used topically is shown in Table 25.7.

Cryotherapy

Many benign and some malignant skin lesions can be quickly and successfully treated by accurately applied low temperature. The most satisfactory agent is liquid

Table 25.7 Some topical preparations used in skin diseases

Topical drug	Use
Tars	Chronic eczema, psoriasis
Dithranol	Psoriasis
Calcipotriol	Psoriasis
Benzoyl peroxide	Acne
Calamine	Pruritus
Aminobenzoic acid esters	Sunscreens
Salicylic acid	Viral warts, other localised hyperkeratotic conditions
Podophyllin	Viral warts
Gamma benzene hexachloride	Scabies
Malathion	Pediculosis (lice)
Compound benzoic acid ointment	Some dermatophyte infections
Antifungal imidazoles	Some dermatophyte and yeast infections
Nystatin and amphotericin B	Candidiasis
Antibiotics, e.g. fusidic acid, mupirocin	Localised superficial Gram-positive bacterial infection
Acyclovir, idoxuridine	Some herpes simplex and zoster infections

nitrogen, whose temperature is −196°C, applied on a cotton-wool swab, by a spray or a probe. The procedure can be painful and is often followed by swelling and blistering, but long-term cosmetic results are generally good. Hypopigmentation and some sensory loss can be troublesome consequences.

BACTERIAL DISEASES

Bacterial infection can produce skin lesions at or near the portal of entry, as in impetigo. Lesions may also be due to organisms deposited in the skin during septicaemia, blood-borne spread of a toxin, and hypersensitivity phenomena, such as the vasculitic Osler nodes and splinter haemorrhages of subacute bacterial endocarditis.

Normal intact skin is colonised by diphtheroids and non-pathogenic staphylococci, and in some sites such as the anterior nares, axilla and perineum, by potentially pathogenic *Staphylococcus aureus*. In moist areas there are often some Gram-negative bacilli.

Overt infection nearly always follows some kind of injury, albeit trivial. If it is associated with some obvious pre-existing skin lesions, such as eczema, it is referred to as secondary infection. Host factors, particularly the immunological status, are important in determining the degree and extent of infection.

Some skin diseases, such as hidradenitis suppurativa, are a non-specific reaction to bacteria, which, although contributory, are not the primary cause.

The types of staphylococcal and streptococcal skin infection are shown in Table 25.8.

Impetigo

Impetigo (Fig. 25.2) is a primary superficial bacterial skin infection, initially vesicular or bullous, later crusted. Impetigo may only involve the openings of hair follicles.

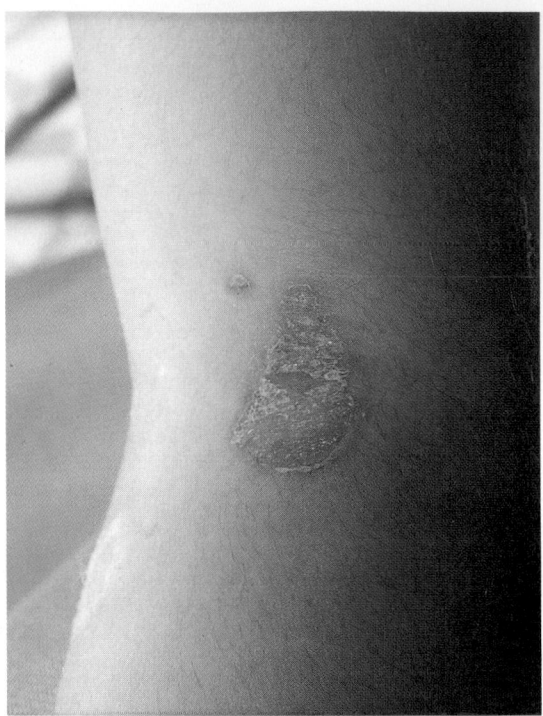

Fig. 25.2 Impetigo: flaccid blisters and crusts on an erythematous base.

It is caused by *Staph. aureus*, *Streptococcus pyogenes* group A, or both. In some tropical regions the streptococci can cause nephritis. Bullous impetigo is usually due to phage group II staphylococci.

Impetigo predominantly occurs among children and is highly contagious. Spread is mainly from skin to skin, although in streptococcal cases infected individuals may acquire the disease from pharyngeal colonisation. Trauma, for example from scratching insect bites, and infestation commonly predispose to the infection.

Exposed parts are mainly affected. The early lesions are clear or turbid blisters which soon become crusts, often golden yellow, with a surrounding zone of erythema. In bullous impetigo there are larger blisters with no erythema. The lesions tend to heal centrally but spread peripherally. Regional lymphadenopathy is common.

Diagnosis is by Gram stain and culture of a swab, which will help to distinguish impetigo from other lesions such as tinea and varicella.

Treatment. Gentle removal of crusts is helpful. If localised, a topical antibiotic, such as fusidic acid or mupirocin, is adequate. For widespread impetigo, oral flucloxacillin (or erythromycin if the patient is allergic to penicillin) is required. Improvement of hygiene may be advisable, e.g. not sharing towels.

Table 25.8 Staphylococcal and streptococcal bacterial infections of the skin

Due to direct bacterial infection	Due to toxin	Due to hypersensitivity
Staphylococcus aureus		
Impetigo	Staphylococcal scalded skin syndrome	
Ecthyma	Toxic shock syndrome	
Follicular infections	Staphylococcal scarlatina	
Streptococcus pyogenes		
Impetigo	Scarlet fever	Erythema
Ecthyma		Vasculitis
Erysipelas		
Cellulitis		
Necrotising fasciitis		

Ecthyma

Ecthyma is a vesiculopurulent condition similar to impetigo, but the infection extends deeper, producing ulceration; it is caused by *Strep. pyogenes*, often with *Staph. aureus*. The condition is common in hot, humid climates, mainly affects children and the elderly, and is often associated with poor hygiene and/or insect bites. The initial vesicular lesion soon becomes a punched-out ulcer with overlying crust. The legs are commonly affected.

The differential diagnosis includes ecthyma gangrenosum, due to *Pseudomonas septicaemia* (see below), and other causes of ulcers (p. 1161).

Treatment is with a penicillinase-resistant antibiotic, such as flucloxacillin or erythromycin. If there is surrounding cellulitis penicillin should be added.

Staphylococcal scalded skin syndrome

Staphylococcal scalded skin syndrome is a generalised skin reaction to blood-borne staphylococcal epidermolytic toxins, which cause a split in the superficial epidermis; unlike impetigo there are no organisms in the accumulating fluid. It is caused by a focus of infection of *Staph. pyogenes* of phage group II which may be cutaneous but can be elsewhere. Children, especially infants, are most susceptible.

Clinical features. A few days after the initiating staphylococcal infection there is a sudden onset of widespread tender erythema with fever. Twelve hours or so later there may be widespread flaccid bullae and the horny layer begins to detach in sheets.

Differential diagnosis. Toxic epidermal necrolysis due to drugs (p. 1150) can be distinguished by the histology of a blister roof, which shows a deeper lever of split in the epidermis in the drug-induced type, and by the history.

Treatment. Treatment is with parenteral flucloxacillin (or equivalent), and careful attention to fluid balance and temperature regulation.

Erysipelas

Erysipelas (Fig. 25.3) is a dermal infection, usually with group A streptococci.

There is often a recognisable portal of entry, such as a fungal infection between the toes or a fissure at the corner of the mouth. There may have been a previous upper respiratory tract streptococcal infection. The onset is often sudden, with fever, malaise and rigors, together with a bright red, tender swelling. The face and lower legs are common sites. The skin becomes oedematous and a well-defined, raised, sometimes blistering edge advances rapidly. There are often red streaks due to lymphangitis.

Diagnosis. Leucocytosis is usual. Surface culture is useless but the organism can sometimes be cultured from

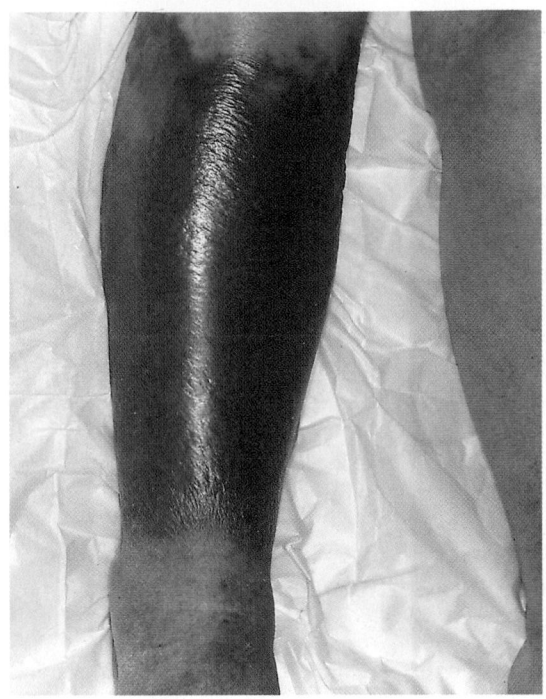

Fig. 25.3 Erysipelas: tender erythema and oedema.

aspirated fluid. There is usually an antibody response to streptococcal proteins with rising titres of antideoxyribonuclease B; anti-streptolysin O is less often elevated.

Differential diagnosis. Acute contact dermatitis and angio-oedema of the face may simulate erysipelas but do not produce fever. Herpes zoster, before the outbreak of vesicles, is associated with pain or paraesthesiae. Erysipeloid (p. 1126) occurs in meat- and fish-handlers and systemic symptoms are much less severe.

Complications. Erysipelas is usually self-limited but can produce suppurative and widespread infection. There is involvement of lymphatics, and this predisposes to persistent swelling (lymphoedema) and recurrent attacks.

Treatment. The treatment of choice is penicillin, parenterally in severe infections, unless contraindicated by hypersensitivity.

Cellulitis

Cellulitis is a deeper dermal/subcutaneous infection than erysipelas, usually with group A streptococci. In practice there is no absolute distinction between erysipelas and cellulitis. There is usually an obvious portal, e.g. a leg ulcer or wound, or oedema of lymphatic, venous or renal origin.

There is spreading erythematous oedema as in erysipelas but without the sharply defined edge or vesiculation. There may be similar constitutional symptoms and lymphangitis. Untreated, gangrene may occur.

Treatment is the same as for erysipelas.

Necrotising fasciitis

Necrotising fasciitis (streptococcal gangrene) is a necrotising process usually due to group A streptococci, involving the deep fascia and vessels within it, with secondary death of overlying skin.

This uncommon process can occur in healthy subjects, but arterial insufficiency and diabetes predispose. Necrotising fasciitis usually begins like cellulitis, but after about 2 days the area becomes purplish, haemorrhagic bullae appear and there is evident tissue death. Untreated, there is a high mortality.

The diagnosis is often based on clinical suspicion alone, but streptococci can often be found in exudate or the blood.

Treatment by urgent and adequate surgical debridement is essential, together with parenteral penicillin or erythromycin if there is penicillin hypersensitivity.

Progressive bacterial synergistic gangrene

Progressive bacterial synergistic gangrene is gangrenous ulceration due to synergistic infection, with micro-aerophilic streptococci and *Staph. aureus*, usually associated with an abdominal or thoracic operation wound.

One to two weeks after surgery there is a slowly spreading area of ulceration which has a rim of gangrenous skin surrounded by purplish erythema. The main differential diagnosis is pyoderma gangrenosum (see p. 1142).

Treatment is by surgical debridement plus antibiotic therapy based on sensitivity tests.

Follicular infections

A furuncle (boil) is an acute necrotising infection of a follicle. A carbuncle is more extensive, involving contiguous follicles and the tissues around them. Infection of the hair follicle opening is termed superficial folliculitis.

The usual infecting organism is *Staph. aureus*, and there is often nasal, axillary or perineal carriage of the organism. Friction, as at the nape of the neck, and moisture, as in the flexures, are important predisposing factors. Obesity, poor hygiene, widespread skin disease, immune deficiency and diabetes mellitus may predispose in severe cases. Superficial folliculitis can be non-infective; causes include contact with oils and other irritant chemicals.

Furuncles are tender red papules or nodules, which become pustular centrally and often heal with some scarring. Furunculosis may be chronic, as in sycosis barbae, a pustular eruption due to *Staph. aureus* occurring on the male face. Carbuncles are often associated with fever and malaise, and with an underlying systemic illness such as diabetes or immune suppression.

Follicular infections can produce bacteraemia and, rarely, bony and cerebral abscesses, and endocarditis.

Swabs should be taken from pus and from the anterior nares, axilla and perineum of the patient and household contacts (potential reservoirs of infection) in chronic cases.

Differential diagnosis. The differential diagnosis includes dermatophyte infection (the fungi can be demonstrated by microscopy and culture of hairs) and pseudofolliculitis, a non-infective papulopustular condition on the face and neck, due to cut hairs growing back into the skin. The latter is very common in black people because their hair is tightly curled. Acne vulgaris (p. 1161) can usually be distinguished by the presence of comedones, and the pustules are sterile. Hidradenitis suppurativa is discussed on page 1161. In anthrax (see Ch. 11) there is a haemorrhagic crust and vesicular margin and a swab will establish the diagnosis.

Treatment. Furuncles and carbuncles may need incision and drainage. Superficial staphylococcal folliculitis should respond to flucloxacillin (or equivalent) for 1–2 weeks, but chronic cases may need treatment for longer, and treatment of reservoir sites, e.g. chlorhexidine for the skin and mupirocin for the nose.

Erythrasma

Erythrasma (Fig. 25.4) is a common surface infection caused by *Corynebacterium minutissimum*. Sharply defined red or reddish-brown patches, sometimes with slight scaling, are seen in the axillae, groins, toe webs and sometimes other body folds. There are usually no symptoms.

The diagnosis is readily made with Wood's light; the affected skin fluoresces pink.

Most cases respond to a topical imidazole, e.g. clotrimazole, but if widespread, oral erythromycin for 10 days may be more effective.

Erysipeloid

Erysipeloid is an acute cutaneous infection with *Erysipelothrix insidiosa*. This Gram-positive bacillus causes infection in several animals and salt-water fish. Transfer to the skin occurs mainly to veterinary-surgeons, butchers, fish-handlers and housewives.

The hand is the common site. A few days after inoculation there is a well-defined, slowly spreading, dusky erythematous oedema with little or no general upset (in contrast with erysipelas).

Treatment is with penicillin or tetracycline.

Pseudomonas infection of the skin

Pseudomonas aeruginosa is not normally found on the skin, but can become pathogenic, with production of a characteristic bluish-green pus and a fruity odour in circum-

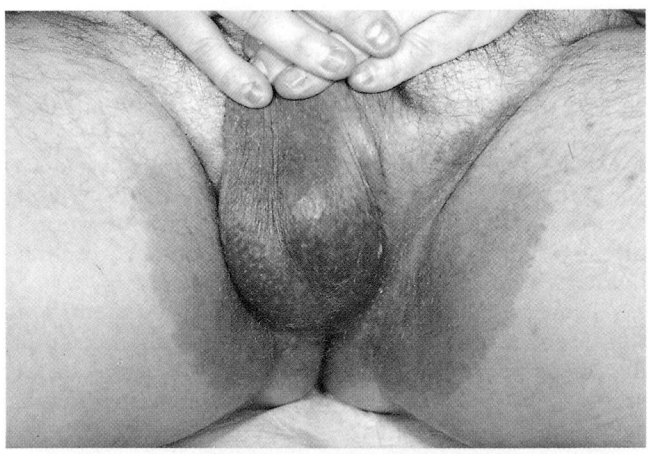

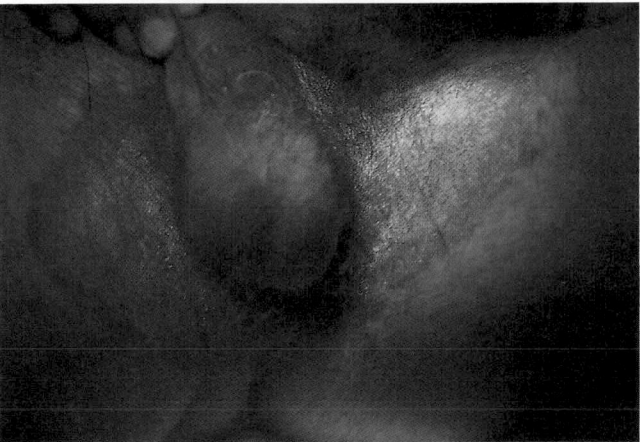

Fig. 25.4 Erythrasma. Well-defined brownish erythema which fluoresces pink by Wood's light.

stances of increased moisture. Examples may be found at the base of the nail in those whose hands are often immersed in water, toe spaces, beneath dressings for ulcers, and very importantly on raw surfaces following burns. Prior eradication of Gram-positive flora may also predispose. A pruritic pseudomonas folliculitis can be acquired from contaminated whirlpools. Localised infection usually responds to simple antiseptic measures, such as acetic acid, silver nitrate or silver sulphadiazine, together with drying.

Pseudomonas septicaemia can produce solitary or widespread vesicles with surrounding red haloes. Subsequent necrosis, often with haemorrhage into the tissues producing black crusts, is known as ecthyma gangrenosum. The lesions, as well as the blood, should yield *Pseudomonas* on culture, and prompt treatment can be life-saving.

Kawasaki's disease

Kawasaki's disease (mucocutaneous lymph node syndrome), described by Kawasaki in 1967, is most common

in parts of Japan but probably has a worldwide distribution. The natural history of the illness suggests an infective aetiology but none has been identified. It is most common in toddlers and rare after 8 years of age; there is a slight male predominance among cases (1.6:1).

Clinical features. Characteristically the child is irritable and febrile and the limbs are tender peripherally. The rash is variable and may look like a severe measles eruption, but the sequence of appearance – on the head, followed by trunk and then limbs – is absent, and the swelling and tenderness of the hands and feet are not compatible with measles. Desquamation of a thick layer of skin starting around the nails and sometimes involving the whole hand and foot occurs later and is a distinctive feature. It differs from staphylococcal toxin-induced desquamation in the thickness of the layer involved, and from streptococcal desquamation, which is flaky. The disease resolves after 6–10 weeks.

About 20% of patients have some cardiac involvement, and myocarditis, with or without aneurysm of the proximal part of the coronary arteries, causes a mortality of 2% in Japanese series. Although small aneurysms have been demonstrated in 17% of patients investigated by coronary angiography, most of these resolve spontaneously. Postmortem pathology shows a small vessel angiitis with thrombus formation as the initiating lesion.

Treatment. Aspirin has been shown to cause early resolution of symptoms and fever; it is used in low dose to inhibit platelet aggregation if thrombocytosis develops. Corticosteroids are not indicated; they may encourage aneurysm formation.

Mycobacterial and treponemal diseases

Tuberculosis (p. 471), leprosy (p. 270) and syphilis (p. 273) all have important cutaneous manifestations.

SUPERFICIAL FUNGAL DISEASES

Fungal infections involving the skin are broadly classified into superficial and deep. The former include the ringworm fungi (dermatophytes), candidiasis and pityriasis versicolor. Except for *Candida*, these fungi rarely invade deeper than the horny layer of the epidermis. Nails and hair, as well as the skin surface, may be involved (Fig. 25.5). The clinical manifestations depend partly on the infecting species, on the body part affected and on the host response to substances diffusing from the fungi into the skin. Deep fungal infections are discussed in Chapter 11.

Diagnosis. Diagnosis is by microscopic examination of scrapings to show fungal hyphae, and species identification is by culture. The dermatophytes are grown on Sabouraud's medium. With skin lesions scale is collected

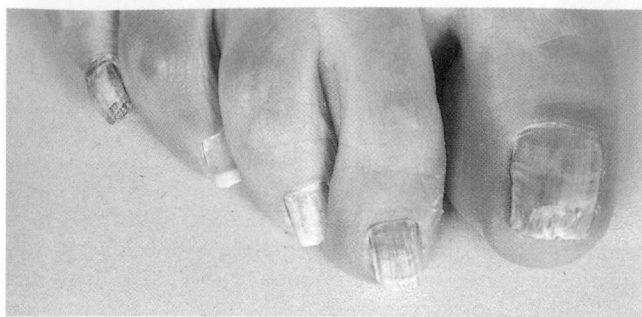

Fig. 25.5 Distal thickening and yellow discoloration due to fungal infection.

by scraping with a blade, hair is plucked and clippings taken from nails. Material is sent to the laboratory dry in folded paper. Microscopy is performed on small samples after clearing with a few drops of 30% potassium hydroxide. For some species of scalp dermatophyte infection and for pityriasis versicolor the Wood's light is valuable (p. 1122).

Tinea

The fungi causing the characteristic annular lesions known as tinea or ringworm (Fig. 25.6) are also known as the dermatophytes, for they have the ability to digest keratin. There are three genera – *Trichophyton*, *Microsporum* and *Epidermophyton* – and numerous species which are recognised by their culture characteristics. Humans are the primary host for some (the anthropophilic species), but with others the fungi are incidental pathogens to man,

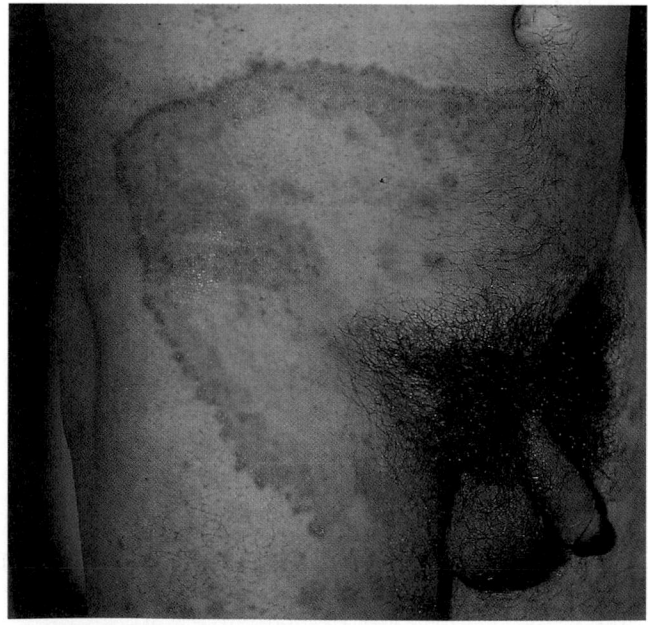

Fig. 25.6 The annular lesions of tinea (ringworm).

being primarily animal parasites (zoophilic) or found in soil (geophilic). The immune response is most marked against zoophilic species and these tend not to recur. With very inflammatory ringworm there can be so-called 'id' reactions, due to the immune response. These are widespread, often follicular, papular lesions which do not contain fungi. Probably for similar reasons, a vesicular eruption on the hands can be associated with ringworm of the feet. The distinctive appearance of ringworm infections can be greatly modified by topical steroids.

Treatment. Successful treatment requires attention to sources of reinfection and measures to deal with acutely inflamed macerated skin, such as aluminium acetate soaks, as well as specific antifungal preparations. Topical agents, including Whitfield's ointment, and various imidazoles are suitable for localised skin infection. Oral terbinafine is the treatment of choice for hair, nail, widespread and chronic skin infections but is not yet licensed in the UK for use in children. Itraconazole and griseofulvin are alternatives. A weak topical steroid, together with antifungal therapy, may be useful if there is much inflammation.

Tinea pedis

Tinea pedis is a dermatophyte infection of the feet, sometimes with concurrent bacterial infection. This very common, often chronic condition is frequently acquired where bathing facilities are shared, and infection is favoured by maceration. It is much commoner in males.

The most common pattern is an itchy, inflamed, fissured, moist toe space, usually between the fourth and fifth toes. It is often unilateral. A vesicular pattern may occur involving the instep, dorsum of the foot or sides of the toes. A very chronic pattern may be seen, with hyperkeratosis and fine white scaling accentuating skin creases on the soles. Tinea pedis may be accompanied by cellulitis.

Tinea pedis can resemble eczema, contact dermatitis, candidal infection and psoriasis. Endogenous eczema and psoriasis are more likely to be bilateral.

Most toe space infections respond to a topical antifungal agent, but extensive involvement of the soles needs oral treatment. Regular cleansing of communal bathing facilities and prophylactic use of antifungal powders help reduce transmission of infection.

Tinea cruris

Tinea cruris is a dermatophyte infection of the groins and adjacent skin. Like tinea pedis, with which it is often associated, tinea cruris is much more common in males.

Itching is very common. There is inflammation with a well-defined margin which is scaly, vesicular or occasionally pustular, often with central clearing.

The differential diagnosis includes candidiasis, in which there is a less well-defined edge and outlying tiny pustules. Erythrasma is not usually inflammatory. Intertrigo, an inflammatory process common in the obese, in which friction sweating and minor bacterial infection cause erythema in body folds, can mimic tinea cruris, but scrapings will be negative. Eczema and psoriasis can usually be recognised by their characteristic appearances on non-flexural skin elsewhere.

For limited infection treatment with a topical imidazole is sufficient. For extensive involvement, topical steroid treated cases or when therapy fails, however, oral therapy is needed for 3–6 weeks.

Tinea corporis

Tinea corporis is often of animal origin, and is then self-limiting. Lesions are usually multiple and often, but not always, ring-shaped. Because the appearances are so variable, scrapings should be taken from any red, scaly rash that cannot be readily diagnosed. If the disease is limited in extent, a topical agent is usually sufficient; if widespread, then oral terbinafine or itraconazole are preferable.

Tinea capitis

Many different fungal species can infect hair and scalp skin (Table 25.9). Affected hairs may break off a few millimetres above the scalp, producing short stubble, or flush with the scalp, giving bald patches with black dots in dark-haired patients. When there is a marked degree of inflammation, producing an appearance like that of a carbuncle, the lesion is called a *kerion*, and in this circumstance there may be concurrent staphylococcal infection. An appearance known as *favus* is now very rare in the UK. In this form yellowish cup-shaped crusts develop, together with hair loss. Both kerion and favus can produce permanent alopecia.

Distinction of fungal infection from other causes of patchy hair loss can be made by microscopy and culture.

Tinea of the hand

A diffuse hyperkeratosis with fine powdery accentuation of the palmar creases, usually of only one hand, is the commonest pattern of tinea of the hand. If there is diagnostic doubt, scrapings should be taken.

Tinea of nails

In many cases nail infection (onychomycosis) occurs in conjunction with fungal disease elsewhere. Predisposing factors include previous trauma and poor peripheral circulation. The toenails are more commonly affected than fingernails. The changes spread proximally from the free edge. The nail plate becomes discoloured and usually thickened, and may crumble away. It may also separate from the nail bed (onycholysis) (Fig. 25.5).

Confirmation of the diagnosis by microscopy and culture of clippings should precede treatment. The differential diagnosis includes psoriasis, in which there is often a distinctive pattern of fine pitting. Candidal infection produces changes that begin proximally. Eczema can simulate fungal infection.

Treatment is with oral terbinafine or griseofulvin.

Candidiasis

Most human candidal infection is caused by *Candida albicans* (Fig. 25.7). This yeast is a common commensal in the gastrointestinal tract, mouth and vagina, but not on

Table 25.9 Types of tinea capitis

Clinical pattern	Representative species	Wood's light fluorescence	Source
Patchy baldness, with broken-off hairs and scaling of the scalp	*Microsporum canis*	Blue-green	Puppies, kittens
	Microsporum audouini	Green	Humans
Patchy baldness with black dots	*Trichophyton tonsurans*	–	Humans
	Trichophyton violaceum	–	Humans
Kerion	*Trichophyton verrucosum*	–	Cattle
Favus	*Trichophyton schoenleinii*	Dull green	Humans

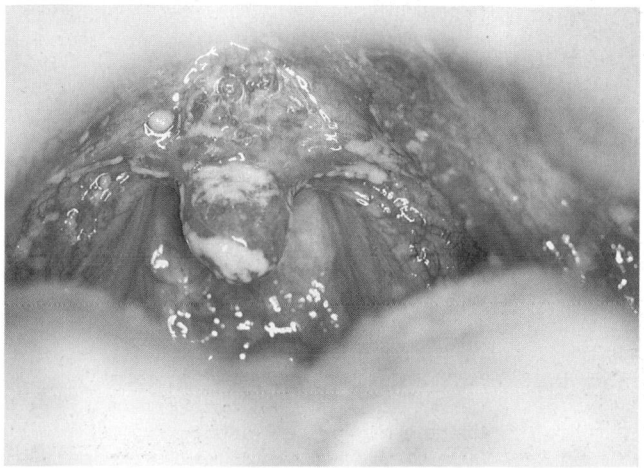

Fig. 25.7 Candidiasis, a superficial fungal infection.

Table 25.10 Some factors facilitating candidal infection

Local	General
Maceration of skin	Debility
Topical steroids	Extremes of age
Dentures	Immunosuppression by drugs or
Poor oral hygiene	disease, particularly HIV
High oral carbohydrate levels	Broad-spectrum antibiotics
	Corticosteroids
	Diabetes mellitus
	Iron deficiency
	Cushing's syndrome
	Hypocalcaemia/hypoparathyroidism
	Pregnancy

the skin. However, it may become pathogenic (Table 25.10).

Unlike the dermatophyte fungi, *Candida* invades living tissue. In some circumstances serious systemic infection can occur (see also p. 279). Some of the clinical patterns of candidal infection of the skin and mucosal surfaces are shown in Table 25.11.

When infection is widespread and refractory to treatment this may be due to an immune deficiency. The skin

Table 25.11 Clinical patterns of *Candida* infection

Type	Pattern of infection	Features
Oral		
Thrush	White patches (Fig. 25.7)	Can be scraped off to reveal inflamed mucous membrane
Atrophic candidiasis	Painful red atrophic mucous membrane	Common with antibiotic treatment and dentures
Chronic hyperplastic candidiasis	Thickened white adherent plaques	Needs differentiating from leukoplakia
Angular stomatitis	Soreness and fissuring at the angles	Occurs in folds, usually due to ill-fitting old dentures
Skin		
Flexural	Sore, red, marginated skin, often with outlying pustules	Due to maceration
Ano-genital		
Vulvo-vaginitis	Itchy, sore with curd-like discharge	Commoner in pregnancy
Balanitis	Tiny red papules and pustules on glans and prepuce	Usually from sexual partner
Nails		
Paronychia	Painful swollen nail folds with loss of adhesion of cuticle	Maceration predisposes. May have poor peripheral circulation
Onychia	Thickened, discoloured nails	Uncommon, often associated with immune defects

lesions in such patients often resemble ringworm, and nails as well as nail folds tend to be affected. There are several clinical/genetic types.

In *group I* there is a well-defined major primary immune defect, e.g. Swiss type agammaglobulinaemia. *Group II* comprises those cases without such a clear-cut primary immune defect. Subgroups include:

- the *Candida* endocrinopathy syndrome, with hypoparathyroidism and Addison's disease being the commoner associated organ-specific autoimmune diseases
- autosomal recessive
- autosomal dominant
- diffuse (severe) mucocutaneous candidiasis
- late-onset candidiasis, in which thymoma and HIV infections should be considered.

Treatment of Candida *infections*

Any remediable predisposing factors should be dealt with. Locally active agents include nystatin, amphotericin B and the imidazoles. For chronic oral candidiasis prolonged treatment is often necessary. Oral agents, including itraconazole and fluconazole, are usually required for chronic mucocutaneous candidiasis, a common problem in patients with symptomatic HIV infection.

Pityriasis versicolor

Pityriasis (tinea) versicolor (Fig. 25.8) is a superficial infection caused by the mycelial form of the commensal yeast *Pityrosporum orbiculare* (also known as *Malassezia furfur*).

For most patients who have the disorder it is assumed that there has been a change in the pathogenicity of their surface commensal yeasts. Young adults are the most affected and it is seen more in the tropics and subtropics. The distinctive hyper- and hypopigmentation is due to the diffusion into the epidermis of azelaic acid, a fatty acid from the fungus, which affects the melanocytes.

Clinical features. The upper trunk, arms and neck are the commonest sites. Lesions are macular and sharply demarcated, and have fine scaling. They may become confluent over large areas. On sun-protected 'white' skin the patches are skin-coloured or pale brown, but after sun exposure and in darker races they are hypopigmented.

Scrapings show a mixture of clustered spherical yeasts and short mycelia. By Wood's light the affected areas fluoresce and it is often apparent that the infection is more widespread than can be seen by visible light.

Treatment. Treatment by 2.5% selenium sulphide in a detergent base applied to affected areas and the scalp (a reservoir of yeasts) left on overnight and repeated a week later, usually clears the condition. Alternatives include topical imidazoles and oral itraconazole.

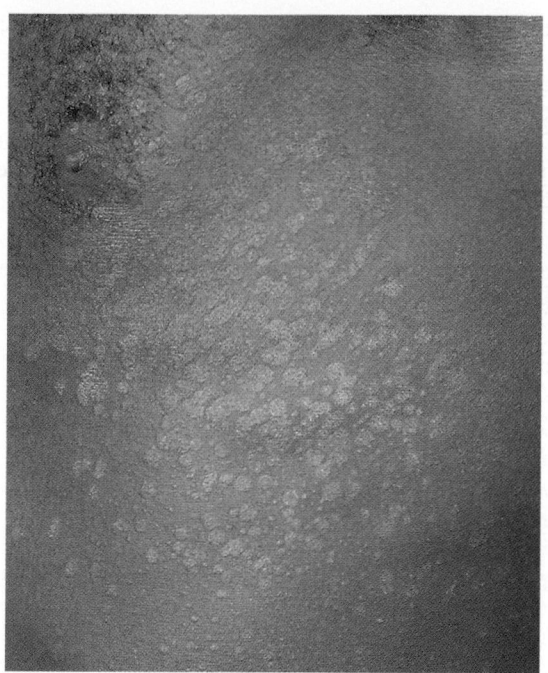

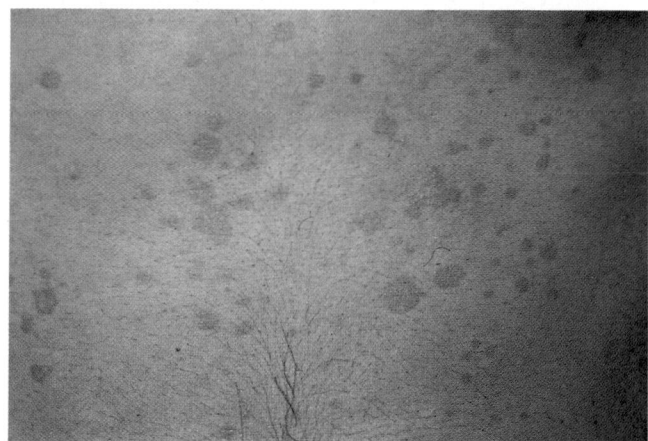

Fig. 25.8 Slightly scaly macules of pityriasis versicolor; brown on a white skin and pale on a tanned skin.

VIRAL DISEASES

Skin lesions are a common feature of many viral infections and may represent the direct consequences of virus replication (e.g. warts), the immune response to a virus, or interaction of the two. Only those where the skin or adjacent mucous membranes are the sole target are discussed here; the remainder, including herpes simplex and zoster, are considered in Chapter 11.

Table 25.12 Viral warts

Type of wart	Main site	Appearance
Common	Hand	Dome-shaped, papilliferous surface
Plane (flat)	Face and backs of hands	Flat-topped; smooth papules
Filiform	Face and neck	Elongated
Digitate	Scalp and neck	Elongated with horny cap
Plantar (verruca)	Soles	Circumscribed, often painful papules or nodules with altered surface pattern, sometimes with black dots
Mosaic plantar	Soles	Aggregation of numerous adjacent plantar warts
Ano-genital	Anal and genital regions	Soft, velvety, vegetative papules and plaques

Warts

Warts arise because of hypertrophy of the prickle cell layer of the skin (or adjacent mucous membranes) induced by human papilloma virus. Warts are transmissible, inoculation being favoured by mild trauma. They are commoner in children and young adults, and are usually self-limiting and benign. However, some subtypes of virus (defined by DNA hybridisation techniques), particularly those found in the genital tract and the rare condition epidermodysplasia verruciformis, predispose to squamous carcinoma.

The hands, feet, face, around the knees, peri-anal and genital skin are the commonest sites (Table 25.12).

Because most warts resolve spontaneously, caution is needed in assessing therapy, and methods such as scalpel surgery and radiotherapy should be abandoned. For many non-genital warts, salicylic acid paints (or plasters for large plantar warts) are effective. Cryotherapy (p. 1123) is uncomfortable but often more rapidly successful. Recently, intralesional bleomycin has proved effective. In selected cases curettage and minimal cautery may be needed.

Venereal warts are frequently associated with other sexually transmitted diseases, requiring appropriate investigations. These lesions usually respond to liquid nitrogen cryotherapy or careful applications of podophyllin paint at weekly intervals, but this agent should be avoided during pregnancy because of the enhanced risk of absorption and fetal damage.

Molluscum contagiosum

Molluscum contagiosum (Fig. 25.9) is a contagious papular eruption caused by a DNA pox virus. It mainly

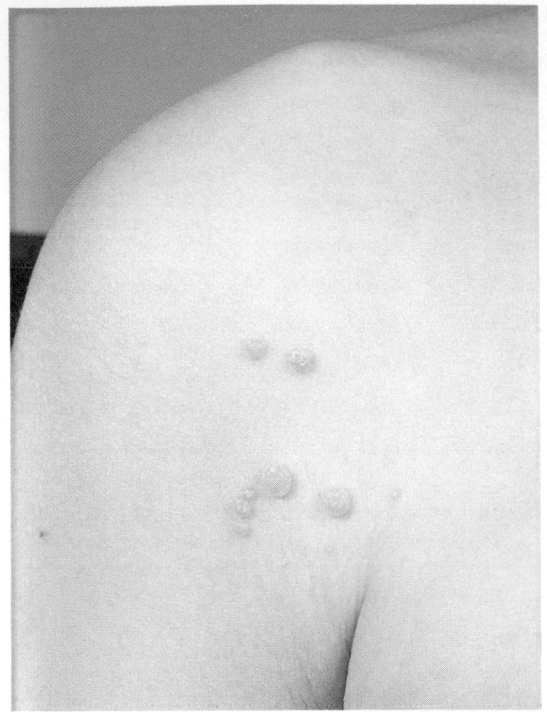

Fig. 25.9 Domed umbilicated papules of molluscum contagiosum.

occurs in children but is also common in AIDS patients. The lesions are smooth, dome-shaped papules, often crater-like with a central keratinous plug or depression. When multiple, they are typically in groups. Lesions are ultimately self-limiting.

Direct microscopic examination of the cheesy contents or an entire curetted lesion reveals the characteristic egg-shaped molluscum bodies. (These are epidermal cells filled with virus particles.) Electron microscopy can also be used.

Single lesions can mimic benign or malignant epithelial tumours, e.g. keratoacanthoma or basal cell carcinoma.

In young children it is often best to leave the lesions. Treatment is local destruction, e.g. with liquid nitrogen or by mildly traumatising the papules and then painting with iodine.

Orf and milkers' nodules

Orf is a pox viral disease of sheep, usually acquired directly from the peri-oral lesions occurring on lambs. Milkers' nodule is a similar condition acquired from infection of teats of cows and ulcers in the mouths of calves. It is caused by a parapox virus.

Several days after animal contact, a red papule appears, and evolves into a 1–2 cm diameter smooth, bluish-red nodule, the centre of which may develop a crusted surface. There is often a whitish ring around the central crust with orf nodules. There may be lymphangitis and lymphadenopathy, and sometimes a rash on the limbs resembling erythema multiforme (p. 1141). Resolution occurs in 3–4 weeks.

Diagnosis is usually evident from the history. Electron microscopy can confirm the diagnosis. No treatment is required.

ARTHROPODS AND THE SKIN

Numerous arthropods can inflict skin lesions on man, by the mechanisms listed below:

- *mechanical trauma* (e.g. horse-fly, tungiasis)
- *injection of toxins* (e.g. some spiders, bees, wasps, ants)
- *hypersensitivity* (local and generalised) to injected materials (e.g. many arthropods, such as fleas, bed-bugs); contact reactions (e.g. locusts); to an invading parasite (e.g. scabies); to retained mouth-parts, etc. (e.g. tick bite granulomas)
- *secondary infection* (e.g. many insect bites, scabies)
- *transmission of disease* (e.g. leishmaniasis, erythema chronicum migrans – caused by a spirochaete.

Insect bite reactions should be suspected when there are grouped or linear arrays of itchy weals or papules. The lesions last longer than urticaria. Fleas and mites, often from domestic pets, mosquitoes, gnats, midges and bedbugs, are frequent causes of this common problem. A careful history and examination of brushings from pets, their bedding, and house dust can help identify the cause.

Scabies

Scabies (Fig. 25.10) is an itchy dermatosis caused by the human mite *Sarcoptes scabiei*.

Clinical features. The female mite, just visible to the naked eye, makes the necessary journey from one human

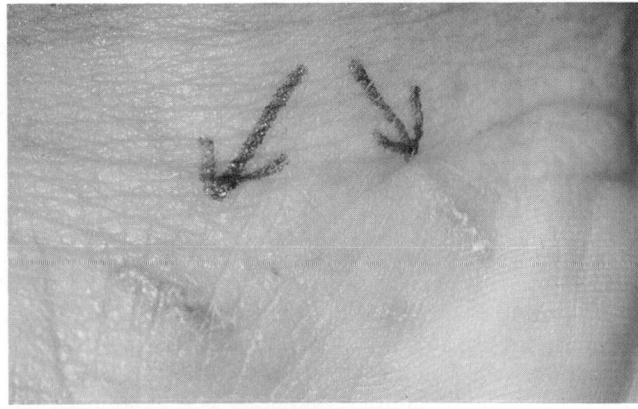

Fig. 25.10 Scabies burrows on wrists.

to another during close bodily contact and burrows into the horny layer, producing a serpiginous greyish elevation 1–10 mm long. Burrows are most commonly seen on the finger webs, wrists, elbows, around the nipples in women and on the male genitalia. In children the palms, soles and even face may be colonised and vesicles and pustules may be evident. In addition there is a widespread papular rash and extensive excoriation, probably the result of an allergic reaction to mite products.

Generally there are only a few burrows at a time, but in so-called crusted or Norwegian scabies there are vast numbers, particularly on the hands. This mainly occurs in mental defectives, the immunosuppressed, the elderly and those who are unable to scratch.

With an initial attack there is a latent period of about 2 months before itching begins, but this is much less with subsequent episodes. The itching is often severe and tends to be worse at night. The distinctive burrows are usually overshadowed by widespread excoriations, eczematisation and secondary infection.

Diagnosis. Mites can be extracted from burrows with a needle; somewhat easier is scraping the area after applying a drop of mineral oil or 30% potassium hydroxide and viewing the material microscopically for mites, eggs, faeces, etc.

Treatment. The patient and all close contacts should be treated with a scabicide such as lindane, malathion, benzyl benzoate or permethrin, from the neck downwards. When properly applied, one dose is usually curative, but sometimes two applications 3 days apart are needed. Pruritus may continue for up to 2 weeks and can be helped by crotamiton (a less effective scabicide which also has antipruritic properties) or a topical steroid.

Other mites

Dogs, cats, birds, grain and stored foodstuffs are sometimes sources of mites that can attack man, producing itchy papules, often topped by tiny vesicles, and weals. Harvest mites, minute red creatures found in grass and other low vegetation, can produce similar and often very florid lesions. Diagnosis involves finding the offending mite, e.g. from brushings of pets.

Fleas

Fleas include varieties that can burrow into skin (e.g. *Tunga penetrans*, found only in the tropics) and those that feed on the skin. In general the human flea is unusual, but occurs in overcrowded communities with poor hygiene. Bites from fleas living on pets, birds and occasionally wild animals, such as hedgehogs, are very common.

The reaction to a flea bite is a hypersensitivity response. Individual lesions are like urticaria but often have a haemorrhagic central punctum and last a week or two.

They characteristically occur in groups, and often leave hyperpigmentation as they resolve. Troublesome itching can be treated with an oral antihistamine and secondary infection with an antibiotic.

When the domestic pet is the source, the diagnosis can often be confirmed by examination of brushings from the animal. Flea faeces in this material stain damp white blotting paper red. The pet, and often the environment, need appropriate treatment.

Bedbugs

Bedbugs (*Cimex lectularius*) are nocturnal, wingless, blood-sucking insects, live in crevices in the walls, floor and furniture and can best be seen in the middle of the night. The lesions following their bites often do not appear until well into the next day. They mainly occur on the face and upper limbs. The environment should be treated with an insecticide.

Lice

Lice are obligate human parasitic wingless insects. The itchy reactions are a result of sensitisation. There are two species: *Pediculus humanus*, which occurs in two varieties – the head and body louse, and *Phthirus pubis* – the pubic or crab louse.

Head lice

Head louse infection is very common in children, presenting as intense irritation, particularly at the back of the scalp. Secondary infection is frequent and may be mistakenly diagnosed as impetigo of the scalp. The insect is 3–4 mm long but usually the eggs and egg cases (nits) are much more easily seen, firmly cemented to the hairs. Treatment is with malathion or carbaryl. Contacts should also be treated.

Body lice

The body louse is rare in developed countries, except in cases of self-neglect. There is widespread irritation with papules and excoriation. The lice and their eggs are best found on the clothing, particularly the seams, and are best treated by hot tumble drying.

Pubic lice

Pubic lice have legs somewhat like crabs' pincers with which they are often found clinging to hairs. Secondary infection is common, and since these creatures are often acquired during sexual intercourse other venereal disease should be excluded. Treatment is with lindane or malathion.

PSORIASIS

Psoriasis is a non-infective, usually chronic inflammatory skin disease with a number of clinical manifestations, the most common of which is red plaques covered by silvery scales (Fig. 25.11). A distinctive arthritis may occur and nails are often involved. Genetic and environmental factors interact to account for the capricious natural history.

Aetiology

Psoriasis occurs in about 2% of the population in Britain, but is less common in other countries, notably West Africa and Japan. The condition may present at any age but onset is most common at puberty and the menopause. Additional triggering factors, both of onset and recurrence, are *infection*, especially streptococcal pharyngitis which characteristically provokes guttate psoriasis; *trauma* to the skin, generating new psoriatic lesions (the Koebner phenomenon, see below); and some *drugs*, notably lithium salts, systemic corticosteroids followed by their rapid withdrawal, and antimalarials. In some subjects UV radiation can initiate psoriasis on exposed skin. Rarely, hypocalcaemia provokes psoriasis. The importance of stress is disputed but sudden psychological trauma can play a part in initiating the disease and causing relapse.

The tendency to develop psoriasis is genetically determined but the mode of inheritance remains unclear. There is a close association with HLA-CW6 and HLA-DR7, the former conferring a 5–10-fold increased risk. HLA-B27 is seen in 70% of those patients with psoriasis and an ankylosing spondylitis pattern of spinal arthritis.

Pathology and pathogenesis

In the well-established psoriatic lesion there is epidermal thickening with increased mitoses, retention of nuclei in

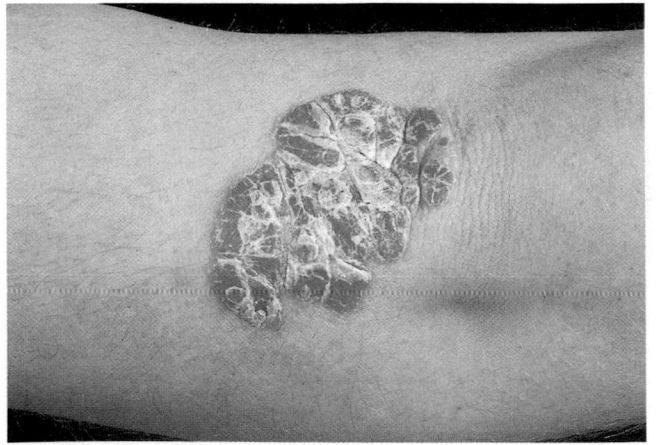

Fig. 25.11 Psoriasis: Well-defined red plaque with silvery scales.

the horny layer (parakeratosis) accounting for the silvery scales, small collections of neutrophil polymorphs in the epidermis, tortuous dilated dermal capillaries and a dermal inflammatory infiltrate. Cell kinetic studies show that epidermal turnover occurs in 5–7 days, compared with the normal 30–45 days. Epidermal maturation is also abnormal, not just as a consequence of the rapid throughput. There is no comprehensive theory to account for the many abnormalities demonstrated in the epidermis, dermis, circulating granulocytes and lymphocytes, and the humoral immune system. From work in which psoriatic skin is explanted on to athymic nude mice it seems that the increased proliferation is intrinsic to the skin. It is likely that circulating factors determine the overall activity of psoriasis and maintain the inflammatory process in the plaques.

Clinical features

The different patterns of psoriasis result from variations in expression of the disease (guttate, erythrodermic and pustular types) and modification of the features at certain sites, notably the scalp, flexures, palms and soles. The extent and duration are usually unpredictable, although some patterns are more likely to improve spontaneously, e.g. guttate psoriasis. Psoriasis means a condition (-iasis) of itching (psor-), but pruritus is not inevitable.

Discoid or plaque psoriasis. The well-defined, silvery-scaled red plaques may be found on any site, but knees, elbows, extensor surfaces of limbs and the lower back are commonly affected. Scratching the scales reveals many tiny bleeding points.

Flexural psoriasis. Psoriasis of the axillae, groins and beneath breasts is less readily recognised because the plaques are smooth, but usually remain more sharply defined than eczema. Lesions are typically symmetrical.

Scalp psoriasis. Scaling often becomes very thick, beneath which are tell-tale areas of well-defined erythema.

Psoriasis of palms and soles. This may be more hyperkeratotic, without the silvery scale, but usually remains well defined.

Guttate psoriasis. There are numerous scaly papules and small plaques. This type of psoriasis mainly occurs in children and adolescents.

Erythrodermic psoriasis. Total involvement of the skin can cause hypothermia and hypoproteinaemia (see also p. 1144).

Pustular psoriasis. Pustules occur when the neutrophil collections become clinically visible. The main varieties are a form localised to palms and soles, in which yellow, white or greenish pustules (sterile) arise on erythematous scaly skin (Fig. 25.12), and a generalised type. In the

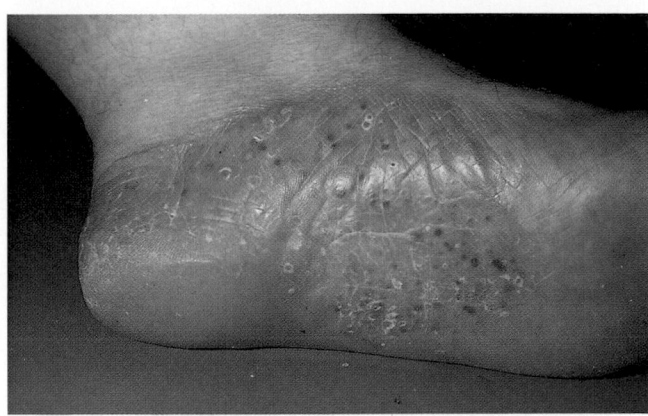

Fig. 25.12 Pustular psoriasis of the sole.

latter the patient is ill, with fever and leucocytosis, and large areas of erythema develop myriads of small sterile pustules which soon dry up and desquamate, to be followed by further waves of pustules. As with erythroderma, management entails rest, prevention of hypothermia, and maintenance of fluid, electrolyte and protein balance, as well as controlling the disease process. Localised pustular psoriasis of palms and soles is probably genetically distinct, there being no association with HLA-CW6 or HLA-DR7, and the condition often occurs without psoriasis elsewhere. Tar and dithranol are contraindicated in generalised pustular psoriasis and generally unhelpful in palmo-plantar pustular psoriasis.

Psoriatic nail changes. Common patterns are:

- multiple small pits, resembling a thimble (Fig. 25.13)
- onycholysis (separation of nail), often with an adjacent zone of orange discoloration
- subungual (nail bed) keratosis
- thickening and distortion of nails.

Nail changes are very common with psoriatic arthropathy involving the fingers.

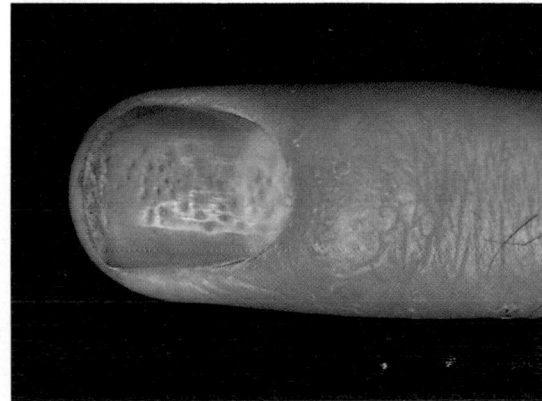

Fig. 25.13 Psoriatic nails showing thimble-like pitting.

Psoriatic arthropathy

Probably about 5% of psoriatics have a seronegative arthritis, although a much higher proportion have abnormalities detected by isotopic bone scans. Different patterns include:

- distal arthritis – terminal interphalangeal joints of fingers and interphalangeal joints of toes
- simulation of rheumatoid arthritis, but more asymmetrical
- sacro-iliitis and ankylosing spondylitis
- arthritis mutilans, involving multiple joints with marked bone resorption.

Diagnosis and management is discussed on page 1008.

Management

The choice of treatment will depend on many factors. These include the capabilities and lifestyle of the patient as well as the type, location, extent and severity of the psoriasis. The options shown in Table 25.13 will not be appropriate for every patient, and are often used in combination. Some patients will prefer not to have any treatment. Nails do not respond well to topical therapy, but may improve with the rest of the psoriasis, especially when systemic treatments are used.

Topical therapy

Rest and bland applications are important in acutely inflamed psoriasis, erythrodermic and generalised pustular psoriasis. Many cases with discoid lesions respond well to tar and dithranol preparations, although, particularly with the latter, it is wise to begin with a weak preparation and gradually increase the potency to minimise irritation. Topical steroids are less likely to clear psoriasis completely, but with due attention to their potential hazards they are useful for areas readily irritated, such as the flexures, genitalia, ears and face; they are often more effective on the palms and soles. The most potent preparations are best avoided, except on palms and soles, and even there they should be restricted to short courses.

The new vitamin D analogue Calcipotriol is effective and provides an effective alternative to tar and dithranol.

Ultraviolet (UV) radiation and photochemotherapy

UVB (p. 1157) is used both alone, e.g. for guttate psoriasis, and together with other modalities. Photochemotherapy (also known as PUVA) is the combination of long-wave UVA and the photosensitising drug psoralen, usually taken orally 2 hours previously. It is a powerful

Table 25.13 Treatment choices in psoriasis

Form	Site	First choice	Second choice	Third choice
Plaque	Face, flexures, genitalia	Topical steroid	Mild tar or weak dithranol	
	Scalp	Tar gel or pomade	Dithranol	Topical steroid
	Trunk, limbs: few plaques	Dithranol	Tar or Calcipotriol	Topical steroid
	Trunk, limbs: many plaques	Dithranol ± UVB UVB	Calcipotriol or PUVA	Systemic therapy, e.g. methotrexate
	Palms and soles	Topical steroid Tar Dithranol	PUVA	Oral retinoid
Guttate		Mild tar ± UVB	UVB	Topical steroid
Erythrodermic with systemic complications		Oral retinoid	Methotrexate	Systemic steroid
Pustular psoriasis	Palms and soles	Topical steroid	PUVA	Oral retinoid
	Generalised	Oral retinoid	Methotrexate	Other systemic therapy

treatment for psoriasis but prolonged use is likely to age the skin prematurely and to induce non-melanoma skin cancer. Photochemotherapy is valuable for extensive plaque psoriasis when topical therapy is poorly tolerated or has failed, and can be successful for erythrodermic and pustular forms.

Systemic therapy

For the most severe forms of psoriasis, antimitotic and immunosuppressant drugs are used. Methotrexate is effective and reasonably safe. In long-term use hepatic fibrosis can occur and liver biopsies are recommended every 1–2 years to identify this before it is irreversible. Alcohol should be avoided. Cyclosporin A has recently been introduced for the treatment of cases where methotrexate is unsuitable. This drug is not antimitotic, and probably works by modulating the immune system. The main hazard is nephrotoxicity. Vitamin A derivatives (retinoids) with less toxicity than vitamin A itself have been found of value in pustular and erythrodermic psoriasis, and useful in combination with other treatments, e.g. photochemotherapy. Retinoids have a number of side-effects and, like methotrexate, are teratogenic, but they are not cytotoxic or immunosuppressant. They probably influence the disturbed maturation of the epidermis in psoriasis.

ECZEMA AND DERMATITIS

Eczema is a pattern of inflammation with many possible causes, rather than a disease. The different types are unified histopathologically by the presence of spongiosis in the epidermis.

The term 'dermatitis' is often used to imply an eczema of external origin, but it should always be qualified, as in 'contact allergic dermatitis', since 'dermatitis' is used in many other contexts, e.g. dermatitis artefacta, dermatitis herpetiformis, etc.

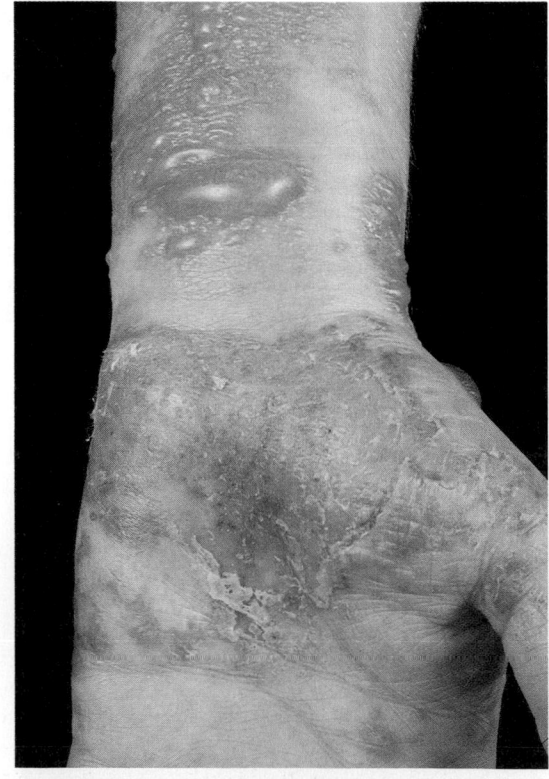

Fig. 25.14 Eczema. With intense inflammation there are vesicles and oozing; if the process continues, scaling and thickening occur.

Eczema is usually itchy and red; when the inflammation is intense, vesicles are seen and there is oozing from the surface (Fig. 25.14). If the process continues, scaling and thickening occur, and with rubbing and scratching lichenification (development of leather-like plaques) is common.

The earliest and most distinctive pathological change is spongiosis, the accumulation of oedema fluid within and between keratinocytes. Viewed in microscopic section, this produces an appearance somewhat like a sponge. In acute eczema the process extends to produce intra-epidermal vesicles. In the dermis, and to a lesser extent the epidermis, there is an inflammatory infiltrate in which lymphocytes are prominent. With time, both the epidermis and dermis become thickened.

Aetiological factors in eczema include:

- skin irritants
- contact allergens
- friction, low humidity, UV light
- infections (bacterial, dermatophytes, yeasts)
- atopic constitution
- drugs and foods
- local factors: venous stasis, ichthyosis.

Several factors may act in concert, particularly with eczema of the hand and lower leg, and not infrequently treatment is an inadvertent contributory factor. A careful history is essential in the evaluation of eczema. Several different clinical patterns of eczema and dermatitis (with eczematous features) are recognised. The basis for these patterns is well understood in some instances (e.g. contact allergic dermatitis) but obscure in others (e.g. discoid eczema). Since successful management depends on recognising external factors that are contributing to the skin disease, it is helpful to classify according to whether the disease process is primarily exogenous or endogenous, although these distinctions are somewhat artificial.

Whatever the cause, while active, eczema tends to spread, often beyond any recognisable stimulus such as a contact allergen. The face is often affected, even when not directly exposed to a causative agent.

EXOGENOUS ECZEMA

Irritant contact dermatitis

When the skin changes are a direct result of exposure and allergic mechanisms are not involved, the rash is termed irritant contact dermatitis. Not all reactions to irritants are eczematous; for example, the agent may produce necrosis or urticaria. Because obvious irritants tend to be avoided, the main problems occur with those which require prolonged and repeated contact, e.g. detergents, alkalis, mineral oils and organic solvents. Atopic individuals are particularly susceptible, as are housewives, hair-dressers and those in a number of industrial occupations. Even when a period of avoidance produces healing, chronic irritant dermatitis tends to recur readily with re-exposure.

Allergic contact dermatitis

Allergic contact dermatitis is the response to a substance to which the individual has become sensitised. Most such substances are of low molecular weight and penetrate the skin to behave as haptens. After conjugation with a skin protein the complete antigen is taken up by Langerhans cells, which migrate to regional lymph nodes and act as antigen-presenting cells in a T lymphocyte mediated (type IV) immune response. All subsequent contact with the sensitiser results in an acute eczematous reaction. This type of response is uncommon in children, although contact urticaria is frequent in atopics (see below).

Contact allergic dermatitis usually begins at the site of contact, but the clinical picture can at times be deceptive, e.g. nail varnish resin which causes no trouble locally but gives rise to eczematous patches when it is transferred to the face and neck by the fingers.

Many factors determine the acquisition of contact allergy. Some substances, e.g. epoxy resin and poison ivy, are inherently more likely to sensitise. Occlusion (e.g. a hand in a glove) and skin damage (e.g. from irritants) enhance penetration. It is possible that some individuals are more likely than others to be sensitised. The thick horny layer of the palms renders them less likely than the dorsa of the hands to be affected.

Once initiated, repeated exposure tends to produce increasingly severe and widespread dermatitis, and sites far removed, such as the eyelids, can be involved. The allergic state usually persists for life. Some common sensitisers are listed in Table 25.14.

Table 25.14 Some common sensitisers

Chemical	Source
Nickel	Jewellery, watch bands, silver coins
Chromate	Wet cement, many engineering processes, leather
Epoxy resin	Two-part glues
Paraphenylenediamine	Hair dyes
Rubber anti-oxidants	Gloves, shoes
Preservatives	Cosmetics and medicaments
Lanolin	Cosmetics and medicaments
Perfumes	Cosmetics and medicaments
Topical drugs	Neomycin, antihistamines, sulphonamides, some local anaesthetics
Colophony	Sticking plasters

The allergic state is reproduced in miniature by the application of a non-irritating dose of a suspected chemical beneath an occluding disc or patch placed on the back for 48 hours. Because some allergens are ubiquitous, a selection of common sensitisers is tested as well as any chosen on the basis of the patient's history. A positive reaction does not prove the cause of a patient's rash, but does help confirm suspicions and suggest unsuspected materials. Positive reactions may be only of past relevance.

Light-induced eczema

Eczema on light-exposed skin may be due to:

- *photo-contact allergy*, e.g. musk ambrette (a perfume in after-shave lotions); sunscreen medicaments – the essential role of UV radiation is shown by patch testing with and without UVR
- *photosensitive drug eruption*, e.g. chlorpromazine; sulphonamide; thiazide
- *exacerbation of existing eczema*, e.g. atopic dermatitis.

Phototoxic reactions, which resemble sunburn rather than eczema, can occur following contact with tar and its derivatives, some dyes and plants, and with drugs (p. 1150).

Sensitivity to airborne allergens can closely mimic light reactions, but areas normally spared from sun exposure, such as the skin beneath the ears, under the chin and around the eyes, are involved. Dermatomyositis may occasionally mimic a light-induced eruption.

ENDOGENOUS ECZEMA

Atopic eczema/dermatitis

Atopic eczema/dermatitis (Fig. 25.15) is closely associated with asthma, hay fever, urticaria and dry skin. There is usually a family history of one or more of these. The separate condition ichthyosis vulgaris (p. 1140) is probably more common in atopic individuals than the rest of the population. The skin readily becomes itchy in response to a number of allergic and non-allergic stimuli, and the pruritus may be disproportionate to the physical signs. High levels of circulating IgE antibodies are very common, as are multiple positive prick tests.

The disorder is very common, most cases beginning in infancy, and at least 10% of the population is affected to some degree. There is often a fluctuating course, but most cases clear up by adulthood, the majority within the first 5 years of life.

Aetiology

There is much evidence for a genetic basis for the atopic state, although how this is translated into the various clini-

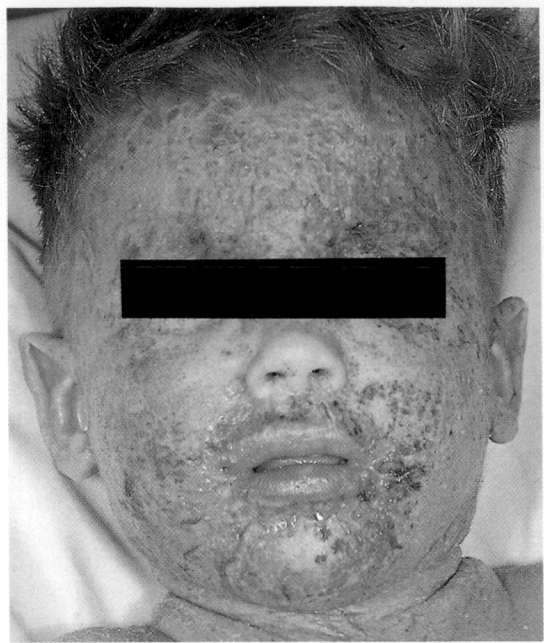

Fig. 25.15 Atopic dermatitis in a young child: erythema, weeping and crusting.

cal manifestations is unknown. A number of immunological abnormalities have been described, including the overproduction of IgE, reduced numbers of suppressor/cytotoxic T lymphocytes, and cutaneous basophil hypersensitivity, e.g. to house dust mite antigen.

Environmental factors are important determinants of fluctuations. These include ingested proteins (e.g. dairy products and eggs), and exposure to house dust mites, pollens and pet hair. Wool next to the skin frequently causes irritation. Extremes of climate often worsen the disease. Beyond a certain level of colonisation, *Staph. aureus* may produce flares of erythema and pruritus.

Clinical features

Onset is often in the first 3 months of life. Itching is the major symptom and at times there may be little rash. In infancy the skin is often patchily dry and red, with episodes of vesiculation and crusting. By 1–2 years the elbow and knee flexures, wrists, hands and tops of the feet are typically involved. With prolonged rubbing and scratching, papules and then leathery plaques (lichenification) are seen. At any stage secondary infection may occur with superimposition of impetigo and follicular pustules. Urticaria from contact, e.g. with a pet or foods, is also common.

Complications

Eczema may be complicated by erythroderma (p. 1144). Severely affected children are often growth-retarded.

Herpes simplex infection can be widespread (eczema herpeticum) and, particularly in the very young, may be disseminated to internal organs.

When eczema begins in infancy or early childhood the prognosis for recovery is generally good. Adults can be affected, especially when the skin is exposed to irritants, e.g. in nursing and hairdressing.

Management

The mainstays of management are avoidance of irritants such as bubble bath, *mild* topical steroids, plentiful use of emollients when the skin is dry, antibiotics when necessary, tar preparations for the more chronic and less inflamed lesions, and a sedative antihistamine at night. Cotton clothes and use of a soap substitute, e.g. emulsifying ointment or aqueous cream BP, are helpful. Current evidence suggests that children of atopic families should be breast-fed, at least up to 3 months if possible. Subsequent supervised dietary manipulation may be helpful.

Discoid eczema

Discoid (nummular) eczema consists of discrete rounded patches of eczema, usually symmetrically distributed, for which there is no apparent cause. The aetiology is unknown, and treatment is symptomatic.

Seborrhoeic eczema/dermatitis

Seborrhoeic eczema/dermatitis (Fig. 25.16) is of distinctive appearance and location. The cause is unknown but *Pityrosporum* yeasts play a part. There is usually no correlation with sebaceous activity although it is a disorder of areas where sebaceous glands are plentiful. Severe seborrhoeic dermatitis is an early feature in about one-third of AIDS patients.

There is less itching than with other eczemas. The lesions are yellowish-red, scaly away from flexures, and involve some or all of the following sites: scalp, eyelids, eyebrows, sides of nose, ears, axillae and groins, beneath the breasts, front of the chest, and upper back.

The differential diagnosis will depend on the sites affected. In the scalp, psoriasis can be very similar. In the flexures, psoriasis, contact allergic dermatitis, dermatophyte infections and candidiasis may need to be excluded; the truncal form can resemble pityriasis rosea and pityriasis versicolor (the latter diagnosed from a scraping). Methyldopa can produce a seborrhoeic dermatitis-like drug eruption.

The addition of sulphur, a mild tar, salicylic acid or an imidazole to a suitable topical steroid is often helpful. Shampoos containing ketoconazole, selenium sulphide or zinc pyrithione are useful for scalp involvement.

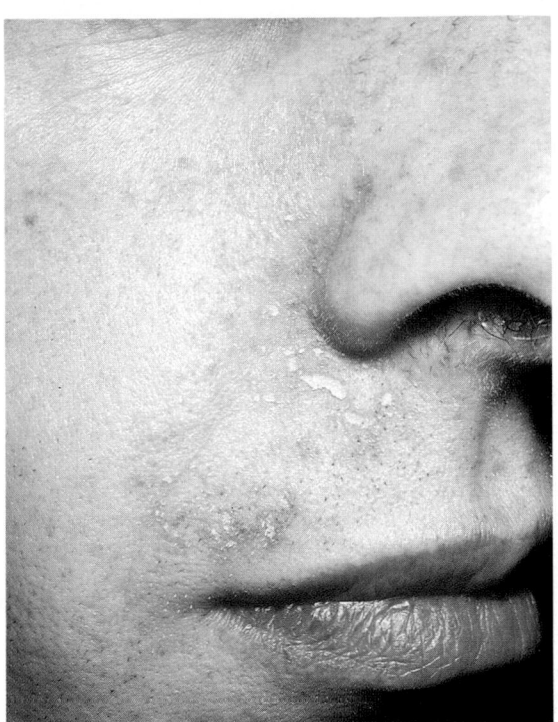

Fig. 25.16 Naso-labial erythema and scaling of seborrhoeic dermatitis.

Pompholyx

Pompholyx is an eruption of vesicles on the sides of fingers, palms and soles. Itching may be severe. The condition is usually episodic. Causes of pompholyx include: onset of warm weather, dermatitis or fungal infection of the feet (producing pompholyx of hands); ingestion of a contact allergen, e.g. nickel; and stress. Often no cause can be found. Treatment is symptomatic.

Asteatotic eczema

Asteatotic eczema is a mildly inflammatory condition which occurs mainly in the elderly on the shins, as erythema with a crazy paving-like pattern of superficial fissuring and scaling. It may be a result of reduced epidermal lipids. Hypothyroidism, uraemia, dehydration, low humidity and overzealous cleansing may contribute.

It often responds to less bathing and to emollients. A mild topical steroid ointment can be added if necessary.

Gravitational eczema

Eczema often occurs on the lower legs as a response to chronic venous hypertension, in association with haemosiderin staining, patchy atrophy, sclerosis, oedema and perhaps ulceration. It is particularly common near the medial malleolus in patients with previous deep vein thrombosis, but may also be seen in relation to varicose veins and incompetent perforating veins (p. 1161). Patches indistinguishable from discoid eczema may spread elsewhere.

Important in management are improvement of the venous hypertension, e.g. with support hosiery, and avoidance of potent topical steroids and potential sensitisers, such as neomycin, lanolin and preservatives.

Symptomatic treatment of eczema

Any causative and aggravating factors should be removed if at all possible. Acute weeping eczema can be soothed with wet compresses, e.g. aluminium acetate lotion BNF or 1:10 000 potassium permanganate solution, followed by a topical steroid cream. In some cases, particularly contact allergy, when a cause has been recognised and dealt with, a short course of systemic steroids is justified. For less acute eczema, a topical steroid of lowest effective potency is needed, often in a greasy base. If the surface is dry, additional applications of an emollient are helpful and reduce the likelihood of overuse of steroid. For chronic lichenification, tar preparations (e.g. as impregnated bandages) are valuable. Secondary infection is usually best treated with a systemic antibiotic, e.g. flucloxacillin or erythromycin.

ICHTHYOSIS

The term ichthyosis is used for a number of conditions in which there is either a disorder of keratinisation or shedding of the horny layer producing persistent, generalised, scaly skin (Fig. 25.17). Most types of ichthyosis are inherited and present in infancy or childhood. Onset in adulthood can be associated with an underlying neoplasm (p. 1153).

Ichthyosis vulgaris is the only common type, occurring in about 1 per 300 of the population. It is inherited as an autosomal dominant trait, and has distinctive histology: absence of the granular cell layer of the epidermis. Individuals have rough skin with white scales, maximal on the extensor surfaces and sparing the antecubital and popliteal fossae. There are often rough follicular papules

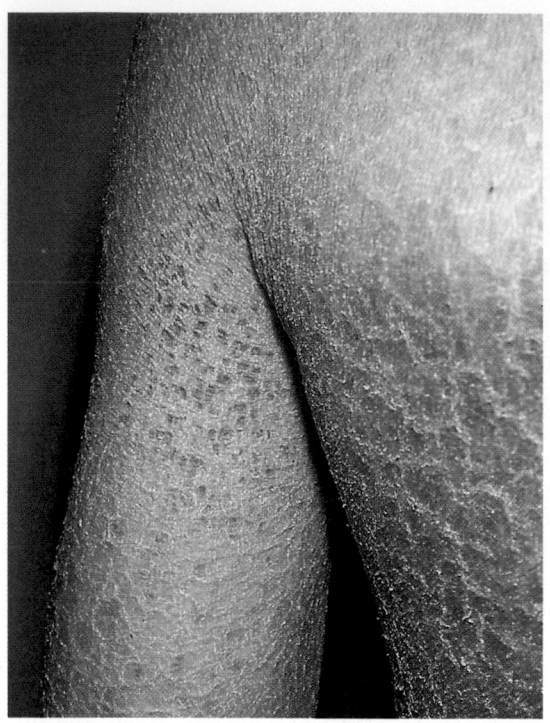

Fig. 25.17 Rough skin and scaling of ichthyosis.

(keratosis pilaris) on the upper arms and thighs. The physical signs are worse in winter. Avoidance of soap and regular use of emollients are helpful measures.

Sex-linked recessive ichthyosis occurs in about 1 per 6000. The female carrier may show mild changes, but the fully developed condition, as seen in the male, is more severe than ichthyosis vulgaris, with large brownish scales; the flexures are involved. The condition is characterised by steroid sulphatase deficiency.

Acquired ichthyosis has a similar clinical pattern to ichthyosis vulgaris. As well as being associated with neoplasis, particularly Hodgkin's disease, it can occur in gross nutritional deficiency.

REACTION PATTERNS

Despite the large number of named diseases, as an organ the skin has a limited range of reactions to noxious stimuli such as circulating immune complexes and infections. Some of these reaction patterns have sufficiently few common causes that their recognition can be a helpful step in arriving at a diagnosis. This may be particularly true when the patient has other symptoms, e.g. cough or malaise, for which there is no obvious cause.

A single aetiological factor may produce one or more of the reaction patterns described below. For example, the hepatitis B virus may lead to urticaria if the effect on dermal blood vessels is fully reversible, but purpuric vasculitis if the damage is more profound.

URTICARIA AND ANGIO-OEDEMA

The characteristic lesion in urticaria is a weal (Fig. 25.18). This is due to oedema in the dermis, so weals are raised and often pallid, but surrounded by a zone of erythema. Urticaria is evanescent, usually lasting from minutes to a few hours (rarely more than 24 hours) and fades without trace. Itching may be severe. Lesions initially like urticaria may occur in vasculitis, arthropod bites and stings, and lupus erythematosus, but in these circumstances they are more long-lasting. If there is doubt, a skin biopsy can be helpful in distinguishing these conditions. Urticaria lasting more than 3 months is regarded as chronic and in most cases no cause is found.

Angio-oedema occurs in the subcutaneous tissues, particularly where they are rather loosely organised such as in and around the mouth, around the eyes and on the

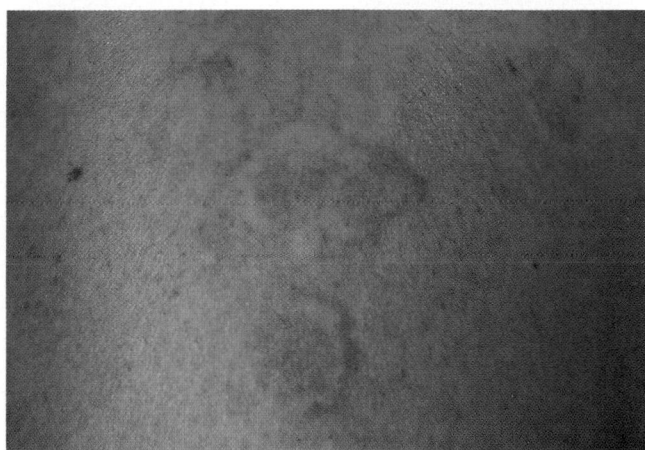

Fig. 25.18 Urticaria: arcuate weals.

Table 25.15 Common causes of urticaria and angio-oedema

Drugs Penicillin, aspirin, X-ray contrast medium	**Plants** Stinging nettles
Foods Azodyes, benzoate preservatives (chronic urticaria)	**Systemic disease** Hepatitis B, other virus infections, systemic lupus erythematosus
Arthropod reactions	**Contact urticaria** Some foods and pet saliva on atopics
Transfusion of blood products and foreign proteins	**Inhalants** Grass pollens, house dust
Physical stimuli Light pressure (dermographism), cold, light, increase in body temperature (cholinergic urticaria)	

Summary 2 Reaction patterns

- Urticaria and angio-oedema
- Erythema multiforme
- Erythema nodosum
- Pyoderma gangrenosum
- Cutaneous vasculitis
- Erythroderma

scrotum. The lesions are larger, less well defined and not necessarily itchy.

Common causes of urticaria and angio-oedema are listed in Table 25.15.

The basis for urticaria and angio-oedema is vasodilatation and extravasation of fluid due to release of mediators from mast cells and/or basophils. In some circumstances the mediators responsible can cause hypotension and bronchospasm, constituting anaphylactic shock (p. 94). Mechanisms include IgE and immune-complex-mediated reactions, and direct effects of chemicals, e.g. toxins and drugs. Symptomatic treatment is with H_1 antihistamines.

Hereditary angio-oedema is a rare but potentially life-threatening condition, in which non-pruritic swellings occur in the gastrointestinal and respiratory tracts as well as the skin and adjacent mucous membranes. A careful family history may suggest the diagnosis. There is either deficiency or an abnormality of the inhibitor of activated complement component C1. The best laboratory investigation is the measurement of C1 esterase inhibitor by antigenic activity or functional assay. Also useful is the demonstration of low C4 and C2, the substrates of activated and unopposed C1. Acute episodes may respond to C1 esterase inhibitor concentrate, and danazol can be used to suppress attacks.

ERYTHEMA MULTIFORME

The causes of erythema multiforme include:

- herpes simplex
- other infections, e.g. mycoplasma
- drugs, e.g. sulphonamides
- pregnancy
- collagen vascular disease, e.g. SLE.

The distinctive features of erythema multiforme are the target lesion (Fig. 25.19), the distribution of the rash and the histology. It is an acute eruption usually lasting about 3 weeks, maximally involving the hands and feet, forearms, elbows and knees. Among a variety of erythematous lesions there are usually some target lesions. These have a purplish or blistering centre inside one or more red rings. The mucosae of the mouth, genitalia and eyes may be

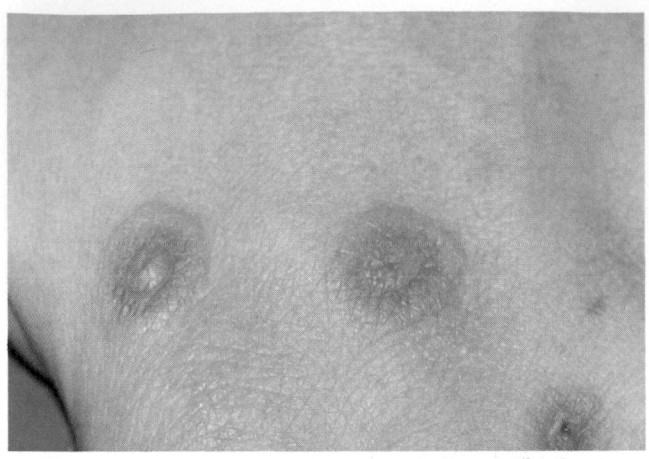

Fig. 25.19 Erythema multiforme: target lesions with central blisters.

- sarcoidosis
- streptococcal infection
- ulcerative colitis and Crohn's disease
- tuberculosis
- other infections, e.g. yersinia, deep mycoses (where prevalent), chlamydia psittaci and lymphogranuloma venereum
- drugs (uncommon), e.g. oral contraceptives, sulphonamides
- leukaemia and Hodgkin's disease.

Similar but smaller nodules are seen in Behçet's disease (p. 1010). Erythema nodosum leprosum is clinically and histologically quite different (p. 271). The lesions of nodular vasculitis are more persistent and occur more on the calves.

Bed rest is advisable at first, and a non-steroidal anti-inflammatory drug may be helpful. Further management will depend on the cause.

PYODERMA GANGRENOSUM

Pyoderma gangrenosum (Fig. 25.21) is an uncommon, non-infective ulcerating condition frequently associated with an underlying systemic disease. The lower limbs and face are the most common sites but any part of the body may be affected. The necrotic area often begins as a sterile pustule which breaks down and spreads, sometimes to form a huge ulcer, with a characteristic ragged, purplish overhanging edge. Lesions may be multiple.

The pathogenesis is unclear, but many patients have evidence of a depressed immune system. Causes include:

- ulcerative colitis
- Crohn's disease
- rheumatoid arthritis
- other forms of arthritis
- leukaemia, lymphomas, monoclonal gammopathies and myeloma.

involved (Stevens-Johnson syndrome) with blistering and haemorrhage. Sometimes internal organs, e.g. the kidney and lungs, are affected. There is an interval of about a week between the stimulus and the eruption, but this is shorter with recurrences. The pathogenesis is not fully understood.

When erythema multiforme is recurrent, the most common cause is herpes simplex.

The condition is self-limiting, but supportive care is needed, especially if there is eye and oral involvement.

ERYTHEMA NODOSUM

The plaques and nodules of erythema nodosum (Fig. 25.20) are red, hot and tender. They typically occur over the shins but may be more widespread on the legs, on the outer aspect of the arms and sides of the neck. Erythema nodosum is often accompanied by fever, malaise and painful joints. Lesions disappear over 3–6 weeks, with the same colour changes as in a resolving bruise. It is mainly a condition of young adults.

Probably most cases are due to circulating immune complexes lodging in or near the venules in the deep dermis and subcutaneous fat. Causes include:

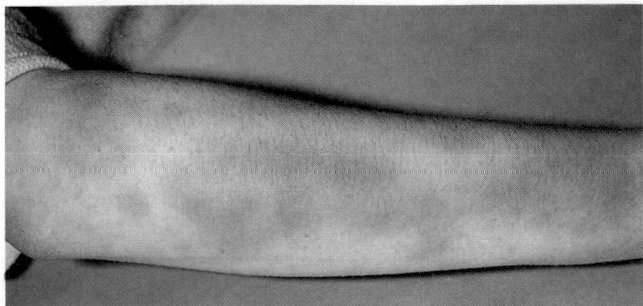

Fig. 25.20 Erythema nodosum.

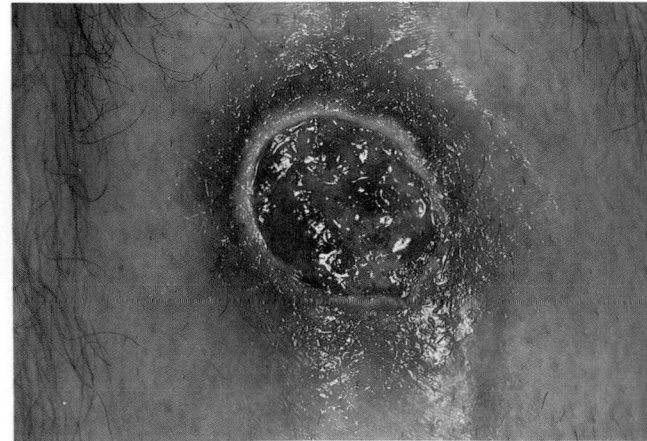

Fig. 25.21 Pyoderma gangrenosum: ulcer with purplish undermined edge.

The differential diagnosis includes infective causes of ulceration (e.g. postoperative gangrene, p. 1126) and vasculitic disorders (e.g. Wegener's granulomatosis). Cultures for aerobic and anaerobic bacteria and other organisms, and a biopsy should be taken before treatment.

Treatment is with high-dose corticosteroids, although for small lesions topical and intra-lesional corticosteroids can be effective; minocycline can be a valuable agent in milder cases.

CUTANEOUS VASCULITIS

Palpable purpura is the hallmark of cutaneous vasculitis (Fig. 25.22), but depending on the type and degree of vessel wall damage, other lesions, not all of which are purpuric, may occur; these include livedo reticularis, weals, papules, pustules, infarcts and ulcers.

Aetiological factors of cutaneous vasculitis include:

- bacteria, e.g. streptococci, gonococci, *Mycobacterium tuberculosis* (erythema induratum) and *M. leprae* (erythema nodosum leprosum)
- viruses, e.g. hepatitis B
- neoplasia, e.g. lymphoma
- drugs, e.g. sulphonamides, thiazides, captopril (see p. 1150)

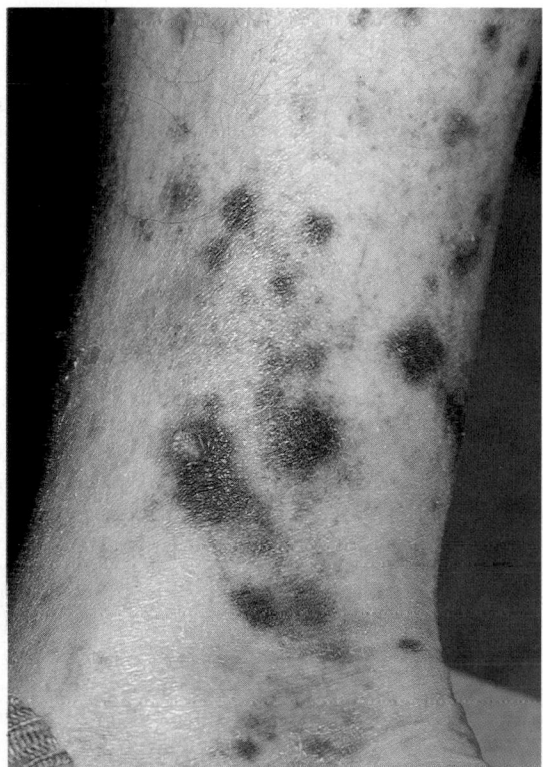

Fig. 25.22 Vasculitis: purpuric papules and nodules.

Table 25.16 Some multisystem vasculitides that may involve the skin

Clinical patterns	Other organs commonly involved
Henoch-Schönlein purpura	Joints, gut, kidney
Polyarteritis nodosa	Kidneys, gut, cardiovascular system, nervous system, muscles and joints
Temporal arteritis	Eyes
Wegener's granulomatosis	Kidneys and respiratory tract
Malignant atrophic papulosis (Degos' disease)	Gut and brain
Lupus erythematosus	Widespread

- food additives, e.g. tartrazine
- autoimmune diseases, e.g. lupus erythematosus, polyarteritis nodosa, scleroderma.

The initial event is damage to the endothelium of the vessel. Both circulating and resident extravascular inflammatory cells are then activated to release mediators, some of which have destructive effects, while others contribute to repair. The net result depends on many factors: these include the nature of the initial insult, the type and location of the vessels affected and the adequacy of the collateral blood supply. One of the most common histological appearances is accumulation of neutrophils, their breakdown products, and nuclear debris around damaged venules, an appearance termed *leucocytoclastic vasculitis*. Sometimes vasculitis occurs because there is inadequate clearance of a potential cause, such as circulating immune complexes, from the circulation, or there is a deficiency in repair mechanisms, e.g. removal of fibrin is too slow to maintain patency of affected vessels. A defect in the reticulo-endothelial system may account for the occurrence of vasculitis in lymphomas, other malignancies and sarcoidosis. Sometimes the localisation of vasculitic lesions can be explained by circumstances that slow blood flow, e.g. in the lower limbs and where skin is cooled by overlying fat.

As well as attempting to find the cause, it is of clinical importance to know whether other organs are being affected, especially the brain, heart, kidneys, lungs and gut.

There is no entirely satisfactory classification of multisystem vasculitis (see Ch. 23, p. 1030 for a further account of the vasculitides).

Most multisystem vasculitides can involve the skin (Table 25.16).

Clinical features

Henoch-Schönlein purpura

Henoch-Schönlein purpura comprises arthralgia, abdominal pain and vasculitic rash, often with renal involvement (see p. 823). Children are predominantly affected. Streptococcal sore throat and upper respiratory virus infections are the most common recognisable causes. The rash is mainly on the buttocks and extensor surfaces of the limbs. As well as purpura there are usually erythematous macules and papules, and urticarial weals. The lesions are characterised by a leucocytoclastic vasculitis, and in many cases there is deposition of IgA around venules.

There is no specific treatment but some authorities use high-dose corticosteroids if there is severe renal disease.

Polyarteritis nodosa

Polyarteritis nodosa, or PAN (see pp. 823, 1031), is a multisystem disorder in which there is necrotising vasculitis of small and medium-sized arteries. The distinctive feature in the skin is the occurrence of nodules along the course of subcutaneous arteries, best felt on the lower limb. In addition to nodules there are often purpuric papules, weals, or plaques of gangrene. Livedo reticularis, a net-like arrangement of bluish venules, is common.

Malignant atrophic papulosis

Malignant atrophic papulosis (Degos' disease) is a rare but very distinctive condition in which insignificant-looking red papules become slowly necrotic with a greyish-white central scale and heal with porcelain-like white scars.

Similar lesions occur internally, particularly in the intestine, and much of the high mortality is due to perforation or haemorrhage. The brain and kidney may also be affected.

Rheumatoid disease

Small purple or black spots around the nail folds are very characteristic of rheumatoid disease (p. 999), although also seen in other vasculitic diseases.

ERYTHRODERMA

Erythroderma, or exfoliative dermatitis, is redness of all or nearly all the skin. There is usually some degree of scaling. Most cases of erythroderma evolve from more limited eczema or psoriasis.

The principal causes include eczema; psoriasis; drugs, especially gold, allopurinol and sulphonamides (see p. 1150); and lymphoma and leukaemia. The cause can usually be determined from the history and a skin biopsy, but in some cases no aetiology is found.

The skin is red, hot to the touch and often oedematous; itching can be severe and scaling is variable. Patients feel uncomfortably cold and shiver.

Summary 3 Causes of erythroderma

- Eczema/dermatitis
- Psoriasis
- Drugs, e.g. gold, allopurinol
- Lymphoreticular neoplasia, e.g. mycosis fungoides
- Miscellaneous

Erythroderma can have serious metabolic consequences, particularly in the elderly. The greatly increased blood flow through the skin, with loss of normal capacity for vasoconstriction, leads to hypothermia in a cold environment and can cause high output cardiac failure. Blood flow to other organs can be greatly diminished. There is increased fluid loss from the skin surface, with compensatory thirst and oliguria. Anaemia is common, and in part is due to a state of malabsorption secondary to the skin disease (dermatogenic enteropathy). Serum albumin falls due to loss from shed skin scales and reduced synthesis. The skin is more prone to infection and thrombophlebitis is common. Lymphadenopathy is usual.

Systemic corticosteroids are needed for severe cases. Maintenance of fluid balance and body temperature is important and use of appropriate emollients can be helpful (p. 1122). More specific treatment will depend on the underlying cause.

BLISTERING DISEASES

Blisters are focal collections of free fluid in the skin. By convention small ones are called vesicles and larger ones bullae. They are the result of a defect or disturbance in the normal mechanisms that hold the components of the skin together. Extensive blistering produces a serious loss of normal skin function, and before effective treatment was available some of the bullous diseases had a high mortality.

Many different pathological processes can result in the clinical appearance of a blister. The diagnosis may be obvious from the history, such as in an insect bite reaction, but often there is a differential diagnosis and investigations are necessary. Light microscopy of an early blister, preferably one less than 24 hours old (before re-epithelialisation has begun), will provide useful evidence of the level of the split in the skin and sometimes details of the pathogenetic mechanism, e.g. spongiosis (Fig. 25.23). Electron microscopy allows a much more detailed analysis of blister formation and is of particular importance in the accurate diagnosis of epidermolysis bullosa, a heterogeneous group of inherited blistering disorders. Immunological phenomena are central to some of

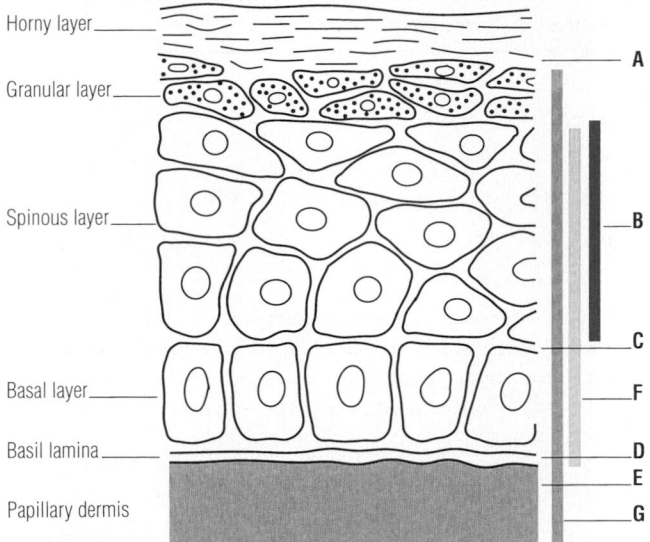

Horny layer
Granular layer
Spinous layer
Basal layer
Basil lamina
Papillary dermis

A
B
C
F
D
E
G

A Sub corneal: impetigo
B Mid epidermal: viral infections (e.g. herpes simplex, varicella zoster),eczema, friction blister
C Supra-basal: pemphigus vulgaris
D Basal lamina: pemphigoid, dermatitis herpetiformis
E Sub-basal: porphyria
F Variable: erythema multiforme, epidermolysis bullosa, blistering drug reactions
G Variable: thermal burns (depends on severity of burn)

Fig. 25.23 Examples of blistering diseases at different levels in the skin.

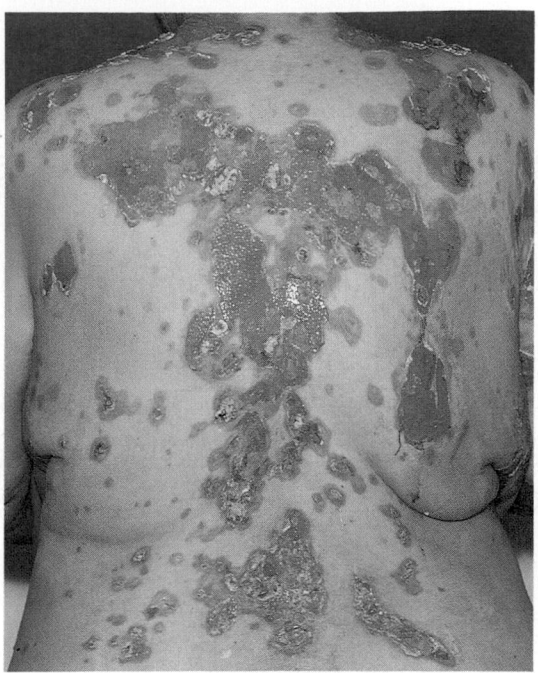

Fig. 25.24 Erosions due to pemphigus vulgaris.

the bullous diseases, particularly pemphigus, pemphigoid and dermatitis herpetiformis, and these are best demonstrated on a sample of unfixed skin from just beyond the edge of a blister (peribullous skin). Other tests that may be indicated include serum for antibodies (see below), bacteriological and viral studies on blister fluid, and when appropriate porphyrin estimations and patch testing.

Pemphigus vulgaris

Pemphigus vulgaris (Fig. 25.24) is an uncommon, chronic, intra-epidermal blistering disease of unknown aetiology, characterised by the presence in affected skin and mucosa of an IgG antibody, which localises to the cell wall of keratinocytes (Fig. 25.25). A split forms within the epidermis.

Aetiology and pathogenesis. The disease is most common in middle age and the Jewish race. The characteristic antibody is usually found in the bloodstream, and antibody titres approximately correlate with disease activity. Relapse is sometimes shown to be preceded by an increased titre. The pemphigus antibody probably brings about separation of keratinocytes by activating proteinases. Occasionally pemphigus is associated with other immunological diseases: thymoma, myasthenia gravis and SLE.

Clinical features. Pemphigus often begins in the mouth and sometimes other mucous membranes, with non-healing erosions. Blisters appear sooner or later on previously normal-looking skin, and when the disease is active, sideways pressure with a finger on unblistered skin can produce new blisters (Nikolsky sign). Increasing numbers of flaccid blisters appear, and when they burst, leave erosions. The resultant problems of infections and fluid loss are similar to the consequences of extensive burns.

Diagnosis. The diagnosis is made from characteristic histology, showing a suprabasal split and free-floating keratinocytes (acantholysis). Immunohistochemical techniques show that the keratinocytes are coated with IgG. In all but localised or treated disease the pemphigus antibody can be demonstrated in the serum.

Treatment. Treatment is with high doses of corticosteroids (about 80 mg prednisolone daily), together with an immunosuppressant agent such as azathioprine, with subsequent gradual reduction of the steroid. Gold salts have also been used with success but toxicity is a problem. Even with treatment, pemphigus remains a serious disorder, up to 25% of patients dying from the disease or consequences of treatment. Most patients need maintenance therapy for lengthy periods, although in some a true remission occurs.

Bullous pemphigoid

Bullous pemphigoid (Fig. 25.26) is a fairly common subepidermal blistering disease characterised by an anti-

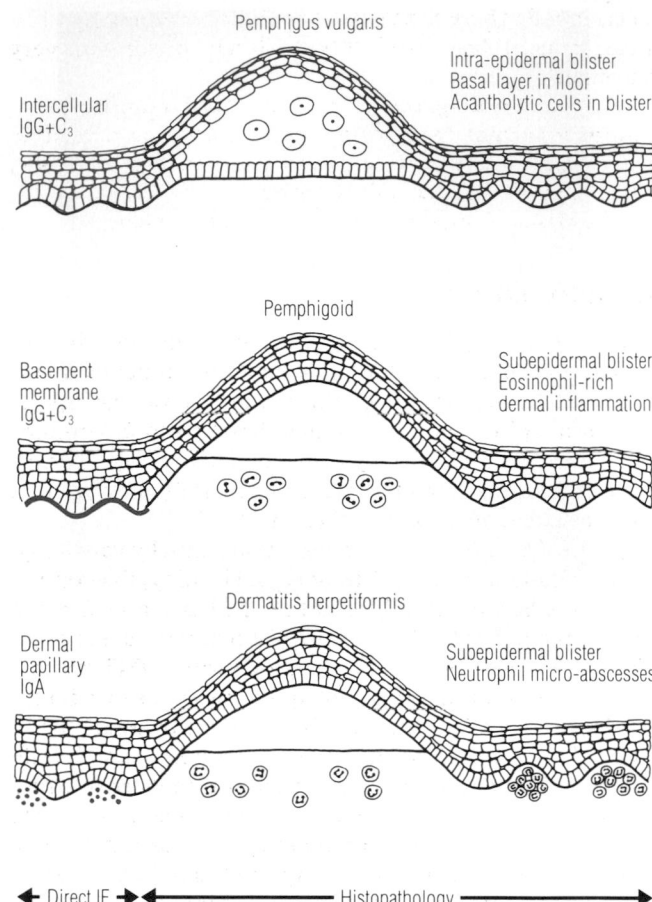

Pemphigus vulgaris

Intercellular IgG+C₃

Intra-epidermal blister
Basal layer in floor
Acantholytic cells in blister

Pemphigoid

Basement membrane IgG+C₃

Subepidermal blister
Eosinophil-rich dermal inflammation

Dermatitis herpetiformis

Dermal papillary IgA

Subepidermal blister
Neutrophil micro-abscesses

◄ Direct IF ►◄————— Histopathology —————►

Fig. 25.25 The lesions of pemphigus vulgaris (A), pemphigoid (B) and dermatitis herpetiformis (C). (IF = immunofluorescence).

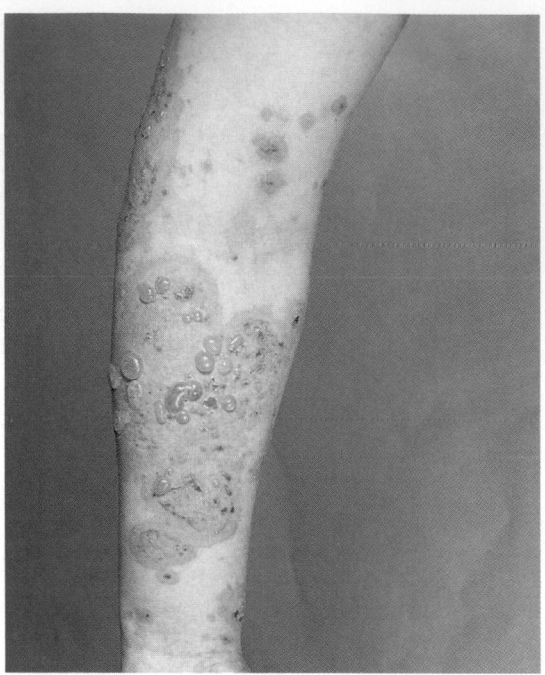

Fig. 25.26 The blisters of bullous pemphigoid are tense, clear or blood-stained, and often remain intact for several days.

Dermatitis herpetiformis

Dermatitis herpetiformis is an uncommon, chronic, intensely itchy disorder in which subepidermal blistering usually occurs.

body which localises to the lamina lucida of the basement membrane (Fig. 25.25).

Pathology. In pemphigoid the complement system is activated, and C3a and C5a attract and activate eosinophils. Eosinophil products and mast cell mediators contribute to the split which occurs in the basement membrane and the clinically evident inflammatory reaction.

Clinical features. Pemphigoid is mainly a disease of the elderly. It is usually preceded by an erythematous itchy rash, which can be mistaken for urticaria or eczema. It may be localised for some weeks before becoming generalised. The blisters are tense, clear or bloodstained, and often remain intact for several days. Unlike pemphigus, pemphigoid does not usually involve the mucous membranes. When blisters do break, the skin usually heals, and the prognosis is better than that of pemphigus. There is a localised variant of pemphigoid involving the mucous membranes in which scarring occurs.

Treatment. Treatment of pemphigoid is with prednisolone and azathioprine to facilitate steroid withdrawal.

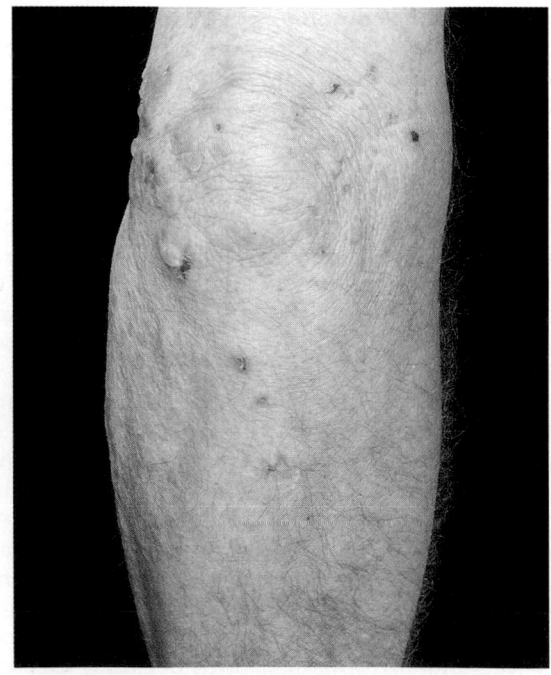

Fig. 25.27 Dermatitis herpetiformis: itchy papules and vesicles.

Aetiology and pathogenesis. There is a close association with HLA-B8 and DRW3, gluten-sensitive enteropathy and deposition of IgA in the dermal papillae throughout the skin. The enteropathy may not be symptomatic but it is likely that absorbed products derived from gluten are important in the pathogenesis of the skin lesions. Abnormal immunity in patients with dermatitis herpetiformis is suggested by an increased incidence of organ-specific autoimmune disease, and a few patients (as with coeliac disease) develop small bowel lymphoma. The skin lesions are a result of activation of dense clusters of neutrophils in the dermal papillae, producing damage and then fluid accumulation.

Clinical features. Dermatitis herpetiformis usually begins in young adults and can persist indefinitely. Initial lesions are very itchy grouped weals or papules, on which arise small blisters (Fig. 25.27). Extensor surfaces are the characteristic sites, especially elbows, knees, shoulders, buttocks and scalp. Oral lesions are sometimes seen.

Diagnosis. The diagnosis is best made from finding typical histology in an early lesion and IgA deposition in unaffected skin. (In the lesions the IgA can disappear as a result of the inflammatory infiltrate.) A jejunal biopsy usually shows subtotal villous atrophy. Potassium iodide, both systemically and topically, provokes dermatitis herpetiformis and has occasionally been used as a diagnostic test.

Treatment. Dapsone has a dramatic beneficial effect in this condition, probably by modulation of the neutrophil myeloperoxidase enzyme system, and/or of the alternate pathway of complement activation. Haemolytic anaemia can occur. A gluten-free diet is helpful in most patients, and may reduce the likelihood of intestinal lymphoma.

MISCELLANEOUS DISORDERS OF UNKNOWN CAUSE

Pityriasis rosea

Pityriasis rosea, a common self-limiting disorder, occurs mainly in children and young adults. Clustering of cases suggests an infective cause and a viral aetiology is likely but unproven.

Clinical features. The first lesion to appear, known as the herald patch, is red, circumscribed, slightly scaly and larger than those that will follow about 10 days later. The generalised eruption is maximal on the trunk and proximal aspects of the limbs, and usually includes distinctive ovoid patches whose long axes are parallel to the major skin creases. This produces a pattern somewhat like a Christmas tree on the back. The pink borders of these lesions are separated from the slightly brown centres by collarettes of scale. There is usually an admixture of smaller pink papules. Itching may occur, and occasionally there is malaise and lymphadenopathy. The rash usually lasts 4–6 weeks. Recurrences are very unusual.

Differential diagnosis. There are no diagnostic tests. Conditions that may resemble pityriasis rosea include drug eruption, seborrhoeic dermatitis, guttate psoriasis, tinea corporis and secondary syphilis.

Treatment. A mild topical steroid may be helpful.

Lichen planus

Lichen planus (Fig. 25.28) is a fairly common disease which may affect the skin, hair, nails and mucous membranes. The histology is distinctive and shows damage to the basal epidermal cells, with a dense band of lymphocytic infiltrate immediately beneath. There are close similarities to the skin changes seen in graft versus host disease and some drug reactions (p. 1151).

Clinical features. The skin lesions are usually very itchy, and typically form purplish, polygonal, shiny, flat-topped papules. They are usually found on the flexor aspect of the wrists, the lower back and shins. Individual lesions often show distinctive fine white lacy patterning (Wickham's striae). Larger, more warty plaques are sometimes found on the lower legs. Induction of new lesions by injury to the skin, the Koebner phenomenon, is often seen. In the mouth lichen planus is mainly seen as a network of white lines on the buccal mucosa and white patches on the tongue, but occasionally can cause chronic ulceration. The scalp may be involved, producing patches of inflammation from which hair fall is usually permanent. Nails can also be affected, usually with longitudinal areas of thinning; in some cases nails also can be permanently lost.

Lichen planus often lasts a year or more and to some extent it is steroid-responsive. Postinflammatory hyperpigmentation is common.

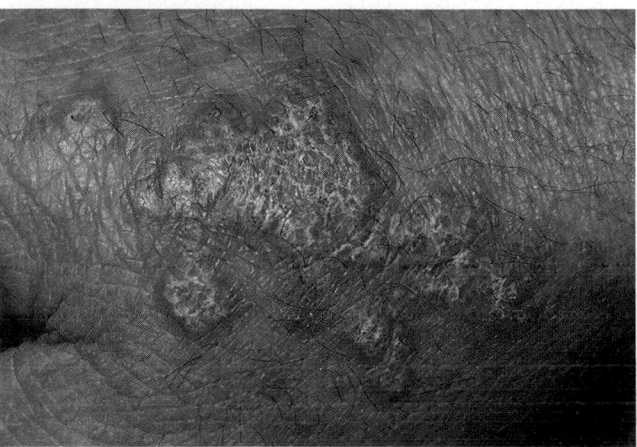

Fig. 25.28 The lesions of lichen planus typically form purplish, polygonal, shiny, flat-topped papules.

Granuloma annulare

There are two forms of granuloma annulare (Fig. 25.29), localised and generalised; both as a rule are asymptomatic. Histologically there is palisading granuloma formation around focal areas of dermal necrosis.

Localised granuloma annulare presents as rings of smooth firm papules. The backs of the hands and the tops of the feet are common sites. The commonest misdiagnoses are warts and fungal infection, in which epidermal changes are prominent in contrast to the smooth surface of granuloma annulare.

In generalised granuloma annulare the papules are much more widespread and not necessarily in ring-shaped configurations. This is often associated with diabetes mellitus. Diagnosis is confirmed by biopsy.

Necrobiosis lipoidica

This condition (Fig. 25.30) occurs in about 3 per 1000 diabetics, and more than half of patients with necrobiosis lipoidica are overtly diabetic (see Ch. 19). The pathology is similar to granuloma annulare but with more pronounced dermal necrosis.

The most common site is the shin. The lesion begins as a purplish plaque, which gradually enlarges and becomes atrophic with yellowish areas centrally. Ulceration is quite common. The condition is chronic, and

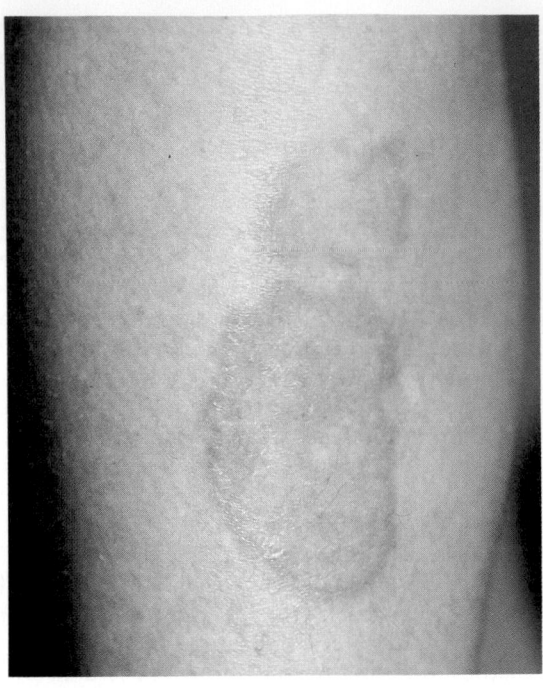

Fig. 25.30 Necrobiosis lipoidica: subcutaneous vein visible due to central atrophy, bordered by dermal inflammation.

when there is associated diabetes, careful control of blood glucose has no effect on the progress of the skin lesions.

SKIN CHANGES IN DIABETES

There are a number of cutaneous problems that occur in diabetics.

One of the commonest is recurrent infections. Mucosal candidal infections may occur, as may recurrent staphylococcal boils (p. 1126). Indeed in developed societies, the carbuncle (p. 1126) is only seen with any frequency in diabetics. Injection sites may become infected, and occasionally deep abscesses may form.

With sensory neuropathy patients may fail to notice repetitive trauma (usually from footwear). This predisposes to ulceration, commonly on the sole (p. 772).

Necrobiosis lipoidica (Fig. 25.30) and granuloma annulare (Fig. 25.29) have histological features in common, and both occur in diabetics (see above).

The term 'diabetic dermopathy' refers to small, dusky-brown, scar-like lesions that often appear on the shins in diabetics. The patients usually have microangiopathy. 'Diabetic sclerosis' or 'cheiroarthropathy' occurs in at least 30% of juvenile-onset, insulin-dependent diabetics. The fingers and toes become stiffened and sclerodermatous. The patients are unable to straighten their fingers completely, and cannot place them flat on a table. A rarer condition is scleredema, in which the skin of the neck and

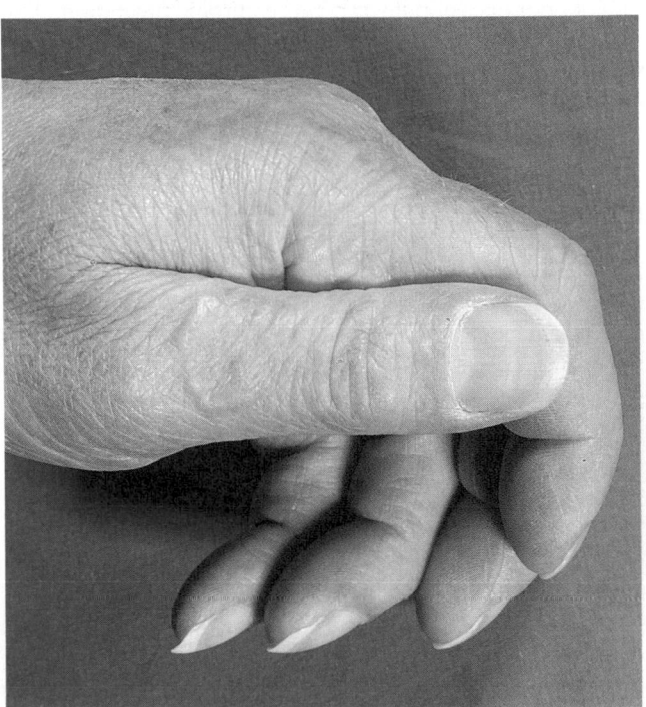

Fig. 25.29 Granuloma annulare, localised form: note the ring-shaped arrangement of dermal papules.

- Cutaneous infections – candidiasis
  – staphylococcal infections
  – injection site infection
- Neuropathic ulcers
- Necrobiosis lipoidica (diabeticorum)
- Disseminated granuloma annulare
- Diabetic 'dermopathy'
- Diabetic sclerosis (cheiroarthropathy)
- Scleredema adultorum (of Buschke)
- Bullae (bullosis diabeticorum)
- Xanthomata and xanthelasmata
- Effects of insulin injections – lipoatrophy
  – lipohypertrophy ('insulin tumours')
  – infections and abscesses
- Generalised lipodystrophy
  (lipoatrophy not due to insulin injection)*
- Acanthosis nigricans*
- Vitiligo

* When these cutaneous signs accompany diabetes, there is usually gross insulin resistance

Table 25.17 Pathogenesis of drug eruptions – some examples

Mechanism	Drug	Clinical pattern
Direct effects		
Immunological		
IgE-mediated	Penicillin	Urticaria
Immune complex	Sulphonamides	Vasculitis
Effector pathway stimulation	Acetyl salicylic acid	Urticaria
Side-effect	Cytotoxic drugs	Alopecia
Overdosage	Anticoagulants	Purpura
Cumulative toxicity	Corticosteroids	Striae
Indirect effects		
Drug interaction	Aspirin-displacing warfarin	Purpura
Metabolic effects	Isoniazid	Pellagra
Ecological disturbance	Broad-spectrum antibiotics	Candidiasis
Exacerbation of existing disease	Hydralazine	Lupus erythematosus
	Lithium	Psoriasis

upper back suddenly becomes stiff and thickened. These changes gradually spread on to the face, trunk and upper arms. Rarely, diabetics develop distinctive non-inflammatory blisters on the extremities.

Hyperlipidaemia is a common complication of diabetes and lipid deposits in the skin may occur in the form of eruptive xanthomata, most commonly on the buttocks and extensor surfaces. Palpebral xanthelasmata may also be seen in diabetics. Injection-site lipoatrophy and lipohypertrophy are discussed on page 750. Rarely glucose intolerance and diabetes are part of a constellation of changes including generalised fat reduction (lipodystrophy) and acanthosis nigricans. Such patients often have marked insulin resistance. There is an association between vitiligo and maturity-onset as well as insulin-dependent diabetes.

DRUG ERUPTIONS

Drug eruptions are a frequent occurrence in hospital practice and can produce skin changes in many ways (Table 25.17). Some of these, such as the predisposition to candidal infection by a broad-spectrum antibiotic are not direct effects of drugs on the skin, but are none the less a consequence of drug exposure. Often the exact mechanism of a drug eruption is unknown.

Some drugs, such as antibiotics, thiazides and sulphonamides, gold, allopurinol, phenylbutazone and other non-steroidal anti-inflammatory drugs, are relatively common causes of rashes; others very rare, but in all patients who develop a rash the drug history is of great importance. Not only prescribed drugs, but also medicines and tablets bought over the counter must be considered.

Types of drug eruption

Urticaria

The mechanisms whereby a drug can cause urticaria include IgE-mediated immediate hypersensitivity, immune complex-mediated generation of activated complement components (serum sickness), a direct action on mast cells causing them to release histamine, and modulation of arachidonic acid metabolism. The drugs commonly implicated in urticaria are:

- penicillin and related antibiotics
- X-ray contrast media
- enzymes
- blood products
- opiates
- non-steroidal anti-inflammatory drugs
- pollen vaccines
- iodides.

Angio-oedema and anaphylaxis may accompany urticaria, particularly when the drug has been injected, and can be life-threatening.

Urticaria usually begins within minutes or hours of the drug being given, but with immune complex-related urticaria it occurs several days after the challenge, and is often associated with fever, lymphadenopathy, joint symptoms and haematuria due to renal damage.

Morbilliform eruption

A widespread, symmetrical, blotchy, maculopapular, erythematous rash is probably the commonest drug eruption. There is often a mild fever, but serious consequences are uncommon. The mechanism is usually obscure but does involve delayed hypersensitivity in some cases, especially when the onset is within a few days of the drug being started. Morbilliform eruptions usually begin within a week of the onset of the drug, and may progress to erythroderma if the drug is continued.

Ampicillin, amoxycillin and derivatives, e.g. talampicillin, are common causes, especially when the patient has infectious mononucleosis or lymphatic leukaemia, or is also taking allopurinol, and can begin up to a few days after the antibiotic has been stopped. The common causes of morbilliform (exanthematic) drug eruptions are:

- allopurinol
- antituberculous drugs
- captopril
- carbamazepine
- gold salts
- H_2 antihistamines
- penicillamine
- penicillins
- phenothiazines
- phenylbutazone
- sulphonamides
- thiazides.

Erythroderma

When due to a drug, erythroderma, or exfoliative dermatitis (p. 1144), tends to begin several weeks after the drug has been started. Common causes of drug-induced erythroderma are:

- allopurinol
- carbamazepine
- phenytoin
- isoniazid
- lithium
- gold salts
- chloroquine
- barbiturates
- P-aminosalicylic acid
- captopril
- sulphonamides
- methyldopa.

Erythema multiforme

Erythema multiforme (p. 1141) is a reaction distinguished by target lesions. Most cases are not due to drugs. The commonest drugs to cause erythema multiforme are:

- sulphonamides
- phenytoin
- phenylbutazone
- barbiturates
- penicillins
- carbamazepine
- rifampicin
- gold salts.

Toxic epidermal necrolysis

Toxic epidermal necrolysis is a rare drug reaction which has a high mortality. There is often a brief prodrome of malaise and fever, followed by widespread, tender, erythe-matous areas which then blister. Large sheets of epidermis readily rub off with light pressure to leave painful denuded dermis. Mucous membranes as well as skin may be involved. Fluid imbalance, septicaemia and pneumonia are the most common problems.

Differentiation from staphylococcal scalded skin syndrome (p. 1125) can be made histologically on a blister roof because in toxic epidermal necrolysis the roof consists of the whole epidermis. Butazones, sulphonamides, allopurinol, gold salts and phenytoin are examples of drugs which can cause the syndrome, which can also be due to infections, graft versus host disease and lymphoma.

Management is similar to that of widespread burns with treatment of fluid and protein loss and of infection.

Photosensitivity

The most common photosensitivity drug reaction resembles sunburn and is usually phototoxic, i.e. does not involve immunological mechanisms. Occasionally drugs produce photo-allergic reactions which may look like eczema on light-exposed skin. Drugs which can induce phototoxic and photo-allergic reactions include:

- phenothiazines
- thiazides
- sulphonamides
- tetracyclines
- sulphonylureas
- nalidixic acid (bullous)
- amiodarone
- azapropazone
- protriptyline
- psoralens.

Drugs can also induce photosensitive diseases, e.g. procainamide can induce lupus erythematosus, and isoniazid, pellagra.

Fixed drug eruption

The characteristic feature of a fixed drug eruption is that inflammation occurs in exactly the same place or few places each time the drug is taken. The reaction is usually a round red patch, which may blister (Fig. 25.31), and after the inflammation has subsided there is often prolonged hyperpigmentation.

One of the commonest causes is phenolphthalein, widely used as a non-prescription laxative, and thus easily missed in the history. Sulphonamides, tetracyclines, barbiturates, phenylbutazone, chlordiazepoxide, quinine and dapsone are other common causes.

Vasculitis

Drug-induced vasculitis (p. 1143), usually in the form of palpable purpura, and often with urticarial and blistering lesions, can be accompanied by similar lesions in other organs and may be a serious illness. The commonest drugs to cause allergic vasculitis are:

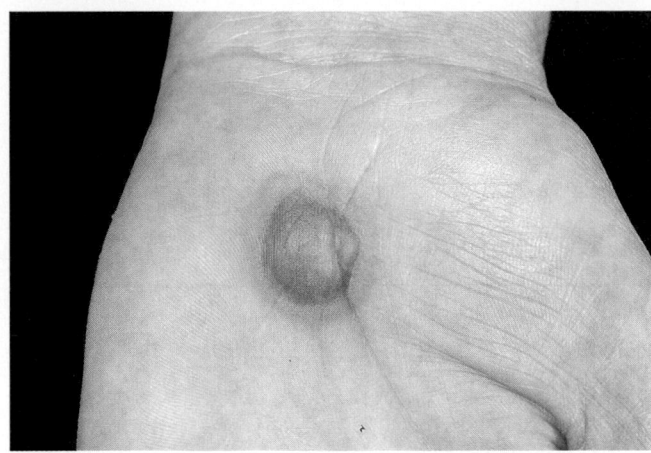

Fig. 25.31 Fixed drug eruption: dusky erythema with central blister.

- allopurinol
- thiazides
- phenytoin
- thiouracil
- non-steroidal anti-inflammatory drugs
- sulphonamides
- hydralazine
- quinidine
- captopril.

Erythema nodosum

Drugs are rarely responsible for erythema nodosum and other causes should be sought (p. 1142). Oral contraceptives and sulphonamides are the drugs most likely to be involved.

Pigmentation changes induced by drugs

Colour change (Table 25.18) can be produced by deposition of the drug in the skin and mucous membranes, stimulation of melanin production and alteration of the distribution of pigment so as to make it more apparent, as in postinflammatory hyperpigmentation (p. 1158). The hyperpigmentation after fixed drug eruption may be the presenting feature. In some situations the pigmentation is only evident in light-exposed skin. In many examples of drug-related pigment change, the mechanism is unknown.

Lichenoid drug eruption

The rash in lichenoid drug eruption is similar to lichen planus (p. 1147). It usually begins weeks to months after the drug is started. As in idiopathic lichen planus, hyperpigmentation is common. Common causes of lichenoid drug eruptions are:

- gold salts
- antimalarials
- thiazides
- frusemide
- beta-blockers
- penicillamine

Table 25.18 Pigmentation caused by drugs

Patterns	Drug
Brown	
Similar to Addison's disease	ACTH
Similar to chloasma	Phenytoin
	Oral contraceptives
Light-exposed areas	Phenothiazines
	Psoralens
	Cytotoxics
Generalised	Cytotoxics, e.g. busulphan
	Pyrimethamine
Generalised, with patchy pigmentation	Arsenic
Blue-grey	
Light-exposed areas	Minocycline
	Amiodarone
	Phenothiazines
Generalised, maximal on light-exposed areas	Gold
	Silver
	Bismuth
Shins, nails and palate (and sometimes light-exposed areas)	Antimalarials
Yellow	
Generalised	Mepacrine
Red	
Generalised	Clofazimine
	Methysergide

- phenothiazines
- methyldopa
- chlorpropamide.

Drug-induced lupus erythematosus

Drug-induced lupus erythematosus has some differences from the naturally occurring condition (p. 1023). It is likely that affected individuals have a genetic predisposition. This has been best documented in association with hydralazine and procainamide. With hydralazine the disorder is broadly dose-related, being seen in 5% on 100 mg daily, 10% on 200 mg daily, but not in patients on 50 mg daily. Other common causes include penicillamine, phenytoin, methyldopa, beta-blockers, sulphasalazine and oral contraceptives. In most cases drug-induced lupus erythematosus occurs after the drug has been taken for at least a few months. On discontinuation, the disease resolves in most cases, but can persist for years.

The condition is relatively less common in black people and more common in the elderly; renal and central nervous system disease are less likely to occur than in idiopathic lupus erythematosus. Antihistone antibodies are characteristic, and antinative DNA antibodies are not found. Complement levels remain normal.

Purpura

When caused by a drug, purpura is usually a result of thrombocytopenia, vascular damage or both. Mechanisms include both toxic and allergic effects.

Pruritus

Itching without a rash is considered on page 1163. Drugs can cause generalised pruritus and the most common causes are:

- opiates
- CNS stimulants
- antidepressants
- oral contraceptives
- hepatotoxic drugs
- chloroquine.

For many drugs the mechanism is unknown, but some drugs produce intrahepatic cholestasis.

Acne and acneform eruption

In true acne there are comedones, papules and pustules in a characteristic distribution (p. 1161). Drugs exerting an androgenic stimulus, such as testosterone and some progestogens, can exacerbate or induce acne.

An acne-like eruption, in which there are follicular lesions but in which the morphology or the distribution differ from true acne, is seen with a number of drugs, including corticosteroids and ACTH, halogens, anti-epileptic drugs, isoniazid and lithium salts.

Alopecia

Partial or complete hair loss is very common and appears early with cytotoxic drugs, but can occur, rarely and late, with other drugs;

- cytotoxic agents (especially cyclo-phosphamide and anthracyclines)
- retinoids
- anticoagulants
- oral contraceptives
- antithyroid drugs
- phenytoin
- valproate.

Hypertrichosis

Corticosteroids and androgenic steroids can produce hirsutism, but some drugs can induce increased hair growth on areas not dependent on a sex hormone stimulus. Minoxidil, cyclosporin A, diazoxide, phenytoin and penicillamine are the main causes.

Eczema

If sensitised via the skin to a 'drug' and then 'challenged' by an internal route, the patient can develop an often widespread eczematous eruption. Examples are given in Table 25.19.

Table 25.19 Eczema induced by topical drugs

Eliciting drug	Source of topical exposure
Antibiotics, e.g. penicillin, streptomycin	Contents of medical and veterinary ampoules
Antihistamines	In antipruritic creams, e.g. mepyramine
Aminophylline	Cross-reaction with ethylenediamine in Tri-adcortyl cream

Vesicular and bullous drug eruptions

Blistering can occur in several different types of drug eruption already described, e.g. fixed eruption, erythema multiforme, photosensitivity and vasculitis. Bullae are common at sites subjected to prolonged pressure in drug-induced coma. Porphyria (p. 780) can be precipitated by drugs, as occasionally can pemphigus (e.g. rifampicin) and acquired epidermolysis bullosa (e.g. frusemide).

Investigation and treatment of drug reaction

The evaluation of a possible drug reaction should include the following:

- *A careful assessment of the risk to the patient*, from the rash itself and involvement of other organs, e.g. kidneys and brain in a vasculitis. An assessment of the airway and maintenance of adequate circulation in urticaria/anaphylaxis.
- *A full drug history*, including all present and recently completed treatments (tablets, mixtures, injections, suppositories, etc.) and their timing in relation to the onset of the rash. Some drugs can cause a rash several days after they were last given, e.g. ampicillin, gold and depot preparations.
- *Past drug history and associated rashes.*
- *Other possible explanations* for the rash, e.g. a virus infection.
- *Consideration of which drugs can be stopped.* Non-essential drugs should be stopped and essential drugs changed to structurally different ones if possible.
- *Laboratory investigations.* Except for the investigation of drug-induced blood dyscrasias, these are disappointing. Blood eosinophilia, if present, is supportive of drug eruption.
- *A skin biopsy* may help in some cases.
- *Treatment.* The most immediately serious drug reaction is anaphylaxis. Emergency treatment is with 1:1000 adrenaline, 1 ml i.m., or slowly i.v. if the patient is moribund. Parenteral antihistamine and hydrocortisone are also given, and if necessary the patient is intubated and managed on ICU.

Depending on severity, some patients with erythroderma, bullous erythema multiforme, toxic epidermal necrolysis and vasculitis will require treatment with systemic corticosteroids.

INTERNAL MALIGNANCY AND THE SKIN

Skin abnormalities may be the first indicator of a systemic malignancy (Table 25.20).

The cause of many other skin disorders associated with malignancy is unknown. Some are:

- *Generalised pruritus* without a primary rash (p. 1163).
- *Dermatomyositis*, adult onset (p. 1029).
- *Acanthosis nigricans* (Fig. 25.32). The skin becomes hyperpigmented and warty, but feels soft. Body folds, e.g. axillae, are affected. There are other causes, such as obesity, some drugs and some inherited syndromes, but onset in a lean adult is highly likely to be associated with an adenocarcinoma or lymphoma.
- *Acquired hypertrichosis lanuginosa*. This is a rare condition but one that has a strong association with malignancy, especially Hodgkin's disease. The patient develops blond downy hair over the whole face and then elsewhere.
- *Erythema gyratum repens*. Here the skin develops irregular wavy bands of erythema, the overall appearance resembling wood grain. Nearly all cases have an associated malignancy.
- *Acquired ichthyosis*. The unexplained occurrence of dry, scaly but non-inflamed skin is often associated with lymphoma (p. 1140).
- *Pachydermoperiostosis with finger clubbing*. The skin becomes thickened, with extra folds; the hands, elbows, knees and tongue enlarge and there may be painful periosteal new bone formation (see hypertrophic pulmonary osteoarthropathy, p. 453). These changes are associated with bronchial carcinoma.

Table 25.20 Skin manifestations of malignancy

Direct involvement
e.g. Direct spread from breast carcinoma; plaques and nodules from lymphoma

Genetic predisposition
e.g. Multiple cysts and benign skin tumours occurring with colonic carcinoma (Gardner's syndrome) with autosomal dominant inheritance

Carcinogen (also causing skin disease)
e.g. Vinyl chloride skin eruption and angiosarcoma of the liver following exposure to vinyl chloride monomer (used in plastic manufacture)

Metabolic products of tumour
e.g. Flushing due to malignant carcinoid; migratory necrolytic erythema with glucagonoma – partly due to essential amino acid deficiencies induced by metabolic abnormality

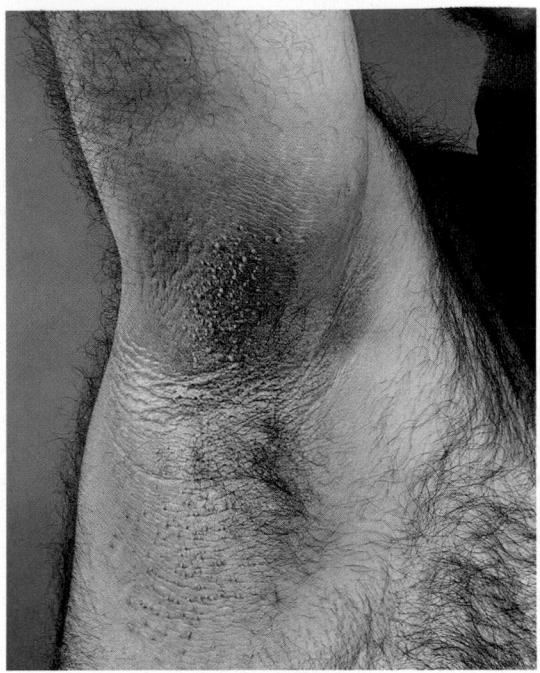

Fig. 25.32 Hyperpigmentation and velvety thickening due to acanthosis nigricans.

- *Pancreatic panniculitis*. Tender red nodules of distinctive histology, due to the effect on subcutaneous fat of circulating lipases from the pancreas, indicate either malignancy or inflammation in that organ. There is often arthritis and eosinophilia.

NAEVI AND TUMOURS OF THE SKIN

Most primary tumours are either clearly benign or malignant, but occasionally some benign lesions evolve into malignant patterns of behaviour and are termed premalignant. Some of the known causes are listed in Table 25.22 (p. 1155). A naevus is a circumscribed developmental defect, and the term has a similar meaning to hamartoma. Naevi are often, but not necessarily, evident at birth. There may be more than one cell type involved in the process.

Each of the cell types in the skin can proliferate to produce a tumour and the exact diagnosis usually rests with the pathologist.

Many benign tumours and naevi are of little more than cosmetic importance, but in some instances they are pointers towards a genetic syndrome or multisystem disorder.

Malignant skin tumours can be fatal, and often come to attention during a routine medical examination. Malignant metastases in the skin can occasionally be the presenting feature of a cancer elsewhere and the histology can provide a valuable indication of the organ of origin.

Naevi

Pigmented naevi

Pigmented (melanocytic) naevi, or common moles, are occasionally evident at birth, but more commonly appear in childhood or adolescence. The naevus is initially brown, with clusters of proliferating melanocytes at the base of the epidermis. Melanocytic naevi that develop after birth are usually symmetrical in shape and colour and rarely grow to more than 1 cm in diameter. In time the cells migrate into the dermis and the lesion often becomes a flesh-coloured nodule.

The blue naevus is a slate-coloured lesion composed of a localised proliferation of melanocytes in the dermis which never reached the epidermis during development.

Malignant melanoma (p. 1156) may arise from a seemingly benign melanocytic naevus, but this is rare except from giant congenital pigmented naevi.

Vascular naevi

There are several types of vascular naevi, some of which resolve in infancy or childhood (e.g. the salmon patch and strawberry naevus). The port wine stain is an area of permanent vascular dilatation, often on the face, where it may produce a disfiguring purplish discoloration. When the area affected is in the distribution of the ophthalmic division of the trigeminal nerve, there may be an associated vascular anomaly in the brain or meninges which can cause epilepsy, hemiplegia or retardation (Sturge-Weber syndrome).

Epithelial naevi

Developmental malformations involving epidermal keratinocytes affect at least 1 in 1000 live births. They are usually circumscribed verrucous plaques which are often linear on the limbs, but may assume quite bizarre, whorled configurations, especially on the trunk. Occasionally lesions may be widespread. Such multiple lesions may be associated with developmental defects in the CNS and skeleton.

Naevi and multisystem disease

Tuberous sclerosis

Tuberous sclerosis is an autosomal dominantly inherited disorder in which mental deficiency is associated with abnormality of many other organs. The first skin lesions to appear, often in early infancy, are the 'ash leaf' macules. These well-circumscribed, often irregularly shaped, pale patches are best seen with Wood's light. From later childhood onwards, one or more of the following may appear: red angiofibromatous papules on the face (misnamed adenoma sebaceum), thickened plaques

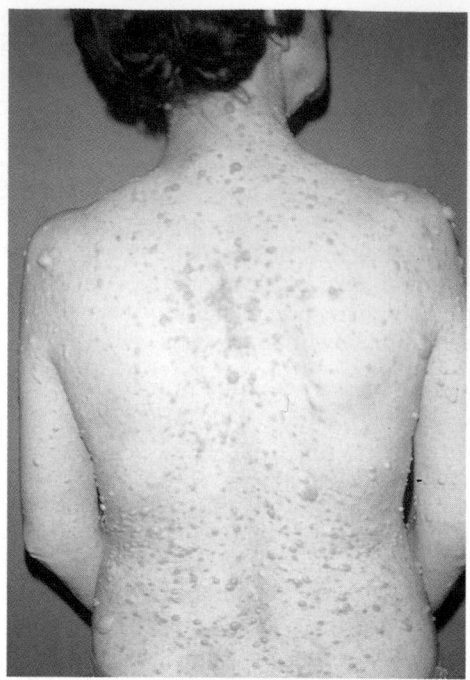

Fig. 25.33 Neurofibromatosis is associated with localised areas of hyperpigmentation.

on the trunk (shagreen patches) and peri-ungual fibromas (smooth nodules beside the nails). The skin lesions can be important in recognising carriers of the gene.

Von Recklinghausen's disease (neurofibromatosis)

The many features of von Recklinghausen's disease, or neurofibromatosis (Fig. 25.33), an autosomal dominantly inherited condition, include acoustic neuroma, gliomas, spinal deformities and phaeochromocytoma. The skin shows multiple pale brown patches (café au lait macules), especially in the axillae (a pathognomonic sign), and soft nodules (neurofibromas) composed of nerve sheath cells.

Benign tumours and cysts

The growth of these is usually slow, does not destroy normal tissues, and is eventually self-limiting. The lesion produced is usually symmetrical in shape. A classification is given in Table 25.21.

Precursors to squamous carcinoma

Actinic keratosis

Actinic (solar) keratosis is a lesion which arises on skin chronically damaged by the harmful effects of UV radiation, in particular UVB (p. 1157). The face, bald scalp, backs of hands and forearms are common sites. Actinic

Table 25.21 Some benign skin tumours

Tumour	Clinical features
Seborrhoeic wart (basal cell papilloma)	Onset from mid-adult life Pale brown through to black (due to melanin) Stuck-on appearance, with finely clefted surface Often multiple
Histiocytoma (dermatofibroma, sclerosing angioma)	May follow trauma, e.g. insect bite Reddish-brown (due to iron pigment) Hard, feels like a lentil in the skin
Pyogenic granuloma	Often follows trauma Rapidly growing, may regress if not treated Red, easily bleeds
Skin tag	Usually on the sides of the neck and in major flexures Soft, pedunculated outpouchings of skin
Lipoma	Soft, often lobulated subcutaneous nodule May be multiple
Keratoacanthoma	Middle age onwards Sunlight, tar and mineral oil may be causes Rapidly growing Smooth nodule with keratin-filled centre Will resolve, with scarring
Keratinising cysts (epidermoid and pilar)	Smooth, firm swelling(s) within the skin May become inflamed and rupture When multiple, may be feature of Gardner's syndrome (colonic polyposis)

Table 25.22 Factors predisposing to primary skin malignancy

- Ultraviolet radiation
- X-rays
- Chemicals, e.g. hydrocarbons in mineral oil, inorganic arsenic
- Immunosuppression
- Genetic, e.g. xeroderma pigmentosum
- Scars, e.g. old burn scar
- Long-standing skin disease, e.g. lupus vulgaris, chronic leg ulcer
- Some human papilloma viruses (rare)

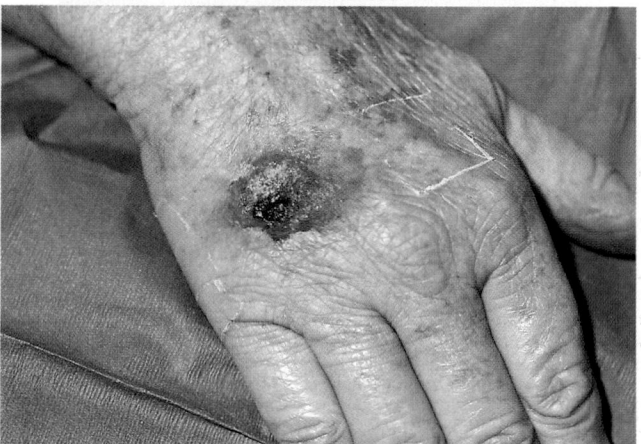

Fig. 25.34 Squamous carcinoma is characterised by induration of the base of the tumour and eventual ulceration.

keratoses are often multiple; they are more likely on the blue-eyed, fair or red-haired, and rare in dark-skinned people. The individual lesion usually presents as a papule or plaque of hard, often brownish keratin. Transformation to squamous carcinoma is uncommon.

Actinic keratoses can be treated by a number of modalities, e.g. cryotherapy, curettage and 5-fluorouracil cream.

Bowen's disease

Bowen's disease can be a consequence of previous ingestion of inorganic arsenic, usually given as a tonic many years ago. It is more common on covered than exposed sites. There is an association in some cases with internal malignancy. Bowen's disease presents as a slow-growing, well-defined, red scaly or crusted patch. It is often solitary, although it can be multiple. The major differential diagnosis is psoriasis.

Small lesions can be treated as for actinic keratosis, but excision is preferable for larger lesions.

Malignant and premalignant tumours

Squamous carcinoma

More than in other skin malignancies, there is likely to be an identifiable cause (Table 25.22) for squamous carci-

noma (Fig. 25.34). The tumour often arises from a premalignant condition and is distinguished clinically by induration of the base and surrounding normal tissues. With growth, ulceration usually occurs.

Squamous carcinoma is more liable to metastasise to regional lymph nodes than is basal carcinoma, and distant metastases can occur.

Diagnosis is by biopsy. Keratoacanthoma can be difficult to distinguish both clinically and histologically from squamous cell carcinoma.

Treatment will usually be by surgical excision, although in some circumstances radiotherapy may be preferable.

Basal cell carcinoma

Basal cell carcinoma (BCC), or rodent ulcer (Fig. 25.35), arises from cells which resemble the basal layer of the epidermis, and may have its origin from skin appendage epithelium.

It is the commonest malignant skin tumour in white races, and although sunlight exposure is clearly a major aetiological factor, unlike squamous cell carcinoma it is not often seen on the backs of the hands. The face is the commonest site, although when there has been exposure

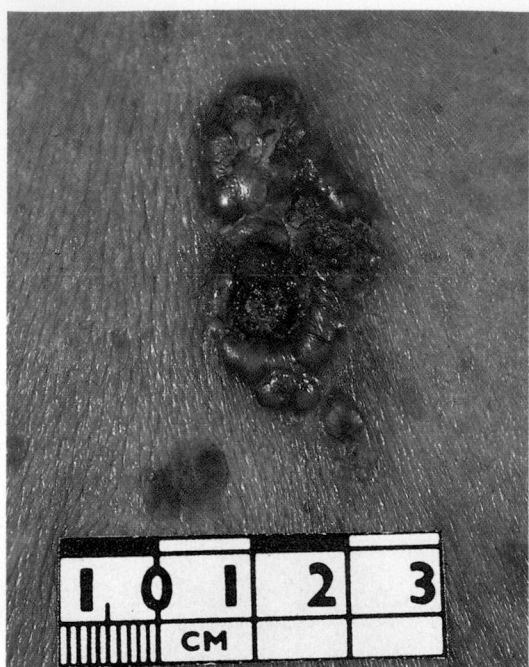

Fig. 25.35 Basal cell carcinoma is often translucent with overlying telangiectatic vessels.

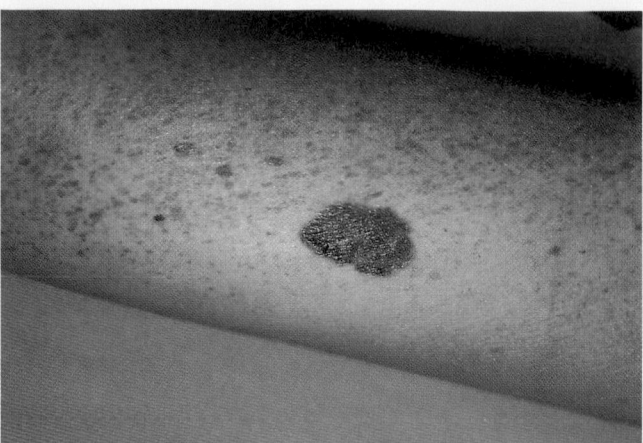

Fig. 25.36 Superficial speading malignant melanoma usually grows with an irregular edge and variable pigmentation.

to a systemic carcinogen such as inorganic arsenic, BCC can be multiple and widespread.

The tumour is usually slow-growing, evolving from a translucent papule. Various growth patterns may occur, e.g. superficial spreading, nodular, infiltrative and sclerosing. Most nodular and infiltrative tumours ulcerate. Except for the sclerosing variety, BCC tends to retain a translucent raised margin as it extends into surrounding tissues. Telangiectatic vessels are often visible on the surface and may bleed on contact. In some tumours there is an admixture of melanocytes and the resultant lesion can simulate malignant melanoma. Local destruction can be extreme, and very rarely BCC metastasises.

Treatment is usually by excision, radiotherapy, curettage or cryotherapy.

Malignant melanoma

Malignant melanoma (Fig. 25.36) usually arises either from previously normal-looking skin, or a benign melanocytic naevus. It may also arise from a naevus in a nail bed, in a mucous membrane or from the choroid or the iris.

At present there is a rapidly rising incidence among white people and, aetiologically, short bursts of sun exposure, as during a hot, sunny holiday, may be important. There is not the same association with chronic sun damage as with squamous cell carcinoma and to a lesser extent BCC. Conditions which can give rise to melanoma are lentigo maligna (Hutchinson's freckle) and dysplastic

naevus. Lentigo maligna evolves as a flat, brown, variably pigmented patch, which slowly spreads on markedly sun-damaged skin. Dysplastic naevi are unusual-looking naevi, often larger than average, with a distinctive histology; they are sporadic or inherited as an autosomal dominant characteristic, and may be a precursor to melanoma.

Melanoma is often suspected when an enlarging pigmented lesion has one or more of the following: irregular notched border, irregular pigmentation, often with red and white as well as brown/black areas, itching or prickling sensation, inflammatory halo, ulceration and bleeding.

The malignant cells spread laterally, in and just beneath the epidermis, and inwards. The prognosis depends on the depth of invasion, being excellent for completely excised, very superficial tumours. Metastasis occurs to both regional lymph nodes and distantly.

Lymphoma and leukaemia in the skin

B cell lymphoma, Hodgkin's disease and leukaemia may occasionally metastasise to the skin, or rarely present with cutaneous nodules. The skin is usually involved rather late in the course of the disease. The diagnosis is made from biopsy and other characteristic features of these diseases.

T lymphocytes have an affinity for the epidermis and its appendages, and therefore T cell neoplasia often involves the skin from the outset and may appear to be localised to the skin in some cases.

Mycosis fungoides is the best characterised T cell cutaneous neoplasm. There is often a long phase of poikilodermatous patches (poikiloderma is a combination of erythema, atrophy and reticulate pigmentation) before plaques and tumours appear. Itching usually occurs. Erythroderma (p. 1144) can develop, and if there are circulating neoplastic T cells, this constitutes the Sézary syndrome. Lymphadenopathy and visceral involvement occur late and indicate a poor prognosis.

Metastatic malignancy

Nodules, often ulcerating, may occur with many visceral malignancies.

Paget's disease of the nipple

The epidermis of the nipple becomes invaded by malignant cells arising from an underlying intraduct carcinoma of the breast tissue. The lesion is red, crusted and well defined, like Bowen's disease.

Kaposi's sarcoma

Kaposi's sarcoma (Fig. 25.37) may well have a viral aetiology. The lesions of this multicentric vascular neoplasm are usually purplish patches, plaques or nodules. Leakage of blood readily produces purpura and brown staining of the skin. The lymphatics can be affected producing lymphoedema.

Initially the lesions may be insignificant-looking, flat, reddish-brown or purple patches. A distinctive feature of AIDS-related Kaposi's sarcoma (p. 245) is a tendency for ovoid lesions to orientate along major skin creases, which on the trunk resembles the arrangement seen in pityriasis rosea.

Treatment, when indicated, is radiotherapy for localised lesions and, in some cases, cytotoxic chemotherapy for extensive disease.

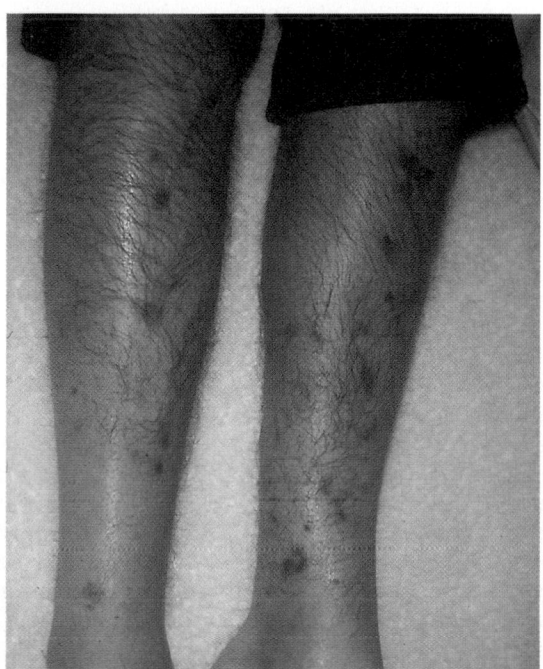

Fig. 25.37 Kaposi's sarcoma in an AIDS patient: multiple purple plaques and nodules.

Table 25.23 Skin and oral lesions in AIDS

Seborrhoeic dermatitis (early feature in 30%)	Severe drug eruptions
Itchy folliculitis	Exacerbation of psoriasis
Kaposi's sarcoma	Vasculitis
Infections	Diffuse alopecia
Molluscum contagiosum	Dry skin (late)
Peri-anal warts	Oral hairy leukoplakia (Fig. 25.38)
Superficial fungal infection	Oral candidiasis
Herpes zoster and simplex	Oral Kaposi's sarcoma
Atypical mycobacteria	

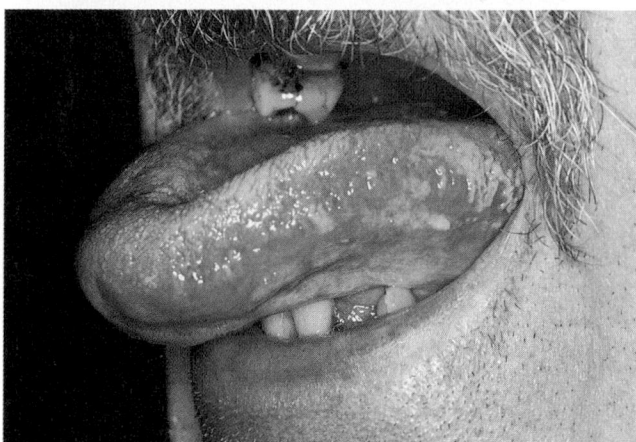

Fig. 25.38 Vertically-oriented white frond-like lesions of oral hairy leucoplakia.

Primary sarcomas

Malignant tumours arising from the various mesenchymal elements in the skin are all rare and present as enlarging masses.

AIDS AND THE SKIN

Skin and oral lesions are common features of patients with symptomatic HIV infection (Table 25.23).

SUNLIGHT AND THE SKIN

For descriptive purposes, the continuum of electro-magnetic radiation emitted by the sun is divided into segments according to wavelengths (Table 25.24).

Of the energy reaching the earth's surface 99% is ultraviolet through to middle infra-red. The shorter wavelengths of ultraviolet are filtered out by ozone in the stratosphere and by the atmosphere. The response of skin to solar radiation depends on the wavelength and on natural defences, the most important being melanin deposition. Ultraviolet B (UVB) is responsible for acute

Table 25.24 Electromagnetic spectrum

Type	Wavelength
Gamma	0.1–100 Å
Vacuum UV	10–200 nm
Ultraviolet C (UVC)	200–290 nm
Ultraviolet B (UVB)	290–320 nm
Ultraviolet A (UVA)	320–400 nm
Visible light	400–760 nm
Near infra-red	0.74–1.5 m
Middle infra-red	1.5–5.6 m
Far infra-red	5.6–1000 m
Microwaves and radiowaves	>1 mm

sunburn and the chronic changes of sun exposure: atrophy, dryness, blotchy pigmentation and wrinkling, solar keratoses and many skin cancers. The consequences of failure to repair damage inflicted on cellular DNA by UVB are seen in the rare autosomal recessively inherited condition xeroderma pigmentosum, in which sun-exposed skin becomes prematurely aged and skin cancers can appear in childhood. UVA has a much less obvious effect on normal skin, but is often responsible for photosensitive drug reactions and polymorphic light eruption. A clinical clue that UVA is playing a part is the provocation of a sun-related skin disorder behind window glass, since this filters out UVB. The action spectrum, i.e. the determination of exactly which wavelengths are responsible for a photosensitivity disorder, is only known for a few diseases. Visible light does not produce reactions on normal skin, but is responsible for photosensitivity in some diseases, notably the porphyrias, where the maximal reactivity is around 400 nm.

Although most of the consequences of solar radiation on the skin appear harmful, one benefit is the synthesis of vitamin D_3. UV light is essential to break the steroid B ring and convert 7-dihydrocholesterol to pre-vitamin D_3 which then isomerises spontaneously to vitamin D_3.

The immune system in the skin is modified by UV exposure, which may be important in development of skin cancer.

Polymorphic light eruption

Polymorphic light eruption is a common disorder which mainly occurs in females. Usually in spring, a day or so after sun exposure, itchy red papules, plaques and sometimes vesicles appear on sun-exposed sites. The condition gradually settles with continued sun exposure.

Drug photosensitivity

It is usually not known whether allergic or toxic mechanisms are involved in drug photosensitivity. The drugs commonly responsible are given on page 1150.

Phytophotodermatitis

Psoralens, a group of chemicals found in many plants, can be activated by UVA to produce inflammation and hyperpigmentation; 8-methoxypsoralen with UVA is used therapeutically as PUVA (p. 1135). Contact with a plant containing a psoralen (e.g. common rue, giant hogweed), together with sun exposure, produces erythema, often blistering, and then considerable hyperpigmentation.

Photo-allergic contact dermatitis

A number of cosmetics and even sunscreens contain chemicals which are activated by UV and, in combination with skin constituents, generate photo-allergy. Investigation is by patch testing, using two sets of patches, one of which is exposed to UV after a period of contact with the skin. Photocontact allergy produces positive results only in the set which has been irradiated. In some patients the state of photosensitivity persists long after the allergen has been withdrawn.

Metabolic disorders with light sensitivity

Skin sensitivity to sunlight may occur in porphyrias (except the acute intermittent variety), pellagra, carcinoid syndrome and Hartnup disease.

Disorders aggravated by sunlight

Many skin diseases may be worsened or triggered by sunlight. Common examples are lupus erythematosus and recurrent facial herpes simplex. Careful use of sunscreens can be helpful.

PIGMENTATION

Normal skin colour is determined by haemoglobin, both oxygenated (red) and reduced (blue), carotenoids (yellow) and melanin (brown).

Melanin is a polymer, synthesised from tyrosine in the melanocytes and distributed in cellular organelles called melanosomes via cell processes (dendrites) to the keratinocytes of the skin and hair. All races have the same number of melanocytes, about 1 per 10 basal keratinocytes, the differences in skin colour being due to the amount of melanin formation in the melanosomes (maximal in dark races) and the way these are dispersed (single in black people; in membrane-bound packages in white people). Apart from genetic factors, melanin production is stimulated by UV radiation and certain hormones, e.g. melanocyte stimulating hormones (MSH), the chemically related ACTH, and female sex hormones. Hyperpigmentation is a common sequel to many inflammatory skin diseases, especially those in which the lower epidermis is damaged. There is both stimulation of melanogenesis and passage of melanin into dermal macrophages. Sometimes hyperpigmentation is due to substances other than melanin, e.g. haemosiderin (brownish-red) and drugs, e.g. amiodarone (grey).

Many conditions associated with localised areas of hyperpigmentation are described elsewhere. These include neurofibromatosis (Fig. 25.18), xeroderma pigmentosum and Peutz-Jeghers disease. In practice the commonest are freckles, benign melanocytic naevi and postinflammatory hyperpigmentation. The causes of generalised or extensive hyperpigmentation are given in Table 25.25.

Loss of pigment

Complete or partial loss of melanin pigment can have many causes. It is helpful to consider localised and generalised loss of pigment separately (Table 25.26).

Vitiligo

Vitiligo (Fig. 25.39) is an acquired disorder in which melanocytes are lost from the basal layer of the epidermis. It occurs in about 0.4% of the population. A genetic basis is likely since about 40% have a family history. In the individuals and their families there is an increased frequency of organ-specific autoimmune diseases. The precise pathogenesis is unknown.

Clinical features. Vitiligo has often begun by the age of 20. It is characterised by sharply defined areas of pigment loss, sometimes with mild hyperpigmentation of the adja-

Table 25.25 Causes of widespread hyperpigmentation

Condition	Cause	Pattern
Hypoadrenalism Cushing's syndrome	ACTH excess	Maximal in flexures, creases of palms and soles, sites of friction and pressure, and buccal mucous membranes
Renal failure	MSH Carotenoids	Diffuse, maximal on hands and face
Haemochromatosis	Melanin Haemosiderin	Exposed skin and flexures
Vitamin B$_{12}$ deficiency	Melanin	Widespread, accentuated over knuckles Hypomelanosis of hair
Any debilitating disease	Melanin	Generalised or Addisonian
Drugs	Melanin and sometimes the drug	See p. 1151, Table 25.18
Acanthosis nigricans	Keratin	Flexures, sides of the neck

Table 25.26 Localised and generalised pigment loss

Condition	Cause	Clinical features
Localised hypopigmentation		
Vitiligo	Loss of melanocytes	Well-defined white patches, often with hyperpigmentation of the bordering skin Personal or family history of organ-specific auto-immune disease common
Pityriasis versicolor	Toxic effect on melanocytes	Slightly scaly macules mainly on the trunk, paler after sun exposure
Postinflammatory (i)	Faulty melanin transfer to keratinocytes	Pale patches with or after inflammation, e.g. Eczema
(ii)	Loss of melanocytes	e.g. Scarring after lupus erythematosus
Tuberous sclerosis	Poorly developed melanosomes	Leaf-shaped, pale macules
Leprosy	Decreased melanocytic activity	Pale patches are anaesthetic
Generalised pigment loss		
Albinism	Faulty production of melanin in skin, hair and eyes	Pale skin and hair, pink irises
Phenylketonuria	Competitive inhibition of tyrosinase by phenylalanine	Pale skin with mental deficiency
Hypopituitarism	ACTH and MSH deficiency	Associated endocrine deficiencies

cent normal skin. The texture is normal and there is no scaling. In pale-skinned individuals their first awareness may be sunburn in the depigmented skin. Any site can be affected and symmetrical involvement is common. Occasionally vitiligo follows a dermatomal pattern. The face, axillae, groins, backs of hands, knees and elbows, and genitalia are common sites. The condition is usually progressive, but repigmentation can occur spontaneously.

Diagnosis. Diagnosis is usually straightforward. By Wood's light pityriasis versicolor (which is scaly) fluoresces yellow, and vitiligo is more strikingly white than the other causes of hypopigmentation (Table 25.26). The pale macules of leprosy are hypoaesthetic.

Treatment. No treatment is entirely satisfactory. Cosmetic camouflage is helpful in a few. Sunscreens should be used on exposed areas to prevent burning and chronic sun damage, and in the pale-skinned this measure can improve the appearance by reducing tanning of surrounding normal skin. Other measures used include psoralen and UVA (see PUVA treatment of psoriasis, p. 1135) and short-term application of potent topical corticosteroids.

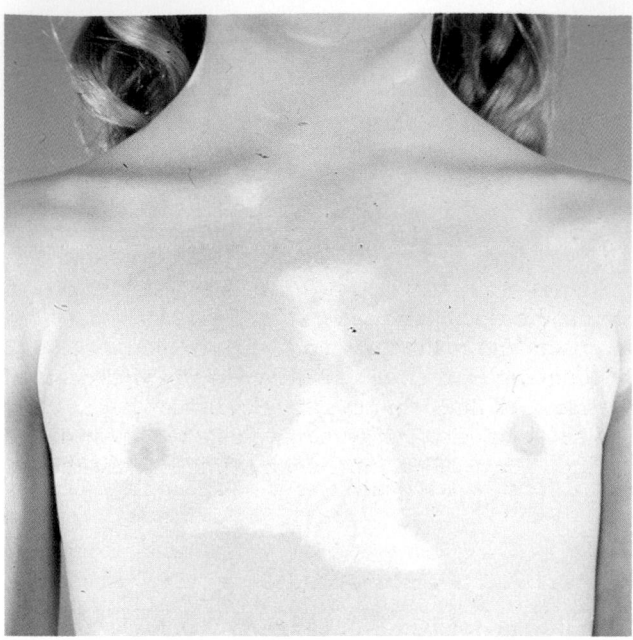

Fig. 25.39 Vitiligo shows sharply outlined areas of pigment loss.

PRESSURE SORES

A pressure sore (synonyms: bed sore, decubitus ulcer) is the consequence of sustained pressure to the tissues and is usually seen over a bony prominence, such as the ischial tuberosity, greater trochanter and elbow. The normal response to sustained pressure is movement to relieve that pressure. If discomfort is not felt or movement is not possible, then ischaemia is likely to occur. Friction (lateral pressure) exacerbates the tissue damage. Because fat and muscle are more susceptible, subcutaneous necrosis may be much greater than the surface changes suggest. Factors responsible for pressure sores are listed in Table 25.27.

The earliest clinical sign is redness on an area subjected to pressure, the erythema not fading within 30 minutes. Action at this stage may prevent further damage. Progressive damage is manifested by blistering, ulceration and formation of slough.

Management

For any patient at risk, prevention is the chief aim. Frequent changes of position, with care not to exert friction by dragging the skin, and careful choice of the surface on which the patient is lying or sitting, are crucial. For the established pressure sore, these measures are equally important. In addition, anaemia and malnutrition should be corrected, slough should be removed and the sore kept scrupulously clean. In some cases excision of the entire necrotic area, with closure or grafting, should be considered.

Table 25.27 Pathogenesis of pressure sores

Major factors	Contributory factors
Prolonged immobility	Anaemia
e.g. Paraplegia	Hypoproteinaemia
Arthritis	Severe weight loss
Operations and intensive care	
Plaster casts	
Apathy	
Loss of sensory stimuli	
e.g. Coma	
Multiple sclerosis	
Vascular disease	
e.g. Atherosclerosis	

LEG ULCERATION

Ulceration of the lower leg can have many causes, some of which are shown in Table 25.28. In the developed world most cases of leg ulceration are wholly or partly due to disorders of the venous system, but arterial insufficiency often co-exists and may be the major factor in many patients. In the tropics, infective causes are much more important. Particularly in the elderly there can be multiple aetiological factors.

VENOUS LEG ULCERATION

Venous leg ulceration is also known as stasis or gravitational ulceration. The skin changes are due to the consequences of raised pressure in the venous system.

Table 25.28 Causes of leg ulceration

Cause	Example
Venous hypertension	Venous thrombosis
Arterial diseases	Atherosclerosis, diabetes mellitus
Vasculitis	Rheumatoid disease, Wegener's granulomatosis
Pyoderma gangrenosum	See p. 1142
Trauma	Mechanical injury, burns, bites
Infections	Ecthyma, tuberculosis, syphilis, deep fungal infection
Neuropathy	Leprosy, diabetes mellitus
Blood disorders	Disseminated intravascular coagulation, platelet disorders, sickle cell anaemia and spherocytosis, polycythaemia
Plasma protein disorders	Cryoglobulinaemia
Scarring disorders	Radiodermatitis
Neoplasia	Cutaneous carcinomas, Kaposi's sarcoma

Aetiology and pathogenesis

In most cases venous return is compromised by previous deep vein thrombosis. In a few cases ulceration is associated with varicosity of the superficial veins, or defective communicating veins. Pressure in the venous system is raised because the valves are absent or destroyed, and this increased pressure is transmitted back to the capillary bed in the skin. There is extravascular deposition of fibrin, followed by fibrosis, and these changes are thought to impair transfer of oxygen and nutrients to the skin. It is also likely that venous distension produces reflex arteriolar constriction. This phenomenon occurs in normal individuals when standing still, but is promptly relieved in them by exercise, but not in those with persistently raised venous pressure. Patients who develop leg ulcers may also have decreased ability to lyse the fibrin and this may contribute to the pathogenesis.

Clinical features

Venous ulceration is most common in middle-aged and elderly women. Interestingly, leg ulcers occur frequently and early in Klinefelter's syndrome (p. 75).

Venous ulcers are usually preceded by varying combinations of oedema, prominent venules around the ankle, brown discoloration due to extravasation of red blood cells, eczema (p. 1139), fibrotic thickening of the dermis and subcutaneous fat, and white plaques stippled with telangiectases (*atrophie blanche*). These signs occur most commonly near the medial malleolus, but may be seen also on the lateral aspect of the ankle and over communicating veins. Another characteristic site is over the dorsum of the foot near the base of the toes. Ulceration may occur spontaneously or after trauma, which is often trivial. Unlike ulceration due to arterial disease or vasculitis, venous ulcers are often painless. The base of the ulcer usually shows red granulation tissue and the edge is oedematous. The ulcer may be complicated by infection; cellulitis, usually due to *Staph. aureus* and/or *Strep. pyogenes*, can develop rapidly. Another common complication is contact allergic dermatitis due to medicaments applied to the ulcer, e.g. antibiotics and antiseptics (p. 1137). In time the fibrotic process causes lymphoedema, and loss of movement at the ankle joint often occurs. Rarely, squamous and basal cell carcinoma can develop in chronic venous leg ulcers.

Management

Patients with venous leg ulcers often have other disorders, correction of which facilitates healing. These include nutritional deficiency, anaemia, diabetes, obesity, hypertension, cardiac and renal disease, myxoedema, and any disease causing immobility. It is most important to assess the arterial system in the legs, since the compression that is valuable for venous insufficiency can be harmful if there is a poor arterial inflow.

Raised venous pressure can be counteracted by elevation of the legs at night and for periods of time during the day, and careful use of compression bandages combined with exercise. If the ulcer is due to incompetent superficial or communicating veins rather than deep vein thrombosis, surgical treatment may be indicated. Numerous treatments are available for the ulcer itself, and in most circumstances materials which do not contain potential sensitisers and maintain a moist surface should be used. Desloughing is often best achieved with a hydrocolloid dressing. Cellulitis requires systemic antibiotics.

When venous ulceration has healed, the patient should continue to exercise and maintain compression with suitable stockings indefinitely.

ARTERIAL ULCERATION

When the arteriolar supply to a region of skin is insufficient or interrupted, necrosis occurs with resultant ulceration. The more profound process of gangrene is discussed on page 441. In general, vascular occlusion can occur because of changes outside the vessel wall, within the wall itself (as in atherosclerosis and vasculitis), and due to changes in the blood (as in cryoglobulinaemia and platelet thrombi). The symptoms and signs will be determined by the size of the ischaemic area and the speed with which the process occurs. The most common cause of arterial ulceration is atheromatous disease of the aorta and its tributaries.

Clinical features of ulceration due to atherosclerosis

Arterial ulcers tend to be painful, sometimes severely so. There may be coldness, and pallor exaggerated by elevation of the limb, but cyanosis and blotchy erythema are also seen. Chronic ischaemia results in dryness and atrophy of the skin, loss of hair and thickened, distorted nails. Intermittent claudication may be present (p. 441). Common sites for arterial ulceration due to atherosclerosis are the front or lateral aspect of the ankle, and the toes. The ulcer tends to be well demarcated with a grey slough-covered base, which may expose deeper structures such as tendons.

The management of arterial ulceration is usually in the province of the vascular surgeon.

ACNE VULGARIS

Acne vulgaris primarily involves the pilosebaceous follicles, i.e. the sebaceous glands, ducts and the distal part of the hair follicles into which they open. The lesions include keratinous plugs in the ducts (comedones), inflammatory papules, pustules, nodules, cysts and scars.

Pathogenesis

The best defined factors that determine the occurrence of acne vulgaris are androgenic stimulation of the sebaceous glands and the commensal anaerobic bacterium *Propionibacterium acnes* which heavily colonises active pilosebaceous follicles. Although the onset of acne around puberty is explained by the increased output of androgens at that time, it is much less clear why the disease becomes quiescent without any measurable change in the hormonal milieu or numbers of propionibacteria. The basis for the disorder of keratinisation in the sebaceous ducts which produces the comedones is uncertain. Inflammatory lesions are mainly derived from closed comedones (see below). Possible mediators of inflammation include free fatty acids, bacterial cell wall components and enzymes, and the patient's complement system. The pus in acne lesions is sterile and a consequence of inflammation, which is often so severe that scarring results.

Clinical features

Acne can occur in infants, but is usually mild and due to the influence of transplacental hormonal stimulus. In older children, acne often represents the beginnings of puberty but may not occur until the mid-teens or beyond. The areas affected are those with maximal numbers of pilosebaceous follicles: the face, upper trunk and shoulders. Comedones are either open (blackheads) or closed (small whitish papules). The inflammatory lesions are erythematous, varying from papules through pustules to nodules and large collections of pus (wrongly) called cysts. The more destructive lesions heal with scarring, which is usually pitted, but hypertrophic or keloidal in those so predisposed. The course of acne can be erratic and there are often premenstrual exacerbations.

Lesions resembling acne can be provoked by halogenated hydrocarbons, mineral oils, tars, greasy cosmetics, and drugs (p. 1152).

Management

Acne can have serious psychological effects and should not be ignored on the basis that it will get better sooner or later. Mild cases often respond to topical agents alone, e.g. benzoyl peroxide, 2.5–10% gel, or topical retinoic acid. The latter is more irritant, but often more effective when comedones are the predominant feature. If there is insufficient response after a few weeks' treatment, or if the acne is of moderate severity, an oral antibiotic should be used in addition (or instead, if topical therapy proves too irritant). Tetracyclines and erythromycin are equally effective, usually in a dose of 0.5 g twice daily for several months. Topical antibiotics, e.g. 1% clindamycin, can also be effective. For females with moderate acne, hormonal modulation with the antiandrogen cyproterone acetate may be more effective. This drug must be given with an oestrogen, for mild cases in the form of a low-dose oral contraceptive pill. Patients with severe and destructive acne usually need treatment with oral isotretinoin. This vitamin A analogue is highly effective, but has a number of adverse effects, notably teratogenicity, and is restricted to hospital use in the UK.

Other measures sometimes used include intralesional corticosteroids for inflammatory nodules and cysts, and dermabrasion, a surgical technique to improve scarring.

HIDRADENITIS SUPPURATIVA

Hidradenitis suppurative is a chronic suppurative, inflammatory and scarring condition of blocked apocrine glands. There may be a genetic basis for this disorder, which has some similarity to acne vulgaris and may be associated with it. Following keratinous plugging of the apocrine glands there is bacterial infection, subsequent gland rupture, damage to surrounding tissues and healing with scarring and sinus tracts. The areas affected are the axillae, anogenital area and breasts. Tender inflammatory nodules, which discharge pus, are seen and blackheads are often present early on.

Because bacteria are playing a perpetuating role in this disorder, courses of antibiotics (if possible governed by sensitivity testing) are helpful but not curative. Incision, marsupialisation and even wide excision may be needed in chronic cases. Hormonal modulation, e.g. with antiandrogens in females, may have a role in treatment.

ROSACEA

Rosacea is a common condition of the middle-aged and elderly, in which there are varying combinations of redness of the face with telangiectasia, papules and sterile pustules (Fig. 25.40). The facial erythema is often easily exacerbated by spicy foods, alcohol and emotional upset; chronic UV exposure may have an aetiological role. Unlike acne there are no comedones and no elevation of sebum excretion rate. Common associations are eye disorders (e.g. conjunctivitis and keratitis), facial lymphoedema and rhinophyma, a hypertrophy of the nasal

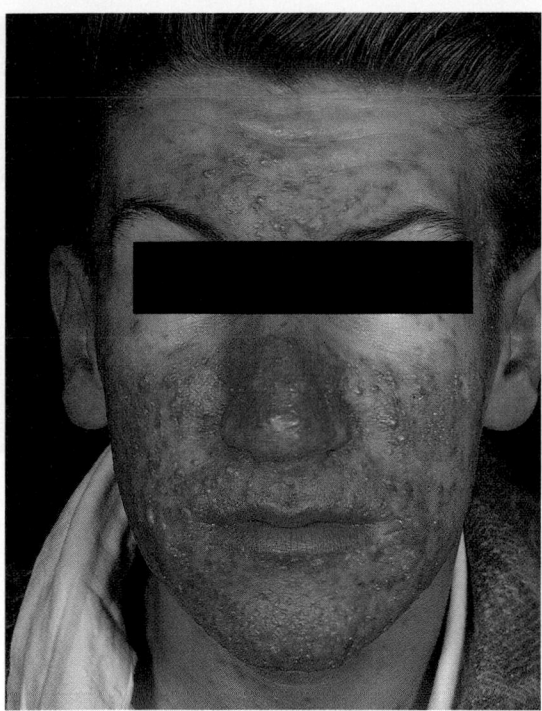

Fig. 25.40 Rosacea is characterised by erythema, papules and pustules but there are no comedones.

Table 25.29 Systemic causes of generalised pruritus

Hepatic disease	Haematological
Obstructive biliary disease	Iron deficiency
Pregnancy: oestrogen-induced cholestasis	Drugs
	Opiates
Endocrine disease	Subclinical drug sensitivity
Hyper- and hypothyroidism	
Diabetes mellitus (rare)	Psychiatric
	Neurosis
Renal	Psychosis, e.g. delusion of
Chronic renal failure	parasitosis
Parasitic	
Trichinosis	
Onchocerciasis	
Malignancy	
Hodgkin's disease	
Leukaemia and lymphoma	
Polycythaemia rubra vera	
Other neoplasms	

skin and its appendages. Despite the cause remaining unknown, treatment with oral oxytetracycline is effectively suppressive in most cases. Topical metronidazole is also helpful. It is usually helpful to minimise the effects of sun exposure.

Rosacea is slowly worsened by the use of topical steroids on the face, and a similar condition, *peri-oral dermatitis*, can be initiated by the more potent topical steroid preparations.

PRURITUS

Pruritus, or itching, is the distinctive sensation whose outward manifestation is the act of scratching. Except for the role of histamine in some disorders, and bile salts in obstructive liver disease, we know disappointingly little about the mechanisms of this common symptom. When severe, pruritus can surpass pain in the distress it can cause.

Many skin diseases can be itchy, and some, such as scabies, dermatitis herpetiformis, lichen planus and urticaria, severely so. Dry skin of whatever cause tends to be itchy, and this is a particularly common problem in the elderly and one of the reasons for pruritus in the atopic individual. Occasionally an external cause (such as fibre-

glass or scabies) can produce widespread pruritus with little to see. Itching can occur without any primary rash, the skin changes, if any, being those due to rubbing and scratching. Generalised pruritus may be a pointer to systemic disease (Table 25.29).

Wherever possible, the underlying cause of generalised pruritus should be treated. When symptomatic measures are called for, the use of emollients can be helpful, probably because dry skin has a lower threshold for pruritus. Oral H_1 antagonists can provide some relief, particularly when sedative anti-histamines are used. Uraemic pruritus can be helped by UVB. Pruritus due to cholestatic liver disease often responds to cholestyramine or colestipol. The itch in polycythaemia vera may respond to anti-serotonin agents, cyproheptadine or pizotifen.

Localised pruritus without primary signs of skin disease is common in the peri-anal (Table 25.30) and vulval areas (Table 25.31). Sometimes there is a psychological basis for this.

Table 25.30 Causes of pruritus ani

Ano-rectal disease	Infection
Fissure	Candidiasis
Haemorrhoids	
Rectal carcinoma	Infestation
Faecal soiling	Threadworms
Skin disease	Psychogenic
Psoriasis	Anxiety
Atopic dermatitis	Depression
Irritant and allergic contact dermatitis (especially medicaments)	Unknown

Table 25.31 Causes of pruritus vulvae

Diseases special to vulval skin	Infection
Lichen sclerosus et atrophicus	Candidiasis
Leukoplakia	Trichomonas
Carcinoma	
	Infestation
Skin disease	Pediculosis
Psoriasis	
Atopic dermatitis	Psychogenic
Irritant and allergic contact	Anxiety
dermatitis (especially medicaments)	Depression

ALOPECIA

The evaluation of alopecia, or hair loss, takes account of:

- the distribution
- any abnormalities of the hair shafts
- the scalp.

Androgenic alopecia (common baldness)

The prerequisites for this very common condition are: an inherited tendency; some degree of ageing; and post-pubertal androgen levels. The longer, coarser, pigmented terminal hairs on the scalp are progressively replaced by small, fine vellus hairs. In males there is recession of the anterior hairline and thinning over the crown, and ultimately terminal hair may only be present at the back and sides of the scalp. In an endocrinologically normal female there is thinning over the top of the scalp, but baldness to the extent seen in males is uncommon, except in the elderly, and if present warrants careful evaluation.

Diffuse alopecia

Diffuse alopecia is a decrease in hair density over the whole scalp without change in the skin or hair morphology. In some instances, e.g. a febrile illness, childbirth and severe emotional upset, the causative factor synchronises a proportion of the follicles so that hairs are shed 2–3 months later, a phenomenon called telogen effluvium. Regrowth usually takes place in about 6 months.

Normal hair growth requires an adequate nutrition, and diffuse alopecia accompanies malnutrition and wasting conditions. Iron deficiency, even in the absence of anaemia, has been associated with hair loss. Dry and progressively sparse hair is a feature of hypothyroidism. Many drugs (p. 1152) can produce diffuse alopecia, sometimes (as with cytotoxic agents) within days of administration, or after several weeks (as with anticoagulants, antithyroid drugs and the retinoids). Stopping the

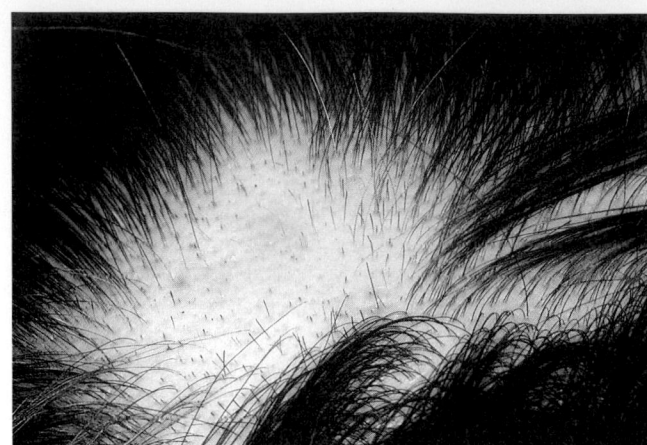

Fig. 25.41 A distinctive feature of alopecia areata is the presence of shortened 'exclamation mark' hairs which taper markedly where they emerge from the scalp.

oral contraceptive has been associated with mild hair loss, similar to the effect of childbirth.

Alopecia areata

Alopecia areata (Fig. 25.41) is a common condition in which there is loss of hair in patches, typically with no skin changes. Hair on the face and body as well as scalp may be affected. A distinctive feature is the presence of shortened hairs which taper markedly where they emerge from the scalp (exclamation mark hairs). White hairs tend to be spared the process causing the hair loss. Alopecia areata is usually reversible, and when hair grows back it is often initially white. When the entire scalp becomes affected the condition is called *alopecia totalis*, and if all the body hair is lost as well the term *alopecia universalis* is applied. Regrowth usually occurs but is less likely with these more severe forms. Nails may show a distinctive pattern of pitting and ridging. There is sometimes an association with one or more organ-specific autoimmune diseases in the patient or family, such as vitiligo. The cause of alopecia areata is not known. Topical and intradermal corticosteroids can be helpful in selected cases. Treatment by induced contact allergic dermatitis, e.g. to diphencyprone, can be helpful.

Inflammatory alopecia

Fungal (p. 1129) and bacterial infection can cause patchy hair loss with varying degrees of erythema, oedema and pustules. Lichen planus (p. 1147) and lupus erythematosus (p. 1023) may affect the scalp, and characteristically produce atrophy. Occasionally metastatic neoplasia presents as inflammatory alopecia.

Traumatic alopecia

Hair can be damaged by chemicals, e.g. those used in permanent waving, and physical trauma such as twisting between the fingers and pulling.

NAILS AND DISEASE

The nail is a specialised sheet of keratin largely produced by an invagination of the epidermis called the matrix, which is located beneath the posterior nail fold and extends beneath the nail plate as the lunule (half-moon). Disorders of the nails may result from local causes such as psoriasis, fungal infection and lesions beneath the nail (e.g. melanoma), or reflect a systemic disorder (see below).

Clubbing

Normally the angle between the nail and the posterior nail fold is less than 180°. In clubbing this angle increases, often becoming greater than 180°. The causes are discussed on page 452.

Koilonychia

Koilonychia is flattening or even depression of the normal slight convexity of the nail, and is usually due to iron deficiency.

Beau's lines

Beau's lines are transverse grooves in all the nails, reflecting a transient reduction in nail growth due to a severe illness. They may also occur after childbirth.

Yellow nail syndrome

In yellow nail syndrome the nails become yellow, thickened and excessively curved and virtually stop growing. Cuticular attachment is lost and there is usually some separation of nail from nail bed. The nail changes are associated with lymphoedema, bronchiectasis and pleural effusions.

It is more common to find yellow nails in circumstances such as psoriasis and dermatophyte fungal infection, these conditions being recognised by the associated skin changes and mycological investigations.

Splinter haemorrhages

Splinter haemorrhages are usually longitudinal or dot-shaped areas of haemorrhage beneath nails. Most are the result of minor trauma, are painless and appear beneath the distal third of the nail. Psoriasis and fungal infection of the nails may be associated with similar distal splinters. Painful and proximal splinter haemorrhages are much more likely to be associated with medical causes, of which the best established are subacute bacterial endocarditis, trichinosis, chronic mountain sickness and indwelling radial arterial catheters.

Paronychia

Paronychia is a painful swelling of the posterior nail fold. When acute, staphylococcal infection is likely. A more gradual onset and chronic course is usually associated with *Candida albicans*. Women are especially prone to chronic paronychia. Common predisposing factors are occupations in which the hands are frequently wet, diabetes mellitus and poor peripheral circulation.

PSYCHOLOGICAL CAUSES OF SKIN DISEASE

Many bona fide skin diseases, such as eczema and psoriasis, may worsen or be precipitated during periods of psychological stress. Similarly, anxiety and depression commonly accompany distressing skin disease, and can often be ameliorated by explanation, reassurance and encouragement.

There is a direct psychological cause with dermatitis artefacta, many cases of delusions of infestation and psychogenic pruritus. A diagnosis of psychogenic pruritus rests on exclusion of an organic cause as well as association with other psychoneurotic symptoms and signs.

Dermatitis artefacta

Dermatitis artefacta is mainly seen in females. The lesions are self-inflicted but this is denied and they may indeed be produced subconsciously. They are often bizarre in appearance, resistant to therapy (except occlusive dressings, in which case lesions may appear at new sites), and often regarded with indifference. The patients tend to be immature or insecure but the motivation behind dermatitis artefacta is often difficult to elucidate, and the condition can be protracted.

Self-inflicted damage is also seen in psychotics and the Lesch Nyhan syndrome, a rare X-linked inherited disorder of purine metabolism associated with mental retardation and spasticity.

Delusions of infestation

This is the conviction that there are parasites on or in the skin, often supported by offerings of excoriated skin fragments. Such a delusion may be one element in a broader presentation of psychosis, including that due to organic disorders such as vitamin B_{12} deficiency, but can present in an isolated form (monosymptomatic delusional hypochondriasis). It is of course essential to exclude infestation such as scabies and pests in the home.

The monodelusional state often responds well to the psychotropic drug pimozide.

Dermatological non-disease

The term 'dermatological non-disease' describes a disproportionate anxiety about minor and often physiological skin changes. Such patients are difficult to manage, but can be seriously disturbed and at risk of suicide.

FURTHER READING

Braverman I M 1981 Skin signs of systemic disease. 2nd edn. W B Saunders, Philadelphia. *Single author, easy to read and well illustrated*

Fitzpatrick T B, Eisen A Z, Wolff K, Freedberg I W, Austen K F 1993 Dermatology in general medicine. 4th edn. McGraw-Hill, New York. *A major, predominantly US text*

Graham-Brown R A C, Burns D A 1990 Lecture notes on dermatology. 6th edn. Blackwell, Oxford. *Excellent value, common-sense dermatology, with humorous touches*

Levene G M, Calnan C D 1984 A colour atlas of dermatology. Wolfe Medical, London. *Minimal text, beautifully illustrated*

Rook A J, Wilkinson D S, Ebling F J G, Champion R H, Burton J L 1991 Textbook of dermatology. 5th edn. Blackwell, Oxford. *The comprehensive British textbook*

Du Vivier A 1987 Atlas of clinical dermatology. Churchill Livingstone, Edinburgh. *A good illustrated introduction*

Index

Index

1168

Index

Index

Index

Index

Index

Index

Index

Index

Index

Index

Index

Index

Index

Index

Index

Index

Index

Index

LONGMAN STUDY GUIDES

GCSE

French

Alasdair McKeane

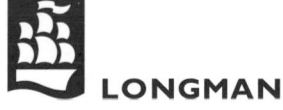

LONGMAN

LONGMAN STUDY GUIDES

SERIES EDITORS: **Geoff Black and Stuart Wall**

Titles available

Biology
Business Studies
Chemistry
Design and Technology
Economics
English
English Literature
French
Geography
German
Information Technology

Mathematics
Mathematics: Higher Level
Music
Physics
Psychology
Religious Studies
Science
Sociology
Spanish
World History

Addison Wesley Longman Limited,
Edinburgh Gate,
Harlow,
Essex CM20 2JE, England
and Associated Companies throughout the World.

© Addison Wesley Longman 1997

First published 1997

ISBN 0582–30485–7

British Library Cataloguing-in-Publication Data
A catalogue record for this book is available from the British Library.

Set by 16 in 9.75/12pt Sabon
Printed in Great Britain by Henry Ling Ltd.
at the Dorset Press, Dorchester, Dorset

▶ CONTENTS

► ### EDITORS' PREFACE

Longman Study Guides have been written by the people who set and mark the exams – the examiners. Examiners are aware that, because of lack of practice and poor preparation, some students achieve only the lowest grades: they are not able effectively to show the examiner what they know. These books give excellent advice about examination practice and preparation, and about organising a structured revision programme, all of which are essential for examination success. Remember: the examiners are looking for opportunities to **give** you marks, not take them away!

Longman Study Guides are designed to be used throughout the course. The self-contained chapters can be read in any order appropriate to the stage you have reached in your course. The examiner guides you through the essential parts of each topic, making helpful comments throughout.

We believe that this book, and the series as a whole, will help you establish and build your basic knowledge and examination techniques. For additional help with examination practice and revision techniques, we have published a series called **Longman Exam Kits**, which are available from all good bookshops, or direct from Addison Wesley Longman.

GEOFF BLACK AND STUART WALL

► ### ACKNOWLEDGEMENTS

To the Examining Groups for providing liberal quantities of advice, materials and encouragement, and permission to reproduce questions:

EDEXCEL Foundation (London)
Midland Examining Group (MEG)
Northern Examinations and Assessment Board (NEAB)
Northern Ireland Council for Curriculum and Assessment (NICCEA)
Southern Examining Group (SEG)
Welsh Joint Education Committee (WJEC)
International General Certificate of Secondary Education (IGCSE)

To my wife Anne, for research, many suggested improvements and encouragement. To my sons John, Andrew and James for their patience. To John Connor, for the vocabulary. To Chris Watson, for research. To Monique Skelsey, for acting as Native Speaker Consultant.

Note: The suggested answers provided in this book, while in accordance with the Examining Groups' guidelines, are the author's own and are not 'official answers'. The Examining Groups are unable to enter into any correspondence concerning the suggested answers.

► ### INFORMATION ABOUT THIS BOOK

This book has been written as a course companion for use throughout your GCSE course in French. The first two chapters concentrate on study skills and examination requirements. You should read these chapters carefully as they give invaluable advice about preparing for the examinations in Listening, Reading, Speaking and Writing; about preparing coursework; and details about assessment and grading. This information will be useful to you throughout your GCSE course.

Study the remaining chapters carefully as they give information about what you need to learn to obtain a good grade in GCSE French, including chapters on essential vocabulary; improving your Listening, Reading, Speaking, Writing and coursework (these chapters include practice questions and tasks, as well as sample answers and examiner's comments); a whole chapter on grammar (including a glossary of grammatical terms); and a verb table. Refer to the Appendix at the end of this book for details on the specific requirements of Examining Groups.

The ideal way to use this book is to use it throughout your course as a **study guide**.

- After covering a new topic area at school, for example 'Tourism', learn the vocabulary and phrases for that topic given in Chapter 3 and check if there are any similar topics covered in the role-play phrases in Chapter 6 'Speaking'.
- If you have been taught some new grammar, for example the perfect tense, then check that you understand it fully by reading through the explanations and examples given in Chapter 9 'Grammar' and practise applying it.
- Before attempting any written homework, look through Chapter 7 to see examples of similar questions and styles of writing, and to learn ways of improving your written work.
- Understanding the types of questions you are likely to face and what will be expected of you in the different examinations will help to improve your grade. Read the chapters on Listening, Reading, Speaking and Writing carefully. Look at the sample student answers and examiner's comments to typical questions, and then try the further practice questions at the end of each chapter.
- Fill in the 'Language task list' during your two-year course so that you can see which topics you need to do some more work on.

Alternatively, you could use this book as a quick **revision guide**, and work from it intensively in the period before your examination. Quick revision will help you, but remember that there is no substitute for hard work during your course.

Study skills

▷ **GETTING STARTED**

This chapter is intended to point out two aspects of preparing for GCSE French, namely, study skills enabling you to make the best possible use of your valuable time in the run-up to the GCSE examination, which will also be of general use in preparing for other subjects, and hints and tips to improve your performance in the four language skills tested in GCSE French: Speaking, Listening, Reading and Writing. Because performance in French is a skill, it is improved by practice. And any good musician or sporting star will confirm that the best forms of practice contain variety. *Alors, allons-y*!

▷ **WHAT YOU NEED TO KNOW**

▷ **Your approach to the GCSE course**

The foundations of success in GCSE French are laid early in your course, not so much by your teacher, as by how you personally approach your work. Let us compare a good student and a poor student, seen from the teacher's point of view.

Good student	Poor student
Is a regular attender.	Attends irregularly.
Catches up with work after absence – usually without prompting.	Makes no effort to catch up. Needs to be 'chased'.
Always writes notes in lessons.	Lets teacher's explanations wash over him/her. Has lost notebook and/or pen.
Tries his/her best during pairwork.	Chats in English during pairwork.
Sits with a good view of board and teacher.	Sits at the back or in a corner.
Asks when stuck.	Gives up if stuck. Claims not to understand.
Does homework on time.	Does homework late, or not at all.
Works at a regular time.	Works when he or she feels like it.
Presents work (rough or neat) tidily, with dates, page numbers, titles, etc.	Work is messy.
Writes legibly, with clear accents. Has obviously done a rough draft of homework.	Hard to read. Accents ambiguous. Hands in first draft with altered letters, crossings-out, etc. A pain to mark.
Re-reads corrected homework, notes errors and resolves to act on comments and corrections.	Never looks at anything teacher writes except the mark at the bottom of work.
When no homework is set, finds something extra to do in French.	When no homework set, does nothing except cheer.
Is basically interested in most aspects of the subject.	Only took French because there was no other option.
Quite enjoys French.	Hates French.

The key to a successful approach is **motivation.** You know your reasons for taking GCSE French. Whatever they are, look for ways to succeed.

▷ **Getting organised**

Observation suggests that successful students are organised. Many students fail to reach their full potential because they approach the mechanics of studying the wrong way.

Here are some practical ways you can get yourself organised. Parents, too, may find this useful.

1 **Have set routines for work** If you have a fixed time or times in the day or week when you do homework, then you don't have to spend time deciding when to do it. Your school, after all, has a set timetable for lessons for that very reason. Set times save you time.

2 **Have set times when you do not work** This ensures that you get enough leisure time. 'All work and no play makes Jack a dull boy', runs the proverb. Again, you save time on decision-making.

3 **Do assignments as they are set** This is particularly important in French, where one piece of work often builds on the previous one, and where you need detailed, early feedback from your teacher to support your learning. By doing work immediately, you also save the time you might spend worrying about how and when to do the work. Do it **now**!

4 **Have a suitable place for study** The ideal location is free from distractions. Aim for a table or desk free from clutter, with good lighting, and pens, pencils, paper and reference books within reach (so you don't have to keep getting up).

5 **Do a reasonable amount of study per week** This might, perhaps, be in the range of 35–45 hours weekly, including the 25–27 hours or so spent in lessons in school. Many adults work about that number of hours. You may, of course, work longer if you can do so effectively.

6 **Approach topics on the 'before, during and after' principle**
Before a new topic – read ahead in your textbook to prepare yourself.
During the lesson – take notes or take part, as appropriate.
After the lesson – go over the notes and the textbook material as soon as possible.

Being organised doesn't take any more time than being disorganised. In fact, it saves time. And most importantly, it makes you a more efficient learner who will certainly gain a better grade in GCSE than your disorganised fellow-students.

▶ Revision planning

As I have suggested, being organised produces better results. This applies, of course, to revision as well as normal study. Here are some tips about efficient revision.

1 **Count the weeks** Work out how many weeks there are left before the GCSE examination. For GCSE French, the various examinations are spread over several weeks, so time the run-up to each one individually. There is little point in slaving over your Writing the day before your Speaking Test, for example.

2 **Make a week-by-week revision planner** Write in the topics you wish to revise, week by week and skill by skill. Allow a week near the end for 'slippage' – time to catch up on what you have missed. Make sure you have sufficient variety, and don't be over-ambitious about what you can get done. You may need to decide what is top priority for you.

3 **Know what the examinations involve** In the Appendix at the back of this book you'll find details for each test. Knowing what to expect gives direction and urgency to your revision and prevents your wasting time on irrelevant material.

4 **Check you can do what is required** Chapter 3 'Vocabulary topics' lists all the tasks you are expected to be able to perform, as laid down by the Defined Content of the various Examining Groups. So there's no excuse for not making sure you can do them!

5 **Identify questions** Use the sample and past papers available for GCSE French. The Defined Content makes it possible to work out fairly accurately the sort of question that might be asked, particularly at Foundation level. For example, there are a limited number of things that could be asked of a pump attendant using the vocabulary given in the 'Vocabulary topics' chapter of this book. If you know them, you have nothing to fear from a role-play exercise on that topic.

6 **Analyse your own performance** If you have done a mock examination, work out where your weaknesses are, and do something about them. If you are uncertain where to begin or whether you should enter for Foundation or Higher papers in a particular skill, consult your teacher who, after all, knows your abilities best. When consulting your teacher, be prepared to take his or her advice – after all, he or she will probably have seen some hundreds or even thousands of GCSE candidates over the years and will know what to expect. You, on the other hand, are doing the examination for the first time! Even if you

haven't done a mock examination, you can still give direction to your revision by honestly pinpointing things you don't do well.

Directed revision pays off. Revise early, and revise often!

▶ Revision techniques

The most difficult thing about revision is overcoming boredom. By definition, you have seen things you are revising before, so you need to find ways of compensating for the lack of novelty.

Many students revise ineffectively because they merely read through notes and chapters in the textbook and let the information wash over them. This is almost always a waste of time, certainly after the first half-hour or so. The key is to **do** something. Activity is an aid to concentration. In a skill-based subject such as French, where your performance is measured, you will improve your performance by practice.

Try some or all of the following techniques.

1 **Write notes**   When reading, say, grammar rules again, make yourself skeleton notes which are sufficiently detailed to jog your memory. Some students do this on small pieces of card (index cards or chopped up pieces of cereal packet) which they carry about with them and consult at odd moments. The same goes for vocabulary. Writing a word down with its gender and meaning will help to fix it in your memory. Another hint is to write down a phrase which contains the word and its gender. When reading texts, make a note of every word you had to look up. As time goes on, you will have to look up fewer and fewer.

2 **Work with a friend**   This can relieve the boredom. Pick a friend who is about the same standard as you are. Working with someone a lot better can be good for their ego, but not for yours. Similarly, working with someone a lot weaker doesn't teach you anything new. Testing each other is a good idea. But don't forget to include written testing, which is the ultimate proof of whether you know things. Because of the danger of being side-tracked, don't rely on this method of revision alone.

3 **Set yourself tests**   While learning, make a note of things you found hard, and test yourself later – at the end of your session, then the following day, then the following week. You have to be honest with yourself about how you got on! Keep a chart of your marks as a rough guide to progress.

4 **Tick off what you've done**   Using the revision planner you have made, tick off the topics you have dealt with. Do **not** tick off ones you have missed out! The more you have dealt with, the better you will feel.

5 **Set realistic targets**   Don't try to do too much in one session – you'll end up frustrated and become more and more depressed. Far better to learn, say, 10 irregular verbs and succeed than to try to learn 56 and fail miserably.

6 **Reward yourself**   If you have done a reasonable stint of revision, or done well in a test, give yourself a treat – a sweet, or a coffee break, or the chance to watch a favourite soap opera. Having something to look forward to is a great incentive.

7 **Don't go too long without a break**   45–50 minutes is probably the longest session most people can concentrate for without a break – even if it's only to stretch your legs for 5 minutes.

8 **Give yourself variety**   Vary what you look at – revise different skills in French. Also, vary the subjects you do in any one session – three spells of 45–50 minutes on three different subjects will be more productive than a 3-hour 'slog' on one area.

9 **Don't be fooled by other students**   During the examination season, some fellow-students will be loudly proclaiming either that they 'never do any revision' or that they are 'up till 2 a.m. every evening working'. Ignore them. They are being hysterical, and may well not be telling the truth anyway. What matters to you is not how much or how little revision your friends do, but how much **you** do.

Most important of all, don't kid yourself that you are working when you aren't. You can't revise at all while watching TV, chatting to friends, washing your hair or eating a meal. So don't even attempt it. Instead, use these activities to reward yourself **after** a revision session.

▷ **Examination techniques**

The best cure for examination nerves is the knowledge that you have done all reasonable preparation. There are also various practical things you can do to make sure you can concentrate on the examination paper.

The evening before an examination

▷ Put everything you need the following morning, ready packed, by the front door to eliminate last-minute panic. Include spare pens, pencils and rubbers, your dictionary, and a silent watch.

▷ At the end of the evening, do something other than work to relax you. If you can manage to take the whole evening off, that's even better.

▷ Go to bed at a reasonable hour so you have enough sleep. Set an alarm.

The morning before an examination

▷ Get up in good time to avoid rush and panic.

▷ Dress carefully, possibly even smartly (to take your mind off the examination).

▷ Eat breakfast so you aren't hungry during the examination.

Just before the examination

▷ Be there in good time, but not **too** early.

▷ Read or listen to something **easy** and familiar in French.

In the examination room

▷ Sit as comfortably as possible. If necessary, use folded paper to stop your desk rocking.

▷ Make sure you know which Tier (Foundation or Higher) you have entered for in the skill being tested today, and that you have been given the right paper.

▷ Check the number of questions you have to answer and the time available. Divide up your time and write down 'clock times' for each question.

▷ Read the questions and the settings carefully. In GCSE French the settings can contain vital clues to the answers.

▷ Do the tasks you are asked to do. This is particularly important in Writing papers, where mark schemes reward 'accomplishment of task'.

▷ Pace yourself so you have enough time to answer the more difficult questions at the end of the paper in Reading and Writing. If you can't do a question early in the paper quickly, leave it and come back to it later.

▷ Don't leave blanks – make a sensible guess. This applies especially to multiple-choice and tick-box questions.

▷ Use your common sense in Listening and Reading papers.

▷ If you don't know what happened, think what a sane and rational person might do in identical circumstances.

▷ When you have finished, check your work systematically.

▷ In Reading and Listening examinations, have you given enough details?

▷ In Writing examinations, check verbs, genders and agreements.

▷ Ignore the behaviour of other candidates. Many poor candidates demonstratively sit back or go to sleep having 'finished', or even walk out early. Don't be tempted to imitate them.

▷ After the Speaking Test avoid panicking others by saying how terrible it was, etc. Smile sweetly and wish them good luck.

▷ When it's all over, celebrate moderately.

So much for general revision skills and examination techniques. As the GCSE examination in French tests the four language skills separately, let us take preparing for each test in turn. The tests will in any case take place on several different days over a period of up to three months, so you can certainly prepare for each of the four skills as they are tested in turn. Allow for this when filling in your revision programme on your planner.

◢ **Preparing Speaking**

The first test you will do is Speaking. This test often worries candidates, but this really isn't necessary if you are well prepared. For one thing, the examiner will be your own teacher, who knows what you can do and should be attempting to help you to show off your knowledge. And for another, it is possible to work out from the GCSE syllabus what is likely to come up. A quick look at the 'Vocabulary topics' chapter of this Study Guide will give you an idea.

Let us look at some practical things you can do to improve your performance in the Speaking test.

1 Make sure you know what the requirements are for the test you will be doing. The requirements are different for Foundation and Higher Tier candidates. If you are not sure what is involved, see Chapter 6 on Speaking.

2 Most Speaking Tests will be tape-recorded. So some time beforehand, practise speaking into a cassette recorder in order to get used to the whirring noise it makes, the sight of the microphone, and the sound of your own voice on tape. Many good candidates who haven't tried this are overcome by shyness on the day and do badly.

3 For role-play-type exercises, you can work out from the list of tasks given in the 'Vocabulary topics' chapter what situations could be set. There are, for example, only a few things that you might want to do at a petrol station – ask for petrol, say what type you need, perhaps ask for air, oil and water to be checked, and pay. Once you have worked out the French for that lot, you shouldn't have anything to worry about. You could do this with a friend, making up role-play questions for each other to do. Over time, you could build up quite a range of these to practise from. In addition, you should make sure you know the basic phrases which are useful in many situations, for example:

▷ Je voudrais...   *I would like...*
▷ C'est combien?   *How much is it?*
▷ A quelle heure...?   *At what time...?*
▷ Où est...?   *Where is...?*
▷ Y a-t-il...?   *Is there...?*

4 For general conversation, you can work out again from the list of topics and settings what you are likely to be asked. Remember that you only ever have to be yourself in the GCSE French – you never have to pretend to be another person. So having a few well-prepared sentences to say about, for example, your actual hobbies is a wise precaution, and can make for a good flow in a conversation, which is one of the things examiners are looking for. Prepare at least these topics:

▷ hobbies
▷ school
▷ family
▷ your daily routine
▷ your local area
▷ holidays and visits to French-speaking countries
▷ your future plans

About a couple of minutes' worth on each should be sufficient.

5 If your teacher offers you a practice Speaking exam on your own, be sure to take advantage of it. There is nothing quite like the experience of actually doing the Speaking Test, on your own, to show you what it will be like. And, of course, your teacher will be your examiner for Speaking, so it's an especially valuable opportunity.

6 As well as practising with your teacher, you should also practise with a friend from your class. They could, for example, ask you some questions you had prepared and work a cassette recorder for you.

7 Look carefully at all role-play material in your textbook and make sure you can do it from memory.

8 Textbooks also contain sets of questions about certain topics such as free time, school, etc. Make sure you can do these, too, as preparation for the conversation section.

9 When answering questions, practise avoiding incomplete sentences or answers which are just *oui* and *non* or, say, the name of a British TV programme (*Eastenders*). Look for opportunities to say more than one sentence in reply; you are most unlikely to say too much, but it is very easy to say too little. Practising what you are going to say and how

you are going to say it beforehand will pay dividends. Only the very best candidates can think on their feet and achieve reasonable fluency in French. And even they enhance their performance considerably by preparation.

10   Ask your teacher to play you (anonymous) recordings of previous oral examinations, or of sample oral examinations provided by the Examining Group, with both good and bad performances, and to point out the good and bad features to you. It's very instructive.

> **Preparing Listening**

Let us look now at Listening. This is the most difficult skill to revise on your own, because it isn't always easy to come by suitable materials. However, if you take a little trouble it is surprising how much French you can hear without ever setting foot in France. Let us try to list these opportunities.

1   There are quite a lot of French films on TV, on both BBC and Channel 4. Sometimes they are shown quite late, but if you have access to a video recorder you can probably view them at a reasonable hour. Some of the language on them is difficult, but the advantage for you is that there are subtitles which will help you to absorb the French that you can manage that much more easily. And generally, the films that are shown outside France are good films, quite apart from their value to you as a learner of French. Look for:

> late-night offerings on Channel 4 and BBC2
> *Téléjournal* on BBC2

2   Also on TV, there are beginners' and intermediate courses in French. These are ideal for you. The simpler ones will be well within your grasp, while the more difficult ones may well be at a level comparable with what you are doing in school. You can find out times from the press, *Radio Times* and *TV Times*. Your teacher may know when schools programmes are on. Look for:

> *Ici Paris*   (BBC) Paris seen through the eyes of two teenage presenters.
> *France – Français*   (BBC) Conversations with young people.
> *Le café des rêves*   (BBC) A five-part soap opera about teenagers.
> *La marée et ses secrets*   (BBC) A five-part adventure series with straightforward French.
> *Quinze minutes*   (BBC) Scenes from teenage life.
> *A vous la France*   (BBC) For adult beginners.
> *The French programme*   (ITV).
> *Vidéothèque*   (ITV) Interviews based on GCSE topics, with two levels, *niveau de base* and *niveau supérieur*.
> *Action-télé 2 & 3*   (ITV) Good comprehension materials and lots of role-plays.
> *Le petit monde de Pierre*   (ITV) Whimsical fun.

Schools may well have these recorded. You could ask your teacher to make them available to you in the lunch-hour if they are not already included in your lessons. It may also be possible to find recordings of older broadcasts in school.

3   If you have access to satellite TV, you should be able to receive some French programmes. Occasional doses will do no harm, and may do some good.

4   Most textbooks in use in school for GCSE have cassettes which go with them. You could ask your teacher to make them available to you so you can re-work Listening exercises done in class. You could also ask your school librarian to stock them.

5   There are also courses on sale in booksellers (or – a cheaper option – available in your public library) which are aimed at travellers and tourists, with titles such as *Survive in French* (Longman) or *Get by in French* (BBC Publications) and *Travellers' French* (Hugo). If your local library doesn't have them, you could ask the librarian to get them for you if you can afford to wait a little. Look for the ones with cassettes as a major part of them. These are likely to be useful in preparing for the Foundation Tests as they tend to concentrate on such things as booking hotel rooms, shopping, and dealing with restaurants and filling stations.

6   BBC Schools Radio and their Learning Zone slot on Radio 4 Long Wave on Sunday evening have programmes concerned with French, often concerned specifically with

GCSE. Find out the times of broadcasts from the press, and record them if you can to work over and over. Alternatively, ask your teacher to make them available to you. The radio version of *A vous la France* is one example.

7   In most parts of Britain, French radio stations can be picked up reasonably well in the vicinity of Radio 4 (either side) on Long Wave. These are music stations, but they also carry news bulletins on the hour. A small daily dose will not be harmful, and may even do you some good! Two popular French radio stations are at the following wavelengths:

Europe 1   1647 metres
France Inter   1829 metres

8   If there are French-speaking visitors in your locality (for example an exchange with younger pupils), you will probably find that the young French people are pleased to talk to you in French. Ask them about such things as schools and their family and their journey as a starting point. The teachers accompanying such parties, too, are worth approaching.

9   If your school is fortunate enough to have a French Assistant(e), be sure to take his/her sessions seriously.

10 Finally, there should be opportunities for you to do Listening practice in your lessons. Make very sure that you take those opportunities seriously!

So, we have seen that there are quite a number of ways of hearing lots of French spoken. Some of these are more enjoyable than others. The most important thing is to try to hear as much as you can as often as you can, and not to be put off by the apparent speed at which 'they' speak. The more practice you have, the easier it gets. Use your common sense to help you work out what is being said, and remember to listen out for words that you do understand to help you to make an intelligent guess about the rest.

▶ Preparing Reading

Reading should not be a skill which is too difficult to practise. The more you read, the better. For GCSE, you need to read a variety of texts ranging from train timetables to articles in teenage magazines, so it is unwise to stick to just one sort of reading material. I have given some suggested sources below.

1   The obvious starting point is your French textbook. It will have a large amount of material in it, specifically chosen to meet the range of topics set for GCSE. You will certainly benefit from spending time working through texts you have previously done in class, or those which your teacher has decided to miss out. Use the vocabulary at the back to help you. Make a note of words you don't know without looking up – that is the first step to learning them.

2   Your school or local library may well have a variety of easy books in French. Some are available with English translations of the same stories. Look out for:

▷   Astérix
▷   Tintin
▷   Barbar the elephant
▷   The Mr Men

European Schoolbooks Ltd stock these and a very wide range of other material not easily available elsewhere. For further information, write to: European Schoolbooks Ltd, Ashville Trading Estate, The Runnings, Cheltenham, GL51 9PQ. Tel: (01242) 245252.

3   You could ask your teacher if there are any out-of-date textbooks in the back of the book cupboard. Old-fashioned first-year books can be quite amusing, and will reinforce your knowledge of things you learned long ago.

4   As well as old textbooks, your teacher may have back-numbers of magazines designed for learners of French, or you could subscribe to them direct. Popular suitable titles include, in order of difficulty:

▷   *Bonjour*
▷   *Ça va*
▷   *Chez nous*

These can be obtained from: Mary Glasgow Magazines, Building 1, Kineton Road Industrial Estate, Southam, CV33 0DG. Tel: (01926) 815560. Fax: (01926) 815563.

A more difficult magazine – probably suitable only for the best candidates – is *Authentique*, available from: The Secretary, *Authentique*, 27 Westland Square, Dublin 2, Eire. Tel: 00 353 16 771512. *Authentique* accepts cheques in £ sterling.

5 French newspapers are available in larger towns and cities, often at a newsagent near the railway station. Buy an occasional edition of *France Soir* or the more difficult *Le Figaro*. It's important to be familiar with journalistic style, as some of the texts set in Reading are taken directly from newspapers. Read not only the stories, but also the adverts, large and small. They're very popular with question-setters. French magazines are also available in many public libraries.

As with listening, a little French reading daily will pay dividends. And the more you do, the easier you will find the examination.

▷ **Preparing Writing**

For Writing there is no doubt that a high standard of accuracy will improve your marks no end. However, accuracy can be difficult to improve unless you are systematic. Make sure that you know the fundamentals of **grammar**, for example, how verbs are formed in all tenses and persons, when to use the different tenses and how to make adjectives agree. Revise a grammar topic a week in the run-up to the examination. A skeleton list of the grammar needed for GCSE is given in Chapter 9, together with explanations and examples. The other area to make sure of is vocabulary. Learn not only the word, but also its spelling (including accents) and its gender.

GCSE examiners will be awarding marks not only for accuracy but also for **getting the message across**. So it is **vitally important** to do exactly what the question tells you. You should also be sure to write at least the number of words you have been told to.

You should also make sure of such things as beginnings and ends of letters, and the sorts of phrases which commonly occur in such things as letters booking accommodation, invitations to a penfriend to stay, and so on. Check in Chapter 7 'Writing'.

Finally, you should look back at any written work you have done over the course. Try doing some of the questions again after noting the mistakes you made last time and making your mind up to avoid repeating them.

▷ **Preparing coursework**

Not all syllabuses offer coursework. Those which do, offer it in Writing or Speaking or, in some cases, both. Some of the coursework is done under controlled conditions; other parts may be done over a longer period of time. Your teacher will know how many pieces of coursework you need to submit, and when the final deadline is. In general, your teacher will be able to select the best work from the pieces you have submitted. It is therefore to your advantage to submit more than the minimum number so that you can show the best work you are capable of. However, as coursework is marked to final GCSE standard, it may be that you should aim to complete your best pieces of work in the last couple of terms of your course.

You will probably be able to re-draft some pieces of coursework after your teacher has seen them. The Examination Groups have rules about what a teacher can or cannot say when seeing a first draft. In general, your teacher can say things such as:

'Had you considered checking the adjective agreements?'
'Would some more sequence words improve this?'
'Why don't you write a little more?'
'This is a great deal longer than is necessary – go for quality, not quantity.'

However, your teacher should not point out specific mistakes and should certainly not correct the whole thing.

Your teacher is required to certify that coursework is your own work. This means that you should not seek help from other people – such as the French Assistant(e) or another French teacher in the school – in doing your coursework. It is, actually, quite easy to spot if a native speaker or an adult has helped a GCSE student. Accepting such help could invalidate your entry.

In the case of Speaking coursework, the actual speaking is naturally done by the candidate. Beware of being under-prepared. A reasonable way of proceeding might be to write a series of notes or even connected prose about a coursework topic as a stepping stone to oral fluency. Try to imagine what else the teacher could ask you about the topic. And prepare some strategies for changing back to a part of the topic you feel happier about.

▷ **Conclusion**   Experience shows that students who spend a little extra time on French over and above their lesson and homework time do better than those who don't. Systematic and well-organised students enjoy their studies and their leisure time more, and generally do well. Be one of them!

Examination requirements

 GETTING STARTED

This book sets out to help you to do well as a candidate for GCSE French. It will lay out for you the precise requirements of your examination, and will provide you with necessary tools to give your best performance. No matter which Examining Group's GCSE you are taking, you will find every chapter relevant. You can use the chapters in any order to suit your revision plan and to match your strengths and weaknesses.

If you work your way through each chapter, you will have had the chance to see and try the sorts of questions set by the GCSE Examining Groups and you will have read the examiner's comments on the student answers. Chapter 3 on vocabulary and Chapter 9 on grammar tell you all you need to know for the GCSE, and provide you with help to learn for it.

Buying this book is a proof of your keenness to do well. The other proof of keenness is to work through it conscientiously. *Bon courage, et bonne chance*!

WHAT YOU NEED TO KNOW

▶ Aims of GCSE French

The GCSE National Criteria for Modern Foreign Languages, which is a set of rules laid down by the Education Minister for GCSE which all Examining Groups must follow, gives four aims for modern languages syllabuses. French syllabuses should:

▷ develop pupils' ability to understand and communicate effectively in French
▷ encourage pupils to acquire language-learning skills
▷ encourage pupils to develop an understanding of the grammar and syntax of French
▷ encourage pupils to understand French in its cultural context.

Relax! Not all of these can be tested by the GCSE examination, and the first one is certainly the most important. If, at the end of your GCSE course, you can communicate effectively in French, you need have no worries about the examination.

▶ Novel features of the GCSE

The introduction of the GCSE French examination in 1988 marked the biggest change in Modern Languages examinations this century. Your parents, who may have taken one of the more old-fashioned O-Level and CSE examinations, would hardly recognise it. Several exercises were banned by the National Criteria, and the following will **not** be found in any GCSE:

▷ dictation
▷ translation into French
▷ reading aloud
▷ reproduction tests
▷ listening comprehensions read out by your teacher.

From September 1996, under the National Curriculum order, every student has had to study a modern foreign language in Key Stage 4, which covers Years 10 and 11. Students must take either a **Full Course**, which occupies about 10% of their time in KS4, or a **Short Course**, which occupies about 5% of their KS4 time.

The Short Course can be done in two modes:

▷ short and fat (10% of time for one year)
▷ long and thin (5% of time for two years).

The first examination of the Short Course took place in June 1997, and the first examination of the Full Course is scheduled for 1998. Some Examining Groups have 'bolted' the Short

Course syllabus onto Business Studies. In such syllabuses, the French element is the same as that on stand-alone Short Courses.

The Short Course measures the same standards as GCSE, and reports the same grades from A* to G. Indeed, from 1998 many of the questions set will be common to Full Course and Short Course papers. So do not be misled into thinking that the Short Course is in any way simpler than the Full Course. The only thing that is simplified about it is that the range of topics covered is reduced.

From 1998 new National Criteria apply to GCSE French. These are based on the requirements of the National Curriculum Programme of Study for Modern Foreign Languages. GCSE will have a new look from 1998, including the following major differences:

- The fiction that every candidate is on a visit to a country where the language is spoken has been downgraded.
- There will be very few questions in Reading and Listening where the candidate answers in English.
- The majority of questions in Reading and Listening will require either non-verbal responses (such as a tick in a box) or very brief answers in French.
- All syllabuses must have at least 50% of the marks awarded for the final examination.
- There will be coursework options offered by most of the GCSE Groups. The Writing Test can be replaced by coursework; in some Groups, the Speaking Test can also be replaced by coursework.
- Candidates will have bilingual dictionaries available to them in most parts of the examination.
- Examining Groups will be able to set questions on any vocabulary they like, except in questions targeted at grades E, F and G, for which a Minimum Core Vocabulary of about 750 words has been developed.
- Entry for the examination will be in two tiers: **Foundation** (grades G–C), **Higher** (grades D–A*).
- Candidates can enter for different tiers in each of the four skills.
- The questions in the overlap area (grades D–C) will be identical.

The principle underlying all the exercises in GCSE is that they should be based on the ability to communicate using French. This means that those who take GCSE French should find themselves able to understand and speak French at least well enough to 'get by'. Gone will be the days when people say 'I did French at school, but I can't speak it'.

In the setting and marking of GCSE questions, there is an emphasis on success. Examiners are asked to measure what candidates 'know and can do'. Students are given tasks which are well within their grasp. However, they are expected to score very highly on them at all levels of performance. So candidates who eventually gain grade F will have shown that they can perform the more straightforward tasks in the examination well. The most able candidates no longer have to attempt the most straightforward tasks – they are assumed to be competent at these.

Although the Examining Groups no longer have a vocabulary list covering all grades (but do have a Minimum Core Vocabulary covering grades G–E), they do still publish a Defined Content for the GCSE. This contains:

- a list of the topic areas to be covered
- a list of the grammar students are expected to know
- a list of the tasks students should be able to perform
- the Minimum Core Vocabulary (grades G–E tasks only).

I am sure that there is no need to stress its usefulness to candidates. French candidates (and, perhaps more importantly, their teachers and those setting the examinations) can be absolutely sure that no unforeseen topics or grammar will occur in the GCSE examination. The Defined Contents of the various Examining Groups have been used in preparing the two chapters on vocabulary and grammar in this Longman Study Guide.

Finally, in GCSE French, unlike in O Level and CSE, there is equal weight for performance in each of the four language skills.

- Speaking or Speaking coursework   25%
- Listening   25%
- Reading   25%
- Writing or Writing coursework   25%

This will allow credit to be given to those who understand and speak French well, but find Writing difficult. In some pre-GCSE O-Level syllabuses which your parents may have done, Writing accounted for 60%+ of the marks. Consequently, those who found that hard did badly. The equal weighting of the four skills underlies the teaching methods prescribed by the National Curriculum order.

▶ Assessment in French

The requirements for GCSE French are very similar for most of the examinations set by the different Examining Groups. This is because they have to fit the **National Criteria for French**, that is, the rules laid down for GCSE French examinations by the Secretary of State for Education.

Depending on the entry policy of your school, and which Examining Group your school uses, your GCSE French assessment pattern will follow one of the schemes below:

- All four skills tested at the final examination: 100% examination.
- Writing measured by coursework, Reading, Listening and Speaking measured by final examination   75% examination, 25% coursework.
- Speaking measured by coursework, Reading, Listening and Writing measured by final examination   75% examination, 25% coursework.
- Half of the assessment by tests at the end of each unit   50% modular.
  Half of the assessment by final examination   50% examination.
  (SEG Modular, 1998 onwards)

If you are doing an examination with coursework make sure you know when assignments are due to be handed in. It is definitely a bad idea to be late with coursework!

In French there is a part of the examination for each of the four language skills. So there are tests in Speaking, Listening, Reading, Writing. These are usually arranged to take place on different days.

- **Speaking** will be conducted by your own teacher between March and May, at a time your teacher decides. In most cases the Speaking Test will be tape-recorded.
- **Listening** comes early in the full examination period, in late May. This is so that you do not get too much out of practice in that skill, which is more difficult to revise at home.
- **Reading** and **Writing** are examined in very late May or in June.

Some Examination Groups also run a November examination in French. At the time of writing, these November examinations are under review, as the number of entries has been falling steadily. So don't assume you can have another 'go' in November – your Group may not run an examination at that time. Check the current position with your teacher.

In each of the four skills there is a Foundation Test and a Higher Test. So there are in fact eight tests:

Foundation Speaking	Higher Speaking
Foundation Listening	Higher Listening
Foundation Reading	Higher Reading
Foundation Writing	Higher Writing

You can only do one test in each skill, but you do not have to do **all** Foundation or **all** Higher Tests. Candidates are allowed to mix and match. The more Higher Tests you take (and, of course, do well in), the higher the maximum grade you can obtain. However, if you do not reach a minimum standard in a Higher Test, you get no credit. You should discuss with your teacher what he or she thinks you should enter for and act on that advice. Take especial note of the results of mock examinations.

▶ Points and grades

For each skill the Examining Group determines how many marks are required to achieve a performance worth a particular grade. For each grade a number of points is awarded. An A* performance is worth 8 points, an A performance is worth 7 points, a B performance is worth 6 points, and so on down to G performance, which is worth 1 point. The points for the four skills are added together to give a total out of 32. This total is then converted to a GCSE grade on the following scale:

Points total	GCSE grade awarded
30–32	A*
25–29	A
21–24	B
16–20	C
12–15	D
8–11	E
5–7	F
2–4	G

On the Higher papers there is a 'safety-net' award of 3 points for performance which is below D standard. This gives extra security to those candidates who have decided to enter for the Higher Test but then obtain C, D or E.

Because papers in Listening, Reading and Writing vary in difficulty in different examinations, the exact marks at which points are awarded on each paper changes from year to year. The Principal Examiners for the subject make judgements in consultation with the Chief Examiner based on the quality of candidates' work, statistical evidence, and written reports from the Assistant Examiners.

To summarise: GCSE French has between 50% and 100% of the marks for the final examination. There are four skills, Listening, Reading, Speaking and Writing. Coursework can be an alternative to Writing or Speaking. Each skill is tested at two tiers, Foundation and Higher. You can enter different levels in different skills to suit what you are good at, although the more Higher papers you try, the better the potential grade. There is a safety-net provision on Higher papers.

▶ **Grade descriptions**

The Examining Groups provide descriptions of performance for key grades, F, C and A. These should provide a yardstick for you to judge your own performance by. Those gaining grade G will not be as good as those awarded grade F, and those gaining grade A* will clearly be better than those described under grade A.

Typical Grade Descriptions for each skill in turn are given below:

Listening

▷ **Grade F** Candidates can identify and note the main points and some details from simple language spoken clearly at near-normal speed.
▷ **Grade C** Candidates can identify and note the main points, some details and points of view from language spoken clearly at normal speed. They understand future and past tenses. The subject matter will include familiar language in unfamiliar contexts.
▷ **Grade A** Candidates understand main points and gist in a variety of authentic recordings. They can draw conclusions, and recognise points of view, attitudes and emotions.

Speaking

▷ **Grade F** Candidates take part in simple transactions and conversations. Their pronunciation can be understood, and, despite some grammatical inaccuracy, they can get a message across.
▷ **Grade C** Candidates take part in transactions and conversations. They use past, present and future tenses. They can express their own personal opinion and deal with some unpredictable tasks. Their pronunciation is generally accurate, and despite some grammatical inaccuracy, they can get a clear message across.
▷ **Grade A** Candidates initiate transactions and conversations, and narrate at some length. They express points of view. They speak confidently, with good pronunciation, using a variety of vocabulary. There are still occasional errors in more complex structures, but the message is clear.

Reading

- **Grade F** Candidates can identify and note the main points and some details from simple texts, which may be printed or handwritten. They use a French–English dictionary to find the meaning of unfamiliar words.
- **Grade C** Candidates can identify and note the main points, some details and points of view from authentic printed and handwritten texts. They understand future and past tenses. The subject matter will include familiar language in unfamiliar contexts. They use a French–English dictionary to find the meaning of unfamiliar words.
- **Grade A** Candidates understand main points and gist in a variety of authentic texts. They can draw conclusions, and recognise points of view, attitudes and emotions. They choose and make good use of reference materials.

Writing

- **Grade F** Candidates write short sentences and substitute words and set phrases. Despite some spelling errors and grammatical inaccuracy, they can get a message across.
- **Grade C** Candidates write simple personal or formal letters. They use past, present and future tenses. They can express their own personal opinion. The writing is of a straightforward style, but conveys a clear message.
- **Grade A** Candidates give factual information and narrate at some length. They express points of view. They write confidently, using a variety of vocabulary and linguistic structures. There are still occasional errors in spelling and grammar, but the message is clear. They write in the correct style for the task set.

Examining Group requirements in detail

These are summarised in the Appendix at the end of this Study Guide.

Vocabulary topics

GETTING STARTED

Learning vocabulary is a vital part of learning a foreign language. One of the hardest things is knowing what to learn. For GCSE French, the Examining Groups have published in their Defined Contents complete lists of the topic areas they expect you to know about. They have been arranged in topics in manageable groups in this chapter, so that you don't waste time learning things which the GCSE will never test.

Hints for helping you to learn your vocabulary more effectively are given at the end of the chapter. But the main message is to do a little but often!

WHAT YOU NEED TO KNOW

Topics

For the GCSE in French the Examining Groups have each published in their Defined Contents a list of topics which they require candidates to know about. They are allowed to set questions which depend on knowing words outside the lists, but candidates will be allowed to take a dictionary – any non-electronic dictionary – into the examination with them. This should be regarded as an extra, because, if you look up every word on the examination paper in the dictionary, you will not have time to finish the examination. On the other hand, there will be less chance of being absolutely stuck for a word.

The *topic lists* vary slightly – but only slightly – from one Examining Group to another, and it is not practical to reproduce them all in this book. What I have done is to combine some of the *lists* from major Examining Groups so that, if you learn what is given here, you can be pretty sure you have covered what is necessary.

The Examining Groups do agree on most topics which they expect candidates to know about. This is because the topics to be covered are laid down in the National Curriculum order for Modern Foreign Languages.

Language tasks

A comprehensive list of the language tasks you need to be able to do is provided below, broken down by topics. It may appear a little daunting, but there are many straightforward things in it such as giving your name and age which you have been able to do well for a long time.

To help you chart your progress through the tasks I have provided two columns next to them on which you can tick off items as you learn them, and when you have been tested at a later date (by yourself or by a friend).

LANGUAGE TASKS BY TOPIC

A1 Language problems

	Learned	Tested
▷ Say whether or not you understand.	☐	☐
▷ Ask for and understand the spelling of names, place names, etc.	☐	☐
▷ Ask if someone speaks English or French.	☐	☐
▷ State how well or how little you speak and understand French.	☐	☐
▷ Ask what things are called in French or English.	☐	☐
▷ Ask what words or phrases mean.	☐	☐

▶ Say you do not know (something). ☐ ☐

▶ Say you have forgotten (something). ☐ ☐

▶ Apologise. ☐ ☐

▶ Ask whether, or state that, something is correct. ☐ ☐

▶ Say for how long you have been learning French and any other languages you know. ☐ ☐

▶ Ask someone to explain something, to correct mistakes. ☐ ☐

▶ Ask how something is pronounced. ☐ ☐

A2 School

	Learned	*Tested*
▶ Describe your school/college and its facilities: state the type, size and location of your school and describe the buildings.	☐	☐
▶ Describe daily routines: when school begins, ends; how many lessons there are and how long they last; break times and lunch times; homework; how you travel to and from school.	☐	☐
▶ Discuss your school year and holidays: subjects studied and preferences; clubs, sports, trips and other activities.	☐	☐

A3 Home life

	Learned	*Tested*
▶ Discuss where and under what conditions you and others live.	☐	☐
▶ Say whether you live in a house, flat, etc., and ask others the same.	☐	☐
▶ Describe your house, flat, etc. and its location.	☐	☐
▶ Mention or enquire about availability of the most essential pieces of furniture, amenities, services.	☐	☐
▶ Say whether you have a room of your own and describe your room or the room where you sleep.	☐	☐
▶ Say what jobs you do around the home.	☐	☐
▶ Ask where places and things are in a house.	☐	☐
▶ Say you need soap, toothpaste, or a towel.	☐	☐
▶ Invite someone to come in, sit down.	☐	☐
▶ Thank somebody for hospitality.	☐	☐
▶ Offer and ask for help to do something about the house.	☐	☐
▶ Ask permission to use or do things when you are the guest of a French-speaking family.	☐	☐
▶ Give and seek information about members of the family.	☐	☐
▶ Describe members of the family and their occupations.	☐	☐
▶ Give and seek information about daily routine.	☐	☐
▶ Say what time you usually get up and go to bed, have meals, how you spend your evenings and weekends.	☐	☐
▶ Express hunger and thirst.	☐	☐
▶ Ask about time and place of meals.	☐	☐

	Learned	Tested
▶ Ask for food and table articles (including asking for more, a little, a lot).	☐	☐
▶ React to offers of food (accept, decline, apologise, express pleasure).	☐	☐
▶ Express likes, dislikes and preferences.	☐	☐
▶ Express appreciation and pay compliments.	☐	☐
▶ Respond to a toast (e.g. *A la vôtre*).	☐	☐

A4 Media

	Learned	Tested
▶ Describe different sorts of film, play or concert.	☐	☐
▶ Discuss a performance, giving your opinion.	☐	☐
▶ Know what sorts of TV programme there are.	☐	☐
▶ Discuss your viewing habits.	☐	☐
▶ Give your opinion on different programmes.	☐	☐
▶ Give reasons for your opinions.	☐	☐
▶ Cope at the box office for:		
a play	☐	☐
a sporting event	☐	☐
a concert	☐	☐
a film.	☐	☐

A5 Health, fitness and welfare

	Learned	Tested
General		
▶ Refer to parts of the body where you are in pain or discomfort.	☐	☐
Hygiene		
▶ Obtain toiletries and other things you need.	☐	☐
Illness and injury		
▶ State how you feel (well, ill, better, hot, cold, hungry, thirsty, tired) and ask others how they feel.	☐	☐
▶ Call for help.	☐	☐
▶ Warn about danger.	☐	☐
▶ Say you would like to rest or go to bed.	☐	☐
▶ Report minor ailments (e.g. temperature, cold, sunburn) and injuries.	☐	☐
▶ Say you would like to lie down.	☐	☐
▶ Respond to an enquiry about how long an ailment or symptom has persisted.	☐	☐
▶ Say you would like to see a doctor or dentist.	☐	☐
▶ Deal with contact with the medical services.	☐	☐
▶ Say whether you take medicine regularly, and if so what.	☐	☐
▶ Say whether or not you are insured.	☐	☐
▶ Tell others about medical facilities, surgery hours.	☐	☐

At the chemist's

▷ Report minor ailments (e.g. temperature, cold, sunburn) and injuries. ☐ ☐

▷ Ask for items in a chemist's and ask if they have anything for particular ailments. ☐ ☐

Accidents

▷ Ask or advise someone to phone the doctor, police, fire brigade, ambulance, consulate, acquaintance, etc. ☐ ☐

▷ Ask for someone's name and address. ☐ ☐

▷ Suggest filling in a road-accident form. ☐ ☐

▷ Describe an accident. ☐ ☐

▷ Ask or say whether it is serious. ☐ ☐

▷ Deny responsibility and say whose fault it was. ☐ ☐

A6 Food and drink

	Learned	Tested

General

▷ Discuss your likes, dislikes and preferences and those of others. ☐ ☐

▷ Discuss your typical meals, meal times and eating habits. ☐ ☐

▷ Buy food and drink (see C2 'Shopping'). ☐ ☐

▷ Explain to a visitor what a dish is, or what it contains. ☐ ☐

Café, restaurant and other public places

▷ Attract the attention of the waiter/waitress. ☐ ☐

▷ Order a drink, snack or meal. ☐ ☐

▷ Ask for a particular fixed-price menu. ☐ ☐

▷ Say how many there are in your group. ☐ ☐

▷ Ask for a table (for a certain number). ☐ ☐

▷ Ask about the availability of certain dishes and drinks. ☐ ☐

▷ Ask the cost of dishes and drinks. ☐ ☐

▷ Ask for an explanation or a description of something on the menu. ☐ ☐

▷ Express opinions about a meal or dish. ☐ ☐

▷ Accept or reject suggestions. ☐ ☐

▷ Ask if the service charge is included. ☐ ☐

▷ Ask about the location of facilities (e.g. toilets, telephone). ☐ ☐

B1 Self, family and friends

	Learned	Tested

▷ Give your identity and information about yourself and others (e.g. members of your family or host family). ☐ ☐

▷ Seek information from others on the following points:

    names (including spelling out the name of your home town) ☐ ☐

    address and telephone numbers ☐ ☐

    ages and birthdays ☐ ☐

    nationality ☐ ☐

family and relatives □ □

religion. □ □

▷ Give general descriptions including sex, marital status, physical appearance, character or disposition of yourself and others. □ □

▷ Likes and dislikes (with regard to other people and other topics in the syllabus). □ □

▷ Pets, other livestock and undomesticated creatures. □ □

B2 Spare-time activities

	Learned	Tested
▷ Discuss pocket money and part-time work.	□	□
▷ Talk about hobbies.	□	□
▷ Discuss sporting activities.	□	□

B3 Personal relationships

	Learned	Tested
▷ Greet someone and respond to greetings.	□	□
▷ Ask how someone is and reply to similar enquiries.	□	□
▷ Say you are pleased to meet someone.	□	□
▷ Introduce yourself (see also B1 'Self, family and friends').	□	□
▷ Introduce an acquaintance to someone else.	□	□
▷ Give, receive and exchange gifts.	□	□

B4 Arranging a meeting or an activity

	Learned	Tested
▷ Find out what a friend wants to do.	□	□
▷ Ask what is on TV or at the cinema.	□	□
▷ Express preferences for an activity (e.g. watching TV, going out, visiting a friend).	□	□
▷ Invite someone to go out (stating when and where).	□	□
▷ Suggest going to a particular place, event or on a visit.	□	□
▷ Accept or decline invitations.	□	□
▷ Express pleasure.	□	□
▷ State likes and dislikes.	□	□
▷ State that something is possible, impossible, probable or certain.	□	□
▷ Ask about, suggest or confirm a time and place to meet.	□	□
▷ Ask about and state the cost (of entry, etc.).	□	□

B5 Holidays

	Learned	Tested

General
▷ Say where you normally spend your holidays; how long they last; with whom you go on holiday; what you normally do; and understand others giving the same information. □ □

▷ Describe a previous holiday: where you went; with whom you went; how you went, and for how long; where you stayed; what the weather was like; what you saw and did; what your general impressions were; and understand others giving the same information. ☐ ☐

▷ Describe your holiday plans. ☐ ☐

▷ Say whether you have been abroad (e.g. to a French-speaking country) and give details if applicable. ☐ ☐

▷ Supply information about travel documents. ☐ ☐

Tourist information

▷ Ask for and understand information about a town or region (maps, brochures of hotels and campsites). ☐ ☐

▷ Ask for and understand details of excursions, shows, places of interest (location, costs, times). ☐ ☐

▷ Give information about your own area or one you have visited to others (e.g. prospective tourists). ☐ ☐

▷ React to (i.e. welcome or reject) suggestions about activities and places of interest. ☐ ☐

▷ Write a short letter asking for information and brochures about a town or region and its tourist attractions. ☐ ☐

B6 Festivals and special occasions

(Most of these items are contained in B1.)

	Learned	Tested
▷ Talk about special occasions and anniversaries (e.g. own and other family birthdays, weddings).	☐	☐
▷ Give information and express opinions about festivals / special events in your own locality.	☐	☐
▷ Give information about special excursions and visits.	☐	☐

C1 Home town, local environment

	Learned	Tested
▷ Give information about your home town or village and surrounding areas, and seek information from others, with respect to:		
location	☐	☐
character	☐	☐
amenities, attractions, features of interest, entertainment.	☐	☐
▷ Express a simple opinion about your own town or someone else's town.	☐	☐
▷ Give full descriptions of your home town / village or that of others, and of the surrounding area and region.	☐	☐
▷ Outline possibilities for sightseeing.	☐	☐

C2 Finding the way

	Learned	Tested
▷ Attract the attention of a passer-by.	☐	☐
▷ Ask where a place is.	☐	☐

▷ Ask the way (to a place). ☐ ☐

▷ Ask if it is a long way (to a place). ☐ ☐

▷ Ask if a place is nearby. ☐ ☐

▷ Ask if there is a place or an amenity nearby. ☐ ☐

▷ Understand directions. ☐ ☐

▷ Ask if there is a bus, train, tram or coach. ☐ ☐

▷ Ask someone to repeat what they have said. ☐ ☐

▷ Say you do not understand. ☐ ☐

▷ Thank people. ☐ ☐

▷ Give directions to strangers. ☐ ☐

▷ State and enquire about distances. ☐ ☐

C3 Weather

	Learned	*Tested*
▷ Describe or comment on current weather conditions.	☐	☐
▷ Ask about weather conditions in the country you are visiting.	☐	☐
▷ Describe the general climate of your own country and ask about the climate in another country.	☐	☐
▷ Understand simple predictions about weather conditions.	☐	☐
▷ Understand spoken and written weather forecasts.	☐	☐

C4 Shopping

	Learned	*Tested*

General

▷ Ask for information about supermarkets, shopping centres, markets, shops.	☐	☐
▷ Ask where specific shops and departments are.	☐	☐
▷ Discuss shopping habits.	☐	☐

Shops and markets

▷ Ask whether particular goods are available.	☐	☐
▷ Ask for particular items (mentioning e.g. colour, size, whom it is for).	☐	☐
▷ Find out how much things cost.	☐	☐
▷ Say an item is (not) satisfactory or too expensive, small, big, etc.	☐	☐
▷ Say you prefer something.	☐	☐
▷ Say you will (not) take something.	☐	☐
▷ Express quantity required (including weights, volumes, containers).	☐	☐
▷ Find out opening and closing times.	☐	☐
▷ Say that is all you require.	☐	☐
▷ Enquire about costs and prices.	☐	☐
▷ Pay for items.	☐	☐
▷ State whether you have enough money.	☐	☐

> Understand currencies used in French-speaking countries, including written and printed prices. ☐ ☐

> Ask for small change. ☐ ☐

> Return unsatisfactory goods and ask for a refund or replacement. ☐ ☐

C5 Services

Learned   Tested

Post office

> Ask where a post office or letter box is. ☐ ☐

> Ask how much it costs to send letters, postcards or parcels to a particular country or within the country. ☐ ☐

> Say whether you would like to send letters, postcards or parcels. ☐ ☐

> Buy stamps of a particular value. ☐ ☐

> Find out opening and closing times. ☐ ☐

> Say that is all you require. ☐ ☐

> Give and seek information about where phone calls can be made. ☐ ☐

Bank or foreign-exchange office

> Say you would like to change traveller's cheques or money (including sterling). ☐ ☐

> Ask for coins or notes of a particular denomination. ☐ ☐

> Give proof of identity (e.g. show passport). ☐ ☐

> Cope with any likely eventuality that may arise while using a bank or foreign-exchange office to change currency or cheques. ☐ ☐

Lost property

> Report a loss or theft, stating what you have lost, when and where it was lost or left, describing the item (size, shape, colour, make, contents). ☐ ☐

> Express surprise, pleasure, disappointment, anger. ☐ ☐

Having things repaired or cleaned

> Report an accident, damage done or breakdown. ☐ ☐

> Ask if shoes, clothes, camera, etc. can be repaired. ☐ ☐

> Explain what is wrong. ☐ ☐

> Ask for, and offer, advice about getting something repaired or cleaned. ☐ ☐

> Find out how long it will take, what it will cost, when it will be ready. ☐ ☐

> Thank, complain, express disappointment, pleasure. ☐ ☐

> Suggest the need for repair or cleaning and report or comment on any action taken. ☐ ☐

C6 Getting around

	Learned	*Tested*

Public transport

▶ Ask if there is a train, bus, ship, hovercraft or plane to a particular place. ☐ ☐

▶ Buy tickets, stating:

destination ☐ ☐

single or return ☐ ☐

class of travel ☐ ☐

proposed times of departure and arrival. ☐ ☐

▶ Ask about the cost of tickets. ☐ ☐

▶ Ask about times of departure and arrival. ☐ ☐

▶ Ask and check whether it is:

the right platform ☐ ☐

the right station ☐ ☐

the right line or bus, tram, coach or stop. ☐ ☐

▶ Ask about the location of facilities (e.g. bus stop, waiting room, information office, toilets). ☐ ☐

▶ Ask if and/or where it is necessary to change buses, trains, trams or coaches. ☐ ☐

▶ Ask or state whether a seat is free. ☐ ☐

▶ Understand information given in brochures and tables. ☐ ☐

▶ Write a letter about requirements for travel arrangements and give this information to others. ☐ ☐

▶ Ask how to get to a place by bus, train, tram, tube or coach and give this information to others. ☐ ☐

▶ Reserve a seat. ☐ ☐

▶ Ask for information, timetables or a plan. ☐ ☐

▶ Ask about price reductions and supplements. ☐ ☐

▶ Make arrangements for taking, leaving or sending luggage. ☐ ☐

▶ Deal with an element of the unexpected in travel arrangements (e.g. delayed or cancelled departures, mislaid tickets, documents, lost luggage). ☐ ☐

Travel by air or sea

▶ Buy a ticket. ☐ ☐

▶ Ask about the cost of a flight or crossing. ☐ ☐

▶ Say where you would like to sit. ☐ ☐

▶ Ask about times of departure and arrival. ☐ ☐

▶ Inform someone about your proposed times of arrival and departure. ☐ ☐

▶ Check which is the right flight, ferry or hovercraft. ☐ ☐

▶ Ask about the location of facilities. ☐ ☐

▶ Say whether you wish to declare anything at the customs. ☐ ☐

Private transport

▶ Buy petrol by type, volume and price. ☐ ☐

▶ Ask for the tank to be filled up. ☐ ☐

▶ Ask the cost. ☐ ☐

▶ Ask someone to check oil, water and tyres. ☐ ☐

▶ Ask where facilities are. ☐ ☐

▶ Ask about availability of facilities nearby. ☐ ☐

▶ Check on your route. ☐ ☐

▶ Obtain and give information about routes, types of roads, traffic rules, parking facilities. ☐ ☐

▶ Report a breakdown, giving location and other relevant information. ☐ ☐

▶ Report a road accident. ☐ ☐

▶ Ask for technical help. ☐ ☐

▶ Pay and ask for a receipt. ☐ ☐

D1 Further education and training

D2 Careers and employment

	Learned	*Tested*
▶ Discuss what sort of education you have had, propose to continue with, at what types of educational establishment.	☐	☐
▶ Talk about examinations.	☐	☐
▶ Discuss your plans and hopes for the future, including:		
immediate plans for the coming months	☐	☐
plans for the time after the completion of compulsory education	☐	☐
where you would like to work, giving reasons as appropriate	☐	☐
occupations.	☐	☐
▶ Say whether you have a part-time job, if so what job, what working hours, how much you earn (see also B2 'Spare-time activities').	☐	☐

D3 Travel to work and school

	Learned	*Tested*
▶ Say how you get to school/place of work (means of transport, if any; duration of journey).	☐	☐
▶ Understand and give information about other journeys.	☐	☐

D4 Advertising and publicity

	Learned	*Tested*
▶ Understand a range of small ads and posters advertising leisure events.	☐	☐

D5 Communication

	Learned	*Tested*
▶ Ask for a telephone number and give your own telephone number.	☐	☐
▶ Answer a phone call, stating who you are.	☐	☐

- Make a phone call and ask to speak to someone. ☐ ☐
- Ask someone to telephone you. ☐ ☐
- Find out if others can be contacted by phone. ☐ ☐
- Tell others you will telephone them. ☐ ☐
- Ask for coins. ☐ ☐
- Ask for a reversed-charge call. ☐ ☐
- Buy a phone card. ☐ ☐

D6 Language at work
(See also B1.)

	Learned	Tested
Understand instructions and signs in school or the workplace.	☐	☐
Fill in simple forms relating to jobs.	☐	☐
Write a simple letter of application for a job.	☐	☐
Ask someone to repeat what they said.	☐	☐

E1 Life in other countries
(See also E4.)

	Learned	Tested
Understand names of countries, nationalities and languages commonly encountered.	☐	☐
Describe any part of a country where French is spoken.	☐	☐
Describe foodstuffs from other countries (see also A6 'Food and drink').	☐	☐

E2 Tourism

	Learned	Tested
Discuss past and future holidays.	☐	☐
Give opinions.	☐	☐
Deal with the tourist office.	☐	☐

E3 Accommodation

	Learned	Tested

General
Describe accommodation you use or have used.	☐	☐
Write a short letter asking about the availability and price of accommodation at a hotel, campsite or youth hostel and about amenities available.	☐	☐
Write a short letter booking such accommodation.	☐	☐
Read and understand relevant information about accommodation (e.g. brochures).	☐	☐
Make complaints.	☐	☐

Hotel
| Ask if there are rooms available. | ☐ | ☐ |

▶ State when you require a room / rooms and for how long.   ☐ ☐

▶ Say what sort of room is required.   ☐ ☐

▶ Ask the cost (per night, per person, per room).   ☐ ☐

▶ Say it is too expensive.   ☐ ☐

▶ Ask to see the room(s).   ☐ ☐

▶ Accept or reject a room.   ☐ ☐

▶ Check in.   ☐ ☐

▶ Say that you have (not) reserved accommodation.   ☐ ☐

▶ Identify yourself.   ☐ ☐

▶ Ask if there is a particular facility (e.g. restaurant) in or near the hotel.   ☐ ☐

▶ Ask where the facilities are (e.g. telephone, car park, lift, lounge).   ☐ ☐

▶ Ask if meals are included.   ☐ ☐

▶ Ask what meals are available.   ☐ ☐

▶ Ask the times of meals.   ☐ ☐

▶ Ask for the key.   ☐ ☐

▶ Say you would like to pay.   ☐ ☐

Youth hostel

▶ Ask if there is any room.   ☐ ☐

▶ State when and for how long the rooms are required.   ☐ ☐

▶ State how many males and females require accommodation.   ☐ ☐

▶ Say you have (not) reserved.   ☐ ☐

▶ Identify yourself.   ☐ ☐

▶ Ask the cost (per night, per person or facility).   ☐ ☐

▶ Ask if there is a particular facility in or near the hostel.   ☐ ☐

▶ Ask where facilities are.   ☐ ☐

▶ Say you would like to pay.   ☐ ☐

▶ Ask about meal times.   ☐ ☐

▶ Ask about opening and closing times.   ☐ ☐

▶ Say you have a sleeping bag.   ☐ ☐

▶ Say you wish to hire a sleeping bag.   ☐ ☐

Campsite

▶ Ask if there is any room.   ☐ ☐

▶ State when and for how long you will be staying.   ☐ ☐

▶ Say you have (not) reserved.   ☐ ☐

▶ Identify yourself.   ☐ ☐

▶ Say how many tents, caravans, people or vehicles it is for.   ☐ ☐

▶ Say how many children and adults are in the group.   ☐ ☐

▶ Ask the cost (per night, per person, per tent, caravan, vehicle or facility).   ☐ ☐

▶ Say it is too expensive.   ☐ ☐

▶ Ask if there is a particular facility on or near the site. ☐ ☐

▶ Ask where the facilities are. ☐ ☐

▶ Buy essential supplies. ☐ ☐

▶ Ask about rules and regulations. ☐ ☐

Holiday home in France
▶ Give a description. ☐ ☐

▶ Discuss advantages and disadvantages. ☐ ☐

(For reservation problems, see hotel, etc.)

E4 The wider world
☐ ☐

Learned *Tested*

▶ Know the names of French-speaking and other countries. ☐ ☐

▶ Know the names of people and nationalities. ☐ ☐

E5 World events and issues

Learned *Tested*

▶ Follow the recounting or discussion of current issues and events of general news value, and of interest to 16-year-old students, and express your reaction to such items. ☐ ☐

▶ **Vocabulary lists** The vocabulary has been listed under the five National Curriculum Areas of Experience. If you are doing the Full Course GCSE, you will need to know about Areas A–E. If you are doing the Short Course GCSE, you will probably only be tested on Areas B and D. The vocabulary is listed under the same headings as the language tasks in this book.

▶ VOCABULARY BY TOPIC AREAS

▶ A1 Language problems

apprendre *to learn*
avoir raison *to be right*
c'est-à-dire *that's to say*
comprendre *to understand*
demander *to ask*
se dire *to be said*
écouter *to listen (to)*
écrire *to write*
s'écrire *to be written*
excusez-moi *excuse me*
je m'excuse *I'm sorry*
lire *to read*
oublier *to forget*
parler *to speak*
penser *to think*
poser une question *to put a question*
pouvoir *to be able*
regretter *to regret*
répéter *to repeat*
répondre *to reply*
savoir *to know*
vouloir dire *to mean*

correct *correct*
désolé *very sorry*
différent *different*
exact *exact*
excellent *excellent*
faux/fausse *wrong, false*
vite *quickly*
vrai *true*

assez *enough, fairly*
bien *good, well*
bof! *oh well!*
comment *how*
au contraire *on the contrary*
depuis *since*
en général *usually*
lentement *slowly*
longtemps *a long time*
mal *badly*
peu (de) *little*
très *very*
trop (de) *too (much)*

aider *to help*

avoir tort   *to be wrong*
conseiller   *to advise*
corriger   *to correct*
critiquer   *to criticise*
douter   *to doubt*
entendre   *to hear*
épeler   *to spell*
expliquer   *to explain*
faire attention   *to pay attention*
prononcer   *to pronounce*
traduire   *to translate*
se tromper   *to make a mistake*

absolument   *absolutely*
autrement dit   *in other words*
bravo!   *well done!*
couramment   *fluently*
égal   *equal, the same*
quoi?   *what?*

un   accent   *accent*
l'   anglais(m)   *English (language)*
la   chose   *thing*
le   doute   *doubt*
un   exemple   *example*
la   faute   *mistake*
la   fois   *time, occasion*
le   français   *French (language)*
la   langue   *language, tongue*
le   machin   *thing*
le   mot   *word*
la   phrase   *phrase, sentence*
le   progrès   *progress*
la   question   *question*
une   sorte de   *a kind of*
le   truc   *thing*
la   voix   *voice*

▷ A2 School

BUILDINGS AND TYPES OF SCHOOL

la   bibliothèque   *library*
la   cantine   *canteen*
le   CES   *secondary school*
le   collège   *secondary school*
une   école primaire   *primary school*
le   gymnase   *gymnasium*
une   infirmerie   *infirmary*
le   labo(ratoire)   *lab(oratory)*
le   lycée   *15–19 school, 6th form college*
la   salle de classe   *classroom*
la   salle des professeurs   *staffroom*
une   université   *university*
les   vestiaires (m)   *cloakrooms, changing rooms*

loin   *far*
mixte   *mixed*
privé   *private*
public   *public*

un   atelier   *workshop, studio*
la   cour   *playground*
le   foyer des élèves   *pupils' common room*
la   pelouse   *lawn*

SCHOOL ROUTINE

le   bic   *ball-point pen*
le   bulletin   *bulletin*

le   bureau   *office*
le   cahier   *exercise book*
le/la   camarade   *friend*
le   cartable   *school satchel*
le   concert   *concert*
le/la   copain/copine   *friend*
le   cours   *lesson*
le   crayon   *pencil*
le(s)   devoir(s)   *homework*
un   échange   *exchange*
l'   éducation (f)   *education*
un   emploi du temps   *timetable*
l'   enseignement (m)   *teaching*
un(e)   étudiant(e)   *student*
un   exemple   *example*
la   faute   *mistake*
le   livre   *book*
le   livre de classe   *textbook*
le   manuel   *textbook*
la   note   *mark*
un   ordinateur   *computer*
le   papier   *paper*
la   permission   *permission*
la   phrase   *phrase, sentence*
le   problème   *problem*
le/la   prof   *teacher*
le   professeur   *teacher*
la   récréation   *break*
le   repas   *meal*
la   réponse   *answer*
sixième   *Year 7*
le   stylo   *ball-point pen*
le   tableau   *picture, blackboard*
terminale   *Year 13*
un   uniforme   *uniform*
le   vocabulaire   *vocabulary*

apprendre   *to learn*
assister à   *to be present at*
calculer   *to calculate*
chanter   *to sing*
choisir   *to choose*
compter   *to count*
demander   *to ask (for)*
dessiner   *to draw*
durer   *to last*
écouter   *to listen to*
s'entraîner   *to train, to practise*
étudier   *to study*
expliquer   *to explain*
faire des progrès   *to make progress*
faire ses devoirs   *to do one's homework*
faire un exercice   *to do an exercise*
faire une expérience   *to do an experiment*
jouer   *to play*
lire   *to read*
manquer   *to be missing*
nager   *to swim*
oublier   *to forget*
poser une question   *to ask a question*
punir   *to punish*
répéter   *to repeat*
réviser   *to revise*
surveiller   *to supervise*

absent   *absent*
bon/bonne   *good*
classique   *classical*

difficile *difficult*
excellent *excellent*
facile *easy*
présent *present*
sévère *strict*

après *after, later*
en avance *in advance, early*
d'abord *first of all*
ensuite *afterwards*
en retard *late*

le congé *leave, time off*
la craie *chalk*
le/la demi-pensionnaire *pupil taking school lunch*
la gomme *rubber*
le/la pensionnaire *boarder*
la règle *ruler, rule*
les vacances (f) *holidays*

Taisez-vous! *Be quiet!*
Demain, nous avons un jour de congé. *Tomorrow we have a day off.*

SUBJECTS

l' allemand (m) *German*
l' anglais (m) *English (language)*
la biologie *biology*
la chimie *chemistry*
le commerce *commerce*
la couture *needlework*
la cuisine *cookery*
le dessin *drawing*
l' éducation physique (f) *physical education*
l' électronique (f) *electronics*
l' espagnol (m) *Spanish (language)*
les études ménagères (f) *home economics*
le français *French (language)*
la géo(graphie) *geography*
le grec *Greek (language)*
la gymnastique *gymnastics*
l' histoire ancienne (f) *ancient history*
l' histoire moderne (f) *modern history*
l' informatique (f) *information technology*
l' instruction civique (f) *civics, social studies*
l' instruction religieuse (f) *religious education*
l' italien (m) *Italian (language)*
les langues modernes (f) *modern languages*
le latin *Latin (language)*
la littérature *literature*
les mathématiques (f) *mathematics*
les maths (f) *maths*
la matière *subject*
la musique *music*
la physique *physics*
la poterie *pottery*
la religion *religion*
le russe *Russian (language)*
les sciences (f) *science*
les sciences économiques (f) *economics*
le sport *sport*
les travaux manuels (m) *crafts*
les travaux pratiques (m) *crafts*
+ *any other subjects studied by the student*

aimer *to like, to love*
détester *to hate*
préférer *to prefer*

bête *stupid*
chouette *great, marvellous*
compliqué *complicated*
difficile *difficult*
ennuyeux/ennuyeuse *boring*
facile *easy*
intéressant *interesting*
marrant *funny*

Je suis fort(e) en anglais. *I'm good at English.*
Je suis faible en histoire. *I'm weak in history.*
Je suis moyen(ne) en biologie. *I'm average in biology.*

MARKS AND EXAMS

un examen *examination*
le résultat *result*

passer un examen *to take an exam*
rater un examen *to fail an exam*
réussir à *to pass, to succeed*

Je vais passer mes examens cet été. *I will take my exams this summer.*
J'ai réussi à mon examen. *I have passed my exam.*
J'ai raté mon examen de physique. *I have failed my physics exam.*

le brevet *diploma, certificate*
le certificat *certificate*
le diplôme *diploma*

échouer à *to fail*
être reçu à *to pass*
tricher *to cheat*

J'ai échoué au bac. *I have failed my 'bac' (A Level/ GNVQ).*
J'ai été reçu(e) au bac. *I have passed my 'bac' (A Level/ GNVQ).*

▶ A3 Home life

HOUSING

un appartement *flat*
le bâtiment *building*
le bruit *noise*
la clé *key*
le confort *comfort*
une entrée *entrance*
la ferme *farm*
la grange *barn*
une HLM *council flat, housing association flat*
un immeuble *building, block of flats*
la location *situation*
la maison *house*
le pavillon *detached house (suburban)*
le rez-de-chaussée *ground floor*
la terrasse *terrace*
la tour *tower*
la vue *view*

acheter *to buy*
adorer *to love*
agrandir *to increase, to enlarge*
aimer *to like, to love*
décorer *to decorate*
déménager *to move house*
détester *to hate*
frapper (à la porte) *to knock (on the door)*

habiter   *to live*
louer   *to rent, to let, to hire*
sonner   *to ring the doorbell*
venir   *to come*

affreux/affreuse   *awful*
agréable   *pleasant*
ancien/ancienne   *old, ex-, former*
beau/bel/belle   *beautiful, fine*
en bois   *of wood*
en brique   *of brick*
en béton   *of concrete*
calme   *calm, quiet*
cher / pas très cher / pas trop cher   *expensive / not very expensive / not too expensive*
chic   *smart*
confortable   *comfortable*
difficile   *difficult*
élégant   *elegant*
étroit   *narrow*
à l' extérieur   *outside*
facile   *easy*
formidable   *great*
grand   *large*
à l' intérieur   *inside*
joli   *pretty*
laid   *ugly*
de luxe   *luxurious*
en métal   *metal*
moderne   *modern*
nécessaire   *necessary*
neuf/neuve   *new*
nouveau/nouvel/nouvelle   *new*
parfait   *perfect*
petit   *small*
plastique   *plastic*
pratique   *practical*
propre   *clean*
sale   *dirty*
typique   *typical*
utile   *useful*
vieux/vieil/vieille   *old*

chez   *at the home of*
loin de   *far from*
près de   *near*
presque   *almost*

la différence   *difference*
le gratte-ciel   *skyscraper*
le logement   *accommodation*
le loyer   *rent*
le mètre carré   *square metre*
le meuble   *(piece of) furniture*
la peinture   *painting, paint*
le propriétaire   *owner*

en bas   *downstairs, below*
bizarre   *odd, strange*
en bon état   *in good condition*
bruyant   *noisy*
étonnant   *surprising*
en haut   *upstairs, above*
en mauvais état   *in poor condition*
tranquille   *peaceful, calm*

aménager   *to furnish*
critiquer   *to criticise*
loger   *to lodge, to accommodate*
nettoyer   *to clean*

tapisser   *to paper*
vendre   *to sell*

GENERAL

un ascenseur   *lift*
le balcon   *balcony*
la cave   *cellar*
la chambre (à coucher)   *bedroom*
le chauffage central   *central heating*
le couloir   *corridor*
la cuisine   *kitchen*
l' eau (non) potable (f)   *(non-) drinking water*
l' électricité (f)   *electricity*
une entrée   *entrance*
un escalier   *staircase*
un étage   *floor, storey*
la fenêtre   *window*
le garage   *garage*
le gaz   *gas*
le grenier   *loft, attic*
le jardin   *garden*
la lampe   *lamp*
la lumière   *light*
le mur   *wall*
le parking   *parking place, car-park*
la pièce   *room*
le plan   *plan*
la porte   *door*
la salle à manger   *dining room*
la salle de bains   *bathroom*
la salle de séjour   *living room*
le salon   *lounge, sitting room*
le séjour   *lounge, sitting room*
le sous-sol   *basement*
les toilettes (f)   *toilets*
le toit   *roof*
le vestibule   *hall*
le WC   *toilet*

allumer   *to light*
appuyer   *to lean, to press*
couper   *to cut*
fermer   *to close*
ouvrir   *to open*

voici...   *here is...*
voilà...   *there is...*

Appuyez sur le bouton.   *Press the button.*
Fermez la porte, s'il vous plaît.   *Close the door, please.*
Coupez le gaz, s'il vous plaît.   *Turn off the gas, please.*

un aménagement   *furnishings, fittings*
une ampoule électrique   *electric light bulb*
la cour   *courtyard*
le débarras   *lumber room, junk room*
l' entretien (m)   *maintenance*
le palier   *landing*
le plafond   *ceiling*
le plancher   *floor*
la prise de courant   *power point*
le radiateur   *radiator*
la serrure   *lock*
le volet   *shutter*

brancher   *to plug in*
faire du bricolage   *to do odd jobs*
réparer   *to repair*

utiliser *to use*

aménagé *fitted, furnished*

Bedroom

une armoire *wardrobe*
la chaîne stéréo *stereo*
la couverture *blanket*
un électrophone *record player*
la lampe *lamp*
le lit *bed*
le magnétophone (à cassettes) *tape recorder (cassette recorder)*
un oreiller *pillow*
le placard *cupboard*
le poster *poster*
le rideau *curtain*
le tapis *carpet*
le transistor *transistor*

partager *to share*

+ *adjectives of size and colour, etc. (see p. 53)*

plusieurs *several*

J'ai une chambre à moi. *I have a room of my own.*
Je partage ma chambre avec ma sœur / mon frère.
I share my room with my sister / brother.

le drap *sheet*
une étagère *shelf*
le matelas *mattress*
le micro-ordinateur *computer*
le miroir *mirror*
la moquette *fitted carpet*
le réveil *alarm clock*

Kitchen

les allumettes (f) *matches*
un aspirateur *vacuum cleaner*
une assiette *plate*
le bol *bowl*
la bougie *candle*
la casserole *saucepan*
le congélateur *freezer*
le couteau *knife*
la cuillère *spoon*
la cuisinière à gaz *gas cooker*
la cuisinière électrique *electric cooker*
l' eau chaude / froide (f) *hot / cold water*
un évier *sink*
le fer à repasser *iron*
le four *oven*
la fourchette *fork*
le frigidaire / frigo *refrigerator*
le lave-linge *washing machine*
le lave-vaisselle *dishwasher*
le placard *cupboard*
la poêle *frying pan*
la poubelle *dustbin*
le robinet *tap*
la table *table*
la tasse *cup*
la vaisselle *crockery*
le verre *glass*

allumer *to light, to switch on*
éteindre *to extinguish, to put out, to switch off*

faire la lessive *to do the washing*
faire la vaisselle *to do the washing-up*
jeter *to throw (out)*

Bathroom

la baignoire *bath*
le bidet *bidet*
la brosse à dents *toothbrush*
le dentifrice *toothpaste*
la douche *shower*
l' eau froide / chaude (f) *cold / hot water*
une éponge *sponge*
le gant de toilette *flannel*
la glace *mirror*
le lavabo *wash-basin*
la prise-rasoir *electric razor socket*
le rasoir *razor*
le savon *soap*
la serviette *towel*
le shampooing *shampoo*

Dining room

le buffet *sideboard*
le carafe *glass jug, carafe*
la chaise *chair*
la cheminée *fireplace, hearth*
une horloge *clock (grandfather)*
la nappe *tablecloth*
le plat *dish*
la serviette *serviette, napkin*
la table *table*
le tableau *picture*
le vaisselier *dresser*

Living room

la bibliothèque *bookcase*
le canapé *sofa*
le cendrier *ashtray*
la chaîne stéréo *stereo*
le coussin *cushion*
le divan *sofa*
une étagère *shelf*
le fauteuil *armchair*
le magnétophone (à cassettes) *tape recorder (cassette recorder)*
le magnétoscope *video recorder*
la pendule *clock*
la photo *photo*
lc piano *piano*
la plante verte *house plant*
la table basse *coffee table*
le tableau *picture*
la télévision *television*
le vase *vase*

Hall

la clé *key*
le mur *wall*
la porte (d'entrée) *(front) door*
le téléphone *telephone*

Garden

un arbre *tree*
un arbre fruitier *fruit tree*
le buisson *bush*
la fleur *flower*
le fruit *fruit*
l' herbe (f) *grass*
le jardinage *gardening*
le légume *vegetable*
les mauvaises herbes (f) *weeds*
la plante *plant*
le sapin *fir tree*

    arroser *to water*
    cultiver *to grow*
    faire pousser *to grow*
    tondre la pelouse *to mow the lawn*

Je cultive des légumes. *I grow vegetables.*
J'ai tondu la pelouse. *I have mown the lawn.*

DAILY ROUTINE

le déjeuner *lunch, midday meal*
le dîner *dinner, evening meal*
le goûter *afternoon tea, snack*
le petit déjeuner *breakfast*
le week-end *weekend*

    accrocher *to hang up*
    acheter *to buy*
    aider *to help*
    aller aux toilettes *to go to the toilet*
    s'amuser *to enjoy oneself*
    apporter *to bring*
    s'asseoir *to sit down*
    avoir besoin de *to need*
    boire *to drink*
    changer *to change*
    se coucher *to go to bed*
    coudre *to sew*
    couper *to cut*
    débarasser (la table) *to clear (the table)*
    déjeuner *to have lunch*
    se déshabiller *to undress*
    dormir *to sleep*
    écouter de la musique/la radio/des disques *to listen to music/the radio/records*
    écrire *to write*
    s'endormir *to go to sleep*
    être prêt à *to be ready to*
    faire les courses *to do the shopping*
    faire la cuisine *to do the cooking*
    faire le lit *to make the bed*
    faire le ménage *to do the housework*
    faire la vaisselle *to wash up*
    faire ses devoirs *to do one's homework*
    garder les enfants *to look after the children, to babysit*
    s'habiller *to dress*
    jeter *to throw (away)*
    se laver *to get washed*
    se laver les mains, etc. *to wash one's hands, etc.*
    se lever *to get up, to stand up*
    manger *to eat*
    mettre le couvert *to lay the table*
    nettoyer *to clean*
    partager *to share*
    passer l'aspirateur *to do the hoovering*
    prendre un bain *to have a bath*

prendre un café *to have a cup of coffee*
prendre une douche *to have a shower*
prendre le petit déjeuner *to have breakfast*
préparer un repas *to prepare a meal*
quitter *to leave*
recevoir *to receive*
regarder la télévision *to watch television*
rentrer *to return home*
repasser *to iron*
se reposer *to rest*
se réveiller *to wake up*
servir *to serve*
sortir *to go out*
travailler *to work*
tricoter *to knit*

    d'habitude *usually*
    enfin *finally*
    ensuite *afterwards*
    généralement *usually*
    puis *then*

J'ai besoin de me laver. *I need to wash.*
Je me couche normalement à dix heures. *I usually go to bed at 10 o'clock.*
Je me suis déshabillé(e) avant de me coucher. *I undressed before going to bed.*
Peux-tu me faire les courses? *Could you do some shopping for me?*
Je me suis lavé les mains. *I have washed my hands.*
Je voudrais prendre une douche. *I would like to have a shower.*
J'aime regarder la télévision. *I like watching TV.*
Est-ce que tu veux te reposer? *Would you like to rest?*
A quelle heure est-ce que tu te réveilles d'habitude? *What time do you usually wake up?*

    aller chercher *to go and get*
    aller voir *to go and see*
    s'en aller *to go away*
    arrêter de *to stop*
    balayer *to sweep*
    se brosser les cheveux *to brush one's hair*
    se changer *to change*
    déranger *to disturb*
    discuter *to discuss*
    se disputer *to argue*
    éplucher les légumes *to prepare (peel, scrape) the vegetables*
    essuyer *to wipe*
    faire du bricolage *to do odd jobs*
    faire cuire *to cook*
    faire la lessive *to do the washing*
    interdire de *to forbid*
    s'occuper de *to be busy with*
    offrir *to offer*
    prêter *to lend*
    se promener *to go for a walk*
    ranger *to put away*
    se raser *to shave*
    recommencer à *to start again*
    réparer *to repair*
    utiliser *to use*
    vouloir bien *to want to*

Je m'en vais. *I'm going.*
Va-t-en! *Go away!*
Va voir qui est là! *Go and see who is there!*
Je me suis changé(e). *I have changed.*

Veux-tu éplucher les carottes? *Will you please prepare (peel, scrape) the carrots?*

Je vais faire cuire ce lapin dans le four. *I'll cook this rabbit in the oven.*

Est-ce que je peux t'aider à ranger ta chambre? *Can I help you tidy your room?*

Je vais m'en occuper. *I'll do that.*

Est-ce que tu peux me prêter 10 francs? *Can you lend me 10 francs?*

Est-ce que je peux vous donner un coup de main? *Can I give you a hand?*

Mon père m'a interdit de sortir ce soir. *My father has forbidden me to go out this evening.*

▷ A4 Media

un/une	acteur/actrice	*actor/actress*
une	ambiance	*atmosphere*
un	animal sauvage	*wild animal*
une	aventure	*adventure*
le	bal	*ball (dancing)*
le	balcon	*balcony*
le	bandit	*bandit*
le	billet	*ticket*
la	boum	*party*
la	cassette	*cassette*
le	chameau	*camel*
la	chanson	*song*
le/la	chanteur/chanteuse	*singer*
le	cinéma	*cinema*
lc	cirque	*circus*
le	clown	*clown*
le	club	*club*
la	comédie	*comedy (theatre)*
le	concert	*concert*
la	discothèque	*disco*
le	drapeau	*flag*
un	éléphant	*elephant*
l'	espionnage (m)	*spying, espionage*
le	film d'amour	*love film*
le	film d'épouvante	*horror film*
le	film policier	*crime film*
le	film de science-fiction	*science-fiction film*
la	flûte	*flute*
le	groupe	*group*
la	guerre	*war*
la	guitare	*guitar*
l'	information (f)	*information*
la	jeunesse	*youth, young people*
le	lion	*lion*
le	loup	*wolf*
le	magicien	*magician*
la	maison des jeunes	*youth club*
la	matinée	*morning, afternoon performance*
un	opéra	*opera*
un	orchestre	*orchestra*
un	ours	*bear*
le	piano	*piano*
la	pièce de théâtre	*play*
la	réunion	*meeting*
le	rhinocéros	*rhinoceros*
lc	risque	*risk*
la	salle	*room, hall*
la	séance	*performance, session*
le	singe	*monkey*
le	spectacle	*entertainment*
la	surprise-partie	*party*
le	théâtre	*theatre*

le	ticket	*ticket*
la	vedette	*(film) star*
la	version anglaise	*English version*
le	violon	*violin*
le	western	*western*
le	zoo	*zoo*

aller voir *to go and see*
commencer *to begin*
dresser un animal *to train an animal*
enfermer *to lock up*
s'évader *to escape*
fuir *to flee*
payer *to pay (for)*
plaire à *to please*
réserver *to reserve*
se sauver *to run away*

affreux/affreuse *awful*
amusant *amusing*
bien! *good!*
bon/bonne *good*
comique *funny*
drôle *funny*
ennuyeux/ennuyeuse *boring*
excellent *excellent*
extraordinaire *extraordinary*
formidable *great, terrific*
intéressant *interesting*
nouveau/nouvel/nouvelle *new*
pas mal *not bad*
sensationnel/sensationnelle *sensational*
super *terrific, great*
surprenant *surprising*
+ *adjectives for hobbies (see p. 44)*

agréablement *pleasantly*
extrêmement *extremely*
tout à fait *quite, totally*

Il y avait une bonne ambiance. *There was a good atmosphere.*

Nous sommes allé(e)s à la boum chez Marie. C'était sensass! *We went to Marie's party. It was great!*

Le film était en version anglaise. *The film had an English soundtrack.*

Comment as-tu trouvé le concert? *What did you think of the concert?*

les	actualités (f)	*news (cinema)*
le/la	comédien/comédienne	*comedian/comédienne*
le	dessin animé	*cartoon*
le	documentaire	*documentary*
un	entracte	*interval*
le	feuilleton	*serial / soap opera*
les	informations (f)	*news*
le	journal télévisé	*news*
les	nouvelles (f)	*news*
une	ouvreuse	*usherette*
le	pourboire	*tip*
la	réduction	*reduction*
les	sous-titres (m)	*subtitles*
le	succès	*success*
le	tube	*hit record*

annuler *to cancel*
apprécier *to appreciate*
avoir raison *to be right*
conseiller *to advise*
découvrir *to discover*
enregistrer *to record*

être à l'affiche   *to be billed, advertised*
être d'accord   *to agree*
penser   *to think*
protester   *to protest*
se réjouir de   *to be delighted*
tourner un film   *to make a film*
trouver   *to find*

favori/favorite   *favourite*
impressionnant   *impressive*
majeur   *major*
merveilleux/merveilleuse   *marvellous*
passionnant   *exciting*
pire   *worse*
rare   *rare*
ridicule   *ridiculous*

Pendant l'entracte nous avons vu la vedette qui était à
l'affiche.   *During the interval we saw the star who was
on the poster.*
J'ai enregistré cette émission sur magnétoscope parce que je
voulais regarder le feuilleton sur l'autre chaîne.
*I recorded this programme on video because I wanted to
see the soap opera on the other channel.*
J'ai oublié de donner une pourboire à l'ouvreuse. Elle était
furieuse.   *I forgot to give the usherette a tip. She was
furious.*

BOX-OFFICE SCENES

Theatre
Je voudrais réserver des places pour la pièce du
13 juillet.   *I would like to reserve seats for the play on
13 July.*
Il n'y a plus de places pour ce jour-là, mais il en reste
encore pour le lendemain.   *There are no seats left for
that day, but there are some for the following day.*
Alors, trois places pour le lendemain.   *All right, three seats
for the following day.*
Des places à quel prix? Il reste des places à 25F et 30F.
*At what price? There are seats left at 25 francs and 30
francs.*

Sporting event
Je voudrais réserver des places pour le match de samedi, s'il
vous plaît.   *I would like to reserve places for the match
on Saturday, please.*
Oui, combien de places?   *Yes, how many places?*
Deux places, s'il vous plaît.   *Two, please.*

Concert
Je voudrais réserver des places pour le concert du
11 novembre, s'il vous plaît.   *I would like to reserve
seats for the concert on 11 November, please.*
Des places à quel prix? Il reste des places à 45F et à
35F.   *What price seats? There are seats left at 45 francs
and 35 francs.*
Deux places à 35F, s'il vous plaît.   *Two seats at 35 francs,
please.*

Cinema
Je voudrais une place pour *Toy Story*, s'il vous plaît.
I'd like a seat for Toy Story, *please*
Il ne reste plus que des places tout à fait à l'avant ou à
l'arrière. Qu'est-ce que vous préférez?   *The only seats*

left are right at the front and at the back. Which would
you prefer?*
Une place à l'arrière, s'il vous plaît.   *A seat at the back,
please.*
Ça vous fait 40F.   *That'll be 40 francs.*
C'est un film en anglais?   *Is the film in English?*
Non, il est en version française.   *No, it's the French
version.*

▶ A5 Health, fitness and welfare

PARTS OF THE BODY
la   bouche   *mouth*
le   bras   *arm*
la   cheville   *ankle*
le   cœur   *heart*
la   dent   *tooth*
le   doigt   *finger*
le   dos   *back*
une   épaule   *shoulder*
un   estomac   *stomach*
le   genou   *knee*
la   gorge   *throat*
la   jambe   *leg*
la   langue   *tongue*
la   main   *hand*
le   nez   *nose*
un   œil (*plural*: les yeux)   *eye(s)*
une   oreille   *ear*
la   pcau   *skin*
le   pied   *foot*
la   poitrine   *chest*
un   os   *bone*
le   sang   *blood*
la   tête   *head*
le   ventre   *stomach*

HYGIENE
le   bain   *bath*
la   brosse à dents   *toothbrush*
le   dentifrice   *toothpaste*
un   essuie-mains   *hand towel*
le   maquillage   *make-up*
la   pâte dentifrice   *toothpaste*
le   rasoir   *razor*
le   savon   *soap*
la   serviette   *towel*
le   shampooing   *shampoo*

se brosser les dents   *to brush one's teeth*
se laver   *to get washed*
se maquiller   *to put on make-up*
prendre un bain   *to have a bath*
prendre une douche   *to have a shower*
se raser   *to shave*

propre   *clean*
sale   *dirty*

WELL-BEING
aller bien   *to be well*
aller mal   *to be ill*
aller mieux   *to be better*

avoir chaud   *to be warm*
avoir faim   *to be hungry*
avoir froid   *to be cold*
avoir soif   *to be thirsty*
dormir   *to sleep*
se faire mal   *to hurt oneself*
piquer   *to sting, to bite*
se reposer   *to rest*
soulager   *to relieve*

en forme   *in form*
fatigué   *tired*

Je ne vais pas bien.   *I am not well.*
Je vais mieux maintenant.   *I'm feeling better now.*
J'ai chaud.   *I'm warm.*
Il a faim.   *He's hungry.*

ILLNESS AND INJURY

la fièvre   *fever, high temperature*
l' indigestion (f)   *indigestion*
le mal de mer   *sea sickness*
le rhume   *cold*
la santé   *health*
la température   *temperature*

s'allonger   *to lie down*
avaler   *to swallow*
avoir mal à l'estomac   *to have stomach ache*
avoir mal à la gorge   *to have a sore throat*
avoir mal à la jambe   *to have a bad leg*
avoir mal à la tête   *to have a headache*
avoir mal au bras   *to have a bad arm*
avoir mal au cœur   *to feel sick*
avoir mal au dos   *to have a bad back*
avoir mal au ventre   *to have stomach ache*
avoir mal aux dents   *to have toothache*
avoir mal aux oreilles   *to have earache*
avoir mal aux yeux   *to have sore eyes*
se blesser   *to get injured*
se brûler la main   *to burn one's hand*
se casser le bras   *to break one's arm*
se cogner   *to get a knock*
conseiller   *to advise*
consulter   *to consult*
se coucher   *to go to bed, to lie down*
se couper le doigt   *to cut one's finger*
crier   *to shout*
être admis(e) à l'hôpital   *to be admitted to hospital*
être enrhumé   *to have a cold*
se fouler la cheville   *to twist (sprain) one's ankle*
guérir   *to heal, to cure*
s'inquiéter   *to worry*
mordre   *to bite*
mourir   *to die*
se noyer   *to drown*
pleurer   *to weep*
saigner   *to bleed*
se sentir bien   *to feel well*
se sentir mal   *to feel ill*
souffrir   *to suffer*
surveiller sa température   *to take one's temperature*
se taire   *to be silent*
tomber   *to fall*
tousser   *to cough*
vomir   *to vomit*

vouloir   *to want, to wish (to)*

Elle s'est fait mal à la jambe.   *She has hurt her leg.*
Un moustique l'a piqué.   *A mosquito has bitten him.*
J'ai de la fièvre.   *I have a high temperature.*

GETTING TREATED

une   ambulance   *ambulance*
une   aspirine   *aspirin*
une   assurance   *insurance (policy)*
le   cabinet   *consulting room, surgery*
le   cachet   *tablet*
la   clinique   *clinic*
le   comprimé   *tablet*
le   coton hydrophile   *absorbent cotton wool*
le   coup de soleil   *sunburn*
la   crème   *cream*
la   crise   *fit, attack, crisis*
la   cuillerée   *spoonful*
le   dentiste   *dentist*
la   diarhée   *diarrhoea*
le   docteur   *doctor (title)*
la   douleur   *pain*
la   fièvre   *fever, high temperature*
la   fois   *time*
les   frais   *expenses*
le   gonflement   *swelling*
la   grippe   *flu*
une   heure   *hour*
un   hôpital   *hospital*
une   insolation   *sunstroke*
le   jour   *day*
les   lunettes (f)   *spectacles*
le/la   malade   *patient*
la   maladie   *illness*
le   médecin   *doctor*
la   médecine   *medicine (as a subject)*
le   médicament   *medicine, treatment*
la   naissance   *birth*
une   opération   *operation*
un/une   opticien/opticienne   *optician*
une   ordonnance   *prescription*
le   pansement   *dressing, plaster*
la   pastille   *throat pastille*
la   pharmacie   *chemist's shop*
le/la   pharmacien/pharmacienne   *chemist*
la   pilule   *pill*
la   piqûre   *sting, bite*
le   problème   *problem*
le   remède   *remedy*
le   rendez-vous   *appointment*
la   salle de consultation   *consulting room*
la   santé   *health*
le   sirop   *medicine*
le   sparadrap   *plaster, Elastoplast®*
la   sympathie   *sympathy*
le   tube   *tube*
la   voix   *voice*

antiseptique   *antiseptic*
assuré   *insured*
blessé   *injured*
capable   *capable*
constipé   *constipated*
enrhumé   *with a cold*
faible   *weak*
fragile   *delicate*

grave   *serious*
inquiet/inquiète   *anxious*
mort   *dead*
sensible   *sensitive*
souffrant   *ill, suffering*
vivant   *alive*

gravement   *seriously*
mieux   *better*

J'ai mal au cœur.   *I feel sick.*
Je me suis brûlé la main.   *I have burnt my hand.*
Elle s'est cassée le bras.   *She has broken her arm.*
Anne s'est foulé la cheville.   *Anne has twisted her ankle.*
Elle souffre.   *She's not well.*
C'est un beau coup de soleil.   *That's quite a sunburn.*
Une insolation, c'est très dangereux.   *Sunstroke is very dangerous.*

AT THE CHEMIST'S

une   angine   *tonsilitis, sore throat*
le   traitement   *treatment*

se couper   *to cut oneself*
saigner du nez   *to have a nose bleed*

antiseptique   *antiseptic*

J'ai une angine.   *I have tonsilitis.*
J'ai la grippe.   *I have flu.*
Un insecte m'a piqué(e).   *I have been bitten (stung) by an insect.*
Je saigne du nez.   *I have a nose bleed.*
Je viens de tomber.   *I have just had a fall.*
Je n'arrête pas de tousser.   *I can't stop coughing.*
Voilà des comprimés efficaces pour la gorge.   *Here are some tablets which are good for the throat.*
Il vaut mieux rester au lit et attendre que le docteur vous donne une ordonnance pour des médicaments.   *You had better stay in bed and wait for the doctor to give you a prescription for some medicine.*
Voici une crème/un traitement très efficace contre les piqûres d'insecte.   *Here is a very good cream/treatment for insect bites.*
Il vaut mieux vous allonger tout de suite.   *You had better lie down straight away.*
Je vais vous soigner. Voici un flacon d'antiseptique et des pansements/du sparadrap pour protéger votre main.   *I will deal with that. Here is a bottle of antiseptic and some bandages/plasters to protect your hand.*
Voici un bon sirop/remède.   *Here is a good syrup/remedy.*

ACCIDENTS

un   accident   *accident*
une   adresse   *address*
un   agent de police   *policeman*
le   car   *coach*
la   collision   *collision*
le   commissariat   *police station*
le   constat   *statement*
le   consulat   *consulate*
le   cycliste   *cyclist*
le   danger   *danger*
le   dommage   *damage*
une   excuse   *excuse*
la   faute   *fault*
la   gendarmerie   *police station*

le   motocycliste   *motorcyclist*
le   passant   *passer-by*
la   permission   *permission*
le   piéton   *pedestrian*
la   police   *police*
   Police-Secours   *police rescue services*
le   poste de police   *police station*
le   problème   *problem*
la   priorité   *priority*
le/la   responsable   *culprit; group leader*
le   risque   *risk*
le   sapeur-pompier   *fireman*
le   sens   *direction*
le   témoin   *witness*
le   véhicule   *vehicle*

accuser   *to accuse*
aider   *to help*
appeler   *to call*
s'arrêter   *to stop*
attendre   *to wait (for)*
avoir le droit   *to have the right*
avoir peur   *to be afraid*
brûler   *to burn*
courir   *to run*
crier   *to shout*
déclarer   *to declare*
dépasser   *to overtake*
se dépêcher   *to hurry*
s'excuser   *to apologise*
faire attention   *to pay attention*
heurter   *to knock, to bump into*
informer   *to inform*
se mettre en colère   *to get angry*
pardonner   *to forgive*
payer   *to pay (for)*
pleurer   *to weep, to cry*
poser   *to put down*
protester   *to protest*
ralentir   *to slow down*
regarder   *to watch, to look at*
remplir   *to fill*
renverser   *to knock over, to turn over*
réparer   *to repair*
respecter   *to respect*
rouler   *to drive, to move*
tomber   *to fall*
tourner   *to turn*
traverser   *to cross*
tuer   *to kill*

blessé   *injured*
certain   *certain*
désolé   *very sorry*
faux/fausse   *false, wrong*
grave   *serious*
mort   *dead*
mouillé   *wet*
sûr   *certain*
surprenant   *surprising*
urgent   *urgent*
vrai   *true*

d'accord   *agreed*
doucement   *gently*
gravement   *seriously*
là   *there*
plus tard   *later*
pourtant   *however*

presque *almost*
tant mieux *so much the better*
tant pis *never mind*
tout à coup *suddenly*
tout de suite *straight away*
vite *quickly*

Attention! *Look out!*
Au feu! *Fire!*
Au secours! *Help!*
Hélas! *Alas!*
Mon Dieu! *My goodness*
'monsieur l'agent' *'officer'*
Oh là là! *Oh dear!*
Pardon! *Sorry!*
Tiens *Hey!*
+ *vocabulary from Travel (see p. 60)*

A6 Food and drink

MEAT

l' agneau (m) *lamb*
le bifteck *beef steak*
le bœuf *beef*
le canard *duck*
la côte *rib*
le filet *fillet steak*
le jambon *ham*
le lapin *rabbit*
le mouton *mutton*
le porc *pork*
le poulet *chicken*
le rôti *roast meat*
le steak *steak*
le veau *veal*

FISH AND SEAFOOD

le crabe *crab*
la crevette *shrimp*
les fruits de mer (m) *seafood*
une huître *oyster*
le maquereau *mackerel*
la morue *cod*
les moules (f) *mussels*
la sardine *sardine*
la sole *sole*
la truite *trout*

VEGETABLES

un artichaut *artichoke*
la carotte *carrot*
le champignon *mushroom*
le chou *cabbage*
le chou-fleur *cauliflower*
le concombre *cucumber*
les épinards (m) *spinach*
un haricot *bean*
la laitue *lettuce*
un oignon *onion*
les petits pois (m) *peas*
le poireau *leek*
la pomme de terre *potato*
le riz *rice*
la salade *salad, lettuce*
la tomate *tomato*

FRUIT

un abricot *apricot*
un ananas *pineapple*
la banane *banana*
la cerise *cherry*
le citron *lemon*
la fraise *strawberry*
la framboise *raspberry*
la groseille à maquereau *gooseberry*
les groseilles (f) (*usually plural*) *redcurrants*
le melon *melon*
la noix *nut*
la pêche *peach*
la poire *pear*
la pomme *apple*
la prune *plum*
le raisin *grape*

OTHER FOODS

une assiette anglaise *cold meat and salad*
la baguette *stick of bread*
le beurre *butter*
le biscuit *biscuit*
le bonbon *sweet*
les chips (m) *crisps*
le chocolat *chocolate*
la confiture *jam*
la crêpe *pancake*
le croissant *croissant*
le croque-monsieur *toasted cheese and ham sandwich*
les crudités (f) *raw vegetables*
le déjeuner *lunch*
le dessert *dessert*
le dîner *dinner, evening meal*
une épaule de mouton *shoulder of mutton*
les frites (f) *chips*
le fromage *cheese*
le gâteau *cake*
la glace *ice cream*
un hors d'œuvre *starter*
le légume *vegetable*
la mayonnaise *mayonnaise*
la moutarde *mustard*
un œuf *egg*
une omelette *omelette*
le pain *bread*
le pâté *pâté*
la pâtisserie *cake, pastry*
le petit déjeuner *breakfast*
le pique-nique *picnic*
le plat du jour *dish of the day*
le poisson *fish*
le poivre *pepper*
le potage *soup*
les provisions (f) *food*
la purée *mashed potato*
la quiche lorraine *egg and cheese flan*
le repas *meal*
la salade *salad, lettuce*
le sandwich *sandwich*
le saucisson *sausage*
le sel *salt*
la soupe *soup*
le sucre *sugar*
la tarte *flan*
la terrine *potted meat*

la	vanille	*vanilla*
le	vinaigre	*vinegar*
le	yaourt	*yoghurt*

DRINKS

un	apéritif	*aperitif*
la	bière	*beer*
la	boisson	*drink*
le	café	*coffee*
le	café-crème	*white coffee*
le	chocolat	*chocolate, hot chocolate*
le	cidre	*cider*
le	citron pressé	*fresh lemon juice*
le	Coca	*Coca Cola®*
une	eau minérale	*mineral water*
le	jus de fruit	*fruit juice*
le	lait	*milk*
la	limonade	*lemonade*
une	orange pressée	*fresh orange juice*
une	pression	*draught beer*
le	thé	*tea*
le	vin blanc/rouge	*white/red wine*

RESTAURANT

une	addition	*bill*
une	assiette	*plate*
le	bar	*bar*
le	bol	*bowl*
la	bouteille	*bottle*
la	cafetière	*coffee pot*
la	carte	*menu*
le	couteau	*knife*
la	cuillère	*spoon*
le	dîner	*dinner, evening meal*
une	entrée	*main dish*
la	fourchette	*fork*
le	garçon	*waiter*
le	goût	*taste*
le	menu	*fixed-price menu*
une	odeur	*smell*
le	parfum	*flavour*
le	pâté maison	*home-made pâté*
le	patron	*owner*
la	personne	*person*
le	plateau	*tray*
le	quart	*quarter (litre)*
le	resto/restaurant	*restaurant*
le	service	*service*
la	soucoupe	*saucer*
la	spécialité	*speciality*
la	table	*table*
la	tasse	*cup*
le	téléphone	*telephone*
les	toilettes (f)	*toilets*
le	verre	*glass*

adorer	*to love*
aimer	*to like*
avoir faim/soif	*to be hungry/thirsty*
boire	*to drink*
choisir	*to choose*
coûter	*to cost*
désirer	*to want, to wish*
détester	*to hate*
dîner	*to have dinner*
manger	*to eat*

passer	*to pass*
préférer	*to prefer*
prendre	*to take*
préparer	*to prepare*
recommander	*to recommend*
servir	*to serve*
trouver	*to find*
je (ne) voudrais (pas)...	*I would (not) like...*

bien	*good, well*
bien cuit	*well cooked, well done*
bon/bonne	*good*
chaud	*hot*
compris	*included*
délicieux/délicieuse	*delicious*
demi	*half*
excellent	*excellent*
froid	*cold*
malade	*ill*
mauvais	*bad*
à point	*medium (steak)*
rôti	*roast*
seul	*alone*

assez	*enough*
beaucoup	*a lot, many*
combien	*how much, how many*
comme	*as, how*
comment	*how*
encore	*more*
exactement	*exactly*
merci	*thank you*
peu (de)	*little*
sans	*without*
en sus	*in addition*
très	*very*

Voilà!	*There you are!*
A votre/ta santé!	*To your health! Cheers!*
A la vôtre/tienne!	*To your health! Cheers!*

la	carafe	*glass jug, carafe*
le	chef	*cook*
le	couvert	*table place, cover charge*
une	erreur	*mistake*
les	félicitations (f)	*congratulations*
le	gaz	*gas*
le	pichet	*pitcher, jug*
le	pourboire	*tip*
la	recette	*recipe*
le/la	serveur/serveuse	*server, waiter/waitress*
la	théière	*teapot*

apporter	*to bring*
apprécier	*to appreciate*
approuver	*to approve*
avoir envie de	*to wish to*
commander	*to order*
désapprouver	*to disapprove*
devoir	*to owe*
féliciter	*to congratulate*
insulter	*to insult*
se mettre en colère	*to get angry*
offrir	*to offer*
se plaindre	*to complain*
plaire	*to please*
protester	*to protest*
vouloir	*to wish*

appétisant	*appetizing*
doux/douce	*mild, sweet*

piquant   *tart, savoury, spicy*
saignant   *rare, underdone*
salé   *salty*
satisfait   *satisfied*
sucré   *sweet*
varié   *varied*

aussi   *also*
Bravo!   *Well done!*
complètement   *completely*
entièrement   *entirely*
inadmissible   *unforgiveable*
lequel/laquelle   *which*
service (non) compris   *service (not) included*
ça suffit   *that's enough*
TTC (toutes taxes comprises)   *inclusive of tax*

Attracting the waiter's attention
Madame!   *Waiter!*
Mademoiselle!   *Waitress!*
Monsieur!   *Waiter!*

Asking for a table
une table libre   *free table*
    réserver une table   *to reserve a table*
    faire une réservation   *to make a reservation*

Avez-vous une table pour ... personnes?   *Have you a table for ... people?*
Oui, messieurs-dames.   *Yes, ladies and gentlemen.*
Merci bien.   *Thank you very much.*
Au revoir.   *Goodbye.*
Bonne journée / soirée. (etc).   *Have a good day / evening (etc).*
Oui, par ici, s'il vous plaît.   *Yes, over here, please.*
Non, je regrette.   *No, I'm sorry.*

Ordering a meal
    choisir   *to choose*
    à la place de   *in place of*
    au lieu de   *instead of*
    le menu à 55F   *55-franc menu*
    à point   *medium (steak)*
    (bien) cuit   *well done*
    saignant   *rare*

On peut commander?   *May we order?*
Je voudrais le menu, s'il vous plaît.   *I'd like the fixed-price menu, please.*
Je vais prendre...   *I'll have...*
Vous avez choisi?   *Have you chosen?*
Bien sûr, certainement.   *Of course.*
Que désirez-vous?   *What would you like?*
Qu'est-ce que vous prendrez?   *What will you have?*
Pour commencer...   *To begin with...*
Pour suivre...   *To follow...*
Ce sera tout, merci.   *That will be all, thank you.*
Qu'est-ce que tu prendras / vous prendrez?   *What are you having?*
Qu'est-ce que tu veux / vous voulez?   *What do you want?*
Pour lui/elle/eux/elles...   *For him/her/them...*
Je voudrais un steak, s'il vous plaît.   *I'd like a steak, please.*
Je voudrais...   *I would like...*
Quel dommage!   *What a pity!*

Alors, je prendrais...   *Right, I'll have...*
Prenez-vous un apéritif?   *Are you having an aperitif?*
Quelle boisson prendrez-vous?   *What drink would you like?*
Votre commande, s'il vous plaît?   *Your order, please?*
Oui, et ensuite?   *Yes, and after that?*
Et pour terminer?   *And to finish?*
Et pour vous, mademoiselle?   *And for you, miss?*
Pour monsieur, ce sera...   *And you, sir, you'll have...*
Vous le voulez comment, votre steak?   *How would you like your steak?*
Ce sera en supplément.   *That will be extra.*
Désolé(e), il n'en reste plus.   *I'm very sorry, we have none left.*
Café compris.   *Coffee included.*
Boissons en sus.   *Drinks extra.*
Service 15% (non) compris   *Service 15% (not) included.*

Requesting extras
S'il vous plaît, on peut avoir...?   *Could we have...?*
    de l'eau / du vin   *some water / wine*
    de l'huile   *oil*
    du sel   *salt*
    du sucre   *sugar*
Vous pouvez changer...?   *Would you change...?*
    le verre   *the glass*
    l'assiette   *the plate*
Il manque...   *We are short of...*
    un couteau   *a knife*
    une cuillère   *a spoon*
    une fourchette   *a fork*
    une tasse   *a cup*
    un verre   *a glass*
Vous pouvez nettoyer la table, s'il vous plaît?   *Could you clean the table, please?*
Tout va bien?   *Is everything all right?*
Mais oui, certainement.   *Yes, of course.*
Je vais vous en chercher un/une.   *I'll go and get you one.*
Tout de suite.   *Straight away.*
On peut avoir (encore)...?   *Could we have some (more)...?*
    du vinaigre   *vinegar*
    de la moutarde   *mustard*
    du poivre   *pepper*

Requesting clarifications
Qu'est-ce que c'est...?   *What is...?*
Pouvez-vous expliquer ce que c'est?   *Could you explain what it is?*
Qu'est-ce qu'il y a comme...?   *What have you got in the way of...?*
Est-ce que vous avez encore...?   *Have you any more...?*
Reste-t-il des...?   *Are there any ... left?*
Ça prendra combien de temps?   *How long will it take?*
Ça ne sera pas trop long, j'espère.   *I hope it won't be too long.*
Ça sera bientôt prêt?   *Will it be ready soon?*
Le service est-il compris?   *Is service included?*
Le vin est-il compris?   *Is the wine included?*
C'est une sauce.   *It's a sauce.*
C'est un plat servi avec...   *It's a dish served with...*
C'est un vin de la région.   *It's a local wine.*
Oui, bien sûr.   *Yes, of course.*
Il y a des ... et des...   *These are ... and...*
Oui, nous en avons encore.   *Yes, we have some more.*

Non, je suis désolé(e), il ne nous en reste plus.   *No, I'm sorry, we have none left.*
Ça prendra ... minutes.   *It'll take ... minutes.*
Oui, le service est compris.   *Yes, service is included.*
Non, le service n'est pas compris.   *No, service is not included.*
Oui, les boissons sont comprises.   *Yes, drinks are included.*
Non, le vin n'est pas compris.   *No, the wine is not included.*

Requesting the bill and dealing with payment

L'addition, s'il vous plaît.   *The bill, please.*
On peut avoir l'addition, s'il vous plaît?   *Could we have the bill, please?*
Je n'ai pas assez d'argent!   *I haven't got enough money!*
Je voudrais régler l'addition, s'il vous plaît.   *I'd like to settle the bill, please.*
Vous acceptez les cartes de credit?   *Do you accept credit cards?*
Vous faites erreur.   *You are mistaken.*
La note, s'il vous plaît.   *The bill, please.*
Tout de suite.   *Straight away.*
Certainement.   *Certainly.*
Ça vous fait ... francs.   *That makes ... francs.*
Voici votre monnaie.   *Here is your change.*
Nous n'acceptons pas les chèques.   *We don't accept cheques.*

Among friends

Je vous invite.   *I'll treat you.*
C'est moi qui paie.   *I'll pay / This is on me.*

▷ BI Self, family and friends

IDENTITY

une   identité   *identity*
le   nom   *name*
le   nom de jeune fille   *maiden name*
le   prénom   *first name*
la   signature   *signature*

s'appeler   *to be called*
écrire   *to write*
s'écrire   *to be written*
épeler   *to spell*
signer   *to sign*

Madame (Mme)   *Mrs, Ms, madam*
Mademoiselle (Mlle)   *Miss*
Monsieur (M.)   *Mr, sir*
+ *letters of the alphabet (see p. 94)*

Je m'appelle...   *My name is...*
Comment ça s'écrit?   *How do you spell that?*

HOME ADDRESS

une   adresse   *address*
une   allée   *walk, lane, avenue*
un   appartement   *flat*
une   avenue   *avenue*
le   boulevard   *boulevard, wide road*
le   code postal   *postcode*
le   département   *administrative department (= county)*
le   domicile   *home*

une   enveloppe   *envelope*
la   lettre   *letter*
la   maison   *house*
le   numéro   *number*
le   pays   *country*
la   place   *square*
la   route   *road*
la   rue   *road, street*
la   ville   *town*
le   village   *village*

habiter (à)   *to live (at, in)*
chez   *at the home of*

J'habite Bristol.   *I live in Bristol.*
J'habite à Bristol.   *I live in Bristol.*
J'habite au premier étage.   *I live on the first floor.*

le/la concierge   *caretaker*
le   rez-de-chaussée   *ground floor*

demeurer   *to live*
habiter (en / au)   *to live (in)*
vivre   *to live*

en bas   *downstairs, below*
en haut   *upstairs, above*
hors de   *outside*
à proximité de   *near to*

J'habite au rez-de-chaussée.   *I live on the ground floor.*
J'habite en Angleterre.   *I live in England.*
J'habite au Pays de Galles.   *I live in Wales.*

TELEPHONE

un   annuaire   *telephone directory*
un   avantage   *advantage*
le   faux numéro   *wrong number*
un   inconvénient   *disadvantage*
le   téléphone   *telephone*

appeler   *to call*
avoir le téléphone   *to have a phone*
composer   *to dial*
contacter   *to contact*
téléphoner à   *to phone*

Allô?   *Hello?*
pratique   *convenient*
quel/quelle   *which, what*

Jacques Colbert à l'appareil.   *Jacques Colbert speaking.*
Ne quittez pas.   *Please hold.*
Je me suis trompé(e) de numéro.   *I've rung the wrong number.*
Quel est ton numéro de téléphone?   *What is your phone number?*

AGES AND BIRTHDAYS

un   âge   *age*
un   an   *year*
une   année   *year*
un   anniversaire   *birthday*
la   date   *date*
la   date de naissance   *date of birth*
la   grande personne   *adult*
le   lieu de naissance   *place of birth*
le   mois   *month*
la   naissance   *birth*

avoir ... ans *to be ... years old*
naître *to be born*

majeur *18 and over*
mineur *under 18*

Né(e) le ... à ... *Born on the ... at ...*
J'ai seize ans. *I am sixteen.*
Je suis né(e) le vingt février dix-neuf cent soixante-treize à
    Londres. *I was born on 20 February 1973 in London.*
Quelle est la date de ton anniversaire? *What is the date
    of your birthday?*

NATIONALITY

la carte d'identité *identity card*
un étranger *foreigner*
le passeport *passport*
la pièce d'identité *item of identification*

venir *to come from*

où *where*
d'où *where from*

CHARACTER AND DISPOSITION

le caractère *character*
la chance *luck*
une opinion *opinion*

aimer *to like, to love*
croire *to believe*
espérer *to hope*
être de bonne / mauvaise humeur *to be in a
    good / bad mood*
se fâcher *to get angry*
penser *to think*
pleurer *to cry, to weep*
réfléchir *to think, to reflect*
rire *to laugh*
sourire *to smile*

affreux/affreuse *awful*
agréable *pleasant*
amusant *amusing*
bête *bizarre*
calme *calm*
célèbre *famous*
charmant *charming*
en colère *angry*
content *pleased, happy*
drôle *funny*
énervé *nervous*
fâché *angry*
formidable *great*
fou/folle *mad*
gentil/gentille *kind*
heureux/heureuse *happy*
important *important*
inquiet/inquiète *anxious*
malheureux/malheureuse *unhappy*
méchant *naughty*
paresseux/paresseuse *lazy*
pauvre *poor*
poli *polite*
riche *rich*
sérieux/sérieuse *serious*
sûr *certain*
sympa *nice*

timide *shy*
triste *sad*

à mon avis *in my opinion*
assez *fairly*
en général *usually*
plutôt *rather*
toujours *always*
très *very*
vraiment *really*

J'ai peur. *I'm afraid.*
J'en ai marre. *I'm fed up.*
Comment est ... ? *What's ... like?*
Comment trouves-tu ... ? *How do you find ... ?*
J'en ai marre du français. *I'm fed up with French.*
Je suis de bonne humeur aujourd'hui. *I'm in a good
    mood today.*

un amour *love*
la confiance *confidence*
un espoir *hope*
l' humour (m) *humour*
une imagination *imagination*
le sentiment *feeling*
le souci *care, worry*

avoir le droit de *to have the right to*
avoir envie de *to wish to*
avoir honte *to be ashamed*
avoir tort *to be wrong*
conseiller *to advise*
effrayer *to frighten*
s'entendre *to understand one another*
étonner *to amaze*
se méfier de *to distrust*
se mettre en colère *to get angry*
oser *to dare*
paraître *to appear*
prouver *to prove*
sembler *to seem*

actif/active *active*
calme *calm*
capable de *capable of*
déçu *disappointed*
dégoûtant *disgusting*
désagréable *disagreeable*
étrange *strange*
fier/fière *proud*
habile *clever*
honnête *honest*
insupportable *unbearable*
jaloux/jalouse *jealous*
marrant *funny*
naturel/naturelle *natural*
normal *normal*
optimiste *optimistic*
pessimiste *pessimistic*
surprenant *surprising*
têtu *obstinate*
tranquille *quiet*

franchement *frankly*
généralement *generally*
naturellement *naturally*
tellement *so*

Je m'entends bien avec mon frère. *I get on well with my
    brother.*
Le professeur s'est mis en colère. *The teacher got angry.*

Jean me semble tout à fait sympathique. *Jean seems to me to be really nice.*

Je lui fais confiance. *I have confidence in him.*

J'ai envie de manger. *I want to eat.*

J'ai le droit de sortir ce soir. *I have permission to go out this evening.*

Tu as tort. *You are wrong.*

J'ai eu honte. *I was ashamed.*

A mon avis, il faut se méfier de lui. *In my opinion, you can't trust him.*

PHYSICAL APPEARANCE

la barbe *beard*
les cheveux (m) *hair*
les lunettes (f) *spectacles, glasses*
les moustaches (f) *moustache*
les yeux *eyes*

    avoir l'air *to seem*
    porter *to wear, to carry*
    trouver *to find*
    reconnaître *to recognise*
    ressembler à *to resemble*

    beau/bel/belle *handsome, beautiful*
    blanc/blanche *white*
    bleu *blue*
    blond *fair*
    bouclé *curly*
    bronzé *tanned*
    brun *brown*
    court *short*
    fort *strong*
    grand *big, tall*
    gris *grey*
    gros *big, fat*
    jaune *yellow*
    jeune *young*
    joli *pretty*
    laid *ugly*
    long/longue *long*
    marron *chestnut, brown*
    mince *thin*
    noir *black*
    orange *orange*
    pâle *pale*
    petit *small*
    raide *stiff*
    rose *pink*
    roux/rousse *red (hair)*
    sportif/sportive *good at sports, keen on sports*
    vert *green*
    vieux/vieil/vieille *old*

Il a les cheveux longs. *He has long hair.*
Il a l'air sportif. *He looks athletic.*
Elle porte des lunettes. *She wears glasses.*
Je la trouve jolie. *I think she's pretty.*

    sembler *to seem*
    paraître *to appear*

    actif/active *active*
    élégant *elegant*
    fragile *weak, fragile, delicate*
    robuste *tough*
    semblable *alike, similar*
    souple *athletic, supple*

    absolument *absolutely*
    complètement *completely*
    tout à fait *totally, quite*

Elle me semble tout à fait honnête. *She seems to me to be totally honest.*

THE FAMILY AND RELATIVES

le beau-père *father-in-law, step-father*
le bébé *baby*
la belle-fille *daughter-in-law, stepdaughter*
la belle-mère *mother-in-law, stepmother*
le/la cousin/cousine *cousin*
un(e) enfant *child*
une épouse *wife*
un époux *husband*
la famille *family*
la femme *woman, wife*
le/la fiancé/fiancée *fiancé(e)*
la fille *girl, daughter*
le fils *son*
le frère *brother*
le garçon *boy*
le gendre *son-in-law*
les gens *people*
la grand-mère *grandmother*
le grand-père *grandfather*
les grands-parents (m) *grandparents*
un homme *man*
la maman *mummy, mum*
le mari *husband*
la mère *mother*
le neveu *nephew*
la nièce *niece*
un oncle *uncle*
le papa *daddy, dad*
les parents (m) *parents, relatives*
le père *father*
le/la petit ami / petite amie *boyfriend / girlfriend*
le petit-fils *grandson*
la petite-fille *granddaughter*
les petits-enfants *grandchildren*
la sœur *sister*
la tante *aunt*
le veuf *widower*
la veuve *widow*

    divorcer *to divorce*
    se marier avec *to marry*

    aîné *elder*
    cadet/cadette *younger*
    célibataire *single*
    dernier/dernière *last*
    divorcé *divorced*
    familial *of the family*
    séparé *separated*

Je suis enfant unique. *I'm an only child.*
Ian, c'est mon frère aîné. *Ian is my elder brother.*
Je suis allé(e) avec ma mère voir des parents. *I went with my mother to see relations.*
Ma sœur s'est mariée avec un Américain. *My sister has married an American.*
Mon oncle est célibataire. *My uncle is a bachelor.*
Ma grand-mère est veuve. *My grandmother is a widow.*
Mes parents sont séparés / divorcés. *My parents are separated / divorced.*

RELIGION

la   réligion *religion*
      catholique *Catholic*
      hindou *Hindu*
      musulman *Muslim*
      protestant *Protestant*
+ *other religions as appropriate to the student*

LIKES AND DISLIKES

    aimer *to like, to love*
    détester *to hate*
    préférer *to prefer*
    trouver *to find*
+ *material from most other topics in the syllabus*

PETS

un animal *animal*
le chat *cat*
le chien *dog*
le cochon d'Inde *guinea-pig*
un hamster *hamster*
le lapin *rabbit*
un oiseau *bird*
la perruche *budgerigar*
le poisson rouge *goldfish*
la souris *mouse*
la tortue *tortoise*
+ *adjectives for the physical description of people (see p. 42)*

As-tu un animal domestique? *Have you got a pet?*

OTHER LIVESTOCK

un agneau *lamb*
un âne *donkey*
un bœuf *bullock*
un canard *duck*
un cheval *horse*
une chèvre *goat*
un cochon *pig*
un coq *cockerel*
un mouton *sheep*
une oie *goose*
une poule *hen*
une puce *flea*
un taureau *bull*
une vache *cow*
un veau *calf*

UNDOMESTICATED CREATURES

une abeille *bee*
une araignée *spider*
un escargot *snail*
une grenouille *frog*
un insecte *insect*
un moineau *sparrow*
un renard *fox*
un serpent *snake*
la truite *trout*

PARTS OF ANIMALS

la fourrure *fur*

la gueule *mouth, muzzle*
la plume *feather*
la queue *tail*

▶ B2 Spare-time activities

POCKET MONEY AND SPARE-TIME JOBS

un après-midi *afternoon*
l' argent de poche (m) *pocket money*
la journée *day*
le matin *morning*
la monnaie *small change*
le portefeuille *wallet*
le porte-monnaie *purse*
le prix *price*
le soir *evening*
le week-end *weekend*

    acheter *to buy*
    commencer *to begin*
    coûter *to cost*
    faire des économies *to save*
    se faire ... F par semaine / de l'heure
        to make ... francs a week / an hour
    finir *to finish*
    gagner *to earn*
    payer *to pay*
    travailler *to work*

    cher\chère *expensive*
    gratuit *free of charge*
    important *important*
    pauvre *poor*
    riche *rich*

(pas) assez *(not) enough*
    beaucoup *a lot*
    peu de *little*

Je fais des économies pour acheter... *I'm saving to buy...*
Je gagne 20 francs de l'heure. *I earn 20 francs an hour.*
Je travaille le week-end. *I work at weekends.*
Je commence à ... heures, et je finis à ... heures. *I begin at ... o'clock and finish at ... o'clock.*

    appartenir à *to belong to*
    dépenser *to spend*
    déposer *to deposit*
    emprunter (à) *to borrow (from)*
    être à court d'argent *to be short of money*
    prêter (à) *to lend (to)*

Je suis à court d'argent. *I'm short of money.*
Je voudrais emprunter 50 francs. *I'd like to borrow 50 francs.*
J'ai tout dépensé. *I have spent everything.*
Je gagne beaucoup. *I earn a lot.*

HOBBIES

le club *club*
la collection *collection*
le disque *record*
la distraction *entertainment*
un échange *exchange*
les échecs (m) *chess*
une excursion *excursion*
une exposition *exhibition*
un illustré *illustrated magazine*

un instrument *instrument*
le jeu *game*
le journal *newspaper*
les loisirs (m) *free time, pastimes*
le magazine *magazine*
le membre *member*
la musique *music*
le passe-temps *hobby*
la pêche *fishing*
le programme *programme*
la revue *magazine*
la société *society, club*
la soirée *evening out*
le sport *sport*
le téléjournal *TV news*
le temps libre *free time*
les vacances (f) *holidays*
la visite guidée *tour (of museum)*
le week-end *weekend*

aimer beaucoup *to like a lot*
collectionner *to collect*
danser *to dance*
écouter *to listen (to)*
s'ennuyer *to get bored*
exposer *to exhibit*
s'intéresser à *to be interested in*
jouer au football (etc.) *to play football (etc.)*
jouer de la guitare (etc.) *to play the guitar (etc.)*
préférer *to prefer*
réaliser *to realize, to put into practice*
regarder *to watch*
rêver *to dream*
rire *to laugh*
sortir *to go out*
visiter *to visit*
+ *any other activity appropriate to the student*

chouette *great, marvellous*
classique *classical*
mauvais *bad*
moche *rotten, ugly*
passionnant *exciting*
pop *pop*
sensass *great, sensational*
seul *alone*
sportif/sportive *athletic, keen on sports*
+ *adjectives for describing people – see p. 42*

longtemps *a long time*
quelquefois *sometimes*
sauf *except*
souvent *often*
de temps en temps *from time to time*
toujours *always*
tout le monde *everyone*

Je m'intéresse à la photographie. *I'm interested in photography.*
Je joue quelquefois au tennis. *I sometimes play tennis.*
Je joue de la flûte. *I play the flute.*
J'aime visiter les châteaux. *I like going to castles.*
Je suis membre d'un club. *I am a member of a club.*
Quelles distractions y a-t-il ici? *What entertainments are there here?*
Je vais à la pêche assez souvent. *I go fishing quite often.*
On a fait la visite guidée du musée. *We had a guided tour of the museum.*

la bande dessinée *cartoon*

la chorale *choir*
les environs (m) *surroundings*
les festivités (f) *festivities*
la lecture *reading*
le tricot *knitting*

avoir horreur de *to hate*
avoir le temps de *to have the time to*
bricoler *to do odd jobs, to potter*
faire de la peinture *to paint*
s'informer *to learn*
pratiquer un sport *to do a sport*

quotidien/quotidienne *daily*
hebdomadaire *weekly*
mensuel/mensuelle *monthly*
populaire *popular*

J'ai horreur du tennis. *I hate tennis.*
Je lis les journaux pour m'informer. *I read the papers to learn about things.*
Je fais partie d'une chorale. *I am in a choir.*
Ma lecture préférée, ce sont les bandes dessinées. *I like reading cartoons best of all.*

SPORTING ACTIVITIES

le ballon *ball (e.g. football)*
le champion *champion*
le championnat *championship*
la compétition *competition*
le courage *courage, drive*
le cricket *cricket*
une équipe *team*
le football *football*
la gymnastique *gymnastics*
un hobby *hobby*
le hockey *hockey*
le jouet *toy*
le/la joueur/joueuse *player*
le match *match*
le rugby *rugby*
les sports d'hiver (m) *winter sports*
le stade *stadium*
le terrain de sport *sports ground*

se baigner *to swim, to bathe*
courir *to run*
faire du cyclisme *to cycle*
faire de la natation *to swim*
faire une promenade en bateau *to go boating*
faire une promenade à vélo *to go for a bike ride*
faire du ski *to ski*
gagner *to win*
perdre *to lose*
se reposer *to rest*

On a perdu le match de rugby. *We lost the rugby match.*
Je fais souvent du ski. *I often go skiing.*
Je me suis baigné(e) dans la rivière. *I bathed in the river.*
J'adore faire de la natation. *I love swimming.*
Bon courage! *Good luck! Play well!*

un arbitre *referee*
un aviron *oar*
l' équipement (m) *equipment*
le match nul *draw*
le titre *title*

battre *to beat*

critiquer   *to criticise*
défendre   *to defend*
faire une partie de tennis (etc.)   *to play a game of tennis (etc.)*
marquer un but   *to score a goal*
marquer un point   *to score a point*
protester   *to protest*
soutenir une équipe   *to support a team*

▷ B3 Personal relationships

GENERAL

un   ami   *friend*
une   amie   *(girl)friend*
le/la   camarade   *friend*
le   club   *club*
le   copain   *(boy)friend*
la   copine   *(girl)friend*
le   correspondant   *(boy) penfriend*
la   correspondante   *(girl) penfriend*
le   membre   *member*
la   musique   *music*

aimer   *to like*
s'amuser   *to enjoy oneself*
connaître   *to know*
danser   *to dance*
écouter   *to listen (to)*
jouer   *to play*
parler   *to speak*
passer   *to spend (time)*
se passer   *to happen*

aussi   *also*
d'habitude   *usually*
souvent   *often*
toujours   *always*

une   activité   *activity*
une   ambiance   *atmosphere*
la   conférence   *lecture*
la   cotisation   *subscription*
une   équipe   *team*
la   jeunesse   *young people, youth*
les   loisirs (m)   *leisure time, pastimes*
la   maison des jeunes   *youth club*
la   réunion   *meeting*
la   société   *society, club*

apprécier   *to appreciate*
discuter   *to discuss*
s'entendre avec quelqu'un   *to get on well with someone*
fréquenter   *to frequent, to go to, to attend*
s'intéresser à   *to be interested in*
s'occuper à   *to be busy at*
participer à   *to take part in*

Je fréquente la maison des jeunes.   *I go to the youth club.*
Il y a une réunion des jeunes ce soir.   *There is a meeting of young people tonight.*
Je ne m'intéresse pas à la politique.   *I'm not interested in politics.*

GREETINGS, WISHES AND GOODBYES

la bienvenue   *welcome*
A bientôt!   *See you soon!*

A ce soir.   *See you this evening.*
A demain.   *See you tomorrow.*
A samedi. (etc.)   *Till Saturday. (etc.)*
A tout à l'heure.   *See you later.*
Au revoir.   *Goodbye.*
Bon anniversaire.   *Happy birthday.*
Bon voyage!   *Have a good trip!*
Bon week-end!   *Have a good weekend!*
Bonne année.   *Have a good year / Happy New Year.*
Bonne chance!   *Good luck!*
Bonne fête.   *Happy name day.*
Bonne nuit.   *Goodnight.*
Bonjour.   *Good morning. Hello.*
Bonsoir.   *Good evening.*
Comment allez-vous?   *How are you?*
Félicitations!   *Congratulations!*
Joyeux Noël!   *Happy Christmas!*
Salut!   *Hi! Hello!*
A votre santé!   *Cheers! To your good health!*

MAKING ACQUAINTANCES

le/la   camarade   *friend*
un   échange   *exchange*
les   gens (m)   *people*
le   jumelage   *twinning (e.g. town twinning)*
le   plaisir   *pleasure*
la   surprise   *surprise*

accompagner   *to accompany*
aller chercher   *to go and get*
assurer   *to assure, to insure*
présenter   *to present, to introduce*
se présenter   *to introduce oneself*
remercier   *to thank*
rencontrer   *to meet*
revenir   *to return*
souhaiter   *to wish*
se voir   *to see one another*

aimable   *pleasant, friendly, kind*
de retour   *back*
enchanté   *delighted*
insupportable   *unbearable, dreadful*
ravi   *delighted*

Je te présente Marie.   *May I introduce Marie to you?*
Enchanté(e).   *Pleased to meet you.*
Je suis ravi(e) de vous voir.   *I am delighted to see you.*
On va se voir demain, n'est-ce pas?   *We'll meet tomorrow, won't we?*

le/la   collègue   *colleague*
le   discours   *speech*
une   intention   *intention*
la   proposition   *suggestion*
les   relations (f)   *relationships*

contacter   *to make contact with*
étonner   *to amaze*
faire la connaissance de quelqu'un   *to make someone's acquaintance*
féliciter   *to congratulate*
remarquer   *to notice*

Je vous souhaite la bienvenue.   *I welcome you.*
Je trouve ces gens insupportables.   *I find these people unbearable.*
Je suis ravi(e) de faire votre connaissance.   *I am delighted to meet you.*

▶ B4 Arranging a meeting or an activity

une	invitation	*invitation*
le	parc	*park*
la	promenade	*walk*
le	rendez-vous	*meeting*
un	idiot	*fool*

accepter   *to accept*
accompagner   *to accompany*
aimer   *to like*
s'amuser   *to enjoy oneself*
arriver   *to arrive*
attendre   *to wait (for)*
avoir lieu   *to take place*
coûter   *to cost*
danser   *to dance*
décider   *to decide*
demander   *to ask (for)*
devoir   *to owe, ought to*
s'excuser   *to apologise*
inviter   *to invite*
oublier   *to forget*
penser   *to think*
préférer   *to prefer*
prendre rendez-vous   *to arrange to meet*
proposer   *to suggest*
recevoir des amis   *to have friends round*
refuser   *to refuse*
regretter   *to regret*
remercier   *to thank*
rencontrer   *to meet*
rendre visite à quelqu'un   *to visit someone*
rester   *to stay*
venir   *to come*
se voir   *to see one another*

chouette   *great*
désolé   *very sorry*
formidable   *great, terrific*
impossible   *impossible*
libre   *free*
possible   *possible*
urgent   *urgent*

bof!   *oh well!*
certainement   *of course*
d'accord   *agreed, OK*
avec plaisir   *with pleasure*
quel dommage!   *what a shame!*
sur   *on*
zut!   *damn!*

+ *places of entertainment – see p. 33*
+ *times – see p. 218*
+ *locations – see p. 49*

LEISURE AND ENTERTAINMENT

aller voir   *to go and see*
annuler   *to cancel*
avoir le droit de   *to have the right to*
avoir envie de   *to want to*
avoir le temps de   *to have the time to*
bavarder   *to chat*
empêcher   *to prevent*
exagérer   *to exaggerate*
offrir à   *to offer to*
promettre de   *to promise to*
refuser de   *to refuse to*

rejoindre   *to join*
retourner   *to return*
suggérer   *to suggest*
supposer   *to suppose*
se trouver   *to be situated*

de bonne heure   *early*
ensemble   *together*
sans doute   *without doubt*
tant mieux   *all the better*
tant pis   *never mind*
Tiens!   *Hey!*
volontiers   *gladly, yes please*

Si on sortait ce soir?   *Shall we go out this evening?*
Tu veux m'accompagner au cinéma?   *Would you like to come to the cinema with me?*
Qu'est-ce qu'on joue / passe?   *What's on?*
Je l'ai déjà vu(e).   *I've already seen it.*
Je voudrais voir un film d'épouvante.   *I'd like to see a horror film.*
D'accord. Où est-ce qu'on va se rencontrer?   *OK. Where shall we meet?*
Devant le cinéma à huit heures.   *In front of the cinema at 8 o'clock.*
Entendu.   *Agreed.*
C'est en version originale?   *Is it the original soundtrack?*
Non, c'est doublé.   *No, it's dubbed.*
Oui, mais il y a des sous-titres.   *Yes, but there are sub-titles.*
A quelle date?   *What date?*
C'est dommage. J'ai trop de devoirs.   *It's a shame. I have too much homework.*
Ça dépend.   *It depends.*
Ça ne fait rien.   *It doesn't matter.*
Ça suffit.   *That's enough.*
Où est-ce qu'on va se rencontrer?   *Where shall we meet?*
Ça m'est égal, franchement.   *To be honest, I don't mind.*
Je vous en prie.   *Please don't mention it.*
Ce n'est pas la peine.   *It's not worth it.*
Tiens! Le grand bal aura lieu demain!   *Hey! The big dance is tomorrow!*
Comment as-tu trouvé le film / la pièce?   *What did you think of the film / play?*
Le film / concert était merveilleux / intéressant / ennuyeux / affreux.   *The film / concert was marvellous / interesting / boring / awful.*
A mon avis c'était trop long / sérieux.   *In my opinion it was too long / serious.*

▶ B5 Holidays

un	appareil photo	*camera*
le	bateau à voile	*sailing boat*
la	brochure	*brochure*
le	bureau de renseignements	*information office*
le	bureau de tourisme	*tourist office*
le	centre de vacances	*holiday centre*
les	chaussures de ski (f)	*ski boots*
les	chèques de voyage (m)	*traveller's cheques*
le	coquillage	*shellfish*
le	coup de soleil	*sunstroke*
la	crème solaire	*sun cream*
la	crêperie	*pancake shop or stall*
une	école de langues	*language school*
la	falaise	*cliff*
la	forêt	*forest*
le	groupe	*group*
la	liste	*list*

le   monde   *world*
le   monument   *monument*
le   musée   *museum*
le   parapluie   *umbrella*
le   parasol   *parasol*
le   phare   *lighthouse*
la   photo   *photograph*
le   pique-nique   *picnic*
la   piscine   *swimming pool*
la   piste   *track, run*
la   plage   *beach*
le   plan   *plan*
la   planche à voile   *sailboard*
le   port   *port*
la   publicité   *publicity*
la   région   *area*
les   renseignements (m)   *information*
le   sac à dos   *rucksack*
le   séjour   *stay*
les   sports d'hiver (m)   *winter sports*
le/la touriste   *tourist*
les   vacances (f)   *holidays*
la   visite   *visit*
la   visite scolaire   *school trip*
le   voyage   *journey*

s'amuser   *to enjoy oneself*
avoir du beau temps   *to have fine weather*
avoir du mauvais temps   *to have bad weather*
descendre dans un hôtel   *to stay at a hotel*
se détendre   *to relax*
être en vacances   *to be on holiday*
se (faire) bronzer   *to get brown*
faire de l'autostop   *to hitch-hike*
faire de la planche à voile   *to go windsurfing*
faire une promenade en bateau   *to go out in a boat*
faire une promenade à vélo   *to go for a bike ride*
faire du ski   *to ski*
faire du ski nautique   *to water-ski*
faire du stop   *to hitch-hike*
faire de la voile   *to go sailing*
louer   *to hire*
se mettre en route   *to set out*
partir en vacances   *to set out on holiday*
plaire à   *to please*
prendre l'avion   *to take the plane, to fly*
rester   *to stay*
sécher   *to dry*
voyager   *to travel*

à la campagne   *in the country*
à l'étranger   *abroad*
à la mer   *at the sea*
à la montagne   *in the mountains*
à partir de 20 heures   *from 8 p.m. onwards*
au bord de la mer   *by the sea*
au mois de juin   *in June*
déjà   *already*
Douvres   *Dover*
en plein air   *in the open air*
quinze jours   *a fortnight*
pendant les vacances   *during the holidays*
Noël   *Christmas*
Pâques   *Easter*
tellement   *so*
tout le monde   *everyone*

+ *adjectives for describing things and people – see p. 42*
+ *geographical items – see p. 48*

+ *travel and accommodation items as appropriate – see p. 60–1*
+ *weather items as appropriate – see p. 49*
+ *free time and entertainment items as appropriate – see p. 44*

Nous sommes descendu(e)s dans un hôtel à Douvres.   *We stayed in a hotel in Dover.*
J'ai cherché des coquillages au bord de la mer.   *I looked for shells by the sea.*
Nous sommes parti(e)s en vacances au mois d'août.   *We set off on holiday in August.*
Tout le monde était en vacances.   *Everyone was on holiday.*

une   agence de voyages   *travel agency*
l'   archéologie (f)   *archaeology*
la   ceinture de sauvetage   *life belt*
la   chaise longue   *couch, sunbed*
le   congé   *leave, day off*
le   cours d'été   *summer school*
les   curiosités (f)   *curiosities*
le   dépliant   *leaflet, brochure*
les   descriptions (f)   *descriptions*
les   festivités (f)   *festivities*
le   genre   *type*
le   guide   *guide*
l'   hospitalité (f)   *hospitality*
le   jardin zoologique   *zoo*
la   marée basse   *low tide*
la   marée haute   *high tide*
la   pellicule   *film (for camera)*
le   syndicat d'initiative (SI)   *information office*
le   site   *site*
le   son et lumière   *sound and light entertainment*
le   spectacle   *entertainment*
la   terrasse de café   *café terrace*

accueillir   *to welcome*
avoir lieu   *to take place*
faire de la plongée sous-marine   *to do deep-sea diving*
faire des sports nautiques   *to do water sports*
faire les valises   *to pack*
s'informer   *to find out*
montrer   *to show*
organiser   *to organise*
se noyer   *to drown*
se passer   *to take place, to happen*
se souvenir   *to remember*
ramer   *to row*

accueillant   *welcoming*
pittoresque   *picturesque*

+ *proper names of geographical features as appropriate to the student*

Le son et lumière aura lieu à dix heures.   *The 'son et lumière' performance will take place at 10 o'clock.*
Un garçon s'est noyé à marée haute l'année dernière.   *A boy drowned at high tide last year.*
Est-ce que vous avez un dépliant qui montre ce qui se passe dans la région?   *Have you a leaflet showing what is on in the area?*

▷ C1 Home town, local environment

IN TOWN

un   aéroport   *airport*

une agence de voyages *travel agency*
un aéroport *airport*
un arrêt d'autobus *bus stop*
une autoroute *motorway*
la banlieue *suburb*
la banque *bank*
le bâtiment *building*
la bibliothèque *library*
la boîte aux lettres *letter box*
le bruit *noise*
le bureau *office*
la cabine téléphonique *phone box*
le camping *campsite*
la capitale *capital*
la cathédrale *cathedral*
le centre commercial *shopping centre*
le centre-ville *town centre*
le château *castle*
le cinéma *cinema*
la circulation *traffic*
la cité *city / housing estate*
le danger *danger*
une église *church*
un endroit *place*
l' environnement (m) *environment*
les environs (m) *surroundings, neighbourhood*
un espace *open space*
un événement *event*
la fabrique *factory*
la fête *festival*
les feux (m) *traffic lights*
la foire *fair*
la gare *station*
la gendarmerie *police station*
un habitant *inhabitant*
un hôpital *hospital*
un hôtel de ville *town hall (in larger towns)*
une industrie *industry*
le jardin public *park*
le magasin *shop*
la mairie *town hall (in smaller towns)*
le marché *market*
le monument *monument*
le musée *museum*
le panneau *board, sign*
le parc *park*
le parking *car-park*
le passage à niveau *level crossing*
le passage clouté *pedestrian crossing*
le passage souterrain *subway*
la piscine *swimming pool*
la place *square*
le pont *bridge*
le port *port*
la poste *post office*
le quartier *quarter, district*
le siècle *century*
le stade *stadium*
le station-service *service station*
le syndicat d'initiative (SI) *information office*
le terrain de camping *campsite*
la terrasse de café *café terrace*
le théâtre *theatre*
la tour *tower*
le trottoir *pavement*
une usine *factory*
la ville *town*
le/la voisine *neighbour*

la zone piétonnière *pedestrian precinct*

J'habite à Newcastle depuis trois ans. *I've been living in Newcastle for three years.*
J'habite à Norwich depuis toujours. *I've always lived in Norwich.*

IN THE COUNTRYSIDE

le bois *wood*
la campagne *countryside*
les champs (m) *fields*
les environs (m) *surroundings*
la ferme *farm*
le fleuve *river*
la forêt *forest*
une île *island*
le lac *lake*
le lieu *place*
la mer *sea*
le monde *world*
la montagne *mountain*
la nature *nature*
le pays *country, region*
le paysage *countryside*
la plage *beach*
la pollution *pollution*
la province *province, region*
la qualité *quality*
la randonnée *long walk*
la région *region*
la rivière *river*
les specialités locales (f) *local specialities*
la terre *land, earth*
la vallée *valley*
le village *village*

POSITIONS

se trouver *to be situated*

à côté de *next door to, beside*
à droite *on the right*
à gauche *on the left*
au milieu de *in the middle of*
au sommet de *at the top of*

autour de *around*
chez *at the home of*
dehors *outside*
encombré de *congested by*
en bas *downstairs, below*
en face de *opposite*
en plein air *in the open air*
entouré de *surrounded by*
hors de *outside*
loin de *far from*
le long de *along*
n'importe où *anywhere*
près de *near*
relié(e) à *linked to*
situé(e) à *situated (at)*

DESCRIPTIONS

accueillant *welcoming*
agréable *pleasant*
agricole *agricultural*

ancien/ancienne   *old, ex-, former*
animé   *lively*
charmant   *charming*
dangereux/dangereuse   *dangerous*
ennuyeux/ennuyeuse   *boring*
historique   *historical*
important   *important*
industriel/industrielle   *industrial*
intéressant   *interesting*
laid   *ugly*
naturel/naturelle   *natural*
paisible   *peaceful*
pittoresque   *picturesque*
pollué   *polluted*
profond   *deep*
propre   *clean*
rare   *rare*
sale   *dirty*
tranquille   *peaceful, quiet*
triste   *sad*
varié   *varied*
voisin   *neighbouring*

à peine   *hardly, scarcely*

▶ C2 Finding the way

un   agent de police   *policeman*
le   bureau de change   *exchange office*
le   carrefour   *crossroads*
la   carte   *map*
le   chemin   *way*
le   commissariat de police   *police station*
le   coin   *corner*
la   direction   *direction*
la   distance   *distance*
une   église   *church*
les   feux (m)   *traffic lights*
le   milieu   *middle*
le   rond-point   *roundabout*
le   WC   *toilet*
+ *geographical surroundings – see p. 48*

aider   *to help*
arriver   *to arrive*
chercher   *to look for*
continuer   *to continue*
s'égarer   *to get lost*
s'en aller   *to go away*
faire attention   *to pay attention*
monter dans   *to get in / on*
passer   *to pass*
passer devant   *to pass in front of*
se perdre   *to get lost*
pour aller à...   *to get to...*
se renseigner   *to get information, to find out*
retourner   *to return*
recommander   *to recommend*
suivre   *to follow*
se trouver   *to be situated*
traverser   *to cross*

à côté de   *next to*
à droite   *to the right*
à l'est   *to the east*
à gauche   *to the left*
à ... mètres   *...metres away*
à ... minutes   *...minutes away*
à l'ouest   *to the west*

alors   *then*
après   *after*
au bout de   *at the end of*
au nord   *to the north*
au sud   *to the south*
avant   *before*
derrière   *behind*
devant   *in front of*
en face de   *opposite*
ensuite   *afterwards, then*
jusqu'à   *as far as*
là   *there*
là-bas   *over there*
le long de   *along*
n'importe où   *anywhere*
premier, deuxième, etc.   *first, second, etc.*
près de   *near to*
proche de   *near to*
puis   *then*
tout droit   *straight on*
toutes directions   *all routes*

Pour aller à Orléans, s'il vous plaît?   *The way to Orléans, please?*
Prenez la troisième route à droite.   *Take the third road on the right.*
Où est la place Marie Curie, s'il vous plaît?   *Where is Marie Curie Square, please?*
Continuez tout droit.   *Go straight on.*
C'est au centre de la ville.   *It's in the town centre.*
C'est au bout de l'allée Foch.   *It's at the end of the Allée Foch.*
Nous pouvons regarder mon plan de la ville.   *We can look at my town plan.*
C'est à quelle distance d'ici?   *How far is it from here?*
C'est à 20 minutes à pied.   *It's 20 minutes on foot.*
C'est à 5 minutes en voiture.   *It's 5 minutes by car.*
C'est à 800 mètres d'ici.   *It's 800 metres from here.*
Il y a combien de kilomètres jusqu'à la plage?   *How far is it to the beach?*
A peu près 7 kilomètres.   *About 7 kilometres.*
Quel jour est la fête foraine?   *On which day is the travelling fair?*
Le syndicat d'initiative vous le dira.   *The information office will tell you.*
Excusez-moi, où est la sortie de secours?   *Excuse me, where is the emergency exit?*
Vous suivez le couloir jusqu'au panneau 'interdit de fumer' et vous tournez à droite. La sortie est au fond du couloir.   *You go along the corridor as far as the 'no smoking' sign and you turn to the right. The exit is at the end of the corridor.*
Merci beaucoup.   *Thank you very much.*
Il n'y a pas de quoi.   *It's a pleasure.*
De rien.   *Don't mention it.*
Où est-ce que je peux me garer?   *Where can I park?*
N'importe où le long de cette rue.   *Anywhere along this road.*

▶ C3 Weather

un   an   *year*
une   année   *year*
un   après-midi   *afternoon*
l'   automne (m)   *autumn*
une   averse   *shower, downpour*
le   brouillard   *fog*
la   chaleur   *heat*

le   climat   *climate*
le   degré   *degree*
un   éclair   *flash of lightning*
l'   été (m)   *summer*
la   glace   *ice*
l'   hiver (m)   *winter*
le   matin   *morning*
la   mer   *sea*
la   météo   *weather forecast*
le   mois   *month*
la   neige   *snow*
le   nuage   *cloud*
la   nuit   *night*
une   ombre   *shadow*
un   orage   *storm*
la   pluie   *rain*
le   printemps   *spring*
la   saison   *season*
le   soir   *evening*
le   soleil   *sun*
la   température   *temperature*
la   tempête   *storm*
le   temps   *weather*
le   tonnerre   *thunder*
le   vent   *wind*

faire beau / chaud / froid   *to be fine / warm / cold*
faire jour   *to be light*
geler   *to freeze*
neiger   *to snow*
pleuvoir   *to rain*

agréable   *pleasant*
beau/bel/belle   *fine*
bleu   *blue*
chaud   *hot*
couvert   *cloudy*
doux/douce   *mild*
ensoleillé   *sunny*
fort   *strong*
froid   *cold*
humide   *damp*
léger/légère   *light*
lourd   *heavy*
mauvais   *bad*
meilleur   *better*
prochain   *next*
rare   *rare*
sec/sèche   *dry*

à peine   *hardly, scarcely*
aujourd'hui   *today*
demain   *tomorrow*
il y a   *there is*
il y aura   *there will be*
maintenant   *now*
normalement   *normally*
quel/quelle   *what, which*
quelquefois   *sometimes*
rapidement   *quickly*
rarement   *rarely*
souvent   *often*

Quel temps fait-il?   *What's the weather like?*
Il pleut / neige / gèle, etc.   *It's raining / snowing / freezing, etc.*

une   amélioration   *improvement*
la   brume   *mist*
le   coucher du soleil   *sunset*

une   éclaircie   *bright period*
la   grêle   *hail*
le   lever du soleil   *sunrise*
la   marée   *tide*
un   orage   *storm*
le   passage   *passage, passing*
la   précipitation   *precipitation (usually of rain)*
la   prévision   *forecast*
la   visibilité   *visibility*

s'adoucir   *to become mild*
en avoir marre   *to be fed up with*
il fait lourd   *it's close, sultry*
plaire   *to please*
pleuvoir à verse   *to pour with rain*
prévoir   *to forecast*
se refroidir   *to become cold*
souffler   *to blow*
tonner   *to thunder*

brumeux/brumeuse   *misty*
frais/fraîche   *chilly*
maximum   *maximum*
minimum   *minimum*
neigeux/neigeuse   *snowy*
nuageux/nuageuse   *cloudy*
orageux/orageuse   *stormy*
pluvieux/pluvieuse   *rainy*
triste   *sad*
variable   *variable*

après-demain   *the day after tomorrow*
cependant   *however*
dans ce cas   *in this case*
dehors   *outside*
de temps en temps   *from time to time*
en général   *usually*
en plein soleil   *in full sunshine*
généralement   *generally*
grâce à   *thanks to*
malgré   *in spite of*
tout à l'heure   *shortly, soon, a few moments ago*

THE WEATHER FORECAST

le   bulletin météo(rologique)   *weather bulletin*
la   météo marine   *shipping forecast*
la   photo satellite   *satellite photo*
la   pression   *pressure*

éclater   *to burst*
fondre   *to thaw, to melt*

▷ C4 Shopping

SHOP TYPES

la   banque   *bank*
la   boucherie   *butcher's shop*
la   boulangerie   *baker's shop*
la   boutique   *small shop*
le   bureau de tabac   *tobacconist's shop*
le   centre commercial   *shopping centre*
la   charcuterie   *pork butcher's shop, delicatessen*
le   coiffeur   *hairdressing salon*
la   confiserie   *sweet shop*
la   crémerie   *dairy*
une   épicerie   *grocer's shop*
l'   hypermarché (m)   *hypermarket*

la   librairie   *bookshop*
le   magasin   *shop*
le   marché   *market*
la   parfumerie   *perfume shop*
la   pâtisserie   *cake shop*
la   pharmacie   *chemist's shop*
la   poissonnerie   *fish shop*
la   quincaillerie   *hardware shop*
le   supermarché   *supermarket*

SHOP INTERIORS

un   ascenseur   *lift*
le   cadeau   *present*
la   caisse   *cash desk, till*
le   chariot   *trolley*
le   choix   *choice*
le   comptoir   *counter*
une   erreur   *mistake*
un   escalier roulant   *escalator*
un   étage   *floor, storey*
une   étagère   *shelf, set of shelves*
la   faute   *mistake*
le   filet   *net bag*
le   jour férié   *public holiday*
le   libre-service   *self-service (shop)*
la   liste   *list*
      ni repris ni échangé   *no return or exchange*
le   panier   *basket*
la   promotion   *offer*
le   rayon   *shelf, department*
la   réclamation   *complaint*
la   réduction   *reduction*
le   rez-de-chaussée   *ground floor*
le   sac   *bag*
les   soldes (m)   *sale*
la   sorte   *sort, kind*
le   sous-sol   *basement*
la   vitrine   *shop window*

PEOPLE

le   client   *customer*
le/la commerçant/commerçante   *shopkeeper, market trader*
le   gérant   *manager*
le/la marchand/marchande   *salesperson*
le   patron   *boss*
le/la vendeur/vendeuse   *sales assistant*
le   voleur   *thief*

CLOTHES

un   anorak   *anorak*
le   blouson   *jacket*
la   botte   *boot*
le   chapeau   *hat*
la   chaussette   *sock*
la   chaussure   *shoe*
la   chemise   *shirt*
le   chemisier   *blouse*
le   collant   *tights*
le   coton   *cotton*
la   couleur   *colour*
la   cravate   *tie*
le   cuir   *leather*
un   imperméable   *raincoat*
le   jean   *jeans*

la   jupe   *skirt*
la   laine   *wool*
le   maillot de bain   *bathing costume*
le   manteau   *coat*
la   mode   *fashion*
le   mouchoir   *handkerchief*
le   nylon   *nylon*
la   paire (de)   *pair (of)*
le   pantalon   *pair of trousers*
le   parapluie   *umbrella*
le   plastique   *plastic*
la   pointure   *size (shoes)*
le   pull(over)   *pullover*
le   pyjama   *pyjamas*
la   robe   *dress*
la   sandale   *sandal*
le   short   *pair of shorts*
le   slip   *underpants, knickers*
le   tricot   *jumper*
le   veste   *jacket*
les   vêtements (m)   *clothes*

FOOD

l'   alimentation (f)   *food*
la   baguette   *French stick of bread*
la   banane   *banana*
le   beurre   *butter*
le   biscuit   *biscuit*
le   bonbon   *sweet*
le   café   *coffee*
la   carotte   *carrot*
la   cerise   *cherry*
le   chou   *cabbage*
la   confiture   *jam*
la   fraise   *strawberry*
le   fromage   *cheese*
le   fruit   *fruit*
le   gâteau   *cake*
le   haricot   *bean*
le   jambon   *ham*
le   lait   *milk*
la   laitue   *lettuce*
les   légumes (m)   *vegetables*
un   œuf   *egg*
un   oignon   *onion*
une   orange   *orange*
le   pain   *bread*
le   pâté   *pâté*
les   pâtisseries (f)   *cakes, pastries*
la   pêche   *peach*
les   petits pois (m)   *peas*
les   plats cuisinés (m)   *cooked dishes*
la   pomme   *apple*
la   pomme de terre   *potato*
le   produit surgelé   *frozen food*
les   provisions (f)   *food*
le   raisin   *grape*
la   salade   *lettuce, salad*
le   saucisson   *sausage, salami*
le   sel   *salt*
le   sucre   *sugar*
le   thé   *tea*
la   tomate   *tomato*
la   viande   *meat*
le   yaourt   *yoghurt*

DRINKS

la   boisson   *drink*
une eau minérale   *mineral water*
le   jus de fruit   *fruit juice*
le   vin rouge/blanc   *red/white wine*

QUANTITIES

la   boîte   *box, tin, can*
la   bouteille   *bottle*
le   centimètre   *centimetre*
la   chose   *thing*
la   douzaine   *dozen, about twelve*
le   gramme   *gram*
le   kilo   *kilogram*
le   litre   *litre*
la   livre   *pound, 500 grams*
la   mesure   *measure*
le   métal   *metal*
le   mètre   *metre*
la   moitié   *half*
le   morceau   *bit, piece*
le   paquet   *packet, parcel*
un   peu plus   *a little more*
la   pièce   *each one*
le   pot   *jar, pot*
la   qualité   *quality*
la   quantité   *quantity*
     quelque chose de...   *something...*
la   taille   *height, size*
la   tranche   *slice*

     assez   *enough, fairly*
     beaucoup (de)   *a lot, many*
     combien   *how much, how many*
     demi   *half*
     mille   *thousand*
     moins   *less*
     peu (de)   *little*
     plus   *more*
     plusieurs   *several*
     quelque   *some*
     trop (de)   *too, too much*
     zéro   *nil*

NON-FOOD ITEMS

une allumette   *match*
les articles de sport (m)   *sports items*
une aspirine   *aspirin*
le   cachet   *tablet*
la   carte   *card, map*
la   carte postale   *postcard*
le   crayon   *pencil*
le   déodorant   *deodorant*
le   disque   *record*
une enveloppe   *envelope*
le   guide   *guide*
le   jouet   *toy*
le   journal   *newspaper*
le   magazine   *magazine*
le   maquillage   *make-up*
le   médicament   *medicine*
le   papier à lettres   *writing paper*
le   parfum   *perfume*
la   pellicule   *film (for a camera)*
le   souvenir   *souvenir*

le   stylo   *ball-point pen*
le   tabac   *tobacco*

MONEY

l'   argent (m)   *money*
le   billet de cent francs   *100-franc note*
le   carnet de chèques   *cheque book*
la   carte de crédit   *credit card*
le   centime   *centime*
le   chèque   *cheque*
le   franc   *franc*
la   livre sterling   *pound sterling*
la   monnaie   *change, currency*
le   prix   *price*

     bon marché   *cheap*
     cher/chère   *dear, expensive*
     compris   *included*
     gratuit   *free (no charge)*
     juste   *exact*

     ça fait...   *that makes...*
     ça va   *that's all right*
     de rien   *don't mention it*
     merci   *thank you*
     par personne   *per person*
     vaut   *is worth*

SHOPPING VERBS

     accepter   *to accept*
     acheter   *to buy*
     aider   *to help*
     aimer   *to like*
     aimer mieux   *to prefer*
     aller chercher   *to go and get*
     avoir   *to have*
     avoir besoin (de)   *to need*
     compter   *to count*
     conseiller   *to advise*
     coûter   *to cost*
     demander   *to ask (for)*
     désirer   *to want*
     devoir   *to owe*
     distribuer   *to distribute*
     échanger   *to exchange*
     essayer   *to try (on)*
     faire des achats   *to go shopping*
     faire du lèche-vitrines   *to window-shop*
     faire les courses   *to do the shopping*
     fermer   *to close*
     je voudrais   *I would like*
     manquer   *to lack*
     montrer   *to show*
     ne pas marcher   *not to work*
     offrir   *to offer*
     ouvrir   *to open*
     payer   *to pay (for)*
     peser   *to weigh*
     se plaindre   *to complain*
     plaire   *to please*
     porter   *to carry, to wear*
     préférer   *to prefer*
     prendre   *to take*
     rapporter   *to bring back*
     rembourser   *to reimburse*
     remercier   *to thank*

rendre *to give back*
se trouver *to be situated*
vendre *to sell*
se vendre bien/mal *to sell well/badly*
voler *to steal*
vouloir *to want (to)*

QUALITIES

autre *other*
déchiré *torn*
différent *different*
entier/entière *complete*
frais/fraîche *fresh*
léger/légère *light*
lourd *heavy*
même *same*
mieux *better*
mûr *ripe*
neuf/neuve *new*
normal *normal*
par-dessous *underneath*
par-dessus *above*
premier/première *first*

à part *apart from*
à partir de... *from...*
lequel/laquelle *which*
pas de... *no...*
quel/quelle *which, what*
quoi *what*
sauf *except*
tout *all*

COLOURS

blanc/blanche *white*
bleu *blue*
brun *brown*
clair *light (in colour)*
foncé *dark (in colour)*
jaune *yellow*
noir *black*
rose *pink*
rouge *red*
vert *green*

PATTERNS

à carreaux *checked*
pois *polka-dot*
rayé *striped*
uni *plain*

SIZE

court *short*
étroit *narrow*
grand *large*
large *broad*
long/longue *long*
petit *small*

exactement *exactly*
trop *too much*

WHAT THE CUSTOMER SAYS

C'est à moi. *It's my turn/It's mine.*
C'est mon tour. *It's my turn.*
Je voudrais des...et des... *I would like some...and some...*
J'ai aussi besoin de... *I also need.*
Combien coûte ce/cette...? *What does this...cost?*
Combien font ces...? *How much are these...?*
C'est combien, les...? *How much are the...?*
J'en voudrais une demi-livre, s'il vous plaît. *I would like half a pound, please.*
Avec ceci, je vais prendre... *Also I'd like...*
Les plus/moins gros/grosses. *The biggest/smallest.*
Oui, s'il vous plaît. *Yes, please.*
Je voudrais aussi de la/du... *I'd also like some...*
Oui, comme ça. *Yes, like that.*
Est-ce que vous avez des...? *Have you any...?*
Est-ce qu'il y a des...? *Are there any...?*
Oui, ce sera tout. *Yes, that will be all.*
Je vous dois combien? *How much do I owe you?*
Je n'ai qu'un billet de (100) francs. *I only have a (100) franc note.*
Qu'est-ce que vous avez comme...? *What have you got in the way of...?*
Je peux choisir les...? *May I choose the...?*
Je voudrais un morceau de... *I'd like a piece of...*
Un peu plus grand, s'il vous plaît. *A little bigger, please.*
Que me conseillez-vous comme...? *Which...would you recommend?*
Vous pouvez me l'envelopper? *Could you wrap it for me?*
Il me faut aussi des... *I also need...*
Quel(le)s sont les meilleur(e)s? *Which are the best?*
Je les prends. *I'll take them.*
Je vais réfléchir. *I'll think about it.*
Vous n'avez rien de moins cher? *Have you nothing cheaper?*
D'où vient ce...? *Where does this...come from?*
Est-ce que vous vendez du...? *Do you sell...?*
Où pourrais-je en trouver...? *Where could I find some...?*

WHAT THE ASSISTANT SAYS

C'est à qui, maintenant? *Whose turn is it now?*
A qui le tour? *Whose turn is it now?*
On vous sert? *Are you being served?*
Qu'y a-t-il pour votre service? *What would you like?*
Vous désirez? *What would you like?*
Qu'est-ce qu'il vous faut? *What would you like?*
Que voulez-vous? *What would you like?*
Voici. Et ensuite? *There. Anything else?*
Je n'en ai plus. *I haven't any left.*
C'est 8 francs le kilo. *It's 8 francs a kilo.*
Ils sont à 2 francs la pièce. *They are 2 francs each.*
Et avec ceci? *Anything else?*
De quelle sorte? *What kind?*
Celles-ci? *These?*
Comme ça? *Like this?*
Comme ceci? *Like this?*
Oui, j'en ai encore. *Yes, I have some more.*
Et avec ça, ce sera tout? *Is that all?*
Alors, ça fera...francs. *That makes...francs.*
Vous avez la monnaie? *Have you any change?*
Ce n'est pas grave. *It doesn't matter.*
Voici votre monnaie. *Here's your change.*
J'ai ces...et ces... *I have these...and these...*
Oui, certainement. *Yes, of course.*
Non, les clients ne se servent pas. *No, customers do not serve themselves.*

Mais oui, bien sûr. *Yes, of course.*
Il vient de... *It comes from...*
D'habitude, j'en ai, mais il ne m'en reste plus. *Usually I have some, but I've none left.*
Ça se vend au poids. *It's sold by weight.*

▶ C5 Services

POST OFFICE

une	adresse	*address*
la	boîte aux lettres	*letter box*
le	bureau de poste	*post office*
la	carte postale	*postcard*
le	colis	*parcel*
le	courrier	*post, mail*
le	facteur	*postman*
le	formulaire	*form*
le	guichet	*counter position*
la	lettre	*letter*
la	lettre recommandée	*recorded letter*
la	levée du courrier	*postal collection*
le	mandat postal	*postal order*
une	opération de guichet	*counter service*
	P et T / PTT	*Post Office*
le	paquet	*package*
la	poste	*post*
	poste restante	*post to be collected*
le	tabac	*tobacconist*
le	tarif	*price list*
le	télégramme	*telegram*
le	timbre	*stamp*
le	timbre à un franc	*1-franc stamp*

compter *to count*
distribuer le courrier *to deliver the post*
mettre à la poste *to post*
payer au mot *to pay by the word*
poster *to post*
remplir une fiche *to fill in a form*
toucher un chèque / un mandat *to cash a cheque / postal order*

à l'étranger *abroad*
combien *how much*
fragile *fragile*
par avion *by air mail*
urgent *urgent*

Je voudrais envoyer cette lettre. *I would like to send this letter.*
Par avion? *By air?*
Je vais la peser. Voilà. Ça vous fait... francs. *I'll weigh it. There. It costs... francs.*
C'est combien, une lettre pour la Suisse? *How much is a letter to Switzerland?*
Je voudrais aussi envoyer ce paquet à l'étranger. *I would also like to send this package abroad.*
Je voudrais envoyer de l'argent. Qu'est-ce que je dois faire? *I would like to send some money. What should I do?*
Combien voulez-vous envoyer? *How much do you want to send?*
Vous pouvez envoyer un mandat. Il faut remplir ce coupon. *You could send a postal order. You have to fill in this coupon.*
Voilà, il est rempli. Voici l'argent. *There, it's filled in. Here's the money.*
Je voudrais envoyer un télégramme. *I would like to send a telegram.*

Remplissez ce formulaire. *Complete this form.*
Voilà, il est rempli. Il y a dix-sept mots. *There, it's complete. There are 17 words.*

PHONING

un	annuaire	*telephone directory*
la	cabine téléphonique	*telephone box*
la	carte téléphonique	*phonecard*
le	coup de téléphone	*phone call*
la	fente	*slot*
le	jeton	*token*
le	moment	*moment*
le	numéro	*number*
une	opératrice	*(female) operator*
la	pièce	*coin*
la	seconde	*second*
la	sonnerie	*ringing*
la	tonalité	*dialling tone*

s'adresser *to apply to*
appeler *to call*
composer le numéro *to dial the number*
décrocher le combiné *to lift the receiver*
écouter *to listen*
entendre *to hear*
faire erreur *to make a mistake*
se munir de *to provide oneself with*
parler *to speak*
raccrocher *to put the receiver down*
rappeler *to call back*
sonner *to ring (bell)*
téléphoner *to telephone*

en panne *out of order*
en PCV *reversed charges*
libre *free*
occupé *occupied, engaged*

à l'appareil *on the phone, 'speaking'*
allô *hello*
bien *good, well*
de la part de *on behalf of*
ici *here*
mal *bad(ly)*
quand *when*
qui *who*

Je voudrais téléphoner. Où pourrais-je trouver les annuaires? *I would like to ring someone. Where can I find the directories?*
Vous pouvez les consulter ici à la poste. Il sont à côté des cabines téléphoniques. *You can look at them here in the post office. They are next to the phone boxes.*
Je peux téléphoner aux renseignements d'abord? *Can I ring for information first?*
Oui, bien sûr. C'est gratuit. *Yes, of course. It's free.*
Ne quittez pas. *Please hold.*
Pouvez-vous m'expliquer comment on téléphone en Angleterre? *Can you explain how to phone to England?*
Eh bien, il faut composer le 00 et attendre la tonalité. *Well, dial 00 and wait for the tone.*
Après, vous faites le code pour la Grande-Bretagne, le 44, et puis le numéro de votre correspondant, sans oublier l'indicatif de la région sans le zéro. *Then, you dial the code for Great Britain, 44, then the number you require, not forgetting the local code omitting the zero.*

Je peux utiliser la cabine là dehors? *Can I use the box outside?*

Voilà, j'ai fini. *There, I have finished.*

Bien. Ça vous fait ... francs en tout. *Good. That will cost ... francs altogether.*

C'est combien? *How much is it?*

La communication a duré 5 minutes. Ça coûte ... francs. *The call lasted 5 minutes. That costs ... francs.*

BANK OR FOREIGN-EXCHANGE OFFICE

l' argent (m) *money*
la banque *bank*
le billet de cent francs *100-franc note*
le bureau de change *foreign-exchange office*
la caisse *cash desk, till*
la carte bancaire *banker's card*
la carte de crédit *credit card*
le centime *centime*
le chèque *cheque*
le chèque de voyage *traveller's cheque*
la commission *commission*
le cours de change *rate of exchange*
le franc *franc*
le guichet *counter position*
la livre sterling *pound sterling*
la moitié *half*
la monnaie *change*
le numéro de compte *account number*
le passeport *passport*
la pièce *coin*
la pièce d'identité *proof of identity*
pour cent *per cent*

accepter *to accept*
changer *to change*
passer à la caisse *to go on to the cash desk*
prendre une commission *to take a commission*
signer *to sign*
valoir *to be worth*
vaut *is worth*

Combien vaut la livre? *What is the pound worth?*

Je voudrais changer des livres, s'il vous plaît. *I would like to change some pounds, please.*

Un passeport, ça va? *Is a passport all right?*

Voilà. *There.*

Oui, bien sûr. Des billets de banque ou des chèques de voyage? *Of course. Banknotes or traveller's cheques?*

Il y a une commission de trois pour cent sur les chèques de voyage. *There is a commission of 3% on traveller's cheques.*

Donnez-moi vos chèques de voyage et une pièce d'identité. *Give me your traveller's cheques and some proof of identity.*

Oui, naturellement. *Of course.*

Tenez, signez là. *Sign here, please.*

Le cours du change est à ... francs. Voilà votre ticket. Vous pouvez passer à la caisse maintenant. *The rate of exchange is ... francs. Here's your ticket. You can go to the cash desk now.*

Voici votre argent. Bon séjour! *Here's your money. Enjoy your stay!*

LOST PROPERTY

un appareil photo *camera*

un après-midi *afternoon*
la bicyclette *bicycle*
le bureau des objets trouvés *lost-property office*
le cambrioleur *burglar*
la caméra *cine camera*
le carnet de chèques *cheque book*
la ceinture *belt*
le centimètre *centimetre*
la clé *key*
le consulat *consulate*
la couleur *colour*
la date *date*
la description *description*
le dommage *damage*
la fiche *form*
le flash *flash gun (photography)*
la forme *form, shape*
la marque *make, brand name*
le matin *morning*
le métal *metal*
la montre *watch*
le mouchoir *handkerchief*
le moyen *means*
le nom *name*
le parapluie *umbrella*
le passeport *passport*
la pièce d'identité *proof of identity*
la poche *pocket*
le porte-monnaie *purse*
le portefeuille *wallet*
la récompense *reward*
le règlement *regulation, settlement*
le sac à dos *rucksack*
le sac à main *handbag*
une sorte de *a kind of*
la taille *size, height*
la valise *suitcase*
le vélomoteur *motor-assisted bicycle*
le vol *theft*
le voleur *thief*

accuser *to accuse*
il s'agit de *it's a question of, it's about*
appartenir *to belong*
s'arranger *to manage*
cambrioler *to break in*
chercher *to look for*
découvrir *to discover*
décrire *to describe*
devoir *to owe*
disparaître *to disappear*
douter *to doubt*
égarer *to mislead, mislay*
emprunter *to borrow*
étonner *to astonish*
il faut *it is necessary*
laisser *to let, to leave*
marquer *to mark*
oublier *to forget*
pardonner *to forgive*
perdre *to lose*
reconnaître *to recognise*
remplir *to fill, to fill in*
rendre *to give back*
se rendre compte de *to realise*
retrouver *to find*
savoir *to know (a fact)*
signer *to sign*
se souvenir de *to remember*

trouver *to find*
voler *to steal*

aucun *no, none*
carré *square*
certain *certain*
clair *light (colour)*
content *pleased*
court *short*
déçu *disappointed*
différent *different*
étroit *narrow*
fâché *angry*
foncé *dark (colour)*
formidable *great*
furieux/furieuse *furious*
grand *big*
heureux/heureuse *happy, lucky*
impossible *impossible*
jaune *yellow*
large *broad*
long/longue *long*
mince *thin*
neuf/neuve *new*
petit *small*
plein *full*
possible *possible*
rectangulaire *rectangular*
rond *round*
solide *solid*
sûr *sure*
tout neuf *brand new*
vide *empty*
vieux/vieil/vieille *old*

après *after*
aujourd'hui *today*
avant *before*
avant-hier *the day before yesterday*
avec succès *with success*
ceci *this one*
cela *that one*
comme *as, like*
dedans *inside*
dessous *underneath*
dessus *above*
dont *whose, of which*
en train de *in the process of*
hier *yesterday*
lequel/laquelle *which*
nulle part *nowhere*
partout *everywhere*
puisque *since*
sur *on*

J'ai perdu mon portefeuille. *I've lost my wallet.*
Est-ce que vous pouvez me le décrire? *Can you describe it to me?*
Ça ne sert à rien. *That's no use.*
Mon Dieu! *Good heavens!*
Tiens! *Hey!*
Zut! *Damn!*
Pas de chance. *No luck.*
Quoi de neuf? *What's new?*

HAVING THINGS REPAIRED OR CLEANED

la batterie *battery (on a car)*
le bouton *button*

le bruit *noise*
la cordonnerie *shoe repairer's shop*
la critique *criticism, complaint*
un/une électricien/électricienne *electrician*
un embrayage *clutch*
un état *state, condition*
le flash *flash gun (photography)*
le frein *brake*
la fuite *leak*
le garage *garage*
le garagiste *garage owner*
une inondation *flood*
la lampe de poche *torch*
le lave-linge *washing machine*
la laverie automatique *car wash, launderette*
la marque *make, brand*
le/la mécanicien/mécanicienne *mechanic*
le moteur *engine*
le nettoyage à sec *dry cleaning*
la panne *breakdown*
la pièce de rechange *spare part*
la pile *battery*
le plombier *plumber*
le radiateur *radiator*
la réclamation *complaint*
le réparateur *repair man*
la réparation *repair*
la roue de secours *spare wheel*
la sécurité *security*
le trou *hole*
les vitesses (f) *gears*

accepter *to accept*
casser *to break*
critiquer *to criticise*
déchirer *to tear*
devoir *to owe*
échanger *to exchange*
emprunter *to borrow*
faire nettoyer *to have cleaned*
faire réparer *to have repaired*
il faut *it is necessary*
se fier à *to trust*
fixer *to fix*
garantir *to guarantee*
laisser tomber *to drop*
laver *to wash*
marcher *to work, to function*
nettoyer à sec *to dry clean*
se plaindre *to complain*
promettre *to promise*
proposer *to propose*
prouver *to prove*
raccommoder *to mend*
refuser *to refuse*
rembourser *to reimburse*
remercier *to thank*
remplacer *to replace*
rendre *to give back*
renverser *to turn over, to reverse, to knock over*
réparer *to repair*
reprendre *to take back*
revenir *to come back*
suggérer *to suggest*
vérifier *to check*

bizarre *odd, strange*
bon/bonne *good*
capable *capable*

crevé   *punctured*
déçu   *disappointed*
désolé   *very sorry*
en panne   *out of order, broken down*
gentil/gentille   *kind*
impossible   *impossible*
mauvais   *bad*
possible   *possible*
prêt   *ready*
propre   *clean*
reçu   *received*
sale   *dirty*
satisfait   *satisfied*
solide   *solid*

après-demain   *the day after tomorrow*
combien de temps   *how long*
dans ce cas   *in this case*
demain   *tomorrow*
malgré   *in spite of*
naturellement   *of course*

Hélas!   *Alas!*
Pas de quoi.   *Don't mention it.*
Ce n'est pas la peine.   *It's not worth it.*
Je vous en prie.   *Please, not at all.*

▷ C6 Getting around

PUBLIC TRANSPORT

Trains

un   aller simple   *single ticket*
un   aller-retour   *return ticket*
une   arrivée   *arrival*
le   billet   *ticket*
le   buffet   *buffet*
la   'Carte Jeune'   *young person's rail card*
le   chemin de fer   *railway*
le   compartiment   *compartment*
la   consigne   *left-luggage office*
la   correspondance (f)   *connection*
le   départ   *departure*
la   deuxième classe   *second class*
un   express   *express*
le   fumeur   *smoker*
la   gare   *station*
le   guichet   *ticket office*
un   horaire   *timetable*
le   non-fumeur   *non-smoker*
un   omnibus   *slow train*
le   porteur   *porter*
la   première classe   *first class*
le   quai   *platform*
le   rapide   *express*
la   réduction   *reduction*
la   réservation   *reservation*
le   sac   *bag*
le   sac à dos   *rucksack*
la   salle d'attente   *waiting room*
la   SNCF   *French railways*
la   sortie   *exit*
la   station de taxis   *taxi rank*
le   tarif   *price list*
le   train   *train*
la   valise   *suitcase*
la   voie   *track*
le   voyageur   *traveller, passenger*

annoncer   *to announce*
attendre   *to wait for*
changer   *to change*
composter   *to date, to punch (ticket)*
contrôler   *to check*
descendre   *to get out / off*
durer   *to last*
s'installer   *to settle*
manquer   *to miss*
porter   *to carry*
prendre trois heures   *to take three hours*

de   *from*
dernier   *last*
en direction de   *going to*
en provenance de   *coming from*
occupé   *occupied*
prochain   *next*
suivant   *next, following*
supplémentaire   *extra*

Bon voyage!   *Have a good trip!*
Je voudrais un billet pour Paris, s'il vous plaît.   *I'd like a ticket for Paris, please.*
Un aller simple ou un aller-retour?   *Single or return?*
Vous voyagez en première ou en seconde?   *Are you going first or second class?*
Vous voulez faire une réservation?   *Do you want to reserve a seat?*
Ce sera la voiture onze, compartiment trois, place cinq.   *That'll be coach 11, compartment 3, seat 5.*
C'est un omnibus ou un express?   *Is it a slow or a fast train?*
A quelle heure part le train?   *At what time does the train leave?*
A quelle heure arrive le train?   *At what time does the train arrive?*
Vous trouverez les heures de départ et d'arrivée affichées là-bas.   *You'll find departure and arrival times posted over there.*
A quelle heure est le prochain train pour Paris? Et le train suivant?   *At what time is the next train for Paris? And the one after that?*
Où puis-je laisser mes bagages?   *Where can I leave my luggage?*
Vous pouvez les déposer à la consigne ou utiliser la consigne automatique.   *You can put it in the left-luggage office or use the automatic luggage locker.*
La salle d'attente est de l'autre côté.   *The waiting room is on the other side.*
D'où part le train pour Calais?   *Where does the Calais train leave from?*
Du quai numéro quatre.   *From platform number four.*
C'est bien ici, le train pour Calais?   *Am I right here for the Calais train?*
Non, ici a sont les trains de banlieue. Il faut aller au départ des grandes lignes.   *No, these are the suburban trains. You have to go to the main-line departures.*
Mesdames et Messieurs, les passagers sont priés de monter en voiture.   *Ladies and gentlemen, passengers are requested to board the train.*

le   changement d'horaire   *timetable change*
la   couchette   *couchette, sleeper*
la   destination   *destination*
la   portière   *door (train)*
le/la   touriste   *tourist*
le   wagon-restaurant   *dining car*

consulter   *to consult*

indiquer *to show, to indicate*
ralentir *to slow down*
rembourser *to reimburse*
rouler *to travel, to move*

Pouvez-vous m'indiquer le wagon-restaurant? *Can you show me the dining car?*

Buses
un arrêt *stop*
un autobus *bus*
un autocar *coach*
le bus *bus*
le car *coach*
le carnet *booklet*
la gare routière *bus station*
la ligne *line*
le numéro *number*
le ticket *ticket*

lent *slow*

+ *many of the items for trains – see p. 57–8*

Ships and hovercraft
un aéroglisseur *hovercraft*
le bateau *boat*
le car-ferry *car ferry*
la gare maritime *dockside station*
la traversée *crossing*
le ferry *ferry*
un hovercraft *hovercraft*
le port *port*

débarquer *to disembark*
embarquer *to embark*
voler *to fly*

Planes
un avion *aeroplane*
la ceinture de sécurité *safety belt*
le vol *flight*

aterrir *to land*
décoller *to take off*
voler *to fly*

GOING THROUGH CUSTOMS
la douane *customs*
le douanier *customs official*
la frontière *frontier, border*
le passeport *passport*

Avez-vous quelque chose à déclarer? *Have you anything to declare?*
Je n'ai rien à déclarer. *I have nothing to declare.*
Ouvrez vos valises, s'il vous plaît. *Open your cases, please.*
J'ai des cigarettes et de l'alcool à déclarer. *I have some cigarettes and some alcohol to declare.*

PRIVATE TRANSPORT
une aire de repos *picnic area*
une assurance *insurance*
une auto-école *driving school*

le camion *lorry*
la carte routière *road map*
la carte verte *green card*
le casque *helmet*
le chauffeur *driver*
la chaussée *roadway*
le conducteur *driver*
la déviation *diversion*
la fin *end*
le garage *garage*
le/la mécanicien / mécanicienne *mechanic*
la moto *motorbike*
le numéro *number*
le parking *car-park*
le passage protégé *right of way*
le péage *toll*
le permis de conduire *driving licence*
le poids lourd *heavy vehicle*
la route nationale *major road*
le scooter *scooter*
le stationnement *parking*
les travaux (m) *road works*
le vélomoteur *motor-assisted bicycle*
le virage *turn, bend*
la vitesse *speed, gear*

conduire *to drive*
freiner *to brake*
garer *to park*
passer le permis *to take one's test*
rouler *to drive, to move*
stationner *to park*
tourner *to turn*

lent *slow*
obligatoire *obligatory, compulsory*
payant *paying, where one must pay*

Attention! *Look out!*
Il faut freiner avant le virage. *You have to brake before the bend.*
Il est interdit de stationner ici. *It is forbidden to park here.*
Priorité à droite. *Priority from the right.*

une amende *fine*
le camion *lorry*
la camionnette *van*
le code de la route *highway code*
le disque de stationnement *parking disc*
un embouteillage *traffic jam*
les heures d'affluence (f) *rush hours*
les papiers (m) *papers*
le piéton *pedestrian*
la police d'assurance *insurance policy*
le trottoir *pavement*
la zone bleu(e) *blue zone (parking)*

circuler *to move about*
conduire *to drive*
dépasser *to overtake*
louer *to hire*
ralentir *to slow down*
retourner *to return*
rouler au pas *to drive at walking pace*

automatique *automatic*

ROAD ACCIDENTS

un accident *accident*
une ambulance *ambulance*
la clinique *clinic*
la collision *collision*
le docteur *doctor*
le gendarme *gendarme, policeman*
la marque de voiture *make of car*
la police *police*

aider *to help*
s'approcher *to approach*
cogner *to bump*
écraser *to crush*
rentrer dans *to crash into, to bump into*
risquer *to risk*
tuer *to kill*
se tuer *to kill oneself*

blessé *injured*
dangereux/dangereuse *dangerous*

THE CAR

l' arrière (m) *the back*
l' avant (m) *the front*
la batterie *battery*
la ceinture de sécurité *safety belt*
la clé de voiture *car key*
le coffre *boot*
la crevaison *puncture*
un essuie-glace *windscreen wiper*
le frein *brake*
le moteur *engine*
la panne *breakdown*
la panne d'essence *running out of petrol*
le pare-brise *windscreen*
le phare *headlight*
le pneu *tyre*
la portière *door*
le rétroviseur *driving mirror*
le siège *seat*
le volant *steering wheel*

accélérer *to accelerate*
allumer les phares *to put on lights*
s'arrêter *to stop*
démarrer *to start*
dépanner *to repair*
éteindre les phares *to put out lights*
fonctionner *to function, to work*
freiner *to brake*
marcher *to function, to work*
passer une vitesse *to change gear*
réparer *to repair*
tomber en panne *to break down*

J'ai allumé les phares. *I have switched on the headlights.*
Je suis tombé en panne d'essence. *I've run out of petrol.*
Le moteur ne marche pas. *The engine doesn't work.*
Pouvez-vous me dépanner? J'ai une crevaison. *Can you put my car right? I have a puncture.*

AT THE SERVICE STATION

l' air (m) *air*
le deux-temps *two-stroke*
l' eau (f) *water*
l' essence (f) *petrol*

la fumée *smoke*
le gas-oil *diesel*
le gazole *diesel*
l' huile (f) *oil*
le lavage automatique *car wash*
le litre *litre*
le/la pompiste *petrol-pump attendant*
le sans plomb *unleaded petrol*
le super sans plomb *super unleaded petrol*
les toilettes (f) *toilets*
les WC (m) *toilets*

vérifier le niveau d'eau *to check the water level*
vérifier le niveau d'huile *to check the oil level*
vérifier la pression / des pneus *to check tyre pressure*

Faites le plein! *Fill it up!*
Le plein de sans plomb, s'il vous plaît. *Fill it up with unleaded, please.*
Le plein de super, s'il vous plaît. *Fill it up with 4 star, please.*
C'est un self-service ici. *It's self-service here.*
Est-ce que vous pouvez laver le pare-brise, s'il vous plaît? *Can you wash the windscreen, please?*
Je voudrais aussi acheter une carte routière. *I would also like to buy a road map.*
Il me faut de l'huile. *I need oil.*
Voulez-vous vérifier le niveau d'eau, s'il vous plaît? *Would you check the water level, please?*

▶ DI Further education and training

J'ai l'intention de faire une licence. *I intend to take a degree.*
Je vais faire mes études à l'université. *I am going to study at university.*
Je préparerai mon bac. *I will take my 'bac' (A Levels / GNVQ).*

▶ D2 Careers and employment

Je voudrais être... *I would like to be...*
un/une acteur/actrice *actor/actress*
une administration *administration*
une agence de voyages *travel agency*
un/une animateur/animatrice *organiser*
un/une avocat/avocate *lawyer*
le/la boucher/bouchère *butcher*
le/la boulanger/boulangère *baker*
le bureau de change *foreign-exchange office*
le/la charcutier/charcutière *pork butcher*
le chef *cook*
le/la chirurgien/chirurgienne *surgeon*
le/la chômeur/chômeuse *unemployed man/woman*
le/la coiffeur/coiffeuse *hairdresser*
le/la commerçant/commerçante *salesperson, market trader*
le/la comptable *accountant*
le/la cuisinier/cuisinière *cook*
la dactylo *shorthand typist*
le/la décorateur/décoratrice *decorator*
le/la dentiste *dentist*
le/la dessinateur/dessinatrice *designer*
le/la directeur/directrice *director, headmaster/ headmistress*
le docteur *doctor*
un/une électricien/électricienne *electrician*
un emploi *job*

un/une	employée	*employee*
un/une	épicier/épicière	*grocer*
un/une	étudiant/étudiante	*student*
le/la	facteur/factrice	*postman/postwoman*
la	femme d'affaires	*businesswoman*
la	femme de chambre	*housemaid*
le/la	fermier/fermière	*farmer*
le	garçon de café	*waiter*
le	gendarme	*policeman*
un	homme d'affaires	*businessman*
une	hôtesse de l'air	*air hostess*
une	industrie	*industry*
un/une	infirmier/infirmière	*nurse*
le/la	jardinier/jardinière	*gardener*
le/la	journaliste	*journalist*
le	laboratoire	*laboratory*
le/la	maçon/maçonne	*builder, bricklayer*
le/le	mécanicien/mécanicienne	*mechanic*
le	médecin	*doctor*
le	métier	*occupation*
le	militaire	*soldier*
le/la	musicien/musicienne	*musician*
un/une	ouvrier/ouvrière	*worker*
le/la	pâtissier/pâtissière	*pastrycook*
le/le	patron/patronne (de restaurant)	*(restaurant) owner*
le	pilote	*pilot*
le	pompier	*fireman*
le	poste	*job*
le	professeur	*teacher*
la	profession libérale	*profession*
le/la	programmeur/programmeuse	*programmer*
la	réception	*reception*
le/la	secrétaire	*secretary*
le/la	serveur/serveuse	*barman/barmaid, shop assistant*
la	société	*company*
le/la	technicien/technicienne	*technician*
une	usine	*factory*
la	vedette	*film star*
le	vétérinaire	*veterinary surgeon*

Je voudrais travailler... *I would like to work...*
....dans une usine. *....in a factory.*
....dans un bureau. *....in an office.*
....dans un magasin. *....in a shop.*
....dans un collège. *....in a school.*
....dans un hôpital. *....in a hospital.*
....en plein air. *....in the open air.*
....dans un hôtel. *....in a hotel.*
....avec des animaux. *....with animals.*
....avec des enfants. *....with children.*
....avec des ordinateurs. *....with computers.*
Mon père est mécanicien. *My father is a mechanic.*
Ma mère est femme au foyer. *My mother is a housewife.*
Je suis attiré(e) par les professions libérales. *I am attracted to professional work.*
J'aimerais être vétérinaire. *I would like to be a vet.*
Je serai au chômage sinon. *Otherwise I shall be unemployed.*
J'aimerais travailler à l'étranger. *I would like to work abroad.*
J'aimerais être professeur. *I'd like to be a teacher.*
C'est un travail important. *It's an important job.*
C'est un travail varié. *It's a varied job.*
C'est assez bien payé. *It's quite well paid.*
J'aimerais habiter une grande ville/une petite ville. *I'd like to live in a large/small town.*
Parce que c'est intéressant/calme. *Because it's interesting/ quiet.*

▶ **D3 Travel to work and school**

la	distance	*distance*
la	gare	*station*
le	moyen de transport	*means of transport*
la	station	*tube station, stop, taxi-rank*
le	transport	*transport*

amener quelqu'un en voiture *to take someone by car*
s'arrêter *to stop*
arriver à neuf heures *to arrive at 9 o'clock*
conduire *to drive*
se dépêcher *to hurry*
déposer quelqu'un en voiture *to drop someone by car*
descendre d'une voiture *to get out of a car*
durer *to last*
entrer *to enter*
être de retour *to be back*
marcher *to walk*
mettre vingt minutes *to take 20 minutes*
se mettre en route *to set out*
monter dans une voiture *to get into a car*
partir *to leave*
préférer *to prefer*
prendre le train *to go by train*
quitter *to leave*
rater *to miss*
rentrer *to return*
renverser *to turn back or knock over*
rester *to remain*
revenir *to come back*
sortir *to go out*
traverser *to cross*
utiliser *to use*
voyager en train *to go by train*

lent *slow*
ponctuel/ponctuelle *punctual*
rapide *fast*
tard *late*
tôt *early*
valable pendant un mois *valid for a month*
à bicyclette *by bicycle*
à l'heure *on time*
à pied *on foot*
à vélo *by bike*
à vélomoteur *by moped*
chez moi *at my home, at my house*
de bonne heure *early*
d'habitude *usually*
en autobus *by bus*
en autocar *by coach*
en avance *in advance*
en métro *by tube*
en retard *late*
par le train *by train*
rapidement *quickly*
toujours *always*

Ma mère m'amène en voiture. *My mother takes/brings me in the car.*
Elle me dépose devant le collège. *She drops me outside school.*
Mon père me conduit le soir. *My father drives me in the evening.*
Je mets vingt minutes pour arriver au collège. *It takes me 20 minutes to get to school.*
Je me mets en route vers huit heures. *I start off at about 8 o'clock .*
Je préfère arriver de bonne heure. *I prefer arriving early.*

Je suis de retour vers cinq heures. *I am back home at about 5 o'clock.*
Je monte dans le train. *I get into the train.*

+school items – see p. 28

+school items – see p. 28

▶ D4 Advertising and publicity

une affiche *poster*
une annonce *small ad*
l' audition (f) *recital, audition*
le bal *ball (dance)*
le balcon *balcony, circle*
le ballet *ballet*
le billet *ticket*
le chœur *choir*
le cinéma *cinema*
le cirque *circus*
la comédie *comedy (theatre)*
le concert *concert*
le dessin animé *cartoon*
la discothèque *disco*
un entracte *interval*
un film *film*
le film d'amour *love film*
le film d'épouvante *horror film*
le film de science-fiction *science-fiction film*
le film policier *police, crime film*
la galerie *gallery*
l' information (f) *information*
la maison des jeunes *youth club*
le match de foot *football match*
la matinée *morning, afternoon performance*
la mise en scène *direction (of play, film)*
le musée *museum*
l' opéra (m) *opera*
un orchestre *orchestra*
la patinoire *skating rink*
la pièce (de théâtre) *play*
un poster *poster*
la réduction *reduction*
la salle *room, hall*
la salle polyvalente *multi-use hall*
la séance *showing, screening, performance*
le spectacle *show, entertainment*
le succès *success*
le théâtre *theatre*
le tube *hit record*
le western *western*
le zoo *zoo*

annuler *to cancel*
aura lieu *will take place*
avoir raison *to be right*
commencer *to begin*
être à l'affiche *to be billed, advertised*
être d'accord *to agree*
penser *to think*
réserver *to reserve*
trouver *to find*

affreux/affreuse *awful*
amusant *amusing*
bien! *good!*
bon/bonne *good*
comique *funny*
drôle *funny*
en version anglaise *with English soundtrack*

en version française *with French soundtrack*
ennuyeux/ennuyeuse *boring*
excellent *excellent*
extra(ordinaire) *extraordinary, great*
formidable *great, terrific*
intéressant *interesting*
nouveau/nouvel/nouvelle *new*
nul/nulle *terrible, awful*
pas mal *not bad*
sensationnel/sensationnelle *sensational*
sous-titré *subtitled*
super *terrific, great*
surprenant *surprising*

agréablement *agreeably*
extrêmement *extremely*
tout à fait *quite, totally*

Interdit aux moins de dix-huit ans. *Under-18s prohibited.*

▶ D5 Communication

le cadran *dial*
le combiné *handset*
la ligne *line*
la monnaie *change*
le numéro de téléphone *telephone number*
les pièces de ... francs *...-franc coins*
le poste *phone extension*
une télécarte *phonecard*

composer *to dial*
décrocher *to pick up (the receiver)*
raccrocher *to hang up (the receiver)*

à l'appareil *on the phone, 'speaking'*
allô *hello*
occupé *busy, engaged*

C'est de la part de qui? *Who's calling?*
Ne quittez pas. *Hold the line.*
Je vous le/la passe. *I'll put you through to him/her.*
Comment? *Pardon?*
Pardon? *Sorry?*
Comment ça s'écrit? *How do you spell that?*
Pourriez-vous répéter? *Could you repeat that?*
Pourriez-vous épeler votre nom, s'il vous plaît? *Could you spell your name, please?*
Lui-même. *'Speaking'. (a man)*
Elle-même. *'Speaking'. (a woman)*
Veuillez patienter. *Wait a moment, please.*
Voulez-vous rappeler? *Would you like to ring back?*
Je rappellerai plus tard. *I'll call back later.*
Vous avez fait un faux numéro. *You have dialled the wrong number.*
Je vous prie de m'excuser. *I'm sorry to have troubled you.*
Voulez-vous laisser un message? *Would you like to leave a message?*
Je peux laisser un message? *Can I leave a message?*
Dites-lui que... *Tell him/her that...*
Demandez-lui de... *Ask him/her to...*
Attendez, je note. *Just a moment, I'll write that down.*
La ligne est mauvaise. *The line is bad.*
A quelle heure? *At what time?*
Demain (matin). *Tomorrow (morning).*
Vous pouvez me contacter par... *You can contact me by...*
...téléphone *...telephone*
...télécopie *...fax*

...télémessage ...*E-mail*

+ *French alphabet (see p. 94)*

▶ EI Life in other countries
COINAGE

un franc *franc*
un centime *centime*

FOOD

une boîte *box, tin*
le casse-croûte *snack*
le déjeuner *lunch*
un demi-kilo *half a kilogram*
le dîner *dinner, evening meal*
le goûter *tea*
l' huile (f) *oil*
un kilo *kilogram*
un morceau *piece*
un paquet *packet*
le petit déjeuner *breakfast*
le poivre *pepper*
le sel *salt*
une sorte de (+ food items) *a kind of*
une tranche *slice*

battre *to beat*
bouillir *to boil*
couper *to cut, to chop*
éplucher *to peel*
frire *to fry*
griller (au feu de bois) *to grill (on a barbecue)*
mélanger *to mix*
(faire) rôtir *to roast*

Ça consiste en quoi? *What is it made of?*
C'est quoi exactement, le/la... *What is ... exactly?*

ADDRESSING PEOPLE

Madame *Madam, Mrs*
Mademoiselle *Miss*
Monsieur *Sir, Mr*

tutoyer *to speak to someone in familiar mode, to address someone as* tu
vouvoyer *to speak to someone in formal mode, to address someone as* vous

▶ E2 Tourism

le bureau de renseignements *information office*
le départ *departure*
le dépliant *leaflet, brochure*
la durée *length (of time), duration*
l' excursion (f) *excursion, trip*
  en autocar *by coach*
  en bateau *by boat*
un horaire *timetable*
la liste des hôtels / campings *list of hotels / campsites*
l' office de tourisme (m) *tourist office*
le plan de la ville *town plan*
le prix *price*
le syndicat d'initiative (SI) *information office*
le tarif *price list*

aller en vacances *to go on holiday*

impressionant *impressive*
intéressant *interesting*
tranquille *restful*
ennuyeux/ennuyeuse *boring*
nul/nulle *terrible*
affreux/affreuse *awful*
moche *ugly*
merveilleux/merveilleuse *marvellous*
sale *dirty*
propre *clean*
moderne *modern*

Où êtes-vous allé(e)(s) en vacances? *Where did you go on holiday?*
Avec qui êtes-vous allé(e)(s)? *Who did you go with?*
Vous êtes allé(e)(s) pendant combien de temps? *How long did you go for?*
Quel temps faisait-il là-bas? *What was the weather like there?*
Qu'est-ce que vous avez fait pendant le séjour? *What did you do while you were there?*
Nous sommes allé(e)s en Turquie. *We went to Turkey.*
Je suis allé(e) avec ma famille. *I went with my family.*
Nous y avons passé quinze jours. *We spent a fortnight there.*
Il faisait très chaud. *It was very hot.*
Nous avons visité les monuments historiques. *We visited historic monuments.*
Nous avons fait de la randonnée en montagne. *We went walking in the mountains.*
Nous avons fait des excursions en bateau. *We took boat trips.*
C'était intéressant / tranquille, etc. *It was interesting / restful, etc.*
Donnez-moi une brochure, s'il vous plaît. *Give me a brochure, please.*
L'année prochaine j'irai aux Etats-Unis. *Next year I'm going to the United States.*
Je ferai du camping. *I'll go camping.*
Je prendrai l'avion. *I'll go by plane.*
Je resterai avec des copains. *I'll stay with friends.*
Je préfère les vacances actives. *I prefer active holidays.*
J'aime beaucoup me bronzer à la plage. *I like sunbathing at the beach.*
Je n'aime pas tellement les sites historiques. *I'm not too keen on historic sites.*

+ *items of leisure activity (see p. 43–5)*

▶ E3 Accommodation
HOTEL

un ascenseur *lift*
le bain *bath*
la clé *key*
la douche *shower*
une entrée *entrance*
un escalier *staircase*
un étage *floor, storey*
un hôtel *hotel*
la porte d'entrée *front door*
la réception *reception*
le restaurant *restaurant*
le rez-de-chaussée *ground floor*
la salle de bains *bathroom*
la sortie *exit*

la   sortie de secours   *emergency exit*
le   sous-sol   *basement*
le   téléphone   *telephone*
la   télévision   *TV*
les   toilettes (f)   *toilets*
la   vue   *view*

bruyant   *noisy*
confortable   *comfortable*
de grand confort   *very comfortable*
de grande luxe   *luxurious*
grand   *big*
moderne   *modern*
pas cher   *not expensive*
pas trop cher   *not too expensive*
petit   *small*
privé   *private*
solide   *solid*

Use of the hotel

les   arrhes (f)   *deposit*
le   chèque   *cheque*
le   cintre   *coat-hanger*
la   date   *date*
la   demi-pension   *half-board*
la   femme de chambre   *maid*
le   garçon   *waiter*
un   incendie   *fire*
le   patron   *manager*
la   pension   *board, guest house*
la   pension complète   *full board*
le   petit déjeuner   *breakfast*
le   prix maximum   *maximum price*
le   prix minimum   *minimum price*
le/la   réceptionniste   *receptionist*
la   valise   *suitcase*

apprécier   *to appreciate*
appuyer/APPUYEZ   *to press/PRESS*
arriver   *to arrive*
déranger   *to disturb*
partir   *to leave*
se plaindre   *to complain*
pousser/POUSSEZ   *to push/PUSH*
prendre un repas   *to have a meal*
regretter   *to regret*
remplacer   *to replace*
réserver   *to reserve*
réveiller   *to wake up*
revenir   *to return*
stationner   *to park*
téléphoner à   *to telephone*
tirer/TIREZ   *to pull/PULL*
trouver   *to find*
vouloir   *to want, to wish*

autre   *other*
disponible   *available*
en supplément   *extra*
inclus   *included*
non compris   *not included*
occupé   *occupied*
satisfait   *satisfied*
seul   *alone*

avec   *with*
pour   *for*
sans   *without*

Est-ce qu'il vous reste des chambres libres?   *Have you any free rooms left?*
Non, je regrette, tout est occupé.   *No, I'm afraid not, we are full.*
Pour combien de personnes et pour combien de temps?   *For how many people and for how long?*
Une grande chambre avec deux lits, ça vous convient?   *A big room with two beds, is that all right for you?*
Ça coûte combien?   *How much does it cost?*
Vous n'avez rien de moins cher?   *Have you anything cheaper?*
Ça ira très bien. Nous les prenons.   *That'll do fine. We'll take them.*
Est-ce que le petit déjeuner est compris?   *Is breakfast included?*
Le petit déjeuner est servi à partir de huit heures jusqu'à dix heures.   *Breakfast is served from 8.00 to 10.00 a.m.*
Puis-je monter mes bagages maintenant?   *May I take my luggage up now?*
Avant, il faut remplir la fiche.   *Before that you must fill in the form.*
Votre passeport, s'il vous plaît.   *Your passport, please.*
Voici votre clé. Chambre numéro vingt-deux.   *Here is your key. Room number 22.*
Il y a un parking à l'arrière.   *There is a car-park at the back.*
Je voudrais réserver une chambre pour trois nuits.   *I'd like to reserve a room for three nights.*
Je voudrais une chambre qui donne sur la mer.   *I'd like a room overlooking the sea.*
Vous avez une chambre avec salle de bains?   *Have you a room with a bathroom?*
Malheureusement, ça ne me convient pas. Au revoir, madame.   *I'm afraid that doesn't suit me. Goodbye, madam.*
Tant pis, je prends la chambre.   *Never mind, I'll take the room.*
C'est cent cinquante francs pour la chambre, service et taxes compris.   *It's 150 francs for the room, service and VAT included.*

Reservation problems

J'ai fait une réservation par téléphone.   *I made a reservation by phone.*
C'est à quel nom?   *What name?*
C'est bien ça?   *Is that it?*
Vous êtes sûr(e)?   *Are you sure?*
Qu'est-ce que je vais faire?   *What shall I do?*
Je suis très déçu(e).   *I am very disappointed.*
Je vous prie de bien vouloir nous excuser.   *Please do accept our apologies.*

Asking for extras

Je voudrais des cintres, s'il vous plaît.   *I'd like some coat-hangers, please.*
Est-ce que je peux avoir une serviette de bain?   *May I have a bath towel?*
Il manque un oreiller.   *There's a pillow missing.*
On va vous en apporter un tout de suite.   *We'll bring you one straight away.*

Complaints

Je voudrais avoir une autre chambre.   *I would like another room.*
La lampe ne marche pas.   *The lamp does not work.*

Le lavabo est bouché.   *The washbasin is blocked.*
Il n'y a plus de papier hygiénique.   *There is no more toilet paper.*
Il ne reste plus de savon.   *There is no soap left.*
Le robinet d'eau froide a une fuite.   *The cold-water tap leaks.*
La douche ne marche pas.   *The shower doesn't work.*
On va arranger ça tout de suite.   *We'll deal with that straight away.*
On va s'en occuper immédiatement.   *We'll see to that immediately.*

YOUTH HOSTEL

une auberge de jeunesse   *youth hostel*
un   avantage   *advantage, facility*
la   bienvenue   *welcome*
le   bureau   *office*
la   carte   *card*
la   carte d'adhérent   *member's card*
la   couverture   *blanket*
la   cuisine   *kitchen*
le   dortoir   *dormitory*
le   drap-sac   *sheet sleeping bag*
l'   eau chaude (f)   *hot water*
un   inconvénient   *drawback*
le   linge   *linen*
la   nuit   *night*
une paire de draps   *a pair of sheets*
la   poubelle   *dustbin*
les provisions (f)   *food*
le   responsable   *organiser, leader*
le   sac de couchage   *sleeping bag*
la   salle à manger   *dining room*
la   salle de jeux   *games room*
le   séjour   *stay*
le   silence   *silence*
le   tarif   *price list*
le   visiteur   *visitor*

aider   *to help*
balayer   *to sweep*
fermer   *to close*
garder   *to keep*
louer   *to hire*
organiser   *to organise*
ouvrir   *to open*
payer   *to pay*
ranger   *to tidy, to put away*
remercier   *to thank*

complet/complète   *full*
défendu   *forbidden*
obligatoire   *obligatory, compulsory*

toute l'année   *all year round*
sauf   *except*

CAMPING

les allumettes (f)   *matches*
le   bac à vaisselle   *washing-up sink*
le   bloc sanitaire   *toilet block*
la   bouteille de gaz   *gas cylinder*
le   campeur   *camper*
le   camping   *campsite*
la   caravane   *caravan*
le   carnet de camping   *camping card*
la   cuisinière à gaz   *gas cooker*

la   cuvette   *washing-up bowl*
l'   eau non-potable (f)   *non-drinking water*
l'   électricité (f)   *electricity*
un   emplacement   *site, pitch*
le   feu de camp   *camp-fire*
les installations sanitaires (f)   *toilets*
le   journal   *newspaper, diary*
la   lampe électrique   *torch*
le   lave-linge   *washing machine*
la   laverie   *launderette*
la   lessive   *washing (clothes), washing powder*
le   lit de camp   *camp bed*
le   matériel de camping   *camping equipment*
la   prise de courant   *power point*
les provisions (f)   *food*
le   supplément   *extra payment*
la   tente   *tent*
le   terrain de camping   *campsite*
le   véhicule   *vehicle*

camper   *to camp*
chercher   *to look for*
coûter   *to cost*
débarrasser   *to clear*
faire du camping   *to go camping*
faire la cuisine   *to cook*
indiquer   *to indicate, to show*
se laver   *to get washed*
monter la tente   *to put up the tent*
payer   *to pay*
plier   *to fold*
surveiller   *to supervise*

à emporter   *to take away*
à proximité de   *near to*
complet/complète   *full*
froid   *cold*
loin   *far*
moderne   *modern*
municipal   *of the town*
propre   *clean*
quand même   *all the same*
sale   *dirty*
serré   *crowded*
simple   *simple*

Est-ce qu'il vous reste de la place pour une caravane?   *Have you room left for a caravan?*
Combien de personnes?   *How many people?*
Nous avons besoin d'un tire-bouchon et des piles.   *We need a corkscrew and some batteries.*
Le camp est éclairé la nuit?   *Is the camp lit up at night?*
Il y a un gardien toute la nuit.   *There is a warden all night.*
L'eau est potable.   *The water is drinkable.*
Je vais vous montrer votre emplacement.   *I will show you your pitch.*
Est-ce qu'il est à l'ombre?   *Is it in the shade?*
Est-ce qu'il est permis d'allumer un barbecue?   *Are we allowed to light a barbecue?*
Il est interdit de faire du feu dans le camp.   *It is forbidden to light a fire in the camp.*
Est-ce que le camp est fermé la nuit?   *Is the camp closed at night?*

HOLIDAY HOME IN FRANCE

la   chambre d'hôte   *guest room, B + B*
la   chasse   *hunting*

un   ensemble de bâtiments   *group of buildings*
le   gîte   *gîte, simple self-catering house*
la   grange   *barn*
la   location de vélos   *cycle hire*
la   réclamation   *complaint, claim*
le   terrain   *plot, area of land*
le   vendange   *grape picking*
le   vigneron   *vine grower*
le   vignoble   *vineyard*

améliorer   *to improve*
aménager   *to furnish, to equip*
attendre   *to wait (for)*
cueillir des fruits   *to pick fruit*
cultiver   *to cultivate, to grow*
demander   *to ask (for)*
égarer   *to lead astray*

faire la récolte   *to reap the harvest*
louer   *to hire*
se plaindre   *to complain*
se présenter   *to introduce oneself*
rendre   *to give back*
transformer   *to change*
vouloir voir   *to want to see*

ailleurs   *elsewhere*
au mois de   *in the month of*
en bon état   *in good condition*
en mauvais état   *in bad condition*
hors saison   *out of season*
indépendant   *independent*
libre   *free*
occupé   *occupied*
provisoire   *temporary*

▷ E4 The wider world

FRENCH-SPEAKING AND OTHER COUNTRIES

country		adjective	inhabitant
l' Europe (f)	*Europe*	européen/européenne	un(e) Européen(ne)
l' Allemagne (f)	*Germany*	allemand	un(e) Allemand(e)
l' Angleterre (f)	*England*	anglais	un(e) Anglais(e)
la Grande-Bretagne	*GB*	britannique	un(e) Britannique
le Royaume-Uni	*UK*		
la Belgique	*Belgium*	belge	un(e) Belge
le Canada	*Canada*	canadien/canadienne	un(e) Canadien(ne)
le Danemark	*Denmark*	danois	un(e) Danois(e)
l' Espagne (f)	*Spain*	espagnol	un(e) Espagnol(e)
la France	*France*	français	un(e) Français(e)
la Grèce	*Greece*	grec/greque	un Grec, une Greque
la Hollande	*Holland*	hollandais	un(e) Hollandais(e)
les Pays Bas	*Netherlands*	néerlandais	un(e) Néerlandais(e)
l' Italie (f)	*Italy*	italien/italienne	un(e) Italien(ne)
le Luxembourg	*Luxembourg*	luxembourgeois	un(e) Luxembourgeois(e)
le Portugal	*Portugal*	portugais	un(e) Portugais(e)
la Suisse	*Switzerland*	suisse	un(e) Suisse

Other countries

l' Amérique (f)	*America*	américain	un(e) Américain(e)
les Etats-Unis	*USA*	américain	un(e) Américain(e)
la Chine	*China*	chinois	un(e) Chinois(e)
l' Ecosse (f)	*Scotland*	écossais	un(e) Ecossais(e)
l' Inde (f)	*India*	indien/indienne	un(e) Indien(ne)
l' Irlande du Nord (f)	*Northern Ireland*	irlandais	un(e) Irlandais(e)
l' Irlande du Sud (f)	*Eire*	irlandais	un(e) Irlandais(e)
le Japon	*Japan*	japonais	un(e) Japonais(e)
le Pays de Galles	*Wales*	gallois	un(e) Gallois(e)
la Russie	*Russia*	russe	un(e) Russe

D'où venez-vous?   *Where do you come from?*
Où êtes-vous né(e)?   *Where were you born?*
Je suis anglais(e).   *I am English.*
Je suis de nationalité britannique.   *I am British. (or other nationality)*

PEOPLE

un/une adolescent/adolescente   *adolescent*
les   ados (m/f)   *kids, teenagers*
un   adulte   *adult*
le/la   célibataire   *bachelor/spinster*

la   dame   *lady*
     Dames   *Ladies*
le/la   divorcé/divorcée   *divorcee*
un/une   étranger/étrangère   *foreigner*
la   femme   *woman, wife*
la   (jeune) fille   *girl*
le   garçon   *boy*
les   gens (m)   *people*
l'   homme (m)   *man*
     Hommes   *Gentlemen*
le   jeune homme   *young man*
une   jeune personne   *young person*

le	mari	*husband*
	Messieurs	*Gentlemen*
le	pays d'origine	*country of origin*
le	veuf	*widower*
la	veuve	*widow*

+ *nationalities - see table on p. 65*

féminin	*feminine*
fiancé	*engaged*
marié	*married*
masculin	*masculine*
séparé	*separated*

▶ E5 World events and issues

une	actualité	*piece of news*
les	armements (m)	*armaments, arms*
un	article	*article*
le	braconnage	*poaching*
le	cas	*case*
le	catastrophe	*disaster*
la	chasse	*hunting*
le	réchauffement général	*global warming*
le	chômage	*unemployment*
la	crise	*crisis*
le	développement	*development*
la	disparition de la forêt	*deforestation*
l'	eau (f)	*water*
l'	effet de serre (m)	*greenhouse effect*
une	élection	*election*
un	employeur	*employer*
l'	énergie (f)	*energy*
une	enquête	*enquiry*
l'	environnement (m)	*environment*
une	époque	*period of time*
une	espèce	*species*
un	événement	*event*
la	faim	*hunger, famine*
le	gouvernement	*government*
la	grève	*strike*
la	guerre	*war*
l'	habitat (m)	*habitat*
un	immigré	*immigrant*
un	impôt	*tax*
une	information	*piece of news*
les	informations (f)	*news*
le	maire	*mayor*
la	maladie	*disease*
la	manif(estation)	*demo(nstration)*

le	niveau de vie	*standard of living*
la	nourriture	*food, nutrition*
une	nouvelle	*piece of news*
une	opération	*operation*
la	pauvreté	*poverty*
la	pluie acide	*acid rain*
la	politique	*policy*
la	pollution	*pollution*
le	premier ministre	*prime minister*
le	président	*president*
le	problème	*problem*
la	question	*question*
la	richesse	*wealth*
la	sécheresse	*drought*
la	securité sociale	*social security*
le	SIDA	*AIDS*
la	solution	*solution*
le	syndicat	*trade union*
le	Tiers Monde	*Third World*
le	titre	*title*
la	violence	*violence*
la	vivisection	*vivisection*

admirer	*to admire*
améliorer	*to improve*
augmenter	*to increase, to augment*
avoir lieu	*to take place*
déclarer	*to declare*
défendre	*to defend, to forbid*
diminuer	*to diminish*
fondre	*to melt*
se passer	*to happen*
persuader	*to persuade*
se produire	*to happen*
promettre	*to promise*
protester	*to protest*
remarquer	*to notice*

à cause de	*because of*
de droite	*on the political right*
de gauche	*on the political left*
étonnant	*surprising*
grave	*serious*
important	*important*
menacé	*threatened*
nucléaire	*nuclear*
probable	*probable*
récent	*recent*
social	*social*

▶ **Learning vocabulary**

This is one of the chores of learning a foreign language. One thing is certain. If you sit down the night before your first examination and attempt to learn 2000 words you will know very few indeed the next morning. You would be far better to have a regular time of day (or perhaps two occasions in the day) when you sit down and spend 10–15 minutes learning vocabulary. And the sooner you start, the better – so start today! This really requires somewhere private, or at least somewhere where you won't be disturbed. So your room, somewhere quiet in school at break or lunch-time, or even on public transport would be suitable. What isn't suitable is trying to do it while talking or listening to someone else, or watching *Neighbours*. Don't kid yourself you are working when you aren't.

As well as having a good place to do it, it's as well to be methodical. Work through the vocabulary topics, changing them daily. Don't try to learn too many words at once. And try to relate them to a situation, rather than just working through an alphabetical list. It's more interesting to learn, say, everything to do with changing money than just 40 words which happen to begin with the same letter.

Begin your sessions with a written test on what you did last time. This could be half and half French-English, English-French. Don't cheat, but check your test afterwards with the vocabulary lists. If you did well, reward yourself with a sweet or something. Keep a record of how you have done so you can see your progress.

While you are learning vocabulary, I strongly recommend *doing* something. The best is to write out each word or phrase two or three times. (It doesn't matter if you can't read it afterwards. Go for speed!) Make sure of accents. Include the gender for nouns, and the past participle for verbs.

If you haven't anywhere to write, you can still test yourself using a piece of card or paper cut or folded as shown below:

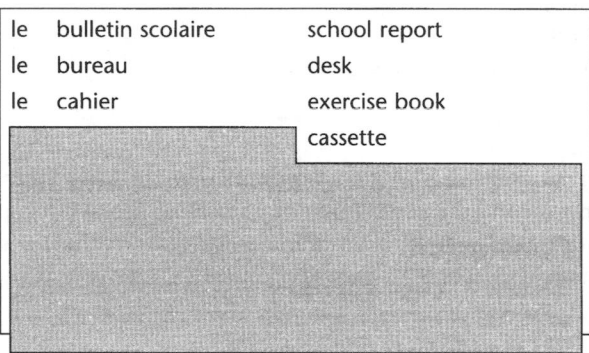

le	bulletin scolaire	school report
le	bureau	desk
le	cahier	exercise book
la	cassette	cassette
la	chaise	chair
le	cours	lesson
la	craie	chalk

1 Select a vocabulary topic to learn.

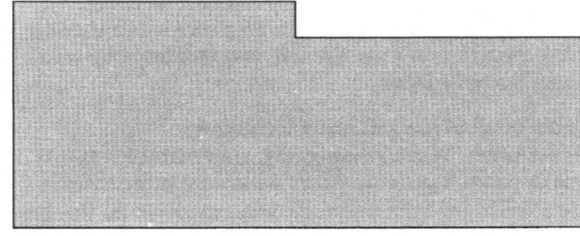

2 Cut out the shape **blind** as shown above out of card or paper.

le	bulletin scolaire	school report
le	bureau	desk
le	cahier	exercise book
		cassette

3 Place blind over the list so that the next English word is shown. Try to remember what the word should be in French.

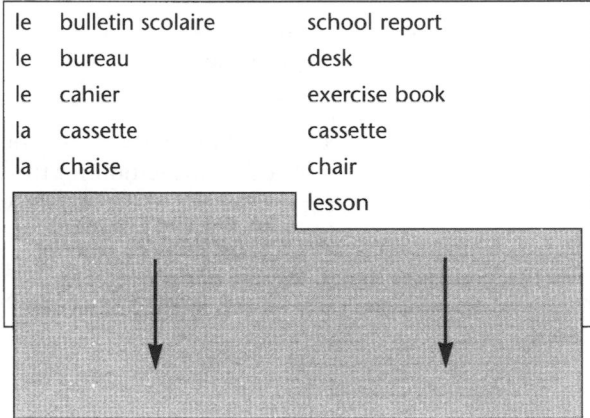

le	bulletin scolaire	school report
le	bureau	desk
le	cahier	exercise book
la	cassette	cassette
la	chaise	chair
		lesson

4 Move the blind down the list. This will reveal the correct French word; check if you were right. Now try the next English word.

le	bulletin scolaire	school report
le	bureau	desk
le	cahier	

5 When you have finished testing yourself on remembering the French words, you can turn the blind over so that the English words are covered up and see if you know what the English translations are.

First cover the English column on your list and see if you can say what the French words mean. Then turn the blind over and see if you can say what the French should be (including gender or past participle, as before). You can also use the blind to give yourself a written test. You immediately find out if you were right as you move it down to the next word. No peeping!

Students often like to learn vocabulary with a friend. This is fine as a way of learning what the English version of French words is, and for checking gender and past participles. However, unless someone is writing, then spelling accuracy is not likely to be improved. You will know that certain sounds in French can be spelt in several ways (e.g. *manger, mangeais, mangé,* and the similar *mon jet*). This makes precise personal proficiency very important. It's no help to you in the exam if your friend can do it. Make sure *you* can do it!

▶ A STEP FURTHER

Some people find it useful to learn ten words about a particular subject. For example, you could write down ten words about transport.

la voiture	l'avion
le vélo	la moto
l'autobus	le ferry
le taxi	le bateau
le train	l'aéroglisseur

Now make up a sentence for each one, for example:

Je vais à Calais en voiture.

Other topics which lend themselves to this treatment include:

clothes	vegetables
weather	food in general
school subjects	sports
furniture	hobbies
shops	buildings
professions	feelings and opinions
fruit	

There are many other possibilities.

Another suggestion for the vocabulary fiend is to get a box similar to an After Eights box, eat the mints and discard the wrappers, and then cut up bits of card from cereal packets to fit in. You then write the French on one side at the top and the English on the other, gradually replacing words you know with new ones. You can then test yourself, and make the tests as easy or as difficult as suits you.

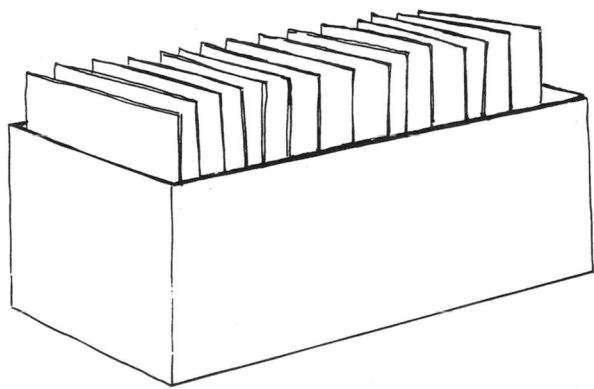

As well as formal learning of vocabulary, the more French you read and listen to, the better your understanding will become. So do follow the hints given in Chapter 1 'Study skills'.

If you have the chance to pay a visit to a French-speaking country, remember to make the most of it by trying out what you have learned. Even if you are only making a day trip, it is surprising how much reading matter you can pick up free or very cheaply from the tourist office and handouts in shops, etc. Much of that will be very helpful for the topics tested in GCSE French.

In any case, learn a little but often, with variety, testing yourself as you go, and writing things down to improve your writing. The more French you read and listen to, the better.

Listening

 GETTING STARTED

Listening comprehension in GCSE is something everyone has to do. There is no doubt that it is a test which worries a lot of students. However, there is a great deal you can do to make it a little easier on the day. As elsewhere in GCSE French, knowing what to expect is half the battle.

Candidates will be required to show their ability to understand genuine French in a range of straightforward 'survival' situations, such as shopping and using hotels and restaurants, and to understand some more complex pieces. Those who have made good use of the practice their teacher has given them in these skills should not find it hard to score high marks.

This chapter contains information about things which seem to be tested particularly frequently, based on an analysis of the Examining Groups' sample papers and on experience of what has been tested in previous GCSE papers. Forewarned is forearmed!

And finally, this chapter refers to the tape which comes with this book, which has extracts from GCSE-type Listening Tests on it. There are transcripts of the passages chosen in the chapter, which should help a great deal when you are preparing for the test. You will find, for example, that you can get used to the sort of speed and accents the Examining Groups use, and to the level of sound effects they insert.

 WHAT YOU NEED TO KNOW

The Listening Test

Listening is a test which is taken by all GCSE candidates, no matter how good or weak they are. Whichever category you fall into, make sure that you gain the maximum credit for your efforts.

All the Examining Groups set Listening Tests which involve the texts you hear being pre-recorded on cassette by native speakers of French. They also agree that you should hear each bit of French twice. There will also be a limited amount of background noise to add to the realism of the situation. Normally these recordings will be played back to you in a smallish room or through a language laboratory if your school has one. It is probably wise, therefore, to check that you know exactly where your Listening Test will be held, as it's not safe to assume it will be in the school hall, gym or canteen like other written examinations.

A related point is that there are two different tests, one for Foundation Tier candidates, and one for Higher Tier candidates. These will go on in different rooms at the same time, so make sure you go to the right place.

If your school has a large number of candidates, it is possible that there will be two 'sittings' for the Listening Test. Again, make sure you go to the right place. There will also be arrangements preventing those who have taken the test from communicating with those who haven't yet done so. Don't lay yourself open to accusations of cheating by trying to talk to people in another 'sitting' for the Listening Test.

Listening comprehension in the form used by the GCSE Examining Groups is a rather unnatural activity. Few of us sit at home answering questions in answer booklets while listening to the weather forecast on a daily basis – and virtually none of us record the weather forecast so we can hear it again a few moments later! And when we do listen to a foreign language and need to understand it, we are usually in a situation where there are other clues such as facial expression, location and gesture to help us to understand. It is therefore as well to gain a little practice in doing it in the manner the Examining Groups use before the actual examination – not even a visit to France can simulate the GCSE examination situation for you!

There is some variation in the length of the Foundation Tier Listening Test. Check the Appendix at the end of this book to see what your Examining Group does.

▷ **Examining Group requirements**

There is a broad measure of agreement among the Examining Groups as to what should be tested, and how. All Groups stress that Listening involves language that is meant to be heard, for example:

▷ conversations
▷ interviews and discussions
▷ arguments
▷ public announcements (shops, campsites, train stations)
▷ advertisements
▷ verbal instructions and requests
▷ news broadcasts, weather forecasts and traffic reports
▷ monologues (one person talking on his/her own)
▷ telephone calls.

They specifically exclude language which was **not** intended to be read out loud, for example:

▷ extracts from novels
▷ extracts from magazines and newspapers.

The Examining Groups also agree on the following points.

1   You shouldn't be at a disadvantage in the tests if your memory isn't very good. This means that the passages of French you have to listen to are kept short, and in some cases, very short. Longer passages are often broken up with a pause. In recent papers passages have not greatly exceeded 150 words without a break, and many will be rather shorter. 150 words take about two minutes to read.
2   The French stimulus should:

▷ be pre-recorded on cassette by native speakers of French
▷ give each bit of French twice
▷ have a limited amount of background noise
▷ have some limited sound effects to add to the realism of the situation.

3   Between 80% and 90% of the marks will be for questions and answers in French. The remaining questions and answers will be in English. Some Examining Groups use the English questions at the very easy and very difficult ends of the papers, and others use them in the middle area. Check with your teacher what your board does.
4   They will print a booklet for you to write your answers under the question. This has the advantage that you are less likely to miss out a question.

Foundation Tier

The Foundation Tier allows performances between grades G and C. For assessment purposes, the Examining Groups distinguish between grade G, F, E tasks and performances and grade D, C tasks and performances.

Grade G, F, E tasks will be set using a limited range of vocabulary. Every Examining Group publishes a **Minimum Core Vocabulary** of about 1500 words. The questions targeting these grades will only be drawn from the Minimum Core Vocabulary. Most of the vocabulary will have been covered in the early years of learning French. Because dictionaries are either not allowed at all or only allowed in limited circumstances (see below) it is likely that the questions and answers will be based virtually entirely on these straightforward vocabulary items.

The tasks set will require candidates:

▷ to identify and note the main points of what they have heard
▷ to extract specific details.

Some Groups set some easy questions in English, with English answers, for these target grades. Others will use mainly objective-type questions involving box-ticking, multiple choice or matching descriptions.

Grade D, C tasks will usually involve listening to longer passages of French, and most of the questions will be in French, requiring answers in French. As well as objective-type tests, there may be a requirement to write a few words in French. The vocabulary covered in this section will not be limited to the words in the Minimum Core Vocabulary.

The tasks set will require candidates:

- to identify and note the main points of what they have read
- to extract specific details
- to identify points of view
- to show some understanding of unfamiliar language
- to show some understanding of familiar language in unfamiliar contexts
- to understand references to past, present and future events.

Higher Tier

The Higher Tier allows performances between grades D and A*. For assessment purposes, the Examining Groups distinguish between grade D, C tasks and performances and grade B, A, A* tasks and performances.

Grade D, C tasks and the type of listening skills expected are identical with those in Foundation Tier at these grades.

Grade B, A, A* tasks will involve listening to longer passages in French. Again, the vocabulary used will be considerably more extensive than that listed in the Minimum Core Vocabulary. Some answers may involve your writing in French.

The tasks set will require candidates:

- to identify and note the main points and themes of what they have heard
- to listen for the gist of a passage
- to extract specific details
- to identify points of view
- to recognise attitudes and emotions
- to show some understanding of unfamiliar language
- to show some understanding of familiar language in unfamiliar contexts
- to understand references to past, present and future events
- to infer meaning from context
- to come to conclusions from what is said.

Apart from the candidate's ability to deal with a longer passage, there are some other additional things which the examiners are looking for in questions targeted at Grades D and above. These are outlined below.

In questions targeted at grades D and above, the French you hear will be rather more natural than that targeted at grades E, F and G, in that it will contain many of the features of ordinary speakers. Listen to a tape recording of someone who is not a professional speaker in English – a friend of yours, for example – and you will find that they hesitate, they repeat themselves, they rephrase things, they say 'um' rather a lot, and generally are not as polished as, say, a newsreader. The French for Higher Listening will contain these features of speech, although not to such an extent as to render it unreasonably difficult.

In addition, there will be a variety of 'registers'. In English, you will know that there is a difference between the way, say, a lawyer speaks and the way teenagers speak. This is 'register'. People also use different registers on different occasions, choosing different vocabulary when, say, addressing a public meeting or talking to their best friend. This difference will be reflected in the GCSE. Examples of registers which may be used include:

- TV and radio
- the language used in the family
- the language used by young people of your age
- the language used on such formal occasions as, for example, official town-twinning receptions.

Dictionary use

Most examining groups do not allow the use of dictionaries during the Listening Test. This is because their use can distract both the user and the other candidates. However, NEAB and WJEC/CBAC do allow use of a bilingual dictionary in the 5 minutes before the tape is played and in the 5 minutes after the tape has finished. Check with your teacher beforehand whether this applies to you, and come prepared.

▶ **Effective answers**

Let us now look at how to answer the questions most effectively. First of all, as everywhere in this examination, you must read the question carefully. This includes the setting given with each text, which will give you valuable clues as to what to expect. These clues are absolutely vital to you in Listening, as they may well contain proper names written out, which might otherwise put you off if you only heard them. The importance of reading the setting cannot be emphasised too strongly. Too many candidates don't even look at it and make silly mistakes as a result. If the questions require answers in French, the setting will be in simple French.

All Examining Groups print a booklet for you to write your answers under the question. This has the advantage that you are less likely to miss out a question.

It is important that you answer the questions in the correct language. Most of the answers to questions in French will be of the objective tick-box type. But if they require you to write a word or phrase in French, you will get no marks if you answer in English, even if you have understood the passage. This may seem somewhat alarming. However, as long as your French is comprehensible (i.e. gets the message across), you will get your mark.

Questions in English will more often require you to write a few words. It is **vital** that you write in English. There will be **no** credit given for answers in French to questions in English, however devastatingly excellent the French you write. Examiners have been fairly tolerant of errors in English spelling in the past, so that should not be a worry if your spelling is poor. WJEC gives the option of answering in Welsh.

Before you hear each piece of French, you will have a few moments to read the questions. Make sure you do so, because only then will you know which details to listen out for.

During the first hearing of the French, you should try to form a theory as to what the answers to the questions are. If you are allowed to take notes during the playing of the French (and most Examining Groups do allow this), make sure they are very brief. It's really much better to write telegram-style notes than to attempt to scribble down a complete sentence.

For example, if there is a question asking about when the train arrives, write:

arr 16.00.

If you attempt to write *Le train arrive à 16.00*, by the time you have done so the second playing of the extract will already be over and you will have no means of checking your theory.

During the second playing of the French you should then attempt to check your theory, before writing the answer you have decided on in the space provided.

The answers need not be in full sentences, so don't waste time writing lengthy sentences in English (or French, for that matter). For example, if the question is 'When does the train arrive?' there is no need to write: 'According to the recording I have just heard, the time of arrival of the train is 16.00'. By the time you have written that, you will have missed the next three questions! And in Listening, there is no chance of hearing the French more than twice. Your primary school and first and second year secondary teachers may have insisted on the sort of answer which 'contains the question'. You can forget that now! The ideal GCSE French answer to that question is: '16.00'. Go for short answers, although not so short that they don't fully answer the question!

If you have to give a time or a price, write it clearly in figures, saying what units you are using.

Most candidates write very clearly. There is, however, no doubt that a near illegible or messy script runs the risk of prejudicing an intolerant examiner against you. So if you have made notes or alterations, cross out clearly what is not needed, and make sure that there is no doubt about what you intend to be marked.

It is worth knowing that questions on longer passages are usually set in sequence. So the third question on a passage, for example, will refer to a point later in the passage than the second, and so on. This knowledge is particularly helpful if you are struggling with a passage and only understand some of it!

Another point worth knowing is that, if there is more than one mark allocated for a question, it is highly likely that there is more than one piece of information or detail required. Look for extra things to say – as long as you can find them in the French! On the other hand, the two marks may be given for saying that there is , for example, *un vieux* (1 mark) *chien* (1 mark) – so make sure you include all the details.

Some Examining Groups have set questions where there are, say, two marks, but four possible answers. Practice among Examination Groups has differed where candidates have given more answers than the minimum. But on objective-type questions there is always a penalty for ticking more boxes than requested. On the other hand, if you are faced with multiple-choice questions, or true/false questions for Listening, remember this tip: even if you aren't sure of the answer, be sure to tick one of the boxes – you could be right!

The objective-type questions which will be very common in GCSE French after 1998 will inevitably test such things as:

- tables to fill in
- charts
- lists to complete
- simple maps to interpret and with perhaps a route to shade
- pictures to compare
- simple arithmetic.

Despite what the Examining Groups say, these skills will be tested in addition to French. Examiners do attempt to keep things as simple as possible, but do ask to try as many sample papers as possible.

▷ Which vocabulary topics?

Many of the questions will be seeking an answer about:

Who?	How long?
What?	How many?
Where?	How much?
When?	Why?

A moment's thought will point you towards the vocabulary topics which are most likely to be covered by each of those questions:

Who?	family and friends
	professions
	descriptions: physical appearance, size, age, character
What?	virtually all objects, prices, and instructions and activities
	food and drink, shopping, free time and entertainment
Where?	positions and prepositions
	location of buildings in town and country
	countries, directions and distances
When?	time by the 12-hour and 24-hour clocks
	time in relation to other events
How long?	time, especially duration
How many?	numbers
How much?	quantity, numbers
Why?	reasons

The questions targeted at grades D and above, but most particularly those measuring grades B, A and A*, test your ability to pick out attitudes and emotions. So it is clear that adjectives which describe opinions and characteristics of things and people will repay some special study.

A little time spent in directed preparation will not go amiss.

Analysis of the sample papers suggests that there are some matters which seem to be measured rather often by Listening papers. It is clear that the following will be well worth making sure of:

1 Telling the time, using the everyday, 12-hour clock, way (*il est deux heures et demie*, etc.) and the timetable, 24-hour clock, way (*le train arrive à quatorze heures trente*, etc.). You can practise this with a friend, setting each other times to write down and seeing how well you do.

2 Dates and days of the week crop up a lot. These, too, can be practised with the help of a friend.

3 Money, particularly French money (but there are also Swiss and Belgian francs, not to mention Canadian dollars). Make sure you know, and can write down from normal

French speech, all the variations. Some examiners are still prone to giving you a choice between 2F 60 and 2F 16 as the correct meaning of *deux francs soixante* (when 2F 60 is the correct answer). So you need to be absolutely certain of the numbers to 100, especially the tens. Again, practise with a friend.

4   Directions (*tournez à droite, à gauche, passez le pont*, etc.), and positions (*en face de, à côté de, près de*, etc.). If you have trouble with left and right on maps, you should put in a bit of practice.

5   School subjects seem to appear more often than might be expected. So make sure you know them.

▶ EXAMINATION QUESTIONS

Every extract in this chapter is recorded on the audio tape. You are recommended to try the questions before checking with the student answers.

In case of difficulty, I have included transcripts of the passages at the end of the chapter so that you can refer to them to see where the answers came from.

Foundation Tier G, F, E grade tasks

In the case of the shorter extracts, I have put a short series of questions together on the tape, so that you will get a flavour of what a section of the examination paper will be like.

Find extract 1 on the audio tape, then attempt to do the questions set on it before looking at the student answer I have reproduced. Remember to read the question and the setting for the question beforehand. The setting is intended to help you by giving you a few clues as to what might occur.

▷ **Extract I**   *Vous êtes chez votre correspondante française, Janine.*
Janine vous montre la maison.

1   Indiquez la salle à manger sur le plan (avec un X).   *(1)*

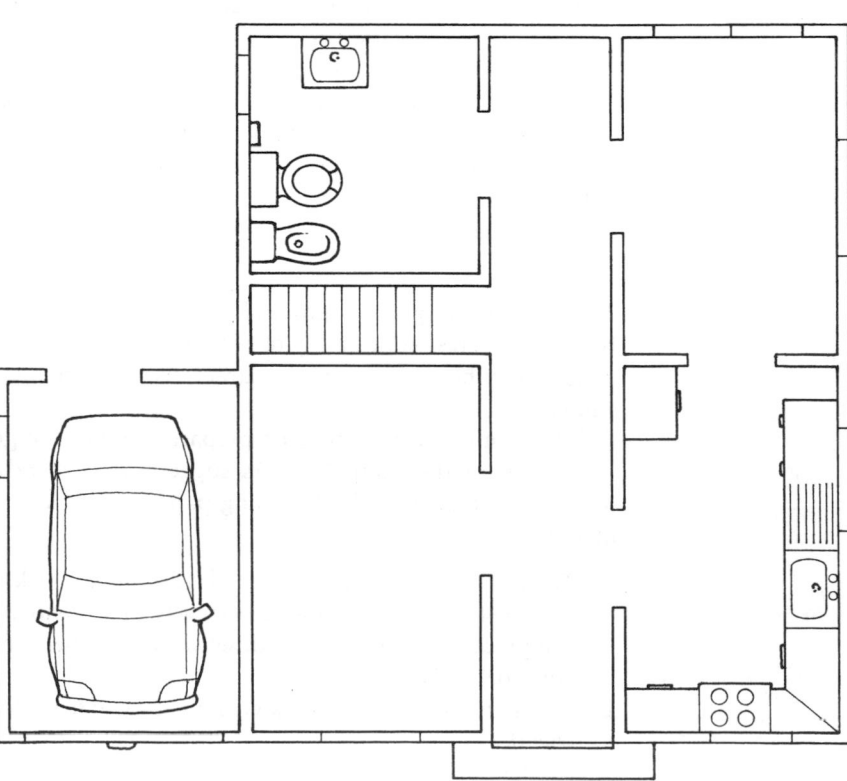

2   Vous regardez l'emploi du temps de Janine au collège.
    Janine, qu'est-ce qu'elle a le vendredi matin?
    Remplissez les cases vides.

jeudi		vendredi	
9h	Anglais	9h	
10h	Sciences	10h	Histoire
11h	Français	11h	

(2)

3   Janine vous parle du déjeuner au collège.
    Qu'est-ce que c'est?
    Cochez la bonne case.   *(1)*

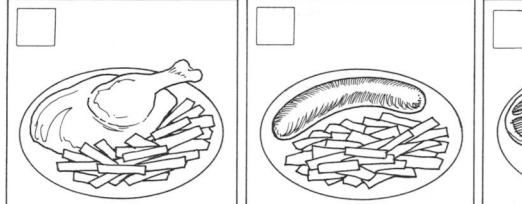 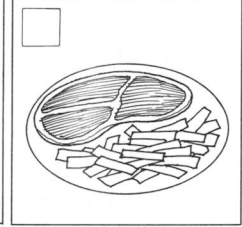 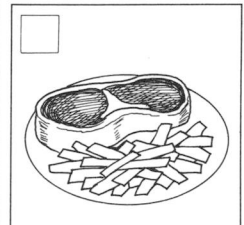

4   A quelle heure est-ce que vous allez manger?
    Ecrivez l'heure en chiffres.   *(1)*

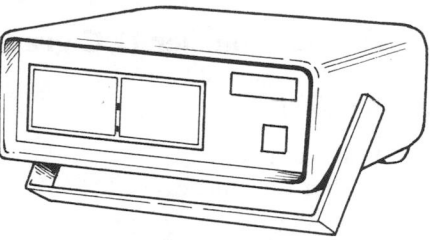

5   Qu'est-ce que vous allez faire après le collège?
    Cochez la bonne case.   *(1)*

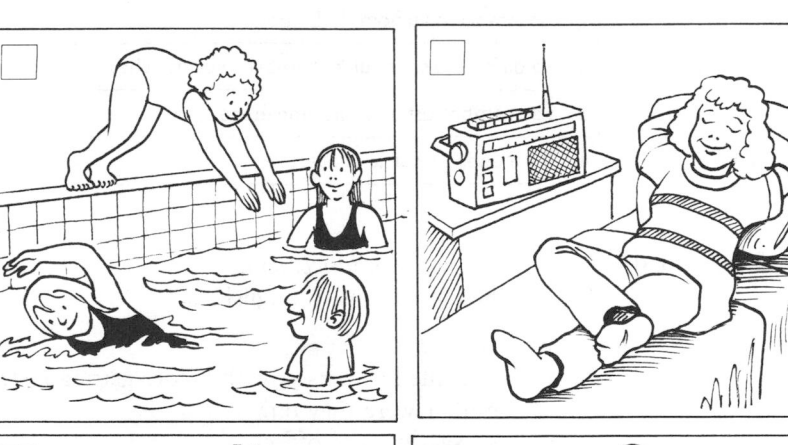

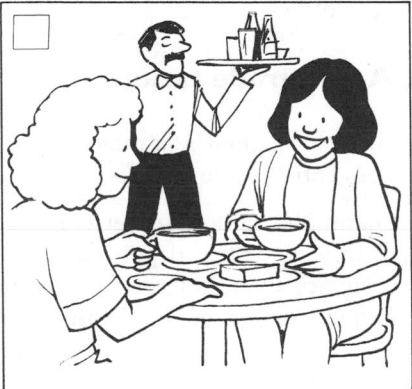 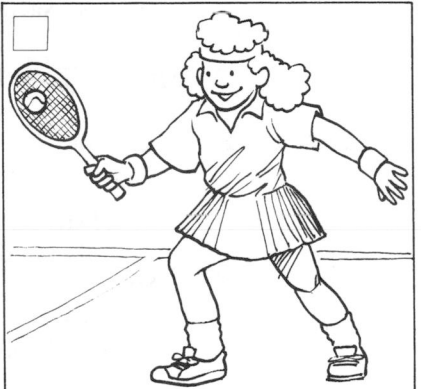

▷ **Extract 2**   *Vous écoutez la radio. Il y a la météo. Quel temps fait-il? Regardez les dessins.*

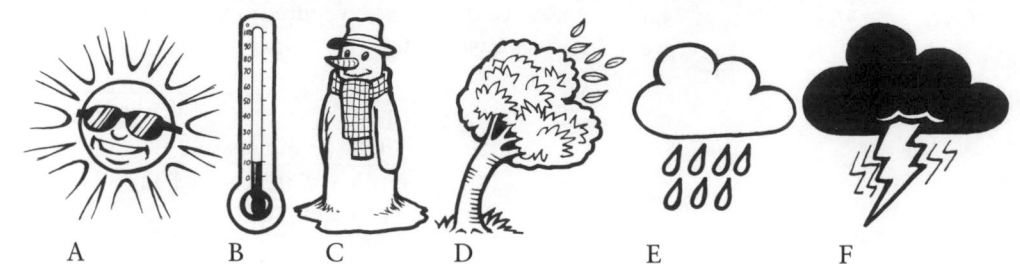

A   B   C   D   E   F

Ecoutez la météo.
Choisissez le dessin qui correspond à la météo pour chaque ville.
Ecrivez la bonne lettre dans la case.

ville	lettre
Exemple: Paris	$\boxed{E}$
1 Bordeaux	☐
2 Nantes	☐
3 Clermont-Ferrand	☐
4 Grenoble	☐
5 Calais	☐

(5)

Foundation Tier D, C grade tasks, Higher Tier D, C grade tasks

▷ **Extract 3**   *A l'hôtel*

Vrai ou faux?
Cochez la bonne case   *(4)*

	vrai	faux
Exemple: Hôtel de la Poste.	✓	
1 Réservation au nom de Dubois.		
2 La dame a réservé une chambre avec douche.		
3 La chambre est au troisième étage.		
4 Il y a une vue sur le château.		

▷ **Extract 4**   *Listen to a shop announcement.*
Answer these questions **in English**.

1   Who is lost?   *(1)*
2   Who was the lost person with before getting lost?   *(1)*
3   Which floor were they on?   *(1)*
4   Where exactly is the office?   *(2)*

Higher Tier B, A, A* grade tasks

▷ **Extract 5**   Voici les gros titres des informations à la radio.
<u>Soulignez</u> les différences entre ce que vous lisez et ce que vous entendez.

Périphérique: Ce matin 8h. Autocar renversé. Pas de blessés.
Paris: Grève des chauffeurs de taxi depuis 6h ce matin.
Sondage: 5% des femmes adultes ont arrêté de fumer en 1997.
Foot: Défaite de l'équipe de France. Les Ecossais triomphent 4 à 2.
Nantes: Biscuiterie LU double sa production de gauffres.

(4)

▶ **Extract 6** *You have interviewed a French lady about health.*
Answer these questions **in English**.

1 What comment does she make about weighing 70 kilos? *(2)*
Give two details.

. . . .

. . . .

2 Who encouraged her to do something about it? *(1)*

. . . .

3 Name two foods she gave up. *(2)*

. . . .

. . . .

4 What other change did she make in her lifestyle? *(1)*

. . . .

5 What general criticism of machines does she imply? *(1)*

. . . .

6 How have cars changed people's habits, according to her? *(1)*

. . . .

▶ **STUDENT ANSWERS WITH EXAMINER'S COMMENTS**

▶ **Extract 1**

1

'Correct.'

'Correct. Even though **anglais** is not correctly spelled, it is quite clear what the candidate intended, so a mark is awarded.'

2

jeudi		vendredi	
9h	Anglais	9h	Maths
10h	Sciences	10h	Histoire
11h	Français	11h	Anglaise

'Correct. The candidate has first eliminated two items, **steak** and **saucisse**, which are easy, and has then correctly selected **jambon** as ham.'

3

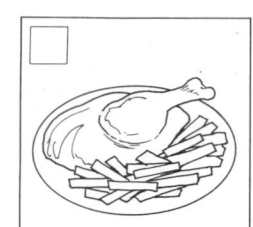 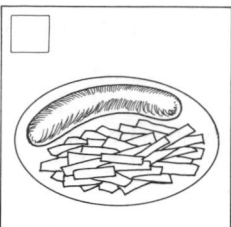 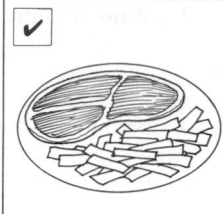 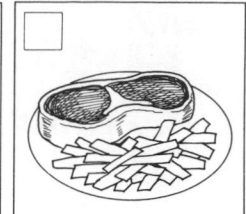

'No mark for this (the correct answer is **12.30**) because the candidate has not completely filled in the clock blank.'

4

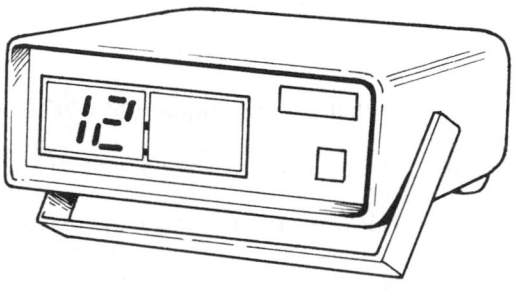

5

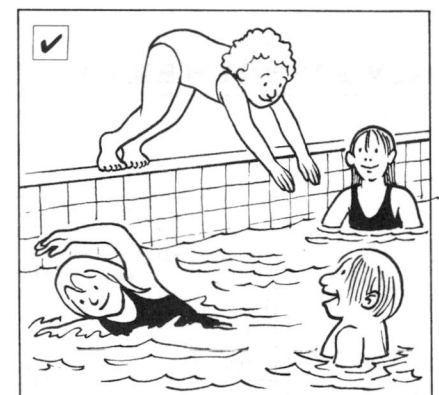 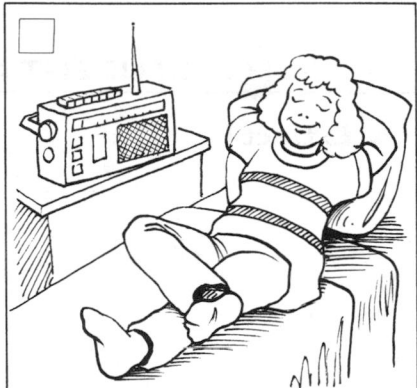

'Correct.'

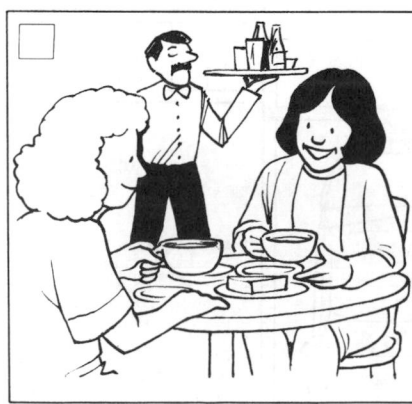 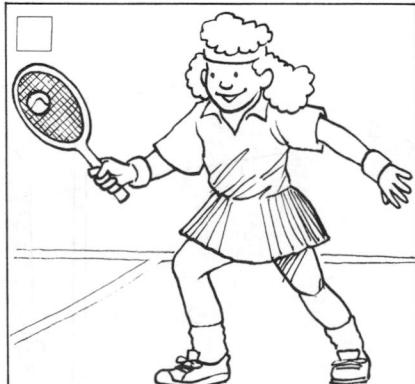

▶ **Extract 2**

ville		lettre
Exemple: Paris		E
1	Bordeaux	D
2	Nantes	B
3	Clermont-Ferrand	☐
4	Grenoble	C
5	Calais	B

Examiner's comment

Nos. 1, 2 and 4 are correct. In this sort of exercise it is unusual for the same answer to crop up twice, which should have alerted the candidate to change either 2 or 5 to something else. The word **degrés** cropped up for both towns, but the answer to 5 should have been A. Leaving a blank, as in no. 3, could never be right. The correct answer was F.

▶ **Extract 3**

	vrai	faux
Exemple: Hôtel de la Poste.	✓	
1 Réservation au nom de Dubois.	✔	
2 La dame a réservé une chambre avec douche.	✔	
3 La chambre est au troisième étage.	✔	
4 Il y a une vue sur le château.	✔	

Examiner's comment

Q1 is pretty easy, as Dubois is repeated several times. Q2 is answered wrongly. Examiners seem unreasonably interested in the plumbing arrangements of hotels, and usually distinguish between baths and showers. Q3 is correct. Q4 is not answered correctly. The château is much mentioned, but is on the other side of the building.

It might be worth knowing that the pattern of having all the answers **vrai** is very rarely set. An alert candidate might have smelt a rat here.

▶ **Extract 4**

1	Who is lost?	*a little girl*
2	Who was the lost person with before getting lost?	*her mum*
3	Which floor were they on?	*1st*
4	Where exactly is the office?	*next to the café*

Examiner's comment

There are 4 marks here for correct answers. However, the candidate has not noticed that more details are required for Q4. Because there are 2 marks available, there should be two details given. So the answer to Q4 should include: 'on the fourth floor'.

Just because questions are in English does not mean you no longer have to be careful!

▶ **Extract 5**

Périphérique: Ce matin 8h. Autocar renversé. <u>Pas de</u> blessés.
Paris: Grève des chauffeurs de taxi depuis 6h <u>ce matin.</u>
Sondage: 5% des femmes adultes ont <u>arrêté</u> de fumer en 1997.
Foot: Défaite de l'équipe de France. Les Ecossais triomphent 4 à 2.
Nantes: Biscuiterie LU <u>double</u> sa production de gauffres.

Examiner's comment

This student has done well. If there are 4 marks, there will be four errors to find. All answers were correct.

Extract 6

1   What comment does she make about weighing 70 kilos?
Give two details.
too much for her age and height
....

2   Who encouraged her to do something about it?
her mother
....

3   Name two foods she gave up.
pastries
....

4   What other change did she make in her lifestyle?
joined a sports club
....

5   What general criticism of machines does she imply?
They make us lazy
....

6   How have cars changed people's habits, according to her?

....

Examiner's comment

Q1 and Q2 are correct. The candidate has only given one answer for Q3. The other two possible ones are 'cheese' and 'meat in sauce'. The candidate could have attempted an informed guess here. Q4 and the difficult Q5 are both correct. However, the candidate has failed to answer Q6. This is difficult, too, but the examiner needs to be told that 'people use their cars instead of going for walks'.

FURTHER SPECIMEN QUESTIONS

Foundation Tier G, F, E grade tasks

Extract 7   *Au café*

Vous êtes au café avec vos amis.
Notez les commandes de vos amis **en français**.

	à manger	à boire
Magali		
Pierre		

(4)

Extract 8   *Au supermarché*

Vous êtes au supermarché. Ecoutez la publicité.

1   Remplissez.
Café ....F le paquet   *(1)*

2   Remplissez.
Camembert en promotion: .... F   *(1)*

3 Où est-ce qu'il y a une promotion? Cochez la case.

    A boulangerie   ☐

    B charcuterie   ☐

    C fruits et légumes   ☐

    D poissonnerie   ☐   *(1)*

4 Quels articles d'hygiène sont en promotion? Cochez la case.

    A brosses à dents   ☐

    B déodorant   ☐

    C savon   ☐

    D brosses à cheveux   ☐   *(1)*

5 C'est quelle sorte de sac en promotion? Cochez la case.

    A en cuir   ☐

    B en coton   ☐

    C en papier   ☐

    D en plastique   ☐   *(1)*

▶ **Extract 9** *You are on holiday in France with a friend. Your friend does not speak French.*
Answer each question by ticking one box only.

1 At the station you ask when the next train for Nantes leaves. When does it leave? *(1)*

2 When you arrive in Nantes you ask for a room at a hotel. How much does a room cost per night?

    A 100F   ☐

    B 150F   ☐

    C 200F   ☐

    D 300F   ☐   *(1)*

3 You ask what facilities the rooms have. What type of rooms are they? *(1)*

4 You ask when the evening meal is served. What time is it served? *(1)*

A ☐   `18:00`   B ☐   `19:00`   C ☐   `19:30`   D ☐   `20:00`

5 You ask the best way to get to the cinema. How does the manager suggest going? *(1)*

A ☐   B ☐   C ☐   D ☐

▷ **Extract 10**   Indiquez les modifications annoncées par téléphone.

> **Hôtel du Port**
> **9 chambres tout confort**
> **Prix à partir de 150 F par chambre par nuit**
> **Bar**
> **Tél: 02.40.56.92.63**

(3)

Foundation Tier D, C grade tasks, Higher Tier D, C grade tasks

▷ **Extract 11**   *Francine a acheté des cadeaux.*
Qu'est-ce qu'elle a acheté pour qui?
Remplissez les blancs.

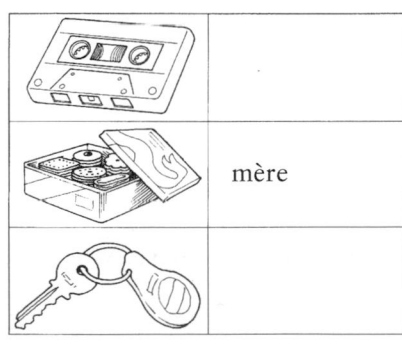

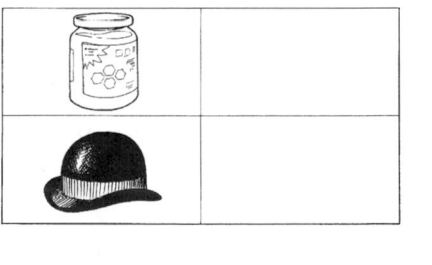

(4)

▷ **Extract 12**   *A Paris on a ouvert un restaurant anglais qui se spécialise dans la cuisine anglaise.*

1 Depuis combien de temps existe ce restaurant?
Cochez la bonne case. *(1)*

Depuis

trois ans	
trois mois	
trois semaines	
trente ans	

2   Comment est-ce qu'on crée une ambiance anglaise?
    Cochez trois cases.

Avec

des meubles	
des musiciens	
du rosbif	
des Français	
des photos	
des danseurs	
la carte	
la cuisine	

(3)

3   Au restaurant on parle français:

A   à tous les clients   ☐

B   le dimanche   ☐

C   avec difficulté   ☐

D   aux clients français   ☐   *(1)*

4   A quelle heure ferme-t-on le dimanche?

    . . . . *(1)*

▶ **Extract 13**   *You are staying with your French friend Marianne. She leaves an answerphone message for you.*
Write down the details **in English**.

1   What has delayed Marianne?

    . . . . *(1)*

2   What has she not done?

    . . . . *(1)*

3   Fill in the details of what she has asked you to buy.

shop	item	details
butcher's		tender
market		1 kilo
grocer's	wine	

(3)

4   What two things should be done to the potatoes?

    (a) . . . . *(1)*

    (b) . . . . *(1)*

5   What else does Marianne ask you to do?

    . . . . *(1)*

Extract 14 *On a demandé à des lycéens de parler de leurs carrières.*
Remplissez la grille **en français**.

nom	métier choisi	pourquoi	inconvénient
Marise			
Jean-Yves			
Joëlle			

(9)

Higher Tier B, A, A* grade tasks

Extract 15 *Un jeune couple, Henri et Elisabeth, parlent du ménage.*
Remplissez la grille **en français**.

	Elisabeth	Henri
une fois par semaine		
tous les jours		
jamais		

(6)

Extract 16 *Vous êtes dans une voiture qui a eu un accident. L'autre conducteur est furieux.*
Cochez la case.

		vrai	faux	pas mentionné
1	L'accident est arrivé à un carrefour.			
2	Le conducteur n'a pas de permis de conduire.			
3	Les voitures ont des crevaisons.			
4	Un conducteur saigne.			
5	La police est déjà sur place.			

(5)

Extract 17 *Le tunnel*

Monsieur Duroc, sa fille Hélène et son fils Eric vont en Angleterre en vacances.
Qui exprime quelle opinion?

		M. Duroc	Hélène	Eric
1	A horreur de la mer.			
2	Se rappelle d'un accident.			
3	Trouve que l'avion serait une nouvelle expérience.			
4	Va faire des recherches.			

Quelles sont leur attitude à ce sujet?
Cochez les trois bonnes cases.

		M. Duroc	Hélène	Eric
5	Favorise le tunnel.			
6	A peur de voyager sous la mer.			
7	N'a pas d'opinion très forte.			

(7)

▷ **Extract 18** *Vous écoutez une émission à la radio au sujet des expériences personnelles. Deux personnes parlent de leur expérience.*
Cochez la case appropriée ou répondez aux questions **en français.**

1 Jacques, comment est-il?

A paresseux ☐

B malheureux ☐

C occupé ☐

D assez content ☐ *(1)*

2 Quelles difficultés a-t-il? Donnez deux exemples.

. . . . *(1)*

. . . . *(1)*

3 Josianne, que pense-t-elle de sa visite?

A Elle en est contente. ☐

B Elle en est au désespoir. ☐

C Elle est sans opinion. ☐

D Elle en est malade. ☐ *(1)*

4 Donnez deux raisons pour son opinion

. . . . *(1)*

. . . . *(1)*

▷ **ANSWERS TO SPECIMEN QUESTIONS**

▷ **Extract 7**

	à manger	à boire
Magali	sandwich au jambon	Orangina®
Pierre	glace au chocolat	Coca®

▷ **Extract 8** *Au supermarché*

1 10F
2 5F 50
3 C
4 A
5 D

▷ **Extract 9** 1 D
2 C
3 B
4 B
5 C

▷ **Extract 10**

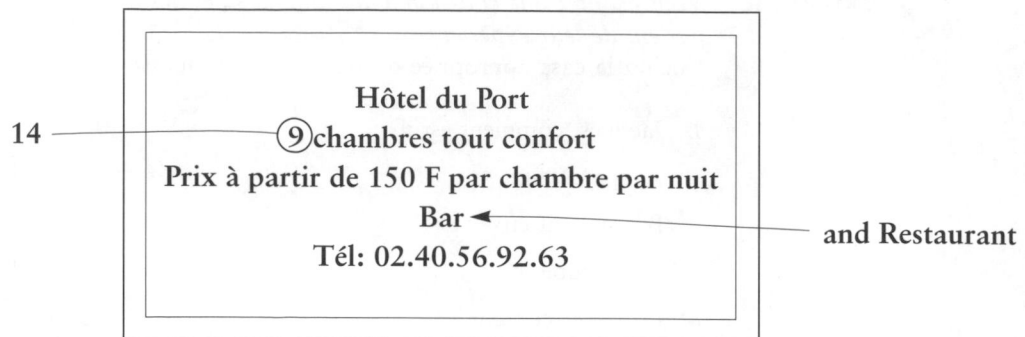

14 ——

Hôtel du Port
⑨ chambres tout confort
Prix à partir de 150 F par chambre par nuit
Bar ◄ ————————— and Restaurant
Tél: 02.40.56.92.63

▷ **Extract 11**

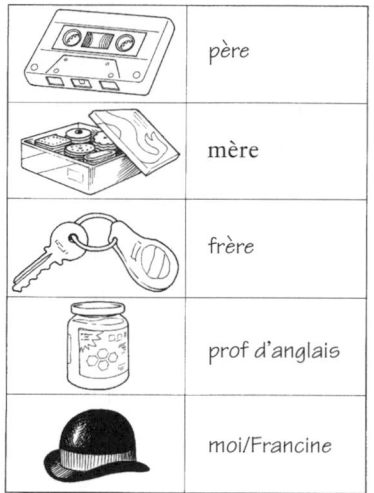

	père
	mère
	frère
	prof d'anglais
	moi/Francine

▷ **Extract 12**   1
Depuis

trois ans	✔
trois mois	
trois semaines	
trente ans	

2
Avec

des meubles	✔
des musiciens	
du rosbif	
des Français	
des photos	
des danseurs	
la carte	✔
la cuisine	✔

3 D
4 23h

▷ **Extract 13**   1 A problem at the office.
2 Prepared the evening meal.

3

shop	item	details
butcher's	*steak*	tender
market	*green beans*	I kilo
grocer's	wine	*red*

4 (a) peeled
  (b) put in cold water
5 Lay the table.

Extract 14

nom	métier choisi	pourquoi	inconvénient
Marise	*dans un hôpital*	*pour aider les gens*	*pas très bien payé*
Jean-Yves	*mécanicien*	*passionné de motos*	*mains sales*
Joëlle	*journaliste*	*aime voyager* or: *aime rencontrer les gens* or: *aime écrire*	*dangereux*

Extract 15

	Elisabeth	Henri
une fois par semaine	*tond le gazon*	*passe l'aspirateur*
tous les jours	*prépare le dîner*	*fait la vaisselle*
jamais	*passe l'aspirateur*	*lave la voiture*

Extract 16

		vrai	faux	pas mentionné
I	L'accident est arrivé à un carrefour.	✔		
2	Le conducteur n'a pas de permis de conduire.		✔	
3	Les voitures ont des crevaisons.			✔
4	Un conducteur saigne.	✔		
5	La police est déjà sur place.		✔	

Extract 17

		M. Duroc	Hélène	Eric
I	A horreur de la mer.		✔	
2	Se rappelle d'un accident.			✔
3	Trouve que l'avion serait une nouvelle expérience.			✔
4	Va faire des recherches.	✔		

		M. Duroc	Hélène	Eric
5	Favorise le tunnel.		✔	
6	A peur de voyager sous la mer.			✔
7	N'a pas d'opinion très forte.	✔		

▷ **Extract 18**
  1 B
  2 Any two of (in French):

  lost job
  sold car
  can only get low-paid / temporary work
  tension with wife
  children don't respect him

  3 A
  4 Any two of (in French):

  has difficulty in paying for his flat
  excellent hotel
  good food
  nice people
  nice weather
  lots to do / see

▷ **TRANSCRIPTS**

▷ **Extract 1**

Announcer:	Vous êtes chez votre correspondante française, Janine.
Announcer:	Numéro 1 Janine vous montre la maison. Indiquez la salle à manger sur le plan (avec un X).
F:	*Alors, voilà la salle à manger, entre la cuisine et le garage.** [repeat from * to ** after a brief pause]
Announcer:	Numéro 2 Vous regardez l'emploi du temps de Janine au collège. Janine, qu'est-ce qu'elle a le vendredi matin? Remplissez les cases vides.
F:	*Euh, vendredi matin, à 9 heures j'ai maths, puis histoire, et à 11 heures j'ai anglais.** [repeat from * to ** after a brief pause]
Announcer:	Numéro 3 Janine vous parle du déjeuner au collège. Qu'est-ce que c'est? Cochez la bonne case.
F:	*Aujourd'hui pour le déjeuner il y a du jambon avec des frites.** [repeat from * to ** after a brief pause]
Announcer:	Numéro 4 A quelle heure est-ce que vous allez manger? Ecrivez l'heure en chiffres.
F:	*Au collège on mange à midi et demi.** [repeat from * to ** after a brief pause]
Announcer:	Numéro 5 Qu'est-ce que vous allez faire après le collège? Cochez la bonne case.
F:	*Alors, cet après-midi après les classes on va aller à la piscine, n'est-ce pas?** [repeat from * to ** after a brief pause]

▷ **Extract 2**

Announcer:	Ecoutez la météo.
M:	*Voici la météo pour demain, jeudi 20 février. On va commencer avec Paris. A Paris, il pleut aujourd'hui, et demain, il va pleuvoir toute la journée. Alors, pour Paris, c'est de la pluie. [pause]

A Bordeaux il y aura des vents très forts avec des températures entre 5 et 8 degrés.

[pause]

Un peu plus au nord, à Nantes, il fera un peu plus chaud, vers 10 degrés.

[pause]

Au centre de la France, à Clermont-Ferrand, il y aura des orages, surtout le soir. Alors, à Clermont-Ferrand, des orages.

[pause]

Au sud-est de la France, à Grenoble, pour les amateurs de ski il y a de bonnes nouvelles: il y aura de la neige. Oui, il va neiger beaucoup.

[pause]

Par contre, à Calais il y a le beau temps avec de soleil et 20 degrés. Alors, une journée ensoleillée à Calais.**

Announcer: Maintenant, écoutez la météo une deuxième fois.

[repeat from * to **]

▶ **Extract 3**   *A l'hôtel*

M: *Bonsoir, Madame. Bienvenue à l'hôtel de la Poste. Qu'y a-t-il pour votre service?
F: Bien, j'ai réservé une chambre au nom de Dubois, D U B O I S.
M: Dubois, Dubois... oui, une chambre avec salle de bains.
F: Oui, c'est ça.
M: Alors, c'est la chambre numéro 36, au troisième étage. Il y a une jolie vue sur la place du marché et la mairie.
F: Est-ce qu'on peut voir le château de la chambre?
M: Le château? Euh, non, le château est de l'autre côté.
F: Tant pis. Ce n'est pas grave.
M: Alors, Madame, je vais vous montrer la chambre. Suivez-moi, s'il vous plaît.**

[repeat from * to **]

▶ **Extract 4**   M: *Mesdames, Messieurs, votre attention s'il vous plaît. Au bureau nous avons une petite fille qui a perdu sa maman. Elle était avec sa mère au rayon des articles de sport au premier étage. Elle attend sa maman au bureau au quatrième étage à côté de la cafétéria.**

[repeat from * to **]

▶ **Extract 5**   M: *Bonjour, chers auditeurs. Les informations.

Sur le périphérique ce matin à 8 heures un accident d'autocar. Le véhicule s'est renversé. Heureusement il n'y avait que le chauffeur à bord. Il en est sorti avec un bras cassé.

A partir de 6 heures demain matin il n'y aura pas de taxis dans les rues de la capitale. Les chauffeurs de taxi protestent contre des problèmes administratifs à Paris.

Cigarettes: D'après un sondage, plus de 5% des femmes françaises ont commencé à fumer des cigarettes en 1997. Par contre, le taux d'hommes fumeurs a diminué légèrement.

Hier soir l'équipe écossaise a gagné son match de la coupe d'Europe contre la France. Ce résultat inattendu était grâce à deux grosses erreurs du gardien français.

A Nantes la grande joie: la biscuiterie LU a annoncé une augmentation de 10% de la production de gauffres. Apparemment, on en mange d'avantage cette année.**

[repeat from * to **]

▶ **Extract 6** *La santé*

F: *Il est très important pour la santé d'être en bonne forme. Il y a trois ans je pesais 70 kilos. C'est beaucoup trop pour une femme de mon âge et de ma taille. J'étais fatiguée tout le temps et j'étais essoufflée quand je montais l'escalier pour aller chez ma mère qui habite au troisième étage. C'est ma mère qui m'a fait des remarques à ce sujet. Elle m'a montré une photo de moi avec mon fils il y a cinq ans. Je pesais beaucoup moins!

C'est alors que j'ai décidé de m'occuper de moi-même. J'ai changé ce que je mangeais. J'ai commencé à manger plus de légumes et de fruits et j'ai complètement arrêté de manger des pâtisseries et des fromages. J'ai mangé beaucoup moins de viande, et toujours des grillades, jamais avec de la sauce. Je me suis inscrite dans un club sportif et j'ai commencé à faire du sport – même assez sérieusement. Je fais attention à ce que je mange, et je fais du sport tous les jours. Comme tu vois, je pèse beaucoup moins que 70 kilos maintenant, et je me sens mieux.

[pause]

Aujourd'hui les gens mangent trop, et ne font pas assez d'exercice. C'est la technologie qui nous a rendu paresseux. Ce sont les machines qui font tout et nous, nous sommes devenus vraiment paresseux. Par exemple, presque tout le monde a une voiture. Autrefois on se promenait en famille le dimanche – souvent on marchait deux bonnes heures. De nos jours si on se promène, c'est en voiture. Dans les pays pauvres il est rare de trouver des gens trop gros.**

[repeat from * to **]

▶ **Extract 7** Announcer: Vous êtes au café avec vos amis.
Notez les commandes de vos amis.

M: *Alors Magali, qu'est-ce que tu prends?
F: Je prends un sandwich et un Orangina®.
M: Quelle sorte de sandwich?
F: Un sandwich au jambon, s'il te plaît.
M: Bon. Et toi, Pierre, qu'est-ce tu prends?
M2: Pour moi simplement une glace au chocolat et un coca.**

[repeat from * to **]

▶ **Extract 8** *Au supermarché*

Announcer: Vous êtes au supermarché. Ecoutez la publicité.

Announcer: Numéro 1

F: *Messieurs, Mesdames, offre spéciale sur le café. Le café est à 10F le paquet. Notre café à 10F le paquet.**

[repeat from * to **]

Announcer: Numéro 2

F: *Pour vous, du camembert en promotion à 5F 50. Le fromage du jour, c'est du camembert à 5F 50. N'hésitez pas!**

[repeat from * to **]

Announcer: Numéro 3

F: *Au rayon des fruits et légumes, promotion sur les tomates. Promotion des tomates au rayon des fruits et légumes.**

[repeat from * to **]

Announcer: Numéro 4

F: *Profitez de nos promotions sur les articles d'hygiène. Les brosses à dents, le dentifrice, le shampooing en promotion aujourd'hui avec de grandes réductions.**

[repeat from * to **]

Announcer:	Numéro 5
F:	*N'oubliez pas nos sacs en plastique très solides à 1F. En promotion, les sacs en plastique, 1F la pièce.**
	[repeat from * to **]

▷ **Extract 9**

Announcer:	You are on holiday in France with a friend. Your friend does not speak French.
	Answer each question by ticking one box only.
	1 At the station you ask when the next train for Nantes leaves. When does it leave?
F:	*Le train pour Nantes, oui, il part à 11h 10.**
	[repeat from * to **]
Announcer:	2 When you arrive in Nantes you ask for a room at a hotel. How much does a room cost per night?
M:	*Une chambre, oui, pas de problème. Ça fait 200F la chambre pour une nuit.**
	[repeat from * to **]
Announcer:	3 You ask what facilities the rooms have. What type of rooms are they?
M:	*Toutes nos chambres sont pour deux personnes, avec douche.**
	[repeat from * to **]
Announcer:	4 You ask when the evening meal is served. What time is it served?
M:	*Le dîner est servi à partir de 19 heures.**
	[repeat from * to **]
Announcer:	5 You ask the best way to get to the cinema. How does the manager suggest going?
M:	*Pour aller en ville, le plus facile, c'est de prendre le bus.**
	[repeat from * to **]

▷ **Extract 10**

Announcer:	Indiquez les modifications annoncés par téléphone.
M:	*L'hôtel du Port vous annonce la construction d'une annexe avec 5 chambres. Il y a maintenant 14 chambres au total. Les chambres sont à partir de 150F. Le bar comprend maintenant un petit restaurant intime.**
	[repeat from * to **]

▷ **Extract 11**

Announcer:	Francine a acheté des cadeaux. Qu'est-ce qu'elle acheté pour qui?
	Remplissez les blancs.
F:	*Je vais te montrer les cadeaux que j'ai achetés pendant ma visite à Cardiff. D'abord cette cassette, c'est pour mon père. Il adore les chorales galloises. Pour ma mère j'ai acheté des biscuits de luxe. Elle les adores. Le porte-clés avec le dragon gallois, c'est pour mon frère. Il collectionne les porte-clés. Pour mon prof d'anglais j'ai acheté un pot de miel. Et ce chapeau-melon, c'est pour moi. Ça fait très chic, n'est-ce pas?**
	[repeat from * to **]

▷ **Extract 12**

Announcer:	A Paris on a ouvert un restaurant anglais qui se spécialise dans la cuisine anglaise.
M:	*Depuis combien de temps existe votre restaurant?

F: Depuis trois ans. Oui, on a fêté notre troisième anniversaire avant-hier.

M: Félicitations! Comment faites-vous pour créer une ambiance anglaise?

F: Il y a toutes sortes de petits trucs. D'abord, tout le personnel est anglais. A Paris il y a beaucoup de jeunes Anglais. Les meubles sont anglais, les tableaux sont des copies de peintures anglaises, et, bien sûr, la carte est en anglais et la cuisine est anglaise.

M: Vous parlez anglais aux clients?

F: Normalement nous parlons français aux clients français. C'est comme ça que nous faisons des progrès en français.

M: Quelles sont vos heures d'ouverture?

F: Du mardi au vendredi on est ouvert entre 19 heures et 22 heures le soir. Samedi et dimanche on est ouvert jusqu'à 23 heures. Le lundi on est fermé.**

[repeat from * to **]

▷ **Extract 13** F: *Allô, c'est Marianne. Alors, écoute. Il y a eu un problème au bureau et je serai en retard. Je ne rentrerai qu'à 8 heures. Pour le dîner ce soir, c'est difficile, parce que je n'ai rien préparé. Alors je te demande de m'aider, s'il te plaît.

[pause]

D'abord il faut faire les courses. A la boucherie tu achètes des steaks bien tendres pour tout le monde. Ensuite, au marché tu prends 5 kilos de pommes de terre – je n'en ai plus à la maison – et 1 kilo de haricots verts. A l'épicerie il faut acheter à boire – du vin rouge, de l'eau minérale et une bouteille d'Orangina®.

[pause]

Quand tu rentres à la maison, est-ce que tu peux préparer les légumes? Si tu épluches les pommes de terre, n'oublie pas de les mettre dans de l'eau froide. Ensuite, veux-tu mettre la table? Alors, je te remercie d'avance. En tout cas, je serai là à 8 heures, et puis on dînera.**

[repeat from * to **]

▷ **Extract 14** Announcer: On a demandé à des lycéens de parler de leur carrière.

M: *Qu'est-ce que tu voudrais faire quand tu quittes le lycée, Marise?

F: Je n'ai pas encore décidé, mais j'aimerais bien aider les gens. Peut-être – je ne sais pas – mais peut-être que j'aimerais travailler dans un hôpital. Mais le travail n'est pas très bien payé.

M: Et toi, Jean-Yves, qu'est-ce que tu veux faire?

M2: Moi, je suis passionné de motos, alors j'aimerais peut-être travailler comme mécanicien de motos.

M: C'est chouette, ça.

M2: Oui, mais c'est un travail difficile et on a toujours les mains sales.

M: Et toi, Joëlle?

F2: Moi, j'aimerais voyager, rencontrer des gens, écrire. Alors, peut-être journaliste.

M: C'est intéressant comme travail.

F2: C'est vrai. Mais quelquefois c'est un travail dangereux. Il y a des pays où on n'hésite pas à assassiner certains journalistes s'ils gênent.**

[repeat from * to **]

▶ **Extract 15** Announcer: Un jeune couple, Henri et Elisabeth, parlent du ménage.

M: *Tu ne fais absolument rien pour le ménage.

F: Alors, je t'en prie. Tous les samedis je tonds le gazon. Ce n'est pas un grand plaisir, tu sais.

M: Une fois par semaine, ce n'est pas grande chose. Moi, je fais la vaisselle tous les jours après le dîner. Ce n'est pas amusant, tu sais.

F: Oui, mais qui prépare le dîner? C'est moi. Et encore une chose: tu ne laves jamais la voiture.

M: Oui, c'est vrai. Mais je ne t'ai jamais vue passer l'aspirateur.

F: Ah, non, j'ai horreur de ça. Ça, c'est une travail de garçons.

M: C'est bon alors que je passe l'aspirateur tous les samedis.

F: A chacun son travail!**

[repeat from * to **]

▶ **Extract 16** M: *Mais enfin, ça ne va pas? Vous ne savez pas conduire peut-être? Vous ne savez pas qu'on s'arrête quand il y a un feu rouge? Vous avez trouvé votre permis de conduire dans une pochette surprise, à ce que je vois. Regardez tous ces dégâts – le pare-chocs est cassé, mon phare ne marche plus.

Qui va payer les réparations? Ça va coûter une vrai fortune. Il ne faut pas dormir quand on conduit, vous savez. Et regardez – mon manteau est couvert de sang – et il était tout neuf. Ah non! J'ai du sang partout. Appelez un médecin et la police, mais vite! Qu'attendez-vous?**

[repeat from * to **]

▶ **Extract 17** M1:   *Alors, les enfants, comment est-ce qu'on va faire pour aller en Angleterre? Il y a un grand choix de possibilités, vous savez.

F: Papa, moi, je n'aime pas la mer. Tu sais, j'ai toujours le mal de mer.
Alors, moi, j'aimerais prendre le tunnel sous la Manche. C'est très rapide et il n'est pas nécessaire de réserver sa place. Et puis, c'est quelque chose de nouveau.

M2:   Alors là, moi, j'ai peur de ce tunnel. Il y a eu cet incendie en 1996. Et puis on est obligé de rester avec sa voiture dans le train. Ce n'est pas reposant du tout.

M1:   Moi, j'ai toujours pris le bateau. C'est calme, on peut se promener, on peut manger au restaurant à bord et on peut même prendre une douche si on veut.

M2:   On pourrait prendre l'avion! Ça aussi, ce serait une nouveauté pour nous.

F: Mais non! C'est horriblement cher et c'est dangereux, à mon avis.

M1:   Ça suffit, les enfants. Je vais chercher des brochures à l'agence de voyages et comparer les prix et les horaires. Ensuite on décidera.**

[repeat from * to **]

▶ **Extract 18** M: Bonjour, Jacques. Dites-nous quelques mots, s'il vous plaît.

M2:   Bonjour. Je voulais vous dire que chez moi tout va mal. J'ai 45 ans et j'ai perdu mon emploi au bureau il y a un an. Depuis, que de problèmes. On a du mal à payer notre appartement. J'ai été obligé de vendre ma voiture. Je ne trouve que du travail mal payé, et temporaire. Ma femme et moi, on se dispute très souvent. Et mes enfants ont perdu un peu de respect pour leur papa. Tout ça, ce n'est pas très amusant. Franchement, je ne sais pas quoi faire.

M: Merci, Jacques, et bon courage.
      Et maintenant, Josianne. Josianne, dites-nous quelque chose, s'il vous plaît.

F: Moi, j'ai quelque chose de plus amusant à vous confier. J'ai gagné un prix au club de sport, et c'était un week-end au centre de l'Angleterre. Alors, vous savez, l'Angleterre au mois de février, ce n'est pas le premier endroit qu'on aurait choisi. Mais je vous avoue qu'on s'est très bien amusé. L'hôtel était excellent, la cuisine délicieuse, les gens aimables, il faisait un temps superbe, et il y avait beaucoup de choses à faire et à voir. Vraiment, je vous dis, on a vraiment tendance à sous-estimer l'Angleterre comme pays touristique. J'y retournerai bientôt.

M: Merci, Josianne, de partager vos impressions avec nous.**

      [repeat from * to **]

▷ **Extract 19**   *L'alphabet français*

*a b c d e f g h i j k l m n o p q r s t u v w x y z
accent aigu (´), accent grave (`), accent circonflexe (ˆ), c cédille (ç), e tréma (ë), deux p (pp), deux l (ll), deux r (rr), deux s (ss)**

[repeat from * to **]

▶ **A STEP FURTHER**

There is no doubt that the more you listen, the better you will become at understanding French. So make sure that you take every opportunity to listen to material of about the right level:

▷ at school
▷ using the extracts on the audio tape
▷ using video of language courses
▷ viewing the French-language satellite channels (TV5 and Arte) which do not require specialised decoding equipment
▷ meeting and listening to French-speaking visitors.

You should also gain some practice in prices, numbers, times and days of the week. This can easily be done with a friend or a friendly native speaker by getting them to say half a dozen times or dates for you, while you write them down in figures. They can then check them afterwards. The more often you can get this sort of practice, the better, and, if it is an area in which you are weak, it has to be top priority in preparing for Listening.

It is as well to be able to understand common abbreviations such as HLM, SNCF, TF1, P et T, RER, ZUP, and so on. Keep a list of them. (See also 'Public signs and notices' in Chapter 5 on Reading.)

The ability to understand spellings given in French is also important. It is also a good idea to be able to spell out such things as your own name, address and place of birth for the Speaking Test. We have therefore recorded the French alphabet on the tape as Extract 19. Use it to make sure you can spell fluently and can write down from others spelling in French.

Reading

 GETTING STARTED

Reading is the skill area which is often done least well. This is probably because students think it is easier than it actually is, and therefore spend less time on it.

From 1998, Reading comprehension will be tested mainly in French. However, although this sounds alarming, in practice it isn't a big problem, because most of the Examining Groups have decided to go for the sort of questions where you tick boxes, or where you only have to write figures or a couple of words in French. There will also be a small number of questions which require an answer in English.

A structured approach to the sorts of questions you will meet, together with some understanding of how the questions are set, should make sure that you can approach this skill with confidence.

Remember that Reading is a skill which is relatively easy to practise, which doesn't require special equipment, and which can be conveniently done in long or short sessions and in virtually any place. So don't neglect it!

WHAT YOU NEED TO KNOW

Examining Group requirements

There are many common features among the Examining Groups in their Reading Tests. The only matter on which they differ is how long the tests should take, so check the table below to see how long your Examining Group allows for this part of the GCSE.

Examining Group	NICCEA	EDEXCEL	MEG	NEAB	SEG	WJEC
Foundation	40 mins.	30 mins.	50 mins.	30 mins.		45 mins.
Higher	40 mins.	45 mins.	50 mins.	50 mins.		45 mins.
Module 1					varies	
Module 2					30 mins.	
Module 4					30 mins.	

So much for the major difference among the Examining Groups – time. Let us look at what all the Groups do require of their candidates.

Foundation and Higher Tiers

1 First the bad news. There is no choice of questions.
2 And now the good news. You are allowed access to a French–English, English–French dictionary in both Foundation and Higher Tier papers. Make sure you have a dictionary with which you are familiar and which is not too complicated.
3 Between 80% and 90% of the marks will be for questions and answers in French. The remaining questions and answers will be in English. Some Examining Groups use the English questions at the very easy and very difficult ends of the papers, and others use them in the middle area. Check with your teacher what your Group does.
4 You are required to read French which was intended to be read (not, for example, a transcript of a conversation).
5 All Examining Groups will print a booklet for you to write your answers under the question. This has the advantage that you are less likely to miss out a question.

Foundation Tier

The Foundation Tier allows performances between grades G and C. For assessment purposes, the Examining Groups distinguish between grade G, F, E tasks and performances and grade D, C tasks and performances.

Grade G, F, E tasks will be set using a limited range of vocabulary. Every Examining Group publishes a **Minimum Core Vocabulary** of about 1500 words. The questions targeting these grades will only be drawn from the Minimum Core Vocabulary. Most of this vocabulary will have been covered in the early years of learning French.

The tasks set will require candidates:

- to identify and note the main points of what they have read
- to extract specific details.

Some Groups set some easy questions in English, with English answers, for these target grades. Others will use mainly objective-type questions involving box-ticking, multiple choice or matching descriptions.

Grade D, C tasks will usually involve reading longer passages of French, and most of the questions will be in French, requiring answers in French. As well as objective-type tests, there may be a requirement to write a few words in French. The vocabulary covered in this section is not limited to the words in the Minimum Core Vocabulary.

The tasks set will require candidates:

- to identify and note the main points of what they have read
- to extract specific details
- to identify points of view
- to show some understanding of unfamiliar language
- to show some understanding of familiar language in unfamiliar contexts
- to understand references to past, present and future events.

Higher Tier

The Higher Tier allows performances between grades D and A*. For assessment purposes, the Examining Groups distinguish between grade D, C tasks and performances and grade B, A, A* tasks and performances.

Grade D, C tasks and the type of reading expected are identical to those in Foundation Tier at these grades.

Grade B, A, A* tasks will involve reading longer passages in French. It is possible that some of these will be handwritten. Again, the vocabulary used will be considerably more extensive than that listed in the Minimum Core Vocabulary.

The tasks set will require candidates:

- to identify and note the main points of what they have read
- to extract specific details
- to identify points of view
- to recognise attitudes and emotions
- to show some understanding of unfamiliar language
- to show some understanding of familiar language in unfamiliar contexts
- to understand references to past, present and future events
- to infer meaning from context.

▶ **Text types** The types of text you can expect to read are listed below, roughly in order of difficulty, with the easiest first:

- public signs and notices
- road signs
- tickets, town plans, road maps
- simple instructions (e.g. how to use a telephone)
- menus, labels on food and drink
- timetables (school and public transport)
- notes left by other people
- advertisements and special offers; handbills

⫸ guides and brochures concerning entertainment, sport, and tourist attractions, etc.

⫸ informal letters from a French-speaking correspondant; invitations

⫸ formal letters (e.g. confirming reservations, replying to job applications)

⫸ newspaper and magazine articles

⫸ imaginative writing.

⫸ **Effective answers**

Let us now look at how to answer the questions most effectively. First of all, as everywhere in this examination, you must read the question carefully. This includes the setting given with each text, which may give you valuable clues as to what to expect.

For objective-type questions, check how many choices you have, and make that number of choices only. Making too many or too few choices will reduce your mark. Even if you aren't absolutely sure of the right answer, you have nothing to lose by having a go.

If you have to write answers in English, the answers need not be in full sentences – so don't waste time writing pretty sentences in English. For example, if the question is 'What does the hotel cost per night?', there is no need to write: 'According to the text the cost of the hotel per night is 35 francs.' Your primary and Year 7 and 8 secondary teachers may have insisted on that sort of answer. You can forget that now! The ideal GCSE French answer to that question is: '35 francs'. Go for short answers, although not so short that they don't fully answer the question!

If the text requires answers in French, the Examining Groups all state that the marks are to be awarded for demonstrating understanding of the text. So as long as your French answer communicates the right answer, you will get the mark even if there are some errors in your French. So you can heave a sigh of relief!

It is worth knowing that questions on longer texts are usually set in sequence. So the third question on a text, for example, will refer to a point later in the text than the second, and so on. This knowledge is particularly helpful if you are struggling with a text and only understand some of it! However, the first or last question or two may refer to the whole text if, for example, there is a question about the 'attitude of the author of the text' in general, or a question such as 'What is the text about?'

Another point worth knowing is that, if there is more than one mark allocated for a question, it is highly likely that there is more than one piece of information or detail required. Look for extra things to say – as long as you can find them in the text! On the other hand, the 2 marks may be given for saying that there is *une grande* (1 mark) *maison* (1 mark) – so make sure you include all the details.

Some Examining Groups set questions where there are, say, 2 marks, but three possible answers. They will generally mark the first two answers given, so make sure that you have put the one you are most certain of first.

In Higher Tier you will need to develop strategies for dealing with unfamiliar words. The application of common sense is the most useful one, but the section on pp. 100–102 about strategies for reading French may help. If faced with an unfamiliar word, don't forget to consider the possibility that it could be a place-name or a person's name. That possibility is especially likely if you can't find the word in your dictionary.

Higher Tier questions which are testing attitudes, emotions and ideas and which ask you to infer things will nevertheless have a logical basis. So you do need to use common sense coupled with the French to deal with these. And if you don't know a word, you should make a sensible guess as to what might come in the gap in your understanding. Many candidates seem to think that, because it's French, the normal rules of logic no longer apply! Examiners at GCSE try very much not to set 'trick' questions – they are more interested in French for 'practical communication', and to allow you to show what you 'know and can do'.

⫸ **Which vocabulary topics?**

Many of the questions will be seeking an answer about:

Who?	How long?
What?	How many?
Where?	How much?
When?	Why?

A moment's thought will point you towards the vocabulary topics which are most likely to be covered by each of those questions:

Who?	family and friends
	professions
	descriptions: physical appearance, size, age, character
What?	virtually all objects, prices, and instructions and activities
	food and drink, shopping, free time and entertainment
Where?	positions and prepositions
	location of buildings in town and country
	countries, directions and distances
When?	time by the 12-hour and 24-hour clocks
	in relation to other events
How long?	time, especially duration
How many?	numbers
How much?	quantity, numbers
Why?	reasons

Topics which might be found more frequently in Higher Tier Reading include:

▶ current affairs
▶ more complicated instructions and adverts
▶ longer notices from shops, banks and post offices.

A little time spent in directed preparation will not go amiss.

▶ Public signs and notices

Public signs and notices have a language all of their own.

I have given below a list – by no means exhaustive – of common ones which may well be tested in GCSE. Of course you may find it very daunting to learn them all. If that is the case, learn some of the most obvious ones from each setting.

General public notices

Appuyer *Press*
Appuyez *Push*
Défense de... *It is forbidden to...*
Entrée *Entrance*
Fermé *Closed*
Hors service *Out of order*
Interdiction de... *Forbidden*
Interdit *Forbidden*
Ne pas... *Don't...*
Ouvert *Open*
Pousser *Push*
Poussez *Push*
Sortie *Exit*
SVP (S'il vous plaît) *Please*
Tirer *Pull*
Tirez *Pull*

Fin de zone bleue *End of disc parking zone*
Parking gratuit *Free parking*
Parking souterrain *Underground parking*
Passez piétons *Cross now*
Péage *Toll*
Priorité à droite *Priority to the right*
Privé *Private*
Roulez au pas *Drive at walking pace*
Sens unique *One-way street*
Serrez à droite *Keep to the right*
Sortie de camions *Lorry exit*
Stationnement interdit *No parking*
Vous n'avez pas la priorité *Give way*
Zone bleue – disque obligatoire
     Disc parking zone
Zone piétonne *Pedestrian zone*

+ *names of shops and buildings – see pp. 48 and 50–1*

Home

Attention au chien *Beware of the dog*
Chien dangereux *Dangerous dog*
Libre *Vacant (on loo door)*
Occupé *Engaged (on loo door)*

Public toilets

Dames *Ladies*
Femmes *Women*
Hommes *Men*
Messieurs *Gents*
Toilettes *Toilets*
W.C. Publics *Public toilets*

Town

Attendez *Wait (at pelican crossing)*
Cédez le passage *Give way*
Centre commercial *Shopping centre*
Côté de stationnement *Parking on this side of the street only*
Défense de stationner *No parking*
Déviation obligatoire pour poids lourds
     Lorry route

School

CES *Secondary school*
Bibliothèque *Library*
Bureau d'administration *School office*
Cantine *Canteen*
Censeur *Head of Discipline*
Concierge *Caretaker*

Directeur *Headteacher*
Laboratoire *Laboratory*
Réfectoire *Canteen*
Salle des professeurs *Staffroom*
Surveillants *(Room for) supervisors*

Places of entertainment
Caisse *Cash desk*
Défense de fumer *No smoking*
Heures d'ouverture *Opening hours*
Vestiaires *Cloakrooms*

Public transport
Accès aux quais *To the platforms*
Arrêt *Bus stop*
Arrêt facultatif *Request stop*
Arrivées *Arrivals*
Autocars *Coaches*
Banlieue *Suburbs*
Billets *Tickets*
Consigne *Left luggage*
Consigne automatique *Luggage lockers*
Correspondances *Connections*
Départs *Departures*
Douane *Customs*
Horaires *Timetables*
RATP *Paris suburban rail network*
Renseignements *Information*
SNCF *French railways*
Vol *Flight*
Voyageurs *Passengers*

Shops
Alimentation générale *Grocer's*
Bricolage *DIY*
Caisse *Cash desk / Pay here*
la dixaine *per ten*
la douzaine *per dozen*
à l'intérieur *inside*
jour de marché *market day*
Libre service *Self-service*
Maison de la presse *Newsagent's*
Mode féminine *Ladies' fashions*
Ne pas toucher *Don't touch*
du pays *local*
la pièce *each*
Prêt-à-porter *Ready-to-wear*
Prière de ne pas toucher *Please don't touch*

Prix chocs *Amazing prices*
Prix réduits *Reduced prices*
Servez-vous *Help yourself*
Soldes *Sales*
Sous-sol *Basement*
TVA *VAT*
à vendre *for sale*
en vente ici *on sale here*

Cafés and restaurants
TTC *taxes included*
Service compris *Service included*
Service non compris *Service not included*

Hotels
Accueil *Reception*
S'adresser à la réception *Ask at the reception desk*
Ascenseur *Lift*
Chambres libres *Rooms available*
Chambres à louer *Rooms available*
Chambres tout confort *Modern rooms*
Complet *Full*
Prise-rasoir *Shaver socket*

Campsites
Bloc sanitaire *Washrooms*
Eau potable *Drinking water*
Eau non potable *Non-drinking water*
Emplacement *Pitch*
Pour ordures *For rubbish*

Garage
Dépannage *Breakdown service*
Lavage *Car wash*
Libre-service *Self-service*
Pose pare-brise *Windscreen replacement service*
Prix au litre *Price per litre*

Post office
Autres destinations *Other destinations (for letters)*
Cabine téléphonique *Phone cubicle*
Heures des levées *Collection times*
Imprimés *Printed matter*
P et T *Post office*
Timbres-poste *Postage stamps*

▷ **False friends** There are many words in French which look like English ones, but which have different meanings. Make sure you are aware of them! Check the lists below.

Straightforward false friends
le car *coach (**not** car)*
la cave *cellar (**not** cave)*
     complet *full, no vacancies (**not** finished)*
la correspondance *place to change trains (**not** letters)*
un hôtel de ville *town hall (**not** hotel)*
la journée *day (**not** journey)*

large   *wide* (**not** *large*)
la monnaie   *change* (**not** *money*)
le parfum   *flavour* (**not** *perfume*)
passer   *to spend time, to take exam* (**not** *to pass*)
la pension   *board in hotel* (**not** *pension!*)
la place   *square* (**not only** *place*)
le quai   *platform* (**not only** *quay*)

Some more difficult false friends

assister à   *to be present at* (**not** *to assist*)
causer   *to chat* (**not** *to cause*)
la chance   *good luck* (**not always** *chance*)
le courrier   *letters, mail* (**not** *courier*)
doubler   *to overtake* (**not** *to double*)
se dresser   *to rise up* (**not** *to get dressed*)
la figure   *face* (**not** *figure*)
la lecture   *reading* (**not** *lecture*)
la librairie   *bookshop* (**not** *library*)
la licence   *university degree* (**not** *licence*)
la location   *hiring* (**not** *location*)
le médecin   *doctor* (**not** *medecine*)
le mouton   *sheep* (**not only** *mutton*)
la note   *bill* (**not** *note*)
un omnibus   *stopping train* (**not** *bus*)
le pétrole   *crude oil* (**not** *petrol*)
le plat   *culinary dish* (**not** *plate*)
la promotion   *special offer* (**not** *promotion*)
la prune   *plum* (**not** *prune*)
rester   *to stay* (**not** *to rest*)
sensible   *sensitive* (**not** *sensible*)
le stage   *course of instruction* (**not** *stage*)
le wagon   *railway coach* (**not** *waggon*)

There are others. Add them to the list as you come across them.

▶ STRATEGIES FOR READING FRENCH

Because English and French are historically related to each other (1066 and all that...), there are many patterns of similarity which English speakers can exploit when reading French.

 Conversion strategies
These include the following:

▷ adverbs changing from -*ment* in French to '-ly' in English, e.g. c*omplètement, rarement*
▷ verbs removing the final -*r* in French to give the English, e.g. *admirer, compléter, arriver*
▷ verbs ending in -*er* in French changing to '-ate' in English, e.g. *décorer*
▷ words ending in -*el* in French changing to '-al' in English, e.g. *officiel, individuel*
▷ words ending in -*aire* in French changing to '-ar' or '-ary', e.g. *populaire, militaire*
▷ words ending in -*ie*, -*é* or -*ée* in French changing to '-y'. e.g. *économie, partie, liberté, armée*
▷ words ending in -*e* in French lose it in English, e.g. *branche, signe, vaste, uniforme*
▷ words gain an '-*e*' in English, e.g. *pur, futur, feminin*
▷ present participles ending in -*ant* in French change to '-ing' in English, e.g. *allant, arrivant.*

▷ **Prefixes**   There are many clues to meaning to be found in prefixes (which are added to the beginnings of words). Look at the examples below and add your own.

French prefix	English prefix	examples	meaning
dé-	*dis-, des-*	décourager	*to discourage*
		découvrir	*to discover*
		déçu	*disappointed*
		dégoutant	*disgusting*
		déguiser	*to disguise*
		détruire	*to destroy*
dé-, dés-	*de-, un-*	déformé	*deformed, damaged*
		démodé	*unfashionable*
		se déshabiller	*to get undressed*
éc-	*sc-, sq-*	école	*school*
		Écosse	*Scotland*
		échelle	*musical scale, ladder*
		écran	*screen*
		écraser	*to squash, to run over*
ép-	*sp-*	épeler	*to spell*
		épice	*spice*
		éponge	*sponge*
		époux, épouse	*spouse*
ét-	*st-, -st-*	établissement	*establishment*
		état	*state*
		s'étonner	*to be astonished*
		étranger	*stranger*
		étudiant	*student*
im-, in-	*un-, in-, im-,*	impoli	*impolite*
		inconnu	*unknown person, stranger*
		incroyable	*unbelievable*
pré-	*fore-*	prédire	*to fortell, to predict*
		prénom	*forename, first name*
		prévision	*forecast*
		prévoir	*to foresee*
re-	*re-, again*	recommencer	*to begin again*
		redevenir	*to become again*
		rentrer	*to return*
		reprendre	*to take back*
		retrouver	*to meet, find again*
		revenir	*to come back*
sous-, sou-	*under-, sub-*	souterrain	*underground*
		sous-marin	*submarine*

▷ **Suffixes**   There are also many clues contained in suffixes (which are found at the ends of words).

French suffix	English suffix	examples	meaning
-aine	*about*	dixaine	*about 10*
		douzaine	*dozen*
		centaine	*about 100*
-é	*-ed*	enlevé	*removed*
		fatigué	*tired*
		situé	*situated*
-er, -ier	*profession/ classification*	boucher	*butcher*
		pâtissier	*pastry-cook, confectioner*

		vacancier	*holiday-maker*
		voilier	*sailing-boat*
-eur	*-er, -or*	acteur	*actor*
		chanteur	*singer*
		directeur	*director*
		mineur	*miner*
-eur	*-ness*	blancheur	*whiteness*
		douceur	*sweetness*
		hauteur	*highness, height*
-eux	*-ous*	curieux	*curious*
		désastreux	*disastrous*
		ingénieux	*ingenious*
		merveilleux	*marvellous*
		précieux	*precious*
-ier	*tree*	bananier	*banana tree*
		cerisier	*cherry tree*
		pommier	*apple tree*
-ir	*-ish*	abolir	*to abolish*
		finir	*to finish*
		punir	*to punish*
-oire	*-ory*	gloire	*glory*
		laboratoire	*laboratory*
		réfectoire	*refectory, canteen*
-té	*-ty*	beauté	*beauty*
		cité	*city; student hall of residence*
		difficulté	*difficulty*
		facilité	*facility*

▶ **The circumflex and the 's'**   It may be worth noting that where there is a circumflex in French, there is often an 's' in English. For example:

août *August*   île *isle, island*
coûter *to cost*   intérêt *interest*
degoûtant *disgusting*   pâte *pasta, paste*
forêt *forest*   prêtre *priest*
hôtel *hotel* (compare: *hostel*)   rôti roast

▷ **EXAMINATION QUESTIONS**

Foundation Tier G, F, E grade tasks

Exercises with questions and answers in English

Answer each question by ticking **one** box only.

Example
Your friend wants to post a letter. Which sign should he follow?

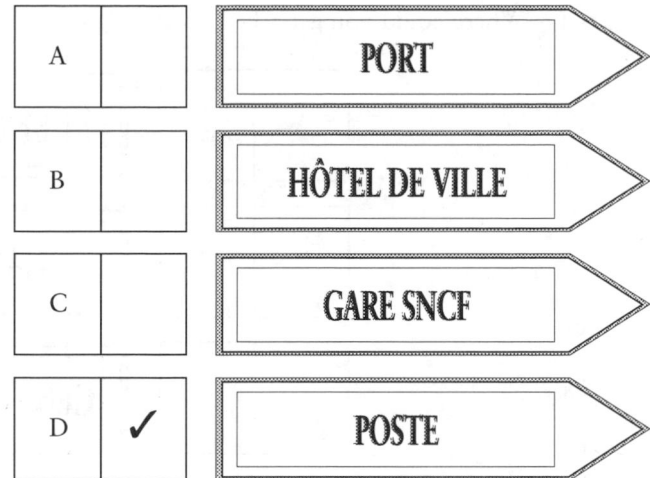

'The correct answer is D.'

▷ **Question 1**   You want to catch a train. Which sign should you follow?

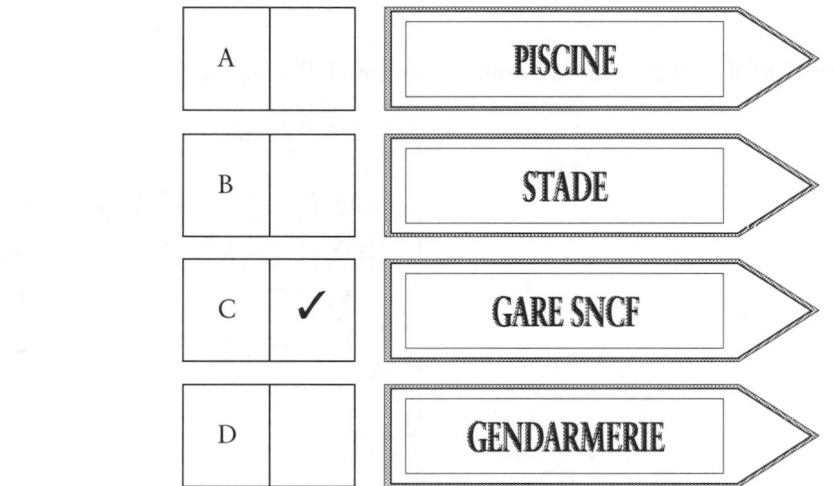

'Correct.'

(1)

▷ **Question 2**   Which shop sells envelopes?

'The student has mixed up
papeterie (stationer's)
with **pâtisserie** (cake
shop).'

A	✓	PÂTISSERIE
B		EPICERIE
C		PAPETERIE
D		BOULANGERIE

(1)

▷ **Question 3**   Where could you get a bed for the night?

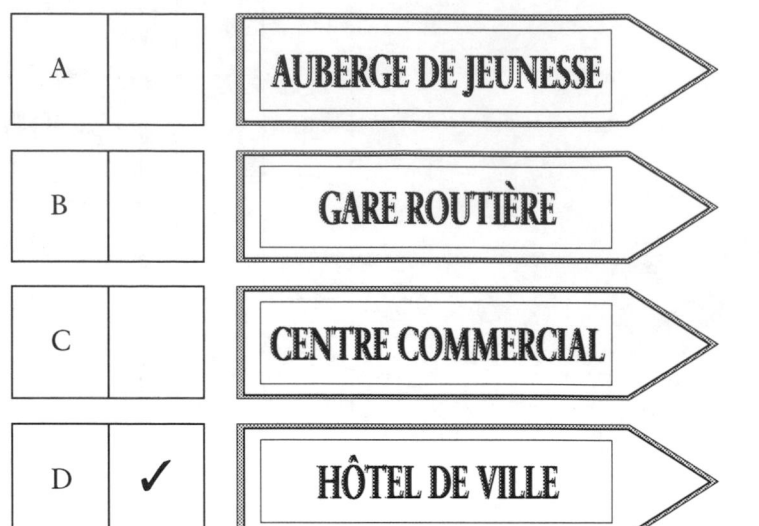

A		AUBERGE DE JEUNESSE
B		GARE ROUTIÈRE
C		CENTRE COMMERCIAL
D	✓	HÔTEL DE VILLE

(1)

'The student has fallen for the **hôtel de ville** distractor, which is, of course, the town hall. The correct answer is the **auberge de jeunesse**, the youth hostel.'

▷ **Question 4**   In your hotel room you see the following notice about the emergency meeting point.

> EN CAS DE DANGER,
> RASSEMBLEZ-VOUS
> SUR LE PARKING
> DEVANT L'HÔTEL

'Correct.'

Where should you meet? *in front of the hotel*   *(1)*

▷ **Question 5**   You see a sign which says:

> STATIONNEMENT
> INTERDIT

What are you not allowed to do there? *station*   *(1)*

Examiner's comment
Wrong. The word **stationnement** means 'parking', so parking is forbidden here. Simple use of a dictionary could have avoided this!

Simple exercise with questions in French

▷ **Question 5**   Où est-ce que je peux trouver......? Ecrivez la bonne lettre dans la case.

1 de l'aspirine? $\boxed{F}$

2 du mouton? $\boxed{}$

3 du pain? $\boxed{A}$

4 du fromage? $\boxed{E}$

5 une carte postale? $\boxed{C}$ (5)

'Correct, apart from no. 2, where the student left a blank. Leaving a blank is always wrong: there was a 50% chance of getting it right in this case!'

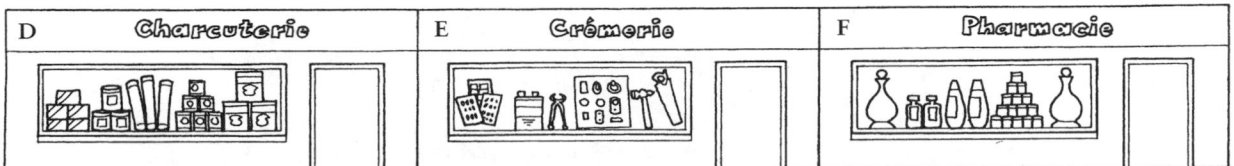

| A Boulangerie | B Boucherie | C Librairie |
| D Charcuterie | E Crêmerie | F Pharmacie |

Longer passages

▷ **Question 6**   Lisez la brochure *Gîtes normands*.
Coche la case *vrai* ou *faux*.   (4)

Les Gîtes normands

En Normandie vous trouverez toutes sortes de gîtes à votre service.

☐ **Les gîtes ruraux**   *Les gîtes ruraux vous invitent à passer un séjour calme et rustique en pleine campagne.*

☐ **Les gîtes d'enfants**   *Les gîtes d'enfants proposent aux enfants des programmes d'activités pendant les vacances scolaires.*

☐ **Les gîtes d'étape**   *Les gîtes d'étape sont à l'intention des groupes qui font des randonnées.*

☐ **Les campings à la ferme**   *Les campings à la ferme vous offrent la possibilité de camper en pleine nature, mais pas trop loin d'une douche et des toilettes.*

☐ **Les chambres d'hôtes**   *L'acceuil des chambres d'hôtes comprend le repas du soir, la chambre, et le petit déjeuner. On prend ses repas avec ses hôtes.*

'Nos. 1 and 2 are both wrong. It is important to make sure you have spent time on understanding the question!'

	vrai	faux
Exemple: Les campings à la ferme sont en ville.		✔
1 Les gîtes d'enfants fonctionnent pendant toute l'année.	✔	
2 Dans les chambres d'hôtes on mange seul.	✔	
3 Les gîtes d'étape sont pour les groupes.	✔	
4 Les gîtes ruraux sont calmes.	✔	

▷ **Question 7**   Lisez l'annonce pour l'hôtel FIMOTEL.

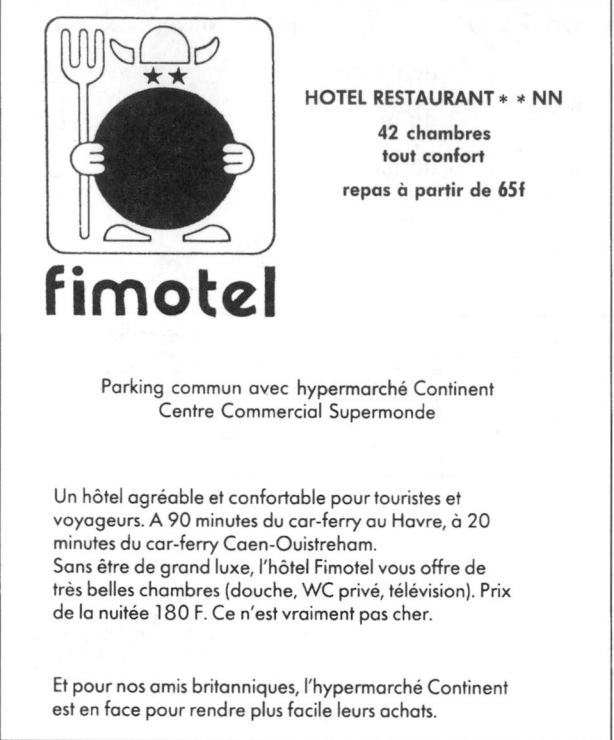

HOTEL RESTAURANT ∗ ∗ NN
**42 chambres
tout confort**
repas à partir de 65f

Parking commun avec hypermarché Continent
Centre Commercial Supermonde

Un hôtel agréable et confortable pour touristes et
voyageurs. A 90 minutes du car-ferry au Havre, à 20
minutes du car-ferry Caen-Ouistreham.
Sans être de grand luxe, l'hôtel Fimotel vous offre de
très belles chambres (douche, WC privé, télévision). Prix
de la nuitée 180 F. Ce n'est vraiment pas cher.

Et pour nos amis britanniques, l'hypermarché Continent
est en face pour rendre plus facile leurs achats.

C'est vrai? Cochez les bonnes cases.

1   Il y a un parking à 20 minutes.   ✔

2   L'hôtel n'accepte pas les touristes.   ☐

'All correct apart from no. 1. Common sense should tell you that a car-park is unlikely to be 20 minutes away from the hotel!'

3   L'hôtel FIMOTEL est près du car-ferry à Caen-Ouistreham.   ✔

4   Il y a une salle de télévision.   ☐

5   Il y a un magasin dans l'hôtel.   ☐

6   Les chambres ont des douches.   ✔   *(3)*

Foundation Tier D, C grade tasks, Higher Tier D, C grade tasks

▷ **Question 8**   Lisez cette lettre d'une Française à sa correspondante.

> Amiens, le 7 avril
>
> Chère Nicola,
>
> Ça va? J'ai une triste nouvelle – je ne peux pas venir te voir à Pâques. Je sais que nous avons tout arrangé – je suis désolée. Mais nous avons des problèmes dans la famille.
>
> C'est que ma mère s'est cassé le pied, et elle doit se reposer pendant quelques semaines. Comme tu sais, j'ai mes deux petits frères et ma petite sœur et les deux chiens. Papa est souvent absent en voyage pour son travail, alors je suis obligée de faire beaucoup pour aider ma mère.
>
> J'apprends beaucoup de choses. Je fais la vaisselle, je fais les courses, je fais la cuisine, je fais la lessive. C'est fatiguant! Et j'ai aussi mes devoirs.
>
> Alors, est-ce qu'il serait possible de venir te voir au mois de juillet? J'aimerais beaucoup te revoir.

Dis bonjour à tes parents de ma part. Je suis très déçue de ne pas pouvoir venir. Ecris-moi vite avec des dates pour l'été.

Amitiés

Marie-Christine

Complètez les phrases. Choisissez la bonne lettre et cochez la case.

Exemple: Marie-Christine
A habite Londres ☐
B habite Amiens ☑
C habite Edimbourg ☐

1 Marie-Christine
A ne peut pas venir à Noël ☐
B ne veut pas venir à Pâques ☑
C ne peut pas venir comme prévu ☐

'Correct. A nice easy question to start the exercises.'

2 Sa mère
A a mal à l'estomac ☐
B est malade ☑
C ne peut pas facilement marcher ☐

'Wrong. A broken foot is not a disease. C is much closer to the truth.'

3 Marie-Christine
A aime son papa ☐
B a deux sœurs ☐
C aide sa mère ☑

'Correct. Although A may well be true, it is not stated in the text.'

4 Elle
A prépare les repas ☐
B change les lits ☑
C achète des vêtements ☐

'Wrong. The correct answer is A, because she says **je fais la cuisine**.'

5 Elle veut venir
A dans quelques mois ☑
B l'année prochaine ☐
C avec sa mère ☐ *(5)*

'Correct. Well deduced.'

▷ **Question 9** Voici des détails de jeunes qui cherchent un correspondant ou une correspondante.

SVEN HARDRADA
U-Thant-Ring 67, 10057
Helsinki, Finlande
Je suis passionné d' animaux.
J'aime les hamsters, les cobayes,
les rats, les chiens et les chats.
Je voudrais correspondre avec
des amis des animaux en France.

JOHANNA BECKER
Alte Schloßstraße 4, 30577
Marienheide, Allemagne
J'ai 15 ans, et je voudrais
correspondre avec des garçons
de 16 ans.

FLORENCE MCNALLY
23 Antrim Road, Belfast
BT23 4SJ, Irlande du Nord
Je suis une fille de 12 ans. J'aime
la danse et le hockey. Je voudrais
correspondre avec des garçons
ou des filles du monde entier.

ROSSANA PAGLIOLICO
via Appia 46, 10124
Turin, Italie
Je cherche des correspondants
qui utiliseront l'internet en
français ou en italien.

FREDERICO GUSTO
31849 Yanci Navarra, Espagne
Je cherche des garçons ou des
filles entre 13 et 15 ans pour
échanger des cartes postales et
des timbres que je collectionne.

MAUD HILDE
avenue de la Liberté 84, 1195
Bruxelles, Belgique
Je m'intéresse aux
correspondants qui parlent
anglais, français, néerlandais
ou allemand et qui, eux
s'intéressent à la musique.

MARIE-CHRISTINE LEBLANC
2324 South Forest, MI 48103
Ann Arbor, USA
Je suis française et j'habite au
nord des Etats-Unis. J'aimerais
correspondre avec des jeunes
français(es) qui s'intéressent à
la littérature française ou
américaine.

HERVÉ LA CHARRETTE
97 Alberta Avenue,
Montréal 3, Canada
Je désire correspondre avec
de jeunes françaises entre 13
et 16 ans. Ma sœur, elle aussi,
cherche des correspondants.

Ecrivez le nom de la personne qui: (6)

	NOM
Exemple: adore les animaux	Sven
1 est sportive	Florence
2 aime la lecture	Sven
3 a une sœur qui aime écrire des lettres	Hervé
4 veut correspondre avec des garçons plus âgés	
5 s'intéresse à l'informatique	Rossana
6 parle quatre langues	Maud

Examiner's comment

Most of these answers are correct. However, it is very unlikely that the same name will be the answer to the example **and** one of the questions, so no. 2 is wrong. If the candidate had looked up **lecture**, which was the difficult word, he or she would know that it meant 'reading', and that **littérature** would give away the correct answer, Marie-Christine. The candidate has also left a blank for no. 4. A blank is never right! Guess if forced to!

Higher Tier B, A, A* grade tasks

▶ **Question 10** Lisez ce texte et répondez aux questions **en français**.

L'éternal combat de l'homme et du loup

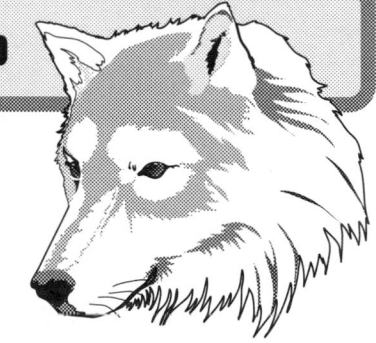

Il semble que, d'abord, l'homme et le loup cohabitaient sans problème. Mais l'habitude humain d'élever le bétail, et l'habitude du loup de le tuer, a causé, avec le temps, des conflits d'intérêts.

Ainsi a commencé une chasse sans merci. Le mépris du loup, aggravé par la superstition et l'ignorance, est à l'origine de la disparition progressive des loups. Aux Etats-Unis ils n'existent que dans 3 des 48 états. En Ecosse, le dernier loup a été tué au 18ème siècle. En France, le dernier loup sauvage a été abattu en 1937. Depuis on a eu parfois des problèmes avec des loups échappés des collections zoologiques.

Sur le plan mondial, le loup n'est pas menacé. Mais il a disparu de la plupart des pays dont la densité de la population est importante. Il a effectivement disparu de l'Europe occidentale. En Russie, par contre, on a pu abattre 50 000 loups par an sans menacer la population.

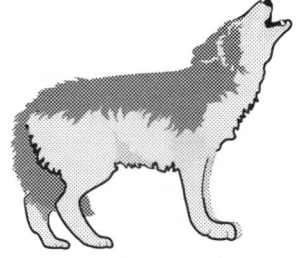

1 Quelle habitude humaine a causé le conflit entre l'homme et le loup?
2 Pourquoi est-ce qu'il y a une chasse sans merci?
3 Dans quelles régions du monde y a-t-il peu de loups, selon le texte?
4 Depuis quand n'y a-t-il plus de loups sauvages en France?
5 Pourquoi y a-t-il parfois des problèmes avec des loups en France aujourd'hui?
6 Qu'est-ce qui indique que, en Russie, il y a encore beaucoup de loups? (6)

Student answers with examiner's comments

'Correct.'
'Not correct. It's cattle they eat.'

'Wrong. There are none there: right answer is US and/or western Europe.'

'Correct. No need to write the date in words.'

'Not the best French, but the meaning is clear.'

'Not an answer. It's the fact that they kill 50 000 a year that makes it clear they have plenty.'

1   L'habitude d'élever le bétail.

2   Les loups mangent les humains.

3   Ecosse

4   1937

5   Des loups quittent des zoos.

6   Il y a beaucoup de loups.

▷ **Question II**   Lisez ce texte.

J'AI HONTE DE RONFLER

Je m'adresse à vous pour que vous m'aidiez à résoudre mon problème. Voilà: il se trouve que je ronfle!

J'ai trente ans et je n'ai jamais parlé de cela à personne. Je n'ai même pas consulté mon médecin, tellement j'en ai honte. Quand j'étais plus jeune, je n'osais même pas dormir chez des amies. Il y a longtemps que j'ai ce problème qui me gâche la vie.

Je suis mariée et, bien sûr, mon mari sait bien que je ronfle. La nuit, ça le gêne et le réveille. Quand je commence à ronfler, il me réveille et me fait remarquer que je l'empêche de dormir. C'est insupportable pour lui, mais que faire?

Quand nous partons en vacances, je n'aime pas l'idée d'aller dormir dans la famille de mon mari ou dans la mienne, car mes ronflements sont si forts que je réveille tout le monde. Il me semble que ça s'entend dans toute la maison.

Le soir devant la télé, quand je suis fatiguée, il m'arrive de m'endormir pendant une émission et là, je commence à ronfler. Souvent ma famille rigole de moi. Ils ne comprennent pas que leurs plaisanteries me font terriblement mal. Je suis gênée.

Maintenant, j'ai des complexes. Quand le moment arrive d'aller se coucher, je me sens mal. J'ai peur.

Mais comment contrôler ce qui se passe quand on dort? Je ferais n'importe quoi pour être guérie. Mais le ronflement, est-il une maladie?

S'il vous plaît, aidez-moi: y a-t-il un remède miracle?

Christelle

Student answer with examiner's comments

Cochez les bonnes cases.

1   Quel est le problème principal de Christelle?

'Incorrect. It is others who can't sleep when Christelle is sleeping. The correct answer is D.'

    A   Elle dort mal.   ☑

    B   Elle ne peut pas se réveiller.   ☐

    C   Elle a honte de son mari.   ☐

    D   Elle fait du bruit en dormant.   ☐

2   Qu'est-ce qu'elle ne faisait jamais quand elle était plus jeune?

'Correct'

    A   Elle ne dormait pas chez ses camarades.   ☑

B Elle n'allait jamais voir ses camarades. ☐

C Elle ne consultait jamais son médecin. ☐

D Elle ne parlait jamais à personne. ☐

3 De quoi se plaint son mari?

A Des gens. ☐

'Correct – an easy question as there is an "echo" of the title.'

B Du ronflement de sa femme. ☑

C Du lit. ☐

D De tout ce qu'elle fait. ☐

4 En vacances, où préfère-t-elle dormir?

A Chez ses parents. ☐

'Correct. This required quite a bit of deduction. Well done.'

B Chez les parents de son mari. ☐

C Dans un hôtel. ☑

D Dans la voiture. ☐

5 Quelle réaction de sa famille la gêne?

'Incorrect. There is no mention of any sympathy from her family. It is their laughs which she finds annoying. B is the correct answer.'

A Leur pitié. ☑

B Leurs rires. ☐

C Leur habitude de la laisser seule devant la télé. ☐

D Leur habitude de la critiquer tout le temps. ☐

6 Comment se manifestent ses complexes?

'Correct. The candidate has found a synonym for **angoissée** in the text. Checking for words with similar meanings to those in the question is a sound technique.'

A Elle est angoissée en fin de soirée. ☑

B Elle a peur de l'obscurité. ☐

C Elle est toujours malade la nuit. ☐

D Elle a du mal à s'endormir. ☐

7 Que demande-t-elle?

A Une solution. ☑

'Correct.'

B Un médicament. ☐

C Une consolation. ☐

D Un miracle. ☐

(7)

▶ **FURTHER SPECIMEN QUESTIONS**

The questions have been laid out so that you can write the answers in the book. Test yourself! The answers are given at the end of the chapter. I have provided a variety of text and test types. You should also ask your teacher if you can see the sample papers and any past papers for your Examining Group. At the time of writing (early 1997) the Examining Groups are very much feeling their way when testing comprehension of French in French, and are certain to learn from experience of 'live' candidates doing 'live' papers.

Foundation Tier G, F, E grade tasks

▶ **Exercise I**   What do these signs mean? Write your answers in the spaces provided.

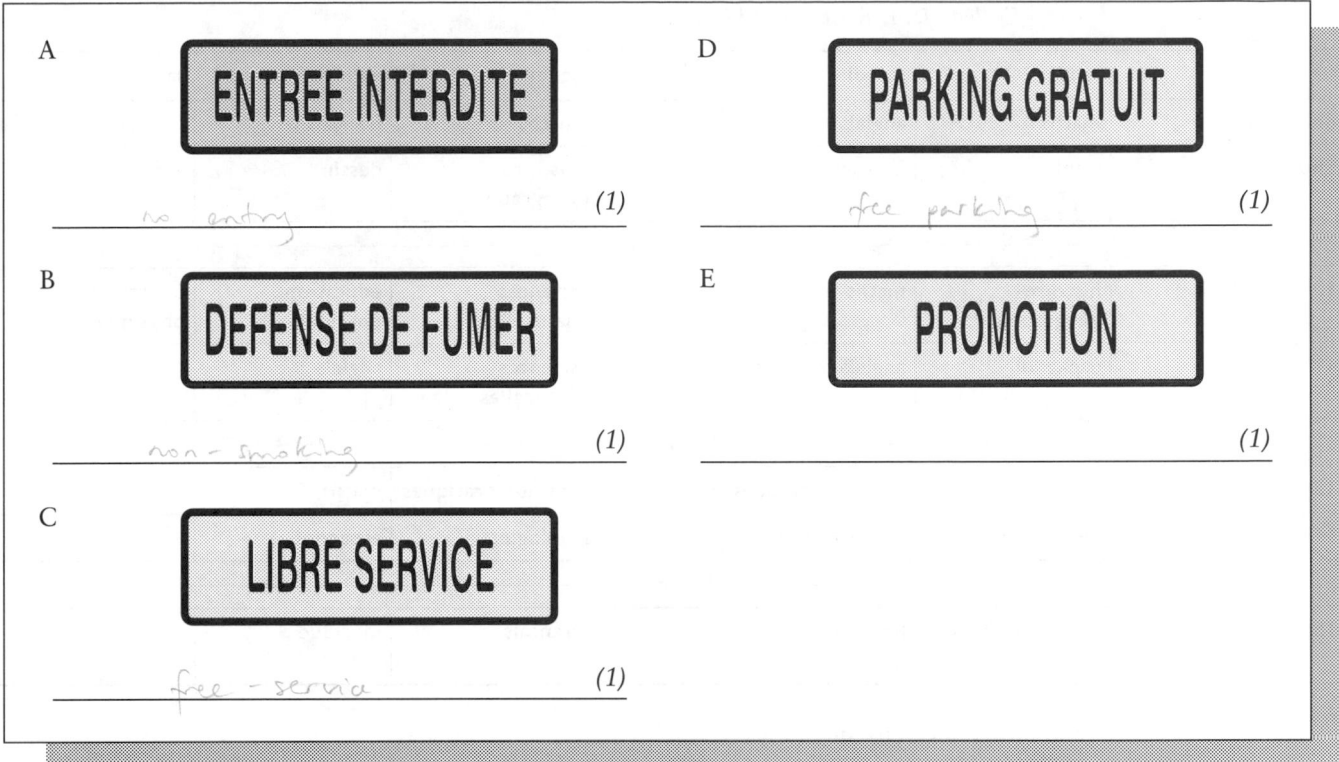

A   ENTREE INTERDITE

_____no entry_____ *(1)*

B   DEFENSE DE FUMER

_____non - smoking_____ *(1)*

C   LIBRE SERVICE

_____free - service_____ *(1)*

D   PARKING GRATUIT

_____free parking_____ *(1)*

E   PROMOTION

_____ *(1)*

▶ **Exercise 2**

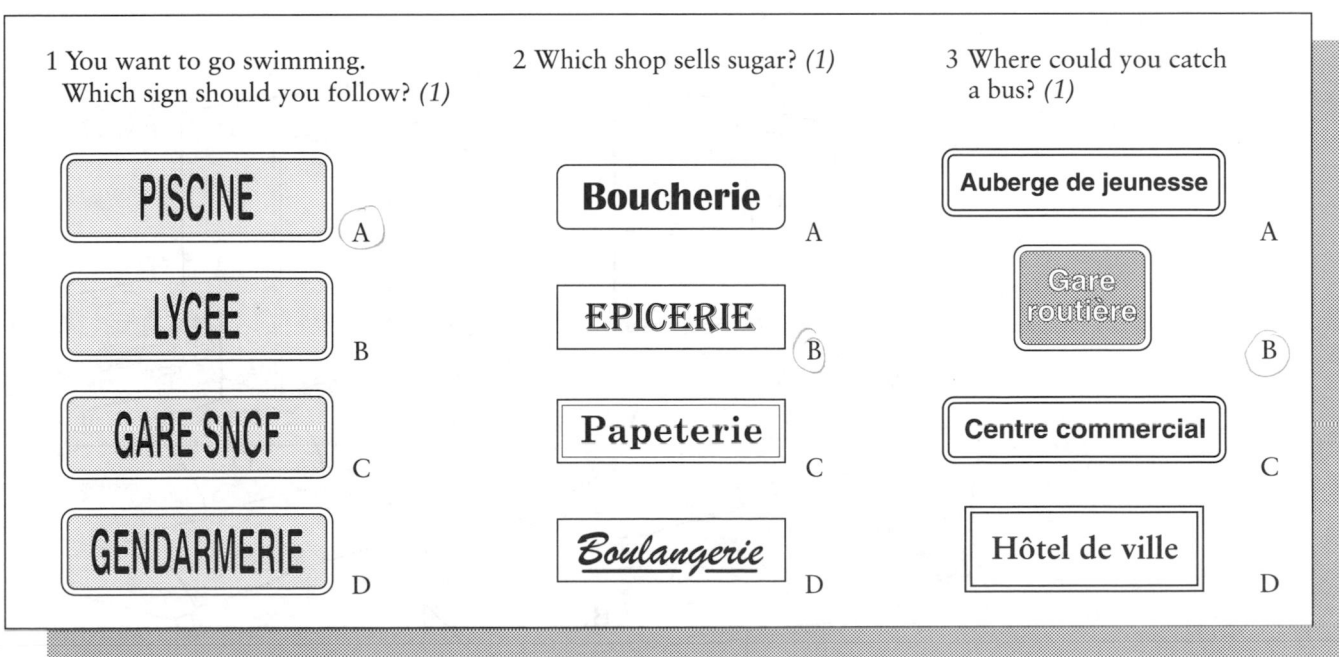

1 You want to go swimming. Which sign should you follow? *(1)*

PISCINE   A

LYCEE   B

GARE SNCF   C

GENDARMERIE   D

2 Which shop sells sugar? *(1)*

Boucherie   A

EPICERIE   B

Papeterie   C

Boulangerie   D

3 Where could you catch a bus? *(1)*

Auberge de jeunesse   A

Gare routière   B

Centre commercial   C

Hôtel de ville   D

▶ **Exercise 3**   Regardez cet emploi du temps d'Alain Legrand

Emploi du temps
Classe 3e A
Collège Jean Rostand, 44700 Orvault

	lundi	mardi	mercredi	jeudi	vendredi	samedi
8h 30–9h 25	maths	anglais		maths	français	français
9h 25–10h 20	étude	français		histoire-géographie	dessin	anglais
	←————————————————— récréation —————————————————→					
10h 35–11h 30	histoire-géographie	maths		sciences naturelles	éducation physique	éducation physique
11h 30–12h 25	espagnol	anglais renforcé		sciences naturelles	anglais	
	←————————————————— déjeuner —————————————————→					
13h 30–14h 25	français	travaux pratiques		travaux pratiques	maths	
14h 25–15h 20	anglais	travaux pratiques		biologie	espagnol	
	←————————————————— récréation —————————————————→					
15h 35–16h 30	anglais renforcé	histoire–géographie		français	musique	

Répondez aux questions.

1   A quelle heure commencent les classes?. . 8h 30 . . . . *(1)*
2   Combien de leçons de maths a-t-il par semaine?. . quatre . . . . *(1)*
3   Qu'est-ce qu'il a le vendredi après l'espagnol? . . musique . . . . *(1)*
4   Combien de langues étrangères est-ce qu'il apprend? . deux . . . . *(1)*
5   Quels jours y a-t-il de l'éducation physique? . . . . . . deux vendredi, samedi . . . *(2)*

▶ **Exercise 4**

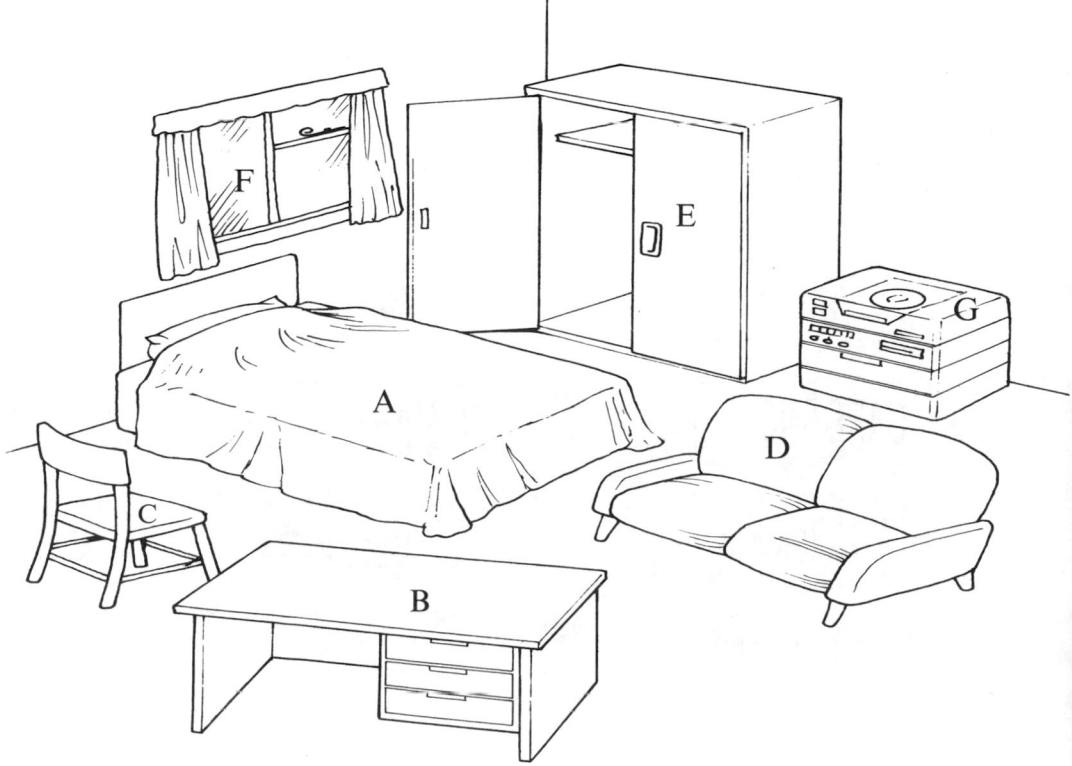

Trouvez les objets sur le dessin.

Ecrivez les 5 bonnes lettres à côté.

Exemple: chaîne stéréo	G
table	B
lampe	
canapé	
fauteuil	E
baskets	
fenêtre	F
lit	A
armoire	D

(5)

▷ **Exercise 5**

Casse-croûte;
boissons fraîches

Qu'est-ce qu'il y a ici?
Cochez (✓) les 3 bonnes cases.

des frites	
du chocolat froid	✓
du thé	✓
du café	✓
un menu à 85F	
un croque-monsieur	

(3)

▷ **Exercise 6**

	Etage
ménager	4 étage
vêtements dames	3 étage
vêtements messiers	2 étage
chaussures	1 étage
articles de sport	rez-de-chaussée
alimentation	sous-sol

Ascenseur

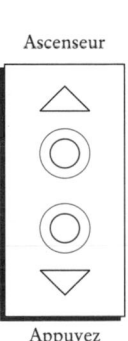

Appuyez

Vous voulez acheter:	Etage?
Exemple: du sel	*sous-sol*
un couteau de cuisine	4 / sous-sol
un pantalon pour ton père	2
des balles de ping-pong	rez-de-ch.
des sandales	1
du beurre	sous sol.

(5)

Foundation Tier D, C grade tasks, Higher Tier D, C grade tasks

▷ **Exercise 7**   Vous lisez cette lettre dans un magazine local pour la jeunesse.

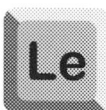 **courrier des lecteurs**

Chers amis

Je recherche une fille que j'ai rencontrée dans le car à destination de Marseille le 5 juillet dernier. Elle est de taille moyenne vers 1m 65. Elle à les cheveux châtaines, et elle a les yeux bruns. Elle portait un blue-jean, un sweat vert et des baskets. Nous avons discuté pendant tout le voyage, mais je ne sais pas son nom. Si quelqu'un la connaît, montrez-lui ce message, et dîtes-lui de me téléphoner au 02.40.23.56.81. Merci.

Bernard Lepeureux

Remplissez les blancs pour donner le sens de la lettre.
Choisissez parmi les mots dans la case.

> un peu; fille; femme; s'habille; blonds; juin; de téléphone; juillet; août; s'appelle; d'immatriculation; beaucoup; de téléphone; bruns

Bernard a rencontré cette ......fille........ au mois de ....juillet........ Elle a les cheveux
.......chatains....... Il a parlé ......beaucoup...... avec cette fille, mais il ne sait pas comment elle
......s'appelle...... Il a donné son numéro ......de téléphone......

(5)

▷ **Exercise 8**   Voici un programme pour une semaine de vacances.

UNE SEMAINE ACTIVE POUR CHACUN

Dimanche	Arrivée en fin d'après-midi. Pot d'accueil à 19h 30 avant le dîner.
Lundi	Matinée libre. Après-midi: randonnée VTT ou initiation planche à voile.
Mardi	Matinée: tournoi de volley. Après-midi: randonnée pédestre dans les collines.
Mercredi	Excursion en car au parc historique du Puy du Fou.
Jeudi	Promenade en mer en bateau de pêche. Après-midi: visite du château de Noirmoutier. A marée basse, retour de l'île de Noirmoutier à pied par le Gouat (3km de marche).
Vendredi	Matinée: baignade en mer ou à la piscine, selon le temps. Après-midi: visite au sous-marin Espadon à St-Nazaire. Soirée: grand bal folklorique.
Samedi	Matinée libre. Départ dans l'après-midi.

Un moniteur accompagne toutes les activités

Ecrivez le jour correct pour chaque activité.

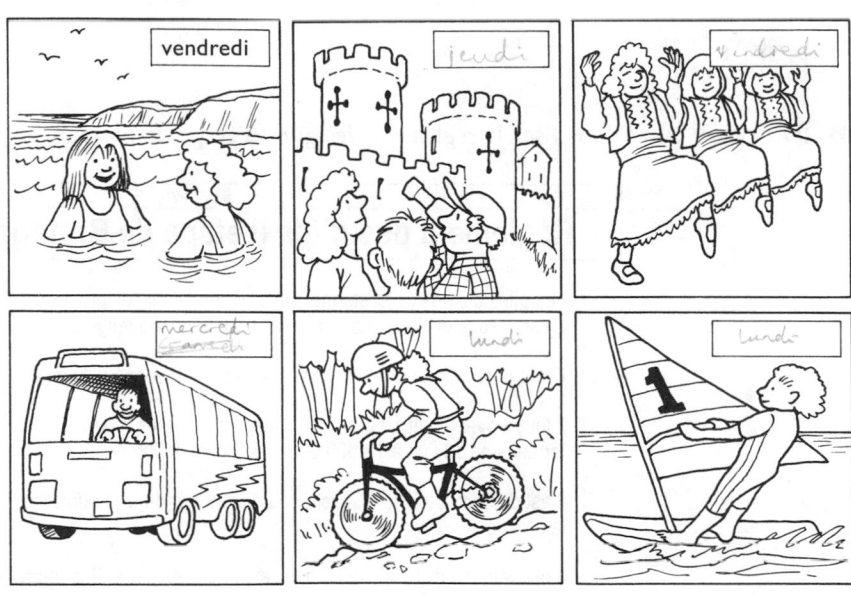

(5)

▷ **Exercise 9**   Lisez ces trois extraits de lettres sur les vacances.

Jean-Yves

Pendant les grandes vacances je suis allé passer deux semaines chez ma tante à Martel, près de la Dordogne. Il faisait très chaud, et nous avons nagé dans la rivière. Mon oncle a une petite barque et nous avons fait beaucoup de bateau. J'ai aussi pêché dans la rivière. Enfin, je me suis bronzé. Le soir je retrouvais mes copains sur la grande place après le dîner et nous bavardions souvent jusqu'à minuit.

Marie-Laure

J'ai passé deux semaines de vacances en colonie de vacances. C'était extra! J'étais seule, c'est-à-dire sans ma famille, mais les autres étaient sympa. Nous avons fait un peu de tout. Il y avait des promenades, des excursions, des visites à la plage, des jeux, des sports, on a fait de la voile. Bref, il y avait toujours quelque chose de différent à faire. Ce qui était vraiment étonnant, c'est qu'on a vraiment bien mangé.

Victoire

Pendant les grandes vacances je suis allée passer une semaine à Paris avec mes parents. Ils ont insisté qu'on visite à peu près tout (ennuyeux), alors nous avons passé deux ou trois jours dans des musées, des églises et des monuments. Heureusement, après trois jours on a commencé à faire des choses plus amusantes et moins fatiguantes. J'ai aimé visiter les magasins chics de place Vendôme, et papa m'a acheté un sac super-chouette. On a assez bien mangé, mais le plus amusant c'était le restaurant Chartier où on écrit sa commande sur la nappe.

Indiquez ensuite la personne ou les personnes pour qui ces phrases sont vraies.

	Jean-Yves	Marie-Laure	Victoire
1 J'ai passé mes vacances près de la rivière.	✓		
2 J'étais dans une grande ville.			✓
3 Je n'étais pas avec mes parents.	✓	✓	
4 J'ai tout aimé.	✓	✓	
5 J'ai discuté avec mes camarades en plein air.		✓	
6 J'ai bien mangé.	✓	✓	✓
7 J'ai visité un magasin de luxe.			✓
8 Il a fait beau.	✓	✓	

(9)

▷ **Exercise 10**   Vous lisez le règlement des gîtes d'étape de Bretagne.

Règlement des gîtes d'étape de Bretagne

☐ Les gîtes d'étape de Bretagne sont ouverts à tous les groupes de jeunes âgés de moins de 25 ans, sans distinction de nationalité, de race, de religion ou d'opinion politique.

☐ Il faut faire une réservation par écrit ou par téléphone à l'avance.

☐ Il faut arriver avant 19.00h. Les gîtes sont fermées à partir de 22.00h. Pour le nettoyage, les gîtes restent fermées de 10.00h à 12.00h et de 14.00h à 16.00h.

☐ Il est défendu de faire la cuisine ou de manger dans les dortoirs. On a le droit de préparer des repas dans la cuisine.

☐ Il est défendu d'utiliser des radios, etc. dans les gîtes. Par contre, les instruments de musique sont bienvenus.

☐ Il est strictement défendu de consommer des boissons alcoolisées et de fumer à l'intérieur des gîtes.

☐ Chaque usager est obligé de se servir à table, et de rincer sa vaisselle après le repas.

☐ Il est recommandé aux usagers de déposer tout objet de valeur au bureau du gîte.

☐ Le jour du départ, il faut nettoyer les dortoirs avant 10.00h.

☐ On n'a pas le droit de partir avant 07.00h.

Remplissez la grille **en français**.

Exemple: Age maximum pour l'usage des gîtes d'étape	24
Deux possibilités de réservation	*par écrit ou téléphone*
Limite de l'heure d'arrivée	*avant 19.00h*
Possibilité de faire la cuisine où?	*dans les cuisine*
Bruit interdit dans le gîte	*des radios, etc.*
Bruit permis dans le gîte	*les instruments de musique*
Fumer	*défendu*
Service des repas	*c'est obligé de se servir*
Nettoyage des dortoirs le jour du départ	*fa avant. 10.00h*

(9)

Higher Tier B, A, A* grade tasks

▷ **Exercise II**   Lisez cet article

Les vacances, c'est casse-pieds pour les enfants!

Demain, c'est le grand départ en vacances. Maman est en train de surveiller le contenu des bagages, de nettoyer la maison, de faire la lessive, de veiller aux besoins de nos cochons d'Inde, et de laisser tout en ordre. Papa s'occupe de la voiture, des papiers, du courrier, du gazon. Chez nous, on est très traditionnel. Mais, moi, je ne veux pas partir en vacances. Pourquoi? Parce que nous allons toujours à la même station balnéaire, toujours dans le même appartement, toujours pour la même quinzaine. Et le programme est toujours identique. Le matin, petit déjeuner sur le balcon, face à la mer. On se promène une heure le long de la plage. On rentre manger à midi, et on fait la sieste jusqu'à trois heures.

On fait ses commissions, on va au spectacle du soir (peu de variation d'une année à l'autre), on mange dans les mêmes restaurants que l'année dernière. C'est calme, c'est trop calme. Moi, je préférais passer des vacances avec mes copines. Comme ça, il y aurait un peu d'animation. On rigolerait. Comme je suis enfant unique, deux semaines en compagnie de mes parents me tuent. Bref, j'en ai ras le bol de ces vacances calmes en famille. Maman, par contre, vante les avantages du climat maritime, de ses restaurants favoris, des promenades le long de la plage. J'avais voulu invité une copine cette année, mais maman n'a pas voulu. Au moins, dans quinze jours je serai rentrée et j'aurai ma liberté personnelle de nouveau.

Gaëlle

Répondez aux questions **en français**.

1 Qui s'occupe des animaux de la famille?
2 Qui s'occupe des lettres?
3 Comment trouve-t-elle ses vacances?
4 Pourquoi?
5 Comment trouverait-t-elle des vacances avec ses copines?
6 Comment a réagi maman à l'idée d'inviter une copine de Gaëlle?
7 Qu'attend Gaëlle avec impatience?

(7)

▷ **Exercise 12**   Lisez ce dépliant.

La Ligue contre le Cancer vous informe

Soleil sourire

Il est là, il vient d'arriver: le soleil, symbole de l'été, des vacances et des plaisirs. Mais pourquoi jouer les biftecks grillés quand il suffit de savoir quoi faire? Le soleil est important pour le bien-être physique et moral, mais quelques sages précautions s'imposent pour en profiter sans risque.

Le résultat immédiat d'un excès d'exposition est le trop connu 'coup de soleil', caractérisé par rougeur, chaleur, gonflement, parfois fièvre.

A long terme, le risque majeur, c'est le cancer de la peau. L'Australie, pays très ensoleillé, peuplé surtout de britanniques à peau claire, est la région du monde où les cancers de la peau sont les plus nombreux. Ce qui montre bien la nécessité d'une protection efficace surtout lorsqu'on est dans la catégorie des peaux claires.

Le bronzage n'a pas toujours été à la mode. Jusqu'au début du 20ème siècle la beauté s'exprimait dans la blancheur de la peau chez les femmes. Les femmes du 19ème cultivaient le teint pâle en se protégeant par des ombrelles ou des chapeaux.

Conseils

Evitez les expositions brutales, les coups de soleil, l'exposition entre 12h et 16h, et soyez très vigilants vis à vis de l'exposition des enfants.

Portez des tee-shirts, des chapeaux ou des casquettes et des lunettes de soleil pour protéger les yeux.

Mettez régulièrement des crèmes-écran avec un bon indice de protection.

N'oubliez jamais qu'au soleil il fait chaud et qu'il faut boire souvent pour éviter de se déshydrater, en particulier chez les enfants.

Vrai ou faux?

1   Le soleil n'a pas d'avantages pour nous.
2   Un coup de soleil peut être assez sérieux.
3   L'expérience des Australiens prouve que le cancer de la peau est un risque réel.
4   On a toujours voulu être bronzé.
5   Au soleil, les enfants ne risquent pas plus que les adultes.
6   Il faut toujours avoir une boisson à la main.

(7)

▷ **Exercise 13**   Lisez cet extrait d'un livre d'histoire.

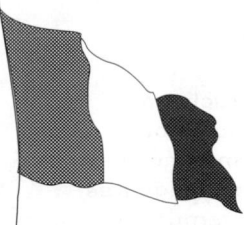

1789 La révolution française

14 juillet   PRISE DE LA BASTILLE

Les Parisiens pillent l'Arsenal pour armer la Garde Nationale. Ils volent 30 000 fusils et 12 canons. Ensuite, ils marchent sur la Bastille où ils pensent trouver des munitions.

La Bastille est une énorme forteresse transformée en prison. Ce jour-là il n'y a que sept prisonniers. Pour la défendre il n'y a qu'une centaine d'hommes. La construction de la Bastille, par contre, très solide.

Le gouverneur de la Bastille refuse de livrer des munitions. La bataille commence, et la Garde Nationale utilise les canons. Après quatre heures de bataille, le gouverneur de la Bastille capitule. La Bastille est prise.

Le Roi, en recevant la nouvelle de ces événements, demande:

– C'est donc une révolte?

– Non, Sire, c'est une révolution.

17 juillet   LE ROI VIENT A PARIS

Le Roi est venu se réconcilier avec les Parisiens. Il met à son chapeau les couleurs bleu, blanc et rouge.

Bleu et rouge sont les couleurs de Paris, et blanc est la couleur du Roi.

Le 14 juillet, date anniversaire de la Prise de la Bastille, a été déclaré Fête Nationale en 1880.

Mettez ces affirmations dans le bon ordre.

Exemple: Les Parisiens ont volé des armes.	1
La Bastille est une prison presque vide.	
On a commencé à commémorer la bataille de la Bastille 91 ans plus tard.	
Le tricolore français date du juillet 1789.	
Le Roi ne sait pas que c'est sérieux.	
On refuse des munitions aux Parisiens.	
Après quelques heures la Bastille tombe.	
Ils cherchent de la poudre et des balles à la Bastille.	

(7)

▶ **Exercise 14**

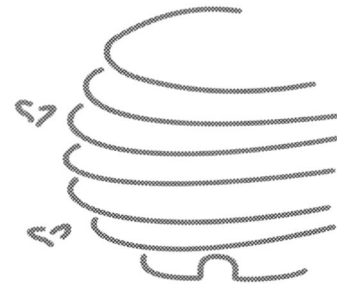

12 août

Suivons une abeille qui est active dans un champ fleuri. Elle se gorge de nectar délicieux et rentre vite dans sa ruche, à un kilomètre de distance. Elle se pose à l'entrée de la ruche, puis elle dépose son chargement de nectar. Ensuite, elle commence une danse étrange. Elle fait une série de cercles étroits. Elle change très souvent de direction en coupant les cercles. En peu de temps cette danse mystérieuse fascine d'autres abeilles. Bientôt elles entourent la danseuse. C'est que l'abeille qui danse est en train d'expliquer aux autres où se trouve le champ fleuri. Elle a gardé en mémoire la direction du champ par rapport à la ruche et au soleil. Sa danse donne ces informations avec précision. C'est comme si on traçait la direction dans le sable avec un bâton. Les abeilles partent vers le champ de fleurs et commencent à travailler, à récolter du pollen.

Répondez aux questions.

1   Pourquoi l'abeille est-elle contente?

. . . .(1)

2   En rentrant à la ruche, que fait-elle d'abord?

. . . .(1)

3   Pourquoi est-ce qu'elle commence à tourner en rond?

. . . .(1)

4   Quels sont les deux points de repère qu'elle utilise

. . . .(2)

5   Que cherchent les abeilles?

. . . .(1)

▶ **Exercise 15**   Read these two newspaper articles about the same event.

Mère et fille réunies après 13 jours d'angoisse

Ermont, le 12 juin

Christine Campagnard a reçu des centaines de cartes et beaucoup de fleurs hier soir. Elle a retrouvé sa fille Natasha (9 mois) qui avait disparu de sa poussette le 31 mai à Ermont.

Mme Campagnard avait laissé le bébé devant la pharmacie Phoque quand elle faisait des courses. Plus de 150 policiers l'ont cherché dans toute la banlieue près d'Ermont, et ils ont trouvé Natasha saine et sauve hier soir dans le village de Creysse. On questionne une femme de 42 ans qui habite Creysse.

Mme Campagnard nous a dit: 'Je n'ai pas dormi pendant ces 13 jours. Aujord'hui, c'est mon anniversaire. Retrouver Natasha—pour moi, c'est le meilleur cadeau de ma vie!'

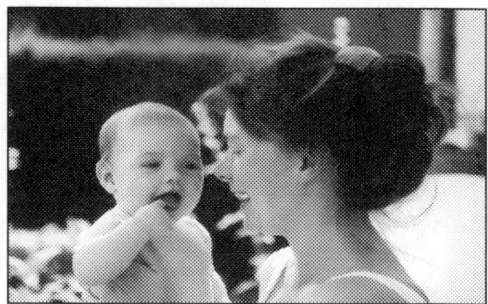

Quel cadeau!

Réunies après 13 jours d'enfer.
Natasha, volée par une maniaque le 31 mai, a souri pour notre photographe. Christine, 30 ans aujourd'hui: 'Mon bébé—quel cadeau d'anniversaire!'

Answer these questions **in English**.

1   What had happened to Natasha?

....(1)

2   How long ago?

....(1)

3   How did the police react?

....(1)

4   With whom was the baby found?

....(1)

5   How had people expressed their sympathy for Christine?

....(1)

6   Why is Natasha's return especially appropriate today?

....(1)

7   Which newspaper account do you prefer and why?

....(1)

▷ ANSWERS TO SPECIMEN QUESTIONS

Foundation Tier G, F, E grade tasks

▷ **Exercise 1**   A   No entry
              B   No smoking
              C   Self-service
              D   Free parking
              E   Special offer

▷ **Exercise 2**   1   A
              2   B
              3   B

▷ **Exercise 3**   1   8h 30
              2   4
              3   musique
              4   2
              5   vendredi, samedi

▷ **Exercise 4**

table	B
lampe	
canapé	D
fauteuil	
baskets	
fenêtre	F
lit	A
armoire	E

▷ **Exercise 5**

des frites	✔
du chocolat froid	✔
du thé	
du café	
un menu à 85F	
un croque-monsieur	✔

▷ **Exercise 6**

Vous voulez acheter:	Etage?
un couteau de cuisine	4
un pantalon pour ton père	2
des balles de ping-pong	rez-de-chaussée
des sandales	1
du beurre	sous-sol

Foundation Tier D, C grade tasks, Higher Tier D, C grade tasks

▷ **Exercise 7**   Bernard a rencontré cette *fille* au mois de *juillet*. Elle a les cheveux *bruns*. Il a parlé *beaucoup* avec cette fille, mais il ne sait pas comment elle *s'appelle*. Il a donné son numéro *de téléphone*.

▷ **Exercise 8**

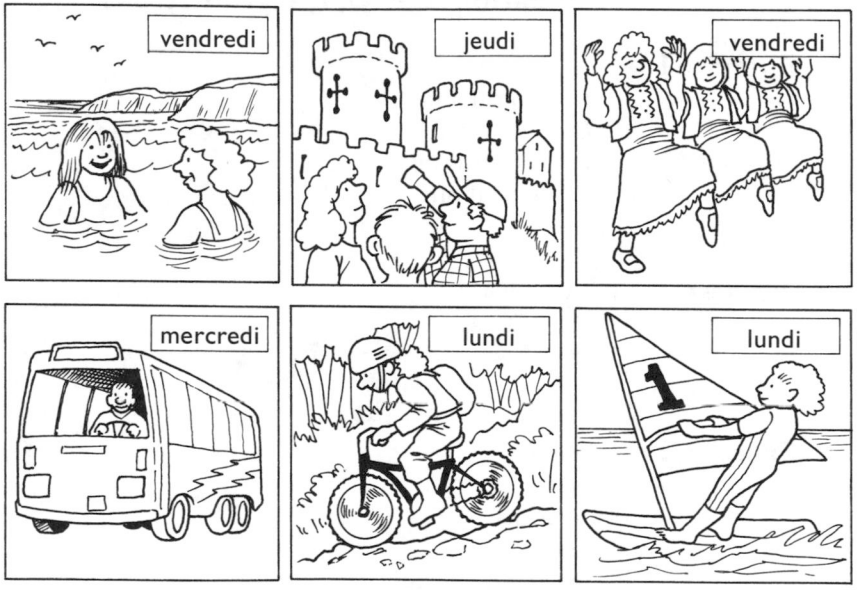

▷ **Exercise 9**

		Jean-Yves	Marie-Laure	Victoire
1	J'ai passé mes vacances près de la rivière.	✔		
2	J'étais dans une grande ville.			✔
3	Je n'étais pas avec mes parents.	✔	✔	
4	J'ai tout aimé.		✔	
5	J'ai discuté avec mes camarades en plein air.	✔		
6	J'ai bien mangé.		✔	
7	J'ai visité un magasin de luxe.			✔
8	Il a fait beau.	✔		

▶ **Exercise 10**

Exemple: Age maximum pour l'usage des gîtes d'étape	*25*
Deux possibilités de réservation	*téléphone; lettre*
Limite de l'heure d'arrivée	*19.00h*
Possibilité de faire la cuisine où?	*dans la cuisine*
Bruit interdit dans le gîte	*radio*
Bruit permis dans le gîte	*instruments de musique*
Fumer	*interdit*
Service des repas	*self-service*
Nettoyage des dortoirs le jour du départ	*avant 10.00h*

Higher Tier B, A, A* grade tasks

▶ **Exercise 11**
1 Maman.
2 Papa.
3 Casse-pieds.
4 C'est toujours la même chose.
5 Amusant.
6 Ne l'a pas permis.
7 Rentrer chez elle / la fin des vacances.

▶ **Exercise 12**
1 faux
2 vrai
3 vrai
4 faux
5 faux
6 faux

▶ **Exercise 13**

Les Parisiens ont volé des armes.	1
La Bastille est une prison presque vide.	3
On a commencé à commémorer la bataille de la Bastille 91 ans plus tard.	8
Le tricolore français date du juillet 1789.	7
Le Roi ne sait pas que c'est sérieux.	6
On refuse des munitions aux Parisiens.	4
Après quelques heures la Bastille tombe.	5
Ils cherchent de la poudre et des balles à la Bastille.	2

▶ **Exercise 14**
1 Elle a trouvé du nectar / un champ fleuri.
2 Elle dépose son chargement de nectar.
3 Pour attirer les autres abeilles / pour dire aux autres où se trouve le champ.
4 Le soleil et la ruche.
5 Du pollen.

▶ **Exercise 15**
1 She had been abducted.
2 13 days.
3 Big search / 150 officers.
4 A 42-year old woman in the village of Creysse.
5 Flowers and cards.
6 It's her mother's (30th) birthday.

7   Either: The first one, because there are more details.
    Or: The second one, because it communicates more snappily.

▶ A STEP FURTHER

Further hints for improving your performance in Reading include the following:

» Learn to take clues from the context given to you in English, and from other parts of the passage. Use your common sense. Speakers of French are just as logical as you are. It sometimes pays to remind yourself of that!

» It is worth being sure about all the variations of French plurals, and making a point of looking whether words are singular or plural. This, too, will help the finer understanding of detail in texts.

» In Higher Tier, it is also important to revise carefully the endings of verbs, the 'tense markers'. So there is a vital difference in meaning between *j'aimerai* (I will like…), *j'aimerais* (I would like…), and *j'aimais* (I used to like…, I was liking…). The same is true of most verbs, and you can be certain that the examiners will be interested in discovering whether you can tell the difference between them. So make sure of those tenses!

» A common problem is candidates' failure to distinguish between the pluperfect and the perfect tenses. Yet the difference between *j'étais allé* and *je suis allé* could well give the clue, for example, to the order in which events happened. Be aware!

Chapter 6

Speaking

GETTING STARTED

Everybody has to take a Speaking Test. It's worth 25% of your final marks, so it's important to make a good job of it. The most important characteristic of Speaking Tests at GCSE are that they are predictable: they should hold few surprises for anyone who has prepared well. Some elements, such as the topic presentations some Examining Groups specify, can be rehearsed and prepared at home. Most of the other elements are either straightforward or follow a clearly laid-out format. Experience shows that a majority of candidates perform better on Speaking than on some of their other skills. Make sure you are one of that majority by being better prepared!

Candidates who gain good marks in Foundation Speaking will be able to manage in straightforward situations encountered by a visitor to a French-speaking country. They will also be able to present a simple topic and answer simple questions about themselves and their own lives and routines. They will pronounce French well enough to be understood by a French speaker who is making an effort to understand them.

Candidates who gain good marks in Higher Speaking will be able to cope in more complex situations, and will be able to talk at greater length on a range of topics. They will be comfortable in discussing past, present and future events and will be able to give their opinions and justify them. They will pronounce French reasonably well, although it will be possible to gain full marks without perfect reproduction of a native speaker's accent.

WHAT YOU NEED TO KNOW

▶ Format of the examination

The Examining Groups, although they have minor differences, agree broadly about the shape of the final Speaking Test. If you are taking the SEG Modular syllabus, you will do part of your Speaking as coursework. EDEXCEL also offers the possibility of taking Speaking as coursework as an option: see Chapter 8 on coursework.

- It will be done between March and May at a time to be decided by your teacher.
- It will be conducted by your own teacher.
- It will almost certainly be recorded on cassette, so that the Examining Group can check it has been properly conducted. This is for your protection.
- Your teacher may well mark what you have done; alternatively, the recording may be sent away to be marked.
- It will typically take about 8–10 minutes for Foundation Tier, and 10–12 minutes for Higher Tier.
- You will have the same length of time to prepare the role-play beforehand, usually while the previous candidate is taking his/her test. During the preparation period you will be allowed access to an English–French, French–English dictionary. If you wish, you can bring a dictionary you own. Some Examining Groups (but not all) allow you to make notes during the preparation period and take them in with you to refer to during the Speaking Test. Check with your teacher the exact regulations for the examination you will be taking. Once you have entered the examination room, you will not be able to refer to a dictionary.

▶ Examining Group requirements

For **Foundation Tier** you will usually have to do two role-play tasks, and conduct a conversation on one or more than one topic with your teacher. In some GCSEs you may also have to present a topic which you have prepared beforehand.

In SEG Modular you will do two presentations, one at the end of Module 1, in February of Year 10, and the other at the end of Module 3, in December of Year 11. For these, you are required to make a short recording. You may be able to do this at home, but the recordings should be made on one occasion without editing.

Detailed Examining Group requirements are given in the table below.

Examining Group	role-play	presentation	conversation
NICCEA	*details not available*	*details not available*	*details not available*
EDEXCEL	2		two topics
MEG	2	yes	three topics
NEAB	2	yes	two topics
WJEC	2		two topics
SEG Modular	Module 4: 1	Module 1 & Module 3 home recording	Module 4

For **Higher Tier** the requirements are usually similar for all the Examining Groups. One of the role-plays will be the same as one of those offered at Foundation Tier. This will be the role-play which is designed to measure grades D and C. It will include some elements of unpredictability. That will normally mean that the teacher will ask you a question which is not written on the card, and will require an instant response. These need not be frightening: they are often quite straightforward as long as you have understood the question.

The Higher Tier conversation will include references to past, present and future events. You should also be able to give and justify and explain your opinion on the topics under discussion. If your Examining Group requires a presentation, the mark scheme will reward the same features, particularly opinions.

The role-plays will require you to take the initiative (for example asking for something in a shop) and may also require you to answer questions from strangers and friends.

Some role-plays will have five things for you to say, while others have three or four. But the technique of dealing with them is the same.

Your pronunciation must be good enough for a sympathetic native speaker who is making an effort to understand. It does not, therefore, have to be perfect in every detail. Indeed, as long as you attempt a French accent and don't mumble overmuch, you need not concern yourself further with pronunciation.

▶ How to do role-plays

Role-plays are of two types. They will either have pictures which tell you what to do, or they will have instructions in French. You will have a few minutes to prepare the role-play, and you are likely to be allowed a dictionary. Not all Examining Groups allow you to take notes into the test room.

The **picture stimulus role-plays** are usually for Foundation Tier candidates only. They are quite simple, and will look something like this:

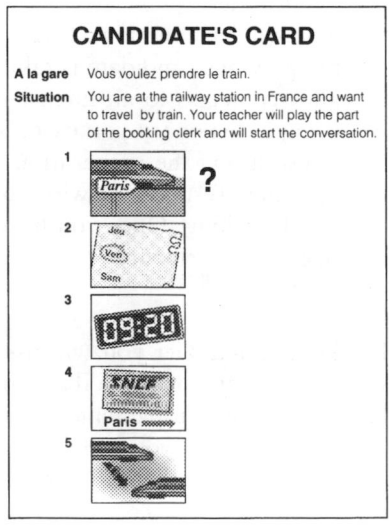

The important thing is to get across the message of what you want. So for this role-play the conversation might sound like this:

Teacher:	Vous désirez?
Pupil:	**Est-ce qu'il y a un train pour Paris?**
Teacher:	Quand voulez-vous aller à Paris?
Pupil:	**Vendredi.**
Teacher:	A quelle heure?
Pupil:	**A neuf heures vingt.**
Teacher:	C'est bon. Il y a un train à neuf heures vingt.
Pupil:	**Un aller simple pour Paris, s'il vous plaît.**
Teacher:	Alors, ça fait 50F.
Pupil:	**C'est direct?**
Teacher:	Oui, c'est direct.

It's important to remember that the exact form of what you say doesn't matter as long as you 'get the message across'. The marking schemes mainly reward the skill of getting what you want. So for the fourth task in the example above, it would have been perfectly acceptable to say *Paris, simple*. You would still have been given the right ticket, so it's worth full marks. Another example is:

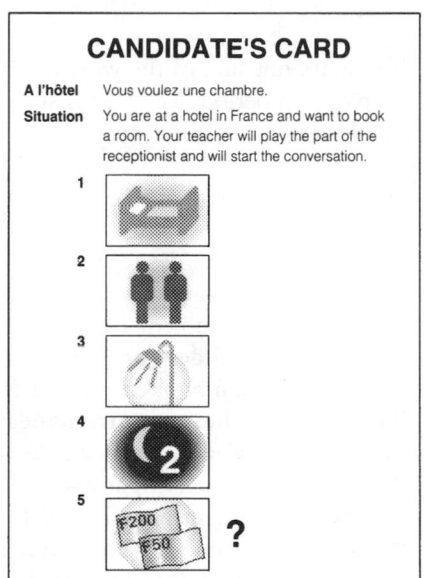

For this role-play the conversation might sound like this:

Teacher:	Vous désirez?
Pupil:	**Je voudrais une chambre.**
Teacher:	C'est pour combien de personnes?
Pupil:	**Pour deux personnes.**
Teacher:	Avec bain?
Pupil:	**Avec douche.**
Teacher:	Pour combien de nuits?
Pupil:	**Pour deux nuits, s'il vous plaît.**
Teacher:	Bon. Pas de problème.
Pupil:	**C'est combien?**
Teacher:	Alors, ça fait 250F par nuit.

Role-plays with instructions in French are for both Foundation and Higher Tier candidates. They may look something like this:

A LA BANQUE

Situation   You go into a bank in France. You want to change some traveller's cheques. Your teacher will play the part of the bank clerk and will begin the conversation.

1   Vous avez des chèques de voyage. Qu'est que vous dites?
2   Dites combien, et quelle sorte de travellers vous avez.
3   Répondez à la question.   *(the unpreparable task)*
4   Vous n'avez pas votre passeport. Dites où il est.
5   Demandez les heures d'ouverture de la banque.

If you are not sure of the words in the task, you will need to use your dictionary during the preparation period. Key words such as *Dites, Demandez* and *Répondez* are worth knowing in advance.

For this role-play the conversation might sound like this:

Teacher:	Vous désirez?
Pupil:	**Je voudrais changer des chèques de voyage.**
Teacher:	Combien? Et c'est quelle sorte de chèques de voyage?
Pupil:	**J'ai des American Express pour cinq cent francs.**
Teacher:	Où habitez-vous en France?
Pupil:	**Chez ma correspondante.**
Teacher:	Votre passeport, s'il vous plaît.
Pupil:	**Je ne l'ai pas avec moi. Il est à la maison.**
Teacher:	Il faut revenir avec le passeport.
Pupil:	**A quelle heure ferme la banque?**
Teacher:	A 18 heures, monsieur/mademoiselle.

'Note that the unpreparable question for task 3 is not a very difficult one.'

Another example is:

AU TÉLÉPHONE

Situation   You are looking for a job in France. You are speaking to an employer on the phone. Your teacher will play the part of the employer and will begin the conversation.

1   Dites qui vous êtes et d'où vous venez.
2   Répondez à la question.   *(the unpreparable task)*
3   Vous n'avez pas votre passeport. Dites où il est.
4   Dites quel travail vous avez déjà fait.
5   Dites pour combien de temps vous voudriez travailler.
6   Demandez s'il y a un logement.

For this role-play the conversation might sound like this:

Teacher:	Allô. C'est qui?
Pupil:	**Je m'appelle Anne Cambridge et je viens de Harlow en Angleterre.**
Teacher:	Vous parlez bien français. Depuis combien de temps apprenez-vous le français?
Pupil:	**Depuis cinq ans.**
Teacher:	Où avez-vous déjà travaillé?
Pupil:	**J'ai travaillé à Woolworth.**
Teacher:	Pendant combien de temps voulez-vous travailler?
Pupil:	**Je voudrais travailler pendant quatre semaines.**
Teacher:	Nous avons un poste pour vous au camping. Avez-vous d'autres questions?
Pupil:	**Est-ce qu'il y a un logement?**

> 'Note that the unpreparable question for task 2 is again not a very difficult one.'

Don't be put off by not knowing the exact best way of saying something. As long as you communicate something suggested by the pictures on the card, you will get your marks. One of the major aims of the GCSE is to use the language for the purposes of practical communication.

You should also remember that there is no one right answer to the role-plays, and that you can certainly improvise if you happen to have forgotten an item of vocabulary. I once had a candidate who had been told to buy cherries. He couldn't remember the word for cherries, but managed to describe *des petits fruits noirs qui se trouvent souvent dans les gâteaux de la forêt noire*. He got his mark for communicating.

▶ Role-play topics

The topics covered by role-plays will include:

▷ directions	▷ post office	▷ minor illness
▷ shopping for food	▷ tourist office	(a) at the doctor's
▷ shopping for clothes	▷ petrol stations	(b) at the dentist's
▷ cafés	▷ garages	(c) at the chemist's
▷ restaurants	▷ cinema / theatre	▷ lost property
▷ hotels	▷ arranging to go out	▷ repairs
▷ youth hostels	▷ party	▷ complaints
▷ campsites	▷ staying with a French	(a) shopping
▷ trains	family / receiving a	(b) eating out
▷ buses and trams	French guest	▷ telephoning
▷ air travel	▷ school	▷ accidents
▷ banks		▷ applying for a job

Make sure you have worked out likely role-plays for these. You can do this with a friend, and check the results with the various chapters in your textbook. Remember not to make them too difficult.

▶ Role-play phrases

Most of the role-play situations are predictable. There are only so many things you need to know when asking the way, for example. Listed below are essential phrases for every likely role-play situation.

General phrases
These can be used in many situations.
The first four are the most common.

Je voudrais... *I would like...*
C'est combien? *How much is it?*
A quelle heure...? *At what time...?*
Y a-t-il...? *Is there...?*

Attendez! *Wait!*

Avec plaisir. *It's a pleasure.*
D'accord. *OK.*
Entendu. *Agreed.*
Excusez-moi. *Excuse me.*
Il me faut... *I need...*
J'ai besoin de... *I need...*
Je dois... *I need to...*
Je peux...? *Can I...?*
Je ne peux pas... *I can't...*
Je veux... *I want to...*

Je ne veux pas...   *I don't want...*
Je suis désolé(e).   *I'm sorry.*
Où est...?   *Where is...?*
Où se trouve...?   *Where is...?*
Pour aller à...?   *How do I get to...?*
Pouvez-vous m'aider?   *Can you help me?*
Pouvez-vous me dire...?   *Can you tell me...?*

Question words

Pourquoi?   *Why?*
Quand?   *When?*
Où?   *Where?*
Qu'est-ce qui...? Qu'est-ce que...?   *What?*
Qui?   *Who?*
Combien (de)?   *How much / how many?*
Comment?   *How?*
Comment est...?   *What is ... like?*

Directions

Pour aller à la gare, s'il vous plaît?   *How do I get to the station, please?*
Où est la place Royale, s'il vous plaît?   *Where is the place Royale, please?*
Y a-t-il une banque près d'ici?   *Is there a bank near here?*
Tournez à droite au rond-point.   *Turn right at the roundabout.*
C'est à gauche après le musée.   *It's on your left after the museum.*
Continuez tout droit (jusqu'aux feux).   *Go straight on (as far as the lights).*
Prenez la première / deuxième / troisième à gauche.   *Take the first / second / third on the left.*
C'est à dix minutes à pied.   *It's a 10-minute walk.*
Vous êtes à pied ou en voiture?   *Are you on foot or in a car?*
Vous pouvez prendre l'autobus.   *You can get there by bus.*
C'est à trois kilomètres d'ici.   *It's 3 kilometres from here.*
A gauche du cinéma, en face du musée   *On the left of the cinema opposite the museum.*
C'est au premier / deuxième étage.   *On the first / second floor.*

Shopping for food

Vous désirez?   *Can I help you?*
Je voudrais trois pommes, s'il vous plaît.   *I'd like three apples, please.*
Et avec ça?   *Anything else?*
Un kilo de pommes de terre.   *A kilo of potatoes.*
Un demi-kilo de tomates.   *Half a kilo of tomatoes.*
Une boîte / un paquet de biscuits.   *A tin / box / packet of biscuits.*
Une tranche de jambon / de gâteau.   *A slice of ham / cake.*
C'est combien, les melons?   *How much are the melons?*
Les melons coûtent 10 francs la pièce.   *The melons cost 10 francs each.*
C'est tout, merci.   *That's all, thank you.*
J'ai seulement un billet de cent francs.   *I have only got a 100–franc note.*

Avez-vous la monnaie de cent francs?   *Have you change for 100 francs?*

Shopping for clothes

Some of the same phrases as in **Shopping for food** can be used here. See also **Complaints** (below).

Je regarde seulement.   *I'm just looking.*
Ce tee-shirt coûte combien, s'il vous plaît?   *How much does that T-shirt cost?*
Vous l'avez d'une autre couleur?   *Do you have it in a different colour?*
Est-ce que je peux essayer le pullover bleu, s'il vous plaît?   *May I try on the blue pullover, please?*
C'est trop petit / grand / cher.   *It's too small / big / expensive.*
Quelle est votre taille?   *What is your size? (clothes)*
Quelle est votre pointure?   *What size do you take? (shoes)*

Cafés

Je te paie un verre.   *I'll buy you a drink.*
Qu'est-ce que tu prends?   *What will you have?*
Vous voulez commander quelque chose?   *Do you wish to order?*
Je voudrais un Orangina®, s'il vous plaît.   *I would like an Orangina®, please.*
C'est tout?   *Anything else?*
Vendez-vous des sandwichs?   *Do you sell sandwiches?*
C'est combien un sandwich au jambon?   *How much is a ham sandwich?*
Je vous dois combien?   *How much do I owe you?*
Le service est compris?   *Is service included?*

Restaurants

See also **Complaints** (below).

Avez vous une table pour trois personnes?   *Have you a table for three?*
Je voudrais une table près de la fenêtre, s'il vous plaît.   *I'd like a table near the window, please.*
J'ai réservé une table au nom de Marsden.   *I've reserved a table in the name of Marsden.*
Je voudrais la carte, s'il vous plaît.   *I'd like to see the menu, please.*
Je voudrais commander maintenant.   *I'd like to order now.*
Vous avez décidé?   *Have you decided?*
Je prendrai le menu à 85 francs.   *I'll have the 85-franc meal.*
Comme hors d'œuvre, je prendrai des œufs mayonnnaise.   *To start with, I'll have egg mayonnaise.*
Comme plat principal, je voudrais poulet-frites.   *For the main course, I'd like chicken and chips.*
Qu'est-ce que vous avez comme légumes?   *What sort of vegetables do you have?*
Je prendrai des carottes, s'il vous plaît.   *I'll have carrots, please.*

Comme dessert, je prendrai une glace. *For dessert I'll have ice cream.*

Quels parfums avez-vous? *Which flavours do you have?*

Comme boisson, je prendrai de l'eau minérale. *I'll have mineral water to drink.*

L'addition, s'il vous plaît? *May I have the bill, please?*

Hotels

Avez-vous des chambres libres? *Have you any rooms available?*

Non, je regrette, c'est complet. *No, I'm sorry, the hotel is full.*

Y a-t-il un autre hôtel près d'ici? *Is there another hotel nearby?*

Je voudrais une chambre à un lit. *I would like a single room.*

Je voudrais une chambre pour deux personnes. *I would like a double room.*

Avec douche / avec salle de bains. *With shower / bathroom.*

Pour combien de nuits? *For how many nights?*

On va rester trois nuits. *We shall be staying for three nights.*

Quel est le prix de la chambre par nuit? *What is the price per room per night?*

Est-ce que le petit déjeuner est compris? *Is breakfast included?*

A quelle heure peut-on prendre le petit déjeuner? *When is breakfast?*

On peut prendre le petit déjeuner entre sept heures et dix heures. *You can have breakfast between 7.00 and 10.00.*

A quelle heure est le dîner? *At what time is dinner?*

Vous pouvez dîner entre sept heures et dix heures du soir. *Dinner is served from 7.00 until 10.00 p.m.*

Je voudrais des serviettes et du savon pour la chambre 3, s'il vous plaît. *May I have towels and soap for room 3, please?*

La note, s'il vous plaît. *The bill, please.*

Youth hostels

Some of the phrases in **Hotels** can also be used here.

Où est l'auberge de jeunesse, s'il vous plaît? *Where is the youth hostel, please?*

Je voudrais voir le père aubergiste, s'il vous plaît. *May I see the warden, please?*

Est-ce que vous avez des lits pour cette nuit? *Have you any beds available for tonight?*

Nous sommes quatre, deux filles et deux garçons. *There are four of us, two girls and two boys.*

C'est combien par nuit? *How much is it per night?*

Est-ce que je peux louer des draps? *Can I hire sheets?*

Où est le dortoir des filles / des garçons, s'il vous plaît? *Where is the girls' / boys' dormitory please?*

Le dortoir des filles est au deuxième étage. *The girls' dormitory is on the second floor.*

La salle commune est au rez-de-chaussée. *The day room is on the ground floor.*

Campsites

Some of the phrases in **Hotels** and **Youth hostels** can also be used here.

Avez-vous de la place pour une tente? *Have you room for a tent?*

Avez-vous un emplacement pour une caravane, s'il vous plaît. *Have you a pitch for a caravan, please?*

Vous êtes combien de personnes? *How many people are there?*

Nous sommes cinq, deux adultes, trois enfants. *There are five of us, two adults, three children.*

Le bloc sanitaire est au centre du camping. *The toilet block is in the middle of the site.*

Les poubelles sont à côté du bloc sanitaire. *The dustbins are next to the toilet block.*

C'est combien, la prise électrique pour les caravanes? *How much is electric connection for caravans?*

Où est-ce que je peux acheter du Camping Gaz? *Where can I buy Camping Gaz?*

Trains

Le train pour Paris part à quelle heure? *When does the train for Paris leave?*

A quelle heure est-ce qu'il arrive? *At what time does it arrive there?*

Le train part de quel quai? *From which platform does the train go?*

C'est direct? *Is it a through train?*

Le train en provenance de Calais arrive à quelle heure? *When does the train from Calais arrive?*

Un aller simple pour Bruxelles, s'il vous plaît. *A single ticket to Brussels, please.*

Un aller-retour, deuxième classe, pour Toulouse, s'il vous plaît. *A second-class return to Toulouse, please.*

Je voudrais réserver une place (non-fumeurs). *I'd like to reserve a (non-smoking) seat.*

Le voyage dure combien de temps? *How long does the journey take?*

Vous avez raté le train. *You have missed the train.*

Le prochain train pour Le Havre part à quelle heure? *When does the next train for Le Havre leave?*

Buses and trams

Some of the phrases in **Trains** can also be used here.

Où est l'arrêt d'autobus? *Where is the bus stop?*

Un carnet, s'il vous plaît. *A book of tickets, please.*

Il y a un autobus tous les combien? *How often do the buses run?*

J'attends déjà depuis dix minutes. *I've been waiting 10 minutes already.*

N'oubliez pas de composter votre billet. *Don't forget to stamp your ticket.*

C'est bien l'autobus pour le centre-ville? *Is this the right bus for the town centre?*

Vous descendez au musée. *You get off at the museum.*

Air travel

Some of the phrases in **Trains** can also be used here.

A quelle heure part le prochain vol pour Manchester? *When does the next plane for Manchester leave?*

Y a-t-il un vol pour Paris ce matin / ce soir / aujourd'hui? *Is there a flight to Paris this morning / this evening / today?*

Je voudrais un billet de classe touriste. *I'd like a tourist-class ticket.*

Je voudrais partir demain. *I would like to leave tomorrow.*

Je voudrais changer de vol. *I'd like to change flights.*

Il n'y a plus de places. *There are no more seats available.*

Où est la boutique hors-taxes? *Where is the duty-free shop?*

Attachez vos ceintures. *Fasten your belts.*

Banks

C'est quel guichet pour changer de l'argent? *Which is the counter for changing money?*

Je voudrais changer des chèques de voyage, s'il vous plaît. *I would like to change some traveller's cheques please.*

Y a-t-il une commission? *Is there a commission?*

Quel est le taux de change pour la livre sterling? *What is the exchange rate for the pound?*

Avez-vous une pièce d'identité? *Have you any means of identification?*

Où est-ce que je dois signer? *Where do I have to sign?*

Quelle est la date aujourd'hui? *What is today's date?*

A quelle heure ferme la banque? *At what time does the bank close?*

Post office

Some of the phrases in **Shopping for food** can also be used here.

C'est combien pour envoyer une carte postale en Grande Bretagne, s'il vous plaît? *How much does it cost to send a postcard to Britain, please?*

Je voudrais expédier ce paquet à Londres. *I would like to send this parcel to London.*

Voulez-vous me faire peser ce paquet? *Will you weigh this parcel, please?*

Il prendra combien de temps pour arriver? *How long will it take?*

Pour les lettres il faut d'habitude quatre jours. *Letters usually take four days.*

Six timbres à deux francs quatre-vingt, s'il vous plaît. *Six stamps at 2F 80, please.*

Où est la boîte aux lettres? *Where is the letter box?*

A droite de la cabine téléphonique. *On the right of the phone box.*

La prochaine levée est à quelle heure? *What time is the next collection?*

Tourist office

Je voudrais un plan de la ville, s'il vous plaît. *I would like a town plan, please.*

Je voudrais une carte de la région, s'il vous plaît. *I would like a map of the area, please.*

Je voudrais un horaire d'autobus. *I would like a bus timetable.*

Pouvez-vous me donner une liste des terrains de camping / des hôtels? *Can you give me a list of campsites / hotels?*

Où est-ce que je peux louer un vélo? *Where can I hire a bike?*

Avez-vous des dépliants sur la ville? *Have you any brochures about the town?*

Y a-t-il des visites guidées de la ville? *Do you do guided tours of the town?*

Nous restons ici pour deux jours. *We are spending two days here.*

Qu'est-ce qu'il faut voir en ville? *What should we see in the town?*

Petrol stations

Vingt litres de sans plomb, s'il vous plaît. *20 litres of lead-free, please.*

Le plein, s'il vous plaît. *Fill it up, please.*

Vérifiez les pneus / le niveau de l'huile / le niveau de l'eau, s'il vous plaît. *Please check the tyres / oil / water.*

Acceptez-vous des cartes de crédit? *Do you take credit cards?*

Est-ce que vous vendez des cartes / des boissons? *Do you sell maps / drinks?*

Là-bas, à côté de la caisse. *Over there by the cash desk.*

Y a-t-il des toilettes ici? *Are there any toilets here?*

Garages

Je suis en panne. *My car has broken down.*

Je suis en panne d'essence. *I've run out of petrol.*

Le moteur ne marche pas. *The engine won't work.*

Les phares / les freins ne marchent pas. *The lights / brakes are not working.*

La batterie est morte. *The battery is dead.*

C'est quelle marque de voiture? *What make of car is it?*

C'est une Ford Escort break rouge. *It's a red Ford Escort estate.*

Quel est votre numéro d'immatriculation? *What is your registration number?*

Où êtes-vous exactement? *Where are you exactly?*

Je suis sur la N12 à six kilomètres de Rennes. *I'm on the N12 6 kilometres from Rennes.*

Cinema/Theatre

Si on allait au cinéma / au théâtre? *How about going to the cinema / theatre?*

Qu'est-ce qu'on joue/passe? *What's on?*

C'est en version anglaise? *Is it in English?*

Non, mais il y a des sous-titres. *No, but there are subtitles.*

Est-ce qu'il y a un tarif réduit pour les étudiants? *Are there reductions for students?*

C'est combien au balcon / à l'orchestre? *How much is it in the balcony / stalls?*

Trois balcons, s'il vous plaît. *Three tickets for the balcony, please.*

La séance commence à quelle heure? *What time does the performance start?*

Ça dure combien de temps? *How long does it last?*

Le film finit à quelle heure? *What time does the film end?*

Comment as-tu trouvé le film / la pièce? *What did you think of the film / play?*

Le film / concert était excellent/intéressant / ennuyeux / affreux. *The film / concert was excellent / interesting / boring / awful.*

C'était trop long / sérieux. *It was too long / serious.*

Arranging to go out

Tu veux sortir ce soir? *Do you want to go out tonight?*

Oui, je veux bien. *Yes, I'd like to.*

Non, je dois faire mes devoirs. *No, I have to do my homework.*

Où est-ce qu'on va se rencontrer? *Where shall we meet?*

Devant le cinéma. *In front of the cinema.*

A quelle heure est-ce qu'on va se rencontrer? *At what time shall we meet?*

A huit heures. *At 8 o'clock.*

A plus tard. *See you later.*

Party

Il y aura une boum chez Chris samedi. *Chris is having a party on Saturday.*

Veux-tu venir à la boum avec moi? *Will you come to the party with me?*

Avec le plus grand plaisir. *Yes, I'd love to.*

Il faut que je demande à mon correspondant/ ma correspondante. *I must ask my penfriend.*

Desolé(e), mais je ne suis pas libre. *Sorry, I'm not free.*

Desolé(e), mais j'y vais avec Michel/ Michelle. *Sorry, I'm going with Michel/ Michelle.*

Malheureusement je dois faire mes devoirs. *Unfortunately I have to do my homework.*

Staying with a French family / Receiving a French guest

As-tu fait un bon voyage? *Have you had a good journey?*

Le voyage était très long. *The journey was very long.*

La traversée était calme / mauvaise. *The crossing was calm / bad.*

J'ai eu le mal de mer. *I was sea-sick.*

Je suis fatigué(e). *I am tired.*

J'ai oublié ma brosse à dents. *I have forgotten my toothbrush.*

Fais comme chez toi. *Make yourself at home.*

Veux-tu écouter des cassettes / la radio? *Would you like to listen to cassettes / the radio?*

Veux-tu regarder la télévision / une vidéo? *Would you like to watch TV / a video?*

Veux-tu sortir ce soir? *Would you like to go out this evening?*

Qu'est-ce qu'il y a à voir à Lorient? *What is there to see in Lorient?*

Qu'est-ce qu'on peut faire à Lyon? *What is there to do in Lyons?*

Puis-je vous aider / t'aider? *May I help you?*

Si on mettait / débarrassait la table? *Shall we set / clear the table?*

Je dois ranger ma chambre. *I have to tidy up my room.*

Je vais faire mes devoirs. *I am going to do my homework.*

Merci pour tout. *Thank you for everything.*

J'ai passé des vacances merveilleuses. *I've had a wonderful holiday.*

A bientôt / A l'année prochaine. *See you soon / next year.*

School

A quelle heure quittes-tu la maison le matin? *What time do you leave home in the morning?*

Je quitte la maison à huit heures et demie. *I leave home at 8.30.*

Comment viens-tu à l'école? *How do you come to school?*

En car / à pied / en voiture / par le train / à vélo. *By bus / on foot / by car / by train / by bike.*

Nous habitons à deux kilomètres de l'école. *We live 2 kilometres from school.*

Il me faut vingt minutes pour y aller à pied. *It takes me 20 minutes to walk there.*

A quelle heure commence / finit l'école? *What time does school start / finish?*

L'école finit à quatre heures moins vingt. *School finishes at 3.40 p.m.*

Tu as combien de cours par jour? *How many lessons do you have each day?*

Nous avons six cours par jour. *We have six lessons a day.*

Combien de temps durent tes cours? *How long do your lessons last?*

Nos cours durent cinquante-cinq minutes. *Our lessons last 55 minutes.*

Quelle est ta matière préférée? *What is your favourite subject?*

Ma matière préférée est le français. *My favourite lesson is French.*

Quelle matière n'aimes-tu pas? *Which subject don't you like?*

Je déteste l'anglais. *I can't stand English.*

Est-ce que tu manges à la cantine à midi? *Do you eat in the canteen at midday?*

Combien de semaines de vacances as-tu en
été? *How many weeks' holiday do you
have in summer?*
Nous avons cinq semaines de vacances en
été. *We have five weeks' holiday in
summer.*
C'est quand, la rentrée? *When do you go
back to school?*
Pour nous la rentrée est le 3 septembre. *We
go back on 3 September.*
As-tu beaucoup de devoirs? *Do you have a
lot of homework?*
Oui, j'ai deux heures de devoirs. *Yes, I have
two hours' homework.*

Minor illness

(a) At the doctor's
Qu'est-ce qui ne va pas? *What's the matter?*
Je me sens malade. *I feel ill.*
J'ai mal à la tête / à l'oreille / au ventre. *I've
got a headache / earache / stomach ache.*
Je me suis fait mal à la main. *I have hurt
hand.*
Je voudrais un analgésique. *I'd like something
for the pain.*
J'ai été piqué(e) par une abeille / une
guêpe. *I've been stung by a bee / wasp.*
Je suis allergique au fromage / aux
guêpes. *I'm allergic to cheese / wasps.*
J'ai de la fièvre. *I have a temperature.*
Voici une ordonnance pour des
comprimés. *Here is a prescription for some
tablets.*
Ma mère est tombée malade. *My mother has
been taken ill.*
Veuillez venir la voir, s'il vous plaît. *Will you
come and see her, please.*
C'est la première fois que ça m'arrive. *It's the
first time that this has happened to me.*
Je viens de vomir. *I've just been sick.*

(b) At the dentist's
Je voudrais un rendez-vous avec le
dentiste. *I'd like to see the dentist.*
J'ai mal aux dents. *I have toothache.*
Un plombage a sauté. *I've lost a filling.*
Vous payez à la réception. *Pay at reception.*

(c) At the chemist's
Avez-vous quelque chose contre un
rhume? *Have you something for a cold?*
J'ai besoin de mouchoirs en papier. *I need
some tissues.*
Mon frère a pris un coup de soleil. *My
brother is suffering from sunburn.*
Je voudrais du coton hydrophile / du
sparadrap. *I would like some cotton
wool / plasters.*
Je voudrais du sirop pour la toux. *I would
like some cough mixture.*
Une grande bouteille ou une petite? *A large
bottle or a small one?*
Ce n'est pas grave. *It is not serious.*

Lost property
J'ai perdu mon passeport / mon appareil-
photo. *I've lost my passport / camera.*
Où est-ce que vous avez perdu votre
sac? *Where did you lose your bag?*
Je l'ai laissé dans l'autobus. *I left it on the
bus.*
Où est-ce que vous l'avez cherché(e)? *Where
have you looked for it?*
J'ai cherché dans ma valise / ma
chambre. *I've looked in my case / in my
room.*
Quand avez-vous perdu votre porte-
monnaie? *When did you lose your purse?*
Hier / ce matin / samedi dernier. *Yesterday /
last week / last Saturday.*
On m'a volé mon argent. *My money has
been stolen.*
Il faut aller au commissariat de police. *You
must go to the police station.*

Repairs
J'ai de l'huile sur mon pantalon. *I've got oil
on my trousers.*
Pouvez-vous me le nettoyer, s'il vous
plaît? *Can you clean it for me, please?*
Ma montre ne marche pas. *My watch is
broken.*
Est-ce que vous pouvez la réparer? *Can you
repair it?*
Pouvez-vous revenir vendredi? *Can you come
back on Friday?*
Ce n'est pas possible. *That's not possible.*
Je retourne en Grande-Bretagne demain. *I go
home to Britain tomorrow.*

Complaints

(a) Shopping
J'ai acheté ceci hier / la semaine dernière. *I
bought this yesterday / last week.*
Ça ne marche pas. *It doesn't work.*
Je voudrais me faire rembourser. *I'd like a
refund.*
Voici le reçu. *Here's the receipt.*

(b) Eating out
Je regrette, mais j'ai un petit problème. *I'm
sorry, but I have a little problem.*
La fourchette est sale. *The fork is dirty.*
J'en voudrais une autre, s'il vous plaît. *I'd
like another, please.*
Le poisson est froid. *The fish is cold.*
Le steak n'est pas assez cuit pour moi. *The
steak is not well-enough cooked for me.*
Je voudrais parler au gérant. *I'd like to speak
to the manager.*

Telephoning
Allô, David à l'appareil. *Hello, David
speaking.*
Ici chez Lenoir. *This is the Lenoirs' house.*
Je suis le correspondant britannique / la
correspondante britannique de Sylvie. *I am
Sylvie's British penfriend.*
Voulez-vous laisser un message? *Can I take a
message?*

Répétez, s'il vous plaît. Je n'ai pas compris. *Say that again, please. I didn't understand.*

Comment écrit-on ça, s'il vous plaît? *Will you spell that, please.*

Est-ce que je peux téléphoner d'ici? *Can I phone from here?*

Je dois téléphoner en Grande-Bretagne. Qu'est-ce qu'il faut faire? *I need to phone Britain. What do I have to do?*

Attendez la tonalité. *Wait for the dialling tone.*

Ne quittez pas. *Hold the line.*

J'ai été coupé(e). *I've been cut off.*

Pouvez-vous me dire le numéro de téléphone de l'hôpital, s'il vous plaît? *Can you tell me the number of the hospital, please?*

Laissez votre message après le bip sonore. *Leave your message after the tone.*

Accidents

Au secours! *Help!*

Il y a eu un accident. *There has been an accident.*

Il y a des blessés. *There are injured people.*

Téléphonez aux pompiers. *Ring the fire brigade.*

Cherchez la police. *Fetch the police.*

Appelez un médecin. *Call a doctor.*

Applying for a job

Je m'appelle Chris Seaton. *My name is Chris Seaton.*

J'ai seize ans. *I'm 16.*

Je viens de Grande-Bretagne. *I come from the UK.*

Je cherche un emploi. *I am looking for a job.*

Je voudrais travailler pendant trois semaines au mois de juillet. *I'd like to work for three weeks in July.*

J'ai déjà travaillé dans un supermarché. *I have already worked in a supermarket.*

Avez-vous du travail pour moi? *Have you got a job for me?*

▷ MEG Narrator role-play

MEG asks candidates to tell a story suggested by a series of notes in French, or by pictures and notes combined. This task is usually intended to be done using past tenses, particularly the perfect tense. Normally you will have to keep going for about 5 minutes. This is easier with practice!

As well as making sure of common verbs in the past tenses, you need to have a repertoire of things you can say in order to keep going.

Prepare the following:

- ▷ a description of the weather
- ▷ a variety of reasons for doing something
- ▷ descriptions of people
- ▷ a description of a picnic and a restaurant meal
- ▷ opinions about how good something was or was not and why
- ▷ a number of things you did when visiting a town / spending a day in the country / spending a day by the seaside
- ▷ some summing-up phrases.

▷ Phrases for telling stories

Time phrases

plus tard que d'habitude *later than usual*

aussitôt que possible *as soon as possible*

un peu plus tard *a little later*

à ce moment-là *at that moment*

ce matin-là / cet après-midi-là / ce soir-là *that morning / that afternoon / that evening*

le lendemain *the next day*

vendredi dernier *last Friday*

la semaine dernière *last week*

pendant les grandes vacances *during the summer holidays*

à la fin de la journée *at the end of the day*

une demi-heure / trois jours plus tard *half an hour / three days later*

pendant trois heures *for three hours*

(tout de suite) après le déjeuner *(immediately) after lunch*

pendant son séjour à l'hôpital *during his stay in hospital*

How

rapidement / vite *quickly*

aussi vite que possible *as quickly as possible*

lentement *slowly*

sans hésiter *without hesitation*

sans rien dire *without speaking*

(mal)heureusement *(un)fortunately*

à ma grande surprise *to my great surprise*

sans perdre du temps *without wasting any time*

pour la première / deuxième / dernière fois *for the first / second / last time*

quand tout était prêt *when everything was ready*

par hasard *by chance*

soudain *suddenly*

Sequences

d'abord *at first*

puis / alors *then*

ensuite / après cela *after that*

après un certain temps *after a while*

quelques minutes plus tard   *a few minutes later*

plus tard dans la journée / soirée   *later that day / evening*

une fois arrivé(e)(s) à Douvres   *after arriving in Dover*

le premier / dernier jour des vacances   *on the first / last day of the holiday*

à une heure et demie   *at half past one*

au cours de la matinée / de l'après-midi / de la soirée   *during the morning / afternoon / evening*

pendant la nuit   *during the night*

à la fin de la journée / de l'excursion / du spectacle   *at the end of the day / outing / show*

à la fin / finalement   *finally*

enfin   *at last*

Example

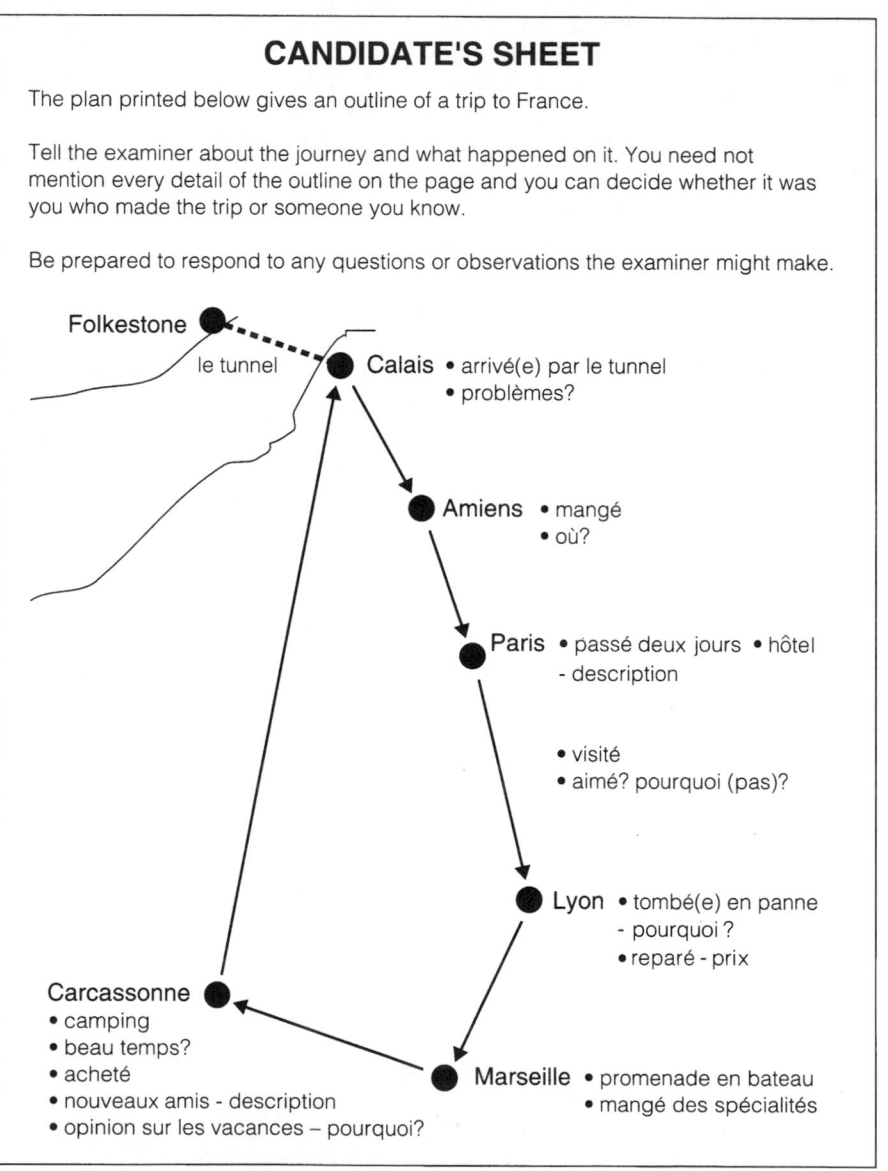

> **Account of a film or book**
>
> Some GCSE Examining Groups may ask you to narrate the story of a book you have read or a film you have seen, or talk about some event you have attended. If you are going to attempt this task, you will need to be at home with past tenses, particularly the perfect tense, and with techniques of story-telling. Clearly it will be necessary to prepare such tasks carefully, making sure you know any specialised vocabulary beforehand. The techniques needed are similar to the narration of a story.

> **How to do the conversation**
>
> Normally your teacher will have cards on which topics of conversation are specified. You will either choose one 'blind' from a number of cards kept face-down, or your teacher will

choose the topic so that it is different from the subject matter of your presentation. Check with your teacher the exact details for your Speaking Test.

Whether you are doing Foundation or Higher Speaking, try to keep going as much as possible. At Foundation Level, try to avoid one-word answers such as *oui* or *non*, or the name of a British TV Programme (*EastEnders*). Look for opportunities to say at least one sentence in reply to each question.

For both Foundation and Higher Tier, try to refer to past, present and future events and notice when the teacher's questioning is trying to get you to use a range of tenses.

The teacher's questioning may be along the lines of:

> *Qu'est-ce que **tu fais** le weekend **normalement**?* (*normalement* suggests a present-tense answer)
> *Qu'est-ce que **tu as fait** le weekend **dernier**?* (perfect tense and *dernier* in the question suggest a perfect-tense answer)
> *Qu'est-ce que **tu vas faire** le weekend **prochain**?* (future tense and *prochain* in the question suggest a future-tense answer)

In French, it isn't vital which future tense (future with *aller* or future proper) you use in the Speaking Test. For Higher Tier, try to give your opinion about the topic under discussion, and say why you hold that opinion. Again, try to notice when the teacher is trying to get you to do this.

Your teacher should be asking you questions which do not have a yes/no answer. However, if you are aware that the situation is ideal for you to show off a little of what you can do, you can avoid the pitfall of the one-word answer. So, for example, if you are asked *Avez-vous un frère?*, it is much more sensible to reply, *Non, mais j'ai une sœur* than just plain *Non*.

If you are a good-ish Foundation Tier candidate or a Higher Tier candidate, your teacher should be asking you open-ended questions. These are questions which have more complex answers, and about which you can say a little more. Quite often they will be along the lines of *Décris ta routine matinale* or *Parle-moi de ton collège*. These more open-ended questions are much easier to do if you have prepared them beforehand. So make sure you have done so.

Another important thing to remember is that your teacher is more interested in your French than in the strict truth. He or she is hardly likely to send a private detective round to check whether or not you own a dog if he or she asks you about pets. So if you are asked about something and you don't have the specialist vocabulary ready (if, for example, you keep a budgie at home but you can only remember *chien*), then fib a little. Too many candidates stumble over such details and clam up – doing considerable harm to their mark. That said, of course, it is even better if you do know the French for your budgie (*une perruche*).

▶ Topics and settings for conversation

The topics you are likely to be asked about will include:

▶ yourself, home and family
▶ your school
▶ holidays, a visit abroad
▶ free time, entertainment, the media, sport and hobbies
▶ morning and evening routines
▶ your home town, village or area
▶ your friends
▶ shopping
▶ future plans
▶ the world of work, careers and employment
▶ pocket money
▶ food and drink
▶ special occasions.

Make sure you have something prepared to say about each of these, even if it is only a few sentences.

▶ **Sample conversation questions and skeleton answers**

I have given below some questions which might well be asked. I have given them in the *vous* form, but your teacher may well use the *tu* form. Check beforehand. Of course, if your teacher gives you a list to learn from, make sure you work through it, because, after all, he or she will actually be doing the Speaking Test with you!

After each question I have given a possible answer. However, common sense will tell you that some details will need to be altered to tailor things to suit your own circumstances.

Yourself, home and family

1 **Comment vous appelez-vous?**
Je m'appelle Ian Wilkinson.
My name is...

2 **Quel âge avez-vous?**
J'ai seize ans.
I'm 16.
Mon anniversaire, c'est le trois septembre.
My birthday is on the...

3 **Avez-vous des frères ou des sœurs?**
Oui, j'ai deux frères et une sœur.
Yes, I have two brothers and a sister.
Non, je suis enfant unique.
No, I am an only child.

4 **Que fait votre père / votre mère dans la vie?**
Mon père est mécanicien. Ma mère est femme au foyer.
My father is a mechanic. My mother is a housewife.

5 **Est-ce que vous avez un animal à la maison?**
J'ai deux cochons d'Inde qui s'appellent Pudding et Littleone, et un chat qui s'appelle Micia.
I've got two guinea pigs called Pudding and Littleone and a cat called Micia.
Non. Je n'en ai pas. Mon père n'aime pas les animaux.
No, I haven't got any. Dad doesn't like animals.

6 **Est-ce que vous avez une chambre individuelle à la maison?**
Oui, j'ai une chambre à moi.
Yes, I've got my own room.
Non, je partage ma chambre avec mon frère.
No, I share a room with my brother.
Non, je partage ma chambre avec ma sœur.
No, I share a room with my sister.

These may be combined to give a longer version in response to an open-ended question:

7 **Décrivez votre famille.**
On est cinq dans la famille. J'ai un frère, Wayne, qui a dix ans et qui s'intéresse beaucoup à l'informatique, et une sœur, Mandy, qui a treize ans. Elle est collégienne. Mon père est mécanicien et ma mère est femme au foyer. Je m'entends bien avec ma sœur, mais mon frère m'ennuie tout le temps avec son ordinateur. Nous sommes tous blonds, à part mon père, qui a perdu la plupart de ses cheveux! Mon père est normalement gentil, mais il se fâche quand je rentre tard le soir. Maman nous aide beaucoup, et elle fait des études..., etc.

There are five of us in my family. I have a brother, Wayne, who is 10 years old and who is very interested in computers, and a sister, Mandy, who is 13. She is at secondary school. My father is a mechanic and my mother is a housewife. I get on well with my sister, but my brother is always annoying me with his computer. We are all blond, except for my Dad, who has lost most of his hair! My Dad is usually nice, but he gets angry if I am late home in the evening. Mum helps us a lot. She is doing a course..., etc.

Your school

1 **Qu'est-ce que vous étudiez au collège?**
J'apprends le français, l'anglais, les maths, la géographie, l'histoire, les sciences et les sports.
I do French, English, maths, geography, history, science and games.

2 **Quelle est votre matière préférée?**
Je préfère le français, naturellement!
My favourite subject is French, of course!

3   **Depuis combien de temps apprenez-vous le français?**
    J'apprends le français depuis cinq ans.   *I have been learning French for five years.*

4   **A quelle heure commencent les cours à votre collège, le matin?**
    Au collège, les cours commencent à neuf heures.   *At school, lessons start at 9.00.*

These may be combined to give a longer version in response to open-ended questions. Other possible open-ended questions include:

5   **Décrivez votre collège.**
    Mon collège est assez grand, avec mille élèves. C'est un collège mixte. Les bâtiments sont assez vieux, mais on les a repeints il y a deux ans. Normalement on est obligé de porter un uniforme – des chaussures noires, des chaussettes blanches, un pantalon gris ou une jupe grise, un pullover bleu et une chemise blanche. Il y a une cravate rouge et bleu pour les garçons.

    My school is quite big, with 1000 pupils. It's a mixed school. The buildings are quite old, but they were repainted two years ago. Usually we have to wear a uniform – black shoes, white socks, grey trousers or a grey skirt, a blue pullover and a white shirt. There is a blue and red tie for the boys.

6   **Qu'est-ce que vous aimez au collège?**
    J'aime bien les leçons d'anglais et de physique, parce que je trouve ces sujets-là intéressants. Le français – je ne l'aime pas tellement. Le professeur est trop stricte.

    I like English and physics lessons, because I find those subjects interesting. I don't like French much. The teacher is too strict.

Holidays, a visit abroad

1   **Où est-ce que vous avez passé vos vacances, l'année dernière?**
    J'ai passé mes vacances en Cornouailles, à Truro.   *I spent my holidays in Cornwall, at Truro.*

2   **Quel temps faisait-il?**
    La plupart du temps, il faisait chaud, mais il a plu pendant deux jours.   *Most of the time it was hot, but it rained for two days.*

3   **Qu'est-ce que vous avez fait en vacances?**
    J'ai nagé dans la mer, je me suis bronzé(e), j'ai fréquenté des discothèques, etc.   *I swam in the sea, sunbathed and went to discos, etc.*

4   **Quels projets de vacances avez-vous pour cette année?**
    J'ai l'intention de visiter la Belgique.   *I intend going to Belgium.*

5   **Est-ce que vous avez déjà visité la France?**
    Oui, j'ai déjà visité la France. J'ai passé deux jours à Bayeux il y a deux ans.   *Yes, I have been to France. I spent two days at Bayeux two years ago.*
    Non, pas encore. Peut-être l'année prochaine.   *No, not yet. Perhaps next year.*

Again, these could be combined to form the basis of a longer reply to a question such as: *Décrivez vos dernières vacances.* This topic is especially likely to be used as it gives the teacher the chance to use past, present and future tenses

Free time, entertainment, the media, sport and hobbies

1   **Quels sont vos passe-temps?**
    Je lis beaucoup, j'écoute des disques, je joue au tennis et je joue de la guitare.   *I read a lot, I listen to records, I play tennis and I play the guitar.*

2   **Qu'est-ce que vous faites le week-end?**
    Le samedi, je travaille dans un magasin. Le soir, je sors avec des amis. Le dimanche, je fais mes devoirs.

    On Saturdays I work in a shop. In the evening I go out with friends. On Sundays I do my homework.

3   **Qu'est-ce que vous avez vu à la télé hier soir?**
    J'ai vu *Neighbours*. C'est un feuilleton.

    I saw Neighbours. *It's a soap opera.*

4   **Faites-vous du sport? Où? Quand? Est-ce que vous y jouez bien?**
    Oui, je joue au tennis et je fais du cyclisme. Je joue normalement au club de tennis, ou au centre sportif. J'y joue assez bien.
    Non, je ne suis pas sportif (sportive).

    Yes, I play tennis and go cycling. I normally play at the tennis club or at the sports centre. I play quite well. No, I'm not sporty.

Open-ended questions on this topic might include:

5   **Qu'est-ce que vous avez fait le week-end dernier?**
    Le samedi je me suis levé(e) tard, car j'étais fatigué(e). J'ai pris le petit déjeuner, et puis je suis allé(e) en ville où j'avais rendez-vous avec mon camarade Sam. Nous avons acheté des CD ensemble, et puis nous sommes rentré(e)s. Vers quatre heures j'ai regardé une émission favorite à la télé. Le soir, je suis sorti(e). Je suis allé(e) à une boum chez Mary. C'était extra. Je suis rentré(e) très tard à la maison. Le dimanche, je n'ai rien fait. Mais j'ai preparé mon examen de français!

    On Saturday I got up late because I was tired. I had breakfast and then I went into town, where I had arranged to meet my friend Sam. We bought some CDs together and then came back home. Around 4 o'clock I watched a favourite programme on TV. In the evening I went out. I went to a party at Mary's. It was excellent. I came home very late. On Sunday I did nothing. But I did prepare my French exam!

6   **Qu'est-ce que vous allez faire le week-end prochain?**
    J'irai en ville, et j'ai l'intention d'acheter un nouveau pantalon. Après cela, je vais rencontrer des amis, et nous irons voir le nouveau film qui passe au cinéma. C'est un film policier. Le soir, j'ai invité mon copain à passer la soirée chez moi.

    I'm going to go into town, and I intend to buy some new trousers. After that I shall meet my friends and we are going to see the new film at the cinema. It's a whodunnit. (In the evening,) I've invited my friend to spend the evening with me.

Morning and evening routines

1   **A quelle heure est-ce que vous vous levez normalement?**
    Je me lève normalement à sept heures et demie.

    I normally get up at 7.30.

2   **Qu'est-ce que vous mangez comme petit déjeuner?**
    Je mange du pain grillé, des cornflakes, et une pomme.

    I eat toast, cornflakes and an apple.

3   **Venez-vous au collège à pied?**
    Oui, je viens à pied.
    Non, je viens en autobus, et quelquefois à bicyclette.
    Non, mon père m'amène en voiture.

    Yes I walk here.
    No, I come by bus, and sometimes by bike.
    No, my Dad brings me by car.

4   **A quelle heure quittez-vous la maison le matin?**
    Je quitte la maison à huit heures et quart.

    I leave the house at 8.15.

5   **A quelle heure est-ce que vous mangez, le soir?**
    Chez nous, on mange à cinq heures et demie.

    At our house, we eat at 5.30.

6   **A quelle heure est-ce que vous vous couchez, d'habitude?**
    D'habitude je me couche à dix heures.

    I generally go to bed at 10.

An open-ended question on this topic might be:

7 **Décrivez votre routine matinale.**
Bon, alors, je me lève à sept heures, je mets la radio, et puis je vais prendre une douche dans la salle de bain. Après m'être seché(e), je m'habille. Normalement, je mets mon uniforme scolaire – que je n'aime pas du tout – mais le week-end je m'habille en jeans avec un pull. Je viens de m'acheter un pull tout à fait chouette. Je me prépare du pain grillé et une tasse de thé comme petit déjeuner, et dans la semaine je quitte la maison vers huit heures et quart. Normalement, j'oublie quelque chose, et je reviens le chercher. Je vais au collège à vélo.

Right, well, I get up at 7, I put the radio on, and then I go and take a shower in the bathroom. After getting dried, I get dressed. Usually I put on my school uniform – which I don't like at all – but at the weekend I put on jeans and a pullover. I've just bought a really smashing pullover. I make myself some toast and a cup of tea for breakfast, and in the week I leave the house around 8.15. Usually I forget something and I come back for it. I go to school by bike.

Your home town, village or area

1 **Où habitez-vous?**
J'habite Preston.
I live in Preston.

2 **C'est où exactement, Preston?**
C'est dans le nord-ouest de l'Angleterre.
It's in the north-west of England.

3 **Est-ce que c'est une grande ville?**
Oui, c'est une ville assez grande. Il y a cent mille habitants.
Yes, it's quite a big town. There are 100,000 inhabitants.
Non, Sudbury est assez petit. Il y a vingt-cinq mille habitants.
No, Sudbury's quite small. There are 25,000 inhabitants.

4 **Qu'est-ce qu'il y a à voir dans votre région?**
Il y a les montagnes, un musée industriel, un beau château, et des villages pittoresques.
There are the hills, an industrial museum, a nice stately home and picturesque villages.

More open-ended questions on this topic might include the following:

5 **Où se trouve Banbury exactement?**
Banbury se trouve au centre de l'Angleterre. C'est à deux cents kilomètres de Londres, et c'est assez près d'Oxford.

Banbury is in the centre of England. It's 120 miles from London and fairly close to Oxford.

6 **Qu'est-ce qu'il y a à faire à Banbury?**
A Banbury il y a un complexè sportif avec piscine, gymnase, etc. Il y aussi une maison de la culture, où il y a aussi un foyer des jeunes. Au collège il y a beaucoup d'activités – des sports, des orchestres, un groupe de théâtre, etc. Et les jeunes participent souvent aux activités du jumelage avec Ermont, près de Paris, et Hennef, près de Bonn, en Allemagne. Comme distractions il y a un cinéma, beaucoup de cafés, et une discothèque en ville.

At Banbury there is a sports centre with a swimming pool, gym, etc. There is also an arts centre, where there is also a youth centre. At school there are lots of activities – sport, orchestras, drama, etc. And the young people often take part in town-twinning activities with Ermont, near Paris, and Hennef, near Bonn in Germany. For entertainment there is a cinema, lots of cafés and a disco in town.

7 **Quelles sont les industries principales?**
Les industries principales sont l'alimentation – la production de café et de desserts – et il y a des laboratoires qui developpent la technologie de l'aluminium. Il y a aussi uns grand marché de bétail et beaucoup d'artisans.

The main industries are food – producing coffee and desserts – and there are laboratories which develop aluminium technology. There is also a large cattle market and lots of tradespeople.

8 **Quelles sont les attractions touristiques?**
Il y a la croix célèbre, qui forme un rond-point au centre de la ville. La place du marché est très pittoresque, et on trouve beaucoup de tavernes traditionnelles. L'église du 18ᵉ siècle est remarquable pour ses dimensions et sa tour.

There is the famous Banbury Cross, which forms a roundabout in the middle of town. The market square is very picturesque and there are lots of traditional pubs. The 18th-century church is famous for its size and its tower.

9 **Quelles excursions pourrait-on faire dans la région?**
On pourrait visiter Oxford, ville universitaire, et très pittoresque. Ou on pourrait faire une belle promenade en voiture dans les Cotswolds – c'est le nom d'une région vraiment jolie qui est à une demi-heure d'ici en voiture. Autrement, on pourrait visiter Stratford. C'est la ville natale de Shakespeare, notre poète national. Aujourd'hui il y a beaucoup de distractions pour les touristes, trois théâtres et de très bons magasins.

You could visit Oxford, a picturesque university town. Or else you could go for a nice drive in the Cotswolds – it's a really pretty area about half an hour's drive from here. Otherwise you would visit Stratford. It's the birthplace of Shakespeare, our national poet. Nowadays there is lots for tourists to do there; there are three theatres and some really good shops.

Your friends

1 **Comment s'appelle votre meilleur ami (votre meilleure amie)?**
Il/Elle s'appelle Chris.   *He/She is called Chris.*

2 **Qu'est ce que vous faites ensemble?**
Nous allons au cinéma et à la piscine ensemble, nous faisons du sport, et nous allons en ville ensemble.   *We go to the cinema and the swimming pool together, we play sport, and we go to town together.*

3 **Comment est-il / Comment est-elle?**
Il est assez grand, avec les cheveux bruns. Il porte toujours un jean et un sweatshirt Adidas®. Il est gentil et très amusant.
Elle est grande, avec les cheveux blonds. Elle porte toujours un caleçon et un pull. Elle est très sympathique.   *He is fairly tall, with brown hair. He always wears jeans and an Adidas® sweatshirt. He is kind and amusing. She is tall, with blonde hair. She always wears leggings and a pullover. She's very nice.*

These may be combined to give a longer version in response to an open-ended question.

Shopping

1 **Où est-ce que vous aller acheter des vêtements?**
Normalement je vais en ville.   *I usually go to town.*
Quelquefois je vais à Londres en train avec mes ami(e)s.   *Sometimes I go to London on the train with my friends.*

2 **Quelle sorte de magasin préférez-vous?**
Je préfère les grands magasins / les petites boutiques.   *I prefer department stores / small boutiques.*

3 **Qui paie vos vêtements, vous ou vos parents?**
C'est moi qui paie / Ce sont mes parents qui paient.   *I pay / My parents pay.*

4 **Est-que que vous vous intéressez à la mode?**
Oui, c'est passionnant.   *Yes, it's fascinating.*
Non, pas tellement.   *No, not much.*

These may be combined to give a longer version in response to an open-ended question.

Future plans

1 **Qu'est-ce vous avez prévu pour le week-end prochain?**
   Je vais faire des courses en ville.
   Je vais voir un match de foot à Liverpool.

   Je vais à une boum samedi soir.

   Je vais passer le dimanche chez Sam, mon copin / ma copine.

   I am going shopping in town.
   I'm going to watch a football match in Liverpool.
   I'm going to a party on Saturday night.
   I'm going to spend Sunday at my friend Sam's.

2 **Quels sont vos projets pour l'été?**
   Je vais travailler dans un magasin.
   Je vais passer mes vacances en Grèce.

   Je vais faire du camping dans le Devon.
   Je vais me reposer après les examens!

   I am going to work in a shop.
   I am going to spend my holidays in Greece.
   I am going camping in Devon.
   I'm going to have a rest after the exams.

3 **Quels sont vos projets pour l'année prochaine?**
   J'ai l'intention d'aller au lycée technique.
   J'ai l'intention de préparer mon bac.
   Je vais faire un apprentissage moderne.

   Je vais trouver un emploi.

   I intend to go to technical college.
   I intend to do A Levels.
   I am going to do a modern apprenticeship.
   I am going to get a job.

4 **Qu'est-ce que vous comptez faire après le bac / après le lycée technique?**
   Je voudrais aller à l'université.
   Je voudrais trouver un emploi.
   Je ne sais pas encore.

   I would like to go to university.
   I would like to get a job.
   I don't know yet.

5 **Où voudriez-vous habitez à l'âge de vingt-cinq ans?**
   J'aimerais habiter à Londres / à la campagne / ici dans la région.

   I'd like to live in London / in the country / round here.

6 **Est-ce que vous comptez avoir des enfants?**
   Oui, un, deux ou trois – j'aime les enfants.

   Non. Je n'aime pas les enfants.
   Ça dépend.

   Yes, one, two or three – I like children.
   No. I don't like children.
   It depends.

7 **Quelle profession aimeriez-vous faire?**
   J'aimerais être professeur de français. C'est un travail varié, intéressant et important.
   Je ne sais pas encore.

   I'd like to be a French teacher. It's a varied, interesting and important job.
   I don't know yet.

   More open-ended questions on this topic might include the following:

8 **Quels sont vos projets pour l'avenir?**
   Je vais continuer mes études l'année prochaine. Je vais faire de la géographie, des maths, et de l'allemand. Ces matières m'intéressent beaucoup. Je passerai mon bac dans deux ans. Après cela, j'espère faire ma licence, mais je ne sais pas où. Je voudrais peut-être devenir journaliste, mais ce n'est pas certain pour le moment.

   I am going to continue my studies next year. I am going to do geography, maths and German. Those subjects interest me a lot. I shall take my A Levels in two years. After that, I hope to do a degree, but I don't know where. I would perhaps like to become a journalist, but it's not certain just now.

The world of work, careers and employment

1 **Avez-vous un emploi?**
   Oui, je travaille chez un coiffeur / dans un supermarché.

   Yes, I work in a hairdresser's / at a supermarket.

Non, je n'ai pas le temps.	*No, I haven't got time.*
Non, j'ai cherché un emploi, mais je n'en ai pas trouvé.	*No, I looked for a job but I didn't find one.*

2 **Combien d'heures travaillez-vous par semaine?**
Je travaille six heures par semaine.   *I work six hours a week.*

3 **Combien gagnez-vous?**
Je gagne £20 par semaine.   *I earn £20 a week.*

4 **Quels jours travaillez-vous?**
Je travaille le vendredi soir et le samedi matin.   *I work Friday evenings and Saturday mornings.*

5 **Comment trouvez-vous votre emploi?**
Je le trouve supportable / intéressant / casse-pieds.   *I find it bearable / interesting / boring.*

6 **Pourquoi?**
Parce que les collègues sont aimables.   *Because my fellow-workers are friendly.*

Parce que le travail est pénible.   *Because the work is boring.*
Parce qu'on s'amuse.   *Because we have a laugh.*

These answers could be combined to produce a longer response to an open-ended question.

Pocket money

1 **Combien d'argent de poche recevez-vous?**
Je reçois £5 par semaine.   *I get £5 a week.*
Mes parents ne me donnent pas d'argent de poche.   *My parents don't give me any pocket money.*

2 **Qu'est-ce que vous achetez avec votre argent de poche?**
J'achète des vêtements, des CD et des magazines.   *I buy clothes, CDs and magazines.*

3 **Est-ce que vous faites des économies?**
Je fais des économies pour acheter un caméscope / une voiture.   *I'm saving up for a video camera / a car.*
Je fais des économies pour les vacances.   *I'm saving up for the holidays.*

Food and drink

1 **Qu'est-ce que vous aimez manger?**
J'aime les frites, les salades, les pizzas.   *I like chips, salad, pizza.*

2 **Qu'est-ce que vous n'aimez pas manger?**
J'ai horreur des épinards.   *I can't stand spinach.*

3 **Qu'est-ce que vous préférez, le thé ou le café?**
Je préfère le thé.   *I prefer tea.*

4 **Qu'est-ce que vous avez mangé hier soir?**
Hier soir, j'ai mangé du poisson avec des pommes de terre et des petits pois.   *Yesterday evening I had fish, potatoes and peas.*

5 **Quel est votre plat préféré?**
Mon plat préféré, c'est les spaghettis à la bolognaise.   *My favourite dish is spaghetti bolognaise.*

6 **Quel repas aimez-vous préparer?**
J'aime préparer du poulet rôti avec des pommes de terre sautées.   *I like cooking roast chicken with sauté potatoes.*

7 **Est-ce que vous aimez manger au restaurant?**
J'aime manger la nourriture chinoise ou l'indienne.   *I like Chinese or Indian.*

This topic is well worth preparing carefully, at it is one which lends itself to questions about past, present and future events.

Special occasions

1   **Quelle est la date de ton anniversaire?**
    Mon anniversaire, c'est le 20 février.   *My birthday is 20 February.*
2   **Comment est-ce que vous célébrez votre anniversaire?**
    Je sors avec mes ami(e)s.   *I go out with my friends.*
    Je mange un gâteau à la maison.   *I eat a cake at home.*
3   **Quelles traditions avez-vous pour Noël?**
    On mange de la dinde aux canneberges.   *We eat turkey with cranberry sauce.*
    On donne des cadeaux le matin du 25 décembre.   *We give presents on the morning of 25 December.*
4   **Comment fêtez-vous le Nouvel An?**
    Normalement il y a une boum.   *Normally there is a party.*

You could also prepare a longer piece describing a particular festival in which you take part. But beware of doing this if you have not prepared it: you won't be able to think of the words on the spot!

▶ Presentations

Presentations are not required for all Examining Groups. However, if you are doing NEAB or MEG, you can expect to present a topic you have chosen and discuss it. In general, you should have about a minute's worth of material prepared, and then be ready to discuss the topic further for another couple of minutes. Many of the possible topics will be descriptive, so the present tense will be all you need. Indeed, if your past tenses are not strong, you should consider concealing that fact by choosing a descriptive topic.

Although the choice of topic is yours, and experience suggests that some students will choose off-beat topics, research them carefully and perform well in them, there is no obligation to go to so much trouble. Unless you are very confident, you would be well advised to stick to one of the conversation topics and perform well in that. However, do beware of choosing a topic that is **too** easy. The topic **Moi** does not allow for very much linguistic challenge and is probably best avoided.

You will be allowed to bring in cue cards or skeleton notes to help you remember the sequence of your presentation. However, you will not be allowed to read out a prepared script. You may also be allowed to bring in materials which you might wish to show, such as a map or photos. Check the exact rules with your teacher.

▶ A STEP FURTHER

There are many ways of improving your fluency. Most of them boil down to actually doing some speaking.

▶   Practise reading out loud. This can improve your ability to get your tongue round the sounds of French.
▶   Talk in French to the cat or your teddy or the goldfish. They may not respond much, but at least you get the feeling of talking to someone. (NB This is not as good as practice with a human!)
▶   Prepare the conversation topics thoroughly, so that you know the French for your parents' professions, your specialised hobbies, etc. Ask your teacher or the French Assistant(e) for specific words. They are employed to tell you such things!
▶   Make sure you have worked through role-plays for all topics. Use ones in this book, but don't neglect your textbook. Your teacher may have textbooks and past papers which contain lots of them.
▶   Take advantage of any mock Speaking Test which is offered to you at school. The chances are you will only have one opportunity to practise individually with your teacher. Don't be so foolish as not to prepare thoroughly for it. After all, it is your teacher who will be doing the Speaking Test with you!

Practice and Preparation lead to Proficiency. But knowledge of what is to come is very useful, too. I have reproduced below the two sides of an appointment sheet given to candidates at a school which uses the MEG syllabus. If you do a different syllabus, amend it to suit your circumstances. And follow the advice it gives!

THE CHASE SCHOOL MODERN LANGUAGES DEPARTMENT
GCSE Speaking Test Appointment–French

Name... Teacher............................

Your appointment for the Speaking Test is on

.... (day)................. (date)

at..................... (time) in room..............

NB You should arrive in the Languages Block 15 minutes before your appointment. Do NOT talk to people who are already preparing material. Quiet is essential, as all Speaking Tests are tape-recorded.

When you have been brought into the preparation area, you may use a bilingual dictionary. You may NOT use any other reference materials such as textbooks, etc. You are NOT allowed to write anything down.

PTO

FORMAT OF THE TEST

Foundation candidates

Role-play 1

5 pictures which suggest 5 things to say.
The marks are for 'getting the message across' to the examiner. So if you can't remember a particular word and you haven't found it in the dictionary, describe what it is.

Role-play 2

Written instructions in French with 5 points to make. Marks as above, with some marks for communicating accurately. There will be one item which requires you to 'think on your feet' and which you cannot prepare.

Presentation

You talk about a prepared topic for a minute. You are allowed to bring in a cue card with 5 short headings in French. You can, if you wish, bring in photos and other material to illustrate your talk. After your presentation, your teacher will ask you questions related to your presentation for another 2 minutes.

Conversation

Your teacher will ask you questions on 3 topics for a total of about 5 minutes. You will not know the topics in advance.

Higher candidates

You will start with role-play 2.

Role-play 2

Written instructions in French with 5 points to make. Marks as above, with some marks for communicating accurately. There will be one item which requires you to 'think on your feet' and which you cannot prepare.

Role-play 3 (about 5 minutes) (Narration exercise)

One situation which will have visual and written clues which you intend to develop in French. The more you say, the better. There will be some items in bold which you ought to include in your story. The mark schemes reward the level of interest and elaboration which you put in. You can always say what you saw, ate, drank, how you felt, what the weather was like, etc. Normally you should use past tenses. It is important to use past tenses and to give your opinion and the reasons for your opinion. Be prepared to be interrupted by your teacher occasionally.

Presentation

You talk about a prepared topic for a minute. You are allowed to bring in a cue card with 5 short headings in French. You can, if you wish, bring in photos and other material to illustrate your talk. After your presentation, your teacher will ask you questions related to your presentation for another 2 minutes.

Conversation

Your teacher will ask you questions on three topics for a total of about 5 minutes. You will not know the topics in advance.

Bonne chance!

Writing

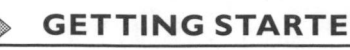 **GETTING STARTED**

Writing is worth 25% of the marks for GCSE. From 1998 it is a compulsory element of the examination. The end-of-course examination in Writing is reasonably straightforward, but certainly not a pushover. If you are very weak in Writing, you should discuss with your teacher whether you should choose the Writing Coursework option, which might involve you in writing less.

There is some variation amongst GCSE Examining Groups about what should be set for Writing, and it pays to know what to expect! What doesn't vary much between Examining Groups is the way that they seek to reward 'getting the message across'. It's vitally important to do the tasks set in order to do well.

WHAT YOU NEED TO KNOW

> **Introduction**

Writing can be seen as the most difficult skill to get absolutely right. Mistakes which would hardly be noticed in Speaking will show up in Writing. Writing really reveals if you know exactly how the language works in every detail.

The Examining Groups are well aware of the difficulty of this skill. They therefore organise the way they assess it to take account of what candidates of differing abilities can be expected to manage.

They measure three aspects of your writing:

> communication
> accuracy
> range and variety of language.

When measuring grade G, F, E performances in Foundation Tier, most of the marks are given for **communication**.

When measuring grade D, C performances in Foundation Tier, some marks are given for **communication**, some for **accuracy**, and some for **range and variety of language**.

In Higher Tier, the D, C performance tasks are the same as in Foundation Tier, and the marks are allocated in exactly the same way.

When measuring grade B, A, A* performance in Higher Tier, the main emphasis is on **accuracy** and **variety of language**.

> **Examining Group requirements**

There is some variation in what each Examining Group requires for Writing, as detailed below. However, the Examining Groups do agree on the features of the Writing examination listed below.

Foundation Tier

The Foundation Tier allows performances between grades G and C. For assessment purposes, the Examining Groups distinguish between grade G, F, E tasks and performances and grade D, C tasks and performances.

Grade G, F, E tasks will consist of list-writing, diary-entry, form-completion and gap-filling exercises. Many of these will require no more than 20 words. In addition, there will usually be a message or a postcard requiring about 40 words or so. In the message or postcard there will be a number of things you will have to say. It is possible that you may have to reply to a postcard in French.

Much of the writing at this level of achievement will consist of single words, short phrases and simple sentences.

Grade D, C tasks will usually consist of letter-writing, sometimes in reply to a stimulus letter in French. The letters may be informal letters (to friends) or formal letters (to businesses). They usually require you to write about 100 words or so, and there will be a number of things you will have to say.

The writing at this level of achievement will consist of connected sentences, and candidates will be expected to be able to refer to past, present and future events. Candidates will be expected to give their opinions, and to express simple emotions.

Higher Tier

The Higher Tier allows performances between grades D and A*. For assessment purposes, the Examining Groups distinguish between grade D, C tasks and performances and grade B, A, A* tasks and performances.

Grade D, C tasks and the type of writing expected are identical to those in Foundation Tier at these grades.

Grade B, A, A* tasks will consist of writing an essay, a report, a letter, publicity material or an imaginative account. There may be either a written stimulus in French or a visual stimulus. You will usually have to write about 120–150 words.

The writing at this level of achievement will consist of connected sentences, and candidates will be expected to be able to refer to past, present and future events. Candidates will be expected to give and justify their opinions, and to express a range of emotions. In practice, you will not do well at this level of performance if you do not use a wide range of idiom, structures and vocabulary, especially a good range of adjectives and adverbs.

Dictionaries

The Examining Groups all agree that you may use a French–English, English–French dictionary during the Writing Test. This should not be seen as a substitute for learning French – it is much better to regard it as a last resort, or a checking tool when you have completed a task.

For an analysis of the Examining Group requirements, see the Appendix at the end of the book.

▷ **Mark schemes**   The mark schemes that the Examining Groups will use are designed to reward 'communication', that is, 'getting the message across'. As long as you can write French well enough to be understood by a sympathetic native speaker of French, you should be OK as far as communication is concerned.

However, because the mark schemes reward communication, they also depend on your doing what the question tells you to do. For example, the question may tell you to give the **time** and **date** of your arrival. There will be so many marks for 'getting the message across'. So obviously, if you fail to mention the **date** of your arrival, you cannot get the marks allocated to that question. To put it another way: if the question gives you tasks to complete, then complete them!

In addition, for the letter question, there are marks to be gained for the form of the letter. So be sure you have put in, correctly, the address, the date, the salutation (*Cher Monsieur, Chère Marie*, etc.) and the closing formula (*Amitiés, A bientôt* or, for a business letter, *Je vous prie d'agréer, monsieur, l'assurance de mes sentiments distingués*). Here is an opportunity to be sure of gaining marks in advance. Don't miss it.

▷ **The form of informal letters**

General

Informal letters (to a friend) are usually written in the *tu* form.

Your address

This is usually written in full on the back of the envelope after *Exp:-* (= *expéditeur*).

Inside, at the top **right-hand** corner of the letter, you write the name of the town you are writing from, with the date.

Example

Scunthorpe, le 12 juin 1998.

Openings

Cher Jean, *(to a male)*
Chère Jeanne, *(to a female)*
Chers amis, *(to more than one person)*

Drawing to a close

Maintenant, je dois faire mes devoirs. *Now I have to do my homework.*
Maintenant, je dois sortir avec ma mère. *Now I have to go out with my mother.*
Maintenant je dois me coucher. *Now it's time to go to bed.*
En attendant de tes nouvelles... *Looking forward to hearing from you...*
Ecris-moi bientôt! *Write soon!*
A bientôt! *See you soon!*

Signing off

These are listed with increasing degrees of affection.
Amicalement...
Amitiés...
Bien cordialement...
Ton ami... *(if you are male)*
Ton amie... *(if you are female)*
Ton correspondant... *(if you are male)*
Ta correspondante... *(if you are female)*
Grosses bises...

If your Examining Group sets a letter or note in French for you to reply to, this may be written in a French handwriting style. Use every opportunity to practise reading the handwriting of French native speakers. Your textbook should have examples in it, and you could also ask friends with penfriends in France to show you their letters so that you get the hang of reading it.

▷ The form of formal letters

General

Formal letters (to a business or an organisation) are written in the *vous* form.

Your address

This is usually written in full on the back of the envelope after *Exp:-* (= *expéditeur*).
   Inside, on the letter, you write your own name and address on the top **left-hand** corner of the page.
   The date is written in the top right-hand corner, together with the town you are writing from.

Example

Scunthorpe, le 12 juin 1998.

The address you are writing to

This is written under the date in the top **right-hand** corner of the page.

Openings

Monsieur, *(Dear Sir)*
Madame, *(Dear Madam)*
Messieurs, *(Dear Sirs)*

Acknowledging receipt

J'accuse réception de votre lettre du 6 juin.   *I acknowledge receipt of your letter of 6 June.*
Je vous remercie de votre lettre du 6 juin.   *Thank you for your letter of 6 June.*

Requesting something

Je vous prie de me réserver deux chambres...   *Please reserve two rooms for me...*
Veuillez m'envoyer un dépliant sur votre région.   *Please send me a brochure about your area.*
Je serais très reconnaissant(e) si vous pouviez me réserver...   *I would be very grateful if you could reserve me...*

Enclosing something

Veuillez trouver ci-joint un eurochèque de ... F à titre d'arrhes.   *Please find enclosed a Eurocheque for ... F as a deposit.*
Veuillez trouver ci-joint un mandat de réponse international.   *Please find attached an international reply coupon.*

Apologising

Je regrette de vous faire savoir que...   *I am sorry to have to tell you that...*
Veuillez accepter mes excuses.   *Please accept my apologies.*

Signing off

Business letters normally end with one of the following two *formules*, both meaning 'Yours sincerely' or 'Yours faithfully'.

Veuillez agréer, Monsieur, l'expression de mes sentiments distingués.
Je vous prie d'agréer, Monsieur, l'expression de mes sentiments distingués.

▶ Phrases to improve essays and reports

Writing with variety will be made much easier with a little work on learning suitable vocabulary to enrich your essays and reports, especially in Higher Tier exercises. The list given here is by no means exhaustive. Most textbooks will contain a list of useful vocabulary and phrases for writing essays and stories, perhaps in a reference section at the back. Do take the opportunity to compare them with the ones I have given below. You will gain from doing so. Try them out in your homework before the examination so that you are sure how they work for the 'real thing'.

à ce moment-là *at that moment*	en mangeant *while eating*
à sa grande surprise *to his/her astonishment*	finalement *finally*
ainsi *thus*	heureusement *fortunately*
alors *then, so*	malgré *despite*
après avoir fait cela *after having done that*	malheureusement *unfortunately*
après y être arrivé(e)(s) *after arriving there*	naturellement *naturally*
cependant *but, however*	parce que *because*
c'est-à-dire *that is to say*	peut-être *perhaps*
complètement *completely*	puis *then*
d'abord *first of all*	quand *when*
déjà *already*	quand même *all the same*
de toute façon *anyway*	simplement *simply*
donc *therefore, so*	soudain *suddenly*
en effet *as a matter of fact*	tandis que *while, whilst*
en fait *in fact*	tout à coup, *suddenly*
enfin *at last*	tout à fait *entirely, completely*
ensuite *after that*	tout de suite *immediately*

Alternatives for *avoir* and *être*:

posséder   *to possess*
se trouver   *to be situated*

▷ **Examples of question types**   Let us now look at examples of the sort of question that you might find. All questions will be set in French. Although the Examining Groups try to keep the language as simple as possible, it may be that you will need to look up some expressions in the dictionary.

A list of common rubrics for Writing is given below.

Choississez thème 1 ou thème 2.   *Choose title 1 or title 2.*

Dans votre lettre vous devez...   *In your letter you should...*

Donnez les renseignements.   *Give information.*

Demandez des conseils.   *Ask for advice.*

Demandez les détails suivants.   *Ask for the following details.*

Ecrivez votre avis avec les raisons.   *Write your opinion and the reasons for it.*

Ecrivez une lettre.   *Write a letter.*

Ecrivez une carte postale.   *Write a postcard.*

Ecrivez une réponse.   *Write a reply.*

Ecrivez un article.   *Write an article.*

Ecrivez environ 150 mots.   *Write about 150 words.*

Expliquez pourquoi.   *Explain why.*

Expliquez comment.   *Explain how.*

Faites une comparaison.   *Make a comparison.*

Faites une description de...   *Describe, write a description of...*

Faites une liste.   *Write a list.*

Imaginez que...   *Imagine that...*

Mentionnez...   *Mention...*

Préparez les tâches suivantes en français.   *Prepare the following tasks in French.*

Présentez-vous.   *Introduce yourself.*

Racontez ce que vous avez fait.   *Say what you did.*

Racontez les choses que vous avez faites.   *Say what you did.*

Racontez vos impressions.   *Give your impressions.*

Remplissez la fiche / le formulaire.   *Fill in the form.*

Répondez à la lettre.   *Reply to the letter.*

Répondez aux questions posées dans la lettre.   *Answer the questions asked in the letter.*

Vous pouvez employer un dictionnaire.   *You can use a dictionary.*

Source: *Your French Dictionary* (Malvern Language Guides) Tel. 01684 577433.

▶ **EXAMINATION QUESTIONS WITH STUDENT ANSWERS AND EXAMINER'S COMMENTS**

Foundation Tier G, F, E grade tasks

▷ **Lists of things**   Faites une liste de 10 choses à acheter pour faire un pique-nique

Student answer with examiner's comments

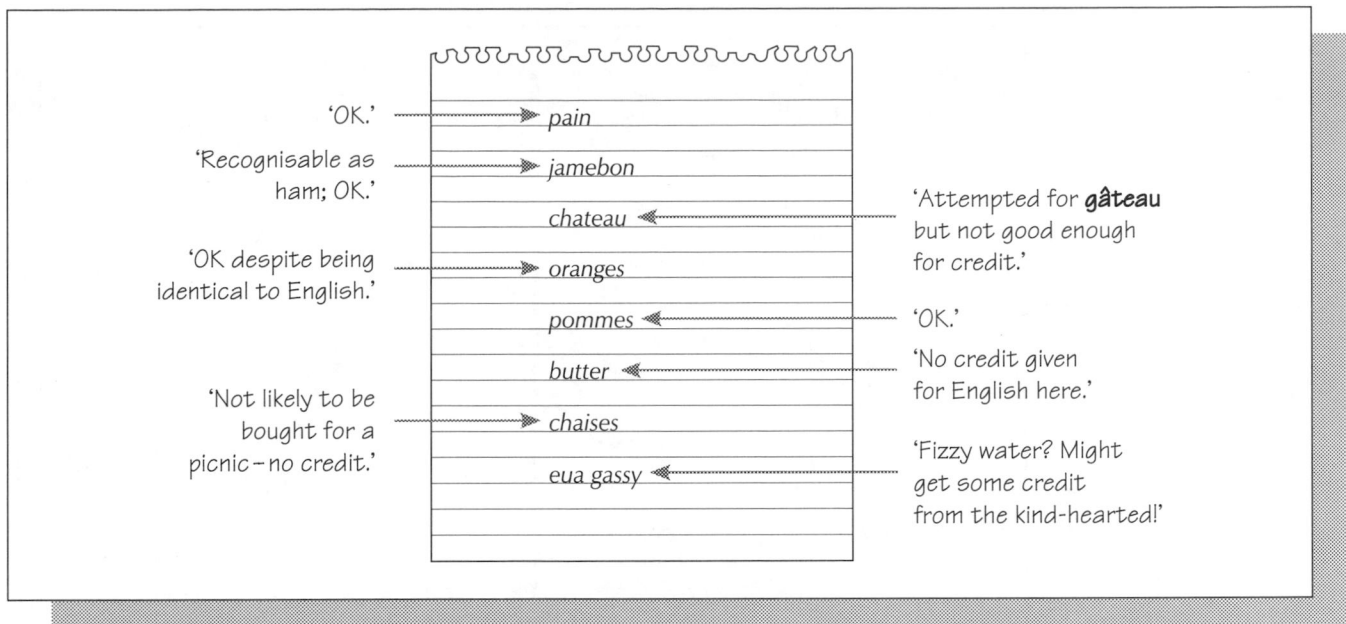

'OK.' → *pain*

'Recognisable as ham; OK.' → *jamebon*

chateau ← 'Attempted for **gâteau** but not good enough for credit.'

'OK despite being identical to English.' → *oranges*

pommes ← 'OK.'

butter ← 'No credit given for English here.'

'Not likely to be bought for a picnic – no credit.' → *chaises*

eua gassy ← 'Fizzy water? Might get some credit from the kind-hearted!'

'The candidate has only answered 8 of the 10 tasks, has one answer which was dubious, and two which were wrong. The mark would be about 5 out of 10. Moral: answer the question!'

▶ **Messages/Notes**   *Vous êtes à la maison. Le téléphone a sonné. Laissez un message en français.*
Dites:

> qui a téléphoné
> à quelle heure
> où il/elle est
> pourquoi
> quand il/elle va téléphoner encore.

Student answer with examiner's comment

'An excellent response. Full marks!'

Ton père a téléphoné à deux heures.

Il est en ville.

Il cherche un cadeau.

Il téléphone encore à cinq heures.

▷ **Diary entries**   Faites une liste de cinq activités différentes pour la visite d'un ami.

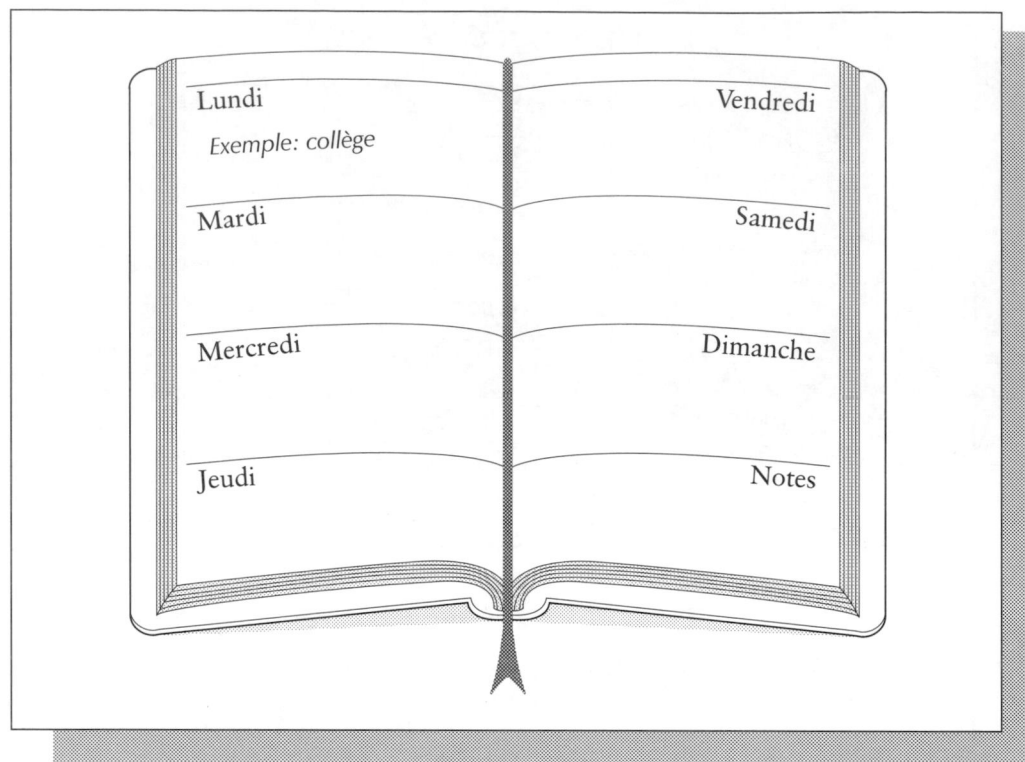

Student answer with examiner's comments

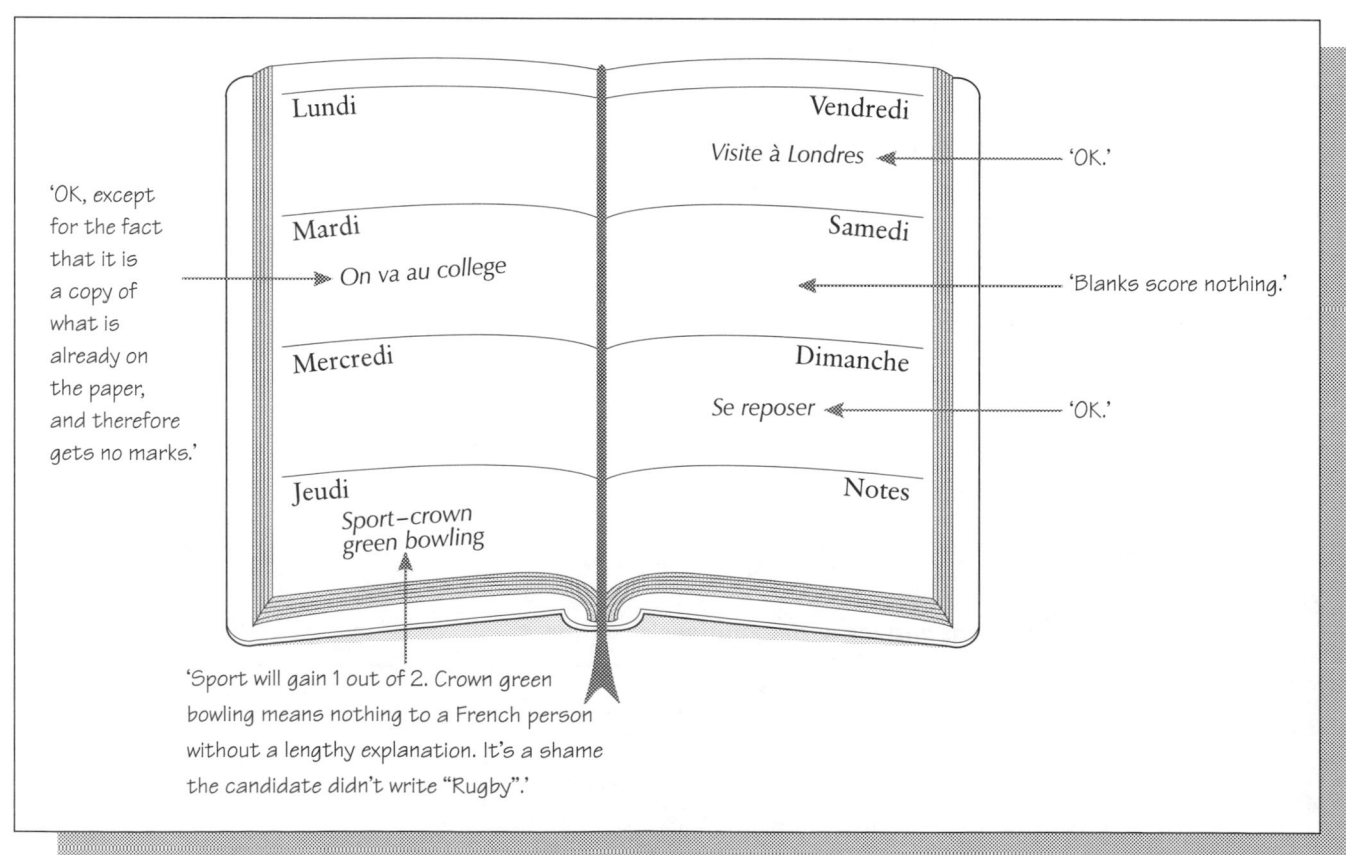

'This fair attempt gains 5/10'.

▷ **Form-filling** *You have contacted an agency in France which organises pen-friendships. They have sent you the following form to fill in.*

Nom	Prénom(s) ....
Age .... ans	
Famille	
....	
....	
Nom du collège	....
Matières préférées	1 ....
	2 ....
	3 ....
J'apprends le français depuis	....
Sports préférés	1 ....
	2 ....
Autres intérêts	1 ....
	2 ....

Student answer with examiner's comments

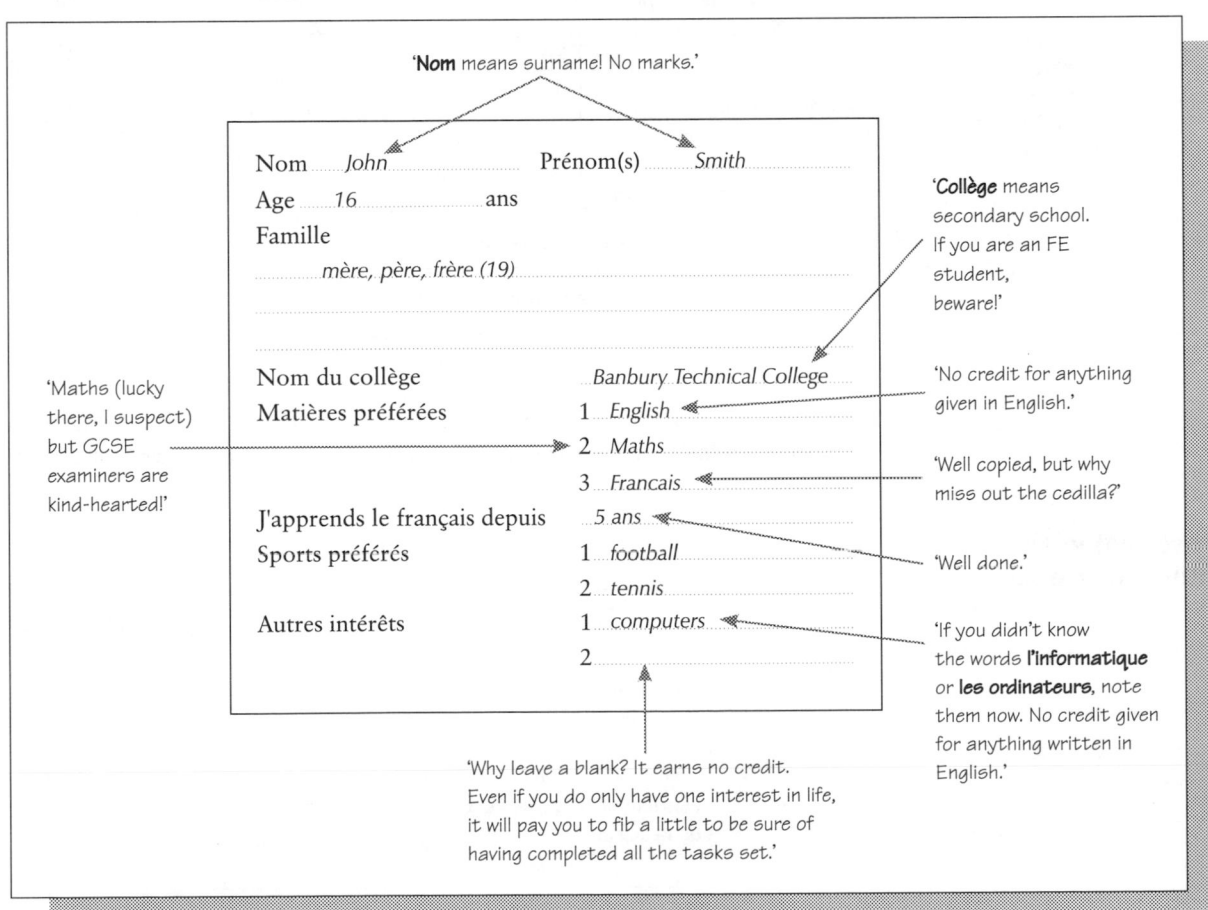

'**Nom** means surname! No marks.'

Nom *John*	Prénom(s) *Smith*
Age *16* ans	
Famille	
mère, père, frère (19)	
Nom du collège	*Banbury Technical College*
Matières préférées	1 *English*
	2 *Maths*
	3 *Francais*
J'apprends le français depuis	*5 ans*
Sports préférés	1 *football*
	2 *tennis*
Autres intérêts	1 *computers*
	2

'**Collège** means secondary school. If you are an FE student, beware!'

'Maths (lucky there, I suspect) but GCSE examiners are kind-hearted!'

'No credit for anything given in English.'

'Well copied, but why miss out the cedilla?'

'Well done.'

'If you didn't know the words **l'informatique** or **les ordinateurs**, note them now. No credit given for anything written in English.'

'Why leave a blank? It earns no credit. Even if you do only have one interest in life, it will pay you to fib a little to be sure of having completed all the tasks set.'

▶ **Postcards**   Ecrivez une carte postale à votre copain / à votre copine.
Mentionnez:

le temps qu'il fait
où vous logez
ce que vous mangez
deux choses que vous avez faites

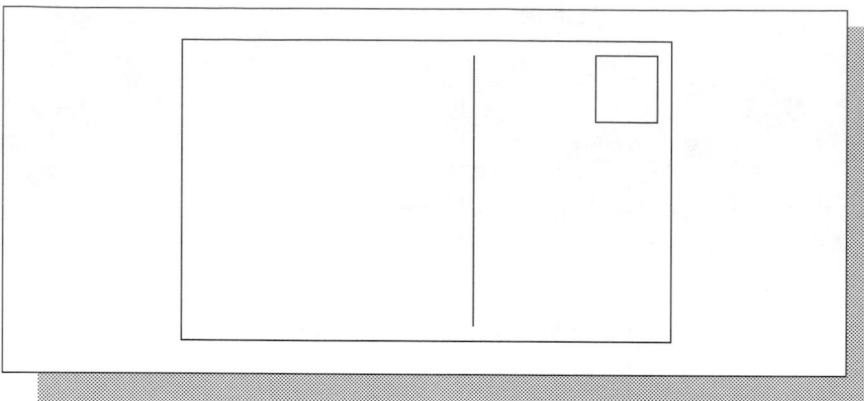

Student answer with examiner's comments

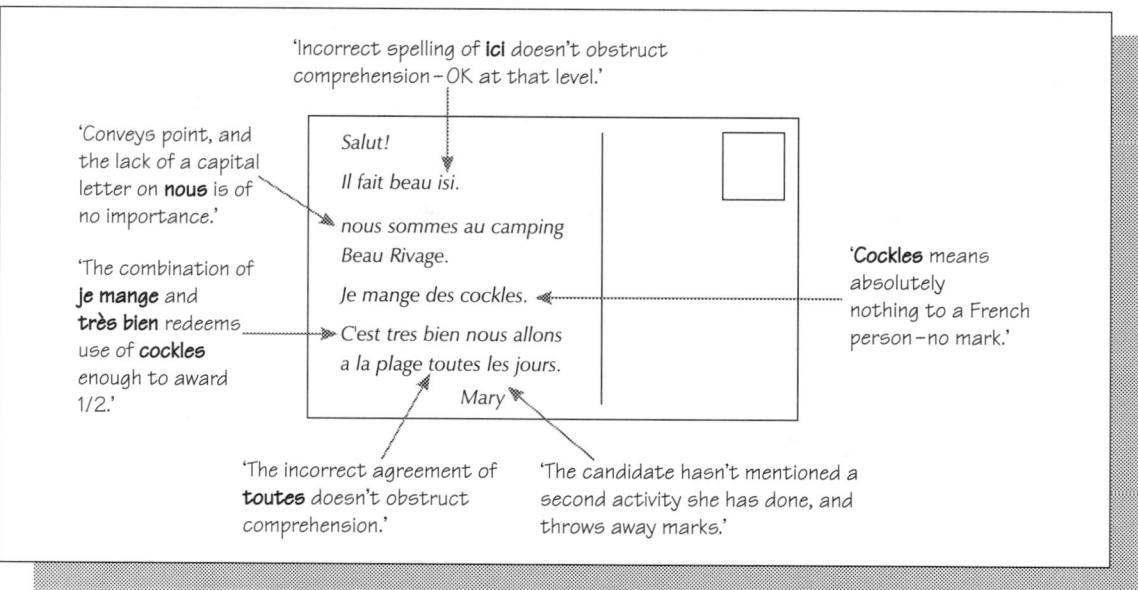

'Incorrect spelling of **ici** doesn't obstruct comprehension – OK at that level.'

'Conveys point, and the lack of a capital letter on **nous** is of no importance.'

'The combination of **je mange** and **très bien** redeems use of **cockles** enough to award 1/2.'

'Cockles means absolutely nothing to a French person – no mark.'

'The incorrect agreement of **toutes** doesn't obstruct comprehension.'

'The candidate hasn't mentioned a second activity she has done, and throws away marks.'

> Salut!
> Il fait beau isi.
> nous sommes au camping Beau Rivage.
> Je mange des cockles.
> C'est tres bien nous allons a la plage toutes les jours.
>   Mary

'The candidate has only answered 4 of the 5 points, but did them reasonably well. The mark would be 7/10. Once again, failing to answer the question fully reduces the final mark quite drastically.'

▶ **Postcard with a stimulus in French**

> Nantes, le trois juillet
> Arrivé à midi. Il fait chaud ici.
> Nantes est une grande ville dans l'ouest de la France.
>
> Demain je vais visiter le château et la tour de Bretagne. Ce soir on va au cinéma.
>   Claude

Lisez la carte postale. Ecrivez une carte postale.
Donnez les détails suivants:

quand vous êtes arrivé(e)
comment vous avez voyagé
où vous êtes
le temps qu'il fait
ce que vous allez faire ce soir.

Student answer with examiner's comments

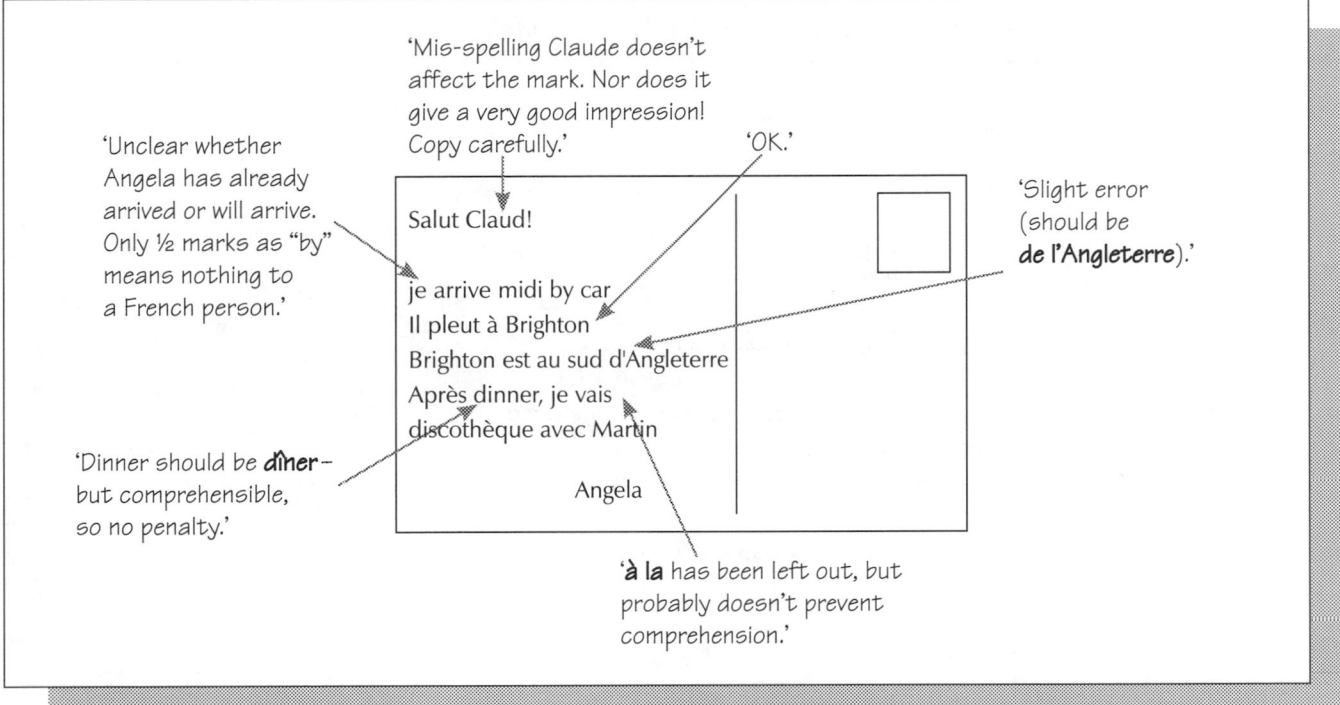

'Mis-spelling Claude doesn't affect the mark. Nor does it give a very good impression! Copy carefully.'

'OK.'

'Unclear whether Angela has already arrived or will arrive. Only ½ marks as "by" means nothing to a French person.'

'Slight error (should be *de l'Angleterre*).'

Salut Claud!

je arrive midi by car
Il pleut à Brighton
Brighton est au sud d'Angleterre
Après dinner, je vais
discothèque avec Martin

Angela

'Dinner should be **dîner** – but comprehensible, so no penalty.'

'**à la** has been left out, but probably doesn't prevent comprehension.'

'This attempt is worth 6/8. Once again, missing things out has reduced the candidate's mark.'

Foundation Tier D, C grade tasks, Higher Tier D, C grade tasks

The tasks are identical in the two tiers.

▷ **Informal letter**   Lisez cette annonce d'un magazine de jeunesse.

Jeune fille de 15 ans veut correspondre avec des jeunes anglais du même âge.
J'aime voyager et nager.

Chantal Daugé, 2 rue Pasteur, 17000 La Rochelle, France

Répondez à l'annonce.
Donnez les détails suivants:

votre nom
votre âge
votre domicile
votre famille
vos intérêts.

Ecrivez 70 mots.

Student answer with examiner's comments

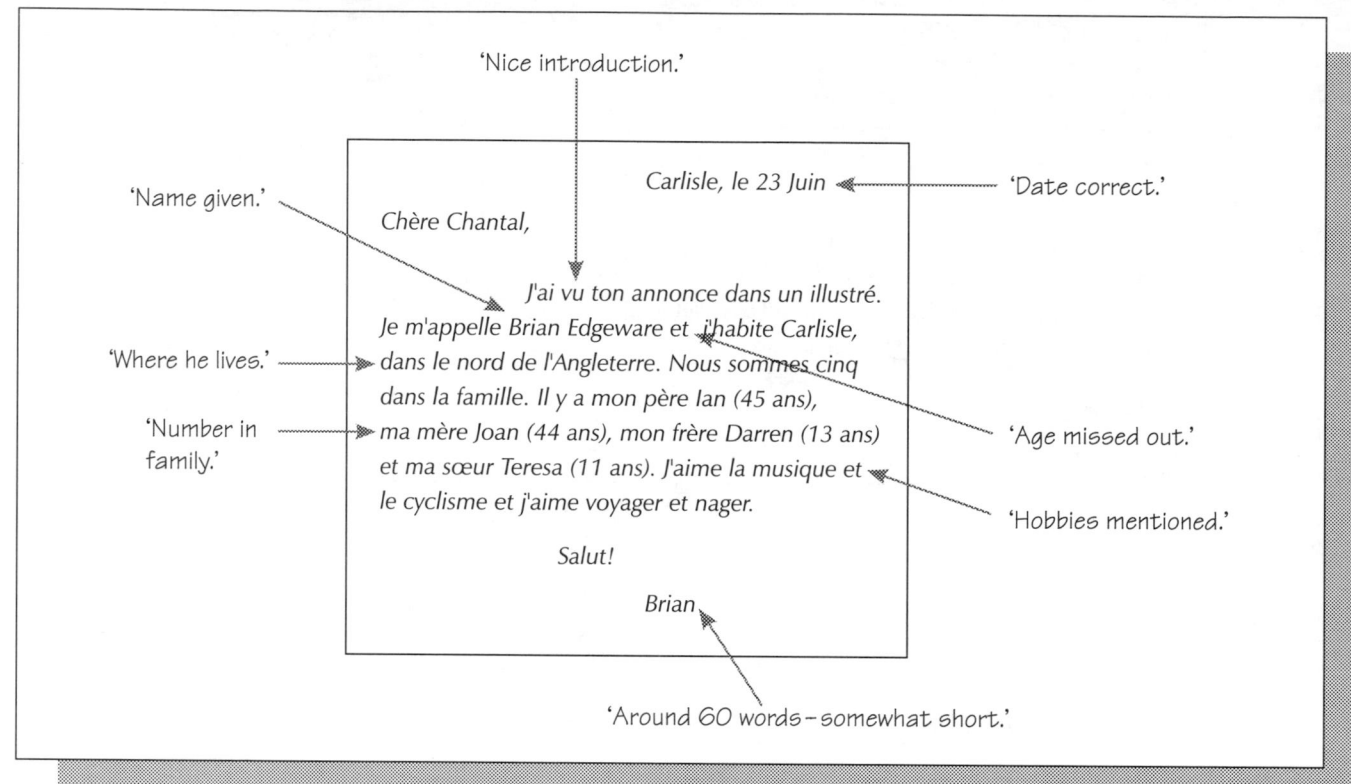

'Nice introduction.'

'Name given.'

'Date correct.'

Carlisle, le 23 Juin

Chère Chantal,

J'ai vu ton annonce dans un illustré.
Je m'appelle Brian Edgeware et j'habite Carlisle,
dans le nord de l'Angleterre. Nous sommes cinq
dans la famille. Il y a mon père Ian (45 ans),
ma mère Joan (44 ans), mon frère Darren (13 ans)
et ma sœur Teresa (11 ans). J'aime la musique et
le cyclisme et j'aime voyager et nager.

Salut!

Brian

'Where he lives.'

'Number in family.'

'Age missed out.'

'Hobbies mentioned.'

'Around 60 words – somewhat short.'

'This student has managed all 5 tasks well, using very simple French. However, he has missed out his age, and has not written quite enough. Otherwise this is a very sound attempt. Answering the question carefully pays, no matter how good your French is!'

▶ **Formal letter**   Ecrivez une lettre à un hôtel français où vous voulez aller visiter avec des ami(e)s.

Donnez les dates de votre séjour.
Dites quelles chambres il vous faut.
Demandez confirmation de la réservation.
Dites pourquoi vous avez choisi cet hôtel.
Demandez des renseignements au sujet d'excursions possibles.

Ecrivez environ 100 mots.

Student answer with examiner's comments

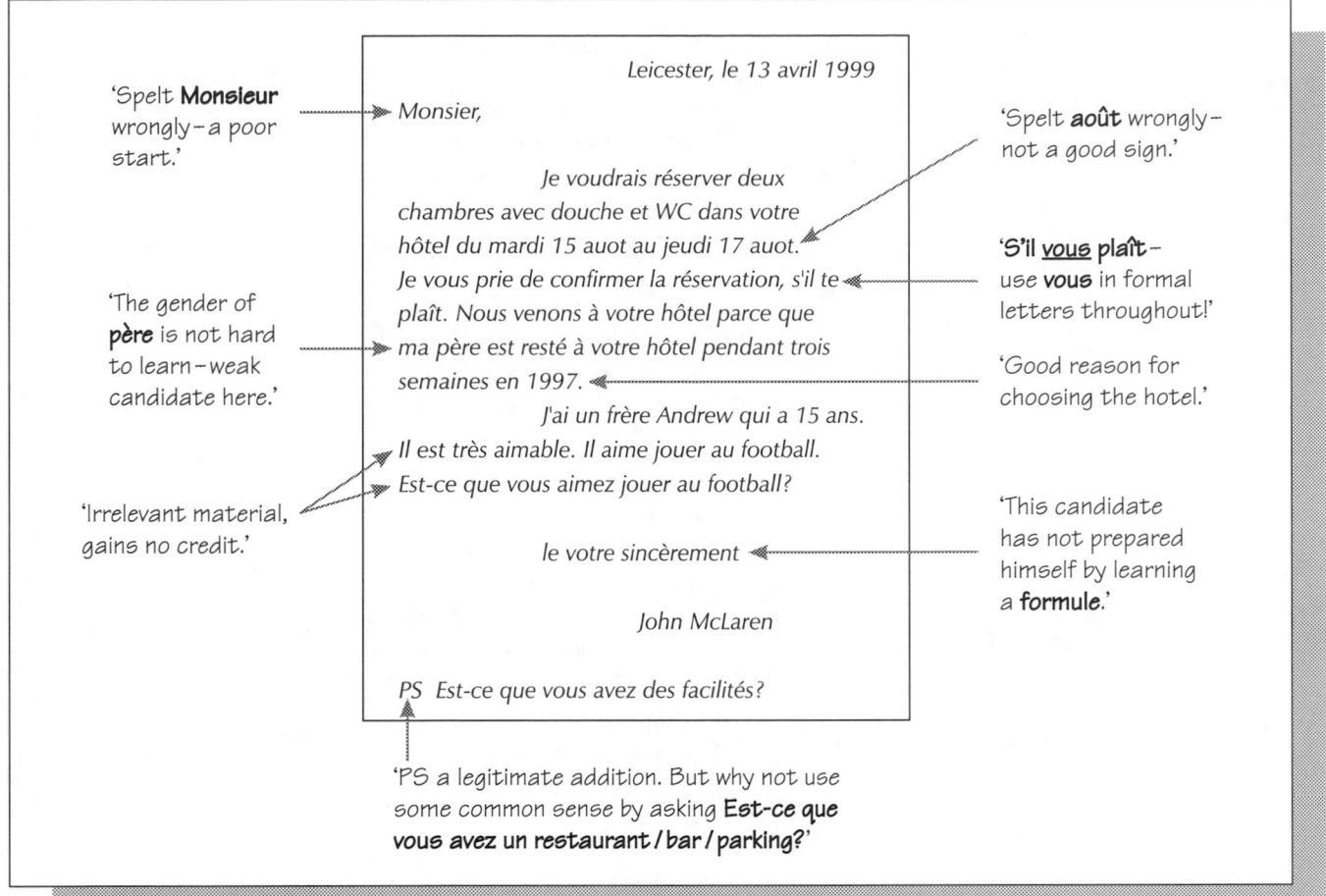

'Spelt **Monsieur** wrongly – a poor start.'

'The gender of **père** is not hard to learn – weak candidate here.'

'Irrelevant material, gains no credit.'

Leicester, le 13 avril 1999

Monsier,

Je voudrais réserver deux chambres avec douche et WC dans votre hôtel du mardi 15 auot au jeudi 17 auot. Je vous prie de confirmer la réservation, s'il te plaît. Nous venons à votre hôtel parce que ma père est resté à votre hôtel pendant trois semaines en 1997.

J'ai un frère Andrew qui a 15 ans. Il est très aimable. Il aime jouer au football. Est-ce que vous aimez jouer au football?

le votre sincèrement

John McLaren

PS Est-ce que vous avez des facilités?

'Spelt **août** wrongly – not a good sign.'

'**S'il vous plaît** – use **vous** in formal letters throughout!'

'Good reason for choosing the hotel.'

'This candidate has not prepared himself by learning a **formule**.'

'PS a legitimate addition. But why not use some common sense by asking **Est-ce que vous avez un restaurant / bar / parking?**'

'The candidate has not made a very good job of this.

"Getting the message across": he has fulfilled only 3 tasks of the 5 set. Has included a lot of irrelevant material more suited to an informal letter. The PS enquiry about "facilities" doesn't really communicate anything. But the inclusion in a PS of a point you may have missed out is allowable.

"Accuracy": not good. Spells all sorts of things poorly, even elementary words such as **Monsieur** and **août**. Mixes **tu** and **vous**.

"Variety of expression": not good. Has little "feel" for French, as shown by the attempt to translate "Yours sincerely".'

Higher Tier B, A, A* tasks

▷ **Essay**   *Vous avez passé des vacances en France avec votre famille. Vous êtes tombé(e) en panne. Décrivez la journée.*

Student answer with examiner's comments

'PDO agreement – good!'

'Nice setting of the scene.'

'Irregular feminine form of the adjective and correct gender of car types.'

'Good idiom.'

'Nice and idiomatic.'

'Good conjunction.'

'Useful adverb.'

'Nice ending – could be used elsewhere.'

'Good knowledge of French terminology for owner.'

Le deuxième jour de notre séjour en France ne nous a pas amusés. Tu sais que mon père conduit une vieille Morris. Vingt kilomètres avant Villeneuve nous sommes tombés en panne. Papa a mis trois heures pour réparer la voiture. C'était casse-pieds, je t'assure! Nous sommes arrivés enfin à Villeneuve le soir, vers huit heures. Le camping était complet car nous étions arrivés trop tard. Alors on a demandé à l'hôtel de France, mais malheureusement il n'y avait plus de chambres libres. A ce moment–là maman commençait à devenir furieuse. Elle a annoncé son intention de vendre la Morris. A la station-service papa a raconté notre histoire au patron. Il nous a offert un endroit pour camper dans son jardin. Enfin nous avions trouvé un endroit pour dormir. Tout est bien qui finit bien.

'A very good attempt!'

▷ **Verbal stimulus in French**

Ecrivez l'histoire sugérée par cet article du journal.

La voiture est toujours là mais les pneus ont disparu

En retrouvant l'autre matin sa voiture qu'il avait garée dans le boulevard Saint-Michel, M. Andrew Anderson, vacancier britannique, a eu la désagréable surprise de constater que les quatre pneus de sa voiture avaient tout simplement disparu!

Student answer with examiner's comments

'Careless use of incorrect past participle.'

'PDO doesn't apply here, so no extra **e** on **garé** – one of the dangers of lifting material.'

'Wrong tense – should be perfect, as in the cutting.'

'**le prochain matin** should be **le lendemain matin**.'

'PDO missing here **les avait volés**.'

'Good use of stock essay phrase – agreement right!'

En vacances en France, quelque chose de très choquant est arrivé. Papa avait garée la voiture dans le boulevard Saint-Michel. Quand il est aller chercher la voiture le prochain matin il avait une surprise désagréable. Les quatre pneus avaient tout simplement disparu! Quelqu'un les avait volé. 'Merde!' a-t-il dit. 'On ne peut pas rouler sans pneus!' Il a appelé la police. Après être arrivés les policiers ont cherché les pneus, mais ils ne les ont pas trouvés. Papa n'etait pas content. Il était obligé d'acheter de nouveaux pneus!

'A successful piece of lifting from the stimulus.'

'Good inversion after speech. Direct speech can sometimes improve a banal essay if it's not overdone.'

'Chance for linking two short sentences with **parce que** missed.'

'Correct position of object pronoun with negative – good

'This is a fair attempt at dealing with quite a difficult stimulus. Fairly intelligent use has been made of the French text, although this answer also shows some of the pitfalls which can result from "lifting" text. However, good candidates could probably be expected to improve on some of the grammatical niceties which have defeated this candidate.'

▷ **Report** Ecrivez 100 mots au sujet d'une excursion que votre famille a faite. Donnez vos opinions sur ce que vous avez fait.

Student answer with examiner's comment

La semaine dernière mes parents ont décidé de faire une excursion. Nous nous sommes levés de bonne heure et après avoir pris notre petit déjeuner, nous sommes montés dans la voiture et nous nous sommes mis en route pour la côte.

Une fois arrivés, nous avons visité le musée que j'ai trouvé très intéressant, et puis, vers midi, nous nous sommes baignés dans la mer.

A une heure nous avons déjeuné. Maman avait apporté un pique-nique magnifique, du poulet rôti et du jambon fumé, et de la salade. L'après-midi nous sommes restés au soleil sur la plage. C'était une journée vraiment agréable!

Examiner's comment

This is nearly as good an answer as could be expected from a GCSE candidate. I have ringed the features which enhance its quality – the variety of vocabulary, the use of adjectives, the varied sentence structure. The only feature lacking is justification of the opinions given.

FURTHER SPECIMEN QUESTIONS

Because such a wide variety of answers is possible, specimen answers have not been provided for these questions.

Foundation Tier G, F, E grade tasks

▷ **Lists of things**   *Vous avez oublié votre valise dans un hôtel suisse.*
Ecrivez la liste des choses dans votre valise.

    1 _____
    2 _____
    3 _____
    4 _____
    5 _____
    6 _____
    7 _____
    8 _____
    9 _____
    10 _____

▷ **Form-filling**   *Vous allez faire un échange.*
Remplissez cette fiche.

    Nom .... Prénom(s) ....
    Age .... ans .... mois
    Famille
    ....
    ....
    Nom du collège ....
    Matières étudiées au collège:
    1 ....   4 ....
    2 ....   5 ....
    3 ....   6 ....
    Langues parlées:
    1 ....   2 ....
    Sports préférés:
    1 ....   2 ....
    Autres intérêts:
    1 ....   3 ....
    2 ....

▷ **Messages/Notes** Laissez un message pour votre correspondant français. Il veut aller à la piscine en autobus. Donnez les détails suivants:

Quel numéro?
Où est l'arrêt d'autobus?
Ça coûte combien?
Ça prend combien de temps?
Où descendre du bus?

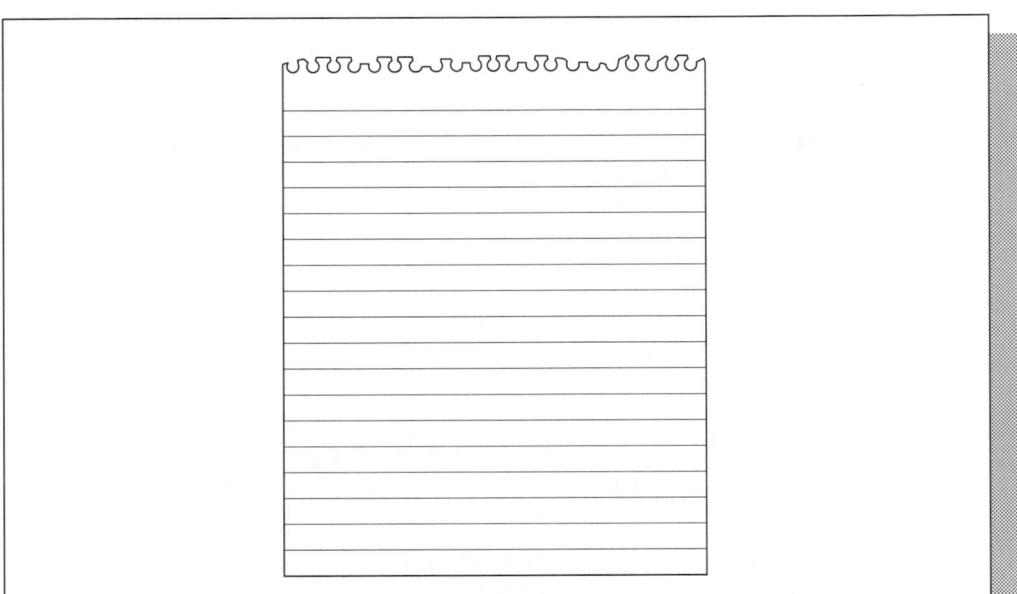

▷ **Diary entries** Complétez ce journal avec 10 activités.

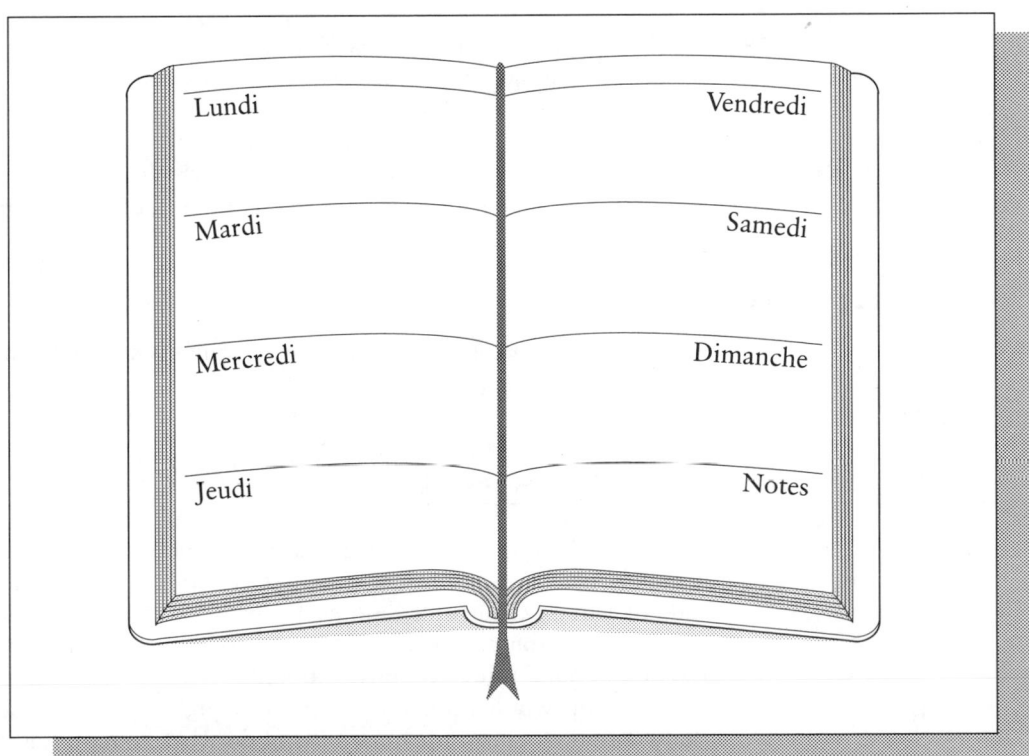

▶ **Postcards**   Ecrivez une carte postale à un(e) camarade.

> Dites où vous êtes.
> Décrivez le temps qu'il fait.
> Dites ce que vous avez mangé.
> Mentionnez **deux** activités.

FoundationTier D, C grade tasks, HigherTier D, C grade tasks

The tasks are identical in the two tiers.

▶ **Informal letter**   Ecrivez une lettre à un(e) camarade français(e).
Mentionnez:

> le week-end dernier
> un problème dans votre famille
> le collège
> vos projets pour l'été
> une invitation

▶ **Formal letter**   *Vous cherchez un travail.*
Ecrivez une lettre.
Mentionnez:

> vos détails personnels
> vos expériences
> quand vous voulez travailler
> pendant combien de temps vous voulez travailler.

Demandez un logement.

HigherTier B, A, A* tasks

▶ **Essay**   1   Décrivez un week-end désastreux. Ecrivez environ 150 mots.
2   La meilleure journée de ma vie. Ecrivez environ 150 mots.

▶ **Report**   1   Vous avez vu un vol dans votre supermarché local. Ecrivez un rapport pour la police.
2   Vous avez vu un accident dans la rue. Ecrivez un rapport pour la police.

▶ **Imaginative**   Continuez ce thème:

Il faisait noir. Dans la gare déserte une forme mystérieuse avançait, un pistolet à la main.
Alors,.......

▶ A STEP FURTHER

The most obvious one is to make sure that you know those things for which there are definitely marks and which will almost certainly come up. These include beginnings and ends of letters, commands, and such things as dates and times of arrival and departure, and activities you or a penfriend would like to do during an exchange visit. All of these should be found readily in most textbooks.

Something which cannot be stressed enough is to make sure that, on the day of the examination, you read the question and do what you are told to do.

Finally, develop strategies for checking your work. There is no doubt that a good standard of accuracy will improve your marks no end. However, accuracy can be difficult to improve unless you are systematic.

Use this checklist for your written work by ticking off the checks you have carried out:

1 **Check genders**
   ▶ by looking up individual words ☐
   ▶ by applying gender rules ☐

2 **Check adjectives**
   ▶ do they have the correct ending for: ☐
      – the gender of the noun
      – singular or plural?
   ▶ do they come before or after the noun? ☐

3 **Check verbs**
   ▶ is the tense right in each instance? ☐
   ▶ is it regular or irregular? ☐
   ▶ is the form of the verb right? ☐
   ▶ does it need *avoir* or *être*? ☐
   ▶ if *être*, does the past participle agree? ☐

4 **Check spelling**
   ▶ accents where needed? ☐
   ▶ accents pointing the right way? ☐

Coursework

▷ **GETTING STARTED**

Coursework is a feature of many GCSE subjects. The principal advantage for students is that they can work at their own pace, and, over time, produce considered pieces of work. Many students find coursework challenging, but rise to the challenge and produce excellent work. Other students find examinations nerve-wracking and prefer to work at coursework where they can be certain to have marks 'in the bag' before the final examination. In French, coursework is not compulsory unless you are taking the SEG Modular syllabus.

▷ **WHAT YOU NEED TO KNOW**

▷ **Introduction**

Coursework in French will be available to many students for the first time in 1998. For practical reasons, it is only available to students in schools and colleges. Private candidates are not allowed to enter for it.

Four Examining Groups, EDEXCEL, MEG, NEAB and WJEC, offer the **option** of Writing coursework in place of the Writing examination.

EDEXCEL has the additional possibility of doing Speaking coursework. However, EDEXCEL candidates are only allowed to do **one** type of coursework, either Speaking or Writing.

In the SEG Modular examination there is some Speaking coursework at the end of Module 1 (February of Year 10) and some in Module 3 (December of Year 11). Additionally, there is Writing coursework in Module 3 (December of Year 11). In the SEG Modular scheme, there is no choice about coursework; you have to do it.

CCEA does not offer coursework.

▷ **Advantages and disadvantages of coursework**

Coursework does have a number of advantages, which may be listed as follows:

▷ You have more control over the final standard of your work.
▷ You are not vulnerable to feeling unwell or ill-prepared on the day of the examination.
▷ You can take as much time as you like over pieces which are done at home.
▷ You can use a range of reference materials to ensure that your work is good.
▷ You can take pleasure in working up a piece of work from idea to draft to final version.
▷ You can often do tasks which interest you particularly.

On the other hand, there are snags to coursework:

▷ You may find it difficult getting down to work.
▷ You may not find it easy to write and research pieces of original work.
▷ You may not be organised enough to ensure that stages of the work are completed on time.
▷ Your workload may become unpredictable with lots of coursework due from a range of subjects at the same time (February in Year 11 can be a busy time).
▷ You may move school.
▷ Your teacher may move school or be ill for an extended period.

▷ **Different types of Writing coursework**

Most of the Examining Groups require that you submit three items of Writing coursework, the exception being SEG, which requires two pieces. Of the three pieces of writing, two may be done at home in your own time, but at least one must be done under controlled conditions (see below). In practice, many teachers will ask you to do more than the minimum number of pieces of coursework and will then select the best three pieces to send in as your final mark. This should be comforting, as it means that any last-minute disasters are less serious for you.

The Examining Groups vary slightly in their regulations about how coursework should be approached, but a typical approach is outlined below.

Task training

Your teacher will cover a topic or a unit of work, and let you know that it provides an opportunity for a piece of coursework to be written. The teacher may then wish to do some work on the sort of thing which you might produce – a description of your home area, for example. This might include reading and listening to descriptions of other areas in French, and some work on, say, useful adjectives for this topic.

Discussion of task choice

Your teacher may ask you to choose a task, and will then discuss with you how practical your choice is. There is no requirement for all tasks done in a class to be different; indeed it may be that many of you complete the same task or similar ones.

After discussing your choice, your teacher will set you a deadline for either a first draft or an outline. Make sure you have done something about the task by this date so that the next stage is useful.

Discussion of first draft or outline

Your teacher will want to see, and probably take in to read at home, your first draft. This should be as good-quality an effort as you can manage, because then the teacher can concentrate on recommending improvements which you could not have thought up yourself. Your teacher is not allowed to mark the work in detail at this stage. However, he or she will be making comments of a general nature, such as:

'This is not long enough to be assessed for grades A*, A or B, although the quality is good.'
'Have you thought of checking the gender of the nouns in the dictionary so that you get them right?'
'Have you remembered to check which verbs take *être* in the perfect tense?'
'This piece doesn't refer to past, present and future events as it stands.'
'You haven't given enough opinions; *bon* and *excellent* are not enough on their own. Justify your opinions by using *parce que*.'

Production of the final piece of coursework

You should re-write your first draft after doing all the checking that your teacher has suggested, as well as any other things that you can think of. It is quite possible, for example, to look up the gender of every noun in a 150-word piece of writing to check that you got it right, and that the adjective that goes with it agrees properly. The final piece of coursework should be written on A4-sized paper.

Certificate of authentication

When you hand in the final piece of coursework, you will be asked to sign a statement that the piece of work is your own unaided effort. Your teacher will also have to countersign that statement. In practice, this means that you will have to do without using human reference sources such as other teachers, older brothers and sisters, parents, the French Assistant(e) and so on.

Reference materials and other help

All Examining Groups allow you to use a French–English, English–French dictionary throughout the preparation of coursework. At home, you will also be able to use your textbook, glossaries, exercise books, notebooks, grammars, etc. If you are able to use IT, this can improve the presentation. You will also be able to use a French spell-checker if you have one. But you should be aware that French spell-checkers require you to have a reasonable knowledge of spelling and of patterns of adjective agreement. Human help, however, should be avoided.

▶ Controlled conditions Writing

As mentioned above, most Examining Groups require you to produce at least one of your three pieces of coursework under controlled conditions. This means that the work is produced under the direct supervision of your teacher, in formal test-type conditons. The work should be done in one sitting.

Some of the rules about reference materials are stricter. You will not be allowed to use IT, and some Groups restrict your use of reference materials to an English–French, French–English dictionary only. Check with your teacher beforehand what your Group allows.

You will not necessarily know the title of the piece of work you are going to be asked to do beforehand, although your teacher will have given you some indication, such as 'you are going to write a formal letter'. Again, practice varies slightly from Group to Group, so check carefully with your teacher.

There is no opportunity to have your teacher's comments on your work before you hand it in, and there is limited time available to draft and check the draft. Do make sure you know how much time you have been allowed so that you can complete your work and produce a neat version on A4 paper at the end of the session.

▶ Writing coursework tasks

Coursework tasks vary somewhat from Group to Group. Some Groups, notably NEAB, have a list of coursework tasks in the syllabus from which all candidates must choose. Other Groups give suggestions, but do not insist that you follow them. Because the rules vary somewhat among different Groups, it is important that you make your choice in consultation with your teacher.

The tasks are divided into three categories, depending on which grade you are aiming for. **Grade G, F, E tasks** are usually short, and require between 20 and about 100 words. Examples might include:

- make a shopping list
- fill in a campsite form
- make a list of foods you have eaten this week
- make a packing list for a walking holiday.

Slightly more ambitious tasks, but still in the grade G, F, E category, might include:

- write a postcard home
- design a poster about your local area
- comment on your school uniform and design a better one
- write about a well-known French entertainer

Grade D, C tasks will typically require between 90 and 120 words.

They could include some of the more ambitious tasks for Grades G, F, E, written at greater length. Other possibilities include:

- my work experience
- my ideal job
- a diary of a real or imagined visit to a French-speaking country
- a job application letter
- a letter reserving hotel accommodation
- a diary of a memorable weekend
- a journey: planning, advantages and disadvantages.

Grade B, A, A* tasks will typically require between 150 and 170 words.

They could include some of the more ambitious tasks for Grades D, C, written at greater length. Other possibilities include:

- an account of a play, film, or book you have enjoyed
- a report on the structure of French TV, satellite TV and radio
- a comparison of festivals in France and UK (e.g. Christmas)
- an account of an incident you have seen in the street
- a plan of campaign to tackle an environmental or social issue

▶ **Marking of Writing coursework**

Your teacher will mark your coursework usually using grids which measure two or three features of your writing.

These are:

▷ communication
▷ accuracy
▷ range and variety of language

Communication is most important at Grades G, F, E, while accuracy and range and variety of language are most important for grades B, A, A*.

At the simplest level, marks will be awarded for communicating your message, even if the French has many errors.

At the highest level, teachers will be looking for French which is more or less accurate, which uses a range of appropriate tenses, and uses a wide range of adjectives and adverbs. The writing will include your personal opinions, expressed in a mature way, and the justification of those opinions. So if you are aiming for a high grade in your coursework, make sure you include those components.

▶ **Speaking coursework**

EDEXCEL

EDEXCEL offers the chance to choose Speaking coursework.

The EDEXCEL coursework option requires you to submit three units of work, each drawn from a different National Curriculum Area of Experience. For each unit you will have to do a role-play-type task and a presentation of a topic. These will be recorded and may be sent off to the Examining Group after being marked. The tasks have to be completed by the end of April in the year of the examination, but your teacher may get you to do them at any time during your course.

EDEXCEL provides example tasks in its syllabus, which your teacher will have a copy of.

If you are a **Foundation** candidate, for each unit you can expect to do a simple role-play, say, in a shop, similar to those used in end-of-course Speaking Tests (see Chapter 6 on Speaking). In addition, you can expect to do a presentation and then discuss your presentation. Again, this is similar to the final examination version.

If you are a **Higher** candidate, for each unit you can expect to do a more complicated role-play, which might be a survey, a negotiation, or a presentation of, say, a radio broadcast. In addition, you can expect to do a presentation and then discuss your presentation. This is similar to the final examination version.

SEG Modular

SEG Modular has compulsory Speaking coursework in Modules 1 and 3.

Module 1 is assessed in February of Year 10. You are asked to produce a short tape-recorded monologue on some aspect of the work you have done. You are not allowed to read from a prepared script, but you can use prompts. You can pause the tape, but it must be recorded on a single occasion.

Module 3 involves the same procedure as Module 1, and is assessed in December of Year 11.

For Speaking coursework, the advice given in Chapter 6 on Speaking should help with most tasks.

WRITING COURSEWORK WITH STUDENT ANSWERS AND EXAMINER'S COMMENTS

G, F, E task   Tu vas faire du camping avec ton ami(e) français(e). Fais une liste des choses qu'il/elle doit mettre dans son sac à dos.

1	un torch
2	chateau
3	tente
4	montre
5	gaz
6	une paire de chaussetes
7	une paire de gants
8	un walkman
9	un sack de dormir
10	un costume de natation

Examiner's comment

This is not a very carefully checked effort. The first item is not French at all. The second one is half-remembered **chapeau**, I presume — it could easily have been checked in a dictionary. Most of the remaining items are OK, even **un walkman**, but the last two items seem to have been looked up in a dictionary but to have given the wrong answer: *un sack* should be spelt **un sac** and *de dormir* is presumably a version of 'to sleep'. It should have been **un sac de couchage**. The *costume de natation* is the product of looking up 'suit' and 'swimming. The correct version is **un maillot de bain**.

▶ **D, C task**   Tu as fait un voyage en France. Ecris une lettre à ton copain/ta copine pour décrire ce voyage.

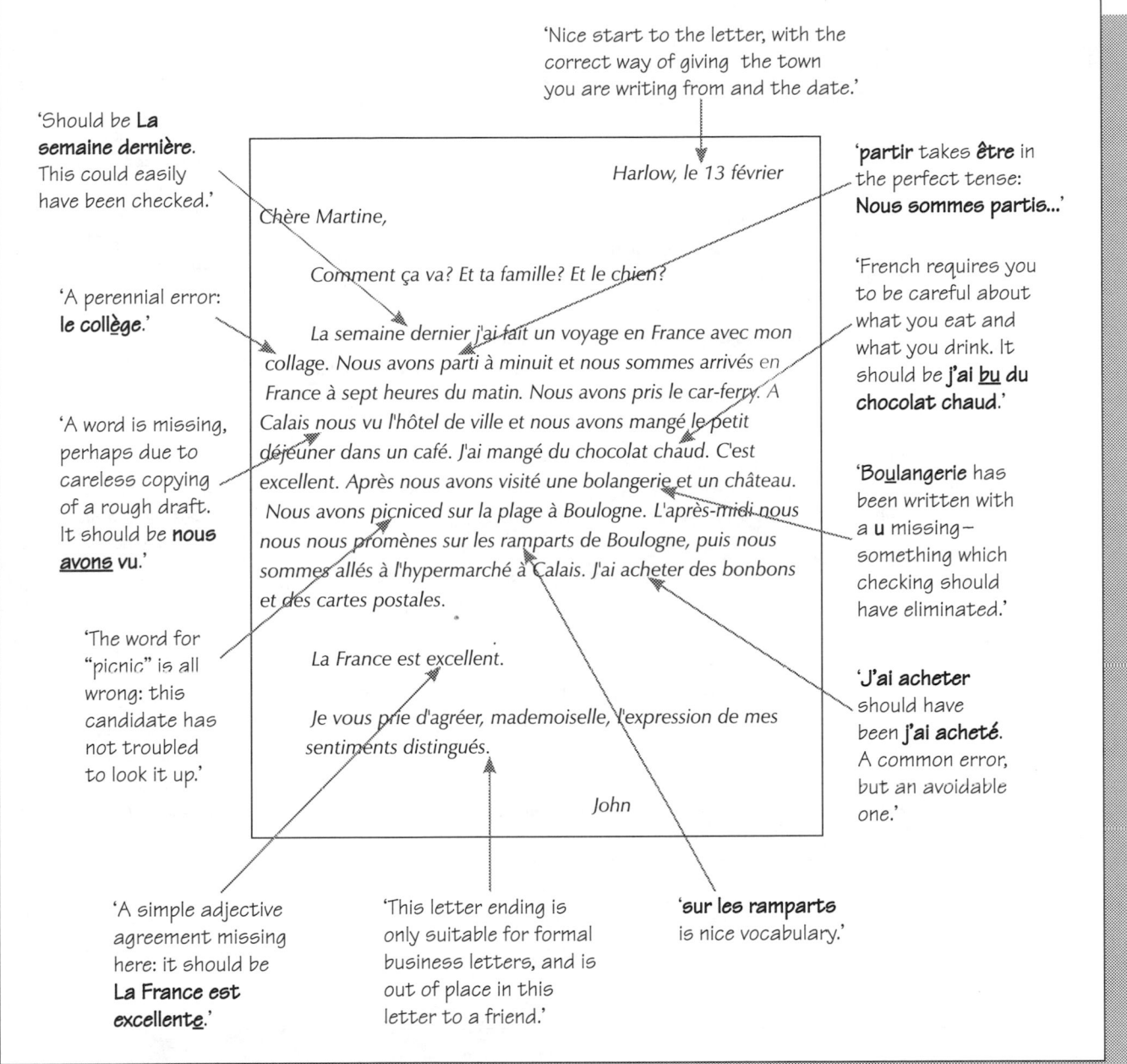

'Nice start to the letter, with the correct way of giving the town you are writing from and the date.'

'Should be **La semaine dernière**. This could easily have been checked.'

'A perennial error: **le collège**.'

'A word is missing, perhaps due to careless copying of a rough draft. It should be **nous avons vu**.'

'The word for "picnic" is all wrong: this candidate has not troubled to look it up.'

'partir takes **être** in the perfect tense: **Nous sommes partis...**'

'French requires you to be careful about what you eat and what you drink. It should be **j'ai bu du chocolat chaud**.'

'**Boulangerie** has been written with a **u** missing – something which checking should have eliminated.'

'**J'ai acheter** should have been **j'ai acheté**. A common error, but an avoidable one.'

> Harlow, le 13 février
>
> Chère Martine,
>
> Comment ça va? Et ta famille? Et le chien?
>
> La semaine dernier j'ai fait un voyage en France avec mon collage. Nous avons parti à minuit et nous sommes arrivés en France à sept heures du matin. Nous avons pris le car-ferry. A Calais nous vu l'hôtel de ville et nous avons mangé le petit déjeuner dans un café. J'ai mangé du chocolat chaud. C'est excellent. Après nous avons visité une bolangerie et un château. Nous avons picniced sur la plage à Boulogne. L'après-midi nous nous nous promèns sur les ramparts de Boulogne, puis nous sommes allés à l'hypermarché à Calais. J'ai acheter des bonbons et des cartes postales.
>
> La France est excellent.
>
> Je vous prie d'agréer, mademoiselle, l'expression de mes sentiments distingués.
>
> John

'A simple adjective agreement missing here: it should be **La France est excellente**.'

'This letter ending is only suitable for formal business letters, and is out of place in this letter to a friend.'

'**sur les ramparts** is nice vocabulary.'

Examiner's comment
Overall this candidate's work is somewhere in the middle of this range. However, with a little more forethought and some more careful checking and copying, this piece of work could have been very definitely in the C range. It answers the question, communicates well, and has a fair range of vocabulary and structure.

▷ **B, A, A* task**   'Les parents et les jeunes ne s'entendent jamais très bien.' Commentez.

'Not quite on target, but a very nice try at complicated language.'

'Asking yourself a question and answering it is a good essay technique.'

'The ability to be sarcastic in a foreign language shows a good command of it.'

'A nice play on words showing good command of idiom.'

Les parents et les jeunes se disputent toujours. Mais il ne faut pas oublier, ils se sont toujours disputés! Les grands animaux rejettent les jeunes dans le monde, et c'est comme ça aussi avec les humains.

Sur pour quoi se disputent-ils? Chez moi, on se dispute au sujet du téléphone, de la télé, des vêtements, de l'argent de poche, l'heure pour retourner à la maison le soir, des amis, de la musique, du désordre, de tout.

Ma mère se met toujours en colère quand je téléphone avec mes amis. Elle me demande qui va payer la facture. (Si ce n'est pas moi, c'est bien, à mon avis!)

Quand je rentre le soir avec un petit peu de retard, mes parents sont fâchés. Ils pensent que les criminels attendent 11.00h du soir pour commencer leur travail!

Ma mère n'aime pas ma chambre. Il y a trop de désordre. C'est peut-être vrai, mais j'ai trop de devoirs à faire. Et puis, les personnes qui aiment l'ordre sont toutes ennuyeux.

Finalement, mes parents ne sont pas parfaits! C'est vrai! Mon père fume – sale habitude. Ma mère passe trop de temps dans la baignoire – habitude moins sale mais ennuyeuse pour le reste de la famille.

Après tout, on ne choisit pas ses parents. Mais la plupart du temps je les aime (un peu).

'A good analogy for the introduction to this piece.'

'A good list of points of conflict, the result probably of brainstorming, then refining into this final draft.'

'Personal opinion – good (even if the sentiments are not very noble!)'

Personal opinion again. The agreement should be **ennuyeuses** because **personne** is feminine, a point which is often overlooked.'

'A nice conclusion.'

'Going on the offensive is another good essay technique.'

Examiner's comment
Overall, this is the sort of work which could expect to achieve A or A*, depending on the absolute level of accuracy. It is a pleasure to read, and the candidate is sufficiently in control of events to write with wry humour.

▷ **CONCLUSION**

Coursework has a number of benefits, and, if you take advantage of the extra time in which to do the work, you should be able to produce the grade you deserve with less worry. On the other hand, you should remember that there is much less excuse for poorly planned, inaccurate work when you have had all the time in the world and all possible reference materials to hand. So when you hand a first draft in, make sure it is good, so that the second draft truly is a polished version.

Grammar

▷ **Learning grammar**

Improving your knowledge of grammar isn't difficult if you take a little at a time, beginning with things you think you know. When you have made sure of them, you can look at the more exotic parts of the list. Don't be put off if you don't understand the grammatical terms. Check the example and see if you have seen something like it in your textbook.

For verbs, check you can write out the various tenses from memory. Then do it a little longer after you last looked at them, and then longer still, until you are foolproof. I once had a successful student who used to write out the present and imperfect tense of *avoir*, *être*, and one *-er*, *-ir* and *-re* verb on her rough paper before she started her essays. She then used them to check her work against. (NB This method only works if your memory is good!)

Grammar is often seen as boring and irrelevant. It isn't, as it allows you to generate sentences which you have not come across before, and helps your reading and listening comprehension. Find out how it works and you have the key to more French than you can possibly expect to learn by heart.

▷ **Glossary of grammatical terms**

Not all students are taught using formal grammar in their English or French lessons nowadays. There is nothing to be frightened of in the use of grammatical terms. After all, mechanics wouldn't attempt to describe what a spanner is every time they wanted to have one passed to them. They just use the technical term, which is 'spanner'. These grammatical terms are the technical 'jargon' of language-learning, which give you access to the patterns of French and other languages to enable you to learn them more quickly.

I have attempted to define them simply, and give examples. There are further examples and explanations later on in the chapter.

Adjective

This is a word which describes a noun or pronoun. It gives information about such things as colour, type, disposition, etc.

Example
le garçon **aimable**   *the **pleasant** boy*

Adverb

This is a word which describes a verb (adds to the verb). It gives information about how something is done.

Example
Il court **vite**.   *He runs **quickly**.*

Adverbs can also be used to add to adjectives or other adverbs.

Examples
le garçon **très** aimable   *the **very** pleasant boy*
Il court **très** vite.   *He runs **very** quickly.*

Agreement

Adjectives in French alter their spelling to agree with, or conform to, or 'match' the noun they describe.

Examples
C'est un **beau** jardin et une **belle** maison avec de **beaux** arbres et de **belles** fleurs.
*It's a **beautiful** garden and a **beautiful** house with **beautiful** trees and **beautiful** flowers.*

Past participles agree, too. Look up the rules (see p. 187).

Articles

There are three sorts of article:

definite	le, la, les	*the*
indefinite	un, une	*a*
partitive	du, de la, des	*some, any*

Clause

This is a part of a sentence which contains a subject and a verb which agrees with that subject. There are main clauses and subordinate clauses. Main clauses tell you most of the message of the sentence.

Example
Le garçon court très vite. *The boy runs very quickly.*

Subordinate clauses tell you something more about some other part of the sentence.

Examples
Le garçon **qui habite Lyon** court très vite. *The boy **who lives in Lyons** runs very quickly.*

Comparatives

A way of using adjectives and adverbs to compare two people or things.

Examples
Je suis **plus fort** que toi. *I am **stronger** than you.*
Il court **plus vit**e que moi. *He runs **faster** than me.*

Conjugation

The name given to the pattern that verbs follow. Regular verbs in French belong to the *-er*, *-ir* and *-re* conjugations. But unfortunately there are lots of exceptions!

Conjunction

Conjunctions join sentences and clauses.

Examples
et, mais, parce que *and, for, because*

Gender

In French there are two grammatical genders. All nouns are either masculine (*le*, *un*) or feminine (*la*, *une*).

Imperatives

These are the command forms of verbs, and are used when telling people to do something. They include the 'Let's...' sort of command, which is a way of telling yourself and one or more other people to do something.

Examples
Ecoute! *Listen!*
Ecoutez! *Listen!*
Ecoutons! *Let's listen!*

Infinitive

This is the part of the verb you find when you look it up in a vocabulary list, and which means 'to...' It doesn't agree with a subject. They may be found in combination with other verbs.

Example
manger *to eat*

Interrogative pronouns

These are questions words. Their English equivalents mostly begin with 'wh'.

Examples
Qui? *Who?*
Quoi? *What?*

Irregular verbs

These are verbs which don't follow one of the set patterns. They are written out for you in the verb table on pp. 224–35. They tend to be common verbs.

Nouns

These are the names of people, places and things.

Number

Things can be **singular** (one only) or **plural** (more than one).

Object

This is the thing or the person affected by the action of a verb. An object can be either a noun or a pronoun.

Examples
Je regarde **la télé**. *I watch **TV**.*
Je **l'**aime. *I like **it**.*

Past participle

This is part of the verb which is used with *avoir* and *être* to form the perfect and pluperfect tenses. Irregular verbs commonly have irregular past participles. Be aware of rules about agreement of past participles (see p. 187).

Examples
J'ai dormi. *I slept / I have slept.*
Nous sommes arrivé(e)s. *We arrived / We have arrived.*
Ils se sont lavés. *They got washed / They have got washed.*

Prepositions

These are words which are placed in front of nouns and pronouns to show position and other relationships.

Examples
Le bol est **dans** l'évier.   *The bowl is in the sink.*
Marie vient **chez** moi.   *Marie is coming to my house.*

Present participle

This is part of a verb which is expressed by '...ing' in English, and in French is usually found in combination with *en*.

Example
en mangeant   *while eating*

Pronouns

These are words which are used to avoid repeating a noun or proper name.

Examples
je, il, me, etc.

Reflexive verbs

These are verbs where the person does the action to himself or herself. There are rather more of them in French than in English, and you would do well to familiarise yourself with the list given in the grammar reference section.

Example
se laver – je **me** lave   *I wash myself*

Relative pronouns

These introduce a relative clause, which is a clause which tells you something more about another part of the sentence. They can often be omitted in English, but never in French.

Example
Voilà l'homme **que** je cherche.   *There's the man I am looking for.*
                                     There's the man that I am looking for.
                                     There's the man who I am looking for.
C'est un homme **qui** est très fort.   *He's a man who is very strong.*

Subject

This is the thing or the person performing the action of the verb. A subject can be either a noun or a pronoun.

Examples
La dame aime la musique classique. **Elle** l'écoute à la radio.
The lady likes classical music. She listens to it on the radio.

Superlative

This is a way of using adjectives and adverbs to say who is the best, the fastest, etc.

Examples

Je suis **le plus fort** de tous.   *I am **the strongest** of all.*
Il court **le plus vite** de tous.   *He runs **the fastest** of all.*

Tenses

These are the different forms of verbs which describe mainly **when** something takes place, took place, will take place, etc.

There are some differences in the use of tenses between French and English, but future tenses refer to the future, present tenses refer to now or to regular events which are still going on, and past tenses refer to events which have already taken place. The conditonal is used for conditions, while the French subjunctive has no direct equivalent in English. Look them up in the grammar (see p. 202 and p. 203).

▷ GRAMMAR IN GCSE FRENCH

The grammar you need to know for GCSE French is laid down by the Examining Groups in their Defined Contents. They have divided what you need to know into four categories, two at each of the Foundation and Higher Tiers.

At each Tier they list:

▷ productive skills (things you have to be able to say and write)
▷ receptive skills (things you need to understand, but are not necessarily able to say or write from memory).

This is just the same as in English, where you will understand many words and some items of grammar which you wouldn't necessarily use yourself.

▷ **Grammar list**   To simplify matters, I am going to list grammar under Foundation and Higher Tiers.

Anything which is listed with an (R) against it is for receptive use only.

Items which have an (R) in the Foundation lists will be used productively at Higher Tier.

Space does not allow many examples in the list. However, I have given the correct grammatical terms for structures so that you can look them up in the grammar reference section of this chapter (see pp. 180–223). If you do have to set a priority on the most important things to revise, go for the forms of verbs in the various tenses first, followed by the agreement of adjectives.

Put a tick in the box alongside this list when you have revised the grammar items, and a tick in the second box when you have been tested (successfully!) by a friend.

You will find for most items of grammar a note of common mistakes, with both the mistake, and, more importantly, the correct answer. This is a unique feature of this book, appropriate because it is a study guide.

Verbs – Foundation Tier

		Learned	*Tested*
▷ present tense	*je joue, je finis, je réponds*	☐	☐
▷ perfect tense (also called *passé composé*) with *avoir* and *être*	*j'ai joué, je suis arrivé(e), j'ai répondu, j'ai fini*	☐	☐
▷ imperfect tense	*je jouais, je finissais, je répondais*	☐	☐
▷ future using *aller* + infinitive	*je vais manger*	☐	☐
▷ future tense	*je jouerai, je finirai, je répondrai*	☐	☐

			Learned	*Tested*
▷	reflexive verbs	*Je m'appelle Anne. Papa se lève.*	☐	☐
▷	question forms		☐	☐
▷	command forms (imperative)	*Joue! Jouons! Jouez!*	☐	☐
▷	infinitive	*jouer, répondre, finir*	☐	☐
▷	infinitive + *pour, sans, avant de, il faut*	*Il faut jouer. C'est pour manger.*	☐	☐
▷	common verb + *à* or *de* + infinitive	*Il a demandé à sortir. Il a décidé de manger en ville.*	☐	☐
▷	(R) perfect infinitive	*après avoir fini, après être venu(e)*	☐	☐
▷	use of tenses with *depuis*	*J'habite à Blackpool depuis deux ans.*	☐	☐
▷	negatives	*ne ... pas, ne ... jamais, ne ... rien, ne ... aucun, ne ... nulle part, ne ... personne, ne ... plus, ne ... que, ne ... ni ... ni ...*	☐	☐
▷	present participle + *en*	*en jouant, en finissant, en répondant*	☐	☐

Verbs – Higher Tier

			Learned	*Tested*
▷	pluperfect tense	*j'avais acheté, j'étais arrivé(e)*	☐	☐
▷	agreement of past participle with preceding direct object (PDO)	*Je les ai achetées, les montrés.*	☐	☐
▷	*venir de* + infinitive	*je viens d'arriver, je venais d'arriver*	☐	☐
▷	*être en train de* + infinitive	*Je suis en train de manger.*	☐	☐
▷	conditional	*J'aimerais voir tes dessins. Si j'étais plus âgée, je conduirais une belle voiture.*	☐	☐
▷	(R) passive	*Il a été mordu.*	☐	☐
▷	agreement of past participle with *être*	*elles sont arrivées*	☐	☐
▷	(R) present subjunctive of regular *-er*, *-ir* and *-re* verbs and of *avoir, être, aller, faire, pouvoir, savoir, prendre, venir*	*Il faut que je fasse mes devoirs. Il faut qu'ils soient bien faits.*	☐	☐
▷	(R) past historic	*Il regarda Napoléon. Ils se regardèrent.*	☐	☐

Adjectives – Foundation and Higher Tiers

			Learned	Tested
▸	agreement		☐	☐
▸	position		☐	☐
▸	certain masculine adjectives before a vowel	*bel, nouvel, vieil*	☐	☐
▸	possessive adjectives	*mon, ma, mes, etc.*	☐	☐
▸	comparative	*Je suis plus grand que toi.*	☐	☐
▸	superlative	*Je suis la plus belle de toutes.*	☐	☐

Adverbs – Foundation and Higher Tiers

			Learned	Tested
▸	regular formation ending in *-ment, -emment, -ement*		☐	☐
▸	irregular adverbs	*bien, mal*	☐	☐
▸	comparison of adverbs	*Il joue mieux que toi. Il court plus vite que toi.*	☐	☐
▸	superlative of adverbs	*Elle chante le mieux.*	☐	☐

Nouns – Foundation and Higher Tiers

			Learned	Tested
▸	gender	*le* or *la, un* or *une*	☐	☐
▸	number (singular or plural)		☐	☐
▸	plurals, including the irregular ones	*chevaux*	☐	☐

Pronouns – Foundation Tier

			Learned	Tested
▸	subject and object pronouns	*je, me, etc.*	☐	☐
▸	emphatic (also known as stressed or disjunctive) pronouns	*moi, toi, lui, elle, etc.*	☐	☐
▸	position of pronouns		☐	☐
▸	(R) order of pronouns	*Il me l'a donné.*	☐	☐
▸	relative pronouns	*qui* and *que*	☐	☐
▸	(R) relative pronoun	*dont*	☐	☐
▸	indefinite pronouns	*quelque chose, quelqu'un, tout, tous, tout le monde*	☐	☐

Pronouns – Higher Tier

As for Foundation, plus:

			Learned	Tested
⫸	relative pronouns	*lequel, lesquels*	☐	☐

Word order – Foundation Tier

			Learned	Tested
⫸	(R) inversion after direct speech	*'Je mange', a-t-elle dit.*	☐	☐
⫸	(R) inversion after *peut-être*	*Peut-être arrivera-t-il.*	☐	☐
⫸	(R) inversion in certain subordinate clauses	*Le collège où travaille mon cousin.*	☐	☐

Word order – Higher Tier

As for Foundation Tier, but all for productive use.

Numbers and time – Foundation and Higher Tiers

			Learned	Tested
⫸	cardinal numbers	*un, deux, trois, etc.*	☐	☐
⫸	ordinal numbers	*premier, deuxième, troisième, etc.*	☐	☐
⫸	telling the time on 24-hour clock and on 12-hour clock		☐	☐
⫸	dates		☐	☐

Conjunctions

			Learned	Tested
⫸	common conjunctions	*et, parce que*	☐	☐

Prepositions

			Learned	Tested
⫸	common prepositions	*dans, pour, chez*	☐	☐

▶ GRAMMAR REFERENCE

Use the grammar list (above) to find out which grammatical features you are expected to know for either Foundation or Higher Tier, and whether you should know them actively or passively. In practice, the more you know the better, and there is a strong case for ignoring the Examining Groups' rather arbitrary divisons into Foundation and Higher and concentrating on mastering the fundamentals of French grammar outlined below.

The items appear in the same order as on the grammar list.

▷ **Verbs** French verbs are notoriously difficult. Many of the common ones are irregular, i.e. they do not follow a rule. In all of them the spelling changes depending on who is speaking, but the pronunciation does not always change to match. If you can master them, you have the key to success. So do make every attempt to get to grips with them. Take a few at a time. Make a point of checking the spelling, including the accents.

Present tense

There is only one form of the present tense for each French verb. In English there are three: 'I eat', 'I am eating' and 'I do eat'. The French form *je mange* is used as an equivalent for all three. (You will probably have noticed that French speakers often mix up the English forms.)

1 **Use of the present tense**   The present tense is used
   ▷ to describe events that happen regularly, for example:
      Je mange beaucoup de bonbons.   *I eat a lot of sweets.*
   ▷ to describe what is happening now, for example:
      Je lis un excellent livre.   *I am reading an excellent book.*
   ▷ after *depuis* (see below).

2 **Formation of the present tense**   Regular verbs are identified by the last two letters of their infinitive: *-er*, *-ir*, and *-re*. They form the present tense in different ways. You will also need to learn the formation of irregular verbs carefully.

Regular -er verbs
Regular *-er* verbs in French follow this pattern:

parler   *to talk or speak*

je parle	*I speak / I am speaking*
tu parles	*you speak / you are speaking*
il parle	*he speaks / he is speaking*
elle parle	*she speaks / she is speaking*
on parle	*we speak / we are speaking (one speaks, etc.)*
nous parlons	*we speak / we are speaking*
vous parlez	*you speak / you are speaking*
ils parlent	*they speak / they are speaking*
elles parlent	*they speak / they are speaking.*

The endings for *-er* verbs are:
je	**-e**
tu	**-es**
il/elle/on	**-e**
nous	**-ons**
vous	**-ez**
ils/elles	**-ent**

These endings are added to the **stem** of the verb, *parl-*, that is the infinitive *parler* minus its *-er* ending.

Other common regular *-er* verbs include:

aider	aimer	arriver*	casser	chercher
compter	danser	déjeuner	désirer	dessiner
détester	donner	durer	écouter	entrer*
fumer	gagner	inviter	jouer	laver

louer	marcher	monter*	montrer	oublier
penser	pleurer	porter	poser	pousser
quitter	préparer	regarder	rencontrer	rentrer*
réserver	réparer	rester*	retourner*	rouler
sauter	sonner	tomber*	toucher	tourner
trouver	travailler	traverser	visiter	voler
voyager				

Note: verbs marked * take *être* in the perfect tense.

This list is by no means exhaustive. Add new verbs to it as you come across them.

Irregular -er verbs
The most irregular *-er* verb is *aller* (to go):
je vais
tu vas
il va
elle va
on va

nous allons
vous allez
ils vont
elles vont

A number of common *-er* verbs have very slight irregularities. Their endings are **not**, however, irregular, as the examples below show.

(a)   *Manger* and other verbs ending *-ger* have irregular *nous* forms for phonetic reasons (to make the *g* soft by following it with an *e*). These verbs follow this pattern:

manger   *to eat*
je mange
tu manges
il mange
elle mange
on mange

nous mangeons
vous mangez
ils mangent
elles mangent

Other verbs in this category include: *changer, échanger, loger, nager, obliger, partager* and *ranger*.

(b)   *Commencer* and other verbs ending in *-cer* have irregular *nous* forms for phonetic reasons (to make the final *c* soft by giving it a cedilla (*ç*)). These verbs follow this pattern:

commencer   *to begin*
je commence
tu commences
il commence
elle commence
on commence

nous commençons
vous commencez
ils commencent
elles commencent

Other verbs in this category include: *avancer, lancer, menacer, prononcer* and *remplacer*.

(c) Verbs ending in *-eler* and *-eter* double the *-l* or the *-t* in some persons of the verb.

s'appeler *to be called*	**jeter** *to throw*
je m'appelle	je jette
tu t'appelles	tu jettes
il s'appelle	il jette
elle s'appelle	elle jette
on s'appelle	on jette
nous nous appelons	nous jetons
vous vous appelez	vous jetez
ils s'appellent	ils jettent
elles s'appellent	elles jettent

Other verbs in this category include: *appeler*. NB *acheter* and *geler* follow the same pattern as *lever* (see *(d)* below).

(d) Verbs ending in *-e* + consonant + *-er* follow this pattern:

lever to lift

je lève
tu lèves
il lève
elle lève
on lève

nous levons
vous levez
ils lèvent
elles lèvent

Other verbs in this category include: *acheter*, *geler*, *mener*, *peser* and *se promener*.

(e) Verbs ending in *-é-er* follow this pattern:

considérer *to consider*

je considère
tu considères
il considère
elle considère
on considère

nous considérons
vous considérez
ils considèrent
elles considèrent

Other verbs in this category include: *espérer*, *s'inquiéter*, *répéter*, *révéler* and *préférer*.

(f) Verbs ending in *-yer* follow this pattern. (The *y* becomes an *i* if it is followed by an *e*).

nettoyer *to clean*

je nettoie
tu nettoies
il nettoie
elle nettoie
on nettoie

nous nettoyons
vous nettoyez
ils nettoient
elles nettoient

Other verbs in this category include: *appuyer*, *employer*, *ennuyer*, *essayer* and *payer*.

Regular -ir verbs

Regular *-ir* verbs in French follow this pattern:

finir *to finish*

je finis	*I finish / I am finishing*
tu finis	*you finish / you are finishing*
il finit	*he finishes / he is finishing*
elle finit	*she finishes / she is finishing*
on finit	*we finish / we are finishing (one finishes, etc.)*
nous finissons	*we finish / we are finishing*
vous finissez	*you finish / you are finishing*
ils finissent	*they finish / they are finishing*
elles finissent	*they finish / they are finishing*

The endings for *-ir* verbs are:

je	**-is**
tu	**-is**
il/elle/on	**-it**
nous	**-issons**
vous	**-issez**
ils/elles	**-issent**

These endings are added to the **stem** of the verb, *fin-*, that is the infinitive *finir* minus its *-ir* ending.

Other common regular *-ir* verbs include:

applaudir	atterir	bâtir	choisir	démolir
remplir	se sentir*			

Note: verbs marked* take *être* in the perfect tense.

This list is by no means exhaustive. Add new verbs to it as you come across them.

Irregular -ir verbs

Irregular *-ir* verbs include a group which have a present tense just like an *-er* verb. They follow this pattern:

ouvrir *to open*

j'ouvre
tu ouvres
il ouvre
elle ouvre
on ouvre

nous ouvrons
vous ouvrez
ils ouvrent
elles ouvrent

Other verbs in this category include: *couvrir, découvrir, offrir* and *souffrir*. Check the verb table for other tenses of these verbs.

There are many other irregular *-ir* verbs. The following are also included in the verb table:

contenir	convenir	courir	devenir*	dormir
s'endormir	entretenir	mourir*	obtenir	partir*
prévenir	repartir	retenir	revenir*	se sentir*
servir	sortir*	tenir	venir*	

Note: verbs marked * take *être* in the perfect tense.

Regular -re verbs

Regular *-re* verbs in French follow this pattern:

vendre   *to sell*

je vends	*I sell / I am selling*
tu vends	*you sell / you are selling*
il vend	*he sells / he is selling*
elle vend	*she sells / she is selling*
on vend	*we sell / we are selling (one sells, etc.)*
nous vendons	*we sell / we are selling*
vous vendez	*you sell / you are selling*
ils vendent	*they sell / they are selling*
elles vendent	*they sell / they are selling*

The endings for *-re* verbs are:

je	**-s**
tu	**-s**
il/elle/on	**-**
nous	**-ons**
vous	**-ez**
ils/elles	**-ent**

These endings are added to the stem of the verb, *vend-*, that is the infinitive *vendre* minus its *-re* ending.

Other common regular *-re* verbs include:

attendre	entendre	perdre	rendre	répondre

This list is by no means exhaustive. Add new verbs to it as you come across them.

Irregular -re verbs

Irregular *-re* verbs are numerous. The following are included in the verb table:

apprendre	battre	boire	comprendre	conduire
connaître	construire	coudre	craindre	croire
descendre*	détruire	dire	disparaître	écrire
entendre	éteindre	être*	faire	lire
mettre	naitre*	paraître	prendre	reconnaître
reprendre	rire	suivre	surprendre	vivre

Note: verbs marked * take *être* in the perfect tense.

-oir verbs

There is a group of verbs ending in *-oir* which are all irregular. The following are included in the verb table:

s'asseoir*	avoir	devoir	falloir	pleuvoir
pouvoir	recevoir	savoir	voir	vouloir

Note: verbs marked * take *être* in the perfect tense.

Common errors with the present tense

- Spelling, especially with *-er* verbs with accents.
- Failing to use any ending at all, for example:
  je regarder (**correct version:** je regarde).
- Using the wrong ending, for example:
  il vends (**correct version:** il vend).
- Trying to translate 'I am drinking' literally, for example:
  je suis boire (**correct version:** je bois).

Students who do this haven't appreciated that there is only one form of the present tense for each verb in French.

▶   Getting confused between present and perfect, for example:
     Je allé au college tous les jours. (**correct version:** Je vais au collège tous les jours.).

Perfect tense (also known as the passé composé)

In French, the perfect tense is used to express the English 'have done' and 'did'.
So *j'ai mangé une pomme* could mean any of the following: I ate an apple; I have eaten an apple; I did eat an apple.

(You will probably have noticed that French speakers often mix up the English forms.)

1 **Use of the perfect tense**   The perfect tense is used in conversation and letters:

▶   to describe an action in the past which is completed and is no longer happening
▶   to describe an action in the past which happened once only.

2 **Formation of the perfect tense**   The perfect tense is made up of two parts, the auxiliary verb, which is the present tense of either *avoir* or *être*, and the past participle. Most verbs have *avoir* as their auxiliary.

Perfect tense with avoir – regular verbs

The past participles of regular verbs (including those -er verbs with minor changes in spelling in the present tense) are formed by removing *-er*, *-ir* or *-re* from the infinitive, and adding *-é*, *-i,* or *-u*. For example:

parler   →   parlé
finir   →   fini
vendre   →   vendu

The past participles are then combined with the auxiliary, the present tense of *avoir*, as follows:

j'ai parlé	j'ai fini	j'ai vendu
tu as parlé	tu as fini	tu as vendu
il a parlé	il a fini	il a vendu
elle a parlé	elle a fini	elle a vendu
on a parlé	on a fini	on a vendu
nous avons parlé	nous avons fini	nous avons vendu
vous avez parlé	vous avez fini	vous avez vendu
ils ont parlé	ils ont fini	ils ont vendu
elles ont parlé	elles ont fini	elles ont vendu

Perfect tense with avoir – irregular verbs

Many common verbs are irregular. The formation of the perfect tense follows the same principle as for regular verbs, that there is an auxiliary – the present tense of *avoir* – and the past participle, as shown in the example below (*lire*). The only problem is that the past participles have to be learned, as irregular verbs naturally don't obey set rules.

lire   past participle **lu**
j'ai lu
tu as lu
il a lu
elle a lu
on a lu

nous avons lu
vous avez lu
ils ont lu
elles ont lu

Here are 25 of the most commonly used verbs with their past participles. These and other irregular verbs can be checked in the verb table. If you don't know them already, make it a top priority to master them.

infinitive	past participle	infinitive	past participle
avoir	eu	mettre	mis
boire	bu	ouvrir	ouvert
comprendre	compris	pleuvoir	plu
conduire	conduit	pouvoir	pu
connaître	connu	prendre	pris
courir	couru	recevoir	reçu
croire	cru	rire	ri
devoir	dû	savoir	su
dire	dit	tenir	tenu
écrire	écrit	vivre	vécu
être	été	voir	vu
faire	fait	vouloir	voulu
lire	lu		

Perfect tense with être – reflexive verbs

All reflexive verbs have the present tense of *être* as their auxiliary. Their past participles may be either regular or irregular – check the verb table. The past participle agrees (like an adjective) with the subject, as shown in the following example.

se laver   *to wash oneself*
je me suis lavé(e)
tu t'es lavé(e)
il s'est lavé
elle s'est lavée
on s'est lavé(e)(s)

nous nous sommes lavé(e)s
vous vous êtes lavé(e)(s)
ils se sont lavés
elles se sont lavées

If the *(e)* is in brackets, it is only added if the subject is feminine. If the *(s)* is in brackets, it is only added if the subject is plural.

Where an irregular past participle ends in *-s*, (e.g. *assis*), no further *s* is required for the masculine plural agreement, for example:

Les garçons se sont assis.   *The boys sat down.*

Perfect tense with être – 16 verbs

Sixteen common verbs which are not reflexive also form the perfect tense with *être* as the auxiliary. Most of them can be remembered in 6 pairs which are (or are nearly) opposite in meaning. Make it a top priority to master them.

infinitive	past participle	infinitive	past participle
aller	allé	monter	monté
venir	venu	descendre	descendu
arriver	arrivé	rester	resté
partir	parti	tomber	tombé
entrer	entré	naître	né
sortir	sorti	mourir	mort

The others are:

infinitive	past participle	infinitive	past participle
retourner	retourné	devenir	devenu
revenir	revenu	rentrer	rentré

As with reflexive verbs, the past participles of these verbs have to agree with the subject, as shown in the following example.

retourner   *to return, go back*
je suis retourné(e)
tu es retourné(e)
il est retourné
elle est retournée
on est retourné(e)(s)

nous sommes retourné(e)s
vous êtes retourné(e)(s)
ils sont retournés
elles sont retournées

If the *(e)* is in brackets, it is only added if the subject is feminine. If the *(s)* is in brackets, it is only added if the subject is plural.

Common errors with the perfect tense

▶ Incorrect form of past participle, usually caused by not knowing which verbs are irregular. A big help is knowing that all -*er* verbs except *aller* are regular and no -*oir* verbs are regular.

▶ Using a verb form which sounds the same, but isn't perfect at all, for example:
    j'ai regarder (**correct version:** j'ai regardé)
    or: j'ai regardez (**correct version:** j'ai regardé).

▶ Using the wrong auxiliary verb, for example:
    il a venu (**correct version:** il est venu).

▶ Getting confused between imperfect, and perfect, for example:
    Il a traversé la rue quand une voiture le tuait.
    He was crossing the road when a car killed him.
    Correct version: Il traversait la rue quand une voiture l'a tué.

▶ Failing to make the past participles of verbs which take *être* agree with the subject. This is particularly common with feminine and/or plural subjects, for example:
    Elles sont allé à Paris.   *They went to Paris.*
    Correct version: Elles sont allées à Paris.

Imperfect tense

The imperfect tense refers to events in the past. It is usually found in combination with the perfect tense.

1   **Use of the imperfect tense:**   The imperfect tense in French is used:

▶ to set the scene in the past (to say what was happening when something else happened), for example:
    Il traversait la rue quand une voiture l'a tué.
    He was crossing the road (imperfect tense) when a car killed him (perfect tense).

▶ for description in the past, for example:
    Il faisait beau. Le soleil brillait. Jeanne était contente.

▶ *The weather was good. The sun was shining. Jeanne was happy.*

▶ for something that happened frequently in the past, or used to happen, for example:
    Quand j'habitais à Londres, j'allais acheter mes cadeaux chez Harrods.
    When I lived in London I used to buy my presents at Harrods.

▶ in reported speech (also known as indirect speech) to report the present tense, for example:
    What the person actually said: 'Je viens d'Angleterre.'
    'I come from England.' (present tense).

▶ Reported speech: Il a dit qu'il venait d'Angleterre.
    (He said (perfect tense) he came (imperfect tense) from England.)

See also pluperfect tense – reported speech (p. 200).

2 **Formation of the imperfect tense**   Most verbs form the imperfect tense in a similar way, the exception is *être*. However, you will need to note the differences with formation of *manger*, *changer*, etc. and *commencer*, *avancer*, etc.

Most verbs
Nearly all verbs, *-er*, *-ir*, *-re* and *-oir*, form the imperfect tense in the following way:

First find the *nous* form of the present tense.
Then remove the *-ons* to leave the imperfect stem.
Finally add the imperfect endings listed below and shown in the example (*faire*).

je	-ais
tu	-ais
il	-ait
elle	-ait
on	-ait
nous	-ions
vous	-iez
ils	-aient
elles	-aient

faire   *to make, to do*

Nous form of present tense:	faisons
Imperfect stem (*faisons* minus *-ons*):	fais-
Imperfect tense:	je faisais
	tu faisais
	il faisait
	elle faisait
	on faisait
	nous faisions
	vous faisiez
	ils faisaient
	elles faisaient

The verb être
There is one irregular verb in the imperfect tense, *être*.
j'étais
tu étais
il était
elle était
on était

nous étions
vous étiez
ils étaient
elles étaient

If you look carefully, you will see that it is only the imperfect stem, *ét-*, which is irregular. The endings are what you would expect.

Manger, changer, etc.
The *-er* verbs which have an extra *e* inserted into the *nous* form to soften a *g* don't need the extra *e* in the *nous* and *vous* forms in the imperfect because the *g* is softened by the *i* in the endings *-ions* and *-iez*. These verbs follow this pattern:

je mangeais
tu mangeais
il mangeait
elle mangeait
on mangeait

nous mangions
vous mangiez
ils mangeaient
elles mangeaient

Other verbs in this category include: *changer, échanger, loger, nager, obliger, partager* and *ranger*.

Commencer, avancer, etc.

The *-er* verbs which have a cedilla inserted into the *nous* form to soften a *c* don't need one in the *nous* and *vous* forms in the imperfect because the *c* is softened by the *i* in the endings *-ions* and *-iez*. These verbs follow this pattern:

je commençais
tu commençais
il commençait
elle commençait
on commençait

nous commencions
vous commenciez
ils commençaient
elles commençaient

Other verbs in this category include: *avancer, lancer, menacer, prononcer* and *remplacer*.

Common errors with the imperfect tense

▷ Spelling, especially of the *-er* verbs which have either the extra *e* or the cedilla, for example:
   je nagais (**correct version:** je nageais).
▷ Using an ending which sounds the same, but isn't imperfect at all, for example:
   je regarder (**correct version:** je regardais)
   or: je regardé (**correct version:** je regardais).
▷ Using the wrong ending, for example:
   il vendais (**correct version:** il vendait).
▷ Getting confused between imperfect and perfect, for example:
   Il a traversé la rue quand une voiture l'a tué.
   He was crossing the road when a car killed him.
   Correct version: Il traversait la rue quand une voiture l'a tué.
▷ Translating 'would' meaning 'used to' with the French conditional when in fact the imperfect is correct, for example:
   Il viendrait chaque été à Paris.   *He would come to Paris each summer.*
   Correct version: Il venait chaque été à Paris.

Future using aller + infinitive

This is the simplest way of talking about events in the future, and is similar to the English 'I am going to...'.

1 **Use of the future with *aller* + infinitive**   This is used to talk about events in the immediate future, for example:
   Je vais regarder la télévision ce soir.   *I am going to watch TV tonight.*

2   **Formation of the future with *aller* + infinitive**   Take the present tense of *aller*. Add the infinitive of any verb, regular or irregular, as shown in the following example.

je vais acheter
tu vas acheter
il va acheter
elle va acheter
on va acheter

nous allons acheter
vous allez acheter
ils vont acheter
elles vont acheter

Common error with aller + *infinitive*

▶   Using the wrong part of *aller*, for example:
     Vous aller acheter une pomme. **Correct version:** Vous allez acheter une pomme.

Future tense

1   **Use of the future tense**
The future tense is used:

▶   to express firm intention, for example:
     Je regarderai la télé ce soir.   *I shall watch TV this evening.*
▶   to refer to events further ahead than the short term, for example:
     Dans cinq ans j'aurai 21 ans.   *I shall be 21 in five years' time.*

2   **Formation of the future tense**   Regular and irregular verbs form the future tense by adding common endings to a future stem. You will need to learn the future stems for irregular verbs.

Regular -er and -ir verbs
Add the following endings to the infinitive, as shown in the examples below (*parler* and *finir*).

je   **-ai**
tu   **-as**
il   **-a**
elle   **-a**
on   **-a**

nous   **-ons**
vous   **-ez**
ils   **-ont**
elles   **-ont**

parler *to speak*	**finir** *to finish*
je parlerai	je finirai
tu parleras	tu finiras
il parlera	il finira
elle parlera	elle finira
on parlera	on finira
nous parlerons	nous finirons
vous parlerez	vous finirez
ils parleront	ils finiront
elles parleront	elles finiront

Regular -re verbs

Remove the final *-e* from the infinitive. Add the same endings as for all other verbs. For example:

vendre *to sell*
je vendrai
tu vendras
il vendra
elle vendra
on vendra

nous vendrons
vous vendrez
ils vendront
elles vendront

Irregular verbs

Irregular verbs have the same future endings as all other verbs. However, the future stem needs to be learned. Listed below are the future tenses of 21 of the most common irregular verbs. Note that this list contains some *-er* verbs which are not irregular in other parts.

infinitive	future tense	infinitive	future tense
acheter	j'achèterai	jeter	je jetterai
aller	j'irai	mourir	je mourrai
appeler	j'appellerai	pleuvoir	il pleuvra
s'asseoir	je m'assiérai	pouvoir	je pourrai
avoir	j'aurai	recevoir	je recevrai
courir	je courrai	répéter	je répéterai
devoir	je devrai	savoir	je saurai
envoyer	j'ennverrai	tenir	je tiendrai
être	je serai	venir	je viendrai
faire	je ferai	voir	je verrai
falloir	il faudra		

The future in French but not in English

The future must be used in French to refer to events in the future. This is not immediately obvious to an English speaker, and needs to be watched out for. For example:

Quand elle viendra, je lui donnerai ta lettre.
When she comes (present in English, future in French) I'll give her your letter.
Elle viendra quand l'émission sera finie.
She will come when the programme is over (present in English, future in French).

Common errors with the future tense

▷ Using the wrong endings, for example:
  Je serer là. **Correct version:** Je serai là.
▷ Confusion with the conditional, which sounds similar, for example:
  Je serais là. **Correct version:** Je serai là.

Reflexive verbs

These verbs have *se* or *s'* in front of the infinitive when you look them up.

1 **Use of reflexive verbs**

▷ They are part of the normal vocabulary of French. They can be used in the same way as any normal verb. There are many more in French than there are in English, and some of the meanings are, at first, confusing.
▷ They are often used when referring to a part of the body, for example:
  Je me suis coupé le doigt. *I have cut my finger.*
  Elle se lave les dents. *She is cleaning her teeth.*

2 **Formation of reflexive verbs**   Add the reflexive pronoun between the subject and the verb. This applies in all tenses. If in doubt, check the verb table at the back of this book.

se laver   *to get washed*
je **me** lave
tu **te** laves
il **se** lave
elle **se** lave
on **se** lave

nous **nous** lavons
vous **vous** lavez
ils **se** lavent
elles **se** lavent

Where the reflexive verb is used as an infinitive, the reflexive pronoun agrees with the subject of the verb, for example:
   Je suis obligé(e) de **me** coucher à neuf heures.
   Nous sommes obligés de **nous** coucher à neuf heures.
   Elle est obligée de **se** coucher à neuf heures.

In the perfect and pluperfect tenses:

▶ all reflexive verbs have *être* as the auxiliary verb
▶ the past participles of reflexive verbs agree with the subject, as shown in the following example.

se laver   *to get washed*
je me suis lavé(e)
tu t'es lavé(e)
il s'est lavé
elle s'est lavée
on s'est lavé(e)(s)

nous nous sommes lavé(e)s
vous vous êtes lavé(e)s
ils se sont lavés
elles se sont lavées

If the (*e*) is in brackets, it is only added if the subject is feminine. If the (*s*) is in brackets, it is only added if the subject is plural.

Where an irregular past participle ends in -*s*, (e.g. *assis*) no further *s* is required for the masculine plural agreement, for example:
Les garçons se sont assis.

Common reflexive verbs

s'amuser *to enjoy oneself*	s'habiller *to get dressed*
s'appeler *to be called*	s'intéresser à *to be interested in*
s'approcher de *to approach*	se laver *to get washed*
s'arrêter *to stop*	se lever *to get up*
se baigner *to bathe*	se mettre à *to begin*
se brosser (les cheveux) *to brush (one's hair)*	se peigner *to comb one's hair*
se coucher *to go to bed*	se promener *to go for a walk*
se débrouiller *to manage, to get on with something*	se raser *to shave*
se dépêcher *to hurry*	se reposer *to rest*
se déshabiller *to undress*	se réveiller *to wake up*
se disputer avec *to have an argument with*	se sauver *to run away*
s'entendre avec *to get on with*	se sentir *to feel*
se fâcher *to get angry*	se taire *to be silent*
se faire mal *to hurt oneself*	se trouver *to be situated*

Verbs not in the above list can be made reflexive to express the idea of 'each other'. They then behave like reflexives in the perfect tense. For example:

Quand est-ce qu'on va se voir?   *When shall we see each other?*

Quand est-ce que nous nous sommes vu(e)s la dernière fois?   *When did we last see each other?*

Common errors with reflexives

▶ Failure to recognise that there is a reflexive verb needed, for example:

Je sens triste.   *I feel sad.*

Correct version: Je me sens triste.

▶ Forgetting to use *être* in the perfect tense, for example:

Nous nous avons lavé ce matin.   *We got washed this morning.*

Correct version: Nous nous sommes lavé(e)s ce matin.

▶ Forgetting to make the past participle agree with the subject, for example:

Elles se sont lavé.   *They got washed.*

Correct version: Elles se sont lavées.

▶ Wrong choice of reflexive pronoun when a reflexive verb is used in the infinitive, for example:

J'ai décidé de se laver.   *I have decided to get washed.*

Correct version: J'ai décidé de me laver.

Question forms

These are sometimes known as **interrogatives**. There are four ways of asking a question in French.

By tone of voice

A rising tone of voice at the end of a statement turns it into a question, for example:

Ton frère habite à Londres?   *Does your brother live in London?*

If you are writing, you obviously can't use tone of voice.

By adding n'est-ce pas?

Add *n'est-ce pas?* to the end of any statement to convert it into a question. It's similar to 'isn't it?', 'doesn't he?', etc. in English. There is only one French form for all the English ones. For example:

Ton frère habite à Londres, n'est-ce pas?   *Your brother lives in London, doesn't he?*

By beginning with Est-ce que

Add *Est-ce que* to the beginning of any statement to convert it into a question, for example:

Est-ce que ton frère habite à Londres?   *Does your brother live in London?*

By inverting (swapping round) the subject and verb

For example:

Habites-tu à Londres?   *Do you live in London?*

If the verb ends in a vowel in the 3rd person singular, you should add an extra *-t-* to make it easier to pronounce, for example:

Votre frère, habite-t-il à Londres?   *Does your brother live in London?*

Question words

Question words can be used in front of *est-ce que*. For example:

Où est-ce que ton frère habite?   *Where does your brother live?*

They can also be used in front of the verb, using the following pattern:

Où habite ton frère?   *Where does your brother live?*

Here is a list of question words:

Combien? *How much?*
Comment? *How? (sometimes: What?)*
Où? *Where?*
D'où? *Where from?*
Lequel... ?* *Which one?*
Pourquoi? *Why?*

Quand? *When?*
Qu'est-ce que... ? *What?*
Quel... ?* *Which? What?*
Qui? *Who?*
Quoi? *Pardon?, What? (only used on its own)*

Note: * *Lequel* and *quel* are adjectives and agree with the noun being asked about, for example:

Quelles chaussettes as-tu perdues? *Which socks have you lost?*

Common errors with questions

▶ Attempting to translate the English 'do' in 'Do you live in London?', for example:
  Fais tu habiter à Londres?
  Correct version: Habites-tu à Londres? **or** Est-ce que tu habites à Londres?

▶ Using the wrong question word. It's best to learn such idiomatic questions as:
  Comment t'appelles-tu? *What's your name?*
  D'où viens-tu? *Where do you come from?*

▶ Replying in the wrong tense. You should mirror the tense of the question you are asked in your reply. For example:
  Question: Quand est-ce que tu as quitté l'Angleterre? *When did you leave England?*
  Answer: Je quitte l'Angleterre hier soir. *I left England yesterday evening.*
  Correct version: J'ai quitté l'Angleterre hier soir.

Command forms

These are also known as **imperatives.** French verbs have three command forms, which are derived from *tu*, *vous* and *nous* forms of the present tense in most cases.

1 **Use of command forms**

The form derived from the *tu* form is used when talking to one person who is
▶ a good friend
▶ a member of the family or a pet
▶ a young person.

The form derived from the *vous* form is used when talking to two or more people who are
▶ good friends
▶ members of the family or pets
▶ young people,
or to one person who is
▶ an adult who doesn't fit any of the categories above.

The form derived from the *nous* form is used to translate 'Let's do something'.

Formation of commands

-ir *and* -re *verbs*

Miss out *tu* or *vous* or *nous* and just use the verb itself. For example:

Finis ce livre! *Finish that book!*
Finissez ce livre! *Finish that book!*
Finissons ce livre! *Let's finish that book!*

Vends ce livre! *Sell that book!*
Vendez ce livre! *Sell that book!*
Vendons ce livre! *Let's sell that book!*

-er verbs
The principle is the same. But miss the -s off the *tu* form. For example:

Parle! *Talk!*
Parlez! *Talk!*
Parlons! *Let's talk!*

Irregular forms
The following verbs have irregular command forms:

avoir	être	savoir	vouloir
aie	sois	sache	veuille
ayez	soyez	sachez	veuillez
ayons	soyons	sachons	veuillons

Aller has a modified form in the phrase *Vas-y* – (*Go to it / On you go.*)

Reflexive verbs
They have the following command forms:

Réveille-toi!
Réveillez-vous!
Réveillons-nous!

Common errors in command forms

▶ Forming the command incorrectly.
▶ Adding reflexive pronouns for verbs which are not reflexive, for example:
   Viens-toi ici! **Correct version:** Viens ici!.
▶ Failing to realise that 'let's' is a command and not using the -*ons* command form at all.

The infinitive

In French there are often two verbs in a sentence, the second of which is in the infinitive form. This is often the case in English, too, for example: 'I prefer to swim.'
   There are four ways in which French uses two verbs in a sentence. Unfortunately you have to learn which way each verb operates.

Verbs followed directly by the infinitive
Some verbs are followed directly by the infinitive, for example:
   J'aime jouer au tennis. *I like playing tennis.*

These verbs include:

adorer *to love*	il faut *you need to*
aimer *to like, to love*	monter *to go upstairs (in order to)*
aller *to go*	penser *to intend to do something*
compter *to intend to*	pouvoir *to be able to (to 'can')*
désirer *to want, to wish*	préférer *to prefer*
détester *to hate*	savoir *to know how to*
devoir *to have to (to 'must')*	venir *to come (in order to)*
entendre *to hear*	voir *to see*
espérer *to hope to*	vouloir *to want to*
faillir *to nearly do something*	

Verbs followed by à + infinitive
Some verbs are followed by *à* and an infinitive. For example:
   Il s'est decidé à acheter une Renault. *He decided to buy a Renault.*

These verbs include:

aider quelqu'un à   *to help someone to*
apprendre à   *to learn to*
commencer à   *to begin to*
consentir à   *to agree to*
continuer à   *to continue to*
se décider à   *to decide to*
demander à   *to ask to*
hésiter à   *to hesitate to*

s'intéresser à   *to be interested in*
inviter quelqu'un à   *to invite someone to*
se mettre à   *to begin to*
obliger quelqu'un à   *to make someone do something*
passer du temps à   *to spend time*
ressembler à   *to look like*
réussir à   *to succeed in*

Verbs followed by de + infinitive

Some verbs are followed by *de* and an infinitive. For example:

Il a cessé de pleuvoir.   *It stopped raining.*

These verbs include:

s'arrêter de   *to stop (doing something)*
cesser de   *to stop (doing something)*
décider de   *to decide to*
se dépêcher de   *to hurry to*
dire de   *to tell to*
essayer de   *to try to*

finir de   *to finish (doing something)*
offrir de   *to offer*
oublier de   *to forget*
permettre de   *to allow to*
refuser de   *to refuse to*
regretter de   *to be sorry to*

Expressions with avoir which are followed by de + infinitive

For example:

J'ai envie de manger.   *I wish to eat.*

These expressions include:

avoir besoin de   *to need to*
avoir le droit de   *to have the right to, to be allowed to*
avoir envie de   *to wish to*
avoir l'intention de   *to intend to*
avoir peur de   *to be afraid of (doing something)*
avoir le temps de   *to have time to*

The preposition *pour* can also be used to introduce an infinitive, for example:

Il est allé au café pour boire une bière.   *He went to the café to drink a beer.*
Il est trop jeune pour boire du vin.   *He is too young to drink wine.*

Similarly, the prepositions *sans, avant de* and *au lieu de* can introduce an infinitive. For example:

Sans hésiter, il est parti.   *Without hesitating, he left.*
Avant d'arriver à la gare il a écrit une lettre.
Before arriving at the station he wrote a letter.
Au lieu de travailler il a joué au flipper.   *Instead of working he played pinball.*

Perfect infinitive

A perfect infinitive is used after *après* to express 'after having done something'. The perfect infinitive is formed by using *avoir* or *être* as appropriate, plus the past participle of the verb in question.

Après être arrivés en France, ils sont allés à Paris.
After arriving in France, they went to Paris.
Après avoir acheté une pomme, elle l'a mangée.   *After buying an apple, she ate it.*
Après s'être rasés, ils se sont habillés.   *After having shaved, they got dressed.*

Common errors with infinitives

▶ Wrong choice of *à* or *de*, for example:
Il a fini à lire son journal. **Correct version:** Il a fini de lire son journal.

▶ Mixing up *se decider à* and *decider de*. The meaning is the same, but you have to be clear about which one you are using. For example:
Je me suis décidé de partir. **Correct version:** Je me suis décidé à partir.

Use of tenses with depuis

Depuis, meaning 'since', or 'for', uses different tenses in French than you might expect.
If the action is still continuing, the **present** tense is used after *depuis*. For example:
J'habite à Londres depuis cinq ans.
I have lived in London for five years. (Implied: ... and I still do.)

If the action lasted for some time, but is now over, the **imperfect** tense is used after **depuis**. For example:
J'habitais à Londres depuis cinq ans quand je me suis décidé à quitter la grande ville.
I had been living in London for five years when I decided to leave the big city.

Common error with depuis

▶ Using the wrong tenses, for example:
J'ai joué du violon depuis cinq ans.   *I have played the violin for five years.*
Correct version: Je joue du violon depuis cinq ans.

Negatives

There are various negatives in French. They have two parts, *ne* and one other, which varies according to meaning.

ne ... pas *not*	ne ... nulle part *nowhere*
ne ... jamais *never*	ne ... plus *no more, no longer*
ne ... rien *nothing*	ne ... que *only*
ne ... personne *nobody*	ne ... ni ... ni ... *neither ... nor ... nor ...*
ne ... aucun* *no, not one*	

Note: **aucun* agrees like an adjective.

Word order and negatives

1 Generally, the negative forms a 'sandwich' round the verb, the *ne* going before the verb and the second part of the negative following it. For example:
Je ne parle pas italien.   *I don't speak Italian.*

2 In the perfect tense, the 'sandwich' is made round the auxiliary verb. For example:
Je ne suis pas sortie ce matin.   *I didn't go out this morning.*
Je n'ai pas vu le journal.   *I haven't seen the newspaper.*

3 With reflexive verbs, the reflexive pronoun is included within the 'sandwich'. For example:
Je ne me lave pas très souvent.   *I don't wash very often.*
Je ne me suis pas lavé très souvent.   *I didn't wash very often.*

4 If there is a pronoun or pronouns before the verb, they are included inside the 'sandwich'. For example:
Je ne les regarde pas.   *I don't look at them.*
Je ne les ai pas regardé(e)s.   *I didn't look at them.*
Je ne les lui ai pas donné(e)s.   *I didn't give them to him.*

Other features of negatives

1 Negatives are usually followed by *de*, in the same way as 'any' follows negatives in English. For example:
Je n'ai pas de fromage.   *I haven't any cheese.*
Je n'ai pas mangé de fromage.   *I haven't eaten any cheese.*

2 *Aucun*, *personne* and *rien* can be used as the subject of a sentence. They still require the *ne*. For example:

Aucune voiture n'est arrivée.   *No car arrived.*

Personne n'a acheté de gâteau.   *Nobody bought any cake.*

Rien n'est arrivé.   *Nothing happened.*

3 *Jamais*, *personne* and *rien* can be used on their own in answer to questions. For example:

Est-ce que tu joues au tennis? Jamais.   *Do you play tennis? Never.*

Qui est là? Personne.   *Who is there? No-one.*

Qu'est-ce que tu as acheté? Rien.   *What did you buy? Nothing.*

4 More than one negative can be combined in the following pairs:
   ▷ *jamais* and *personne*:
      Je ne vois jamais personne.   *I never see anybody.*
   ▷ *jamais* and *rien*:
      Je n'achète jamais rien.   *I never buy anything.*
   ▷ *plus* and *personne*:
      Je ne vois plus personne.   *I never see anybody any more.*
   ▷ *plus* and *rien*:
      Jean ne fait plus rien.   *Jean doesn't do anything any more.*

5 All negatives except *ne ... personne* come before the infinitive. For example:

On m'a demandé de ne plus chanter au club.

I have been asked not to sing at the club any more.

J'ai décidé de ne jamais acheter de cigarettes.   *I've decided never to buy any cigarettes.*

Ne ... personne works like this:

J'ai l'intention de ne voir personne du collège.   *I intend to not see anyone from school.*

Common errors with negatives

▷ Wrong positioning of the two parts of the negative, for example:
   Il n'est venu pas.   *He didn't come.*
   Correct version: Il n'est pas venu.
▷ Missing out the *ne*. This is understandable, as it's often skipped over in speech. On paper, it can't be omitted.
   Il est jamais à l'heure.   *He's never on time.*
   Correct version: Il n'est jamais à l'heure.

Present participle

1 **Present participle + *en*** The construction *en* + present participle has two uses:
   ▷ to describe two actions which happen more or less at the same time, rendering 'while -ing', for example:
      Je me suis cassé la jambe en jouant au hockey.   *I broke my leg (while) playing hockey.*
   ▷ to explain how something can be done, rendering 'by -ing', for example:
      En lisant ce livre, vous réussirez à votre examen.   *By reading this book you will pass your exam.*

The present participle can only be used when the subject of both verbs is the same. Where it differs, use *pendant que* + the imperfect tense.

2 **Formation of the present participle** For most verbs, take the *nous* form of the present tense, remove *-ons*, and add *-ant*.

Examples

parlons → parlant

finissons → finissant

vendons → vendant

There are three exceptions:

avoir → ayant
être → étant
savoir → sachant

Common errors with en + present participle

▶   Trying to use the construction when there is a change of subject, for example:
        Example: Anne-Marie a chanté, Alain en jouant du piano.
        Anne-Marie sang while Alain played the piano.
        Correct version: Anne-Marie a chanté pendant qu'Alain jouait du piano.
▶   Ignorance of the irregular forms, which are very common.

From this point on, verb items are only required for Higher Tier.
Check in the grammar list (see p. 177) which are for active, and which for receptive, use.

Pluperfect tense

1   **Use of the pluperfect tense**   The pluperfect tense is used:
    ▶   to talk about events in the past which had occurred before other events took place
    ▶   in reported (indirect) speech to report things which were originally said in the perfect or imperfect tense.

2   **Formation of the pluperfect tense**   The pluperfect tense is formed in the same way as the **perfect tense**, except that the imperfect tense of the auxiliary verb (*avoir* or *être*) is used, as shown in the examples. The same rules about the agreement of past participles apply.

Examples

j'avais parlé	j'étais venu(e)	je m'étais lavé(e)
tu avais parlé	tu étais venu(e)	tu t'étais lavé(e)
il avait parlé	il était venu	il s'était lavé
elle avait parlé	elle était venue	elle s'était lavée
on avait parlé	on était venu(e)(s)	on s'était lavé(e)(s)
nous avions parlé	nous étions venu(e)s	nous nous étions lavé(e)s
vous aviez parlé	vous étiez venu(e)(s)	vous vous étiez lavé(e)(s)
ils avaient parlé	ils étaient venus	ils s'étaient lavés
elles avaient parlé	elles étaient venues	elles s'étaient lavées

If the *(e)* is in brackets, it is only added if the subject is feminine. If the *(s)* is in brackets, it is only added if the subject is plural.

Where an irregular past participle ends in *-s*, (e.g. *assis*) no further s is required for the masculine plural agreement, for example:
    Les garçons se sont assis.

Talking about past events which preceded others
    Avant d'arriver en Amérique, il avait vendu son magasin.   *Before arriving in America, he had sold his shop.*

Using the pluperfect in reported speech
If the original speaker used the imperfect or perfect tenses, the report of that speech is made in the pluperfect. For example:
    What the person actually said: 'Il faisait beau ce jour-là.'
    'It was (imperfect tense) nice that day.'

Reported speech: Il a dit qu'il avait fait beau ce jour-là.
He said (perfect tense) it had been nice that day (pluperfect tense).
What the person actually said: 'J'ai acheté une pomme.'
'I bought (perfect tense) an apple.'
Reported speech: Il a dit qu'il avait acheté une pomme.
He said (perfect tense) he had bought (pluperfect tense) an apple.

Common errors with the pluperfect tense

▷ Incorrect form of past participle, usually caused by not knowing which verbs are irregular. A big help is knowing that all -*er* verbs except *aller* are regular.
▷ Using the wrong auxiliary verb, for example:
Il avait venu. **Correct version:** Il était venu.
▷ Failing to make the past participles of verbs which take *être* agree with the subject. This is particularly common with feminine and/or plural subjects, For example:
Elles étaient allé à Paris.   They had gone to Paris.
Correct version: Elles étaient allées à Paris.

Agreement of past participle with preceding direct object (PDO)

Verbs which have *avoir* in the perfect tense do not agree with the subject. (Unlike verbs using *être* as an auxiliary, which do!) However, where the direct object comes before (precedes) the verb, the past participle of any verb using *avoir* as an auxiliary **does** agree. For example:
J'ai acheté une banane.
Comment: no agreement, as no PDO – the direct object comes after the verb.

But:
Voici une banane – je l'ai achetée.
Comment: *l'* is the direct object, the pronoun for *une banane*. It comes before the verb, so the past participle agrees.

Also:
Voici les bananes que j'ai achetées.
Comment: *les bananes* are the direct object and come before the verb, so the past participle has to agree.

Common error with PDO

▷ Failing to notice it and not making the agreement!

Venir de + *infinitive*

This construction renders 'just'. The present tense of *venir* + *de* + infinitive is used to mean 'I/you (etc.) **have just** ...-ed'. For example:
Vous venez d'arriver à l'aéroport de Toulouse.   *You have just arrived at Toulouse airport.*
Il vient de partir.   *He has just left.*

Similarly, the imperfect tense of *venir* + *de* + infinitive is used to mean 'I/you (etc.) **had just** ...-ed'. For example:

Vous veniez d'arriver à l'aéroport de Toulouse.   *You had just arrived at Toulouse airport.*
Il venait de partir.   *He had just left.*

Être en train de + *infinitive*

This construction renders the English continuous present and continuous past. For example:
Je suis en train de manger.   *I am (in the act of) eating.*
Vous êtes en train de partir?   *Are you (in the act of) leaving?*
J'étais en train de manger.   *I was (in the act of) eating.*
Vous étiez en train de partir?   *Were you (in the act of) leaving?*

Conditional

Some forms of the conditional such as *je voudrais* will be well known to all learners of French.

1   **Use of the conditional**   The conditional is used:
▶ as a politer alternative to the present tense when making requests, for example:
   Je voudrais une bière, s'il vous plaît.   *I would like a beer, please.*
   Contrast: Je veux une bière.   *I want a beer.*
▶ as a way of expressing what you would do if something else happened, of expressing conditions, for example:
   Si j'étais (*imperfect*) très riche, je ne travaillerais (*conditional*) plus.   *If I was very rich, I would not work any more.*

2   **Formation of the conditional**   The conditional is formed in the same way for *all* verbs. Take the future stem of the verb and add the imperfect endings.
Check the section on the future tense if you are unsure about the future stem. I have contrasted the future and the conditional of the same verb – *avoir* – below.

Examples

future tense	conditional
j'aurai	j'aurais
tu auras	tu aurais
il aura	il aurait
elle aura	elle aurait
on aura	on aurait
nous aurons	nous aurions
vous aurez	vous auriez
ils auront	ils auraient
elles auront	elles auraient.

Use of tenses after si

The tenses used after *si* are as follows:

1   *Si* + present tense is followed by the future tense. This is the same as English. For example:
   S'il fait beau, j'irai au parc zoologique.   *If the weather's good, I'll go to the zoo.*

2   *Si* + imperfect tense is followed by the conditional. This is similar to English, too. For example:
   S'il faisait beau, j'irais au parc zoologique.   *If the weather was good, I would go to the zoo.*

The passive

The passive is used in sentences where the subject of the sentence suffers the action of the verb. The French passive is formed by using any tense of *être* + the past participle. The past participle agrees with the subject. For example:
   Elle a été piquée par un moustique.   *She was bitten by a mosquito.*
   Cette usine a été construite l'année dernière.   *This factory was built last year.*

Generally, the passive is avoided by:

▶ 'turning the sentence round', for example:
   Un moustique l'a piquée.
▶ using *on* as the subject, for example:
   On a construit cette usine l'année dernière.

English students are strongly recommended not to use the passive – they often get it wrong! (It has been given here for recognition purposes only.)

Present subjunctive

At GCSE level, students will only be required to recognise the subjunctive.

1   **Use of the subjunctive**   At GCSE, the following uses may be found in Reading and Listening passages:

▷   After *il faut que*
   For example:
      Il faut que je vienne.   *I have to come.*

▷   After certain verbs + *que*
   These verbs + *que* are followed by the subjunctive:

   désirer que
   préférer que
   regretter que
   vouloir que
   il est possible que

   Examples:
      Tu veux que je fasse la vaisselle?   *Do you want me to do the washing up?*
      Je préfère que tu y ailles en autobus.   *I prefer you to go there by bus.*
      Je regrette que ma fille ne soit pas plus forte en anglais.
      I'm sorry my daughter isn't better at English.
      Il est possible qu'ils puissent venir.   *It's possible they are able to come.*

The present subjunctive is formed from the *ils* form of the present tense. Remove the *-ent* and add *-e* to gain the *je* form of the subjunctive.

Examples

parler → ils parlent → je parle
finir → ils finissent → je finisse
vendre → ils vendent → je vende

The endings for the present subjunctive are as below and as in the example (*finir*).

je	-e	je finisse	
tu	-es	tu finisses	
il	-e	il finisse	
elle	-e	elle finisse	
on	-e	on finisse	
nous	-ions	nous finissions	
vous	-iez	vous finissiez	
ils	-ent	ils finissent	
elles	-ent	elles finissent	

Irregular forms of the subjunctive
The following common verbs have irregular forms:

aller	j'aille, nous allions, ils aillent
avoir	j'aie, il ait, nous ayons, ils aient
être	je sois, il soit, nous soyons, ils soient
faire	je fasse (*follows regular pattern*)
pouvoir	je puisse (*follows regular pattern*)
savoir	je sache (*follows regular pattern*)
vouloir	je veuille, nous voulions, ils veuillent

Past historic

This tense is also known as the **passé simple**. At GCSE level, students will only be required to recognise the past historic in Reading tests.

1 **Use of the past historic**   It is an alternative to the perfect tense which is only used in formal written French:

 ▶ in newspaper articles
 ▶ in stories
 ▶ in novels
 ▶ in history books.

 It is **not** used in conversation or in letters.

The most common form of the past historic is the third person, i.e. *il, elle, on, ils* and *elles*.

2 **Formation of the past historic**   For regular verbs remove *-er, -ir* or *-re* from the infinitive and add the endings appropriate to the verb type (whether *-er, -ir* or *-re* verb). You should also be familiar with the irregular verbs.

-er *verbs*

Remove the *-er* from the infinitive, and add the following endings, as shown in the example:

je	-ai	je parlai
tu	-as	tu parlas
il	-a	il parla
elle	-a	elle parla
on	-a	on parla
nous	-âmes	nous parlâmes
vous	-âtes	vous parlâtes
ils	-èrent	ils parlèrent
elles	-èrent	elles parlèrent

-ir *verbs*

Remove the *-ir* from the infinitive and add the following endings, as shown in the example:

je	-is	je finis
tu	-is	tu finis
il	-it	il finit
elle	-it	elle finit
on	-it	on finit
nous	-îmes	nous finîmes
vous	-îtes	vous finîtes
ils	-irent	ils finirent
elles	-irent	elles finirent

-re *verbs*

Remove the *-re* from the infinitive and add the following endings, as shown in the example:

je	-is	je vendis
tu	-is	tu vendis
il	-it	il vendit
elle	-it	elle vendit
on	-it	on vendit
nous	-îmes	nous vendîmes
vous	-ites	vous vendîtes
ils	-irent	ils vendirent
elles	-irent	elles vendirent

Irregular verbs

Irregular verbs follow two main patterns, and there are some exceptions. There is often a similarity with the past participle, which should help you to spot and understand them.

1   The following group have the same endings as regular *-ir* and *-re* verbs. But the first part of the verb is different from the infinitive:

infinitive	past historic	example – voir
s'asseoir	il s'assit	je vis
comprendre	il comprit	tu vis
conduire	il conduisit	il vit
dire	il dit	elle vit
écrire	il écrit	on vit
faire	il fit	
mettre	il mit	nous vîmes
naître	il naquit	vous vîtes
prendre	il prit	ils virent
rire	il rit	elles virent
voir	il vit	

2   The second group of verbs, most of which have a past participle ending in *-u*, take the following endings:

je	**-us**
tu	**-us**
il	**-ut**
elle	**-ut**
on	**-ut**
nous	**-ûmes**
vous	**-ûtes**
ils	**-urent**
elles	**-urent**

infinitive	past historic	example – être
avoir	il eut	je fus
boire	il but	tu fus
connaître	il connut	il fut
courir	il courut	elle fut
croire	il crut	on fut
devoir	il dut	
être	il fut	nous fûmes
falloir	il fallut	vous fûtes
lire	il lut	ils furent
mourir	il mourut	elles furent
pouvoir	il put	
recevoir	il reçut	
savoir	il sut	
vivre	il vécut	
vouloir	il voulut	

3   There are some exceptions.

Venir and its compounds *convenir*, *devenir* and *revenir*, and *tenir* and its compounds *contenir*, *obtenir* and *retenir* follow this pattern:

je revins
tu revins
il revint
elle revint
on revint

nous revînmes
vous revîntes
ils revinrent
elles revinrent

▶ **Adjectives**   *Agreement of adjectives*

Adjectives change their spelling to agree with the noun they describe. They often have a different spelling for masculine and feminine, and always for the plural. The changes may or may not be heard in speech, but they are always made in writing. Some GCSE Examining Groups have Higher Writing mark schemes which particularly reward good use of adjective agreements.

Patterns of adjective agreement
French adjectives have different patterns for showing agreement.

1   Many adjectives follow this pattern:

masculine singular	feminine singular	masculine plural	feminine plural
noir	noire	noirs	noires

Others which follow this pattern include: *anglais, grand, fort, français, intelligent, intéressant, petit* and *vert*. There are many more. Add them to this list as you come across them.

2   Adjectives which already end in *-e* (without an accent!) have no different feminine form. They are actually following the same logic as in 1 above.

masculine singular	feminine singular	masculine plural	feminine plural
jeune	jeune	jeunes	jeunes

Others which follow this pattern include: *bête, célèbre, jaune, mince, orange, propre, rouge* and *stupide*. There are many more. Add them to this list as you come across them.

3   Adjectives which end in *-u, -i* and *-é* follow the same logic as in 1, although the extra *e* in the feminine form does not affect pronunciation.

masculine singular	feminine singular	masculine plural	feminine plural
bleu	bleue	bleus	bleues
joli	jolie	jolis	jolies
cassé	cassée	cassés	cassées

Others which follow this pattern include: *âgé, fatigué, perdu* and *trouvé*. Many of these adjectives are in fact past participles. There are many more. Add them to this list as you come across them.

4   Adjectives which end in *-x* follow this pattern:

masculine singular	feminine singular	masculine plural	feminine plural
joyeux	joyeuse	joyeux	joyeuses

Others which follow this pattern include: *délicieux, heureux, malheureux* and *merveilleux*. There are more. Add them to this list as you come across them.

5   Adjectives which end in *-er* follow this pattern:

masculine singular	feminine singular	masculine plural	feminine plural
premier	première	premiers	premières

Others which follow this pattern include: *cher, dernier, entier* and *régulier*.

6   Some adjectives double the last consonant when changing to the feminine form.

masculine singular	feminine singular	masculine plural	feminine plural
bon	bonne	bons	bonnes

Others which follow this pattern include: *ancien, gentil, gras* and *gros*.

7   Many common adjectives are irregular.

masculine singular	feminine singular	masculine plural	feminine plural
blanc	blanche	blancs	blanches
doux	douce	doux	douces
favori	favorite	favoris	favorites
jaloux	jalouse	jaloux	jalouses
long	longue	longs	longues
neuf	neuve	neufs	neuves
public	publique	publics	publiques
roux	rousse	roux	rousses
sec	sèche	secs	sèches
vif	vive	vifs	vives

8   Four adjectives have extra masculine forms which are used when the adjective is followed by a vowel or a silent *h*.

masculine singular	feminine singular	masculine plural	feminine plural
beau *or* bel	belle	beaux	belles
fou *or* fol	folle	fous	folles
nouveau *or* nouvel	nouvelle	nouveaux	nouvelles
vieux *or* vieil	vieille	vieux	vieilles

9   *Demi* does not agree when it is joined to another word. For example:
une demi-heure **but:** Il est une heure et demie.

Common errors with adjective agreement

▶ Failure to spot the gender of the noun the adjective agrees with and therefore missing the agreement, for example:
J'ai deux pommes énorme.   *I have two enormous apples.*
Correct version: J'ai deux pommes énormes.

▶ Treating an irregular adjective as if it was regular, for example:
J'ai une voiture neufe.   *I have a new car.*
Correct version: J'ai une voiture neuve.

Position of adjectives

Adjectives in French, unlike in English, usually follow the noun to which they refer. For example:
J'ai un pullover noir et un pantalon jaune.   *I have a black pullover and a yellow pair of trousers.*

A few common adjectives, however, come before the noun. These are:

beau	gentil	jeune	mauvais
bon	grand	joli	petit
court	gros	large	vieux
excellent	haut	long	vilain

For example:
C'est un vilain garçon.   *He's an ugly boy.*

A few adjectives, including *ancien, cher, même, pauvre* and *propre*, change their meaning, depending on whether they come before or after the noun. For example:

C'est mon ancien professeur.   *It's my former teacher.*
C'est un professeur ancien.   *It's an ancient teacher.*

C'est ma chère amie.   *It's my dear friend.*
C'est un restaurant cher.   *It's an expensive restaurant.*

Il porte toujours la même cravate.   *He always wears the same tie.*
Il est arrivé le jour même.   *He arrived that very day.*
Même mon professeur n'aime pas la grammaire.   *Even my teacher doesn't like grammar.*

Le pauvre Fred. Il est mort.   *Poor Fred. He's dead.*
Le Sudan est un pays pauvre.   *The Sudan is a poor country.*

Ma mère a sa propre voiture.   *My mother's got her own car.*
Sa voiture est toujours propre.   *Her car is always clean.*

Common errors with the position of adjectives

▶ Putting them in the wrong position! It's an easy error to make, as so many common adjectives do come before the noun. However, the list I have given above only contains 16 adjectives which always come before the noun, so it ought to be possible to learn them.

▶ Putting one of those with two meanings in the wrong position and achieving an unintended result, for example:

C'est un pauvre garçon.
Intended meaning: He's a poverty-stricken boy.
Correct version: C'est un garçon pauvre.

Possessive adjectives

Possessive adjectives in French are as follows:

masculine singular	feminine singular	plural	meaning
mon	ma	mes	*my*
ton	ta	tes	*your*
son	sa	ses	*his/her*
notre	notre	nos	*our*
votre	votre	vos	*your*
leur	leur	leurs	*their*

They agree with the gender and number of the noun which follows in the singular, and with the number of the noun in the plural. The agreement has nothing to do with the gender of the owner. For example:

mon frère   *my brother*
ma sœur   *my sister*
mes parents   *my parents*

If a feminine word begins with a vowel or a silent *h*, the *mon*, *ton*, etc. form of the possessive is used. For example:

mon amie Giselle   *my friend Giselle*
ton intention   *your intention*
son idée   *her/his idea*

Comparative adjectives

To compare one thing with another, add:

▶ plus   *more*
▶ moins   *less*
▶ aussi   *as ... as*

before the adjective, which agrees as usual. For example:

Ma mère est plus intelligente que mon père.
My mother is more intelligent than my father.
Ma mère est moins intelligente que mon père.
My mother is less intelligent than my father.
Ma mère est aussi intelligente que mon père.
My mother is as intelligent as my father.

There are two irregular forms:

▶ bon becomes *meilleur*
▶ mauvais becomes *pire*.

For example:
> Cette équipe est meilleure que l'autre. *This team is better than the other one.*
> Cette équipe est pire que l'autre. *This team is worse than the other one.*

Common errors with comparative adjectives

▶ Failing to make them agree, for example:
> Ces garçons sont plus grand que mon frère. *These boys are taller than my brother.*
> **Correct version:** Ces garçons sont plus grands que mon frère.

▶ Missing the two irregular forms, for example:
> Ces vins sont plus bons que les autres. *These wines are better than the others.*
> **Correct version:** Ces vins sont meilleurs que les autres.

Superlative adjectives

To say what is 'the biggest', 'the best', 'the greatest', etc., use:

▶ le plus
▶ la plus
▶ les plus

+ the adjective.

For example:
> Le centre Pompidou est le musée le plus amusant de Paris.
> *The Pompidou Centre is the most entertaining museum in Paris.*
> La tapisserie de Bayeux est la plus vieille du monde.
> *The Bayeux tapestry is the oldest in the world.*
> Les Renaults sont les voitures françaises les plus vendues.
> *Renaults are the French cars with the highest sales.*

The same can be done with *le/la/les moins*. For example:
> Le français est la langue la moins difficile pour moi.
> *French is the least difficult language for me.*

Once again, there are two irregular forms:

▶ *bon* becomes *le meilleur*
▶ *mauvais* becomes *le pire*.

For example:
> Cette équipe est la meilleure. *This team is the best.*
> Cette équipe est la pire. *This team is the worst.*
> C'est le meilleur film de tous. *It's the best film of all.*
> C'est la pire équipe de toutes. *It's the worst team of all.*

Common errors with superlatives

▶ Failing to make them agree, for example:
> Ces garçons sont les plus grand. *These boys are the tallest.*
> **Correct version:** Ces garçons sont les plus grands.

▶ Missing the two irregular forms, for example:
> Ces vins sont les plus bons. *These wines are the best.*
> **Correct version:** Ces vins sont les meilleurs.

▶ Adverbs   *Formation of adverbs from adjectives*

1 In most cases, *-ment* is added to the feminine singular form of the adjective. For example:

masculine adjective	feminine adjective	adverb
doux	douce	doucement
heureux	heureuse	heureusement
entier	entière	entièrement

2   If the masculine singular form ends in a vowel (usually *-e* or *-i*) *-ment* is added straight onto that. For example:

masculine adjective	adverb
vrai	vraiment
difficile	difficilement

3   If the adjective ends in *-ant* in the masculine singular form, the adverb ends in *-amment*. If it ends in *-ent*, the adverb ends in *-emment*. For example:

masculine adjective	adverb
constant	constamment
évident	évidemment

4   Exceptions which end in *-ment*. The rules given above have the following common exceptions:

énormément
gentiment
lentement
précisément
profondément

5   Some adverbs are irregular in that they are adjectives being used as adverbs. These include *bon*, *cher*, *faux* and *fort*. For example:
   Ils chantent faux.   *They are singing out of tune.*

6   Other adverbs are just plain irregular. As these are the most common adverbs, it would be well worth learning this list!

beaucoup	souvent
bien	tard
loin	tôt
longtemps	trop
mal	vite
peu	

Position of adverbs

The adverb generally goes after the verb, unlike in English – beware! For example:
   Il va souvent au collège.   *He often goes to school.*

In the perfect and pluperfect tenses it comes after the auxiliary verb. For example:
   Il n'a pas bien dormi.   *He didn't sleep well.*

Common errors with adverbs

▶   Attempting to put a *-ment* ending on an adverb that doesn't have one, for example:
      Il conduisait vitement.   *He was driving quickly.*
      Correct version: Il conduisait vite.
▶   Putting the adverb in the wrong place, for example:
      Il souvent va au collège.   *He often goes to school.*
      Correct version: Il va souvent au collège.

Comparative adverbs

These operate in much the same way as for adjectives. To compare one thing with another, add:

▶   plus   *more*
▶   moins   *less*
▶   aussi   *as ... as*

before the adverb.

For example:

Ma mère court plus vite que mon père.   *My mother runs faster than my father.*
Ma mère court moins vite que mon père.   *My mother runs less fast than my father.*
Ma mère court aussi vite que mon père.   *My mother runs as fast as my father.*

There are two irregular forms:

▷ *bien* becomes *mieux*
▷ *mal* becomes *pire*.

For example:

Cette équipe joue mieux que l'autre.   *This team plays better than the other one.*
Cette équipe joue pire que l'autre.   *This team plays worse than the other one.*

Common errors with comparative adverbs

▷ Missing the two irregular forms, for example:
  Ces garçons chantent plus bien que les autres.   *These boys sing better than the others.*
  Correct version: Ces garçons chantent mieux que les autres.
▷ Confusing *mieux* and *meilleur*, for example:
  Ces garçons chantent meilleur que les autres.
  Correct version: Ces garçons chantent mieux que les autres.

Superlative adverbs

To say what happens the quickest, the least well, etc., use *le plus* + the adverb (regardless of gender). For example:
  Annette est arrivée le plus vite.   *Annette arrived the quickest.*

The same can be done with *le moins* + the adverb. For example:
  Annette chante le moins bien.   *Annette sings the least well.*

Once again, there are two irregular forms:

▷ *bien* becomes *le mieux*
▷ *mal* becomes *le pire*.

For example:

L'équipe galloise a joué le mieux.   *The Welsh team played the best.*
Cette équipe a joué le pire.   *This team played worst.*

Common errors with superlative adverbs

▷ Missing the two irregular forms, for example:
  Je vois le plus bien.   *I can see best.*
  Correct version: Je vois le mieux.
▷ Inserting *la* or *les* as for an adjective, for example:
  La chorale galloise a chanté la mieux.   *The Welsh choir sang the best.*
  Correct version: La chorale galloise a chanté le mieux.

▷ Nouns   *Gender*

All nouns in French are either masculine (*un, le* or *l'*) or feminine (*une, la* or *l'*). Knowledge of their gender is particularly well rewarded in GCSE Higher Tier Writing, but can help with Reading and Listening comprehension and some aspects of Speaking. With adjective agreements (which depend on a knowledge of the gender of the noun in the first place) and good verb usage, a thorough knowledge of the gender of nouns marks out the very good candidate from the rest.

Number

It is particularly important to take note of whether nouns are singular or plural in order to make sure of adjective agreements and verb forms. Make a habit of it!

Plurals

Where nouns are plural, most French nouns add an -s, as in English. For example:
  une voiture
  deux voitures

There are a few groups of nouns which do not do this:

1   Those ending in -s, -x, and -z remain unchanged. For example:

le fils	les fils
la voix	les voix
le prix	les prix

2   Those ending in -al change the ending to -aux in the plural. For example:

le cheval	les chevaux

3   Those ending in -eau, -eu or -ou add an -x in the plural. For example:

le château	les châteaux
le feu	les feux
un genou	des genoux

4   Common exceptions include:

le ciel	les cieux	la pomme de terre	les pommes de terre
le mal	les maux	le pneu	les pneus
l'œil	les yeux	le timbre-poste	les timbres-poste
la petite-fille	les petites-filles	le travail	les travaux
le petit-fils	les petits-fils	le trou	les trous

Note also:

monsieur	messieurs
mademoiselle	mesdemoiselles
madame	mesdames.

Surnames do not change in the plural in French. For example:
  Nous sommes invités par les Leclerc.   *We've been invited by the Leclercs.*

Common errors with nouns

⯈ Mistakes of gender, for example:
   C'est un voiture.   *It's a car.*
   Correct version: C'est une voiture.
⯈ Incorrect formation of plurals, for example:
   J'ai trois animals à la maison.   *I have three animals at home.*
   Correct version: J'ai trois animaux à la maison.

⯈ Pronouns

Pronouns take the place of a noun which has been referred to earlier.

Subject pronouns

je   *I*
tu   *you*
il   *he, it*
elle   *she, it*
on   *one, we, they, you*

nous   *we*
vous   *you*
ils   *they*
elles   *they*

Use of subject pronouns
Tu is used when talking to one person who is

▶ a good friend
▶ a member of the family or a pet
▶ a young person.

Vous is used when talking to two or more people who are

▶ good friends
▶ members of the family or pets
▶ young people,

or to one person who is

▶ an adult who doesn't fit any of the categories above.

Il and *elle* can mean 'it' when referring to masculine or feminine nouns.

On has a variety of meanings.

▶ 'we', for example:
   On rentre?   *Shall we go home?*
▶ 'one', for example:
   On est obligé de porter une cravate.   *One has to wear a tie.*
▶ 'you' (where the meaning could be rendered more poshly by 'one'), for example:
   On est obligé de porter une cravate.   *You have to wear a tie.*
▶ 'they' (where 'they' are unspecified people in authority), for example:
   On n'accepte pas de chèques chez Montrichard.
   They don't accept cheques at Montrichard's.

Ils is used for 'they' where

▶ all the nouns referred to are masculine
▶ there is a group of nouns referred to of which one is masculine. (It makes no difference how many feminine ones there are!)

Elles is used for 'they' where all the nouns referred to are feminine.

Object pronouns

Direct object pronouns
me   *me*
te   *you*
le   *him, it (masculine)*
la   *her, it (feminine)*

nous   *us*
vous   *you*
les   *them*

Indirect object pronouns
me   *to me*
te   *to you*
lui   *to him, to her, to it*

nous   *to us*
vous   *to you*
leur   *to them*

Position of pronouns

Object pronouns come immediately before the verb, or, in the perfect and pluperfect tenses, immediately before the auxiliary. For example:

Je les vois. *I see them.*

Je les ai vu(e)s. *I have seen them.*

In command forms, where the command is straightforward, the object pronoun follows the verb. For example:

Donnez-le-moi! *Give it to me.* (Note the hyphens!)

Where the command is negative, the following applies:

Ne me le donnez pas! *Don't give it to me.*

Order of pronouns

The normal order of pronouns can be learned by imagining them as a traditional football or hockey team + a reserve.

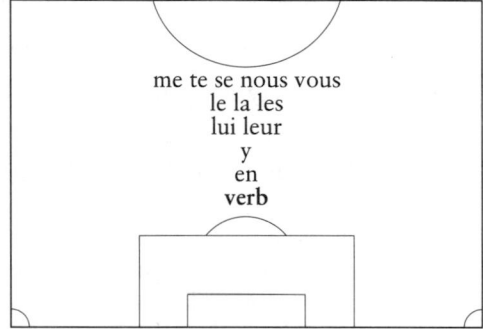

Pronouns from each line, starting with the 'forwards', take a position ahead of the line below. For example:

Il nous les a donnés. *He gave them to us.*

Vous m'en avez déjà offert. *You have already offered me some.*

In straightforward commands, the team is playing a more defensive formation!

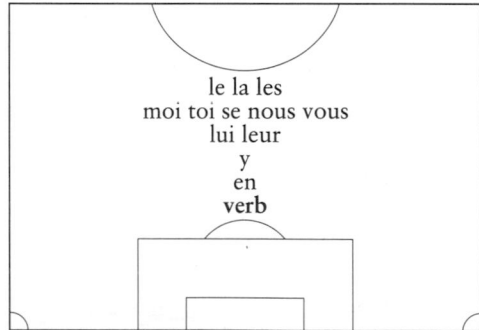

Pronouns from each line, starting with the 'forwards', take a position ahead of the line below. Note also the the change from *me* to *moi* and from *te* to *toi*. For example:

Donnez-les-moi! *Give them to me.* (Note the hyphens!)

Common errors with subject and object pronouns

▷ Failure to recognise that nouns are feminine, and therefore using the wrong subject pronoun for 'it'. For example:

J'ai acheté une voiture. Il est formidable. *I have bought a car. It's great.*

Correct version: J'ai acheté une voiture. Elle est formidable.

▷ Getting the pronouns in the wrong order, for example:

Je lui les ai donné(e)s. *I gave them to him.*

Correct version: Je les lui ai donnés.

Emphatic pronouns

These are also known as **stressed** or **disjunctive** pronouns.

moi *me, I*
toi *you*
lui *him, he*
elle *her, she*

nous *us, we*
vous *you*
eux *them (masculine), they*
elles *them (feminine), they*

Use of emphatic pronouns
1 After prepositions. For example:
   chez moi *at my house*
   devant eux *in front of them*

2 With *c'est* and *ce sont*. For example:
   Ah, c'est toi, Maigret! *Oh! It's you Maigret!*
   Ce sont eux. *It's them.*

3 To emphasise the subject pronoun, for example:
   Toi, tu as de la chance. *You are lucky, you are.*

4 As a one-word answer to a question. For example:
   Qui a mangé mon sandwich?—Moi. *Who ate my sandwich?—Me.*

5 In comparisons. For example:
   Napoléon était plus petit que toi. *Napoleon was smaller than you.*

6 Combined with *-même(s)*: *moi-même* (myself), *toi-même* (yourself), etc.
Soi-même (oneself), also exists and is related to *on*. For example:
   Vous l'avcz vu vous-mêmes. *You saw it yourselves.*
   On peut faire la lessive soi-même. *One can do the washing oneself.*

Relative pronouns

Relative pronouns introduce a clause giving more information about a noun. The correct relative pronoun is determined by its grammatical function within the relative clause.

Relative pronoun as the subject of the clause – qui
Examples:
   La personne qui est arrivée est ma mère. *The person who has arrived is my mother.*
   L'avion qui vole le plus vite s'appelle Concorde.
   The plane which flies fastest is called Concorde.

Relative pronoun as the (direct) object of the clause – que
Clauses of this type will contain a different subject. For example:
   Les personnes que j'aime sont importantes pour moi.
   The people I like are important to me.
   Le travail que je fais est ennuyeux. *The work I am doing is boring.*

Note: In the perfect and pluperfect tenses, the past participle will normally agree in this type of clause, as the direct object *que* **precedes** the verb (PDO rule – see p. 201). For example:
   La jupe que j'ai achetée est rouge. *The skirt that I bought is red.*

Relative pronoun as the indirect object of the clause – à qui
Example:
   Voilà l'homme à qui j'ai donné les clés. *There is the man to whom I gave the keys.*

Relative pronoun expressing 'whose', 'of whom', or 'of which' – dont
Examples:

Voilà l'homme dont le chien est mort.   *There is the man whose dog died.*
Regarde la grammaire dont je parle.
Look at the grammar I am talking about / of which I am talking.

Lequel

Lequel, laquelle, lesquels and *lesquelles* are used as relative pronouns after prepositions. For example:

Il regardait la voiture derrière laquelle se trouvait le chat.
He was looking at the car behind which was the cat.

Common errors with relative pronouns

➤ Wrong choice of pronoun, especially between *qui* and *que*. This is probably caused by the fact that 'that' can be either a subject relative pronoun or an object relative pronoun in English, and that students don't apply the basic rule that *que* is only used where there is another subject in the clause. For example:

Voilà la maison qui j'ai vu.   *Here is the house which I saw.*
Correct version: Voilà la maison que j'ai vue.

➤ Missing out the relative pronoun altogether, as in English. For example:

J'aime la jupe j'ai vue.   *I like the skirt I saw.*
Correct version: J'aime la jupe que j'ai vue.

Indefinite pronouns

There are numbers of these in French. It's probably best to learn them as vocabulary.

autre
Example:

Je n'ai pas vu Jean, mais j'ai vu les autres.   *I didn't see Jean, but I saw the others.*

chacun
Example:

J'ai beaucoup d'amies. Chacune est agréable.
I've lots of (female) friends. Each one is pleasant.

n'importe
This can be combined with various other words to mean 'any ... at all', etc. For example:
n'importe qui   *anybody at all*
n'importe quoi   *anything at all*
n'importe quel(le)   *no matter which*

plusieurs
Example:

As-tu des livres d'Astérix? Oui, j'en ai plusieurs.
Have you any Astérix books. Yes, I've got several.

quelqu'un
Examples:

J'attends quelqu'un.   *I am waiting for someone.*
Quelques-unes de ces photos sont amusantes.   *Some of these photos are entertaining.*

tous
Example:

Il était aimé de tous.   *He was liked by everyone.*

tout
Example:

Il sait tout.   *He knows everything.*

tout le monde

Example:

    Tout le monde est là.   *Everyone is here.*

Note: *tout le monde* is singular, despite its meaning!

> **Word order**   Word order in French is very often similar to that in English. But check the sections above on

>   adjectives   negatives
>   adverbs   pronouns

for various differences.

Inversion after direct speech

After direct speech, the subject and verb are inverted (i.e. swapped round). If the verb form ends with a vowel, a *-t-* is inserted. For example:

    'Je mange', a-t-elle dit.   *'I am eating', she said.*
    'Nous mangeons', ont-ils dit.   *'We are eating', they said.*

Inversion after peut-être

Where *peut-être* begins a sentence, the subject and verb are inverted. Again, if the verb form ends with a vowel, a *-t-* is inserted. For example:

    Peut-être arrivera-t-il ce soir.   *Perhaps he'll arrive this evening.*

Inversion in certain subordinate clauses

In clauses introduced by *où*, the subject and verb are inverted. For example:

    Voici le collège où travaille mon cousin.   *Here is the school where my cousin works.*

> **Numbers and time**

Cardinal numbers

0	zéro	18	dix-huit	80	quatre-vingts
$\frac{1}{4}$	un quart	19	dix-neuf	81	quatre-vingt-un
$\frac{1}{3}$	un tiers	20	vingt	82	quatre-vingt-deux, *etc.*
$\frac{1}{2}$	un demi	21	vingt et un		
$\frac{2}{3}$	deux tiers	22	vingt-deux, *etc.*	90	quatre-vingt-dix
$\frac{3}{4}$	trois quarts			91	quatre-vingt-onze, *etc.*
1	un, une	30	trente		
2	deux	31	trente et un	99	quatre-vingt-dix-neuf
3	trois	32	trente-deux, *etc.*	100	cent
4	quatre			101	cent un
5	cinq	40	quarante	102	cent deux, *etc.*
6	six	41	quarante et un		
7	sept	42	quarante-deux, *etc.*	200	deux cents
8	huit			210	deux cent dix
9	neuf	50	cinquante		
10	dix	51	cinquante et un	1 000	mille
11	onze	52	cinquante-deux, *etc.*	1 311	mille trois cent onze
12	douze				
13	treize	60	soixante	3 000	trois mille
14	quatorze	61	soixante et un		
15	quinze	62	soixante-deux, *etc.*	1 000 000	un million
16	seize				
17	dix-sept	70	soixante-dix	1 000 000 000	un milliard
		71	soixante et onze		
		72	soixante-douze, *etc.*		

Note the following points:

▶ $\frac{1}{2}$ = *un demi* only in arithmetic and orders for beer. Elsewhere it is *une moitié*.
▶ For 1, use either *un* or *une*, depending on the gender of the object.
▶ There are no hyphens in *vingt et un*, *trente et un*, etc.
▶ Note the form *soixante et onze*. Contrast *quatre-vingt-onze*.
▶ *Quatre-vingt-un* and *quatre-vingt-onze* are hyphenated.
▶ *Mille* does not have an s in the plural.

Telephone numbers are read out in groups of two digits and are written 05.58.46.92.17.

Ordinal numbers

1st	premier(1er), première (1e)	12th	douzième (12e)
2nd	deuxième (2e) (second, seconde)	13th	treizième (13e)
3rd	troisième (3e)	14th	quatorzième (14e)
4th	quatrième (4e)	15th	quinzième (15e)
5th	cinquième (5e)	16th	seizième (16e)
6th	sixième (6e)	17th	dix-septième(17^e)
7th	septième (7e)	18th	dix-huitième (18e)
8th	huitième (8e)	19th	dix-neuvième (19e)
9th	neuvième (9e)	20th	vingtième (20e)
10th	dixième (10e)	21st	vingt et unième (21e), *etc.*
11th	onzième (11e)		

Note the following points:
▶ For '1st', use either *premier* or *première*, depending on the gender of the object.
▶ *Seconde* is used to mean 'second' when there are only two items in a series. Note also: Je suis en seconde. *I am in year II.*

Telling the time

Telling the time may seem an elementary thing to be revising before GCSE. However, it is quite clear that it is over-represented in Listening Tests. So you need to to make very certain of it.

Hours
Il est une heure. *It's one o'clock.*
Il est cinq heures. *It's five o'clock.*

Quarters and half hours
Il est deux heures et quart. *It's quarter past two.*
Il est deux heures et demie. *It's half past two.*
Il est trois heures moins le quart. *It's quarter to three.*

Minutes past and to the hour
Il est huit heures dix. *It's ten past eight.*
Il est huit heures moins dix. *It's ten to eight.*

Midnight and midday
Il est minuit. *It's midnight.*
Il est midi. *It's midday.*
Il est midi cinq. *It's five past twelve.*
Il est minuit moins dix. *It's ten to midnight.*
Il est midi et demie. *It's half past twelve.*

24-hour clock

Il est dix-huit heures.	18.00
Il est dix-huit heures quinze.	18.15
Il est dix-huit heures trente.	18.30
Il est dix-huit heures quarante-cinq.	18.45
Il est dix-huit heures cinquante-neuf.	18.59
Il est dix-neuf heures deux.	19.02

Common errors in telling the time
- Confusing *et* and *moins*.
- Missing out *le* in *moins le quart*.

Dates

Like times, days and dates are very common in Listening and Reading Tests. Make sure you can do them!

Days of the week
lundi
mardi
mercredi
jeudi
vendredi
samedi
dimanche

Note: they are not written with capital letters!

Months of the year

janvier	juillet
février	août
mars	septembre
avril	octobre
mai	novembre
juin	décembre

Note: these don't have capital letters either!

The year
Given below are possible years of GCSE students' birth and the years in which they sit the examination, for reference.

It will be acceptable to write dates in figures in the Writing Tests, so they only need to be known for recognition and for Speaking. Either version will do.

1982	mil neuf cent quatre-vingt-deux dix-neuf cent quatre-vingt-deux	1998	mil neuf cent quatre-vingt-dix-huit dix-neuf cent quatre-vingt-dix-huit
1983	mil neuf cent quatre-vingt-trois dix-neuf cent quatre-vingt-trois	1999	mil neuf cent quatre-vingt-dix-neuf dix-neuf cent quatre-vingt-dix-neuf
1984	mil neuf cent quatre-vingt-quatre dix-neuf cent quatre-vingt-quatre	2000	deux mille
1985	mil neuf cent quatre-vingt-cinq dix-neuf cent quatre-vingt-cinq	2001	deux mille un
1986	mil neuf cent quatre-vingt-six dix-neuf cent quatre-vingt-six	2002	deux mille deux

Giving the date

Use the following patterns:

Quel jour sommes-nous?   *What is the date?*
Nous sommes le vingt-neuf février.   *It's the 29th of February.*

Quelle est la date?   *What is the date?*
C'est le vingt-neuf février.   *It's the 29th of February.*

mardi le 29 février *or* le mardi 29 fevrier   *Tuesday 29th February*

▷ **Conjunctions**

French has the following common conjunctions which GCSE candidates need to be familiar with:

alors *so, for that reason*	mais *but, however*
car *for (= because)*	ou *or*
comme *as*	parce que *because*
depuis que *since*	pendant que *while*
dès que *as soon as*	puisque *since*
donc *therefore, so*	quand *when*
et *and*	si *if*
lorsque *when*	tandis que *while*

Most of these are straightforward in their usage. However, studying the following tips and examples will help to improve your French:

alors

This should only be used in the middle of a sentence. For example:

Il avait la grippe, alors il est resté au lit.   *He had flu so he stayed in bed.*

car

This is often confused with *pour* by non-native speakers. If you could use 'because', then it's OK to use *car*. For example:

Il était triste car il avait perdu son porte feuille.
He was sad because he had lost his wallet.

comme

Example:

Tu peux faire comme tu veux.   *You can do as you like.*

depuis que

This only means 'since' in expressions of time. For example:

Il a commencé à pleuvoir depuis que je suis rentré.
It has begun to rain since I came home.

dès que

Example:

Dès que je le regarde, il rougit.   *As soon as I look at him he reddens.*

donc

This should only be used in the middle of a sentence. For example:

Il avait la grippe, donc il est resté au lit.   *He had flu so he stayed in bed.*

et

At the end of a list, there is no comma before the final *et*. For example:

On nous apporte du pain, de la confiture, du beurre et du café.
They bring us bread, jam, butter and coffee.

lorsque

This often refers to the future. When it does, remember that future time requires the future tense in French. For example:

Je t'écrirai lorsque je serai à Londres.   *I'll write to you when I am in London.*

mais
Example:
Je suis intelligent, mais il est stupide.   *I am intelligent but he is stupid.*

ou
Example:
Je te téléphonerai ou tu me téléphoneras.   *I'll phone you or you'll phone me.*

parce que
Spelt without a hyphen! For example:
Je suis content parce que mon frère m'a donné(e) un cadeau.
I am happy because my brother has given me a present.

pendant que
This means 'while', 'whilst', referring to time. For example:
Pendant qu'il écrivait une lettre, le téléphone a sonné.
While he was writing a letter the telephone rang.

puisque
This means 'since' in the sense of 'because'. For example:
Il fait beaucoup de devoirs puisqu'il veut devenir fort en français.
He does lots of homework because he wishes to be good at French.

quand
This often refers to the future. When it does, remember that future time requires the future tense in French. It's more common than *lorsque*. For example:
Je t'écrirai quand je serai à Londres.   *I'll write to you when I am in London.*

si
There are special rules governing the tenses after *si*. Look them up in the section on the conditional (see p. 202).

tandis que
This means 'while, whilst', contrasting two activities. For example:
Jeanne a fait des économies, tandis que Hélène a tout dépensé.
Jeanne has saved up while Hélène has spent everything.

▷ Prepositions

The use of prepositions in French is well rewarded in the accuracy mark scheme used in Higher Writing. This is because there is often no direct, once-and-for-all translation of the English equivalent – the French rendering will vary according to circumstances. In Reading and Listening papers you will have to be aware of the different meanings of various prepositions.

I have given below examples of the use of various prepositions, not all of which behave as you might expect. Study and imitation of these will pay dividends!

à
à droite   *on the right*
à bicyclette   *by bike*
au collège   *at secondary school*
à mon avis   *in my opinion*

à peu près
Je gagne à peu près deux cents francs par jour.   *I earn about 200 francs a day.*

à propos de
à propos de la boum   *about the party*

au-dessus de
Ma chambre est au-dessus du salon.   *My bedroom is above the living room.*
Le ballon est passé au-dessus de ma tête.   *The ball passed over my head.*

au sujet de

au sujet de la boum   *about the party*

avant

avant minuit   *before midnight*

avant d'arriver   *before arriving*

dans

dans le placard   *in the cupboard*

On danse dans la rue.   *They are dancing in the street.*

de

la plume de ma tante   *my aunt's pen*

Il était suivi d'un gendarme.   *He was being followed by a policeman.*

de quoi

De quoi parlez-vous?   *What are you talking about?*

depuis

J'habite ici depuis deux ans.   *I have been living here for two years.*

En 1997 il habitait là depuis deux ans.   *In 1997 he had been living there for two years.*

Depuis Pâques il n'a rien fait.   *He has done nothing since Easter.*

devant

Ils sont devant le café.   *They are in front of the café.*

en

Je suis allé(e) à Paris en voiture.   *I went to Paris by car.*

entre

Entre nous, c'est un idiot.   *Between you and me, he's a fool.*

Nous sommes entre amis.   *We are among friends.*

hors de

hors de danger   *out of danger*

jusqu'à

Nous jouerons jusqu'à trois heures.   *We shall play till 3 o'clock.*

le long de

Il courait le long de la rue.   *He was running along the road.*

par

J'ai été mordu par un chien.   *I've been bitten by a dog.*

Elles regardaient par la fenêtre.   *They were looking out of the window.*

par-dessus

Le chat a sauté par-dessus le mur.   *The cat jumped over the wall.*

parmi

Il cherchait quelque chose parmi les rochers.

He was looking for something among the rocks

pendant

J'ai travaillé pendant quatre heures.   *I have worked for four hours.*

plus de

J'ai plus de vingt livres d'Astérix.   *I have over 20 Astérix books.*

pour

Nous serons en France pour deux jours.   *We shall be in France for two days.*

près de

Assieds-toi près de moi.   *Sit by me.*

sous

J'aime me promener sous la neige.   *I like walking when it's snowing.*

sur

Une personne sur cinq porte des lunettes.   *One person in five wears glasses.*

VERB TABLE

Infinitive / Present participle / Imperative	Present	Perfect	Imperfect	Pluperfect	Future	Conditional	Past historic
Regular verbs							
parler *to speak, talk* parlant	je parle tu parles il parle	j'ai parlé tu as parlé il a parlé	je parlais tu parlais il parlait	j'avais parlé tu avais parlé il avait parlé	je parlerai tu parleras il parlera	je parlerais tu parlerais il parlerait	je parlai tu parlas il parla
parle! parlons! parlez!	nous parlons vous parlez ils parlent	nous avons parlé vous avez parlé ils ont parlé	nous parlions vous parliez ils parlaient	nous avions parlé vous aviez parlé ils avaient parlé	nous parlerons vous parlerez ils parleront	nous parlerions vous parleriez ils parleraient	nous parlâmes vous parlâtes ils parlèrent
finir *to finish* finissant	je finis tu finis il finit	j'ai fini tu as fini il a fini	je finissais tu finissais il finissait	j'avais fini tu avais fini il avait fini	je finirai tu finiras il finira	je finirais tu finirais il finirait	je finis tu finis il finit
finis! finissons! finissez!	nous finissons vous finissez ils finissent	nous avons fini vous avez fini ils ont fini	nous finissions vous finissiez ils finissaient	nous avions fini vous aviez fini ils avaient fini	nous finirons vous finirez ils finiront	nous finirions vous finiriez ils finiraient	nous finîmes vous finîtes ils finirent
vendre *to sell* vendant	je vends tu vends il vend	j'ai vendu tu as vendu il a vendu	je vendais tu vendais il vendait	j'avais vendu tu avais vendu il avait vendu	je vendrai tu vendras il vendra	je vendrais tu vendrais il vendrait	je vendis tu vendis il vendit
vends! vendons! vendez!	nous vendons vous vendez ils vendent	nous avons vendu vous avez vendu ils ont vendu	nous vendions vous vendiez ils vendaient	nous avions vendu vous aviez vendu ils avaient vendu	nous vendrons vous vendrez ils vendront	nous vendrions vous vendriez ils vendraient	nous vendîmes vous vendîtes ils vendirent
se laver *to wash oneself* se lavant	je me lave tu te laves il se lave	je me suis lavé(e) tu t'es lavé(e) il s'est lavé ell s'est lavée	je me lavais tu te lavais il se lavait	je m'étais lavé(e) tu t'étais lavé(e) il s'était lavé elle s'était lavée	je me laverai tu te laveras il se lavera	je me laverais tu te laverais il se laverait	je me lavai tu te lava il se lava
lave-toi! lavons-nous!	nous nous lavons	nous nous sommes lavé(e)s	nous nous lavions	nous nous étions lavé(e)s	nous nous laverons	nous nous laverions	nous nous lavâmes
lavez-vous!	vous vous lavez	vous vous êtes lavé(e)(s)	vous vous laviez	vous vous étiez lavé(e)(s)	vous vous laverez	vous vous laveriez	vous vous lavâtes
	ils se lavent	ils se sont lavés elles se sont lavées	ils se lavaient	ils s'étaient lavés elles s'étaient lavées	ils se laveront	ils se laveraient	ils se lavèrent

VERB TABLE (contd)

Infinitive / Present participle / Imperative	Present	Perfect	Imperfect	Pluperfect	Future	Conditional	Past historic
Irregular verbs							
aller *to go*	je vais	je suis allé(e)	j'allais	j'étais allé(e)	j'irai	j'irais	j'allai
allant	tu vas	tu es allé(e)	tu allais	tu étais allé(e)	tu iras	tu irais	tu allas
	il va	il est allé	il allait	il était allé	il ira	il irait	il alla
va!		elle est allée		elle était allée			
allons!	nous allons	nous sommes allé(e)s	nous allions	nous étions allé(e)s	nous irons	nous irions	nous allâmes
allez!	vous allez	vous êtes allé(e)(s)	vous alliez	vous étiez allé(e)(s)	vous irez	vous iriez	vous allâtes
	ils vont	ils sont allés	ils allaient	ils étaient allés	ils iront	ils iraient	ils allèrent
		elles sont allées		elles étaient allées			
apprendre *to learn* see prendre							
s'asseoir *to sit down*	je m'assieds	je me suis assis(e)	je m'asseyais	je m'étais assis(e)	je m'assiérai	je m'assiérais	je m'assis
s'asseyant	tu t'assieds	tu t'es assis(e)	tu t'asseyais	tu t'étais assis(e)	tu t'assiéras	tu t'assiérais	tu t'assis
	il s'assied	il s'est assis	il s'asseyait	il s'était assis	il s'assiéra	il s'assiérait	il s'assit
assieds-toi!		elle s'est assise		elle s'était assise			
asseyons-nous!	nous nous asseyons	nous nous sommes assis(es)	nous nous asseyions	nous nous étions assis(es)	nous nous assiérons	nous nous assiérions	nous nous assîmes
asseyez-vous!	vous vous asseyez	vous vous êtes assis(es)	vous vous asseyiez	vous vous étiez assis(es)	vous vous assiérez	vous vous assiériez	vous vous assîtes
	ils s'asseyent	ils se sont assis	ils s'asseyaient	ils s'étaient assis	ils s'assiéront	ils s'assiéraient	ils s'assirent
		elles se sont assises		elles s'étaient assises	ils s'assiéront		
avoir *to have*	j'ai	j'ai eu	j'avais	j'avais eu	j'aurai	j'aurais	j'eus
ayant	tu as	tu as eu	tu avais	tu avais eu	tu auras	tu aurais	tu eus
	il a	il a eu	il avait	il avait eu	il aura	il aurait	il eut
aie!							
ayons!	nous avons	nous avons eu	nous avions	nous avions eu	nous aurons	nous aurions	nous eûmes
ayez!	vous avez	vous avez eu	vous aviez	vous aviez eu	vous aurez	vous auriez	vous eûtes
	ils ont	ils ont eu	ils avaient	ils avaient eu	ils auront	ils auraient	ils eurent

VERB TABLE (contd)

Infinitive / Present participle / Imperative	Present	Perfect	Imperfect	Pluperfect	Future	Conditional	Past historic
battre *to beat* battant bats! battons! battez!	je bats tu bats il bat nous battons vous battez ils battent	j'ai battu tu as battu il a battu nous avons battu vous avez battu ils ont battu	je battais tu battais il battait nous battions vous battiez ils battaient	j'avais battu tu avais battu il avait battu nous avions battu vous aviez battu ils avaient battu	je battrai tu battras il battra nous battrons vous battrez ils battront	je battrais tu battrais il battrait nous battrions vous battriez ils battraient	je battis tu battis il battit nous battîmes vous battîtes ils battirent
boire *to drink* buvant bois! buvons! buvez!	je bois tu bois il boit nous buvons vous buvez ils boivent	j'ai bu tu as bu il a bu nous avons bu vous avez bu ils ont bu	je buvais tu buvais il buvait nous buvions vous buviez ils buvaient	j'avais bu tu avais bu il avait bu nous avions bu vous aviez bu ils avaient bu	je boirai tu boiras il boira nous boirons vous boirez ils boiront	je boirais tu boirais il boirait nous boirions vous boiriez ils boiraient	je bus tu bus il but nous bûmes vous bûtes ils burent
comprendre *to understand* see **prendre**							
conduire *to drive* conduisant conduis! conduisons! conduisez!	je conduis tu conduis il conduit nous conduisons vous conduisez ils conduisent	j'ai conduit tu as conduit il a conduit nous avons conduit vous avez conduit ils ont conduit	je conduisais tu conduisais il conduisait nous conduisions vous conduisiez ils conduisaient	j'avais conduit tu avais conduit il avait conduit nous avions conduit vous aviez conduit ils avaient conduit	je conduirai tu conduiras il conduira nous conduirons vous conduirez ils conduiront	je conduirais tu conduirais il conduirait nous conduirions vous conduiriez ils conduiraient	je conduisis tu conduisis il conduisit nous conduisîmes vous conduisîtes ils conduisirent
connaître *to know* connaissant connais! connaissons! connaissez!	je connais tu connais il connaît nous connaissons vous connaissez ils connaissent	j'ai connu tu as connu il a connu nous avons connu vous avez connu ils ont connu	je connaissais tu connaissais il connaissait nous connaissions vous connaissiez ils connaissaient	j'avais connu tu avais connu il avait connu nous avions connu vous aviez connu ils avaient connu	je connaîtrai tu connaîtras il connaîtra nous connaîtrons vous connaîtrez ils connaîtront	je connaîtrais tu connaîtrais il connaîtrait nous connaîtrions vous connaîtriez ils connaîtraient	je connus tu connus il connut nous connûmes vous connûtes ils connurent

Verb table **225**

VERB TABLE (contd)

Infinitive Present participle Imperative	Present	Perfect	Imperfect	Pluperfect	Future	Conditional	Past historic
construire *to build* see **conduire**							
contenir *to contain* see **tenir**							
convenir *to suit* see **venir**, but takes *avoir* in perfect and pluperfect tenses							
coudre *to sew* cousant couds! cousons! cousez!	je couds tu couds il coud nous cousons vous cousez ils cousent	j'ai cousu tu as cousu il a cousu nous avons cousu vous avez cousu ils ont cousu	je cousais tu cousais il cousait nous cousions vous cousiez ils cousaient	j'avais cousu tu avais cousu il avait cousu nous avions cousu vous aviez cousu ils avaient cousu	je coudrai tu coudras il coudra nous coudrons vous coudrez ils coudront	je coudrais tu coudrais il coudrait nous coudrions vous coudriez ils coudraient	je cousis tu cousis il cousit nous cousîmes vous cousîtes ils cousirent
courir *to run* courant cours! courons! courez!	je cours tu cours il court nous courons vous courez ils courent	j'ai couru tu as couru il a couru nous avons couru vous avez couru ils ont couru	je courais tu courais il courait nous courions vous couriez ils couraient	j'avais couru tu avais couru il avait couru nous avions couru vous aviez couru ils avaient couru	je courrai tu courras il courra nous courrons vous courrez ils courront	je courrais tu courrais il courrait nous courrions vous courriez ils courraient	je courus tu courus il courut nous courûmes vous courûtes ils coururent
couvrir *to cover* see **ouvrir**							
craindre *to fear* craignant crains! craignons! craignez!	je crains tu crains il craint nous craignons vous craignez ils craignent	j'ai craint tu as craint il a craint nous avons craint vous avez craint ils ont craint	je craignais tu craignais il craignait nous craignions vous craigniez ils craignaient	j'avais craint tu avais craint il avait craint nous avions craint vous aviez craint ils avaient craint	je craindrai tu craindras il craindra nous craindrons vous craindrez ils craindront	je craindrais tu craindrais il craindrait nous craindrions vous craindriez ils craindraient	je craignis tu craignis il craignit nous craignîmes vous craignîtes ils craignirent
croire *to believe* croyant crois! croyons! croyez!	je crois tu crois il croit nous croyons vous croyez ils croient	j'ai cru tu as cru il a cru nous avons cru vous avez cru ils ont cru	je croyais tu croyais il croyait nous croyions vous croyiez ils croyaient	j'avais cru tu avais cru il avait cru nous avions cru vous aviez cru ils avaient cru	je croirai tu croiras il croira nous croirons vous croirez ils croiront	je croirais tu croirais il croirait nous croirions vous croiriez ils croiraient	je crus tu crus il crut nous crûmes vous crûtes ils crurent

VERB TABLE (contd)

Infinitive / Present participle / Imperative	Present	Perfect	Imperfect	Pluperfect	Future	Conditional	Past historic
découvrir *to discover* see **ouvrir**							
descendre *to go down*	je descends	je suis descendu(e)	je descendais	j'étais descendu(e)	je descendrai	je descendrais	je descendis
descendant	tu descends	tu es descendu(e)	tu descendais	tu étais descendu(e)	tu descendras	tu descendrais	tu descendis
	il descend	il est descendu	il descendait	il était descendu	il descendra	il descendrait	il descendit
descends!		elle est descendue		elle était descendue			
descendons!	nous descendons	nous sommes	nous descendions	nous étions	nous descendrons	nous descendrions	nous descendîmes
descendez!		descendu(e)s		descendu(e)s			
	vous descendez	vous êtes	vous descendiez	vous étiez	vous descendrez	vous descendriez	vous descendîtes
		descendu(e)(s)		descendu(e)(s)			
	ils descendent	ils sont descendus	ils descendaient	ils étaient descendus	ils descendront	ils descendraient	ils descendirent
		elles sont descendues		elles étaient descendues			
détruire *to destroy* see **conduire**							
devenir *to become* see **venir**							
devoir *to have, to*	je dois	j'ai dû	je devais	j'avais dû	je devrai	je devrais	je dus
owe	tu dois	tu as dû	tu devais	tu avais dû	tu devras	tu devrais	tu dus
devant	il doit	il a dû	il devait	il avait dû	il devra	il devrait	il dut
dois!	nous devons	nous avons dû	nous devions	nous avions dû	nous devrons	nous devrions	nous dûmes
devons!	vous devez	vous avez dû	vous deviez	vous aviez dû	vous devrez	vous devriez	vous dûtes
devez!	ils doivent	ils ont dû	ils devaient	ils avaient dû	ils devront	ils devraient	ils durent
dire *to say*	je dis	j'ai dit	je disais	j'avais dit	je dirai	je dirais	je dis
disant	tu dis	tu as dit	tu disais	tu avais dit	tu diras	tu dirais	tu dis
	il dit	il a dit	il disait	il avait dit	il dira	il dirait	il dit
dis!							
disons!	nous disons	nous avons dit	nous disions	nous avions dit	nous dirons	nous dirions	nous dîmes
dites!	vous dites	vous avez dit	vous disiez	vous aviez dit	vous direz	vous diriez	vous dîtes
	ils disent	ils ont dit	ils disaient	ils avaient dit	ils diront	ils diraient	ils dirent

VERB TABLE (contd)

disparaître *to disappear* see **connaître**

Infinitive / Present participle / Imperative	Present	Perfect	Imperfect	Pluperfect	Future	Conditional	Past historic
dormir *to sleep* dormant dors! dormons! dormez!	je dors tu dors il dort nous dormons vous dormez ils dorment	j'ai dormi tu as dormi il a dormi nous avons dormi vous avez dormi ils ont dormi	je dormais tu dormais il dormait nous dormions vous dormiez ils dormaient	j'avais dormi tu avais dormi il avait dormi nous avions dormi vous aviez dormi ils avaient dormi	je dormirai tu dormiras il dormira nous dormirons vous dormirez ils dormiront	je dormirais tu dormirais il dormirait nous dormirions vous dormiriez ils dormiraient	je dormis tu dormis il dormit nous dormîmes vous dormîtes ils dormirent

s'endormir *to go to sleep* see **dormir**, but note: reflexive verb taking *être* in perfect and pluperfect tenses.

Infinitive / Present participle / Imperative	Present	Perfect	Imperfect	Pluperfect	Future	Conditional	Past historic
écrire *to write* écrivant écris! écrivons! écrivez!	j'écris tu écris il écrit nous écrivons vous écrivez ils écrivent	j'ai écrit tu as écrit il a écrit nous avons écrit vous avez écrit ils ont écrit	j'écrivais tu écrivais il écrivait nous écrivions vous écriviez ils écrivaient	j'avais écrit tu avais écrit il avait écrit nous avions écrit vous aviez écrit ils avaient écrit	j'écrirai tu écriras il écrira nous écrirons vous écrirez ils écriront	j'écrirais tu écrirais il écrirait nous écririons vous écririez ils écriraient	j'écrivis tu écrivis il écrivit nous écrivîmes vous écrivîtes ils écrivirent
entendre *to hear* entendant entends! entendons! entendez!	j'entends tu entends il entend nous entendons vous entendez ils entendent	j'ai entendu tu as entendu il a entendu nous avons entendu vous avez entendu ils ont entendu	j'entendais tu entendais il entendait nous entendions vous entendiez ils entendaient	j'avais entendu tu avais entendu il avait entendu nous avions entendu vous aviez entendu ils avaient entendu	j'entendrai tu entendras il entendra nous entendrons vous entendrez ils entendront	j'entendrais tu entendrais il entendrait nous entendrions vous entendriez ils entendraient	j'entendis tu entendis il entendit nous entendîmes vous entendîtes ils entendirent

entretenir *to maintain* see **tenir**

Infinitive / Present participle / Imperative	Present	Perfect	Imperfect	Pluperfect	Future	Conditional	Past historic
envoyer *to send* envoyant envoie! envoyons! envoyez!	j'envoie tu envoies il envoie nous envoyons vous envoyez ils envoient	j'ai envoyé tu as envoyé il a envoyé nous avons envoyé vous avez envoyé ils ont envoyé	j'envoyais tu envoyais il envoyait nous envoyions vous envoyiez ils envoyaient	j'avais envoyé tu avais envoyé il avait envoyé nous avions envoyé vous aviez envoyé ils avaient envoyé	j'enverrai tu enverras il enverra nous enverrons vous enverrez ils enverront	j'enverrais tu enverrais il enverrait nous enverrions vous enverriez ils enverraient	j'envoyai tu envoyas il envoya nous envoyâmes vous envoyâtes ils envoyèrent

VERB TABLE (contd)

Infinitive / Present participle / Imperative	Present	Perfect	Imperfect	Pluperfect	Future	Conditional	Past historic
éteindre *to put out, to switch off* éteignant éteins! éteignons! éteignez!	j'éteins tu éteins il éteint nous éteignons vous éteignez ils éteignent	j'ai éteint tu as éteint il a éteint nous avons éteint vous avez éteint ils ont éteint	j'éteignais tu éteignais il éteignait nous éteignions vous éteigniez ils éteignaient	j'avais éteint tu avais éteint il avait éteint nous avions éteint vous aviez éteint ils avaient éteint	j'éteindrai tu éteindras il éteindra nous éteindrons vous éteindrez ils éteindront	j'éteindrais tu éteindrais il éteindrait nous éteindrions vous éteindriez ils éteindraient	j'éteignis tu éteignis il éteignit nousé éteignîmes vous éteignîtes ils éteignirent
être *to be* étant sois! soyons! soyez!	je suis tu es il est nous sommes vous êtes ils sont	j'ai été tu as été il a été nous avons été vous avez été ils ont été	j'étais tu étais il était nous étions vous étiez ils étaient	j'avais été tu avais été il avait été nous avions été vous aviez été ils avaient été	je serai tu seras il sera nous serons vous serez ils seront	je serais tu serais il serait nous serions vous seriez ils seraient	je fus tu fus il fut nous fûmes vous fûtes ils furent
faire *to do, make* faisant fais! faisons! faites!	je fais tu fais il fait nous faisons vous faites ils font	j'ai fait tu as fait il a fait nous avons fait vous avez fait ils ont fait	je faisais tu faisais il faisait nous faisions vous faisiez ils faisaient	j'avais fait tu avais fait il avait fait nous avions fait vous aviez fait ils avaient fait	je ferai tu feras il fera nous ferons vous ferez ils feront	je ferais tu ferais il ferait nous ferions vous feriez ils feraient	je fis tu fis il fit nous fîmes vous fîtes ils firent
falloir *must, is necessary*	il faut	il a fallu	il fallait	il avait fallu	il faudra	il faudrait	il fallut
lire *to read* lisant lis! lisons! lisez!	je lis tu lis il lit nous lisons vous lisez ils lisent	j'ai lu tu as lu il a lu nous avons lu vous avez lu ils ont lu	je lisais tu lisais il lisait nous lisions vous lisiez ils lisaient	j'avais lu tu avais lu il avait lu nous avions lu vous aviez lu ils avaient lu	je lirai tu liras il lira nous lirons vous lirez ils liront	je lirais tu lirais il lirait nous lirions vous liriez ils liraient	je lus tu lus il lut nous lûmes vous lûtes ils lurent

VERB TABLE (contd)

Infinitive Present participle Imperative	Present	Perfect	Imperfect	Pluperfect	Future	Conditional	Past historic
mettre *to put* (*on*) mettant mets! mettons! mettez!	je mets tu mets il met nous mettons vous mettez ils mettent	j'ai mis tu as mis il a mis nous avons mis vous avez mis ils ont mis	je mettais tu mettais il mettait nous mettions vous mettiez ils mettaient	j'avais mis tu avais mis il avait mis nous avions mis vous aviez mis ils avaient mis	je mettrai tu mettras il mettra nous mettrons vous mettrez ils mettront	je mettrais tu mettrais il mettrait nous mettrions vous mettriez ils mettraient	je mis tu mis il mit nous mîmes vous mîtes ils mirent
mourir *to die* mourant meurs! mourons! mourez!	je meurs tu meurs il meurt nous mourons vous mourez ils meurent	je suis mort(e) tu es mort(e) il est mort elle est morte nous sommes mort(e)s vous êtes mort(e)(s) ils sont morts elles sont mortes	je mourais tu mourais il mourait nous mourions vous mouriez ils mouraient	j'étais mort(e) tu étais mort(e) il était mort elle était morte nous étions mort(e)s vous étiez mort(e)(s) ils étaient morts elles étaient mortes	je mourrai tu mourras il mourra nous mourrons vous mourrez ils mourront	je mourrais tu mourrais il mourrait nous mourrions vous mourriez ils mourraient	je mourus tu mourus il mourut nous mourûmes vous mourûtes ils moururent
naître *to be born* naissant nais! naissons! naissez!	je nais tu nais il naît nous naissons vous naissez ils naissent	je suis né(e) tu es né(e) il est né elle est née nous sommes né(e)s vous êtes né(e)(s) ils sont nés elles sont nées	je naissais tu naissais tu naissait nous naissions vous naissiez ils naissaient	j'étais né(e) tu étais né(e) il était né elle était née nous étions né(e)s vous étiez né(e)(s) ils étaient nés elles étaient nées	je naîtrai tu naîtras il naîtra nous naîtrons vous naîtrez ils naîtront	je naîtrais tu naîtrais il naîtrait nous naîtrions vous naîtriez ils naîtraient	je naquis tu naquis il naquit nous naquîmes vous naquîtes ils naquirent

obtenir *to obtain* see **tenir**

offrir *to offer, give* see **ouvrir**

VERB TABLE (contd)

Infinitive / Present participle / Imperative	Present	Perfect	Imperfect	Pluperfect	Future	Conditional	Past historic
ouvrir *to open* ouvrant ouvre! ouvrons! ouvrez!	j'ouvre tu ouvres il ouvre nous ouvrons vous ouvrez ils ouvrent	j'ai ouvert tu as ouvert il a ouvert nous avons ouvert vous avez ouvert ils ont ouvert	j'ouvrais tu ouvrais il ouvrait nous ouvrions vous ouvriez ils ouvraient	j'avais ouvert tu avais ouvert il avait ouvert nous avions ouvert vous aviez ouvert ils avaient ouvert	j'ouvrirai tu ouvriras il ouvrira nous ouvrirons vous ouvrirez ils ouvriront	je ouvrirais tu ouvrirait il ouvrirait nous ouvririons vous ouvririez ils ouvriraient	j'ouvris tu ouvris il ouvrit nous ouvrîmes vous ouvrîtes ils ouvrirent
paraître *to appear* see **connaître**							
partir *to leave* partant pars! partons! partez!	je pars tu pars il part nous partons vous partez ils partent	je suis parti(e) tu es parti(e) il est parti elle est partie nous sommes parti(e)s vous êtes parti(e)(s) ils sont partis elles sont parties	je partais tu partais il partait nous partions vous partiez ils partaient	j'étais parti(e) tu étais parti(e) il était parti elle était partie nous étions parti(e)s vous étiez parti(e)(s) ils étaient partis elles étaient parties	je partirai tu partiras il partira nous partirons vous partirez ils partiront	je partirais tu partirais il partirait nous partirions vous partiriez ils partiraient	je partis tu partis il partit nous partîmes vous partîtes ils partirent
pleuvoir *to rain* pleuvant	il pleut	il a plu	il pleuvait	il avait plu	il pleuvra	il pleuvrait	il plut
pouvoir *to be able, can*	je peux tu peux il peut nous pouvons vous pouvez ils peuvent	j'ai pu tu as pu il a pu nous avons pu vous avez pu ils ont pu	je pouvais tu pouvais il pouvait nous pouvions ovus pouviez ils pouvaient	j'avais pu tu avais pu il avait pu nous avions pu vous aviez pu ils avaient pu	je pourrai tu pourras il pourra nous pourrons vous pourrez ils pourront	je pourrais to pourrais il pourrait nous pourrions vous pourriez ils pourraient	je pus tu pus il put nous pûmes vous pûtes ils pureît
prendre *to take* prenant prends! prenons! prenez!	je prends tu prends il prend nous prenons vous prenez ils prennent	j'ai pris tu as pris il a pris nous avons pris vous avez pris ils ont pris	je prenais tu prenais il prenait nous prenions vous preniez ils prenaient	j'avais pris tu avais pris il avait pris nous avions pris vous aviez pris ils avaient pris	je prendrai tu prendras il prendra nous prendrons vous prendrez ils prendront	je prendrais tu prendrais il prendrait nous prendrions vous prendriez ils prendraient	je pris tu pris il prit nous prîmes vous prîtes ils prirent

VERB TABLE (contd)

prévenir *to warn* see **venir**, but takes *avoir* in perfect and pluperfect tenses

Infinitive / Present participle / Imperative	Present	Perfect	Imperfect	Pluperfect	Future	Conditional	Past historic
recevoir *to receive* recevant	je reçois tu reçois il reçoit	j'ai reçu tu as reçu il a reçu	je recevais tu recevais il recevait	j'avais reçu tu avais reçu il avait reçu	je recevrai tu recevras il recevra	je recevrais tu recevrais il recevrait	je reçus tu reçus il reçut
reçois!	nous recevons vous recevez ils reçoivent	nous avons reçu vous avez reçu ils ont reçu	nous recevions vous receviez ils recevaient	nous avions reçu vous aviez reçu ils avaient reçu	nous recevrons vous recevrez ils recevront	nous recevrions vous recevriez ils recevraient	nous reçûmes vous reçûtes ils reçurent
recevons! recevez!							

reconnaître *to recognise* see **connaître**
repartir *to set out again, to go away again* see **partir**
reprendre *to take again, to resume* see **prendre**

retenir *to hold back, to retain* see **tenir**
revenir *to come back, return* see **venir**

Infinitive / Present participle / Imperative	Present	Perfect	Imperfect	Pluperfect	Future	Conditional	Past historic
rire *to laugh* riant	je ris tu ris il rit	j'ai ri tu as ri il a ri	je riais tu riais il riait	j'avais ri tu avais ri il avait ri	je rirai tu riras il rira	je rirais tu rirais il rirait	je ris tu ris il rit
ris!	nous rions vous riez ils rient	nous avons ri vous avez ri ils ont ri	nous riions vous riiez ils riaient	nous avions ri vous aviez ri ils avaient ri	nous rirons vous rirez ils riront	nous ririons vous ririez ils riraient	nous rîmes vous rîtes ils rirent
rions! riez!							
savoir *to know* sachant	je sais tu sais il sait	j'ai su tu as su il a su	je savais tu savais il savait	j'avais su tu avais su il avait su	je saurai tu sauras il saura	je saurais tu saurais il saurait	je sus tu sus il sut
sache!	nous savons vous savez ils savent	nous avons su vous avez su ils ont su	nous savions vous saviez ils savaient	nous avions su vous aviez su ils avaient su	nous saurons vous saurez ils sauront	nous saurions vous sauriez ils sauraient	nous sûmes vous sûtes ils surent
sachons! sachez!							

se sentir *to feel* see **partir**
servir *to serve* see **partir**, but takes *avoir* in perfect and pluperfect tenses.

sortir *to go out* see **partir**

VERB TABLE (contd)

Infinitive / Present participle / Imperative	Present	Perfect	Imperfect	Pluperfect	Future	Conditional	Past historic
souffrir *to suffer* souffrant souffre! souffrons! souffrez!	je souffre tu souffres il souffre nous souffrons vous souffrez ils souffrent	j'ai souffert tu as souffert il a souffert nous avons souffert vous avez souffert ils ont souffert	je souffrais tu souffrais il souffrait nous souffrions vous souffriez ils souffraient	j'avais souffert tu avais souffert il avait souffert nous avions souffert vous aviez souffert ils avaient souffert	je souffrirai tu souffriras il souffrira nous souffrirons vous souffrirez ils souffriront	je souffrirais tu souffrirais il souffrirait nous souffririons vous souffririez ils souffriraient	je souffris tu souffris il souffrit nous souffrîmes vous souffrîtes ils souffrirent
suivre *to follow* suivant suis! suivons! suivez!	je suis tu suis il suit nous suivons vous suivez ils suivent	j'ai suivi tu as suivi il a suivi nous avons suivi vous avez suivi ils ont suivi	je suivais tu suivais il suivait nous suivions vous suiviez ils suivaient	j'avais suivi tu avais suivi il avait suivi nous avions suivi vous aviez suivi ils avaient suivi	je suivrai tu suivras il suivra nous suivrons vous suivrez ils suivront	je suivrais tu suivrais il suivrait nous suivrions vous suivriez ils suivraient	je suivis tu suivis il suivit nous suivîmes vous suivîtes ils suivirent
surprendre *to surprise* see **prendre**							
tenir *to hold* tenant tiens! tenons! tenez!	je tiens tu tiens il tient nous tenons vous tenez ils tiennent	j'ai tenu tu as tenu il a tenu nous avons tenu vous avez tenu ils ont tenu	je tenais tu tenais il tenait nous tenions vous teniez ils tenaient	j'avais tenu tu avais tenu il avait tenu nous avions tenu vous aviez tenu ils avaient tenu	je tiendrai tu tiendras il tiendra nous tiendrons vous tiendrez ils tiendront	je tiendrais tu tiendrais il tiendrait nous tiendrions vous tiendriez ils tiendraient	je tins tu tins il tint nous tînmes vous tîntes ils tinrent
venir *to come* venant viens! venons! venez!	je viens tu viens il vient nous venons vous venez ils viennent	je suis venu(e) tu es venu(e) il est venu elle est venue nous sommes venu(e)s vous êtes venu(e)(s) ils sont venus elles sont venues	je venais tu venais il venait nous venions vous veniez ils venaient	j'étais venu(e) tu étais venu(e)(s) il était venu elle était venue nous étions venu(e)s vous étiez venu(e)(s) ils étaient venus elles étaient venues	je viendrai tu viendras il viendra nous viendrons vous viendrez ils viendront	je viendrais tu viendrais il viendrait nous viendrions vous viendriez ils viendraient	je vins tu vins il vint nous vînmes vous vîntes ils vinrent

VERB TABLE (contd)

Infinitive / Present participle / Imperative	Present	Perfect	Imperfect	Pluperfect	Future	Conditional	Past historic
vivre *to live* vivant vis! vivons! vivez!	je vis tu vis il vit nous vivons vous vivez ils vivent	j'ai vécu tu as vécu il a vécu nous avons vécu vous avez vécu ils ont vécu	je vivais tu vivais il vivait nous vivions vous viviez ils vivaient	j'avais vécu tu avais vécu il avait vécu nous avions vécu vous aviez vécu ils avaient vécu	je vivrai tu vivras il vivra nous vivrons vouv vivrez ils vivraient	je vivrais tu vivrais il vivrait nous vivrions vous vivriez ils vivraient	je vécus tu vécus il vécut nous vécûmes vous vécûtes ils vécurent
voir *to see* voyant vois! voyons! voyez!	je vois tu vois il voit nous voyons vous voyez ils voient	j'ai vu tu as vu il a vu nous avons vu vous avez vu ils ont vu	je voyais tu voyais il voyait nous voyions vous voyiez ils voyaient	j'avais vu tu avais vu il avait vu nous avions vu vous aviez vu ils avaient vu	je verrai tu verras il verra nous verrons vous verrez ils verront	je verrais tu verrais il verrait nous verrions vous verriez ils verraient	je vis tu vis il vit nous vîmes vous vîtes ils virent
vouloir *to want, wish* voulant veuille! veuillons! veuillez!	je veux tu veux il veut nous voulons vous voulez ils veulent	j'ai voulu tu as voulu il a voulu nous avons voulu vous avez voulu ils ont voulu	je voulais tu voulais il voulait nous voulions vous vouliez ils voulaient	j'avais voulu tu avais voulu il avait voulu nous avions voulu vous aviez voulu ils avaient voulu	je voudrai tu voudras il voudra nous voudrons vous voudrez ils voudront	je voudrais tu voudrais il voudrait nous voudrions vous voudriez ils voudraient	je voulus tu voulus il voulut nous voulûmes vous voulûtes ils voulurent

Appendix

GCSE syllabus details, Group by Group.

▶ **EDEXCEL**
Foundation

Publications available from London Examinations/EDEXCEL Foundation, Stewart House, 32 Russell Square, London WC1B 5DN.

EDEXCEL Foundation runs an advice line for syllabus queries on 0171 331 4010.

Full Course 1225

Listening Foundation: 25 minutes
Higher 35 minutes

Papers conform to the usual pattern described in the main text.

Speaking Foundation 8–10 minutes
Higher 10–12 minutes

All candidates do two role-plays. All candidates do two conversation topics. Candidates choose the first topic, the teacher the second.

All Speaking Tests take place in a specified five-week period.

As an alternative to the Speaking Test, candidates may do Speaking coursework – see below.

Reading Foundation 30 minutes
Higher 45 minutes

Papers conform to the usual pattern described in the main text.

Writing Foundation 30 minutes
Higher 50 minutes

Foundation candidates do three exercises:

▷ write a short list or complete a form
▷ write a message, postcard, poster text
▷ write a letter, expand notes or react to other simple stimulus in French (70 words).

Higher candidates do two exercises:

▷ write a letter, expand notes or react to other simple stimulus in French (70 words)
▷ write a descriptive or imaginative piece, for example a letter, an article, etc. (150 words).

Coursework may be offered as an alternative to Writing **or** to Speaking (but not both).

Writing coursework
Candidates submit three pieces of work by the end of the first week in May in the year of the examination. The topics have to be drawn from three different Areas of Experience, one of which must be D or E. One of the three pieces is done in controlled conditions in class time.

Foundation candidates should write a total of 250–350 words over three pieces of work. Higher candidates should write a total of 500–600 words over three pieces of work.

Speaking coursework
Candidates record three mini-speaking tests covering a range of exercises similar to those in the standard Speaking Test.

Short Course 3225

Listening	Foundation	20 minutes
	Higher	25 minutes

Papers conform to the usual pattern described in the main text.

Speaking:	Foundation	6–7 minutes
	Higher	8–9 minutes

All candidates do two role-plays. Candidates choose a conversation topic.
   All Speaking Tests take place in a specified five-week period.
   As an alternative to the Speaking Test, candidates may do Speaking coursework – see below.

Reading	Foundation	25 minutes
	Higher	40 minutes

Papers conform to the usual pattern described in the main text.

Writing	Foundation	30 minutes
	Higher	50 minutes

Foundation candidates do three exercises:

▷ write a short list or complete a form
▷ write a message, postcard, poster text
▷ write a letter, expand notes or react to other simple stimulus in French (70 words).

Higher candidates do two exercises:

▷ write a letter, expand notes or react to other simple stimulus in French (70 words)
▷ write a descriptive or imaginative piece, for example a letter, article, etc. (150 words).

Coursework may be offered as an alternative to Writing **or** to Speaking (but not both).

Writing coursework

Candidates submit two pieces of work by the end of the first week in May in the year of the examination. The topics have to be drawn from Areas of Experience D and E. One of the two pieces is done in controlled conditions in class time.
   Foundation candidates should write a total of 200–250 words over two pieces of work. Higher candidates should write a total of 350–400 words over two pieces of work.

Speaking coursework

Candidates record two mini-speaking tests covering a range of exercises similar to those in the standard Speaking Test.

▷ **MEG**   Publications available from MEG, 1 Hills Road, Cambridge CB1 2EU.

Full Course 1525

Listening	Foundation	40 minutes
	Higher	40 minutes

Papers conform to the usual pattern described in the main text.

Speaking:	Foundation	10–12 minutes
	Higher	10–12 minutes

All candidates do two role-plays. The second role-play at Higher Tier involves re-telling a series of events from pictorial and verbal clues. All candidates do presentation, discussion and general conversation. General conversation covers three topics chosen at random.
   All Speaking Tests take place in a specified six-week period.

Reading	Foundation	50 minutes
	Higher	50 minutes

Papers conform to the usual pattern described in the main text.

Writing	Foundation	50 minutes
	Higher	50 minutes

Foundation candidates do three exercises:

➤ write a short list or complete a form
➤ write a message, postcard, poster text
➤ write a formal or an informal letter (100 words).

Higher candidates do two exercises:

➤ write a formal or informal letter (100 words)
➤ write a descriptive or imaginative piece, for example a letter, an article, etc. (150 words).

Coursework may be offered as an alternative to Writing.

Writing coursework

Candidates submit three pieces of work by early May in the year of the examination. One of the three pieces is done in controlled conditions in class time.

Foundation candidates should write a total of 60–300 words over three pieces of work. Higher candidates should write a total of 300–450 words over three pieces of work

Short Course 3525

Listening	Foundation:	30 minutes
	Higher	30 minutes

Papers conform to the usual pattern described in the main text.

Speaking	Foundation	8–10 minutes
	Higher	8–10 minutes

All candidates do two role-plays. The second role-play at Higher Tier involves re-telling a series of events from pictorial and verbal clues. All candidates do presentation, discussion and general conversation. General conversation covers two topics chosen at random.

All Speaking Tests take place in a specified six-week period.

Reading	Foundation	35 minutes
	Higher	35 minutes

Papers conform to the usual pattern described in the main text.

Writing	Foundation	40 minutes
	Higher	40 minutes

Foundation candidates do three exercises:

➤ write a short list or complete a form
➤ write a message, postcard, poster text
➤ write a formal or an informal letter (70–80 words).

Higher candidates do two exercises:

➤ write a formal or informal letter (70–80 words)
➤ write a descriptive or imaginative piece, for example a letter, an article, etc. (120 words).

Coursework may be offered as an alternative to Writing.

Writing coursework

Candidates submit three pieces of work by early May in the year of the examination. One of the three pieces is done in controlled conditions in class time.

Foundation candidates should write a total of 60–300 words over three pieces of work. Higher candidates should write a total of 300–450 words over three pieces of work.

▷ **NEAB** Publications available from NEAB, 12 Harter Street, Manchester M1 6HL.

Full Course 1211

| Listening | Foundation | 30 minutes |
| | Higher | 40 minutes |

Papers conform to the usual pattern described in the main text.

| Speaking: | Foundation | 8–10 minutes |
| | Higher | 10–12 minutes |

All candidates do two role-plays. All candidates do presentation, discussion and general conversation. General conversation covers two topics out of three shown on a card chosen at random.

All Speaking Tests take place in a specified two-week period.

| Reading | Foundation | 30 minutes |
| | Higher | 50 minutes |

Papers conform to the usual pattern described in the main text and are held in the same session as the Writing paper.

| Writing | Foundation | 40 minutes |
| | Higher | 60 minutes |

Foundation candidates do three exercises:

▷ write a short list or complete a form
▷ write a message, postcard, poster text
▷ write a formal or an informal letter (90 words).

Higher candidates do two exercises:

▷ write a formal or an informal letter (90 words)
▷ write a descriptive or imaginative piece, for example a letter, an article, etc. (120 words).

Coursework may be offered as an alternative to Writing.

Writing coursework
Candidates submit three pieces of work by 30 April in the year of the examination. The topics have to be drawn from three different Areas of Experience. Candidates choose titles from a list set by NEAB. One of the three pieces is done in controlled conditions in class time.

Foundation candidates should write a total of 200–300 words over three pieces of work. Higher candidates should write a total of 300–600 words over three pieces of work

Short Course 2211

Timings and details closely resemble those for the Full Course. The main difference is that the syllabus tests Areas of Experience B and D. For coursework, work must cover at least one title from each Area of Experience.

▷ **NICCEA** Publications available from NICCEA, 29 Clarendon Road, Belfast BT1 3BG.

Full Course 1211

| Listening | Foundation: | 30 minutes |
| | Higher | 30 minutes |

Papers conform to the usual pattern described in the main text.

| Speaking: | Foundation | 10 minutes |
| | Higher | 10 minutes |

Includes role-plays and general conversation.
All speaking tests take place in a specified period.

Reading   Foundation   40 minutes
               Higher   40 minutes

Papers conform to the usual pattern described in the main text.

Writing   Foundation   45 minutes
               Higher   45 minutes

Foundation candidates do exercises including some of the following:

- write a short list or complete a form
- write a message, postcard, poster text
- write a formal or an informal letter.

Higher candidates do two exercises:

- write a formal or informal letter
- write a more substantive letter, report or account.

Coursework is not available.

Short Course

NICCEA does not offer a Short Course in French.

▷ **SEG**   Publications are available from SEG, Stag Hill House, Guildford, GU2 5XJ.

Full Course Modular 2700

SEG only offers a modular Full Course. It is best summarised as below:

Module no:	1	2	3	4
Title	Contact with a French-speaking country	Organising a visit to a French-speaking country	Holidays and travel	The young person in society
When	February, Year 10	June, Year 10	December, Year 11	June, Year 11
How assessed	Coursework	External test	Coursework	Examination
Listening	5%	10% 20 minutes		10% 20 minutes
Speaking	5%		5%	15% Foundation 5 minutes Higher 8 minutes
Reading	5%	10% 30 minutes		10% 30 minutes
Writing			10%	15% 30 minutes

Short Course 1470

The SEG Short Course syllabus is **not** modular. It broadly follows the conventional pattern.

Listening   Foundation: 25 minutes
                 Higher   30 minutes

Papers conform to the usual pattern described in the main text.

| Speaking | Foundation | 5 minutes |
| | Higher | 8 minutes |

All candidates do two role-plays. All candidates do general conversation. G[...] tion may cover the whole syllabus.

All Speaking Tests take place between the start of the summer term and the[...]

| Reading | Foundation | 25 minutes |
| | Higher | 40 minutes |

Papers conform to the usual pattern described in the main text.

Writing is assessed by coursework.

Writing coursework

Candidates submit three pieces of work by early May in the year of the examination. One o[...] the three pieces is done in controlled conditions in class time.

Foundation candidates should write a total of 230–270 words over three pieces of work. Higher candidates should write a total of 300–360 words over three pieces of work.

▶ WJEC/CBAC

Publications available from WJEC/CBAC, 245 Western Avenue, Cardiff, CF5 2YX.

Full Course

| Listening | Foundation | 45 minutes |
| | Higher | 45 minutes |

Papers conform to the usual pattern described in the main text.

| Speaking | Foundation | 10 minutes |
| | Higher | 12 minutes |

All candidates do two role-plays. All candidates do a general conversation. General conversation covers at least two Areas of Experience.

All Speaking Tests take place in a specified period.

| Reading | Foundation | 45 minutes |
| | Higher | 45 minutes |

Papers conform to the usual pattern described in the main text.

| Writing | Foundation | 45 minutes |
| | Higher | 60 minutes |

Coursework may be offered as an alternative to Writing. No further details are available at the time of writing (early 1997).

Short Course

| Listening | Foundation | 25 minutes |
| | Higher | 25 minutes |

Papers conform to the usual pattern described in the main text.

| Speaking | Foundation | 10 minutes |
| | Higher | 12 minutes |

All candidates do two role-plays. All candidates do a general conversation. General conversation covers at least two Areas of Experience.

All Speaking Tests take place in a specified period.

| Reading | Foundation | 30 minutes |
| | Higher | 30 minutes |

Papers conform to the usual pattern described in the main text.

| Writing | Foundation | 30 minutes |
| | Higher | 30 minutes |

Index